369 0073588

Textbook of Pediatric Rheumatology

Textbook of Pediatric Rheumatology

Fourth Edition

James T. Cassidy, MD
Professor of Child Health
Chief, Division of Pediatric Rheumatology
Department of Child Health
University of Missouri Health Sciences Center
and Children's Hospital
Columbia, Missouri, United States

Ross E. Petty, MD, PhD, FRCPC
Professor of Pediatrics
University of British Columbia
Head, Division of Rheumatology
Department of Pediatrics
British Columbia Children's Hospital
Vancouver, British Columbia, Canada

W.B. SAUNDERS COMPANY
A Harcourt Health Sciences Company
Philadelphia London New York St. Louis Sydney Toronto

W.B. SAUNDERS COMPANY
A Harcourt Health Sciences Company

The Curtis Center
Independence Square West
Philadelphia, Pennsylvania 19106

Library of Congress Cataloging-in-Publication Data

Textbook of pediatric rheumatology / [edited by] James T. Cassidy, Ross E. Petty.—4th ed.

p. ; cm.

Includes bibliographical references and index.

ISBN 0–7216–8171–9

1. Pediatric rheumatology. 2. Rheumatism in children. I. Cassidy, James T. II. Petty, Ross E.
[DNLM: 1. Rheumatic Diseases—Child. 2. Arthritis—Child. 3. Connective Tissue Diseases—Child. 4. Vasculitis—Child. WE 544 T355 2001]

RJ482.R48 C37 2001

618.92′723—dc21 2001020286

Editor-in-Chief: Richard Zorab
Acquisitions Editor: Cathy Carroll
Project Manager: Mimi McGinnis
Production Manager: Mary Stermel
Illustration Specialist: John Needles
Book Designer: Marie Gardocky-Clifton
Indexer: Dennis Dolan

TEXTBOOK OF PEDIATRIC RHEUMATOLOGY ISBN 0–7216–8171–9

Printed in the United States of America.

Last digit is the print number: 9 8 7 6 5 4 3 2 1

To Nan and Beryl

Contributors

Balu H. Athreya, MD
Professor of Pediatrics, Thomas Jefferson University/ Jefferson Medical College, Philadelphia, Pennsylvania; Senior Physician, DuPont Hospital for Children, Wilmington, Delaware, United States

Elia M. Ayoub, MD
Distinguished Service Professor, Department of Pediatrics, University of Florida College of Medicine, Gainesville, Florida, United States

Arvind Bagga, MD
Associate Professor, Division of Nephrology, Department of Pediatrics, All India Institute of Medical Sciences, New Delhi, India

Rubén Burgos-Vargas, MD
Professor of Medicine, Universidad Nacional Autonóma de México; Director, Research Division, Hospital General de México, Mexico City, Mexico

James T. Cassidy, MD
Professor of Child Health, Chief, Division of Pediatric Rheumatology, Department of Child Health, University of Missouri Health Sciences Center and Children's Hospital, Columbia, Missouri, United States

Michael J. Dillon, MD, MB, BS, FRCP, FRCPCH, DCH
Professor of Paediatric Nephrology, Institute of Child Health, University College London; Consultant Physician and Senior Clinical Nephrologist, Great Ormond Street Hospital for Children, London, United Kingdom

Frank Dressler, Dr. med.
Lecturer, Pediatrician, and Senior Fellow, Department of Pediatrics, Hannover Medical School; Assistenzarzt, Kinderklinik der Medizinischen, Hochschule Hannover, Hannover, Germany

Ciarán M. Duffy, MB, BCh, MSc, FRCPC
Associate Professor of Paediatrics and Director, Division of Paediatric Rheumatology, Montreal Children's Hospital, and McGill University, Montreal, Quebec, Canada

Madlen Gazarian, MBBS, MSc, FRACP
Senior Lecturer, School of Paediatrics, University of New South Wales, Sydney Children's Hospital, Randwick, New South Wales, Australia

Edward H. Giannini, MSc, DrPH
Professor, Division of Rheumatology, Department of Pediatrics, University of Cincinnati College of Medicine and Children's Hospital Medical Center, Cincinnati, Ohio, United States

David N. Glass, MB, ChB, FRCP
Professor of Pediatrics, Department of Pediatrics, University of Cincinnati College of Medicine; Director, William S. Rowe Division of Rheumatology, Children's Hospital Medical Center, Cincinnati, Ohio, United States

Judith G. Hall, OC, MD, FRCPC, FCCMG
Professor, Medical Genetics and Pediatrics, University of British Columbia, Vancouver, British Columbia, Canada

Hans-Iko Huppertz, Dr. med.
Professor of Pediatrics, Head, and Director, Children's Hospital (Professor-Hess-Kinderklinik), Bremen, Germany

Wietse Kuis, MD, PhD
Professor in Pediatrics, University of Utrecht and Department of Pediatrics, University Medical Center, Utrecht, The Netherlands

Ronald M. Laxer, MDCM, FRCPC
Professor of Pediatrics and Medicine and Associate-Chairman, Department of Pediatrics, University of Toronto; Associate Pediatrician-in-Chief and Staff Rheumatologist, The Hospital for Sick Children, Toronto, Ontario, Canada

Carol B. Lindsley, MD
Professor and Chair, Department of Pediatrics, and Chief, Pediatric Rheumatology, University of Kansas Medical Center, Kansas City, Kansas, United States

Daniel J. Lovell, MD, MPH
Professor of Pediatrics, University of Cincinnati College of Medicine; Associate Director, William G. Rowe Division of Rheumatology, Children's Hospital Medical Center, Cincinnati, Ohio, United States

Peter N. Malleson, MBBS, MRCP, FRCPC
Professor of Pediatrics, Division of Pediatric Rheumatology, University of British Columbia, British Columbia Children's Hospital, Vancouver, British Columbia, Canada

Alberto Martini, MD
Professor of Pediatrics, University of Pavia; Director, General Pediatrics and Pediatric Rheumatology, IRCCS Policlinico San Matteo, Pavia, Italy

Audrey M. Nelson, MD
Professor of Medicine, Mayo Medical School; Consultant in Internal Medicine and Rheumatology and Chair, Division of Pediatric Rheumatology, Department of Pediatric and Adolescent Medicine, Mayo Medical Center, Rochester, Minnesota, United States

Ross E. Petty, MD, PhD, FRCPC
Professor of Pediatrics, University of British Columbia; Head, Division of Rheumatology, Department of Pediatrics, British Columbia Children's Hospital, Vancouver, British Columbia, Canada

Anne-Marie Prieur, MD
Praticien Hospitalier Pédiatre, Université Paris V, Médecin des hôpitaux, Unité d'Immunologie-hématologie et Rhumatologie Pédiatriques, Hôpital Necker-Enfants-Malades, Paris, France

Lieke A. M. Sanders, MD, PhD
Associate Professor in Pediatric Immunology, University of Utrecht and Department of Pediatrics, University Medical Center, Utrecht, The Netherlands

David D. Sherry, MD
Associate Professor of Pediatrics, University of Washington; Director, Pediatric Rheumatology, Children's Hospital and Regional Medical Center, Seattle, Washington, United States

Earl D. Silverman, MD, FRCPC
Professor of Pediatrics and Immunology, University of Toronto; Director of Pediatric Systemic Lupus Erythematosus Clinic, Division of Rheumatology, The Hospital for Sick Children, Toronto, Ontario, Canada

Taunton R. Southwood, MD, BM, BS, FRCP, FRCPCH
Professor of Paediatric Rheumatology, Department of Rheumatology, University of Birmingham Medical School, and Birmingham Children's Hospital, Birmingham, United Kingdom

Janitzia Vázquez-Mellado, MD, PhD
Professor of Medicine, Universidad Nacional Autónoma de México; Senior Investigator, Rheumatology Service, Hospital General de México, Mexico City, Mexico

Patricia Woo, PhD, FRCP, FRCPCH
Professor of Paediatric Rheumatology, University College Medical School, London, United Kingdom

Nico M. Wulffraat, MD, PhD
Associate Professor in Pediatric Immunology, University of Utrecht and Department of Pediatrics, University Medical Center, Utrecht, The Netherlands

Preface

Two decades have passed since publication of the first edition of this *Textbook of Pediatric Rheumatology*. The intervening years have encompassed an enormous increase in our understanding of the pathogenic mechanisms of the rheumatic diseases, much of which is specific for the discipline of pediatric rheumatology. These scientific discoveries afford exciting new opportunities for better diagnosis and treatment of our children. Consequently, the present edition follows in the tradition of change established by its predecessors and represents a complete revision of the original text. We hope that it will be a testament to the clinical practice and science of the subspecialty of pediatric rheumatology and the new maturity that it has achieved. These advances in rheumatology are increasingly recognized as an important part of the clinical, investigative, and educational programs of academic institutions of medical training.

We have undertaken this reorganization in order to provide a comprehensive but focused source of information regarding the rheumatic diseases of childhood for physicians concerned with the care of these children. Significant advances in practice and knowledge have been incorporated in this edition, including exhaustive reviews of the major clinical syndromes resulting in rheumatic and inflammatory diseases of childhood and continuing international efforts directed toward their classification and diagnosis. A chapter on health care assessment and the conduct of clinical trials and another on the design and statistical analysis of therapeutic investigations have been added. Most importantly, there has truly been a therapeutic revolution in the field of rheumatology that has required a complete reworking and considerable enlargement of the chapter on pharmacology.

In the process of documenting these changes, references have been extensively updated, retaining those regarded as "classics" or having historic importance and incorporating new publications that specifically contribute to our understanding of the rheumatic diseases. Twenty-seven of our international colleagues have been enlisted in these efforts in what is now a multiauthored text. Their contributions represent expert appraisals of their respective fields of interest; we are incredibly grateful for their enthusiastic cooperation in this endeavor. Their efforts have clarified areas of immunogenetics that emphasize the extensive changes in knowledge that will ultimately result from sequencing the human genome, immunologic mechanisms of inflammatory disease, neuroendocrine dysregulation, and developmental defects contributing to the inflammatory arthropathies.

In addition to our colleagues, we are deeply indebted to our families and close associates, without whose patience and understanding this book would not have been possible, and to W.B. Saunders for encouragement and support throughout the long process of revision. It is therefore our hope that the fourth edition of this *Textbook of Pediatric Rheumatology* will aid physicians caring for children with rheumatic diseases to interpret the complex web of symptoms, signs, and laboratory abnormalities that are characteristic of these disorders; will inspire students of medicine and pediatrics to recognize the challenges and excitement of our discipline; and ultimately will ensure the provision of optimal care to the hundreds of thousands of children and their families around the world who endure the pain and limitations imposed by these disorders.

James T. Cassidy, MD
Ross E. Petty, MD, PhD, FRCPC

NOTICE

Medicine is an ever-changing field. Standard safety precautions must be followed, but as new research and clinical experience broaden our knowledge, changes in treatment and drug therapy may become necessary or appropriate. Readers are advised to check the most current product information provided by the manufacturer of each drug to be administered to verify the recommended dose, the method and duration of administration, and contraindications. It is the responsibility of the treating physician, relying on experience and knowledge of the patient, to determine dosages and the best treatment for each individual patient. Neither the Publisher nor the editor assumes any liability for any injury and/or damage to persons or property arising from this publication.

THE PUBLISHER

Contents

1

Basic Concepts

2

Chronic Arthritis

3

Systemic Connective Tissue Diseases

4

Systemic Vasculitis

5

Arthritis Related to Infection

6

Primary and Acquired Disorders of Bone and Connective Tissue

Basic Concepts

1

1

Introduction to the Study of Rheumatic Diseases in Children

Ross E. Petty and James T. Cassidy

HISTORY

Rheumatic diseases are chronic multisystem disorders that represent the clinical manifestations of acute and chronic inflammation of the tissues of the musculoskeletal system, blood vessels, and skin. *Homo sapiens* has been afflicted with a variety of rheumatic diseases for hundreds, if not thousands, of years. Chronic arthritis-like changes have been observed in the spines of Egyptian mummies dating from 8000 B.C.,[1] and ankylosing spondylitis may be the most ancient of the defined rheumatic diseases, having been diagnosed in the skeletal remains of a person from medieval Europe.[2] However, rheumatoid arthritis is thought to be a much more recent development,[3] at least in Europe, where it was first described in the nineteenth century, although it may have originated much earlier among the aboriginals of North America.[4]

Evolution of Terminology

In 1883, Thomas Barlow, a mentor to George Frederic Still at the Hospital for Sick Children, Great Ormond Street, London, introduced a discussion on "Rheumatism and its allies in childhood" as follows: "The fundamental difficulty in discussing rheumatism consists in defining what we mean by it."[5] The problem of definition has been a persistent one and is being addressed even today in new classification criteria for idiopathic childhood arthritis.[6, 7] The term *rheumatism* is derived from the Greek *rheumatismos*: a flux.[8] The first use of this term has been ascribed to Galen.[9] Its current usage describes inflammatory or degenerative diseases of the joints, bones, muscles, or bursae. The adjective *rheumatic* was used originally to refer to rheumatic fever. Guillaume Baillou (1558–1616) first employed the word *rheumatism* to distinguish acute arthritis from gout.[10]

The word *arthritis* is derived from the Greek *arthron*, meaning joint, and the suffix *-itis*, meaning inflammation.[8] It came into the English language about 1544 when it was used to refer only to gout. Today, objective inflammation of a joint is called arthritis; the term *arthralgia* indicates joint pain without objective evidence of inflammation. Although it is likely that Hippocrates[11] recognized *rheumatoid arthritis* in the fourth century B.C., Sir Alfred Baring Garrod first proposed the term to differentiate it from both gout and rheumatism.[12]

In the absence of knowledge of specific causes, it is not surprising that terminology used to describe and classify rheumatic diseases, including those of childhood, continues to evolve. The discrepancies between the American College of Rheumatology criteria for the classification of juvenile rheumatoid arthritis (JRA)[13] and the European League Against Rheumatism criteria for the classification of juvenile chronic arthritis[14] exemplify this point. Attempts to develop globally acceptable terminology have resulted in the proposed criteria for the classification of the juvenile idiopathic arthritides (see Chapter 11).[6, 7] Terminology for other childhood rheumatic diseases has been less controversial; in large part, the terms used to describe similar or identical diseases in adults have been adopted without consideration for age-related differences in the following disorders: systemic lupus erythematosus (SLE), scleroderma, dermatomyositis, and most of the vasculitides. "New" diseases such as Kawasaki disease, Lyme disease, and parvovirus B19–associated arthritis have been increasingly recognized as their classification criteria have evolved. In recent decades, the chronic noninflammatory pain syndromes such as reflex sympathetic dystrophy (one of its many names) or fibromyalgia have become major components of the field of rheumatology in its broadest sense.

Recognition of Rheumatic Diseases in Childhood

Pediatric rheumatology is a clinical discipline that embraces the study of inflammatory and noninflammatory disorders of the connective tissues in children. The boundaries of the discipline continue to expand, and although inflammatory disorders of joints, muscles, and connective tissues constitute the core of pediatric rheumatology, the differential diagnosis of these diseases necessitates a broad knowledge of potentially confusing disorders.

The first English-language reference to rheumatism in children is contained in the 1545 text *The Regiment of Life Whereunto Is Added a Treatise of the Pestilence, with the Boke of Chyldren*, by Thomas Phaire. In this work, Phaire refers to the "stifnes or starckenes of the Limmes" resulting from exposing a child to cold,[15, 16] a complaint that may not represent any specific rheumatic disease. In 1864, Cornil described a woman in whom polyarthritis had developed when she was 12 years old.[17] The disease pursued a chronic relapsing course and terminated in her death in uremic coma at the age of 28 years. Necropsy documented myocardial degeneration, nephrotic syndrome, and ankylosis of some joints and synovial proliferation with marked destruction of cartilage in others. This girl may have had amyloidosis complicating chronic polyarticular juvenile rheumatoid arthritis. In 1873, Bouchut described chronic rheumatism in six children,[18] and in 1870 Moncorvo,[19] a Brazilian, described childhood arthritis in one of his own patients and eight from the literature.[16] West's *Lectures on the Diseases of Infancy and Childhood*[20] (1881) notes that "chronic rheumatic arthritis in children is a rare occurrence," although some form of chronic arthritis was recognized occasionally in Europe.

In 1883, at the 51st annual meeting of the British Medical Association, Thomas Barlow chaired a discussion on rheumatism in childhood.[5] In this publication, the term *rheumatism* appears to have been used to describe poststreptococcal disease, including rheumatic fever. Barlow recognized the extent and complexity of such disorders in childhood: "For there are in children many affections of joints, and of structures around joints, which do not suppurate, and yet are not rheumatic; and there is much rheumatism in children which does not affect joints."[5] What we would today call toxic synovitis of the hip, acute pyogenic arthritis, syphilitic arthritis, hemophiliac arthropathy, Henoch-Schönlein purpura, poststreptococcal arthritis, and acute rheumatic fever including carditis, arthritis, nodules, erythema marginatum, and chorea are all identifiable in this paper. Barlow is careful to exclude both rickets and scurvy from consideration because he considered that the joint itself was not primarily involved in these conditions.

In 1891, Diamant-Berger published the first detailed account of chronic arthritis in 38 children whom he had seen personally or whose cases had been documented in the literature.[21] He noted the heterogeneity of onset of the disease, its predominance in girls, and the occurrence of cervical spine and temporomandibular joint disease as well as ocular involvement. He also noted that the prognosis of arthritis in children generally was better than in chronic arthritis in adults. The patients in this series had what we would recognize today as JRA, juvenile chronic arthritis, or juvenile idiopathic arthritis rather than rheumatic fever.

Six years later, in 1896, George Frederic Still (1868–1941) described 22 cases of acute and chronic arthritis in children, almost all of whom were observed at the Hospital for Sick Children.[22] This treatise, representing work done under the mentorship of Barlow,[23] carefully documented the clinical characteristics of these children and pointed out the differing modes of onset. Still was the first English physician to confine his practice to diseases of children and was the first Professor of Paediatrics at King's College Hospital Medical School, London. Unfortunately, after his classic study, he rarely returned to the field of pediatric rheumatology, although his scholarly work comprised 108 papers and 5 books, including his *History of Paediatrics* and *Common Diseases in Children*. In the same year, Koplick[24] described the first American child with chronic arthritis. Subsequently, a few case reports of patients with "Still's disease" were published.[25–27]

Although these descriptions of childhood arthritis rank as the most important milestones in the early development of pediatric rheumatology, other rheumatic diseases began to be identified in children in the nineteenth century. The clinical characteristics of leukocytoclastic vasculitis were described by Henoch[28] and Schönlein[29] in the early to mid-1800s. Juvenile dermatomyositis was first described by Unverricht in 1877,[30] although it was not until the mid-1960s that significant experience with this childhood disease was reported. SLE has been recognized in children at least since 1904.[31] The original description of scleroderma was in a 17-year-old girl,[32] but the disease was rarely described in a child until the early 1960s. Ankylosing spondylitis was perhaps first described in a child[33]; it was certainly known to occur in childhood in the 1950s,[34] but specific studies of the disease in children did not emerge until the late 1960s.[35, 36]

More recent additions to the family of childhood rheumatic diseases include Kawasaki disease, which was reported in some detail in 1967,[37] although its clinical characteristics (in infants dying of polyarteritis nodosa) were described by Munro-Faure in 1959.[38] Other childhood-onset rheumatic diseases, such as chronic infantile neurologic, cutaneous, and articular (CINCA) syndrome (also called neonatal-onset multisystem inflammatory disease, or NOMID),[39] neonatal lupus,[40] and Lyme disease,[41] have only recently been identified. Noninflammatory musculoskeletal pain syndromes also are recent additions to the list of disorders that cause musculoskeletal pain and dysfunction in children and adolescents.[42]

Very little further information about childhood rheumatic diseases was published until the last half of the twentieth century. Today, the specialty of pediatric rheumatology is concerned with a diverse group of disorders (Table 1–1), most of which are manifestations of systemic disorders and require the greatest expertise for optimal management. Of all of the specialties, rheumatology may deal with the broadest spectrum of disease, both organ-specific and systemic. It is sometimes considered a "gray area" of medicine because there

Table 1–1

Classification of Rheumatic Diseases in Childhood

Inflammatory Rheumatic Diseases of Childhood

CHRONIC ARTHROPATHIES

- Juvenile rheumatoid arthritis
  - Oligoarticular onset
  - Polyarticular onset
  - Systemic onset
- Spondyloarthropathies
  - Juvenile ankylosing spondylitis
  - Juvenile psoriatic arthritides
  - Arthritides with inflammatory bowel disease
  - Reiter's syndrome
- Arthritis associated with infectious agents
  - Infectious arthritis
    - Spirochetal (Lyme disease)
    - Viral
    - Other
  - Reactive
    - Acute rheumatic fever
    - Post-enteric infection
    - Post-genitourinary infection
    - Other

CONNECTIVE TISSUE DISORDERS

- Systemic lupus erythematosus
- Juvenile dermatomyositis
- The sclerodermas
  - Systemic scleroderma
  - Localized sclerodermas
  - Eosinophilic fasciitis
  - Mixed connective tissue disease
  - Other
- Vasculitis
  - Polyarteritis
    - Polyarteritis nodosa
    - Kawasaki disease
    - Microscopic polyarteritis nodosa
    - Other
  - Leukocytoclastic vasculitis
    - Henoch-Schönlein purpura
    - Hypersensitivity vasculitis
    - Other
  - Granulomatous vasculitis
    - Allergic granulomatosis
    - Wegener's granulomatosis
    - Other
  - Giant cell arteritis
    - Takayasu's arteritis
    - Temporal arteritis
  - Other

ARTHRITIS AND CONNECTIVE TISSUE DISEASES ASSOCIATED WITH IMMUNODEFICIENCIES

- Complement component deficiencies
- Antibody deficiency syndromes
- Cell-mediated deficiencies

Noninflammatory Disorders

BENIGN HYPERMOBILITY SYNDROMES

- Generalized
- Localized

PAIN AMPLIFICATION SYNDROMES AND RELATED DISORDERS

- Growing pains
- Primary fibromyalgia syndrome
- Reflex sympathetic dystrophy
- Acute transient osteoporosis
- Erythromelalgia

OVERUSE SYNDROMES

- Chondromalacia patellae
- Plica syndromes
- Stress fractures
- Shin splints
- Tennis elbow, Little Leaguer's elbow, tenosynovitis

TRAUMA

- Osteochondritis dissecans
- Traumatic arthritis, non-accidental trauma
- Congenital indifference to pain
- Frostbite arthropathy

PAIN SYNDROMES AFFECTING BACK, CHEST OR NECK

- Spondylolysis and spondylolisthesis
- Intervertebral disc herniation
- Slipping rib
- Costochondritis
- Torticollis
- Aneuralgic amyotrophy

Skeletal Dysplasias

OSTEOCHONDRODYSPLASIAS

- Generalized
  - Achondroplasia
  - Diastrophic dwarfism
  - Metatrophic dwarfism
- Epiphyseal dysplasias
  - Spondyloepiphyseal dysplasias
  - Multiple epiphyseal dysplasias

OSTEOCHONDROSES

- Legg-Calvé Perthes disease
- Osgood-Schlatter disease
- Thiemann's disease, Köhler's disease
- Freiberg's infraction
- Scheuermann's disease

Heritable Disorders of Connective Tissue

- Osteogenesis imperfecta
- Ehlers-Danlos syndromes
- Cutis laxa
- Pseudoxanthoma elasticum
- Marfan's syndrome

Storage Diseases

- Mucopolysaccharidoses
- Mucolipidoses
- Sphingolipidoses

Metabolic Disorders

- Osteoporosis
- Rickets
- Scurvy
- Hypervitaminosis A
- Gout
- Ochronosis
- Kashin-Beck disease
- Mseleni disease
- Fluorosis
- Amyloidosis

Systemic Diseases With Musculoskeletal Manifestations

- Hemoglobinopathies
- Hemophilia
- Diabetes mellitus
- Hyperlipoproteinemias
- Pseudohypoparathyroidism
- Secondary hypertrophic osteoarthropathy
- Sarcoidosis

HYPEROSTOSIS

- Infantile cortical hyperostosis (Caffey's disease)
- Other

are few useful diagnostic tests, pathognomonic clinical signs are sparse, and therapy often lacks specificity. This specialty requires patience, careful observation over long periods of time, and the ability to tolerate ambiguity and uncertainty. Sometimes only the passage of time makes diagnosis possible. Nonetheless, pediatric rheumatology is one of the most stimulating and challenging areas in all of medicine.

Emergence of the Specialty of Pediatric Rheumatology

The roots of contemporary pediatric rheumatology are found in internal medicine, orthopedics, and pediatrics; however, as experience with rheumatic diseases in children accumulated, it became apparent that many aspects of these diseases required a uniquely pediatric approach. Furthermore, many of the diseases or their complications were confined to the childhood and adolescent population. These realizations found their early home in the United Kingdom in particular, where the study of rheumatic disease in children was established in earnest in 1947 by the founding of the Rheumatism Research Unit at the Canadian Red Cross Memorial Hospital in Taplow, England.[43]

Until the recognition of the link between infection with group A *Streptococcus* and rheumatic fever and the advent of penicillin to prevent this disease, little attention had been paid to the broad spectrum of the chronic arthritides of childhood. Thus, initially the Taplow unit dealt almost exclusively with rheumatic fever. As the frequency of this disease declined in England during the mid-twentieth century, its focus shifted to chronic rheumatic diseases of childhood, and a small group of physician-scientists, including E. G. L. Bywaters and B. M. Ansell, laid the foundation for the specialty of pediatric rheumatology.

In the United States, a focus on pediatric rheumatology began to develop in the early 1950s. Establishment of centers of pediatric rheumatology in the United States, Canada, Australia, France, Norway, Sweden, Germany, Austria, Holland, Italy, Mexico, Turkey, and many other nations has marked the "coming of age" of the specialty. Reminiscences of five of the pioneers of pediatric rheumatology (J. Sidney Stillman, Virgil Hanson, Joseph E. Levinson, Barbara M. Ansell, and Earl J. Brewer, Jr.) are available to the interested reader.[44–48]

FACTORS THAT MODIFY RHEUMATIC DISEASES IN CHILDREN

One of the fundamental questions that has pervaded research in pediatric rheumatology is the extent to which rheumatic diseases in childhood are the same as, or different from, rheumatic diseases in adults. It is important to differentiate semantic from biologic similarities: The fact that two diseases bear the same name (e.g., juvenile and [adult] rheumatoid arthritis) should not necessarily imply that they are the same diseases biologically. Historically, diseases were usually named in ignorance of epidemiology, genetics, or biology. A complete distinction among diseases based on age at onset alone is arbitrary and unlikely to represent accurately the biologic "truth." *There is no age at which these diseases abruptly change from one to the other,* and yet, if one examines JRA and its subtypes, the age-related associations are clear.[49] There is little doubt that some rheumatic diseases occur only in young children (e.g., oligoarticular JRA with uveitis or Kawasaki disease), and others appear almost exclusively in adults (e.g., gout, osteoarthritis). More commonly, however, diseases with similar names and similar biologic characteristics occur in both pediatric and adult populations (e.g., scleroderma, ankylosing spondylitis, SLE).

Age-related differences in many of the manifestations of these diseases are well recognized. Some of the prominent age-related differences between children and adults that may modify the clinical expression of a rheumatic disease are presented in Table 1–2.

The influence of the degree of skeletal maturity on the expression of rheumatic diseases is poorly understood. It seems probable, however, that physical and biochemical differences between young and older cartilage and bone profoundly influence the effect of an inflammatory process involving these structures. Because physes are not fused in the growing child with arthritis, local growth abnormalities such as leg-length inequality may occur. Short stature is a frequent result of widespread arthritis in the child, but shortness is obviously not an expected development in the skeletally mature adult with arthritis. The anatomy of the blood supply to the physis and epiphysis in the infant is reflected in this age group's predisposition to septic arthritis as a complication of osteomyelitis.

The influence of gonadal immaturity in causing differences in the expression of rheumatic diseases between children and adults is unclear. In some studies of SLE,[50] girls and boys are affected with equal frequency in early childhood; in adulthood, women are affected 8 to 9 times more commonly than men. That this observation may reflect the role of sex hormones in the pathogenesis of SLE is supported by studies of adult males with Klinefelter's syndrome (i.e., males with 2 X chromosomes and 1 Y chromosome), in whom the incidence of SLE is high,[51] and by studies of lupus-like disease in mice.[52] In contrast, the sex ratios in children and adults with ankylosing spondylitis do not appear to be markedly different.

Table 1–2

Factors That Potentially Modify Expression of Rheumatic Diseases in Childhood

- Immaturity of the skeleton and the potential for growth and development
- Immaturity of the gonads and variable hormonal influences
- Immaturity and relative inexperience of the immune system
- Limited antigenic exposure
- Early expression of genetically determined abnormalities

Many genetically determined diseases are expressed very early in life. This is particularly true for the inherited dysplasias of bone and cartilage and for biochemical disorders such as mucopolysaccharidoses and hemophilia. The influence of age on expression of diseases associated with specific histocompatibility antigens is less clear, however. The strongest major histocompatibility complex disease association is that of human leukocyte antigen B27 with ankylosing spondylitis, a disease that begins in childhood in only about 10 percent of cases. The fact that this genetic predisposition does not more frequently result in childhood onset of disease may reflect yet another factor that differentiates the child from the adult: the extent of environmental antigenic experience and the ability of the immune system to respond to that experience.

One argument in support of the significance of antigenic experience and immune reactivity might be exemplified by oligoarticular-onset JRA. This disease has a narrow age-at-onset distribution: In the majority of children, onset of disease occurs between the ages of 1 and 4 years.[45] Another striking age restriction is apparent in Kawasaki disease, which affects most frequently the 1- to 3-year age group in North America.[53] It is tempting to speculate that these diseases reflect the age of initial exposure to an environmental pathogen such as a virus or bacterium, together with the absence of specific protective immunity, in a genetically predisposed individual.

CHILDHOOD RHEUMATIC DISEASES: EXTENT OF THE PROBLEM

It has been difficult to establish the extent of childhood rheumatic disease with any accuracy. In many of the most densely populated areas of the world, incidence and prevalence data for such diseases do not exist. In the developed world, inconsistencies of definition and classification, as well as brevity of follow-up, have prevented accumulation of any substantial body of data from which incidence and prevalence data could be derived. Two fundamental questions require answers: (1) How many children and adolescents have each of the identifiable rheumatic diseases? and (2) What is the outcome for these children?

Three national registries provide some insights concerning prevalence of childhood rheumatic diseases in the United Kingdom,[54] the United States,[55] and Canada[56] (Table 1–3). Conspicuously under-represented in these registries are children with rheumatic fever, which is the major rheumatic disease of childhood in much of the world. A study by Manners and Diepeveen[57] documented that in Western Australia, a great many cases of definite chronic arthritis in children went undiagnosed and untreated. If this is the case in a developed area of the world with readily available expert medical care, the proportion of such children in areas where medical care is less accessible is probably even higher. In Finland, Kunnamo and colleagues[58] surveyed all children under the age of 16 years who had swelling or limitation of motion of a joint, walked with a limp, or had hip pain as determined by a primary care physician, pediatrician, or orthopedic surgeon. All patients were subsequently examined by a single group of pediatric rheumatologists. Overall, the incidence of arthritis was estimated at 109 per 100,000 children per year. Transient synovitis of the hip accounted for 48 percent, other acute transient arthritis (Henoch-Schönlein purpura, serum sickness) for 24 percent, JRA for 17 percent, septic arthritis for 6 percent, and reactive arthritis for 5 percent of cases. Connective tissue diseases such as SLE were not detected in this survey. Estimates of the relative frequencies of adult-onset and childhood-onset rheumatic diseases are shown in Table 1–4. Estimates of the prevalence of chronic diseases of childhood, including those of the musculoskeletal system and connective tissues, are presented in Table 1–5.

Determination of the lifelong "burden of pediatric rheumatic disease" has not been attempted but is an important area of future investigation. The effect of childhood rheumatic diseases on life expectancy, their contribution to morbidity and costs of medical care, and the effect on quality of life are all outcome parameters of importance about which there is very little information, even in Europe and North America; there is no information whatsoever on the global scene. There can be little doubt, however, that a child with, for example, arthritis beginning at the age of 2 or 3 years will carry a lifelong burden in one or more of these areas. The expense and inconvenience for other members of the family are also not inconsequential.

Table 1–3

Relative Frequencies of Rheumatic Diseases in Pediatric Rheumatology Clinics in North America and the United Kingdom

	U.S.A.[55]	U.K.[54]	CANADA[56]
Chronic arthritis	33.1	61.7	50.0
Mechanical/orthopedic	34.9	32.6	40.6
Vasculitis	10.2	1.9	3.0
Systemic lupus erythematosus	7.1	1.3	3.9
Juvenile dermatomyositis	5.2	2.3	1.6
Systemic scleroderma	0.9	0.2	0.2
Rheumatic fever/poststreptococcal arthritis	8.6	0	0.7

Table 1–4

Incidence of the Connective Tissue Diseases

RHEUMATIC DISEASE IN ADULTS	ANNUAL RATE/10^5	SEX RATIO F:M	RACE RATIO W:B	PEAK AGE AT RISK (yr)	CHILDHOOD ONSET (%)
Ankylosing spondylitis	130–1000	1:3	W>B	Young adult	10
Rheumatoid arthritis	40	3:1	Equal	Increases with age (20–30)	5
Systemic lupus erythematosus	6	8:1	1:4	15–45	18
Dermatomyositis/polymyositis	0.8	2:1	1:3	45–65	20
Scleroderma	0.4	3:1	Equal	Increases with age (30–50)	3
Polyarteritis	0.2	1:3	Equal	Midadult	Rare*

*Except for Kawasaki disease.
W, white; B, black.

ADVANCES IN PEDIATRIC RHEUMATOLOGY

It may be premature to consider advances in the understanding of the childhood rheumatic diseases because so much more must be understood. Nevertheless, it is evident that mortality from diseases such as systemic arthritis complicated by amyloidosis, dermatomyositis, and SLE has been dramatically reduced since the 1970s. Disability associated with all forms of chronic arthritis has been minimized: Wheelchair dependence is now rare, the need for aids to ambulation is uncommon, and significant leg-length inequalities are infrequent. Visual outcome in children with JRA and uveitis is much improved.

The reasons for this shift in outcome are multiple; chief among them are the establishment of a body of knowledge and expertise and the involvement of a multidisciplinary team of health professionals in diagnosis and care. Improved application of old techniques and the development of new approaches have been important contributors to improved prognosis. The use of methotrexate and intra-articular glucocorticoid has revolutionized the management of polyarthritis and oligoarthritis, respectively. More judicious use of glucocorticoids and cytotoxic drugs has minimized toxicity and maximized effectiveness in diseases such as SLE and dermatomyositis. Therapeutics is becoming more scientific with the introduction of biologic agents that are designed specifically to interfere with inflammatory mediators. Exciting new treatments for JRA based on fundamental research in inflammation, such as the use of biologic agents that specifically interfere with the action of tumor necrosis factor α, may mark a new dawn in antirheumatic therapy. Although not curative, these agents and their successors promise to revolutionize the management of severe rheumatic diseases of childhood. The identification of Lyme disease, neonatal lupus, and the aggressive treatment of Kawasaki disease represent landmarks of progress. The recognition of the appropriateness of patient and family involvement at all stages of decision-making has enabled individualized treatment options and improved compliance. Family support organizations such as the American Juvenile Arthritis Organization in the United States have helped promote education and research and provide psychosocial support for patients and families.

Table 1–5

Prevalence of Chronic Conditions Among Children Younger Than 17 Years, 1979–1981

CONDITION	PREVALENCE PER 100,000
Diseases of the respiratory system	1079
Mental and nervous system disorders	454
Diseases of the eye and ear	288
Endocrine, nutritional, metabolic, and blood disorders	163
Disease of the circulatory system	151
Certain congenital anomalies and causes of perinatal morbidity	150
Diseases of the musculoskeletal system and connective tissue	132
Diseases of the skin and subcutaneous tissue	114

Reprinted from J Chron Dis, vol 39, Newacheck PW, Halfon N, Budetti P, Prevalence of activity limiting chronic conditions among children based on household interviews, pp 63–71, Copyright 1986, with permission from Elsevier Science.

References

1. Ruffer MA, Rietti A: On osseous lesions in ancient Egyptians. J Pathol Bacteriol 16: 439, 1912.
2. Kramer C: A case of ankylosing spondylitis in mediaeval Geneva. Ossa 8: 115, 1982.
3. Wood PHN: Is rheumatoid arthritis a recent disease? *In* Dumonde DC (ed): Infection and Immunology in the Rheumatic Diseases. Oxford, Blackwell, 1976, p 619.
4. Rothschild BM, Woods RJ: Symmetrical erosive disease in Archaic Indians: the origin of rheumatoid arthritis in the New World? Arthritis Rheum 19: 278, 1990.
5. Barlow T: 51st Annual Meeting of the BMA; Section of Diseases of Children. BMJ 2: 509, 1883.
6. Fink CW: Proposal for the development of classification criteria for idiopathic arthritides of childhood. J Rheumatol 22: 1566, 1995.
7. Petty RE, Southwood TR, Baum J, et al: Revision of the proposed classification criteria for juvenile idiopathic arthritis. J Rheumatol 25: 1991, 1997.
8. The Oxford English Dictionary. London, Oxford University Press, 1955.

9. Dieppe P: Did Galen describe rheumatoid arthritis? Ann Rheum Dis 88: 84, 1988.
10. de Baillou G: The Book on Rheumatism and Back Pain. Paris, 1642.
11. The Genuine Works of Hippocrates. Translated from the Greek by F. Adams. London, The Sydenham Society, 1849.
12. Garrod AB: The nature and treatment of gout and rheumatic gout. London, Walton and Maberly, 1859, p 534. (Cited by Baethge BA [Letter]. J Rheumatol 19: 185, 1992.)
13. Brewer EJ, Bass J, Baum J, et al: Current proposed revision of JRA criteria. Arthritis Rheum 20: 195, 1977.
14. European League Against Rheumatism: EULAR Bulletin No. 4. Nomenclature and classification of arthritis in children. Basel, National Zeitung AG, 1977.
15. Phaire T: The Regiment of Life Whereunto is Added a Treatise of the Pestilence, with the Boke of Chyldren, Newly Corrected and Enlarged. London, Edw. Whitechurch, 1545.
16. Bywaters EGL: The history of pediatric rheumatology. Arthritis Rheum 20(Suppl): 145, 1977.
17. Cornil MV: Memoire sur des coincidences pathologiques du rhumatisme articulaire chronique. C R Soc Ciol (Paris), Series 4, 3: 3, 1964.
18. Bouchut E: Traite pratique des Malades des Enfants, 6th ed. Paris, 1875.
19. Moncorvo: Du Rhumatisme Chronique noueux des enfants. Paris, 1880.
20. West C: Lectures on the Diseases of Infancy and Childhood, 7th ed. Philadelphia, 1881.
21. Diamant-Berger M-S: Du Rhumatisme Noueux (Polyarthrite deformante) Chez les Enfants. Paris, Lecrosnier et Babe, 1891. (Reprinted by Editions Louis Pariente, Paris, 1988.)
22. Still GF: On a form of chronic joint disease in children. Med Chirurg Trans 80: 47, 1897. (Reprinted in Arch Dis Child 132: 195, 1978.)
23. Keen JH: George Frederic Still—Registrar, Great Ormond Street Children's Hospital. Br J Rheumatol 37: 1247, 1998.
24. Koplick H: Arthritis deformans in a child seven years old. Arch Pediatr 13: 161, 1896.
25. Wever F: A case of the form of chronic joint disease in children observed by Still. BMJ 1: 730, 1903.
26. Whitman R: A report of final results in two cases of polyarthritis in children of the type first described by Still together with remarks on rheumatoid arthritis. Med Rec 63: 601, 1903.
27. Litchfield HR, Muson FR: Still's disease (atrophic arthritis). Preliminary report of a case. Arch Pediatr 34: 112, 1922.
28. Henoch EH: About a peculiar form of purpura. Berl Klin Wochschr 11: 641, 1874. (Translated and reprinted in Am J Dis Child 128: 78, 1974.)
29. Schönlein JL: Allgemeine und spezial Pathologie und Therapie, 3rd ed. Herisau Lit Compt. Würzburg, Etlinger, 1837.
30. Unverricht H: Uber eine eigentumliche Form von acuter Muskelentzundung mit einem der Trichinose ahnelnden Krankheitsbilde. Munch Med Wochenschr 34: 488, 1887.
31. Osler W: On the visceral manifestations of the erythema group of skin diseases. Am J Med Sci 127: 1, 1904.
32. Watson R: An account of an extraordinary disease of the skin, and its cure. Extracted from the Italian of Carlo Crusio; accompanied by a letter of the Abbe Nollet, F.R.S. to Mr William Watson F.R.S. Philos Trans R Soc Lond 48: 579, 1754. (Cited by Rodnan GP, Benedeck GT: An historical account of the study of progressive systemic sclerosis [diffuse scleroderma]. Ann Intern Med 57: 305, 1968.)
33. Travers B: Curious case of achylosis of a great part of the vertebral column, probably produced by an ossification of the intervertebral substance. Lancet 5: 254, 1814. (Cited by Bywaters EGL. *In* Moll JMH: Ankylosing Spondylitis. Edinburgh, Churchill Livingstone, 1980, p 14.)
34. Hart FD, McLagan NF: Ankylosing spondylitis: a review of 184 cases. Ann Rheum Dis 14: 77, 1955.
35. Schaller J, Bitnun S, Wedgwood R: Ankylosing spondylitis with childhood onset. J Pediatr 74: 505, 1969.
36. Ladd JR, Cassidy JT, Martel W: Juvenile ankylosing spondylitis. Arthritis Rheum 14: 579, 1971.
37. Kawasaki T: Acute febrile mucocutaneous syndrome with lymphoid involvement with specific desquamation of fingers and toes. Jpn J Allergy 16: 178, 1967.
38. Munro-Faure H: Necrotizing arteritis of the coronary vessels in infants. Pediatrics 23: 914, 1959.
39. Ansell BM, Bywaters EGL, Elderkin FM: Familial arthropathy with rash, uveitis and mental retardation. Proc R Soc Med 68: 584, 1975.
40. Kitridou RC: The neonatal lupus syndrome. *In* Wallace DJ, Hahn BH (eds): Dubois' Lupus Erythematosus, 5th ed. Baltimore, Williams & Wilkins, 1997.
41. Steere AC, Malawista SE, Snydman DR, et al: Lyme arthritis: an epidemic of oligoarticular arthritis in children and adults in three Connecticut communities. Arthritis Rheum 10: 7, 1977.
42. Yunus MB, Masi AT: Juvenile primary fibromyalgia syndrome: a clinical study of thirty-three patients and matched normal controls. Arthritis Rheum 28: 138, 1985.
43. Ansell BM, Bywaters EGL, Spencer PE, Tyler JP: Looking back 1947–1985. The Canadian Red Cross Memorial Hospital. Cliveden, Taplow, England. Gerrards Cross, United Kingdom, BM Ansell, 1997.
44. Stillman JS: The history of pediatric rheumatology in the United States. Rheum Dis Clin North Am 13: 143, 1987.
45. Hanson V: Pediatric rheumatology: a personal perspective. Rheum Dis Clin North Am 13: 155, 1987.
46. Levinson JE: Reflections of a pediatric rheumatologist. Rheum Dis Clin North Am 13: 149, 1987.
47. Ansell BM: Taplow reminiscences. J Rheumatol 19(Suppl 33): 108, 1992.
48. Brewer EJ Jr: The last thirty and the next ten years. J Rheumatol 19(Suppl 33): 108, 1992.
49. Sullivan DB, Cassidy JT, Petty RE: Pathogenic implications of age of onset in juvenile rheumatoid arthritis. Arthritis Rheum 18: 251, 1975.
50. Cassidy JT, Sullivan DB, Petty RE, Ragsdale CG: Lupus nephritis and encephalopathy. Prognosis in 58 children. Arthritis Rheum 20(Suppl): 315, 1977.
51. Ortiz-New C, LeRoy EC: The coincidence of Klinefelter's syndrome and systemic lupus erythematosus. Arthritis Rheum 12: 241, 1969.
52. Roubinian JR, Talal N, Greenspan JS, et al: Sex hormone modulation of autoimmunity in NZB/NZW mice. Arthritis Rheum 22: 1162, 1979.
53. Morens DM, O'Brien RJ: Kawasaki disease in the United States. J Infect Dis 137: 91, 1978.
54. Symmons DPM, Jones M, Osborne J, et al: Pediatric rheumatology in the United Kingdom: data from the British Pediatric Rheumatology Group National Diagnostic Register. J Rheumatol 23: 1975, 1996.
55. Bowyer S, Roettcher P, and the members of the Pediatric Rheumatology Database Research Group: Pediatric rheumatology clinic populations in the United States: results of a 3 year survey. J Rheumatol 23: 1968, 1996.
56. Malleson PN, Fung MY, Rosenberg AM: The incidence of pediatric rheumatic diseases: results from the Canadian Pediatric Rheumatology Association Disease Registry. J Rheumatol 23: 1981, 1996.
57. Manners PJ, Diepeveen DA: Prevalence of juvenile chronic arthritis in a population of 12-year-old children in urban Australia. Pediatrics 98: 84, 1996.
58. Kunnamo I, Kallio P, Pelkonen P: Incidence of arthritis in urban Finnish children. Arthritis Rheum 29: 1232, 1986.

2

Anatomy and Physiology of the Musculoskeletal System

James T. Cassidy and Ross E. Petty

A thorough understanding of the scientific basis of the rheumatic diseases is essential to a working knowledge of their clinical manifestations, diagnosis, and therapy. The fundamentals of anatomy, physiology, biochemistry, pathology, immunology, and genetics now encompass a body of literature well beyond the comprehension of any single physician and an enormous yearly publication of new research data. Therefore, this chapter cannot be intended as a comprehensive review of the basic sciences of rheumatology but rather as an overview and a stimulus for further study.

STRUCTURE AND PHYSIOLOGY

Rheumatic diseases frequently affect many different organ systems. Even so, inflammation of the structures of the musculoskeletal system, particularly joints, connective tissues, and muscles, is common to all rheumatic diseases.[1] This brief discussion focuses on selected aspects of the anatomy, histology, and biochemistry of tissues that are particularly important to the study of rheumatic diseases of childhood.

Joints

Classification of Joints

Joints may be classified as *fibrous, cartilaginous*, or *synovial* (Table 2–1).[2] Fibrous joints are those in which little or no motion occurs and in which the bones are separated by fibrous connective tissue. Cartilaginous joints are those in which little or no motion occurs but the bones are separated by cartilage. Synovial joints are those in which considerable motion occurs and a joint space that is lined with a synovial membrane is present between the bones. It is the synovial joint that is the site of inflammation in most of the chronic arthritides of childhood, such as juvenile rheumatoid arthritis and the seronegative arthropathies. In the latter group, however, cartilaginous joints, such as those at the symphysis pubis and the sternomanubrium, may also be affected.

Development of Joints

In the fetus, diarthrodial joints (joints in which motion occurs) develop by cavitation of the cartilage core of the limb bud.[3] This "cavity" is occupied at first by joint fluid. Further development of the diarthrodial joint apparently depends on fetal movement, which induces formation of cartilage and synovial membrane, and without which the "cavity" regresses and becomes filled with fibrous tissue.[4] The synovial lining begins to form subsequent to cavitation, and the development of other structures—such as bursae, intra-articular fat, tendons, muscle, and capsule—quickly ensues. The whole process takes place from the 4th to 7th weeks of gestation, except for the temporomandibular joint, which develops much later.[5]

Anatomy of Synovial Joints

The anatomy of a typical synovial joint is illustrated in Figure 2–1. The bones of such joints are almost always

Table 2–1

Classification of Joints

TYPE	MOTION	CHARACTERISTICS	EXAMPLES	DISEASE TARGET
Fibrous	No	Bones separated by fibrous connective tissue	Sutures of skull	None
Cartilaginous	No	Bones separated by cartilage	Symphysis pubis	Ankylosing spondylitis
Synovial	Yes	Bones separated by joint space lined with synovial membrane	Joints of extremities	Juvenile rheumatoid arthritis

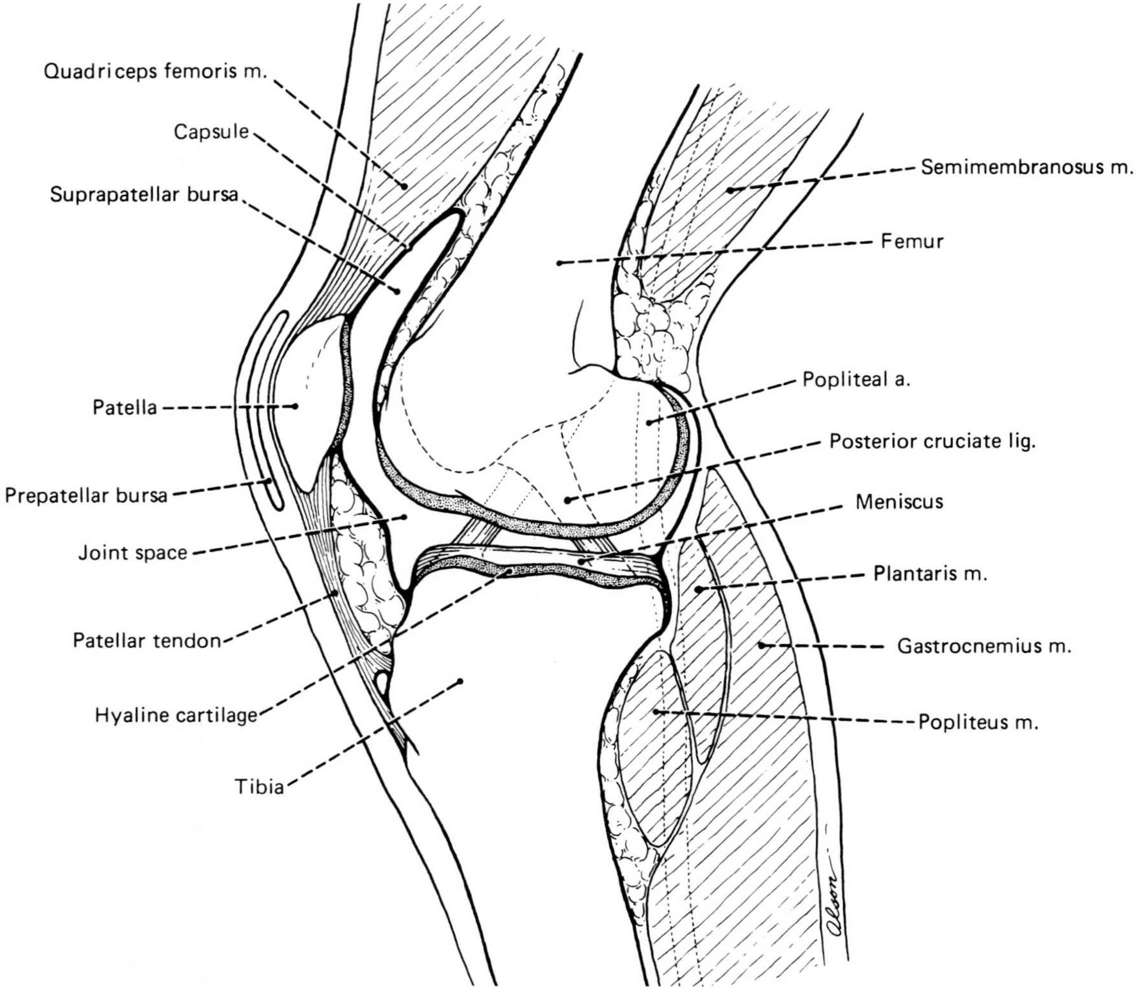

Figure 2–1. Sagittal section of the knee. The distinguishing features of the diarthrodial joint are shown, including bone, hyaline cartilage, synovial space, fibrocartilage, capsule, bursae, ligaments, tendons, muscles, and the vascular and nervous supply. The rheumatic diseases affect all these structures individually or in concert.

covered by hyaline cartilage.[6] The synovial membrane attaches at the cartilage-bone junction so that the entire joint "space" is covered by either hyaline cartilage or synovium. The temporomandibular joint is unusual in that the articular surface of the condyle is covered by fibrocartilage rather than by hyaline cartilage. In some synovial joints, intra-articular fibrocartilage structures are present. Thus, a disk (or meniscus) separates the temporomandibular joint into two spaces; the knee joint contains two menisci that separate the articular surfaces of the tibia and femur, and the triangular fibrocartilage of the wrist joins the distal radioulnar surfaces. Other intra-articular structures include the anterior and posterior cruciate ligaments of the knee, the interosseous ligaments of the talocalcaneal joint, and the triangular ligament of the femoral head. These structures are actually extrasynovial, although they cross through the joint space.

Articular Cartilage

Hyaline cartilage facilitates relatively frictionless motion and absorbs the compressive forces generated by weight bearing.[7–12] The cartilage is firmly fixed to subchondral bone, and its margins blend with the synovial membrane and the periosteum of the metaphysis of the bone. In children, hyaline cartilage is white or slightly blue and is somewhat compressible. It is composed of chondrocytes within an acellular matrix and becomes progressively less cellular throughout the period of growth.[13] The matrix consists of collagen fibers that contribute tensile strength and ground substance composed of water and proteoglycan that contributes resistance to compression.[14–17] The articular cartilage is organized into four zones (Fig. 2–2).[18] Zones 1, 2, and 3 represent a continuum from the most superficial area of zone 1, in which the long axes of the chondrocytes and collagen fibers are tangential to the surface; through zone 2, where the chondrocytes become rounder and the collagen fibers are oblique; to zone 3, where the chondrocytes tend to be arranged in columns perpendicular to the surface. The *tidemark*, a line that stains blue with hematoxylin and eosin (H & E), represents the level at which calcification of the matrix occurs and separates zone 3 from zone 4.

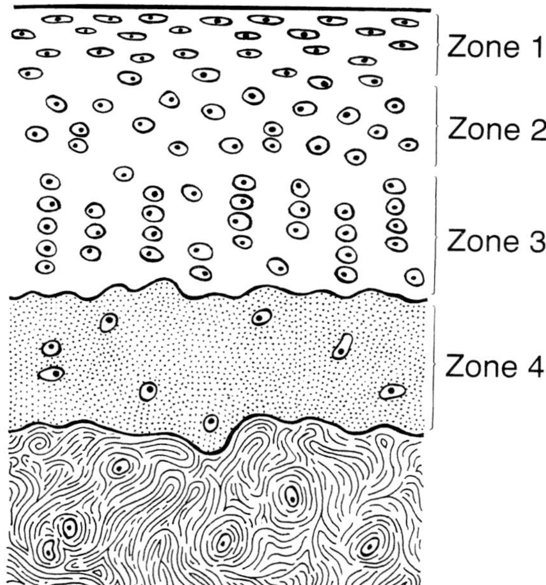

Figure 2–2. Organization of articular cartilage. In zone 1, adjacent to the joint space, the chondrocytes are flattened. In zone 2, the chondrocytes are more rounded, and in zone 3 they are arranged in perpendicular columns. The tide mark separates zone 3 from zone 4, which is impregnated with calcium salts. Bone is beneath zone 4.

Chondrocytes[19] are capable of phagocytosis and are responsible for the synthesis of the two major constituents of the matrix, collagen and proteoglycan, as well as enzymes that have the ability to degrade matrix components (collagenase, neutral proteinases, and cathepsins).[20] This dual function places the chondrocyte in the role of regulating cartilage synthesis and degradation. Whether chondrocytes have any reparative function mediated by cell division is less clear.[21] In the child, end-capillaries proliferate in zone 4, eventually leading to replacement of this area by bone. This is probably how the chondrocytes are nourished, although in the adult, constituent replacement (through the exchange of synovial fluid with cartilage matrix) may play the predominant role.

Synovium

Synovial Membrane

The synovial membrane is a vascular connective tissue structure that lines the capsule of all diarthrodial joints and has important intra-articular regulatory functions.[22, 23] The synovium consists of specialized fibroblasts,[24] one to three cells in depth, overlying a loose meshwork of type I collagen fibers containing blood vessels, lymphatics, fat pads, unmyelinated nerves, and isolated cells such as mast cells.[25, 26] There is no basement membrane separating the joint space from the subsynovial tissues. The synovial membrane is discontinuous, and within the joint space there are so-called *bare areas* between the edge of the cartilage and the attachment of the synovial membrane to the periosteum of the metaphysis.[27] These bare areas are especially vulnerable to damage (erosion) by inflamed synovium in diseases such as juvenile rheumatoid arthritis. Folds, or villi, of synovium provide for unrestricted motion of the joint and for augmented absorptive area. The synoviocytes are of two predominant types, a subdivision that may reflect different functional states rather than different origins. Synovial A cells are capable of phagocytosis and pinocytosis, have numerous microfilopodia and a prominent Golgi apparatus, and may synthesize hyaluronic acid. B cells are more fibroblast-like, have a prominent rough endoplasmic reticulum, and synthesize fibronectin, laminin, and types I and III collagen as well as enzymes (collagenase, neutral proteinases) and catabolin (Fig. 2–3).

Synovial Fluid

Synovial fluid, present in very small quantities in normal synovial joints, has two functions: lubrication and

Figure 2–3. Synovial lining cells. These lining cells from a child with juvenile rheumatoid arthritis show marked phagocytic activity. One lining cell contains a partially degraded cell, probably a neutrophil with lysosomal granules. Another lining cell shows many filopodia (Fp). These cells, which often contain many lysosomal granules and a well-developed Golgi complex, have been called *A (phagocytic) cells.* They are in contrast with *B (synthetic) cells,* which contain well-developed lamellae of the rough endoplasmic reticulum. Cells intermediate between these two principal types are called *C (intermediate) cells.* Another phagocytic cell *(lower left)* contains many lysosomes (L). N, nucleus; Phl, phagolysosome; n, nucleolus. Lead citrate and uranyl acetate × 7260. (Courtesy of Dr. C. R. Wynne-Roberts.)

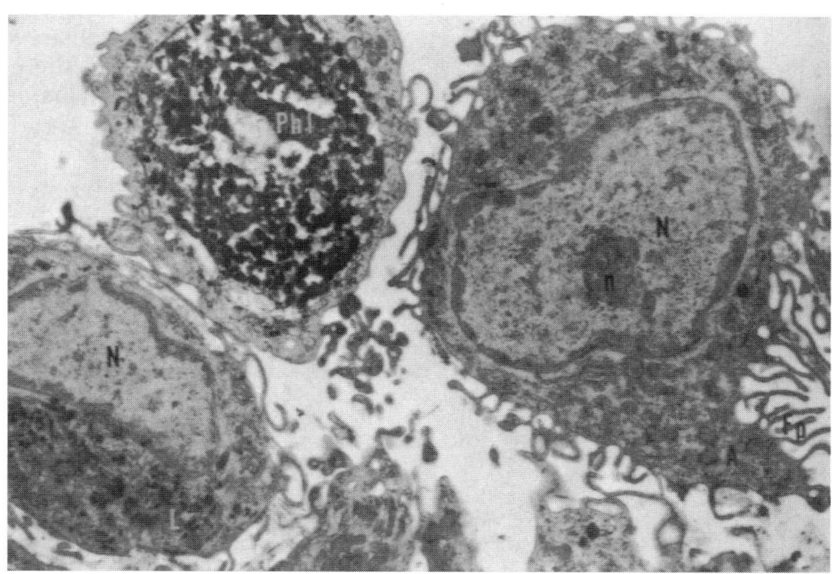

nutrition.[28, 29] Synovial fluid is a combination of a filtrate of plasma, reaching the joint space from the subsynovial capillaries, and hyaluronic acid secreted by the synoviocytes. Hyaluronic acid provides the high viscosity of synovial fluid and, with water, its lubricating properties.[30] Concentrations of small molecules (electrolytes, glucose) are similar to those in plasma, but larger molecules are present in low concentrations relative to plasma (e.g., complement components) unless an inflammatory state alters vasopermeability. Notably absent from synovial fluid are elements of the coagulation pathway (fibrinogen, prothrombin, Factors V and VII, tissue thromboplastin, and antithrombin),[31] thus rendering normal synovial fluid resistant to clotting. There appears to be free exchange of small molecules between synovial fluid of the joint space and water bound to collagen and proteoglycan of cartilage. Characteristics of normal synovial fluid are listed in Table 2–2.[32–40]

Synovial Structures

Synovium lines bursae and tendon sheaths as well as joints.[6] Bursae facilitate frictionless movement between surfaces, such as subcutaneous tissue and bone, or between two tendons. Bursae located near synovial joints frequently communicate with the joint space. This is particularly evident at the shoulder, where the subscapular bursa or recess communicates with the glenohumeral joint; and around the knee, where the suprapatellar pouch, the posterior femoral recess, and occasionally other bursae communicate with the knee joint. Tendon sheaths lined with synovial cells are prominent around tendons as they pass under the extensor retinaculum at the wrist and the ankle. Although closely associated with joints, tendon sheaths do not communicate with the synovial space.

Table 2–2

Normal Synovial Fluid

CHARACTERISTICS	MEAN OR REPRESENTATIVE VALUE*	REFERENCE
Volume	0.13–3.5 ml (adult knee)	32
pH	7.3–7.4	36
Relative viscosity	235	32
Cl, HCO_3	Slightly higher than serum	32
Na, K, Ca, Mg	Slightly lower than serum	32
Glucose	Serum value ± 10%	33
Total protein	1.7–2.1 g/dl	39
Albumin	1.2 g/dl	40
Alpha-1	0.17 g/dl	
Alpha-2	0.15 g/dl	
Beta	0.23 g/dl	
Gamma	0.38 g/dl	
IgG	13% serum value	37
IgM	5% serum value	
IgE	22% serum value	38
α_2-Macroglobulin	3% serum value	37
Transferrin	24% serum value	
Ceruloplasmin	16% serum value	
CH50	30–50% plasma value	35
Hyaluronic acid	300 mg/dl	34
Cholesterol	7.1 mg/dl	40
Phospholipid	13.8 mg/dl	40

*These values represent different adult synovial fluid studies. Similar data are not available for children.

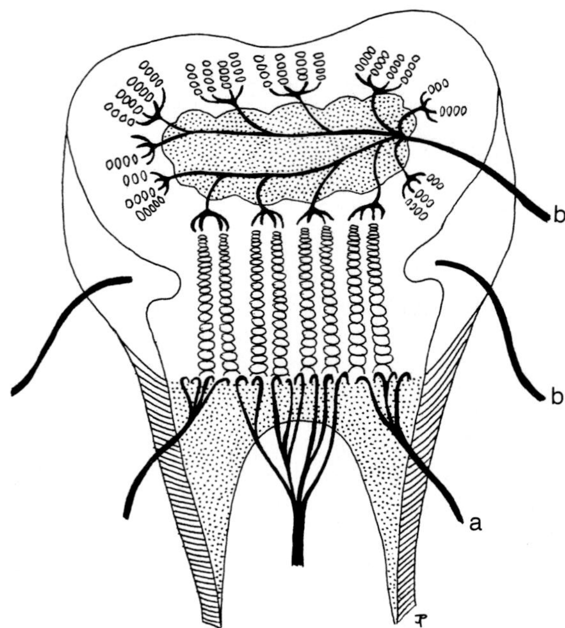

Figure 2–4. Blood supply to the epiphysis and metaphysis. End-arteries (a) at the epiphyseal plate arise from the medullary arteries. Juxta-articular arteries (b) supply epiphysis and synovium.

Vascular System

The arterial supply to the diaphysis and metaphysis of long bones arises from a nutrient artery that penetrates the diaphysis and terminates in the child in end-arteries at the epiphyseal plate.[41] The epiphyseal blood supply arises from juxta-articular arteries that also supply the synovium via a complex network of arterial and arteriovenous anastomoses and capillary beds, called the *circulus articularis vasculosus* by William Harvey. Not until growth has ceased and the epiphyseal plate has ossified is there arterial communication between the metaphyseal and epiphyseal-synovial circulations, a phenomenon of importance in explaining the predisposition of the immature diaphysis to infection and aseptic necrosis after trauma (Fig. 2–4).

Connective Tissues

Collagen

Collagens, the most abundant structural proteins of connective tissues, are glycoproteins with high proline and hydroxyproline content.[42, 43] They are constituted of tough, fibrous proteins that provide structural strength to the tissues of the body.[44] There are at least 19 different types of collagen divided into seven sub-

Table 2–3

Types of Collagen

TYPE	COMPOSITION	TISSUE DISTRIBUTION
Fibril-Forming Collagens		
Type I	α1(I), α2(I)	Most connective tissues; abundant in bone, skin, and tendon
Type II	α1(II)	Cartilage, intervertebral disk, vitreous humor
Type III	α1(III)	Most connective tissues, particularly skin, lung, blood vessels
Type V	α1(V), α2(V), α3(V)	Tissues containing type I collagen, quantitatively minor component
Type XI	α1(XI), α2(XI), α3(XI)	Cartilage, intervertebral disk, vitreous humor
Network-Forming Collagens		
Type IV	α1(IV), α2(IV), α3(IV), α4(IV), α5(IV), α6(IV)	Basement membranes
Type VIII	α1(VIII), α2(VIII)	Several tissues, especially endothelium
Type X	α1(X)	Hypertrophic cartilage
FACIT Collagens		
Type IX	α1(IX), α2(IX), α3(IX)	Cartilage, intervertebral disk, vitreous humor
Type XII	α1(XII)	Tissues containing type I collagen
Type XIV	α1(XIV)	Tissues containing type I collagen
Type XVI	α1(XVI)	Several tissues
Type XIX	α1(XIX)	Rhabdomyosarcoma cells
Beaded Filament-Forming Collagen		
Type VI	α1(VI), α2(VI), α3(VI)	Most connective tissues
Collagen of Anchoring Fibrils		
Type VII	α1(VII)	Skin, oral mucosa, cervix, cornea
Collagens With a Transmembrane Domain		
Type XIII	α1(XIII)	Endomysium, perichondrium, placenta, mucosa of the intestine, meninges
Type XVII	α1(XVII)	Skin, cornea
Collagen Types XV and XVIII		
Type XV	α1(XV)	Many tissues, especially skeletal and heart muscle, placenta
Type XVIII	α1(XVIII)	Many tissues, especially kidney, liver, lung

FACIT, fibril-associated collagens with interrupted triple helices.
From Ala-Kokko L, Prockop DJ: Collagen and elastin. *In* Ruddy S, Harris ED Jr, Sledge CB (eds): Kelley's Textbook of Rheumatology, 6th ed. Philadelphia, WB Saunders, 2000, p 28.

classes (Table 2–3).[45] Types I, II, and III are among the most common proteins in humans (Table 2–4). Only types II and V are found in articular cartilage. Type II collagen, the principal constituent that accounts for more than half the dry weight of cartilage, is a trimer of three identical alpha-helical chains. Type V collagen, a trimer consisting of two alpha-1 chains and one alpha-2 chain (or, in some tissues, one alpha-1, one alpha-2, and one alpha-3 chain), is found in small quantities around chondrocytes. Collagen types VI through X are present in very minute quantities. Collagen synthesis appears to be minimal in the mature animal. The degree of stable crosslinking of collagen fibers increases with advancing age up to the fourth decade of life.[46] This results in increased resistance to pepsin degradation and may contribute to the increased rigidity and decreased tensile strength of old cartilage.[47]

Table 2–4

Composition of Osteoid

Collagens
- Type I (minor amounts of III, V, XI, XIII)

Bone mineral
- Hydroxyapatite

Proteoglycans
- Hyaluronan, etc.

Glycoproteins
- Osteocalcin, osteonectin, osteopontin, thrombospondin, fibronectin

Proteolipids

Enzymes
- Bone-specific alkaline phosphatase, collagenase, proteinases, plasminogen activator

Growth factors
- Transforming growth factor (TGF-β), fibroblast growth factor, insulin-like growth factor (ILGF)

Collagen undergoes extensive changes in primary and tertiary structure after it is secreted from the fibroblast into the extracellular space as a triple helical procollagen (Fig. 2–5).[48] Specific peptidases cleave the amino and carboxyl extension peptides, yielding collagen molecules that in some types form crosslinks and fibrils via lysyl and hydroxylysyl residues. Glycosylation also occurs at this post-translational stage.

Collagen genes are named for the type of collagen (COLI) and the fibril (A1) and code for the large triple-helical domain common to human collagens. Mutations in the collagen genes[49–52] are known to account for human diseases such as Ehlers-Danlos syndrome and osteogenesis imperfecta (see Chapter 37).[53–55] A mutation in the gene for type II procollagen has been linked

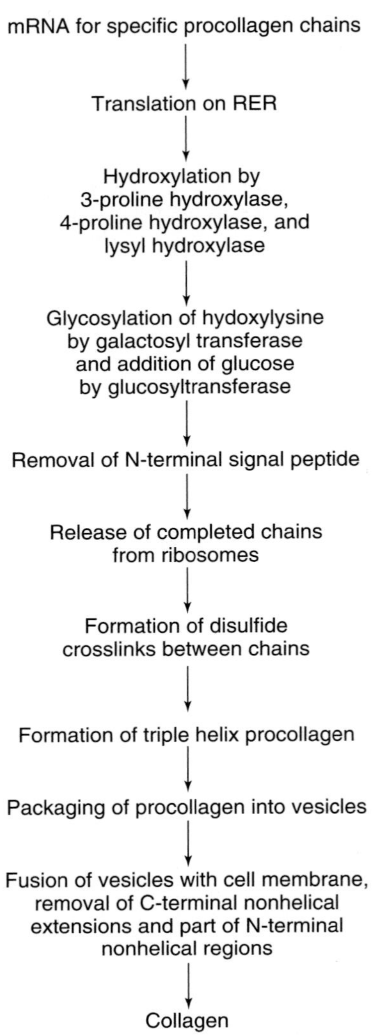

Figure 2–5. Schematic representation of collagen biosynthesis. Triple helical procollagen is secreted from the fibroblast. Specific procollagenases produce collagen by cleaving the ends of the molecules. The collagen molecules (except for type IV collagen) then form fibrils that undergo cross-linking to form collagen fibers. (Adapted from Nimni ME: Collagen: structure, function, and metabolism in normal and fibrotic tissues. Semin Arthritis Rheum 13:1, 1983.)

to osteoarthritis in Finnish kindreds.[56] Another mutation accounts for osteoarthritis in association with a mild form of chondrodysplasia,[57, 58] and another results in severe chondroplasia.[59]

Proteoglycans

Proteoglycans are macromolecules consisting of a protein core to which are attached 50 to 100 unbranched sulfated carbohydrates called *glycosaminoglycans*.[60–62] The structures of the proteoglycans are incompletely understood. At least five different protein cores have been defined. The proteoglycans are attached via a link protein to a nonsulfated glycosaminoglycan, hyaluronic acid, to form large proteoglycan aggregates with molecular weights of several million.[63, 64] This structure is shown schematically in Figure 2–6, and the constituents are listed in Table 2–5. With increasing age, the size of the proteoglycan aggregates increases, the protein and keratan sulfate content increases, and the chondroitin sulfate content decreases.[65, 66] Dermatan sulfate and chondroitin-4-sulfate are the principal mucopolysaccharides in skin, tendon, and aorta; chondroitin-4-sulfate, chondroitin-6-sulfate, and keratan sulfate are in cartilage. Heparan sulfate is found in basal lamina.

A complete description of the functions of matrix glycoproteins and proteoglycans is beyond the scope of this discussion. They are classically organized into a solid phase, a fluid phase, and a cell surface phase. The number and complexity of the constituent species and their interactions are staggering.

Other Connective Tissue Constituents

In addition to collagens, a number of specialized tissues derived from embryonic mesoderm contribute to connective tissue structures. *Elastin* occurs in association with collagen in many tissues, especially in the walls of blood vessels and in certain ligaments.[67] Fibers of elastin lack the tensile strength of collagens but can stretch and return to their original length. Elastin is produced by fibroblasts and smooth muscle cells. *Fibronectin* is a dimeric glycoprotein with a molecular weight of 450,000 that acts as an attachment protein in the extracellular matrix.[68] It is produced by many different cell types, including macrophages, dedifferentiated chondrocytes, and fibroblasts. It has the ability to bind to collagens, proteoglycans, fibrinogen, and actin as well as to cell surfaces and bacteria. Fibronectin is present in plasma and as an insoluble matrix throughout loose connective tissues, especially between basement membranes and cells. *Laminin* is a major constituent of the basement membrane together with type IV collagen.[69] *Reticulin* may be an embryonic form of type III collagen. It is present as a fine branching network of fibers widespread in spleen, liver, bone marrow, and lymph nodes.

Proteinases for Collagen and Cartilage

The proteinases (endopeptidases) are proteolytic enzymes that are active in homeostatic remodeling of the extracellular matrix during health and in its degradation during inflammation.[70] These enzymes occur both intracellularly and extracellularly in tissue fluids and plasma and have been classified into four categories based on functional catalytic groups[71]: the *metalloproteinases* and *serine proteinases,* which are active at neutral to slightly alkaline pH, and the *cysteine* and *aspartic proteinases,* which are most active at acid pH (Table 2–6).

The metalloproteinases are activated by calcium and stabilized by zinc ions and consist of at least 11 well-characterized enzymes found in human tissues.[72] They are active in the degradation or remodeling of collagens and are known to be synthesized by rheumatoid

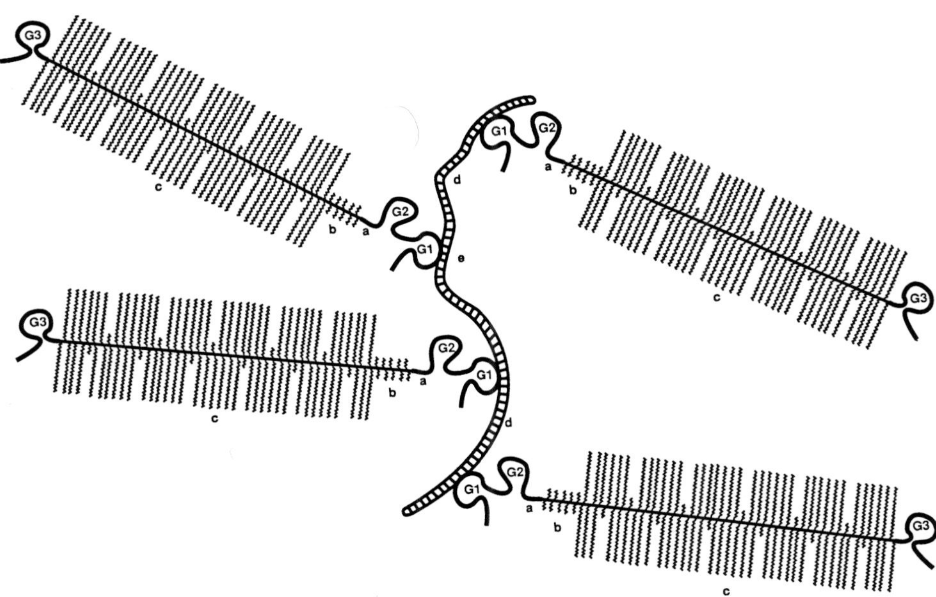

Figure 2–6. The structure of the proteoglycan aggregate of cartilage. The proteoglycan monomer consists of a core protein (a) of variable length that contains three globular domains: G1, located at the NH_2-terminus and containing the hyaluronate binding region; G2; and G3. Link protein (e) stabilizes the aggregate by binding simultaneously to the hyaluronate chain (d) and G1. Glycosaminoglycan molecules are attached to the core protein in specific regions: keratan sulfate (b) and chondroitin sulfate (c).

Table 2–5

Glycosaminoglycans (GAGs)—Composition and Distribution

GAG	AMINO SUGAR	HEXURONIC ACID OR MONOSACCHARIDE	DISTRIBUTION
Hyaluronic acid	NAGlu	D-Glucuronic acid	Most connective tissues
Chondroitin-4-sulfate	NAGal	D-Glucuronic acid	Cartilage, skin, bone
Chondroitin-6-sulfate	NAGal	D-Glucuronic acid	Cartilage, skin, aorta, nucleus pulposus, umbilical cord
Dermatan sulfate	NAGal	D-Glucuronic acid	Heart valves, vessels
		L-Iduronic acid	Skin, tendon, ligament
Heparan sulfate	NAGlu	D-Glucuronic acid	Cell membranes
		L-Iduronic acid	All connective tissue
Heparin	NAGlu	D-Glucuronic acid	An anticoagulant
		L-Iduronic acid	Mast cells, liver capsule
Keratan sulfate	NAGlu	D-Galactose	Cornea, skeletal tissues

NAGlu, *N*-acetyl-D-glucosamine; NAGal, *N*-acetyl-D-galactosamine.

Table 2–6

Proteinases and Inhibitors for Collagen and Cartilage Substrates

ENZYME	SUBSTRATE	INHIBITOR
Metalloproteinase		
Collagenase	Various collagens and GAGs	TIMP
Gelatinase	Denatured collagens	TIMP
Stromelysin	Fibronectin, GAG, elastin, collagens	TIMP
Serine proteinase		
Plasmin	Metalloproteinases	α_2-Antiplasmin
Elastase	Various collagens and GAGs	α_1-Plasminogen inactivator
Cathepsin G	GAGs, type II collagen, elastin, TIMP	α_1-Plasminogen inactivator
Plasminogen activator	Proplasminogen	
Cysteine proteinase		
Cathepsin B	Type II collagen, GAGs, link protein	Cystatins
Cathepsin L	Type I collagen, GAGs, link protein, elastin	Cystatins
Aspartic proteinase		
Cathepsin D	GAGs, type II collagen	α_2-Macroglobulin

GAGs, glycosaminoglycans; TIMP, tissue inhibitor of metalloproteinase.

synovium. Collagenases are inhibited naturally by α_2-macroglobulin and by the *tissue inhibitor of metalloproteinase*. *Stromelysin* is a neutral proteinase synthesized by cultured fibroblasts and synovium. Other members of this family with differing activities have been identified; for example, *gelatinases* are secreted by many cells in culture and are active in the remodeling of collagen-containing tissues.

The serine proteinases are a family of endopeptidases that participate in matrix degradation either directly or by activating precursors of the metalloproteinases. They include many of the enzymes of pathways involving coagulation, fibrinolysis, complement activation, and kinin generation: plasmin, plasminogen activator, kallikrein, and elastase. Serine proteinase inhibitors constitute 10 percent of the plasma proteins. The cysteine proteinases that degrade extracellular matrix include cathepsins B and L, which are lysosomal enzymes associated with inflammatory reactions. The aspartic proteinases are primarily lysosomal proteinases active at acid pH. Cathepsin D is the major representative of this family that degrades proteoglycans and is present in the lysosomes of most cells.

Connective Tissue Structures

Connective tissues have diversified throughout evolution to provide the supporting structures of the body (bone, periosteum, cartilage), to permit the action of muscles on this structure (tendons, ligaments, fasciae), to support internal organs (dermis, capsules, serosal membranes, basement membranes), and to provide support for blood vessels, lymphatics, and the bronchopulmonary tree.

Tendons

Tendons are specialized connective tissue structures that attach muscle to bone.[73] They contain, in addition to water, type I collagen and small amounts of elastin and type III collagen, the latter forming the *epitenon* and *endotenon*. The type III collagen fibers themselves are densely packed in a parallel configuration in a proteoglycan matrix containing elongated fibroblasts.

Ligaments and Fasciae

Ligaments and fasciae join bone to bone and, like tendons, are composed of type I collagen. So-called elastic ligaments, such as the ligamenta flava and ligamentum nuchae, predominantly contain elastin.

Entheses

An enthesis is the site of attachment of tendon, ligament, fascia, or capsule to bone. Unlike tendon or ligament, the enthesis is an active metabolic site, particularly in the child. It includes the *peritenon*, which is continuous with the periosteum; collagen fibers of the tendon or ligament, which insert into the bone (*Sharpey's fibers*); the adjoining cartilage; and bone not covered by periosteum.[74] In 1998, a highly informative and interesting commentary was published on the strongest tendon in the body, the Achilles tendon, and its enthesis.[75]

The Growing Skeleton

An understanding of bone biology is essential to an appreciation of skeletal growth and adaptation to mechanical stresses throughout life.[76–80] Bone can be divided into two primary types: *cortical* bone, which consists of compact bone found in the long bones of the appendicular skeleton; and *trabecular* bone, which is the primary component of vertebral bodies and the flat bones of the skull and pelvis.[81] Bones change remarkably in size, shape, and microstructure throughout the period of growth.[82, 83] Bones of the appendicular and axial skeletons develop initially by ossification of preexisting cartilage that has developed from mesenchymal condensations in the embryo (*enchondral ossification*). In contrast, bones of the face, the skull, and initially the mandible and clavicle develop by ossification of fibrocellular tissue (*membranous ossification*). All axial and appendicular bones also undergo secondary membranous ossification—the diaphyseal cortex is continuously modified by periosteal bone deposition.

Anatomy of Bone

Long bones consist of four parts.[84] The *diaphysis* is the long tubular midportion of bone that ends in the *metaphysis*, the flared portion of bone that is separated from the *epiphysis* by the growth plate or *physis*. At birth, the diaphysis is relatively short. It grows in length by enchondral ossification. Cartilage cells proliferate toward the ends of bone; those closest to the middle of the bone ossify. Periosteal deposition of new bone increases the diameter of the diaphysis. The newborn diaphysis consists of laminar bone that lacks the *haversian canal system* characteristic of mature bone; as the child ages, the intercellular matrix increases, porosity decreases, and hardness of the bone increases.[85] All epiphyses, except that of the distal femur, are completely cartilaginous at birth. The cartilage is gradually replaced by bone until only the articular cartilage remains unossified in the mature person.

The physis is a cellular zone in which mitoses are frequent and new cells are being formed. Factors influencing growth at the physis include thyroxine, growth hormone, and testosterone. Thyroxine and growth hormone act synergistically to induce cell division. Growth hormone and insulin-like growth factor I act together to facilitate achievement of peak bone mass during puberty.[86] Testosterone stimulates the physis to undergo rapid cell division with resultant physeal widening during the growth spurt (the anabolic effect) but eventually slows growth (androgenic effect). Estrogens suppress the growth rate by increasing calcification of the matrix, a prerequisite to epiphyseal closure. There do not appear to be receptors for these steroids on physeal cells, although there are receptors for somatomedin, insulin, and prolactin. It is probably through these molecules and their receptors that the steroid effects are mediated.[87] Hydrocortisone affects physeal physiology indirectly by suppressing growth hormone release.[88–90]

The relative contributions of individual physes to limb length are summarized in Table 2–7. Growth in the bones of the appendicular skeleton ceases with completion of the ossification of the iliac apophyses, although the height of the vertebral bodies may continue to increase and contribute to overall height until the third decade of life.[91] Skeletal bone age can be determined by radiographic identification of the onset of secondary ossification in the long bones and by physeal closure. In general, ossification centers appear earlier and physes fuse earlier in girls than in boys.

Bone Mineral Metabolism

The complex structure and composition of bone is directly related to the two primary functions of the skeleton: support of the tissues of the body in order to permit locomotion and a reservoir of ions critical to body functions.[80, 92, 93] Bone is composed of 70 percent mineral and 30 percent organic constituents. *Hydroxyapatite*, constituted primarily of calcium and phosphorus, accounts for 95 percent of the mineral.[94, 95] The organic component consists of 98 percent matrix, which is predominantly type I collagen. Noncollagenous proteins, such as osteocalcin, fibronectin, osteonectin, and osteopontin, make up 5 percent of the matrix.[96] Cells occupy the remaining 2 percent of the organic component of bone and are responsible for formation, resorption, and maintenance of the remodeling cycle.[97–100] *Osteoclasts* are derived from mononuclear cells and resorb bone.[101] The *osteoblasts* form osteoid and osteoid matrix (see Table 2–4). *Osteocytes* differentiate from osteoblasts and maintain the integrity of bone through a network of canaliculi.

Calcium, phosphate, and magnesium are minerals important in the homeostasis of bone.[102, 103] Although serum concentrations of zinc, copper, and magnesium are often used as controls in studies of bone mineral metabolism,[104] levels of zinc are decreased in chronic inflammation, and those of copper are increased. Magnesium remains unaffected and is often used as an internal control for clinical studies. The urinary magnesium:creatinine ratio is often employed similarly.

Table 2–7

Relative Contributions of Individual Physes to Length of the Bone and Limb

GROWTH AREA		CONTRIBUTION TO TOTAL GROWTH (%) Of Bone	Of Limb
Humerus	Proximal	80	40
	Distal	20	10
Radius/ulna	Proximal	20	10
	Distal	80	40
Femur	Proximal	30	15
	Distal	70	40
Tibia/fibula	Proximal	55	27
	Distal	45	18

Data from Ogden JA: Skeletal Injury in the Child. Philadelphia, Lea & Febiger, 1982.

Biochemical Markers of Bone Formation and Resorption

Studies of bone mineral metabolism generally assay a specific set of markers of *bone formation* and *resorption* performed on blood or urine.[105–108] Measures of bone formation include the activity of *bone-specific alkaline phosphatase,* which is a component of the osteoblast plasma membrane and is released during osteoblastic activity. *Osteocalcin,* derived from osteoblasts, is a vitamin K–dependent gamma carboxylated protein.[96] Its serum concentration reflects that portion of newly synthesized protein that does not bind to the mineral phase of bone and is released into the circulation. The serum *carboxy-terminal propeptide of type I procollagen* (PICP) is also a marker of bone formation.[109] PICP is a globular protein that is cleaved by a specific peptidase at the C-terminal end of the procollagen triple helix. Its concentration in blood directly reflects the number of collagen fibrils that have been formed.

The plasma *tartrate-resistant acid phosphatase* (TRAP) is a marker of bone resorption.[110, 111] It is a labile enzyme that is released during osteoclastic activity. The urinary concentration of the *deoxypyridinoline crosslinked telopeptide domain of type I collagen* represents hydroxylysyl and lysyl post-translational components of the crosslinkage of type I collagen that stabilize the molecule.[112, 113] They are measured in relation to the concentration of creatinine in the urine. These crosslinks are reflective of mature collagen breakdown. Deoxypyridinoline is found in large amounts only in type I collagen; therefore, its urinary excretion reflects the breakdown of that molecule. Urinary hydroxyproline has been used similarly. The *urinary calcium:creatinine ratio* is also a marker of bone resorption. There are many confounding factors in using this measure, however, such as the urinary acidity, various medications, magnesium concentration, and renal function.

Calcium Regulating Hormones

Assessment of bone mineral metabolism would not be complete without assays for the calcium-regulating hormones.[114, 115] These include *parathyroid hormone (PTH), 25-OH vitamin* D_3 *(25-OHD),* and *1,25*$(OH)_2$ *vitamin* D_3 *(1,25*$(OH)_2$*D).*[116–118] The primary function of PTH is to maintain the ionized calcium concentration of the blood within a narrow physiologic range. Hypocalcemia results in stimulation of PTH secretion, whereas hypercalcemia suppresses its secretion. PTH regulates calcium homeostasis by action on the major reservoir of the body's calcium, the skeleton. It stimulates osteoclastic activity and thereby bone resorption. It also stimulates the conversion of 25-OHD to 1,25$(OH)_2$D. The principal source of 25-OHD is vitamin D_2 of the diet.[119] Ultraviolet light also endogenously stimulates the production of D_3 from 7-dehydrocholesterol in the skin. 25-OHD is biologically inactive and is hydroxylated in the kidney to the 1,25$(OH)_2$D hormone (see Fig. 36–1). This hormone, often called *calcitriol*, stimulates intestinal absorption of calcium, thereby elevating the serum calcium concentration. Receptors for 1,25$(OH)_2$D are present on intestinal cells. This hormone also facilitates bone resorption by stimulating the differentiation of osteoclast precursors to mature osteoclasts. 1,25$(OH)_2$D is also judged to have a role in autoimmunity. Measurement of vitamin D hormones must be carefully controlled because diet, malnutrition, the presence of diseases leading to malabsorption or a catabolic state, and season of the year (sun exposure) will alter results.

Absorptiometry

Absorptiometry is a means of assessing bone mineral content or density of various areas of the skeleton. *Single-photon absorptiometry* (SPA) uses an iodine-125 source and is restricted to measuring *bone mineral content* at the one-third and one-tenth distal radial sites of the forearm.[120] This technique is therefore primarily a measure of disturbances in the appendicular skeleton. Although bone width can be calculated in SPA, estimations of *bone mineral density* (g/cm^2) are not accurate. *Dual-photon absorptiometry* employs a gadolinium source with photons of 44 keV and 100 keV measured simultaneously in order to calculate bone mineral content or density of any area of the skeleton by a computerized subtraction of tissue density from that of bone. Although applicable to children and accurate with a variance of less than or equal to 3 percent, measurement time is prolonged over 30 to 45 minutes for a complete skeletal survey. The technique most appropriate for children because of low radiation ($\leq$3 mRem), speed (0.5 to 2.5 minutes), and accuracy is that of *dual-energy x-ray absorptiometry* (DEXA).[121, 122] DEXA employs two beams of 70 keV and 140 keV in order to distinguish soft tissue from bone (Fig. 2–7). The introduction of DEXA has been responsible for adding much new knowledge in pediatrics concerning skeletal maturation and diseases that affect bone metabolism.

Bone mineral content (BMC) is a measurement of total body or site-specific mineralization by absorptiometry. Bone mineral density (BMD) is a measurement of bone mineral content partially corrected for bone

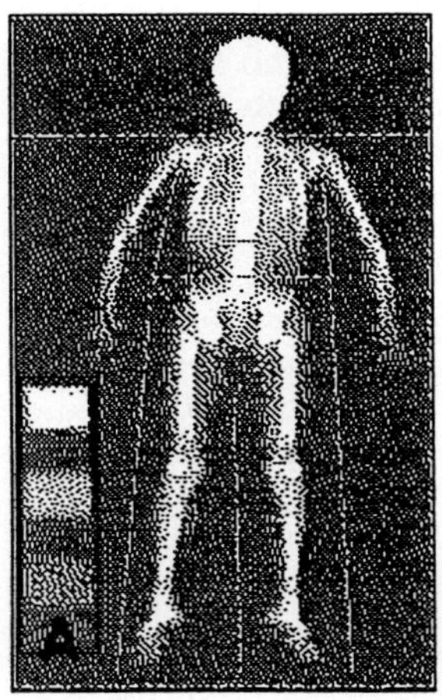

Region	Area (cm2)	BMC (grams)	BMD (gms/cm2)
Head	205.62	269.70	1.312
L Arm	80.80	49.97	0.618
R Arm	82.01	50.14	0.611
L Ribs	65.04	35.65	0.548
R Ribs	81.20	42.24	0.520
T Spine	84.43	52.26	0.619
L Spine	25.85	14.27	0.552
Pelvis	106.25	69.16	0.651
L Leg	210.47	145.69	0.692
R Leg	214.51	145.62	0.679
TOTAL	1156.18	874.69	0.757

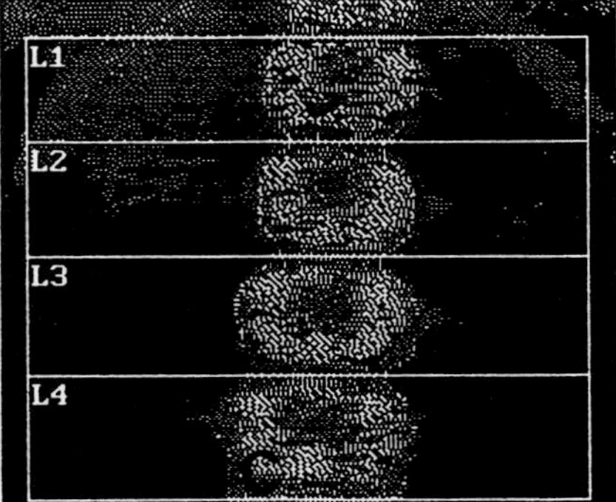

Region	Area (cm2)	BMC (grams)	BMD (gms/cm2)
L1	6.12	3.02	0.494
L2	7.00	3.90	0.557
L3	8.60	5.76	0.670
L4	10.26	7.10	0.692
TOTAL	31.97	19.78	0.619

Figure 2–7. Dual energy x-ray absorptiometry (DEXA) of an 8-year-old girl with juvenile rheumatoid arthritis. *A*, Whole body scan with bone mineral content (BMC) calculations on its right. *B*, Scans of ultradistal (UD) and one-third (mid) distal radius. *C*, L1–L4 vertebral scan with BMC and bone mineral density (BMD) below it.

size (BMC divided by surface area). Because this is only a two-dimensional computation, it is called *areal BMC*.[123] A three-dimensional estimate of skeletal density can be obtained when both AP and lateral measurements are correlated for skeletal size (cubic centimeters), a measurement called *volumetric BMD*. The latter value is seldom available in published data.

Osteoporosis is the parallel loss of bone mineral and matrix. It is defined by the World Health Organization as BMD less than 2.5 S.D. below the mean for young adults.[124] Osteopenia is a low bone mass for age, or more specifically for skeletal age and stage of sexual maturation. In young adults, osteopenia is defined as BMD between 1 and 2.5 S.D. below the mean for young healthy adults. Osteopenia is the primary disorder in children with chronic illness; osteoporosis may be superimposed on this abnormality related to malnutrition, cachexia, and glucocorticoid medication.

The ratio of cortical to trabecular bone differs in various parts of the skeleton. Sites often measured by absorptiometry include the one-third distal radius (95 percent cortical and 5 percent trabecular); the one-tenth distal radius (25 percent cortical and 75 percent trabecular); the lumbar vertebral bodies (5 percent cortical and 95 percent trabecular); the femoral neck (75 percent cortical and 25 percent trabecular); and the greater trochanteric area of the femur (50 percent cortical and 50 percent trabecular).

Physiologic Phases of Skeletal Growth

Of great importance in disability related to the chronic rheumatic diseases of children is the fact that approximately half of the total peak skeletal mass is achieved during the adolescent growth spurt. Complete skeletal maturation for some bones is not reached until the latter part of the third decade of life.[125–128] Determinants of peak bone mass are intrinsic factors such as heredity, sex and hormones, and extrinsic factors such as nutrition (calcium, vitamins, calories, protein) and mechanical influences related to body weight and physical activity.[129, 130] In general, it is estimated that heredity determines 75 to 80 percent of the skeletal mass of the child.[130–132] Environmental variables, including those related to endocrine and nutritional influences, mechanical forces, and risk factors, account for the remainder.

Sexual Maturation

Skeletal growth correlates closely with sexual maturation because epiphyseal closure is under androgenic control. In North America, girls reach puberty at approximately 11.15 years of age (S.D., ±1.10) and have a peak height velocity of approximately 8.3 cm per year at age 12.14 (S.D., ±0.88).[133, 134] Menarche occurs soon after at 13.5 years (S.D., ±1.02), and epiphyseal closure is complete at approximately age 16 years. Puberty in boys begins 1/2 year later at 11.64 years (S.D., ±1.07) and lasts approximately 1 year longer than in girls (until about 15 years in boys).[133, 134] Peak height velocity of approximately 9.5 cm per year is reached at an age of 14.06 years (S.D., ±0.92), and epiphyseal closure occurs at 18 years or soon thereafter.

Skeletal Maturation

Bone mineralization during childhood and adolescence is highly correlated with age, weight, height, and Tanner stage.[135–138] Bone turnover is a linked phenomenon of facilitating bone formation and limiting bone resorption in order for skeletal growth to occur. Peak bone mass is achieved in developed countries by late adolescence or very early in the third decade of life.[121, 135, 139–143] Rapid skeletal accretion occurs during intrauterine growth of the fetus and the early months of infancy. Thereafter, skeletal growth is linear during childhood. Early puberty and adolescence are characterized by accelerated skeletal maturation and account for at least 40 percent of the total skeletal mass.[137, 139, 144, 145] During puberty, sex differences in skeletal maturation appear with varying effects depending on bone site.[146] Trabecular bone is more sensitive to hormonal regulation; and bone size, cortical shell, and trabecular bone are greater in boys than in girls.[147] However, there is essentially no difference in volumetric BMD between the sexes.[148] Total body BMD continues to increase modestly after epiphyseal closure in boys but plateaus in girls.[149] Linear growth and accrual of appendicular skeletal mass (with one exception—the radius) are completed prior to those of the axial skeleton.

Axial Skeleton. Lumbar BMD increases 35 to 70 percent during adolescence in both boys and girls.[135, 144, 147, 148, 150] In general, skeletal maturation of the lumbar spine is completed by the end of the second decade of life. The rate of change in lumbar BMD is greatest in girls between 10 and 15 years and in boys between 13 and 17 years of age.[151–154]

Appendicular Skeleton. The radius is different from other bones in terms of skeletal maturation as assessed by absorptiometry. BMD of the radius increases in both sexes until approximately 15 years of age, at which time it accelerates in boys until the end of the second decade of life.[144] Measurements of radial cortical bone continue to increase gradually into the young adult years in girls.[139, 155] BMD of the femoral neck increases approximately 35 to 40 percent, and BMD of the femoral shaft 40 to 50 percent, during adolescent growth.[135, 144] In girls, peak bone mass of the femoral neck is gained by 14 to 15 years and in the femoral shaft by 17 to 18 years of age. In boys, bone mass of both the femoral shaft and neck continues to increase between the ages of 15 and 18 years.

Extrinsic Factors

An adequate intake of calcium is a relatively important factor in achievement of peak bone mass.[156–161] Calcium, however, is a threshold nutrient.[162] Some studies support the observation that absorption is also influenced by vitamin D receptor alleles[163]; others do not.[164] The influence of adequate calcium intake was greater for the prepubertal skeleton in the twin study of Johnston and colleagues[165]: Addition of calcium citrate malate (approximately 1000 mg/day) to the diet over a 3-year period produced measurable increases in both appendicular and axial bone density in the supplemented twin of 70 pairs of monozygotic twins. In the treatment group, significant incremental bone formation at several measured sites of cortical and trabecular bone was documented in 22 prepubertal children but did not occur in 23 postpubertal or pubertal children. If persistent, such an increase would lead to a peak bone mass that was higher than expected and above the genetic threshold. The inability to document the effects of supplementation to increase bone mass in older children may have been obscured by the rapid gain that occurs during adolescent growth.

Skeletal loading is also a crucial variable associated with body weight that is an independent determinant of peak BMD.[159, 160, 166, 167] This may be most clearly related to lean body mass, which at the end of adolescence averages 90 percent in boys and 75 percent in girls. Physical stress on bones appears to be more influential during the prepubertal phase of growth than during puberty.[146, 168, 169] Weight-bearing activity may be more significant in boys than in girls in achieving maximal BMD.[170] In girls, it is estimated that Tanner stage and weight account for 80 percent of the variance in lumbar BMD and 85 percent of the variance in total-body BMD. In boys, weight and calcium intake explain up to 90 percent of the variance in total body BMD.

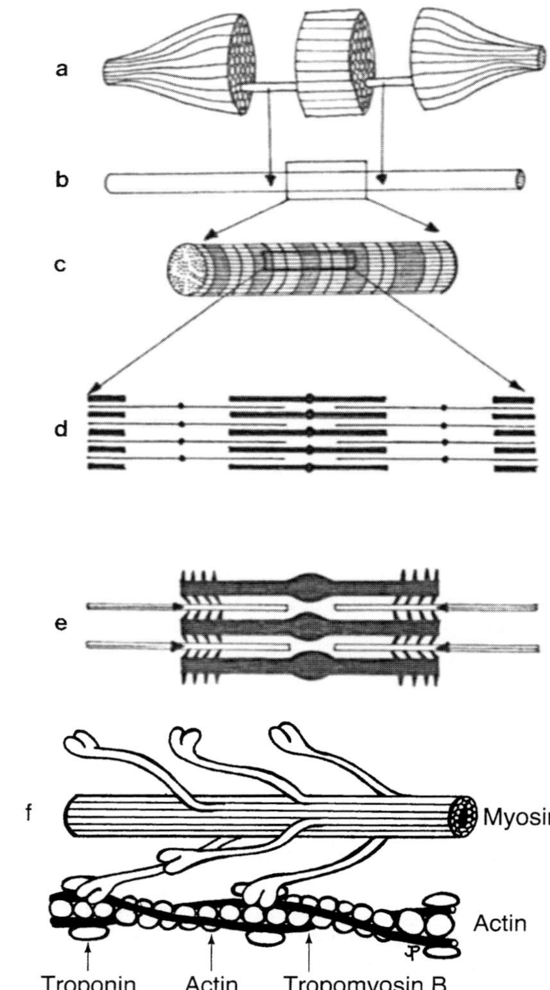

Figure 2–8. Schematic representation of the anatomy of skeletal muscle: a, fascicle; b, fiber; c, myofibrils; d, actin and myosin; e and f, enlargement of actin and myosin filaments showing the actin filaments coiled around each other and associated with tropomyosin B lying in the groove.

Skeletal Muscle

Anatomy

Skeletal muscle makes up approximately 40 percent of the adult body mass and consists of about 640 separate muscles that support the skeleton and permit movement and locomotion. Skeletal muscle is formed during embryogenesis from mesodermal stem cells that differentiate into the various types of muscle, bone, and connective tissue. A skeletal muscle is surrounded by the connective tissue *epimysium*. Within the muscle, *fascicles* are covered by connective tissue *perimysium*.[171] Each fascicle contains many individual muscle *fibers* that are the basic structural units of skeletal muscle (Fig. 2–8). Muscle fibers are elongated multinucleated cells surrounded by connective tissue *endomysium* (reticulin, collagen) that is richly supplied with capillaries. Within each fiber are a large number of *myofibrils*, consisting of highly organized interdigitated *myofilaments* of actin and myosin.[172] Each myofilament has approximately 180 myosin molecules with a molecular weight of 500,000, a long tail, and a double head. The myofilament is composed of the myosin tails; the myosin heads project in a spiral arrangement. Lying parallel to the myosin molecules are *actin filaments* (F-actin) composed of globular subunits of G-actin with a molecular weight of 42,000. Two actin filaments are coiled around each other as a helix, with a second protein, *tropomyosin B*, lying in the groove. A regulatory protein, *troponin*, is located at intervals along this structure. This complex structure is demonstrable by light or electron microscopy as striations.[84] *Creatine kinase* is bound to the myosin filaments at regular intervals.[173]

Muscle Contraction

The functional ability of muscle to produce coordinated movements is governed by the conversion of chemical to mechanical energy by *actomyosin*.[174, 175] Calcium diffusion in the myoplasm and binding to thin-filament regulatory proteins are stimulated by the action potential of the alpha-motor neuron. Variation in the properties of the various types of motor fibers and motor units, and recruitment of motor units, result in the specific patterns of movement. The properties of the motor unit are influenced by the genetic makeup of the

Table 2–8

Classification of Muscle Fiber Types

CHARACTERISTIC	TYPE I	TYPE IIA	TYPE IIB	TYPE IIC
Size	Moderate	Small	Large	Small
Color	Red	White	White	White
Myoglobin content	High	Medium	Low	High
Mitochondria	Many	Intermediate	Few	Intermediate
Blood supply	+ + +	+	+	+
ATPase (pH 4.4)	High	Low	Low	–
ATPase (pH 10.6)	Low	High	High	–
Lipid	High	Low	Low	–
Glycogen	Low	High	High	Variable
Metabolic characteristics				
Oxidative (aerobic)	High	Intermediate	Low	High
Glycolytic (anaerobic)	Moderate	High	High	High
Function				
Contraction time	Slow and sustained	Fast twitch	Fast twitch	Moderate twitch
Resistance to fatigue	High	Moderate	Low	Moderate

individual, muscular conditioning, and the presence of any disease that results in joint pain or immobilization or metabolic, hormonal, or nutritional disturbances.[176]

Types of Muscle Fibers

Muscle fibers constitute 85 percent of muscle tissue. There are two major types of fibers, which differ in structure and biochemistry (Table 2–8).[177–180] Most muscles contain both types: *Type I (slow) fibers* are narrower, have poorly defined myofibrils, are irregular in size, have thick Z bands, and are rich in mitochondria and oxidative enzymes but poor in phosphorylases. *Type II (fast) fibers* have fewer mitochondria and are poor in oxidative enzymes but rich in phosphorylases and glycogen. These fibers have been further subdivided into three types. Type I and II muscle fibers can be differentiated histochemically (Fig. 2–9). Muscles differ in the proportions of each fiber type that they contain; the diaphragm contains predominantly "slow" fibers, and small muscles contain predominantly "fast" fibers.

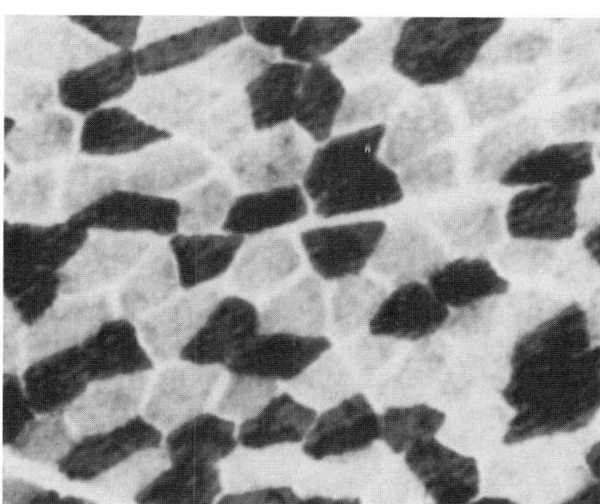

Figure 2–9. Frozen section of normal skeletal muscle stained with ATPase, pH 9.2. Type I fibers are pale, and type II fibers are dark. Magnification × 800. (Courtesy of Dr. M. Norman.)

Muscle conditioning leads to adaptations in the contractile and structural proteins and fiber species within the genetic potential of the individual. Strength training results in hypertrophy of type IIB fibers, and endurance training leads to metabolic alterations in type I and IIA fibers.[176, 181–183]

ANIMAL MODELS OF RHEUMATIC DISEASES

The study of animal models of human disease provides clues about etiology, but it must always be remembered that such models are, at best, approximations of human disease and that fundamental differences in etiology and pathogenesis almost certainly exist and may be difficult to recognize. In spite of these limitations, and because of the obvious difficulties involved in direct study of human rheumatic diseases, a number of spontaneous or induced models of disease in animals have been the focus of an abundance of studies in recent decades (Table 2–9).[184]

Models of Inflammatory Joint Disease

A great many models of inflammatory joint disease in animals may be relevant to human rheumatic diseases. The interested reader is referred to the excellent review by Sokoloff.[185] Several models deserve emphasis in this brief account.

Adjuvant Disease

Intradermal injection of complete Freund's adjuvant (mineral oil, detergent, and *Mycobacterium butyricum*) into the footpad of susceptible strains of rats results in the development of a chronic polyarthritis, sometimes accompanied by lesions of the skin and auricular carti-

Table 2–9

Animal Models of Rheumatic Disease

	SPONTANEOUS	EXPERIMENTAL
Rheumatoid arthritis	*Erysipelothrix* arthritis in pigs Caprine arthritis-encephalitis virus MRL-*lpr/lpr* mice	Adjuvant-induced arthritis in rats (muramyl dipeptide) Type II collagen–induced arthritis in rats and mice Streptococcal cell-wall arthritis in rats and mice (peptidoglycan polysaccharide)
Systemic lupus erythematosus	NZB/W F_1 mice BSXB mice MRL-*lpr/lpr* mice Aleutian disease of mink Outbred household dogs	T-cell engrafted SCID mice 16/6 idiotype immunized mice
Scleroderma	Tight skin (tsk) mice Avian scleroderma	Chronic graft-vs.-host disease Mice injected intraperitoneally with urinary glycosaminoglycans from patients with scleroderma
Dermato/Polymyositis	Familial canine dermatomyositis Coxsackievirus-induced polymyositis ECM virus–induced polymyositis	
Spondyloarthropathy	*Yersinia*-induced arthritis Murine progressive spondylitis	B27-transgenic rat Adjuvant arthritis (some strains) Type II collagen–induced arthritis (some strains)
Vasculitis	Equine encephalitis and anemia in horses Mycoplasmal cerebral arteritis in turkeys	*Lactobacillus*-induced coronary arteritis in mice (Kawasaki disease)

lages, and an anterior uveitis (Fig. 2–10).[186, 187] This disease is adoptively transferable by T lymphocytes, and Cohen and associates demonstrated that the model may be manipulated by T-cell clones capable of inducing, preventing, or ameliorating the disease.[188–191] Antibody appears to have no significant role in pathogenesis. The course of adjuvant arthritis may be intermittent but, when chronic, results in tissue destruction with calcification and ankylosis of joints. The arthritogenic component of the adjuvant is a peptidoglycan dimer, muramyl dipeptide.[192]

Polyarthritis Induced by Type II Collagen

Native type II collagen in incomplete Freund's adjuvant induces chronic polyarthritis in certain strains of rats and mice.[193–198] The disease can be passively transferred with specific antibody to type II collagen.[199] Recent studies have suggested a role for cell-mediated immunity in the pathogenesis of this disease.[200–204]

Arthritis Induced by Infectious Agents

Erysipelothrix rhusiopathiae and *Mycoplasma* are each capable of inducing arthritis in domestic pig,[205–207] and *Mycoplasma* species are arthritogenic in many other species, including rabbit, cow, goat, sheep, mouse, chicken, and turkey.[208] Spontaneous infection with *Chlamydia psittaci* causes polyarthritis in lambs.[209] Reovirus causes synovitis in chicks.[210] Caprine arthritis is caused by infection with a retrovirus.[211–213]

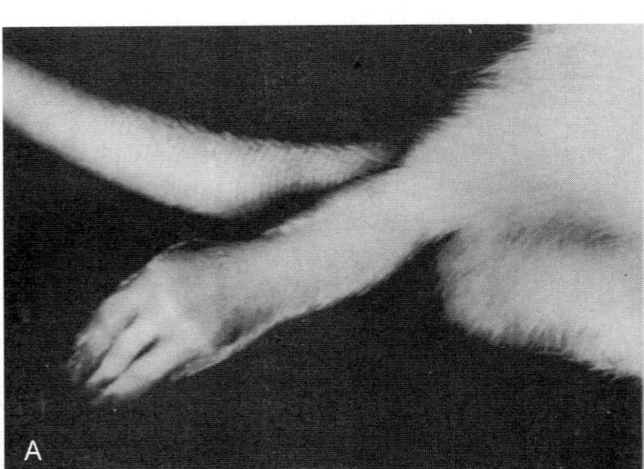

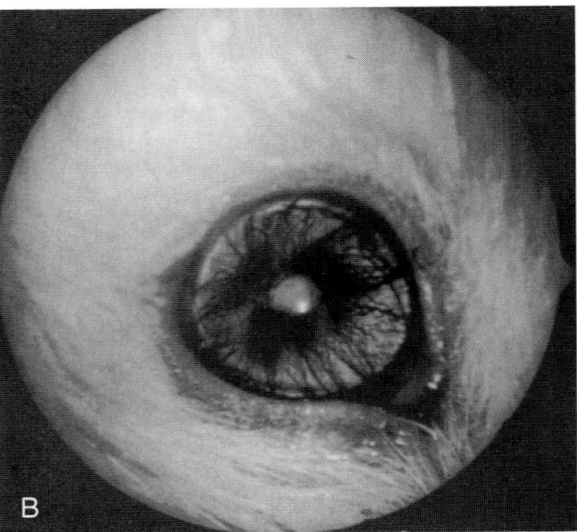

Figure 2–10. This rat was injected in the footpad with complete Freund's adjuvant 21 days previously. *A*, The resultant polyarthritis. *B*, The anterior uveitis.

Spontaneous Rheumatoid-Like Arthritis

A disease resembling rheumatoid arthritis spontaneously occurs in dogs[214] and MRL/l mice[215] but rarely in primates such as monkeys.[216] In the canine and mouse models, rheumatoid factors are demonstrable.[215, 217]

Models of Systemic Lupus Erythematosus

Animal models of lupus-like disease have been extensively studied and have yielded much important information related to human disease. These publications have been extensively reviewed.[218, 219] Only the most frequently studied models are discussed here.

In 1930, a breeding colony of mice was established at the University of Otago Medical School in New Zealand, using stock from the Imperial Cancer Research Fund Laboratories at Mill Hill in England.[220] These mice were maintained in closed colonies by random breeding until, in 1948, pairs of mice from this randomly bred colony were selected solely on the basis of coat color for inbreeding by brother-sister mating.[221] From these lines, the New Zealand Black (NZB) and New Zealand White (NZW) strains were developed. These mice have served as an important source of study of lupus-like disease. Mice of the NZB strain develop hemolytic anemia and thymic lesions characterized by the presence of germinal follicles.[221, 222] The F_1 (first filial generation) hybrids of the cross between NZB and NZW experience a severe lupus-like disease characterized by the production of autoantibodies, glomerulonephritis, lymphoid hyperplasia, hemolytic anemia, hypocomplementemia, and other clinical and laboratory abnormalities. The NZB strain is now known to be deficient in C5, although the relationship of this abnormality to the pathogenesis of the murine disease is not clear.

Other strains of mice have also been used in the study of lupus. BXSB mice and MRL strains were developed at the Jackson Laboratory. BXSB mice are derived from a cross between a C57BL/6J female and a SB/Le male (which has a pigment abnormality and giant lysosomal granules similar to those in Chédiak-Higashi syndrome). The gene associated with the autoimmune features of this strain is carried on the Y chromosome of the BXSB mouse. MRL/l mice were derived from a cross between the leukemia-prone AKR/J mouse and several nonautoimmune strains. These mice develop polyarthritis, glomerulonephritis, lymphoid hyperplasia, and vasculitis.[223] All strains have hypergammaglobulinemia, antinuclear antibody (anti-dsDNA and anti-ssDNA), immune complexes, hypocomplementemia, and cryoglobulinemia. Anti-Sm antibodies, which are highly characteristic of human lupus, are also present in MRL/l mice[224] along with rheumatoid factors.[214]

Spontaneous lupus-like disease has also been observed in mink[225] and dogs.[226] The disease in the Aleutian mink resembles lupus and polyarteritis. It is a chronic viral disease that was first observed in mutants with a gunmetal coat color called Aleutian. It is now known to occur in all genotypes of mink, but homozygous genotypes are most susceptible. This disease is characterized by hemorrhagic phenomena, anemia, and plasma cell proliferation with hypergammaglobulinemia, hepatitis, glomerulonephritis, and segmental arteritis with fibrinoid degeneration. In the Aleutian mink, two factors appear to combine to create clinical disease: a genetic predisposition and an environmental factor (virus).

Lewis and Schwartz have studied a spontaneous multisystem disease in outbred dogs characterized by arthritis, autoimmune hemolytic anemia, thrombocytopenia, proteinuria, diffuse glomerulonephritis, and antibodies to DNA, RNA, and DNA-histone complexes.[226] This canine disease is not strictly genetic and can be transmitted by a cell-free filtrate. The etiologic agent has not been isolated.[227, 228]

Models of Scleroderma

Chronic graft-versus-host disease, first noted in rats[229] and subsequently in humans after bone marrow transplantation, is characterized by scleroderma-like skin changes.[230] Spontaneous, genetically determined scleroderma-like disease has been studied in the tight-skinned mouse[231] and in white Leghorn chickens.[232–234] The tight-skinned mouse forms excessive dermal and subcutaneous collagen. This disorder is transmitted as an autosomal dominant trait. Ishikawa and colleagues reported the induction of sclerodermatous skin changes in normal mice by urinary glycosaminoglycans from patients with scleroderma.[235]

Models of Dermatomyositis

A dermatomyositis-like disease has been described in household cats and dogs.[236, 237] It appears to have a familial basis. A polymyositis-like disease is also induced in mice infected with coxsackievirus[238] or encephalomyocarditis virus.

Models of Spondyloarthropathy

The most important model of spondyloarthropathy resulted from development of the B27 transgenic rat.[239] This animal spontaneously experiences inflammatory disease that bears a striking resemblance to human spondyloarthropathy. One Lewis inbred strain and another inbred Fisher line express HLA-B27 and human β_2-microglobulin; they spontaneously experience chronic inflammatory disease affecting both axial and peripheral joints, the gastrointestinal tract, skin, and nails. The lamina propria of the gut is infiltrated by B27-positive T lymphocytes. It has been postulated that the high density of the B27 molecule on mononuclear cells of the affected rat strains facilitates the presentation of a B27 peptide to a reactive T-lymphocyte population, triggering the inflammatory process. An alternative hypothesis attributes susceptibility to spondyloarthropathy to misfolding of B27 heavy chains in the endoplasmic reticulum.[239a] Maintaining the B27 transgenic rat in a germ-free environment abrogates development of the spondyloarthropathy. Spondylitis in turkeys has been associated with infection with *Pasteurella anatipestifer*.[240]

Models of Vasculitis

Kawasaki Disease

Coronary arteritis that is histologically similar to that of Kawasaki disease is induced in C57BL/6 mice by intraperitoneal injection of cell walls of *Lactobacillus casei*. Arteritis, coronary aneurysms, and thrombosis developed within 3 weeks.[241–243] Potential therapeutic maneuvers in humans have been studied in the mouse model,[244] most recently with an angiogenesis inhibitor.[245] Additional animal models of Kawasaki disease include the cat[246] and the rabbit.[247]

Equine Encephalitis and Anemia

Vasculitis of the media of small arteries occurs in the horse; the vasculitis is of viral origin and is transmitted via an arthropod vector.[248] Principal clinical features include an acute onset with a high fever, conjunctival injection, subcutaneous edema of the extremities, anorexia, diarrhea, and death in two thirds of the animals. Pregnant mares abort. Hemolytic anemia and hypergammaglobulinemia are consistently present, and mild glomerulitis accompanied by immune complexes and depletion of C3 is frequent. The persisting viremia coexists with antibodies to the virus. The gross and microscopic lesions of this disease resemble the fibrinoid lesions of human polyarteritis.

Dermatitis-Nephropathy Syndrome in Swine

Systemic vasculitis that involves the skin and kidneys has been described in swine.[249] It may be secondary to infection with porcine reproductive and respiratory syndrome virus.

Vasculitis in Deer

In 1996, systemic vasculitis associated with high mortality was described in mule deer.[250] Intranuclear adenovirus was identified in all six deer that were examined. This disease was similar to bluetongue virus infection and epizootic hemorrhagic disease virus infection in white-tailed deer.

Central Nervous System Vasculitis in Turkeys

Infectious and fatal vasculitis of turkeys in commercial lots has been associated with *Mycoplasma synoviae*[251] and previously with a toxin elaborated by *Mycoplasma gallisepticum*.[252, 253]

References

1. Edwards JC, Morris V: Joint physiology: relevant to the rheumatologist? Br J Rheumatol 37: 121–125, 1998.
2. Sokoloff L, Boland JH: The Musculoskeletal System. Baltimore, Williams & Wilkins, 1975.
3. Resnick D, Niwayama G: Articular anatomy and histology. *In* Resnick D (ed): Diagnosis of Bone and Joint Disorders, 3rd ed. Philadelphia, WB Saunders, 1995, pp 652–671.
4. Drachman DB, Sokoloff L: The role of movement in embryonic joint development. Dev Biol 14: 401, 1966.
5. O'Rahilly R, Gardner E: The embryology of moveable joints. *In* Sokoloff L (ed): The Joints and Synovial Fluid. New York, Academic Press, 1978, p 49.
6. Ghadially FN: Fine structure of joints. *In* Sokoloff L (ed): The Joints and Synovial Fluid. New York, Academic Press, 1978.
7. Silver FH: Biological Materials: Structure, Mechanical Properties, and Modeling of Soft Tissues. New York, New York University Press, 1987.
8. Mow V, Rosenwasser M: Articular cartilage: biomechanics. *In* Woo SLY, Buckwalter JA (eds): Injury and Repair of the Musculoskeletal Soft Tissues. Park Ridge, IL, American Academy of Orthopaedic Surgeons, 1988, p 427.
9. Hall BK, Newman SA (eds): Cartilage: Molecular Aspects. Boca Raton, FL, CRC Press, 1991.
10. Jasin HE: Structure and function of the articular cartilage surface. Scand J Rheumatol Suppl 10: 51–55, 1995.
11. Dijkgraaf LC, de Bont LG, Boering G, et al: Normal cartilage structure, biochemistry, and metabolism: a review of the literature. J Oral Maxillofac Surg 53: 924–929, 1995.
12. Guilak F, Jones WR, Ting-Beall HP, et al: The deformation behavior and mechanical properties of chondrocytes in articular cartilage. Osteoarthritis Cartilage 7: 59–70, 1999.
13. Mankin HJ, Baron PA: The effect of aging on protein synthesis in articular cartilage of rabbits. Lab Invest 14: 658, 1965.
14. Heinegard D, Oldberg A: Structure and biology of cartilage and bone matrix noncollagenous macromolecules. FASEB J 3: 2042–2051, 1989.
15. Bruckner P, van der Rest M: Structure and function of cartilage collagens. Microsc Res Tech 28: 378–384, 1994.
16. Cohen NP, Foster RJ, Mow VC: Composition and dynamics of articular cartilage: structure, function, and maintaining healthy state. J Orthop Sports Phys Ther 28: 203–215, 1998.
17. Mow VC, Wang CC, Hung CT: The extracellular matrix, interstitial fluid and ions as a mechanical signal transducer in articular cartilage. Osteoarthritis Cartilage 7: 41–58, 1999.
18. Ghadially FN: Structure and function of articular cartilage. Clin Rheum Dis 7: 3, 1981.
19. Stockwell RA, Meachim G: The chondrocytes. *In* Freeman MAR (ed): Adult Articular Cartilage. London, Pitman Medical, 1979, p 69.
20. Ghadially FN, Oryschak AF, Ailsby RL, et al: Electron probe x-ray analysis of siderosomes in haemarthrotic articular cartilage. Virchows Arch B Cell Pathol 16: 43–49, 1974.
21. Malemud CJ, Moskowitz RW: Physiology of articular cartilage. Clin Rheum Dis 7: 29, 1981.
22. Edwards J: Second international meeting on synovium. Cell biology, physiology and pathology. Ann Rheum Dis 54: 389–391, 1995.
23. FitzGerald O, Bresnihan B: Synovial membrane cellularity and vascularity. Ann Rheum Dis 54: 511–515, 1995.
24. Edwards JC: Synovial intimal fibroblasts. Ann Rheum Dis 54: 395–397, 1995.

25. Revell PA, al-Saffar N, Fish S, et al: Extracellular matrix of the synovial intimal cell layer. Ann Rheum Dis 54: 404–407, 1995.
26. Athanasou NA: Synovial macrophages. Ann Rheum Dis 54: 392–394, 1995.
27. Muller-Ladner U, Gay RE, Gay S: Molecular biology of cartilage and bone destruction. Curr Opin Rheumatol 10: 212–219, 1998.
28. McCutchen CW: Lubrication of joints. *In* Sokoloff L (ed): The Joints and Synovial Fluid. New York, Academic Press, 1978, p 437.
29. Simkin PA: Synovial perfusion and synovial fluid solutes. Ann Rheum Dis 54: 424–428, 1995.
30. Levick JR, McDonald JN: Fluid movement across synovium in healthy joints: role of synovial fluid macromolecules. Ann Rheum Dis 54: 417–423, 1995.
31. Cho MH, Neuhaus OW: Absence of blood clotting substances from synovial fluid. Thromb Diath Haemorrh 5: 496, 1960.
32. Ropes MW, Bauer W: Synovial Fluid Changes in Joint Disease. Cambridge, MA, Harvard University Press, 1953.
33. Ropes MW, Muller AF, Bauer W: The entrance of glucose and other sugars into joints. Arthritis Rheum 3: 496, 1960.
34. Hamerman D, Schuster H: Hyaluronate in normal human synovial fluid. J Clin Invest 37: 57, 1958.
35. Pekin TJ, Zvaifler NJ: Hemolytic complement in synovial fluid. J Clin Invest 43: 1372, 1964.
36. Cummings NA, Nordby GL: Measurement of synovial fluid pH in normal and arthritic knees. Arthritis Rheum 9: 47–56, 1966.
37. Kushner I, Somerville JA: Permeability of human synovial membrane to plasma proteins. Relationship to molecular size and inflammation. Arthritis Rheum 14: 560–570, 1971.
38. Hunder GG, Gleich GJ: Immunoglobulin E (IgE) levels in serum and synovial fluid in rheumatoid arthritis. Arthritis Rheum 17: 955–963, 1974.
39. Rose NR, de Marcario EC, Fahey JL, et al (eds): Manual of Clinical Laboratory Immunology, 4th ed. Washington, D.C., American Society for Microbiology, 1992.
40. Gatter RA, Schumacher HR: A Practical Handbook of Joint Fluid Analysis, 2nd ed. Philadelphia, Lea & Febiger, 1992.
41. Liew M, Dick WC: The anatomy and physiology of blood flow in a diarthrodial joint. Clin Rheum Dis 7: 131, 1981.
42. Nimni ME: Collagen: structure, function, and metabolism in normal and fibrotic tissues. Semin Arthritis Rheum 13: 1–86, 1983.
43. van der Rest M, Garrone R: Collagen family of proteins. FASEB J 5: 2814–2823, 1991.
44. Boskey AL, Wright TM, Blank RD: Collagen and bone strength. J Bone Miner Res 14: 330–335, 1999.
45. Uitto J, Murray LW, Blumberg B, et al: UCLA conference. Biochemistry of collagen in diseases. Ann Intern Med 105: 740–756, 1986.
46. Weiss JB, Sedowofia K, Jones C: Collagen degradation: a defended multi-enzyme system. *In* Viidik A, Vuust J (eds): Biology of Collagen. London, Academic Press, 1978, p 113.
47. Muir H, Bullough P, Maroudas A: The distribution of collagen in human articular cartilage with some of its physiological implications. J Bone Joint Surg [Br] 52: 554–563, 1970.
48. Piez K: Molecular and aggregate structures in the collagens. *In* Piez KA, Reddi AH (eds): Extracellular Matrix Biochemistry. New York, Elsevier, 1984, p 1.
49. Prockop DJ, Kivirikko KI: Heritable diseases of collagen. N Engl J Med 311: 376–386, 1984.
50. Kainulainen K, Pulkkinen L, Savolainen A, et al: Location on chromosome 15 of the gene defect causing Marfan syndrome. N Engl J Med 323: 935–939, 1990.
51. Dietz HC, Cutting GR, Pyeritz RE, et al: Marfan syndrome caused by a recurrent de novo missense mutation in the fibrillin gene. Nature 352: 337–339, 1991.
52. Lee B, Godfrey M, Vitale E, et al: Linkage of Marfan syndrome and a phenotypically related disorder to two different fibrillin genes. Nature 352: 330–334, 1991.
53. Prockop DJ, Kivirikko KI: Collagens: molecular biology, diseases, and potentials for therapy. Annu Rev Biochem 64: 403–434, 1995.
54. Raff ML, Byers PH: Joint hypermobility syndromes. Curr Opin Rheumatol 8: 459–466, 1996.
55. Prahalad S, Colbert RA: Genetic diseases with rheumatic manifestations in children. Curr Opin Rheumatol 10: 488–493, 1998.
56. Palotie A, Vaisanen P, Ott J, et al: Predisposition to familial osteoarthrosis linked to type II collagen gene. Lancet 1: 924–927, 1989.
57. Knowlton RG, Katzenstein PL, Moskowitz RW, et al: Genetic linkage of a polymorphism in the type II procollagen gene (COL2A1) to primary osteoarthritis associated with mild chondrodysplasia. N Engl J Med 322: 526–530, 1990.
58. Ala-Kokko L, Baldwin CT, Moskowitz RW, et al: Single base mutation in the type II procollagen gene (COL2A1) as a cause of primary osteoarthritis associated with a mild chondrodysplasia. Proc Natl Acad Sci U S A 87: 6565–6568, 1990.
59. Kuivaniemi H, Tromp G, Prockop DJ: Mutations in fibrillar collagens (types I, II, III, and XI), fibril-associated collagen (type IX), and network-forming collagen (type X) cause a spectrum of diseases of bone, cartilage, and blood vessels. Hum Mutat 9: 300–315, 1997.
60. Gallagher JT: The extended family of proteoglycans: social residents of the pericellular zone. Curr Opin Cell Biol 1: 1201–1218, 1989.
61. Iozzo RV: Matrix proteoglycans: from molecular design to cellular function. Annu Rev Biochem 67: 609–652, 1998.
62. Lander AD: Proteoglycans: master regulators of molecular encounter? Matrix Biol 17: 465–472, 1998.
63. Birk DE, Silver FH, Trelstad RL: Matric assembly. *In* Hay ED (ed): Cell Biology of the Extracellular Matrix. New York, Plenum Press, 1991, p 221.
64. Goetinck P, Winterbottom N: Proteoglycans: modular macromolecules of the extracellular matrix. *In* Goldsmith L (ed): Biochemistry and Physiology of the Skin. New York, Oxford University Press, 1991.
65. Bayliss MT, Ali SY: Age-related changes in the composition and structure of human articular-cartilage proteoglycans. Biochem J 176: 683–693, 1978.
66. Roughley PJ, White RJ: Age-related changes in the structure of the proteoglycan subunits from human articular cartilage. J Biol Chem 255: 217–224, 1980.
67. Sandberg LB, Soskel NT, Leslie JG: Elastin structure, biosynthesis, and relation to disease states. N Engl J Med 304: 566–579, 1981.
68. Ruoslahti E, Engvall E, Hayman EG: Fibronectin: current concepts of its structure and functions. Coll Relat Res 1: 95–128, 1981.
69. Beck K, Hunter I, Engel J: Structure and function of laminin: anatomy of a multidomain glycoprotein. FASEB J 4: 148–160, 1990.
70. Bond JS, Butler PE: Intracellular proteases. Annu Rev Biochem 56: 333–364, 1987.
71. Cawston TE: Proteinases and inhibitors. Br Med Bull 51: 385–401, 1995.
72. Woessner JFJ: Matrix metalloproteinases and their inhibitors in connective tissue remodeling. FASEB J 5: 2145–2154, 1991.
73. Canoso JJ: Bursae, tendons and ligaments. Clin Rheum Dis 7: 189, 1981.
74. Niepel GA, Sit'aj S: Enthesopathy. Clin Rheum Dis 5: 857, 1979.
75. Canoso JJ: The premiere enthesis. J Rheumatol 25: 1254–1256, 1998.
76. Buckwalter JA: Bone Biology. J Bone Joint Surg [Am] 77: 1256–1276, 1995.
77. Buckwalter JA, Glimcher MJ, Cooper RR, et al: Bone biology. I: Structure, blood supply, cells, matrix, and mineralization. Instr Course Lect 45: 371–386, 1996.
78. Buckwalter JA, Glimcher MJ, Cooper RR, et al: Bone biology. II: Formation, form, modeling, remodeling, and regulation of cell function. Instr Course Lect 45: 387–399, 1996.
79. Ng KW, Romas E, Donnan L, et al: Bone biology. Baillieres Clin Endocrinol Metab 11: 1–22, 1997.
80. Eriksen EF, Axelrod DW, Melsen F: Bone Histomorphometry. New York, Raven, 1994.
81. Baron R: Anatomy and ultrastructure of bone. *In* Favus J (ed): Primer on the Metabolic Bone Diseases and Disorders of Mineral Metabolism, 4th ed. Philadelphia, Lippincott Williams & Wilkins, 1999, pp 3–10.
82. Marks SCJ, Popoff SN: Bone cell biology: the regulation of development, structure, and function in the skeleton. Am J Anat 183: 1–44, 1988.

83. Olsen BR: Bone morphogenesis and embryologic development. *In* Favus J (ed): Primer on the Metabolic Bone Diseases and Disorders of Mineral Metabolism, 4th ed. Philadelphia, Lippincott Williams & Wilkins, 1999, pp 11–13.
84. Williams PL, Bannister L: Gray's Anatomy: The Anatomical Basis of Medicine and Surgery, 38th ed. New York, Churchill Livingstone, 1995.
85. Robey PG: The biochemistry of bone. Endocrinol Metab Clin North Am 18: 859, 1989.
86. Clark PA, Rogol AD: Growth hormones and sex steroid interactions at puberty. Endocrinol Metab Clin North Am 25: 665–681, 1996.
87. Kappy MS: Regulation of growth in children with chronic illness. Therapeutic implications for the year 2000. Am J Dis Child 141: 489–493, 1987.
88. Sledge CB: Biochemical events in the epiphyseal plate and their physiologic control. Clin Orthop 61: 37–47, 1968.
89. Balogh KJ, Kunin AS: The effect of cortisone on the metabolism of epiphyseal cartilage. A histochemical study. Clin Orthop 80: 208–215, 1971.
90. Shaw NE, Lacey E: The influence of corticosteriods on the normal and papain-treated epiphysial growth plate in the rabbit. J Bone Joint Surg [Br] 57: 228–233, 1975.
91. Ogden JA: Anatomy and physiology of skeletal development. *In* Ogden JA (ed): Skeletal Injury in the Child, 2nd ed. Philadelphia, WB Saunders, 1990, pp 23–63.
92. Manologas SC, Olefsky JM (eds): Metabolic Bone and Mineral Disorders. New York, Churchill Livingstone, 1988.
93. Avioli LV, Krane SM (eds): Metabolic Bone Disease and Clinically Related Disorders. Philadelphia, WB Saunders, 1990.
94. Posner AS: Crystal chemistry of bone mineral. Physiol Rev 49: 760–792, 1969.
95. Boskey AL: Biomineralization: conflicts, challenges, and opportunities. J Cell Biochem Suppl 30/31: 83–91, 1998.
96. Termine JD: Non-collagen proteins in bone. Ciba Found Symp 136: 178–202, 1988.
97. Owen M: The origin of bone cells in the postnatal organism. Arthritis Rheum 23: 1073–1080, 1980.
98. MacDonald BR, Gowen M: The cell biology of bone. Baillieres Clin Rheumatol 7: 421–443, 1993.
99. Lian JB, Stein GS, Canalis E, et al: Bone formation: osteoblast lineage cells, growth factors, matrix proteins, and the mineralization process. *In* Favus J (ed): Primer on the Metabolic Bone Diseases and Disorders of Mineral Metabolism, 4th ed. Philadelphia, Lippincott Williams & Wilkins, 1999, pp 14–29.
100. Mundy GR: Bone remodeling. *In* Favus J (ed): Primer on the Metabolic Bone Diseases and Disorders of Mineral Metabolism, 4th ed. Philadelphia, Lippincott Williams & Wilkins, 1999, pp 30–38.
101. Rifkin BR, Gay CV (eds): Biology and Physiology of the Osteoclast. Boca Raton, FL, CRC Press, 1992.
102. Broadus AE: Mineral balance and homeostasis. *In* Favus J (ed): Primer on the Metabolic Bone Diseases and Disorders of Mineral Metabolism, 4th ed. Philadelphia, Lippincott Williams & Wilkins, 1999, pp 74–79.
103. Portale AA: Blood calcium, phosphorus, and magnesium. *In* Favus J (ed): Primer on the Metabolic Bone Diseases and Disorders of Mineral Metabolism, 4th ed. Philadelphia, Lippincott Williams & Wilkins, 1999, pp 115–118.
104. Wallwork JC, Sandstead HH: Zinc. *In* Simmons DJ (ed): Nutrition and Bone Development. New York, Oxford University Press, 1990, p 316.
105. Delmas PD: Biochemical assessment of bone turnover in osteoporosis. *In* DeLuca HG, Mazess R (eds): Osteoporosis: Physiologic Basis, Assessment and Treatment. New York, Elsevier, 1990, p 109.
106. Robins SP, New SA: Markers of bone turnover in relation to bone health. Proc Nutr Soc 56: 903–914, 1997.
107. Woitge HW, Seibel MJ: Molecular markers of bone and cartilage metabolism. Curr Opin Rheumatol 11: 218–225, 1999.
108. Khosla S, Kleerekoper M: Biochemical Markers of Bone Turnover. *In* Favus J (ed): Primer on the Metabolic Bone Diseases and Disorders of Mineral Metabolism, 4th ed. Philadelphia, Lippincott Williams & Wilkins, 1999, pp 128–133.
109. Parfitt AM, Simon LS, Villanueva AR, et al: Procollagen type I carboxy-terminal extension peptide in serum as a marker of collagen biosynthesis in bone. Correlation with iliac bone formation rates and comparison with total alkaline phosphatase. J Bone Miner Res 2: 427–436, 1987.
110. Minkin C: Bone acid phosphatase: tartrate-resistant acid phosphatase as a marker of osteoclast function. Calcif Tissue Int 34: 285–290, 1982.
111. DeCastro JAS, Peakcock M, McClintock R: Plasma tartrate-resistant acid phosphatase (TRAP) as a marker of bone resorption. J Bone Miner Res 4(Suppl 1): 171, 1989.
112. Delmas PD, Schlemmer A, Gineyts E, et al: Urinary excretion of pyridinoline crosslinks correlates with bone turnover measured on iliac crest biopsy in patients with vertebral osteoporosis. J Bone Miner Res 6: 639–644, 1991.
113. Robins SP: Biochemical markers for assessing skeletal growth. Eur J Clin Nutr 48(Suppl 1): S199–S209, 1994.
114. Arnaud CD: The calcitropic hormones and metabolic bone disease. *In* Greenspan FS (ed): Basic and Clinical Endocrinology. Norwalk, CT, Appleton & Lange, 1991, p 247.
115. Rizzoli R, Bonjour JP: Hormones and bones. Lancet 349(Suppl 1): S120–S123, 1997.
116. Jüppner H, Brown EM, Kronenberg HM: Parathyroid hormone. *In* Favus J (ed): Primer on the Metabolic Bone Diseases and Disorders of Mineral Metabolism, 4th ed. Philadelphia, Lippincott Williams & Wilkins, 1999, pp 80–87.
117. Blind E, Gagel RF: Assay methods: parathyroid hormone, parathyroid hormone-related protein. *In* Favus J (ed): Primer on the Metabolic Bone Diseases and Disorders of Mineral Metabolism, 4th ed. Philadelphia, Lippincott Williams & Wilkins, 1999, pp 119–123.
118. Hollis BW, Clemens TL, Adams JS: Vitamin D metabolites. *In* Favus J (ed): Primer on the Metabolic Bone Diseases and Disorders of Mineral Metabolism, 4th ed. Philadelphia, Lippincott Williams & Wilkins, 1999, pp 124–127.
119. Holick MF: Vitamin D: photobiology, metabolism, mechanism of action, and clinical applications. *In* Favus J (ed): Primer on the Metabolic Bone Diseases and Disorders of Mineral Metabolism, 4th ed. Philadelphia, Lippincott Williams & Wilkins, 1999, pp 92–98.
120. Barden HS, Mazess RB: Bone densitometry in infants. J Pediatr 113: 172–177, 1988.
121. Glastre C, Braillon P, David L, et al: Measurement of bone mineral content of the lumbar spine by dual energy x-ray absorptiometry in normal children: correlations with growth parameters. J Clin Endocrinol Metab 70: 1330–1333, 1990.
122. Miller PD, Bonnick SL: Clinical application of bone densitometry. *In* Favus J (ed): Primer on the Metabolic Bone Diseases and Disorders of Mineral Metabolism, 4th ed. Philadelphia, Lippincott Williams & Wilkins, 1999, pp 152–159.
123. Prentice A, Parsons TJ, Cole TJ: Uncritical use of bone mineral density in absorptiometry may lead to size-related artifacts in the identification of bone mineral determinants. Am J Clin Nutr 60: 837–842, 1994.
124. Wasnich RD: Epidemiology of osteoporosis. *In* Favus J (ed): Primer on the Metabolic Bone Diseases and Disorders of Mineral Metabolism, 4th ed. Philadelphia, Lippincott Williams & Wilkins, 1999, pp 257–259.
125. McKay CP, Specker BL, Tsang RC, et al: Mineral metabolism during childhood. *In* Coe FL, Favus MJ (eds): Disorders of Bone and Mineral Metabolism. New York, Raven Press, 1992, p 395.
126. Cassidy JT, Langman CB, Allen SH, et al: Bone mineral metabolism in children with juvenile rheumatoid arthritis. Pediatr Clin North Am 42: 1017–1033, 1995.
127. Cassidy JT, Hillman LS: Abnormalities in skeletal growth in children with juvenile rheumatoid arthritis. Rheum Dis Clin North Am 23: 499–522, 1997.
128. Cassidy JT: Osteopenia and osteoporosis in children. Clin Exp Rheumatol 17: 245–250, 1999.
129. Kelly PJ, Hopper JL, Macaskill GT, et al: Genetic factors in bone turnover. J Clin Endocrinol Metab 72: 808–813, 1991.
130. Pocock NA, Eisman JA, Hopper JL, et al: Genetic determinants of bone mass in adults. A twin study. J Clin Invest 80: 706–710, 1987.
131. Sambrook PN, Kelly PJ, White CP, et al: Genetic determinants of bone mass. *In* Marcus R, Feldman D, Kelsey J (eds): Osteoporosis. New York, Academic Press, 1996, pp 477–482.

132. Slemenda CW, Christian JC, Williams CJ, et al: Genetic determinants of bone mass in adult women: a reevaluation of the twin model and the potential importance of gene interaction on heritability estimates. J Bone Miner Res 6: 561–567, 1991.
133. Tanner JM, Davies PS: Clinical longitudinal standards for height and height velocity for North American children. J Pediatr 107: 317–329, 1985.
134. Tanner JM: Growth at Adolescence. Oxford, Blackwell Scientific, 1962, p 32.
135. Bonjour JP, Theintz G, Buchs B, et al: Critical years and stages of puberty for spinal and femoral bone mass accumulation during adolescence. J Clin Endocrinol Metab 73: 555–563, 1991.
136. Mazess RB, Cameron JR: Growth of bone in school children: comparison of radiographic morphometry and photon absorptiometry. Growth 36: 77–92, 1972.
137. DePriester JA, Cole TJ, Bishop NJ: Bone growth and mineralisation in children aged 4 to 10 years. Bone Miner 12: 57–65, 1991.
138. Hillman LS: Bone mineral acquisition in utero and during infancy and childhood. *In* Marcus R, Feldman D, Kelsey J (eds): Osteoporosis. New York, Academic Press, 1996, pp 449–464.
139. Matkovic V, Jelic T, Wardlaw GM, et al: Timing of peak bone mass in Caucasian females and its implication for the prevention of osteoporosis. Inference from a cross-sectional model. J Clin Invest 93: 799–808, 1994.
140. De Schepper J, Derde MP, Van den Broeck M, et al: Normative data for lumbar spine bone mineral content in children: influence of age, height, weight, and pubertal stage. J Nucl Med 32: 216–220, 1991.
141. Katzman DK, Bachrach LK, Carter DR, et al: Clinical and anthropometric correlates of bone mineral acquisition in healthy adolescent girls. J Clin Endocrinol Metab 73: 1332–1339, 1991.
142. Lloyd T, Rollings N, Andon MB, et al: Determinants of bone density in young women. I: Relationships among pubertal development, total body bone mass, and total body bone density in premenarchal females. J Clin Endocrinol Metab 75: 383–387, 1992.
143. Miller JZ, Slemenda CW, Meaney FJ, et al: The relationship of bone mineral density and anthropometric variables in healthy male and female children. Bone Miner 14: 137–152, 1991.
144. Rubin K, Schirduan V, Gendreau P, et al: Predictors of axial and peripheral bone mineral density in healthy children and adolescents, with special attention to the role of puberty. J Pediatr 123: 863–870, 1993.
145. Gertner JM: Childhood and adolescence. *In* Favus J (ed): Primer on the Metabolic Bone Diseases and Disorders of Mineral Metabolism, 4th ed. Philadelphia, Lippincott Williams & Wilkins, 1999, pp 45–49.
146. Slemenda CW, Reister TK, Hui SL, et al: Influences on skeletal mineralization in children and adolescents: evidence for varying effects of sexual maturation and physical activity. J Pediatr 125: 201–207, 1994.
147. Gilsanz V, Gibbens DT, Carlson M, et al: Peak trabecular vertebral density: a comparison of adolescent and adult females. Calcif Tissue Int 43: 260–262, 1988.
148. Genant HK, Gluer CC, Lotz JC: Gender differences in bone density, skeletal geometry, and fracture biomechanics. Radiology 190: 636–640, 1994.
149. Lu PW, Briody JN, Ogle GD, et al: Bone mineral density of total body, spine, and femoral neck in children and young adults: a cross-sectional and longitudinal study. J Bone Miner Res 9: 1451–1458, 1994.
150. Kroger H, Kotaniemi A, Kroger L, et al: Development of bone mass and bone density of the spine and femoral neck—a prospective study of 65 children and adolescents. Bone Miner 23: 171–182, 1993.
151. Theintz G, Buchs B, Rizzoli R, et al: Longitudinal monitoring of bone mass accumulation in healthy adolescents: evidence for a marked reduction after 16 years of age at the levels of lumbar spine and femoral neck in female subjects. J Clin Endocrinol Metab 75: 1060–1065, 1992.
152. Gilsanz V, Boechat MI, Roe TF, et al: Gender differences in vertebral body sizes in children and adolescents. Radiology 190: 673–677, 1994.
153. Sabatier JP, Guaydier-Souquieres G, Laroche D, et al: Bone mineral acquisition during adolescence and early adulthood: a study in 574 healthy females 10–24 years of age. Osteoporos Int 6: 141–148, 1996.
154. Sabatier JP, Guaydier-Souquieres G, Benmalek A, et al: Evolution of lumbar bone mineral content during adolescence and adulthood: a longitudinal study in 395 healthy females 10–24 years of age and 206 premenopausal women. Osteoporos Int 9: 476–482, 1999.
155. Haapasalo H, Kannus P, Sievanen H, et al: Development of mass, density, and estimated mechanical characteristics of bones in Caucasian females. J Bone Miner Res 11: 1751–1760, 1996.
156. Abrams SA, Stuff JE: Calcium metabolism in girls: current dietary intakes lead to low rates of calcium absorption and retention during puberty. Am J Clin Nutr 60: 739–743, 1994.
157. Lloyd T, Martel JK, Rollings N, et al: The effect of calcium supplementation and Tanner stage on bone density, content and area in teenage women. Osteoporos Int 6: 276–283, 1996.
158. Sentipal JM, Wardlaw GM, Mahan J, et al: Influence of calcium intake and growth indexes on vertebral bone mineral density in young females. Am J Clin Nutr 54: 425–428, 1991.
159. Maggioni A: Nutrition and physical activity with particular emphasis on bone health. J Am Coll Nutr 17: 103–104, 1998.
160. Barr SI, McKay HA: Nutrition, exercise, and bone status in youth. Int J Sport Nutr 8: 124–142, 1998.
161. Wang MC, Moorre EC, Crawford PB, et al: Influence of preadolescent diet on quantitative ultrasound measurements of the calcaneus in young adult women. Osteoporos Int 9: 532–535, 1999.
162. Matkovic V, Heaney RP: Calcium balance during human growth: evidence for threshold behavior. Am J Clin Nutr 55: 992–996, 1992.
163. Riggs BL, Nguyen TV, Melton LJ, et al: The contribution of vitamin D receptor gene alleles to the determination of bone mineral density in normal and osteoporotic women. J Bone Miner Res 10: 991–996, 1995.
164. Hustmyer FG, Peacock M, Hui S, et al: Bone mineral density in relation to polymorphism at the vitamin D receptor gene locus. J Clin Invest 94: 2130–2134, 1994.
165. Johnston CCJ, Miller JZ, Slemenda CW, et al: Calcium supplementation and increases in bone mineral density in children. N Engl J Med 327: 82–87, 1992.
166. Welten DC, Kemper HC, Post GB, et al: Weight-bearing activity during youth is a more important factor for peak bone mass than calcium intake. J Bone Miner Res 9: 1089–1096, 1994.
167. Bouxsein ML, Marcus R: Overview of exercise and bone mass. Rheum Dis Clin North Am 20: 787–802, 1994.
168. Kannus P, Haapasalo H, Sankelo M, et al: Effect of starting age of physical activity on bone mass in the dominant arm of tennis and squash players. Ann Intern Med 123: 27–31, 1995.
169. Ruiz JC, Mandel C, Garabedian M: Influence of spontaneous calcium intake and physical exercise on the vertebral and femoral bone mineral density of children and adolescents. J Bone Miner Res 10: 675–682, 1995.
170. Vuori I: Peak bone mass and physical activity: short review. Nutr Rev 54(4 Pt 2): S11–S14, 1996.
171. Goldman YE, Dantzig JA: Structure, function, and disease of muscle. *In* Ruddy S, Harris ED Jr, Sledge CB (eds): Kelley's Textbook of Rheumatology, 6th ed. Philadelphia, WB Saunders, 2000, pp 1261–1272.
172. Gowitzke BA, Milner M: Scientific Basis of Human Movement. Baltimore, Williams & Wilkins, 1988, p 144.
173. Turner DC, Wallimann T, Eppenberger HM: A protein that binds specifically to the M-line of skeletal muscle is identified as the muscle form of creatine kinase. Proc Natl Acad Sci U S A 70: 702–705, 1973.
174. Squire J: The Structural Basis of Muscular Contraction. New York, Plenum Press, 1981.
175. Kelly AM, Rubinstein NA: Development of neuromuscular specialization. Med Sci Sports Exerc 18: 292–298, 1986.
176. Faulkner JA, White TP: Adaptations of skeletal muscle to physical activity. *In* Bouchard C, Shephard RJ, Stephens T, et al (eds): Exercise, Fitness, and Health. Champaign, IL, Human Kinetics, 1990, p 265.
177. Heffner RR Jr (ed): Muscle Pathology. New York, Churchill Livingstone, 1984.
178. Stockdale FE: Mechanisms of formation of muscle fiber types. Cell Struct Funct 22: 37–43, 1997.

179. Staron RS: Human skeletal muscle fiber types: delineation, development, and distribution. Can J Appl Physiol 22: 307–327, 1997.
180. Zhang M, Koishi K, McLennan IS: Skeletal muscle fibre types: detection methods and embryonic determinants. Histol Histopathol 13: 201–207, 1998.
181. Booth FW, Tseng BS, Fluck M, et al: Molecular and cellular adaptation of muscle in response to physical training. Acta Physiol Scand 162: 343–350, 1998.
182. Hargreaves M: 1997 Sir William Refshauge Lecture. Skeletal muscle glucose metabolism during exercise: implications for health and performance. J Sci Med Sport 1: 195–202, 1998.
183. Taylor AW, Bachman L: The effects of endurance training on muscle fibre types and enzyme activities. Can J Appl Physiol 24: 41–53, 1999.
184. Greenwald RA, Diamond HS (eds): CRC Handbook of Animal Models for the Rheumatic Diseases. Boca Raton, FL, CRC Press, 1988.
185. Sokoloff L: Animal models of rheumatoid arthritis. Int Rev Exp Pathol 26: 107–145, 1984.
186. Pearson CM: Development of arthritis, periarthritis and periostitis in rats given adjuvant. Proc Soc Exp Biol Med 91: 95, 1956.
187. Waksman B, Bullington S: Studies of arthritis and other lesions induced in rats by injection of mycobacterial adjuvant. II: lesions of the eye. Arch Ophthalmol 64: 751, 1960.
188. Holoshitz J, Naparstek Y, Ben-Nun A, et al: Lines of T lymphocytes induce or vaccinate against autoimmune arthritis. Science 219: 56–58, 1983.
189. van Eden W, Holoshitz J, Nevo Z, et al: Arthritis induced by a T-lymphocyte clone that responds to Mycobacterium tuberculosis and to cartilage proteoglycans. Proc Natl Acad Sci U S A 82: 5117–5120, 1985.
190. Lider O, Karin N, Shinitzky M, et al: Therapeutic vaccination against adjuvant arthritis using autoimmune T cells treated with hydrostatic pressure. Proc Natl Acad Sci U S A 84: 4577–4580, 1987.
191. Stanescu R, Lider O, van Eden W, et al: Histopathology of arthritis induced in rats by active immunization to mycobacterial antigens or by systemic transfer of T lymphocyte lines. A light and electron microscopic study of the articular surface using cationized ferritin. Arthritis Rheum 30: 779–792, 1987.
192. Zidek Z, Masek K, Jiricka Z: Arthritogenic activity of a synthetic immunoadjuvant, muramyl dipeptide. Infect Immun 35: 674–679, 1982.
193. Moder KG, Nabozny GH, Luthra HS, et al: Immunogenetics of collagen induced arthritis in mice: a model for human polyarthritis. Reg Immunol 4: 305–313, 1992.
194. Staines NA, Wooley PH: Collagen arthritis—what can it teach us? Br J Rheumatol 33: 798–807, 1994.
195. Nabozny GH, David CS: The immunogenetic basis of collagen induced arthritis in mice: an experimental model for the rational design of immunomodulatory treatments of rheumatoid arthritis. Adv Exp Med Biol 347: 55–63, 1994.
196. Cremer MA, Rosloniec EF, Kang AH: The cartilage collagens: a review of their structure, organization, and role in the pathogenesis of experimental arthritis in animals and in human rheumatic disease. J Mol Med 76: 275–288, 1998.
197. Myers LK, Rosloniec EF, Cremer MA, et al: Collagen-induced arthritis, an animal model of autoimmunity. Life Sci 61: 1861–1878, 1997.
198. Anthony DD, Haqqi TM: Collagen-induced arthritis in mice: an animal model to study the pathogenesis of rheumatoid arthritis. Clin Exp Rheumatol 17: 240–244, 1999.
199. Stuart JM, Townes AS, Kang AH: Collagen autoimmune arthritis. Annu Rev Immunol 2: 199–218, 1984.
200. Kakimoto K, Katsuki M, Hirofuji T, et al: Isolation of T cell line capable of protecting mice against collagen-induced arthritis. J Immunol 140: 78–83, 1988.
201. Holmdahl R, Andersson M, Goldschmidt TJ, et al: Type II collagen autoimmunity in animals and provocations leading to arthritis. Immunol Rev 118: 193–232, 1990.
202. Holmdahl R, Malmstrom V, Vuorio E: Autoimmune recognition of cartilage collagens. Ann Med 25: 251–264, 1993.
203. Durie FH, Fava RA, Noelle RJ: Collagen-induced arthritis as a model of rheumatoid arthritis. Clin Immunol Immunopathol 73: 11–18, 1994.
204. Staines NA, Harper N, Ward FJ, et al: Arthritis: animal models of oral tolerance. Ann N Y Acad Sci 778: 297–305, 1996.
205. Sikes D: A rheumatoid-like arthritis in swine. Lab Invest 8: 1406, 1959.
206. Drew RA: Erysipelothrix arthritis in pigs as a comparative model for rheumatoid arthritis. Proc R Soc Med 65: 994–998, 1972.
207. Goudswaard J, Hartman EG, Janmaat A, et al: Erysipelothrix rhusiopathiae strain 7, a causative agent of endocarditis and arthritis in the dog. Tijdschr Diergeneeskd 98: 416–423, 1973.
208. Cole BC: Mycoplasma-induced arthritis in animals: relevance to understanding the etiologies of the human rheumatic diseases. Rev Rhum (Engl Ed) 66: 45S–49S, 1999.
209. Storz J: Chlamydia and chlamydia-induced diseases. Springfield, IL, Charles C Thomas, 1971.
210. Walker ER, Friedman MH, Olson NO, et al: Ultrastructural study of avian synovium infected with an arthrotropic reovirus. Arthritis Rheum 20: 1269–1277, 1977.
211. Crawford TB, Adams DS, Sande RD, et al: The connective tissue component of the caprine arthritis-encephalitis syndrome. Am J Pathol 100: 443–454, 1980.
212. Wilkerson MJ, Davis WC, Baszler TV, et al: Immunopathology of chronic lentivirus-induced arthritis. Am J Pathol 146: 1433–1443, 1995.
213. Hanson J, Hydbring E, Olsson K: A long term study of goats naturally infected with caprine arthritis-encephalitis virus. Acta Vet Scand 37: 31–39, 1996.
214. Pedersen NC, Castles JJ, Weisner K: Noninfectious canine arthritis: rheumatoid arthritis. J Am Vet Med Assoc 169: 295–303, 1976.
215. Hang L, Theofilopoulos AN, Dixon FJ: A spontaneous rheumatoid arthritis-like disease in MRL/1 mice. J Exp Med 155: 1690–1701, 1982.
216. Bywaters EG: Observations on chronic polyarthritis in monkeys. J R Soc Med 74: 794–799, 1981.
217. Schumacher HR, Newton C, Halliwell RE: Synovial pathologic changes in spontaneous canine rheumatoid-like arthritis. Arthritis Rheum 23: 412–423, 1980.
218. Theofilopoulos AN, Dixon FJ: Murine models of systemic lupus erythematosus. Adv Immunol 37: 269–390, 1985.
219. Brey RL, Sakic B, Szechtman H, et al: Animal models for nervous system disease in systemic lupus erythematosus. Ann N Y Acad Sci 823: 97–106, 1997.
220. Bielschowsky M, Goodall CM: Origin of inbred NZ mouse strains. Cancer Res 30: 834–836, 1970.
221. Howie JB, Helyer BJ: The immunology and pathology of NZB mice. Adv Immunol 9: 215–266, 1968.
222. Lambert PH, Dixon FJ: Pathogenesis of the glomerulonephritis of NZB/W mice. J Exp Med 127: 507–522, 1968.
223. Alexander EL, Moyer C, Travlos GS, et al: Two histopathologic types of inflammatory vascular disease in MRL/Mp autoimmune mice. Model for human vasculitis in connective tissue disease. Arthritis Rheum 28: 1146–1155, 1985.
224. Eisenberg RA, Tan EM, Dixon FJ: Presence of anti-Sm reactivity in autoimmune mouse strains. J Exp Med 147: 582–587, 1978.
225. Porter DD, Larsen AE: Aleutian disease of mink: infectious virus antibody complexes in the serum. Proc Soc Exp Biol Med 126: 689, 1967.
226. Lewis RM, Schwartz RS: Canine systemic lupus erythematosus. Genetic analysis of an established breeding colony. J Exp Med 134: 417–438, 1971.
227. Fournel C, Chabanne L, Caux C, et al: Canine systemic lupus erythematosus. I: a study of 75 cases. Lupus 1: 133–139, 1992.
228. Jones DR: Canine systemic lupus erythematosus: new insights and their implications. J Comp Pathol 108: 215–228, 1993.
229. Stastny P, Stembridge VA, Ziff M: Homologous disease in the adult rat, a model for autoimmune disease. I: General features and cutaneous lesions. J Exp Med 118: 635, 1963.
230. Jaffee BD, Claman HN: Chronic graft-versus-host disease (GVHD) as a model for scleroderma. I: Description of model systems. Cell Immunol 77: 1–12, 1983.
231. Jimenez SA, Millan A, Bashey RI, et al: The tight skin (TSK) mouse: an experimental model resembling scleroderma. *In* Black CM, Myers AR (eds): Systemic Sclerosis (Scleroderma). New York, Gower Medical, 1985, pp 145–150.

232. Gershwin ME, Abplanalp H, van de Water J: An avian model for scleroderma. *In* Black CM, Myers AR (eds): Systemic Sclerosis (Scleroderma). New York, Gower Medical, 1985, pp 151–156.
233. Van de Water J, Gershwin ME: Animal model of human disease. Avian scleroderma. An inherited fibrotic disease of white Leghorn chickens resembling progressive systemic sclerosis. Am J Pathol 120: 478–482, 1985.
234. Wilson TJ, van de Water J, Mohr FC, et al: Avian scleroderma: evidence for qualitative and quantitative T cell defects. J Autoimmun 5: 261–276, 1992.
235. Ishikawa H, Tamura T, Kitabatake M, et al: Experimental scleroderma in the mouse induced by urinary glycosaminoglycans isolated from patients with systemic scleroderma. *In* Black CM, Myers AR (eds): Systemic Sclerosis (Scleroderma). New York, Gower Medical, 1985, pp 157–163.
236. Hargis AM, Prieur DJ: Animal models of polymyositis/dermatomyositis. Clin Dermatol 6: 120–124, 1988.
237. Hargis AM, Winkelstein JA, Moore MP, et al: Complement levels in dogs with familial canine dermatomyositis. Vet Immunol Immunopathol 20: 95–100, 1988.
238. Ytterberg SR, Mahowald ML, Messner RP: Coxsackievirus B1–induced polymyositis. Lack of disease expression in nu/nu mice. J Clin Invest 80: 499–506, 1987.
239. Hammer RE, Maika SD, Richardson JA, et al: Spontaneous inflammatory disease in transgenic rats expressing HLA-B27 and human beta 2m: an animal model of HLA-B27-associated human disorders. Cell 63: 1099–1112, 1990.
239a. Mear JP, Schreiber KL, Munz C, et al: Misfolding of HLA-B27 as a result of its B pocket suggests a novel mechanism for its role in susceptibility to spondyloarthropathy. J Immunol 163: 6665–6670, 1999.
240. Cooper GL, Charlton BR: Spondylitis in turkeys associated with experimental Pasteurella anatipestifer infection. Avian Dis 36: 290–295, 1992.
241. Lehman TJ, Walker SM, Mahnovski V, et al: Coronary arteritis in mice following the systemic injection of group B Lactobacillus casei cell walls in aqueous suspension. Arthritis Rheum 28: 652–659, 1985.
242. Lehman TJ, Mahnovski V: Animal models of vasculitis. Lessons we can learn to improve our understanding of Kawasaki disease. Rheum Dis Clin North Am 14: 479–487, 1988.
243. Tomita S, Myones BL, Shulman ST: In vitro correlates of the L. casei animal model of Kawasaki disease. J Rheumatol 20: 362–367, 1993.
244. Lehman TJ: Can we prevent long term cardiac damage in Kawasaki disease? Lessons from Lactobacillus casei cell wall–induced arteritis in mice. Clin Exp Rheumatol 11(Suppl)9: S3–S6, 1993.
245. Brahn E, Lehman TJA, Peacock DJ, et al: Suppression of coronary vasculitis in a murine model of Kawasaki disease using an angiogenesis inhibitor. Clin Immunol 90: 147–151, 1999.
246. Felsburg PJ, HogenEsch H, Somberg RL, et al: Immunologic abnormalities in canine juvenile polyarteritis syndrome: a naturally occurring animal model of Kawasaki disease. Clin Immunol Immunopathol 65: 110–118, 1992.
247. Onouchi Z, Ikuta K, Nagamatsu K, et al: Coronary artery aneurysms develop in weanling rabbits with serum sickness but not in mature rabbits. An experimental model for Kawasaki disease in humans. Angiology 46: 679–687, 1995.
248. Jones TC, Doll ER, Bryans JT: The lesions of equine viral arthritis. Cornell Vet 47: 52, 1957.
249. Thibault S, Drolet R, Germain MC, et al: Cutaneous and systemic necrotizing vasculitis in swine. Vet Pathol 35: 108–116, 1998.
250. Woods LW, Swift PK, Barr BC, et al: Systemic adenovirus infection associated with high mortality in mule deer (Odocoileus hemionus) in California. Vet Pathol 33: 125–132, 1996.
251. Chin RP, Meteyer CU, Yamamoto R, et al: Isolation of Mycoplasma synoviae from the brains of commercial meat turkeys with meningeal vasculitis. Avian Dis 35: 631–637, 1991.
252. Thomas L: The neurotoxins of M. neurolyticum and M. gallisepticum. Trans Assoc Am Physicians 79: 388–398, 1966.
253. Chin RP, Daft BM, Meteyer CU, et al: Meningoencephalitis in commercial meat turkeys associated with Mycoplasma gallisepticum. Avian Dis 35: 986–993, 1991.

3

Anatomy and Pathophysiology of Pain

Peter N. Malleson and David D. Sherry

Musculoskeletal pain in children is common[1] and a frequent cause of referral to pediatric rheumatologists. It is therefore important to understand the mechanisms that underlie such pain.

Pain has been defined by the Committee for Taxonomy of the International Association for the Study of Pain as "an unpleasant sensory and emotional experience associated with actual or potential tissue damage, or described in terms of such damage."[2]

Thus, pain is a child's subjective interpretation of a noxious or apparently noxious stimulus. For most acute pain, the noxious stimulus is obvious; however, for many children with chronic pain syndromes, the origin of the pain is much less clear. What is certain is that perception of pain, whether acute or chronic, is influenced by multiple modulating factors, occurring at all levels of the nervous system from the nociceptors in the muscles and joints to the higher cortical centers.

To understand a child's or adolescent's pain, one must grasp not only the mechanisms underlying noxious transmission and modulation but also those factors that influence how a child perceives pain. One must also know how the child's and the family's concepts of pain affect pain behaviors and coping strategies. Different children react differently to pain, with inherently different degrees of regulation of the focus of attention and arousal to pain.[3,4] Some of these differences are almost certainly genetic, but it is increasingly recognized that noxious events in neonatal and early infancy may play important roles in determining how individuals respond to pain later in life.[5,6] It should be noted that many of the data presented in this chapter have been deduced from animal experiments including animal models of arthritis, but it seems probable that the information is generally applicable to humans.

NOCICEPTIVE MECHANISMS

Peripheral Nociceptor System (Nociceptors and Afferent Nerve Fibers)

Nociceptors are free nerve endings. In the joints, they are present in the capsule, adipose tissues, ligaments, menisci, and periosteum. They are not found in articular cartilage, and their presence in synovium is controversial.[7] In muscle, the nociceptors are typically located in the wall of arterioles and surrounding connective tissue.[8] Nociceptors have high thresholds responding to noxious thermal, chemical, or mechanical forces. Some nociceptors are modality-specific (specific to a single type of stimulus such as mechanical or thermal); others are polymodal. Generally, nociceptors have no spontaneous activity, being activated only by intense, potentially damaging stimuli.[9]

Noxious impulses are transmitted either via thinly myelinated Aδ fibers or by nonmyelinated slow-conducting C fibers. The Aδ fibers are responsible for the well-localized first pain sensation occurring immediately after injury, whereas C fibers carry the more poorly localized, diffuse, burning second pain.[10] These afferent nociceptive fibers have their cell bodies in the dorsal root ganglia and terminate in the spinal cord at second-order neurons in the dorsal horn over several spinal segments.[7]

Neuropeptides, including substance P and calcitonin gene-related peptide, are responsible for the transmission of nociceptive signals from the periphery to the spinal cord neurons. At the same time, these peptides, which are produced in the dorsal root ganglia, are also released into the joint and muscle and thereby modulate the afferent response (see later).[7,8,11]

Spinal Cord and Central Nervous System

The receptive fields of dorsal horn neurons receiving input from afferent fibers from the joint have converging input from adjacent structures such as muscle and skin, and sometimes input from skin distant to the joint.[12] The fact that input from the joint occurs over several spinal segments, and the fact that the spinal neurons have receptive fields from sites other than joints, help explain the relatively poorly localized quality of joint and muscle pain. Dorsal horn neurons responsible for transmitting noxious stimuli from the joint and muscles can be classified as either *nociceptive-*

specific or *wide-range-dynamic*. The wide-range-dynamic neurons respond to both innocuous and noxious stimuli but fire at higher rates in response to noxious inputs. There are also interneurons that are responsible for modulating the ascending progression of nociceptive impulses by the dorsal horn neurons. Interneurons receiving input from small-diameter nociceptive afferents are excitatory, whereas those receiving input from large-diameter non-nociceptive afferents (Aβ) are inhibitory. The summation of excitatory and inhibitory impulses determines whether a nociceptive impulse is projected to the brain.

Noxious stimuli ascend via the spinothalamic, spinoreticular, and spinomesencephalic tracts, which terminate within the thalamus, reticular formation, and periaqueductal gray area in the midbrain.[13] The noxious stimulus as such probably terminates in the thalamus; the sensory cortex is responsible for integrating the sensory message with ongoing cognitive functions and for organizing conscious behavior in response to the stimulus. If thalamofrontal tracts are severed, patients can accurately detect and localize pain, but the pain loses its aversive and motivational components.

Noxious impulses reach the locus ceruleus, a pontine nucleus that is one of the main autonomic (sympathetic) centers and regulates arousal. The locus ceruleus/norepinephrine system is closely related to the hypothalamic-pituitary-adrenal axis; together, these can be considered part of a dedicated stress system responsible for re-establishing homeostasis after all forms of stress, including those associated with pain.[14]

MODULATING (SENSITIZING AND INHIBITING) MECHANISMS

Peripheral Nervous System

Repeated intense stimuli such as occur in joint inflammation lead to long-lasting sensitization of the nociceptive units. The thresholds required to excite the nociceptors become reduced, so they are activated by movements that previously were nonactivating. Sensitization and excitation in injured or inflamed joints is caused by many compounds, acting directly, indirectly, or both, often with synergistic interactions. Release of substance P into the joint after afferent fiber stimulation produces vascular responses such as vasodilatation, thereby contributing to the inflammatory process as well as sensitizing nociceptive units to excitation by inflammatory mediators such as bradykinin, protons, serotonin, and histamine.[7, 11] In addition, prostaglandins, leukotrienes, and adenosine produced by inflammation and tissue damage directly sensitize the nociceptive units. Various cytokines, norepinephrine, and nitric oxide also sensitize nociceptive afferents indirectly.[11, 15] The sympathetic nervous system within the joint probably contributes to the potentiation of pain in arthritis.[16, 17] Hyperesthesia and allodynia (pain to light touch) persisting long after an injury has resolved, as occurs in causalgia or algodystrophy, appear to often be sympathetically mediated (reflex sympathetic dystrophy); however, the explanation for this phenomenon remains speculative.[18]

Spinal Cord

The spinal cord plays a major role in modulating pain. After joint inflammation, the nociceptive input is amplified in the dorsal horn. This central sensitization occurs in several ways. Thresholds of nociceptive-specific neurons with receptive fields for the inflamed joint become lowered so that they can be activated by usually innocuous stimuli, and wide-range-dynamic neurons become more responsive to both innocuous and noxious signals. Spinal cord neurons manifest considerable neuroplasticity, developing expanded receptive fields, thereby becoming responsive to stimuli from areas to which they were previously insensitive. There also appears to be an induction, an increase, or both of spontaneous, ongoing neuronal discharges.[7, 19, 20] Repeated C-fiber afferent stimulation, as occurs in persistent inflammation, leads to a sequential increase in dorsal horn activity, resulting in prolonged neuronal discharges—a phenomenon known as *windup*.[21]

Phantom limb pain (persistence of pain in a limb that has been amputated) is a well-recognized phenomenon.[22] It appears to be largely explained by neuroplasticity of the dorsal horn neurons leading to central sensitization.[23] In 1995, Hogeweg et al[24, 25] demonstrated (1) that children with juvenile chronic arthritis have reduced pain thresholds not only at inflamed joints but also in noninflamed paraspinal areas and (2) that children whose arthritis had resolved had persistently lower thresholds than healthy control subjects (although thresholds in this group were higher than in children with continuing joint inflammation). These findings would appear to indicate that children with chronic arthritis experience central sensitization.

The pathophysiologic explanation for central sensitization remains uncertain. A comprehensive model of how noxious signals produce central sensitization has been proposed by Wilcox[26] and reviewed by Coderre et al.[23] In brief, high levels of afferent input cause the release of excitatory amino acids such as glutamate and aspartate, as well as neuropeptides such as substance P within the dorsal horn. Via actions on *N*-methyl-D-aspartate (NMDA) and non-NMDA neuronal receptors, these neurotransmitters cause intraneuronal changes that last minutes to hours. More long-term changes (hours to days) result from the induction of proto-oncogenes C-*fos* and C-*jun*. This development leads to increased synthesis of dynorphin, causing enhanced excitability and expanded receptive fields, particularly if there is a loss of the usual negative feedback by small inhibitory spinal interneurons on dynorphin-containing neurons.

Aside from central sensitization, another critical role of the spinal cord is pain inhibition. Nociceptive processes are modulated by several descending inhibitory systems, including a serotoninergic system, norepinephrine via α_2-adrenergic receptors, and three genetically distinct families of endogenous opioid polypeptides (enkephalin, β-endorphin, and dynorphin).[11, 27] These tonic descending inhibitory systems probably play a role in determining the size of the receptive fields of the spinal neurons and their excitation thresholds. Concentrations of these inhibitory compounds have been shown to be increased in experimental arthritis, presumably as an attempt to inhibit the forward transmission of nociceptive signals from the inflamed joints.[28–30]

In addition to the descending inhibitory systems just described, there is another form of inhibition known as *heterotopic inhibition*. In this form of inhibition, noxious stimuli applied to areas remote from the nociceptive receptive fields inhibit the initial pain.[31] Interestingly, gentle stimulation of the contralateral inflamed ankle in rats can trigger inhibition of pain in the opposite inflamed ankle.[32] These findings perhaps partly explain why counter-irritants often provide some pain relief.

Brain

Although the spinal cord is now recognized as being important to pain modulation, it is of course the brain that determines the final outcome. The descending inhibitory mechanisms described earlier originate in several different areas, including the periaqueductal gray area, the rostral ventromedial medulla (which includes the nucleus raphe magnus), and the locus ceruleus.

The periaqueductal gray area contains large quantities of opioid peptides. Their analgesic effects are activated by signals from the frontal cortex, amygdala, and hypothalamus. Signals from the periaqueductal gray area then descend and synapse in the nucleus raphe magnus before proceeding down the dorsal lateral funiculus to the dorsal horns, where they synapse with inhibitory interneurons. Noradrenergic impulses from the locus ceruleus pass via the rostral ventromedial medulla. An electrical stimulus of the periaqueductal gray area or the rostral ventromedial medulla can cause analgesia without altering alertness,[33, 34] and destructive lesions or local anesthetics injected into the rostral ventromedial medulla can abolish analgesia produced by stimulation of the periaqueductal gray area.[35] There is some evidence that patients with fibromyalgia have decreased levels of enkephalins and serotonin and increased levels of substance P in the cerebrospinal fluid[36, 37]; this suggests that dysfunction of the central inhibitory systems may contribute to the development of chronic noninflammatory pain syndromes. These findings confirm the importance of subcortical deep brain structures in modulating nociceptive inputs from the periphery.

Cortical structures modulate pain in both excitatory and inhibitory ways. Stressful situations perceived at the cortical level are transmitted to the locus ceruleus and hypothalamic-pituitary-adrenal axis and can lead to either increased pain perception or pain inhibition.[14] Other factors that have been shown to be important in how pain is perceived by children include ability to regulate the focus of attention toward or away from pain, level of arousal in response to noxious stimuli,[3, 4] use of coping strategies,[38, 39] and self-esteem.[40] These factors may be in part genetically determined, but they are significantly modified by exposure to environmental factors, including exposure to pain in early childhood,[41] memories of previous painful episodes,[42] parental responses to pain or painful situations,[43, 44] and the developmental age of the child.[45]

Different children respond very differently to painful medical procedures,[46] and they demonstrate large differences in pain sensitivity and tolerance in the laboratory.[47] A 1997 study of 56 children with juvenile chronic arthritis indicated that only about 50 percent of the pain variability among children could be explained by a model that included demographic, medical status, and coping variables.[39] About 30 percent of the pain variance was explained by disease activity, and approximately 20 percent was explained by coping strategies. The remaining 50 percent of the variability was not explained by the model. It seems likely that many factors interact in a complex manner to modulate the extent to which noxious stimuli are perceived as pain.

CONCLUSIONS

Most children with acute pain do not develop a chronic pain syndrome. What factors cause some children to suffer chronic pain that persists long after any injury has resolved? It is clear that certain children are pain-vulnerable, both because of intrinsic factors present at birth, or soon afterward, and because of exposure to environmental factors during their cognitive development. Modulating factors at all levels of the nervous system are clearly important in determining whether acute pain becomes persistent. A number of these factors have been described, but many remain either unproven or unknown. Importantly, although few if any children have pain that is purely psychogenic, the fact that pain can be modulated centrally indicates that painful conditions can be helped by a number of interventions such as acupuncture, transcutaneous nerve stimulation working at the spinal cord level,[47] or cognitive-behavioral therapies that act at a more central level.[4, 48]

References

1. Goodman JE, McGrath PJ: The epidemiology of pain in children and adolescents: a review. Pain 46: 247–264, 1991.
2. Merksey H: Pain terms: a list with definitions and notes on usage. Recommended by the International Association for the Study of Pain (IASP) Subcommittee on Taxonomy. Pain 6: 249–252, 1979.
3. LeBaron S, Zeltzer L, Fanurik D: An investigation of cold pressor pain in children: Part I. Pain 37: 161–171, 1989.
4. Zeltzer LK, Bursch B, Walco GA: Pain responsiveness and chronic pain: a psychobiological perspective. J Dev Behav Pediatr 18: 413–422, 1998.
5. Fitzgerald M. Development of pain pathways and mechanisms. *In* Anand KJS, McGrath PJ (eds): Pain in Neonates. New York, Elsevier, 1993, p 39.
6. Taddio A, Katz J, Ilersich AL: Effect of neonatal circumcision on

pain response during subsequent routine vaccination. Lancet 349: 599–603, 1997.
7. Schaible H, Grubb BD: Afferent and spinal mechanisms of joint pain. Pain 55: 5–54, 1993.
8. Mense S: Nociception from skeletal muscle in relation to clinical muscle pain. Pain 54: 241–289, 1993.
9. Schaible H, Schmidt RF: Effects of an experimental arthritis on the sensory properties of fine articular afferent units. J Neurophysiol 54: 1109–1122, 1985.
10. Dubner R: Neurophysiology of pain. Dent Clin North Am 22: 11–30, 1978.
11. Markenson JA: Mechanisms of chronic pain. Am J Med 101: 6S–18S, 1996.
12. Schaible H, Schmidt RF, Willis WD: Convergent inputs from articular, cutaneous and muscle receptors onto ascending tract cells in the cat spinal cord. Exp Brain Res 66: 479–488, 1987.
13. Willis WD: The origins and destination of pathways involved in pain transmission. *In* Wall PD, Melzack R (eds): Textbook of Pain. New York, Churchill Livingstone, 1989, p 112.
14. Pillemer SR, Bradley LA, Crofford LJ, et al: The neuroscience and endocrinology of fibromyalgia. Arthritis Rheum 40: 1928–1939, 1997.
15. Konttinen YT, Kemppinnen P, Sergerberg M, et al: Peripheral and spinal neural mechanisms in arthritis, with particular reference to treatment of inflammation and pain. Arthritis Rheum 37: 965–982, 1994.
16. Levine JD, Clark R, Devor M, et al: Contribution of sensory afferents and sympathetic efferents to joint injury in experimental arthritis. J Neurosci 6: 3423–3429, 1986.
17. Levine JD, Fye K, Heller P, et al: Clinical response to regional intravenous guanethidine in patients with rheumatoid arthritis. J Rheumatol 13: 1040–1043, 1986.
18. Roberts WJ: A hypothesis on the physiological basis for causalgia and related pains. Pain 25: 297–311, 1986.
19. Neugebauer V, Schaible H: Evidence for a central component in the sensitization of spinal neurons with joint input during development of acute arthritis in cat's knee. J Neurophysiol 64: 299–311, 1990.
20. Grubb BD, Stiller RU, Schaible H: Dynamic changes in the receptive field properties of spinal cord neurons with ankle-input in rats with unilateral adjuvant-induced inflammation in the ankle region. Exp Brain Res 92: 441–452, 1992.
21. Mendell LM: Physiological properties of unmyelinated fiber projections to the spinal cord. Exp Neurol 16: 316–332, 1966.
22. Melzack R: Phantom limb pain: implications for treatment of pathologic pain. Anesthesiology 35: 409–419, 1971.
23. Coderre TJ, Katz J, Vaccarino AL, Melzack R: Contribution of central neuroplasticity to pathological pain: review of clinical and experimental evidence. Pain 52: 259–285, 1993.
24. Hogeweg JA, Kuis W, Huygen AC, et al: The pain threshold in juvenile chronic arthritis. Br J Rheumatol 34: 61–67, 1995.
25. Hogeweg JA, Kuis W, Oostendorp RA, Helders PJ: General and segmental reduced pain thresholds in juvenile chronic arthritis. Pain 62: 11–17, 1995.
26. Wilcox GL: Excitatory neurotransmitters and pain. *In* Bond MR, Charlton JE, Woolf CJ (eds): Pain Research and Clinical Management. Proceedings of VIth World Congress on Pain. Amsterdam, Elsevier, 1991, p 97.
27. Ruda MA, Bennett GJ, Dubner R: Neurochemistry and neural circuitry in the dorsal horn. *In* Emson PC, Rossor MN, Fonyama M (eds): Progress in Brain Research. Amsterdam, Elsevier, 1986, p 219.
28. Hylden JLK, Thomas DA, Iadarola MJ, et al: Spinal opioid analgesic effects are enhanced in a model of unilateral inflammation/hyperalgesia: possible involvement of noradrenergic mechanisms. Eur J Pharmacol 194: 135–143, 1991.
29. Iadarola MJ, Brady LS, Draisci G, Dubner R: Enhancement of dynorphin gene expression in spinal cord following experimental inflammation: stimulus specificity, behavioural parameters and opioid receptor binding. Pain 35: 313–326, 1988.
30. Godefroy F, Weil-Fugazza J, Besson J: Complex temporal changes in 5-hydroxytryptamine synthesis in the central nervous system induced by experimental polyarthritis in the rat. Pain 28: 223–238, 1987.
31. LeBars D, Dickenson AH, Besson JM: Diffuse noxious inhibitory controls (DNIC). I: Effects on dorsal horn convergent neurones in the rat. Pain 6: 283–304, 1979.
32. Calvino B, Billanueva L, LeBars D: Dorsal horn (convergent) neurones in the intact anaesthetized arthritic rat. II: Heterotopic inhibitory influences. Pain 31: 359–379, 1987.
33. Reynolds DV: Surgery in the rat during electrical analgesia induced by focal brain stimulation. Science 164: 444–445, 1969.
34. Mayer DJ, Liebeskind JC: Pain reduction by focal electrical stimulation of the brain: an anatomical and behavioral analysis. Brain Res 68: 73–93, 1974.
35. Bitz AJ: The sites of origin of brain stem neurotensin and serotonin projections to the rodent nucleus raphe magnus. J Neurosci 2: 819–824, 1982.
36. Russell IJ, Orr MD, Littman B, et al: Elevated cerebrospinal fluid levels of substance P in patients with the fibromyalgia syndrome. Arthritis Rheum 37: 1593–1601, 1994.
37. Russell IJ: Neurochemical pathogenesis of fibromyalgia syndrome. J Musculoskeletal Pain 4: 61–92, 1996.
38. Bédard GB, Reid GJ, McGrath PJ, Chambers CT: Coping and self-medication in a community sample of junior high school students. Pain Res Manage 2: 151–156, 1997.
39. Schanberg LE, Lefebvre JC, Keefe FJ, et al: Pain coping and the pain experience in children with juvenile chronic arthritis. Pain 73: 181–189, 1997.
40. Litt IF, Cuskey WR, Rosenberg BA: Role of self-esteem and autonomy in determining medication compliance among adolescents with juvenile rheumatoid arthritis. Pediatrics 69: 15–17, 1982.
41. Grunau RVE, Whitfield MF, Petrie JH, Fryer EL: Early pain experience, child and family factors, as precursors of somatization: a prospective study of extremely premature and fullterm children. Pain 56: 353–359, 1994.
42. Siegel LJ, Smith KE: Children's strategies for coping with pain. Pediatrician 16: 110–118, 1989.
43. Lumley MA, Ableles LA, Melamed BG, et al: Coping outcomes in children undergoing stressful medical procedures: the role of child-environment variables. Behav Assess 12: 223–238, 1990.
44. Chun DY, Turner JA, Romano JM: Children of chronic pain patients: risk factors for maladjustment. Pain 52: 311–317, 1993.
45. Gaffney A, Dunne EA: Children's understanding of the causality of pain. Pain 29: 91–104, 1986.
46. Jay SM, Ozolins M, Elliott CH, Caldwell S: Assessment of children's distress during painful medical procedures. Health Psychol 2: 133–147, 1983.
47. Eland J: The use of TENS with children. *In* Schechter NL, Berde CB, Yaster M (eds): Pain in Infants, Children, and Adolescents. Baltimore, Williams & Wilkins, 1993.
48. de C Williams AC, Nicholas MK, Richardson PH, et al: Evaluation of a cognitive behavioural programme for rehabilitating patients with chronic pain. Br J Gen Pract 43: 513–518, 1993.

4

The Immune System

Alberto Martini

This chapter provides a concise approach to the function of the immune system; it particularly examines aspects that are relevant to the etiopathogenesis of autoimmune diseases. The effector mechanisms of the immune system leading to inflammation and tissue damage are discussed in Chapter 5.

GENERAL OVERVIEW

The immune system,[1-3] the function of which is to protect against infections, comprises two branches: a more primitive one called *innate* (natural, native) immunity and a highly sophisticated one called *adaptive* (specific) immunity. Innate and adaptive immunity are not two separate compartments but an integrated system of host defense, sharing bidirectional interactions fundamental to both the inductive phase and the effector phase of the immune response. The cells of the immune system originate from the pluripotent hematopoietic stem cells that give rise to stem cells of more limited potential (lymphoid and myeloid precursors) (Fig. 4–1). The immune system functions by means of a complex network of cellular interactions that involve cell surface proteins and soluble mediators such as cytokines.

Innate Immunity

Innate immunity provides the first line of defense against microbes and is a more primitive mechanism of protection. The principal components are (1) physical and chemical barriers such as epithelia and antimi-

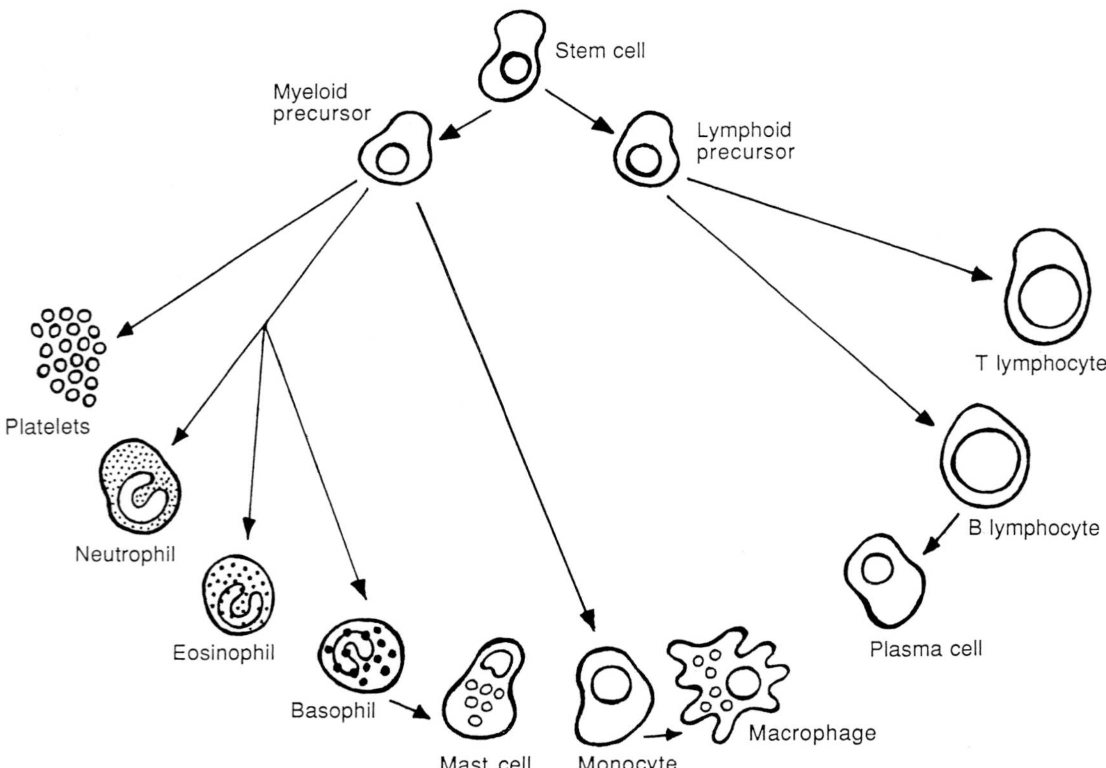

Figure 4–1. Lineage of cells involved in the immune and inflammatory responses. Most of the dendritic cells appear to be related to the mononuclear phagocyte lineage; a subset of them is supposed to be of lymphoid origin.

crobial substances produced at epithelial surfaces, (2) proteins such as the complement components, acute phase proteins, and cytokines, and (3) phagocytes (neutrophils and macrophages) and natural killer (NK) cells.

Phagocytes have surface receptors that have evolved to recognize highly conserved structures characteristic of microbial pathogens but not present in mammalian cells. These structures include bacterial lipopolysaccharide, peptidoglycan, and mannans; they are referred to as *pathogen-associated molecular patterns,* and the receptors of the innate immune system that evolved to recognize them are called *pattern-recognition receptors.* The binding of microbial structures to pattern-recognition receptors triggers the cell to engulf the bacterium and induces cytokines, chemokines, and costimulators that recruit and activate antigen-specific lymphocytes and initiate adaptive immune responses. Thus, innate immunity not only represents an early effective defense mechanism against infection but also provides the "warning" of the presence of an infection against which a subsequent adaptive immune response has to be mounted.[3a] NK cells are non-T, non-B cells (see later) that do not bear specific antigen receptors on their surface. They possess the ability to recognize and kill virus-infected cells.[4, 4a] Moreover, they bear membrane receptors for immunoglobulins and can lyse antibody-coated target cells, a phenomenon known as *antibody-dependent cell-mediated cytotoxicity* (ADCC). Innate immunity represents an effective first line of defense against infections. However, its capacity to recognize infectious agents is limited, and viruses and some bacteria are able to survive and multiply within cells, where they are not accessible to the defense mechanisms of innate immunity.

Adaptive Immunity

Adaptive immunity is a highly sophisticated defense mechanism that has evolved in vertebrates to overcome the limitations of innate immunity. Its main characteristics are the capacity to recognize microbes with a high level of molecular specificity and to remember and respond more promptly and vigorously to subsequent exposure to the same microbe (immunologic memory). Any substance capable of being recognized by the adaptive immune system is called an *antigen.*

Lymphocytes, the cells responsible for adaptive immunity, consist of various cell subsets that are morphologically similar but different in their functions. Subsets of these cells express different membrane proteins with specific functions. The membrane proteins mentioned in this chapter are listed in Table 4–1. On its surface,

Table 4–1
Some Examples of Differentiation Antigens*

CD ANTIGEN COMMON NAMES	MAIN CELLULAR EXPRESSION	KNOWN OR SUPPOSED FUNCTIONS	OTHER COMMON NAMES
CD1 (a,b,c,d)	Thymocytes, dendritic cells	MHC class I–like molecule, presentation of nonpeptide antigens to some T cells	
CD2	T cells, NK cells	Adhesion molecule (binds LFA-3)	LFA-3
CD3	T cells, thymocytes	Associated with the T-cell receptor and involved in signal transduction	
CD4	Helper T cells	Co-receptor for MHC class II molecules	
CD5	T cells, B-cell subset	Signaling molecule	
CD8	Cytotoxic T cells	Co-receptor for MHC class I molecules	
CD11a	Leukocytes	Subunit of LFA-1 (adhesion molecule)	LFA-1 α chain
CD18	Leukocytes	Subunit of LFA-1 (adhesion molecule)	LFA-1 β chain
CD19	B cells	Role in B-cell activation	
CD21	B cells	Role in B-cell activation	CR-2
CD28	T-cell subsets	Receptor for co-stimulatory molecules B7-1, B7-2	
CD34	Precursors of hematopoietic cells, endothelial cells in high endothelial venules	Adhesion molecule (ligand for L-selectin)	
CD40	B cells, macrophages, dendritic cells	Tyrosine phosphatase role in B-cell, macrophage, and dendritic cell activation induced by T cells; binds CD40L (CD154)	
CD44	Leukocytes	Mediates adhesion of leukocytes	
CD45	Leukocytes	Tyrosine phosphatase, role in signal transduction	Leukocyte common antigen
CD80	Antigen-presenting cells	Co-stimulator for T-lymphocyte activation; ligand for CD28 and CTLA-4	B7-1
CD86	Antigen-presenting cells	Co-stimulator for T-lymphocyte activation; ligand for CD28 and CTLA-4	B7-2
CD95	Multiple cell types	Role in activation-induced apoptosis; binds FasL	Fas
CD154	Activated CD4 T cells	Ligand for CD40	CD40L

LFA, leukocyte function-associated antigen; MHC, major histocompatibility complex; NK, natural killer.
*Defined by means of monoclonal antibodies and designed by the abbreviation CD (clusters of differentiation) followed by a number.

each naive lymphocyte bears receptors of only a single specificity; they are generated during lymphocyte maturation through a unique genetic mechanism that occurs independent of and prior to exposure to antigen. Because there are millions of lymphocytes (each with a single, different specificity), the total repertoire of antigen receptors enables the immune system to specifically respond to virtually any antigen. The antigen selects a specific preexisting clone *(clonal selection)* and activates it to proliferate and differentiate into effector and memory cells.

There are two main types of lymphocytes: B lymphocytes (which mature in the bone marrow) and T lymphocytes (which mature in the thymus). B lymphocytes produce antibodies and are responsible for humoral immunity. Their antigen receptors are membrane-bound antibodies that can recognize soluble antigens; cell activation leads to a sequence of events that culminates in the generation of plasma cells that secrete antibodies. T lymphocytes are responsible for cell-mediated immunity. The T-cell receptor (TCR) for antigen recognizes cell surface–associated, but not soluble, antigens. Indeed, the TCR recognizes peptide antigens that are generated inside particular cells (called *antigen-presenting cells*, or APCs) and brought to the cell surface in association with specialized molecules belonging to the major histocompatibility complex (MHC). This allows the immune system to detect intracellular pathogens. There are two functionally distinct populations of T lymphocytes: helper T lymphocytes and cytotoxic T lymphocytes. Helper T lymphocytes play the pivotal role in adaptive immunity and activate other cells such as B lymphocytes, macrophages, and cytotoxic T cells to perform their effector functions. Cytotoxic T lymphocytes lyse cells that are infected by virus or other intracellular microorganisms.

The adaptive immune response can be divided into three phases. The recognition phase consists of the binding of antigens to specific lymphocyte receptors. The activation phase is the sequence of events induced in lymphocytes after specific antigen recognition. Lymphocytes first proliferate and then differentiate into either effector cells (that are aimed at eliminating the antigen) or memory cells (that survive and are ready to respond promptly to antigen re-exposure). In the effector phase, activated lymphocytes perform their function of eliminating the antigen. Many effector functions require the participation of molecules or cells that belong to the innate immune system. For instance, some antibodies activate complement, whereas T lymphocytes release cytokines that stimulate the function of phagocytes and the inflammatory response.

The maturation of lymphocytes occurs in the central lymphoid organs, the bone marrow for B lymphocytes and the thymus for T lymphocytes. Once they have matured, lymphocytes enter the bloodstream. The encounter between foreign antigens and mature naive lymphocytes occurs in the peripheral lymphoid organs (lymph nodes, spleen, and mucosal-associated lymphoid tissues). Indeed, lymphocytes continually recirculate through peripheral lymphoid organs to which antigens are also carried from the site of infection.

The immune system is able to recognize and eliminate a foreign antigen but normally does not react harmfully to self-antigenic molecules (self-tolerance).

B CELLS AND IMMUNOGLOBULINS

Immunoglobulin Molecule

Antibodies are the antigen-specific immunoglobulin (Ig) products of B cells. Once they are produced and released by antigen-activated B cells, immunoglobulins (1) serve as membrane-bound antigen receptors of B cells, (2) bind their specific antigen, and (3) recruit other molecules or cells to destroy the target to which they have bound. These functions are fulfilled as follows: one end of the antibody molecule, the variable region (Fab), binds to the antigen; the other end of the molecule, the constant region (Fc), binds to a limited number of effector molecules and cells.

The basic immunoglobulin structure (Fig. 4–2) is substantially the same for all five main immunoglobulin classes or isotypes (IgM, IgD, IgG, IgA, IgE).[5] Antibodies are Y-shaped molecules composed of two identical heavy (H) chains (each 50 or 70 kD) and two identical light (L) chains (each about 25 kD). In all antibodies, there are only two types of functionally equivalent L chains, which are called lambda (λ) and kappa (κ) chains. The amino-terminal sequence of both L and H chains, which vary greatly among different antibodies (variable, or V, region), pairs to generate two identical antigen-binding sites that lie at the tips of the arms of the Y. The carboxy-terminal sequences are constant (constant, or C, region) among immunoglobulin chains of the same heavy-chain isotype.

Within the variable regions, there are hypervariable (HV) regions. These HV regions, also called the complementarity-determining regions, or CDRs (CDR1, CDR2, CDR3), are localized to a particular part of the surface of the molecule so that when the VH and the VL regions pair in the antibody molecule, the hypervariable regions are brought together, creating a single hypervariable site that forms the binding site for antigens. Thus, final antigen specificity is particularly determined by the juxtaposition of the CDRs. The molecular region that is recognized specifically by an antibody is called the *antigenic determinant*, or *epitope*. On protein surfaces, epitopes may be composed of a single segment of a polypeptide chain of amino acids (continuous or linear epitopes) or by amino acids present in different parts of the primary protein sequence brought together by protein folding (conformational or discontinuous epitopes). The binding between antigen and antibody is a reversible noncovalent interaction.

B Cell Antigen Receptor Complex

On B lymphocytes, immunoglobulins are bound to the membrane, where they serve as specific antigen receptors. Membrane immunoglobulins have a very short cytoplasmic tail that is unable to transduce the signal to the cell once they have reacted with their specific

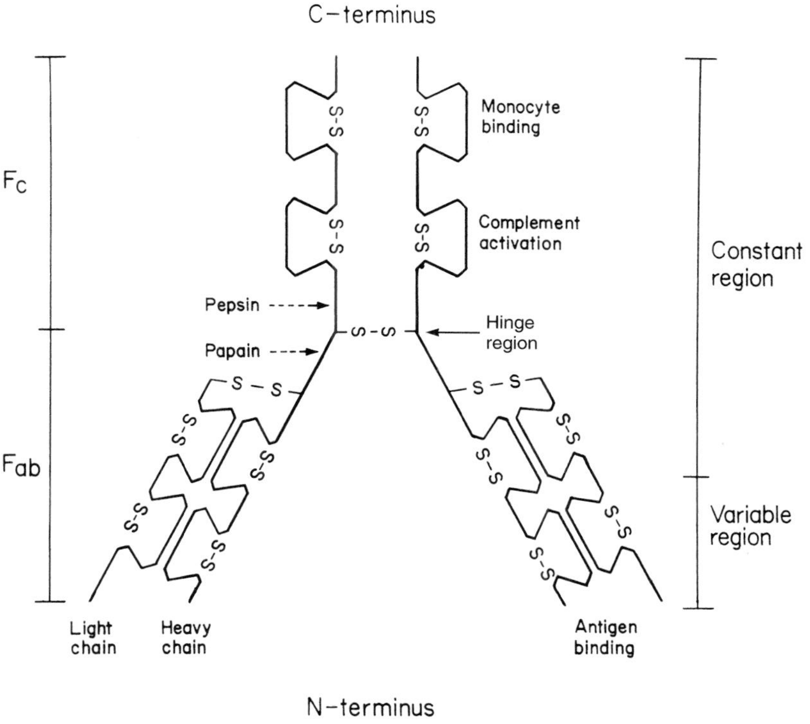

Figure 4–2. Basic immunoglobulin structure. Linear and tertiary structure of a typical immunoglobulin G molecule. The variable regions of the light and heavy chains are shown by the brackets. Each chain can be divided into domains on the basis of sequence similarities; the light chains contain two domains and the heavy chain comprises four. The Fab (fragment antigen binding) and the Fc (fragment crystallizable) regions are defined by analysis with papain and pepsin. Pepsin destroys the larger part of the Fc portion, leaving an F(ab′)2 divalent molecule. The hinge region that links the Fc and Fab portions is flexible and allows independent movement of the two Fab arms.

antigen. Immunoglobulins in the cell membrane, however, are associated with two other chains, Igα and Igβ, to form a receptor complex.[6] The cytoplasmic tail of these two chains contains particular sequence motifs called *immunoreceptor tyrosine activation motifs* (ITAMs), which are common to other signaling molecules of the immune system, including those of the TCR complex. Three tyrosine kinases (Fyn, Blk, and Lyn) are also associated with the receptor complex. The antigen activates the signaling cascade by crosslinking the surface immunoglobulin molecules and therefore bringing receptor-associated tyrosine kinases together with the ITAMs they phosphorylate. When phosphorylated on tyrosine, the ITAMs are recognized by cytoplasmic molecules that activate a cascade of events resulting in cell activation. Surface immunoglobulin function is also modulated by a particular co-receptor complex, present on cell membrane, which contains at least three cell surface molecules, known as CD19, TAPA-1, and (CD21).[7] Co-ligation of the surface immunoglobulins with this co-receptor complex greatly increases the efficiency of cell activation. CR2 is a receptor for the complement protein C3d, generated by the proteolysis of C3, and many microbes activate complement by the alternative pathway in the absence of antibody.[7] Therefore, as for T cell activation, the innate immune response to microbes provides signals that are essential also for B cell activation. In most instances, however, the activation of B cells requires the presence of other additional signals, the most important of which is delivered by helper T cells that recognize antigen on the surface of B cells.

Generation of Antibody Diversity

The heterogeneity of antibodies allows each molecule to recognize a particular antigen. The entire collection of antibody specificities in a given individual (the antibody repertoire) is large enough to ensure that virtually any structure can be recognized. The problem of how this almost infinite range of specificities could be encoded by a finite number of genes was solved with the demonstration that different parts of the variable region are encoded by different sets of gene segments.[8] Indeed, each immunoglobulin chain, both light (κ or λ) and heavy, is coded by distinct genomic regions, one for the variable portion and one for the constant portion. For the light chain, each variable region is encoded in two different DNA segments: the variable (V) chain segment and the joining (J) chain gene segment. In the case of heavy-chain variable regions, in addition to the V and J segments there is a third gene segment called *diversity* (D). There are multiple functional copies of the V, D, and J segments (approximately 40 V_κ, 5 J_κ, 29 V_λ, 4 J_λ, 51 V_H, 27 D_H, and 6 J_H). During the development of a lymphocyte, one copy of each gene segment is joined randomly to the others by irreversible DNA recombination *(somatic recombination)*. This process generates light- and heavy-chain variable regions and is summarized in Figure 4–3. Several enzymes act in concert during somatic gene recombination and include the product of recombination-activating genes (RAG)-1 and -2, terminal deoxynucleotidyl transferase (TdT), and DNA-dependent protein kinase.

Antibody diversity is therefore generated in four main ways. Because variable-region gene segments (V, D, J) are present in multiple copies and only one of these copies is selected during recombination, the resulting sequence depends on both the copy that has been selected and the recombination process that joins together the different gene segments. Additional diversity results from the insertion of a random number of nucleotides in the junctions between gene segments. These insertions may or may not disrupt the reading

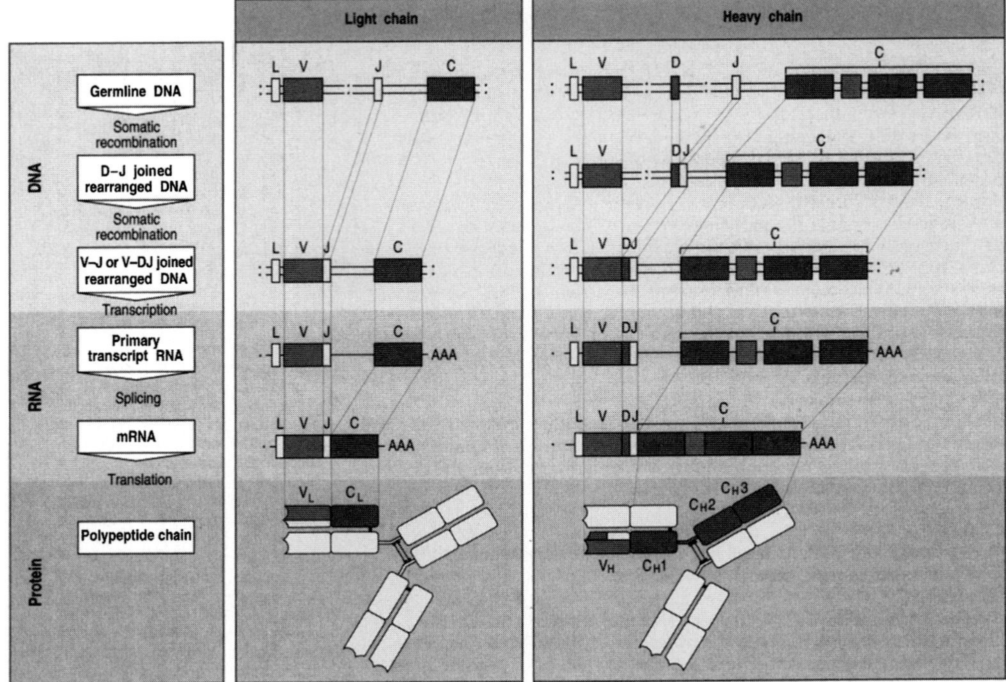

Figure 4–3. Generation of light- and heavy-chain variable regions. Variable regions are constructed by a process of somatic recombination that joins together different gene segments. There are multiple copies of the V and J segments (for light chains) and V, D, and J segments (for heavy chains); only one of these copies is selected during recombination. The constant (C) region of heavy chains is coded by different exons corresponding to the different immunoglobulin classes and subclasses. For the sake of simplicity, only one heavy C region exon is shown. Once formed, the variable region is joined to the constant region by a process of RNA splicing, giving rise to antibodies of any of the five isotypes. The rearrangement of immunoglobulin genes is regulated to ensure that each B lymphocyte expresses only one rearranged light-chain gene and only one rearranged heavy-chain gene. (From Janeway CA, Travers P, Walport M, Capra DJ: Immunobiology. London, Elsevier, 1999.)

frame of the coding sequence, therefore leading to nonproductive or productive rearrangements, respectively. Another mechanism of variability results from the pairing of different combinations of light- and heavy-chain variable regions to form the antigen-binding site. Finally, in mature lymphocytes that respond to antigens, a process known as *somatic hypermutation*[9] introduces a very high rate of point mutations into rearranged variable region genes and generates further variability; some of the mutant immunoglobulin molecules bind antigens better than the original surface immunoglobulin, and B cells expressing them are selected to mature into antibody-secreting cells, a phenomenon called *affinity maturation*.

Immunoglobulin Isotypes

As stated earlier, there are five major classes or isotypes of immunoglobulins (IgM, IgD, IgG, IgE, and IgA).[5] Moreover, there are four subclasses of IgG antibodies (IgG1, IgG2, IgG3, IgG4) and two subclasses of IgA molecules (IgA1, IgA2). The heavy chains that define the isotypes are designated by the Greek letters μ, δ, γ, ϵ, and α. IgM and IgE heavy chains contain an extra constant region domain. IgM molecules are found as pentamers; IgA in mucous secretions, but not in plasma, is present principally as dimers. Pentamers and dimers are formed using the joining (J) chain, a 15-kD polypeptide synthesized by the plasma cell that binds the C-terminal of heavy chains. The structural features that distinguish the heavy-chain constant regions of the various isotypes confer on each of them distinct properties that enable them to activate different effector mechanisms and to be transported across epithelia or the placenta (Table 4–2).

Constant region genes in the same species are polymorphic, and the allelic variants are called *allotypes*. The determinants of the antigen receptor that are specific for a given lymphocyte clone are called *idiotopes*, and the collection of all the idiotopes of a given receptor is called the *idiotype*. The idiotype therefore represents the collection of specific determinants that distinguish each lymphocyte clone from all the others. In the antibody molecule, a given variable region can be associated with any constant region. Indeed, the constant region expressed in a B lymphocyte changes during the maturation of the cell and its subsequent proliferation in the course of the immune response, a phenomenon known as *isotype switch* (see later).

B-Cell Development

The process of gene rearrangement that gives rise to membrane immunoglobulins continually generates new

Table 4–2

Immunoglobulins

	IgG1	IgG2	IgG3	IgG4	IgA1	IgA2	IgM	IgD	IgE
Normal adult serum level (mg/ml)	9	3	1	0.5	3	0.5	1.5	0.03	0.00005
Sedimentation coefficient	7S	7S	7S	7S	7S	7S	19S	7S	8S
Molecular weight (× 10^3)	146	146	170	146	160	160	970	184	188
Carbohydrate (%)	3	3	3	3	8	8	12	10	12
Intravascular (%)	45	45	45	45	40	40	75	75	50
Total circulating pool (mg/kg)	325	115	35	20	80	15	37	1	0.02
Half-life (days)	23	23	9	25	6	6	5	3	3
Synthetic rate (mg/kg/day)	30		4		25		7	0.4	0.02
Biologic function									
Crosses placenta	++	±	+	+	–	–	–	–	–
Complement fixation	++	+	+++	–	–*	–*	+++	±	±
Cell binding									
Mononuclear cells	+++	±	+++	±	–	–	–	–	–
Neutrophils	+++	+	+++	+	+	+	–	–	–
Lymphocytes	+	+	+	+	–	–	+	–	–
Mast cells	–	–	–	–	–	–	–	–	+++
Platelets	+	+	+	+	–	–	–	–	–

Ig, immunoglobulin.
*Alternative pathway fixation.

populations of B cells of highly diverse specificity and provides the material on which clonal selection acts during the adaptive immune response. Nonlymphoid stromal cells of the bone marrow provide the essential microenvironment for B-cell development by means of specific cell-to-cell contacts and release of growth factors. The different stages of B-cell maturation in the bone marrow are summarized in Figure 4–4. The process is characterized by sequential rearrangements and expression of the immunoglobulin genes, which regulate progression from one stage to the next.[10] The generation of an intact immunoglobulin chain by productive somatic gene rearrangement blocks further rearrangement of the set of gene segments specifying that chain and leads to progression to the next developmental step. On the contrary, if rearrangements are not productive, the cell fails to develop and dies. Fully differentiated B cells have only one successfully rearranged light-chain gene and one successfully rearranged heavy-chain gene and therefore an immunoglobulin molecule of only one given specificity.

Several proteins regulate immunoglobulin gene rearrangement and function and are differently expressed in the various stages of B-cell development. Some known immune deficiencies reflect alteration of these proteins; for instance, mutations in Bruton's tyrosine kinase (Btk) gene are responsible for Bruton's X-linked agammaglobulinemia. During development, B

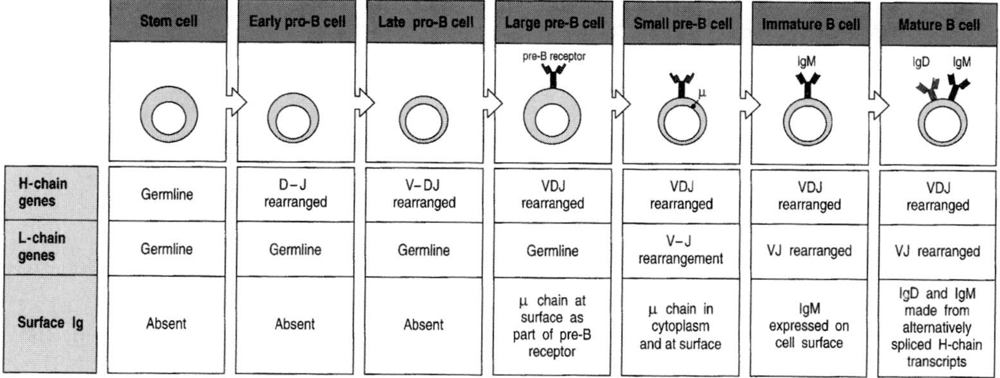

Figure 4–4. Different stages in B-lymphocyte development. The maturation of B cells is characterized by sequential rearrangements and expression of the immunoglobulin genes. In large pre-B cells, productive VDJH joining leads to the production of a chain that is transiently expressed on the cell surface in association with a surrogate light chain to form a pre-B cell receptor whose ligand is unknown. Pre-B cell receptor ligation triggers cell proliferation, which gives rise to small non-dividing pre-B cells in which the μ chain is found intracellularly and in which the L-chain gene rearrangement starts. After successful assembling of a light-chain gene, the cell becomes an immature B cell that expresses surface IgM molecules. Mature B cells are characterized by the additional appearance of IgD on cell membrane. (From Janeway CA, Travers P, Walport M, Capra DJ: Immunobiology. London, Elsevier, 1999.)

cells express stage-specific membrane molecules. Antibodies to these molecules are used to characterize lymphoproliferative diseases or to identify immunodeficiencies affecting B-cell development.

B-Cell Selection

The random generation of the B-cell repertoire gives rise to autoreactive B cells that are eliminated during development in the bone marrow at the stage of immature B cells by two main known mechanisms.[11] Immature B cells express only surface IgM and, in contrast with mature B cells, undergo apoptosis and are removed from the repertoire (clonal deletion) if they bind abundant multivalent antigens such as ubiquitous cell surface molecules. However, a small proportion of these autoreactive immature B cells may escape this fate by replacing their autoreactive receptors with receptors that are not autoreactive. This rescue process is made possible by further gene rearrangement and is known as *receptor editing*.[11a]

Immature B cells that bind to soluble antigens are inactivated but not deleted; this state of nonreactivity is called *anergy*. Because anergic B cells cannot be activated by T cells, they fail to compete with other B cells in the periphery and are rapidly lost. Moreover, because B cells specific for protein antigens need T-cell help in order to be activated, T-cell self-tolerance by itself generally appears to be adequate for preventing the production of high-affinity autoantibodies specific for self-proteins.

Mature B cells leave the bone marrow and enter the peripheral lymphocyte pool as naive B cells. The influx of new mature B cells must compensate for the death of an equal number of peripheral B cells to maintain the steady state of the peripheral pool. Some naive B cells have a half-life of only a few days, probably because they are excluded from the lymphoid follicles. Naive B cells that successfully enter lymphoid follicles have a half-life of several weeks. After encountering the specific antigen, some B cells become nondividing, very-long-lived memory cells.

Some B cells do not follow the developmental pathways so far described and have a distinctive receptor repertoire and functional properties. These cells are called B1 or CD5 B cells (conventional B cells are called B2 B cells)[12] because they were first identified by the surface expression of the protein CD5 (which is also present on T cells). Little is known about their function. They arise early in ontogeny and, in adults, form a self-renewing population that is abundant in pleural and peritoneal cavities. They have a limited diversity in their repertoire; produce low-affinity, polyspecific, and autoreactive antibodies (mainly IgM); and contribute little to the adaptive immune response against protein antigens, but they do contribute to the immune response against some bacterial polysaccharides. All these characteristics suggest that B1 B cells mediate a more primitive, less adaptive immune response than conventional B cells.

T CELLS AND THEIR ANTIGEN RECEPTORS

Immunoglobulins bind antigens in the blood and the extracellular space. However, some bacteria and parasites, and all viruses, replicate inside cells, where they cannot be recognized by antibodies. These pathogens are destroyed by T cells, which are responsible for cell-mediated immunity and recognize only antigens displayed on the cell surface, to where they are delivered by specialized, highly polymorphic molecules encoded by the genes of the MHC. Moreover, T cells are essential in helping B cells; therefore, both cellular and humoral immune responses to protein antigens depend on antigen recognition by T lymphocytes.

Infectious agents may replicate inside the cell either in the cytosol or in the vesicular system (endosomes and lysosomes). Cells infected with viruses or bacteria that live in the cytosol are killed by cytotoxic T cells, which are distinguished by the presence of the cell surface molecule CD8. Pathogens or their products that are internalized by the cell in the vesicular system are detected by T cells that express the cell surface molecule CD4. CD4 T cells, also called helper (T_H) cells, do not directly kill the infected cells but activate other types of effector cells. T_H cells comprise different cell types, the best characterized of which are T_H1 cells (which activate macrophages to kill intravesicular bacteria) and T_H2 cells (which activate B cells to make antibodies). MHC class I molecules deliver peptides from the cytosol to the cell membrane, where the peptide–MHC complex is recognized by CD8 T cells. MHC class II molecules deliver peptides from the vesicular system to the cell surface, where the peptide–MHC complex is recognized by CD4 T cells. Therefore, depending on the type of the MHC molecule that presents the peptide, the immune system can recognize the intracellular compartment in which the infectious agent is localized and activate different and appropriate effector mechanisms.

Antigen Recognition

The MHC is also described in Chapter 6. For the purpose of this discussion, recall that MHC class I molecules are heterodimers composed of a membrane-spanning α chain noncovalently linked with β_2-microglobulin. The α chain has three domains. The α_1 and α_2 domains fold together to form a cleft that represents the peptide-binding site. MHC class II molecules are heterodimers composed of two noncovalently joined transmembrane glycoproteins α and β. Each chain has two domains. The α_1 and β_1 domains join together to form the peptide-binding cleft.

Anchor Residues

Unlike antibodies that can recognize both conformational and continuous epitopes on a protein surface,

T cells respond only to continuous short amino acid sequences that bind to the cleft of the outer surface of the MHC molecule.[13] Because the composition of the MHC peptide-binding cleft is highly polymorphic, different allelic variants of MHC molecules bind preferentially to different peptides. Amino acids that are critical for the binding of a peptide to a given MHC molecule (the peptide-binding motif) are called *anchor residues*. Changing anchor residues may prevent the peptide from binding, whereas peptides with the same anchor residues bind the appropriate MHC molecule irrespective of the sequence of the peptides at other positions. The anchor residues binding a given MHC molecule need not be identical but are always related (e.g., aromatic or hydrophobic amino acids).

Peptides that bind to MHC class I molecules are about 8 to 10 amino acids long; because of the open ends of the peptide-binding cleft of MHC class II molecules, peptides that bind MHC class II molecules are usually longer (13 amino acids or more). The peptide-binding clefts of MHC class II molecules are generally more permissive than those of the MHC class I molecules, and therefore it is more difficult to detect a peptide-binding motif for MHC class II than for MHC class I molecules. In summary, MHC molecules are able to bind a variety of different peptides of suitable length that share common anchor residues. MHC molecules bind peptides as an integral part of their structure and are unstable in the absence of peptides. This phenomenon prevents peptide exchange at cell surfaces that would impair the efficiency of intracellular antigen recognition.

MHC class I and class II molecules have different functions and are differently expressed on cells. MHC class I molecules present peptides to cytotoxic T cells. Viruses can infect any nucleated cell, and MHC class I molecules are expressed with variable intensity on all cells except erythrocytes. The main function of CD4 T cells is to activate other cells of the immune system. Therefore, MHC class II molecules are normally present on these effector cells. Class II molecules are also abundant on cells that are specialized to present antigen to T cells in lymphoid tissues (B lymphocytes and macrophages). The expression of MHC molecules of both classes is enhanced by some cytokines (particularly interferons)—which, moreover, can induce MHC class II molecules on several cells that normally do not express them.

Antigen Processing and Presentation

Complex intracytoplasmic machinery, which differs for class I and class II molecules, is responsible for peptide formation and loading on MHC molecules as well as the delivery of the peptide–MHC complex to the cell surface. All proteins, including viral proteins, are formed in the cytosol. Proteins such as the MHC molecules that have to be delivered to the cell surface are translocated into the lumen of the endoplasmic reticulum. For both MHC class I and class II molecules, loading of the specific peptide into the peptide-binding groove occurs in the vesicular system.[14, 15]

Proteins in the cell are continuously being degraded and replaced by new ones. A protease complex, the *proteasome*, plays a major role in cytosolic protein degradation (Fig. 4–5). Two subunits of the proteasome (LMP2 and LMP7) are encoded in the MHC. Proteins are targeted for proteasomal degradation by covalent linkage of several copies of a small polypeptide called *ubiquitin*. Peptides generated by the proteasome are actively transported into the endoplasmic reticulum by two proteins (also encoded in the MHC) called *transporters associated with antigen processing 1* and *2* (TAP-1 and TAP-2) that associate to form a heterodimer. MHC class I molecules are assembled in the endoplasmic reticulum and are associated with various chaperoning proteins (calnexin, calreticulin, tapasin) that maintain these molecules in a partially unfolded state. When TAPs deliver a suitable peptide, complete folding of the MHC molecule occurs and the peptide–MHC complex is transported through the Golgi complex to the cell surface.

Some intracellular pathogens replicate in intracytoplasmic vesicles that may also contain engulfed proteins derived from extracellular pathogens or other proteins that have been internalized by endocytosis (Fig. 4–6). All this material is degraded into peptide fragments by vesicular acid proteases. MHC class II molecules, which present peptides generated in intracellular vesicles, are assembled in the endoplasmic reticulum, where premature peptide binding is prevented by the association with a protein known as the *invariant chain* (Ii). This protein also targets delivery of MHC class II molecules through the Golgi apparatus to the acidified vesicles. Here the invariant chain is cleaved in different stages that involve the formation of a short, invariant, chain-derived peptide called CLIP (class II–associated invariant-chain peptide). Once CLIP is released, the MHC molecule binds the antigenic peptide and is transported to the cell surface. A MHC-encoded class II–like molecule, called human leukocyte antigen (HLA)-DM, that is not expressed on cell membrane appears to catalyze the release of the CLIP fragment from HLA class II molecules and their subsequent binding to the suitable peptide.

Loading of peptides on MHC molecules is a continuous process, and in uninfected cells the peptide-binding cleft is filled by peptides derived from self-proteins. As previously mentioned, MHC molecules are unstable in the absence of peptide and peptide binding is substantially irreversible.

Individuality of the Immune Response

The MHC is not only polygenic but also highly polymorphic because there are many multiple alleles of each gene. All MHC class I and class II molecules are able to present antigens to T cells, and each molecule binds a different range of peptides. The diversity due to polygeny is further increased by the fact that, because of the marked polymorphism, most humans are

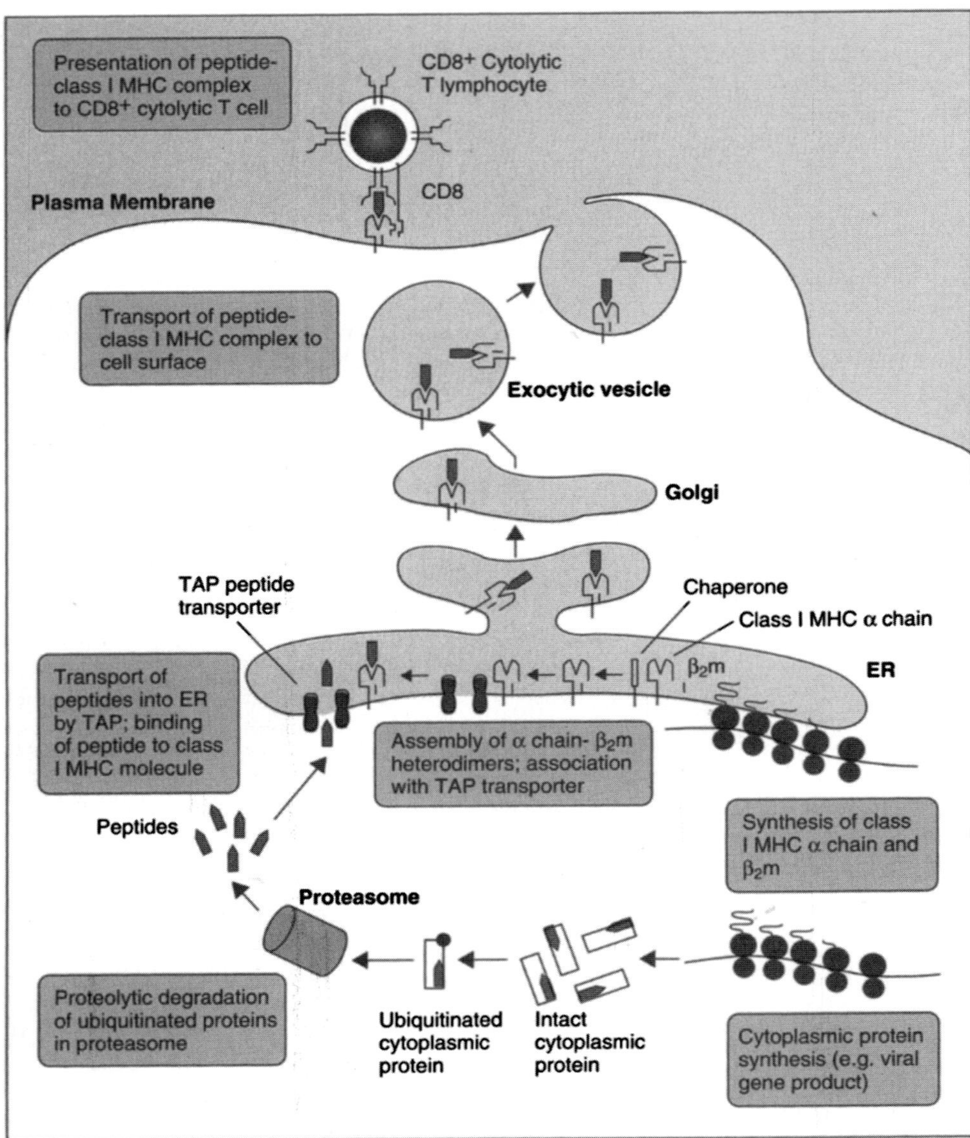

Figure 4–5. The class I major histocompatibility complex (MHC) pathway of antigen presentation. ER, endoplasmic reticulum; β_2m, β_2 microglobulin; TAP, transporters associated with antigen processing. (From Abbas AK, Lichtman AH, Pober JS: Cellular and Molecular Immunology. Philadelphia, WB Saunders, 1997.)

heterozygous at these loci, and the expression of MHC genes is co-dominant; indeed, both alleles are expressed on the same cell, and both can present peptides to T cells.

Because there are three MHC class I genes and four potential sets of MHC class II genes, a heterozygous person expresses six different MHC class I molecules and eight different MHC class II molecules. For MHC class II molecules, the number of different products may be further increased by the combination of α and β chains from different chromosomes. Differences among the various HLA alleles are mainly related to variations in the residues that line the peptide-binding groove and therefore affect the peptide-binding specificity. Because T cells respond to protein antigen by recognizing protein-derived peptides, the expression of several different HLA molecules on cell surfaces, each with different peptide-binding motives, ensures the recognition of at least some of the peptides derived by the proteolysis of the antigen. Therefore, because there is no response to the antigen in the absence of peptides available for HLA binding, HLA polymorphism extends the range of antigens to which the immune system can respond and makes antigen nonresponsiveness unlikely.[16] Allelic differences among MHC molecules also imply that the immune response against a given antigen may differ among individuals and are a major factor in the individuality of the immune response.

The polymorphism of other genes encoded in the MHC and involved in antigen presentation may also affect the immune response. For instance, the products of the two TAP alleles differ in their capacity to transport peptides; therefore, allelic variations in the TAP proteins can affect the repertoire of peptides available for MHC class I binding.

The MHC contains many other genes whose function in the immune response is still not well established or is unknown. Some of these genes are induced in

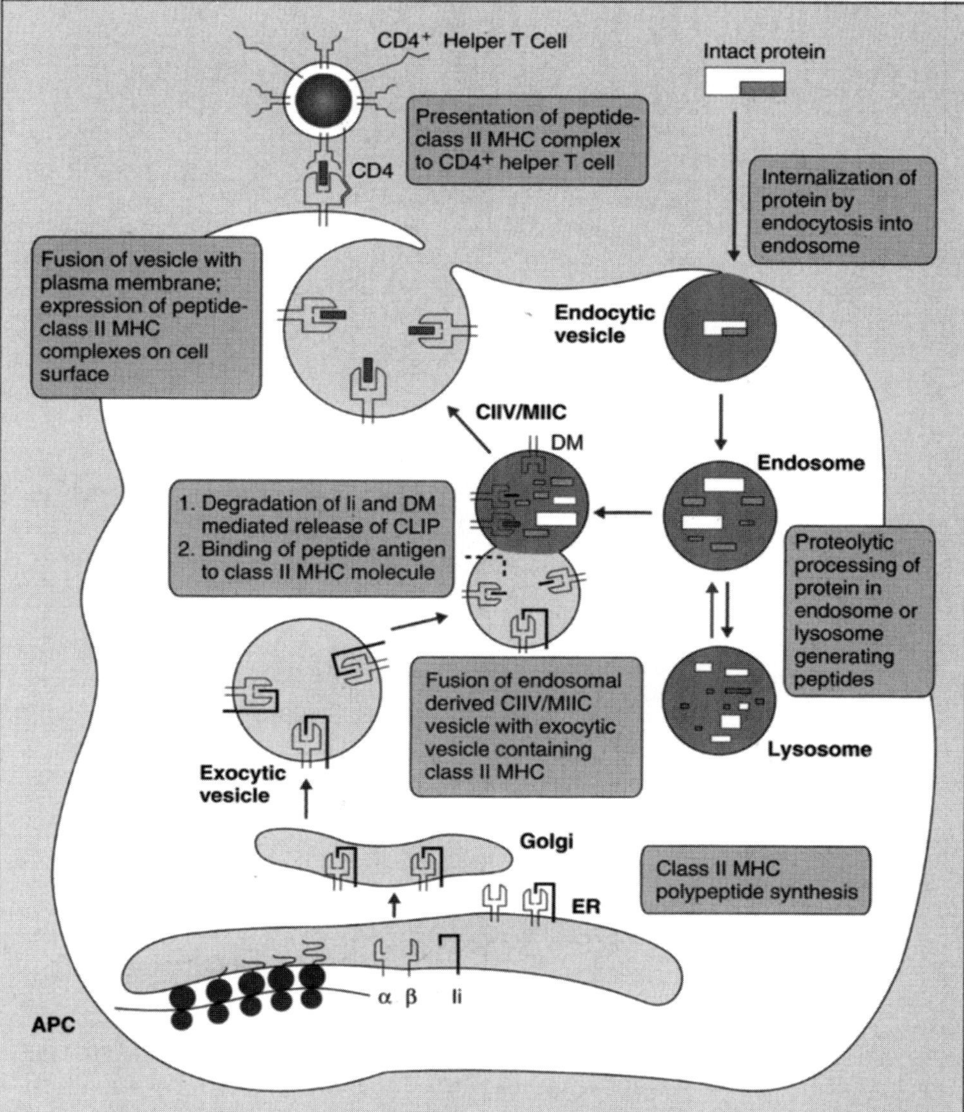

Figure 4–6. The class II major histocompatibility complex (MHC) pathway of antigen presentation. CLIP, class II–associated invariant-chain peptide; DM, HLA-DM; ER, endoplasmic reticulum; Ii, invariant chain; see text for other explanations. (From Abbas AK, Lichtman AH, Pober JS: Cellular and Molecular Immunology. Philadelphia, WB Saunders, 1997.)

response to cellular stress (such as heat shock) and code for a group of molecules, called *heat shock proteins,* which are present in abundant levels even under normal conditions. Heat shock proteins function as chaperones, and several studies suggest that they are relevant in both adaptive and innate immunity.[17]

T-Cell Receptor

The TCR, the antigen receptor of T cells, is a heterodimer composed of two different transmembrane glycoprotein chains (α and β) bound in a structure that is very similar to the Fab fragment of the immunoglobulin molecules (Fig. 4–7).[18] The organization of the gene segments encoding the TCR is very similar to that of immunoglobulins.[19] Each TCR locus consists of variable (V), joining (J), and constant (C) region genes; the β locus also contains the diversity (D) gene segments. As for immunoglobulins, the different gene segments coding for the variable regions of the TCR are present in multiple copies and undergo a process of gene rearrangement that, if successful, leads to the production of a functional TCR. During rearrangement, TCR genes are recognized by the same enzymes that recognize immunoglobulin genes. A further similarity between immunoglobulin and TCR rearrangements is the random addition of nucleotides at gene segment junctions. Because the TCR recognizes antigen but does not directly mediate the effector function, its constant chain is much simpler than that of immunoglobulins. Indeed, there is only one Cα gene and two Cβ genes (whose products appear to be functionally similar).

The TCR recognizes the complex formed by the peptide and the presenting HLA molecule. Moreover, T cells recognize and respond to antigens presented by an APC only if that APC expresses MHC molecules that the T cell recognize as self—in other words, they

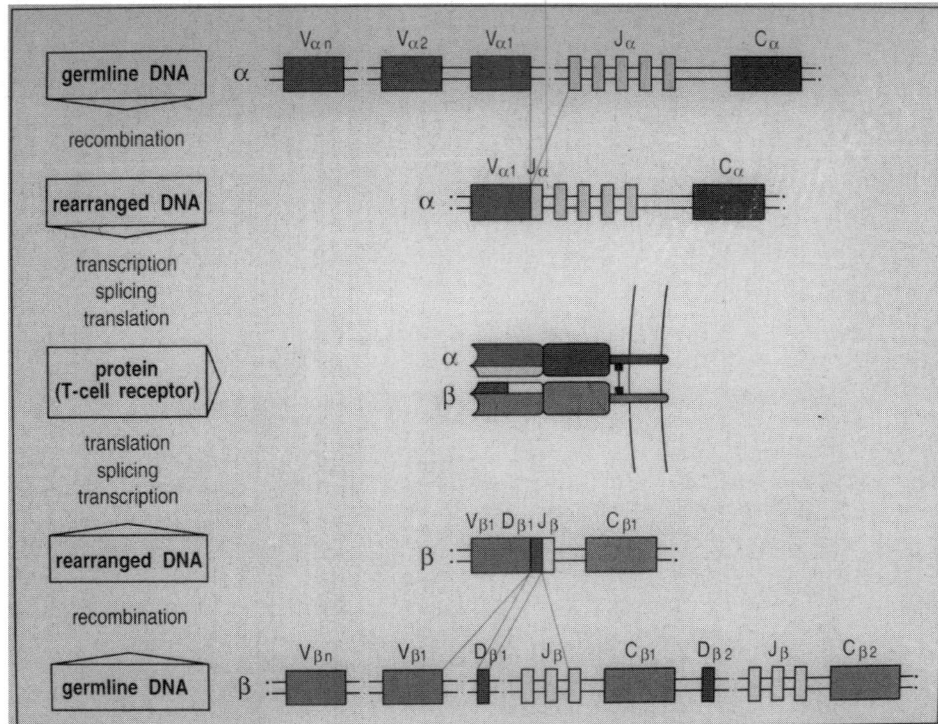

Figure 4–7. Structure of the T-cell receptor. Similar to the case with immunoglobulins, each chain of the T-cell receptor has a constant and a variable region. The juxtaposition of the variable regions forms the antigen-recognition site. Unlike immunoglobulins, the T-cell receptor is monovalent and is never secreted. (From Janeway CA, Travers P, Walport M, Capra DJ: Immunobiology. London, Elsevier, 1999.)

are self–MHC restricted (Fig. 4–8).[20] Like immunoglobulins, the TCR also has three hypervariable regions (CDR1, CDR2, and CDR3). CDR3 is located at the center of the peptide-binding site and is the most variable region, and CDR1 and CDR2 are located at the periphery of the binding site. The center of the TCR lies over the peptide; the periphery of the receptor is in touch with the periphery of the ligand, including amino acid residues present in the α helices of the peptide-binding cleft of the MHC molecules. Unlike immunoglobulins, somatic hypermutation is not a major mechanism for generating diversity in the TCRs. The probable reason for this difference is that somatic hypermutation of the TCR could be very harmful. Indeed, because T cells play the crucial role in the activation of both humoral and cellular immune response, somatic hypermutation could give rise to autoreactive T cells during the course of the immune response and lead to autoimmune disease. On the contrary, if a B cell mutates and becomes self-reactive, it normally fails to make antibodies because of the lack of the appropriate T-cell help.

Although the vast majority of T cells have the earlier-described α:β TCR, some lymphocytes have another type of TCR[21] consisting of a heterodimer formed by γ and δ polypeptide chains (γ:δ TCR). Similar to the

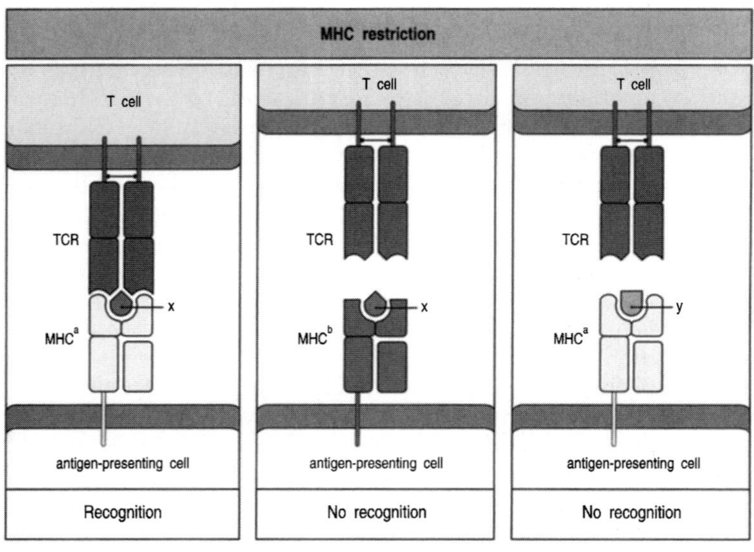

Figure 4–8. T-cell recognition of antigen is major histocompatibility complex (MHC)-restricted. A T-cell receptor (TCR) specific for an x peptide and a particular MHC^a allele will not recognize the complex of peptide x with a different MHC^b allele or the complex of peptide y with MHC^a. The phenomenon that any one lymphocyte is restricted to recognize a peptide antigen only if it is complexed to a single allelic form of an MHC molecule is called *MHC restriction.* (From Janeway CA, Travers P, Walport M, Capra DJ: Immunobiology. London, Elsevier, 1999.)

homologous α:β TCR, γ:δ TCR is associated with a CD3 complex on the cell membrane (see later). The organization of the γ and δ genes is also similar to that of α and β genes, although there are many fewer V region gene segments. The true function of γ:δ T cells is still unknown, but it appears that these cells represent a link between innate and adaptive immunity.[22] They account for less than 5 percent of blood T cells; are present in epithelia of the gut, lungs, and skin; and appear to be able to recognize pathogens as well as stress-associated antigens expressed on cell surfaces. They produce chemokines that recruit inflammatory cells and appear to secrete cytokines that can drive adaptive immunity. Recent findings suggest that stem cells from the bone marrow may home directly to the gut, bypassing the thymus, and develop into a population of precursors of γ:δ T cells. A possible role for these cells in the pathogenesis of autoimmunity has been suggested.[22, 23]

Membrane Co-Receptors

The TCR specifically recognizes the peptide–MHC complex but is independently incapable of activating the T cell. This function is carried out by a complex of proteins—the CD3 complex—which is associated with the TCR on the cell surface.[24] Like the Igα and Igβ chains associated with membrane immunoglobulin, the cytoplasmic domains of the CD3 proteins contain sequences called ITAM that allow them, after receptor stimulation, to associate with tyrosine kinases and signal to the interior of the cell that antigen binding has occurred.[25]

Helper T cells and cytotoxic T cells are characterized by the presence of the cell surface co-receptor proteins CD4 and CD8, respectively. CD4 binds to invariant parts of MHC class II molecules, and CD8 binds to invariant parts of MHC class I molecules. During antigen recognition, they associate on the cell membrane with components of the TCR, participate in signal transduction, and bring about a 100-fold increase in the sensitivity of the T cell to the antigen presented by MHC molecules.[26]

T-Cell Development

T cells originate in the bone marrow and migrate at a very early stage to the thymus, where they undergo TCR gene rearrangement. The thymus consists of multiple lobes, each composed of an outer cortex and an inner medulla. Scattered throughout the thymus are nonlymphoid epithelial cells, which are of ectodermal origin in the cortex and of endodermal origin in the medulla. The thymus is colonized by immature lymphocytes (which in the thymus are called thymocytes) and by other cells of hematopoietic origin such as macrophages and dendritic cells. The cortex contains only immature thymocytes and scattered macrophages, whereas the medulla contains more mature thymocytes, dendritic cells, and most of the macrophages.

The human thymus is fully developed at birth, and until puberty it is the site of a sustained production of T cells. After puberty, the thymus begins to shrink and the production of T cells decreases. However, adult thymectomy is not accompanied by any relevant loss of T-cell function, indicating that once the T-cell repertoire is established, production of large numbers of new T cells is not needed.

In the thymus, thymocytes proliferate and mature into T cells through a series of events characterized by rearrangement of the TCR genes and expression on the cell membrane of the TCR, co-receptors CD4 and CD8, and other surface molecules that reflect the functional maturation of the cell.[27, 28] Thymocytes enter the thymic cortex and, during maturation, migrate from the cortex toward the medulla, coming in contact with epithelial cells, macrophages, and dendritic cells. Thus, the medulla contains mostly mature T cells, and only mature CD4-positive or CD8-positive T cells exit the thymus and enter the blood. The main steps of thymocyte maturation are illustrated in Figure 4–9.

Thymocytes initially begin to express some markers of T-cell developmental lineage but do not express the TCR or the co-receptor molecules CD4 and CD8. For this reason, they are called *double-negative thymocytes*. A minority of these cells have rearranged and are expressing the genes encoding the γ:δ TCR. The majority of double-negative thymocytes are committed to develop into α:β TCR–bearing mature T cells. During their further development, these cells rearrange their TCR β-chain genes; if the rearrangement is successful, the β chain reaches the cell surface in association with a surrogate α chain called the pTα (pre-T cell α) together with the CD3 molecules. Expression of this complex leads to cell proliferation and expression of both CD4 and CD8 (double-positive thymocytes). Once proliferation ceases, α-chain genes rearrange, eventually producing a complete α:β TCR.

The next fundamental step in thymocyte maturation (after expression of the TCR, CD4, and CD8 molecules) is the selection of cells that will make up the repertoire of mature T cells in the periphery. Mature T cells recognize only peptides bound to MHC molecules. As previously discussed, T cells are self-restricted, which means that only those T cells that recognize the body's own MHC molecules will be able to contribute to the adaptive immune response. On the other hand, the random generation of TCR can give rise not only to lymphocytes that do not recognize self-MHC molecules (and are therefore useless) but also to lymphocytes that recognize complexes of self-peptides/self-MHC molecules with high affinity (and are therefore potentially harmful). The dual need of selecting only cells that recognize self-MHC molecules and eliminating autoreactive cells is accomplished through processes of positive and negative selection (Fig. 4–10) that occur once thymocytes have rearranged their α:β TCR genes.[29, 30] Evidence from fetal thymic organ cultures suggests that these processes, which shape the future immunologic repertoire, are driven by the differential avidity for self-peptide/self-MHC complexes.[31] Thymocytes that express a TCR with low but measurable avidity for a

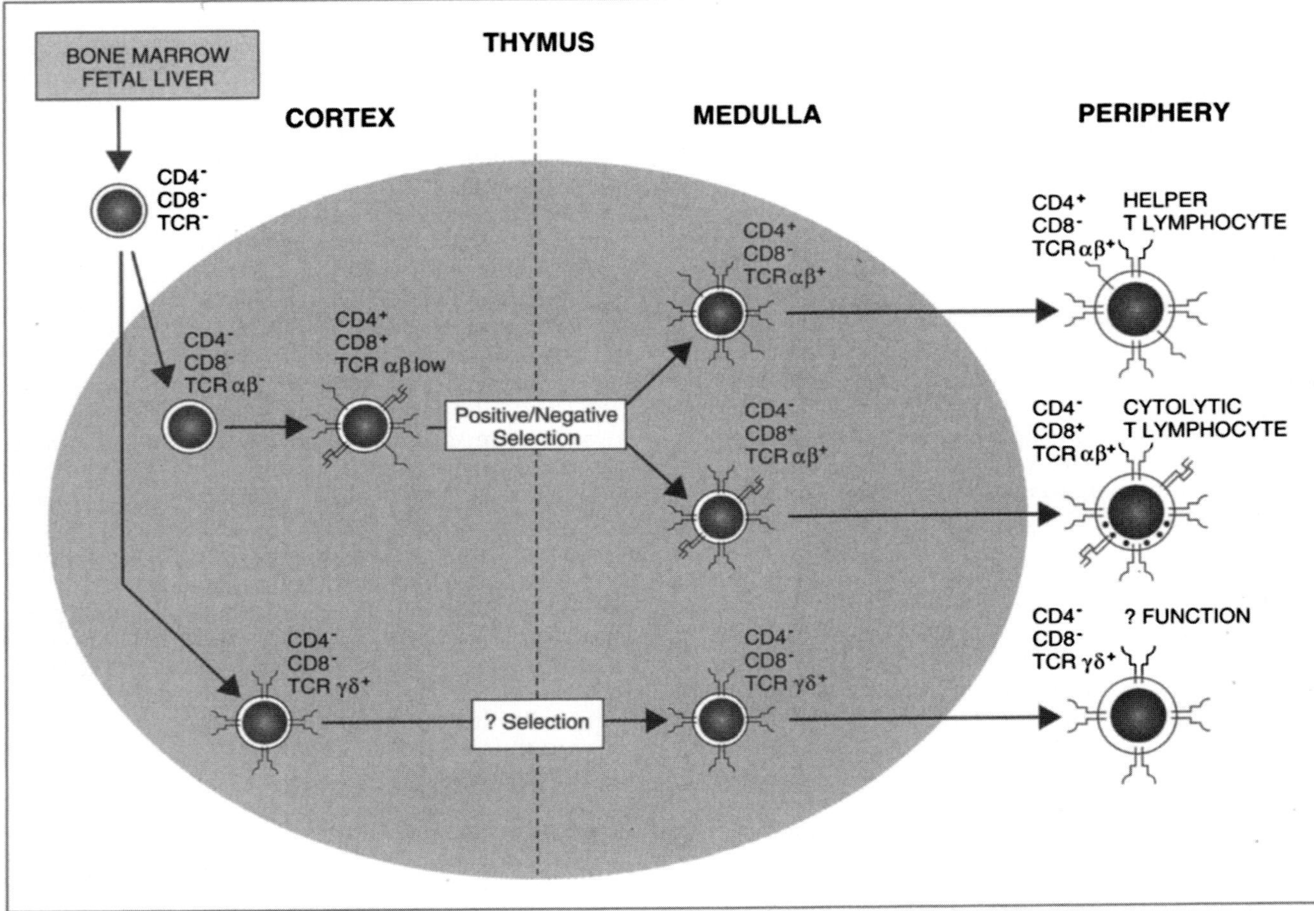

Figure 4–9. Thymocyte maturation. The stage of the expression of pTα is not shown. See text for explanation. TCR, T-cell receptor. (From Abbas AK, Lichtman AH, Pober JS: Cellular and Molecular Immunology. Philadelphia, WB Saunders, 1997.)

self-peptide/self-MHC complex are allowed to differentiate into mature T cells, whereas immature lymphocytes that express TCRs that have no or strong avidity for self-peptide/self-MHC complexes die by apoptosis. Avidity is determined by both the TCR affinity for its peptide–MHC ligand and the number of TCR-peptide-MHC ligand pairs formed at the time of antigen recognition.

Those thymocytes that recognize self-MHC with low avidity and are positively selected mature. They extinguish further TCR α-chain gene rearrangement (so that their specificity becomes fixed) and stop the expression of one or other of the two co-receptor molecules to become either CD4 or CD8 single-positive lymphocytes, depending on the MHC class molecule that they have recognized on thymic epithelial cells (see Fig. 4–9). The process of negative selection, which eliminates those T cells that recognize self-MHC with high avidity via apoptosis (clonal deletion), occurs during and after the double-positive stage of development. More than 95 percent of developing thymocytes are thought to die in the thymus by apoptosis because they do not recognize self-MHC molecules or undergo negative selection. Cells that survive this dual selection process leave the thymus as mature naive T cells. Like B cells, naive T cells may survive for long periods (up to several months in mice) in the absence of overt antigen exposure. It appears that the maintenance of the pool of naive lymphocytes requires antigen receptor–mediated signals. The nature of these signals is unknown. They could include environmental or even self-antigens that are recognized with low affinity.

LYMPHOCYTE ACTIVATION

T Lymphocytes

Two Signals

The TCR's recognition of the specific peptide presented in the context of MHC molecules is necessary but not sufficient to activate T cells. In order to induce cell activation, TCR recognition must be simultaneously accompanied by the delivery of a second, co-stimulatory signal. This may occur when T cells interact with APCs. There are three main types of APCs: dendritic cells, macrophages, and B cells. Although dendritic cells appear to function exclusively as APCs, macrophages and B cells are also targets of activated T cells.

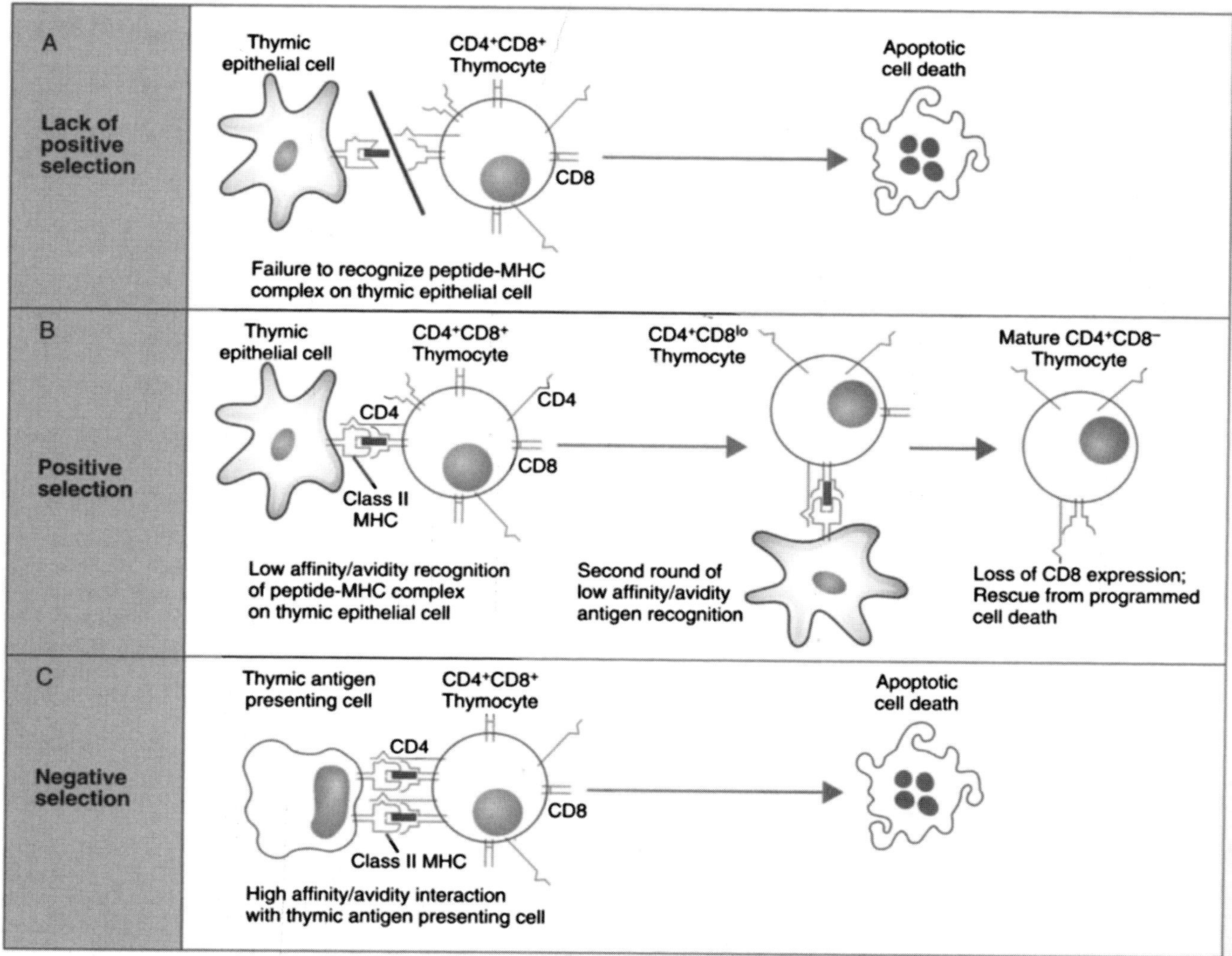

Figure 4–10. Selection processes during thymocyte maturation. The three possible fates of a $CD4^+CD8^+$ double-positive thymocyte. See text for explanation. MHC, major histocompatibility complex. (From Abbas AK, Lichtman AH, Pober JS: Cellular and Molecular Immunology. Philadelphia, WB Saunders, 1997.)

The activation of T cells upon the initial encounter with the specific peptide on the surface of an APC (priming) occurs in peripheral lymphoid organs.

The initial interaction between naive T cells and APCs is mediated by adhesion molecules (Fig. 4–11). If the naive T cell recognizes its specific peptide–MHC complex on the surface of an APC, signaling through the TCR induces conformational changes in the adhesion molecules that enhance the adhesiveness between the two cells. On the contrary, if no recognition takes place, the T cell dissociates from that APC and samples other APCs. The binding of the TCR and of the co-receptors (CD4 or CD8) transmits a first signal to the cell indicating that the specific antigen has been recognized. The second, co-stimulatory signal is delivered through specialized molecules called *co-stimulatory molecules,*[32, 33] the best known of which are two structurally related molecules known as B7.1 (CD80) and B7.2 (CD86). The receptors for B7 molecules on T cells are two similar molecules called CD28 (which is constitutively expressed on most T cells) and CTLA-4. Once the first signal has been provided, ligation of CD28 by B7 molecules induces lymphocyte activation. T-cell activation also induces the expression on cell surface of CTLA-4, which has a higher affinity for B7 molecules than CD28 and delivers a negative signal to the cell, thereby limiting the proliferative response of activated T cells. The CD28/CTLA-4 and B7-1/B7-2 interactions therefore provide a regulation system that ensures that immune responses are turned on when needed and turned off when not needed (Fig. 4–12). Recent data suggest that co-stimulation acts by modulating the signaling environment around the engaged TCR[34, 34a] rather than by providing independent signals that are integrated in the nucleus to regulate transcription.

Approximately 100 specific peptide–MHC complexes are required on a target cell to trigger a T cell. Then, TCR aggregation initiates the events that lead to T-cell activation. One of these events involves a cytoplasmic phosphatase, called *calcineurin,* which activates *NAFT* (nuclear activation factor of T cells), which binds to the promoter region of the IL-2 gene and is

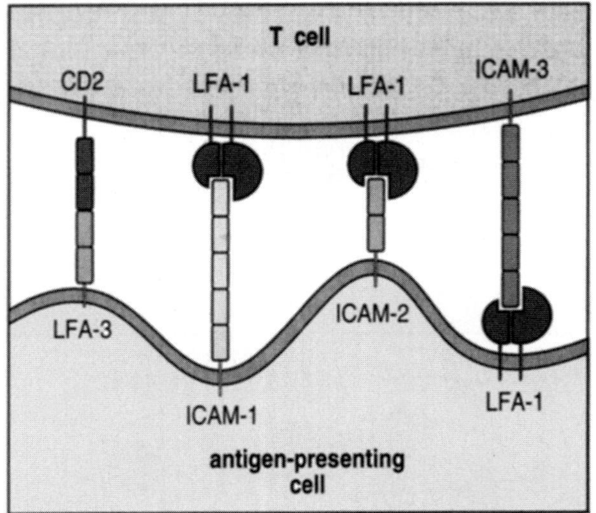

Figure 4–11. Adhesion molecules involved in the interactions of T cells with antigen-presenting cells. ICAM, intracellular adhesion molecule 1; LFA, leukocyte function-associated antigen. (From Janeway CA, Travers P, Walport M, Capra DJ: Immunobiology. London, Elsevier, 1999.)

necessary to activate transcription. Because NAFT is a T-cell–specific factor, blockade of the signaling pathway leading to NAFT is a way to specifically inhibit the T-cell response. Both cyclosporin and FK506 inhibit calcineurin and therefore prevent the activation of NAFT.

T-cell activation leads to a 100-fold increase in IL-2 production, to the expression of anti-apoptotic proteins of the Bcl family, and to the synthesis of the α chain of the IL-2 receptor. Resting T cells express a low-affinity IL-2 receptor composed of a β and a γ chain. The association of the α chain with the β and γ chains generates a receptor with a much higher affinity. Interaction of IL-2 with its receptor activates cell proliferation, which leads to the production of many T cells, all bearing an identical TCR (clonal expansion). Activation also induces the expression of CD40 ligand (CD40L),[35] which binds to CD40. This interaction induces expression of B7 molecules, thereby further driving the T-cell response.

CD45 (T-200, leukocyte common antigen) is a cell surface protein that plays a critical role in T-cell activation, with an intrinsic tyrosine phosphatase in its cytoplasmic tail. During the process of activation and maturation of T cells, different forms of CD45 are expressed on cell membrane. Naive T cells express CD45RA; activated and memory T cells induced by prior exposure to antigen express the isoform CD45RO. CD45 isoforms are therefore useful markers to differentiate naive from activated T cells (Table 4–3).

Once activated, CD4 T lymphocytes can differentiate into either T_H1 or T_H2 cells (see later). Naive CD8 T cells, because of their highly destructive effects, are kept under strict control and require high levels of co-stimulatory activity to be activated by APCs. This high level of co-stimulation may be induced on APCs by inflammatory cytokines or by the previous interaction of the APC with antigen-specific CD4 cells. It has been shown[36] that CD40L expressed on antigen-stimulated T-helper cells can activate APC by interacting with CD40 on APCs. This activation allows APCs to activate antigen-specific cytotoxic T cells in a subsequent encounter.

The delivery to the naive T cell of signal 1 alone not only fails to activate the cell but also induces a state of unresponsiveness (anergy) in which the T cell is refractory to activation. The most important change induced in anergic T cells is their inability to produce IL-2. The need of the second co-stimulatory signal for T-cell activation and the fact that this signal is provided only by APCs is important in preventing autoimmune diseases because not all potentially self-reactive T cells are deleted in the thymus.

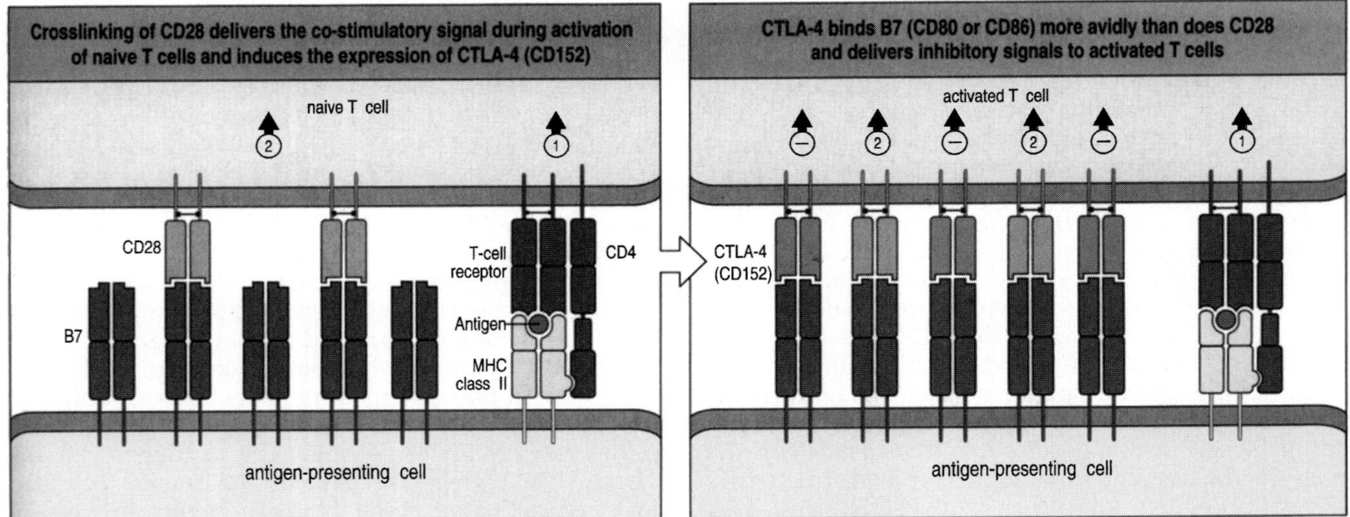

Figure 4–12. CD28 and CTLA-4 expression during lymphocyte activation. T-cell activation through the T-cell receptor and CD28 leads to increased expression of CTLA-4, which binds to B7 molecules and inhibits T-cell activation. (From Janeway CA, Travers P, Walport M, Capra DJ: Immunobiology. London, Elsevier, 1999.)

Table 4–3

Differences in the Expression of Cell-Surface Molecules Between Resting and Activated CD4 T Cells

	CELL SURFACE MOLECULES							
	CD4	TCR	CD2	L-selectin	LFA-1	VLA-4	CD45RA	CD45RO
Resting	+	+	+	+	+	–	+	–
Activated	+	+	++	–	++	+	–	+

LFA, leukocyte function associated antigen; TCR, T-cell receptor; VLA, very late appearing antigen.

Antigen-Presenting Cells

As previously mentioned, there are three main types of APC: macrophages, dendritic cells, and B cells. Macrophages normally express few MHC class II and no B7 molecules on their surface. Both molecules are expressed when macrophages engulf microbial constituents and are activated. Macrophages, as well as dendritic cells and B cells, have a number of receptors for common microbial constituents, and the presence of these receptors is important in allowing the immune system to distinguish antigens that are derived from infectious agents from those derived from innocuous proteins.[37] Antigens derived from infectious agents, but not those associated with innocuous proteins, induce co-stimulatory molecules. Indeed, innocuous proteins administered in conjunction with bacterial products (the so-called adjuvants) may elicit an immune response because bacterial products induce co-stimulatory activity in APCs that have ingested the protein. Experimental autoimmune diseases are also induced in susceptible animals by the administration of antigens mixed with bacterial adjuvants, a phenomenon that underscores the importance of co-stimulatory activity in the process of self/nonself discrimination.

Not all infectious agents effectively induce MHC class II and co-stimulatory molecules on the surface of macrophages. This is particularly true for viruses that replicate inside the cell. Dendritic cells, which are present in the lymph nodes and constitutively express large quantities of MHC class II and co-stimulatory molecules, are thought to have a major role in presenting viral peptides to naive T cells and to prime both CD4 and CD8 T cells.[38] An immature form of lymphoid dendritic cells found mainly in surface epithelia includes Langerhans' cells in the skin. These cells are able to ingest microbes and lack co-stimulatory molecules on their surface. Tissue dendritic cells, once triggered by infection, transport the antigen from epithelia to lymph nodes, where they differentiate into mature dendritic cells, lose their phagocytic properties, and express co-stimulatory molecules. Recent evidence suggests the presence of different subsets of dendritic cells with different functions in the regulation of the type of T cell–mediated immune response as well as in tolerance induction.[38]

B cells internalize soluble antigens bound to their surface immunoglobulins; peptide fragments generated from these antigens are displayed on the cell surface in association with constitutively expressed MHC class II molecules.[39] This is the pathway by which B cells can be the target of antigen-specific helper CD4 T cells. However, in circumstances in which peptide display is associated with the induction of co-stimulatory activity, B cells may act as APCs. The importance of B cells in priming naive T cells is unclear.

T-Cell Receptor Degeneracy

Studies have shown that the same TCR may be activated by different peptides that share relatively little primary sequence homology (TCR degeneracy).[40] Unlike the case with antibodies, there is no affinity maturation process that improves the fit of a TCR for a given peptide–MHC molecule complex during an ongoing immune response. Therefore, specificity of the TCR repertoire likely represents a balance between two possible extremes (Fig. 4–13): highly specific TCRs and highly degenerated TCRs. The former recognize particular amino acids at many positions of the MHC-bound peptide; the latter recognize only certain sequence features and therefore may cross-react, although with different affinity, with many different microbial peptides. The highly specific TCR has a low probability of meeting the corresponding antigen and may never be engaged in the immune response; the highly degenerated TCR has a higher probability of being engaged but may also theoretically cross-react with self-peptide and induce an autoimmune response.[41] Further elucidation of the crystal structure of the TCR/peptide–MHC complex[42, 43] will provide important insights into the structural basis of TCR specificity and degeneracy.

TCR engagement by different peptide ligands may lead to different functional outcomes that depend on whether the peptide acts as an agonist, partial agonist, or antagonist. Indeed, the functional consequences of T-cell antigen recognition may vary depending on the nature of the peptide that contacts the TCR. It has been shown that peptides in which one or two TCR contact residues have been changed (known as *altered peptide ligands*, or APLs) induce only a subset of the functional changes induced by the wild-type peptide or may even induce a state of T-cell anergy that prevents response upon secondary exposure to the wild-type peptide. The APLs appear to induce different intracellular pathways with respect to those induced by the usual T-cell activation. These differences may depend on differences in affinity or conformational changes of the TCR. By these mechanisms, antigen receptors may translate quantitative differences in ligand

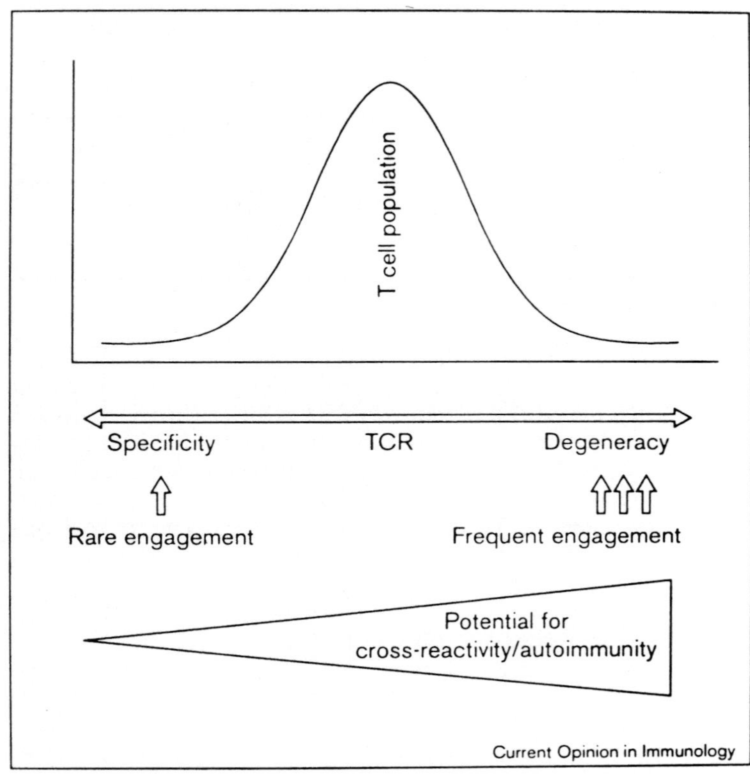

Figure 4–13. Distribution of T-cell receptor (TCR) specificity and degeneracy. Schematic representation of the distribution of peripheral T cells with respect to the degree of specificity/degeneracy of their TCR. Degenerate T cells are engaged more frequently and have a higher potential for causing autoimmunity with respect to more specific TCR. (Reprinted from Curr Opin Immunol, Vol 9, Hausmann S, Wucherpfennig W, Activation of autoreactive T cells by peptides from human pathogens, pp 831–838, Copyright 1997, with permission from Elsevier Science.)

binding into qualitatively different biologic responses.[44] T-cell anergy may therefore be induced not only by antigen recognition in the absence of co-stimulation but also when, despite the availability of adequate co-stimulation, the antigen receptor signal is suboptimal—as for example when a T cell encounters an APL that does not optimally bind to the TCR. APLs have been successfully used to prevent experimental autoimmune diseases.[45]

Alloreactivity

Transplanted tissues from donors bearing MHC molecules that differ from those of the recipients are rejected by a rapid and very potent T-cell immune response. Before the discovery of the role of MHC in antigen presentation, it was a mystery why such a potent immune response was evoked by nonself MHC molecules because there was no reason for the immune system to have evolved a defense against tissue transplants. There is now consistent evidence that this response (alloreactivity) results from cross-reactivity of TCRs normally specific for a variety of self-peptides bound to self-MHC molecules.

Superantigens

Some products of bacteria, mycoplasma, and viruses induce a potent polyclonal and potentially harmful immune response. These superantigens bind to the outer surface of both the MHC class II molecules and the V_β region of the TCR, outside the peptide-binding site, and lead to T-cell activation.[46] Each superantigen may activate all the T cells that express a particular set or family of V_β TCR genes. This stimulation does not prime an adaptive specific immune response against the pathogen but may cause massive production of inflammatory cytokines such as IL-1 and tumor necrosis factor (TNF) and may lead to septic shock, the most severe cytokine-induced complication of infection by gram-negative and some gram-positive bacteria. Bacterial superantigens include the staphylococcal enterotoxins, the most common cause of food poisoning in humans, and the toxic shock syndrome toxin 1.

Heterogeneity of Helper T Cells

The two best characterized subsets of helper T cells are called T_H1 and T_H2 and are distinguished on the basis of the cytokines they produce: IL-2, interferon-γ (IFN-γ), and TNF-β for T_H1 cells and IL-4, IL-5, IL-10, and IL-13 for T_H2 cells.[47, 48] It is increasingly evident, however, that many T cells cannot easily be classified into T_H1 or T_H2 cells and that some (called T_H0) have quite a heterogeneous pattern of cytokine secretion. Nevertheless, the differentiation of naive CD4 T cells into either T_H1 or T_H2 cells appears to be a fundamental step for the subsequent evolution of the immune response. Production of T_H1 cells induces cell-mediated immunity; production of T_H2 cells leads to humoral immunity, a phenomenon that profoundly influences disease outcome, as exemplified by infections with intracellular pathogens such as leprosy.

Mycobacterium leprae grows in macrophage vesicles, and effective host defense requires macrophage activation by T_H1

cells. In patients with tuberculoid leprosy, which is characterized by a prevalent T_H1 response, the infection is controlled and the patient usually survives. In lepromatous leprosy, which is characterized by a prevalent T_H2 response, the main response is represented by antibody production; these antibodies cannot kill the intracellular bacteria, and patients eventually die.

T_H1 and T_H2 Development

The mechanisms controlling helper T-cell differentiation are not fully understood but involve several factors, including the type of released cytokines, the amount and sequence of the antigenic peptide, and possibly the nature of the APC.[47, 48]

IL-12 is the most important cytokine that stimulates the development of T_H1 cells and is produced by macrophages and NK cells. IFN-γ, which is produced by macrophages, NK cells, and T_H1 cells themselves, enhances IL-12 secretion by macrophages, probably has a direct T_H1-inducing effect, and inhibits the development of T_H2.

IL-4, produced by T_H2 cells, stimulates T_H2 development; both IL-4 and IL-10 inhibit the generation of T_H1 cells. It has been hypothesized that activated CD4 cells produce small amounts of IL-4 leading to T_H2 differentiation unless they are counteracted by the presence of T_H1-inducing cytokines. The differing capacity of pathogens to interact with macrophages and NK cells may therefore influence the overall balance of cytokines produced early during the immune response and thus determine the preferential development of T_H1 or T_H2 cells.

Another factor influencing the differentiation of CD4 T cells is the amount and the sequence of the antigenic peptide. Peptides presented in high density on the surface of APCs tend to stimulate T_H1 responses, whereas low-density presentation favors T_H2 responses. Moreover, peptides that interact strongly with the TCR tend to elicit T_H1 responses, whereas weak bonds tend to stimulate T_H2 responses. Extracellular pathogens, which normally elicit a strong T_H2-dependent antibody response, do not multiply inside the APCs that present them; thus, their peptides tend to be presented at relatively low density. On the contrary, intracellular pathogens, such as viruses that elicit a strong T_H1-mediated cellular response, multiply inside the APCs and therefore tend to be presented in higher density on cell surface by MHC molecules.

Timing and levels of co-stimulation may also critically affect functional differentiation of CD4 T cells, but the mechanisms are still not well defined. Some experiments have suggested that dendritic cells exist as functionally distinct subsets able to provide T cells with selective signals leading to either T_H1 or T_H2 responses.[38, 49] In inbred mice, a genetic influence on T_H1/T_H2 development has been demonstrated, but the mechanisms are unknown.

Each T-cell subset produces cytokines that serve as its own autocrine growth factor and promote differentiation of naive T cells to that subset. Moreover, the two subsets produce cytokines that cross-regulate each other's development and activity (Fig. 4–14). Indeed, as previously mentioned, IFN-γ produced by T_H1 cells

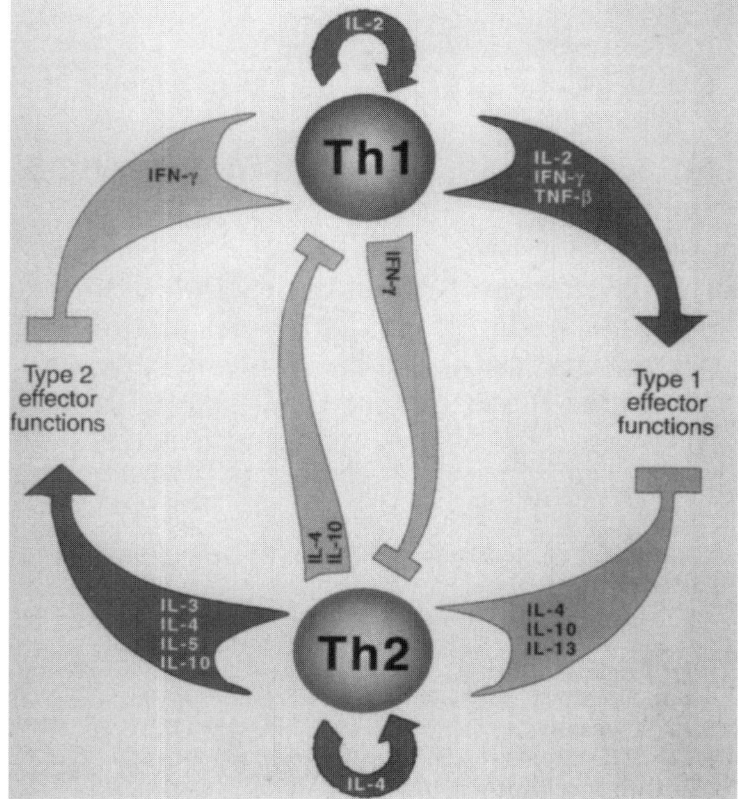

Figure 4–14. Helper T cells (T_H1 and T_H2) and their cytokines. Effector (black) and inhibitor (gray) functions of the cytokines produced by T_H1 and T_H2 cells. Interleukin-2 (IL-2) and IL-4 are shown as autocrine growth factors for T_H1 and T_H2 cells, respectively. IFN, interferon; TNF, tumor necrosis factor. (From Abbas AK, Murphy KM, Sher A: Functional diversity of helper T lymphocytes. Reprinted with permission from Nature 383:787, copyright 1996 Macmillan Magazines Limited.)

amplifies T_H1 development and inhibits proliferation of T_H2 cells, whereas IL-10 produced by T_H2 cells blocks activation of T_H1 cells and suppresses numerous macrophage responses. This is probably the reason that T_H1 and T_H2 cells may be interconvertible early in their development and, later on, during the immune response, appear to be irreversibly committed. Also, CD8 T cells can respond to antigen by secreting cytokines typical of either T_H1 or T_H2 cells.

T_H1 and T_H2 cells express different chemokine receptors[50] and therefore can be differentially attracted to the site of inflammation. Chemokine receptor antagonism thus appears to be a promising approach for future treatment of autoimmune and allergic disorders.

T_H1 and T_H2 Effector Functions

T_H1 cells are very important for activating macrophages; T_H2 cells are the most effective activators of B cells, particularly in primary responses (Fig. 4–15). The principal T_H1 effector cytokine is IFN-γ, which not only inhibits the development of T_H2 cells but also has two other main functions: It activates macrophages to phagocytose and destroy microbes, and it stimulates the production of IgG antibody subclasses that bind to complement and high-affinity Fcγ receptors and are the principal antibodies involved in microbe opsonization and phagocytosis.

T_H2 cells act as B-cell helpers and induce the production of IgM and non–complement-fixing IgG subclasses. IL-4 is the main inducer of B-cell switching to IgE production, and IL-5 is the principal cytokine that activates eosinophils. The net result of T_H2 activation is also to inhibit inflammation through the release of anti-inflammatory cytokines. IL-4 and IL-13 antagonize the macrophage-activation effect of IFN-γ, IL-10 suppresses various macrophage responses, and transforming growth factor (TGF)-β (produced by some T_H2 cells and other cell types) inhibits leukocyte proliferation and activation. The T_H2 response therefore might also be a way to limit the potentially dangerous consequence of uncontrolled T_H1-mediated immunity.

T-Cell Homing

The adaptive immune response is initiated by the activation of specific T cells in the peripheral lymphoid organs. Antigens reach the lymph nodes through the lymph draining the infectious site either passively or transported by immature APCs (such as Langherans' cells). Otherwise, if antigens reach the bloodstream directly, they are picked up by APCs in the spleen. T lymphocytes continuously recirculate between blood and the peripheral lymphoid organs. Depending on their state of activation, they express different adhesion molecules and chemokine receptors that bind to complementary ligands expressed on cells with which leukocytes interact.[51, 51a]

Naive T cells express L-selectin, which binds to the vascular addressins GlyCAM-1 and CD34 expressed on the walls of specialized venules (high endothelial venules, or HEVs) present in lymph nodes. This first interaction is weak but allows rolling of lymphocytes on the endothelial surface and their stimulation by chemokines bound to extracellular matrix that leads to activation on the lymphocyte surface of the integrin

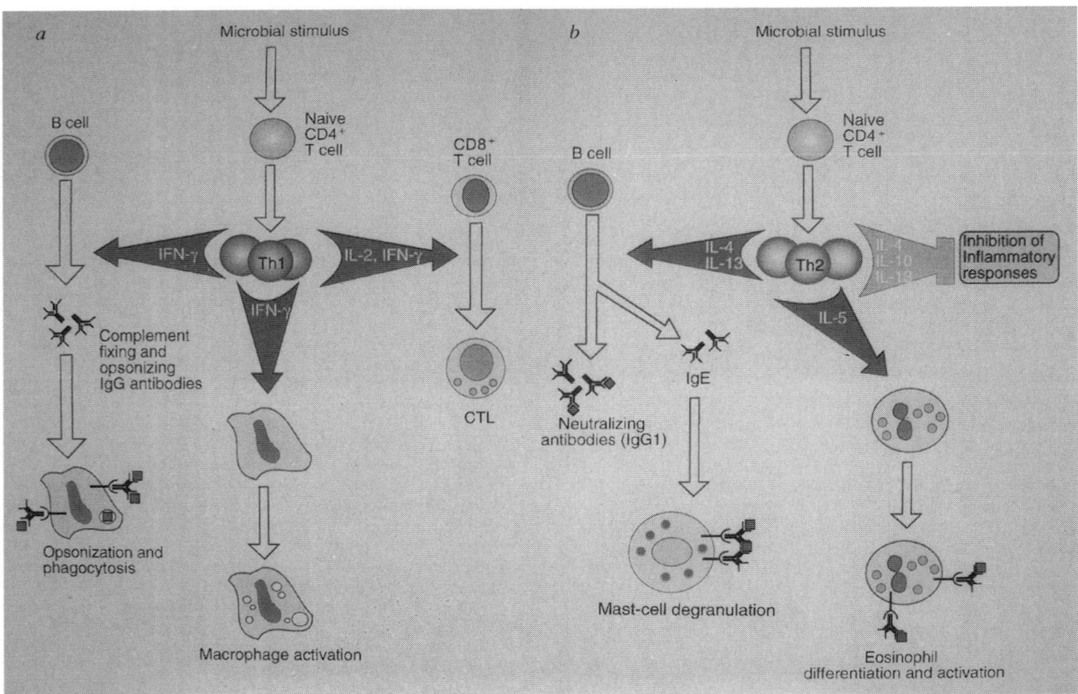

Figure 4–15. Effector functions of helper T cells (T_H1 and T_H2). CTL, cytotoxic T lymphocytes; IgG, immunoglobulin G; IL, interleukin. (From Abbas AK, Murphy KM, Sher A: Functional diversity of helper T lymphocytes. Reprinted with permission from Nature 383:787, copyright 1996 Macmillan Magazines Limited.)

leukocyte function-associated antigen (LFA)-1 (CD11a/CD18). LFA-1 binds to intercellular adhesion molecule (ICAM)-2, which is expressed on all endothelial cells, and ICAM-1, which, in the absence of inflammation, is expressed only on HEVs. This tight adhesion allows the migration of the naive T cell through the vessel wall into the T cell–rich zone of the lymph node, where APCs are present. The mechanisms of lymphocyte homing to the spleen are less well understood. If the T cells that have entered the lymph node fail to recognize their specific antigen on APCs, they exit through an efferent lymphatic vessel and return to the blood via the thoracic duct. On the contrary, if the T cell recognizes its specific peptide–MHC complex on the surface of APCs, signaling through the TCR induces conformational changes in the adhesion molecules that enhance the adhesiveness between the two cells and initiate lymphocyte activation.

Activation of T cells in the lymph node is accompanied by changes in cell surface adhesion molecules. Most effector T cells lose surface L-selectin that mediates homing to the lymph nodes and express other molecules, particularly the α4 integrin *very late activation antigen* (VLA)-4, which binds to *vascular adhesion molecule* (VCAM)-1, the expression of which is induced on the endothelium by cytokines released at the site of inflammation. These modifications in adhesion molecules allow the effector T cell (T_H1 cells and cytotoxic CD8 T cells) to reach the site where infection is taking place. Many of the cells in afferent lymph draining peripheral tissues are memory and effector cells that express CD45RO and lack L-selectin (see Table 4–3). They appear to be committed to migration to potential sites of infection.

Differential expression of adhesion molecules also directs effector T cells to different tissues. For instance, homing to Peyer's patches and the lamina propria of the gut involves the binding of both T-cell L-selectin, and the α4β7 integrin to separate sites on mucosal addressin cell adhesion molecule (MAdCAM)-1, whereas lymphocytes that home to the skin express the cutaneous lymphocyte antigen and bind E-selectin. Also in experimental autoimmune diseases, it appears that different adhesion molecules are involved in homing to different target organs, a finding that may have therapeutic implications.[52]

Some infections do not trigger innate immunity that in turn activates endothelial cells. However, effector T cells appear to randomly enter all tissues in very small numbers, possibly through binding with LFA-1 and ICAM-2, which are expressed on all endothelial cells. If they recognize specific antigen in the tissue, they produce cytokines, such as TNF-α, which activates endothelial cells to express adhesion molecules with consequent recruitment of further effector cells and other inflammatory cells. Thus, one or a few specific effector T cells encountering their specific antigen in a tissue can initiate a potent inflammatory response.

B Lymphocytes

Similar to T cells, the simple binding of surface immunoglobulin to its specific antigen is not sufficient to activate B cells. A second signal is required that is sometimes provided by the pathogen itself (thymus-independent, or TI, antigens) but is usually delivered by an already-primed CD4 cell (thymus-dependent, or TD, antigens).

Thymus-Independent Antigens

The so-called TI antigens[53] are nonprotein antigens that stimulate antibody production in athymic persons. The most important TI antigens are polymeric polysaccharides or glycolipids that induce maximal crosslinking of membrane immunoglobulins on B cells, leading to activation without the requirement of T-cell help. However, responses to TI antigens, which are frequent among CD5 B cells, need some form of T-cell help because they are markedly reduced in animals completely lacking T cells. Possible candidates are those T cells, such as γ:δ T cells, that may recognize nonprotein antigens and develop outside the thymus. Responses to TI antigens, which are components of bacterial cell wall, are important in defending against several extracellular pathogens because cell-wall polysaccharides allow bacteria to resist ingestion by phagocytes.

Although rigorous depletion of T cells greatly affects the response to some TI antigens (also known as *TI-2 antigens*), other TI antigens (known as *TI-1 antigens*) stimulate B cells without the requirement of any other cell type. At high concentrations, these TI-1 antigens cause the proliferation and differentiation of most B cells regardless of their antigenic specificity. Because they cause a polyclonal activation of B cells, TI-1 antigens are also known as *B-cell mitogens*. The prototypic TI-1 antigen in mice is lipopolysaccharide (*endotoxin*), which is a component of the cell wall of many gram-negative bacteria. Lipopolysaccharide is also a potent activator of macrophages.

Thymus-Dependent Antigens

Antibody responses to protein antigens require antigen-specific T-cell help. Antigen-specific helper T cells must therefore have been primed earlier during the course of the immune response by macrophages or dendritic cells. B cells internalize the antigen bound to their surface immunoglobulin, degrade it, and present peptides on the cell surface in association with MHC class II molecules for recognition by specific helper T cells. The two cells do not need to recognize the same epitopes. What is crucial is that the epitope recognized by the T cell is part of the antigen that has been recognized and internalized by the B cell; this allows the B cell to present on the cell surface the peptide to which the T cell is specific.

This linked recognition explains the immune response to the so-called haptens, small chemical groups that are unable to elicit an immune response because they are not recognized by T cells. However, haptens coupled to a protein can elicit an immune response because T cells recognize the protein-derived peptides and provide the necessary help. This phenomenon is responsible for antibody production against substances such as penicillin that interact with host proteins and become able to induce an immune response.

B-Cell/T-Cell Interactions

CD4 T cells that provide help for B-cell activation in response to TD antigens belong to the T_H2 subset.[54] Naive T cells enter the T-cell zone of peripheral lymphoid tissues (Fig. 4–16) through HEVs and become activated if they recognize their specific antigen on APCs. B cells migrate through HEVs in the same T-cell zone. If they interact with an activated CD4 T cell that is specific for the peptide–MHC complex presented on the B cells, they form a primary focus. Recognition of the specific peptide–MHC complex on the surface of B cells activates T_H2 cells both to express the cell surface molecule CD40 ligand (which binds to the B-cell surface molecule CD40) and to secrete IL-4. CD40 ligand and IL-4 synergize in driving clonal expansion of the B cell. Later stages of B-cell activation involve isotype switching,[55] a DNA recombination process during which the same variable region of the clonally expanded B cell is associated with different constant regions. B cells initially express IgM and IgD; later in the immune response, the same variable region may be associated with other constant portions, giving rise to IgG, IgA, or IgE. Unlike variable-gene segment recombination, switch recombination occurs only after antigen stimulation and not during B-cell development. B cells undergo isotype switching to express transmembrane immunoglobulins of a different isotype before initiating the production of the secreted corresponding antibody. In the mouse, IL-4 preferentially induces switching to IgG1 and IgE, whereas TGF-β induces switching to IgG2b and IgA. IL-5 augments IgA production by cells that have already undergone switching. Although T_H1 cells are poor inducers of antibody production, they release IFN-γ, which in mice induces switching to IgG2a and IgG3 subclasses that bind to high-affinity Fcγ receptors and complement.

Germinal Centers

B cells that have been activated by T cells follow one of two patterns. Some migrate to the medullary cords and differentiate into short-lived plasma cells secreting IgM or IgG, thus providing an early immune response. Others migrate together with the specific helper T cells into the primary follicles, where they divide and form germinal centers (Fig. 4–17).[56] Primary follicles contain resting B cells clustered around a network of processes extending from a specialized cell, the *follicular dendritic cell,* that plays a central role in the selection process during an antibody response. Although they have similar morphology, follicular dendritic cells are unrelated to the dendritic cells that present antigens to the T cells. They do not derive from the hematopoietic stem cell, lack MHC class II expression, and express membrane receptors for complement and the Fc portion of immunoglobulins. Follicular dendritic cells play an important role in driving the maturation of the humoral immune system through their capacity to bind antigen–antibody complexes by their Fc receptor and to retain antigens on their surface for long periods. The early antibodies secreted by B cells of the medullary cord not only provide early protection but also trap antigen, in the form of immune complexes, on the surface of follicular dendritic cells.

B cells rapidly proliferate in the germinal center and assume the appearance of blast cells (called *centroblasts*). They then stop dividing and become centrocytes, which make contact with the dense network of follicular dendritic cell processes. Helper T cells also undergo some clonal expansion in the germinal center and are mingled with centrocytes. B cells

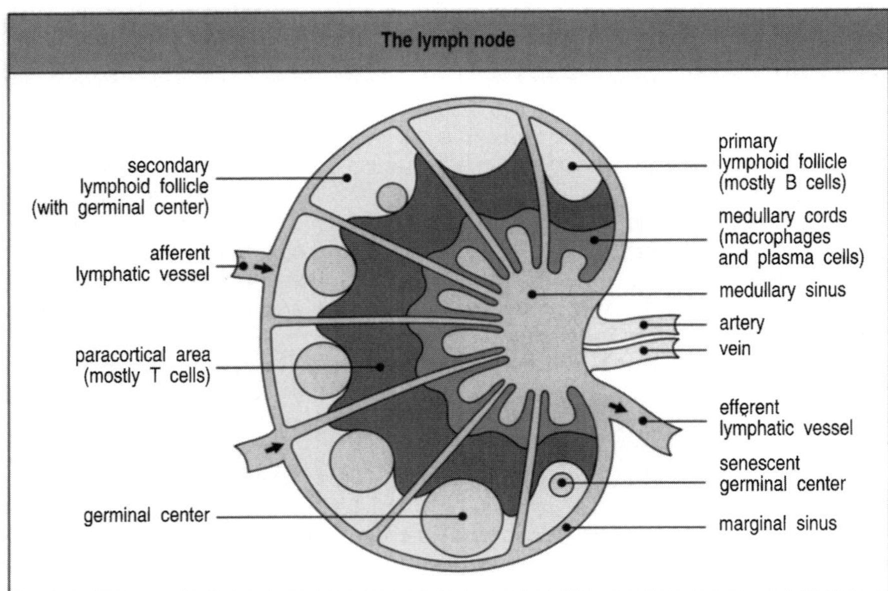

Figure 4–16. A lymph node. A lymph node is composed of an outer cortex and an inner medulla. The cortex consists of an outer cortex of B lymphocytes organized into lymphoid follicles and a deep or paracortical area composed mainly of T lymphocytes and dendritic cells. Some B-cell follicles (known as secondary follicles) contain central areas of intense B-cell proliferation called germinal centers. The medulla consists of strings of macrophages and plasma cells (medullary cords). Naive lymphocytes enter the lymph node from the bloodstream through the high endothelial venules and leave with the lymph through the efferent lymphatic. (From Janeway CA, Travers P, Walport M, Capra DJ: Immunobiology. London, Elsevier, 1999.)

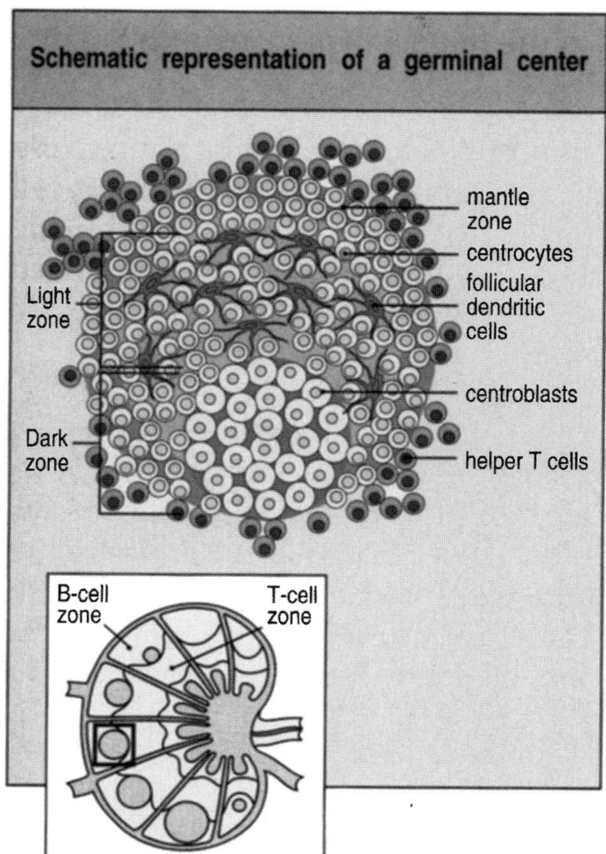

Figure 4–17. Germinal center. See text for explanation. (From Janeway CA, Travers P, Walport M, Capra DJ: Immunobiology. London, Elsevier, 1999.)

that are not specific for antigen are pushed outside and form the mantle zone. Most germinal centers are therefore derived from only one or a few founder cells. Somatic hypermutation of the immunoglobulin variable-domain genes occurs in the rapidly dividing centroblasts and generates different surface immunoglobulins with variable affinity for the antigen.

Selection of B cells that bear surface immunoglobulins with the highest affinity for the antigen occurs at the surface of follicular dendritic cells. This process is called *affinity maturation.* B cells that lose their ability to bind the antigen die by apoptosis. On the contrary, those with the highest affinity take up antigen from follicular dendritic cells, internalize it, and move to the outer edge of the light zone where helper T cells expressing CD40 ligand are concentrated. Interaction with helper T cells induces B cells to become plasma cells or memory cells and prevents the selection of B cells that have acquired self-reactivity during somatic hypermutation.

Some B cells leave germinal centers as pre-plasma cells (plasmablasts) and migrate to distant sites where they differentiate into plasma cells that have a life span of about 1 month. Those originating from lymph nodes and spleen migrate to the bone marrow; those originating from the mucosa-associated lymphoid tissue migrate to the lamina propria of epithelial surfaces. Plasma cells are terminally differentiated B cells that produce immunoglobulins, no longer interact with helper T cells, and are unable to change isotypes or undergo somatic hypermutation. Germinal centers last about 3 to 4 weeks after the supply of extrafollicular antigen is exhausted. Small numbers of B cells continue to proliferate in the follicles for months, however; these B cells are likely the precursors of antigen-specific plasma cells in the mucosa and bone marrow.

IMMUNOLOGIC MEMORY

Immunologic memory is one of the most important characteristics of the adaptive immune response. It allows rapid and effective response to antigens that have been encountered previously and represents the presence of an already clonally expanded population of specific lymphocytes. These responses are called *secondary, tertiary,* and so on, depending on the number of antigen exposures. Several hypotheses have been proposed to explain immunologic memory. It may depend on the persistence of long-lived lymphocytes in a resting state. Alternatively, lymphocytes activated by the original exposure to antigen may be restimulated repetitively in the absence of further encounters with the original antigen. This may depend on the persistence of a small amount of antigen (possibly at the level of follicular dendritic cells), from stimulation with cross-reactive antigens, or from the release, during subsequent immune responses to other antigens, of soluble mediators that restimulate memory cells.[57–59]

B Cells

Secondary antibody responses due to the stimulation of memory B cells differ in several aspects from primary immune responses. Memory cells not only have been clonally expanded but also have undergone somatic mutation, affinity maturation, and isotype switching; they therefore express high-affinity immunoglobulins of different, predominantly IgG, isotypes on their membrane. The antibody response is therefore more intense, and the antibodies are of different isotypes (mainly IgG) and of high affinity. Secondary and subsequent responses lead to increasing affinity of antibody by a mechanism similar to that observed in a primary response and based on further somatic hypermutation and selection by antigen on follicular dendritic cells in germinal centers.

T Cells

Long-lived effector T cells are difficult to distinguish from memory cells. The identification of memory T cells rests largely on the existence of a population of cells with the surface characteristics of activated effector T cells but distinct from them in that they require additional stimulation before acting on target cells.

Changes in three cell surface proteins—L-selectin, CD44, and CD45—are particularly significant after exposure to antigen. L-selectin is lost on most memory cells, whereas CD44 levels increase on all memory cells and CD45 changes from a high (CD45RA) to a low (CD45RO) molecular weight isoform. These changes are characteristic of all cells that have been activated to effector T cells, yet some of the cells in which these changes have occurred have many characteristics of resting T cells, suggesting that they are memory CD4 T cells.

Original Antigenic Sin

In an immunized person, antibody and effector T cells prevent the activation of naive B and T cells by the same antigen. This inhibition explains a phenomenon called *original antigenic sin*.[60] This means that in a person previously immunized with, for instance, a virus, there tends to be a response to the same epitopes recognized during the primary immune response even if the person was infected with a variant of the virus that carries different immunogenic epitopes. This does not occur if the variant lacks the epitopes present in the microorganism responsible for the original infection.

MUCOSAL IMMUNE SYSTEM

The mucosal immune system is important in the defense against infection.[61] Much of the current knowledge of mucosal immunity is based on studies of the gastrointestinal tract, but it is likely that the general features of mucosal immunity are similar in all mucosa-associated lymphoid tissues. Immune response to antigens delivered by the oral route differs from those to antigens encountered in other sites in two main respects: (1) the predominant production of IgA in mucosal tissues and (2) the tendency of oral immunization with protein antigens to induce systemic T-cell tolerance rather than activation, a phenomenon that is particularly appealing for the possible induction of tolerance to autoantigens in autoimmune diseases.

Gut-Associated Lymphoid Tissue

In the intestinal mucosa (Fig. 4–18), lymphocytes are scattered both among epithelial cells (intraepithelial lymphocytes) and in the lamina propria. Ten percent of intraepithelial lymphocytes bear the γ:δ TCR; both γ:δ and α:β intraepithelial T cells show a limited diversity of antigen receptors and are thought to have evolved to recognize commonly encountered intraluminal antigens. The small intestine contains organized mucosal lymphoid follicles (Peyer's patches). Similar follicles are found along the gastrointestinal and respiratory tract (such as pharyngeal tonsils). Peyer's patches have B cell–rich areas that often contain germinal centers and CD4 T cells mainly located in the interfollicular regions. The epithelium overlying Peyer's patches contains specialized cells, called *membranous* (M) *cells*, that lack microvilli and engulf and transport macromolecules from the intestinal lumen into subepithelial tissues. M cells are thought to be important in delivering antigens to Peyer's patches. Lymphocyte homing to Peyer's patches and the lamina propria of the gut has particular characteristics (see T-Cell Homing).

Most of the orally administered antigens are carried by lymphatics to the draining mesenteric lymph nodes, where an immune response is initiated. Some protein antigens are transported by M cells into Peyer's patches, where they can stimulate both T and B cells. Lymphocytes derived from both the mesenteric lymph nodes and Peyer's patches may then populate the lamina propria or reach the bloodstream. IgA is the main class of antibody secreted through epithelia.[62] B cells differentiate into IgA-producing cells principally under the influence of TGF-β and IL-5. IgA-expressing B cells tend to home to Peyer's patches and the lamina propria. In the lamina propria, IgA is held in the form of a dimer by a coordinately synthesized J chain; the complex interacts with a receptor (poly-Ig receptor) on

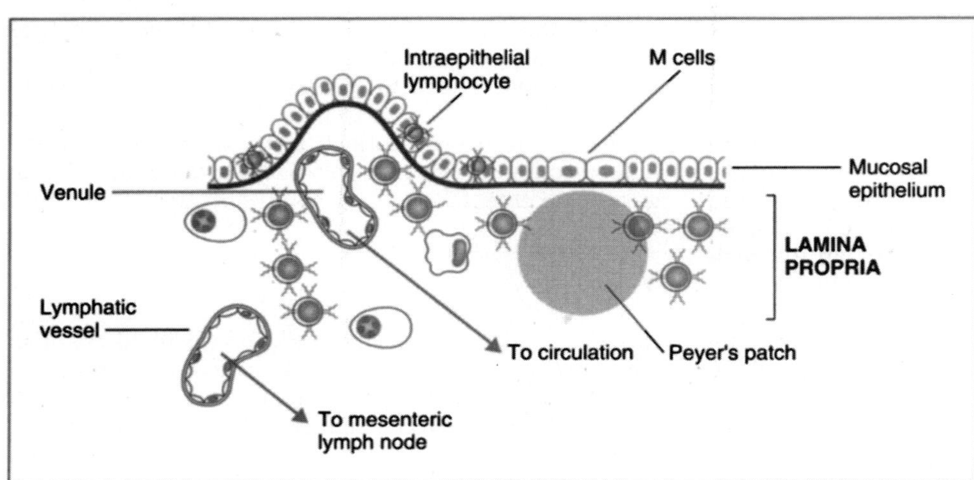

Figure 4–18. Components of the mucosal immune system. (From Abbas AK, Lichtman AH, Pober JS: Cellular and Molecular Immunology. Philadelphia, WB Saunders, 1997.)

the basal surface of epithelia. The complex is transported in a vesicle across the cell to the apical surface and released into the lumen in association with the secretory component, which is a cleaved fragment of the poly-Ig receptor. Molecules of dimeric IgA that diffuse from the lamina propria to the blood are excreted into the gut via the bile. IgA is also produced in other lymphoid tissues and in the bone marrow, giving rise to serum IgA, which is monomeric.

Oral Tolerance

Oral tolerization[63] is a phenomenon in which the oral (or, more generally, the mucosal) administration of an antigen induces a marked suppression of systemic humoral and cell-mediated immune responses to immunization with the same antigen without affecting the response to other antigens. It is presumed that this mechanism has evolved to prevent systemic immune responses to ingested proteins and to bacteria that normally reside in the intestinal lumen.

The reason why some protein antigens induce oral tolerance while others elicit effective immunity is not known. As in other instances, one possible explanation may be the capacity of infectious organisms to activate APCs to express co-stimulatory molecules. The phenomenon of oral tolerance appears to be induced by multiple mechanisms that are only partly understood. These include deletion mechanisms, the induction of a state of anergy, and active immunosuppression through the release of immunosuppressive cytokines such as TGF-β. The dose of the fed antigen seems to influence the mechanism involved: low doses favor active suppression, and high doses favor deletion or anergy. Active suppression seems to depend on a subset of CD4 T cells, also called *T_H3 cells,* that primarily secrete TGF-β. These cells are similar to another described subset (T regulatory cell, or Tr1) that secretes the immunosuppressive cytokine IL-10.[64] They are part of a more general "dominant" control mechanism that seems to be involved in the maintenance of self-tolerance. Mucosal tolerance can also be induced by administration of antigen via the nasal or respiratory route.

Several studies have shown that oral administration of the specific autoantigen is effective in treating experimental autoimmune diseases, including experimental allergic encephalomyelitis and collagen-induced arthritis.[65] Oral tolerance could be an interesting therapeutic option for human autoimmune diseases, such as rheumatoid arthritis, in which the relevant eliciting antigen is unknown. The cytokines secreted by T cells induced in the gut-associated lymphoid tissue by oral antigen administration suppress inflammation in an antigen-nonspecific way *(bystander immunosuppression)* in the microenvironment where the fed antigen is localized. Therefore, the induction of oral tolerance to an antigen present, for instance, in the joint could theoretically result in suppression of joint inflammation when the elicited regulatory cells migrate to the joint, meet the specific antigen, and release suppressive cytokines. The first antigen tested in the treatment of rheumatoid arthritis was collagen type II, but the results have been disappointing thus far.[66]

EFFECTOR MECHANISMS

Cell-Mediated Immunity

The three types of effector T cells are shown in Figure 4–19. Like the initial binding of naive T cells to APCs, the first interaction between effector T cells and their targets is mediated through nonspecific adhesion molecules (LFA-1 and CD2 on T cells and ICAMs and LFA-3 on target cells). If no antigen-specific interaction occurs, the cells separate. If antigen recognition occurs, changes are triggered that enhance the affinity of adhesion molecules and more tightly bind the T cell to its target. This is followed by the release of antigen-nonspecific effector molecules that are highly focused onto the antigen-bearing target.

T Cell–Mediated Cytotoxicity

Upon antigen recognition, cytotoxic T cells exert their effector function through the release of specialized cytoplasmic lytic granules containing two main classes of cytotoxins: *perforins* and *granzymes.*[67] Perforins polymerize and insert into the membrane of the target cell to form pores that allow water and salt to pass rapidly into the cell. Granzymes are serine proteases that induce apoptosis once they have reached the cytoplasm of the target cell. Induction of apoptosis appears to be the most important mechanism by which cytotoxic T cells kill their targets. The nucleases that are activated during the apoptotic process not only destroy the cellular DNA but degrade viral DNA, thus preventing viral release and infection of adjacent cells. Cytotoxic T cells rapidly synthesize their cytotoxins de novo and therefore may kill many targets in succession. Other effector mechanisms of cytotoxic T lymphocytes include the membrane expression of Fas ligand (which induces apoptosis by activating the Fas molecule expressed in the target cell membrane) and release of cytokines such as IFN-γ, TNF-α, and TNF-β.

Macrophage Activation

Intracellular microorganisms that grow in the phagolysosomes of macrophages are protected from the effector mechanisms of both antibodies and cytotoxic T cells. Macrophages act as APCs and prime T cells that are specific for the peptides derived from the microorganism that has been engulfed by the macrophages. These primed effector CD4 T cells in turn enhance the antimicrobial effects of macrophages.[68] Macrophage activation, the principal effector function of T_H1 cells, occurs through two main mechanisms: (1) the secretion by T_H1 cells of IFN-γ and (2) the expression on T_H1 cells of CD40 ligand, which activates the CD40 molecule on the surface of macrophages. Activated macrophages

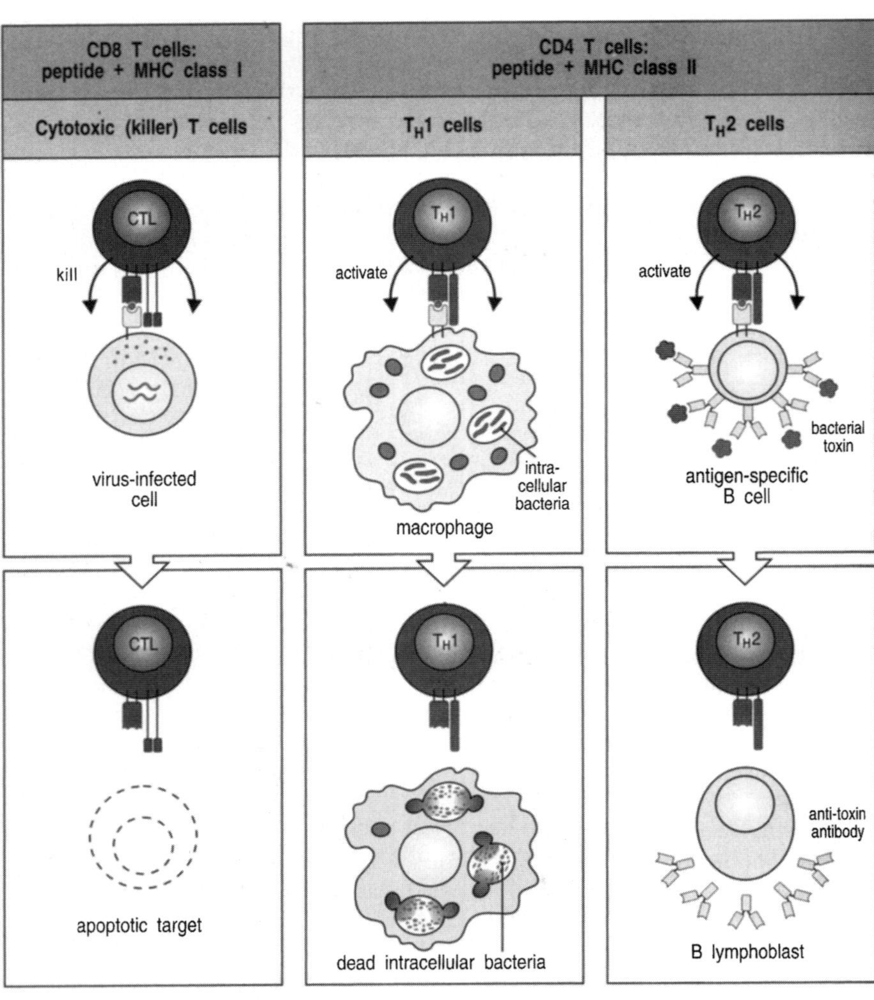

Figure 4–19. The three types of effector T cells. CD8 cytotoxic T cells *(left)* kill target cells that display peptide derived from cytosolic pathogens (mainly viruses) and presented on the cell surface by major histocompatibility complex (MHC) class I molecules. Helper T cells, T_H1 *(middle)* and T_H2 *(right)*, recognize peptides derived from antigens degraded within intracellular vesicles and presented on the cell surface in the context of MHC class II molecules. T_H1 cells activate macrophages to more efficiently destroy intracellular pathogens; moreover, they activate B cells to produce opsonizing antibodies. T_H2 cells, which drive B cells to produce immunoglobulins of all types, initiate B-cell response by activating B cells to proliferate and secrete IgM. (From Janeway CA, Travers P, Walport M, Capra DJ: Immunobiology. London, Elsevier, 1999.)

undergo several changes that augment their antimicrobial capacity and potentiate the immune response (e.g., upregulation of B7 molecules, further IL-12 secretion). T_H1 cells also are fundamental in recruiting macrophages to the site of infection. This occurs through the secretion by T_H1 cells of several additional different cytokines, which include (1) IL-3 and granulocyte/macrophage colony-stimulating factor (GM-CSF), which stimulate the production of new phagocytic cells in the bone marrow; (2) TNF-α and TNF-β, which induce the expression of adhesion molecules on endothelial cells; and (3) macrophage chemotactic factor (MCF) and other chemokines that direct the migration of macrophages from the endothelium to the site of infection. Other cytokines, such as TGF-β, IL-4, IL-10, and IL-13, inhibit macrophage functions. Many of these cytokines are produced by T_H2 cells, which therefore are important in controlling the effector function of macrophages during the immune response.

Antibody-Mediated Immunity

The first humoral response is characterized by the production of low-affinity IgM. IgM is also produced in the secondary immune response and after somatic hypermutation, but other isotypes dominate the later phases of the response. IgG is the principal immunoglobulin in the blood and extracellular fluid, whereas IgA is the principal immunoglobulin in mucosal secretions.

The different immunoglobulin isotypes have distinct properties (see Table 4–2) that enable them to induce different effector mechanisms such as complement[69] or cell activation. Antibodies can activate a variety of effector cells that bear a receptor for their Fc portion.[70] *Fc receptors* make up a family of related molecules with different affinities for different isotypes; the isotype therefore determines which effector cell is preferentially activated. Only Fc portions of immunoglobulins that have interacted with their antigens can activate Fc receptors. This occurs because of aggregation of immunoglobulin on the pathogen surface or because of conformational changes in the Fc portion occurring after antigen binding or both.

Fc receptor activation may induce phagocytosis; activate phagocytes, mast cells, basophils, and eosinophils; and initiate ADCC. ADCC is carried out by NK cells that recognize antibody-coated infected cells and destroy them by a mechanism similar to that used by cytotoxic T lymphocytes.

IMMUNE HOMEOSTASIS

Lymphocyte activation triggers feedback mechanisms that limit their proliferation and differentiation. During the course of a normal immune response, after the eliciting foreign antigen has been eliminated, the immune system must terminate its activation and return to a state of rest. Moreover, because lymphocytes bearing receptors capable of recognizing self-antigens are generated constantly, the immune system must be able to prevent or abort potentially self-reactive responses. Several mechanisms, only partly understood, fulfill these control functions (Fig. 4–20).[71] The disruption of these mechanisms may theoretically lead to autoimmune reactions.

Apoptosis

Upon exposure to the antigen, clonal expansion of specific lymphocytes may increase their frequency by more than 1000-fold within a week. After 1 to 3 months, the number of specific lymphocytes returns to baseline levels, leaving long-lived, functionally quiescent memory cells (Fig. 4–21). This rapid decline in antigen-specific lymphocyte numbers is due to their elimination by apoptosis.

Cells can die because of injury that causes cell necrosis. Apoptosis, another type of cell death, is a normal cellular response that is crucial in many physiologic conditions, such as tissue remodeling that occurs during development. The destruction of the cell in this case is a programmed event, the hallmark of which is the fragmentation of nuclear DNA through the activation of endogenous nucleases. The cell shrinks by shedding membrane-bound vesicles that are then taken-up by macrophages. Interestingly, surface "blebs" released by apoptotic cells contain the type of self-antigens to which patients with systemic lupus erythematosus develop autoantibodies.[72]

Passive Cell Death

Apoptosis occurs by two main pathways. Lymphocytes that are deprived of survival stimuli, such as co-stimulators and cytokines, lose expression of specialized antiapoptotic proteins, mainly belonging to the Bcl family,[73] and die "by neglect." This mechanism leading to apoptosis is called *passive cell death* and is probably the most important mechanism that downregulates the immune response once the eliciting antigen has been eliminated and the innate immunity reaction to antigen exposure subsides. The stimuli that maintain quiescent and viable naive and memory cells are probably sufficient to maintain the expression of antiapoptotic proteins and therefore to prevent cell death. Passive cell death has to be distinguished from the other mechanism, *activation-induced cell death,* in which apoptosis is actively induced. Although these two mechanisms are distinct in their induction and function, they share the same terminal biochemical pathway.

Activation-Induced Cell Death

Activation-induced cell death[74, 75] is important in preventing uncontrolled T-cell activation and as an effector

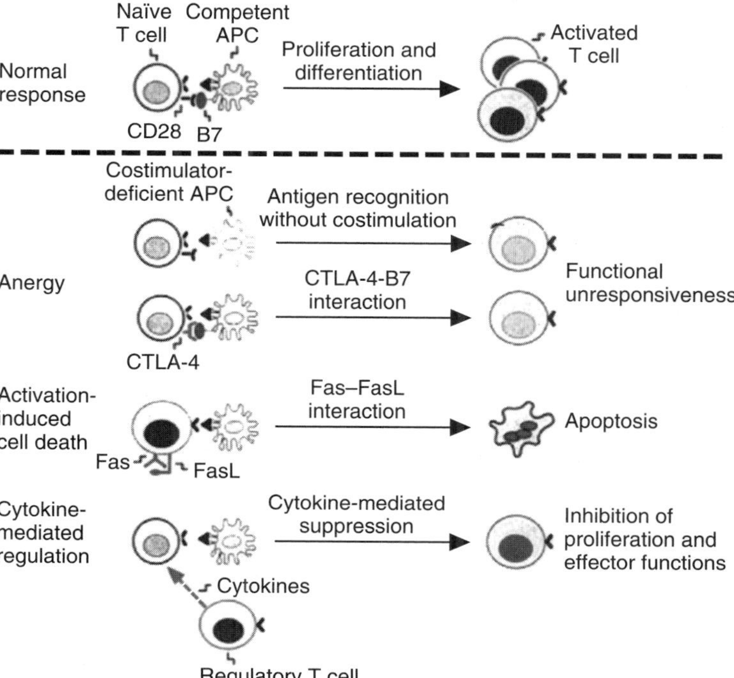

Figure 4–20. Mechanisms of active termination of the immune response. T-cell activation *(top)* is triggered by the recognition of the antigen in association with the delivery of second signals. Antigen recognition without co-stimulation leads to a state of anergy while multiple mechanisms may inhibit the expansion or the effector function (or both) of T lymphocytes. APC, antigen-presenting cell. (Reprinted with permission from Van Parijs L, Abbas AK: Homeostasis and self-tolerance in the immune system: turning lymphocytes off. Science 280:243, 1998. Copyright 1998 American Association for the Advancement of Science.)

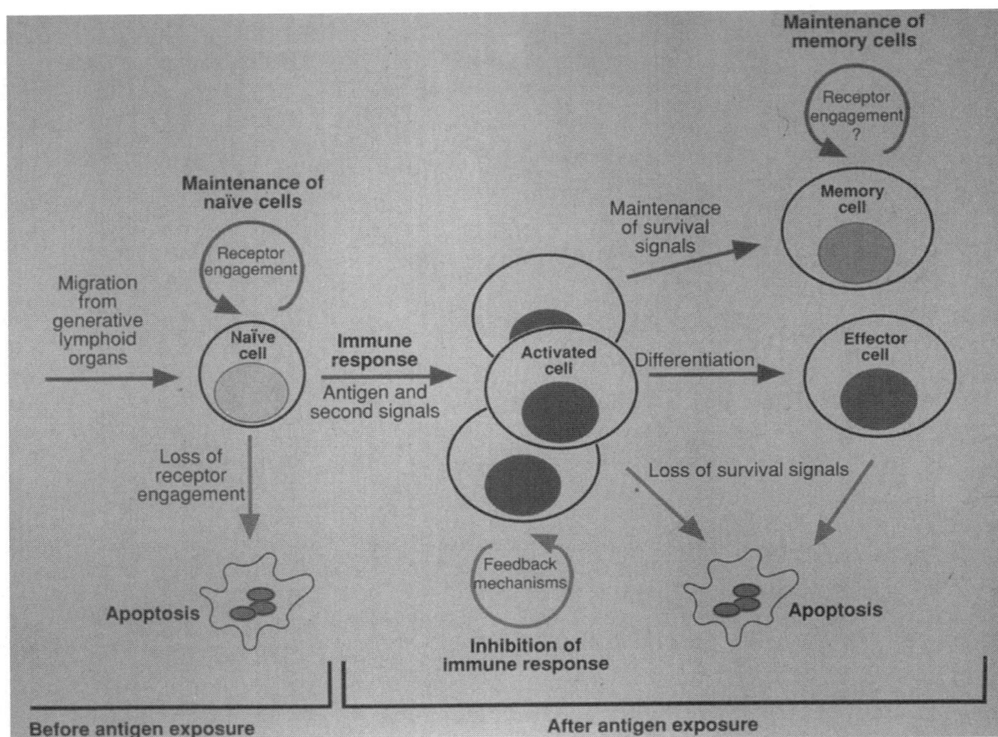

Figure 4–21. Stages in the development and homeostasis of an immune response. (Reprinted with permission from Van Parijs L, Abbas AK: Homeostasis and self-tolerance in the immune system: turning lymphocytes off. Science 280:243, 1998. Copyright 1998 American Association for the Advancement of Science.)

mechanism of CD8 cytotoxic T cells and NK cells. It is usually the result of the interaction of two molecules that are co-expressed on activated cells: the surface receptor Fas (CD95) and its ligand (Fas ligand or CD95L). Fas belongs to a family of proteins that includes TNF receptors (TNF-R) I and II and the B cell–activating molecule CD40. This family of proteins dictates signals that can induce cell survival and proliferation or apoptotic death.

Fas is expressed on different cell types, and in lymphocytes its levels increase after antigen stimulation. Fas ligand is expressed on activated T lymphocytes; therefore, activated, mature T cells express both Fas and Fas ligand. The interaction of Fas ligand with Fas induces a series of intracellular events that lead to apoptosis. These events are initiated by the cytoplasmic region of Fas, which contains a sequence called the *death domain* and involves a proteolytic system, the central component of which is represented by a family of proteases called *caspases*.[76] The activation of TNF-RI probably triggers a pathway of events similar to those triggered by Fas activation. The expression in the cell of antiapoptotic proteins (such as those belonging to the Bcl family) protects against passive cell death but does not prevent activation-induced apoptosis. Fas appears to be a major mediator of apoptosis in CD4 T cells; apoptosis induced by TNF-R is more relevant for CD8 T cells.

In mice, mutations in the Fas receptor (lpr, lymphoproliferation phenotype) or its ligand (gld, generalized lymphoproliferative disease) are associated with massive lymphadenopathy and lupus-like autoimmunity.[77] In humans, Fas mutations cause the *Canale-Smith syndrome*,[78] characterized by lymphadenopathy and autoimmunity. Most patients are heterozygous for the Fas mutation; other family members, although affected by the same heterozygous mutation and showing defective in vitro apoptosis, do not develop disease. Therefore, besides the Fas mutation, additional genetic factors are required for disease development. In humans, a FasL mutation associated with autoimmunity has also been reported,[79] as well as an autoimmune lymphoproliferative syndrome (type II) due to caspase 10 mutations.[79a]

Fas-mediated apoptosis is likely to be important mainly for eliminating cells that are specific for persistent antigens such as self-antigens. Indeed, mutations in Fas and Fas ligand genes cause autoimmune diseases but not prolonged responses to foreign antigens. On the contrary, a prolonged immune response occurs with the constitutive expression of Bcl-2 as a transgene in B or T cells,[80] a phenomenon that underlines the importance of passive cell death in the termination of responses to foreign antigens.

In lymphocyte development in the thymus, apoptosis that occurs from a lack of positive selection appears to be secondary to lack of a rescue signal by the TCR, leading to passive cell death. On the contrary, apoptosis during negative selection is actively induced (activation-induced cell death) but does not appear to be secondary to Fas–Fas ligand interactions, as occur in peripheral deletion mechanisms.

CTLA-4

As previously discussed, T-cell activation induces the expression of the membrane-associated molecule CTLA-4, which, upon binding B7, transduces signals that inhibit the transcription of IL-2 and the progression of T cells through the cell cycle. The targeted disruption of the CTLA-4 gene in mice results in massive accumulation of activated lymphocytes in lymph nodes and spleen and in infiltration of multiple tissues by activated lymphocytes.[81–83]

Interleukin-2

Although IL-2 is an important T-cell growth factor that stimulates clonal expansion of antigen-stimulated lymphocytes, mice lacking IL-2 or the α or β chain of the IL-2 receptor develop lymphadenopathy and various manifestations of autoimmunity.[84–86] This suggests that although the function of IL-2 as a growth factor can be supplanted by other cytokines, IL-2 is part of a necessary feedback mechanism that controls lymphocyte responses.

Cytokine-Mediated Suppression

Cytokines (IL-4, IL-10, IL-13) released by T_H2 cells inhibit macrophage activation and therefore might represent a way to control T_H1-mediated immunity. Moreover, IFN-γ, released by T_H1 cells, inhibits IL-4–stimulated B-cell switching to IgE. Therefore, cytokines released by different T-cell populations are able to suppress different types of immune responses.

Regulatory T cells can release suppressive cytokines such as TGF-β or IL-10 upon specific antigen stimulation.[87] Mice with targeted disruption of TGF-β have inflammatory lesions in heart, liver, and lungs[88]; mice with targeted disruption of IL-10 experience chronic enterocolitis.[89] If autoreactive lymphocytes are held in check by suppressive lymphocytes, depletion of these cells may result in autoimmunity. In mice, selective depletion of a subset of T cells with an activated phenotype allows the development of multiorgan autoimmune lesions.[90]

Several basic issues regarding the homeostasis of the immune response remain to be solved. As pointed out by Van Parijs and Abbas,[71] although it is clear that the same molecules (such as B7 and IL-2) may function to amplify or terminate immune responses, what regulates these opposing functional effects is still unknown. Moreover, it is not known whether the different feedback mechanisms operate together to terminate all immune responses or they became operative in different conditions. Alteration of the mechanisms that control immune homeostasis are an important area of research for autoimmune diseases because uncontrolled inflammation may theoretically lead to abnormal presentation of self-antigens. The fact that disruption of any one of the different homeostatic mechanisms leads to autoimmunity in animals suggests that these mechanisms are not redundant and cannot compensate for one another.[71]

SELF-TOLERANCE

Immunologic tolerance is the antigen-induced functional inactivation or death of specific lymphocytes that results both in the inability to respond to that antigen and in the inhibition of lymphocyte activation during subsequent administration of the same antigen in an immunogenic form. Antigens that induce an immune response are called *immunogens,* whereas antigens that induce tolerance are called *tolerogens.* Self-antigens are normally tolerogens; many foreign antigens, depending on their physicochemical form, dose, and route of administration, may act as immunogens, tolerogens, or both. For instance, protein antigens administered subcutaneously or intradermally are usually immunogenic, whereas large amounts of protein antigens administered intravenously or orally often induce unresponsiveness.

The need to avoid self-aggression during the immune response to foreign antigens has been a determinant factor during the evolution of the immune system. The persistence of autoimmune diseases could be explained by the fact that they more frequently affect people after they have reached the reproductive age and therefore no longer represent a serious threat to the survival of the species. Although the question concerning the balance between immunity and tolerance, including self-tolerance, has yet to be resolved, many observations are yielding a general framework.[91–93]

The random generation of antigen receptors during lymphocyte maturation can give rise to lymphocytes that are specific for self-antigens. As we have seen, lymphocytes with high avidity for abundant self-antigens constitutively expressed in all cells (and therefore present in high concentration in the thymus and the bone marrow) are deleted during their development in central lymphoid organs *(central tolerance).* Although clonal deletion of self-reactive lymphocytes in central lymphoid organs is an efficient process, not all self-antigens are expressed in central lymphoid organs or gain access to it. Examples of such antigens are those specifically expressed in parenchymal tissues (although some of these antigens have been shown to be expressed in the thymus[94]) or those that are expressed only at certain stages, such as puberty. Lymphocytes that are specific for these antigens therefore survive and must be eliminated or held in check by other mechanisms. These mechanisms, only partly understood, are responsible for peripheral tolerance and include not only clonal deletion but also clonal anergy, active suppression, and ignorance.

Self-antigen–specific T lymphocytes may be clonally deleted by apoptosis. As previously discussed, antigen binding to the TCR in the absence of co-stimulation not only fails to activate T cells but also may lead to a state of anergy in which the cell becomes refractory to activation. Therefore, self-antigens may not elicit an autoimmune response because they are presented to T cells in the absence of inflammation-induced co-stimulation. In some experimental models of tolerance, specific T cells actively suppress *(dominant tolerance)* the activity of other self-reactive T cells capable of inducing tissue damage.[90, 93] Dominant tolerance also appears to be involved in mucosal tolerance. Moreover, in some experimental systems of peripheral tolerance, the induction and responses of T_H1 cells are preferentially blocked. The finding that T_H2 responses are often unaffected or even stimulated raises the possibility that the state of immunologic unresponsiveness is at least partially due to the immunosuppressive cytokines produced by T_H2 cells. Although preferential T_H2 differentiation is not immunologic tolerance in its strict sense, the result is functional suppression of T_H1-mediated (auto)immunity. Indeed, one of the present aims in the treatment of some autoimmune diseases is to convert a potentially harmful T_H1 response into a possibly protective T_H2 response, a process called *immune deviation*.

Finally, several studies suggest that many self-proteins are presented too poorly to T cells to be recognized. These self-antigens are called *cryptic epitopes* and collectively referred to as *cryptic self*. T cells that are specific for these epitopes are not tolerant because they can respond if the antigen is presented appropriately. They are considered ignorant because they are not aware of the existence of the self-antigen they are able to recognize. Given the number of self-protein epitopes, an immune system in which all potential self-reactivity has been removed would probably not respond to foreign antigens.[95] It is therefore likely that a large number of potentially autoreactive T cells reside in the immune system in a resting state without causing disease because they ignore their respective self-antigens. Strictly speaking, ignorance is not a mechanism of tolerance because it represents a lack of response rather than an actively induced immunologic unresponsiveness. Ignorance may also be related to the difficulty of T cells to gain access to some tissues such as brain, gonads, and eye ("immunologically privileged sites") because of the existence of blood–tissue barriers. It is now apparent that the "immune privilege" of these tissues is a complex and active phenomenon that includes local production of immunosuppressive neuropeptides and cytokines, limited MHC antigen expression, and in the eye and testis, constitutive expression of Fas ligand, which promotes the death of invading Fas-positive cells during viral infections.[96]

Which characteristics of self-antigens determine which mechanism of self-tolerance is activated is largely unknown. There do not appear to be fundamental differences in the acquisition of tolerance to self-antigens or nonself-antigens. Rather, the mechanisms by which foreign antigens shut off rather than stimulate specific lymphocytes are the same as those that evolved to maintain unresponsiveness to self-antigens and to many otherwise innocuous environmental proteins in the air and food.

In this respect, several interesting theories have been proposed. Janeway[97] has suggested that the immune system evolved to discriminate infectious nonself from noninfectious self. This process is allowed by the presence, on cells of the innate immune system, of germ-line–encoded receptors that recognize particular molecular structures that are produced only by microbes and not by the host organism. Activation of these receptors, which signals the presence of pathogen-associated nonself, induces the expression of co-stimulatory molecules on APCs and initiates the immune response. According to this theory, therefore, the innate immune system instructs lymphocytes on the nature (infectious or not) of the antigen for which they are specific, thus preventing harmful responses against self-antigens.

A similar theory has been proposed by Matzinger–the *danger hypothesis*.[98] In this model, it is not the pathogen by itself but the damage that is induced by the infectious agent that leads to co-stimulation, possibly through the release of molecules during cell stress or lysis.

Zinkernagel and associates[99] have proposed that there is no need to discriminate between self and nonself and that localization, dose, and time of availability of antigen are the elements that determine whether an immune response is induced.

TOLERANCE BREAKDOWN AND AUTOIMMUNITY

Several systemic or organ-specific chronic inflammatory diseases are, or are thought to be, autoimmune in origin, but the mechanisms leading to self-tolerance breakdown are unknown. Autoimmune diseases are multigenic and multifactorial; the importance of environmental factors in eliciting disease is indicated by the relatively low disease concordance in monozygotic twins and by the fact that migrant populations tend to acquire the disease prevalence of the geographic area to which they move.[100]

Despite the great number of potential autoantigens, there are relatively few distinct autoimmune diseases and, in persons with a particular autoimmune disease, the same autoantigens tend to be recognized. This suggests that only a small fraction of self-proteins can actually serve as autoantigens. It is also conceivable that lymphocytes that mediate autoimmune responses do not undergo clonal deletion in central lymphoid organs but rather are present in a tolerant or ignorant state in all normal persons and may be activated only in particular circumstances.

Genetic Predisposition

The human and animal genomes contain a pool of allelic variants or DNA mutations that affect the control of the immune response. Although the complex genetic mechanisms that predispose to autoimmune diseases have not yet been elucidated, it appears that some of these genetic variants in combination with other genes confer increased susceptibility to autoimmunity. That these allelic variants act in combination explains both the difficulty in mapping them and the observation that autoimmune diseases are not inherited in a simple mendelian way.

In human autoimmune diseases, and particularly in animal models, almost 40 genes that predispose to autoimmunity have been localized. There appear to be both genes that cause general defects in immune regulation and are shared between different diseases and genes that are unique to a given disease and may confer susceptibility of the target organ to the autoimmune process. Some conclusions have been drawn from the analysis of murine autoimmune disease models[100]: (1) no single allele but rather a combination of genes causes the disease, and more than one combination may exist; (2) the risk of the disease depends on the number of susceptibility alleles at unlinked loci; (3) some alleles have a greater effect than others; and (4) several predisposing alleles have a weak effect and are therefore difficult to map.

As discussed elsewhere, a major genetic predisposing factor in both experimental and human autoimmune diseases is represented by the MHC haplotype. Alterations in Fas or FasL genes are associated with autoimmunity both in animals and in humans. The gene of the autosomal recessive disease *autoimmune polyendocrinopathy-candidiasis-ectodermal dystrophy* (APECED) has been localized on chromosome 21;[101] its identification will provide important clues for understanding autoimmunity.

Infection and Autoimmunity

Infection appears to be the most important exogenous factor in the induction of autoimmunity. However, how infections can trigger in vivo the activation of autoaggressive T cells and cause tissue destruction is unknown. New insights have been provided by the observations that a single TCR may bind different peptides (TCR degeneracy) and that autoreactive "ignorant" T cells are present in the circulation of normal persons.

Another important finding has been the description of *epitope spreading* during an autoimmune response. This phenomenon was initially demonstrated in experimental allergic encephalomyelitis.[102] Experimental allergic encephalomyelitis can be induced in susceptible strains by immunization with myelin basic protein (MBP) or its immunogenic peptides. During the course of the disease, a T-cell response developed not only to the original immunizing peptide but also to some cryptic epitopes within MBP; the T-cell response against these cryptic epitopes was also encephalitogenic. Subsequent work in other experimental models such as nonobese diabetic (NOD) mice[103] confirmed these results and showed that epitope spreading can be both intramolecular and intermolecular because determinants of other antigens at the site of inflammation, including heat shock proteins, can also become targets of the autoimmune response. Thus, these results have shown that during the course of the disease, a sequence of pathogenic autoimmune responses to several cryptic epitopes develops, probably as a consequence of upregulation of processing and presentation of self-molecules in the context of inflammation.

The activation of autoimmune T-cell clones is necessary but not sufficient to cause autoimmune diseases, the development of which depends on several other factors,[41] including the following:

- A sufficient clonal expansion of autoreactive T cells
- A sufficient expression of MHC and co-stimulatory molecules in the target organ
- Development of an effector immune response that is pathogenic
- The possibility for autoreactive lymphocytes to reach the target organ

Indeed, although self-reactive lymphocytes may invade their target tissue and form inflammatory cell infiltrates upon activation, cell infiltration per se is not sufficient to produce tissue damage.[104]

Co-administration of a microbial adjuvant together with the relevant antigen or peptide is necessary for inducing experimental autoimmune disease. Exposure to microbial agents is important for the development of some spontaneous autoimmunity models in transgenic mice.[41] Therefore, the presence of autoreactive lymphocytes per se does not appear to be sufficient to trigger the disease; additional factors, such as infections and/or cytokine release, seem to be needed in order to activate self-reactive anergic or ignorant T cells. For instance, tolerance could be broken if anergic T cells were exposed to high concentrations of IL-2 (which may theoretically occur if adjacent T cells are stimulated by another antigen) or if the inflammatory process causes efficient presentation of cryptic self-antigen on activated APCs. Thus, the development of autoimmune diseases probably is a multistep process involving various components.

Various mechanisms, not necessarily mutually exclusive, have been hypothesized to explain how infection can trigger autoimmune diseases. Three of them (molecular mimicry, bystander activation, and superantigen activation) have been the subject of considerable attention in recent years.

Molecular Mimicry

According to this theory, microbial antigens that share structural similarities with self-antigens are able to elicit an immune response that cross-reacts with self-tissue antigens. Many experimental autoimmune models are generated by hyperimmunization of genetically susceptible strains with foreign proteins that are homologous to tissue-specific self-proteins. Although in this case the triggering antigen is a homologous nonmicrobial antigen, the mechanism is equivalent to that which occurs after infection with a pathogen whose antigens, although nonhomologous, share structurally related epitopes with self-antigens.

In experimental autoimmune uveitis and experimental ovarian autoimmune disease, microbial peptides have been identified that induce tissue-specific autoimmunity.[41] Immunization with heat-killed *Mycobacterium tuberculosis* in mineral oils (complete Freund's adjuvant) induces arthritis in Lewis rats. The disease can be transferred to naive, irradiated recipients with a T-cell clone specific for the mycobacterial heat shock protein 65 peptide 180–188.[105] Activation of human autoreactive T-cell clones by viral and bacterial peptides has been reported. In insulin-dependent diabetes mellitus, molecular mimicry at the T-cell level between glutamate decarboxylase (a pancreatic-islet autoantigen) and a coxsackie virus antigen has been shown.[106] In multiple sclerosis, seven viral and a single bacterial peptide were found to stimulate at least one of seven autoimmune T-cell clones specific for MBP.[107] In patients with Lyme disease who develop chronic arthritis that is resistant to antibiotic treatment, Gross and colleagues[108] demonstrated cross-reactivity between a peptide of OspA, the major surface antigen of *Borrelia burgdorferi*, and the self-protein LFA-1.

These studies have demonstrated that microbial peptides with limited sequence homology are effective activators of autoreactive T cells. Moreover, the studies suggest the possibility that epitopes present on different microbial peptides may all be responsible for the activation of autoreactive T cells in a given autoimmune disease. In diseases in which a single pathogen has not been implicated, cross-reactive epitopes that are common to various pathogens may be important.

HLA–disease association is usually explained by the fact that the HLA molecule associated with a given disease is involved in the presentation of the pathogenic peptide. However, another function of the MHC class II molecules is to present self-peptides to developing T cells in the thymus in order to shape the T-cell repertoire.

An alternative explanation for the role of HLA in predisposing to autoimmune diseases has been formulated. Based on the fact that peptides derived from MHC class II molecules themselves are among the self-peptides presented by MHC molecules in the thymus, this explanation is known as the *multistep molecular mimicry hypothesis*.[109] According to this model (Fig. 4–22), a peptide of the disease-associated HLA molecule would select the pathogenic TCR during lymphocyte maturation in the thymus (step 1). The selected TCR then is stimulated by a foreign peptide having structural homology with the HLA peptide by which it has been selected in the thymus (step 2). T-cell activation is perpetuated by the TCR's recognition of a third self-peptide, which also is structurally homologous to the two previous peptides and represents the disease target (step 3). Evidence for this model has been provided in the setting of adult rheumatoid arthritis.[110]

Although molecular mimicry is an attractive hypothesis to explain the etiology of autoimmunity, its relevance in human diseases is unproven. Surveys of the growing database of protein sequences show many similar sequential alignments between candidate self-antigens and microbial sequences[111]; therefore, functional studies are required to establish whether shared determinants are biologically active T-cell epitopes. It is also possible that peptides that do not show obvious structural similarities on sequential alignment may be cross-reactive if they form similar TCR-accessible surfaces. However, as previously mentioned, a potential cross-reactivity between an infectious agent and a human self-protein per se is not sufficient to cause disease, and other factors are needed to transform autoreactivity into autoaggression.

Bystander Activation

The bystander activation hypothesis postulates that infection-induced local inflammation—by provoking cell death and the release of abundant quantities of self-antigens, potentiating antigen presentation, and perturbing the cytokine balance—leads to bystander activation of a preexisting but controlled autoimmune response.

Support for the bystander activation theory has been provided by the experiments of Horwitz and colleagues.[112] They showed that coxsackie virus infection, which induces exocrine pancreatitis, failed to accelerate the onset of diabetes in NOD mice despite well-established evidence that prediabetic NOD mice respond immunologically to the islet antigen glutamic acid decarboxylase (GAD65) and that this response can cross-react with the P2-C protein of coxsackie virus. Moreover, in these mice the viral-induced T-cell population did not appear to be primed for either of the cross-reactive epitopes, thus calling into question the ability of the cross-reactive sequences to be processed and presented as antigenic epitopes. On the contrary, diabetes developed rapidly in mice with a TCR transgene specific for a different islet autoantigen. It was therefore postulated that local inflammation through the breakdown and release of sequestered antigen and cytokine production may activate a preexisting memory population of autoreactive cells by a bystander mechanism. In human disease, this autoreactive but not pathogenic T-cell population could have been elicited as a consequence of previous viral infections. Other models of virus-induced demyelinating disease suggest

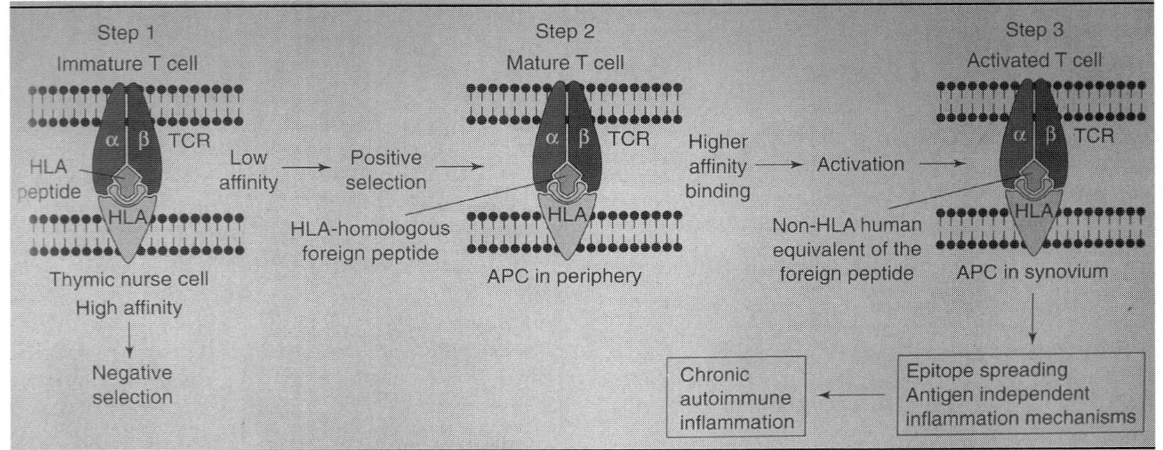

Figure 4–22. Multistep molecular mimicry hypothesis. APC, antigen-presenting cell; HLA, human leukocyte antigen; TCR, T-cell receptor. (Reprinted from Immunol Today, vol 17, Albani S, Carson DA, A multistep molecular mimicry hypothesis for the pathogenesis of rheumatoid arthritis pp 466–470, Copyright 1996, with permission from Elsevier Science.)

that bystander activation of autoreactive T cells previously elicited during viral infections can lead to tissue damage.[113] The work of Horwitz and colleagues also underscores the importance of the tropic role of the pathogen (in their case, infection of the exocrine pancreas).

Superantigens

Superantigens induce a potent polyclonal immune response and could trigger autoimmune diseases either by driving anergic autoreactive T cells out of their nonresponsive state or by facilitating activation of ignorant T cells that are specific for cryptic epitopes.[114] Superantigen-induced immune activation could also be a cause of disease exacerbation in already established autoimmune diseases.

References

1. Abbas AK, Lichtman AH, Pober JS: Cellular and Molecular Immunology, ed 3. Philadelphia, WB Saunders, 1997.
2. Janeway CA, Travers P, Walport M, Capra DJ: Immunobiology. London, Elsevier, 1999.
3. Paul WE (ed): Fundamental Immunology, ed 4. New York, Raven Press, 1998.

3a. Medzhitov R, Janeway C: Innate immunity. N Engl J Med 343: 338, 2000.

4. Moretta A, Biassoni R, Bottino C, et al: Natural cytotoxicity receptors that trigger human NK-cell–mediated cytolysis. Immunol Today 21: 228, 2000.

4a. Seaman WE: Natural killer cells and natural killer T cells. Arthritis Rheum 43: 1204, 2000.

5. Frazer DT, Capra JD: Immunoglobulins: structure and function. *In* Paul WE (ed): Fundamental Immunology, ed 4. New York, Raven Press, 1998.
6. Gold MR, DeFranco AL: Biochemistry of B lymphocyte activation. Adv Immunol 55: 221, 1994.
7. Fearon DT, Carroll MC: Regulation of B lymphocyte responses to foreign and self-antigens by the CD19/CD21 complex. Annu Rev Immunol 18: 393, 2000.
8. Max EE: Immunogobulins: molecular genetics. *In* Paul WE (ed): Fundamental Immunology, ed 4. New York, Raven Press, 1998.
9. Wagner SD, Neuberger MS: Somatic hypermutation of immunoglobulin genes. Annu Rev Immunol 14: 441, 1996.
10. Cumano A, Kee BL, Ramsden DA, et al: Development of B-lymphocytes from lymphoid committed and uncommitted progenitors. Immunol Rev 137: 5, 1994.
11. Cornall RJ, Goodnow CC, Cyster JG: The regulation of self-reactive B cells. Curr Opin Immunol 7: 804, 1995.

11a. Nemazee D: Receptor selection in B and T lymphocytes. Annu Rev Immunol 18: 19, 2000.

12. Murakami M, Honjo T: Involvement of B-1 cells in mucosal immunity and autoimmunity. Immunol Today 16: 534, 1995.
13. Rammensee HG: Chemistry of peptides associated with MHC class I and II molecules. Curr Opin Immunol 7: 85, 1995.
14. Germain RN: MHC-dependent antigen processing and peptide presentation: providing ligands for T lymphocyte activation. Cell 76: 287, 1994.
15. York IA, Rock KL: Antigen processing and presentation by the class I major histocompatibility complex. Annu Rev Immunol 14: 369, 1996.
16. Franco A, Ferrari C, Sette A et al: Viral mutations, TCR antagonism and escape from the immune system. Curr Opin Immunol 7: 524, 1995.
17. Srivastava PK, Menoret A, Basu S, et al: Heat shock proteins come of age: primitive functions acquire new roles in an adaptive world. Immunity 8: 657, 1998.
18. Ashwell JD, Klausner RD: Genetic and mutational analysis of the T-cell antigen receptor. Annu Rev Immunol 8: 139, 1990.
19. Rowen L, Koop BF, Hood L: The complete 685-kilobase DNA sequence of the human bT cell receptor locus. Science 272: 1755, 1996.
20. Zinkernagel RM, Doherty PC: Restriction of in vivo T-cell mediated cytotoxicity in lymphocytic choriomeningitis within a syngeneic or semiallogeneic system. Nature 248: 701, 1974.
21. Li H, Lebedeva MI, Llera AS, et al: Structure of the Vd domain of a human g:d T-cell antigen receptor. Nature 391: 502, 1998.
22. Hayday A: γδ cells: a right time and a right place for a conserved third way of protection. Annu Rev Immunol 18: 975, 2000.
23. Hayday A, Geng L: γδ cells regulate autoimmunity. Curr Opin Immunol 9: 884, 1997.
24. Malisson B, Malisson M: Functions of TCR and preTCR subunits: lessons from gene ablation. Curr Opin Immunol 8: 394, 1996.
25. Peterson EJ, Koretzky GA: Signal transduction in T lymphocytes. Clin Exp Rheumatol 17: 107, 1999.
26. Zamoyska R: CD4 and CD8: modulators of T cell receptor recognition of antigen and of immune response? Curr Opin Immunol 10: 82, 1998.
27. Anderson G, Moore NC, Owen JJ, et al: Cellular interactions in thymic development. Annu Rev Immunol 14: 73, 1996.
28. Shortman K, Wu L: Early T lymphocyte progenitors. Annu Rev Immunol 14: 29, 1996.
29. Von Boehmer H: Positive selection of lymphocytes. Cell 76: 219, 1994.
30. Nossal GJV: Negative selection of lymphocytes. Cell 76: 229, 1994.
31. Ashton-Rickardt PG, Bandeira A, Delaney JR, et al: Evidence for a differential avidity model of T-cell selection in the thymus. Cell 74: 577, 1994.
32. Lenschow DJ, Walunas TL, Bluestone JA: CD28/B7 system of T cell costimulation. Annu Rev Immunol 14: 233, 1996.
33. Rudd CE: Upstream-downstream: CD28 cosignaling pathways and T cell function. Immunity 4: 527, 1996.
34. Lanzavecchia A, Lezzi G, Viola A, et al: From TCR engagement to T cell activation: a kinetic view of T cell behaviour. Cell 96: 1, 1999.

34a. Dustin ML, Cooper JA: The immunological synapse and the actin cytoskeleton: molecular hardware for T cell signaling. Nat Immunol 1: 23, 2000.

35. Banchereau J, Bazan F, Blanchard D, et al: The CD40 antigen and its ligand. Annu Rev Immunol 12: 881, 1994.
36. Lanzavecchia A: License to kill. Nature 393: 413, 1998.
37. Medzhitov R, Janeway CA Jr: Innate immunity: the virtues of a nonclonal system of recognition. Cell 91: 295, 1997.
38. Banchereau J, Briere F, Caux C, et al: Immunobiology of dendritic cells. Annu Rev Immunol 18: 767, 2000.
39. Lanzavecchia A: Receptor-mediated antigen uptake and its effect on antigen presentation to class II-restricted T lymphocytes. Annu Rev Immunol 8: 773, 1993.
40. Kersh GJ, Allen PM: Essential flexibility in the T-cell recognition of antigen. Nature 380: 495, 1996.
41. Hausmann S, Wucherpfennig W: Activation of autoreactive T cells by peptides from human pathogens. Curr Opin Immunol 9: 831, 1997.
42. Garboczi DN, Ghosh P, Utz U, et al: Structure of the complex between human T-cell receptor, viral peptide and HLA-A2. Nature 384: 134, 1996.
43. Garcia KC, Degano M, Stanfield RL, et al: An αβ T cell receptor structure at 2.5 Å and its orientation in the TCR-MHC complex. Science 274: 209, 1996.
44. Malissen B: Translating affinity into response. Science 281: 528, 1998.
45. Nicholson LB, Greer JM, Sobel RA, et al: An altered peptide ligand mediates immune deviation and prevents autoimmune encephalomyelitis. Immunity 3: 397, 1995.
46. Herman A, Kappler JW, Marrack P, et al: Superantigens: mechanisms of T-cell stimulation and role in immune responses. Annu Rev Immunol 9: 745, 1991.
47. Abbas AK, Murphy KM, Sher A: Functional diversity of helper T lymphocytes. Nature 383: 787, 1996.

48. Romagnani S: The Th1/Th2 paradigm. Immunol Today 18: 263, 1997.
49. Bottomly K: T cells and dendritic cells get intimate. Science 283: 1124, 1999.
50. Sallusto F, Lanzavecchia A, Mackay CR: Chemokines and chemochine receptors in T-cell priming and Th1/Th2-mediated responses. Immunol Today 19: 568, 1998.
51. von Andrian UH, Mackay CR: T-cell function and migration. N Engl J Med 343: 1020, 2000.
51a. Rossi D, Zlotnik A: The biology of chemokines and their receptors. Annu Rev Immunol 18: 217, 2000.
52. Steinman L: Escape from "horror autotoxicus": pathogenesis and treatment of autoimmune disease. Cell 80: 7, 1995.
53. Mond JJ, Lees A, Snapper CM: T cell-independent antigens type 2. Annu Rev Immunol 13: 655, 1995.
54. Parker DC: T cell-dependent B-cell activation. Annu Rev Immunol 11: 331, 1993.
55. Stavnezer J: Immunoglobulin class switching. Curr Opin Immunol 8: 199, 1996.
56. MacLennan ICM: Germinal centers. Annu Rev Immunol 12: 117, 1994.
57. Ahmed R, Gray D: Immunological memory and protective immunity: understanding their relation. Science 272: 54, 1996.
58. Ahmed R: Tickling memory T cells. Science 272: 1904, 1996.
59. Dutton RW, Bradley LM, Swain SL: T cell memory. Annu Rev Immunol 16: 201, 1998.
60. McMichael AJ: The original sin of killer T cells. Nature 394: 421, 1998.
61. Neutra MR, Pringault E, Kraehenbuhl J-P: Antigen sampling across epithelial barriers and induction of mucosal immune responses. Annu Rev Immunol 14: 275, 1996.
62. Brandtzaeg P, Baekkevold ES, Farstad IN, et al: Regional specialization in the mucosal immune system: what happens in the microcompartments? Immunol Today 20: 141, 1999.
63. Strobel S, Mowat AM: Immune responses to dietary antigens: oral tolerance. Immunol Today 19: 173, 1998
64. Groux H, O'Garra A, Bigler M, et al: A CD4+T-cell subset inhibits antigen-specific T-cell responses and prevents colitis. Nature 389: 737, 1997.
65. Weiner HL: Oral tolerance: immune mechanisms and treatment of autoimmune diseases. Immunol Today 18: 335, 1997.
66. Kalden JR, Sieper J: Oral collagen in the treatment of rheumatoid arthritis. Arthritis Rheum 41: 191, 1998.
67. Squier MKT, Cohen JJ: Cell-mediated cytotoxic mechanisms. Curr Opin Immunol 6: 447, 1994.
68. Paulnock DM: Macrophage activation by T cells. Curr Opin Immunol 4: 344, 1992.
69. Liszewski MK, Farries TC, Lublin DM, et al: Control of the complement system. Adv Immunol 61: 201, 1996.
70. Ravetch JV, Kinet J: Fc receptors. Annu Rev Immunol 9: 457, 1993.
71. Van Parijs L, Abbas AK: Homeostasis and self-tolerance in the immune system: turning lymphocytes off. Science 280: 243, 1998.
72. Casciola-Rosen LA, Anhalt G, Rosen A: Autoantigens targeted in systemic lupus erythematosus are clustered in two populations of surface structures on apoptotic keratinocytes. J Exp Med 179: 1317, 1994.
73. Chao DT, Korsmeyer SJ: BCL-2 family: regulators of cell death. Annu Rev Immunol 16: 395, 1998.
74. Nagata S: Apoptosis by death factor. Cell 88: 355, 1997.
75. Ashkenazi A, Dixit VM: Death receptors: signaling and modulation. Science 281: 1305, 1998.
76. Thornberry NA, Lazebnik Y: Caspases: enemies within. Science 281: 1312, 1998.
77. Nagata S, Suda T: Fas and Fas ligand: lpr and gld mutations. Immunol Today 16: 39, 1995.
78. Drappa J, Vaishnaw AK, Sullivan KE, et al: Fas gene mutations in the Canale-Smith syndrome, an inherited lymphoproliferative disorder associated with autoimmunity. N Engl J Med 335: 1643, 1996.
79. Wu J, Wilson J, He J, et al: Fas ligand mutation in a patient with systemic lupus erythematosus and lymphoproliferative disease. J Clin Invest 98: 1107, 1996.
79a. Wang J, Zheng L, Lobito A, et al: Inherited human caspase 10 mutations underlie defective lymphocyte and dendritic cell apoptosis in autoimmune lymphoproliferative syndrome type II. Cell 98: 47, 1999.
80. Van Parijs L, Peterson DA, Abbas AK: The Fas/Fas ligand pathways and bcl-2 regulate T cell responses to model self and foreign antigens. Immunity 8: 265, 1998.
81. Tivol EA, Borriello F, Schweitzer AN, et al: Loss of CTLA-4 leads to massive lymphoproliferation and fatal multiorgan tissue destruction, revealing a critical negative regulatory role of CTLA-4. Immunity 3: 541, 1995.
82. Waterhouse P, Penninger JM, Timms E, et al: Lymphoproliferative disorders with early lethality in mice deficient in CTLA-4. Science 270: 98, 1995.
83. Chambers CA, Sullivan TJ, Allison JP: Lymphoproliferation in CTLA-4-deficient mice is mediated by costimulation-dependent activation of CD4+ T cells. Immunity 7: 885, 1997.
84. Sadlack B, Merz H, Schorle H, et al: Ulcerative colitis-like disease in mice with a disrupted interleukin-2 gene. Cell 75: 253, 1993.
85. Willerford DM, Chen J, Ferry JA, et al: Interleukin-2 receptor alpha chain regulates the size and content of the peripheral lymphoid compartment. Immunity 3: 521, 1995.
86. Suzuki H, Kundin TM, Furlonger C, et al: Deregulated T cell activation and autoimmunity in mice lacking interleukin-2. Science 268: 1472, 1995.
87. Mason D, Powrie F: Control of immune pathology by regulatory T cells. Curr Opin Immunol 10: 649, 1998.
88. Shull MM, Ormsby I, Kier AB, et al: Targeted disruption of the mouse transforming growth factor-beta 1 gene results in multifocal inflammatory disease. Nature 359: 693, 1992.
89. Kuhn R, Lohler J, Rennick D, et al: Interleukin-10–deficient mice develop chronic enterocolitis. Cell 75: 263, 1993.
90. Gleeson PA, Ban-Hock T, van Driel IR: Organ-specific autoimmunity induced by lymphopenia. Immunol Rev 149: 97, 1996.
91. Goodnow CC: Balancing immunity and tolerance: deleting and tuning lymphocyte repertoires. Proc Natl Acad Sci U S A 93: 2264, 1996.
92. Mondino A, Khoruts A, Jenkins MK: The anatomy of T-cell activation and tolerance. Proc Natl Acad Sci U S A 93: 2245, 1996.
93. Sakaguchi S: Regulatory T cells: key controllers of immunologic self-tolerance. Cell 101: 455, 2000.
94. Hanahan D: Peripheral-antigen-expressing cells in thymic medulla: factors in self-tolerance and autoimmunity. Curr Opin Immunol 10: 656, 1998.
95. Benoist C, Mathis D: The pathogen connection. Nature 394: 227, 1998.
96. Griffith TS, Ferguson TA: The role of Fas-L induced apoptosis in immune privilege. Immunol Today 18: 240, 1997.
97. Janeway CA Jr: The immune system evolved to discriminate infectious nonself from noninfectious self. Immunol Today 13: 11, 1992.
98. Matzinger P: Tolerance, danger, and the extended family: Annu Rev Immunol 12: 1045, 1994.
99. Zinkernagel RF, Ehl S, Aichele P, et al: Antigen localisation regulates immune response in a dose-and time-dependent fashion: a geographical view of immune reactivity. Immunol Rev 156: 199, 1997.
100. Vyse TJ, Todd JA: Genetic analysis of autoimmune disease. Cell 85: 311, 1996.
101. Peterson P, Nagamine K, Scott A, et al: APECED: a monogenic autoimmune disease providing new clues to self-tolerance. Immunol Today 19: 384, 1998.
102. Miller SD, McRae BL, Vanderlugt CL, et al: Evolution of the T-cell repertoire during the course of experimental immune-mediated demyelinating disease. Immunol Rev 144: 225, 1995.
103. Kaufman DL, Clare-Salzler M, Tian J, et al: Spontaneous loss of T cell tolerance to glutamic acid decarboxylase in murine insulin-dependent diabetes. Nature 366: 69, 1993.
104. Wekerle H: The viral triggering of autoimmune disease. Nature Med 4: 770, 1998.
105. Holoshitz J, Naparstek Y, Ben-Nun A, et al: Lines of T lymphocytes induce or vaccinate against autoimmune arthritis. Science 219: 56, 1983.
106. McLaren NK, Atkinson MA: Insulin-dependent diabetes melli-

tus: the hypothesis of molecular mimicry between islet cell antigens and microorganisms. Mol Med Today 2: 76, 1997.
107. Wucherpfennig KW, Strominger JL: Molecular mimicry in T-cell mediated autoimmunity: viral peptides activate human T cell clones specific for myelin basic protein. Cell 80: 695, 1995.
108. Gross DM, Forsthuber T, Tary-Lehmann M, et al: Identification of LFA-1 as a candidate autoantigen in treatment-resistant Lyme arthritis. Science 281: 703, 1998.
109. Albani S, Carson DA: A multistep molecular mimicry hypothesis for the pathogenesis of rheumatoid arthritis. Immunol Today 17: 466, 1996.
110. Albani S, Keystone EC, Ollier WER, et al: Positive selection in autoimmunity: abnormal immune responses to a bacterial dnaJ antigenic determinant in patients with early rheumatoid arthritis. Nat Med 1: 448, 1995.
111. Parry SL, Hall FC, Olson J, et al: Autoreactivity versus autoaggression: a different perspective on human autoantigens. Curr Opin Immunol 10: 663, 1998.
112. Horwitz MS, Bradley LM, Harbertson J, et al: Diabetes induced by Coxsackie virus: initiation by bystander damage and not molecular mimicry. Nat Med 4: 781, 1998.
113. Segal BM, Dwyer BK, Shevach EM: An interleukin (IL)-10/IL-12 immunoregulatory circuit controls susceptibility to autoimmune disease. J Exp Med 187: 537, 1998.
114. Behar SM, Porcelli SA: Mechanisms of autoimmune disease induction. Arthritis Rheum 38: 458, 1995.

5

Mediators of Inflammation

Patricia Woo

Inflammation is essential to protect one's integrity against physical, chemical, and infective attacks. A large number of physiologic changes occur during the process of inflammation. Cells are recruited and soluble mediators are secreted in response to the external insult. The effect is the elimination of the insult and repair of the tissues involved. These changes have positive and negative feedback mechanisms so that resolution is achieved or homeostasis is maintained. Inflammation can cause disease when it becomes chronic because of failure of the normal mechanisms for resolution of inflammation or persistence of the stimulus.

This chapter reviews some of the basic physiology and pathophysiology of inflammation and how the normal regulation of inflammation is disturbed in rheumatic diseases. Variation in host defenses may be important in disease development as well as in disease resolution; this is illustrated by genetic variations in cytokine genes and association with different types of chronic arthritis.

ACUTE VERSUS CHRONIC INFLAMMATION

Acute inflammation is a normal reaction to an external insult. The classic triad of dolor, rubor, and calor (pain, redness, and heat) is the standard by which the clinician diagnoses inflammation. There is a marked systemic acute-phase response. Histologic examination of the lesion typically demonstrates accumulation of leukocytes, predominantly neutrophils, and exudation of fluid and plasma proteins. Examples include all infectious episodes, trauma, and acute reactive arthritis in children. The processes are sequential and complex, initiated by vascular permeability, extravasation of inflammatory cells, matrix deposition, and tissue repair.

The lesion of chronic inflammation is typified by the infiltration of lymphocytes and monocytes/macrophages and by activation and proliferation of connective tissue. It is thought to be either the result of persistence of the agent, such as *Staphylococcus aureus* in osteomyelitis, or the failure of regulation of inflammation due to genetic variations in the molecules that mediate the innate and adaptive immune responses. Thus, the same agent can produce a spectrum of disease phenotypes depending on the genetic makeup of the individual. Furthermore, genetic polymorphisms can influence a person's susceptibility to as well as the pattern of inflammatory damage. Malignant clones of cells can also cause inflammation, as in Castleman's disease, in which cytokine-secreting tumors produce predominantly interleukin-6, thereby causing multisystem inflammation.

GENETICS OF INFLAMMATION

Human Leukocyte Antigen Associations

The adaptive immune response is described in Chapter 4. The role of human leukocyte antigen (HLA) molecules in disease susceptibility is discussed in Chapters 4 and 6. The most fascinating aspect is that chronic arthritides presenting at different ages have different HLA associations. In particular, HLA-DR8*0801 has been documented to be associated with early onset of oligoarthritis by case-control studies and transmission disequilibrium tests of nuclear families[1]; HLA-B27 is increased in frequency in arthritis beginning in preteen boys.[2] The "age effect" is also apparent with other effector molecules, such as cytokines (see later). One explanation is that adaptive immune responses require further development during the first 5 to 6 years of life.

Complement Deficiencies

Complement deficiencies are examples of associations between inherited variations in these effector molecules of inflammation and a chronic inflammatory disease, such as systemic lupus erythematosus (SLE). Figure 5–1 presents a simplified diagram of the complement activation cascade. Complement proteins are enzymes that exist in precursor forms and are biologically active only when cleaved. There are two main pathways of complement activation—classical (C1, C4, C2) and alternative (Factor B)—that converge in the activation of C3. A third pathway, the lectin pathway, activates C4 via a mannose-binding protein, which is important in innate immunity of the neonate. The activation of C3 leads to stepwise activation of the "terminal attack complex" and lysis of cell membranes. Cleavage products of C3 (C3bi, C3d) serve as opsonins

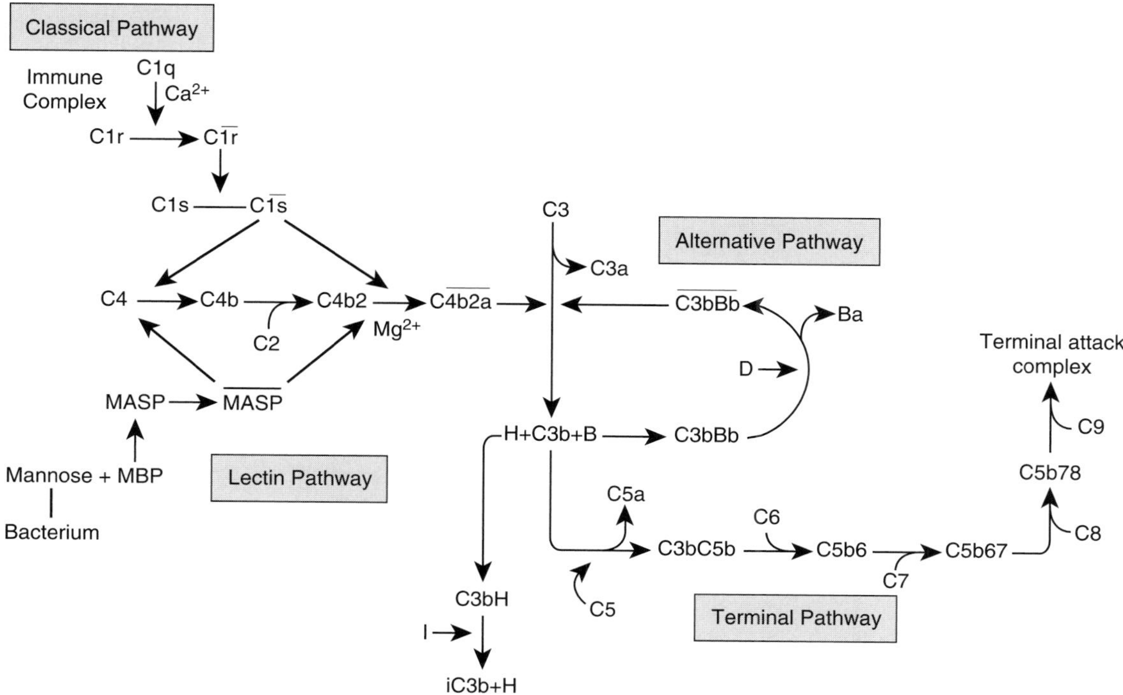

Figure 5–1. Simplified diagram of the complement system. Complement C3 is activated by the classic, lectin, and alternative pathways. The latter is a positive-feedback loop, counterbalanced by inactivation of C3b by factors H and I. The activation of C3 leads to the formation of the terminal attack complex via the "terminal pathway." MASP, mannose binding protein ligand associated proteases; MBP, mannose binding protein.

of immune complexes to cell surface receptors as well as a potent chemotaxin (C3a).

The complement proteins are essential for the clearance of immune complexes. The classical complement pathway proteins maintain immune complexes in a soluble state; the alternative pathway proteins are implicated in the solubilization of preformed immune complexes. Their clearance is achieved via the C3 receptors on phagocytes. There is a hierarchic association of complement component deficiencies with both the prevalence and the severity of the prototypic human immune complex disease SLE.[3] Deficiencies of C1q, C1r, C1s,[4] and C4[5] are associated with a very high prevalence of SLE (>75 percent). Deficiency of C2, the next protein in the classical cascade, is associated with milder disease and lower prevalence (~33 percent).[6] C3 deficiency is mainly associated with pyogenic infections, although 3 of 24 reported patients had an SLE-like illness.[7]

The mechanism for the development of SLE in the complement-deficient person is not yet characterized. It has been reported that C1q deficiency leads to increased apoptosis of cells in the glomerulus[8] and that splenic clearance of immune complexes is defective in complement-deficient persons.[9] How the various features of the clinical disease are produced is still unresolved.

CYTOKINE NETWORK

Cytokines are potent polypeptide mediators secreted by a large variety of cell types to regulate cell growth, differentiation, and activation through specific receptors on target cells. Within the immune system, there are 18 cytokines called *interleukins*. They are produced by leukocytes and mediate the immune response and inflammation. In addition, three other cytokines produced by leukocytes are functionally related to the interleukins: interferon-γ (IFN-γ), tumor necrosis factor α (TNF-α), and tumor necrosis factor β (TNF-β). Interleukins can be divided into those that are largely responsible for immunoregulation—that is, lymphocyte proliferation and differentiation (e.g., interleukin [IL]-2, -3, -4, -5, -9, -10)—and those responsible for the inflammatory response (e.g., IL-1, -6, -8, TNF-α).

The findings that IL-1 and TNF-α have biologic properties that include stimulation of inflammatory prostanoids, activation of vascular endothelial cells, induction of bone and cartilage metabolism, and activation of lymphocytes have helped to explain many aspects of inflammation in joint diseases. Injection of IL-1 into animal joints produces acute arthritis with leukocytes in the synovial fluid and breakdown of proteoglycans in the connective tissue matrix. These pro-inflammatory cytokines potentiate the immune response as well as self-produce during such responses, and they may well contribute to self-perpetuating mechanisms in chronic diseases. The in vivo biologic activity of a cytokine is a net effect determined by its concentration and the presence of specific inhibitory molecules, such as IL-1 receptor antagonist (IL-1ra) and soluble TNF receptors (sTNFR), as well as a general inhibitor of pro-inflammatory cytokine synthesis such as IL-10.

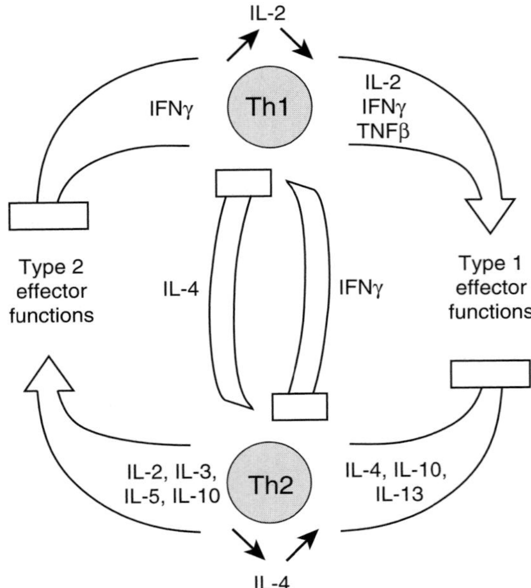

Figure 5–2. Cytokines involved in T-cell differentiation and polarization. IFN, interferon; IL, interleukin; TNF, tumor necrosis factor. (Reprinted with permission from Nature, Abbas AK, Murphy KM, Sher A: Functional diversity of helper T lymphocytes. Copyright 1996 Macmillan Magazines Limited.)

Cytokines and T-Cell Polarization

After exposure to antigen, precursor helper T lymphocytes differentiate into two major types of helper T cells, T_H1 and T_H2, that differ with respect to their function and the range of cytokines they produce (see Chapter 4) (Fig. 5–2).[10] The degree of differentiation or polarization and heterogeneity of T lymphocytes may reflect the nature of the antigenic and environmental stimuli to which the cells have been exposed. This is particularly true of responses to persistent infections with microbes such as *Leishmania, Listeria,* mycobacteria, and helminths or to noninfectious, persistent antigens such as those in allergies and autoimmune diseases, wherein T_H1 or T_H2 polarization is found in the tissues. Furthermore, the degree of polarization increases with the chronicity of immune responses.

These types of cells differentiate mainly under the influence of two cytokines. IL-12 is produced by monocytic antigen-presenting cells (APCs), including the dendritic cells. In conjunction with co-stimulatory molecules, IL-12 promotes differentiation of potential T helper cells (T_H0) to a T_H1 phenotype, which is responsible for cell-mediated immunity. IL-4 is the cytokine that promotes T cells to differentiate into the T_H2 phenotype, which is mainly responsible for antibody responses. The cytokines produced by T_H1 cells are IL-2, IL-3, IFN-γ, granulocyte/macrophage colony-stimulating factor (GM-CSF), and TNF-α and -β. T_H2 cells secrete IL-3, -4, -5, -6, and -10, GM-CSF, and TNF-α. These two major pathways of T-cell differentiation are mutually antagonistic.

The preferential expression of the T_H1 cells in autoimmune diseases such as diabetes, rheumatoid arthritis, and multiple sclerosis[11–13] led to the hypothesis that the prolonged imbalance of T helper subtypes can lead to pathology.[10] In a study of five patients with oligoarticular juvenile arthritis who were positive for antinuclear antibody, negative for rheumatoid factor, and negative for HLA-B27, the T-cell clones were of the T_H1 or T_H0 phenotype.[14] Further analysis of different subgroups of patients not using T-cell clones also showed T_H1 polarization of cells in the synovial fluid but not in the paired blood sample.[15] This is in contrast to the findings in rheumatoid arthritis, in which polarization of T_H1 cells occurs in the peripheral blood.[13]

Study of the inflamed synovium in childhood arthritis revealed differences among disease types, with more IL-2R–positive cells and a lower CD4:CD8 ratio in oligoarticular than in polyarticular disease. Analysis by reverse transcriptase polymerase chain reaction of the cytokine mRNA in synovial tissues documented that IL-4 is mainly found in oligoarthritis and juvenile spondyloarthropathy (i.e., restricted disease with a better articular outcome than polyarticular arthritis, systemic arthritis, or rheumatoid arthritis). There was also a relative absence of IL-4 and IL-10 in the more erosive disease.[16] The biologic reasons for these findings are still unclear and may relate to the persistence of pathogens in the child with oligoarthritis or spondyloarthropathy. Thus, any therapeutic application of the approach of changing the polarization of T-cell phenotypes from T_H1 to T_H2 in autoimmune diseases may well be premature in childhood arthritides.

Cytokines and Inflammation

Monocyte-derived cytokines are important in the inflammatory process. IL-1 and TNF-α have direct effects on tissues as well as the ability to potentiate immune responses. In considering the process of inflammation, the concept of imbalance between pro-inflammatory and anti-inflammatory cytokines (or cytokine inhibitors) is crucial to both the induction and resolution of inflammation. Examples of pro-inflammatory and anti-inflammatory cytokines are given in Table 5–1. Some

Table 5–1

Examples of Pro- and Anti-Inflammatory Cytokines

PRO-INFLAMMATORY CYTOKINES	ANTI-INFLAMMATORY CYTOKINES
Interferon-γ (IFN-γ)	Interleukin-1 receptor antagonist (IL-1ra)
Interleukin-1 (IL-1)	Interleukin-4 (IL-4)
Tumor necrosis factor-α (TNF-α)	Interleukin-10 (IL-10)
Interleukin-6 (IL-6)	Interleukin-13 (IL-13)
	Transforming growth factor-β (TGF-β)
	Soluble tumor necrosis factor receptors (sTNFRs)
	Interleukin-6 (IL-6)

Note: IL-6 is inflammatory in producing fever and multisystem disease in transgenic animals. It is also thought to be anti-inflammatory because it can induce metalloproteinase inhibitors.

cytokines (IL-4 and IL-6) can be either pro- or anti-inflammatory, depending on the concentration and site of secretion.

Polarization toward pro-inflammatory cytokines is induced by infectious agents. Thus, there is a major increase in the pro-inflammatory cytokines IL-1 and TNF-α but very little IL-1ra when peripheral blood mononuclear cells (PBMCs) are cultured with the Lyme agent *Borrelia burgdorferi*.[17] Resolution occurs when the balance is reversed. In autoimmune diseases, however, there is a persistent imbalance favoring a pro-inflammatory state. This could result from antigen persistence or a genetic imbalance in the cytokine network so that homeostasis is not readily restored.

Research in many laboratories on the role of cytokines in arthritis has been based on the hypothesis that the cytokine response is imbalanced. Both pro-inflammatory and anti-inflammatory cytokines are in the peripheral blood of children with chronic arthritis,[18–21] and there is no obvious cytokine deficiency. However, Madson and colleagues[19] found that the ratio of IL-1ra to IL-1 was higher in the synovial fluid of patients with oligoarticular juvenile rheumatoid arthritis (JRA) than in patients with polyarticular JRA. Molar ratios of sTNFR:TNF in the synovial fluid of patients with oligoarticular juvenile chronic arthritis (JCA) and spondyloarthropathies were significantly higher than those of patients with polyarticular JCA, consistent with the fact that the latter is a more erosive disease.[22]

As mentioned earlier, the net biologic effect of a cytokine depends on its concentration in relation to the concentration of its inhibitors. Because proliferation of T_H1 cells depends on IL-2, a number of studies have examined IL-2 and its soluble IL-2 receptor (IL-2R) in children with chronic arthritis, but they have yielded contradictory results, probably reflecting the heterogeneity in the patient population and variations in the different assay methods employed. Examination of synovial biopsies by Murray and colleagues[16] has documented that IL-4 mRNA was found only in the oligoarticular subtype, implying that the polarization to T_H1 may not be as marked, but these experimental results could also reflect the disease duration.

In a 2-year prospective study, Mangge and colleagues[20] examined the usefulness of measuring serum levels of cytokines as an indicator of disease activity in different subgroups of JRA. They found that sTNFR and sIL-2R are more sensitive markers of active disease than C-reactive protein (CRP) and erythrocyte sedimentation rate (ESR), especially in oligoarticular JRA, consistent with the hypothesis that T-cell involvement is pathogenic, at least in this type of chronic arthritis. Measurement of cytokine concentrations in synovial fluids of subgroups of JRA and adult rheumatoid arthritis have indicated that these arthritides are different biologically.[23] IL-6 levels are highest in the synovial fluids of systemic JRA, and IL-1α is present in a significant proportion of those with oligoarticular JRA but not in those with rheumatoid arthritis or systemic JRA.

The earliest study of cytokine balance in systemic JRA, by Prieur and colleagues,[24] found undetectable levels of IL-1β in serum but high levels of IL-1ra inhibitory substance in the serum and urine, especially during the febrile episodes. This finding was confirmed by Rooney and colleagues,[21] who also demonstrated that the IL-1ra concentration fluctuates with fever, lagging approximately 1 hour behind the rise and fall of the fever. In contrast, plasma IL-6 levels rose and fell with fever. Thus, IL-6 is at least one of the stimuli for IL-1ra production in systemic JCA. There was no detectable rise and fall of IL-1β in this study. Because it is unclear whether IL-1β was degraded before it was assayed, it remains possible that IL-1β is the stimulus for the increase in IL-6.

TNF-α is also a stimulus of IL-6 synthesis, and serum TNF-α levels have also been detected, although not in temporal relationship to the rise and fall of IL-6.[21] Finally, the soluble receptors of TNF (sTNFR-I and -II) have been found to parallel disease activity in patients with systemic JRA,[18–20, 25, 26] and sTNFR-II was found to parallel fever.[27] TNF:sTNFR ratios in systemic or other types of JRA have not been compared, nor have they been compared with levels in children with febrile infections.

Because anti-inflammatory cytokines are induced by an increased level of pro-inflammatory cytokines, there will always be an oscillating phenomenon if measurements are continuous. The amplitude of the oscillation would depend on the amount of pro-inflammatory cytokines. In systemic JRA, the pulsatile nature of IL-6 levels and the corresponding fever could be due to extremely high levels of IL-6 in the plasma. Exceptionally high levels of IL-6 in systemic JRA have been recorded by many laboratories and may be the result of genetic deregulation of IL-6.

An additional level of complexity is conferred by the function of the IL-6 soluble receptor. There are two receptors for Il-6: the binding receptor IL-6R and the signaling receptor gp130, which signals intracellularly after it binds to the IL-6/IL-6R complex. Many cells such as neurons possess only gp130 and respond only to the complex. Thus soluble IL-6R is an agonist for IL-6. The disease phenotype of systemic JRA involves not only cells expressing both receptors but also cells expressing only gp130. De Benedetti and colleagues[28] demonstrated higher levels of complexes containing IL-6 during the febrile period in these patients. The levels of sIL-6R measured by enzyme-linked immunosorbent assay (ELISA) decreased during the fever peak, probably the result of the binding site to the sIL-6R antibody being masked by sIL-6R complexed with IL-6. Using antibodies that detected complexed IL-6 and sIL-6R, Keul and associates[29] reported that there was a slight increase of sIL-6R during fever but generally high serum sIL-6R levels in systemic compared with other types of JCA. The case for systemic JRA being mediated by IL-6 was well argued in a 1998 editorial by de Benedetti and Martini.[30] Many of the clinical features (fever, hypergammaglobulinemia, thrombocytosis, anemia, and stunted growth) are typical of excessive IL-6 production. In the only study of regulatory cytokine production in systemic JRA, whole blood cultures suggested that IL-10 production was reduced in these patients.[31]

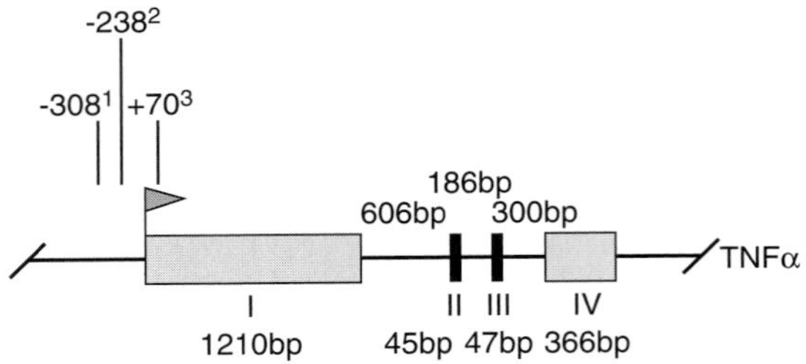

Figure 5–3. Polymorphisms within the *TNFA* locus (6p21). TNF, tumor necrosis factor. Superscripts (1, 2, 3) refer to single nucleotide polymorphisms. (From Walport JM, Duff GW: Cells and mediators of inflammation. *In* Maddison PJ, Isenberg DA, Woo P, Glass DN [eds]: Oxford Textbook of Rheumatology, 2nd ed. Oxford, Oxford University Press, 1998, p 505.)

Cytokine Genes

The cytokine genes themselves may also contribute to disease phenotype. Single-nucleotide polymorphisms in the TNF, IL-1, IL-4, IL-6, and IL-10 genes have been described. The haplotype B8, DR3 is in linkage disequilibrium with a rare allele of TNF-α (TNFA2), which confers high expression of TNF-α.[32] Furthermore, persons who are high producers of TNF-α (TNFA2) have an eightfold increased risk of susceptibility and death from cerebral malaria (Fig. 5–3).[33] Thus, polymorphisms of the regulatory region of cytokine genes can alter pathologic outcomes of diseases. McDowell and colleagues[34] have reported that the IL-1A2 polymorphism is associated with a higher risk of uveitis in Norwegian children with oligoarticular JRA. This observation was not confirmed by Donn and colleagues[35] in English children with comparable disease. However, further studies are needed to determine whether the IL-1 locus influences the development of uveitis in children with oligoarticular JRA.

Current research has identified polymorphisms in the regulatory regions of the IL-6 gene. In particular, a single G/C polymorphism at position −174 determines variable IL-6 gene transcription (Fig. 5–4). There is a significant decrease in the frequency of the protective genotype (CC: low producer of IL-6 on stimulation) in patients in whom the onset of systemic JCA occurs before the age of 5 years.[36] In addition, the single-nucleotide polymorphic haplotype ATA of the

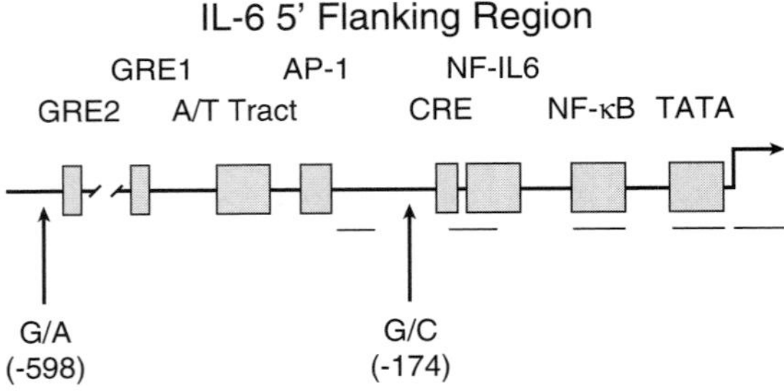

Figure 5–4. Polymorphisms in the 5′ flanking region of the gene of interleukin-6. AP-1, activating protein 1; CRE, cyclic AMP response element; GRE, glucocorticoid receptor response element; IL, interleukin; NF, nuclear factor.

polymorphic IL-10 gene that is associated with low in vitro IL-10 production is associated with more severe inflammation (extended compared with persistent oligoarticular JRA,[37] and severe compared with mild asthma) (Fig. 5–5).[38] A separate study has also indicated that oligoarticular-onset JCA is associated with IL-10; the study used analysis of the microsatellite cluster at 1 kb, which is in linkage disequilibrium with the haplotypes mentioned earlier (R. Donn, personal communication, 1999). Experiments to confirm these genetic associations with the transmission disequilibrium test of nuclear families are in progress. These studies represent a new perspective on effector molecules. More work in this area should yield a "map" of the potential points of deregulation within individual cytokine networks.

Molecular Events Induced by Cytokines

Mechanisms regulating genes concerned with inflammation, such as cytokine genes, could affect the outcome of an encounter with an infectious agent. Defining these factors would allow the development of interventions to remedy undesirable effects. Functional polymorphisms of the responsible genes are only a partial explanation. Cytokines signal by way of their receptors on the cell surface to activate cytoplasmic transcription factors that migrate into the nucleus and bind to DNA, thus initiating the transcription of DNA. Polymorphisms or mutations of the signaling/binding domains of these receptors can result in pathology. For example, mutation in the receptors for IFN-γ and IL-12 can lead to disseminated mycobacterial infections.[39, 40]

Intracellular signaling is a complex, overlapping, multistep process, often involving kinases. The target genes, however, are so far known to be activated by only four transcription factor families. These are: NFkB, C/EPB, STAT, and c-FOS/JUN. The pleiotropism or overlapping functions of many of these cytokines can be explained by the fact that they activate the same transcription factor families. Subtle variations are conferred by whether the cytokines activate homodimers or heterodimers, which have differing affinities for the same DNA binding site on the gene. The DNA structure of the gene in question is important, and a number of the cytokine-inducible factors alter the DNA structure to facilitate binding by factors that are responsible for activating gene transcription (sequestration and ac-

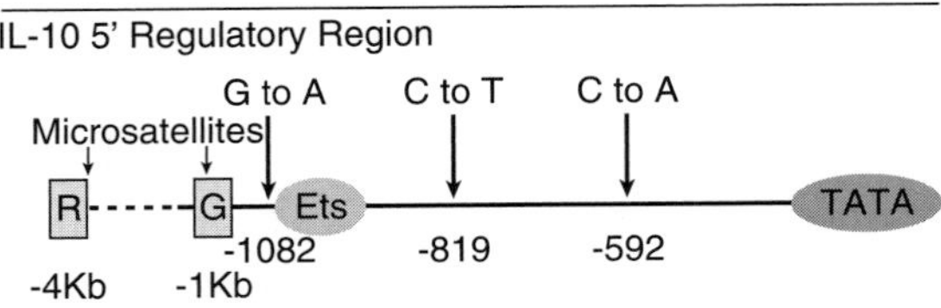

Figure 5–5. Polymorphisms in the 5′ flanking region of the interleukin-10 (IL-10) gene. Microsatellite clusters are at −1 kb and −4 kb. The single-nucleotide polymorphisms are shown by arrows. Caucasians have three haplotypes: GCC, ACC, and ATA.

tivation of RNA polymerase II). Cell specificity is conferred by the fact that the cells may make only one of the transcription factors. Furthermore, synergism between cytokines can occur when transcription factor family members interact.[41] If synergism is downregulated, homeostasis may be more readily restored. It is of interest that some of the most effective anti-inflammatory drugs, such as glucocorticoids and cyclosporin, act intracellularly and interfere with the availability of transcription factors for DNA binding and activation. Glucocorticoids stimulate production of the inhibitor of NFkB, thus preventing its activation[42] as well as interfering with the binding of activated NFkB to DNA.[43] Cyclosporin acts by inhibition of the phosphatase calcineurin, thus preventing nuclear translocation of a component of the transcription factor NFAT1[44] as well as preventing dephosphorylation of NFAT, thereby affecting its binding to DNA.[45] In order to design more rational and specific therapy, the relevant molecules in specific cells must be targeted. Gene delivery systems currently offer the best chance of achieving this targeting.

CHEMOKINES

One area of important research is that of the chemokines. There are many nonspecific leukocyte chemotactic factors: activated complement components C3a/5a, bacteria-derived peptides such as F-Met-Leu-Phe, platelet-activating factor, and lipid metabolites such as leukotrienes. Chemokines, in contrast, have specific actions on leukocytes of particular lineages.[46] They have important functions in the migration of lymphocytes, monocytes, and neutrophils to sites of inflammation. They are released by leukocytes in response to cytokines such as IL-1 and TNF-α. Chemokines are proteins that bind to glycosaminoglycans, thus participating in the regulation of movement of leukocytes along a "bound chemoattractant gradient" (see later). The interaction with their receptors is mediated via the N-terminal region and the exposed loop of the backbone of the molecule between the third and fourth cysteines. The chemokine family has over 40 members. They are small proteins of 8 to 10 kD, with four conserved cysteines forming two essential disulfide bonds. Their classification depends on the proximity of the first two cysteines: CXC, CC, or CX3C. Five receptors for CXC chemokines and eight receptors for CC chemokines have been characterized (Table 5–2). There is redundancy in this system, as there is in the cytokine network (Fig. 5–6).

In allergic inflammation, cells possessing CCR3 chemokine receptors are recruited; they include basophils and eosinophils as well as T_H2 cells (known to be pathogenic in allergic inflammation). T lymphocytes express different chemokine receptors during differentiation and activation. Thus, T_H1-like T cells preferentially express CCR5 and CXCR3, and T_H2-like T cells express CCR2, CCR4, and CXCR2. This division is not absolute; nevertheless, the implication is that the different cells traffic differently and influence the course of the local immune response. For example, CCR5-positive T cells (T_H1-like phenotype) accumulate selectively in the rheumatoid joint (compared with the peripheral blood[47]) and in oligoarticular juvenile idiopathic arthritis (JIA).[15] This could be a selective recruitment due to surface receptors on endothelial cells[48] or the result of the chemokines present in the synovium and synovial fluid. In support of the latter mechanism is the finding that the CCR5 ligands regulated upon activation normal T cell expressed and secreted (RANTES) and macrophage inflammatory protein 1α (MIP-1α) are found at high levels in the synovial fluid in rheumatoid arthritis.

Table 5–2

Human Chemokine Receptors and Their Ligands*

RECEPTOR	CHEMOKINE
CXCR1	IL-8, GCP-2
CXCR2	IL-8, GROα/β/λ, NAP-2, ENA78, GCP-2
CXCR3	IP10, Mig
CXCR4	SDF-1
CXCR5	BCA-1/BLC
CCR1	RANTES, MIP-1α, MCP-2, MCP-3
CCR2	MCP-1, MCP-2, MCP-3, MCP-4
CCR3	Eotaxin, eotaxin-2, RANTES, MCP-2, MCP-3, MCP-4
CCR4†	TARC, RANTES, MIP-1α, MCP-1
CCR5	RANTES, MIP-1α, MIP-1β
CCR6	LARC/MIP-3α/exodus
CCR7	ELC/MIP-3β
CCR8	I-309‡
CX_3CR1	Fraktalkine/neurotacin

IL, interleukin; MCP, monocyte chemotactic protein; MIP, macrophage inflammatory protein; RANTES, regulated upon activation normal T cell expressed and secreted.

*The receptors for the lymphocyte-specific chemokines SLC/6Ckine/exodus-2 and DC-CK1/PARK are unknown.

†There is a disagreement about the selectivity of CCR4, which was first described as a receptor for RANTES, MIP-1α, and MCP-1 and was later shown to be specific for TARC.[48]

‡See references Tiffany HL, Lautrens LL, Gao JL, et al: Identification of CCR8: a human monocyte and thymus receptor for the CC chemokine 1-309. J Exp Med 186: 165–170, 1997; and Roos RS, Loetscher M, Legler DF, et al: Identification of CCR8, the receptor for the human CC chemokine 1-309. J Biol Chem 272: 17251–17254, 1997.

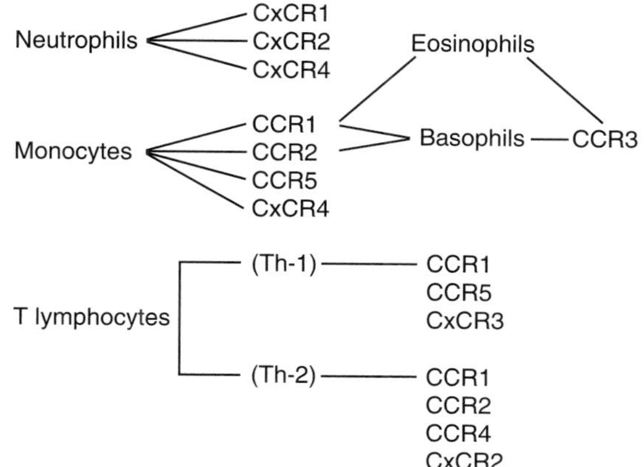

Figure 5–6. Redundancy and specificity of chemokine receptors in different cell types. Th, helper T cells.

Finally, chemokines are involved in homeostatic function in lymphoid tissues. The traffic of T and B lymphocytes through the different tissue compartments is regulated by constitutive tissue expression of chemokines, and the maturation of B lymphocytes, for example, appears to depend at least in part on the presence of specific chemokines such as stromal derived factor 1 (SDF-1).

OTHER HUMORAL PATHWAYS OF INFLAMMATION

Coagulation and Kinin Systems

The coagulation, fibrinolysis, and kinin systems are independent enzyme cascades important in the process of inflammation. They are triggered during recognition of foreign antigens or altered self-antigens and amplify and localize the recognition response. All of these have been found to contribute to tissue injury during inflammation. Activation of the coagulation pathway in particular has been described for systemic JRA,[25, 49] indicating a pro-coagulant state—the precursor for the development of disseminated intravascular coagulopathy.

Neuroendocrine Influence

The endocrine, nervous, and immune systems are interdependent. The important effector molecules in each system have overlapping activities in the other systems. For example, lymphocytes have α-adrenergic receptors.[50] Cytokines are mediators for immune cells, phagocytes, and cells of the nervous system. Nitric oxide is a neurotransmitter, an endothelial relaxant as well as an inducer of inflammatory mediators such as cyclo-oxygenase 2.[51]

Endocrine System and Inflammation

Sex Hormones

Sex steroids or the sensitivity response to sex steroids may contribute to disease. In Caucasian populations, there is a predominantly female distribution of oligoarticular JRA under the age of 5 years and a characteristic association with silent uveitis. There is a predominance of females with SLE over the age of 10 years, and in most patients with SLE, the disease develops between puberty and menopause. Lahita[52] observed several abnormalities of sex hormone metabolism in patients with SLE, including the fact that such patients are hyperestrogenic, with low serum levels of testosterone. In the NZB × NZW F_1 murine model of SLE, androgen protects against the disease, whereas estrogen accelerates its onset and severity. There are relatively more male patients with SLE younger than 10 years and kindreds with multiple male members,[53] so perhaps a Y chromosome gene also confers susceptibility, with effects other than those on sex steroid levels.

Hypothalamic-Pituitary-Adrenal Axis

A number of pro-inflammatory cytokines—IL-1, TNF-α, and IL-6—stimulate the production of corticotropin-releasing hormone (CRH) by the hypothalamus by stimulation of prostanoids.[54, 55] There is positive feedback between CRH and IL-1 and IL-6. CRH stimulates the release of adrenocorticotropic hormone (ACTH) by the pituitary, which in turn stimulates the production of glucocorticoids by the adrenal glands. Because an increase of glucocorticoids downregulates the inflammatory response, defects in this regulatory pathway could lead to persistence of inflammation, a possibility that is supported by evidence from animal models of experimental arthritis. The Lewis rat has an increased susceptibility to antigen-induced arthritis; Fischer rats are resistant. This difference can be attributed to the fact that the CRH response in the Lewis rat is diminished, with a lower level of plasma glucocorticoids after stress.[56] Furthermore, adrenalectomy/hypophysectomy of Fischer rats increases their susceptibility to disease. As far as human rheumatic diseases are concerned, there is preliminary evidence that patients with rheumatoid arthritis may have a blunted cortisol response to surgical stress.[57]

Peripheral release of CRH at sites of inflammation has been described.[58] In contrast to CRH's inhibitory role when produced centrally, local levels of CRH are increased in association with pro-inflammatory effects.[59] Receptors for this hormone can be found on lymphocytes and monocytes.

Neural Influences

The synovium is richly innervated.[60] The normal extension of the fibers to the surface is altered in the inflamed synovium, where the fibers are buried deeper. There is a network of small, unmyelinated afferent C-fibers containing many neurotransmitters, including substance P, neurokinin A, and calcitonin gene–related peptide. Efferent noradrenergic sympathetic fibers surrounding blood vessels also contain neurotransmitters, including neuropeptide Y, which is found mainly in the blood vessels of the synovium and periosteal tissue. Evidence that a neuronal stimulus can induce an inflammatory reaction was first reported by Bayliss in 1901 and Lewis in 1927. They observed that antidromic conduction in sensory neurones was observed for the triple response (redness, flare, and wheal) seen in physical injury to the skin. This reaction was found to be largely mediated by substance P via its vasodilatory activities.[61] The neurotransmitters are analogous to cytokines in the sense that they have pleiotropic effects on a variety of cell types and can stimulate leukocytes and synoviocytes to produce inflammatory compounds.[62] The effects of substance P are summarized in Table 5–3. These effects illustrate how a nociceptive stimulus can initiate acute inflammation.

Other neural influences include reflex inhibition of the musculature around the inflamed joint, leading to rapid wasting of these muscles. The joint is richly innervated by efferent sympathetic nerve fibers that exhibit ongoing and reflex discharges. A high level of systemic sympathetic nervous system activity may influence the severity of arthritis,[63] and blockade of the postsynaptic effects by antagonists at the adrenergic receptors in the tissues partially reduced the severity of the lesions in polyarthritic rats.[64] This may help to explain the anecdotal reports of the effects of stress on the flares of inflammatory disease.

Vascular Changes: Angiogenesis and Nitric Oxide

New blood vessel formation occurs in inflammatory arthritis, in which vessels invade cartilage and bone. The vessels are buried deeper in the synovium, similar to the nervous supply. Many peptides promote angiogenesis: growth factors such as fibroblast growth factors, transforming growth factors α and β, platelet-derived growth factor, the family of endothelial growth factors, and cytokines and chemokines such as TNF-α and IL-8. Although there are no similar published data on childhood inflammatory arthritides, the cytokines found in the joint are similar, and it is likely that neoangiogenesis also occurs.

Nitric oxide is a short-lived free radical with an impressive range of activities (Table 5–4). It was initially described as an endothelium-derived relaxing factor. The effect is extravasation of plasma proteins and fluid. It is synthesized from arginine by the constitutive and inducible nitric oxide synthetases.[65] The inducible synthetases respond to pro-inflammatory cytokines and are responsible for the production of nitric oxide at sites of inflammation. There is evidence that nitric oxide synthesis is increased in human inflammatory arthritis,[66] in adjuvant arthritis in rats,[67] and in the MRL-lpr/lpr mice.[68] The osteoporosis associated with inflammatory rheumatic diseases could also be attributed to the effect of the stimulation of nitric oxide production from osteoblasts by cytokines.[69]

Table 5–3

Pleiotropic Effects of Substance P

TARGET CELL	EFFECT OF SUBSTANCE P
Synoviocyte	Prostaglandin E_2 synthesis Collagenase synthesis Cell division
Neutrophil	Promotion of chemotaxis Degranulation Promotion of phagocytosis
Mast cell	Degranulation
Macrophage	Thromboxane B_2 synthesis
T lymphocyte	Proliferation

Table 5–4

Biologic Effects of Nitric Oxide

SYSTEM/CELLS	EFFECT
Cardiovascular	Endothelium-dependent relaxation
Central nervous system	Neurotransmitter, memory
Peripheral nervous system	Sensory transmission, noradrenergic mediator of vasodilation
Gastrointestinal/genitourinary	Dilator tone
Platelets	Inhibit aggregation and adhesion
Macrophages/neutrophils	Cytostatic/cytotoxic (in conjunction with respiratory cycle enzymes)

CELLULAR COMPONENTS OF INFLAMMATION

Endothelium

Traditional discussions of the cellular components of inflammation describe the neutrophil as the major player, but the endothelium is worthy of first consideration because it presents a barrier between the circulation and the synovium and extracellular connective tissues. It is important in the delivery of blood to sites of inflammation and in the regulation of cell traffic and plasma proteins from the circulation. Adhesion of leukocytes to the luminal surface of the vascular endothelial cells is the first step in their transmigration from the blood to the tissues. Such interactions regulate the number and type of cells and thus the nature and the progression of the inflammatory response. Leukocytes normally roll along the endothelial surface, and adhesion occurs via the expression of adhesion molecules, or integrins, on both cell types.

There are three classes of adhesion molecules. The first consists of the selectin family, single-chain integral membrane glycoproteins that bind oligosaccharide motifs expressed on glycoproteins and glycolipids; these molecules are responsible for tethering of leukocytes to endothelial cells (Table 5–5). The second group comprises the integrins, which are heterodimeric glycoproteins connecting the cytoskeleton to the extracellular environment (Table 5–6). The third group comprises the immunoglobulin superfamily molecules such as intercellular adhesion molecules (ICAM)-1, -2, and -3; vascular cell adhesion molecule (VCAM)-1; and mucosal addressin cell adhesion molecule (MAdCAM)-1, all of which act as adhesion ligands for integrins. The concept of the "adhesion cascade" has been proposed

Table 5–5

The Selectin Family

TYPE	CELL DISTRIBUTION
L-Selectin	Leukocytes
P-Selectin	Endothelial cells Platelets
E-Selectin	Endothelial cells

Table 5–6

The Integrins

TYPE	CELL DISTRIBUTION	LIGANDS
LFA-1 ($\alpha^L\beta_2$)	All leukocytes	ICAM-1, -2, -3
CR3 ($\alpha^M\beta_2$)	PMN, Mo, LGL, Bp, Eo	ICAM-1, iC3b fibrinogen, factor X, β-glucan
VLA1-6	Mainly different subtypes of T lymphocytes + EC	Collagens I and IV, fibronectin
Vitronectin receptor	Activated T, Mo, NK, EC	Vitronectin, fibronectin, laminin, VWF, thrombospondin, fibrinogen

Bp, basophils; CR3, complement receptor 3; EC, endothelial cells; Eo, eosinophils; ICAM, intercellular adhesion molecule; LFA-1, leukocyte function–associated antigen-1; LGL, large granular lymphocytes; Mo, monocytes; NK, natural killer cells; PMN, polymorphonuclear leukocytes; VLA, very late activation antigen; VWF, von Willebrand factor.

to account for the specificity of leukocytes migrating into different tissues. Whether the leukocyte migrates depends on its participation in a series of selective adhesion and activation events.[70, 71]

The rolling leukocyte is thought to be stimulated by molecules on the endothelial surface, such as selectins, or chemokines bound to membrane glycosaminoglycans.[72] Rapid stimulation of endothelial cells by histamine, thrombin, C3a/5a, or the terminal complement complex leads to secretion of prostacyclin and nitric oxide, decreasing vascular tone, and surface expression of platelet-derived growth factor and P-selectin, which are thought to initiate the early phases of leukocyte adhesion. Firm integrin-mediated adhesion to the immunoglobulin superfamily molecules (such as ICAM-1, ICAM-2, and VCAM-1) follows. Transmigration through the endothelial basement membrane[73] occurs by mechanisms that are incompletely understood.

One of the steps for granulocytes and monocytes appears to be the enzymatic cleavage of L-selectin to the leukocyte cell surface, leading to de-adhesion from the endothelial luminal surface. What signal(s) guides the migrating leukocyte is also unclear, but two-way signaling events and a chemoattractant gradient appear to be involved. The latter is enhanced by prior activation of endothelial cells by cytokines. Cytokines such as IL-1, TNF-α, and lipopolysaccharide (LPS) stimulate the expression of adhesion molecules involved in the "adhesion cascade": E-selectin, P-selectin, ICAM-1, VCAM-1, and MAdCAM-1. The endothelial cell is stimulated to secrete cytokines (IL-1 and -6, granulocyte colony-stimulating factor [G-CSF], GM-CSF, and macrophage colony-stimulating factor [M-CSF]), platelet-derived growth factor, and chemokines such as IL-8 and monocyte chemotactic protein 1 (MCP-1). An example of two-way signaling is that the T-cell cytokines IFN-γ and IL-4 can further modify the expression of these chemokines (e.g., IFN-γ increases IL-8 synthesis but has no effect on MCP-1). Endothelial cells may express HLA class II and function as APCs. They utilize a different set of accessory molecules than bone marrow–derived APCs, thereby activating a different subset of T cells (CD45RO-positive, B7-independent).[74]

The adhesion molecules involved in the transmigration through the endothelium are similar to those needed for the initial firm adhesion to the luminal surfaces. A role for CD31 has also been proposed.[75, 76] Finally, the penetration of the basal lamina, which is composed of collagen and matrix proteins, is not well understood but probably involves the secretion of degradative enzymes.[77]

Granulocytes

Neutrophils, eosinophils, basophils, and mast cells collectively provide a vital mechanism for the removal of bacteria and parasites. Genetic deficiencies of neutrophil function lead to pyogenic, opportunistic, and fungal infections. The respiratory burst and release of enzymes from granules are the effector mechanisms of the neutrophil. They are triggered by a signal transmitted via neutrophil receptors. Characteristics of the four classes of neutrophil receptors are summarized in Table 5–7. Multivalent binding appears to be necessary to induce the full neutrophil response.

The cytoplasmic granules contain densely packed proteases assembled in a mucopolysaccharide matrix that participate in cell migration and bacterial killing. They include general proteases such as elastase, cathepsin G, lysozyme, gelatinase, myeloperoxidase, and collagenase. They also include enzymes directly toxic to bacteria and parasites, such as defensins, bactericidal/permeability-increasing protein, lactoferrin, and B_{12}-binding protein. These granules also act as stores for other membrane receptors such as complement receptors CR1 and CR3. The precise signal for degranulation is unknown.

Granulocytes, in common with other phagocytic cells such as macrophages, require extra consumption

Table 5–7

Neutrophil Receptors

RECEPTOR	LIGANDS
Growth	
Colony-stimulating factors	Granulocytes, monocytes
Cytokine receptors	IL-1, IFN-γ, TNF-α, TNF-β
Opsonic receptors	
Fc	Immune-complexed IgG
CR1 and CR3	Complement C3b and iC3b
Chemotaxis	
C5a receptor	C5a
f-Met-Leu-Phe	Bacterial products

Ig, immunoglobulin; IL, interleukin; TNF, tumor necrosis factor.

of oxygen after engulfing bacteria: the *respiratory burst*. Without this respiratory burst, killing of ingested organisms does not take place, as in chronic granulomatous disease. The consumption of oxygen generates free radicals, myeloperoxidase-catalyzed halogenation, and alkalization of the phagocytic vacuole. Degranulation and release of enzymes follow, but the mechanism is unclear. In chronic granulomatous disease, there is a genetic deficiency of the NADPH (reduced form of nicotinamide adenine dinucleotide phosphate) oxidase system, a membrane-bound electron transport complex that feeds electrons across the phagocytic vacuole to molecular oxygen and generates superoxide radicals.[78] Thus, it appears that the generation of superoxide radicals is intimately related to the final killing of the engulfed bacteria.

In chronic arthritides, neutrophils are present in large numbers at sites of inflammation. The half-life of a neutrophil is 7 hours, and the production rate is 1.63 $\times$ 10^9 cells/kg/day. Therefore, phagocytosis of dead cells without further stimulation of the macrophage is critical. Programmed cell death (apoptosis) is the mechanism whereby dead neutrophils are phagocytosed without stimulating the phagocyte. Defects in apoptosis could lead to inflammation; such defects have been found in autoimmune animal models: lpr mice (mutations of the Fas gene) and gld mice (mutations of the FasL gene). The result is an inflammatory multisystem lymphoproliferative syndrome. Human lymphoproliferative syndromes (Canale-Smith syndrome and subgroups of SLE) also carry mutations in Fas.[79, 80]

Monocytes and Macrophages

The activities of these cells overlap those of the granulocytes in that they are phagocytic cells that require the respiratory burst to kill organisms. These cells do not have granules but are nevertheless cytolytic. In addition, they synthesize a large number of pro-inflammatory and regulatory cytokines and chemokines as well as C2, C3, C1 inhibitor and Factor B of the complement pathways. Because the cytokine network is crucial to the process of inflammation, monocytes are key cells in the regulation of the inflammatory process. In addition, they express HLA molecules and can act as APCs. These cells are long-lived and exist at different stages of activation and differentiation, depending on their location. The synovium, for example, is composed of fibroblasts and resident macrophages known as *type-A lining cells*. Monocytes are recruited to sites of inflammation by a number of factors. The T-cell cytokine IFN-γ is a potent monocyte activator and differentiator. IFN-γ also primes the macrophage to respond to other activating agents, such as LPS or immune complexes containing C3.

In systemic JRA, there is clinical and laboratory evidence of high levels of pro-inflammatory cytokine release, and the term *macrophage activation syndrome* has been coined to describe an acute systemic flare, often after a viral infection, with derangement of liver function and a procoagulant state.[81] The term *hemophagocytic syndrome* is also applied to this state because hemophagocytosis is present in the bone marrow aspirate.

Fibroblasts

The second cell type in the synovium is a fibroblast, the *type-B lining cell*. These cells also participate in inflammatory arthritis by secreting prostanoids, cytokines, matrix proteinases such as metalloproteinases, and their inhibitors. They also secrete matrix components such as hyaluronan. These cells are susceptible to stimulation not only by soluble cytokines but also by membrane-associated cytokines from direct contact with T lymphocytes.[82]

MECHANISMS OF JOINT DAMAGE

A variety of effector mechanisms lead to a number of damaging consequences in children with chronic arthritis. These are the release of free radicals, proteinases, prostaglandins, and leukotrienes.

Free Radicals

Free radicals derived from oxygen include superoxide ($O^-{}_2$), hydroxyl (OH), and hydrogen peroxide (H_2O_2). They are generated during oxidative metabolism, and their existence is transient, both extracellularly and intracellularly. The evidence that they contribute to inflammation is based on demonstration of molecular and tissue injury that is compatible with the effects of free radicals, as shown by in vitro experiments.[83] Free radicals are strong candidates for mediators of extracellular degradation of hyaluronic acid, immunoglobulin aggregation, and collagen degradation. They can inactivate enzymes such as α_1-proteinase inhibitor (previously known as α_1-antitrypsin) by oxidation of its methionine residue; this results in pro-inflammatory phenomena because its substrates (e.g., elastase) are not inactivated.

The main source of free radicals in the joint is the phagocyte, stimulated by adherence to matrix proteins or ligand binding of its receptor molecules such as Fc receptors. A second potential source of free radicals in the joint is hypoxic reperfusion injury.[84] How much the transient free radicals generated within the joint contribute to inflammation remains unresolved at this time.[83]

Metalloproteinases, Other Neutral Proteinases, and Their Inhibitors

Native and denatured collagen is degraded by a family of matrix metalloproteinases: collagenases and gelatinases, respectively.[85, 86] Stromelysins cleave core proteoglycan, laminin, and fibronectin. They are secreted by fibroblasts, osteoblasts, chondrocytes, neutrophils, macrophages, and endothelium. Thus, similar to the case with other inflammatory systems, the balance between these enzymes and their inhibitors determines the amount of tissue damage and repair. Metalloproteinase inhibitors have been used therapeutically in animal models of inflammation.

Overlap with the cytokine network has been described.[87, 88] A metalloproteinase is responsible for cleavage of TNFR from the cell surface to produce soluble TNFR, an antagonist of TNF-α. Thus, these enzymes have an indirect anti-inflammatory effect. Neutral proteinases of neutrophils such as cathepsin G and elastase may be potential mediators of tissue damage. However, beige mice, deficient in both of these enzymes, do not show any diminution of antigen-induced synovitis.

Prostaglandins and Leukotrienes

The importance of these eicosanoids in joint pathology is implied by the widespread efficacy of drugs that interfere with their production, the cyclo-oxygenase inhibitors. Membrane phospholipids are converted into arachidonic acid by phospholipase A_2, which is induced by pro-inflammatory cytokines such as IL-1. Cyclo-oxygenases 1 and 2 (COX-1 and COX-2) catalyze the cleavage of arachidonic acid into prostaglandin H_2, the precursor of prostaglandins and thromboxane. Arachidonic acid also gives rise to leukotrienes via the lipoxygenase pathway (Fig. 5–7). Although cyclo-oxygenases are ubiquitous, lipoxygenases are restricted to monocytes, macrophages, and granulocytes. Lipoxygenases also catalyze the cleavage of eicosapentaenoic acid, resulting in the production of pentanoic leukotrienes, which are biologically less potent than leukotrienes from arachidonic acid. This could form the basis of the reported anti-inflammatory effects of diets rich in fish oils. Products of both pathways are potentially pro-inflammatory, however. Prostaglandins cause vasodilatation of the microcirculation; amplify edema caused by other agents, such as bradykinin; and sensitize pain receptors. Leukotriene B_4 acts as a chemotaxin for neutrophils and increases their adhesion to endothelial cells. However, prostaglandins can also be anti-inflammatory by suppressing the synthesis of IL-1 and TNF,[89] another example of a negative feedback within the cytokine network.

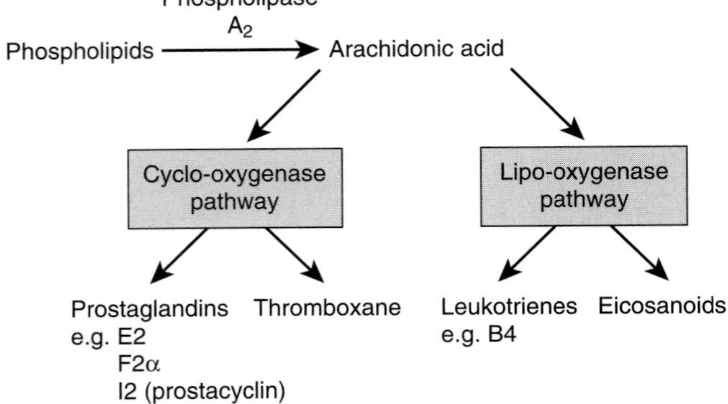

Figure 5–7. Arachidonic acid metabolism.

Recent interest has focused on inhibition of COX-1 or -2 in the therapy of inflammatory arthritis. COX-1 is constitutively expressed in many cells, including the gastric mucosa; COX-2 is expressed selectively at sites of inflammation because it is inducible by cytokines.[90] The first COX-1 inhibitor, aspirin, was followed by the great variety of nonsteroidal anti-inflammatory drugs currently on the market. These have variable effects on the gastric mucosa. Selective COX-2 inhibitors are reported to have anti-inflammatory effects without producing gastrointestinal side effects (see Chapter 7).

CONCLUSIONS

The complexity of the mechanisms of inflammation is daunting. They exhibit a high degree of redundancy and interactive positive and negative feedback mechanisms. Characterization of genetic deficiencies and the new technology, such as production of "gene knockout" animals, will greatly contribute to understanding pivotal points within the cascades or networks of inflammatory mediators and cells. Until such pivotal compounds are identified, it is unlikely that pharmacologic manipulation will fully address the therapeutic challenge of the control of inflammation.

References

1. Moroldo MB, Donnelly P, Saunders J, et al: Transmission disequilibrium as a test of linkage and association between HLA alleles and pauciarticular-onset juvenile rheumatoid arthritis. Arthritis Rheum 41: 1620, 1998.
2. Murray KJ, Moroldo MB, Donnelly P, et al: Age specific effects of JRA-associated HLA alleles. Arthritis Rheum 42: 1843–1853, 1999.
3. Morgan BP, Walport MJ: Complement deficiency and disease. Immunol Today 12: 301, 1991.
4. Bowness P, Davies KA, Norsworthy PJ, et al: Hereditary C1q deficiency and systemic lupus erythematosus. Q J Med 87: 455, 1994.
5. Hauptmann G, Goetz J, Uring-Lambert B, et al: Component deficiencies. 2: The fourth component. Prog Allergy 39: 232, 1986.
6. Ruddy S: Component deficiencies. 3: The second component. Prog Allergy 39: 250, 1986.
7. Botto M, Alport MJ: Hereditary deficiency of C3 in animals and humans. Int Rev Immunol 10: 37, 1993.
8. Botto M, Dell'Agnola C, Bygrave AE, et al: Homozygous C1q deficiency causes glomerulonephritis associated with multiple apoptotic bodies. Nat Genet 19: 56, 1998.
9. Davies KA, Erlendsson K, Beynon HL, et al: Splenic uptake of immune complexes in man is complement-dependent. J Immunol 151: 3866, 1993.
10. Abbas AK, Murphy KM, Sher A: Functional diversity of helper T lymphocytes. Nature 383: 787, 1996.
11. Katz JD, Benoist C, Mathis D: T helper cell subsets in insulin-dependent diabetes. Science 268: 1185, 1995.
12. Miller SD, McRae BL, Vanderlugt CL, et al: Evolution of the T-cell repertoire during the course of experimental immune-mediated demyelinating diseases. Immunol Rev 144: 225, 1995.
13. Schulze-Koops H, Lipsky PE, Kavanaugh AF, et al: Elevated Th1- or Th0-like cytokine mRNA in peripheral circulation of patients with rheumatoid arthritis. Modulation by treatment with anti-

ICAM-1 correlates with clinical benefit. J Immunol 155: 5029, 1995.
14. Gattorno M, Facchetti P, Ghiotto F, et al: Synovial fluid T cell clones from oligoarticular juvenile arthritis patients display a prevalent Th1/Th0-type pattern of cytokine secretion irrespective of immunophenotype. Clin Exp Immunol 109: 4, 1997.
15. Wedderburn LR, Robinson N, Patel A, et al: Selective recruitment of polarized T cells expressing CCR5 and CXCR3 to the inflamed joints of children with juvenile idiopathic arthritis. Arthritis Rheum 43:765–774, 2000.
16. Murray KJ, Grom AA, Thompson SD, et al: Contrasting cytokine profiles in the synovium of different forms of juvenile rheumatoid arthritis and juvenile spondyloarthropathy: prominence of interleukin 4 in restricted disease. J Rheumatol 25: 1388, 1998.
17. Miller LC, Isa S, Vannier E, et al: Live *Borrelia burgdorferi* preferentially activate interleukin-1 beta gene expression and protein synthesis over the interleukin-1 receptor antagonist. J Clin Invest 90: 906, 1992.
18. Lepore L, Pennesi M, Saletta S, et al: Study of IL-2, IL-6, TNF alpha, IFN gamma and beta in the serum and synovial fluid of patients with juvenile chronic arthritis. Clin Exp Rheumatol 12: 561, 1994.
19. Madson KL, Moore TL, Lawrence JM, et al: Cytokine levels in serum and synovial fluid of patients with juvenile rheumatoid arthritis. J Rheumatol 21: 2359, 1994.
20. Mangge H, Kenzian H, Gallistl S, et al: Serum cytokines in juvenile rheumatoid arthritis. Correlation with conventional inflammation parameters and clinical subtypes. Arthritis Rheum 38: 211, 1995.
21. Rooney M, David J, Symmons J, et al: Inflammatory cytokine responses in juvenile chronic arthritis. Br J Rheumatol 34: 454, 1995.
22. Rooney M, Varsani H, Martin K, et al: Tumour necrosis factor alpha (TNFα) and its soluble receptors in juvenile chronic arthritis (JCA). Rheumatology 39: 432–438, 2000.
23. de Benedetti F, Pignatti P, Gerloni V, et al: Differences in synovial fluid cytokine levels between juvenile and adult rheumatoid arthritis. J Rheumatol 24: 1403, 1997.
24. Prieur AM, Kaufmann MT, Griscelli C, et al: Specific interleukin-1 inhibitor in serum and urine of children with systemic juvenile chronic arthritis. Lancet 2: 1240, 1987.
25. de Benedetti F, Pignatti P, Massa M, et al: Soluble tumour necrosis factor receptor levels reflect coagulation abnormalities in systemic juvenile chronic arthritis. Br J Rheumatol 36: 581, 1997.
26. Gattorno M, Picco P, Buoncompagni A, et al: Serum p55 and p75 tumour necrosis factor receptors as markers of disease activity in juvenile chronic arthritis. Ann Rheum Dis 55: 243, 1996.
27. Prieur AM, Roux-Lombard P, Dayer JM: Dynamics of fever and the cytokine network in systemic juvenile arthritis. Rev Rheum Engl Ed 63: 163, 1996.
28. de Benedetti F, Massa M, Pignatti P, et al: Serum soluble interleukin 6 (IL-6) receptor and IL-6/soluble IL-6 receptor complex in systemic juvenile rheumatoid arthritis. J Clin Invest 93: 2114, 1994.
29. Keul R, Heinrich PC, Muller-Newen G, et al: A possible role for soluble IL-6 receptor in the pathogenesis of systemic-onset juvenile chronic arthritis. Cytokine 10: 729, 1998.
30. de Benedetti F, Martini A: Is systemic juvenile rheumatoid arthritis an interleukin 6 mediated disease? J Rheumatol 25: 203, 1998.
31. Müller K, Herner EB, Stagg A, et al: Inflammatory cytokines and cytokine antagonists in whole blood cultures of patients with systemic juvenile rheumatoid arthritis. Br J Rheumatol 37: 562, 1998.
32. Wilson AG, di Giovine FS, Duff GW: Genetics of tumour necrosis factor-alpha in autoimmune, infectious, and neoplastic diseases. J Inflamm 45: 1, 1995.
33. McGuire W, Hill AV, Allsopp CE, et al: Variation in the TNF-alpha promoter region associated with susceptibility to cerebral malaria. Nature 371: 508, 1994.
34. McDowell TL, Symons JA, Ploski R, et al: A genetic association between juvenile rheumatoid arthritis and a novel interleukin-1 alpha polymorphism. Arthritis Rheum 38: 221, 1995.
35. Donn RP, Farhan AJ, Barrett JH, et al: Absence of association between interleukin 1 alpha and oligoarticular juvenile chronic arthritis in UK patients. Rheumatology (Oxford) 38: 171, 1999.
36. Fishman D, Faulds G, Jeffery R, et al: The effect of novel polymorphisms in the interleukin-6 (IL-6) gene on IL-6 transcription and plasma IL-6 levels, and an association with systemic-onset juvenile chronic arthritis. J Clin Invest 102: 1369, 1998.
37. Crawley E, Kay R, Sillibourne J, et al: Polymorphic haplotypes of the interleukin-10 5′ flanking region determine variable interleukin-10 transcription and are associated with particular phenotypes of juvenile rheumatoid arthritis. Arthritis Rheum 42: 1101, 1999.
38. Lim S, Crawley E, Woo P, et al: A haplotype associated with low IL-10 production is more common in patients with severe asthma. Lancet 352: 113, 1998.
39. Jouanguy E, Altare F, Lamhamedi S, et al: Interferon-gamma-receptor deficiency in an infant with fatal bacille Calmette-Guérin infection. N Engl J Med 335: 1956, 1996.
40. de Jong E, Altare F, Haagen IA, et al: Severe mycobacterial and salmonella infections in interleukin-12-receptor-deficient patients. Science 280: 1435, 1998.
41. Betts JC, Cheshire J, Akira S, et al: The role of NFκB and NFIL6 transactivating factors in the synergistic activation of human serum amyloid A gene expression by interleukin 1 and interleukin 6. J Biol Chem 268: 25624, 1993.
42. Scheinman RI, Cogswell PC, Lofquist AK, et al: Role of transcriptional activation of I kappa B alpha in mediation of immunosuppression by glucocorticoids. Science 270: 283, 1995.
43. Liden J, Delaunay F, Rafter I, et al: A new function for the C-terminal zinc finger of the glucocorticoid receptor. Repression of RelA transactivation. J Biol Chem 272: 21467, 1997.
44. Luo C, Burgeon E, Carew JA, et al: Recombinant NFAT1 (NFATp) is regulated by calcineurin in T cells and mediates transcription of several cytokine genes. Mol Cell Biol 16: 3955, 1996.
45. Park J, Yaseen NR, Hogan PG, et al: Phosphorylation of the transcription factor NFATp inhibits its DNA binding activity in cyclosporin A-treated human B and T cells. J Biol Chem 270: 20653, 1995.
46. Baggiolini M: Chemokines and leukocyte traffic. Nature 392: 565, 1998.
47. Suzuki N, Nakajima A, Yoshino S, et al: Selective accumulation of CCR5+ T lymphocytes into inflamed joints of rheumatoid arthritis. Int Immunol 11: 553, 1999.
48. Gerszten RE, Garcia-Zepeda EA, Lim YC, et al: MCP-1 and IL-8 trigger firm adhesion of monocytes to vascular endothelium under flow conditions. Nature 398: 718, 1999.
49. Inamo Y, Pemberton S, Tuddenham EG, et al: Increase of activated factor VIIA and haemostatic molecular markers in juvenile chronic arthritis. Br J Rheumatol 34: 466, 1995.
50. Heijnen CJ, Rouppe VD, Wulffraat N, et al: Functional alpha 1-adrenergic receptors on leukocytes of patients with polyarticular juvenile rheumatoid arthritis. J Neuroimmunol 71: 223, 1996.
51. Salvemini D, Misko TP, Masferrer JL, et al: Nitric oxide activates cyclooxygenase enzymes. Proc Natl Acad Sci U S A 90: 7240, 1993.
52. Lahita RG: Sex hormones as immunomodulators of disease. Ann N Y Acad Sci 685: 278, 1993.
53. Lahita RG, Chiorazzi N, Gibofsky A, et al: Familial systemic lupus erythematosus in males. Arthritis Rheum 26: 39, 1983.
54. Buller KM, Xu Y, Day TA: Indomethacin attenuates oxytocin and hypothalamic-pituitary-adrenal axis responses to systemic interleukin-1 beta. J Neuroendocrinol 10: 519, 1998.
55. van der Meer MJ, Sweep CG, Rijnkels CE, et al: Acute stimulation of the hypothalamic-pituitary-adrenal axis by IL-1 beta, TNF alpha and IL-6: a dose response study. J Endocrinol Invest 19: 175, 1996.
56. Wilder RL: Hormones and autoimmunity: animal models of arthritis. Baillieres Clin Rheumatol 10: 259, 1996.
57. Chikanza IC, Petrou P, Kingsley G, et al: Defective hypothalamic response to immune and inflammatory stimuli in patients with rheumatoid arthritis. Arthritis Rheum 35: 1281, 1992.
58. Karalis K, Sano H, Redwine J, et al: Autocrine or paracrine inflammatory actions of corticotrophin-releasing hormone in vivo. Science 254: 421, 1991.
59. Crofford LJ, Sano H, Karalis K, et al: Corticotrophin-releasing hormone in synovial fluids and tissues of patients with rheumatoid arthritis and osteoarthritis. J Immunol 151: 1587, 1993.
60. Kidd BL, Mapp PI, Blake DR, et al: Neurogenic influences in arthritis. Ann Rheum Dis 49: 649, 1990.

61. Garrett NE, Mapp PI, Cruwys SC, et al: Role of substance P in inflammatory arthritis. Ann Rheum Dis 51: 1014, 1992.
62. Levine JD, Goetzl EJ, Basbaum AI: Contribution of the nervous system to the pathophysiology of rheumatoid arthritis and other polyarthritides. Rheum Dis Clin North Am 13: 369, 1987.
63. Kidd BL, Cruwys S, Mapp PI, et al: Role of the sympathetic nervous system in chronic joint pain and inflammation. Ann Rheum Dis 51: 1188, 1992.
64. Schaible HG, Grubb BD: Afferent and spinal mechanisms of joint pain. Pain 55: 5, 1993.
65. Moncada S, Higgs A: The L-arginine-nitric oxide pathway. N Engl J Med 329: 2002, 1993.
66. Kaur H, Halliwell B: Evidence for nitric oxide-mediated oxidative damage in chronic inflammation. Nitrotyrosine in serum and synovial fluid from rheumatoid patients. FEBS Lett 350: 9, 1994.
67. Stefanovic-Racic M, Meyers K, Meschter C, et al: N-monomethyl arginine, an inhibitor of nitric oxide synthase, suppresses the development of adjuvant arthritis in rats. Arthritis Rheum 37: 1062, 1994.
68. Weinberg JB, Granger DL, Pisetsky DS, et al: The role of nitric oxide in the pathogenesis of spontaneous murine autoimmune disease: increased nitric oxide production and nitric oxide synthase expression in MRL-lpr/lpr mice, and reduction of spontaneous glomerulonephritis and arthritis by orally administered NG-monomethyl-L-arginine. J Exp Med 179: 651, 1994.
69. Ralston SH, Todd D, Helfrich M, et al: Human osteoblast-like cells produce nitric oxide and express inducible nitric oxide synthase. Endocrinology 135: 330, 1994.
70. Butcher EC: Leukocyte-endothelial cell recognition: three (or more) steps to specificity and diversity. Cell 67: 1033, 1991.
71. Springer TA: Traffic signals for lymphocyte recirculation and leukocyte emigration: the multistep paradigm. Cell 76: 301, 1994.
72. Webb LM, Ehrengruber MU, Clark-Lewis I, et al: Binding to heparan sulfate or heparin enhances neutrophil responses to interleukin 8. Proc Natl Acad Sci U S A 90: 7158, 1993.
73. Smith ME, Ford WL: The recirculating lymphocyte pool of the rat: a systematic description of the migratory behaviour of recirculating lymphocytes. Immunology 49: 83, 1983.
74. Rose ML: Endothelial cells as antigen-presenting cells: role in human transplant rejection. Cell Mol Life Sci 54: 965, 1998.
75. Vaporciyan AA, DeLisser HM, Yan HC, et al: Involvement of platelet-endothelial cell adhesion molecule-1 in neutrophil recruitment in vivo. Science 262: 1580, 1993.
76. Bogen S, Pak J, Garifallou M, et al: Monoclonal antibody to murine PECAM-1 (CD31) blocks acute inflammation in vivo. J Exp Med 179: 1059, 1994.
77. Romanic AM, Madri JA: The induction of 72-kD gelatinase in T cells upon adhesion to endothelial cells is VCAM-1 dependent. J Cell Biol 125: 1165, 1994.
78. Segal AW: The NADPH oxidase and chronic granulomatous disease. Mol Med Today 2: 129, 1996.
79. Nagata S: Human autoimmune lymphoproliferative syndrome, a defect in the apoptosis-inducing Fas receptor: a lesson from the mouse model. J Hum Genet 43: 2, 1998.
80. Wu J, Wilson J, He J, et al: Fas ligand mutation in a patient with systemic lupus erythematosus and lymphoproliferative disease. J Clin Invest 98: 1107, 1996.
81. Mouy R, Stephan JL, Pillet P, et al: Efficacy of cyclosporine A in the treatment of macrophage activation syndrome in juvenile arthritis: report of five cases. J Pediatr 129: 750, 1996.
82. Burger D, Rezzonico R, Li JM, et al: Imbalance between interstitial collagenase and tissue inhibitor of metalloproteinase 1 in synoviocytes and fibroblasts upon direct contact with stimulated T lymphocytes: involvement of membrane-associated cytokines. Arthritis Rheum 41: 1748, 1998.
83. Hogg N: Free radicals in disease. Semin Reprod Endocrinol 16: 241, 1998.
84. McCord JM: Oxygen-derived free radicals in postischemic tissue injury. N Engl J Med 312: 159, 1985.
85. Docherty AJ, Murphy G: The tissue metalloproteinase family and the inhibitor TIMP: a study using cDNAs and recombinant proteins. Ann Rheum Dis 49: 469, 1990.
86. Murphy G, Willenbrock F: Tissue inhibitors of matrix metalloendopeptidases. Methods Enzymol 248: 496, 1995.
87. Gearing AJ, Beckett P, Christodoulou M, et al: Processing of tumour necrosis factor-alpha precursor by metalloproteinases. Nature 370: 555, 1994.
88. Mohler KM, Sleath PR, Fitzner JN, et al: Protection against a lethal dose of endotoxin by an inhibitor of tumour necrosis factor processing. Nature 370: 218, 1994.
89. Pettifer ER, Higgs GA, Salmon JA: Eicosanoids (prostaglandins and leukotrienes). *In* Whicher J, Evans S (eds): Biochemistry of Inflammation. Dordrecht, The Netherlands, Kluwer, 1992, pp 91–108.
90. Dubois RN, Abramson SB, Crofford L, et al: Cyclooxygenase in biology and disease. FASEB J 12: 1063, 1998.

6

Genomics

David N. Glass

When viewed from the perspective of the pediatric rheumatology clinic, few patients with arthritis appear to have genetically determined diseases. Family histories are rarely positive for the more common diseases, including juvenile rheumatoid arthritis (JRA), and those diseases with a mendelian pattern of inheritance are especially uncommon. Few extended families with chronic pediatric rheumatologic illnesses suitable for traditional linkage studies have been reported. Pediatric rheumatic diseases share this scenario with autoimmune diseases in general, in which the absence of family history is the usual experience. The paradoxical view that these diseases, including the subtypes of JRA, are genetically based is considered in this context; in addition, it is commonly hypothesized that this genetic effect extends not only to a primary predisposition but also to variation in the extent and severity of disease (i.e., many, if not all, aspects of disease phenotype are also genetically determined, whether it be JRA, systemic lupus erythematosus [SLE], scleroderma, or dermatomyositis).

The presence of human leukocyte antigen (HLA) associations in most of these diseases already provides some indication of their genetic nature, although for many years HLA or HLA-linked genes were not necessarily perceived to be central to pathogenesis. It is argued herein that they are a necessary part of genetic predisposition (although only a component) and that other non–major histocompatibility complex (MHC) genes predispose to the disease in a given individual. This does not exclude an environmental component. It is timely to note that the enormous explosion in knowledge from the Human Genome Project and its related technological advances allows questions to be asked and tested about the role of genes in all diseases, not just those traditionally viewed as having a genetic basis.

Current molecular technology not only allows screening of DNA but also can track newly identified genes through to their expressed product and then to their function; thus, the traditional approach, starting from a disease phenotype and then identifying the gene, can be reversed. One must review knowledge of the genome with respect to genes and polymorphic variability before discussing the genetic component in pediatric rheumatic diseases and whether they have traditional mendelian patterns of inheritance.

THE GENOME

The *genome* can be defined as the individual's (or cell's) total genetic information. The related science of mapping, sequencing, and analyzing genomes is known as *genomics*. The Human Genome Project, started in 1990 and proceeding at an accelerating pace, should complete a physical and DNA sequence map of the human genome well ahead of the 2003 target. The working draft announced in spring 2000 reports assembled sequences for approximately 85 percent of the genome.[1] This map will be the basis for understanding gene function and its pathophysiology. A complete description of this project can be found at *http://www.nhgri.nih.gov/HGP/*

Structure

At the DNA level, genetic information consists of over 3×10^9 base pairs organized into three components: paired autosomal chromosomes, two sex chromosomes, and mitochondrial DNA. A large part of this genetic material is aggregated into repetitive sequences that contribute, as either long or short interspersed sequences, to the familiar banding pattern that characterizes the morphology of chromosomes. The remainder is single copy DNA, about 10 percent of the whole, which is primarily organized into genes. The human genome likely has 50,000 to 100,000 genes.

Experimentally, expressed or functional genes are documented as expressed sequence tags (ESTs), which are partially sequenced cDNAs. A cDNA is synthesized DNA that is complementary to RNA and reflects expressed gene products. The number of these genes expressed is probably different in different organs: A metabolically complex one, the liver, may have 50,000; the synovium may well have fewer, perhaps 30,000, varying with stage of development. Genes are divided into coding and noncoding compartments—exons and introns, respectively—with additional promoter and flanking sequences that are much less well defined. The latter are a major part of the regulatory process, which determines when and where specific genes are expressed. Thus, the gene is a complex unit in both its structure and its regulation. Some idea of the concept can be gauged from Table 6–1, which illustrates the variability in structure and the genome-wide location

Table 6–1

Variability in Structure and Genome-Wide Location of Genes Relevant or Potentially Relevant to Arthritis

PROTEIN/GENE LOCUS	CHROMOSOMAL LOCATION	TOTAL SPAN OF CODING SEQUENCE (kilobases)	EXONS	PROTEIN (AMINO ACIDS)	DISEASE
Dystrophin/DMD	Xp21.2	2400	79	3685	Muscular dystrophy (Duchenne and Becker)
β-Myosin heavy chain/ MYH6	14q11.2-13	23	38	1935	Hypertrophic cardiomyopathy
Hypoxanthine-guanine phosphoribosyltransferase/ HPRT1	Xq26.1	40	9	218	Lesch-Nyhan syndrome/gout
HLA-H/HFE	6p21.3	8	6	348	Hemochromatosis
Homogentisate 1,2-dioxygenase/HGD	3q21-q23	54	14	445	Alkaptonuria
Interleukin-4/IL-4	5q31.1	8.5	4	153	
Interleukin-15/IL-15	4q31			162	
Tumor necrosis factor α/TNF	6p21.3	2	4	232	
Tumor necrosis factor β (lymphotoxin-α)/LTA	6p21.3	2	3	205	
Interleukin-1α/(IL-1A)	2q14	10	7	271 precursor, 159 mature protein	
Interleukin-10/IL-10	1q31-q32	3.7	5	178	

using genes with relevance or potential relevance to arthritis.

Polymorphic Elements

It is fundamental to the understanding of human diversity and of disease to recognize that, although the genome and gene structure are broadly the same for all persons, variability is substantial with respect to both ethnicity and individual genetic makeup; this can give rise to disease—the focus of this review. This variability may be local (i.e., gene specific) or part of genome-wide polymorphic elements.

Local Variability

Local variability in a given gene or segment of DNA can result from a change or mutation in a single nucleotide due to deletions or translocations or to gene conversion. The resulting functional change can range from deleterious (including fatal), to neutral, or even to a gain in function. Clearly, the nature and site of the change (e.g., coding regions, regulatory regions) are critical in this regard and can be reflected in changed phenotypes and disease. The complement deficiencies are examples of relevance to autoimmunity; the chromosome 22 deletion associated with JRA is another such example.[2]

Genome-Wide Polymorphisms

A key aspect of research in the genetics of disease is associating sequence variations with heritable phenotypes. One of the consequences of this explosion in knowledge relating to the genome has been the identification of polymorphic variants that occur throughout the genome in both coding and noncoding elements of DNA. There are two important broad classes of importance with respect to the science of genomics.

Very Numerous Tandem Repeats

Very numerous tandem repeats (VNTRs) are at present the best documented genome-wide polymorphisms, there being over 10,000 throughout the genome.[3] They appear to be randomly distributed and in coding or noncoding regions and, because they are small, repetitive sequences of DNA, they are commonly called *microsatellites*. These polymorphisms can be distinguished by polymerase chain reaction (PCR)-based methods (see later). Their utility is enhanced by the availability of genome-wide maps and by knowledge of their polymorphic information content (PIC), allowing the selection of polymorphisms likely to optimize any given data set.

Single-Nucleotide Polymorphisms

Single nucleotide polymorphisms (SNPs) are much more common than VNTRs.[4] There may be over 1 million in the genome. SNPs form the basis of restriction fragment length polymorphisms (RFLPs), which are SNPs that happen to be located in an enzyme (endonuclease) cutting site. SNPs located in a coding region are known as *cSNPs*.[5] As of August 2000, over 800,000 SNPs were documented, with about 45,000 of these mapped to the finished human genome sequence.

Overall less is known about their map positions and PIC than for VNTRs, although this situation is changing rapidly as a major effort is being vested in their identification and in establishing their map position.

With regard to SNPs being a tool for genomics, their number will eventually allow a much greater frequency of markers and offset the fact that VNTRs are more polymorphic. The ability to use SNPs will be enhanced by the use of DNA chip technologies, although the very great number of SNPs—as many as perhaps 10 or more in some genes—adds complexity to their analysis.[6] However, their utility in the dissection of complex genetic traits can be illustrated by two SNPs that have been associated with components of a disease phenotype. These SNPs involve a mutation, resulting in a gain of function in the interleukin-4 receptor gene, which is associated with severe asthma, and a mutation in a β_2-adrenergic receptor gene (ADRB2) associated with greater resistance to adrenergic drugs.[7, 8]

Clearly, genome-wide maps are being generated and there are going to be different sources of information for constructing these maps.

Maps

Chromosome Map

Cytochemical approaches have been widely used to generate the familiar chromosome banding pattern. The addition of fluorescent in situ hybridization (FISH) has been a substantial benefit, combining cytochemical and molecular approaches. Although only broad localization is possible, several thousand genes have been mapped by this process to specific chromosomes, albeit with low resolution. Fluorescent tags on intact chromosomes cannot be resolved into separate spots unless they are 2 to 5 million base pairs apart.

Genetic Map

A genetic map, although an extension of the chromosome map described earlier, is a more detailed process in which the relationship of individual genes to each other and their eventual assignments to a chromosome region and linkage group becomes possible. Approximately 30,000 genes or anonymous polymorphic markers are mapped (GeneMap '98). Traditionally, extended kindreds are studied for the co-inheritance of a particular phenotype, whether this is physiologic or pathologic. Genes that co-segregate will be established by this process; two genes can be shown to be closely linked and, therefore, a component of a linkage group. This sometimes involves genes of like function, the linkage group having arisen by gene duplication, but often the cluster of genes is not necessarily a cluster with similar or related functions.

An example of a functional cluster is the HLA and T-cell receptor genes, which form close linkage groups. The statistical analyses used in such situations are logarithm of the odds (LOD) scores in which a score of 3.0 or more is the standard for establishing linkage between two genes. A particular linkage group may be inferred from findings in other species, a process known as *synteny.* Although clustering of a particular set of genes may be shared across species, it may be that the same linkage group is found on a different chromosome in humans. For example, the MHC linkage group is located on chromosome 6 in humans and on chromosome 17 in the mouse.

The recombination rate detected in families is a measure of the closeness of linkage. Recombination may be current or ancestral and translates into map distance, or centimorgans (cM). There are approximately 3500 cM in the human genome. This genetic distance may be different from the physical distance between linkage groups on the same chromosome. The HLA region itself amounts to about 1 cM (i.e., about 0.03 percent of the genome).

Physical Map

The advent of DNA sequencing allows definition of individual genes as well as their relationship to each other in terms of intervening DNA structure. Considerable amounts of genetic information have been generated and entered into sequence databanks, much of which is available to investigators (*www.ncbi.nlm.nih.gov* and *www.nhgri.nih.gov*). This process allows physical mapping of individual stretches of DNA; interim physical maps are based on VNTRs and, more recently, SNPs.[9, 10] For example, the HLA region, with its multiple numbers of genes, has in the order of 3500 kilobases of DNA. The physical map will identify the genes and their location within the total genome but will not determine whether they are functional. There are genes that cannot be expressed because of specific mutations; these genes are known as *pseudogenes.* Pseudogenes need to be differentiated from a gene that, because of mutation, will not function. The nonfunctioning gene is known as a *null gene* and is allelic with functioning variants.

Functional Map

The functional map is based on functional genomics, the analysis of gene function, which is itself based on the structural or physical map.[11] Through the process of identification of expressed genes (i.e., ESTs), assisted now with technological advances using gene arrays,[12] it will be possible not only to identify all expressed genes in a given tissue but also to consider their function. Comparisons between developing and developed tissues, as well as disease and normal states, are now ongoing. This will result in a functional map that should also progress rapidly.

Biotechnology and Bioinfomatics

The Human Genome Project—and with it the potential to establish the genetic basis of disease—would not have been possible without parallel technological advances. The key element includes the PCR. This method allows the expansion of specific segments of DNA to make enough of them available for quantitative analysis, including sequencing. With respect to genomics, the widespread availability of polymorphic markers detectable by PCR for every part of the genome and the commercial availability of the appropriate PCR primers have created great opportunities for scientific advances. These primer pairs are organized into sets that allow a genome-wide approach.[13] Although substantial work is still involved, marker sets are available that allow multiplexing of primer pairs based on product size and fluorescent tag and permit up to 15 genotypes to be determined simultaneously on a single lane of a gel or capillary tube. In parallel, developments of high-throughput genotyping/sequencing machines may now generate more than 20,000 genotypes per week.[14] The newer technologies are now capillary-based rather than gel-based.[15] This advance, combined with robotics for the PCR process, allows a laboratory with one or two technical staff members to complete up to a million genotypes per year. A medium-density genome screen (about every 10 cM) for a given disease may number about 150,000 genotypes.

In parallel with this enormous flow of data is the development of appropriate software to assign genotypes, to validate the accuracy of the genotyping in the context of the family tree, and then to facilitate the analytic process. Automated processes are particularly important for SNPs because they are likely to be used eventually in tenfold or greater numbers than VNTRs. The development of software for large databases has been paralleled by conceptual advances in genetic methods. Of particular relevance are approaches to linkage analysis that do not depend on large kindreds. Two particularly relevant methods are allele sharing using affected sib pairs (ASPs) and transmission disequilibrium testing (TDT) that utilizes family-based controls.[16–19] TDT is an alternative approach to establishing linkage that is valid for either simplex or multiplex families (see discussion under "Genome Screen").

MONOGENIC DISEASE IN PEDIATRIC RHEUMATOLOGY

The diseases inherited in a pattern recognizable as mendelian, primarily autosomal dominant and autosomal recessive, are numerous. More than 10,000 are now listed; of these, hundreds might well involve the musculoskeletal system. A few present directly with a form of arthritis, others with musculoskeletal features. These particular disorders make up a very small portion of the referral base for a pediatric rheumatology clinic but are well recognized. However, with the increasing capacity to identify particular genes and their mutations, as well as the functional consequences that lead to particular phenotypes, molecular analysis becomes more practical and necessary—as is awareness of the phenotypes of these disorders.

The familial categories of inherited disease (dominant, recessive, and X-linked) provide patterns of inheritance that are discernible if typically penetrant. A dominant disease should be evident in every generation, showing vertical transmission; a recessive disease occurs in approximately one of four children and is more likely to occur in offspring of consanguineous marriages. X-linked recessive diseases become evident in male children whose mothers are the carriers, although female carriers may show some features of the disease consistent with the Lyon hypothesis of X-chromosome mosaicism. In 1997, Athreya and colleagues[20] categorized these diseases into three groups: arthritic (e.g., Lesch-Nyhan), those with contractures or stiff joints (e.g., Gaucher's disease), and those with hypermobility (e.g., Ehlers-Danlos syndrome). A total of 75 disorders were identified, probably only a portion of the whole (see Appendix).[21] It is recognized that not all of these disorders would present in the classic or traditional Mendelian manner.

Confounding Variables in the Recognition of Mendelian Inheritance

Monogenic effects may be implicated in a given instance but not recognizable for a variety of reasons. Transmission anomalies include inheritance of two copies of a whole chromosome from the same parent: *uniparental disomy.* Other variances in a monogenic disease may have more subtle bases and are summarized in Table 6–2. In addition, modifier genes may alter a specific phenotype, giving different levels of expression. A disease caused by a single gene could be modified by the function of others on a variable basis. This might be distinguished from complex genetic traits in which a number of genes are required to generate the primary disease phenotype, although the distinction is probably relative.

COMPLEX GENETIC TRAITS

A complex genetic trait may be defined as one dependent on multiple genes and with nonmendelian inheritance patterns. It is likely that the diseases more com-

Table 6–2

Variables in the Recognition of Monogenic Disease

Uniparental disomy
New mutations
Low penetrance
Parental imprinting
Variable phenotype
Mitochondrial genes
Parental reproductive choice or fitness

From Ostrer H: Non-mendelian genetics in humans. *In* Oxford Monographs on Medical Genetics No. 35. Oxford, England, Oxford University Press, 1998.

monly encountered in the pediatric rheumatology clinic are the result of complex genetic traits, although the evidence to support this statement is not yet at hand. However, as is evident from the preceding discussion, the genome-wide approaches needed to validate the concept are available and already tested in insulin-dependent diabetes mellitus (IDDM) and many other autoimmune diseases.[22, 23] Examples of complex genetic traits in this category include ankylosing spondylitis, multiple sclerosis, psoriatic arthritis, scleroderma, and SLE, in addition to IDDM.[24] Other potential complex genetic traits, including hypertension and osteoarthritis, have a metabolic but nonimmunologic basis.

Of most relevance to this discussion is the likelihood that JRA and its various subtypes are complex genetic traits.[25] How are these recognized in the absence of genetic data? Features that suggest a complex genetic trait include a definite but limited family history but with few or no extended affected kindreds; an increased presence of other autoimmune diseases in the family[26]; and HLA disease associations that suggest an immunologically related complex genetic trait. Of these features, HLA associations have been extensively documented and family history has been reported for the disease affecting the proband but less commonly for autoimmune disease in general.

Individual components of the phenotype are likely to be regulated separately such that each component could be called a *quantitative-like trait* [QLT], with its own genetic basis. For example, vasculitis complicating SLE or uveitis complicating early-onset pauciarticular JRA may be viewed as individual QLTs. Some patients have these features in their disease phenotype; others do not. Studies of animal models support this QLT concept in rheumatologic disease.[27] What has also been missing and important to predict is information regarding the likelihood that other non-HLA genes are involved. It is likely that responses to therapy (or failures with therapy) are also QLTs and will prove to be genetically mediated, part of the science of pharmacogenetics.

Quantitation of the Family History

Genomic screens are time-consuming ventures; thus, some quantitation of familial risk for a given disease would help to determine the probability that a given disease is or is not likely to be a complex genetic trait. The standard measure of risk of affected sibs is λs, calculated as the prevalence of the disease in sibs of the patient with the illness in question divided by the prevalence of disease in the general population.[28, 29] For JRA, one estimate of λs is 15, similar to that of IDDM.

Disease-Specific Susceptibility Genes Versus General Autoimmune Genes

Mutations in genes with an immunologic function may relate to a variety of immunologic diseases. This can be the experience in both patients and animal models of autoimmunity, one such example being the *fas* gene defects in mice and in humans that effect cell death or apoptosis.[30, 31] This gives rise to the concept that both general autoimmune-predisposing genes and disease-specific susceptibility confer risk of disease. The number of genes involved in a particular complex trait is likely to be between 5 and 20; confirmation of this concept is being worked out as genome screens are completed in many autoimmune diseases. Analysis of 22 genome screens identified over 13 chromosome regions or genes found in common in different autoimmune diseases[32]; similar evidence is accruing in animal models.[33] Because different autoimmune diseases tend to have different HLA associations, it is likely that disease specificity will partly rest with HLA, whereas a general predisposition would be more related to the other non-HLA susceptibility regions.

Disease Phenotype as a Potential Complex Genetic Trait

Two strategies are commonly used in evaluating a disease as a complex trait. One is a candidate gene approach, including specific genes or chromosome regions that are tested for disease susceptibility; the other is a comprehensive genome screen. As the growing number of comprehensive screens in other autoimmune diseases identify chromosomal loci that confer disease susceptibility, a candidate gene approach for any potential autoimmune complex genetic trait becomes more feasible. Using candidate genes has the potential to reduce the overall workload but may miss loci or decrease the resolution, whereas the genome-wide screen systematically examines every genetic region. However, a conservative approach allows both methods of ascertaining linkage or association to be tried in parallel.

Candidate Genes

With most of the likely autoimmune diseases, the literature supports the involvement of individual genes or polymorphisms in susceptibility. For JRA, a recent review[25] identified 30 such potential genes or chromosome regions (Tables 6–3 and 6–4; see also Table 6–2). Although the data supporting the candidacy of such entities are conflicting at best, the probability that one or more will be shown to be involved in disease susceptibility is high—especially those chromosome regions for which selection is based on meta-analysis of prior genome screens.[32]

Genome Screen

A genome screen searches systematically throughout the genome for individual chromosome regions of susceptibility. The marker density selected for such ap-

Table 6–3

Non-HLA Genes/Loci in JRA

POLYMORPHISM/CHROMOSOME REGION	REFERENCE
IgA deficiency	55
Complement deficiency	56
α_1-Antitrypsin	57
Amyloid P component	58
IL-1α promoter	59
TNF-α/β	60
TCR Vβ6.1 null gene	61
IL-6 promoter	62
IL-10	63
Chromosome 22	2

HLA, human leukocyte antigen; IgA, immunoglobulin A; IL, interleukin; JRA, juvenile rheumatoid arthritis; TCR, T-cell receptor; TNF, tumor necrosis factor.

From Glass DN, Giannini EH: Juvenile rheumatoid arthritis as a complex genetic trait. Arthritis Rheum 42: 2261–2268, Copyright © 1999 Wiley-Liss, Inc. Reprinted by permission of Wiley-Liss, Inc., a subsidiary of John Wiley & Sons, Inc.

proaches has generally been about 10 cM, which necessitates the use of 350+ markers genome-wide. This number being a reasonable compromise between identifying positive areas without excessive workload, a database of 100 sib pairs (screened with all parents included) will result in 150,000 genotypes if the DNA quality is sufficient. As noted earlier, the marker sets now available with PCR primer pairs are organized so that multiple PCR products can be run on a given gel, a process known as *multiplexing*. Appropriately, different fluorescein tags are used to facilitate this process, leading to a high throughput of samples. One marker set has over 800 marker pairs, substantially increasing the density of the screen.

Strategy for an Individual Genome Screen

Although the general approach to genome screening is common to all potential complex genetic traits (i.e., the use of multiple markers in all chromosome regions), the strategy selected for any given disease will be specific. The definition of λs, discussed earlier, may be a good indication that "positive" data should result. Some autoimmune diseases (e.g., SLE) have extensive multiplex kindreds. Most disorders have less extensive kindreds, but almost all autoimmune diseases appear to have ASPs as a common denominator. However, the number of available ASPs differs with each disease and will also have a bearing on the stratagem to be adopted.

Table 6–4

Non-HLA Candidate Genes/Loci of Potential Relevance to Juvenile Rheumatoid Arthritis Based on Experience in Autoimmune Arthropathies

GENES/CHROMOSOME MARKER	DISEASE	REFERENCE
NRAMP1 (2q35)	RA	64
1q41-q42	SLE	50
IL-5R, IFN-γ, IL2	RA	65
3q13	RA	66
IL-10	RA	67
D16S 422	AS	51
TCRB	RA	68

AS, ankylosing spondylitis; IL, interleukin; IFN, interferon; RA, rheumatoid arthritis; SLE, systemic lupus erythematosus; TCRB, T-cell receptor β chain.

From Glass DN, Giannini EH: Juvenile rheumatoid arthritis as a complex genetic trait. Arthritis Rheum 42: 2261–2268, Copyright © 1999 Wiley-Liss, Inc. Reprinted by permission of Wiley-Liss, Inc., a subsidiary of John Wiley & Sons, Inc.

Studies with 800 to 1000 ASPs are ongoing in rheumatoid arthritis, and several hundred ASPs are available for ankylosing spondylitis; in pediatric rheumatology, however, the numbers are relatively modest. On the other hand, in the context of a pediatric patient, both parents are usually available in a very high proportion of sib pairs, which adds considerable analytic power unavailable without parental DNA.[34] Normally, sib pairs share both haplotypes in 25 percent of instances and one haplotype in 50 percent; a deviation from this expected distribution among ASPs indicates linkage.[29] If insufficient ASPs are available, other approaches are needed. An alternative method will be the TDT, which requires parents and a single proband (i.e., a simplex family). It is considered a test of both association and linkage.[18, 19, 35] An example of the use of family-based control genes is preferential transmission of particular genes to the proband, which is compared with the allelic distribution in genes that are not transmitted.[36]

Associations generated through case-control studies have often been confounded by population stratification (founder effects), which indicates the importance of family-based studies for assessment of both linkage and association. Unaffected sibs can be used if a stratagem can be devised to work out an individual's potential to contract the autoimmune disease in question. Availability of information on parents is generally necessary, although the absence of one parent can be compensated for if genetic information in the children is sufficient. ASPs can also be used in the TDT as sib-pair TDT; this doubles the power of the test. There is considerable discussion as to the meaning of the TDT; results probably will not be positive in the absence of linkage, although TDT results also depend on linkage disequilibrium and association.

Which Polymorphisms?

In general, microsatellite repeats have been used most frequently. As noted earlier, they not only have the advantage of being mapped but their polymorphic content is known, so microsatellites with maximum PIC content can be selected to optimize the available family materials and minimize uninformative genotyping. As an alternative, SNPs are less polymorphic and less commonly mapped; however, their much greater number will increasingly offset the present advantages of microsatellites.

Because use of the TDT in simplex families requires

higher-density markers (linkage disequilibrium may rarely extend more than 50 kb), the more densely distributed SNPs are likely to become the method of choice in the TDT. This is especially likely given that the technology is now available to read such polymorphisms from DNA-based chips, which adds another automated step to the process and allows increased volumes of genotypes to be more readily processed.[37] Candidate genes can be tested in ASPs or by the TDT, the latter in either simplex or multiplex families. In this situation, association studies using a family-based pool with controls will also reduce the element of population stratification that has made case-controlled studies problematic.

Replication and Extension of Findings

Initial findings suggestive of linkage in any genome study will need confirmation. Hence, a second set of DNA on a new population would be an asset. The method of approach, whether through sib pairs or through case-controlled studies (see later), need not be identical in design to the first study and could be focused on areas of potential interest (chromosome loci or genes) established in the initial study. Fine mapping then becomes possible with high-density markers. For example, of the markers in most common use, VNTRs (microsatellites), 60 to 80 might be available for a particular chromosome region and could be applied in multipoint linkage or association studies. In this approach, it is possible to define the point of maximum linkage or association and thus more exactly map the gene involved in the disease. Chromosome regions so confirmed will still have the potential to contain many genes, perhaps 20, compared with the larger number in the original region. Such an approach was applied to the mapping of the diastrophic dysplasia and hemochromatosis genes.[38–40] This allows the gene-hunting phase to be applied with greater precision.

PEDIATRIC RHEUMATIC ILLNESSES AS COMPLEX GENETIC TRAITS

To what extent are the common chronic pediatric rheumatic illnesses complex genetic traits? The subtypes of JRA, juvenile dermatomyositis, psoriatic arthropathy, ankylosing spondylitis, SLE, and scleroderma are all candidates. Supportive evidence in children is available (though limited) for some diseases but not at all for others; only data in adult patients are available where disease overlap occurs.

For oligoarticular JRA with onset in young children, the relatively frequent occurrence of this illness has ensured that enough ASPs are available to demonstrate substantial concordance for disease.[41, 42] HLA associations are well documented, although extended multiplex families are not available for linkage studies. HLA and JRA have been shown to be linked through two approaches by the TDT in 103 HLA-typed simplex families[43] and through allele sharing in 53 ASPs.[44] Both of these studies have used fewer numbers of families than has generally been the case in genomic studies in adults, suggesting that a genome-wide screen using the available number of sib pairs will be successful in identifying at least the major susceptibility (if not all of the minor susceptibility) loci. The numbers required to consider other aspects of this form of JRA (e.g., polyarticular course or development of chronic uveitis as a QLT) may not be available, requiring the use of simplex families to resolve some of these additional genetic issues. Both the candidate-gene approach and genome-wide screens are feasible.

The selection of candidate genes can be based on the literature on JRA (see Table 6–3), from the literature on other arthropathies (see Table 6–4), and from candidate loci in other autoimmune diseases in general (Table 6–5), the last being especially useful because such data are oriented toward non-HLA genes. The occurrence of autoimmune diseases in JRA families is reported[45–47] but not well documented, contrasting with the situation in juvenile dermatomyositis in which, in addition to HLA associations, there is stronger evidence of an increased familial prevalence of autoimmune disease.[26, 48] In the instance of juvenile dermatomyositis, the limited occurrence of the disease, 2000 or so patients in the United States, precludes the possibility of enough sib pairs for genome screens, although such sib pairs do occur. In this instance, simplex families will prove to be the most reliable resource, especially if both parents are available. For the other pediatric rheumatic disorders, studies in adults—both those already reported and those under way, especially for rheumatoid arthritis, SLE, and ankylosing spondylitis—will generate candidate genes and loci that can be readily sought in pediatric populations.[49–53]

Table 6–5

Candidate Loci in Other Autoimmune Diseases of Potential Relevance to JRA*

CHROMOSOME	POLYMORPHIC MARKERS	DISEASE
1p21.3	D1S 236	MS/CD
3p13	D3S 1261	MS
4q35.1	D4S 1540	MS, PS
4q35.2	D4S 171	PS
4q35.2	D4S 426	MS
7p15.2	NPY	IDDM, MS, IA
7p15.2	D7S 484	MS, CD, UC
7q21.3-22.1	D5 MIT 43	IDDM
11p15.5	D11S 922	MS, IDDM
11q13.1	FgF3	IDDM
12p13.12	PRH 1	IDDM
17p13.3	D17S513	MS, IDDM
Xp11.1	DX 5991	MS, IDDM

CD, celiac disease; IA, inflammatory arthritis; IDDM, insulin-dependent diabetes mellitus; MS, multiple sclerosis; PS, psoriasis; UC, ulcerative colitis.

*Selected markers reported in more than one autoimmune/inflammatory disease.

Adapted from Becker KG, Simon RM, Bailey-Wilson JE, et al: Clustering of non–major histocompatibility complex susceptibility candidate loci in human autoimmune diseases. Proc Natl Acad Sci U S A 95: 9979–9984, 1998.

CONCLUSIONS

It seems highly likely that the autoimmune diseases most commonly encountered by pediatric rheumatologists are complex genetic traits that can be read from an individual's genome. Eventually, diagnosis and prognosis will be based on such traits. It is also evident that genomic polymorphisms will be used to predict responsiveness to therapy. Ultimately, therapy will be matched to an individual's genomic findings, a science known as *pharmacogenetics*. The methods now being developed to evaluate genomes will also allow gene therapy to be applied to chronic pediatric rheumatic illness.

References

1. Collins FS, Patrinos A, Jordan E, et al: New goals for the US human genome project: 1998–2003. Science 282: 682–689, 1998.
2. Sullivan KE, McDonald-McGinn DM, Driscoll DA, et al: Juvenile rheumatoid arthritis–like polyarthritis in chromosome 22q11.2 deletion syndrome (DiGeorge anomalad/velocardiofacial syndrome/conotruncal anomaly face syndrome). Arthritis Rheum 40: 430–436, 1997.
3. Weber JL, May PE: Abundant class of human DNA polymorphisms which can be typed using the polymerase chain reaction. Am J Hum Genet 44: 388–396, 1989.
4. Kruglyak L: The use of a genetic map of biallelic markers in linkage studies. Nat Genet 17: 21–24, 1997.
5. Beaudet AL: 1998 ASHG presidential address. Making genomic medicine a reality. Am J Hum Genet 64: 1–13, 1999.
6. Pennish E: A closer look at SNPs suggests difficulties. Science 281: 1787–1789, 1998.
7. Martinez FD, Graves PE, Baldini MA, et al: Association between genetic polymorphisms of β2-adrenoreceptor and response to albuterol in children with and without a history of wheezing. J Clin Invest 100: 3184–3188, 1997.
8. Hershey GK, Friedrich MF, Esswein LA, et al: The association of atopy with a gain-of-function mutation in the alpha subunit of the interleukin-4 receptor. N Engl J Med 337: 1720–1725, 1997.
9. Cohen D, Chumakov I, Weissenbach J: A first-generation physical map of the human genome. Nature 366: 698–701, 1993.
10. Dib C, Faure S, Fizames C, et al: A comprehensive genetic map of the human genome based on 5,264 microsatellites. Nature 380: 152, 1996.
11. Strachan T, Abitbol M, Davidson D, Beckmann JS: A new dimension for the human genome project: towards comprehensive expression maps. Nat Genet 16: 126–132, 1997.
12. Heller RA, Schena M, Chai A, et al: Discovery and analysis of inflammatory disease–related genes using cDNA microarrays. Proc Natl Acad Sci U S A 94: 2150–2155, 1997.
13. Reed PW, Davies JL, Copeman JB, et al: Chromosome-specific microsatellite sets for fluorescence-based, semiautomated genome mapping. Nat Genet 7: 390–395, 1994.
14. Ziegle JS, Su Y, Corcoran KP, et al: Application of automated DNA sizing technology for genotyping microsatellite loci. Genomics 14: 1026–1031, 1992.
15. Simpson PC, Roach D, Woolley AT, et al: High-throughput genetic analysis using microfabricated 96-sample capillary array electrophoresis microplates. Proc Natl Acad Sci U S A 95: 2256–2261, 1998.
16. Risch N: Linkage strategies for genetically complex traits. II: The power of affected relative pairs. Am J Hum Genet 46: 229–241, 1990.
17. Spielman RS, McGinnis RE, Ewens WJ: The transmission/disequilibrium test detects cosegregation and linkage. Am J Hum Genet 54: 559–560, 1994.
18. Spielman RS, McGinnis RE, Ewens WJ: Transmission test for linkage disequilibrium: the insulin gene region and insulin-dependent diabetes mellitus (IDDM). Am J Hum Genet 52: 506–516, 1993.
19. Spielman RS, Ewens WJ: A sibship test for linkage in the presence of association: the sib transmission/disequilibrium test. Am J Hum Genet 458, 1998.
20. Chalom EC, Ross J, Athreya BH: Syndromes and arthritis. Rheum Dis Clin North Am 23: 709–727, 1997.
21. Prahalad S, Colbert RA: Genetic diseases with rheumatic manifestations in children. Curr Opin Rheumatol 10: 488–493, 1998.
22. Lander ES, Schork NJ: Genetic dissection of complex traits. Science 265: 2037–2048, 1994.
23. Risch N, Merikangas K: The future of genetic studies of complex human diseases. Science 273: 1516–1517, 1996.
24. Davies JL, Kawaguchi Y, Bennet SI, et al: A genome-wide search for human type 1 diabetes susceptibility genes. Nature 371: 130–136, 1994.
25. Glass DN, Giannini EH: JRA as a complex genetic trait. Arthritis Rheum 42: 2261–2268, 1999.
26. Ginn LR, Lin J-P, Plotz PH, et al: Familial autoimmunity in pedigrees of idiopathic inflammatory myopathy patients suggests common genetic risk factors for many autoimmune diseases. Arthritis Rheum 41: 400–405, 1998.
27. Weis JJ, McCracken BA, Ma Y, et al: Identification of quantitative trait loci governing arthritis severity and humoral responses in the murine model of Lyme disease. J Immunol 162: 948–956, 1999.
28. Risch N: Linkage strategies for genetically complex traits. I: Multilocus models. Am J Hum Genet 46: 222–228, 1990.
29. Risch N: Linkage strategies for genetically complex traits. II: The power of affected relative pairs. Am J Hum Genet 57: 911–919, 1995.
30. Adachi M, Watange-Fukunaga R, Nagata S: Aberrant transcription caused by the insertion of an early transposable element in an intron of the Fas antigen gene of *lpr* mice. Proc Natl Acad Sci U S A 90: 1756–1761, 1993.
31. Fisher G, Rosenberg F, Straus S: Dominant interfering Fas gene mutations impair apoptosis in a human autoimmune lymphoproliferative syndrome. Cell 81: 935–946, 1995.
32. Becker KG, Simon RM, Bailey-Wilson JE, et al: Clustering of non-major histocompatibility complex susceptibility candidate loci in human autoimmune diseases. Proc Natl Acad Sci U S A 95: 9979–9984, 1998.
33. Kawahito Y, Cannon GW, Gulko PS, et al: Localization of quantitative trait loci regulating adjuvant-induced arthritis in rats: evidence for genetic factors common to multiple autoimmune diseases. J Immunol 161: 4411–4419, 1998.
34. Gonzalez-Roces S, Alvarez MV, Gonzalez S, et al: HLA-B27 polymorphism and worldwide susceptibility to ankylosing spondylitis. Tissue Antigens 49: 116–123, 1997.
35. Cleves MA, Olson JM, Jacobs KB: Exact transmission-disequilibrium tests with multiallelic markers. Genet Epidemiol 14: 337–347, 1997.
36. Thomson G: Mapping disease genes: family-based association studies. Am J Hum Genet 57: 487–498, 1995.
37. Scott WK, Pericak-Vance MA: Genetic analysis of complex diseases. Science 275: 1327, 1997.
38. Ajioka RS, Yu P, Gruen JR, et al: Recombinations defining centromeric and telomeric borders for the hereditary haemochromatosis loci. J Med Genet 34: 28–33, 1997.
39. Gandon G, Jouanolle AM, Chauvel B, et al: Linkage disequilibrium and extended haplotypes in the HLA-A to D6S105 region: implications for mapping the hemochromatosis gene (HFE). Hum Genet 97: 103–113, 1996.
40. Hastbacka J, de la Chapelle A, Mahtani MM, et al: The diastrophic dysplasia gene encodes a novel sulfate transporter: positional cloning by fine-structure linkage disequilibrium mapping. Cell 78: 1073–1087, 1994.
41. Clemens LE, Albert E, Ansell BM: Sibling pairs affected by chronic arthritis of childhood: evidence for a genetic predisposition. J Rheumatol 12: 108–113, 1985.
42. Moroldo MB, Tague BL, Shear ES, et al: Juvenile rheumatoid arthritis in affected sibpairs. Arthritis Rheum 40: 1962–1966, 1997.
43. Moroldo MB, Donnelly P, Saunders J, et al: Transmission disequilibrium as a test of linkage and association between HLA alleles and pauciarticular-onset juvenile rheumatoid arthritis. Arthritis Rheum 41: 1620–1624, 1998.
44. Prahalad S, Ryan MH, Shear ES, et al: Juvenile rheumatoid arthritis: linkage to HLA demonstrated by allele sharing in affected sibpairs. Arthritis Rheum 43: 2335–2338, 2000.

45. Rossen RD, Brewer EJ, Sharp RM, et al: Familial rheumatoid arthritis: linkage of HLA to disease susceptibility locus in four families where proband presented with juvenile rheumatoid arthritis. J Clin Invest 65: 629–642, 1980.
46. Rudolph MCJ, Tamborlane WV, Dwyer JM, et al: Juvenile rheumatoid arthritis in children with diabetes mellitus. J Pediatr 99: 519–524, 1981.
47. Firooz A, Mazhar A, Ahmed AR: Prevalence of autoimmune diseases in the family members of patients with pemphigus vulgaris. J Am Acad Dermatol 31: 434–437, 1994.
48. Friedman JM, et al: Immunogenetic studies of juvenile dermatomyositis: HLA-DR antigen frequencies. Arthritis Rheum 26: 214–216, 1983.
49. Cornelis F, Faure S, Martinez M, et al: New susceptibility locus for rheumatoid arthritis suggested by a genome-wide linkage study. Proc Natl Acad Sci U S A 95: 10746–10750, 1998.
50. Tsao BP, Cantor RM, Kalunian KC, et al: Evidence for linkage of a candidate chromosome 1 region to human systemic lupus erythematosus. J Clin Invest 99: 725–731, 1997.
51. Wordsworth P: Genes in the spondyloarthropathies. Rheum Dis Clin North Am 24: 843–862, 1998.
52. Gaffney PM, Kearns GM, Shark KB, et al: A genome-wide search for susceptibility genes in human systemic lupus erythematosus sib-pair families. Proc Natl Acad Sci U S A 95: 14875–14879, 1998.
53. Moser KL, Neas BR, Salmon JE, et al: Genome scan of human systemic lupus erythematosus: evidence for linkage on chromosome 1q in African-American pedigrees. Proc Natl Acad Sci U S A 95: 14869–14874, 1998.
54. Ostrer H: Non-mendelian genetics in humans. *In* Oxford Monographs on Medical Genetics No. 35. Oxford, England, Oxford University Press, 1998.
55. Cassidy JT, Petty RE, Sullivan DB: Occurrence of selective IgA deficiency in children with juvenile rheumatoid arthritis. Arthritis Rheum 20: 181–183, 1977.
56. Glass D, Litvin D, Wallace K, et al: Early-onset pauciarticular juvenile rheumatoid arthritis associated with human leukocyte antigen-DRw5 iritis, and antinuclear antibody. J Clin Invest 66: 426–429, 1980.
57. Aranaud P, Galbraith RM, Faulk WP, Ansell BM: Increased frequency of the MZ phenotype of alpha-1-protease inhibitor in juvenile chronic polyarthritis. J Clin Invest 60: 1442–1444, 1977.
58. Woo P, O'Brien J, Robison M, Ansell BM: A genetic marker for systemic amyloidosis in juvenile arthritis. Lancet 2: 767–769, 1987.
59. McDowell TL, Symons JA, Ploski R, et al: A genetic association between juvenile rheumatoid arthritis and a novel interleukin-1a polymorphism. Arthritis Rheum 38: 221–229, 1995.
60. Epplen C, Rumpf H, Albert E, et al: Immunoprinting excludes many potential susceptibility genes as predisposing to early onset pauciarticular juvenile chronic arthritis except HLA class II and TNF. Eur J Immunogenet 22: 311–322, 1995.
61. Maksymowych WP, Gabriel CA, Luyrink L, et al: Polymorphism in a T cell receptor variable gene is associated with susceptibility to a juvenile rheumatoid arthritis subset. Immunogenetics 35: 258–263, 1992.
62. Fishman D, Faulds G, Jeffery R, et al: The effect of novel polymorphisms in the interleukin-6 (IL-6) gene on IL-6 transcription and plasma IL-6 levels, and an association with systemic-onset juvenile chronic arthritis. J Clin Invest 102: 1369–1376, 1998.
63. Crawley E, Kay R, Sillibourne J, et al: Polymorphic haplotypes of the IL-10 5′ flanking region determine variable IL-10 transcription and are associated with particular phenotypes of juvenile rheumatoid arthritis. Arthritis Rheum 42: 1101–1108, 1999.
64. Shaw M-A, Clayton D, Atkinson SE, et al: Linkage of rheumatoid arthritis to the candidate gene NRAMP1 on 2q35. J Med Genet 33: 672–677, 1996.
65. John S, Myerscough AM, Marlow A, et al: Linkage of cytokine genes to rheumatoid arthritis: evidence of genetic heterogeneity. Ann Rheum Dis 57: 361–365, 1998.
66. Cornelis F, Faure S, Martinez M, et al: New susceptibility locus for rheumatoid arthritis suggested by a genome-wide linkage study. Proc Natl Acad Sci U S A 95: 10746–10750, 1998.
67. Eskdal J, McNicholl J, Wordsworth P, et al: Interleukin-10 microsatellite polymorphisms and IL-10 locus alleles in rheumatoid arthritis susceptibility. Lancet 352: 1282–1283, 1998.
68. McDermott M, Kastner DL, Holloman JD, et al: The role of T cell receptor beta chain genes in susceptibility to rheumatoid arthritis. Arthritis Rheum 38: 91–95, 1995.

7

Pharmacology and Drug Therapy

Ronald M. Laxer and Madlen Gazarian

The therapy of pediatric rheumatic diseases has seen a great deal of progress in recent years, and the potential for rapid advances over the next few years is even greater. Basic research has led to a better understanding of the immunobiology of many of the inflammatory rheumatic diseases, especially rheumatoid arthritis, and allowed for the design of new therapies that are now being evaluated in children with juvenile rheumatoid arthritis (JRA). Coordinating study groups (e.g., Pediatric Rheumatology Collaborative Study Group, Pediatric Rheumatology International Trial Organization) have increased the recruitment of children from an increased number of centers to participate in clinical trials. The development of functional and outcome measures (see Chapter 9),[1–5] which have been translated into different languages and validated in many populations, allows for objective measures of efficacy to be applied across populations. An agreed-upon definition of improvement has brought clinical relevance to many of the outcome measures previously used in trials.[6] Finally, trial designs other than the gold-standard randomized controlled trial have been proposed to address the problems of small patient numbers, lack of interest of pharmaceutical companies, and difficulties with international trials.[7, 8]

The principal drugs used in pediatric rheumatology are those that suppress the inflammatory and immune responses. The targets of their therapeutic effects are predominantly the arachidonic acid metabolic pathways and the cells of the immune system. This chapter outlines some of the most important general principles relating to use of these medications, particularly as they apply to children. The treatment of specific rheumatic disorders is detailed in the chapters dealing with each disease.

CONCEPTS IN PHARMACOLOGY

Although often incomplete, knowledge of the pharmacokinetics of drugs used to treat childhood rheumatic diseases contributes to understanding their clinical application. This brief overview can be supplemented by referring to standard works in the field.[9–11]

Drug Absorption and Bioavailability

Most drugs are given by the oral route and are absorbed through the mucosa of the gastrointestinal (GI) tract, particularly that of the small intestine. GI absorption may be influenced by a number of factors, including the presence or absence of food in the gastric lumen, luminal pH, gastric emptying time, and the coadministration of other drugs. Drug bioavailability, the net result of these factors, is usually determined by sequential measurement of plasma drug concentrations. Three parameters are routinely considered: peak drug concentration, the time necessary to reach peak concentration, and the area under the time-concentration curve. The area under the curve after intravenous (IV) administration is considered equivalent to complete absorption after oral administration. Because the effect of many repeatedly administered drugs is cumulative, except with drugs of extremely short half-life given at infrequent intervals, bioavailability is best determined at the mean steady-state concentration of the drug—that is, the point at which drug intake is equal to drug elimination.

Volume of Distribution

The volume of distribution is the volume of fluid into which a drug would need to be distributed to achieve a concentration equal to the concentration ultimately measured in plasma. If the drug stays in the plasma, its volume of distribution is smaller than if it is distributed widely in tissues.

Drugs in the body are either free or bound to plasma proteins or tissue lipids. The extent and nature of binding affect the volume of distribution of the drug, the rate of renal clearance (because only free drug is filtered by the glomerulus), the drug half-life, and the amount of free drug that reaches the target tissue or receptor.

Most acidic drugs are bound to plasma albumin, whereas the basic drugs are bound to lipoproteins,

α_1-acid glycoproteins, and globulins. In inflammatory states, plasma albumin concentration falls and α_1-acid glycoproteins increase, although the extent of the decrease usually does not require any change in drug therapy. Drugs that are highly protein-bound tend to stay within the vascular compartment and have a relatively limited volume of distribution. Those that are widely bound to lipids in tissues have large volumes of distribution.

Half-Life and Clearance

The *half-life* of a drug is the time necessary for the serum concentration to fall by 50 percent during the elimination phase of a time-concentration curve. *Clearance* is a measure of the removal of a drug from the body as a whole or from a specific part of the body, such as liver or kidney. It is expressed as the volume of body fluid from which a drug is removed per unit of time.

The *first-pass effect* refers to the rapid breakdown of a drug when it passes through the intestinal mucosa or enters the liver for the first time. In this case, the drug reaches the systemic circulation predominantly in the form of metabolites that may be pharmacologically inactive. Avoidance of this effect requires IV administration.

When the rate of elimination of a drug is directly proportional to its concentration in the body, the drug is said to have *first-order kinetics.* Drugs that are eliminated at a constant rate, unrelated to the amount of the agent in the body, are said to follow *zero-order kinetics.* Some drugs obey *capacity-limited kinetics:* at low concentrations, first-order kinetics are observed; at higher concentrations, the enzymes used in metabolism of the drug are saturated, and zero-order kinetics is approached. Salicylate and its metabolites demonstrate this phenomenon. Time-dependent kinetics may be altered by the effect of drug metabolites. For most drugs, a steady state is not reached until the passage of five half-lives. Blood levels measured prior to that time may be erroneous.

Drug Biotransformation

Drug biotransformation or metabolism principally occurs in the liver, kidney, skin, and GI tract. In the liver, biotransformation involves hydrolysis, oxidation, reduction, or demethylation, and conjugation of the metabolite with glycine, glucuronide, sulfate, or hippurate with subsequent secretion into the bile. In the kidney, drugs may be filtered, filtered and secreted, filtered and passively reabsorbed (e.g., acetaminophen), or filtered or actively secreted and passively reabsorbed (e.g., salicylates).[12] Many drugs used to treat rheumatic diseases are active in the form in which they are administered; exceptions include sulindac, salsalate, prednisone, cyclophosphamide, and azathioprine, which require biotransformation before they exert their principal effects.

Because the liver and kidney play such key roles in drug metabolism, dysfunction of these organs may require alteration in drug dose. In general, however, additional toxicity caused by drugs that totally depend on the kidney for their elimination is not a danger unless renal function is diminished by more than 50 percent.[10] In patients with significant renal or hepatic disease, monitoring of drug levels and attention to the potential of drug toxicity become more critical.

ANTIRHEUMATIC DRUGS

The pharmacologic agents used to treat children with rheumatic disorders are grouped into five categories: the nonsteroidal anti-inflammatory drugs (NSAIDs), disease-modifying or slow-acting antirheumatic drugs, glucocorticoids, cytotoxic or immunosuppressive agents, and biologic response modifiers (Table 7–1).

Nonsteroidal Anti-Inflammatory Drugs

The NSAIDs (Fig. 7–1) remain the mainstay of the initial treatment of the chronic arthropathies of childhood and have a role in management of some aspects of the other connective tissue diseases. They provide symptomatic anti-inflammatory relief and are recommended for the majority of patients with JRA. In the United States and Canada, only acetylsalicylic acid (aspirin, ASA), tolmetin, naproxen, and ibuprofen are approved for use in the young child. In Australia, only aspirin, naproxen, and ibuprofen are licensed for use in children. The range of actual NSAID use in childhood is broader in these and many other areas of the world and usually extends beyond the range of drugs approved for use in children and the manufacturer's recommendations in terms of dosage and minimum age for use.[13] In general, ASA is now used much less often because it is associated with a greater frequency of adverse effects (including Reye's syndrome—see later) without any demonstrated superiority in terms of efficacy compared with other NSAIDs for the treatment of arthropathies; however, it continues to have a major role in the treatment of Kawasaki disease. ASA is also less convenient to use because of the need for more frequent dosing, its poor solubility in liquid form, and the need for monitoring serum levels. More recently, a new class of NSAID, the cyclo-oxygenase 2 (COX-2)

Table 7–1

Agents Used to Treat Rheumatic Diseases

Agents
Nonsteroidal anti-inflammatory drugs
Disease-modifying antirheumatic drugs/slow-acting anti-inflammatory drugs
Glucocorticoids
Cytotoxic or immunosuppressive drugs
Biologic immunomodulators

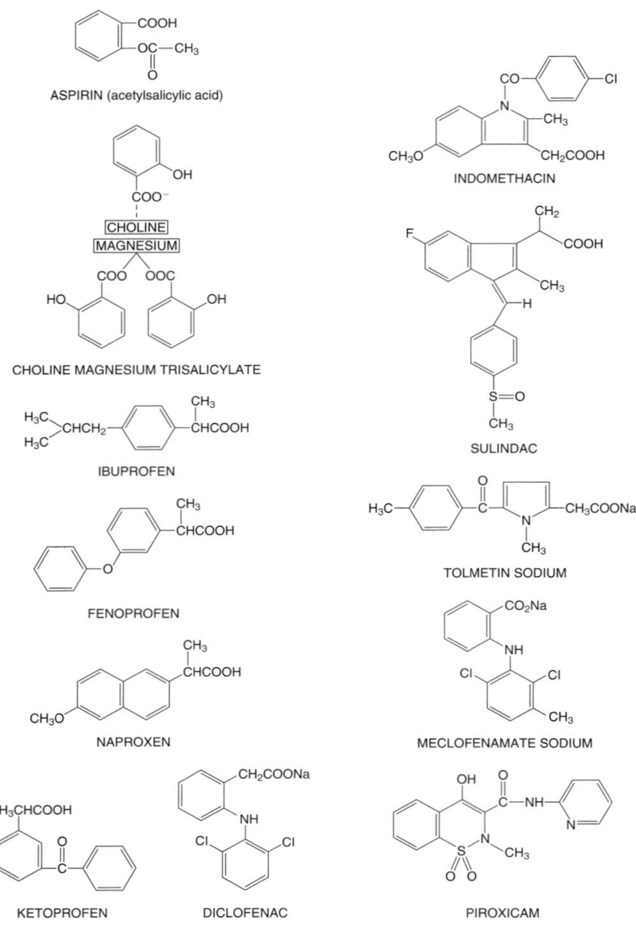

Figure 7–1. NSAID structures.

inhibitors, has emerged as a potentially useful addition to this category of anti-inflammatory drug in adults and may eventually prove useful in children.

Mechanism of Action

NSAIDs inhibit pro-inflammatory pathways that lead to chronic inflammation. The major anti-inflammatory effect of NSAIDs is mediated by inhibition of cyclo-oxygenase in the metabolism of arachidonic acid to prostaglandins, thromboxanes, and prostacyclins (Fig. 7–2; see Chapter 5).[14] Currently available NSAIDs (except diclofenac and indomethacin) have little effect on the lipoxygenase pathway, the other major pathway of arachidonic acid metabolism.[15] The discovery of two related but unique isoforms of the cyclo-oxygenase enzyme, COX-1 and COX-2, has resulted in a greater understanding of the mechanism of action of NSAIDs.[16–19] These enzymes are structurally very similar but are encoded by distinct genes and differ in their distribution and expression in tissues.

The COX-1 isoenzyme has a wide tissue distribution and is constitutively expressed under basal conditions. It appears to have a "housekeeping" function and is associated with the production of prostaglandins resulting in diverse physiologic effects such as gastric cytoprotection, platelet aggregation, vascular homeostasis, and maintenance of renal blood flow (see Fig. 7–2). In contrast, COX-2 is an inducible enzyme that is upregulated at sites of inflammation by various pro-inflammatory mediators, including interleukin-1 (IL-1), tumor necrosis factor α (TNF-α), bacterial endotoxins, and various mitogenic and growth factors. It also appears to be expressed in the central nervous system (CNS) and to have a role in the central mediation of pain and fever.

After the discovery of COX-2 in the early 1990s,[20] it was hypothesized that COX-1 mediated uniquely physiologic prostaglandin production whereas COX-2 mediated uniquely pathologic prostaglandin production; consequently, the anti-inflammatory effects of NSAIDs were considered to result from COX-2 and adverse effects from COX-1 inhibition. However, this appears to be an oversimplification.[21] More recent information suggests that COX-2 may also have a physiologic function in certain tissues; it is expressed constitutively in structures such as the ovary, uterus, brain, kidney, cartilage, and bone.[19] COX-2 knockout mice have severe renal dystrophy, suggesting an important role for this isoenzyme in early renal development. Conversely, COX-1 may have nonphysiologic functions and, like COX-2, may be upregulated at sites of inflammation. Thus, the two isoforms of cyclo-oxygenase each appear to have a role in both physiologic and pathologic prostaglandin production and have more broad and complex functions than originally thought.

Currently available NSAIDs inhibit both isoforms of cyclo-oxygenase, but most inhibit COX-1 preferentially, resulting in undesirable adverse effects such as GI toxicity while producing desirable anti-inflammatory effects through concurrent inhibition of COX-2. Existing NSAIDs are known to differ in the degree of COX-2:COX-1 inhibition they produce. This has been found to correlate with their adverse-effect profiles: NSAIDs that are more selective for COX-2 appear to have more favorable adverse effect profiles.[17]

In light of the differences between the COX-1 and COX-2 isoenzymes and their binding sites for NSAIDs, there has been a profusion of research into a "safer" class of drugs that selectively bind to and inhibit COX-2 activity: the COX-2 inhibitors.[16] However, much of the currently available information on COX-2 selectivity is derived largely from in vitro studies, which may not necessarily correlate with effects in vivo or ultimately with clinical outcomes.[21, 22] Furthermore, the degree of COX-2 suppression needed to produce an anti-inflammatory and analgesic effect in vivo is uncertain—a threshold degree of COX-2 inhibition that must be achieved with no associated COX-1 suppression cannot be clearly defined at this time.[18, 22]

A number of additional concerns remain about specific COX-2 inhibitors: Because COX-1 may also be induced at sites of inflammation, a specific COX-2 inhibitor may be less effective as an anti-inflammatory or analgesic agent.[16, 17, 21] COX-2 appears to be involved in the healing of ulcers and GI inflammation such as with *Helicobacter pylori* gastritis; the safety of specific

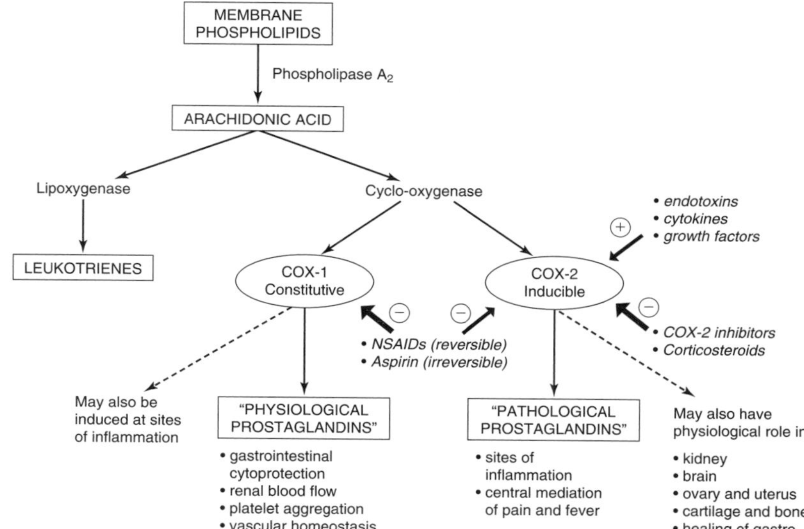

Figure 7–2. Synthesis of prostaglandins and leukotrienes. Sites of action of anti-inflammatory agents and cytokines are highlighted by arrows (−, downregulation; +, upregulation). COX, cyclo-oxygenase.

COX-2 inhibitors in these settings is not known. In addition, the consequences of specific COX-2 inhibition in tissues wherein the COX-2 isoenzyme appears to have a physiologic role, such as the renal medulla, ovary, and uterus, is also unknown.[16, 17] Although many COX-2 inhibitors have been described and are in various stages of development, only two (celecoxib and rofecoxib) have been launched in the United States. Further clinical studies, including those in children, are needed to address these issues.

The doses of existing NSAIDs that are required to reduce inflammation are generally higher than those needed to inhibit prostaglandin formation, suggesting the existence of other mechanisms by which their anti-inflammatory effects are mediated (Table 7–2). In addition to inhibiting prostaglandin production, current NSAIDs inhibit specific proteinases involved in degradation of proteoglycans and collagens of cartilage[23] and inhibit the generation of oxygen radicals, particularly superoxide.[24–26] NSAIDs also have been shown to interfere with bradykinin release, response of lymphocytes to antigenic challenge, phagocytosis, and chemotaxis of granulocytes and monocytes.[27]

Individual NSAIDs may have additional specific mechanisms of action. Indomethacin blocks the action of phosphodiesterase, thus increasing intracellular cyclic adenosine monophosphate.[28] This effect leads to a decrease in the generation of superoxide and hydroxyl radicals.[28–30] Indomethacin also inhibits the mobility of polymorphonuclear neutrophils in inflammatory sites. Like ASA and ibuprofen, indomethacin uncouples oxidative phosphorylation and decreases the synthesis of mucopolysaccharides.[31] Diclofenac and indomethacin also limit the availability of the substrate for prostaglandin and leukotriene synthesis by facilitating incorporation of arachidonic acid into triglycerides.[15, 32] Piroxicam at high concentrations inhibits neutrophil migration, phagocytosis, lysosomal enzyme release,[33] and oxygen radical production by neutrophils.[34] Meclofenamate sodium may inhibit prostaglandin binding at its receptor and inhibits phospholipase A_2.[35] Meclofenamate also inhibits the lipoxygenase pathway of arachidonic acid metabolism.[36] Other differences in the mechanism of action of various NSAIDs have been reviewed.[15, 37]

Table 7–2

Processes Influenced by NSAIDs

Prostaglandin production
Leukotriene synthesis
Superoxide generation
Lysosomal enzyme release
Neutrophil aggregation and adhesion
Cell-membrane functions
  Enzyme activity (NADPH oxidase, phospholipase C)
  Transmembrane anion transport
  Oxidative phosphorylation
  Uptake of arachidonate
Lymphocyte function
Rheumatoid factor production
Cartilage metabolism

NADPH, nicotinamide adenine dinucleotide phosphate, reduced form; NSAIDs, nonsteroidal anti-inflammatory drugs.

From Brooks PM, O'Day RO: Nonsteroidal antiinflammatory drugs—differences and similarities. N Engl J Med 324: 1716–1725, Copyright © 1991 Massachusetts Medical Society. All rights reserved.

Pharmacology

The pharmacokinetic evaluation of NSAIDs in children with JRA has been variable, ranging from extensive for the salicylates to minimal or none with the newer agents; the interested reader is referred to reviews on the subject.[38, 39] However, studies in adults indicate that most NSAIDs share similar pharmacokinetic properties. They are weakly acidic drugs that are rapidly absorbed after oral administration, with most of the absorption taking place in the stomach and upper small intestine. Circadian rhythms in gastric pH and intestinal motility may lead to variability in NSAID absorption, with reduced absorption of a dose given at night compared with that given in the morning.[40]

The majority of NSAIDs are strongly protein bound, primarily to albumin, leading to a potential for drug–disease and drug–drug interactions. Hypoalbuminemia may occur as a manifestation of disease activity in JRA, especially with systemic-onset disease, and may be one of the most important factors influencing the pharmacokinetics of NSAIDs in these children. Because clinical effects are determined by unbound or free drug levels, states of hypoalbuminemia may be associated with a corresponding increase in the unbound fraction and hence potential for increased toxicity. Interestingly, however, most of the studies of NSAID pharmacokinetics in children do not report the level of disease activity.[39] Protein binding may also be reduced with renal or hepatic disease.

Although the strong plasma-protein binding of NSAIDs also makes possible drug–drug interactions with other highly protein-bound drugs, significant clinical interactions are rare.[41, 42] Furthermore, children rarely need to be prescribed drugs that have a potential for interacting with NSAIDs. However, NSAIDs may potentially interact with methotrexate (MTX) through several mechanisms, including displacement from plasma protein binding sites, competition for renal secretion, and impairment of renal function. Although the impact of NSAIDs on MTX clearance varies widely and the potential for clinically significant interactions exists in some children,[43] MTX–NSAID interactions are rarely of clinical significance.

The kinetics of NSAIDs at their anti-inflammatory sites of action, such as in synovial fluid, may be more clinically relevant than their kinetics in plasma. The comparative kinetics of NSAIDs in plasma and synovial fluid are related to the drug's half-life and differences in protein binding at these sites. Studies in adults indicate that NSAIDs with short half-lives have less fluctuation in synovial fluid concentrations than plasma concentrations over a given dosage interval.[41] This phenomenon may partially account for the dosage interval of these drugs being longer than their plasma half-lives. In addition, because synovial fluid albumin concentrations are lower than in plasma, the free fraction of NSAIDs in synovial fluid can be significantly higher than in plasma and has been shown to correlate with clinical effectiveness.[40] This may account for clinical effects being observed with relatively low plasma drug levels. Except for naproxen and ASA, plasma concentrations correlate poorly with anti-inflammatory activity.[44]

NSAIDs are eliminated predominantly by hepatic metabolism; only small amounts are excreted unchanged in urine. Some NSAIDs, such as sulindac or indomethacin, are also secreted in significant amounts in bile and undergo enterohepatic recirculation.[41] Most NSAIDs are metabolized by first-order or linear kinetics, whereas salicylate is metabolized by zero-order or nonlinear kinetics. Thus, dosage adjustments are frequently required with ASA therapy, and small changes in dose may lead to large fluctuations in serum levels of ASA at the higher end of the therapeutic range.[39] Naproxen may also demonstrate nonlinear pharmacokinetics at doses above 500 mg/day in adults because of saturation of plasma protein binding sites and associated increase in clearance.[39, 40] Interpatient differences in the metabolic clearances of individual NSAIDs may be marked, resulting in considerable variation in the extent of their accumulation at all sites throughout the body.[41] In children, NSAIDs may be eliminated more rapidly than in adults; thus, children may require more frequent doses to maintain a clinical response.[45]

Differences in pharmacokinetics between short- and long-term administration may be significant, but this has not been studied systematically.[38] Abnormalities of hepatic function are common in children with JRA, particularly those with systemic-onset disease. Because hepatic metabolism plays a major role in NSAID elimination, it is necessary to assess hepatic function prior to institution of NSAID therapy in these children. NSAIDs should not be started if there is significant elevation of transaminase levels (e.g., three times normal or higher).

General Principles of NSAID Therapy

The NSAIDs are generally good analgesic and antipyretic drugs and weak anti-inflammatory agents. They provide good symptomatic relief but have traditionally not been considered to influence the underlying disease process or to significantly affect long-term outcomes. The analgesic effect of NSAIDs is rapid, but the anti-inflammatory effect takes longer and requires doses up to twice as large as those needed for analgesia.[46, 47] NSAIDs are relatively safe for long-term use. Toxicity, although not infrequent, especially for GI side effects, is seldom serious.[48–50] Given the wide variety of available NSAIDs, a few general principles can be applied in the selection of a particular NSAID for therapy in an individual patient (Table 7–3).

First, according to empirical evidence from clinical experience and some studies in adults, response to the NSAIDs appears to have some disease specificity. Indomethacin, one of the more potent NSAIDs, may be more useful in treating manifestations of systemic

Table 7–3

General Principles of NSAID Use

A specific diagnosis should be established.
The objectives of therapy (analgesia or suppression of inflammation) should be understood.
The objectives of therapy must be balanced against the risks of toxicity and cost of the drug.
An adequate trial (appropriate dose for at least 6 to 8 wk) is needed before assessing efficacy.
Use of combinations of NSAIDs should be avoided.
Clinical and laboratory evidence of effect and toxicity should be objectively monitored.

NSAID, nonsteroidal anti-inflammatory drug.

JRA, such as fever and pericarditis, and in managing the spondyloarthropathies. Ibuprofen is also a very effective antipyretic agent in systemic-onset JRA. Sustained-release preparations of naproxen or, in the older child, indomethacin, given at night may be effective in reducing night pain or prolonged morning stiffness. Recent studies, however, suggest that differences in the effectiveness of NSAIDs are small but that some NSAIDs, such as ASA or indomethacin, are more toxic than others.[46]

Second, individual patient response to NSAIDs is variable and often relatively unpredictable; a child may fail to respond to one drug and yet respond to another. Similarly, the frequency of toxicity may also vary widely. A favorable initial response occurs in more than 50 percent of patients on the first NSAID chosen; of those showing an inadequate response to the first NSAID, a further 50 percent improve when given another drug of the same class.[39] Therefore, in the child whose condition has not responded to one NSAID or who is experiencing significant toxicity, a subsequent trial with another agent is usually warranted. An adequate trial of any NSAID should not be less than about 8 weeks[13, 51]; although about 50 percent of children who respond favorably to an NSAID do so by 2 weeks of therapy, mean time to therapeutic response can be 4 weeks, and up to 25 percent may not respond until after approximately 12 weeks of therapy.[52]

Third, additional factors such as the availability in liquid form, frequency of dosing, cost, and tolerability of any given NSAID may influence patient preference. These factors may have a major impact on patient adherence to a particular treatment regimen and so should be carefully evaluated when making therapeutic choices. Choosing an NSAID that has a favorable toxicity-efficacy profile, that can be taken on a convenient schedule (such as once or twice daily), that is not too expensive and, for young children, is available in a liquid formulation that is palatable seems to be a reasonable initial approach. For these reasons, naproxen has become the initial drug of choice for children with arthritis because it is generally well tolerated and safe, is administered twice daily, and is available in a palatable liquid form.[53]

Generally, therapy should commence with the NSAID of choice at the lowest recommended dose, which can then be titrated to the patient's clinical response. Use of multiple NSAIDs is not recommended because this approach has no documented benefit in terms of efficacy and can be associated with a greater potential for drug interactions and organ toxicity. The dose range and schedule of administration vary with the individual NSAID (Table 7–4). Patients who are on long-term NSAID therapy should have monitoring of liver and renal function and a complete blood count at least every 6 months. Patients with active systemic disease should have more frequent monitoring of liver function, including serum albumin, particularly with any changes in dose. Once a patient has responded and is considered to be in clinical remission, withdrawal of NSAID therapy can be considered. Although there are no good studies of NSAID discontinuation in children with JRA to guide recommendations, most pediatric rheumatologists would consider it reasonable to attempt gradual withdrawal of therapy after remission has been maintained for at least 6 months.

Toxicity

Serious toxicity associated with the use of NSAIDs appears to be rare in children.[47] Much of the available information, however, is derived from case reports, case series, or retrospective cohort studies, thus making it difficult to derive accurate figures for the incidence and prevalence of various toxicities, particularly for children. Prospective studies using standardized approaches to measuring drug-related toxicities are needed to allow a better quantification of the magnitude of risk for the various adverse effects associated with NSAID therapy. In general, however, most toxicities are shared to a greater or lesser degree by all NSAIDs (Table 7–5), although individual patients may have fewer side effects with one drug than with another.[29, 48, 49, 54, 55]

Gastrointestinal Toxicity

GI tract toxicity is common to all NSAIDs. The pathogenesis of gastroduodenal mucosal injury involves multiple mechanisms with both local and systemic effects due to NSAIDs.[56] The systemic effects appear to have a predominant role and are largely the result of inhibition of prostaglandin synthesis, which leads to impairment of many cytoprotective actions such as epithelial mucus production, secretion of bicarbonate, mucosal blood flow, epithelial proliferation, and mucosal resistance to injury.[56] The associated symptoms range from mild epigastric discomfort immediately after taking the medication to symptomatic or asymptomatic peptic ulceration.[57]

The incidence of symptomatic ulcers and potentially life-threatening ulcer complications, such as upper GI bleeding, perforation, and gastric outlet obstruction, is about 2 to 4 percent in adults taking NSAIDs for 1 year.[58] The relative risk of upper GI bleeding and perforation associated with current NSAID use is estimated to be 4.7 overall, with variability in the magnitude of risk associated with individual NSAIDs.[59] Complication-related hospitalization and death rates are estimated to be less than 1.5 percent per annum in adults.[60] However, many of the studies on which these figures are based have limitations in ascertainment as well as attribution of adverse effects to NSAIDs, resulting in the potential for substantial under- or over-ascertainment of NSAID adverse effects. Furthermore, differences in patient populations, drugs used, dosages, and periods of exposure add to the variability in estimates of prevalence.

Data from a randomized, placebo-controlled study of the efficacy of a cytoprotective agent, misoprostol, in 8843 patients with rheumatoid arthritis treated with NSAIDs determined that the incidence of definite serious GI complications was 0.95 percent in the placebo group over the 6-month trial period.[61] Possible risk factors for GI complications during NSAID therapy include advanced age, past history of GI

Table 7–4

NSAIDs Commonly Used in Children

DRUG	DOSE (mg/kg/d)	MAX DOSE (mg/d)	DOSES/D	COMMENTS
Salicylates				
Acetylsalicylic acid	ANTI-INFLAMMATORY DOSE 80–100 (<25 kg) 2500 mg/m² (>25 kg) ANTIPLATELET DOSE 5	4900	2–4	Kawasaki disease: high dose for initial and low dose for subsequent treatment Therapeutic serum levels (for anti-inflammatory therapy) = 15–25 mg/dl (measure 5 days after initiation of therapy or alteration of dose) Nonlinear (zero order) kinetics (*see text*) LFT abnormalities common (stop ASA if LFTs more than 3 times normal) Association with Reye's syndrome (*see text*) Watch for salicylism
Propionic Acid Group				
Naproxen*	10–20	1000	2	Most frequently used initial NSAID Overall favorable toxicity:efficacy profile Pseudoporphyria in fair-skinned children (*see text*) May have nonlinear pharmacokinetics at higher doses
Ibuprofen*	30–40	2400	3–4	Most favorable toxicity:efficacy profile Association with aseptic meningitis in patients with SLE
Ketoprofen	2–4	300	3–4	Least favorable toxicity:efficacy profile
Fenoprofen	35		4	Significant risk of nephrotoxicity
Acetic Acid Derivatives				
Indomethacin*	1.5–3.0	200	3	Useful in spondyloarthropathies and treatment of fever or pericarditis in systemic-onset JRA Less favorable toxicity profile Headache common at initiation and may diminish with continuation of therapy
Tolmetin	20–30	1800	3–4	Least favorable toxicity:efficacy profile May cause false-positive result for urinary protein
Sulindac	4–6	400	2	Absorbed as a prodrug and converted to active metabolite Significant enterohepatic recirculation May be less nephrotoxic than other NSAIDs
Diclofenac	2–3	150	3	Similar potency to indomethacin Reports of significant hepatotoxicity
Oxicams				
Piroxicam	0.2–0.3	20	1	Least favorable toxicity:efficacy profile Once-daily dosing possible: may be useful in older children or adolescents with poor medication compliance

ASA, acetylsalicylic acid; JRA, juvenile rheumatoid arthritis; LFT, liver function tests; NSAIDs, nonsteroidal anti-inflammatory drug; SLE, systemic lupus erythematosus.

*Available in liquid form.

Table 7–5

Relative Toxicities of NSAIDs

TOXICITY	ASA	IBUPROFEN	FENOPROFEN	NAPROXEN	INDOMETHACIN	SULINDAC	TOLMETIN	MECLOFENAMATE
GI irritation	+ + +	+	+ +	+ +	+ + + +	+ +	+ +	+ +
Peptic ulcer	+ +	+	+	+ +	+ + +	+	+	+
CNS	+	±	+ +	+	+ + + +	+	+	±
Tinnitus	+ + +	+	+ + +	+	+	+	+	±
Hepatitis	+ +	+	+	+	+	+	?	+
Asthma	+ +	+	+	+	+	+	+	+
Renal function	+	+	+	+	+ +	±	+ +	+
Bone marrow	−	+	+	+	+	+	+	+

ASA, acetylsalicylic acid; CNS, central nervous system; GI, gastrointestinal; NSAIDs, nonsteroidal anti-inflammatory drugs.

bleeding, or peptic ulcer disease and cardiovascular disease.[61] Most patients who have a serious GI complication requiring hospitalization, however, have not had prior GI side effects.[56, 57] Additional risk factors may include longer disease duration, higher NSAID dose, the use of more than one NSAID, longer duration of NSAID therapy, concomitant glucocorticoid or anticoagulant use, and serious underlying systemic disorders.[56, 57] Many of the studies on which these conclusions are based, however, do not account for the interaction of multiple factors or confounding by coexisting conditions.[56] It appears that infection with *H. pylori* increases the risk of gastroduodenal mucosal injury associated with NSAID use only minimally, if at all.[62]

The magnitude of this problem in children is poorly documented but has traditionally been thought to be considerably less than in adults, partly because of the absence of the associated risk factors identified in the adult population. *H. pylori* has not been reported to be an important pathogen in children with JRA treated with NSAIDs.[63] Studies in children confirm that although mild GI disturbances are frequently associated with NSAID therapy, the number of children who develop clinically significant gastropathy appears to be low.[50] In many children who develop GI symptoms while receiving NSAIDs, alternative causes, such as the underlying disease process, psychosocial factors, and other concomitant medications, may account for their symptoms. The rigor with which these have been systematically evaluated and the way that "clinically significant" gastropathy has been defined varies considerably among studies, resulting in variability in reported rates for this complication.

A retrospective study of a cohort of 702 children receiving NSAID therapy for JRA followed for at least 1 year found 5 children (0.7 percent) with clinically significant gastropathy defined as esophagitis, gastritis, or peptic ulcer disease.[64] The retrospective nature of this study may have resulted in a substantial underestimation of the prevalence of NSAID-associated gastropathy. A more recent prospective study of a cohort of 203 children found that although 135 children (66.5 percent) had documented GI symptoms at some stage during NSAID therapy, only 9 children (4.4 percent) had endoscopically detected ulcers or erosions; the most commonly reported GI symptoms were abdominal pain (49.7 percent) and appetite loss (32.0 percent).[65] Factors frequently associated with clinically significant gastropathy in children are abdominal pain at night, melanotic stools, and a previous history of gastropathy.[64] Endoscopic studies in very small numbers of highly selected groups of children with JRA receiving NSAIDs have reported a higher frequency of abnormalities.[66, 67] However, these endoscopic lesions, which are usually mild, have not been found to correlate well with symptoms, and their clinical significance is not clear.[66, 67] Further prospective studies are needed.

A number of studies have shown differences in rates of serious GI complications associated with different NSAIDs. Systematic reviews have found that ibuprofen was associated with the lowest risk; indomethacin, naproxen, sulindac, and aspirin with moderate risk; and tolmetin, ketoprofen, and piroxicam with the highest risk.[59, 68] Studies in children have also found that tolmetin may be associated with higher risk.[64, 65] Thus, a reasonable approach to therapy would be to initially choose an NSAID with a lower risk of GI complications. GI symptoms can be further minimized by ensuring that NSAIDs are always given with food. Although some studies in healthy volunteers suggest that enteric coating may reduce acute gastric mucosal injury,[69] the use of enteric-coated preparations and parenteral or rectal administration of NSAIDs aimed at preventing topical mucosal injury have not been shown to prevent gastric ulceration.[56] The development of "safer" NSAIDs, such as the highly selective COX-2 inhibitors or NSAIDs containing nitric oxide, offers considerable promise, but the clinical utility of these agents remains to be determined.[56]

The utility of antacids and H_2 antagonists for prophylaxis against serious NSAID-induced GI complications is controversial. Although these medications suppress symptoms, they do not prevent significant GI events such as endoscopically documented gastric ulcers; in fact, asymptomatic patients on acid-reduction therapies appear to be at greater risk for serious GI complications than patients not taking these medications, so their routine use in asymptomatic patients taking NSAIDs cannot be recommended.[56, 57] Sucralfate also does not appear to offer any significant benefit in the prophylaxis of NSAID-induced gastric ulcers.[70]

Misoprostol, a synthetic prostaglandin E_1 analogue, has been shown in adults to be effective in both prophylaxis[61, 71] and treatment of NSAID-induced gastroduodenal damage, allowing continuation of NSAID therapy while achieving ulcer healing.[72, 73] Studies of misoprostol co-therapy in children are limited but also suggest that it may be effective in the treatment of gastrointestinal toxicity symptoms in children receiving NSAIDs.[66, 74] Misoprostol may also be associated with a protective effect on hemoglobin values in NSAID-treated patients.[74, 75] Omeprazole, a proton pump inhibitor, has been shown to be superior to ranitidine and misoprostol for the prevention and treatment of NSAID-related gastroduodenal ulcers in adults.[76, 77] Currently, there are no good data regarding omeprazole use in children. Prospective studies are needed to further evaluate the role of misoprostol and omeprazole co-therapy in children.

Recommendations for the treatment of established dyspeptic symptoms or active gastroduodenal ulceration, with or without continuation of NSAIDs, differ from those for the prophylaxis of gastroduodenal injury. Symptoms of active gastroduodenal ulceration when NSAIDs have been discontinued can be treated empirically with an H_2-receptor antagonist or a proton pump inhibitor. If an ulcer develops, discontinuation of the NSAID is generally preferred, but if NSAID therapy needs to be continued, proton pump inhibitors are recommended.[56]

Hepatotoxicity

Hepatitis with elevation of transaminase levels can occur with any NSAID but has most commonly been reported in children with JRA receiving ASA; up to 50 percent of these children may have some elevation of enzyme levels,[78] and up to 15 percent may require discontinuation of therapy for this reason.[48] In one retrospective study, transaminase levels were increased in 6 percent of children receiving naproxen.[48] One of the confounding factors is that transaminases can be elevated in untreated JRA, particularly in the systemic-onset subtype, and in systemic lupus erythematosus (SLE). Elevated transaminase levels are rarely of clinical significance and often resolve spontaneously but may require lowering of the dose or temporary cessation of therapy. Rarely, hepatotoxicity is severe; NSAIDs have been associated with a poorly understood severe multisystem disorder, now called the *macrophage activation syndrome*, consisting of macrophage activation, hepatic involvement, consumptive coagulopathy, and neurologic manifestations.[79, 80] Thus, liver function should be carefully monitored in children taking NSAIDs, particularly those with systemic-onset JRA.

Renal Toxicity

Several types of renal complications have been associated with NSAID therapy. These include reversible renal insufficiency and acute renal failure; acute interstitial nephritis; nephrotic syndrome; papillary necrosis; and sodium, potassium, and water retention.[81–84] Although these complications are more often reported in the adult population, with an estimated prevalence of 1 to 2 percent, a number of cases have also been described in children.[81, 85–88] The limited data on the prevalence of these complications in children indicate that it is considerably lower than that reported in adults.

A 4-year prospective study of 226 children with JRA treated with NSAIDs found the prevalence of renal and urinary abnormalities attributable to NSAID therapy to be only 0.4 percent[89]; an even lower prevalence of 0.2 percent was reported in another cohort of 433 children.[90] Several studies have demonstrated subclinical abnormalities of renal glomerular or tubular function in children with JRA receiving NSAIDs by measuring the urinary excretion of selected glomerular (albumin, transferrin, immunoglobulin G, or IgG) and tubular protein (α_1- and β_2-microglobulin) or enzyme markers (*N*-acetyl-β-glucosaminidase).[91, 92] However, the clinical relevance of these abnormalities as potential markers for the development of more serious renal complications is not yet clear because no long-term data are available to correlate these abnormalities with important clinical outcomes.

The various renal syndromes associated with NSAID therapy differ in their pathophysiologic basis, clinical presentation, frequency, and predisposing risk factors. The most commonly reported complication is reversible renal insufficiency, mediated through the effect of NSAIDs on prostaglandin synthesis. Inhibition of renal prostaglandin synthesis has little effect on renal function in healthy persons. However, in states of hypovolemia or salt depletion, the adrenergic and renin-angiotensin system is activated, resulting in renal vasoconstriction. Prostaglandins are needed to maintain renal perfusion under such conditions by producing local vasodilatation. Inhibition of prostaglandin synthesis with NSAID therapy may suppress this protective autoregulatory mechanism, resulting in unopposed vasoconstrictor activity and renal hypoperfusion.[82, 83] This type of renal insufficiency is generally reversible within 24 to 72 hours.[81] Risk factors include underlying renal disease (such as SLE) or states of hypovolemia and salt depletion with high plasma renin activity (e.g., gastroenteritis, sepsis, congestive cardiac failure, cirrhosis, or diuretic treatment) in normal persons. Indomethacin is the NSAID most often implicated with this complication.[82, 93] In addition to impairment of renal function, some children show signs of fluid retention, such as congestive heart failure, edema, or hypertension, when treated with NSAIDs. A modest drop in hematocrit value with ASA or other NSAIDs may result from mild degrees of sodium retention and hemodilution rather than from anemia related to GI bleeding.[47]

Acute interstitial nephritis with nephrotic syndrome is far less commonly reported with NSAIDs. It occurs sporadically and is thought to represent a hypersensitivity type reaction.[83] It typically has a more abrupt onset with hematuria, heavy proteinuria, and flank pain. Unlike classic drug-induced allergic nephritis, however, fever, rash, eosinophilia, and eosinophiluria are generally not present. Onset may be from 2 weeks to 18 months after initiation of NSAID therapy, and resolution may take from 1 month to almost a year after discontinuation of the NSAID.[83] Renal failure may be severe enough to require temporary dialysis support. Glucocorticoids have been used to treat this complication, but their efficacy is unproven. Interstitial nephritis with and without nephrotic syndrome has also been described in a small number of children.[47] This complication is more commonly reported with propionic acid (naproxen, fenoprofen) and acetic acid (tolmetin, indomethacin, sulindac) derivatives.[83, 84]

Papillary necrosis is a chronic renal injury that has been most commonly associated with long-term analgesic abuse, particularly those containing phenacetin.[83, 94] It has also been reported to occur with several NSAIDs, including ibuprofen, fenoprofen, phenylbutazone, and mefenamic acid. Medullary ischemia is thought to be the initiating factor in the production of papillary necrosis.[83] The syndrome is usually characterized by painless leukocyturia and hematuria, without impairment of renal function, and by demonstration of changes on the IV pyelogram.[83, 86, 87, 95–99] Combination NSAID therapy appears to be a risk factor in both adults and children.[81, 99]

Central Nervous System Effects

Three general categories of CNS side effects have been reported in association with NSAID therapy in adults: aseptic meningitis, psychosis, and cognitive dysfunction.[100] The NSAID most commonly reported to cause aseptic meningitis has been ibuprofen; susceptibility appears to be greater in patients with SLE. However, there does not seem to be any cross-reactivity between NSAIDs for this complication. Indomethacin and sulindac have been reported to induce psychotic symptoms, including paranoid delusions, depersonalization, and hallucinations, in a small number of patients.[100] More subtle CNS effects such as cognitive dysfunction and depression can also occur and are probably under-recognized and under-reported. Tinnitus may occur with any NSAID but particularly with ASA.[47] A prospective study of 203 children with JRA found that CNS symptoms occurred in 55 percent of patients on NSAIDs; the most common symptom was headache, occurring in about one third of children.[101] Other reported symptoms included fatigue, sleep disturbance, and hyperactivity. Seizures were noted in two patients, both of whom were on indomethacin.

Cutaneous Toxicity

A diverse group of skin reactions, including pruritus, urticaria, morbilliform rashes, erythema multiforme, and phototoxic reactions, have been described.[47, 102] Initially described in Australia,[103] the syndrome of pseudoporphyria occurring in association with naproxen therapy in children with JRA has now been reported in several case series.[104–107] It is a distinctive photodermatitis marked by erythema, vesiculation, and in-

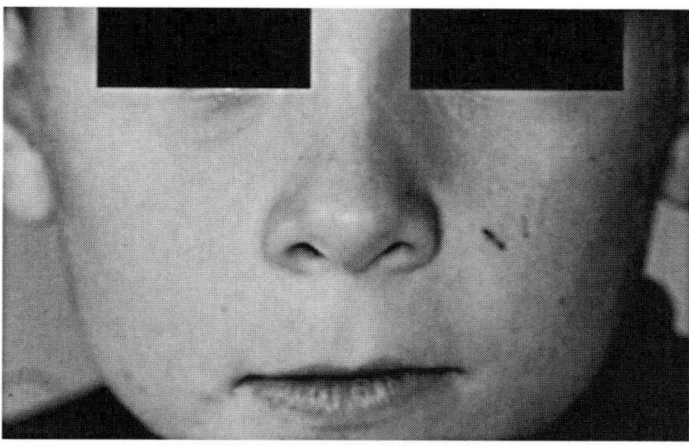

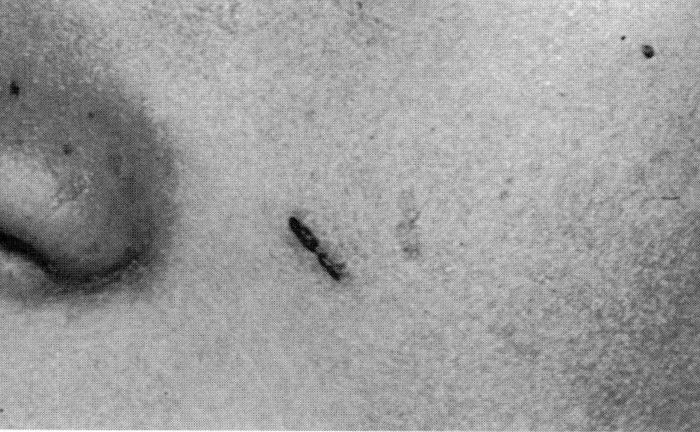

Figure 7–3. Distant and close-up views of the face of an 8-year-old boy with pseudoporphyria who was taking naproxen. Note a blistered lesion adjacent to a superficial scar. Superficial scars are also visible on the nose.

creased skin fragility characterized by easy scarring of sun-exposed skin (Fig. 7–3). Porphyrin metabolism is normal. All findings except scarring resolve with discontinuation of naproxen. Children with fair skin and blue eyes are particularly susceptible. Pseudoporphyria appears to be a common side effect even in geographic areas without high sun exposure; a 6-month prospective study of children seen in a rheumatology clinic in Halifax, Nova Scotia, reported a prevalence of 12 percent in those treated with naproxen.[106] Although this complication has most often been reported with naproxen, other NSAIDs have also been implicated.

Effects on Coagulation

The NSAIDs decrease platelet adhesiveness by interfering with platelet prostaglandin synthesis, such as thromboxane B_2, which promotes platelet aggregation. This inhibition is reversible in the case of all NSAIDs except ASA, which irreversibly acetylates and inactivates cyclo-oxygenase (see Fig. 7–2), an effect that persists for the life of the platelet; bleeding time returns to normal only as new platelets are released into the circulation.[47] The NSAIDs also displace anticoagulants from protein-binding sites, thereby potentiating their pharmacologic effect. These effects of NSAIDs must be considered when planning any surgical procedure.

Reye's Syndrome

Reye's syndrome was first described in Australia in 1963 as a distinct clinicopathologic entity by Reye and associates.[108] An association with salicylate therapy was later demonstrated in the early 1980s.[109] Reye's syndrome is an acute illness characterized by encephalopathy and fatty degeneration of the liver occurring almost exclusively in children and usually in association with a viral-like prodromal illness, the most common being influenza or other respiratory illnesses, varicella, or gastroenteritis.[110]

The onset of the illness is characterized by profuse vomiting and varying degrees of neurologic impairment: Initially, there may be fluctuating personality changes and deterioration in consciousness, followed by extreme irritability, agitation, confusion, delirium, and coma as the encephalopathy progresses. Associated metabolic abnormalities include hyperammonemia and elevated levels of hepatic transaminases, with consequences of hepatic dysfunction such as prolongation of the prothrombin time and severe hypoglycemia. Characteristic liver histopathologic abnormalities include microvesicular fat accumulation in hepatocytes on light microscopy and mitochondrial disorganization and proliferation of smooth endoplasmic reticulum on electron miscroscopy.[110]

The illness can be fatal, with an overall case-fatality rate of 31 percent and significantly higher rates in children less than 5 years of age and those with serum ammonia level greater than 45 μg/dl.[110] Reye's syndrome appears to be a heterogeneous condition; in recent years, a proportion of children presenting with Reye-like illnesses have been found to have various inborn metabolic disorders. This subgroup is characterized by features such as younger age, recurrent episodes, family history of similar illness, frequent hypoglycemia, cardiac enlargement, muscle weakness, and lack of mitochondrial disorganization in liver tissue.[110]

The association between Reye's syndrome and salicylate therapy was first reported in a small case-control study.[111] Although this study initially was a source of controversy, its findings were later confirmed by larger and more rigorously designed studies.[109] The association between salicylate use and Reye's syndrome is consistent among different studies and is very strong, with odds ratios as high as 35 to 40 in the larger studies.[112, 113] Although demonstration of an epidemiologic association alone is not sufficient to prove causation, there is further evidence in support of an etiologic role for salicylates in Reye's syndrome: The finding of a dose-response relationship, with higher doses of salicylate used in case subjects than in controls, and more recent epidemiologic evidence from the United States and United Kingdom indicate that there has been a dramatic decline in the incidence of Reye's syndrome concurrent with a decline in the use of salicylates in children since public health warnings in the mid-1980s.[110, 114]

In a large epidemiologic study in the United States, 14 of 361 patients with Reye's syndrome for whom data on aspirin use were available had taken salicylate-containing medications for illnesses such as JRA and Kawasaki disease.[110] Other studies have reported higher rates of Reye's syndrome in children taking salicylates for JRA.[115, 116] None of the studies to date has reported any association with other NSAIDs.[109] Physicians and others caring for children requiring long-term salicylate therapy should be aware of the risk of Reye's syndrome and be able to recognize the early symptoms so that salicylate therapy can be promptly withdrawn. These children should be offered varicella vaccine and annual vaccination against influenza in accordance with the recommendations of the Advisory Committee on Immunization Practices.[117]

Hypersensitivity and Miscellaneous Effects

The precipitation of asthma or anaphylaxis with NSAIDs has been reported in adults as a unique syndrome associated with nasal polyps; 15 to 40 percent of patients with nasal polyps may experience bronchospasm when given aspirin.[118, 119] Although this syndrome can theoretically be provoked by any NSAID, it has most commonly been reported with ASA or tolmetin; cross-reactivity between NSAIDs may occur.[47] However, there appears to be a correlation with the strength of cyclo-oxygenase inhibition so that more potent NSAIDs such as indomethacin induce bronchospasm at smaller doses than less potent ones such as ibuprofen.[120] Although "allergy" to ASA is often reported by patients or parents, true hypersensitivity to the drug is exceedingly rare in childhood. ASA hypersensitivity occurs in about 0.3 to 0.9 percent of the general population, 20 percent of patients with chronic urticaria, and 3 to 4 percent of patients with chronic asthma and nasal polyps.[121–123] It should be noted that such patients are often hypersensitive to the other NSAIDs.[124]

Effects on the bone marrow, including aplastic anemia, agranulocytosis, leukopenia, and thrombocytopenia have been reported but are rare.[47] Mild anemia occurs in about 2 to 14 percent of children[48] and may be partly due to hemodilution, hemolysis,[125] or occult GI blood loss due to NSAID therapy.[74]

Salicylates

The salicylates are a group of related drugs, differing by the nature of the substitutions on the carboxyl or hydroxyl groups of the molecule: acetylsalicylic acid, salsalate, choline salicylate, magnesium salicylate, and sodium salicylate. They are hydrolyzed in vivo to salicylic acid. Related compounds such as salicylamide and diflunisal are not hydrolyzed to salicylic acid and so are not considered salicylates.[126]

ASA is the oldest NSAID and has been used to treat the articular manifestations of rheumatic diseases for many years.[126–132] Although newer NSAIDs have largely replaced ASA as the mainstay of anti-inflammatory drug therapy in pediatric rheumatology, ASA continues to have a role in the management of Kawasaki disease (see Table 7–4). The general principles of NSAID mechanism of action and pharmacology, as well as the principles of therapy and spectrum of known adverse effects, have already been addressed with reference to salicylates where relevant. However, the salicylates differ from other NSAIDs in a number of specific aspects; these are addressed in the following paragraphs.

Mechanism of Action

ASA exerts its anti-inflammatory, analgesic, and antipyretic effects in part by irreversibly acetylating and inactivating cyclo-oxygenase, thus inhibiting the biosynthesis and release of the prostaglandins (see Fig. 7–2; see Chapter 5).[119, 133, 134] Other salicylates also inactivate this enzyme, but not irreversibly. A dose-dependent effect of ASA on the inhibition of prostacyclin (prostaglandin I_2) production by endothelial cells and of thromboxane A_2 production by platelets has also been noted and may be relevant in the management of Kawasaki disease or other types of vasculitis in children (see Chapter 27).[135, 136] Large doses of ASA increase urinary excretion and lower the serum concentration of urate; low doses have the opposite effect.[137] This phenomenon must not be confused with hyperuricemia or with gout, which is extremely rare in children.

Pharmacology

The plasma level of salicylate (ASA and salicylate ion) peaks 1 to 2 hours after a single dose, and the drug is virtually undetectable at 6 hours. ASA itself is bound very little to plasma protein, but salicylic acid binds extensively to albumin and erythrocytes. Salicylic acid is found in most body fluids (including the cerebrospinal fluid, saliva, synovial fluid, and breast milk), and it crosses the placenta.

ASA is metabolized by hepatic microsomal enzymes by conjugation with glycine to form salicyluric acid and, to a lesser extent, by conjugation with the phenolic and acyl glucuronides, which are in turn excreted by the kidneys. Renal clearance of these metabolites, which have longer half-lives than the parent drug, is augmented by alkalinization of the urine.

Administration

ASA is quickly absorbed from the stomach and proximal small intestine.[138, 139] Some salicylates (methyl salicylate, salicylic acid) are well absorbed through the skin. The systemic anti-inflammatory effects of ASA are maximal, and in most cases they are achieved only when serum steady-state levels are 15 to 25 mg/dl (1.09 to 1.81 mmol/L).[140, 141] Below 15 mg/dl, ASA does not function effectively as an anti-inflammatory agent; above 30 mg/dl (2.17 mmol/L), it is likely to be toxic. The dosage necessary to reach these concentrations is usually 75 to 90 mg/kg/day, divided into four doses given with food. Lower doses suffice in the child weighing more than 25 kg. The plasma half-life of salicylate increases as the plasma concentration of the drug increases (capacity-limited kinetics). For example, at a plasma concentration of 26 mg/dl, the half-life of ASA can be as long as 16 hours, whereas at a plasma level of 4 mg/dl, the half-life may be as short as 2.5 hours.[39] Consequently, the drug need not be given as frequently once plasma concentrations are high, and toxic concentrations of the drug take much longer to decrease than would otherwise be anticipated.

Therapeutic levels are not reliably attained before 2 to 5 days of administration. Serum salicylate and serum liver enzyme levels should be checked 5 days after initiation of therapy or after any dose adjustment. Although it is our practice to monitor salicylate concentrations in serum taken 2 hours after the morning dose, one study indicated that the timing of blood sampling was not critical if the interval between doses was 8 hours or less and a steady state had been achieved after 5 days of therapy.[142]

Toxicity—Salicylism

Salicylism (acute or chronic salicylate intoxication) may occur rapidly in the young child, and early signs such as drowsiness, irritability, or hyperpnea can easily be overlooked. In the very young child, metabolic acidosis and ketosis occur, whereas the older child may first experience respiratory alkalosis by direct action of ASA on the hypothalamus. Abdominal pain or vomiting may occur in some children. The child with fever and dehydration is prone to salicylism: in the child with intercurrent illness and nausea, vomiting, or diarrhea, the drug should be immediately discontinued.

Symptoms of salicylism include tinnitus, deafness, nausea, and vomiting (Table 7–6). Early, there is CNS stimulation (hyperkinetic agitation, excitement, maniacal behavior, slurred speech, disorientation, delirium, convulsions). Later, CNS depression (stupor and coma) supervenes. The young child, in whom there is a narrow margin between therapeutic and toxic levels,[143–145] may not effectively communicate symptoms of salicylism; therefore, the family must be thoroughly schooled in the signs of overdose.

Mild salicylate toxicity requires no treatment and often only a minor decrease in salicylate dose. In a child with persisting symptoms, evidence of CNS stimulation, or depression, the drug must be discontinued. The child should be monitored for evidence of acute salicylate toxicity: fever, acute renal failure, CNS depression, pulmonary edema, bleeding, and hypoglycemia. In situations of severe chronic salicylism or acute overdose, the stomach contents should be emptied, and activated charcoal (0.5 to 1.0 g/kg) should be administered. Urine output, body temperature, serum electrolytes, and glucose should be monitored, and glucose-containing IV fluids should be given as required. Alkaline diuresis induced with sodium bicarbonate and furosemide increases the rate of salicylate excretion in the urine but must be carefully titrated in the presence of rapidly changing metabolic or respiratory function. Peritoneal dialysis or hemodialysis may be necessary. The reader is referred to the recommendations of Mofenson and Caraccio[146] for details of the management of the child with severe salicylate poisoning.

Table 7–6

Toxicity of Salicylates

Gastric irritation (50%)
Tinnitus and/or diminished hearing (15%)
Hepatotoxicity (2%)
Reye's syndrome (rare)
Hypersensitivity (in asthma) (rare)
Salicylism
  Mild: lethargy, dizziness, headache, diaphoresis, nausea
  Moderate: confusion, hyperpnea, metabolic acidosis, respiratory alkalosis
  Severe: hyperpyrexia, convulsions, cardiovascular collapse

Contraindications

ASA leads to hemolysis in children with the enzyme defects glucose-6-phosphate dehydrogenase and pyruvate kinase deficiency. It should be avoided in children with bleeding disorders, such as hemophilia or von Willebrand's disease, and in patients receiving thrombolytic agents or anticoagulants. ASA should not be given during the last trimester of pregnancy because of the effects on coagulation and platelet function.

Drug Interactions

ASA should be used with caution in children taking certain other drugs. Levels of methotrexate,[43] valproic acid,[147] phenytoin,[148] and other NSAIDs (tolmetin, diclofenac)[142, 149] may be increased in children who are also receiving aspirin. ASA decreases the bioavailability of other NSAIDs by 20 to 50 percent[142] and increases the digitalis concentration by 30 percent,[148] although the clinical significance of this interaction is uncertain. Glucocorticoids increase the rate of excretion of aspirin,[150] and salicylism may occur if glucocorticoid drugs are abruptly discontinued in a child taking therapeutic amounts of ASA.

Disease-Modifying Antirheumatic Drugs

A number of drugs used to treat JRA and certain other rheumatic diseases do not produce an immediate analgesic or anti-inflammatory effect but exert their beneficial effects weeks to months after initiation of therapy. These compounds, called *disease-modifying antirheumatic drugs* (DMARDs) or *slow-acting antirheumatic drugs* (SAARDs), currently include MTX, the antimalarials, sulfasalazine, gold compounds and D-penicillamine.[151]

Historically, there was reluctance to start DMARD treatment until relatively late in the course of disease. Standard practice had been to use one, two, or even three NSAIDs sequentially (or occasionally even in combination) before starting DMARD therapy. Much of this delay had to do with the potential serious toxicities of DMARDs (principally gold and D-penicillamine), the fact that JRA was not a fatal disease and therefore thought not to warrant treatment with drugs of such potentially significant toxicities, and a belief that most children would eventually "outgrow" the disease. However, in recent years, there has been a philosophical shift in therapeutic approach. This shift has been based on an appreciation that irreversible damage occurs early; that active disease, leading to deleterious long-term effects, persists for many years[152]; and that MTX, the most frequently prescribed drug in this class, is both safe and effective.[153–155] Therefore, there has been a tendency to pursue a more aggressive approach than in the past and to start DMARDs early in the course of the disease to prevent irreversible joint damage, rather than wait for significant damage to declare itself. Furthermore, experience with combination therapy in adult rheumatoid arthritis has led to use of a variety of combinations in JRA as well.

MTX is the most commonly used DMARD for JRA. Gold and D-penicillamine now are rarely used for JRA. Several DMARDs are also used to treat other rheumatic diseases (e.g., hydroxychloroquine in the management of SLE and, occasionally, juvenile dermatomyositis [JDM]; sulfasalazine in therapy of the spondyloarthropathies). In the treatment of arthritis, DMARDs are usually given in addition to an NSAID. The goal of treatment is to achieve disease control with drugs from this class and then to stop other treatments (e.g., NSAIDs and prednisone).

Methotrexate

Low-dose weekly MTX has emerged as one of the most useful agents in the therapeutic armamentarium for the management of children with rheumatic diseases. It is one among only a small number of agents that has been demonstrated to be efficacious in a randomized controlled trial in children; this drug is now often the first-choice second-line agent in childhood arthritis.[156] Although it has been most extensively studied in adult rheumatoid arthritis and in children with JRA, its use is growing in many other chronic inflammatory disorders.[157]

Mechanism of Action

MTX (Fig. 7–4) is a folic acid analogue and a potent competitive inhibitor of dihydrofolate reductase (DHFR) (Fig. 7–5). It may also inhibit thymidylate synthase and interfere with the metabolic transfer of single carbon units in methylation reactions, especially those involved in synthesis of thymidylate and purine deoxynucleosides, which are essential components of DNA.[158] It may also interfere with de novo purine biosynthesis by inhibition of 5-aminoimidazole-4-carboxamide ribonucleotide (AICAR) transformylase, an enzyme in the purine biosynthetic pathway. MTX-induced inhibition of AICAR transformylase and secondary inhibition of adenosine deaminase may also lead to accumulation and enhanced release of adenosine, a potent inhibitor of neutrophil adherence.[159, 160] It is now thought that the effects of MTX are in fact mediated primarily through the anti-inflammatory action of adenosine.[161]

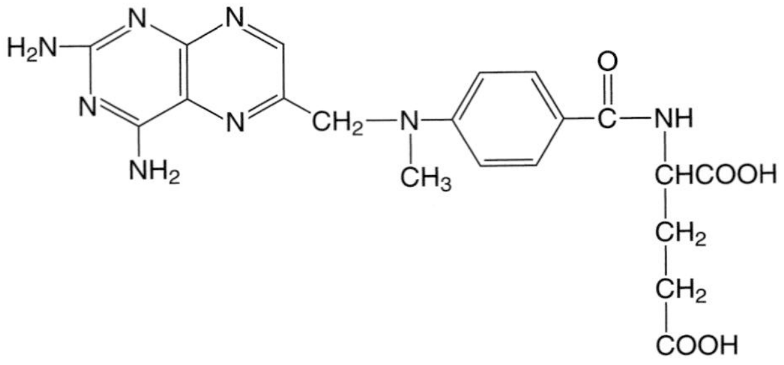

Figure 7–4. Structure of methotrexate.

The mechanism of action of MTX in JRA or adult rheumatoid arthritis is not clearly elucidated, although MTX is known to act at a number of intracellular levels. In addition to its action as an antimetabolite, it acts as an anti-inflammatory and immunomodulatory agent. MTX modulates the function of many of the cells involved in inflammation and affects the production of a variety of cytokines, thus acting as a potent inhibitor of cell-mediated immunity.[158, 161, 162] It may also have more direct effects in inflamed joints by inhibiting the proliferation of synovial cells and synovial collagenase gene expression.[163] Although the exact mechanism of action is the subject of intense study, it is not yet possible to clearly distinguish which of the many cellular and immune effects demonstrated in vitro and in vivo are of particular relevance to MTX's clinical effects. The reader is referred to reviews that explore this issue in greater detail.[158, 161, 162] The widespread biologic effects of MTX may in fact account for its observed efficacy in a wide variety of diseases with disparate

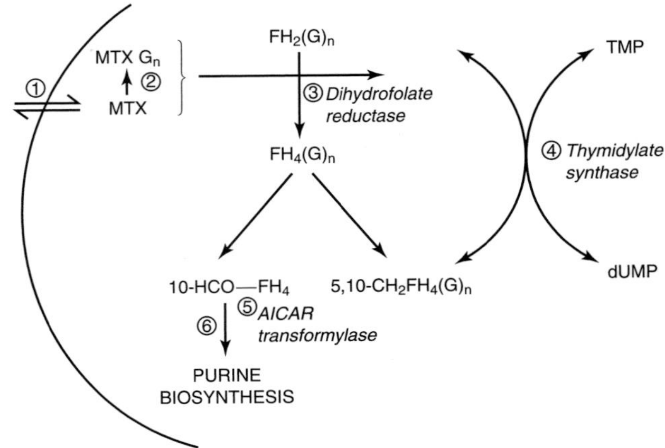

Figure 7–5. Steps in methotrexate intracellular metabolism and possible sites of action. AICAR, 5-aminoimidazole-4-carboxamide ribonucleotide; dUMP, deoxyuridylate monophosphate; MTX, methotrexate; TMP, thymidylate monophosphate. (From Kremer J: Mechanism of action of MTX in RA. Rheumatology 34[Suppl 2]: 26–29, 1995. By permission of Oxford University Press.)

pathogeneses such as cancer, psoriasis, and the various rheumatic and other chronic inflammatory diseases.

Pharmacology

There is significant intraindividual and interindividual variability in the absorption and pharmacokinetics of MTX after oral administration.[164] Although the average oral bioavailability is about 0.70 (compared with IV dosing), the range may be quite wide (0.25 to 1.49), with 25 percent of subjects in one study absorbing less than half their dose.[165] Factors such as age-related differences, the influence of food, and the effects of concurrently administered medications contribute to this variability. The effect of food on the oral bioavailability of MTX has been controversial.[166] However, a pharmacokinetic study demonstrated that factors such as age, body weight, creatinine clearance, sex, dose, and fed-versus-fasted state significantly influenced the disposition of MTX in adults with rheumatoid arthritis.[167] The bioavailability of MTX has also been demonstrated to be greater in the fasting state in children with JRA.[168] We currently recommend that MTX be given on an empty stomach with water or clear citrus beverages. In general, oral bioavailability is about 15 percent less than after intramuscular (IM) administration. Bioavailability of IM and subcutaneous administration is similar,[169] with the latter being generally more acceptable for children who require parenteral MTX.

After a single dose of MTX, the drug is present in the circulation for a relatively short period of time before redistribution to the tissues (Fig. 7–6). Peak serum levels are reached in approximately 1.5 hours (range, 0.25 to 6 hours), with elimination half-life being approximately 7 hours in subjects with normal renal function.[170] Circulating levels fall rapidly as the drug is distributed into tissue and eliminated. The predominant route of elimination is renal, with more than 80 percent of the drug eliminated unchanged via glomerular filtration and tubular secretion within 8 to 48 hours. A smaller but significant route of elimination is the biliary tract. The pharmacokinetics of MTX are triphasic. The initial rapid phase represents tissue distribution and renal clearance; the second phase is prolonged because of slow release from tissues, tubular reabsorption, and enterohepatic recirculation; the third phase is flat between weekly doses, reflecting the gradual release of tissue MTX.[170]

Most MTX is delivered to cells as the parent compound, with 3 to 11 percent being hydroxylated in the liver to 7-OH-MTX. A portion of intracellular MTX and 7-OH-MTX is metabolized to MTX polyglutamates, long-lived derivatives that retain biochemical and biologic activity within the cell.[170] These intracellular, polyglutamated MTX derivatives may in fact be the active anti-inflammatory agents.[161] This may explain why plasma drug levels do not correlate well with clinical effects and so are not useful in routine monitoring of MTX therapy.[164] Measurement of MTX levels in saliva has also not been helpful.[170, 171] The pharmacokinetics of oral MTX in JRA appear to be age dependent, with more extensive metabolism of MTX in younger children.[172] This difference may account for the observation that children require higher doses of MTX than adults to obtain similar therapeutic effects.[173, 174]

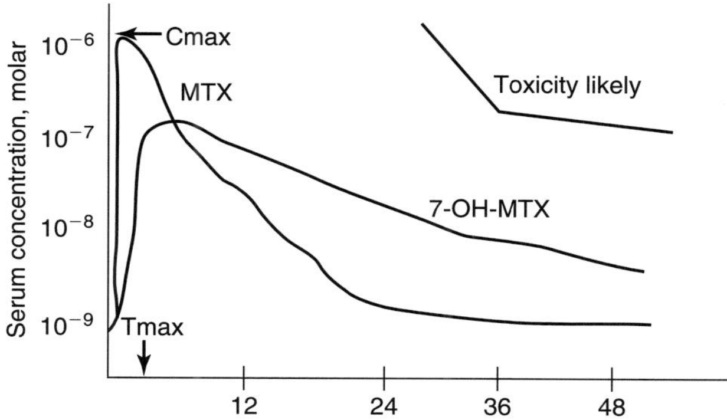

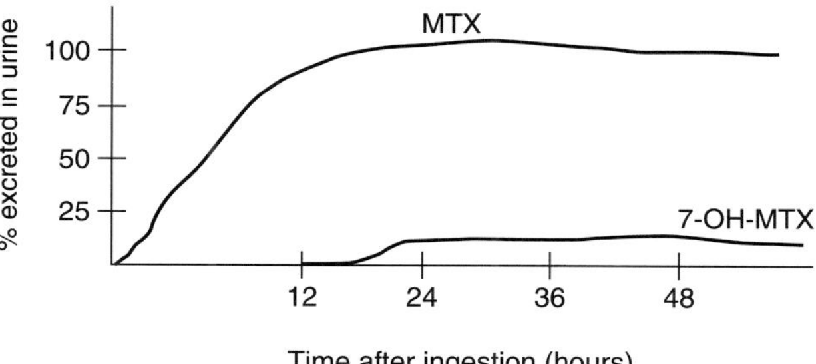

Figure 7–6. Time course of methotrexate (MTX) and 7-OH-methotrexate (7-OH-MTX) after an oral dose of 15 mg. (From Hillson JL, Furst DE: Pharmacology and pharmacokinetics of methotrexate in rheumatic disease. Practical issues in treatment and design. Rheum Dis Clin North Am 23[4]: 757–778, 1997.)

At low doses, MTX is only moderately protein bound (11 to 57 percent), and so the potential for interactions with other protein-bound drugs is small and usually not clinically significant.[170] Studies in adults have not shown a consistent or clinically important interaction between MTX and NSAIDs. However, several studies in children have demonstrated an interaction between MTX and NSAIDs that may be clinically significant in individual patients, particularly those with any renal dysfunction.[43, 175] It is thought that this interaction may be mediated through competition for protein-binding sites and through alteration of renal clearance.[157] The combination of MTX and trimethoprim-sulfamethoxazole should be avoided because it may lead to hematologic toxicity through the synergistic effects of these drugs on DHFR. Although the potential for interaction between MTX and various other drugs such as sulfasalazine, glucocorticoids, and folate supplementation exists, current clinical data do not support general avoidance of these combinations.[170]

Efficacy

The short- to medium-term efficacy of MTX in children with JRA is now well established.[157, 176] Benefits in initial retrospective and uncontrolled studies were subsequently confirmed in a combined USA-USSR placebo-controlled, randomized controlled clinical trial.[153] In this 6-month study of 127 children with resistant JRA (mean age, 10.1 years; mean disease duration, 5.1 years), 63 percent of the group treated with 10 mg/M² of MTX improved compared with only 32 percent of those treated with 5 mg/M² and 36 percent of the placebo group. The assessment of efficacy was based on a composite of clinical and laboratory parameters and subjective global assessment by physician and parent but did not include any functional assessments or radiographic examinations.

Several subsequent studies have suggested that MTX may also slow the radiologic progression of disease in JRA, although the available data are not conclusive.[177, 178] Some authors suggest that earlier treatment with MTX, possibly before the appearance of radiographic changes, may favorably influence the outcome of MTX treatment in children with systemic-onset disease.[179] Similar results have been found with early "aggressive" treatment in adults with recent-onset rheumatoid arthritis.[180] However, there appears to be a plateau effect in MTX efficacy after about 6 months and worsening of disease in some children with systemic-onset JRA.[181] The longer-term efficacy of MTX in JRA and its impact on function and quality of life need further study.

There is also accumulating experience with the use of MTX in many other pediatric rheumatic disorders, including JDM, SLE, various vasculitides, spondyloarthropathies, sarcoidosis, scleroderma, and idiopathic uveitis.[157] However, the evidence for the efficacy of MTX in these conditions is less strong and often based on open, uncontrolled studies or extrapolated from the larger experience in adults, which is not always valid. The reader is referred to the chapters dealing with these conditions for a fuller discussion of the role of MTX in their overall management.

Dosage, Route of Administration, and Duration of MTX Therapy

Standard effective doses of MTX in children with JRA are in the range of 10 to 15 mg/M²/week or 0.3 to 0.6 mg/kg/week. However, children seem to tolerate much higher doses than adults, and some series have described using up to 20 to 25 mg/M²/week or up to 1.1 mg/kg/week in children with resistant disease with relative safety in the short term.[173, 174] The longer-term safety of MTX therapy at these doses is not known.

Parenteral MTX administration should be considered in those children who (1) have a poor clinical response to orally administered MTX (this may be due to poor compliance or to reduced oral bioavailability for a variety of reasons), (2) need a dose in excess of about 10 to 15 mg/M²/week in order to achieve maximum clinical response—oral MTX absorption is a saturable process, whereas subcutaneous administration is not (Fig. 7–7),[182, 183] and (3) develop significant GI toxicity with orally administered MTX because there is some anecdotal experience that patients complain of less GI irritation when the drug is given parenterally.[51, 157] Some pediatric rheumatologists even advocate using parenteral MTX at initiation of treatment to ensure complete absorption and achievement of early disease remission.[157, 184]

The issue of when, how, and by what criteria to attempt withdrawal of MTX therapy in JRA is currently undecided. There have been a number of studies in children who have been treated with variable doses of MTX for variable periods of time in whom discontinuation of MTX has been attempted after clinical "remission" of variable length was achieved.[185–187] The criteria for "remission" or "relapse" have usually not been well defined or standardized among various studies, and the assessment of outcomes has been nonblinded. Given these limitations, no firm conclusions can be drawn about the optimal time and mode of MTX discontinuation in children with JRA. MTX withdrawal may result in disease flare in more than 50 percent of patients; this rate may be even higher in younger children.[185, 187] There are conflicting data about the ease with which remission can be re-established when MTX is restarted after disease relapse, which may be related to the different doses of MTX used and the differing lengths of follow-up in the studies reported to date. Prospective studies with more standardized assessments of outcome and durations of follow-up are needed to address these issues.

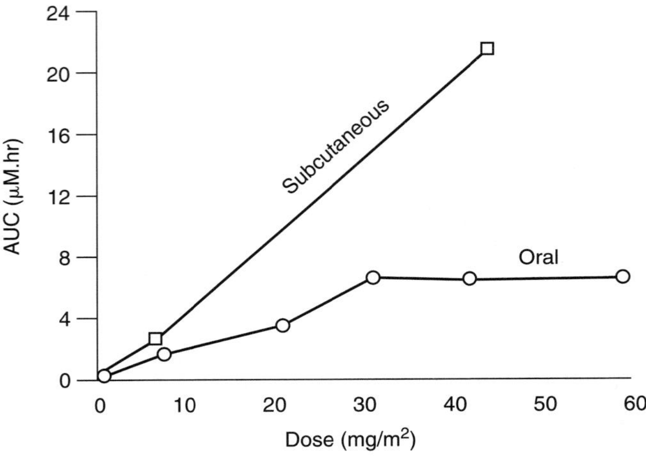

Figure 7–7. Bioavailability of oral and subcutaneously administered methotrexate. AUC, area under the curve. (Adapted from Wallace CA: New uses of methotrexate. Contemp Pediatr 11: 43–53, 1994.)

Safety

MTX is currently considered the second-line agent with the best efficacy-toxicity profile for the treatment of various rheumatic diseases in children and adults.[176, 188] Although MTX is associated with a number of potential toxicities, the documented overall frequency and severity of adverse effects in children with arthritis have been low (Table 7–7).[155, 157, 189] Most side effects are mild and reversible and can be treated conservatively. The two areas of greatest concern and debate, especially in children, have been the potential increased risk of hepatic cirrhosis in patients exposed to large cumulative doses of MTX and a possible increased risk of malignancies. Although the precise mechanism of all MTX-related toxicities is not yet clearly understood, at least some of its adverse effects are directly related to its folate antagonism and its cytostatic effects.[190] This is especially evident in tissues with a high cell turnover, such as the GI tract and bone marrow, which have a high requirement for purines, thymidine, and methionine. Supplementation with folic or folinic acid may diminish these but not other types of toxicities which, along with MTX efficacy, may be mediated by different mechanisms (see later).[190]

Table 7–7

Reported Adverse Effects in Children Treated with Methotrexate*

	1	2	3	4	5	6	7	8	TOTALS
Patients (n)	19	23	12	19	30	62	86	27	277
Treatment duration									
Mean (mo)	10.5	19.2	6	18.5		27	6		
Range (mo)	4–10	6–52	6	8–39	6–30	19–65		6–72	4–72
Methotrexate dose									
($mg/M^2/wk$)	4–17		8–25	5–15		5–20	5 or 10	10–15	
(mg/kg/wk)		0.1–0.6			0.4–0.8				
Adverse Effects									
Gastrointestinal symptoms	2	0	1	2	6	14	8	0	33
Peptic ulcer	0	0	ND	0	0	4	0	1	5
Stomatitis	1	0	ND	1	0	0	2	1	5
Mouth ulcers	1	0	1	0	2	0	1	0	4
Rashes	0	0	ND	0	ND	0	1	0	1
Alopecia	ND	0	ND	0	ND	2	0	0	2
Jaundice	0	0	ND	0	ND	ND	0	1	1
Bacterial infections	0	0	ND	ND	ND	4	0	ND	4
Herpes zoster	1	0	0	0	1	1	0	ND	3
Mood changes	0	ND	1	ND	ND	ND	0	ND	1
Liver function test elevations	3	10	1	1	3	9	1	4	25
Hematuria	0	0	0	0	0	0	0	0	0
Leukopenia	0	0	0	0	1	0	0	0	1
Anemia	0	0	0	0	0	1	0	0	1
Proteinuria	3	0	0	0	0	0	0	0	3

ND, not determined.

*References of studies 1 through 8:

1. Truckenbrodt H, Hafner R: Methotrexate therapy in juvenile rheumatoid arthritis: a retrospective study. Arthritis Rheum 29(6): 801–807, 1986.
2. Wallace CA, Bleyer WA, Sherry DD, et al: Toxicity and serum levels of methotrexate in children with juvenile rheumatoid arthritis. Arthritis Rheum 32: 677–681, 1989.
3. Speckmaier M, Findeisen J, Woo P, et al: Low-dose methotrexate in systemic onset juvenile chronic arthritis. Clin Exp Rheumatol 7: 647–650, 1989.
4. Rose CD, Singsen BH, Eichenfield AH, et al: Safety and efficacy of methotrexate therapy for juvenile rheumatoid arthritis. J Pediatr 117: 653–659, 1990.
5. Halle F, Prieur AM: Evaluation of methotrexate in the treatment of juvenile chronic arthritis according to the subtype. Clin Exp Rheumatol 9: 297–302, 1991.
6. Graham LD, Myones BL, Rivas-Chacon RF, Pachman LM: Morbidity associated with long-term methotrexate therapy in juvenile rheumatoid arthritis. J Pediatr 120: 468–473, 1992.
7. Giannini EH, Brewer EJ, Kuzmina N, et al: Methotrexate in resistant juvenile rheumatoid arthritis. Results of the USA-USSR double-blind, placebo-controlled trial. The Pediatric Rheumatology Collaborative Study Group and The Cooperative Children's Study Group. N Engl J Med 326: 1043–1049, 1992.
8. Huang JL: Methotrexate in the treatment of children with chronic arthritis—long-term observations of efficacy and safety. Br J Clin Pract 50: 311–314, 1996.

Modified from Singsen BH, Goldbach-Mansky R: Methotrexate in the treatment of juvenile rheumatoid arthritis and other pediatric rheumatic and nonrheumatic disorders. Rheum Dis Clin North Am 23(4): 811–841, 1997.

Gastrointestinal Toxicity. Abdominal discomfort and nausea are the most frequently reported symptoms, occurring in about 12 percent of children with JRA who receive MTX. Stomatitis or oral ulcers are reported in about 3 percent of children.[157] Higher rates are reported in adults, with up to 60 percent of patients on low-dose MTX developing GI adverse events in the form of stomatitis, anorexia, abdominal pain, indigestion, dyspepsia, nausea, vomiting, weight loss, or diarrhea.[191, 192] MTX-related abdominal discomfort, anorexia, nausea, or oral ulcers usually occur within 24 to 36 hours of the weekly dose and can be diminished by the addition of folic acid supplementation (see later), dose reduction or, in some troublesome cases, conversion to subcutaneous MTX administration, although the evidence for the effectiveness of the latter strategy is only anecdotal.[157]

Liver Toxicity. The effect of MTX on liver function and the development of hepatic fibrosis remains a major concern and has been extensively reviewed.[193] MTX is associated with the potential for both acute and chronic hepatotoxicity; mild acute toxicity, with elevations of transaminases, is common, occurring in about 9 percent of MTX-treated children with JRA.[157] These elevations are usually transient and resolve with either MTX discontinuation or lowered dose after a brief interval off treatment.[153, 155] In some of these cases, concurrent administration of NSAIDs may be contributing to the elevation in transaminases, and discontinuing NSAID treatment may allow normalization of liver function.[194]

The issue of greatest concern with the long-term use of low-dose MTX in children has been the potential for significant liver fibrosis or cirrhosis. However, the risk of this complication in children with JRA may differ from that in adults with rheumatoid arthritis or psoriasis treated with low-dose MTX. Long-term studies of MTX use in adult patients with rheumatoid arthritis have found a much lower incidence of liver fibrosis and cirrhosis than that initially reported in psoriatic patients; one retrospective study of 16,000 patients with rheumatoid arthritis reported a 5-year cumulative incidence of liver cirrhosis or failure of 1 in 1000 MTX-treated patients.[195]

Another study has suggested that the incidence may be higher, with a 5-year cumulative incidence of cirrhosis of 9.4 in 1000 MTX-treated patients with rheumatoid arthritis.[196] A meta-analysis of patients with rheumatoid arthritis and psoriasis found that higher cumulative dose of MTX, heavy alcohol consumption, and the presence of psoriasis were associated with higher risk of progressive liver histologic abnormalities.[197] Other risk factors include preexisting liver disease, obesity, insulin-dependent diabetes mellitus, and renal insufficiency.[193, 198]

The American College of Rheumatology has suggested guidelines for monitoring liver toxicity in patients with rheumatoid arthritis based on regular measurement of liver enzymes and performance of liver biopsy in selected cases with persistent abnormalities of liver enzymes (Table 7–8).[199] These guidelines were developed by expert consensus and subsequently evaluated for their usefulness; they were found to be cost effective and clinically useful, with a sensitivity of 80 percent and specificity of 82 percent but a low positive predictive value of 27 percent.[198] Although a similar level of consensus does not exist for monitoring MTX-treated children with JRA, most pediatric rheumatologists tend to follow these guidelines or a variation of these recommendations.[157] A study examining the relationship between hepatotoxic risk factors and liver histopathology in MTX-treated children with JRA found that serial biochemical abnormalities were significantly associated with Roenigk grade and the presence of liver fibrosis, suggesting that the guidelines for monitoring MTX hepatotoxicity in rheumatoid arthritis may also be applicable to patients with JRA.[200] It must be remembered, however, that even close monitoring of liver function tests does not eliminate the possibility of progressive hepatic fibrosis. Erickson and colleagues[198] reported one patient in a series who developed cirrhosis despite normal results on liver function tests. Furthermore, these guidelines may not apply to patients receiving more than 25 mg/week or a cumulative dose of greater than 10 g; surveillance liver biopsies may be indicated for these patients.[193]

Table 7–8

Recommendations for Monitoring for Hepatic Safety in Rheumatoid Arthritis (RA) Patients Receiving Methotrexate (MTX)

A. Baseline
   1. Tests for all patients
      a. Liver blood tests (aspartate aminotransferase [AST], alanine aminotransferase [ALT], alkaline phosphatase, albumin, bilirubin), hepatitis B and C serologic studies
      b. Other standard tests, including complete blood cell count and serum creatinine
   2. Pretreatment liver biopsy (Menghini suction-type needle) only for patients with:
      a. Prior excessive alcohol consumption
      b. Persistently abnormal baseline AST values
      c. Chronic hepatitis B or C infection

B. Monitor AST, ALT, albumin at 4- to 8-week intervals

C. Perform liver biopsy if:
   1. Five of 9 determinations of AST within a given 12-month interval (6 of 12 if tests are performed monthly) are abnormal (defined as an elevation above the upper limit of normal)
   2. There is a decrease in serum albumin below the normal range (in the setting of well-controlled RA)

D. If results of liver biopsy are:
   1. Roenigk grade I, II, or IIIA: resume MTX and monitor as in B, C1 and C2 above
   2. Roenigk grade IIIB or IV: discontinue MTX

E. Discontinue MTX in patient with persistent liver test abnormalities, as defined in C1 and C2 above, who refuses liver biopsy

From Kremer JM, et al: Methotrexate for rheumatoid arthritis: suggested guidelines for monitoring liver toxicity. Arthritis Rheum 37: 316–328, Copyright © 1994 Wiley-Liss, Inc. Reprinted by permission of Wiley-Liss, Inc., a subsidiary of John Wiley & Sons, Inc.

In a number of small studies in children, liver biopsies were performed after cumulative doses of up to 3000 mg had been reached; none has shown any cirrhosis.[155, 201, 202] More recently, a cross-sectional study has reported on results of liver histology in children exposed to even higher cumulative doses of MTX (>3000 mg or >4000 mg/1.73 M²), with mean duration of treatment being about 6 years (some children being treated for up to 10 years).[203] No significant fibrosis or cirrhosis was found. However, 13 of 14 biopsies (93 percent) showed some histologic abnormality, with only one being graded as Roenigk grade II.

Although these data are encouraging, their interpretation requires some caution: First, the number of children studied is small, and so the statistical power for detection of infrequent events, such as cirrhosis, is low (type II error); second, only 58 percent of eligible MTX-treated patients underwent biopsy, and so selection bias may have occurred; and third, the clinical significance, if any, of the minor histologic abnormalities detected in the majority of biopsies is not known; there were no control biopsies to help distinguish the effects of disease (e.g., systemic-onset JRA) or concomitant medications (e.g., NSAIDs) on liver histology.

A follow-up study from the same group reported the results of 33 liver biopsies in 25 patients; 27 biopsies (82 percent) were classified as Roenigk grade I; 4 (12 percent) as grade II; and 2 (6 percent) as grade IIIA; none demonstrated significant fibrosis. The frequency of biochemical abnormalities and body mass index were the only risk factors found to significantly relate to the Roenigk grade.[203] However, the same limitations as with the earlier study apply, particularly with respect to the small numbers of patients studied (possibility of type II error) and the unknown significance of the minor histologic abnormalities observed in the majority of patients. Further long-term prospective studies in larger numbers of MTX-treated children are needed to define more accurately the risk of MTX-related liver fibrosis or cirrhosis and to develop appropriate guidelines for monitoring therapy in JRA.

Infection. Although MTX may potentially increase the risk for common bacterial infections, herpes zoster, and opportunistic infections, these complications are infrequently reported in treated patients. One study of 62 children with JRA treated for a mean of 161 weeks reported only two cases of recurrent cellulitis, one of osteomyelitis, and one of an infected Hickman catheter site; there were eight viral infections including one case of herpes zoster, one case of mononucleosis, and six cases of primary varicella. Many of the patients with varicella infection were also concurrently receiving glucocorticoids.[155] The randomized controlled clinical trial of MTX treatment in JRA did not document an increased frequency of infection in the children treated with MTX compared with placebo.[153]

Although the overall risk of infection appears to be low, it has not been precisely quantitated in adults or children. Infections in MTX-treated patients are usually common bacterial infections (e.g., lungs or skin) or herpes zoster. Opportunistic infections associated with MTX treatment are rare unless there is concurrent treatment with high-dose glucocorticoids.[204] Immunization with inactivated vaccines is not contraindicated in MTX-treated children, but immunization with live attenuated vaccines should be avoided.[51, 205] There are currently no generally accepted guidelines regarding varicella immunization in these children. However, one may need to consider active varicella immunization of susceptible children and family members prior to initiation of MTX therapy.[205] Family members of MTX-treated patients who require polio immunization should receive inactivated vaccine.

Hematologic Toxicity. Hematologic toxicity may include macrocytic anemia, leukopenia, thrombocytopenia, and pancytopenia. In adult patients with rheumatoid arthritis, pancytopenia has been reported in about 1 to 2 percent of MTX-treated patients.[206] Identified risk factors in this population include impaired renal function, advanced age, concurrent viral infection, alcohol ingestion, folate deficiency, hypoalbuminemia, or drug interactions (e.g., trimethoprim/sulfamethoxazole). MTX-associated pancytopenia has not been reported in children, and hematologic toxicity is uncommon overall; a 1997 review of published studies, including a total of 277 MTX-treated children, found only one case of leukopenia and one case of macrocytic anemia in this population.[157] Although supplemental folate treatment results in lowering of the mean corpuscular volume in MTX-treated patients, whether this will prevent pancytopenia is not yet known. Spontaneous recovery is usual within 2 weeks of withdrawal of MTX in patients with mild bone marrow suppression. Patients with moderate to severe bone marrow suppression may require folinic acid rescue and supportive therapy such as with colony-stimulating factors.[192]

Malignancy. The issue of whether MTX treatment is an independent risk factor for various malignancies is controversial and remains unresolved. Although in vitro studies have shown that MTX has mutagenic and carcinogenic potential, in vivo studies in animal models (mice, rats, hamsters) have failed to demonstrate any carcinogenicity. In humans, low-dose weekly MTX therapy has not been convincingly linked to malignancy.[204, 207] However, there have been a number of case reports of an association between MTX treatment and lymphoproliferative diseases in adult patients with rheumatoid arthritis[208, 209]; it has not been possible to determine whether these observations were merely coincidental or causally linked to MTX or to the underlying disease process.[207] Rheumatoid arthritis is known to be associated with an increased risk of hematologic malignancy.[210]

More recently, there have been several cases of Epstein-Barr virus–associated lymphoma presenting during the course of MTX treatment for rheumatoid arthritis or dermatomyositis that regresses with discontinuation of MTX.[211] Some of the reported cases have also demonstrated features typical of immunosuppression-induced lymphoproliferation, including extranodal location, large cell or polymorphous histology, geographic areas of necrosis, and the presence of Epstein-Barr virus.[212] The association of MTX with reversible lymphoproliferation suggests a causative role.[213, 214] However, it is also important to note that MTX has not been shown to increase the risk of lymphoproliferative disorders when used in other diseases such as psoriasis[215, 216] or in bone marrow transplantation.[207] To date, there has only been one case report of Hodgkin's lymphoma occurring in a child with JRA treated with MTX: a 6-year-old girl with systemic-onset JRA who was treated with low-dose MTX for 18 months (total dose, 370 mg).[217] Long-term prospective cohort studies, with appropriate controls, are needed to define the risk of hematologic or other malignancies in MTX-treated patients.

Pulmonary Toxicity. Significant pulmonary toxicity occurring during the course of treatment with low-dose weekly MTX has been described in adult patients with rheumatoid arthritis; reported prevalence rates in published studies range from 0.3 to 18 percent, with a mean prevalence of 3.3 percent.[218] However, the actual frequency of this complication is difficult to estimate because the literature has not been clear in defining toxicity related to the drug itself rather than to secondary problems associated with MTX therapy, such as opportunistic lung infections. The issue is clouded further by the fact that rheumatoid arthritis itself is associated with interstitial lung disease. The mechanism of this toxicity and the risk factors for its development are poorly defined, although a number of studies implicate preexisting lung disease as an important predisposing factor in the development of MTX pneumonitis.[192, 218, 219] Interestingly, MTX-associated pneumonitis is rarely reported in psoriatic patients.

In 1998, the first pediatric case of possible MTX-induced pneumonitis was reported in an 11-year-old girl with rheumatoid factor (RF)-positive, antinuclear antibody–negative polyarticular JRA.[220] However, the clinical course of lung disease in this case was not typical of that described in adults with MTX pneumonitis, clinical and laboratory information was insufficient to satisfactorily exclude alternative causes, and no biopsy was performed. Prospective studies of lung function in children with various types of JRA have not demonstrated any significant abnormalities in pulmonary function test results in those treated with MTX.[154, 155, 221]

Accelerated Nodulosis. MTX has been associated with a syndrome of "accelerated nodulosis," with an estimated prevalence of 8 percent in adult patients with rheumatoid arthritis.[191] More recently, this association was described in two teenagers with RF-positive JRA[222] and one 3-year-old girl with systemic-onset JRA.[223] These nodules are similar in distribution and size to those reported in adults and developed within 6 months of the initiation of MTX treatment in these children. Although discontinuation of MTX is associated with regression of nodulosis, some patients have been successfully treated with hydroxychloroquine[222] or colchicine,[224] allowing stabilization of nodulosis with continued MTX treatment of the underlying disease. Although the exact mechanism of MTX-associated nodulosis is not known, it is thought to be mediated by MTX-enhanced adenosine production; therapies that inhibit adenosine production or interfere with adenosine A_1 receptor function may thus be effective in treating MTX-associated nodulosis.[191]

Other Adverse Effects

CENTRAL NERVOUS SYSTEM. Various CNS symptoms, including headaches, mood alterations, change in sleep patterns, irritability, fatigue, and impaired academic performance, have been reported by some pediatric rheumatologists to occur transiently in the 12 to 48 hours following the weekly dose of MTX.[157] These problems may be subtle and need to be differentiated from effects of underlying disease and from various psychosocial issues that may coexist.

OSTEOPATHY. Animal studies have shown that prolonged administration of low-dose MTX is associated with suppression of osteoblast activity and stimulation of osteoblast recruitment, resulting in increased bone resorption and osteopenia.[225] Similar effects have been described in a small number of case reports in adults with rheumatoid arthritis or psoriasis treated with low-dose weekly MTX.[226, 227] Although leg pain and spontaneous fractures attributed to MTX therapy in pediatric oncology has been recognized for some time,[191] this phenomenon has so far not been described in children with JRA treated with low-dose MTX.

TERATOGENICITY. MTX therapy is associated with spontaneous abortions.[228] In 1997, a case of multiple congenital abnormalities in a baby whose mother was treated with low-dose MTX for JRA was reported.[229] Although it is difficult to quantitate the risk of teratogenicity with low-dose weekly MTX treatment, women of child-bearing age should be counseled to practice effective contraception during the course of treatment. Patients should be informed that past MTX use does not predispose to congenital abnormalities and that, ideally, MTX should be discontinued prior to attempts at conception. There have not been any reports of azoospermia due to low-dose MTX treatment of JRA.[157]

Folate Supplementation. A number of recent studies have examined the issue of minimizing MTX toxicities with the use of concurrent folic or folinic acid (leucovorin) supplementation in adults with rheumatoid arthritis.[230–233] These studies have evaluated the effect of folate supplementation on both the efficacy and the toxicity of low-dose weekly MTX therapy. Although the doses and regimens of folic and folinic acid used in the various trials, the doses of concurrent MTX therapy, and the assessment of "toxicity" have not been standardized, there is evidence for overall effectiveness of folate supplementation.

A 1998 systematic review of all published clinical trials found that folic acid supplementation was associated with a significant reduction in mucosal and GI toxicity in MTX-treated adults with rheumatoid arthritis.[234] There was no adverse effect on efficacy except with high-dose folinic acid supplementation. Currently, data are insufficient to assess the effect of long-term folate supplementation on hepatic or hematologic toxicities. It is also not clear whether folate supplementation should be commenced as prophylaxis with initiation of MTX therapy in all patients or as treatment when specific toxicities develop. There has not been any formal cost-benefit study to address this issue. Folic acid is cheaper and has a greater margin of safety in dosing compared with folinic acid. However, the two agents have not been directly compared for their clinical effectiveness and cost.

Studies in children are limited. A short-term, randomized, double-blind, placebo-controlled, crossover trial of folic acid (1 mg/day) added to a stable dose of MTX (mean, 9–9.7 mg/week) in 19 children with JRA showed no effect on clinical efficacy.[235] There were no observable abnormalities of liver function, but no information about other toxicities is available from this small study. High-dose folinic acid supplementation has been used effectively to treat manifestations of MTX toxicity in children with JRA but is associated with disease flares.[236] At present, it is not possible to make firm recommendations about routine folate supplementation in MTX-treated children. However, based on the information from adult studies and the small trial in children with JRA, it appears that low-dose (1 mg/day) folic acid supplementation does not have any detrimental effect on disease control and confers a beneficial effect in terms of GI and mucosal toxicities associated with low-dose weekly MTX treatment. Folic acid supplementation should be considered at least in symptomatic patients. High-dose folinic acid rescue should be reserved for those with severe, life-threatening toxicity such as aplastic anemia.

Antimalarials

Hydroxychloroquine sulfate (Fig. 7–8) is the least toxic of the 4-aminoquinolone drugs and has generally supplanted chloroquine in rheumatologic practice,[237–239] although other antimalarials are occasionally used for recalcitrant skin disease in SLE. Hydroxychloroquine is rapidly absorbed from the intestine. Equilibrium concentrations are reached after 2 to 6 months of a constant daily dose, and the half-life exceeds 40 days.[240] Tissue levels are much greater than plasma concentrations, and there is increased affinity of the drug for melanin as well as for the liver, pituitary, spleen, kidney, lung, and adrenals. Excretion is primarily via the kidney, although hepatic oxidative deamination accounts for part of the excretion.

The antimalarial drugs inhibit the synthesis of DNA, RNA, and protein by interacting with nucleic acid.[237] These drugs alter lysosomal pH, thereby interfering with ligand-receptor dissociation and antigen processing; stabilize lysosomal membranes[241]; inhibit antigen-antibody reactions[242]; suppress lymphocyte responses to mitogens; act as antioxidants[241]; inhibit phospholipase activity[243]; and inhibit neutrophil chemotaxis and phagocytosis.[237] They may also antagonize the action of some of the prostaglandins.[244] Antimalari-

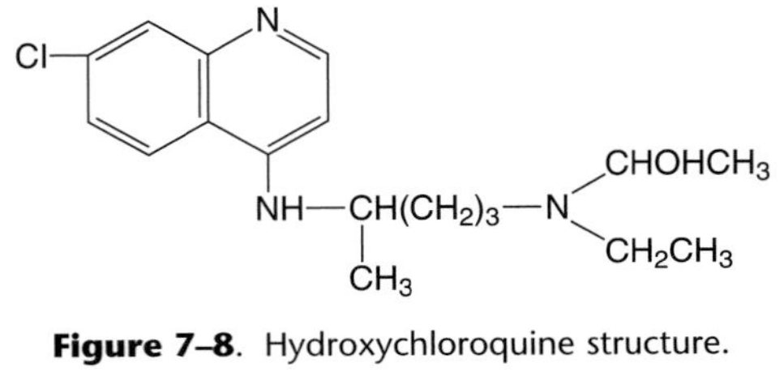

Figure 7–8. Hydroxychloroquine structure.

als interfere with IL-1 release by monocytes[242]; interfere with TNF-α, IL-6, and interferon γ (IFN-γ) production[245]; inhibit natural killer activity[246]; and induce apoptosis.[247] They also have antiplatelet and antihyperlipidemic effects that are extremely important in patients with SLE.[248]

Antimalarials are important in many rheumatic diseases. In JRA, the therapeutic efficacy has never been established, and the only placebo-controlled study did not prove antimalarials to be better than placebo.[249] However, recent work in adult rheumatoid arthritis has demonstrated them to be effective, especially in early disease.[250, 251] Antimalarials are also effective in combination with other DMARDs in adult rheumatoid arthritis.[252] Hydroxychloroquine reduces some MTX-related toxicity, such as elevated liver enzymes and nodulosis.[253, 254]

Studies in adult SLE have also provided proof of efficacy for hydroxychloroquine, especially in preventing flares of disease.[255] Its role in SLE is primarily for treatment of dermatitis, arthritis, and serositis. It may have particular benefit as a result of its lipid-lowering effect in steroid-treated SLE patients.[256] It has also been used in dermatomyositis, especially for skin disease, but the results are not clear.[257, 258]

When used at recommended doses, the antimalarials are considered extremely safe. However, at least four young children have died from respiratory failure after accidental ingestion of large doses (1 to 3 g) of chloroquine,[259] and it is recommended that antimalarials be used with great caution in the very young child because there is no antidote.

GI intolerance occurs in 10 percent of adults but is probably less common in children. Antimalarials occasionally cause bleaching of the skin and hair. Rarely, neuropathy or myopathy occurs. CNS side effects are common, may be reversible with dose reduction, and may remit spontaneously. These include headache, lightheadedness, tinnitus, insomnia, and increased nervousness. Myasthenia and muscle weakness have been described.[260]

The major side effect of concern is retinal toxicity.[261–263] Antimalarials accumulate in the pigmented cells of the retina and persist for long periods of time after they have been discontinued; however, the binding to melanin may not be predictive of ocular damage. Retinal toxicity, though rare, may cause blindness, even after the medication has been stopped. Retinitis is sometimes, but not always, reversible.[262] Recent evidence in adults suggests that retinal toxicity will not occur if the dose of hydroxychloroquine is maintained at <6.5 mg/kg/day, even if used for as long as 7 years.[264] Early detection of pre-maculopathy prevents visual loss if the medication is discontinued, and forms the basis for routine ophthalmologic monitoring (every 6 months) with visual field testing, color vision testing, corneal examination, and visual acuity testing. A progressive loss of color vision may signify early retinopathy and is an indication for stopping the drug. Corneal deposits are not visually limiting but are also probably an indication to lower the dose.

Debate continues as to whether an initial ocular examination, as well as 6-month examinations, is necessary. Our current policy is to continue to perform these examinations every 6 months but not to perform a baseline examination. Each examination should include visual acuity, color vision testing, visual field corneal examination,[264, 265] and retinoscopy. Retinal abnormalities or interference with vision, especially with foveal recognition of red,[266] is an absolute indication for discontinuing the medication. Use of hydroxychloroquine in children under 7 years of age may be limited by difficulty in obtaining satisfactory evaluation of color vision in this age group.

The dose of antimalarials is limited by retinal toxicity. For hydroxychloroquine, the recommended dose is ≤ 6.5 mg/kg/day to a maximum of 400 mg/day. The overall retinal toxicity seems to be related to daily dose rather than to cumulative dose. One study of children with JRA did correlate outcome with serum levels of hydroxychloroquine,[267] but levels are not measured in clinical practice.

Sulfasalazine

Sulfasalazine is an analogue of 5-aminosalicylic acid linked by an azo bond to sulfapyridine, a sulfonamide (Fig. 7–9). Its development was based on the concept that rheumatoid arthritis might be an infectious disease and would respond to combination therapy with an antibacterial and an anti-inflammatory drug.[268, 269] Sulfasalazine has become a primary therapeutic choice in the treatment of mild to moderate inflammatory bowel disease, and it has been reported to be beneficial in the management of childhood arthritis,[270–275] psoriatic arthritis,[276] and reactive arthritis.[277] Its role in ankylosing spondylitis is controversial.[278–280]

Sulfasalazine is poorly absorbed from the GI tract.[281–283] Peak serum concentrations are reached after 5 days of therapy. The half-life of the drug is 10 hours. Approximately one third of the dose is absorbed in the small intestine and excreted unchanged in the bile. The remaining 70 percent enters the colon intact, where the azo linkage is split by bacterial enzymes to sulfapyridine, which is absorbed and excreted in the urine, and 5-aminosalicylate, which reaches high concentrations in the feces. Approximately 90 percent of the sulfapyridine is absorbed from the colon. Sulfapyridine is tightly protein bound and acetylated, hydroxylated, and conjugated with glucuronic acid in the liver. Both sulfasalazine and sulfapyridine reach synovial fluid in concentrations comparable to those in serum. About one third of the 5-aminosalicylic acid is absorbed, acetylated, and excreted in the urine. The rest is eliminated unchanged in the stool. The small amount of salicylate absorbed is not sufficient to reach anti-inflammatory levels in the plasma.

Several mechanisms of action may explain the anti-

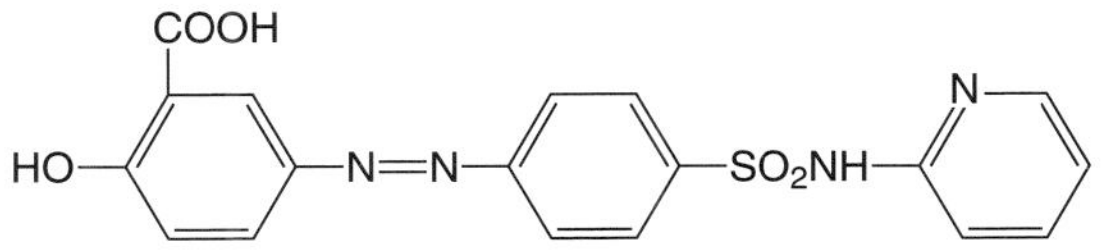

Figure 7–9. Sulfasalazine structure.

inflammatory effect of sulfasalazine. Bacterial growth is reduced by sulfasalazine and sulfapyridine, and thus the bacterial antigenic load delivered to the gut-associated lymphoid tissue may be reduced. This may be important for patients with spondyloarthropathies in whom bacteria may gain access through inflamed gut mucosa and stimulate the immune system. Sulfasalazine interferes with a number of enzymes that are important in inflammation in the formation of leukotrienes and prostaglandins.[284] Sulfasalazine is a potent inhibitor of AICAR transformylase; as a result, there is an accumulation of extracellular adenosine with a consequent reduction in inflammation via occupancy of A_2 receptors on inflammatory cells.[285] Sulfasalazine reduces the release of IL-1, IL-2, TNF-α, IL-6, and IFN-γ.[286–288] This effect is likely mediated by inhibition of I-kappa-B degradation, resulting in an inhibition of NF-kappa-B upregulation of gene transcription.[289] Sulfasalazine decreases natural killer cell activity and induces neutrophil apoptosis in vitro.[290] Sulfasalazine may also have anti-angiogenic properties.[291, 292]

Intolerance and toxic reactions occur with sulfasalazine in approximately 20 percent of adults with rheumatoid arthritis (range, 5 to 55 percent).[293–317] In a placebo-controlled study of children with JRA, 29 percent of 35 patients developed adverse effects that led to discontinuation of the drug.[273] Toxicity may be more common in patients with a slow acetylator phenotype, but there is no clinical indication to document a patient's acetylator status prior to starting sulfasalazine. Enteric-coated preparations probably cause fewer GI side effects (anorexia, nausea, vomiting, dyspepsia, diarrhea). Rashes occur in 1 to 5 percent of patients. A maculopapular rash occurring within 2 days of institution of therapy, especially on sun-exposed skin, is the most common dermatologic complication.[293] In patients who develop hypersensitivity reactions (usually early), desensitization protocols can be carried out. Oral ulcers[294] and the Stevens-Johnson syndrome[295] are uncommon but important complications. Neutropenia occurs in up to 4.4 percent of patients treated with sulfasalazine.[296] Sulfasalazine-induced thrombocytopenia has also been reported,[297] and pancytopenia[298] and macrocytic anemia[299] may occur. It is important to note that serious hematologic toxicity can develop many months after starting treatment. Drug-induced SLE,[300] Raynaud's phenomenon,[301] interstitial pneumonitis, fibrosis, alveolitis,[302, 303] and hepatitis (granulomatous hepatitis, elevated transaminases)[304] are rare complications of sulfasalazine therapy. Hypogammaglobulinemia and IgA deficiency have been reported in up to 10 percent of patients, and immunoglobulin levels should be monitored. However, serious infections have not been reported. A reversible decrease in sperm count has been observed,[305] but there are no reports of increased fetal wastage or abnormalities.

The drug should not be used in infants or in those with known hypersensitivity to sulfa drugs or salicylates, impaired renal or hepatic function, or specific disease contraindications (e.g., porphyria, glucose-6-phosphate dehydrogenase deficiency). Most authors also think that sulfasalazine is contraindicated in patients with systemic-onset JRA because of an apparent increased risk of diffuse intravascular coagulation (DIC)-like reactions.[272, 318]

The suggested dosage in children is 30 to 50 mg/kg/day in two to three divided doses, usually taken with food or milk.[270, 319] Treatment is initiated at a lower dose (10 to 15 mg/kg/day) and increased weekly over 4 weeks to achieve maintenance levels. A satisfactory clinical response may occur within 4 to 8 weeks. Sulfasalazine should probably be continued for at least 1 year after disappearance of clinical disease before tapering is begun (Table 7–9).

Table 7–9

Guidelines for Use of Sulfasalazine

Dose

Initially, 12.5 mg/kg/d (maximum 500 mg) given in one dose; increase to maintenance dose over 4 wk

Maintenance dose: 50 mg/kg/d to a maximum of 2 g/d for 1 yr or more

Clinical Monitoring

After first month, then every 2–3 mo to follow disease course; discontinue if rash appears

Laboratory Monitoring

CBC with WBCC differential and platelet count, hepatic enzymes, and urinalysis every week until maintenance dose is achieved, then monthly for 2 mo; then every 3 mo. Immunoglobulin levels every 6 mo.

Discontinue if persistent neutropenia, thrombocytopenia, elevated hepatic enzymes, decreased immunoglobulins

CBC, complete blood count; WBCC, white blood cell count.

Gold Compounds

Sulfhydryl-containing organic gold compounds have been prescribed for treatment of rheumatoid arthritis since the 1920s, following the observations of Forestier.[320, 321] The place of gold treatment in the management of children with JRA has essentially been replaced by MTX and sulfasalazine, except perhaps for patients with RF-positive disease.

Pharmacology

The mechanisms of action of gold compounds are not entirely clear[322] but appear to depend on the sulfhydryl bond, which is also thought to be responsible in part for the beneficial effects of D-penicillamine. Gold compounds may diminish vascular permeability, reduce the number of inflammatory cells in rheumatoid foci, and impair phagocytosis. They stabilize lysosomal membranes and suppress enzymatic activity in general. They may prevent denaturation of proteins induced by free oxygen radicals. In vitro lymphocyte responses to mitogens and specific antigens are inhibited, and monocyte interaction in cell-mediated immune function is impaired.[323–325]

The IM preparations are 50 percent gold by weight

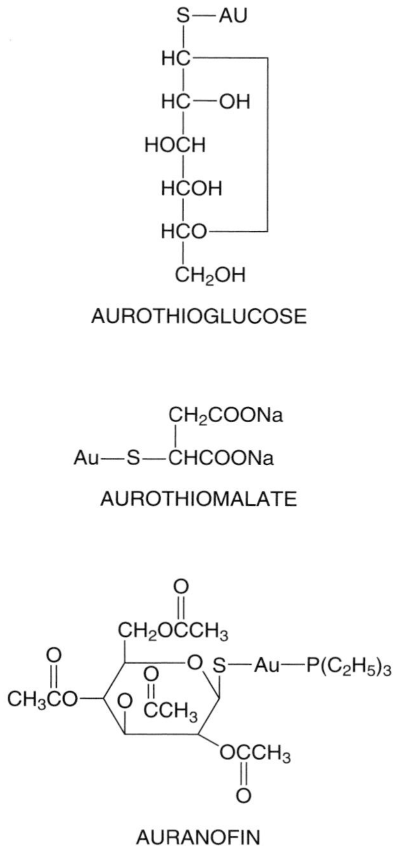

AUROTHIOGLUCOSE

AUROTHIOMALATE

AURANOFIN

Figure 7–10. Structure of gold compounds.

(Fig. 7–10).[326] The oral gold compound auranofin is 30 percent gold by weight and is lipid soluble. With aurothiomalate, the gold is predominantly bound to serum albumin; however, with auranofin, approximately 50 percent of the gold is bound to leukocytes and erythrocytes. Gold compounds are excreted in both urine and stool. They cross the placenta in substantial concentrations, apparently without harm to the fetus, and the level in breast milk is low. The gold concentration in synovial fluid is approximately half of that in blood. Gold is concentrated in organs rich in mononuclear phagocytes and in synovial type A cells. The initial half-life of IM administered gold is approximately 7 days but increases with chronic administration.[143] After discontinuation of gold injections, plasma concentration falls to undetectable levels by 40 to 80 days, but gold is still excreted in the urine for up to a year.[327]

Auranofin is more hydrophobic than the IM gold compounds and is readily absorbed orally.[328, 329] The tissue half-life of gold is approximately 80 days. Plasma gold concentrations in patients treated with auranofin take longer to reach plateau levels and are only 20 percent of those achieved with aurothiomalate.[143, 329–331] However, no direct relationship has been observed between plasma gold concentrations and either clinical benefit or toxicity with any gold compound. The drug is principally excreted in the urine.

Intramuscular Gold Administration and Toxicity

Two IM-administered gold preparations are available in North America: aurothioglucose and sodium aurothiomalate.[331] Neither preparation has a clear-cut advantage over the other. Aurothioglucose is more viscous and requires a larger-bore needle for administration. Hypersensitivity reactions after aurothioglucose administration are sometimes related to the oil vehicle. Aurothiomalate may rarely induce a nitritoid reaction (flushing, tachycardia, occasionally transient hypotension).

Although IM-administered gold compounds are reasonably safe (Table 7–10),[332, 333] a complete blood count and urinalysis should be obtained before each injection in order to detect early signs of toxicity. Toxicity requiring discontinuation of the drug occurs in 25 percent of children,[334–344] pruritic dermatitis in approximately 15 percent, and stomatitis in approximately 5 to 10 percent. Pigmentation (chrysiasis) of the skin and mucous membranes may occur.

Although rashes and mouth ulcers may be the most common side effects of gold therapy, the greatest difficulty we have encountered in maintaining children with JRA on gold is the development of an abnormal urinary sediment,[345, 346] which is related to damage to the proximal tubules or, rarely, glomerulonephritis. Because children with JRA may have minimal, transient microscopic hematuria and proteinuria unrelated to drug intake, a thorough renal evaluation is important prior to gold therapy. During gold therapy, renal function should remain normal, and microscopic hematuria should be minimal and intermittent at most and unaccompanied by significant proteinuria (≤300 mg/24 hours). If any question of toxicity arises, the drug should be discontinued and the child should be re-

Table 7–10

Guidelines for Use of Aurothiomalate or Aurothioglucose

Initial Course

0.75–1.0 mg/kg/wk

Test doses of 5 mg, then 10 mg, then 25 mg weekly; maximum of 50 mg/wk for at least 20 weeks

Maintenance

1 mg/kg (max, 50 mg) every 2 wk for 3 mo; then q 3 wk for 3 mo, then q 4 wk thereafter

Clinical Monitoring

Clinical evaluation prior to every injection: dermatitis, pruritus, stomatitis, vasomotor (nitritoid) reaction

Laboratory Monitoring

Weekly before each dose: CBC, WBCC differential and platelet count, urinalysis. Monthly: hepatic enzymes, BUN, creatinine

Discontinue drug if WBCC < 3500/mm³ (<3.5 × 10^9/L), platelet count <100,000/mm³ (<100 × 10^9/L), persistent proteinuria (>0.5 g/24 hr) or hematuria

BUN, blood urea nitrogen; CBC, complete blood count; WBCC, white blood cell count.

evaluated a week later before readministration of the drug is considered, perhaps at a lower dose.

An immune complex–mediated membranous glomerulonephritis, heralded by proteinuria, accounts for 10 to 20 percent of renal toxicity and may result in the nephrotic syndrome.[347] Significant proteinuria is an absolute contraindication to reinstitution of gold therapy. Hematologic abnormalities, including leukopenia, eosinophilia, and thrombocytopenia, occur in only 1 to 2 percent of gold-treated patients: Aplastic anemia is rare but may be fatal.[348] The risk of mucocutaneous, hematologic, or renal toxicity from gold compounds in adults with rheumatoid arthritis is increased in patients with HLA-DR3.[349]

Other toxic reactions that have been reported specifically in children with JRA include DIC,[80, 350] intrahepatic cholestasis and liver disease,[351, 352] and hypogammaglobulinemia.[353] Pulmonary injury induced by gold compounds is uncommon and to our knowledge has not been reported in children.[354, 355] In adults, pulmonary toxicity is characterized by cough, dyspnea, fever, pleuritic pain, eosinophilia, and skin rash. Neurologic complications of gold therapy include psychiatric syndromes and focal, central, and peripheral nerve abnormalities.[356]

Occasionally, glucocorticoids or chelating agents are prescribed for severe gold-induced reactions such as neutropenia or exfoliative dermatitis.[356] Reports of accidental overdose of injectable gold compounds (500 mg twice in 1 week) noted no significant ill effects,[357] but other reports of acute toxicity have been published,[358] including one in a child with JRA.[359] One study indicated that 7 surviving infants of 10 pregnancies (there were two abortions and one stillbirth) who had been exposed in utero to maternal gold administration had no long-term adverse effects.[360] No teratogenic or embryopathic effects were encountered.

Oral Gold Administration and Toxicity

Triethylphosphine gold, auranofin, was effective in the treatment of adults with rheumatoid arthritis.[361] Preliminary, open-label, noncontrolled studies in children with JRA indicated that nearly all patients sustained some improvement after 6 months at dosages between 0.1 and 0.2 mg/kg/day.[362–366] However, a subsequent double-blind trial demonstrated no significant advantage of auranofin over placebo.[367]

Orally administered gold appears to be better tolerated than the injectable compounds. Auranofin therapy is associated with loose stools in approximately 10 percent of patients, a side effect that can often be controlled by decreasing the dose. Proteinuria and hematologic toxicity appear to be less common than with IM-administered gold. Stomatitis and dermatitis are about equally frequent with both the oral and the injectable compounds.

D-Penicillamine

```
        CH3
        |
  CH3—C—CH—COOH
        |   |
        SH  NH2
```

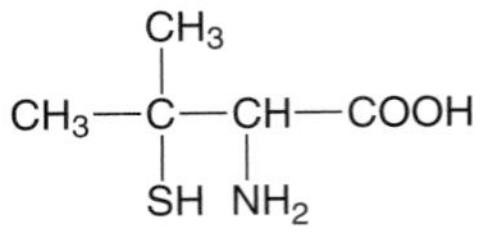

Figure 7–11. Penicillamine structure.

D-Penicillamine (D-b,b-dimethylcysteine) (Fig. 7–11) is now rarely used in the treatment of JRA because safer and more effective agents have replaced it. Its role in the treatment of scleroderma has recently been questioned.[368] It has three major biochemical effects.[369] It influences the formation of disulfide bonds with other sulfhydryl compounds by either an oxidation or an exchange reaction; it undergoes condensation with aldehydes and ketones to give substituted thiazolidinedione carboxylic acids, causing inhibition of collagen crosslinking and dissociation of macroglobulins; and it chelates, or forms complexes with metals. D-Penicillamine has been used in the treatment of rheumatic diseases (rheumatoid arthritis, scleroderma),[370, 371] in Wilson's disease to reduce tissue concentrations of copper, in lead and mercury poisoning, and in patients with cystinuria.

D-Penicillamine is absorbed orally, with peak blood levels achieved by approximately 1 to 4 hours. Absorption of the drug is significantly diminished by food, antacids, and iron. Oxidation of D-penicillamine in the presence of transition metals such as copper results in the formation of poorly absorbed disulfides. The D-penicillamine–albumin disulfide bond is quantitatively the most important during chronic therapy because the drug tends to accumulate in this form and only slowly dissociates from albumin.[372] The disulfide metabolites are excreted in urine and stool. Little unmetabolized drug can be detected in the blood 2 days after a dose. D-Penicillamine is usually started at a low dose and increased as tolerated according to a schedule such as the one in Table 7–11.

The mechanisms whereby D-penicillamine and its metabolites influence inflammation in chronic arthritis or scleroderma are uncertain.[373] D-Penicillamine–induced reduction of sulfhydryl groups on macrophages, and possibly other cells, may influence their function. Oxidation of D-penicillamine results in the production of reactive oxygen species that inhibit the reactivity of T cells. D-Penicillamine also directly inhib-

Table 7–11

Guidelines for Use of D-Penicillamine

Dose

Initially 5 mg/kg/d (maximum 250 mg/d) for 3 mo; then 10 mg/kg/d for 3 mo; then 15 mg/kg/d (maximum 1 g/d) for 1–3 yr

Clinical Monitoring

Clinical evaluation every month: dermatitis, pruritus, bruising

Laboratory Monitoring

CBC with differential WBCC, platelet count, and urinalysis every 2 wk until dose is stable, then monthly

Discontinue drug if: WBCC $< 3500/mm^3$ ($< 3.5 \times 10^9/L$), platelets $< 100{,}000/mm^3$ ($< 100 \times 10^9/L$), persistent proteinuria (> 0.5 g/24 hr) or hematuria

CBC, complete blood count; WBCC, white blood cell count.

its myeloperoxidase, thereby reducing the production of hypochlorite, which is toxic to tissue.[374] By complexing with trace metals such as copper, D-penicillamine may interfere with the action of superoxide dismutase and may thereby influence the production and scavenging of oxygen-derived free radicals.[375, 376] It also inhibits carboxypeptidase and angiotensin II converting enzymes that are involved in the kinin pathways,[377] although the concentrations required to achieve this effect considerably exceed those achieved in vivo. It may interfere with immune complex formation[378, 379] and may block the replication of viral RNA.[369, 380]

The toxicity of D-penicillamine is unusually similar to that of gold,[381–387] and monitoring should be carried out in the same manner as for gold toxicity. However, autoimmune diseases, including SLE, polymyositis, Goodpasture's syndrome, and myasthenia gravis, may develop after D-penicillamine therapy.[388–390] A child who has a toxic reaction to a gold compound may develop toxicity to D-penicillamine, in many cases even with the same manifestations. In adults, at least, this predisposition may be associated with HLA-DR3 (DW33) and the C4 null allele.[348, 391]

Colchicine

The primary use of colchicine (Fig. 7–12) in pediatrics is for treatment of familial Mediterranean fever (FMF), wherein it has been shown to reduce not only the frequency of attacks but also the development of amyloidosis. Colchicine is also occasionally used for recurrent aphthous stomatitis, Behçet's disease, and cutaneous vasculitis. Peak plasma levels are reached 1 to 3 hours after oral administration. The drug is metabolized extensively in the liver by the cytochrome-P450 system.[392] Its half-life after oral administration is 9 ± 4 hours.[393] Its action is thought to depend on binding of two of its rings to cellular microtubules, inhibiting the movement of intracellular granules and preventing secretion of various components to the cell exterior.[394] Interaction with endothelial cells and neutrophils is inhibited by reducing the expression of adhesion molecules on the neutrophil membrane.[395] The drug is present in granulocytes to a much greater extent than lymphocytes and monocytes, perhaps because of reduced activity of the p-glycoprotein efflux pump in these two cell types.[394] Drug interactions may occur either at the level of the intestine (reduced absorption[396]) or through the cytochrome-P450 system. Agents that inhibit this system may lead to colchicine toxicity; alternatively, drugs that are metabolized by this system may compete with colchicine, leading to a buildup of both agents.

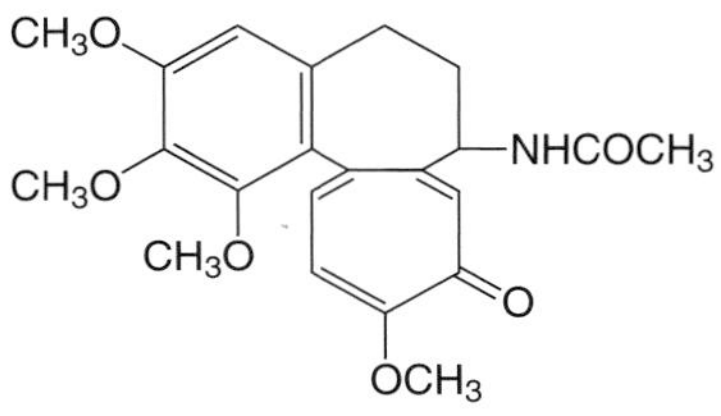

CH_3O CH_3O CH_3O $NHCOCH_3$ O OCH_3

Figure 7–12. Colchicine structure.

The effect of colchicine on microtubules has raised concern about chromosomal and gonadal aberrations. In a group of patients with FMF on long-term treatment with colchicine, there were no differences between patients and controls in lymphocyte mitotic rate, percentage of tetraploidy, or chromosomal breakage.[397]

The amount of colchicine needed to reduce sperm motility is much greater than that used with standard therapy.[398] Azoospermia and oligospermia are more common in patients with Behçet's disease than FMF, which suggests that genetic makeup or the underlying disease may contribute to reduced sperm production.[399] Concerns regarding growth delay in children are unfounded.[400, 401]

The therapeutic dose of colchicine ranges from 0.5 to 2.0 mg/day as needed to prevent or significantly reduce the frequency of FMF attacks. Toxicity is extremely rare with oral administration and is generally limited to the GI tract (nausea, vomiting, abdominal pain, diarrhea). However, severe toxicity can result in dehydration, multiorgan failure, and a DIC-like syndrome.[394]

Thalidomide

Thalidomide (*N*-α-phthalimidoglutarimide) has acquired a well-deserved reputation as a major teratogen. However, it has been shown to be effective in a variety of immune-mediated disorders. Its immunosuppressive effects include inhibition of neutrophil chemotaxis,[402] decreased monocyte phagocytosis,[403] decrease in the ratio of helper T cells to suppressor T cells,[404] inhibition of expression of TNF-α and IL-6 mRNA,[405] and inhibition of angiogenesis.[406, 407] Its structure includes two ring systems (Fig. 7–13). Mean peak plasma concentrations occur 4.39 ± 1.27 hours after a 200-mg dose.[408] It is metabolized by the cytochrome-P450 system.

Although no randomized controlled clinical trials with thalidomide have been conducted, multiple case series have reported improvement in patients with the following disorders[409]: cutaneous lupus, aphthous stomatitis, Behçet's syndrome with stomatitis, and graft-versus-host disease. Single series or case reports have documented improvement in patients with palmoplantar pustulosis, sarcoidosis, rheumatoid arthritis, pyoderma gangrenosum, erythema multiforme, Weber-Christian disease, pemphigoid, and adult-onset Still's disease.[410]

In addition to embryopathy (which can occur with as small a dose as 100 mg given between 34 and 50 days of gestation), the major side effects of thalidomide include peripheral neuropathy and drowsiness. The neuropathy is predominantly sensory and presents as painful paresthesias in a glove-and-stocking distribution.[411] The neuropathy can progress despite discontinuation of thalidomide and may or may not be dose related; it has been reported in 1 to 70 percent of

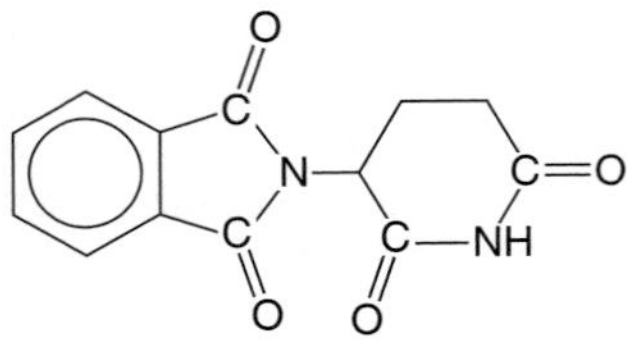

Figure 7–13. Thalidomide structure.

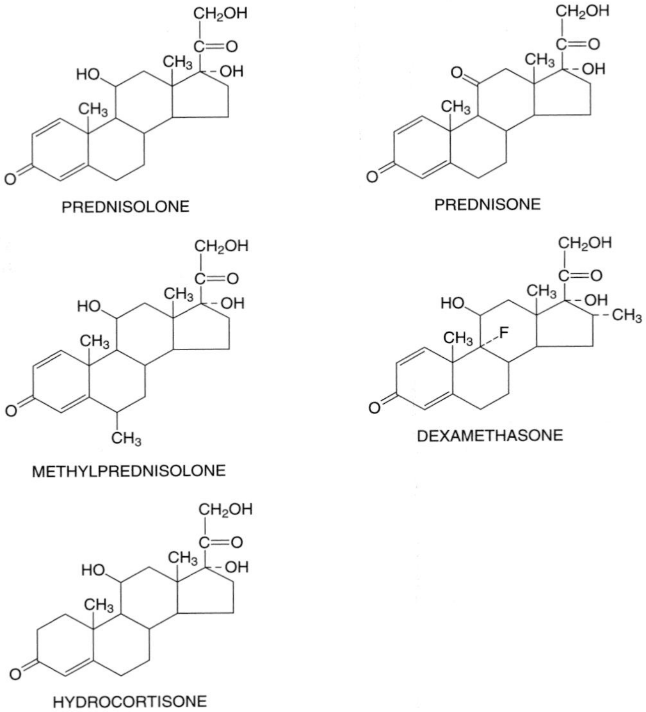

patients. Even after discontinuation of the drug, recovery may be delayed for several years. Baseline and routine follow-up electrophysiologic testing should be performed, and the dose should be reduced or discontinued upon detection of abnormalities.[412] A variety of other neurologic effects, including carpal tunnel syndrome, muscle weakness and cramps, and signs of pyramidal tract involvement, may occur. Endocrine effects include hypothyroidism, hypoglycemia, and stimulation of adrenocorticotropic hormone (ACTH) and prolactin production or secretion.[413]

The dose of thalidomide varies between 100 and 400 mg/day. Doses of 4 mg/kg/day have been suggested for children with SLE.[414, 415] Birth control must be practiced. Women who are prescribed thalidomide should sign a consent form indicating knowledge of potential birth defects and agreeing to adequate methods of birth control.

PREDNISOLONE PREDNISONE METHYLPREDNISOLONE DEXAMETHASONE HYDROCORTISONE

Figure 7–14. Structure of the glucocorticoids.

Glucocorticoid Drugs

Glucocorticoid drugs are the most potent anti-inflammatory agents in the treatment of rheumatic diseases.[416] Reports of their use in children with rheumatic diseases, especially rheumatic fever, JRA, and SLE, began to appear in the 1950s and 1960s.[417–420] Specific aspects of therapy are discussed in the chapters on individual diseases and in reviews.[421–427] Here we review more general aspects such as the pharmacology, physiology, and mechanism of action of glucocorticoids as well as the indications and contraindications for systemic and local glucocorticoid therapy and their associated adverse effects.

Pharmacology

The glucocorticoid drugs are modeled on the principal naturally occurring glucocorticoid, hydrocortisone (cortisol). They are 21-carbon molecules, which in active form have a hydroxyl group at C11. Synthetic preparations such as prednisone and cortisone must be metabolized to the active forms (prednisolone and hydrocortisone, respectively) (Fig. 7–14). Glucocorticoids that are used topically (e.g., dexamethasone) or given by intra-articular injection (e.g., triamcinolone hexacetonide [THA]) have a hydroxyl group at C11 and are therefore already in active form.[428] The different relative potencies and durations of biologic action of the various synthetic analogues are outlined in Table 7–12.

Orally administered glucocorticoids (prednisone, prednisolone) are rapidly absorbed. Prednisone is converted to prednisolone in the liver and reaches a peak plasma concentration within 2 hours. Hydrocortisone and prednisolone bind to the serum proteins transcor-

Table 7–12

Relative Doses and Equivalent Potencies of Glucocorticoids

	POTENCY RELATIVE TO HYDROCORTISONE		
GLUCOCORTICOID	Equivalent Dose§ (mg)	Relative Anti-Inflammatory Potency	Relative Sodium-Retaining Potency
Short-Acting*			
Hydrocortisone	20	1	1
Deflazacort	6	4	1
Intermediate-Acting†			
Prednisone	5	4	0.8
Prednisolone	5	4	0.8
Methylprednisolone	4	5	0.5
Long-Acting‡			
Dexamethasone	0.75	25	0

*Short-acting: 8–12 hr biologic half-life (deflazacort half life ~ 1.5 hr)
†Intermediate-acting: 12–36 hr biologic half-life
‡Long-acting: 36–72 hr biologic half-life
§These dose relationships apply only to oral or IV administration.
Adapted from Goodman LS, Gilman A (eds): Goodman and Gilman's The Pharmacological Basis of Therapeutics, 8th ed. New York, Pergamon Press, 1990. Reproduced with permission of The McGraw-Hill Companies.

tin (high affinity) and albumin (low affinity). Methylprednisolone and dexamethasone are bound primarily to albumin.[428] Prednisolone has a large volume of distribution; about two thirds is taken up by muscle. After metabolism in the liver, excretion occurs principally by way of the bile.

Physiologic and Pharmacologic Effects

Glucocorticoids are unique among the pharmacologic agents given to treat rheumatic diseases in that they are synthetic analogues of chemicals produced by the body and thus have a *physiologic*, as well as a *pharmacologic*, role. Glucocorticoids enter cells passively and bind to mineralocorticoid (type I) and glucocorticoid (type II) receptors. Type I receptors have highest affinity for aldosterone and are found principally in cells of the CNS, especially the hippocampus. Type II receptors have highest affinity for dexamethasone and are present in virtually all cells, including those of the immune system. The receptors are present in the cytoplasm and consist of a hormone-binding portion, a DNA-binding portion, and an immunogenic region. Binding of the hormone to the receptor causes translocation of the complex to the nucleus, where the DNA-binding portion binds to glucocorticoid-responsive elements of the DNA. This induces mRNA transcription of specific genes that encode for proteins of importance in the inflammatory and immune responses, such as phospholipase A_2 inhibitory protein. The effect is reflected indirectly in decreased prostaglandin production.[429, 430] This mechanism of glucocorticoid effect, mediated via binding to a cytosolic receptor, reflects traditional understanding of the therapeutic effects of glucocorticoids and can be categorized as "genomic" action.

However, a new hypothesis has been proposed to describe the therapeutic effects of glucocorticoids occurring in a modular fashion via both "genomic" and "nongenomic" mechanisms (Table 7–13).[431] This new modular hypothesis postulates the following:

- At very low dosages of glucocorticoids, genomic effects occur (module 1). These include the classic receptor-mediated actions resulting in increase in the transcription of certain genes (such as those coding for lipocortin) and decrease in the transcription of others (such as those coding for various cytokines), resulting in net anti-inflammatory and immunosuppressive effects.
- As the dosage is increased (up to a dose of about 200 to 300 mg of prednisone equivalent per day), greater occupation of receptors results in increased genomic effects. However, it is postulated that a further increase in dosage may affect pharmacodynamics (e.g., receptor off-loading and reoccupancy), receptor synthesis, and receptor expression as well as bring additional therapeutic benefit via other mechanisms (module 2). In contrast with genomic actions, these receptor-mediated actions are rapid, occurring within seconds to minutes of glucocorticoid administration. The clinical correlates of these rapid effects may include the negative feedback of ACTH production, behavioral changes, cardiovascular effects, programmed cell death (apoptosis) and, possibly, antianaphylactic glucocorticoid action.
- The assumed additional therapeutic effects of higher dosages could be obtained predominantly via nongenomic mechanisms, mediated by membrane-bound receptors (module 2) or initiated by even more rapid effects through physicochemical interactions with cellular membranes (module 3).[431]

Thus, this hypothesis provides a modular system of increasing therapeutic effect with increasing dosage, occurring through recruitment of a number of nongenomic actions, with increasingly more rapid onset of effect than the classic genomic actions of glucocorticoids.

The actions of glucocorticoids at physiologic levels are summarized in Table 7–14. Glucocorticoids are essential for normal vascular integrity and responsiveness; they suppress leukocyte migration and immune reactions and stabilize cell membranes.[432–443] Glucocorticoids influence protein, carbohydrate, fat, and purine metabolism; electrolyte and water homeostasis; cardiovascular, nervous, and renal function; and bone and muscle integrity.

Table 7–13

Dose-Effect Relationships of Glucocorticoids

	PREDNISONE EQUIVALENT (MOLES/L)	MECHANISMS	ONSET OF ACTION
Module 1	$>10^{-12}$	*Genomic* actions	After at least 30 min
Module 2	$>10^{-9}$	Additional nongenomic, *receptor-mediated* actions	Seconds to 1–2 min
Module 3	$>10^{-4}$	Additional nongenomic, *physicochemical* actions	Within seconds

From Buttgereit F, Wehling M, Burmester GR: A new hypothesis of modular glucocorticoid actions. Steroid treatment of rheumatic diseases revisited. Arthritis Rheum 41: 761–767, Copyright © 1998. Reprinted by permission of Wiley-Liss, Inc., a subsidiary of John Wiley & Sons, Inc.

Table 7–14

Actions of Glucocorticoids at Physiologic Levels

Negative feedback modulation of corticotropin-releasing factor and adrenocorticotropic hormone
Maintenance of blood glucose and liver glycogen levels
Maintenance of cardiovascular function, blood pressure, and muscle work capacity
Excretion of a water load
Permissive effects on pressor, lipolytic, and gluconeogenic activities of hormones
Protection against moderate stress

Adapted from Munck A, Guyre PM: Glucocorticoid physiology and homeostasis in relation to anti-inflammatory actions. *In* Scheimer RP, Claman HN, Oronsky A (eds): Anti-Inflammatory Steroid Action: Basic and Clinical Aspects. San Diego, Academic Press, 1989.

Carbohydrate, Protein, and Lipid Metabolism

Glucocorticoids stimulate the synthesis of glucose, diminish its peripheral use, and promote its storage as glycogen. They increase secretion of insulin by pancreatic islet cells. In the periphery, they mobilize amino acids from tissues that are then diverted in the liver to the production of glucose and glycogen. This catabolic action results in lymphoid and muscular atrophy, osteoporosis, thinning of the skin, and negative nitrogen balance. Glucocorticoids stimulate fat cell differentiation and, in high doses, redistribution of fat in a typical "Cushing's" distribution. Various other effects on lipids have been reported, but most have not been conclusively demonstrated to result from the direct actions of glucocorticoids themselves. There is no consistent alteration in plasma lipids in either hypercorticism or hypocorticism.[444]

Electrolyte and Water Balance

The glucocorticoid analogues used in the treatment of rheumatic diseases have been modified to decrease their mineralocorticoid potency. In that manner, increased resorption of sodium ions from the distal renal tubules is moderated, as is increased urinary excretion of potassium and hydrogen ions. Patients on long-term therapy are nonetheless in positive sodium balance, have an increased extracellular fluid volume, and have a tendency toward hypokalemia and alkalosis. However, in practice, these changes are only moderate in severity, reflecting the relatively weak effect of glucocorticoids on electrolyte balance. Glucocorticoids also decrease the absorption of calcium from the intestine and increase its renal excretion, thus producing a negative calcium balance (discussed later).

Anti-Inflammatory and Immunosuppressive Actions

Glucocorticoids have both anti-inflammatory and immunosuppressive effects.[424–427, 432–443] These effects are largely mediated by the inhibition of specific functions of leukocytes such as the elaboration or the action of a variety of lymphokines.

Anti-Inflammatory Actions. Steroids inhibit both the early stages of inflammation (such as edema, fibrin deposition, capillary dilatation, migration of lymphocytes into inflamed areas, and phagocytic activity) and the later manifestations (such as proliferation of capillaries and fibroblasts and deposition of collagen).[444] Many of these effects are mediated by inhibition of the elaboration of a number of chemokines and cytokines, including:

- Arachidonic acid and its metabolites (e.g., prostaglandins and leukotrienes)—glucocorticoids induce synthesis of lipocortins by macrophages and other cells.[442, 443, 445] Lipocortins inhibit the binding of phospholipase A_2 to its substrate and thus reduce the generation of arachidonic acid, the substrate for the cyclo-oxygenase–mediated synthesis of prostaglandins and leukotrienes
- Platelet-activating factor (PAF), also mediated by the induction of lipocortin[446]
- TNF
- IL-1, which exerts a number of inflammatory actions including stimulation of the production of prostaglandin E_2 and collagenase, activation of T lymphocytes, stimulation of fibroblast proliferation, and enhanced hepatic synthesis of acute phase proteins

In addition, glucocorticoids can inhibit the action of humoral regulators of inflammation such as PAF and macrophage migration inhibition factor (MIF).[444] The reader who is interested in the subject of the anti-inflammatory effects of glucocorticoids is referred to the extensive review by Schleimer and colleagues.[447]

Immunosuppressive Actions. The glucocorticoid effects on the immune system are mediated principally through T lymphocytes.[435] Acute administration of hydrocortisone produces a 70 percent decline in circulating lymphocytes. T lymphocytes are affected more than B lymphocytes, and T helper cells are affected more than T suppressor cells. The lymphocytopenia is probably a result of sequestration of cells in the bone marrow rather than cell lysis, although drug-induced apoptotic cell death may also be involved.[448] The most pronounced lymphopenia occurs 4 to 8 hours after a single dose of glucocorticoid and disappears by 24 hours. There is also a 90 percent decline in circulating monocytes within the initial 6 hours. Proliferative T-cell responses to antigens (streptodornase-streptokinase), mitogens (concanavalin A), and cell surface antigens (as in the mixed leukocyte reaction) are reduced by glucocorticoids. IL-2 production by T cells in vitro is also reduced.[449]

Glucocorticoids cause an increase in the numbers of blood neutrophils by increasing the release of cells from the marginated neutrophil pool, prolonging their stay in the circulation, and reducing chemotaxis of neutrophils to sites of inflammation.[450] Another effect of the decreased action of phospholipase A_2 is reduction of neutrophil chemotaxis, thereby decreasing accumulation of these cells at inflammatory sites.[439] However, no consistent effect of glucocorticoids on neutrophil phagocytosis or bacterial killing has been demonstrated.[450]

IV glucocorticoid causes a fall in circulating immunoglobulin G (IgG) but little discernible effect on the serum titer of specific antibodies. However, the protein catabolic effects of long-term administration may have consequences on the humoral immune system. Endothelial secretion of C3 and factor B of the complement cascade is inhibited by glucocorticoid.[451]

Indications for Systemic Glucocorticoid Therapy

When considering the use of glucocorticoids in children with rheumatic diseases, one must carefully

Table 7–15

Adverse Effects of Glucocorticoid Drugs

Cushing's syndrome
Growth suppression
Effects on bone
  Osteoporosis
  Avascular necrosis of bone
Immunosuppression
Lymphopenia and neutrophilia
Central nervous system effects
  Psychosis
  Mood and behavioral disturbances
Cardiovascular system effects
  Hypertension
  Dyslipoproteinemia
Cataracts and glaucoma
Metabolic effects
  Impaired carbohydrate tolerance
  Protein wasting
  Metabolic alkalosis
Myopathy

weigh the risk:benefit ratio because these agents are associated with substantial toxicity when used systemically in the long term (Table 7–15). Clinicians must review the specific indications for which glucocorticoids are to be used and the outcomes that will be monitored in order to measure response and consequently determine the duration of therapy. The overall aim is to limit the dose and duration of steroid therapy to the lowest possible while achieving disease control. Administration of a single dose in the morning and alternate-day regimens, which have been shown to minimize the suppression of linear growth in children, should be used whenever possible.[452] The child who is being treated with these drugs should be under the care of a physician who is experienced in management of the disease and in minimizing the adverse effects of glucocorticoids.[453–455]

For example, in JRA the use of systemic glucocorticoids is mainly limited to treating the extra-articular features of systemic-onset disease. These include systemic "toxicity" and fevers unresponsive to NSAID therapy, severe anemia, myocarditis or pericarditis, and the rare DIC syndromes associated with systemic-onset JRA.[79, 80] The presence of fever or arthritis alone in systemic-onset JRA is not sufficient indication for systemic glucocorticoid therapy. Low-dose, short-term systemic glucocorticoids may also be indicated in severe forms of polyarticular JRA with significant functional impairment and for chronic uveitis unresponsive to local therapy. High-dose systemic glucocorticoids are used in children with other inflammatory conditions such as JDM, vasculitis, and SLE.

Adverse Effects

Two broad categories of adverse effects occur with the therapeutic use of systemic glucocorticoids: those resulting from prolonged use of large doses and those resulting from withdrawal of therapy. The major manifestation of the latter is acute adrenal insufficiency following too-rapid withdrawal after prolonged therapy (see "Preventing Acute Adrenal Insufficiency [Addisonian Crisis]"). The adverse effects of glucocorticoid excess are many (see Table 7–15).

Cushing's Syndrome. Cushing's syndrome, a term used originally to identify the effects of idiopathic hypercorticism, may also be induced by prolonged glucocorticoid administration (Table 7–16). It is characterized biochemically by high plasma glucocorticoid levels and suppression of the hypothalamic-pituitary-adrenal axis. The syndrome is characterized clinically by a number of features, including truncal obesity, osteoporosis, thinning of the subcutaneous tissues, and hypertension.

In Cushing's syndrome, the distribution of fat is predominantly in the subcutaneous tissue of the abdomen and upper back (buffalo hump) and in the face (moon facies). Weight gain reflects both fluid retention and increased caloric intake: Children taking prednisone are often ravenously hungry. Attempts to minimize weight gain by limiting caloric and sodium intake may be useful but difficult. Skin changes, in addition to the characteristic purple striae on the lower abdomen, lower legs, upper arms, and chest, include hirsutism and acne. Hypertension is usually mild but occasionally requires treatment or reduction of the glucocorticoid dose. Osteoporosis is one of the most troublesome consequences of long-term, high-dose glucocorticoid therapy and is further discussed later.[456]

Few side effects occur at the start of therapy; the major manifestations of iatrogenic Cushing's syndrome and other toxicities are related more directly to the total dose administered than to the length of time that the patient has been on the drug. Cushingoid effects supervene when the long-term daily dose in a child (25 kg) exceeds approximately 5 mg of prednisone. Cushingoid appearance is an important source of distortion of body image and can affect self-esteem and psychological well-being, particularly in adolescents and young adults. However, with the exception of skin striae, all of the physical features contributing to the Cushingoid appearance are reversible after cessation of glucocorticoid therapy.

Growth Suppression. Growth suppression is one of the most worrisome long-term adverse effects. It occurs in young children who are receiving prolonged therapy

Table 7–16

Comparison of Idiopathic and Iatrogenic Cushing's Syndromes

PROMINENT IN IDIOPATHIC CUSHING'S SYNDROME	EQUAL FREQUENCY	PROMINENT IN IATROGENIC CUSHING'S SYNDROME
Hypertension	Obesity	Avascular necrosis
Menstrual irregularities	Psychosis	Cataract, glaucoma
Impotence	Edema	Pseudotumor cerebri
Hirsutism		Pancreatitis
Acne, striae		Panniculitis
Purpura, plethora		

in dosages equivalent to 3 mg/day of prednisone and increases with higher doses.[457, 458] However, there may be substantial interindividual variability in the severity of growth suppression and the minimal dose required to suppress growth. The mechanism of glucocorticoid-associated growth suppression in children with arthritis is controversial.[423] Glucocorticoids have been shown to inhibit production of insulin-like growth factor I (somatomedin C).[459, 460] In addition, the general inhibitory effect of glucocorticoids on cell growth and division probably contributes to growth failure.[457] However, the glucocorticoid-induced inhibition of growth in children cannot be overcome by the administration of human growth hormone, suggesting that other mechanisms may be contributing.[461]

Growth suppression may in fact be a consequence of the underlying disease process, as in JRA.[462] Evidence suggests that when glucocorticoids are used, growth retardation is more severe in patients with JRA than in those with SLE receiving equivalent doses.[463] Furthermore, growth suppression appears to be worse in patients with systemic-onset disease compared with those with polyarticular- or oligoarticular-onset disease.[463] Although alternate-day regimens have been shown to minimize this adverse effect,[464, 465] the usefulness of such regimens for controlling the actual disease remains unclear.[423]

Effects on Bone: Osteoporosis and Avascular Necrosis. Osteoporosis is another serious consequence of long-term glucocorticoid therapy in children with rheumatic disease. There are multiple other contributing factors, including inadequate dietary intake of calcium and vitamin D, the underlying disease activity (e.g., in children with polyarticular- or systemic-onset JRA),[466–468] reduced physical activity,[469] reduced exposure to sunlight (e.g., in children with JDM or SLE), and low body weight.[470]

Glucocorticoids are associated with both a reduction in bone formation and an increase in bone resorption. Reduced bone formation is due to a direct inhibitory effect on osteoblasts. Glucocorticoids also directly inhibit gut absorption of calcium and cause increased urinary calcium excretion, resulting in secondary hyperparathyroidism and hence increased bone resorption.[471, 472] The extent of bone loss appears to be related to both the dose and the duration of glucocorticoid therapy, although these do not necessarily have a consistent relationship with fracture risk. Significant trabecular bone loss occurs with doses ≥7.5 mg/day in most adults.[473, 474] Bone loss appears to occur rapidly within the first 6 to 12 months of therapy and then reaches a plateau.[473] Alternate-day glucocorticoid therapy may not be protective.[475] In adults, bone loss is predominantly trabecular (e.g., spine and ribs) rather than cortical, whereas in children the osteoporotic effect of glucocorticoids is more generalized. Not all patients exposed to long-term glucocorticoids develop bone loss.[476] However, there are no reliable biochemical markers that can be used to predict which glucocorticoid-treated children will undergo significant bone loss.[477] Bone densitometry may be used to screen children at high risk for osteoporosis. Approaches to the prevention and treatment of glucocorticoid associated osteoporosis are discussed later (see "Minimizing Toxicity").

High-dose glucocorticoids have also been associated with avascular necrosis of bone (AVN), although the mechanism is not known.[478] Many sites can be involved, but the most common and clinically significant location for AVN is the femoral head. This complication is more frequently reported in SLE (in which the underlying disease process can be a contributing factor) and possibly also after high-dose IV methylprednisolone therapy, although the data to support the latter association are not strong.[479, 480]

Infection and Immunity. Glucocorticoids interfere with the ability to resist infection through two main mechanisms. They act as immunosuppressives and unpredictably decrease the patient's resistance to viral and bacterial infections. They are also anti-inflammatory agents and hence may mask the signs and symptoms of infection. These may include important signs such as fever or abdominal pain in peritonitis, for example. Susceptibility to infections in general is related to the dose and duration of glucocorticoid administration. However, the minimal amount of systemic steroids and the duration of administration sufficient to cause immunosuppression in an otherwise healthy child are not well defined.[205] Additional factors that may affect the overall extent of immunosuppression in steroid-treated children with rheumatic diseases include the effects of the underlying disease and concurrent immunosuppressive therapies.

The most profound effect of glucocorticoid administration is on cell-mediated immune reactions, including delayed hypersensitivity and allograft rejection. Patients receiving high doses of glucocorticoid over a prolonged period are prone to infections that are associated with defects of delayed hypersensitivity, such as tuberculosis. If possible, the Mantoux test (purified protein derivative, 5 tuberculin units) should be performed before glucocorticoids are started. If the result is positive at 72 hours, further investigations for tuberculosis should be carried out. The risk of complications of varicella infection must also be considered. The susceptible glucocorticoid-treated child who is exposed to chickenpox should receive zoster immune globulin within 96 hours (for maximum effectiveness, as soon as possible after exposure or ideally within 72 hours) or acyclovir during the infectious illness itself.[205]

There is little information to guide decisions about the glucocorticoid regimen in varicella-infected children who have been on chronic steroid therapy; it would seem reasonable to try to minimize doses while maintaining disease control during the course of such an infection. If bacterial infection develops in a child treated with glucocorticoids, the dose may be maintained or increased and the best available treatment for the infection vigorously administered. In those with *Pneumocystis carinii* pneumonia (PCP), early adjunctive treatment with glucocorticoids has been demonstrated to have a beneficial effect on the clinical course and outcome, at least in adult patients with AIDS and moderate to severe PCP.[481] Although no controlled trials of glucocorticoids in young children have been performed, most experts would recommend glucocorticoids as part of therapy for children with moderate to severe PCP.[205] The impact of glucocorticoids in the immunocompromised host without AIDS appears to be similar to that in patients with AIDS.[482]

Hematologic System. Glucocorticoids decrease the number of circulating lymphocytes, monocytes, basophils, and eosinophils but increase the number of circulating neutrophils.[483] Excess glucocorticoid may also cause polycythemia.

Central Nervous System. The effect of glucocorticoids on the CNS results from changes in the concentration of plasma glucose, circulatory dynamics, and electrolyte balance. These effects are reflected by changes in mood, behavior, and electroencephalographic studies.[484] Pseudotumor cerebri is rare but may follow rapid reduction of glucocorticoid dose.[485]

Most glucocorticoid-induced psychoses have an acute onset, are related to high doses, and occur within 96 hours of initiation of medication.[486, 487] Psychosis is more common in idiopathic Cushing's syndrome than in iatrogenic disease. Early, there may be euphoria and mania; later in Cushing's syndrome, depression tends to predominate. Other types of mood and behavioral disturbances such as anxiety and insomnia may occur.

A prospective cohort study of the adverse effects of high-dose intermittent IV glucocorticoids in 213 children with rheumatic diseases found behavioral changes in 21 (10 percent).[488] These abnormalities included altered mood in 14, hyperactivity in 4, sleep disturbance in 3, and psychosis in 2 children. In some cases, CNS effects may be related to the underlying disease such as SLE. Abnormalities of behavior usually disappear when glucocorticoids are withdrawn. However, there are anecdotal reports of depression lasting for several weeks in some children treated with short-term steroids in the form of intra-articular triamcinolone hexacetonide or high-dose IV pulse methylprednisolone.

Cardiovascular System. The major effect of glucocorticoids on the cardiovascular system is mediated by their influence on the regulation of renal sodium excretion, sometimes leading to hypertension. However, this complication is uncommon in children with JRA who do not have underlying renal disease. The actual mechanism of glucocorticoid-induced hypertension is not fully explained. Although sodium retention plays a role, additional factors such as increased plasma renin activity or antidiuretic hormone may be involved.[444] Glucocorticoids also exert an important effect on capillaries, arterioles, and myocardium.[444] These influences are relevant in acute relative steroid deficiency when patients treated with long-term glucocorticoids are subject to physiologic stress (see "Preventing Acute Adrenal Insufficiency [Addisonian Crisis]")

Other important possible long-term effects of chronic glucocorticoid administration include hyperlipemia and accelerated coronary atherosclerosis.[489] Patients with SLE, who are often treated with large doses of glucocorticoids for prolonged periods, are at increased risk for dyslipoproteinemia and coronary artery disease (CAD) after about 10 years of disease. Although the pathogenesis of CAD in these patients is multifactorial, some studies have suggested that a long duration of glucocorticoid therapy may be an important risk factor.[490]

A cross-sectional study of 40 children with SLE did not find steroids to be an independent risk factor for CAD.[491] These children had a median age of 15.9 years and median disease duration of 1.4 years at the time of study. In contrast to adults, children with abnormalities in coronary perfusion tended to have shorter median duration of prednisone use as well as lower cumulative dose of steroids and fewer IV pulsed doses of steroids. Although the study was small and these were only observed trends and not statistically significant differences, they raise the possibility that CAD may be more a manifestation of the underlying disease process rather than the glucocorticoid therapy used to treat it.

Cataracts and Glaucoma. Subcapsular cataracts[485, 492, 493] are more common with glucocorticoid therapy than in idiopathic Cushing's syndrome. The risk of cataract development becomes significant when a dose of prednisone equal to or greater than 9 mg/M^2/day has been maintained for longer than 1 year. Most children who have been treated with doses of glucocorticoid equivalent to 20 mg/day of prednisone for 4 years or more develop cataracts.[485] These cataracts often do not progress, are functionally benign, and rarely affect vision. Children on long-term glucocorticoids should also be monitored for glaucoma, especially if they have a history of uveitis.

Muscle Disease. The muscle wasting that results from high-dose glucocorticoid administration is associated with atrophy of muscle fibers, especially type IIB fibers. Steroid myopathy can complicate the clinical assessment of a patient with SLE or JDM (see Chapters 18 and 20). Myopathy induced by glucocorticoids usually affects proximal muscles, is seldom painful, and is usually associated with normal serum levels of muscle enzymes and an electromyogram suggestive of myopathy. However, a muscle biopsy may be needed to differentiate between steroid myopathy and active myositis. Glucocorticoid-induced hypokalemia may also lead to muscular weakness and fatigue. Recovery from steroid myopathy may be slow and incomplete.[494]

Other Side Effects. Glucose intolerance and glycosuria may occur after prolonged exposure to large doses of glucocorticoids, particularly if there is a genetic predisposition to diabetes.[495] Such intolerance can usually be managed with diet or insulin; such side effects should not be important to the decision to continue glucocorticoid therapy or to initiate it in diabetic patients who need it.

The role of glucocorticoids in peptic ulceration is controversial. Although some have suggested an increased risk, current evidence does not support a definitive association between peptic ulceration and glucocorticoid therapy independent of any other factors such as NSAID therapy or concomitant illness.[496]

Minimizing Toxicity

The deleterious effects of glucocorticoids can be minimized by choosing a drug with a relatively short half-

Table 7–17

Systemic Administration of Glucocorticoid Drugs

SCHEDULE	ADVANTAGES	DISADVANTAGES
Divided daily doses	Better disease control	More side effects
Single daily dose	Good disease control	Fewer side effects May not control severe disease
Alternate-day dose	Fewer side effects	Less disease control
IV pulse therapy	Less long-term toxicity	Acute toxicities

life (see Table 7–12).[497] Prednisone is the drug most often given for oral therapy. Its enhanced glucocorticoid and minimal mineralocorticoid actions give it the lowest risk:benefit ratio of any of the analogues in general use.[498] Adherence to the use of a single synthetic analogue simplifies communications with the patient, parents, and medical personnel and lessens the risk of an error in dose.

Deflazacort, an oxazoline derivative of prednisone with anti-inflammatory and immunosuppressive activity, may have a bone-sparing effect compared with prednisone.[499–501] However, there are at least two case reports of children who developed symptomatic vertebral collapse while receiving deflazacort for vasculitis and a lupus-like syndrome.[502] Thus, the long-term efficacy and safety of deflazacort in children with rheumatic diseases need further study before it can be recommended for general use.

The anti-inflammatory effect and toxicity of glucocorticoids increase with larger doses and more frequent administration (Table 7–17). Four-times-daily administration is more effective than twice-daily administration of the same dose. Daily administration is more effective than the same total dose every other day.[464, 501, 503–505] Glucocorticoid administration should be as infrequent as is consistent with achieving disease control. Short-acting glucocorticoids given in the morning (upon waking) have less capacity to suppress the pituitary than those given later in the day (which suppress the normal surge of ACTH that occurs during sleep).[444]

Reduction in glucocorticoid dose must be gradual and should be individualized for the child and the disease. At high doses (e.g., 60 mg/day) reductions of 10 mg are usually well tolerated; at lower doses (e.g., 10 mg/day), reductions of only 1 or 2 mg may be necessary. The dose can be tapered on every second day so that an alternate-day regimen is established as early as possible. Glucocorticoid dose tapering is often fraught with difficulty because of the adaptation of the patient's metabolism to chronic steroid excess.[506, 507] *Steroid pseudorheumatism* may result from a rapid dose decrease in some children.[507] Signs and symptoms include increased stiffness and pain in the joints, malaise, fever, and irritability. *Pseudotumor cerebri* may occur under similar conditions.[485] It is characterized by headache, vomiting, and papilledema. It must be differentiated from other causes of increased intracranial pressure. These withdrawal effects gradually resolve over 1 or 2 weeks and are minimized if each decrement in daily prednisone is 1 mg or less per week (at the lower dose levels).

A number of approaches for the prevention and treatment of corticosteroid-associated *osteoporosis* have been studied in adults (Fig. 7–15). These have included vitamin D and its analogues, calcitonin, and various bisphosphonates. Calcitriol (vitamin D_3) or cholecalciferol (vitamin D), with or without calcitonin, has been shown to prevent bone loss from the lumbar spine better than calcium alone in several randomized controlled clinical trials of adult patients starting long-term glucocorticoid therapy.[508, 509] A 1998 meta-analysis also concluded that treatment with calcium and vitamin D in adult patients on glucocorticoids effectively retards lumbar and forearm bone loss.[510] The reported adverse effects include mainly constipation (calcium) and hypercalcemia and hypercalciuria (calcitriol), although these may be less frequent with physiologic doses. However, the clinical significance of these findings needs interpretation in light of the fact that none of the studies was able to demonstrate any significant decrease in fracture incidence. This is likely due to the lack of power for the detection of infrequent events in these relatively small studies. Furthermore, none of the controlled studies included children with rheumatic diseases; hence, the generalizability of results to this group of patients also requires caution. However, several open studies suggest that some children with rheumatic disease receiving glucocorticoids may also benefit from calcium and vitamin D supplementation.[511, 512]

The bisphosphonates have also been studied as a potential treatment for glucocorticoid-induced osteoporosis. Etidro-

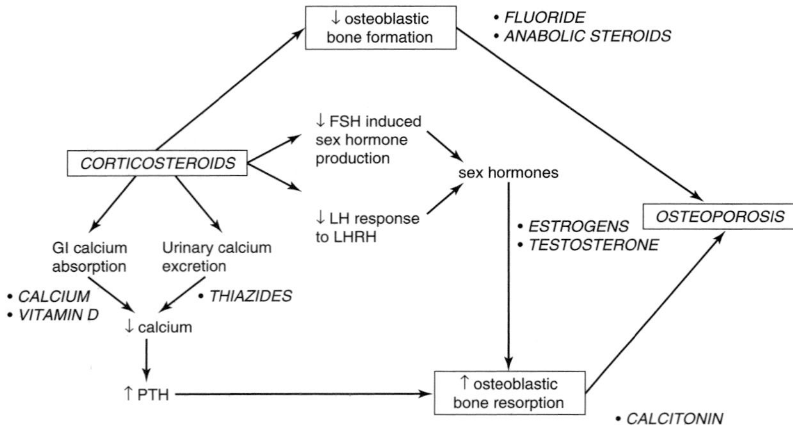

Figure 7–15. Approaches to the prevention and treatment of steroid-induced osteoporosis. FSH, follicle-stimulating hormone; GI, gastrointestinal; LH, luteinizing hormone; LHRH, luteinizing hormone–releasing hormone; PTH, parathyroid hormone.

nate, pamidronate, and more recently, alendronate have been shown in randomized controlled trials to increase lumbar spine bone mineral density in adult patients receiving long-term glucocorticoids for a variety of diseases.[513–516] However, once again, these trials did not include children and did not demonstrate any significant reduction in fracture incidence, which is the most clinically relevant outcome. Bisphosphonates have been studied in children with severe osteogenesis imperfecta and appear to be of benefit in reducing bone resorption, increasing bone density, and reducing the chronic bone pain associated with this condition.[517, 518]

In summary, although much is known about the mechanisms of glucocorticoid-induced osteoporosis, our knowledge about how best to prevent and treat this complication, particularly in children, is somewhat limited. Although it has been suggested that all patients initiating steroids should perhaps receive preventative therapy (calcium, vitamin D, or bisphosphonates), this is not yet common practice. Prospective trials evaluating these therapies in children are also needed. While awaiting the results of more definitive studies, it seems reasonable to recommend that all children who are at risk should at least maintain an adequate daily dietary intake of calcium (1000 to 1500 mg) and vitamin D (400 units) and satisfactory levels of mobility to prevent osteoporosis.

Preventing Acute Adrenal Insufficiency (Addisonian Crisis)

The short-term use of glucocorticoids for days or a few weeks does not lead to adrenal insufficiency upon cessation of treatment. However, prolonged therapy may lead to suppression of pituitary-adrenal function that can be slow in returning to normal. This is potentially the most serious and life-threatening adverse effect associated with glucocorticoid therapy. The magnitude of the effect on adrenal function of relatively low amounts of glucocorticoid, especially if given over prolonged periods, is often underestimated (Table 7–18). However, the actual doses and duration of therapy that are associated with this suppression and the length of the recovery period after cessation of therapy are not well defined.[519] Furthermore, some evidence suggests that a component of adrenal insufficiency may be due to the underlying inflammatory process in some patients.[520]

If not recognized, suppression of the hypothalamic-pituitary-adrenal axis as a consequence of chronic glucocorticoid administration places the child at risk for vascular collapse, adrenal crisis, and death in situations that demand increased availability of cortisol.[521] Under conditions of stress (serious infection, trauma, surgery), all children who may be at risk for hypothalamic-pituitary-adrenal axis suppression require additional glucocorticoids.

Glucocorticoid supplementation should be prescribed prior to surgery in any patient who has received significant amounts of glucocorticoids at any time during the preceding 12 months (possibly as long as 36 months).[521] For an elective procedure, a "steroid prep" consists of dexamethasone (0.05 to 0.15 mg/kg/24 hours) prior to the procedure in four divided IM doses given 6 hours apart, and hydrocortisone (1.5 to 4.0 mg/kg/24 hours) as a continuous IV infusion beginning at the time of surgery and continuing for 24 hours postoperatively or until the child has recovered or is able to take prednisone again by mouth.

This regimen is based on requirements for hydrocortisone during stress. Hydrocortisone (0.36 mg/kg/24 hours) is needed for physiologic maintenance. During maximal stress, 1.5 to 4.0 mg/kg/24 hours is required. Dexamethasone sodium phosphate (0.75 mg has a mineralocorticoid effect approximately equivalent to 20 mg hydrocortisone) is given preoperatively because of its long half-life; hydrocortisone is used during the procedure because of its immediate biologic availability. These recommended doses should be modified according to the magnitude of the stress and the severity and duration of suppression of the hypothalamic-pituitary-adrenal axis by exogenous steroid administration.

The requirement of increased amounts of glucocorticoid during acute stress should be explained to the parents. In addition, each child should carry a card or wear a necklace or bracelet indicating that glucocorticoid medication is being taken. Such a warning can be of great value to emergency medical teams if the patient is involved in an accident.

Table 7–18

Suppression of the Hypothalamic-Pituitary-Adrenal Axis by Glucocorticoid Drugs

In a 70-kg (1.73 M^2) adult, prednisone in a daily dose of:
- ≤5 mg given in the morning does not suppress; same dose given at night may suppress
- 7.5–15 mg for 1 mo causes variable suppression
- >15 mg for 1 wk or more causes suppression

High-Dose Intravenous Glucocorticoid Therapy

IV glucocorticoid "pulse" therapy is sometimes used to treat the more severe, acute, systemic connective tissue diseases such as SLE, JDM, and vasculitis.[522–524] It has also been used to treat the refractory systemic features of systemic-onset JRA.[525–527] The rationale of this approach is to achieve an immediate, profound anti-inflammatory effect and to minimize toxicity related to long-term continuous therapy in moderate to high daily doses. The main benefit appears to be rapid clinical improvement that lasts for about 3 weeks after a single bolus. This may be useful in the context of concurrent treatment with a disease-modifying agent, which may take several weeks or months to begin to exert its effect.[422] Although oral pulse regimens have been reported,[528] most publications deal with studies in which IV pulse therapy has been used. Methylprednisolone has been the drug of choice, given in a dose of 10 to 30 mg/kg/pulse up to a maximum of 1 g, administered according to a variety of protocols (Table 7–19). These have consisted of a single administration repeated as clinical circumstances warrant, a pulse each day for 3 to 5 days, or alternate-day pulses for three

Table 7–19

Suggested Protocol for Administration of Intravenous Methylprednisone

Dose

Methylprednisolone up to 30 mg/kg (maximum 1 g)

Preparation

Prepare drug with diluent provided with package
Calculated dose is added to 100 ml 5% dextrose in water and infused over 1–3 hr

Monitoring

Temperature, pulse rate, respiratory rate, blood pressure prior to beginning infusion
Pulse and blood pressure every 15 min for 1st hr, every 30 min thereafter
Slow rate or discontinue infusion, and increase frequency of monitoring if there are significant changes in blood pressure or pulse rate

Side Effects

Hypertension or hypotension, tachycardia, blurring of vision, flushing, sweating, metallic taste in mouth

doses. IV glucocorticoid pulse therapy, although perhaps efficacious in selected circumstances (no controlled trials have been reported in children), may be associated with potentially serious complications (Table 7–20).

The most frequently reported short-term adverse effect in children is abnormal behavior in up to 10 percent.[488] These behavioral changes include altered mood, hyperactivity, psychosis, disorientation, and sleep disturbances. Nonbehavioral adverse effects include headache, abdominal complaints, pruritus, vomiting, hives, hypertension, bone pain, dizziness, fatigue, lethargy, hypotension, tachycardia, and hyperglycemia.[488] Potential longer-term effects, such as influences on bone metabolism and risk of AVN, have not been systematically studied. Although there have been a number of reports of AVN associated with IV-pulse methylprednisolone,[529, 530] a retrospective cohort study of patients with rheumatoid arthritis did not find an increased risk of AVN in those treated with pulse methylprednisolone.[531]

Intra-Articular Steroids

Injection of long-acting glucocorticoids directly into inflamed joints has emerged as a major advance in the management of children with various types of arthritis. Although intra-articular steroid (IAS) therapy has not been studied in the randomized controlled clinical trial setting, there is accumulating evidence for its efficacy and safety in children (i.e., a number of uncontrolled, prospective cohort studies).[532–536] However, summarizing the results of the available studies is difficult because of the variability in the populations studied; the type, dose, and frequency of steroids used; the lack of control groups; and the variability in the assessment of outcomes, which are often not blinded and do not use standard outcome measures or lengths of follow-up.

IAS therapy has been most often used in children with oligoarticular disease when indications for use have included lack of response to NSAIDs given in optimal dosage for 3 months or more; significant NSAID toxicity; and the presence of joint deformity, growth disturbance, or muscle wasting.[532, 534–536] IASs may also have a role as an alternative to NSAIDs in children with oligoarticular disease.[536] In polyarticular disease, multiple IAS injections can be used as a temporizing measure while one is awaiting response to second-line agents given systemically. IASs may also be useful as an alternative to increasing systemic therapy in children with polyarticular disease who have significant inflammation in only a few joints.

Virtually all patients experience rapid resolution of symptoms and signs of joint inflammation within a few days of injection. About two thirds achieve remission for 12 months or more after a single injection.[533, 534] The duration of response seems to be longer in children with oligoarticular JRA than in those with polyarticular- or systemic-onset disease and in those with other forms of arthritis (e.g., spondyloarthropathies).[537] Younger patients and those with shorter disease duration also seem to achieve longer remissions after IAS injection.[532]

Type of Steroid, Dosage, and Frequency of Injection. A variety of preparations are available for intra-articular injection. The most frequently studied agents in children are the least soluble and hence longest-acting forms of injectable steroid: THA[532, 533, 536] and triamcinolone acetonide.[534] These agents are completely absorbed from the site of injection over a period of 2 to 3 weeks. Because of its lower solubility, THA is absorbed slower than triamcinolone acetonide, thus maintaining synovial levels for a longer time and creating lower systemic glucocorticoid levels.[538] Although THA is preferred by most pediatric rheumatologists, the efficacy and safety of the two agents have not been evaluated in comparative studies. Intra-articular THA, however, is superior to betamethasone[539] and methylprednisolone.[535]

The dose of THA that has been used in various clinical studies has varied: Some data indicate that higher doses (about 1 mg/kg) may be associated with a better response.[532] Although there are no hard and fast rules regarding the choice of steroid, the dosage and frequency of injection have been outlined.[51] Children who weigh less than 20 kg receive 20 mg THA in large joints. Those above 20 kg receive 30 to 40 mg THA in the hips, knees, and shoulders and 10 to 20 mg in the ankles and elbows. In smaller joints such as the wrist, midtarsal, and subtalar joints, 10 mg THA is used. For injections into tendon sheaths and small

Table 7–20

Potential Acute Toxicities of Intravenous Glucocorticoid Pulse Therapy

Cardiac arrhythmia secondary to potassium depletion
Hypertension secondary to sodium retention
Acute psychosis, convulsions
Hyperglycemia with or without ketosis
Anaphylaxis
Infection
Osteonecrosis

joints of the hands and feet, 0.25 to 0.50 ml of a combination of methylprednisolone acetate mixed 1:1 with preservative-free 1 percent lidocaine (Xylocaine) is recommended. The shorter-acting steroid is associated with less risk of damage to tendon sheaths or local soft tissue atrophy as a result of leakage of steroid from the smaller-volume joints. Repeated injections into the same joint are not performed more than three times per year, although there are few data on which to base this recommendation. There are also no controlled studies in children about whether postinjection rest has a role. Although immobilization of the injected joint is common practice in some clinics, our recommendation is to allow normal ambulation but to avoid high-impact physical activity in the 24 to 48 hours following joint injections.

Adverse Effects. Despite initial reservations about the safety of intra-articular steroid injections in children, clinical studies indicate an overall favorable adverse-effect profile. Iatrogenic septic arthritis is always a potential risk but has never been reported in children. It occurs very rarely in adults and can be avoided with aseptic precautions.[540] Transient crystal synovitis occurs in a small proportion of patients.[534] It is very similar to gouty arthritis and is self-limited, with resolution of symptoms within 3 to 5 days in most cases without any intervention.[536] The most frequent adverse effects are atrophic skin changes at the site of injection, particularly of small joints such as wrists and ankles in young children, and asymptomatic calcifications on radiographs in joints after multiple injections.[541] The frequency of these skin changes ranges from 5.6 percent of knees to 16 percent of ankles, 22 percent of wrists, and 50 percent of metatarsophalangeal joints injected.[541] The skin changes are attributed to the leakage of long-acting steroids into subcutaneous tissues and can be minimized by clearing the needle track with injection of saline or local anesthetic as the needle is withdrawn from the joint. Most skin changes eventually resolve.[533, 541] Radiographic reviews have demonstrated joint calcifications in 6 to 50 percent of injected joints.[542, 543] These are usually asymptomatic, but in one case surgical removal was required because of the size of the calcification.[544]

One of the main reservations about the use of IAS in young children was based on the theoretical potential for cartilage toxicity. Cartilage damage occurred after intra-articular injection of steroids in the rabbit model but was not reproduced in higher species.[540] Clinical MRI studies in children to assess cartilage integrity up to 13 months after steroid injection of single joints have demonstrated no toxic effects on cartilage and no detrimental effects on statural growth.[545, 546] Some children with multiple steroid injections (more than five per joint) followed for longer periods (6 to 18 years) may have nonspecific abnormalities of cartilage on MRI.[547] The clinical significance of these findings is not clear.

Although the majority of adverse effects associated with IAS injections are local, they are also associated with some systemic effects. Children develop transient suppression of endogenous cortisol production lasting 10 to 30 days after IAS injection.[548, 549] Younger children may undergo a more prolonged period of suppression.[548] However, the clinical significance of this finding in terms of effects on linear growth or actual risk of adrenal crisis at times of stress is not known. Although these complications have not been reported after single injections, whether there is any risk after multiple injections, particularly in younger children, needs further study. The systemic absorption of steroid may also be associated with altered salicylate kinetics, resulting in a transient fall in serum salicylate levels. Diabetic children may require a transient increase in insulin requirements.

Cytotoxic Agents

Cytotoxic drugs prevent cell division or cause cell death. They act primarily on rapidly dividing cells such as those of the immune system, particularly T lymphocytes, and are therefore immunosuppressive. Thus, cytotoxic drugs have both immediate anti-inflammatory actions and delayed immunosuppressive effects. Specific pharmacologic actions are usually considered specific for the cell cycle or not specific for the cell cycle. The cell cycle consists of the G_1 presynthetic phase, the S phase (synthesis of DNA), the G_2 resting (or postsynthetic) phase, and mitosis. 6-Mercaptopurine and azathioprine inhibit biosynthesis of purine and nucleotide interconversions and act during the G_1 and S phases in proliferating cells. Mycophenolate mofetil (MMF) reduces the pool of guanine nucleotide, thus interfering with purine biosynthesis; it also acts in the G_1 and S phases. Alkylating agents crosslink DNA and act during all phases of the cell cycle whether or not a cell is replicating. These agents are maximally effective in inhibiting immunologic responses when their administration coincides with the period of proliferation of the specific immunologically competent cells.

Although cytotoxic drugs have been used to treat children who are seriously ill with rheumatic diseases when other modes of therapy have proved ineffective, there have been no adequately controlled trials in the childhood rheumatic diseases. In most instances, the effects of these drugs are delayed and they have therefore proved more valuable in moderate- to long-term therapy than in an acute crisis. The potential toxicity of these drugs is substantial. Extensive experience has been accumulating with the use of these agents; nevertheless, each child's illness must be considered thoroughly before drugs from this class are recommended. These agents are not approved for unrestricted use in children with rheumatic diseases and should be used only by physicians who are familiar with their administration, toxicity, and expected benefits. Occasionally, a cytotoxic agent is used for its steroid-sparing effect.

Azathioprine

Azathioprine (Fig. 7–16), a purine analogue, is inactive until it is metabolized to 6-mercaptopurine by the liver

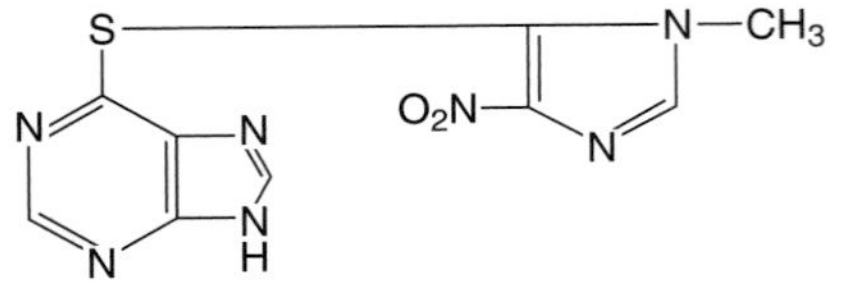

Figure 7–16. Azathioprine structure.

and erythrocytes.[550] Hypoxanthine phosphoribosyl transferase metabolizes 6-mercaptopurine to 6-thioinosinic acid, which suppresses the synthesis of adenine and guanine, thereby interfering with DNA synthesis. Furthermore, 6-inosinic acid inhibits phosphoribosyl pyrophosphate conversion in purine nucleotide synthesis, conversion of inosinic acid to xanthylic acid by purine nucleoside phosphorylase, and incorporation of nucleotide triphosphates into DNA.

Azathioprine suppresses cell-mediated immune functions and inhibits monocyte functions.[551–554] These immunosuppressive effects are related primarily to inhibition of T-cell growth during the S phase of cell division. A measurable decrease in antibody synthesis occurs with long-term administration; occasionally a decrease in serum antibody concentration occurs.

Approximately 50 percent of the drug is absorbed after oral administration, of which one third is protein bound.[129] The plasma half-life is approximately 75 minutes. The kidneys are the major route of excretion. Azathioprine crosses the placenta and may cause severe disease in the fetus.[555]

Toxicity to the GI tract (oral ulcers, nausea, vomiting, diarrhea, epigastric pain) is common.[556] Toxicity to the liver (mild elevation of serum levels of liver enzymes or cholestatic jaundice), lung (interstitial pneumonitis), pancreas (pancreatitis), or skin (maculopapular rash) is uncommonly associated with azathioprine therapy. Dose-related toxicity to the bone marrow results in leukopenia and, less commonly, thrombocytopenia and anemia. An idiosyncratic arrest of granulocyte maturation that occurs shortly after initiation of therapy has been described and results from reduced activity of the enzyme thiopurine methyltransferase.[557, 558] The bone marrow effects of azathioprine may be increased by concomitant use of trimethoprim.[559] Although the risk of malignancy theoretically increases in patients treated with azathioprine, the long-term data are not conclusive. Data are insufficient with respect to childhood rheumatic diseases, but in adults with rheumatoid arthritis treated with azathioprine, the risk of malignancy does not appear to be greater than that in similar patients who did not receive azathioprine.[560–562]

The use of azathioprine has been reported anecdotally in many pediatric rheumatic diseases and in series of patients with JRA or SLE.[563, 564] Starting doses should be 1 to 1.5 mg/kg/day, increasing as needed and tolerated to 2 to 2.5 mg/kg/day (Table 7–21).

Mycophenolate Mofetil

MMF has been used successfully in patients with solid organ transplants and with anecdotal success in inflammatory diseases (Fig. 7–17). Mycophenolic acid (MPA), a fermentation product of *Penicillium stoloniferum,* is the active immunosuppressant species, and MMF was developed to increase the oral bioavailability of MPA. Its major effect is on T and B lymphocytes, for which it is relatively selective. Action of MPA is mediated through noncompetitive binding to inosine monophosphate dehydrogenase, an enzyme critical for de novo synthesis of guanine nucleotide, a pathway on which T and B lymphocytes are primarily dependent.

In vitro MPA inhibits T- and B-cell mitogen proliferation,[565–567] antigen-specific antibody response of memory B cells,[568, 569] suppression of the humoral immune response,[570] the proliferative response of fibroblast and endothelial cells,[565] and attachment of monocytes to endothelial cells.[571] However, MPA enhances vascular cell adhesion molecules induced by TNF-α and E-selectin surface expression on endothelial cells.[572] It does not inhibit IL-2 production, Il-2 receptor expression, phagocytic activity, or secretion of T_H1 cytokines. Because its effect appears to be at a late stage of T-cell activation, it can be used safely with cyclosporin and tacrolimus.

MMF is rapidly absorbed after oral administration and hydrolyzed in the liver to the biologically active MPA. MPA is 8 percent albumin bound, and the activity of the drug results from the unbound MPA. Peak plasma levels occur 1 to 3 hours after a single dose, with a second peak at 6 to 12 hours as a result of enterohepatic circulation. The oral bioavailability is approximately 94 percent. The elimination half-life is ap-

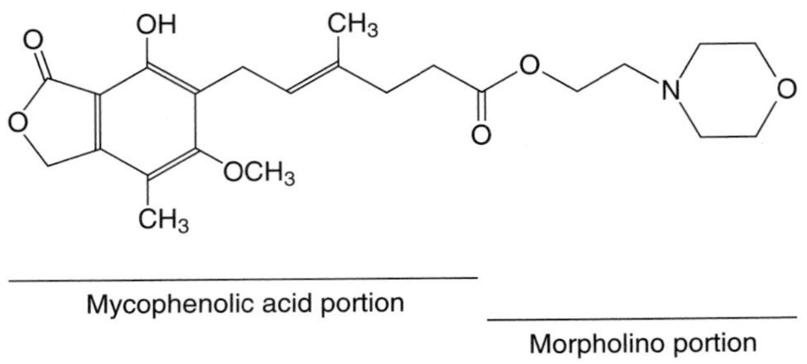

Table 7–21

Guidelines for Azathioprine Use

Dose

0.5–2.5 mg/kg/d in a single dose (taken with food) for 1 yr or more

Clinical Monitoring

Clinical evaluation every 1–2 mo

Laboratory Monitoring

CBC with WBCC differential and platelet count weekly until stable dose is achieved, then monthly

Hepatic enzymes, BUN, serum creatinine initially and then monthly

Discontinue if WBCC <3500/mm³, platelet count <100,000/mm³, elevated liver enzymes

BUN, blood urea nitrogen; CBC, complete blood count; WBCC, white blood cell count.

Figure 7–17. Mycophenolate mofetil structure.

proximately 17 hours after oral administration.[573] The effective adult dose in solid organ transplantation is 2 g/day in two divided doses. The dose used in children has been 46 mg/kg/day.[573] Because of its extensive binding to albumin, MMF may interact with other albumin-bound drugs. Antacids containing aluminum and magnesium decrease absorption and so should not be administered simultaneously. There may be competition for renal tubular secretion with acyclovir.

Adverse effects of MMF include toxicity on the GI tract, hematologic effects (leukopenia, anemia, thrombocytopenia, pancytopenia), and opportunistic infections. The GI side effects generally improve by giving the dose three or four times instead of twice a day, or by reducing it. Hematologic toxicity usually responds to therapy cessation within 1 week. The incidence of lymphoma has been reported at 0.6 percent, similar to that of azathioprine.[574]

Although the majority of studies are in the solid organ transplant literature, preliminary reports show promise in patients with rheumatoid arthritis,[575] SLE,[576, 577] vasculitis,[574] and inflammatory eye disease.[578]

Cyclophosphamide

Cyclophosphamide, an alkylating agent, is a nitrogen mustard derivative (Fig. 7–18). It is well absorbed after oral administration and may also be given intravenously (Table 7–22). It is inactive until metabolized, principally in the liver, by the cytochrome-P450 mixed-function oxidase system to inactive intermediates and the active metabolite phosphoramide mustard. Phosphoramide mustard covalently binds to guanine in DNA, destroying the purine ring and thereby preventing cell replication.[579, 580] Cyclophosphamide potentially acts on all cells, including those that are mitotically inactive (G_0 interphase) at the time of administration—for example, memory T cells.[581, 582] Excretion of the drug is primarily by the kidney; the dose must therefore be reduced in patients with renal impairment (Table 7–23). Acrolein, the other principal metabolite, is thought to be therapeutically inactive but is responsible for bladder toxicity. The half-life of cyclophosphamide is approximately 7 hours.

Cyclophosphamide exerts anti-inflammatory actions by its effects on mononuclear cells and cellular immunity. Alkylating agents cause B- and T-cell lymphopenia. B cells appear to be more sensitive than T cells to the effects of cyclophosphamide.[583] It has been suggested that the route of administration influences the nature of the effects of this drug; daily oral low-dose therapy may more profoundly affect cell-mediated immunity, whereas intermittent high-dose IV therapy predominantly affects B-cell immunity.[584, 585] In humans,

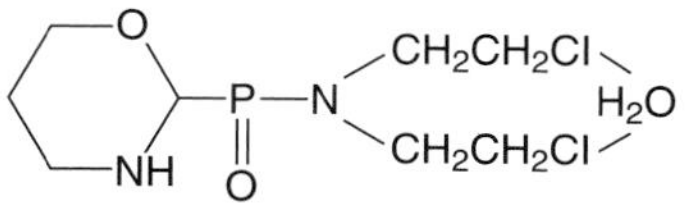

O, NH, P, O, N, CH_2CH_2Cl, CH_2CH_2Cl, H_2O

Figure 7–18. Cyclophosphamide structure.

Table 7–22

Guidelines for Daily Cyclophosphamide Use

Dose

0.5–2.0 mg/kg/d in a single oral dose
0.5–2.0 mg/kg/d as an IV pulse (with ample IV fluids for 24 hr)
Encourage fluid intake to minimize risk to bladder
Encourage frequent emptying of bladder

Clinical Monitoring

Clinical evaluation every month

Laboratory Monitoring

CBC with WBCC, differential and platelet counts, urinalysis every week until stable dose is achieved, then every month
Hepatic enzymes, BUN, serum creatinine initially and then every month
Discontinue drug if: WBCC <1500/mm³ (1.5 × 10⁹/L), platelet count <100,000/mm³ (100 × 10⁹/L), hematuria

BUN, blood urea nitrogen; CBC, complete blood count; WBCC, white blood cell count.

IgG and IgM synthesis is depressed and there is a measurable decrease of serum antibody concentration after chronic administration.[581, 582]

The alkylating agents have prominent toxic effects.[586–594] Short-term side effects are common; although troublesome to the child, they are seldom serious. These include anorexia, nausea and vomiting, and alopecia. Alopecia appears to be related to dose and duration of treatment and is usually reversible. Pulmonary fibrosis has been reported in a small number of patients on daily cyclophosphamide therapy.

Leukopenia and thrombocytopenia are the most common adverse reactions, although with careful monitoring, they are seldom of clinical significance. The cyclophosphamide dose should be adjusted to maintain the total granulocyte count at 1500/mm³ or higher (≥1.5 × 10⁹/L). The nadir of granulocytopenia with IV therapy occurs between the first and the second weeks of therapy, and the dose should be adjusted accordingly based on the complete blood count and differential white blood cell count obtained on days 7, 10, and 14 after IV cyclophosphamide administration. Lymphocyte counts less than 500/mm³ (<0.5 × 10⁹/L) are also an indication to lower the dose. Glucocorti-

Table 7–23

Recommended Reductions of Cyclophosphamide Dose in Patients With Impaired Renal Function

SERUM CREATININE (μM/L)	ORAL CYCLOPHOSPHAMIDE DOSE
<250	2 mg/kg/d
250–500	1.75 mg/kg/d
>500	1.5 mg/kg/d

Adapted from Luqmani RA, Palmer RG, Bacon PA: Azathioprine, cyclophosphamide, and chlorambucil. Clin Rheumatol 4: 595, 1990.

Table 7–24

Suggested Protocol for the Administration of Intravenous Cyclophosphamide

Dose

0.5–1.0 g/M² cyclophosphamide

Preparation

Start IV with 5% dextrose in water

Administer 2 L/M² of IV fluid as 5% dextrose in water or 2/3 + 1/3 over next 24 hr, start hydration 4 hr prior to administration of cyclophosphamide

MESNA injection (30% of cyclophosphamide dose) IV in 240 mg of 0.2 normal saline at 10 ml/hr over 24 hr, start immediately after cyclophosphamide

Ondansetron (0.15 mg/kg/dose) IV/PO 30 min prior to cyclophosphamide and every 8 hr until infusion complete

Dilute cyclophosphamide to 10 mg/ml in 5% dextrose in water and infuse prescribed dose over at least 1 hr (to minimize nausea and vomiting)

Monitoring

Pulse, blood pressure, and respiratory rate every 30 min during infusion, then every 4 hr for next 24 hr

Urinalysis pre and post infusion

Monitor urinary output: Empty bladder every 2–4 hr. If urinary output falls to less than 50% of IV input over any 4-hr period, give furosemide 1 mg/kg IV. Repeat at 2–4 mg/kg in 2 hr, if necessary.

coids probably aid in protecting the bone marrow from the neutropenia-inducing effects of cyclophosphamide.

Cyclophosphamide is administered in one of two ways: either orally each day or by IV bolus every 2 to 4 weeks (Table 7–24). IV pulse is less toxic and at least as efficacious for lupus nephritis[595]; in some systemic vasculitides, it is not clear whether the IV route is as effective as oral administration.[585]

Bladder toxicity (cystitis, fibrosis, transitional cell carcinoma) is a major risk of cyclophosphamide and results from prolonged contact of acrolein with the bladder mucosa.[589–591] To prevent cystitis, one must emphasize adequate hydration and frequent voiding for children on daily cyclophosphamide. Persistent nonglomerular hematuria is an indication for cystoscopy, and if cystitis is observed, the dose should be reduced or the drug stopped. IV pulse therapy reduces the risk of toxicity, including hemorrhagic cystitis, and confines those risks to a short period each month instead of every day. Prophylactic 2-mercaptoethanesulfonic acid (MESNA) should be considered a part of any IV cyclophosphamide protocol to minimize contact of acrolein with the bladder mucosa.

The syndrome of inappropriate antidiuretic hormone secretion has been reported in patients receiving large doses of cyclophosphamide and is exacerbated by the large fluid load that must be administered.[596] It does not matter which hydration solution is used.[597] With the large doses of cyclophosphamide administered by IV bolus, children must be encouraged to empty their bladders every 2 hours and awakened during the night to do so; if not, furosemide should be given and catheterization considered to prevent significant contact of the bladder mucosa with acrolein. Nausea and vomiting can be a significant problem; prophylactic use of a potent antiemetic (e.g., ondansetron) is encouraged as part of IV protocols.

An important consideration with the use of alkylating agents is the effect on fertility for both males and females. The stage of sexual maturity is critical in terms of inducing gonadal dysfunction; the further beyond puberty, the greater the chance of infertility on an equivalent dose of cyclophosphamide.[598] In females with lupus nephritis, amenorrhea and oligomenorrhea occur more frequently with higher total dose and increased age at administration.[599, 600] Use of IV bolus at current recommended doses results in a much lower total cumulative dose than daily oral administration and thus should be the preferred route, presuming equivalent effectiveness. Ovarian destruction attributable to cyclophosphamide was reported in one child.[586] In rhesus monkeys, luteinizing hormone–releasing hormone may protect the ovary against cyclophosphamide-induced damage and may be effective in patients treated with cyclophosphamide, as demonstrated in a study of women with lymphoma who received gonadotropin-releasing hormone agonist.[601, 602] Protocols using leuprorelin in young women treated with cyclophosphamide are now being evaluated.[603]

Cyclophosphamide is associated with an increased risk of malignancy in adults with rheumatoid arthritis, a risk that is dose-related and increases with duration of follow-up. One case-control study demonstrated a fourfold elevation of myeloproliferative disorders,[593] and a more recent study showed an increased risk of bladder and skin cancer.[604] The incidence of bladder cancer in adults with Wegener's granulomatosis treated with cyclophosphamide is 5 percent at 10 years and 16 percent at 15 years; the incidence is related to both total dose and duration of treatment. Nonglomerular hematuria identified a subgroup of patients at high risk for bladder cancer.[605] More recently, short courses of very high doses of cyclophosphamide have been used either as primary therapy in myeloablative doses for SLE and aplastic anemia[606] or as part of a transplantation protocol for patients with autoimmune disease.

Cyclophosphamide is used commonly in patients with severe lupus nephritis (World Health Organization class IV) and other life-threatening complications of lupus. In addition, cyclophosphamide is well accepted in the treatment of severe necrotizing and granulomatous vasculitis.

Chlorambucil

Chlorambucil (Fig. 7–19), like cyclophosphamide, is an alkylating agent that preferentially reduces B-cell numbers, with less effect on memory T cells and natural killer cells, and acts by crosslinking macromole-

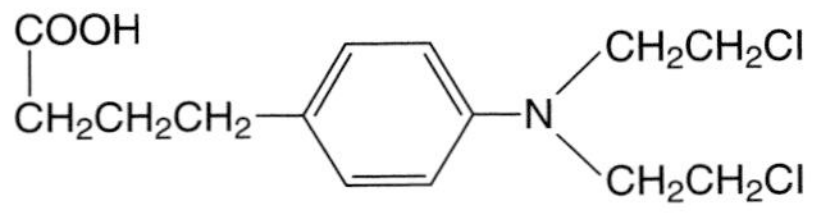

$$\mathrm{HOOC{-}CH_2CH_2CH_2{-}C_6H_4{-}N(CH_2CH_2Cl)_2}$$

Figure 7–19. Chlorambucil structure.

cules, thereby interfering with several cellular functions. It is generally prescribed orally at a dose of 0.1 to 0.2 mg/kg/day but can be given intravenously as well. Because of serious toxicity, use of chlorambucil is reserved for very narrow indications. It is the drug of choice for amyloidosis complicating inflammatory disease and occasionally for severe uveitis.[607] However, the very high risk of malignancy, ranging up to 7.5 percent,[608] precludes its use in all but the most severe cases. In addition to the risk of malignancy, male infertility is very common once total doses of 25 mg/kg are reached.[609] Thrombocytopenia and infection are also common.[607]

Cyclosporin

Cyclosporin (Fig. 7–20), a cyclic peptide of fungal origin, and tacrolimus (FK506), another fungal macrolide, have been shown to have profound effects on the immune system. The observation that cyclosporin could virtually eliminate mitogen-induced proliferation by T cells but had little effect on other cell types[610] indicated the potential of this drug in the treatment of immunologically mediated disease. Both drugs have had a major impact on the prevention of solid organ transplant rejection.

Cyclosporin is inactive until complexed with its intracellular receptor, cyclophilin. In the process of T- or B-cell activation, cell receptor signaling leads to a release of intracellular calcium, which binds to calmodulin, activating serine-threonine phosphatase calcineurin.[611] Once activated, calcineurin stimulates the translocation of the transcription factor NF-ATc, which is an important stimulus for IL-2 gene transcription,[612] and cell-mediated immune responses.[610, 613–615] The cyclosporin-cyclophilin complex binds to calcineurin, thus inhibiting the early phase of T-cell activation and IL-2 production. Cyclosporin also inhibits the production of IL-3, IL-4, and IFN-γ,[616] and it enhances the production of transforming growth factor β_1 protein.[617]

Cyclosporin may also result in immune suppression by inhibiting degradation of I-kappa-B.[618] In addition, it may modulate anti-inflammatory effects by inhibiting monocyte production of tissue factor, a potential stimulus of the coagulation cascade via inhibition of NF-kappa-B.[619] It may also result in apoptosis of T and B cells.[620]

Whether cyclosporin affects antigen presentation is uncertain. Some studies have shown that the drug has no effect on macrophage function in antigen presentation,[621] whereas others have suggested that the drug interferes with antigen presentation by dendritic cells[622] and Langerhans' cells.[623]

Cyclosporin is incompletely and variably absorbed from the GI tract, bound principally to serum albumin and erythrocytes, metabolized by the liver, and excreted in the bile. It has a half-life of approximately 18 hours. A microemulsion formulation of cyclosporin has been developed to improve absorption and bioavailability.[624] This preparation has more consistent interpatient and intrapatient pharmacokinetics. Cyclosporin crosses the placenta and is present in breast milk. It is important to note the several significant drug interactions associated with cyclosporin[415] and the considerable toxicity associated with the use of this drug: impaired renal function,[625, 626] hypertension, hepatic toxicity,[627] tremor, mucous membrane lesions, and nausea and vomiting. Hypertrichosis, paresthesias, and gingival hyperplasia have been observed. Renal toxicity may result in hypertension from interstitial fibrosis or tubular atrophy, even in adults treated with relatively low dosages (3 to 5 mg/kg/day orally). Concomitant use of NSAIDs may exacerbate this toxic effect of the drug.

Several open trials have shown improvement in children with JRA,[628, 629] dermatomyositis,[630] and uveitis.[631, 632] Cyclosporin has been reported to have dramatic beneficial effects in patients with the macrophage activation syndrome.[633] In the largest series reported[629] (17 patients with JRA, 5 patients with JDM), 6 children experienced a doubling of serum creatinine (although no level was beyond the normal range), 4 developed anemia (normochromic, normocytic), and 6 experienced infections (varicella-zoster in 3, PCP in 1, and a urinary tract infection in 2). Despite concern of an increased incidence of malignancy, a case-control series[634] did not show

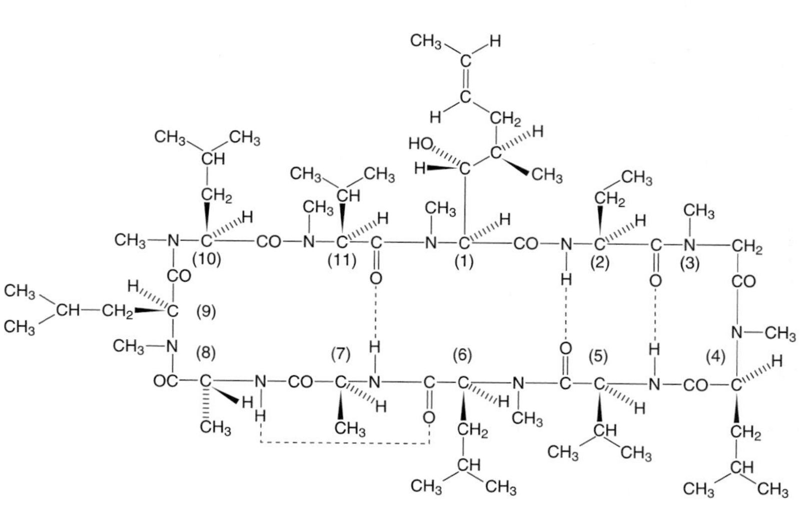

Figure 7–20. Cyclosporin structure.

Table 7–25

Guidelines for Cyclosporin Use

Dose	
3–5 mg/kg/d orally	
Clinical Monitoring	
Blood pressure every week for first month, then monthly	
Laboratory Monitoring	
Renal function studies (BUN, creatinine, urinalysis) at start of therapy and every month	
Hepatic enzymes, CBC with WBCC differential, and platelet count every month	
Maintain 12 hr whole-blood trough drug levels between 125 and 175 ng/ml (RIA method)	
Reduce dose if serum creatinine increases by ≥30%	

BUN, blood urea nitrogen; CBC, complete blood count; WBCC, white blood cell count.

any increased risk of malignancy over a 5-year follow-up period in adult patients treated with cyclosporin compared with controls.

Current guidelines for cyclosporin use are outlined in Table 7–25. Factors that most commonly limit clinical use of cyclosporin are hypertension and a rise in serum creatinine of greater than 30 percent from baseline. Unfortunately, long-term renal damage can occur despite normal serum creatinine levels during the course of therapy.[624] In the rheumatic diseases, the goal has been to achieve a whole blood trough level between 125 and 175 μg/ml. It is important to note that grapefruit juice increases cyclosporin and cyclosporin metabolite levels significantly.[635]

Leflunomide

Leflunomide (Fig. 7–21) is an immunomodulatory agent that, through its active plasma metabolite, A77-1766, inhibits de novo pyrimidine synthesis by inhibiting the enzyme dihydro-orotate dehydrogenase.[636] As a result, p53 in the cytoplasm translocates to the nucleus and initiates cellular arrest in the G_1 phase of the cell cycle. It also inhibits tyrosine kinase,[637] inhibits leukocyte-endothelial adhesion,[638] and affects cytokine production leading to immunosuppression.[639] Because its actions are similar to those of methotrexate, it might be better classified as a DMARD.

Initial studies in adults with rheumatoid arthritis have shown that at daily doses of 10 and 25 mg, leflunomide is more effective than placebo[640, 641] and as effective as sulfasalazine over 24 weeks.[641] After a 3-day loading dose of 100 mg, daily doses of 10, 20, and 25 mg have shown benefit as early as 4 weeks and continuing improvement for up to 20 weeks, after

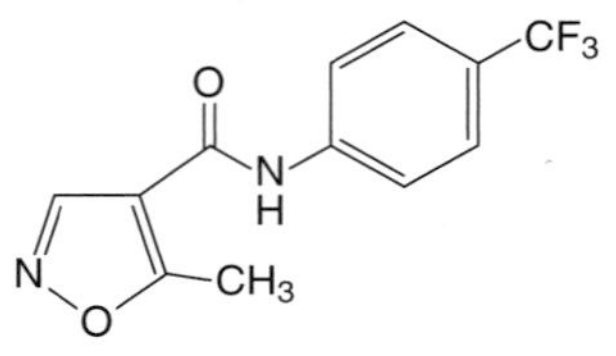

Figure 7–21. Leflunomide structure.

which the clinical improvements are maintained. Side effects from leflunomide have been mild and dose-related. These include GI side effects (abdominal pain, dyspepsia, anorexia, diarrhea, gastritis), allergic rash, reversible alopecia, mild weight loss, and elevation of liver function test results.[641, 642] No increase in infection has been reported. No studies have been reported yet in pediatrics.

Combination Therapies

In the past, there was a reluctance to use combinations of DMARDs for arthritis because of concerns about increased toxicity of agents with similar toxicity profiles. However, a number of factors support the use of combination therapies. In adult rheumatoid arthritis, single agents seem to lose efficacy over time[643]; furthermore, these agents rarely induce sustained long-term remissions. An increased appreciation of the long-term morbidity of both rheumatoid arthritis and JRA supports a more "aggressive" approach to medical management.[152] A better understanding of the mechanisms of action of these agents, and recent well-designed studies of combination therapy in adults that demonstrate efficacy without a significant increase in toxicity, support the use of this approach. In adult rheumatoid arthritis, studies demonstrate the efficacy of triple therapy with sulfasalazine, MTX, and hydroxychloroquine versus treatment with any two drugs alone[252]: MTX and cyclosporin versus MTX or placebo[644, 645]; chloroquine and MTX versus MTX[646]; and sulfasalazine-leflunomide versus sulfasalazine or placebo.[641] In addition, the improvement noted with biologic therapy can be enhanced when combined with MTX.[647, 648] In JRA, combination therapy has included IV methylprednisolone, IV cyclophosphamide, and MTX.[525, 649] Combination therapy would seem particularly appropriate in severe systemic-onset JRA. However, well-designed studies in JRA are necessary before embarking on such a course of therapy. Important questions to address include which patients are most at risk for long-term damage and thus most "deserving" of combination therapy; whether therapy should be started in combination or medication added only with a partial inadequate response; and whether full or reduced doses of each agent should be used.

Antibiotics

The concept that rheumatoid arthritis was caused by microbial pathogens led to early treatment with antimicrobial therapy. In fact, it was for that reason that gold was first introduced as a treatment for rheumatoid arthritis. Sulfasalazine was synthesized to take advantage of its antimicrobial properties. Recently, antibiotics have again been considered in the treatment of inflammatory rheumatic disease.

Penicillin plays a key prophylactic role in preventing the recurrence of acute rheumatic fever and perhaps in the prevention of poststreptococcal arthritis.[650] Cutaneous polyarteritis, which may be a streptococcus-related disease, is also often treated with prophylactic penicillin.[651] In Wegener's granulomatosis, treatment with trimethoprim-sulfamethoxazole may prevent disease relapses.[652]

Studies in rheumatoid arthritis have suggested a

role for synthetic tetracycline antibiotics.[653, 654] In early disease, minocycline was more effective than placebo.[655] The mechanism of action may depend more on the biochemical than on the antimicrobial effect of these agents. Antibiotics do not seem to be effective in enteric reactive arthritis but may have a role in urogenital reactive arthritis.[656]

Biologic Therapies

Intravenous Immunoglobulin

Intravenous immunoglobulin (IVIG) is prepared from pooled human plasma. Its effectiveness in the treatment of Kawasaki disease has encouraged its use in a number of other childhood rheumatic diseases. It is also reported to be of benefit in some cases of JDM[657] and systemic-onset JRA,[658] although placebo-controlled randomized trials did not show benefit in either systemic- or polyarticular-onset JRA.[659, 660] Although IVIG has a good record of safety, anaphylactoid reaction is a risk. Other potential side effects include myalgia, fever, and headache during the infusion, and aseptic meningitis 24 to 48 hours afterward.[661] Although current preparation protocols purify the product so that it is free from contamination with HIV, hepatitis C, and other known viruses, there is a potential theoretical risk of transmission of Creutzfeldt-Jacob disease as well as other, yet-unidentified pathogens. Guidelines for IVIG administration are listed in Table 7–26.

The mechanisms whereby IVIG exerts its therapeutic effect are not clear and may differ in different situations. Its action may be mediated by specific antibodies that neutralize an as-yet unknown causative agent such as a virus. IVIG contains anti-idiotype antibodies that may bind to the idiotype of an antibody involved in the pathogenesis of the disease.[662] Such anti-idiotype antibodies have been shown to suppress autoimmune disease in animal models.[663] Antibodies to inflammatory mediators, including cytokines, may also have important therapeutic roles. The rapid defervescence that occurs after IVIG administration in Kawasaki disease suggests that interleukins, particularly IL-1 and IL-6, are removed from the circulation or neutralized, or that their production is stopped by some constituent of the IVIG. It is known that normal serum contains antibodies to IL-1α,[664] IL-6,[665] TNF-α,[666] IFN-α2b, and IFN-γ.[667] Normalization of T-cell numbers and function has also occurred after administration of IVIG.[668] IVIG can neutralize superantigens, which may be involved in Kawasaki disease.[669] Another mechanism of action whereby IVIG might exert its beneficial anti-inflammatory effects is a reduction in the expression of adhesion molecules. In JDM, IVIG can decrease the activity of the membrane attack complex.[670]

Table 7–26

Guidelines for the Use of Intravenous Immunoglobulin

Dose

Up to 2 g/kg

Preparation

Start IV with normal saline

Administration

Give IVIG at rate of 0.5 ml/hr every 30 min, then 1.0 ml/kg/hr every 30 min, then 2.0 ml/kg/hr for the remainder

Monitor

Blood pressure and pulse rate every 15 min for first hr, 30 min for second hr, 60 min thereafter

Observe

Sudden fall in blood pressure (anaphylaxis)
Headache, vomiting 18–36 hr after infusion (aseptic meningitis)

Specific Biologic Agents

Elucidation of some of the basic mechanisms involved in rheumatoid arthritis has resulted in an understanding of many of the cellular and effector mechanisms that participate in inflammatory states. Specific biologic agents have been developed that can target one or several steps involved in the immune response. Strategies for intervention (adapted from Wallis and associates[671]) can be grouped as follows:

- Tolerance induction
- Inhibition of major histocompatibility complex (MHC) antigen/T-cell receptor interaction
- Inhibition of cellular function and cell–cell interaction
- Interference with cytokines
- Apoptosis

Although the initial excitement regarding biologic therapy was tempered by either lack of efficacy or severe toxicity, more recent developments justify a great deal of optimism for the development of new, more focused and targeted therapies over the next few years.

Induction of Tolerance

Autoreactive T cells that escape thymic deletion during ontogeny can be deleted by at least two peripheral mechanisms of tolerance.[672] If the T cells interact with antigen but are not activated, T-cell dormancy, or *anergy,* develops. If T_H2 cells have the same T-cell receptor as the autoreactive clone, cytokines with an anti-inflammatory profile will be released, which can suppress an antigen-specific T_H1 response. This is the principle behind attempts to achieve oral tolerance to an antigen. Reactive T_H2 cells can leave the gut and migrate to sites in which the antigen may be localized and are stimulated to release anti-inflammatory cytokines, thereby mediating local immune suppression. Trials of oral administration of type II collagen have been attempted because of the high incidence of autoimmunity to type II collagen in adult rheumatoid arthritis (and in approximately 25 percent of children with JRA), as well as the success of this approach in a variety of animal models of arthritis in which type II collagen autoimmunity occurred.[673] Studies in humans have shown varying results, but results seem to be better when lower doses of collagen are administered.[674] In an open trial involving 10 patients with JRA who were treated with type II chick collagen, 8 responded; no adverse effects were observed.[675] Placebo studies are required.

Inhibition of Major Histocompatibility Complex/Antigen/T-Cell Receptor Interaction

The immune response is driven by the interaction between antigen-presenting cells processing and presenting an antigenic peptide to a specific T-cell receptor in the context of a specific MHC molecule. Any component of this trimolecular complex could theoretically be targeted for biologic modulation. If the initiating antigen were known, an immunization program could be developed to prevent disease, and this is the principle behind oral tolerance (see earlier). T-cell receptor vaccines may be one way to prevent or reduce activity of synovial inflammation, as shown in animal models. This strategy would work only if specific V_β region subtypes could be shown to predominate in synovitis and did not change over time. Early studies in patients with rheumatoid arthritis who were vaccinated with several V_β subtypes show promise and are continuing.[676] Data in children with JRA and spondyloarthropathies suggest that this approach may have some merit.[677] Another possible route of attack is to block the MHC site by anti-MHC antibodies.

Inhibition of Cellular Function and Cell–Cell Interaction

T cells appear to play a central role in initiating the rheumatoid process in adult disease and in JRA, but their role in continuing to drive the inflammatory process is less clear. Results of initial studies using monoclonal T-cell–depleting antibodies were disappointing. Initial clinical improvements, if they occurred at all, were short lived or associated with profound lymphopenia, thus precluding further treatment.[678, 679] These included studies with anti-CD7 monoclonal antibodies (mAbs), CD-5 PLUS (immunotoxin composed of murine anti-CD5 mAbs conjugated to the toxin ricin),[680] CAMPATH (humanized α-CDw52 mAb),[681, 682] and cM-T412, an anti-CD4 mAb.[683, 684] Possible explanations for the lack of efficacy in these studies are that T cells are not necessarily critical for the perpetuation of synovitis; the specific T cells targeted by monoclonal antibodies may not be the ones involved in synovitis; targets are too nonspecific; and although peripheral T cells may be affected, synovial T cells may not be.[685] Early results in adult rheumatoid arthritis with nondepleting anti-CD4 mAbs, including one placebo-controlled trial, are encouraging.[686]

Generation of the immune response involves not only antigen processing and T-cell receptor/MHC interactions but also interactions between molecules expressed on the surface of T cells and antigen-presenting cells, as well as various adhesion molecules and their companion receptors. Although preclinical studies in animals are encouraging, no studies have been reported to date in humans.[687, 688]

Interactions between activated endothelium and leukocytes via adhesion molecules allow leukocytes to leave the peripheral circulation to enter sites of inflammation (e.g., the synovium). The results of early studies using a murine IgG2 anti-intercellular adhesion molecule mAb to inhibit this interaction in rheumatoid arthritis were encouraging,[689] but retreatment frequently resulted in allergic side effects,[690] which suggested that repeated treatment would not be a useful strategy.

Interference With Cytokines

The biologic effects of T-cell and monocyte-derived cytokines can explain much of the clinical syndrome of synovitis as well as the systemic manifestation associated with JRA.[691–693] Cytokines are critical in perpetuating and damping the immune response and, as such, important targets for therapeutic manipulation.

A great deal of evidence supports the role of TNF-α in the initiation and perpetuation of the rheumatoid process. A chimeric mouse/human mAb, cA_2 (infliximab), has been studied in adult rheumatoid arthritis with impressive benefit in clinical, laboratory, and synovial histologic features.[694, 695] The duration of response after a single IV infusion is prolonged with increasing doses; the clinical response is also improved by concomitant use of MTX.[647] One patient with JRA experienced improvement with this treatment.[696] Administration of this agent will be limited by the development of antibodies to the mouse component, and the development of a completely humanized TNF-α mAb will be an improvement.[697] Although short-term toxicity was mild (headache, nausea, minor infection), the development of autoantibodies (ANA, anti-dsDNA) as well as lymphoproliferative disorders is cause for concern. This agent has been approved in the United States for the treatment of Crohn's disease.

Another agent that neutralizes the effect of TNF-α is etanercept, a compound containing the extracellular domain of the human p75 TNF receptor fused to the Fc region of human IgG1 (Fig. 7–22). Administered twice weekly subcutaneously at a dose of 25 mg in adults, etanercept has been effective in controlling synovitis in patients with rheumatoid arthritis in whom MTX and other second-line agents had failed.[676] Etanercept is also effective in combination with MTX in patients who have had only a partial response to MTX.[648] Side effects to date have been limited to local reactions and symptoms of upper respiratory tract infections. In a placebo-controlled clinical trial, etanercept was also effective in children with polyarticular arthritis at a subcutaneous dose of 0.4 mg/kg twice per week.[698]

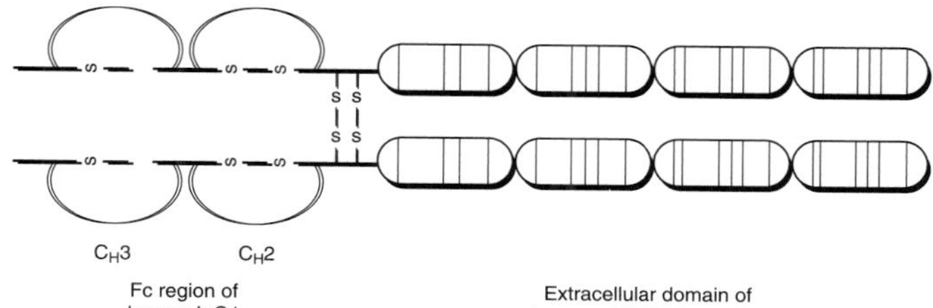

Figure 7–22. Etanercept structure.

Studies with soluble IL-1 receptor and IL-1 receptor antagonists have been carried out in adult rheumatoid arthritis and show initial promise. To date, there have been no studies in JRA. Similarly, studies with anti-IL-6, recombinant IL-4, IL-10, and IL-11 are under way.[671] Anti-IL-6 will be particularly relevant for systemic-onset JRA because early phase I studies have demonstrated some clinical improvement.

Specific cytokine production is regulated by the nuclear transcription factor NFκB and its inhibitor I-kappa-B. A reduction of NFκB binding to DNA may prevent the synthesis of inflammatory cytokines TNF-α, IL-1, and Il-6. Manipulation of this system has inhibited the development of collagen-induced arthritis in the rat model and holds promise for human disease.[699] Stimulation of the T-cell response from a T_H1 (proinflammatory) to a T_H2 (anti-inflammatory) mode can be achieved with cytokine therapy and may be another way that cytokine production can be affected to dampen the immune response.[671]

Apoptosis

Apoptosis (programmed cell death) is a process whereby normal tissue growth is maintained and controlled by the expression of oncogenes. Inflammatory cytokines in rheumatoid arthritis synovial fluid upregulate the expression of apoptosis factors, but apoptosis per se appears to be defective,[700] possibly because of a defect in the interaction between the oncogene fas and its ligand. Strategies to correct defective apoptosis include monoclonal anti-fas antibodies and administration of fas ligand; this approach may be amenable to gene therapy (see the following discussion).

Gene Therapy

Studies with immunotherapy have supported a potential role for gene therapy in patients with arthritis. The strongest argument in support of this approach is the ability of gene therapy to deliver sustained concentrations of therapeutic macromolecules in a defined anatomic location. It might be ideal for oligoarticular JRA once its safety is established. It also eliminates the need for repeated administration of a therapeutic agent that has limited therapy with some biologics.

Gene therapy has been applied to rheumatoid arthritis patients[701] in the form of autologous synovial cell implants containing IL-1Ra in a retroviral vector. There is great potential for gene therapy to control gene expression (e.g., IL-10 to change a T_H1 to a T_H2 response; administration of fas ligand to correct defective apoptosis); the impact on systemic manifestation awaits clinical trials, which are under way.

High-Dose Immunotherapy With Transplantation

Cures of adjuvant arthritis in animal models by either syngeneic[702] or autologous bone marrow transplantation,[703] together with "experiments in nature" in which patients with rheumatoid arthritis who required bone marrow transplantation for other disorders and were noted to experience an improvement in their rheumatoid arthritis, have paved the way for new approaches to the treatment of autoimmune disease (i.e., autologous transplantation). The principles behind this treatment are that high-dose myeloablative therapy will destroy the autoreactive clones that initiate the autoimmune process, and the marrow can be repopulated with a "naive" population of stem cells. As the immune system redevelops after transplantation, immune cells may become "tolerized" to the putative antigens that are involved in the autoimmune process. In fact, allogeneic matched bone marrow transplantation for patients with RF-positive rheumatoid arthritis and associated aplastic anemia has led to remission of the arthritis. However, the length of the remission varied, from as short as 1 year to as long as 13 years.[704, 705]

Allogeneic bone marrow transplantation carries a significant risk of both mortality (15 to 35 percent) and subsequent development of graft-versus-host-disease (GVHD). The use of an autologous transplant, from either marrow or peripheral blood stem cells (autologous stem cell transplantation—ASCT), reduces the mortality from the procedure to 1 to 5 percent and is not associated with GVHD. Thus, high-dose immunotherapy with ASCT has become a method that is undergoing evaluation for treating several autoimmune diseases; protocols are currently being developed and refined.

Initial studies in patients with autoimmune diseases and associated malignancies who underwent ASCT showed recurrence of disease within 5 weeks to 1 year.[706] In these initial studies, the "retransplanted" stem cells were not manipulated in either a positive way (selection for CD34-positive stem cells) or a negative way (removal of T cells with potential autoreactivity). Relapses may also occur because (1) the putative autoantigen(s) responsible for the disease are not eliminated, (2) the HLA status of the host has not changed and thus a predisposition to selecting arthritogenic peptides and a limited number of T-cell developmental pathways persists, and (3) autoreactive T cells may not have been completely eliminated prior to transplantation. Preliminary studies of ASCT have been described in children with JRA and scleroderma with excellent outcomes in most but not all.[707, 708]

Many questions remain regarding this treatment and the crucial variables in the protocols. The intensive immunotherapy (high-dose cyclophosphamide ± irradiation ± antithymocyte globulin) itself may result in disease remission, as described in several cases of aplastic anemia and SLE.[606, 709] It is not clear whether irradiation is necessary, particularly because it may significantly increase the risk of malignancy. It is likely that manipulation of the "graft" is required prior to reinfusion. The number of stem cells required must be defined.

If this treatment proves effective, patient selection will be critical to its success. Patients should be chosen whose disease can be predicted to have a severe outcome but who are not yet at the stage of severe, irreversible damage. The development of prognostic markers thus is critical for proper selection of candidates.[710] The ethical issues of attempting a procedure with a 5 percent mortality rate in children with chronic diseases, but much lower predicted mortality rates, are monumental. The long-term risk of immunosuppression (cyclophosphamide ± lymphoid irradiation) is significant, and safer ways to provide immunosuppression need to be developed.

References

1. Howe S, Levinson J, Shear E, et al: Development of a disability measurement tool for juvenile rheumatoid arthritis: the Juvenile Arthritis Functional Assessment Report for Children and their Parents. Arthritis Rheum 34: 873–880, 1991.
2. Singh G, Athreya BH, Fries JF, Goldsmith DP: Measurement of health status in children with juvenile rheumatoid arthritis. Arthritis Rheum 37: 1761–1769, 1994.
3. Wright FV, Kimber JL, Law M, et al: The Juvenile Arthritis Functional Status Index (JASI): a validation study. J Rheumatol 23: 1066–1079, 1996.
4. Feldman BM, Ayling-Campos A, Luy L, et al: Measuring disability in juvenile dermatomyositis: validity of the childhood health assessment questionnaire. J Rheumatol 22: 326–331, 1995.
5. Duffy CM, Arsenault L, Duffy KN, et al: The Juvenile Arthritis Quality of Life Questionnaire—development of a new responsive index for juvenile rheumatoid arthritis and juvenile spondyloarthritides. J Rheumatol 24: 738–746, 1997.
6. Giannini EH, Ruperto N, Ravelli A, et al: Preliminary definition of improvement in juvenile arthritis. Arthritis Rheum 40: 1202–1209, 1997.
7. Giannini EH: Can non-fundable trials be conducted anyway? The case for open, randomised, actively controlled trials in rheumatology. Ann Rheum Dis 57: 128–130, 1998.
8. Feldman BM, Giannini EH: Where's the evidence? Putting clinical science into pediatric rheumatology. J Rheumatol 23: 1502–1504, 1996.
9. Gilman AG, Rall TW, Nies AS, Taylor P (eds): The Pharmacologic Basis of Therapeutics, 8th ed. New York, Pergamon Press, 1990.
10. Spino M: Pediatric dosing rules and nomograms. *In* MacLeod SM, Radde IC (eds): Textbook of Pediatric Clinical Pharmacology. Littleton, MA, PSG, 1985.
11. Hardman JG, Limbird LE, Molinoff PB, et al: Goodman and Gilman's The Pharmacological Basis of Therapeutics, 9th ed. New York, McGraw-Hill, 1996.
12. Radde IC: Renal elimination of drugs during development. *In* MacLeod SM, Radde IC (eds): Textbook of Pediatric Clinical Pharmacology. Littleton, MA, PSG, 1985.
13. Hollingworth P: The use of non-steroidal anti-inflammatory drugs in paediatric rheumatic diseases. Br J Rheumatol 32: 73–77, 1993.
14. Vane JR, Botting RM: The mode of action of anti-inflammatory drugs. Postgrad Med J 66: S2, 1990.
15. Brooks PM, O'Day RO: Nonsteroidal antiinflammatory drugs—differences and similarities. N Engl J Med 324: 1716–1725, 1991.
16. Hawkey CJ: COX-2 inhibitors. Lancet 353: 307–314, 1999.
17. Donnelly MT, Hawkey CJ: Review article: COX-II inhibitors—a new generation of safer NSAIDs? Aliment Pharmacol Ther 11: 227–236, 1997.
18. Bolten WW: Scientific rationale for specific inhibition of COX-2. J Rheumatol 25(Suppl 51): 2–7, 1998.
19. Crofford LJ: COX-1 and COX-2 tissue expression: implications and predictions. J Rheumatol 24(Suppl 49): 15–19, 1997.
20. Needleman P, Isakson PC: The discovery and function of COX-2. J Rheumatol 24(Suppl 49): 6–8, 1997.
21. Wallace JL, Reuter BK, McKnight W, Bak A: Selective inhibitors of cyclooxygenase-2: are they really effective, selective, and GI-safe? J Clin Gastroenterol 27(Suppl): S28–S34, 1998.
22. Lipsky PE, Abramson SB, Crofford L, et al: The classification of cyclooxygenase inhibitors. J Rheumatol 25: 2298–2303, 1998.
23. Lentini A, Ternai B, Ghosh P: Synthetic inhibitors of human leucocyte elastase 4. Inhibition of human granulocyte elastase and cathepsin G by non-steroidal anti-inflammatory drugs (NSAIDs). Biochem Int 15: 1069, 1987.
24. Haggag AA, Mohamed HF, Eldawy MA, Elbahrawy H: Biochemical studies on anti-inflammatory activity of salicylates as superoxide radical scavengers. IRCS Med Sci Biochem 14: 1104, 1986.
25. Minta JO, Williams MD: Some nonsteroidal antiinflammatory drugs inhibit the generation of superoxide anions by activated polymorphs by blocking ligand-receptor interactions. J Rheumatol 12: 751, 1985.
26. Biemond P, Swaak AJ, Penders JMA, et al: Superoxide production by polymorphonuclear leucocytes in rheumatoid arthritis and osteoarthritis: in vivo inhibition by the antirheumatic drug piroxicam due to interference with the activation of the NADPH-oxidase. Ann Rheum Dis 17: 170, 1986.
27. Paulus HE: Pharmacological considerations. *In* Roth SH (ed): Handbook of Drug Therapy in Rheumatology. Littleton, MA, PSG, 1985.
28. Weiss B, Hait WN: Selective cyclic nucleotidephosphodiesterase inhibitors as potential therapeutic agents. Annu Rev Pharmacol Toxicol 17: 441, 1977.
29. Simon LS, Mills JA: Nonsteroidal antiinflammatory drugs. N Engl J Med 302: 1179, 1980.
30. Mielke K, Otto P, Platz CM: Current Concepts of Antiinflammatory Drugs. New York, Biomedical Information, 1980.
31. Kanton TG: Ibuprofen. Ann Intern Med 91: 877, 1979.
32. Liauw HL, Moscaritola JD, Burcher J: Diclofenac sodium (Voltaren). *In* Lewis AJ, Furst DE (eds): Anti-Inflammatory Agents. New York, Marcel Dekker, 1987.
33. Dahl SI, Ward JR: Pharmacology, clinical efficacy and adverse effects of piroxicam, a new nonsteroidal anti-inflammatory agent. Pharmacotherapy 2: 80, 1982.
34. Montecucco C, Mazzone A, Pasotti D, et al: Effects of piroxicam therapy on granulocyte function and granulocyte elastase concentration in peripheral blood and synovial fluid of rheumatoid arthritis patients. Inflammation 13: 211, 1989.
35. Maclean JR, Gluckman MI: On the mechanism of the pharmacologic activity of meclofenamate sodium. Arzneimittelforschung 33: 627, 1983.
36. Boctor AM, Eickholt M, Pugsley TA: Meclofenamate sodium is an inhibitor of both the 5-lipoxygenase and cylooxygenase pathways of the arachidonic acid cascade in vitro. Prostaglandins Leukot Med 23: 229, 1986.

37. Furst D: Are there differences among nonsteroidal antiiflammatory drugs? Arthritis Rheum 37: 1–9, 1994.
38. Walson PD, Mortensen ME: Pharmacokinetics of common analgesics, anti-inflammatories and antipyretics in children. Clinical Pharmacokinetics 17(Suppl 1): 116–137, 1989.
39. Skeith KJ, Jamali F: Clinical pharmacokinetics of drugs used in juvenile arthritis. Clin Pharmacokinet 21: 129–149, 1991.
40. Davies NM, Anderson KE: Clinical Pharmacokinetics of naproxen. Clin Pharmacokinet 32: 268–293, 1997.
41. Graham GG: Pharmacokinetics and metabolism of non-steroidal anti-inflammatory drugs. Med J Aust 147: 597–602, 1987.
42. Sellers EM: Plasma protein displacement reactions are rarely of clinical significance. Pharmacology 18: 225–227, 1979.
43. Dupuis LL, Koren G, Shore A, et al: Methotrexate–nonsteroidal antiinflammatory drug interaction in children with arthritis. J Rheumatol 17: 1469–1473, 1990.
44. American Medical Association: Antiarthritic Drugs. Drug Evaluation Annual. Chicago, American Medical Association, 1992.
45. Wells TG, Mortensen ME, Dietrich A, et al: Comparison of the pharmacokinetics of naproxen tablets and suspension in children. J Clin Pharmacol 34: 30–33, 1994.
46. Giannini EH, Cawkwell GD: Drug treatment in children with juvenile rheumatoid arthritis. Pediatr Rheumatol 42: 1099–1125, 1995.
47. Lindsley CB: Uses of nonsteroidal anti-inflammatory drugs in pediatrics. Am J Dis Child 147: 229–236, 1993.
48. Barron KS, Person DA, Brewer EJ: The toxicity of nonsteroidal antiinflammatory drugs in juvenile arthritis. J Rheumatol 9: 149–155, 1982.
49. O'Brien WM, Bagby GF: Rare adverse reactions to nonsteroidal antiinflammatory drugs. J Rheumatol 12: 13–20, 1985.
50. Dowd JE, Cimaz R, Fink CW: Nonsteroidal antiinflammatory drug-induced gastroduodenal injury in children. Arthritis Rheum 38: 1225–1231, 1995.
51. Laxer RM, Silverman ED: The pharmacological management of juvenile chronic arthritis. Bailliere's Clin Paediatr 1: 3825–3873, 1993.
52. Lovell DJ, Giannini EH, Brewer EJ: Time course of response to nonsteroidal antiinflammatory drugs in juvenile rheumatoid arthritis. Arthritis Rheum 27: 1433–1437, 1984.
53. Szer IS: Chronic arthritis in children. Comp Ther 23: 124–129, 1997.
54. Schlegel SI, Paulus HE: Nonsteroidal antiinflammatory drugs—use in rheumatic disease, side effects and interactions. Bull Rheum Dis 36: 1, 1986.
55. Bombardier C, Chalmers A, Jamali F: Proceedings of workshops. The monitoring of clinical and pharmacological effects of antiinflammatory drugs in populations. J Rheumatol 15: 17, 1988.
56. Wolfe MM, Lichtenstein DR, Singh G: Gastrointestinal toxicity of nonsteroidal antiinflammatory drugs. N Engl J Med 340: 1888–1899, 1999.
57. Singh G, Ramey DR: NSAID induced gastrointestinal complications: The ARAMIS perspective—1997. J Rheumatol 51: 8–16, 1998.
58. Paulus HE: FDA arthritis advisory committee meeting: serious gastrointestinal toxicity of nonsteroidal antiinflammatory drugs. Arthritis Rheum 31: 1450–1451, 1988.
59. Garcia Rodriguez LA, Jick H: Risk of upper gastrointestinal bleeding and perforation associated with individual non-steroidal anti-inflammatory drugs. Lancet 343: 769–772, 1994.
60. Fries JF: NSAID gastropathy: the second most deadly rheumatic disease? J Rheumatol 18: 6–10, 1991.
61. Silverstein FE, Graham DY, Senior JR, et al: Misoprostol reduces serious gastrointestinal complications in patients with rheumatoid arthritis receiving nonsteroidal anti-inflammatory drugs: a randomized, double-blind, placebo-controlled trial. Ann Intern Med 123: 241–249, 1995.
62. Barkin J: The relation between Helicobacter pylori and nonsteroidal anti-inflammatory drugs. Am J Med 105: 22S–27S, 1998.
63. Shabib S, Laxer R, Silverman E, et al: Seroprevalence of Helicobacter pylori infection is not increased in pediatric inflammatory arthritides. J Rheumatol 21: 1548–1552, 1994.
64. Keenan GF, Giannini EH, Athreya BH: Clinically significant gastropathy associated with nonsteroidal antiinflammatory drug use in children with juvenile rheumatoid arthritis. J Rheumatol 22: 1149–1151, 1995.
65. Duffy CM, Gibbon M, Yang H, et al: Non-steroidal anti-inflammatory drug-induced gastrointestinal toxicity in a practice-based cohort of children with juvenile arthritis. J Rheumatol 27(Suppl 58): 73, 2000.
66. Mulberg AE, Linz C, Bern E, et al: Identification of nonsteroidal antiinflammatory drug-induced gastroduodenal injury in children with juvenile rheumatoid arthritis. J Pediatr 122: 647–649, 1993.
67. Hermaszewski R, Hayllar J, Woo P: Gastro-duodenal damage due to non-steroidal anti-inflammatory drugs in children. Br J Rheumatol 32: 69–72, 1993.
68. Henry D, Lim L, Garcia Rodriguez LA, et al: Variability in risk of gastrointestinal complications with individual non-steroidal anti-inflammatory drugs: results of a collaborative meta-analysis. BMJ 312: 1563–1566, 1996.
69. Cole AT, Hudson N, Liew LCW, et al: Protection of human gastric mucosa against aspirin-enteric coating or dose reduction? Aliment Pharmacol Ther 13: 187–193, 1999.
70. Agrawal NM, Roth S, Graham DY, et al: Misoprostol compared with sucralfate in the prevention of nonsteroidal anti-inflammatory drug induced gastric ulcer. Ann Intern Med 115: 195–200, 1991.
71. Agrawal NM, Aziz K: Prevention of gastrointestinal complications associated with nonsteroidal antiinflammatory drugs. J Rheumatol 51: 17–20, 1998.
72. Roth S, Agrawal N, Mahowald M, et al: Misoprostol heals gastroduodenal injury in patients with rheumatoid arthritis receiving aspirin. Arch Intern Med 149: 775–779, 1989.
73. Ballinger AB, Kumar PJ, Scott DL: Misoprostol in the prevention of gastroduodenal damage in rheumatology. Ann Rheum Dis 51: 1089–1093, 1992.
74. Gazarian M, Berkovitch M, Koren G, et al: Experience with misoprostol therapy for NSAID gastropathy in children. Ann Rheum Dis 54: 277–280, 1995.
75. Shield MJ: Diclofenac/Misoprostol: Novel findings and their clinical potential. J Rheumatol 51: 31–41, 1998.
76. Hawkey CJ, Karrasch J, Szczepanski L, et al: Omeprazole compared with misoprostol for ulcers associated with nonsteroidal antiinflammatory drugs. N Engl J Med 338: 727–734, 1998.
77. Yeomans ND, Tulassay Z, Juhasz L, et al: A comparison of omeprazole with ranitidine for ulcers associated with nonsteroidal antiinflammatory drugs. N Engl J Med 338: 719–726, 1998.
78. Bernstein BH, Singsen BH, King KK, Hanson V: Aspirin-induced hepatotoxicity and its effect on juvenile rheumatoid arthritis. Am J Dis Child 131: 659–663, 1977.
79. Hadchouel M, Prieur A-M, Griscelli C: Acute hemorrhagic, hepatic and neurologic manifestations in juvenile rheumatoid arthritis: possible relationship to drugs or infection. J Pediatr 106: 561–566, 1985.
80. Silverman ED, Miller JJ, Bernstein B, Shafai T: Consumptive coagulopathy associated with juvenile rheumatoid arthritis. J Pediatr 103: 872–876, 1983.
81. Lindsley CB, Warady BA: Nonsteroidal antiinflammatory drugs. Renal toxicity. Review of pediatric issues. Clin Pediatr 29: 10–13, 1990.
82. Carmichael J, Shankel SW: Effects of nonsteroidal anti-inflammatory drugs on prostaglandins and renal function. Am J Med 78: 992–1000, 1985.
83. Clive DM, Stoff JS: Renal syndromes associated with nonsteroidal anti-inflammatory drugs. N Engl J Med 310: 563, 1984.
84. Schrier RW, Henrich WL: Nonsteroidal anti-inflammatory drugs. Caution still indicated. JAMA 251: 1301–1302, 1984.
85. Laxer RM, Silverman ED, Balfe JW, et al: Naproxen associated renal failure in a child with arthritis and inflammatory bowel disease. Pediatrics 80: 904–908, 1987.
86. Allen RC, Petty RE, Lirenman DS, et al: Renal papillary necrosis in children with chronic arthritis. J Pediatr 97: 37, 1986.
87. Ray PE, Rigolizzo D, Wara DR, Piel CF: Naproxen nephrotoxicity in a 2 year old child. Am J Dis Child 142: 524–525, 1988.
88. Robinson J, Malleson P, Lirenman D, Carter J: Nephrotic syndrome associated with nonsteroidal anti-inflammatory drug use in two children. Pediatrics 85: 844–847, 1990.
89. Szer IS, Goldstein-Schainberg C, Kurtin PS: Paucity of renal

complications associated with nonsteroidal antiinflammatory drugs in children with chronic arthritis. J Pediatr 119: 815–817, 1991.

90. Haftel HM, Mitchell JM, Adams BS: Incidence of renal toxicity from anti-inflammatory medications in a pediatric rheumatology population: role of routine screening of urine. J Rheumatol 27(Suppl 58): 73, 2000.
91. Kordonouri O, Dracou C, Papadellis F, et al: Glomerular microproteinuria in children treated with nonsteroidal anti-inflammatory drugs for juvenile chronic arthritis. Clin Exp Rheumatol 12: 567–571, 1994.
92. Malleson PN, Lockitch G, Mackinnon M, et al: Renal disease in chronic arthritis of childhood: a study of urinary N-acetyl-beta-glucosaminidase and beta2-microglobulin excretion. Arthritis Rheum 33: 1560–1566, 1990.
93. Garella S, Matarese RA: Renal effects of prostaglandins and clinical adverse effects of nonsteroidal anti-inflammatory agents. Medicine 63: 165, 1984.
94. De Broe ME, Elseviers MM: Analgesic nephropathy. N Engl J Med 338: 446–452, 1998.
95. Dunn MJ, Patrono C: Renal effects of nonsteroidal antiinflammatory drugs. Proceedings of a Symposium. Am J Med 81: 2B, 1986.
96. Husserl FE, Lange RK, Kantrow CM: Renal papillary necrosis and pyelonephritis accompanying fenoprofen therapy. JAMA 242: 1896, 1979.
97. Whelton A, Hamilton CW: Nonsteroidal anti-inflammatory drugs: effects on kidney function. J Clin Pharmacol 31: 588, 1991.
98. Sedor JR, Davidson EW, Dunn MJ: Renal effects of nonsteroidal antiinflammatory drugs in healthy subjects. Am J Med 81: 58, 1986.
99. Wortmann DW, Kelsch RC, Kuhns L, et al: Renal papillary necrosis in juvenile rheumatoid arthritis. J Pediatr 97: 37–40, 1980.
100. Hoppmann RA, Peden JG, Ober SK: Central nervous system side effects of nonsteroidal anti-inflammatory drugs. J Intern Med 151: 1309–1313, 1991.
101. Duffy CM, Gibbon M, Yang H, et al: Non-steroidal anti-inflammatory drug-induced central nervous system toxicity in a practice-based cohort of children with juvenile arthritis. J Rheumatol 27(Suppl 58): 73, 2000.
102. Bigby M, Stern R: Cutaneous reactions to nonsteroidal anti-inflammatory drugs. J Am Acad Dermatol 12: 866–876, 1985.
103. Howard AM, Dowling J, Varigos G: Pseudoporphyria due to naproxen. Lancet 2: 819–820, 1985.
104. Allen R, Rogers M, Humphrey I: Naproxen induced pseudoporphyria in juvenile chronic arthritis. J Rheumatol 18: 893–896, 1991.
105. Creemers MCW, Chang A, Franssen MJ, et al: Pseudoporphyria due to Naproxen. Scand J Rheumatol 24: 185–187, 1995.
106. Lang BA, Finlayson LA: Naproxen-induced pseudoporphyria in patients with juvenile rheumatoid arthritis. J Pediatr 124: 639–642, 1994.
107. Levy ML, Barron KS, Eichenfield A, Honig PJ: Naproxen-induced pseudoporphyria: a distinctive photodermatitis. J Pediatr 117: 660–664, 1990.
108. Reye RDK, Morgan G, Baral J, et al: Encephalopathy and fatty degeneration of the viscera: a disease entity in childhood. Lancet 2: 749–752, 1963.
109. Kauffman RE: Commentary: Reye's syndrome and salicylate use, by Karen M. Starko, MD, et al, Pediatrics 66:859–864, 1980, and National patterns of aspirin use and Reye syndrome reporting, United States, 1980–1985, by Janet B. Arrowsmith et al, Pediatrics 79:858–863, 1987. Pediatrics 102: 259–262, 1998.
110. Belay ED, Bresee JS, Holman RC, et al: Reye's syndrome in the United States from 1981 through 1997. N Engl J Med 340: 1377–1382, 1999.
111. Starko KM, Ray CG, Dominguez LB, et al: Reye's syndrome and salicylate use. Pediatrics 66: 859–864, 1980.
112. Forsyth BW, Horwitz RI, Acampora D, et al: New epidemiological evidence confirming that bias does not explain the aspirin/Reye's syndrome association. JAMA 261: 2517–2524, 1989.
113. Hurwitz ES, Barrett MJ, Bregman D, et al: Public Health Service study of Reye's syndrome and medications, report of main study. N Engl J Med 257: 1905–1911, 1987.
114. Hardie RM, Newton LH, Bruce JC, et al: The changing clinical pattern of Reye's syndrome 1982–1990. Arch Dis Child 74: 400–405, 1996.
115. Remington PL, Shabino CL, McGee H, et al: Reye syndrome and juvenile rheumatoid arthritis in Michigan. Am J Dis Child 139: 870–872, 1985.
116. Rennebohm RM, Heubi JE, Daugherty CC, Daniels SR: Reye syndrome in children receiving salicylate therapy for connective tissue disease. J Pediatr 107: 877–880, 1985.
117. MMWR: Prevention and control of influenza: recommendations of the Advisory Committee on Immunization Practices (ACIP). MMWR 47(RR-6): 1–26, 1998.
118. Morassut P, Yang W, Karsh J: Aspirin intolerance. Semin Arthritis Rheum 19(22–30):1989.
119. Oates JA, Fitzgerald GA, Branch RA, et al: Clinical implications of prostaglandin and thromboxane A_2 formation. N Engl J Med 319: 689–698, 1988.
120. Furst DE: Toxicity of antirheumatic medications in children with juvenile arthritis. J Rheumatol 33: 11–15, 1992.
121. Slepian IK, Mathews KP, McLean JA: Aspirin-sensitive asthma. Chest 87: 386, 1985.
122. Rachelefsky GS, Coulson A, Siegel SC, Stiehm ER: Aspirin intolerance in chronic childhood asthma: detected by oral challenge. Pediatrics 56: 443, 1975.
123. Fischer TJ, Guilfoile TD, Kesarwala HH, et al: Adverse pulmonary responses to aspirin and acetaminophen in chronic childhood asthma. Pediatrics 71: 313, 1983.
124. Szceklik A: Analgesics, allergy, and asthma. Drugs 32(Suppl 4): 148–163, 1986.
125. Squires JE, Mintz PD, Clark S: Tolmetin-induced haemolysis. Transfusion 25: 410–412, 1985.
126. American Hospital Formulary Service: Drug Information 88. Bethesda, MD: American Society of Hospital Pharmacy, 1988.
127. Lindsley CB: Pharmacotherapy of juvenile rheumatoid arthritis. Pediatr Clin North Am 28: 161, 1981.
128. Laxer RM, Shore AD, Silverman ED: Drug therapy in juvenile rheumatoid arthritis. *In* Kean WF (ed): Sulfasalazine in Rheumatic Disease. Proceedings of the International Rheumatology Conference. Quebec, Medicopea, 1987.
129. Huskisson EC: Azathioprine. Clin Rheum Dis 10: 325, 1984.
130. Furst DE: Salicylates in pediatric rheumatology. *In* Moore TD (ed): Arthritis in Childhood. Report of the Eightieth Ross Conference in Pediatric Research. Columbus, OH, Ross Laboratories, 1981, pp 104–114.
131. Hollister JR: Aspirin in juvenile rheumatoid arthritis. Am J Dis Child 139: 866, 1985.
132. Dromgoole SH, Furst DE, Paulus HE: Rational approaches to the use of salicylates in the treatment of rheumatoid arthritis. Semin Arthritis Rheum 11: 257, 1981.
133. Lasagna L, McMahon FG (eds): New perspectives on aspirin therapy. Proceedings of a Symposium. Am J Med 18(Suppl), 1983.
134. Burch JW, Stanford N, Majerus PW: Inhibition of platelet prostaglandin synthetase by oral aspirin. J Clin Invest 61: 314, 1978.
135. Preston FE, Whipps S, Jackson CA, et al: Inhibition of prostacyclin and platelet thromboxane A2 after low-dose aspirin. N Engl J Med 304: 76, 1981.
136. Pedersen AK, Fitzgerald GA: Dose-related kinetics of aspirin. Presystemic acetylation of platelet cyclooxygenase. N Engl J Med 311: 1206, 1984.
137. Yu T-F, Gutman AB: Study of the paradoxical effects of salicylate in low, intermediate and high dosage on the renal mechanisms for excretion of urate in man. J Clin Invest 38: 1298, 1959.
138. Levy G: Clinical pharmacokinetics of aspirin. Pediatrics 62: 867, 1978.
139. Done AK, Yaffe SJ, Clayton JM: Aspirin dosage for infants and children. J Pediatr 95: 617, 1979.
140. Mandelli M, Tognoni G: Monitoring plasma concentration of salicylate. Clin Pharmacokinet 5: 424, 1980.
141. Kvien TK, Olsson B, Hoyeraal HM: Acetylsalicylic acid and juvenile rheumatoid arthritis. Effect of dosage interval on the serum salicylic acid level. Acta Paediatr Scand 74: 755, 1985.
142. Pachman LM, Olufs R, Procknal JA, et al: Pharmacokinetic monitoring of salicylate therapy in children with juvenile rheumatoid arthritis. Arthritis Rheum 22: 826, 1979.

143. Makela A-L, Peltola OL, Makela P: Gold serum levels in children with juvenile rheumatoid arthritis. Scand J Rheumatol 7: 161, 1978.
144. Poe TE, Mutchie KD, Saunders GH, et al: Total and free salicylate concentrations in juvenile rheumatoid arthritis. J Rheumatol 7: 717, 1980.
145. Bardara M, Cislaghi GU, Mandelli M, et al: Value of monitoring plasma salicylate levels in treating juvenile rheumatoid arthritis. Arch Dis Child 53: 381, 1978.
146. Mofenson HC, Caraccio RE: Salicylate poisoning. *In* Gellis SS, Kagan BM (eds): Current Pediatric Therapy. Philadelphia, WB Saunders, 1990.
147. Goulden KJ, Dooley JM, Camfield PR, Fraser AD: Clinical valproate toxicity induced by acetylsalicylic acid. Neurology 37: 1392, 1987.
148. Verbeeck RK: Pharmacokinetic drug interactions with nonsteroidal anti-inflammatory drugs. Clin Pharmacokinet 19: 44, 1990.
149. Marsh CC, Schuna AA, Sundstrom WR: A review of selected investigational nonsteroidal anti-inflammatory drugs in the 1980's. Pharmacotherapy 6: 10, 1986.
150. Needs CJ, Brooks PM: Clinical pharmacokinetics of the salicylates. Clin Pharmacokinet 10: 164, 1985.
151. Bunch TW, O'Duffy ID: Disease modifying drugs for progressive rheumatoid arthritis. Mayo Clin Proc 55: 161, 1980.
152. Wallace CA, Levinson JE: Juvenile rheumatoid arthritis: outcome and treatment for the 1990s. Rheum Dis Clin North Am 17: 891–905, 1991.
153. Giannini E, Brewer E, Kuzmina N, et al, for the Pediatric Rheumatology Collaborative Study Group and the Cooperative Children's Study Group: Methotrexate in resistant juvenile rheumatoid arthritis: Results of the USA-USSR double-blind, placebo-controlled trial. N Engl J Med 326: 1043–1049, 1992.
154. Rose C, Singsen B, Eichenfield A, et al: Safety and efficacy of methotrexate therapy in juvenile rheumatoid arthritis. J Pediatr 117: 653, 1990.
155. Graham LD, Myones BL, Rivas-Chacon RF, Pachman LM: Morbidity associated with long-term methotrexate therapy in juvenile rheumatoid arthritis. J Pediatr 120: 468–473, 1992.
156. Bowyer SL, Roettcher PA, Lovell D, et al: Initial medication choices made by pediatric rheumatologists in the United States for patients with JRA. J Rheumatol 27(Suppl 58): 72, 2000.
157. Singsen BH, Goldbach-Mansky R: Methotrexate in the treatment of juvenile rheumatoid arthritis and other pediatric rheumatic and nonrheumatic disorders. Rheum Dis Clin North Am 23:811–841, 1997.
158. Kremer JM: The mechanism of action of methotrexate in rheumatoid arthritis: the search continues. J Rheumatol 21: 1–5, 1994.
159. Baggott JE, Morgan SL, Ha T-S, et al: Antifolates in rheumatoid arthritis: a hypothetical mechanism of action. Clin Exp Rheumatol 11(Suppl 8): S101–S105, 1993.
160. Cronstein BN, Eberle MA, Gruber HE, et al: Methotrexate inhibits neutrophil function by stimulating adenosine release from connective tissue cells. Proc Natl Acad Sci U S A 88: 241–245, 1991.
161. Cronstein BN: The mechanism of action of methotrexate. Rheum Dis Clin North Am 23: 739–751, 1997.
162. Kremer JM: Possible mechanisms of action of methotrexate in patients with rheumatoid arthritis. Br J Rheumatol 34(Suppl 2): 26–29, 1995.
163. Firestein GS, Paine MM, Boyle DL: Mechanisms of methotrexate action in rheumatoid arthritis. Selective decrease in synovial collagenase gene expression. Arthritis Rheum 37: 193–200, 1994.
164. Ravelli A, Di Fuccia G, Molinaro M, et al: Plasma levels after oral methotrexate in children with juvenile rheumatoid arthritis. J Rheumatol 20: 1573–1577, 1993.
165. Herman RA, Veng-Pedersen P, Hoffman J, et al: Pharmacokinetics of low dose methotrexate in rheumatoid arthritis patients. J Pharm Sci 78: 165, 1989.
166. Furst DE: Practical clinical pharmacology and drug interactions of low-dose methotrexate therapy in rheumatoid arthritis. Br J Rheumatol 34(Suppl 2): 20–25, 1995.
167. Godfrey C, Sweeney K, Miller K, et al: The population pharmacokinetics of long-term methotrexate in rheumatoid arthritis. Br J Clin Pharmacol 46: 369–376, 1998.
168. Dupuis LL, Koren G, Silverman ED, Laxer RM: Influence of food on the bioavailability of oral methotrexate in children. J Rheumatol 22: 1570–1573, 1995.
169. Jundt JW, Browne BA, Fiocco GP, et al: A comparison of low dose methotrexate bioavailability: oral solution, oral tablet, subcutaneous and intramuscular dosing. J Rheumatol 20: 1845–1849, 1993.
170. Hillson JL, Furst DE: Pharmacology and pharmacokinetics of methotrexate in rheumatic disease. Practical issues in treatment and design. Rheum Dis Clin North Am 23: 757–778, 1997.
171. Press J, Berkovitch M, Laxer R, et al: Evaluation of therapeutic drug monitoring of methotrexate in saliva of children with rheumatic diseases. Ther Drug Monit 17: 247, 1995.
172. Albertioni F, Flato B, Seideman P, et al: Methotrexate in juvenile rheumatoid arthritis. Evidence of age dependent pharmacokinetics. Eur J Clin Pharmacol 47: 507–511, 1995.
173. Reiff A, Shaham B, Wood BP, et al: High dose methotrexate in the treatment of refractory juvenile rheumatoid arthritis. Clin Exp Rheumatol 13: 113–118, 1995.
174. Wallace CA, Sherry DD: Preliminary report of higher dose methotrexate treatment in juvenile rheumatoid arthritis. J Rheumatol 19: 1604–1607, 1992.
175. Wallace CA, Smith AL, Sherry DD: Pilot investigation of naproxen/methotrexate interaction in patients with juvenile rheumatoid arthritis. J Rheumatol 20: 1764–1768, 1993.
176. Giannini E, Cassidy J, Brewer E, et al: Comparative efficacy and safety of advanced drug therapy in children with juvenile rheumatoid arthritis. Semin Arthritis Rheum 23: 34, 1993.
177. Harel L, Wagner-Weiner L, Poznanski AK, et al: Effects of methotrexate on radiologic progression in juvenile rheumatoid arthritis. Arthritis Rheum 36: 1370–1374, 1993.
178. Ravelli A, Viola S, Ramenghi B: Radiographic progression in juvenile rheumatoid arthritis patients treated with methotrexate. Arthritis Rheum 39(Suppl): S59, 1996.
179. Ravelli A, Ramenghi B, Di Fuccia G, et al: Factors associated with response to methotrexate in systemic-onset juvenile chronic arthritis. Acta Paediatr 83: 428–432, 1994.
180. Stenger AA, Van Leeuwen MA, Houtman PM, et al: Early effective suppression of inflammation in rheumatoid arthritis reduces radiographic progression. Br J Rheumatol 37: 1157–1163, 1998.
181. Halle F, Prieur AM: Evaluation of methotrexate in the treatment of juvenile chronic arthritis according to the subtype. Clin Exp Rheumatol 9: 297–302, 1991.
182. Balis FM, Savitch JL, Bleyer WA: Pharmacokinetics of oral methotrexate in children. Cancer Res 43: 2342–2345, 1983.
183. Balis FM, Mirro J, Reaman GH, et al: Pharmacokinetics of subcutaneous methotrexate. J Clin Oncol 6: 1882–1886, 1988.
184. Wallace CA, Sherry DD: A practical approach to avoidance of methotrexate toxicity. J Rheumatol 22: 1009–1012, 1995.
185. Ravelli A, Viola S, Ramenghi B, et al: Evaluation of response to methotrexate by a functional index in juvenile chronic arthritis. Clin Rheumatol 14: 322, 1995.
186. Wallace CA, Sherry DD, Mellins ED, Aiken RP: Predicting remission in juvenile rheumatoid arthritis with methotrexate treatment. J Rheumatol 20: 118–122, 1993.
187. Gottlieb BS, Keenan GF, Lu T, Ilowite NT: Discontinuation of methotrexate treatment in juvenile rheumatoid arthritis. Pediatrics 100: 994–997, 1997.
188. Felson DT, Anderson JJ, Meenan RF: Use of short-term efficacy/toxicity tradeoffs to select second-line drugs in rheumatoid arthritis. A metaanalysis of published clinical trials. Arthritis Rheum 35: 1117–1125, 1992.
189. Hunt P, Rose C, Singsen B: Long-term safety and efficacy of methotrexate in juvenile rheumatoid arthritis. Arthritis Rheum 36: S61, 1993.
190. van Ede AE, Laan RFJM, Blom HJ, et al: Methotrexate in rheumatoid arthritis: an update with focus on mechanisms involved in toxicity. Semin Arthritis Rheum 27: 277–292, 1998.
191. McKendry RJR: The remarkable spectrum of methotrexate toxicities. Rheum Dis Clin North Am 23: 939–954, 1997.
192. Sandoval DM, Alarcon GS, Morgan SL: Adverse events in methotrexate-treated rheumatoid arthritis patients. Br J Rheumatol 34(Suppl 2): 49–56, 1995.
193. West SG: Methotrexate hepatotoxicity. Rheum Dis Clin North Am 23: 883–915, 1997.

194. Wallace CA, Smith AL, Aronson H, Sherry DD: Methotrexate and naproxen kinetics in patients with juvenile rheumatoid arthritis. J Rheumatol 19(Suppl 33): 112, 1992.
195. Walker AM, Funch D, Dreyer NA, et al: Determinants of serious liver disease among patients receiving low-dose methotrexate for rheumatoid arthritis. Arthritis Rheum 36: 329–335, 1993.
196. Chandran G, Ahern MJ, Hall PM, et al: Cirrhosis in patients with rheumatoid arthritis receiving low-dose methotrexate. Br J Rheumatol 33: 981, 1994.
197. Whiting-O'Keefe QE, Fye KH, Sack KD: Methotrexate and histological abnormalities: a meta-analysis. Am J Med 90: 711–716, 1991.
198. Erickson AR, Reddy V, Vogelgesang SA, West SG: Usefulness of the American College of Rheumatology recommendations for liver biopsy in methotrexate-treated rheumatoid arthritis patients. Arthritis Rheum 38: 1115–1119, 1995.
199. Kremer JM, Alarcon GS, Lightfoot RW, et al: Methotrexate for rheumatoid arthritis. Suggested guidelines for monitoring liver toxicity. Arthritis Rheum 37: 316–328, 1994.
200. Hashkes PJ, Balistreri WF, Bove KE, et al: The relationship of hepatotoxic risk factors and liver histology in methotrexate therapy for juvenile rheumatoid arthritis. J Pediatr 134: 47–52, 1999.
201. Keim D, Ragsdale C, Heidelberger K, Sullivan D: Hepatic fibrosis with the use of methotrexate for juvenile rheumatoid arthritis. J Rheumatol 17: 846–848, 1990.
202. Kugathasan S, Newman AJ, Dahms BB, Boyle T: Liver biopsy findings in patients with juvenile rheumatoid arthritis receiving long-term, weekly methotrexate therapy. J Pediatr 128: 149–151, 1996.
203. Hashkes PJ, Balistreri WF, Bove KE, et al: The long-term effect of methotrexate therapy on the liver in patients with juvenile rheumatoid arthritis. Arthritis Rheum 40: 2226–2234, 1997.
204. Kanik KS, Cash JM: Does methotrexate increase the risk of infection or malignancy. Rheum Dis Clin North Am 23: 955–967, 1997.
205. Peter G (ed): 1997 Redbook: Report of the Committee on Infectious Diseases, 24th ed. Elk Grove Village, IL, American Academy of Pediatrics, 1997.
206. Guiterrez-Urena S, Molina JF, Garcia CO, et al: Pancytopenia secondary to methotrexate therapy in rheumatoid arthritis. Arthritis Rheum 39: 272, 1996.
207. Bleyer WA: Methotrexate induced lymphoma? J Rheumatol 25: 404–407, 1998.
208. Shiroky JB, Frost A, Skelton JD, et al: Complications of immunosuppression associated with weekly low-dose methotrexate. J Rheumatol 18: 1172–1175, 1991.
209. Kingsmore SF, Hall BD, Allen NB, et al: Association of methotrexate, rheumatoid arthritis and lymphoma: report of two cases and literature review. J Rheumatol 19: 1462–1465, 1992.
210. Tennis P, Andrews E, Bombardier C: Record linkage to conduct an epidemiologic study on the association of rheumatoid arthritis and lymphoma in the province of Saskatchewan, Canada. J Clin Epidemiol 46: 685–695, 1993.
211. Kamel OW, van de Rijn M, Weiss LM, et al: Reversible lymphomas associated with Epstein-Barr virus occurring during methotrexate therapy for rheumatoid arthritis and dermatomyositis. N Engl J Med 328: 1317–1321, 1993.
212. Kamel OW, van de Rijn M, LeBrun DP, et al: Lymphoid neoplasms in patients with rheumatoid arthritis and dermatomyositis: frequency of Epstein-Barr virus and other features associated with immunosuppression. Hum Pathol 25: 638–643, 1994.
213. Georgescu L, Quinn GC, Schwartzman S, Paget SA: Lymphoma in patients with rheumatoid arthritis: association with the disease state or methotrexate treatment. Semin Arthritis Rheum 26: 794–804, 1997.
214. Salloum E, Cooper DL, Howe G, et al: Spontaneous regression of lymphoproliferative disorders in patients treated with methotrexate for rheumatoid arthritides and other rheumatic diseases. J Clin Oncol 14: 1943–1949, 1996.
215. Bailin PL, Tindall JP, Roenigk HH, et al: Is methotrexate therapy for psoriasis carcinogenic? A modified retrospective prospective analysis. JAMA 232: 359–362, 1975.
216. Nysfors A, Jensen H: Frequency of malignant neoplasms in 248 long-term methotrexate-treated psoriatics: a preliminary study. Dermatologica 167: 260–261, 1983.
217. Padeh S, Sharon N, Schiby G, et al: Hodgkin's lymphoma in systemic onset juvenile rheumatoid arthritis after treatment with low dose methotrexate. J Rheumatol 24: 2035–2037, 1997.
218. Salaffi F, Manganelli P, Carotti M, et al: Methotrexate-induced pneumonitis in patients with rheumatoid arthritis and psoriatic arthritis: report of five cases and review of the literature. Clin Rheumatol 16: 296–304, 1997.
219. Carroll GJ, Thomas R, Phatouros CC, et al: Incidence, prevalence and possible risk factors for pneumonitis in patients with rheumatoid arthritis receiving methotrexate. J Rheumatol 21: 51–54, 1994.
220. Cron RQ, Sherry DD, Wallace CA: Methotrexate-induced hypersensitivity pneumonitis in a child with juvenile rheumatoid arthritis. J Pediatr 132: 901–902, 1998.
221. Pelucchi A, Lomater C, Gerloni V, et al: Lung function and diffusing capacity for carbon monoxide in patients with juvenile chronic arthritis: effect of disease activity and low dose methotrexate therapy. Clin Exp Rheumatol 12: 675–679, 1994.
222. Muzaffer MA, Schneider R, Cameron B, et al: Accelerated nodulosis during methotrexate therapy for juvenile rheumatoid arthritis. J Pediatr 128: 698–700, 1996.
223. Falcini F, Taccetti G, Ermini M, et al: Methotrexate-associated appearance and rapid progression of rheumatoid nodules in systemic-onset juvenile rheumatoid arthritis. Arthritis Rheum 40: 175–178, 1997.
224. Merrill JT, Cronstein BN, Shen C, et al: Reversal of new but not old rheumatoid nodules by colchicine: evidence from an in vitro model and case reports of 14 patients. Arthritis Rheum 39: S240, 1996.
225. May KP, West SG, McDermott MT, Huffer WE: The effect of low-dose methotrexate on bone metabolism and histomorphometry in rats. Arthritis Rheum 37: 201–206, 1994.
226. Zonneveld IM, Bakker WK, Dijkstra PF, et al: Methotrexate osteopathy in long term, low-dose methotrexate treatment for psoriasis and rheumatoid arthritis. Arch Dermatol 132: 184, 1996.
227. Preston SJ, Diamond T, Scott A, Laurent MR: Methotrexate osteopathy in rheumatic disease. Ann Rheum Dis 52: 582–585, 1993.
228. Kozlowski RD, Steinbrunner JV, Mackenzie AH, et al: Outcome of first-trimester exposure to low-dose methotrexate in eight patients with rheumatic disease. Am J Med 88: 589–592, 1990.
229. Buckley LM, Bullaboy CA, Leichtman L, Marquez M: Multiple congenital anomalies associated with weekly low-dose methotrexate treatment of the mother. Arthritis Rheum 40: 971–973, 1997.
230. Morgan SL, Baggott JE, Vaughn WH, et al: The effect of folic acid supplementation on the toxicity of low-dose methotrexate in patients with rheumatoid arthritis. Arthritis Rheum 33: 9–18, 1990.
231. Morgan SL, Baggott JE, Vaughn WH, et al: Supplementation with folic acid during methotrexate therapy for rheumatoid arthritis. A double-blind, placebo-controlled trial. Ann Intern Med 121: 833–841, 1994.
232. Shiroky JB, Neville C, Esdaile JM, et al: Low-dose methotrexate with leucovorin (folinic acid) in the management of rheumatoid arthritis. Results of a multicenter randomized, double-blind, placebo-controlled trial. Arthritis Rheum 36: 795–803, 1993.
233. Weinblatt ME, Maier AL, Coblyn JS: Low dose leucovorin does not interfere with the efficacy of methotrexate in rheumatoid arthritis: an 8 week randomized placebo controlled trial. J Rheumatol 20: 950–952, 1993.
234. Ortiz Z, Shea B, Suarez-Almazor ME, et al: The efficacy of folic acid and folinic acid in reducing methotrexate gastrointestinal toxicity in rheumatoid arthritis. A metaanalysis of randomized controlled trials. J Rheumatol 25: 36–43, 1998.
235. Hunt PG, Rose CD, McIlvain-Simpson G, Tejani S: The effects of daily intake of folic acid on the efficacy of methotrexate therapy in children with juvenile rheumatoid arthritis. A controlled study. J Rheumatol 24: 2230–2232, 1997.
236. Modesto C, Castro L: Folinic acid supplementation in patients with juvenile rheumatoid arthritis treated with methotrexate. J Rheumatol 23: 403–404, 1996.
237. Proceedings of a Symposium: A reassessment of plaquenil in the treatment of rheumatoid arthritis. Am J Med 75(Suppl), 1983.

238. Maksymowych W, Russell AS: Antimalarials in rheumatology: efficacy and safety. Semin Arthritis Rheum 16: 206, 1987.
239. Hughes GRV, Rynes RI: Antimalarials in rheumatic disease: opportunity for an expanding role? Br J Clin Pract 41(Suppl): 52, 1987.
240. Tett SE, Cutler DJ, Day RO, Brown KF: Bioavailability of hydroxychloroquine tablets in healthy volunteers. Br J Clin Pharmacol 27: 771, 1989.
241. Miyachi Y, Yoshioka A, Imamura S, et al: Antioxidant action of anti-malarials. Ann Rheum Dis 45: 244, 1986.
242. Salmeron G, Lipsky PE: Immunosuppressive potential of antimalarials. Am J Med 75: 19, 1983.
243. Matsuzawa Y, Hostetler KY: Inhibition of lysosomal phospholipase A and phospholipase C by chloroquine and 4c-bis-(diethylaminoethyoxy)b-diethyldiphenylethane. J Biol Chem 255: 5190, 1980.
244. Greaves MW, McDonald-Gibson W: Effect of non-steroidal anti-inflammatory drugs and antipyretic drugs on prostaglandin biosynthesis by human skin. J Invest Dermatol 61: 127, 1973.
245. van den Borne BE, Dijkmans BA, de Rooij HH, le Cessie S, Verweij CL: Chloroquine and hydroxychloroquine equally affect tumor necrosis factor-alpha, interleukin 6, and interferon-gamma production by peripheral blood mononuclear cells. J Rheumatol 24: 55–60, 1997.
246. Wallace DJ: Antimalarial agents and lupus. Rheum Dis Clin North Am 20: 243–263, 1994.
247. Meng XW, Feller JM, Ziegler JB, et al: Induction of apoptosis in pheripheral blood lymphocytes following treatment in vitro with hydroxychloroquine. Arthritis Rheum 40: 927–935, 1997.
248. Petri M: Hydroxychloroquine use in the Baltimore Lupus Cohort: effects on lipids, glucose and thrombosis. Lupus 5(Suppl 1): S16–S22, 1996.
249. Brewer EJ, Giannini EH, Kuzmina N, Alekseev L: Penicillamine and hydroxychloroquine in the treatment of severe juvenile rheumatoid arthritis. Results of the U.S.A.-U.S.S.R. double-blind placebo-controlled trial. N Engl J Med 314: 1269–1276, 1986.
250. Clark P, Casas E, Tugwell P, et al: Hydroxychloroquine compared with placebo in rheumatoid arthritis. A randomized controlled trial. Ann Intern Med 119: 1067–1071, 1993.
251. A randomized trial of hydroxychloroquine in early rheumatoid arthritis: the HERA Study. Am J Med 98: 156–168, 1995.
252. O'Dell JR, Haire CE, Erikson N, et al: Treatment of rheumatoid arthritis with methotrexate alone, sulfasalazine and hydroxychloroquine, or a combination of all three medications. N Engl J Med 334: 1287–1291, 1996.
253. Fries JF, Singh G, Lenert L, Furst DE: Aspirin, hydroxychloroquine, and hepatic enzyme abnormalities with methotrexate in rheumatoid arthritis. Arthritis Rheum 33: 1611–1619, 1990.
254. Combe B, Guttierrez M, Anaya JM, Sany J: Possible efficacy of hydroxychloroquine on accelerated nodulosis during methotrexate therapy for rheumatoid arthritis. J Rheumatol 20: 755–756, 1993.
255. Tsakonas E, Joseph L, Esdaile JM, et al: A long-term study of hydroxychloroquine withdrawal on exacerbations in systemic lupus erythematosus. The Canadian Hydroxychloroquine Study Group. Lupus 7: 80–85, 1998.
256. Hodis HN, Quismorio FPJ, Wickham E, Blankenhorn DH: The lipid, lipoprotein, and apolipoprotein effect of hydroxychloroquine in patients with systemic lupus erythematosus. J Rheumatol 20: 661–665, 1993.
257. Woo TY, Callan JP, Voorhees JJ, et al: Cutaneous lesions of dermatomyositis are improved by hydroxychloroquine. J Am Acad Dermatol 10: 592–600, 1984.
258. Olson NY, Lindsley CB: Adjunctive use of hydroxychloroquine in childhood dermatomyositis. J Rheumatol 16: 1545–1547, 1989.
259. Markowitz HA, McGrinley JM: Chloroquine poisoning in a child. JAMA 189: 950, 1964.
260. Dubois E: Antimalarials in the management of discoid and systemic lupus erythematosus. Semin Arthritis Rheum 8: 33, 1978.
261. Henkind P, Rothfield NF: Ocular abnormalities in patients treated with synthetic antimalarial drugs. N Engl J Med 269: 433, 1963.
262. Rynes RI, Krohel G, Falbo A, et al: Ophthalmologic safety of long-term hydroxychloroquine treatment. Arthritis Rheum 22: 832, 1979.
263. Rynes RI: Side effects of antimalarial therapy. Br J Clin Pract 41(Suppl 52): 42, 1987.
264. Easterbrook M: Current concepts in monitoring patients on antimalarials. Aust N Z J Ophthalmol 26: 101–103, 1998.
265. Grierson DJ: Hydroxychloroquine and visual screening in a rheumatology outpatient clinic. Ann Rheum Dis 56: 188–190, 1997.
266. Sassaman FW, Cassidy JT, Alpern M, et al: Electroretinography in patients with connective tissue diseases treated with hydroxychloroquine. Am J Ophthalmol 70: 515, 1970.
267. Laaksonen A-L, Koshiadhe V, Juva K: Dosage of antimalarial drugs for children with juvenile rheumatoid arthritis and systemic lupus erythematosus. A clinical study with determination of serum concentrations of chloroquine and hydroxychloroquine. Scand J Rheumatol 3: 103–108, 1974.
268. Svartz N: Salazopyrin, a new sulfanilamide preparation. Acta Med Scand 60: 577, 1942.
269. Svartz N: The treatment of rheumatoid arthritis with acid azo compounds. Rheumatism 4: 56, 1948.
270. Ozdogan H, Turunc M, Deringol B, et al: Sulphasalazine in the treatment of juvenile rheumatoid arthritis: a preliminary open trial. J Rheumatol 13: 124–125, 1986.
271. Huang JL, Chen LC: Sulphasalazine in the treatment of children with chronic arthritis. Clin Rheumatol 17: 359–363, 1998.
272. Ansell BM, Hall MA, Loftus JK, et al: A multicentre pilot study of sulphasalazine in juvenile chronic arthritis. Clin Exp Rheumatol 9: 201–203, 1991.
273. van Rossum MA, Fiselier TJ, Franssen MJ, et al: Sulfasalazine in the treatment of juvenile chronic arthritis: a randomized, double-blind, placebo-controlled, multicenter study. Dutch Juvenile Chronic Arthritis Study Group. Arthritis Rheum 41: 808–816, 1998.
274. Sinclair RJG, Duthie JRR: Salazopyrin in the treatment of rheumatoid arthritis. Ann Rheum Dis 8: 226, 1948.
275. Mielants H, Veys EM: HLA-B27 related arthritis and bowel inflammation. Part 1: Sulfasalazine (salazopyrin) in HLA-B27 related reactive arthritis. J Rheumatol 12: 287, 1985.
276. Clegg DO, Reda DJ, Mejias E, et al: Comparison of sulfasalazine and placebo in the treatment of psoriatic arthritis. A Department of Veterans Affairs Cooperative Study. Arthritis Rheum 39: 2013–2020, 1996.
277. Clegg DO, Reda DJ, Weisman MH, et al: Comparison of sulfasalazine and placebo in the treatment of reactive arthritis (Reiter's syndrome). A Department of Veterans Affairs Cooperative Study. Arthritis Rheum 39: 2021–2027, 1996.
278. Clegg DO, Reda DJ, Weisman MH, et al: Comparison of sulfasalazine and placebo in the treatment of ankylosing spondylitis. A Department of Veterans Affairs Cooperative Study. Arthritis Rheum 39: 2004–2012, 1996.
279. Dougados M, van der Linden S, Seirisalo-Repo M, et al: Sulfasalazine in the treatment of spondylarthropathy. A randomized, multicenter, double-blind, placebo-controlled study. Arthritis Rheum 38: 618–627, 1995.
280. Ferraz MB, Tugwell P, Goldsmith CH, Atra E: Meta-analysis of sulfasalazine in ankylosing spondylitis. J Rheumatol 17: 1482–1486, 1990.
281. Schroeder H, Campbell DES: Absorption, metabolism and excretion of salicylazosulfapyridine in man. Clin Pharmacol Ther 13: 36, 1972.
282. Bird HA, Dixon JS, Pickup ME, et al: A biochemical assessment of sulfasalazine in rheumatoid arthritis. J Rheumatol 9: 36, 1982.
283. Peppercorn MA: Sulfasalazine, pharmacology, clinical use, toxicities and related new drug development. Ann Intern Med 101: 377, 1984.
284. Stenson WF, Lobos E: Sulfasalazine inhibits the synthesis of chemotactic lipids by neutrophils. J Clin Invest 69: 494, 1982.
285. Gadangi P, Longaker M, Naime D: The anti-inflammatory mechanism of sulfasalazine is related to adenosine release at inflamed sites. J Immunol 156: 1937, 1996.
286. Carlin G, Nyman AK, Gronberg A: Effects of sulfasalazine on cytokine production by mitogen-stimulated human T cells. Arthritis Rheum 37: S783, 1994.
287. Gronenberg A, Isaksson P, Smedegard G: Inhibitory effect of sulfasalazine on production of IL-1B, IL-6, and TNFa [Abstract]. Arthritis Rheum 37: S383, 1994.

288. Aono H, Hasunuma T, Fujisawa K, et al: Direct suppression of human synovial cell proliferation *in vitro* by salazosulfapyridine and bucillamine. J Rheumatol 22: 65–70, 1995.
289. Wahl C, Liptay S, Adler G, Schmid RM: Sulfasalazine: a potent and specific inhibitor of nuclear factor kappa B. J Clin Invest 101: 1163–1174, 1998.
290. Akahoshi T, Namai R, Sekiyama N, et al: Rapid induction of neutrophil apoptosis by sulfasalazine: implications of reactive oxygen species in the apoptotic process. J Leukoc Biol 62: 817–826, 1997.
291. Sharon P, Drab EA, Linder JS, et al: The effect of sulfasalazine on bovine endothelial cell proliferation and cell cycle phase distribution. Comparison with olsalazine, 5-aminosalicylic acid, and sulfapyridine. J Lab Clin Med 119: 99–107, 1992.
292. Madhok R, Wijelath E, Smith J, et al: Is the beneficial effect of sulfasalazine due to inhibition of synovial neovascularization? J Rheumatol 18: 199–202, 1991.
293. Taffet SL, Das KM: Sulfasalazine: adverse effects and desensitization. Dig Dis Sci 28: 833, 1983.
294. Amos RS, Pullar T, Bax DE, et al: Sulphasalazine for rheumatoid arthritis: toxicity in 774 patients monitored for one to 11 years. BMJ 293: 420, 1986.
295. Raforth R: Systemic granulomatous reaction to salicylazosulfapyridine in a patient with Crohn's disease. Am J Dig Dis 19: 465, 1974.
296. Capell HA, Pullar T, Hunter JA: Comparison of white blood cell dyscrasias during sulfasalazine therapy of rheumatoid arthritis and inflammatory bowel disease. Drugs 32(Suppl 1): 44, 1986.
297. Wijnands MJ, Allebes WA, Boerbooms AMT, et al: Thrombocytopenia due to aurothioglucose, sulfasalazine, and hydroxychloroquine. Ann Rheum Dis 49: 798, 1990.
298. Logan EC, Williamson LM, Ryrie DR: Sulfasalazine associated pancytopenia may be caused by acute folate deficiency. Gut 27: 868, 1986.
299. Prouse PJ, Shawe D, Gumpel JM: Macrocytic anaemia in patients treated with sulfasalazine for rheumatoid arthritis. BMJ 293: 1407, 1986.
300. Clementz GL, Dolin BJ: Sulfasalazine-induced lupus erythematosus. Am J Med 84: 535, 1988.
301. Reid J, Holt S, Housley E, Sneddon DJC: Raynaud's phenomenon induced by sulphasalazine. Postgrad Med J 56: 106, 1980.
302. Averbuch M, Halpern Z, Hallak A, et al: Sulfasalazine pneumonitis. Am J Gastroenterol 80: 343, 1985.
303. Hamadeh MA, Atkinson J, Smith LJ: Sulfasalazine-induced pulmonary disease. Chest 101: 1033, 1992.
304. Caspi D, Fuchs D, Yaron M: Sulphasalazine induced hepatitis in juvenile rheumatoid arthritis. Ann Rheum Dis 51: 275, 1992.
305. Toth A: Reversible toxic effect of salicylazosulfapyridine on semen quality. Fertil Steril 31: 538, 1979.
306. Pullar T, Hunter JA, Capell HA: Sulfasalazine in rheumatoid arthritis. A double blind comparison of sulfasalazine with placebo and sodium aurothiomalate. BMJ 287: 1102, 1983.
307. Neumann VC, Grindulis KA, Hubball S, et al: A comparison between penicillamine and sulfasalazine in rheumatoid arthritis. BMJ 287: 1099, 1983.
308. Pullar T, Capell HA: Sulphasalazine: a "new" antirheumatic drug. Br J Rheumatol 23: 26, 1984.
309. Neumann VC, Grindulis KA: Sulphasalazine in rheumatoid arthritis: an old drug revived. J R Soc Med 77: 169, 1984.
310. Grindulis K, McConkey B: Outcome of attempts to treat rheumatoid arthritis patients with gold, penicillamine, sulfasalazine or dapsone. Ann Rheum Dis 43: 398, 1984.
311. Bax DE, Amos RS: Sulfasalazine: a safe, effective agent for prolonged control of rheumatoid arthritis. A comparison with sodium aurothiomalate. Ann Rheum Dis 44: 194, 1985.
312. Watkinson G: Sulphasalazine: a review of 40 years experience. Drugs 32: 1, 1986.
313. Kean WF: Sulfasalazine in rheumatic disease. International Rheumatology Conference, Quebec, Medicopea, 1987.
314. Proceedings: Sulfasalazine in rheumatic diseases. J Rheumatol 16, 1988.
315. Williams HJ, Ward JL, Dahl DL: A controlled trial comparing sulfasalazine, gold sodium thiomalate, and placebo in rheumatoid arthritis. Arthritis Rheum 31: 702, 1988.
316. Farr M, Scott DG, Bacon PA: Side effect profile of 200 patients with inflammatory arthritides treated with sulfasalazine. Drugs 32: 49, 1986.
317. Scott DL, Dacre JE: Adverse reactions to sulfasalazine: the British experience. J Rheumatol 15: 17, 1988.
318. Hertzberger-ten Cate R, Cats A: Toxicity of sulfasalazine in systemic juvenile chronic arthritis. Clin Exp Rheumatol 9: 85–88, 1991.
319. Suschke HJ: Sulfasalazin bei juveniler chronishcher Arthritis. Pediatr Prax 33: 681, 1986.
320. Forestier J: L'aurotherapie dans les rheumatismes chroniques. Bull Soc Med Hop Paris 53: 323, 1929.
321. Forestier J: Rheumatoid arthritis and its treatment with gold salts. J Lab Clin Med 20: 827, 1935.
322. Lewis AJ, Walz DT: Immunopharmacology of Gold, vol 19. *In* Ellis JP (ed): Progress in Medicinal Chemistry. New York, Elsevier Biomedical Press, 1982.
323. Lipsky PE, Ugai K, Ziff M: Alterations in human monocyte structure and function induced by incubation with gold sodium thiomalate. J Rheumatol 6(Suppl 5): 130, 1979.
324. Martini A, De Amici M, Visconti L, et al: Immunological evaluation in children with juvenile chronic arthritis treated with auranofin. Int J Clin Pharmacol Res 5: 149, 1985.
325. Fantini F, Corvaglia G, Bergomi P, et al: Validation of the Italian version of the Stanford Childhood Health Assessment Questionnaire for measuring functional status in children with chronic arthritis. Clin Exp Rheumatol 13: 785–791, 1995.
326. Sadler PJ: The comparative evaluation of the physical and chemical properties of gold compounds. J Rheumatol 9(Suppl 8): 71, 1982.
327. Gottlieb NL: Comparative pharmacokinetics of parenteral and oral gold compounds. J Rheumatol 9(Suppl 8): 99, 1982.
328. Blocka K, Furst D, Landau E, et al: Single dose pharmacokinetics of auranofin in rheumatoid arthritis. J Rheumatol 9(Suppl 8): 110, 1982.
329. Giannini EH, Brewer EJ, Person DA: Blood gold concentrations in children with juvenile rheumatoid arthritis undergoing long-term oral gold therapy. Ann Rheum Dis 43: 228, 1984.
330. Giannini EH, Person DA, Brewer EJ Jr, et al: Blood and serum concentration of gold after a single dose of auranofin in children with juvenile rheumatoid arthritis. J Rheumatol 10: 496, 1983.
331. Nuki G, Gumpel JM: Myocrisin. 50 Years Experience. London, Medi-Cine Communications International, Proceedings of an International Symposium, 1985.
332. Sairanen E, Laaksonen A-L: The toxicity of gold therapy in children suffering from rheumatoid arthritis. Ann Paediatr Fenn 8: 105, 1962.
333. Kean WF, Anastassiades TP: Long-term chrysotherapy: incidence of toxicity and efficacy during sequential time periods. Arthritis Rheum 22: 495, 1979.
334. Sairanen E, Laaksonen A-L: The results of gold therapy in juvenile rheumatoid arthritis. Ann Paediatr Fenn 10: 274, 1963.
335. Hicks RM, Hanson V, Kornreich HK: The use of gold in the treatment of juvenile rheumatoid arthritis. Arthritis Rheum 13: 323, 1970.
336. DeBenedetti C, Tretbar H, Corrigan JJ: Gold therapy in juvenile rheumatoid arthritis. Ariz Med 33: 373, 1976.
337. Levinson JF, Balz GP, Bondi S: Gold therapy. Arthritis Rheum 20: 531, 1977.
338. Brewer EJ Jr, Giannini EH, Barkley E: Gold therapy in the management of juvenile rheumatoid arthritis. Arthritis Rheum 23: 404, 1980.
339. Levinson JE: Gold salts in the rheumatic diseases. *In* Moore TD (ed): Arthritis in Childhood. Report of the Eightieth Ross Conference in Pediatric Research. Columbus, OH, Ross Laboratories, 1981, pp 120–124.
340. Kvien TK, Hoyeraal HM, Sandstad B: Slow acting antirheumatic drugs in patients with juvenile rheumatoid arthritis-evaluated in a randomized, parallel 50-week clinical trial. J Rheumatol 12: 533, 1985.
341. Kvien TK, Hoyeraal HM, Sandstad B: Gold sodium thiomalate and D-penicillamine. A controlled, comparative study in patients with pauciarticular and polyarticular juvenile rheumatoid arthritis. Scand J Rheumatol 14: 346, 1985.
342. Manners PJ, Ansell BM: Slow-acting antirheumatic drug use in systemic onset juvenile chronic arthritis. Pediatrics 77: 99, 1986.

343. Malleson PN, Grondin C, Petty RE, et al: Outcome of gold therapy in juvenile rheumatoid arthritis. Arthritis Rheum 30: 528, 1987.
344. Grondin C, Malleson P, Petty RE: Slow-acting antirheumatic drugs in chronic arthritis of childhood. Semin Arthritis Rheum 18: 38, 1988.
345. Husserl FE, Shuler SE: Gold nephropathy in juvenile rheumatoid arthritis. Am J Dis Child 133: 50, 1979.
346. Merle LJ, Reidenberg MM, Camacho MT, et al: Renal injury in patients with rheumatoid arthritis treated with gold. Clin Pharmacol Ther 28: 216, 1980.
347. Rothermich NO: Chrysotherapy in rheumatoid arthritis. Clin Rheum Dis 5: 631, 1979.
348. Aaron S, Davis P, Percy J: Neutropenia occurring during the course of chrysotherapy. A review of 25 cases. J Rheumatol 12: 897, 1985.
349. Wooley PH, Griffin J, Panayi GS: HLA-DR antigens and toxic reaction to sodium aurothiomalate and D-penicillamine in patients with rheumatoid arthritis. N Engl J Med 303: 300, 1980.
350. Jacobs JC, Gorin LJ, Hanissian AS, et al: Consumption coagulopathy after gold therapy for JRA. J Pediatr 105: 674, 1984.
351. Favreau M, Tannenbaum H, Lough J: Hepatic toxicity associated with gold therapy. Ann Intern Med 87: 717, 1977.
352. Harats N, Shalit M, Ehrenfeld M, et al: Gold-induced granulomatous hepatitis. Isr J Med Sci 21: 753, 1985.
353. Olsen JL, Lovell DJ, Levinson JE: Hypogammaglobulinemia associated with gold therapy in a patient with juvenile rheumatoid arthritis. J Rheumatol 13: 224, 1986.
354. Winterbauer RH, Wilski KR, Wheelis RF: Diffuse pulmonary injury associated with gold treatment. N Engl J Med 294: 919, 1976.
355. Gould PW, McCormack PL, Palmer DG: Pulmonary damage associated with sodium aurothiomalate therapy. J Rheumatol 4: 252, 1977.
356. Fam AG, Gordon DA, Sarkozi J, et al: Neurologic complications associated with gold therapy for rheumatoid arthritis. J Rheumatol 11: 700, 1984.
357. Pik A, Cohen N, Yona E, et al: Should acute gold overdose be invariably treated? J Rheumatol 12: 1174, 1984.
358. Gambari P, Ostuni P, Lazzarin P, et al: Neurotoxicity following a very high dose of oral gold (auranofin). Arthritis Rheum 27: 1316, 1984.
359. Garland JS, Sheth KJ, Wortmann DW: Poor clearance of gold using peritoneal dialysis for the treatment of gold toxicity. Arthritis Rheum 29: 450, 1986.
360. Tarp U, Graudal H: A follow-up study of children exposed to gold compounds in utero. Arthritis Rheum 28: 235, 1986.
361. Paulus HE: Government affairs: FDA Arthritis Advisory Committee meeting: Auranofin. Arthritis Rheum 28: 450, 1985.
362. Giannini EH, Brewer EJ, Person DA: Auranofin in the treatment of juvenile rheumatoid arthritis. J Pediatr 102: 450, 1983.
363. Giannini EH, Brewer EJ, Person DA, et al: Longterm auranofin therapy in patients with juvenile rheumatoid arthritis. J Rheumatol 13: 768, 1986.
364. Garcia-Morteo O, Suarez-Almazor ME, Maldonado-Cocco JA, et al: Auranofin in juvenile rheumatoid arthritis: an open label, non-controlled study. Clin Rheumatol 3: 223, 1984.
365. Kvien TL, Hoyraal HM, Sandstad B, et al: Auranofin therapy in juvenile rheumatoid arthritis: a 48-week phase II study. Scand J Rheumatol 63: 79, 1986.
366. Marcolongo R, Mathieu A, Pala R, et al: The efficacy and safety of auranofin in the treatment of juvenile rheumatoid arthritis. A long-term open study. Arthritis Rheum 31: 979, 1988.
367. Giannini EH, Brewer EJ, Kuzmina N, et al: Auranofin in the treatment of juvenile rheumatoid arthritis: results of the U.S.A.-U.S.S.R. double-blind, placebo-controlled trial. Arthritis Rheum 33: 466, 1989.
368. Clements PJ, Furst DE, Wong WK, et al: High-dose versus low-dose D-penicillamine in early diffuse systemic sclerosis: analysis of a two-year, double-blind, randomized, controlled clinical trial. Arthritis Rheum 42: 1194, 1999.
369. Howard-Lock HE, Lock CJL, Mewa A, et al: D-Penicillamine: chemistry and clinical use in rheumatic disease. Semin Arthritis Rheum 15: 261, 1978.
370. Jaffe IA: D-Penicillamine. Bull Rheum Dis 28: 948, 1978.
371. Multicenter Trial Group: Controlled trial of D-penicillamine in severe rheumatoid arthritis. Lancet 1: 275, 1980.
372. Joyce DA: D-Penicillamine pharmacokinetics and action. Agents Actions (Suppl)24: 197–206, 1988.
373. Joyce DA: D-Penicillamine. Clin Rheumatol 4: 553, 1990.
374. Cuperus RA, Hoogland H, Wever R, Juijsers AOL: The effect of D-penicillamine on myeloperoxidase: formation of compound III and inhibition of the chlorinating activity. Biochim Biophys Acta 912: 124, 1987.
375. Theyboom RHB, Jaffe IA: Metal antagonists. Side Effects Drugs Annu 11: 211, 1987.
376. Lipsky PE: Immunosuppression by D-penicillamine in vitro. Inhibition of human T lymphocyte proliferation by copper- or ceruloplasmin-dependent generation of hydrogen peroxide and protection by monocytes. J Clin Invest 73: 53, 1984.
377. Sheikh IA, Kaplan AP: Assessment of kinases in rheumatic diseases and the effects of therapeutic agents. Arthritis Rheum 30: 138, 1987.
378. Bresnihan GP, Ansell BM: Effect of penicillamine treatment on immune complexes in two cases of seropositive juvenile rheumatoid arthritis. Ann Rheum Dis 35: 463, 1976.
379. Sim E, Dodds AW, Goldin A: Inhibition of the covalent binding reaction of complement component C4 by penicillamine, an anti-rheumatic drug. Biochem J 259: 415, 1989.
380. Chandra P, Sarin PS: Selective inhibition of the AIDS-associated virus HTLV-III/LAV by synthetic D-penicillamine. Arzneimittelforschung 36: 184, 1986.
381. Bourke B, Maini RN, Griffiths ID, et al: Fatal marrow aplasia in patient on penicillamine. Lancet 2: 515, 1976.
382. Blasberg B, Dorey JL, Stein HB, et al: Lichenoid lesions of the oral mucosa in rheumatoid arthritis patients treated with penicillamine. J Rheumatol 11: 348, 1984.
383. Dische FE, Swinson DR, Hamilton EBD, et al: Immunopathology of penicillamine-induced glomerular disease. J Rheumatol 11: 584, 1984.
384. Stein HB, Schroeder M-L, Dillon AM: Penicillamine-induced proteinuria: risk factors. Semin Arthritis Rheum 15: 282, 1986.
385. Kay A: European League Against Rheumatism Study of adverse reactions to D-penicillamine. Br J Rheumatol 25: 193, 1986.
386. Steen VD, Blair S, Medsgar A: The toxicity of D-penicillamine in systemic sclerosis. Ann Intern Med 104: 699, 1986.
387. Baum J: The use of penicillamine in the treatment of rheumatoid arthritis and scleroderma. Scand J Rheumatol 28: 65, 1979.
388. Forre O, Munthe E, Kass E: Side-effects and autoimmunogenicity of D-penicillamine treatment in rheumatic diseases. Adv Inflamm Res 6: 251, 1984.
389. Takahashi K, Ogita T, Okudaira H, et al: D-Penicillamine–induced polymyositis in patients with rheumatoid arthritis. Arthritis Rheum 29: 560, 1986.
390. Kuncl RW, Pestronk A, Drachman DB, Rechthand E: The pathophysiology of penicillamine-induced myasthenia gravis. Ann Neurol 20: 740, 1986.
391. Perrier P, Raffoux C, Thomas P, et al: HLA antigens and toxic reactions to sodium aurothiopropanol sulphonate and D-penicillamine in patients with rheumatoid arthritis. Ann Rheum Dis 44: 621, 1985.
392. Hunter AL, Klaasen CD: Biliary excretion of colchicine. J Pharmacol Exp Ther 192: 605–617, 1975.
393. Ben-Chetrit E, Scherrmann JM, Zylber-Katz E, Levy M: Colchicine disposition in patients with familial Mediterranean fever with renal impairment. J Rheumatol 21: 710, 1994.
394. Ben-Chetrit E, Levy M: Colchicine: 1998 update. Semin Arthritis Rheum 28: 48, 1998.
395. Molad Y, Reibman J, Levin RI, Cronstein BN: A new mode of action for an old drug: colchicine decreases surface expression of adhesion molecule on both neutrophils (PMNs) and endothelium [Abstract]. Arthritis Rheum 35(Suppl): S35, 1992.
396. Venho VM, Koivuniemi A: Effect of colchicine on drug absorption from the rat small intestine in situ and in vitro. Acta Pharmacol Toxicol (Copenh) 43: 251, 1978.
397. Cohen MM, Levy M, Eliakim M: A cytogenic evaluation of long-term colchicine therapy in the treatment of familial Mediterranean fever (FMF). Am J Med Sci 274: 147, 1977.
398. Ben-Chetrit A, Ben-Chetrit E, Nitzan R, Ron M: Colchicine inhibits spermatozoal motility in vitro. Int J Fertil Menopausal Stud 38: 301–304, 1993.

399. Haimov-Kochman R, Ben-Chetrit E: The effect of colchicine on sperm production and function: a review. Hum Reprod 13: 360–362, 1998.
400. Zemer D, Livneh A, Danon YL, et al: Long-term colchicine treatment in children with familial Mediterranean fever. Arthritis Rheum 34: 973, 1991.
401. Majeed HA, Carroll JE, Khuffash FA, Hijazi Z: Long-term colchicine prophylaxis in children with familial Mediterranean fever. J Pediatr 116: 997, 1990.
402. Faure M, Thivolet J, Gaucherand M: Inhibition of PMN leukocytes chemotaxis by thalidomide. Arch Dermatol Res 269: 275–280, 1980.
403. Barnhill RL, Doll NJ, Millikan LE, Hastings RC: Studies on the anti-inflammatory properties of thalidomide: effects on polymorphonuclear leukocytes and monocytes. J Am Acad Dermatol 11: 814, 1984.
404. Gad SM, Shannon EJ, Krotoski WA, Hastings RC: Thalidomide induces imbalances in T-lymphocyte sub-populations in the circulating blood of healthy males. Lepr Rev 56: 35, 1985.
405. Rowland TL, McHugh SM, Deighton J, et al: Differential regulation by thalidomide and dexamethasone of cytokine expression in human peripheral blood mononuclear cells. Immunopharmacology 40: 11, 1998.
406. D'Amato RJ, Loughnan MS, Flynn E, Folkman J: Thalidomide is an inhibitor of angiogenesis. Proc Natl Acad Sci U S A 91: 4082, 1994.
407. Bauer KS, Dixon SC, Figg WD: Inhibition of angiogenesis by thalidomide requires metabolic activation, which is species-dependent. Biochem Pharmacol 55: 1827, 1998.
408. Chen TL, Vogelsang GB, Petty BG, et al: Plasma pharmacokinetics and urinary excretion of thalidomide after oral dosing in healthy male volunteers. Drug Metab Dispos 17: 402, 1989.
409. Tseng S, Pak G, Washenik K, et al: Rediscovering thalidomide: a review of its mechanism of action, side effects, and potential uses. J Am Acad Dermatol 35: 969, 1996.
410. Stambe C, Wicks IP: TNF alpha and response of treatment-resistant adult-onset Still's disease to thalidomide. Lancet 352: 544, 1998.
411. Ochonisky S, Verroust J, Bastuji-Garin S, et al: Thalidomide neuropathy incidence and clinico-electrophysiologic findings in 42 patients. Arch Dermatol 130: 66, 1994.
412. Lagueny A, Rommel A, Vignolly B, et al: Thalidomide neuropathy: an electrophysiologic study. Muscle Nerve 9: 837, 1986.
413. Locker D, Superstine E, Sulmar FG: The mechanism of the push and pull principle. 8: Endocrine effects of thalidomide and its analogues. Arch Int Pharmacodyn Ther 194: 39, 1971.
414. Atra E, Sato EI: Treatment of the cutaneous lesions of systemic lupus erythematosus with thalidomide. Clin Exp Rheumatol 11: 487–493, 1993.
415. American Medical Association: Drug Evaluation Annual. Chicago, American Medical Association: 1992, p 1729.
416. Hench PS: The potential reversibility of rheumatoid arthritis. Mayo Clin Proc 24: 167, 1949.
417. Ansell BM, Bywaters EGL, Isdale IC: Comparison of cortisone and aspirin in the treatment of juvenile rheumatoid arthritis. BMJ 1: 1075, 1956.
418. Schaller JG: Corticosteroids in juvenile rheumatoid arthritis (Still's disease). J Rheumatol 1: 137, 1974.
419. Schaller JG: Corticosteroids in juvenile rheumatoid arthritis. Arthritis Rheum 20: 537, 1977.
420. Stoeber E: Corticosteroid treatment of juvenile chronic polyarthritis over 22 years. Eur J Pediatr 121: 141, 1976.
421. Prieur A-M: The place of corticosteroid therapy in juvenile chronic arthritis in 1992. J Rheumatol 20(Suppl 7): 32–34, 1993.
422. Kimberly RP: Steroids. Curr Opin Rheumatol 2: 510, 1990.
423. Southwood TR: Report from a symposium on corticosteroid therapy in juvenile chronic arthritis. Clin Exp Rheumatol 11: 91, 1993.
424. Thompson EB, Lippman ME: Mechanism of action of glucocorticoids. Metabolism 23: 159, 1974.
425. Fauci AS, Dale DC, Balow JE: Glucocorticosteroid therapy: mechanisms of action and clinical considerations. Ann Intern Med 84: 304, 1976.
426. Axelrod L: Glucocorticoid therapy. Medicine (Baltimore) 55: 39, 1976.
427. Baxter JD: Glucocorticoid hormone action. Pharmacol Ther B2: 605, 1976.
428. Szefler SJ: General pharmacology of glucocorticoids. *In* Schleimer RP, Claman HN, Oronsky A (eds): Anti-Inflammatory Steroid Action. Basic and Clinical Aspects. San Diego, Academic Press, 1990.
429. Burnstein KL, Cidlowski JA: Regulation of gene expression by glucocorticoids. Annu Rev Physiol 51: 683, 1989.
430. LaPointe MC, Baxter JD: Molecular biology of glucocorticoid hormone action. *In* Schleimer RP, Claman HN, Oronsky A (eds): Anti-Inflammatory Steroid Action. Basic and Chemical Aspects. San Diego, Academic Press, 1989, p 3.
431. Buttgereit F, Wehling M, Burmester G-R: A new hypothesis of modular glucocorticoid actions. Steroid treatment of rheumatic diseases revisited. Arthritis Rheum 41:761–767, 1998.
432. Parillo JE, Fauci AS: Mechanisms of glucocorticoid action on immune processes. Annu Rev Pharmacol Toxicol 19: 179, 1979.
433. Claman HN: Corticosteroids and lymphoid cells. N Engl J Med 287: 388, 1972.
434. Fauci AS, Dale DC: Effect of hydrocortisone on the kinetics of normal human lymphocytes. Blood 46: 235, 1975.
435. Weston WL, Claman HN, Krueger GG: Site and action of cortisol in cellular immunity. J Immunol 110: 880, 1973.
436. Rinehart JJ, Balcerzak SP, Sagone AL, LoBuglio AF: Effects of corticosteroids on human monocyte function. J Clin Invest 54: 1337, 1974.
437. Balow JE, Rosenthal AS: Glucocorticoid suppression of macrophage migration inhibitory factor. J Exp Med 137: 1031, 1973.
438. Schreiber AD, Parsons J, McDermott P, Cooper A: Effect of corticosteroids on the human monocyte IgG and complement receptors. J Clin Invest 56: 1189, 1975.
439. MacGregor RR: Granulocyte adherence changes induced by hemodialysis, endotoxin, epinephrine, and glucocorticoids. Ann Intern Med 86: 35, 1977.
440. Granelli-Piperano A, Vassali JD, Reich E: Secretion of plasminogen activator by human polymorphonuclear leukocytes. Modulation by glucocorticoids and other effectors. J Exp Med 146: 1693, 1977.
441. Priestly GC, Brown JC: Effects of corticosteroids on the proliferation of normal and abnormal human connective tissue cells. Br J Dermatol 102: 35, 1980.
442. Hirata F, Schiffmann E, Venkatasubramanian K, et al: A phospholipase A2 inhibitory protein in rabbit neutrophils induced by glucocorticoids. Proc Natl Acad Sci U S A 77: 2533, 1980.
443. Blackwell GJ, Carnuccio R, DiRosa M, et al: Macrocortin: a polypeptide causing the antiphospholipase effect of glucocorticoids. Nature 287: 147, 1980.
444. Haynes RC: Adrenocorticotrophic hormone; adrenocortical steroids and their synthetic analogs; inhibitors of the synthesis and actions of adrenocortical hormones. *In* Goodman Gilman A, Rall TW, Nies AS, et al (eds): Goodman and Gilman's The Pharmacological Basis of Therapeutics, 8th ed. New York, Pergamon Press, 1990.
445. Flower RJ: Glucocorticoids and the inhibition of phospholipase A2. *In* Schleimer RP, Claman HN, Oronsky A (eds): Anti-Inflammatory Steroid Action. Basic and Clinical Aspects. San Diego, Academic Press, 1989, p 48.
446. Parente L, Flower RJ: Hydrocortisone and "macrocortin" inhibit the zymosan-induced release of lyso-PAF from rat peritoneal leucocytes. Life Sci 36: 1225–1231, 1985.
447. Schleimer RP, Claman HN, Oronsky A (eds): Anti-Inflammatory Steroid Action. Basic and Clinical Aspects. San Diego, Academic Press, 1989.
448. Cohen JJ: Lymphocyte death induced by glucocorticoids. *In* Schleimer RP, Claman HN, Oronsky A (eds): Anti-Inflammatory Steroid Action. Basic and Clinical Aspects. San Diego, Academic Press, 1989, p 110.
449. Cupps TR: Effects of glucocorticoids on lymphocyte function. *In* Schleimer RP, Claman HN, Oronsky A (eds): Anti-Inflammatory Steroid Action. Basic and Clinical Aspects. San Diego, Academic Press, 1989, p 132.
450. Butterfield JH, Gleich GJ: Anti-inflammatory effects of glucocorticoids on eosinophils and neutrophils. *In* Schleimer RP, Claman HN, Oronsky A (eds): Anti-Inflammatory Steroid Action. Basic and Clinical Aspects. San Diego, Academic Press, 1989, p 151.

451. Dauchel H, Julen N, Lemercier C, et al: Expression of complement alternative path proteins by endothelial cells. Different regulation by interleukin 1 and glucocorticoids. Eur J Immunol 20: 1669, 1990.
452. Hyams JS, Carey DE: Corticosteroids and growth. J Paediatr 113: 249–254, 1988.
453. Good RA, Vernier RL, Smith RT: Serious untoward reactions to therapy with cortisone and A.C.T.H. in pediatric practice. Pediatrics 19: 95, 1957.
454. Ansell BM: Problems of corticosteroid therapy in the young. Proc R Soc Med 61: 281, 1968.
455. Reimer LG, Morris HG, Ellis EF: Growth of asthmatic children during treatment with alternate-day steroids. J Allergy Clin Immunol 55: 224, 1975.
456. Hahn TJ, Hahn BJ: Osteopenia in patients with rheumatoid diseases: Principles of diagnosis and therapy. Semin Arthritis Rheum 6: 165, 1976.
457. Loeb JN: Corticosteroids and growth. N Engl J Med 295: 547, 1976.
458. Brouhard B, Travis LB, Cunningham RJ, et al: Inhibition of linear growth using alternate day steroids. J Pediatr 91: 343, 1977.
459. McCarthy TL, Centrella M, Canalis E: Cortisol inhibits the synthesis of insulin-like growth factor 1 in skeletal cells. Endocrinology 126: 1569, 1990.
460. Bennett AE, Silverman ED, Miller JJ III, Hintz RL: Insulin-like growth factors in children with systemic onset juvenile arthritis. J Rheumatol 15: 655–658, 1988.
461. Morris HG, Jorgensen JR, Elrick H, Goldsmith RE: Metabolic effects of human growth hormone in corticosteroid-treated children. J Clin Invest 47: 436, 1968.
462. Ansell BM, Bywaters EGL: Growth in Still's disease. Ann Rheum Dis 15: 295–319, 1956.
463. Bernstein BH, Stobie D, Singsen BH, et al: Growth retardation in juvenile rheumatoid arthritis (JRA). Arthritis Rheum 20(Suppl): 212–216, 1977.
464. Ansell BM, Bywaters EGL: Alternate-day corticosteroid therapy in juvenile chronic polyarthritis. J Rheumatol 1: 176, 1974.
465. Byron MA, Jackson J, Ansell BM: Effect of different corticosteroid regimens on hypothalamic-pituitary-adrenal axis and growth in juvenile chronic arthritis. J R Soc Med 76: 452–457, 1983.
466. Falcini F, Trapani S, Civinini R, et al: The primary role of steroids on the osteoporosis in juvenile rheumatoid arthritis patients evaluated by dual energy X-ray absorptiometry. J Endocrinol Invest 19: 165–169, 1996.
467. Bianchi ML, Bardare M, Caraceni MP, et al: Bone metabolism in juvenile rheumatoid arthritis. Bone Mineral 9: 153–162, 1990.
468. Reed AM, Haugen M, Pachman LM, Langman CB: Repair of osteopenia in children with juvenile rheumatoid arthritis. J Paediatr 122: 693–696, 1993.
469. Rabinovich CE, Wagner-Weiner L, Wuellner J, Spencer C: Osteoporosis in juvenile rheumatoid arthritis. Arthritis Rheum 40: S323, 1997.
470. Kotaniemi A, Savolainen A, Kautiainen H, Kroger H: Estimation of central osteopenia in children with chronic polyarthritis treated with glucocorticoids. Pediatrics 91: 1127–1130, 1993.
471. Adachi JD, Bensen WG, Hodsman AB: Corticosteroid-induced osteoporosis. Semin Arthritis Rheum 22: 375–384, 1993.
472. Sambrook PN: Corticosteroid induced osteoporosis. J Rheumatol 23(Suppl 45): 19–22, 1996.
473. Adachi JD, Bensen WG, Bell MJ, et al: Corticosteroid induced osteoporosis: followup over 3 years. Third International Symposium on Osteoporosis, Copenhagen, 1990.
474. Ruegsegger P, Medici TC, Anliker M: A longitudinal study of alternate day therapy in patients with bronchial asthma using quantitative computed tomography. Eur J Clin Pharmacol 25: 615–620, 1983.
475. Gluck OS, Murphy WA, Hahn TJ, et al: Bone loss in adults receiving alternate day glucocorticoid therapy. Arthritis Rheum 24: 892–898, 1981.
476. Sambrook PN, Kelly PJ, Fontana D, et al: Mechanism of rapid bone loss following cardiac transplantation. Osteoporosis Int 4: 273–276, 1994.
477. Reeve J, Loftus J, Hesp R, et al: Biochemical prediction of changes in spinal bone mass in juvenile chronic (or rheumatoid) arthritis treated with glucocorticoids. J Rheumatol 20: 1189–1195, 1993.
478. Zizic TM, Marcoux C, Hungerford DS, et al: Corticosteroid therapy associated with ischemic necrosis of bone in systemic lupus erythematosus. Am J Med 79: 596–604, 1985.
479. Bergstein JM, Wiens C, Fish AJ, et al: Avascular necrosis of bone in systemic lupus erythematosus. J Paediatr 85: 31–35, 1974.
480. Ansell BM: Overview of the side effects of corticosteroid therapy. Clin Exp Rheumatol 9: 19–20, 1991.
481. Bozzette SA, Sattler FR, Chiu J, et al: A controlled trial of early adjunctive treatment with corticosteroids for Pneumocystis carinii pneumonia in the acquired immunodeficiency syndrome. N Engl J Med 323: 1451–1457, 1990.
482. Fishman JA: Treatment of infection due to Pneumocystis carinii. Antimicrob Agents Chemother 42: 1309–1314, 1998.
483. Schleimer RP: Effects of glucocorticosteroids on inflammatory cells relevant to their therapeutic application in asthma. Am Rev Respir Dis 141: 559, 1990.
484. Lewis DA, Smith RE: Steroid-induced psychiatric syndromes. J Affective Disord 5: 319–332, 1983.
485. Levine SB, Leopold IH: Advances in ocular corticosteroid therapy. Med Clin North Am 57: 1167–1177, 1973.
486. Rogers MP: Psychiatric aspects. *In* Schur PH (ed): The Clinical Management of Systemic Lupus Erythematosus. New York, Grune & Stratton, 1983, p 189.
487. Ling MH, Perry PJ, Tsuang MT: Side effects of corticosteroid therapy. Arch Gen Psych 38: 371, 1981.
488. Klein-Gitelman MS, Pachman LM: Intravenous corticosteroids: adverse reactions are more variable than expected in children. J Rheumatol 25: 1995–2002, 1998.
489. Ilowite NT, Samuel P, Ginzler E, Jacobson MS: Dyslipoproteinemia in pediatric systemic lupus erythematosus. Arthritis Rheum 31: 859, 1988.
490. Petri M, Perez-Gutthann S, Spence D, Hochberg MC: Risk factors for coronary artery disease in patients with systemic lupus erythematosus. Am J Med 93: 513–519, 1992.
491. Gazarian M, Feldman BM, Benson LN, et al: Assessment of myocardial perfusion and function in childhood systemic lupus erythematosus. J Pediatr 132: 109–116, 1998.
492. Lubkin VL: Steroid cataract—a review and conclusion. J Asthma Res 14: 55, 1997.
493. Urban RC, Cotlier E: Corticosteroid-induced cataracts. Surv Opthalmol 31: 102–110, 1986.
494. Knox AJ, Mascie-Taylor BH, Muers MF: Acute hydrocortisone myopathy in severe asthma. Thorax 41: 411–412, 1986.
495. Perlman K, Ehrlich RM: Steroid diabetes in childhood. Am J Dis Child 136: 64–68, 1982.
496. Conn HO, Poynard T: Corticosteroids and peptic ulcer: meta-analysis of adverse events during steroid therapy. J Intern Med 236: 619–632, 1994.
497. Gambertoglio JG, Amend WJ Jr, Benet LZ: Pharmacokinetics and bioavailability of prednisone and prednisolone in healthy volunteers and patients. A review. J Pharmacokinet Biopharm 8: 1, 1980.
498. Myles AB, Schiller LF, Glass D, Daly JR: Single daily dose of corticosteroid treatment. Ann Rheum Dis 35: 73, 1976.
499. Loftus J, Allen R, Hesp R, et al: Randomized, double-blind trial of deflazacort versus prednisone in juvenile chronic (or rheumatoid) arthritis: a relatively bone-sparing effect of deflazacort. Pediatrics 88: 428–436, 1991.
500. Markham A, Bryson HM: Deflazacort: a review of its pharmacological properties and therapeutic efficacy. Drugs 50: 317–333, 1995.
501. David J, Loftus J, Hesp R, et al: Spinal and somatic growth in patients with juvenile chronic arthritis treated for up to 2 years with deflazacort. Clin Exp Rheumatol 10: 621, 1992.
502. Falcini F, Trapani S, Ermini M, Bartolozzi G: Deflazacort in paediatric rheumatic diseases needs a frequent follow-up of bone densitometry [Letter]. Pediatrics 95: 318, 1995.
503. MacGregor RR, Sheagren JN, Lipsett MB, Wolff SM: Alternate-day prednisone therapy. Evaluation of delayed hypersensitivity responses, control of disease and steroid side effects. N Engl J Med 280: 1427, 1969.
504. Dale DC, Fauci AS, Wolff SM: Alternate day prednisone. Leuko-

cyte kinetics and susceptibility to infection. N Engl J Med 291: 1154, 1974.
505. Dixon RB, Christy NP: On the various forms of corticosteroid withdrawal syndrome. Am J Med 68: 224, 1980.
506. Amatruda TT Jr, Hollingsworth DR, D'Esopo ND, et al: A study of the mechanism of the steroid withdrawal syndrome. J Clin Endocrinol Metab 20: 339, 1960.
507. Laaksonen A-L, Sunell JE, Westeren H, Mulder J: Adrenocortical function in children with juvenile rheumatoid arthritis and other connective tissue disorders. Scand J Rheumatol 3: 137, 1974.
508. Buckley LM, Leib ES, Cartularo KS, et al: Calcium and vitamin D3 supplementation prevents bone loss in the spine secondary to low dose corticosteroids in patients with rheumatoid arthritis. A randomized, double-blind, placebo-controlled trial. Ann Intern Med 126: 961–968, 1996.
509. Sambrook P, Birmingham J, Kelly P, et al: Prevention of corticosteroid osteoporosis. A comparison of calcium, calcitriol, and calcitonin. N Engl J Med 328: 1747–1752, 1993.
510. Homik J, Suarez-Almazor ME, Shea B, et al: Osteoporosis (OP): Calcium (Ca) and Vitamin D for the treatment of corticosteroid-induced osteoporosis (Cochrane Review). The Cochrane Library, vol 3. Oxford, Update Software, 1998.
511. Warady BD, Lindsley CB, Robinson RG, Lukert BP: Effects of nutritional supplementation on bone mineral status of children with rheumatic diseases receiving corticosteroid therapy. J Rheumatol 21: 530–535, 1994.
512. Reed A, Haugen M, Pachman LM, Langman CB: 25-Hydroxyvitamin D therapy in children with active juvenile rheumatoid arthritis: short term effects on serum osteocalcin levels and bone mineral density. J Pediatr 119: 657–660, 1991.
513. Reid IR, King AR, Alexander CJ, Ibbertson HK: Prevention of steroid-induced osteoporosis with (3-amino-1-hydroxypropylidene)-1, 1-bisphosphonate (APD). Lancet 1: 143–146, 1988.
514. Roux C, Oriente P, Laan R, et al: Randomized trial of effect of cyclical etidronate in the prevention of corticosteroid-induced bone loss. J Clin Endocrinol Metab 83: 1128–1133, 1998.
515. Adachi JD, Bensen WG, Brown J, et al: Intermittent etidronate therapy to prevent corticosteroid-induced osteoporosis. N Engl J Med 337: 382–387, 1997.
516. Saag KG, Emkey R, Schnitzer TJ, et al: Alendronate for the prevention and treatment of glucocorticoid-induced osteoporosis. N Engl J Med 339: 292–299, 1998.
517. Brumsen C, Hamdy NAT, Papapoulos SE: Long-term effects of bisphosphonates on the growing skeleton. Studies of young patients with severe osteoporosis. Medicine 76: 266–283, 1997.
518. Glorieux FH, Bishop NJ, Plotkin H, et al: Cyclic administration of pamidronate in children with severe osteogenesis imperfecta. N Engl J Med 339: 947–952, 1998.
519. Christy NP: Pituitary-adrenal function during corticosteroid therapy: learning to live with uncertainty. N Engl J Med 326: 266–267, 1992.
520. Gundbjornsson B, Skogseid B, Oberg K, et al: Intact adrenocorticotropic hormone secretion but impaired cortisol response in patients with active rheumatoid arthritis. Effect of glucocorticoids. J Rheumatol 23: 596–602, 1996.
521. Graber AL, Ney RE, Nicholson WE, et al: Natural history of pituitary-adrenal recovery following long term suppression with corticosteroids. J Clin Endocrinol Metab 25: 11, 1965.
522. Cathcart ES, Idelson BA, Scheinberg MA, et al: Beneficial effects of methylprednisolone "pulse" therapy in diffuse proliferative lupus nephritis. Lancet 1: 163, 1976.
523. Miller JJ III: Prolonged use of large intravenous steroid pulses in the rheumatic diseases of children. Pediatrics 65: 989–994, 1980.
524. Laxer RM, Stein L, Petty RE: Intravenous pulse methylprednisolone treatment of juvenile dermatomyositis. Arthritis Rheum 30: 328, 1989.
525. Shaikov AV, Maximov AA, Speransky AI, et al: Repetitive use of pulse therapy with methylprednisolone and cyclophosphamide in addition to oral methotrexate in children with systemic juvenile rheumatoid arthritis—preliminary results of a long term study. J Rheumatol 19: 612–616, 1992.
526. Picco P, Gattorno M, Buoncompagni A, et al: 6-Methylprednisolone "mini-pulses": a new modality of chronic glucocorticoid treatment in systemic onset juvenile chronic arthritis. Scand J Rheumatol 25: 24–27, 1996.
527. Job-Deslandre C, Menkes CJ: Administration of methylprednisolone pulse in chronic arthritis in children. Clin Exp Rheumatol 9(Suppl 6): 15–18, 1991.
528. Hayball PJ, Cosh DG, Ahern MJ, et al: High dose oral methylprednisolone in patients with rheumatoid arthritis: pharmacokinetics and clinical response. Eur J Clin Pharmacol 42: 85, 1992.
529. Shipley ME, Bacon PA, Hazleman BL, et al: Pulsed methylprednisolone in active early rheumatoid disease: a dose-ranging study. Br J Rheumatol 27: 211–214, 1988.
530. Walters MT, Cawley MID: Combined suppressive drug treatment in severe refractory rheumatoid disease: an analysis of the relative effects of parenteral methylprednisolone, cyclophosphamide, and sodium aurothiomalate. Ann Rheum Dis 47: 924–929, 1988.
531. Williams IA, Mitchell AD, Rothman W, et al: Survey of the long term incidence of osteonecrosis of the hip and adverse medical events in rheumatoid arthritis after high dose intravenous methylprednisolone. Ann Rheum Dis 47: 930–933, 1988.
532. Allen RC, Gross KR, Laxer RM, et al: Intraarticular triamcinolone hexacetonide in the management of chronic arthritis in children. Arthritis Rheum 29: 997–1001, 1986.
533. Earley A, Cuttica RJ, McCullogh C, Ansell BM: Triamcinolone into the knee joint in juvenile chronic arthritis. Clin Exp Rheumatol 6: 153–155, 1988.
534. Hertzberger-ten Cate R, de Vries-van der Vlugt BCM, van Suijlekom-Smit LWA, Cats A: Intra-articular steroids in pauciarticular juvenile chronic arthritis, type 1. Eur J Pediatr 150: 170–172, 1991.
535. Honkanen VEA, Rautonen JK, Pelkonen PM: Intra-articular glucocorticoids in early juvenile chronic arthritis. Acta Paediatr 82: 1072–1074, 1993.
536. Padeh S, Passwell JH: Intraarticular corticosteroid injection in the management of children with chronic arthritis. Arthritis Rheum 41: 1210–1214, 1998.
537. Smith J, Scuccimari R, Gibbon M, et al: Efficacy of intra-articular triamcinolone hexacetonide in a practice-based cohort of children with juvenile arthritis. J Rheumatol 27(Suppl 58): 95, 2000.
538. Derendorf H, Mollmann H, Gruner A, et al: Pharmacokinetics and pharmacodynamics of glucocorticoid suspensions after intra-articular administration. Clin Pharmacol Ther 39: 313–317, 1986.
539. Balogh Z, Ruzsonyi E: Triamcinolone hexacetonide versus betamethasone. A double blind comparative study of the long-term effects of intra-articular steroids in patients with juvenile chronic arthritis. Scand J Rheumatol 67(Suppl): 80–82, 1987.
540. Grillet B, Dequeker J: Intra-articular steroid injection. A risk-benefit assessment. Drug Safety 5: 205–211, 1990.
541. Job-Deslandre C, Menkes CJ: Complications of intra-articular injections of triamcinolone hexacetonide in chronic arthritis in children. Clin Exp Rheumatol 8: 413–416, 1990.
542. Sparling M, Malleson P, Wood B, Petty R: Radiographic followup of joints injected with triamcinolone hexacetonide for the management of childhood arthritis. Arthritis Rheum 33: 821–826, 1990.
543. Gilsanz V, Bernstein BH: Joint calcification following intraarticular corticosteroid therapy. Radiology 151: 647–649, 1984.
544. Jalavas S, Haapasaari J, Isomaki H: Peri-articular calcification after intraarticular triamcinolone hexacetonide. Scand J Rheumatol 9: 190–192, 1980.
545. Eich GF, Halle F, Hodler J, et al: Juvenile chronic arthritis: imaging of the knees and hips before and after intraarticular steroid injection. Pediatr Radiol 24: 558–563, 1994.
546. Huppertz H-I, Tschammler A, Horwitz AE, Schwab KO: Intraarticular corticosteroids for chronic arthritis in children: efficacy and effects on cartilage and growth. J Pediatr 127: 317–321, 1995.
547. Hagelberg S, Magnusson B, Jenner G, Andersson U: Do frequent corticosteroid injections in the knee cause cartilage damage in juvenile chronic arthritis? Long-term follow-up with MRI. J Rheumatol 27(Suppl 58): 95, 2000.
548. Huppertz H-I, Pfuller H: Transient suppression of endogenous cortisol production after intraarticular steroid therapy for chronic arthritis in children. J Rheumatol 24: 1833–1837, 1997.
549. Lazarevic MB, Djordjevic-Denic G, Mladenovic V, et al: Adrenocortical suppression after single intra-articular or intra-muscular injection of 40 mg of methylprednisolone acetate. Arthritis Rheum 34: S128, 1991.

550. Elion GB: Biochemistry and pharmacology of purine analogues. Fed Proc 26: 898, 1967.
551. Maibach HI, Epstein WL: Immunologic responses of healthy volunteers receiving azathioprine (Imuran). Int Arch Allergy Appl Immunol 27: 102, 1965.
552. Abdou NI, Sweiman B, Casella SR: Effects of azathioprine therapy on bone marrow-dependent and thymus-dependent cells in man. Clin Exp Immunol 13: 55, 1973.
553. Sharbaugh RJ, Ainsworth SK, Fitts CK: Lack of effect of azathioprine on phytohemagglutinin-induced lymphocyte transformation and established delayed cutaneous hypersensitivity. Int Arch Allergy Appl Immunol 51: 681, 1976.
554. Fox DA, McCune WJ: Immunologic and clinical effects of cytotoxic drugs used in the treatment of rheumatoid arthritis and systemic lupus erythematosus. Concepts Immunopathol 7: 20, 1989.
555. De Witte DB, Buick MK, Cyran SE, Maisels MJ: Neonatal pancytopenia and severe combined immunodeficiency associated with antenatal administration of azathioprine and prednisone. J Pediatr 105: 625, 1984.
556. Singh G, Fries JF, Williams CA, et al: Toxicity profiles of disease modifying antirheumatic drugs in rheumatoid arthritis. J Rheumatol 18: 188, 1991.
557. Leipold G, Schutz E, Haas JP, Oellerich M: Azathioprine-induced severe pancytopenia dur to a homozygous two-point mutation of the thiopurine methyltransferase gene in a patient with juvenile HLA-B27-associated spondylarthritis. Arthritis Rheum 40: 1896–1898, 1997.
558. Stolk JN, Boerbooms AM, de Abreu RA, et al: Reduced thiopurine methyltransferase activity and development of side effects of azathioprine treatment in patients with rheumatoid arthritis. Arthritis Rheum 41: 1858–1866, 1998.
559. Bailey RR: Leukopenia due to trimethoprim-azathioprine interaction. N Z Med J 97: 739, 1984.
560. Prior P, Symmons DPM, Hawkins CF, Scott DL: Cancer morbidity in rheumatoid arthritis. Ann Rheum Dis 43: 522, 1984.
561. Silman AJ, Petrie J, Hazleman B, Evans SJW: Lymphoproliferative cancer and other malignancy in patients with rheumatoid arthritis treated with azathioprine: a 20 year follow up study. Ann Rheum Dis 47: 988, 1988.
562. Singh G, Fries JF, Spitz P, Williams CA: Toxic effects of azathioprine in rheumatoid arthritis. Arthritis Rheum 32: 837, 1989.
563. Savolainen HA, Kautiainen H, Isomaki H, et al: Azathioprine in patients with juvenile chronic arthritis: a longterm followup study. J Rheumatol 24: 2444–2450, 1997.
564. Mah G, Laxer RM, Bargman JM, et al: Long-term outcome in pediatric systemic lupus erythematosus. Arthritis Rheum 37: S319, 1994.
565. Eugui EM, Almquist SJ, Muller CD, Allison AC: Lymphocyte-selective cytostatic and immunosuppressive effects of mycophenolic acid in vitro: role of deoxyguanosine nucleotide depletion. Scand J Immunol 33: 161–173, 1991.
566. Platz KP, Sollinger HW, Hullett DA, et al: RS-61443—a new, potent immunosuppressive agent. Transplantation 51: 27–31, 1991.
567. Grailer A, Nichols J, Hullett D, et al: Inhibition of human B cell responses in vitro by RS-61443, cyclosporine A and DAB486 IL-2. Transplant Proc 23: 314–315, 1991.
568. Burlingham WJ, Grailer AP, Hullett DA, Sollinger HW: Inhibition of both MLC and in vitro IgG memory response to tetanus toxoid by RS-61443. Transplantation 51: 545–547, 1991.
569. Woo J, Zeevi A, Yao GZ, et al: Effects of FK 506, mycophenolic acid, and bredinin on OKT-3-, PMA-, and alloantigen-induced activation molecule expression on cultured CD4+ and CD8+ human lymphocytes. Transplant Proc 23: 2939–2940, 1991.
570. Smith KG, Isbel NM, Catton MG, et al: Suppression of the humoral immune response by mycophenolate mofetil. Nephrol Dial Transplant 13: 160–164, 1998.
571. Laurent AF, Dumont S, Poindron P, Muller CD: Mycophenolic acid suppresses protein N-linked glycosylation in human monocytes and their adhesion to endothelial cells and to some substrates. Exp Hematol 24: 59–67, 1996.
572. Hauser IA, Johnson DR, Thevenod F, Goppelt-Strube M: Effect of mycophenolic acid on TNF alpha-induced expression of cell adhesion molecules in human venous endothelial cells in vitro. Br J Pharmacol 122: 1315–1322, 1997.
573. Sievers TM, Rossi SJ, Ghobrial RM, et al: Mycophenolate mofetil. Pharmacotherapy 17: 1178–1197, 1997.
574. Nowack R, Birck R, van der Woude FJ: Mycophenolate mofetil for systemic vasculitis and IgA nephropathy. Lancet 349: 774, 1997.
575. Goldblum R: Therapy of rheumatoid arthritis with mycophenolate mofetil. Clin Exp Rheumatol 11(Suppl 8): S117–S119, 1993.
576. McMurray RW, Elbourne KB, Lagoo A, Lal S: Mycophenolate mofetil suppresses autoimmunity and mortality in the female NZB × NZW F1 mouse model of systemic lupus erythematosus. J Rheumatol 25: 2364–2370, 1998.
577. Glicklich D, Acharya A: Mycophenolate mofetil therapy for lupus nephritis refractory to intravenous cyclophosphamide. Am J Kidney Dis 32: 318–322, 1998.
578. Larkin G, Lightman S: Mycophenolate mofetil. A useful immunosuppressive in inflammatory eye disease. Ophthalmology 106: 370–374, 1999.
579. Fischer DS: Alkylating agents. *In* Fischer DS, Marsh JC (ed): Cancer Therapy. Boston, GK Hall, 1972.
580. Kovarsky J: Clinical pharmacology and toxicology of cyclophosphamide: emphasis on use in rheumatic disease. Semin Arthritis Rheum 12: 359, 1983.
581. Cupps TR, Edgar LC, Fauci AS: Suppression of human B lymphocyte function by cyclophosphamide. J Immunol 128: 2453, 1982.
582. Turk JL, Parker D: Effect of cyclophosphamide on immunological control mechanisms. Immunol Rev 65: 99, 1982.
583. Stockman GD, Heim LR, South MA: Differential effects of cyclophosphamide in B and T cell compartments of adult mice. J Immunol 110: 277, 1973.
584. Hersh EM, Wong VG, Freireich EJ: Inhibition of the local inflammatory response in man by antimetabolites. Blood 27: 38, 1966.
585. Hoffman GS, Leavitt RY, Fleischer TA, et al: Treatment of Wegener's granulomatosis with intermittent high-dose intravenous cyclophosphamide. Am J Med 89: 403–410, 1990.
586. Miller JJ 3rd, Williams GF, Leissring JC: Multiple late complications of therapy with cyclophosphamide including ovarian destruction. Am J Med 50: 530, 1971.
587. Warne GL, Fairley KF, Hobbs JB, et al: Cyclophosphamide-induced ovarian failure. N Engl J Med 289: 1159, 1973.
588. DeFronzo RA, Braine H, Colvin OM, et al: Water intoxication in man after cyclophosphamide therapy: time course and relation to drug activation. Ann Intern Med 78: 861, 1973.
589. Wall RL, Clausen KP: Carcinoma of the urinary bladder in patients receiving cyclophosphamide. N Engl J Med 293: 271, 1975.
590. Plotz PH, Klippel JH, Decker JL, et al: Bladder complications in patients receiving cyclophosphamide for systemic lupus erythematosus or rheumatoid arthritis. Ann Intern Med 91: 221, 1979.
591. Trompeter RS, Evans PR, Barratt TM: Gonadal function in boys with steroid-responsive nephrotic syndrome treated with cyclophosphamide for short periods. Lancet 1: 1177, 1981.
592. Devries CR, Freiha FS: Hemorrhagic cystitis: a review. J Urol 143: 1, 1990.
593. Baltus JAM, Boersma JW, Hartman AP, Vandenbroucke JP: The occurrence of malignancies in patients with rheumatoid arthritis treated with cyclophosphamide: a controlled retrospective follow-up. Ann Rheum Dis 42: 368, 1983.
594. Bradley JD, Brandt KD, Katz BP: Infectious complications of cyclophosphamide treatment for vasculitis. Arthritis Rheum 32: 45, 1989.
595. Dooley MA, Falk RJ: Immunosuppressive therapy of lupus nephritis. Lupus 7: 630–634, 1998.
596. Harlow PJ, DeClerck YA, Shore NA, et al: A fatal case of inappropriate ADH secretion induced by cyclophosphamide therapy. Cancer 44: 896–898, 1979.
597. Spital A, Ristow S: Cyclophosphamide induced water intoxication in a woman with Sjögren's syndrome. J Rheumatol 24: 2473–2475, 1997.
598. Rivkees SA, Crawford JD: The relationship of gonadal activity and chemotherapy-induced gonadal damage. JAMA 259: 2123–2125, 1988.
599. Mok CC, Lau CS, Wong RW: Risk factors for ovarian failure in patients with systemic lupus erythematosus receiving cyclophosphamide therapy. Arthritis Rheum 41: 831–837, 1998.

600. Boumpas DT, Austin HA 3rd, Vaughan EM, et al: Risk for sustained amenorrhea in patients with systemic lupus erythematosus receiving intermittent pulse cyclophosphamide therapy. Ann Intern Med 119: 366–369, 1993.
601. Blumenfeld Z, Haim N: Prevention of gonadal damage during cytotoxic therapy. Ann Med 29: 199–206, 1997.
602. Blumenfeld Z, Avivi I, Linn S, et al: Prevention of irreversible chemotherapy-induced ovarian damage in young women with lymphoma by a gonadotropin-releasing hormone agonist in parallel to chemotherapy. Hum Reprod 11: 1620–1626, 1996.
603. Slater CA, Liang MH, McCune JW, et al: Preserving ovarian function in patients receiving cyclophosphamide. Lupus 8: 3–10, 1999.
604. Radis CD, Kahl LE, Baker GL, et al: Effects of cyclophosphamide on the development of malignancy and on long-term survival of patients with rheumatoid arthritis. A 20-year followup study. Arthritis Rheum 38: 1120–1127, 1995.
605. Talar-Williams C, Hijazi YM, Walther MM, et al: Cyclophosphamide-induced cystitis and bladder cancer in patients with Wegener granulomatosis. Ann Intern Med 124: 477–484, 1996.
606. Brodsky RA, Petrie M, Smith BD, et al: Immunoablative high-dose cyclophosphamide without stem-cell rescue for refractory, severe autoimmune disease. Ann Intern Med 129: 1031–1035, 1998.
607. David J, Vouyiouka O, Ansell BM, et al: Amyloidosis in juvenile chronic arthritis: a morbidity and mortality study. Clin Exp Rheumatol 11: 85–90, 1993.
608. Buriot D, Prieue AM, Lebranchu Y, et al: Acute leukemia in 3 children with chronic juvenile arthritis treated with chlorambucil. Arch Fr Pediatr 36: 592–598, 1979.
609. Guesry P, Lenoir G, Broyer M: Gonadal effects of chlorambucil given to prepubertal and pubertal boys for nephrotic syndrome. J Pediatr 92: 299–303, 1978.
610. Borel J, Feurer C, Magnee C, Stahelin H: Effects of the new anti-lymphocyte cyclosporin A in animals. Immunology 32: 1017, 1977.
611. Fruman DA, Klee CB, Bierer BE, Burakoff SJ: Calcineurin phosphatase activity in T lymphocytes is inhibited by FK 506 and cyclosporin A. Proc Natl Acad Sci U S A 89: 3686–3690, 1992.
612. Schreiber SL, Crabtree JR: The mechanisms of action of cyclosporin A and FK506. Immunol Today 13: 136, 1992.
613. Bunjes D, Hardt C, Rollinghoff M, Wagner H: Cyclosporin A mediates immunosuppression of primary cytotoxic T cell responses by impairing the release of interleukin 1 and interleukin 2. Eur J Immunol 11: 657, 1981.
614. Navarro J, Touraine JL: Comparative study of cycloimmune cyclosporin A on human lymphocyte proliferation in vitro: the lack of an immunosuppressive effect by specific clonal deletion. Int J Immunopharmacol 5: 157, 1983.
615. Kronke M, Leonard WJ, Depper JM, et al: Cyclosporin A inhibits T-cell growth factor gene expression at the level of mRNA transcription. Proc Natl Acad Sci U S A 81: 5214, 1984.
616. Reem GH, Cook LA, Vilcek J: Gamma interferon synthesis by human thymocytes and T lymphocytes inhibited by cyclosporin A. Science 221: 63–65, 1983.
617. Ahuja SS, Shrivastav S, Danielpour D, et al: Regulation of transforming growth factor-beta 1 and its receptor by cyclosporine in human T lymphocytes. Transplantation 60: 718–723, 1995.
618. Meyer S, Kohler NG, Joly A: Cyclosporine A is an uncompetitive inhibitor of proteasome activity and prevents NF-kB activation. FEBS Lett 413: 354–358, 1997.
619. Holschermann H, Durfeld F, Maus U, et al: Cyclosporine A inhibits tissue factor expression in monocytes/macrophages. Blood 88: 3837–3845, 1996.
620. Andjelic S, Khanna A, Suthanthiran M, Nikolic-Zugic J: Intracellular Ca^{2+} elevation and cyclosporine A synergistically induce TGF-beta 1-mediated apoptosis in lymphocytes. J Immunol 158: 2527–2534, 1997.
621. Muller S, Adorini L, Appella E, Nagy ZA: Lack of influence of cyclosporine on antigen presentation to lysozyme-specific T cell hybridomas. Transplantation 46(Suppl 2): 44S–48S, 1988.
622. Knight SC, Roberts M, Macatonia SE, et al: Blocking of acquisition and presentation of antigen by dendritic cells with cyclosporine. Transplantation 46(Suppl 2): 48S–53S, 1988.
623. Furue M, Katz SI: Cyclosporine A inhibits accessory cell and antigen-presenting cell functions of epidermal Langerhans cells. Transplant Proc 20(2 Suppl 2): 87–91, 1998.
624. Somerville MF, Scott DG: Neoral—new cyclosporin for old? Br J Rheumatol 36: 1113–1115, 1997.
625. Myers BD, Ross J, Newton L, et al: Cyclosporine-associated chronic nephropathy. N Engl J Med 311: 699–705, 1984.
626. Palestine AG, Austin HA, Balow JE, et al: Renal histopathologic alterations in patients treated with cyclosporin for uveitis. N Engl J Med 314: 1293, 1986.
627. Rodger S, Turney JH, Haynes I, et al: Normal liver function in renal allograft recipients treated with cyclosporine. Transplantation 36: 451–452, 1983.
628. Pistoia V, Buoncampagni A, Scribanis R, et al: Cyclosporin A in the treatment of juvenile chronic arthritis and childhood polymyositis-dermatomyositis. Results of a preliminary study. Clin Exp Rheumatol 11: 203–208, 1993.
629. Reiff A, Rawlings DJ, Shaham B, et al: Preliminary evidence for cyclosporin A as an alternative in the treatment of recalcitrant juvenile rheumatoid arthritis and juvenile dermatomyositis. J Rheumatol 24: 2436–2443, 1997.
630. Zeller V, Cohen P, Prieur AM, Guillevin L: Cyclosporin A therapy in refractory juvenile dermatomyositis. Experience and longterm followup of 6 cases. J Rheumatol 23: 1424–1427, 1996.
631. Walton RC, Nussenblatt RB, Whitcup SM: Cyclosporine therapy for severe sight-threatening uveitis in children and adolescents. Ophthalmology 105: 2028–2034, 1998.
632. Kilmartin DJ, Forrester JV, Dick AD: Cyclosporin A therapy in refractory non-infectious childhood uveitis. Br J Ophthalmol 82: 737–742, 1998.
633. Mouy R, Stephan JL, Pillet P, et al: Efficacy of cyclosporine A in the treatment of macrophage activation syndrome in juvenile arthritis: report of five cases. J Pediatr 129: 750–754, 1996.
634. van den Borne BE, Landewe R-B, Houkes I, et al: No increased risk of malignancies and mortality in cyclosporin A-treated patients with rheumatoid arthritis. Arthritis Rheum 41: 1930–1937, 1998.
635. Ioannides-Demos LL, Christophidis N, Ryan P, et al: Dosing implications of a clinical interaction between grapefruit juice and cyclosporine and metabolite concentrations in patients with autoimmune diseases. J Rheumatol 24: 49–54, 1997.
636. Davis JP, Cain CA, Pitts WJ, et al: The immunosuppressive metabolite of leflunomide is a potent inhibitor of human dihydroorotate dehydrogenase. Biochemistry 35: 1270–1273, 1996.
637. Xu X, Blinder L, Shen J, et al: In vivo mechanism by which leflunomide controls lymphoproliferative and autoimmune disease in MRL/MpJ-lpr/lpr mice. J Immunol 159: 167–174, 1997.
638. Dimitrijevic M, Bartlett RR: Leflunomide, a novel immunomodulating drug, inhibits homotypic adhesion of mononuclear cells in rheumatoid arthritis. Transplant Proc 28: 3086–3087, 1996.
639. Cao WW, Kao PN, Aoki Y, et al: A novel mechanism of action of the immunomodulatory drug, leflunomide: augmentation of the immunosuppressive cytokine, TGF-beta 1, and suppression of the immunostimulatory cytokine, IL-2. Transplant Proc 28: 3079–3080, 1996.
640. Mladenovic V, Domljan Z, Rozman B, et al: Safety and effectiveness of leflunomide in the treatment of patients with active rheumatoid arthritis. Arthritis Rheum 38: 1595–1603, 1995.
641. Smolen JS, Kalden JR, Scott DL, et al: Efficacy and safety of leflunomide compared with placebo and sulphasalazine in active rheumatoid arthritis: a double-blind, randomised, multicentre trial. European Leflunomide Study Group. Lancet 353: 259–266, 1999.
642. Rozman B: Clinical experience with leflunomide in rheumatoid arthritis. J Rheumatol 25(Suppl 53): 27–32, 1998.
643. Felson DT, Anderson JJ, Meenan RJ: The comparative efficacy and toxicity of second-line drugs in rheumatoid arthritis. Results of two metaanalyses. Arthritis Rheum 33: 1449–1461, 1990.
644. Tugwell P, Pincus T, Yocum D, et al: Combination therapy with cyclosporine and methotrexate in severe rheumatoid arthritis. The Methotrexate-Cyclosporine Combination Study Group. N Engl J Med 333: 137–141, 1995.
645. Stein CM, Pincus T, Yocum D, et al: Combination treatment of severe rheumatoid arthritis with cyclosporine and methotrexate for forty-eight weeks: an open-label extension study. The Meth-

otrexate-Cyclosporine Combination Study Group. Arthritis Rheum 40: 1843–1851, 1997.
646. Ferraz MB, Pinheiro T, Helfenstein M, et al: Combination therapy with methotrexate and chloroquine in rheumatoid arthritis. A multicenter randomized placebo-controlled trial. Scand J Rheumatol 23: 231–236, 1994.
647. Maini RN, Breedveld FC, Kalden JR, et al: Therapeutic efficacy of multiple intravenous infusions of anti-tumor necrosis factor alpha monoclonal antibody combined with low-dose weekly methotrexate in rheumatoid arthritis. Arthritis Rheum 41: 1552–1563, 1998.
648. Weinblatt ME, Kremer JM, Bankhurst AD, et al: A trial of etanercept, a recombinant tumor necrosis factor receptor: Fc fusion protein, in patients with rheumatoid arthritis receiving methotrexate. N Engl J Med 340: 253–259, 1999.
649. Wallace CA, Sherry DD: Trial of intravenous pulse cyclophosphamide and methylprednisolone in the treatment of severe systemic-onset juvenile rheumatoid arthritis. Arthritis Rheum 40: 1852–1855, 1997.
650. Birdi N, Allen U, D'Astous J: Poststreptococcal reactive arthritis mimicking acute septic arthritis: a hospital-based study. J Pediatr Orthop 15: 661–665, 1995.
651. Fink CW: The role of the streptococcus in poststreptococcal reactive arthritis and childhood polyarteritis nodosa. J Rheumatol Suppl 29: 14–20, 1991.
652. Stegeman CA, Tervaert JWC, de Jong PE, Kallenberg CGM: Trimethoprim-sulfamethoxazole (co-trimoxazole) for the prevention of relapses of Wegener's granulomatosis. N Engl J Med 335: 16–20, 1996.
653. Tilley BC, Alarcon GS, Heyse SP, et al: Minocycline in rheumatoid arthritis. A 48-week, double-blind, placebo-controlled trial. MIRA Trial Group. Ann Intern Med 122: 81–89, 1995.
654. Langevitz P, Bank I, Zemer D, et al: Treatment of resistant rheumatoid arthritis with minocycline: an open study. J Rheumatol 19: 1502–1504, 1992.
655. O'Dell JR, Haire CE, Palmer W, et al: Treatment of early rheumatoid arthritis with minocycline or placebo: results of a randomized, double-blind, placebo-controlled trial. Arthritis Rheum 40: 842–848, 1997.
656. Sieper J, Braun J: Treatment of reactive arthritis with antibiotics. Br J Rheumatol 37: 717–720, 1998.
657. Lang BA, Laxer RM, Murphy G, et al: Treatment of dermatomyositis with intravenous gammaglobulin. Am J Med 91: 169–172, 1991.
658. Uziel Y, Laxer RM, Schneider R, Silverman ED: Intravenous immunoglobulin therapy in systemic onset juvenile rheumatoid arthritis: a followup study. J Rheumatol 23: 910–918, 1996.
659. Silverman ED, Cawkwell GD, Lovell DJ, et al: Intravenous immunoglobulin in the treatment of systemic juvenile rheumatoid arthritis: a randomized placebo controlled trial. Pediatr Rheumatol Collaborative Study Group. J Rheumatol 21: 2353–2358, 1994.
660. Giannini EH, Lovell DJ, Silverman ED, et al: Intravenous immunoglobulin in the treatment of polyarticular juvenile rheumatoid arthritis: a phase I/II study. Pediatr Rheumatol Collaborative Study Group. J Rheumatol 23: 919–924, 1996.
661. Duhem C, Dicato MA, Ries F: Side-effects of intravenous immune globulins. Clin Exp Immunol 97(Suppl 1): 79–83, 1994.
662. Nydegger UE, Blaser K, Hassig A: Anti-idiotypic immunosuppression and its treatment with human immunoglobulin preparations. Vox Sang 47: 92, 1984.
663. Hahn BH, Ebling FM: Suppression of murine lupus nephritis by administration of an anti-idiotypic antibody to anti-DNA. J Immunol 132: 1887, 1984.
664. Svenson M, Hansen MB, Bendtzen K: Distribution and characterization of autoantibodies to interleukin 1 alpha in normal human sera. Scand J Immunol 32: 695, 1990.
665. Hansen M, Svenson M, Diamant M, Bendtzen K: Anti-interleukin-6 antibodies in normal human serum. Scand J Immunol 33: 777, 1991.
666. Fomsgaard A, Svenson M, Bendtzen K: Autoantibodies to tumour necrosis factor alpha in healthy humans and patients with inflammatory disease and gram-negative bacterial infections. Scand J Immunol 30: 219, 1989.
667. Ross C, Hansen MB, Schyberg T, Berg K: Autoantibodies to crude human leukocyte IFN, recombinant IFN-alpha 2b, and human IFN gamma in healthy blood donors. Clin Exp Immunol 8: 57, 1990.
668. Saulsbury FT: The effect of intravenous immunoglobulin on lymphocyte populations and activation markers in Kawasaki syndrome. Arthritis Rheum 34: S121, 1991.
669. Takei S, Arora YK, Walker SM: Intravenous immunoglobulin contains specific antibodies inhibitory to activation of T cells by staphylococcal toxin superantigens. J Clin Invest 91: 602–607, 1993.
670. Dalakas MC, Illa I, Dambrosia JM, et al: A controlled trial of high-dose intravenous immune globulin infusions as treatment for dermatomyositis. N Engl J Med 329: 1993–2000, 1993.
671. Wallis WJ, Furst DE, Strand V, Keystone E: Biologic agents and immunotherapy in rheumatoid arthritis. Progress and perspective. Rheum Dis Clin North Am 24: 537–565, 1998.
672. Weiner HL, Friedman A, Miller A, et al: Oral tolerance: immunologic mechanisms and treatment of animal and human organ-specific autoimmune diseases by oral administration of autoantigens. Annu Rev Immunol 12: 809–837, 1994.
673. Trentham DE, Dynesius-Trentham RA, Orav EJ, et al: Effects of oral administration of type II collagen on rheumatoid arthritis. Science 261: 1727–1730, 1993.
674. Barnett ML, Kremer JM, St Clair EW, et al: Results of a multicenter, double-blind, placebo-controlled trial. Arthritis Rheum 41: 290–297, 1998.
675. Barnett ML, Combitchi D, Trentham DE: A pilot trial of oral type II collagen in the treatment of juvenile rheumatoid arthritis. Arthritis Rheum 39: 623–628, 1996.
676. Moreland LW, Baumgartner SW, Schiff MH, et al: Treatment of rheumatoid arthritis with a recombinant human tumor necrosis factor receptor (p75)-Fc fusion protein. N Engl J Med 337: 141–147, 1997.
677. Thompson SD, Murray KJ, Grom AA, et al: Comparative sequence analysis of the human T cell receptor β chain in juvenile rheumatoid arthritis and juvenile spondylarthropathies: evidence for antigenic selection of T cells in the synovium. Arthritis Rheum 41: 482–497, 1998.
678. Kirkham BW, Pitzalis C, Kingsley GH, et al: Monoclonal antibody treatment in rheumatoid arthritis: the clinical and immunological effects of a CD7 monoclonal antibody. Br J Rheumatol 30: 459–463, 1991.
679. Kirkham BW, Thien F, Pelton BK, et al: Chimeric CD7 monoclonal antibody therapy in rheumatoid arthritis. J Rheumatol 19: 1348–1352, 1992.
680. Olsen NJ, Brooks RH, Cush JJ, et al: A double-blind, placebo-controlled study of anti-CD5 immunoconjugate in patients with rheumatoid arthritis. The Xoma RA Investigator Group. Arthritis Rheum 39: 1102–1108, 1996.
681. Isaacs JD, Watts RA, Hazelman BL, et al: Humanised monoclonal antibody therapy for rheumatoid arthritis. Lancet 340: 748–752, 1992.
682. Isaacs JD, Manna VK, Rapson N, et al: CAMPATH-1H in rheumatoid arthritis—an intravenous dose-ranging study. Br J Rheumatol 35: 231–240, 1996.
683. Choy EH, Chicanza IC, Kingsley GH, et al: Treatment of rheumatoid arthritis with single dose or weekly pulses of chimaeric anti-CD4 monoclonal antibody. Scand J Immunol 36: 291–298, 1992.
684. Choy EH, Pitzalis C, Cauli A, et al: Percentage of anti-CD4 monoclonal antibody-coated lymphocytes in the rheumatoid joint is associated with clinical improvement. Implications for the development of immunotherapeutic dosing regimens. Arthritis Rheum 39: 52–56, 1996.
685. Choy EH, Kingsley GH, Panayi GS: Monoclonal antibody therapy in rheumatoid arthritis. Br J Rheumatol 37: 484–490, 1998.
686. Levy R, Weisman M, Wiesenhutter C, et al: Results of a placebo-controlled multicenter trial using a Primitized nondepleting anti-CD4 monoclonal antibody in the treatment of rheumatoid arthritis. Arthritis Rheum 39: S122, 1996.
687. Durie FH, Fava RA, Foy TM, et al: Prevention of collagen-induced arthritis with an antibody to gp39, the ligand for CD40. Science 261: 1328–1330, 1993.
688. Webb LM, Walmsley MJ, Feldmann M: Prevention and amelioration of collagen-induced arthritis by blockade of the CD28 co-

stimulatory pathway: requirement for both B7-1 and B7-2. Eur J Immunol 26: 2320–2328, 1996.
689. Kavanaugh AF, Davis LS, Nichols LA, et al: Treatment of refractory rheumatoid arthritis with a monoclonal antibody to intercellular adhesion molecule 1. Arthritis Rheum 37: 992–999, 1994.
690. Kavanaugh AF, Schulze-Koops S, Davis LS, Lipsky PE: Repeat treatment of rheumatoid arthritis patients with a murine anti-intercellular adhesion molecule 1 monoclonal antibody. Arthritis Rheum 40: 849–853, 1997.
691. De Benedetti F, Ravelli A, Martini A: Cytokines in juvenile rheumatoid arthritis. Curr Opin Rheumatol 9: 428–433, 1997.
692. Muller K, Herner EB, Stagg A, et al: Inflammatory cytokines and cytokine antagonists in whole blood cultures of patients with systemic juvenile chronic arthritis. Br J Rheumatol 37: 562–569, 1998.
693. Mangge H, Schauenstein K: Cytokines in juvenile rheumatoid arthritis (JRA). Cytokine 10: 471–480, 1998.
694. Elliott MJ, Maini RN, Feldmann M, et al: Randomised double-blind comparison of chimeric monoclonal antibody to tumour necrosis factor alpha (cA2) versus placebo in rheumatoid arthritis. Lancet 344: 1105–1110, 1994.
695. Elliott MJ, Maini RN, Feldmann M, et al: Repeated therapy with monoclonal antibody to tumour necrosis factor alpha (cA2) in patients with rheumatoid arthritis. Lancet 344: 1125–1127, 1994.
696. Elliott MJ, Woo P, Charles P, et al: Suppression of fever and the acute-phase response in a patient with juvenile chronic arthritis treated with monoclonal antibody to tumour necrosis factor-alpha (cA2). Br J Rheumatol 36: 589–593, 1997.
697. Kavanaugh AF: Anti-tumor necrosis factor-alpha monoclonal antibody therapy. Rheum Dis Clin North Am 24: 593–614, 1998.
698. Lovell DJ, Giannini EH, Reiff A, et al: Etanercept in children with polyarticular juvenile rheumatoid arthritis. Pediatric Rheumatology Collaborative Study Group. N Engl J Med 16: 763–769, 2000.
699. Tomita T, Takeuchi E, Tomita N, et al: In vivo transfection of NF-KB decoy reduced severity of rat collagen-induced arthritis as a gene therapy. Arthritis Rheum 40: S220, 1997.
700. Nakajima T, Aono H, Hasunuma T, et al: Apoptosis and functional Fas antigen in rheumatoid arthritis synoviocytes. Arthritis Rheum 38: 485–491, 1995.
701. Ghivizzani SC, Kang R, Muzzonigro T, et al: Gene therapy for arthritis—treatment of the first three patients. Arthritis Rheum 40: S223, 1997.
702. van Bekkum DW, Bohre EP, Houben PF, Knaan-Shanzer S: Regression of adjuvant-induced arthritis in rats following bone marrow transplantation. Proc Natl Acad Sci U S A 86: 10090–10094, 1989.
703. Knaan-Shanzer S, Houben PF, Kinwel-Bohre EP, van Bekkum DW: Remission induction of adjuvant arthritis in rats by total body irradiation and autologous bone marrow transplantation. Bone Marrow Transplant 8: 333–338, 1991.
704. McKendry RJ, Huebsch L, Leclair B: Progression of rheumatoid arthritis following bone marrow transplantation. A case report with a 13-year followup. Arthritis Rheum 39: 1246–1253, 1996.
705. Snowden JA, Kearney P, Kearney A, et al: Long-term outcome of autoimmune disease following allogeneic bone marrow transplantation. Arthritis Rheum 41: 453–459, 1998.
706. Euler HH, Marmont AM, Bacigalupo A, et al: Early recurrence or persistence of autoimmune diseases after unmanipulated autologous stem cell transplantation. Blood 88: 3621–3625, 1996.
707. Wulffraat N, van Royen A, Bierings M, et al: Autologous haemopoietic stem-cell transplantation in four patients with refractory juvenile chronic arthritis. Lancet 353: 550–553, 1999.
708. Martini A, Maccario R, Ravelli A, et al: Marked and sustained improvement two years after autologous stem cell transplantation in a girl with systemic sclerosis. Arthritis Rheum 42: 807–811, 1999.
709. Brodsky RA, Sensenbrenner LL, Jones RJ: Complete remission in severe aplastic anemia after high-dose cyclophosphamide without bone marrow transplantation. Blood 87: 491–494, 1996.
710. Schneider R, Lang BA, Reilly BJ, et al: Prognostic indicators of joint destruction in systemic-onset juvenile rheumatoid arthritis. J Pediatr 120: 200–205, 1992.

8

Design, Measurement, and Analysis of Clinical Investigations

Edward H. Giannini

EVIDENCE-BASED MEDICINE AND CLINICAL INVESTIGATION

Today, more than ever, the clinician is encouraged to practice "evidenced-based medicine." That is, the practitioner must be able to access, summarize, and apply information from the literature to day-to-day clinical problems.[1, 1a] But how strong should the evidence be before a clinician modifies his or her practice because of new data in a clinical research report? The same question can be asked of any clinical or biomedical research report whether or not it applies to clinical practice. The strength of evidence depends on many factors, including the rigor of the study design, the selection of patients and appropriate controls, the rigorousness with which the data were gathered, and the appropriateness with which the data were analyzed, interpreted, and reported. In addition, the similarity between the study patients and the patients seen by the particular clinician is of utmost importance in determining the relevance of a study. The reader must be able to judge the quality of the work in order to determine its overall validity and the acceptability of the conclusions. The mere fact that the work has been published (even in a reputable journal) may not be enough of a yardstick whereby one decides that the work is of superior quality. Outstanding "users' guides to the medical literature" have now been published, and the reader is encouraged to supplement the discussion in this chapter with the appropriate guide for a specific topic.[2–21]

This chapter provides readers with enough clinical, epidemiologic, and biostatistical skills to assess the literature critically to determine the "strength of the evidence" independently (i.e., to become more proficient at the practice of evidence-based medicine) and promotes basic skills that will facilitate the design, undertaking, and reporting of clinical research. Although this chapter emphasizes clinical research, many of the concepts discussed here *are easily translated to the realm of basic science*. "Whether it be mice or men," one must understand the basic concepts of, for example, frequency distributions and statistical inferences.

DEFINITION OF CLINICAL RESEARCH

Academicians have argued for years about exactly what is incorporated in the concept of clinical research. The Nathan Report (*www.nih.gov/news/crp/97report/index.htm*) defines clinical research as epidemiologic and behavioral studies, outcomes research and health services research, and patient-oriented research. Research conducted with human subjects (or on material of human origin such as tissues, specimens, and cognitive phenomena) for which an investigator (or colleague) directly interacts with human subjects also qualifies as clinical research. This area of research includes mechanisms of human disease, therapeutic interventions, clinical trials, and development of new technologies. Excluded from this definition are in vitro studies that utilize human tissues but do not deal directly with patients. This definition, however, does not exclude laboratory or *translational* research ("bench-to-bedside"), provided that the identity of the patients from whom the cells or tissues under study are derived is known.

GENERAL TERMINOLOGY AND BASIC CONCEPTS ASSOCIATED WITH CLINICAL STUDIES

To be conversant in clinical study designs and methodology, one needs a working knowledge of the vocabulary and basic concepts relevant to the various approaches. Readers must attempt to *generalize the usage* of common terms from one type of study to the next. For example, "exposure" may mean that the subject was exposed to cigarette smoke in a retrospective case-comparison study, exposed to a drug in a clinical trial, or exposed to human leukocyte antigen (HLA)-B27 in a genetic study.

All clinical investigations may be divided broadly into observational or experimental. In *observational studies,* there is no artificial manipulation of any factor that is to be assessed in the study, nor is there active manipulation of the patient. In observational studies, the subjects have received the "etiologic" agent by mechanisms other than active assignment or randomization. This may include self-imposed exposure (personal habits or nutritional patterns), prescription by a physician, atmospheric pollutants, or occupational toxins. Observational studies may be either retrospective or prospective. *Retrospective* implies that the data already exist and are retrieved using a systematic approach, but missing data are not retrievable. In *prospective* observational studies, a cohort is followed prospectively through time and data are gathered on an ongoing basis. In this case, missing data may possibly be retrieved for purposes of the study.

Experimental studies imply that the experimenter artificially manipulated some study factor—subjects, therapeutic regimen, or some other parameter. In experimental studies, the subjects are followed prospectively, some artificial manipulation is conducted, and the results of this manipulation are then observed.

Meta-analysis is an approach whereby the quantitative evidence from two or more studies bearing on the same question is statistically combined. Usually, the summary statistics rather than the raw data from the various studies are combined. Meta-analysis may be considered a form of a retrospective experimental study in that the data already exist and were gathered during prospective experimental studies.

Hypothesis-Generating Versus Hypothesis-Testing Studies

The design of a clinical investigation depends on whether the study intends to *generate hypotheses* to be tested in future studies or to *test specific hypotheses* for which the investigator has some existing evidence to support the belief that they are true or not true. *Hypothesis-generating studies* are considered *exploratory*; those designed as tests of hypotheses may be called *pivotal* or *confirmatory* studies. A single study may have both confirmatory and exploratory aspects.

Each type of study has distinct advantages and disadvantages. The design chosen is always deeply influenced by reality—what is economically, logistically, ethically, and scientifically possible. A common exercise used by epidemiologists is to design the best theoretical experiment to answer the question being posed—without regard to time, money, ethics, patient availability, or anything else that could cause a lessening in the quality of the study. (A related approach is known as the "infinite data set."[22]) Then, realizing that there is no such thing as the perfect clinical study, the designer eliminates the most unrealistic "requirement" (e.g., it is not likely one can enroll 300 patients with scleroderma who will agree to the possibility of being randomized to placebo for a year). The study is compromised further and further by reality until one arrives at what can be done in consideration of all the issues. If what one ends up with is unacceptable scientifically, perhaps the question cannot (and should not) be answered. The decision to pursue or not pursue the "compromised" study, based in reality, is one of the most difficult in the entire research process.

Main Objectives, Process Objectives, Hypotheses, and Long-Term Goals

The first challenge after identifying a clinical question to be addressed is to clearly establish *main* (or *primary*) and *secondary objectives*. Objectives are statements as to what the investigators plan to learn or accomplish by conducting the study. *Process objectives* then follow the main objectives and are the procedures that must be completed in order to meet the main objectives.

Hypotheses are then developed and are formal statements that declare what the investigator will test and then either reject or fail to reject. As discussed earlier, exploratory (hypothesis-generating) studies may not state hypotheses a priori. Such studies frequently allow the data to drive the hypotheses to be tested in the data-exploration phase.

Finally, longer-term goals are stated that often are to be met only after the main objectives of the current projects are complete; they frequently give a hint as to what future direction the research may take.

Clinical research proposals often misstate hypotheses and mix main objectives (specific aims) with process objectives or longer-term goals. The following example may assist the reader in formulating each of these elements of a research proposal. Suppose the question is, "Does the selective cyclooxygenase-2 inhibitor, celecoxib, produce fewer gastrointestinal (GI) adverse effects in children with juvenile rheumatoid arthritis (JRA) than does naproxen when each drug is given in anti-inflammatory doses for a period of up to 3 months?"

The objectives are typically written nonjudgmentally and are more informal in their language than the hypotheses. A primary objective could be, "To determine the incidence of GI adverse drug events among patients with JRA treated for up to 3 months with celecoxib compared with those treated with naproxen." Equally acceptable (but less distinguishing from the statement of hypothesis) is, "To test the hypothesis that celecoxib produces fewer GI adverse drug effects than does naproxen in children with JRA." A secondary objective could be, "To determine the incidence of GI events requiring pharmacologic intervention in the two groups and compare the differences." The main objective is not, for example, "To enroll 250 patients with JRA in a clinical trial in which half are randomized to celecoxib and half to naproxen." That is a process objective—one of the necessary steps that will be carried out to meet the main objective. Even large studies typically have only one or two main objectives and accompanying hypotheses.

The usual *null hypothesis* (abbreviated H_o) is that the treatments are not different with regard to the primary outcome. H_o can be stated as, "There is no difference in the incidence of GI adverse drug effects among patients treated with naproxen compared with those treated with celecoxib." The *alternative hypothesis* (abbreviated H_a) is, "There is a difference in the incidence of GI adverse drug effects. . . ." As stated, H_a does not specify whether there are more or fewer GI effects with celecoxib. This is a *2-tailed hypothesis.* One could have used a *1-tailed hypothesis* by stating, "Patients with juvenile rheumatoid arthritis (JRA) treated with celecoxib will have a lower incidence of GI adverse drug effects than those treated with naproxen." But statisticians point out that this hypothesis sounds as if one isn't interested in testing to see whether celecoxib produces more GI effects, just less. For this reason, the usual approach is to use 2-tailed hypotheses, at least in early studies when the direction of the difference is not known, if there is a difference. The choice of a 1-tailed as opposed to a 2-tailed hypothesis influences the statistical interpretation of the data, as discussed later. A *secondary null hypothesis* in this example might be, "There is no difference in the incidence of GI adverse drug events that require pharmacologic intervention among patients with JRA treated with celecoxib compared with those treated with naproxen."

Finally, the *longer-term goal* is not, "To complete the study in a 5-year time frame," but, "To provide safer and more effective anti-inflammatory medications to children with JRA."

EPIDEMIOLOGIC AND BEHAVIORAL STUDIES

Clinical epidemiology is a medical science that studies the distribution and determinants of disease frequency in human populations in order to understand why some people contract a disease and others do not. Epidemiology combined with biostatistics makes up the basic tools of the clinical investigator. Epidemiologic methods can be used to answer questions in the following categories.

Descriptive Epidemiology

Studies in descriptive epidemiology typically concern themselves with patterns of disease occurrence with respect to person, place, or time. Descriptive epidemiologic studies serve as hypothesis-generating studies for studies of causation much the same way as small exploratory clinical trials serve as preliminary studies for therapeutic confirmatory trials. The *person* variable is concerned with who experiences the disease. A basic tenet is that the disease does not occur at random and is more likely to develop in some people than in others. Personal factors of potential importance include age, sex, race, ethnicity, socioeconomic status, existing morbidity, health habits, and genetics. The *place* factor is concerned with where the disease develops. Variation in the place of occurrence can be evaluated at the local, regional, or international levels. The *time* variable is concerned with the variation of the occurrence of disease in time and its seasonality or periodicity.

A hypothetical example of a descriptive epidemiologic study is the investigation of a group of workers in a factory who experience what is suspected of being environmentally acquired lupus. The epidemiologist would investigate the detailed characteristics of the workers to determine whether there are patterns among those who do and do not experience lupus. Do all types of workers—management through hourly manufacturing employees—demonstrate the same rates of disease development? Are persons living close to the factory or its effluent also affected? Systematic investigation of the patterns of disease allows a more precise hypothesis of causation, particularly if some exposure or dose level is found to be more strongly associated with the illness.

Frequency of Disease Occurrence

The frequency of disease occurrence is an important aspect of understanding a disease process. This can be measured in a number of ways. *Prevalence* is the number of existing cases in a defined population. Mathematically, prevalence is equal to the number of existing cases divided by the number of persons in the population. It is expressed in different ways: a proportion (0 to 1), a percent (0 to 100), or by actual numbers using a convenient denominator (1 case per 1000 children).

Point prevalence is the number of new and old cases in a defined population at a given "instant" in time. For example, hospital epidemiologists are frequently asked to estimate the point prevalence of nosocomial infections among current inpatients. The epidemiologist then counts all the confirmed and suspected cases of hospital-acquired infections within the hospital on a given day and divides this by the census for that day to obtain the point prevalence.

Period prevalence is the number of new and old cases that exist in a defined population during a given time period (e.g., 1 year).

Incidence is the rate at which newly diagnosed cases develop over time in a population. Mathematically, incidence is equal to the number of new cases divided by the persons at risk in the population multiplied by the time of observation. This rate is expressed in units of *cases/person-time*. Incidence is related to the concept of *risk*, defined as the proportion of unaffected individuals who will, on average, contract the disease over a specific period of time. Therefore, risk is equal to the new cases divided by the persons at risk. Risk has no units and can have values between 0 (no new occurrences) and 1—the entire population becomes affected during the risk period. Epidemiologic theory states that incidence is best estimated from prospective studies; prevalence may be calculated by prospective or retrospective approaches.

Etiology of Disease

In his presidential address to the Royal Society of Medicine in January of 1965, Sir Austin Bradford Hill gave his now famous oration entitled "The Environment and Disease: Association or Causation."[23] In it, he described what have become known as *Koch's postulates for epidemiologists*. That is, what evidence must be present to establish a factor as being causally linked to a disease. These include the following:

- *Strength of the association*. How strong is the association between the factor and the outcome? For example, how significant is the *P* value of the association between dietary intake of calcium and bone mineral density among children with JRA.
- *Consistency of the association*. Does the association between factor and disease persist from one study to the next, even if variations in study design and samples of patients vary substantially?
- *Specificity of the association*. Is the association limited, for example, to specific alleles and to types of disease, with little association between the alleles and other diseases? (As the study of causation, including genetic risk, has advanced, the issue of specificity is considered less important than it once was.)
- *Temporal correctness*. Did the exposure to the factor occur prior to the disease?
- *Biologic gradient*. Is there a dose-response between factor and disease? For example, does increasing the dose or time of exposure to cyclophosphamide result in a consequent increase in frequency of malignancy?
- *Biologic plausibility*. Does the association make sense with what is currently understood about the disease and its pathogenesis?
- *Experiment*. Does the association hold up under experimental conditions? For example, if one reduces the dose or time of exposure to cyclophosphamide, is there a corresponding decrease in the frequency of malignancy?

No one study proves indisputably that any potential etiologic factor causes the disease, complication, or adverse event. It is the accumulating body of knowledge concerning factor and disease, or (to generalize the terms) treatment and outcome, that finally allows the medical community to state that evidence is sufficient to prove a causal link between the two.

An important concept in the study of disease etiology is that of *relative risk*. The relative risk (*risk ratio*) can be defined as the risk of one group (e.g., boys) compared with another group (girls) to develop a disease. Relative risk can range from zero to infinity and has no units. A relative risk of 1 means that there is no difference in risk between the groups. A relative risk greater than 1 means increased risk, and a relative risk less than 1 indicates decreased risk (protection). In pediatric rheumatology, the concept of risk is used frequently to specify increased or decreased risk of disease associated with certain genetic markers.

Table 8–1 presents terms that are relevant to risk and shows how each may be calculated using a 2 × 2 contingency table. Disease state (present or absent) is considered the dependent variable and is usually placed in the columns (x axis). The risk factor (positive or negative) is considered the independent variable and is usually placed in the rows (y axis). Notice that relative risk is calculated differently than the *odds ratio*, although in medicine the two are frequently used synonymously. More correctly, however, relative risk is calculated from incidence studies, whereas odds ratios are calculated from retrospective studies.

Epidemiologic Study Designs Aimed at the Establishment of Associations and Cause-Effect Relationships

The Case-Controlled Retrospective Study

One of the most common types of study designs used to establish an association or cause and effect is the *observational case-controlled, retrospective study*. (The term *case-comparison* is now frequently used because the studies are not controlled in the usual sense.) In this situation, patients who have the disease are compared with those who do not, and data documenting prior

Table 8–1
Terms Associated With Risk Factors and Disease

	DISEASE	
RISK FACTOR	**Present**	**Absent**
Positive	a	b
Negative	c	d

The 2 × 2 table may be used for calculating associations between a risk factor and a disease.

Incidence:	The number of new cases among those at risk. Calculate as: a + c / a + b + c + d.
Absolute risk:	Synonymous with incidence.
Attributable risk:	Incidence among those with the risk factor minus incidence among those without the risk factor. Calculate as: a / a + b minus c / c + d. (This is sometimes expressed as a percentage of the incidence rate among those with the risk factor.)
Relative risk:	Incidence among those exposed ÷ incidence among those not exposed. Calculate as: (a / a + b) ÷ (c / c + d).
Odds ratio:	An approximation to the relative risk used in retrospective studies. Calculate as: (a)(d) / (b)(c).
Case exposure rate:	Among those with the disease, what proportion had the risk factor. Calculate as: a / a + c.
Control exposure rate:	Among those without the disease, what proportion had the risk factor. Calculate as: b / b + d.

exposure to some agent are ascertained retrospectively. The most frequent statistic to come from this type of study is the odds ratio (see Table 8–1). The odds ratio is a fairly good estimate of the relative risk, provided the disease is rare. Patients included in the study are often identified from a search of medical records or a disease registry. However, there are no standard guidelines for selection of control subjects. Control subjects may be hospitalized patients with conditions other than the disease of interest, residential neighbors, a probability sample of the general population, or a combination of these. Advantages of case-controlled studies include efficiency, low cost, quick results, and low risk to study subjects.

The disadvantages of the case-controlled study are several, however. The temporal relationship of exposure and disease may be obscured. Historical information may be incomplete or inaccurate; a detailed study of mechanisms of disease is often not possible; and if the study is not well done, results may be biased.

The Prospective Cohort Study

The observational approach that most closely resembles an experiment is the *prospective cohort study*. In this case, a population is defined from which the sample is drawn. Exposure to some factor is then established and subjects are categorized as having been either "exposed" or "not exposed" to a factor thought to contribute risk of some outcome. Each of the two cohorts is followed prospectively to observe whether the outcome develops. Relative risk is the statistic most commonly used in describing this study. The identification of exposed persons presents several problems. The first is to correctly identify the exposed persons and measure the degree of exposure. This may be done by selecting subjects with some type of unusual occupational or environmental exposure. Another method is selecting those who are available and suitable for the needed investigation or selecting those who offer some special resource that facilitates the study, such as members of a health plan, or a combination of all these factors.

The advantages of a prospective observational cohort study are that a clear temporal relationship between exposure and disease is established, and the study may yield information about the length of induction (incubation) of the disease. Relative risk can be estimated directly. The design facilitates the study for rare exposures (but not rare diseases) and allows calculation of rates of disease occurrence.

The disadvantages of cohort studies may include the potential for loss to follow-up or alteration of behavior because of the long follow-up time that may be necessary. Cohort studies are not particularly good for rare diseases, and they may be very expensive. Detailed studies of the mechanisms of the disease are typically not possible in cohort studies.

A rheumatologic example of a cohort study is the study by Inman and associates,[24] who prospectively followed a cohort of persons "exposed" to *Salmonella typhimurium* infection to determine whether reactive arthritis developed.

Diagnosis of Disease

The diagnosis of disease as it applies to epidemiology refers to the *performance of screening and diagnostic tests* used in populations rather than the process of differential diagnosis of individual patients.

Validity of a Diagnostic or Screening Test

The validity of a diagnostic or screening test involves a variety of parameters, as shown in Table 8–2. The table is constructed with the presence or absence of

Table 8–2
Estimating the Validity of a Diagnostic Test

TEST RESULTS	DISEASE: Present	DISEASE: Absent
Positive	True positives (TP)	False positives (FP)
Negative	False negatives (FN)	True negatives (TN)

Sensitivity:	The proportion (or percentage) of diseased persons who test positive. Calculate as: TP / TP + FN.
Specificity:	The proportion (or percentage) of non-diseased persons who test negative. Calculate as: TN / TN + FP.
Positive Predictive Value:	The proportion (or percentage) of persons who test positive who are diseased. Calculate as: TP / TP + FP.
False-Positive Rate:	The proportion (or percentage) of persons who test positive who are not diseased. Calculate as: FP / TP + FP.
Negative Predictive Value:	The proportion (or percentage) of persons who test negative who are not diseased. Calculate as: TN / TN + FN.
False-Negative Rate:	The proportion (or percentage) of persons who test negative who are diseased. Calculate as: FN / TN + FN.
Reliability (Related term) (sometimes called reproducibility):	The ability of a test to yield the same result on retesting.

disease as the column labels (i.e., x axis), whereas the test results are typically the row values (i.e., dependent variable being shown on the y axis). Those patients in row 1, column 1 are called *true positives*, those in row 1, column 2 are *false positives*, those in row 2, column 1 are *false negatives*, and those in row 2, column 2 are *true negatives. Sensitivity, specificity, positive* and *negative predictive* values, *false-positive* and *false-negative* rates, and *reliability* are terms used to describe the validity of a screening test.

Prognosis of Disease

Prognosis refers to the possible outcomes of a disease and the frequency with which they can be expected to occur. Prognostic factors need not cause the outcome but merely be associated with an outcome strongly enough to predict it. Prognosis is somewhat narrower in focus and more short-term than those consequences of disease and treatment considered in the field of *outcomes research*. For example, the six most frequently measured outcomes in outcomes research are known as the 6 Ds: *death, disease, disability, discomfort, dissatisfaction*, and *dollars*. Many studies of prognosis are cohort studies that prospectively follow large numbers of patients to determine eventual clinical events and then look for certain prognostic factors for the events. At present and in the past, the estimation of prognosis has largely concentrated on clinical variables. Studies of prognosis in JRA, for example, have included the sex of the patient, the age at onset, and a variety of clinical and laboratory variables to estimate outcome.[25–28]

Genetics is being investigated more intensely to delineate its ability to predict outcome. At this writing, pharmacogenetics is just becoming a household word. It is likely that, in the future, much of the determination of outcome will be based on genetic screening for various genetic markers that will be able to predict whether individuals will respond to a particular therapy, whether they will experience an adverse drug effect, and whether their quality of life will be improved after a particular treatment.

Treatment of Disease

For special emphasis, this chapter considers clinical trials separately from epidemiologic studies (see "Clinical Trials—Useful Guidelines").

Behavioral Studies

The National Institutes of Health (NIH) considers behavioral studies as a category of clinical research. This class of studies is not considered here.

OUTCOMES AND HEALTH SERVICES RESEARCH

The terms *clinical effectiveness* and *health services research* are closely related to outcomes research and are considered synonymous here. Outcomes research may be defined as the study of effectiveness, cost effectiveness, and quality of healthcare. The interest in outcomes research has been generated by a more cost-conscious healthcare system. For example, only 10 to 20 percent of medical procedures have been evaluated through randomized controlled trials. Both established and new technologies can be ineffective. Certainly, the outcomes researcher must rely on much evidence-based medicine present in the literature as well as new studies. Outcomes researchers often use randomized controlled trial designs, prospective cohorts, retrospective cohorts, and case-control studies (described later). Chart reviews are frequently used, as are administrative data including local hospital discharge data, insurance claims, and national health survey information. In addition, meta-analysis, decision analysis, and cost-effectiveness analysis are typical study designs employed by the outcomes researcher. There are few reports of "true" outcomes research related to pediatric rheumatology. There are excellent guides for evaluating outcomes research.[13–18]

Decision Analysis

Decision analysis may employ all of the techniques mentioned in the previous section and therefore is discussed in greater detail here. Decision analysis is an analytical formulation of a decision in which uncertainty exists. It incorporates probability of events as well as values for the consequences of action. It is decision oriented (not truth oriented), it is prescriptive (not descriptive), and it enhances, but does not replace, clinical judgment. The premises of decision analysis are that decisions must be made, the consequences of actions are uncertain, the consequences of action include both favorable and unfavorable effects, and healthcare resources are constrained. Decision analysis should enhance the ability to make rational decisions that lead to optimal therapeutic outcomes. Often, the principles of decision-making are obscured by substitution of established protocols. "Decision trees" should not be confused with flow charts presented in clinical practice guidelines for the management of particular diseases such as rheumatoid arthritis (RA)[29] or JRA.[30] The decision trees tend to be more complicated, more branched, and more speculative than flow charts.

Elements of a decision analysis are as follows. Choices are outlined, and the method to assess the overall value of the outcome of each choice is determined. The underlying assumptions are that there is uncertainty about the future and that we value various possible outcomes differently. A decision tree is then constructed. Decision analysis itself includes outlining the problem, laying out the options and possible outcomes in explicit detail, assessing the probabilities and values of each outcome, and selecting the "best choice." In summary, the *elements of decision analysis include choices, outcomes, and utilities.*

The areas of outcome research and decision analysis are in their infancy in pediatric rheumatology. Each should offer a fruitful field for investigators for many years to come because many different "standards of care" exist for most diagnoses that are included under the realm of pediatric rheumatology. Two excellent guides for judging the quality of decision analysis studies are those by Richardson and Detsky.[11, 12]

PATIENT-ORIENTED RESEARCH

The NIH definition of clinical research groups four categories of investigation under the major heading of *patient-oriented research*: mechanisms of human disease, therapeutic interventions, clinical trials, and development of new technologies. This chapter emphasizes clinical trial classification and methods. However, many of the concepts and much of the terminology presented herein can be generalized to the conduct of clinical studies in any of these four areas of clinical research.

Clinical Trials—Useful Guidelines

For simplicity, the generic term *drug* is used in the following discussions. It should be considered synonymous with any medicinal product, vaccine, or biological. The principles discussed can also apply to interventional procedures such as surgery and radiotherapy. Clinical epidemiologists are frequently concerned with evaluating the effectiveness and safety of new therapies.

Numerous useful guidance documents (distinguish from guidelines) are now in the literature. and should be consulted for a more detailed explanation of the principles outlined here. Of particular relevance to the pediatric rheumatologist is the recently available *Guidance for Industry: Clinical Development Programs for Drugs, Devices and Biological Products for the Treatment of Rheumatoid Arthritis*,[31] published in the Federal Register in February 1999[32] (*www.fda.gov/cder/guidance*). This guidance document summarizes the position of the U.S. Food and Drug Administration (FDA) as to what clinical development programs should consist of, and it provides a framework for conducting studies used to obtain regulatory agency approval for a therapy for RA or JRA.

An extremely useful set of guidance documents also available through the FDA's website is the *International Conference on Harmonisation (ICH) of Technical Requirements for Registration of Pharmaceuticals for Human Use*. These documents contain valuable guidance for industry and the clinical investigator as well as definitions of terms related to overall clinical development programs, considerations for individual trials, statistical methods and reporting, and a variety of other topics. The ICH guidance documents seek to establish harmonization of clinical trials in various regions throughout the world. As such, acceptance of the guidance documents is very broad. It is strongly recommended that the designer or reader of clinical trials be familiar with their content.

Particularly relevant ICH documents that are available via the Internet include the following:

- Structure and Content of Clinical Study Reports[33]
- Good Clinical Practice: Consolidated Guidance[34]
- Guidance on General Considerations for Clinical Trials[35]
- Statistical Considerations and Design of Clinical Trials[36]

Before general and specific considerations for individual trials can be discussed, an understanding of the different systems of classification of clinical trials is essential.

Classification of Clinical Trials by the Initiator

Clinical trials may be initiated either by industry or by an individual investigator. Those that are part of *a clinical development program* and conducted under a *sponsor's* (pharmaceutical company) *Investigational New Drug* (*IND*) submission are usually initiated by industry. Trials undertaken under a sponsor's IND are used frequently by the sponsor in its submission to obtain approval for a new drug, known in the United States and elsewhere as a *New Drug Application* (NDA). If the NDA is approved by the regulatory agency, the drug may be marketed and labeled for the specific indication (i.e., disease or conditions) stated in the NDA.

Investigator-initiated protocols are typically, but not always, conducted after the drug is approved for market. The main objective of investigator-initiated protocols may be new dosage regimens or use in diseases other than that for which the drug has obtained an indication. Many such trials are exploratory rather than confirmatory. Funding for investigator-initiated protocols in pediatric rheumatology has come from the manufacturer and from regulatory and nonregulatory agencies.

Classification of Clinical Trials by Phase

Clinical drug development programs are often described as consisting of four temporal phases (*Phase I to Phase IV*). This system of classification, despite its shortcomings, is perhaps the most commonly used today by the pharmaceutical industry and regulatory agencies (Fig. 8–1).

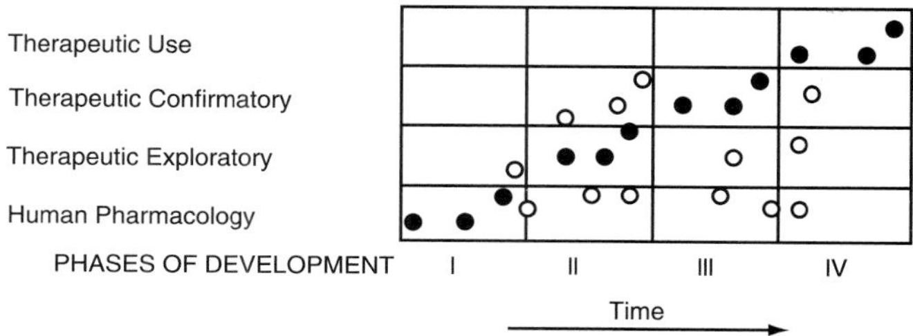

Figure 8–1. This graph indicates that study types are not synonymous with phases of development. (From Fed Reg 62[242], 1997.)

Phase I

Phase I studies are *human pharmacology* trials whose overall aim is to establish preliminary safety and tolerability of the dose range expected to be needed for later clinical studies, and to determine adverse drug effects that can be expected. Studies in this phase include both single- and multiple-dose administration schedules and have one or more of the following aspects:

Pharmacokinetics (PK). PK studies typically determine the drug's absorption, distribution, metabolism, and excretion pathways. PK may progress throughout a clinical development program and be assessed in separate studies or as part of larger trials to determine efficacy and safety. These studies are necessary to assess the clearance of the drug and to anticipate possible accumulation of the drug or its metabolites and potential for drug–drug interactions. Assessing PK in subpopulations, such as those with impaired renal function or hepatic failure, is another important aspect of this phase of studies. Pharmacokinetic data are usually expressed using the following terms:

Area-under-the-concentration curve (AUC, or AUC_{0-24} if done over a 24-hour period) is a measure of the total amount of drug absorbed; it is frequently estimated after the drug has reached *steady-state levels*
Peak concentration (C_{max}) reached at a particular dosage
Time to peak concentration (T_{max}). C_{max} and T_{max} are used together to measure the *rate of absorption*
Cumulative percentage recovered of drug (A_c%) usually relates to urine data and is the cumulative amount of drug recovered over some time period (e.g., 24 hours) divided by the initial dose
Elimination (or terminal) half-life ($t_{1/2}$) is a measure of how long it takes to clear a drug from the system; it can be estimated by dividing 0.693 by the absolute value of the slope of the terminal linear phase of the concentration profile plotted on a semi-log scale[37]

Estimation of Initial Safety and Tolerability. *Drug safety* refers to the frequency of *adverse drug effects* (i.e., physical or laboratory toxicity that could possibly be related to the drug) that are *treatment emergent* (i.e., that emerge during treatment and were not present before treatment or become worse during treatment compared with the pretreatment state). An adverse drug effect is distinguished from an *adverse event* (or *experience*), which refers to any untoward experience that occurs while a patient is receiving the medication, whether or not it is attributable to the drug. The seriousness of an adverse event dictates how quickly it must be reported to regulatory agencies and to others who may have ongoing experimental protocols. A serious adverse event (SAE) is defined as one that results in death, is life-threatening, requires inpatient hospitalization or prolongation of existing hospitalization, results in persistent or significant disability/incapacity, or is a congenital anomaly/birth defect. The term *severity* is distinguished from *serious* in that severity refers to the intensity of a specific event, whereas serious refers to the outcome of the event. *Drug tolerability* refers to how well subjects are able to tolerate overt adverse drug effects.

Assessment of Pharmacodynamics (PD). These studies typically observe the relation of drug blood levels to clinical response or to adverse drug events. They may provide early estimates of drug activity and potential efficacy and help to establish dosage and dose regimen in later phases of drug development.

Early Assessment of Drug Activity. Although not part of human pharmacology, phase I studies may also determine preliminary efficacy as secondary variables that may be confirmed in later studies.

Phase II

Phase II studies are the earliest attempt to establish efficacy in the intended patient population. Many are called *therapeutic exploratory studies* that will form the basis for later trials. The hypotheses may be less well defined than in later studies, and they may be data driven. The designs are flexible so that changes can be made as the data accumulate.

These studies may use a variety of different types of study design, including comparisons with baseline status or concurrent controls. In these studies, the eligibility criteria are typically very narrow, thus leading to a homogeneous population that is carefully monitored for safety. Further studies may establish the drug's safety and efficacy in a broader population once it is determined that a drug does indeed have activity. These studies may also aim to determine more exactly the doses and regimens for later studies. Phase II studies may use *dose-escalation designs* to estimate *dose response,* which may be confirmed in later studies. In phase II, doses of the drug are typically but not always less than the highest doses used in phase I: Another important goal of phase II studies is to determine potential study end-points, therapeutic regimens (including the use of concurrent medications), and subsets of the disease population (mild vs. severe).

Phase III

The primary objective of phase III studies is to confirm a therapeutic benefit. Thus, the most typical kind of study is *therapeutic confirmatory,* which provides firm evidence of an agent's efficacy and safety. This type of trial always has a predefined hypothesis that is tested. These studies also estimate (with substantial precision) the size of the treatment effect attributable to the drug. Studies incorporated in the phase III development include further exploration of the dose-response relationship and study of the drug in a wider population, study of the drug in different stages of the disease, or the effects of adding drugs to the test drugs. These studies continue to add information to the accumulating safety database.

Phase IV

Phase IV studies, sometimes called *postmarketing surveillance studies,* begin after the drug reaches the market. These studies extend the prior demonstration of the drug's safety, efficacy, and dose. The most frequent phase IV study is of *therapeutic use,* which goes beyond the prior demonstration of the drug's safety and efficacy. These studies demonstrate how the drug performs when used in the everyday setting of the clinic, when patients have comorbid conditions, and when patients may be on a host of concurrent medications.

Investigations in Special Populations. Investigations in children typically take place after considerable data have been gathered in an adult population with a similar disease. When clinical development includes children, it is usually appropriate to start with older children before extending the studies to younger children. The exception to the "adults first" rule is when a medication is developed to treat a condition that occurs only in childhood.

Classification of Clinical Trials by Objective

The ICH believes that the classification system based on phases of development is inadequate for classifying clinical trials because one type of trial may occur in several different phases, as shown in Figure 8–1. Table 8–3 presents an alternative classification system based on the objective of the study, using terminology described earlier.

Considerations for Individual Clinical Trials

For special issues relevant to trials in children, please see electronic citation E11 available at www.fda.gov/cder/guidance/index.htm

Objectives

Clearly stated primary and secondary objectives and hypotheses form the backbone around which every clinical trial is developed. These should all be clearly stated in the protocol and study report. Table 8–3 provides a framework for developing appropriate objectives for the various types of study planned. In general, trials tend to have one to three main objectives and numerous process objectives. Be wary of trials with more than a few objectives, although exploratory trials may have objectives less clearly delineated than those of later trials.

Population

The specific population to be studied is delineated by the *inclusion/exclusion criteria*. The development of these criteria is one of the more formidable tasks in the entire process. Developers of trials must attempt to reach a compromise between limiting the heterogeneity of the sample and not making the criteria so strict that recruitment of eligible subjects becomes untenable or threatens to restrict the generalizability of results.

The heterogeneity of the patient population that will be allowed to enroll in the trial is influenced by the

Table 8–3

An Approach to Classifying Clinical Studies According to Objective

TYPE OF STUDY	OBJECTIVE OF STUDY	STUDY EXAMPLES
Human pharmacology	Assess tolerance Define/describe PK and PD Explore drug metabolism and drug interactions Estimate activity	Dose tolerance studies Single- and multiple-dose PK and/or PD studies Drug-interaction studies
Therapeutic exploratory	Explore use for the targeted indication Estimate dosage for subsequent studies Provide basis for confirmatory study design, end-points, methods	Earliest trials of relatively short duration in well-defined narrow patient populations, using surrogate or pharmacology end-points or clinical measures Dose-response exploration studies
Therapeutic confirmatory	Demonstrate/confirm efficacy Establish safety profile Provide an adequate basis for assessing the risk:benefit relationship to support licensing Establish dose-response relationship	Adequate and well-controlled studies to establish efficacy Randomized parallel dose-response studies Clinical safety studies Studies of mortality/morbidity outcomes Large simple trials Comparative studies
Therapeutic use	Refine understanding of risk:benefit relationship in general or special Identify less common adverse reactions Refine dosing recommendation	Comparative effectiveness studies Studies of mortality/morbidity outcomes Studies of additional end-points Large simple trials Pharmacoeconomic studies

PD, pharmacodynamics; PK, pharmacokinetics.

phase of development. Early, exploratory studies are often concerned with whether a drug has any effect whatsoever. Thus, one may use a very narrow subgroup of the total patient population for which the agent may eventually be labeled. Later-phase, confirmatory trials typically relax the eligibility criteria to allow for a broader, more heterogeneous sample of the target population. Still, if the criteria for enrollment are too broad, interpretation of treatment effects becomes difficult.

Design

The study's phase, objectives, ethics, and reality influence the specific design of a trial. New designs have appeared in recent years that reduce the time during which children receive placebo or a known inferior medication.[38] More than one type of design may be used to answer the same question. If the same results and conclusions are reached regardless of the design and analysis used, the results are said to demonstrate *robustness*.

Comparative and Noncomparative Studies

Trials may be classified as either comparative or noncomparative studies. A comparative study implies that some type of comparison is made between the drug under investigation at a particular dosage level and a *placebo*, another dosage level of the investigational drug, or an *active comparator* (an existing drug known to be effective for the specific condition). Noncomparative trials involve no such comparisons with the investigational agent. Studies that compare the agent with placebo or an active comparator are called *controlled studies*. For a discussion and guidance on the proper selection of a control group, please see electronic citation E10 available at www.fda.gov/cder/guidance/index.htm. Studies that involve dose escalation or compare PK and PD of differing dosage levels of the same drug are not considered controlled in the usual sense.

Open Studies

The early human pharmacology studies in the first phase of development and the postmarketing surveillance (phase IV) studies are usually *open label*, meaning that everyone involved with the study, including the patient and physician, knows what the patient is receiving. Studies that occur in phase II and III may have an *open-label extension* phase during which patients who took part in the comparative phase receive the investigational drug openly for an extended period. The chief purpose is to gather longer-term safety and efficacy data. Investigator-initiated protocols may also be open when the intent is simply to gather additional information about an agent in another disease or at a dosage level other than that indicated in the label. As one would expect, the possibility of bias in interpretation of safety and efficacy information with open studies is much greater than with blinded studies.

Blinded, Comparative Studies

Beginning either in late phase I or early phase II, *blinded*, controlled (comparative) studies are performed. Blinding refers to the masking of those involved in the assessment of the patient and, in some situations, of the data analyst. The purpose of blinding is to prevent identification of the treatment until any opportunity for bias has passed. These biases include (but are not limited to) decisions about whether to enroll a patient, allocation of patients, clinical assessment of end-points, and approaches to data analysis and interpretation. Designs in which both the assessor and the patient are blinded are called *double-blind designs*. Designs in which only the patient or only the assessor is blinded to the treatment are called *single-blind designs*. Studies should attempt to maintain the blind until the final patient has completed the study, although this has proven difficult in certain pediatric studies of severe diseases.

Blind Assessor

Certain studies present challenges to the maintenance of blinding because blinding is either unethical or impractical. For example, surgical versus nonsurgical interventions prevent the patient and the surgeon from being blinded because they know whether surgery was performed. In this situation, a *blind assessor* may be used to evaluate the patient's condition. The blind assessor may be a physician, nurse, or other health professional who evaluates the patient's response to treatment but is unaware of the treatment being given.

Double-Dummy Design to Maintain Blinding

Another situation in which blinding of the patient is difficult is when the dosage administration regimen is different for two drugs. An example in rheumatology is the comparison of methotrexate (administered once per week) versus hydroxychloroquine (administered daily). In this case, the *double-dummy* design can be a useful way to maintain the blind. Patients who are to receive methotrexate take active methotrexate once per week, and dummy hydroxychloroquine each day. Patients who are to receive hydroxychloroquine receive active hydroxychloroquine each day and dummy methotrexate once per week.

Randomization

The purpose of randomization is to introduce a deliberate element of chance into patient assignment to the treatment groups. Randomization thus reduces (but

Table 8–4

Example of a Randomization Schedule (Nonstratified, Blocks of 8)*

Randomization Block 1

	Patient Number			
Treatment 1	1	2	6	8
Treatment 2	3	4	5	7

Randomization Block 2

	Patient Number			
Treatment 1	12	13	14	15
Treatment 2	9	10	11	16

*The first patient entering the study would receive treatment 1, the second treatment 1, the third treatment 2, and so on. Note that the sequence of assignments is random, and when the block is full equal numbers of patients will be enrolled into each treatment group. When block 1 is full, the assignment would move to block 2.

does not eliminate) the chance of an unequal distribution of known and unknown prognostic factors among the treatment groups. It also reduces possible bias in the selection and allocation of subjects.

Many randomization schemes are currently employed. The simplest form of randomization is *unrestricted*. Patients are assigned to one of two or more treatment groups by a sequential list of treatments. The list of treatments is known as the *randomization schedule*. *Blocked randomization* is commonly used to ensure that equal numbers of patients are placed in each treatment group (Table 8–4). Note in the table that the assignment to groups is not sequential, but when the block is full an equal number of patients will have been enrolled into each group: If the blocks are too small, one runs the risk of unblinding.

As an extreme example, suppose blocks were only two cells large for a study that planned to compare two drugs. If a clinical investigator knew the block size, enrolled only two patients, and became aware of what one of the patients was receiving through an adverse drug effect, he or she would automatically know what both patients received. If the blocks are too large they may not be completely filled, thus increasing the likelihood of unequal assignment to the groups. In recent pediatric rheumatology studies involving two groups, block sizes of six to eight have been used. Clinical investigators are never made aware of block size during the trial.

Blocks may also be *stratified* by some prognostic factor to ensure equal distribution of the factor among the treatment groups (Table 8–5). In multicentered trials, randomization may be stratified by center such that each center has its own set of blocks. This tends to produce equal numbers of patients in each group at individual centers. In pediatric rheumatology, stratification by center is frequently not possible because only small numbers of patients are enrolled at each center. If multicentered trials use only one randomization schedule for all centers, whether it is unrestricted or stratified, the study is said to be *randomized across all centers*. Typically, a central coordinating center takes responsibility for giving all centers randomization numbers. The use of more than two stratification factors is rare. Such designs are logistically difficult and do little to achieve balance of prognostic factors.

Large trials have a Data Monitoring and Safety Committee to check whether randomization is achieving balance of important prognostic factors while the trial is continuing. If imbalance of one—or at the most two—prognostic factors is found, the randomization scheme may be altered to achieve more balanced groups. This is known as *dynamic randomization*. Table 8–5 demonstrates a form of dynamic randomization. At about the midpoint of the patient enrollment phase of the trial, the statistician detected that, by chance, patients assigned to Treatment 1 were significantly younger than those in Treatment 2. Because age was an independent variable strongly associated with the outcome, the statistician had to attempt to equalize the age of patients in the two treatment groups. This was done by a form of dynamic randomization. In this case, an age-stratified block randomization scheme was developed, as shown in Table 8–5. Notice that, with this scheme, there was a lower (but not zero) probability that patients 11 years of age or older would receive Treatment 2 instead of Treatment 1. With this randomization schedule, the statistician monitored the data on age closely to determine whether the groups equalized. When they did, the trial reverted back to the original (not stratified by age) randomization schedule.

Design Configurations of Comparative Studies

Design configurations refer to treatment group assignments after initial randomization (i.e., whether or not

Table 8–5

Example of a Stratified Block Randomization Schedule, Attempting to Correct for an Imbalance in Age Between Treatment Group 1 and Treatment Group 2

Randomization Block 1*

	Patient Treatment Group					
≥11 years	1†	2	1	1	1	1
<11 years	2†	2	1	2	2	2

Randomization Block 2

	Patient Treatment Group					
≥11 years	1	1	1	2	1	1
<11 years	2	2	2	2	1	2

**Example:* The first patient to be enrolled who is >11 years of age would be given treatment 1 (active agent), the second patient who is >11 years of age would be given treatment 2 (placebo), the third, treatment 1, and so on. The first patient who is <11 years of age would be given treatment 2, the second patient who is <11 years of age would be given treatment 2, the third, treatment 1, and so on.

†Treatment 1, investigational drug; treatment 2, placebo.

patients remain in the same treatment group throughout the study). Keep in mind that all the configurations discussed below may be open, blinded, or both.

If patients remain in the same group to which they are initially randomized, the study is known as a *parallel group design*. In *crossover designs*, patients switch from one treatment to the next, often in a randomized manner, and they act as their own control for purposes of analysis. The crossover design in the trial must be distinguished from the frequently used open-label extension phase (discussed earlier) in which all patients receive active drug. *Factorial designs* allow for the study of the *interaction* of two treatments that are likely to be used in combination. The simplest factorial design is a 2 × 2 design in which patients are assigned to receive drug a, drug b, drug a and drug b, or neither drug a nor drug b. Factorial designs are also used to study dose response when two agents are used together. *Group sequential designs* are particularly well suited to interim analyses. This design implies that the various treatment groups are evaluated for safety and efficacy at periodic intervals during the trial to determine whether the trial should continue or be stopped because of safety or efficacy concerns. Other comparative designs whose basic approach is evident by their name include *dose-escalation* and *fixed-dose dose-response* trials.

A design recently used to study etanercept in the treatment of polyarticular JRA[38] is the *blinded withdrawal design*. In this approach, all patients receive active medication long enough to establish whether patients respond (according to a standard definition). Patients who are not classified as "responders" after the prescribed time period are discontinued from the study and are classified as therapeutic failures. Patients who respond are randomized either (1) to be withdrawn blindly from active medication and given placebo or (2) to continue to receive active medication, but in a blind manner. A common phenomenon in blinded-withdrawal studies is a mild flare of disease among patients who continue to receive (blinded) active medication after randomization. This is called the *reverse placebo effect* because it is the reverse of the beneficial effect often observed when patients are blindly randomized to placebo. The primary outcome among those randomized can be *time-to-flare* or percent who flare (according to a standard definition).

A design that has gained widespread acceptance in oncology and is now being used in pediatric rheumatology is the open-randomized, actively controlled trial. Patients are randomized to one of two or more treatment arms, all of which are active. The trial is open and, in general, no additional trial procedures or visits other than routine care are required. These trials have numerous advantages but also substantial disadvantages, as recently described.[39] This design has gained in popularity as a method to study treatment of rare conditions in which pivotal, confirmatory trials are not possible and for which there is little economic incentive from pharmaceutical companies to develop the product. They are particularly well suited for studying combination therapy, such as pulse therapy in systemic JRA.[40] These trials tend to be more "user-friendly" than studies that are part of a clinical development program. Perhaps their biggest advantage is that they are inexpensive to conduct because third-party payers may be billed for the procedures. They are not used to seek a new label or indication for an agent, and they are considered exploratory.

N *of 1 Design*

This approach repeatedly and randomly crosses over individual patients from one therapy to the next. Thus, the randomization scheme may be A, B, B, A, A, B: Data from numerous N of 1 trials in individuals may be combined to increase the sample size, but this is fraught with difficulties and sources of potential bias. These studies are considered exploratory and are hampered in rheumatology and other diseases by the carryover effects of the treatment, natural fluctuations of the disease state unrelated to therapy, and logistical problems. For a discussion of the usefulness of these designs in rheumatology, see the 1988 article by Giannini.[41]

Intents of Comparative Studies

The type of comparison that one intends to carry out must be decided on before the protocol can be synthesized. Major types of comparisons include trials to show superiority, trials to show equivalence, trials to show noninferiority, and trials to show dose-response relationship. All comparative trials must possess *assay sensitivity*, defined as the ability of a study to distinguish between active and inactive treatments.[41a]

Trials to show superiority are perhaps the most frequent intent of comparative studies. They are designed to show superiority of the investigative agent as compared with either placebo or an active comparator or by demonstrating a dose-response relationship. In pediatric rheumatology, placebo-controlled studies have become more difficult because some existing agents are clearly better than placebo. In such situations, the use of a placebo design is considered unethical and an active comparator is substituted.

Trials to show equivalence do not aim to show superiority but rather equivalence. Equivalence trials (either biologic or clinical equivalence) aim to show that the difference in response to two or more treatment approaches is clinically unimportant. For equivalence trials, the usual statistical approach is to use two-sided confidence intervals (CIs) (explained further later). Equivalence is inferred when the entire CI of the true treatment difference falls within the *equivalence margins*. Stated another way, a statistical test of inference that results in a nonsignificant P value (i.e., no difference between the test drug and the active comparator) is not enough to conclude that the two agents are equivalent.

Trials to show noninferiority are similar to equivalence trials, but the question is asked in only one direction (i.e., no worse than the standard therapy). In this case a 1-tailed CI is used to infer noninferiority. Again, a simple one-sided test of the null hypothesis that finds "no difference" in the treatments is insufficient to make conclusions about noninferiority.

The two aforementioned trial types can be difficult to design, and sample size requirements are often much higher than superiority trials. This is particularly true in active control equivalence or noninferiority trials that do not use placebo or that do not use multiple doses of the new drug.[41a] The lack of internal validity makes external validation necessary. Active comparators should be chosen that have been shown through convincing, confirmatory trials to be efficacious in the particular condition. Further, the same response variables should be used in the equivalence or noninferiority trials that were used in the confirmatory trials of the active comparator, and equivalence margins should be clinically sound.

Trials to show dose-response relationships occur throughout the development phase of a drug and may have numerous objectives, including confirmation of efficacy, establishment of the dose-response curve, estimation of the most appropriate starting dose, strategies for dose adjustment, and estimation of the maximum dose.

Conducting the Clinical Trial

With the advent and widespread use of independent for-profit *clinical research organizations* (CROs), the quality of clinical trial conduct has risen substantially. *Academic research organizations* (AROs) appeared in the 1990s. Although not typically involved in the day-to-day operations of the trial, AROs provide the basic scientific and theoretical background for the trial. These functions may include biologic justification for the selection of the particular therapy, identification of biologic and clinical response variables, development of the protocol, interpretation of the results, and final report preparation.

Pediatric rheumatology clinical trials, with few exceptions, are *multicentered* approaches. This term implies that multiple clinical investigative sites are used to enroll enough patients to meet statistical power requirements. A *coordinating center* (CC) is responsible for coordinating nearly all trial activities. The role of the CC is determined in part by whether a CRO is used and whether the trial is part of a clinical development program or an investigator-initiated protocol. If a CRO is used, the CC performs as an ARO.

Site monitoring may be a function of the CC or the CRO. During visits to clinical sites, site monitors (known throughout industry as clinical research associates [CRAs]) verify the data on the case report forms against *source documentation* (i.e., original reports from the laboratory and clinical records).

Data collection (or capture) is moving to "paperless coordinating centers." Prior to the widespread use of electronic communication, nearly all data were collected during the site-monitoring visit or forms were mailed to the CC or directly to the sponsor. Now, use of e-mail and electronic entry of data via scanning of forms is increasing. The electronic age has drastically reduced the number of patients entered into trials who do not meet the eligibility criteria and the amount of inappropriate, incorrect, or missing data.

Data collation refers to the distillation of data from the case report forms to summary tables and spreadsheets. This step is necessary prior to data analysis and facilitates the review of both safety and efficacy data by the *Independent Data Monitoring and Safety Committee*. This committee is charged with, among other items, determining whether the trial should continue unchanged, be modified, or be stopped early because of safety or efficacy concerns.

Data Analysis Plan

The role of the statistician begins with the planning of the study and not after the data are already in hand. Plans for exploratory studies may not be as formal as those for confirmatory trials because the former permit the use of data-driven hypotheses to be tested. That is, data exploration is encouraged in exploratory, hypothesis-generating, nonpivotal trials. A single study may have both confirmatory and exploratory aspects.

At a minimum, the statistical considerations document includes the following items:

1. Whether descriptive statistics, statistical inference, or both will play a role in the analysis
2. Identification of the primary and secondary response (outcome) variables
3. Calculation of sample size, including assumptions that will be used to justify the sample size, which in turn include the alpha and beta error levels, the difference that one wishes to detect as statistically significant, and how the variance estimate will be obtained
4. How the various *analysis sets* of patients to be used in the analysis will be formed, including the plan for handling dropouts, noncompliant patients, and other sets of patients who do not complete the protocol as written
5. Which statistical tests of inference will be used and the justification for their use
6. Plans for adjustment of P values based on the number of secondary hypotheses to be tested
7. Statement of which aspects of the analysis plan are expected to generate confirmatory data and which are exploratory, including plans for any subgroup analyses
8. Plans for handling covariates
9. The data management and statistical analysis software that will be used

Most of these items are discussed later (see "Understanding and Describing Data" and "Statistical Tests of Inference Commonly Used in Clinical Investigations"); others are self-explanatory. Items 2 and 4 require further attention here.

Primary and Secondary Response Variables

Response variables are defined as those outcomes that will be used as the main evidence of the treatment effect of the investigational drug. *Treatment effect* is defined as an effect that is expected to result from a therapy. In comparative trials, the treatment effect of interest is a comparison of two or more agents. Treatment effect is distinguished from *effect size*, which is a measure of sensitivity to change (responsiveness) of the outcome variable and is defined mathematically as the mean change of the variable among the patient groups divided by the standard deviation (S.D.) of the baseline score. A related term is the *standardized response mean*, which is the mean change in a variable's score from baseline to the follow-up visit divided by the S.D. of this change.[42]

In studies designed primarily to observe safety and tolerability of an agent, the "response" variable relates to adverse events or treatment-emergent adverse drug effects rather than to efficacy. Thus, the choice of primary response variable(s) largely depends on the objectives of the trial and should reflect clinically relevant effects. Secondary response variables are usually (but not always) associated with the exploratory nature of the study. *Surrogate end-points* are outcomes that are intended to relate to a clinically important end-point but do not in themselves measure a clinical benefit. The use of biologic surrogate end-points in rheumatology as primary outcomes is somewhat suspect. For example, a decrease in some targeted T-cell type may not produce clinical benefit even though the desired biologic effect was achieved.

A frequently encountered problem in rheumatology is that of *multiplicity* (i.e., the use of multiple primary end-points with repeated statistical testing). To avoid this problem, the use of *composite variables* has become popular. This strategy involves integration or the combining of multiple relevant variables into a single variable, using a predefined algorithm. Two examples of composite variables that have been accepted by the FDA are the American College of Rheumatology 20 ("ACR20"), developed by Felson and colleagues[43] for use in trials of adults with RA, and the preliminary definition of improvement (PDI) for JRA developed by Giannini and coworkers[44] (Tables 8–6 and 8–7). Each attempts to dichotomously categorize patients as improved or not-improved using a combination of variables. The pediatric definition of improvement, as well as the individual response variables in the core set, has now been shown to be sensitive to change (responsiveness) in prospective validation studies.[45–47] Composite variables avoid the multiplicity problem without requiring adjustment of the type I error level (described later) due to multiple hypothesis testing.

Table 8–6

American College of Rheumatology "20"

Required ≥20% improvement in tender joint count
≥20% improvement in swollen joint count
+
≥20% improvement in three of the following five:
- Patient pain assessment
- Patient global assessment
- Physician global assessment
- Patient self-assessed disability
- Acute-phase reactant (ESR or CRP)

ESR, erythrocyte sedimentation rate; CRP, C-reactive protein.
ACR "70" requires 70% improvement.
From Felson DT, et al: American College of Rheumatology preliminary definition of improvement in rheumatoid arthritis. Arthritis Rheum 38: 727–735, 1995.

Table 8–7

Preliminary Definition of Improvement for Juvenile Rheumatoid Arthritis

At least 30% improvement from baseline in three of any six core-set variables, with no more than one of the remaining variables worsening by greater than 30%.

1. Physician global assessment of overall disease activity
2. Parent or patient global assessment of overall well-being
3. Functional ability
4. Number of joints with active arthritis
5. Number of joints with limited range of motion
6. Erythrocyte sedimentation rate

From Giannini EH, et al: Preliminary definition of improvement in juvenile arthritis. Arthritis Rheum 40: 1202–1209, 1997.

Response Variable Based on Claims Allowed

The claims that the FDA allows for antirheumatic and anti-inflammatory therapies include reduction in signs and symptoms of RA or JRA, major clinical response, complete clinical response, remission, prevention of disability, and prevention of structural damage.

The *reduction in signs and symptoms claim* is usually the first to be granted for marketing approval. This claim is typically established in trials of at least 6 months' duration unless the product belongs to an already well-characterized pharmacologic class, for which trials of 3 months' duration are sufficient to establish efficacy for signs and symptoms. For trials in adults, the FDA recommends that the ACR20 criteria be used. In pediatric rheumatology, the FDA suggests that the PDI for JRA be used.

The *major clinical response claim* is awarded to agents that are able to show a response at the ACR70 rather than the 20 percent improvement needed for signs and symptoms claim. This claim is based on statistically significant improvement response rates by the ACR70 definition compared with background therapy in a randomized controlled group: trial duration should be a minimum of 7 months for an agent that is expected to have a rapid onset of action and longer for agents with less rapid effects.

The *complete clinical response claim* is granted to a drug that produces a remission for at least 6 continuous months by the ACR20 criteria[48] and by radiographic arrest. Thus, complete clinical response indicates that the patient is in remission but is still taking antirheumatic drugs. Typically, trials for a complete clinical response last a minimum of 1 year.

Remission is defined as the same result while off all antirheumatic drugs. The *remission claim* is granted if remission by the ACR definition and radiographic arrest (no radiographic progression by the method of Larsen and colleagues[49] or the modified method of Sharp and associates[50]) are maintained over a continuous 6-month period while off all antirheumatic therapy. A drug need not be a cure to be awarded a remission claim. A remission claim can be granted even if the patient relapses after 6 months or more of remission. Trials aimed at a remission claim should be at least 1 year in duration.

The *prevention of disability claim* is granted to drugs for which the primary outcome is a functional ability measure, such as the Childhood Health Assessment Questionnaire or the Arthritis Impact Measurements Scale. In addition, the full effect of JRA on a patient is not captured without the use of a more general health-related measure of quality of life. For this reason, data from a validated measure such as the Medical Outcome Study Short-Form Health Survey (SF-36)[50a] or the *Childhood Health Questionnaire* should also be gathered and the patient's condition should not worsen on these measures over the duration of the trial.

The *prevention of structural damage claim* is granted to drugs that show either a slowing of radiographic progression or the prevention of new erosions demonstrated by radiography or other measurement tools such as magnetic resonance imaging: these trials should be at least 1 year in duration.

Certainly, other clinical efficacy response variables are possible, and in pediatric rheumatology the preliminary definition of improvement by Giannini and coworkers[44] is likely to be inappropriate for the study of other rheumatic conditions of childhood. Whatever variables are chosen, they must possess a host of validity characteristics. These include *responsiveness* (sensitivity to change within the trial's duration), *face* (clinical sensibility), and *construct* (biologic sensibility) validity. In addition, variables should be *reproducible* (reliability) and, if more than one variable is chosen, *nonredundant* with one another.

Analysis Sets (Patients)

Not all patients who enter a trial complete the protocol as it is written. Thus, the analysis plan must state how subjects who drop out, are noncompliant, or in some other manner do not follow the protocol specifications will be handled. The formation of analysis sets should be aimed at minimizing bias and avoiding an increase in the possibility of an erroneous conclusion that a difference is present between groups when, in fact, it is not (type I error, described later). The *per-protocol set* (also called valid cases set, efficacy sample, and evaluable subjects sample) are those subjects who closely follow and complete the protocol. In practice, consideration of only the per-protocol set results in the loss of valuable information from patients who perhaps completed most of the study or had only one or two major protocol violations related to, for example, concurrent medication. Thus, the *full-analysis set* is also used for the primary analysis. The full-analysis set refers to the *intent-to-treat* approach and is derived from all randomized patients, including those who dropped out early or had a major protocol violation.

Historically, the intent-to-treat analysis meant that all patients, whether they dropped out, were noncompliant, or otherwise deviated from the written protocol, were evaluated for outcome at the time that they would have had their last visit (because one intended to treat them until then). The concept is embodied in the brief saying, "Once randomized, analyzed." However, this results in introduction of substantial bias and is problematic in rheumatology and other specialties wherein patients, once off trial, are lost to follow-up and receive various other medications and procedures. More recently, the intent-to-treat analysis has used the *last-observation-carried-forward* (LOCF) approach. This technique involves using the last value obtained for a response variable (no matter when in the trial it was measured) as if it were measured at the scheduled final visit. In this way, the data from noncompleters who were exposed to the drug long enough to experience treatment effects (if any) can be combined with the data from the per-protocol set. The intent-to-treat approach allows for minimal exclusion of some patients such as those who, after randomization, never received any of the investigational medication.

UNDERSTANDING AND DESCRIBING DATA

In any type of clinical investigation, the investigators collect data and want to be able to summarize, interpret, and convey it to other parties. In order to do this, it is important to understand how measurements are made, how data can be displayed, and how the types of data determine the appropriate statistical test. The types of measurements (variables) determine which statistical test to use.

Scales of Measurement: Categorical, Ordinal, and Continuous Data

The *scale* or *level of data* has important implications for how information is displayed and summarized. All data may be classified into one of the following measurement scales: *categorical* (sometimes called *nominal*, i.e., "in name only"), *ordinal*, or *continuous* (numerical).

Categorical Variables. For categorical (qualitative) variables, each subject can be placed into one of the categories. Variables with two possible outcomes, such as yes/no or male/female, are called dichotomous. Categorical variables are categorized in terms of proportion or percentages (e.g., the study population was 75 percent female and 25 percent male). The best ways to display categorical data include contingency tables and bar charts.

Ordinal Variables. When the variables used have an inherent order, this is called an ordinal scale. Subjects can be placed in "ranked categories." Examples of ordinal variables include the severity scores of swelling (0 to 3+), Apgar scores, and tumor staging. Order exists among the categories, but the difference between adjacent categories is not uniform throughout the scale. Figure 8–2 is an example, below which is the standard method used to grade swelling by pediatric rheumatologists. The difference between a swelling severity score of 0 and 1 is likely not the same magnitude as the difference between 2 and 3. Ordinal variables are best summarized using percentages and proportions. The entire set of data measured as an ordinal scale may be summarized by a median value.

Continuous Variables. Continuous variables are observations in which the differences between numbers have meaning on a numerical scale. These are quantitative measures and examples are age, height, weight, blood pressure, length of time of survival, and laboratory values such as glucose, sodium, and potassium. Although continuous variables all have meaning on a numerical scale, differing degrees of precision are required for different types of studies. For instance, age in a study of adults may be estimated to the closest year; the age of children may have to be estimated to the closest month, and that of neonates to the closest day or hour. Characteristics measured on numerical scales can be displayed in tables and graphs. Means and S.D. (discussed later) are used to summarize continuous variables.

When to Convert Higher Levels of Data to Lower Levels

As a rule, one should work with the highest level of data possible because of increased quantitative precision and because parametric statistics are, in general, more powerful than nonparametric equivalents (see later). Yet, there are times when, for example, numerical data should be converted to ordinal or nominal level data prior to conducting further analyses. Several situations in which "lowering" the level of data may be appropriate are described in the following paragraphs.

In a multicentered study in which different methods are used to generate a numerical value (e.g., erythrocyte sedimentation rate [ESR] performed by the modified Westergren in some centers versus the Panchenkov technique used in Eastern Europe, and the antinuclear antibody [ANA] titer when different substrates are used). In these situations, one may be forced to "dichotomize" patient results into "normal" or "elevated" and conduct the analysis using statistics appropriate for a nominal rather than a continuous variable.

When the experimenter suspects measurement error in the data. An example is compliance with a prescribed drug dosage or with a clinical trial or physical therapy program. One may have to divide the patients dichotomously and classify each as "compliant" or "noncompliant."

When reliability (reproducibility) of the measurement tool is unknown or likely to be poor. In pediatrics, the reliability of measurement on visual analogue scales is suspected to be low in young children. Thus, rather than reading the result in centimeters from the left side of the scale, investigators frequently place a vertical grid that is divided into 10 equal segments over the visual analogue scale line and read the result as 0 to 10. This effectively converts a continuous variable to an ordinal level outcome.

In clinical trials when one wishes to use a set of response variables (that may be of any data level) to dichotomously divide patients into "responders" and "nonresponders." Examples of this have been presented earlier in this chapter.

0 ———— 1+ ———— 2+ ———— 3+

None	Mild	Moderate	Severe
No joint swelling	Mild, definite swelling but with no blurring of normal skeletal outlines	Definite swelling with obscuring of skeletal landmarks	No discernible skeletal landmarks

Figure 8–2. Example of an ordinal level variable assessing the severity of swelling in a joint.

Concepts Related to Measurement of Variables—Validity, Variability, and Bias

In clinical research, it is obvious that not all patients treated identically will experience an identical response. This is known as the variability that is common to virtually all human experimentation. Certain important terms are associated with describing how this variability may have arisen. Thus, its sources in some situations can be minimized or eliminated altogether. Variability is sometimes also called *error.* Error may be broadly classified into *nonrandom* and *random error.* Nonrandom error is also called *bias* or *systematic error.* It results in a lack of validity of a measure and therefore influences the accuracy of the measure. In general, *validity* is equated with *accuracy.* Random error refers to *imprecision.* In Figure 8–3, the different types of random error and systematic error are graphically demonstrated.

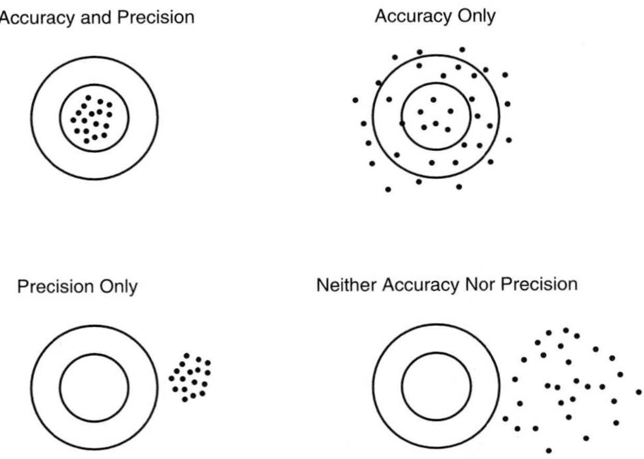

Figure 8–3. Combinations of accuracy and precision in describing a continuous variable.

Potential Sources of Variability in Measurement of Individuals

Variability may arise among individuals from a number of factors, including diurnal variation; changes related to factors such as age, diet, and exercise; and environmental factors, such as season or temperature. Variability may also arise from measurement characteristics, including poor calibration, inherent lack of precision of the instrument, and misreading or misrecording information from the instrument.

External Versus Internal Validity

External validity may be equated with *generalizability.* It determines the population settings to which measurement and treatment variables can be generalized. *Internal validity* defines how valid the conclusions are within the patient sample studied. It is a basic minimum requirement without which any study is uninterpretable. The question of external validity is meaningless without first establishing whether the study is internally valid. Obviously, both types of validity are important. However, they may be at odds in that study design features that increase one may tend to decrease the other.

Bias

There are three major types of bias: selection, information (misclassification), and confounding bias, each of which can be subdivided further.

Selection bias, the distortion of the study effects resulting from the sampling of subjects, includes *volunteer bias*, *nonresponse bias*, and *bias resulting from loss to follow-up*. Two other common subtypes of selection bias are *detection bias* and *Berkson's bias*. Detection bias occurs if an exposure to some potential risk factor is related to increased medical surveillance, thus making it more likely that the disease will be detected. As a consequence, the disease may be falsely associated with the factor. Berkson's bias occurs, for example, if a study is hospital based and hospitalization age differs for different disease groups. The relation between exposure and disease may become distorted.

Information bias is the distortion of the study effect resulting from inaccurate determination of the study variables (either exposure or disease). Information bias may be divided into *nondifferential* and *differential misclassification*. Nondifferential information bias may occur when the exposure is not accurately assessed. This type of bias may occur in occupational research when job titles are used as a surrogate for exposure status.

Another form of nondifferential information bias is *unacceptableness* bias, in which the exposure may be under-reported by patients if it is unacceptable behavior. This is likely to have an impact on all subjects, not just subjects with the disease of interest. Differential misclassification bias includes *recall bias*, in which the recall of information about exposure is influenced by whether the person has the disease (cases have more accurate memory of events leading to disease than controls who have no disease). *Interview bias* may occur when the circumstances under which different groups of subjects are interviewed are not compatible. These circumstances include time from exposure to interview, setting of the interview, person doing the interview, manner in which questions are asked (prompting), and whether the subject has knowledge of the research hypothesis. Case-control studies are particularly vulnerable to information bias.

Confounding bias is a distortion of the study effect resulting from the mixing of the exposure association with the disease, with the effect(s) of extraneous variable(s). The effect of an extraneous variable that wholly or partially accounts for the apparent effect of the exposure or that masks an underlying true association is called confounding. Examples of confounding are (1) an apparent association between an exposure and a disease that may actually be due to another variable and (2) an apparent lack of association between exposure and disease that results from failure to control for the effect of some other factor. A confounding factor must satisfy two conditions:

1. It is a risk factor for the disease under study (i.e., it may cause the disease or be associated with causal factors); the confounder's association with the disease must occur in the absence of the exposure being studied.
2. The confounder must be associated with the exposure being studied but not be a consequence of the exposure.

To assess the possibility of confounding, one may use the standard technique of stratifying the data by the potential confounder. One can then look for an association between the exposure as a possible causal factor and the disease, then compare those who have the confounder with those who do not to see if an association exists. Another common method is to use *Mantel-Haenszel* procedures to calculate an overall relative risk in which the results from each stratum are weighted by the sample size of the stratum.[51]

Only established risk factors for the disease should be investigated as potential confounders. In brief, these can be dealt with in the design of the study (i.e., by matching) or by stratification or multivariate analysis (see later).

Describing Data and the Frequency Distribution of Continuous Variables

Descriptive statistics are commonly used to represent graphically individual data points or summarize groups of data, regardless of the data level. Many exploratory and epidemiologic studies use only descriptive, rather than inferential (tests of hypotheses), statistics. Graphs such as dose-response curves represent descriptive statistics. Rates and ratios are commonly used in epidemiologic studies to describe disease frequency and distribution. A *rate* (or proportion) implies that the numerator is part of the denominator and is usually associated with a time element (e.g., case-fatality rate per year = 11/120, wherein the 11 deaths came from the total of 120 cases). The numerator of a *ratio* is not part of the denominator (e.g., the female:male ratio among patients with oligoarticular-onset JRA is 6:1).

Statisticians employ many types of distributions for describing and analyzing data. These include the binomial (Bernoulli), geometric, chi-square, Poisson, *t*, and F distributions, among others. The *frequency distribution of continuous variables* is most commonly referred to in the medical literature and is the only distribution discussed in detail in this chapter. Its parameters form the basis of much of the descriptive statistics used in the reporting of data from clinical investigations.

A frequency distribution of a continuous variable is simply an x-y plot of the possible values that a variable can take on (x axis) versus the number of observations having the particular values (y axis). If the frequency distribution is *normally distributed* it is called a *gaussian* distribution (Fig. 8–4).

Measures of Central Tendency, Skewness, and Kurtosis

Every distribution of continuous variables has an arithmetic *mean* (average) calculated by adding the observations and dividing by the number of observations. The *median* of any distribution is the centermost value. If the distribution has an even number of observations

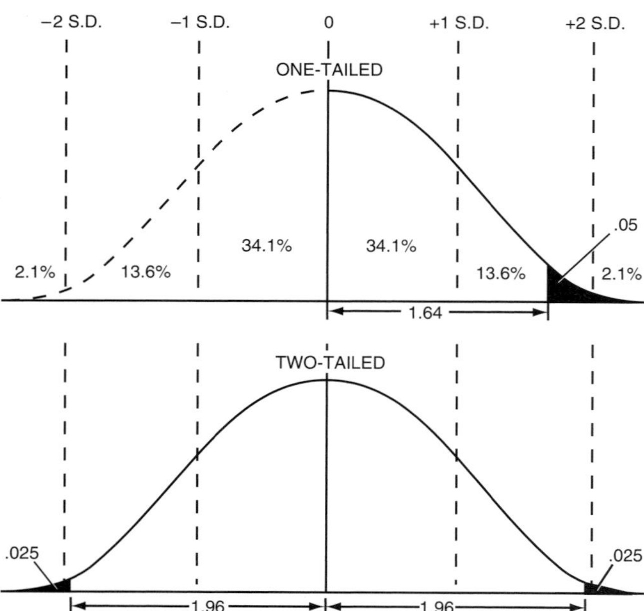

Figure 8–4. The normal or gaussian distribution (bell-shaped curve) showing the approximate percentage of observations expected to be within one and two standard deviations from the mean value. Also note the critical values for one- and two-tailed tests of hypotheses.

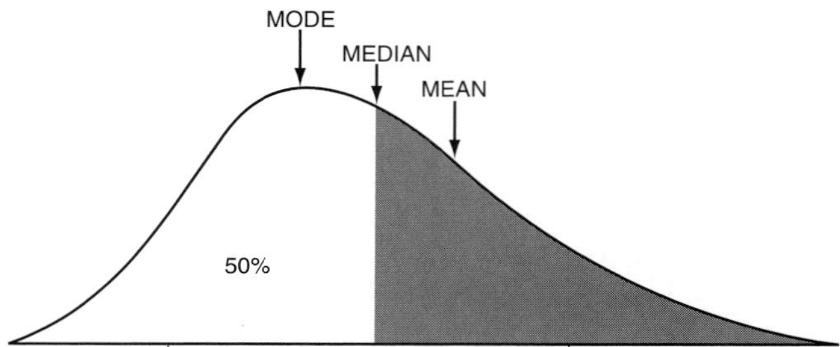

Figure 8–5. Effect of positive skewing on the location of the mean, median, and mode. (The mean and median are skewed to the right.) The effect of negative skewing is the mirror image of this figure.

such that there is no center value, the median is calculated by averaging the two most center values. The median is also the 50th percentile. The *mode* is the most frequently observed value. The mean, median, and mode are all called *measures of central tendency.* A distribution has only one mean and one median, but numerous modes are possible; thus, the terms *bimodal* and *multimodal distributions*.

In a normal distribution, the mean, median, and mode are all the same value. Figure 8–5 demonstrates the effect of *positive skewing* on the measures of central tendency. The skewness is said to be positive because there are too many observations in the upper (shaded) tail (i.e., toward the right side of the distribution). This type of skewing typically occurs in distributions with a fixed lower boundary but without an upper boundary (e.g., results of liver function test). *Negative skewing* is the mirror image of Figure 8–5 and has the opposite effect on central tendency measures. An example is the age at onset of disease among patients with oligoarticular JRA. *Kurtosis* is a measure of the peakedness of a distribution.

Measures of Spread or Variation

The frequency distribution of continuous variables can be described by its mean and by its *standard deviation.* The standard deviation is a measure of the spread of values. Abbreviations in common usage for the mean include x for the sample mean and μ for the underlying population mean from which the sample was drawn. The standard deviation (S.D.) in formulas is designated s for the sample S.D. and σ for the population S.D. It is the square root of the distribution's *variance.* Variance is calculated by subtracting the mean from each of the individual values in the distribution, squaring the differences (to eliminate the negative sign), summing the squares, and dividing the result by the number of observations minus 1. The sample variance is abbreviated "s^2," and the population variance from which the sample was drawn as "σ^2."

If a frequency distribution is normally distributed, ± 1 S.D. from the mean includes 68.3 percent of the observations, ± 2 S.D. includes 95.8 percent of the observations, and ± 3 S.D. includes 99.7 percent of the values. Actual distributions from clinical investigations may include more or less of the observations at the S.D. cutpoints than these theoretical percentages indicate.

To demonstrate an S.D., consider the following example. The mean number of swollen joints among 551 children who have entered into trials of second-line agents is 16.1, with an S.D. of 11.6. Thus, 68.3 percent (376) of the children in these trials should have swollen joint counts between 28 and 4.5 (16.1 ± 11.6). Note that if one were to consider 2 or 3 S.D.s from the mean, the range of values drops below 0, again pointing to the theoretical nature of the S.D. rather than actual numbers of values. The impossible values are an indication that the distribution is not perfectly normal.

Z Scores—Placing a Single Value Within a Distribution of Values

Frequently, clinical investigators find it useful to locate exactly where an individual patient's value for some variable lies within a distribution of values. Because the normal distribution depends on two parameters, the mean and the S.D., there is an infinite number of normal curves, based on the variable being measured. However, all tables of the normal distribution are for the distribution described by a mean of 0 and an S.D. of 1. Therefore, any variable with a mean not equal to 0 and an S.D. equal to 1 must be rescaled so that these parameters are met. The solution is to convert the variable to a standard normal variable Z (also called a standard normal deviate).

For example, eligibility criteria for a clinical trial of calcium supplementation in postpubertal females with JRA may require that, to be eligible for a study, a patient must have a bone mineral content (by dual-energy x-ray absorptiometry) of less than 1.5 S.D. below the mean of the normal population. A Z score can be calculated by subtracting the population mean from the individual's value and dividing by the S.D. of the population (i.e., $Z = [X_i - \mu]/\sigma$, where X_i is the individual's value). One may transform the Z scale back to the original scale by the formula $X_i = \mu + \sigma Z$. Thus, if the population mean is 2143 g and the population S.D. is 308 g, a patient whose bone mineral content is less than 1681 g (i.e., 2143 − [308 × 1.5] respecting the negative direction) qualifies for the study with regard to this eligibility criterion. A Z score also can be calculated using the sample mean and S.D. In addition, two means can be compared to determine whether they are statistically significant via the Z test if the sample size is larger. Any continuous variable can be converted to the Z scale.

Standard Error of the Mean

The standard error of the mean (S.E.M.) represents a different concept than the S.D. Mathematically, it is expressed as $S.E.M. = S.D./\sqrt{n}$. Because each sample drawn from an underlying population will not produce the same mean (but will tend to cluster around the same value), one must calculate the range of where the true (unknown) population mean lies. From the formula, it can be seen that the greater the n (i.e., the larger the denominator), the smaller the S.E.M. Thus, the S.E.M. gives the clinical investigator an idea of how "tightly" the estimated mean from the sample represents the true, underlying mean. Investigators often ask statisticians what should be plotted when presenting the data as a mean and its accompanying measure of variability, the S.D. or the S.E.M. Because the S.E.M. is always less than the S.D., investigators tend to plot it rather than the S.D. A rule of thumb is that the S.D. should be used in comparing values from individual subjects to a population distribution. The S.E.M. is used when plotting mean values of two groups of subjects.

Confidence Intervals

As stated earlier, the S.D. encompasses the variability of individual observations and the S.E.M. indicates the variability of means. The mean ± 1.96 S.D. estimates the range of values in which 95 percent of the observations from subjects can be expected to fall (see Fig. 8–4). Similarly, the mean ± 1.96 S.E.M. estimates the range in which 95 percent of the means of repeated samples from the same population will fall. If the mean and the S.E.M. are known, the 95 percent CIs can easily be estimated. These limits provide an estimate of the range within which the investigator is 95 percent sure that the true mean of the underlying population lies. One can easily calculate any CI level (such as 90 percent or 99 percent) by using the critical values that cut off specific areas of the curve. CIs are frequently used in addition to statistical hypothesis testing. They can be calculated for the chi-square test, the *t* test, regression, and a variety of other tests of statistical inference.

STATISTICAL TESTS OF INFERENCE COMMONLY USED IN CLINICAL INVESTIGATIONS

This chapter does not attempt to describe comprehensively the myriad of statistical procedures that are readily available to the clinical investigator through such computer programs as Statistical Analysis System (SAS) or Statistical Package for Social Sciences (SPSS). The interested reader is referred to more advanced texts on the individual topics.[52–57] Rather, a basic introduction to statistical concepts is provided, followed by a description of the inferential and other procedures found most commonly in the literature. Formulas are not stressed because virtually all statistical procedures are now conducted using computer programs.

Basic Concepts Relevant to Analysis

Statistical approaches may be divided into *frequentist methods* and *bayesian approaches*. Frequentist methods refer to *P* values and CIs, which can be interpreted as the frequency of specific outcomes from the same experimental situation if it is repeated many times.

That is, what are the chances of this outcome—and outcomes even more extreme—if one repeats the experiment many times? Bayesian analysis permits a calculation of the probability that, for example, a treatment is superior according to the observed data *and* prior knowledge. It begins with a *posterior probability distribution* for some parameter, which is derived from the data, and a *prior probability distribution* for that parameter. The posterior distribution is used as the basis for statistical inference.[58] This chapter emphasizes the frequentist school because the majority of statistics in today's literature follow frequentist rather than bayesian theory.

The types of variables in the study and the number of variables studied determine the choice of the appropriate statistical approach. The first step is to determine which variables are independent (predictor or explanatory) and which are dependent (outcome or response) variables. An *independent variable* is the variable that is the explanatory factor or thought to be the cause. A *dependent variable* is one whose value is the outcome in the study or the response or thought to be the effect. The second step is to determine the measurement scale of the variable: categorical (nominal), ordinal (ranked), or continuous numerical, definitions for which are provided earlier. The third step is to determine whether study observations are independent of each other.

In the design of a clinical study, one must determine whether the groups to be compared are independent or paired. Samples for which the values of one group cannot be predicted from the values of the other group are called *independent groups*. In other words, the patient group and the control group represent different individuals rather than the same individual measured at two different times. Paired groups (matched groups) are groups for which the values of one group may be predicted from values in the other group: For instance, a paired experiment may represent either the patient before and after therapy, in which the patient acts as her or his own control, or the patient as paired with another individual who has been matched with respect to all independent variables (e.g., age, duration of disease) that may affect the dependent (response) variable. In animal studies, in which genetically identical animals are frequently used in research, paired experiments are the rule. However, in human clinical studies, it is rare that the two groups can be matched for all independent variables that may influence the outcome variable. An investigator may wish to match the groups as closely as possible to eliminate bias but still treat the groups as if they were independent, thus improving the overall quality of the experimental design as described earlier.

The nature and distribution of the values of the variables also determine whether parametric or nonparametric tests can be used. The use of a parametric test is based on certain assumptions. The major assumption is that the variable of interest follows a normal distribution. It may be possible to *transform* variables that are not normally distributed. This technique expresses the values of observations on another scale such as a natural log scale. This may allow the use of parametric statistical tests when the actual values obtained in the study do not follow a normal distribution. Another alternative is to use a nonparametric test. Nonparametric methods are based on weaker assumptions in that they do not assume a normal distribution or equality of variance between the different groups. There are nonparametric procedures for most statistical needs, but because they are not based on the assumption of normality, nonparametric tests are more conservative. Unfortunately, they are also less powerful (less able to reject the null hypothesis when it is false) than their parametric counterparts.

Two Types of Statistical Error and *P* Values

Type I error is the probability of rejecting a null hypothesis when it is true (i.e., concluding that there is a difference when, in fact, there is not). It is abbreviated as α (alpha error level). The *P* value is the calculated type I error level based on the data and is defined as the likelihood of an observed difference at least as large as a difference having occurred by chance alone. That is, it is analogous to a false-positive result in diagnostic tests (discussed earlier in this chapter). Whether the *P* is capitalized is arbitrary and varies among publishers and journals. *P* values that exceed the predefined type I error level (e.g., $P = .08$ when α was set at .05) are called *not statistically significant*; values at or below the preset type I error level (e.g., .001) are called *statistically significant. The* α *or type I error level is set; the* P *value is calculated.*

The debate about when to adjust *P* values to deal with the issue of *multiplicity*, or multiple hypothesis testing, appears far from resolution.[59, 60] When one is conducting exploratory studies not aimed at establishing definite cause-effect relationships, *P* need not be corrected for fear of missing a possible true association or difference. False-positive results can later be discarded in confirmatory, pivotal studies. In confirmatory studies aimed at adding pivotal evidence to a cause-effect relationship, there is no need to correct the *P* value for the main test of hypothesis (i.e., that on which sample size was based). However, results of secondary, exploratory hypotheses should present both uncorrected and corrected *P* values. An alternative to correcting the *P* value is to set α lower (e.g., at .01 instead of .05) in anticipation of conducting multiple hypothesis testing.

There are numerous techniques for correcting *P* values for multiple comparisons. By far, the most widely used (perhaps because of its simplicity) is the *Bonferroni correction*, despite its conservativeness. To adjust a *P* value using the Bonferroni correction, the *P* value obtained is multiplied by the number of statistical tests. Thus, a *P* value of .05 obtained in a series of 10 tests of hypotheses becomes ($.05 \times 10$), or .5. Alternatively, when the experiment is designed, the α error level can be divided by the number of anticipated tests (in the prior example: $.05 \div 10 = .005$) and refer to values of *P* above this level as nonsignificant.

Type II error is the probability of accepting a false null hypothesis and is commonly abbreviated as β (beta error level). In other words, a type II error is concluding that there is no difference when, in fact, there is a difference. Table 8–8 is a summary of the types of decision errors using the concepts of the null hypothesis and alpha and beta errors.

Power, the ability of a statistical test to identify a true difference if in fact one exists, is expressed mathematically as $1 - \beta$. When designing an experiment, the power of the test will be affected by the sample size. The distribution of the test statistic is divided into two areas: *acceptance* and *rejection*. These concepts are graphically shown in Figure 8–6. If the null hypothesis is rejected, one concludes that the evidence supports a significant difference between the groups. If the null hypothesis is not rejected, one concludes that there is no such difference. The lower the *P* value, the higher the level of significance.

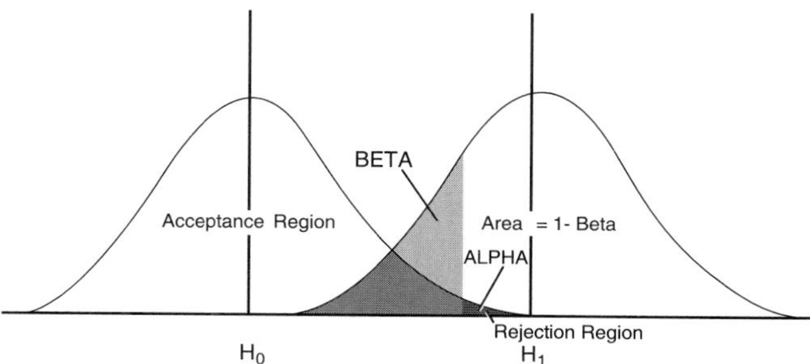

Figure 8–6. Theoretical visual representation of acceptance and rejection regions, alpha and beta error regions, and power. There are four possibilities when one compares the means (or other summary descriptors of a distribution of values) of two (or more) populations or samples. (1) Correctly conclude that there is no difference between the two means (i.e., correctly accept, or fail to reject, the null hypothesis [H_o] of no difference), in which case the mean of, say, the treated group would fall in the distribution on the left anywhere in the acceptance region, but not in the rejection region. This implies that the second mean arose from a population having the same underlying mean as the population that gave rise to the first mean, and the experimenter correctly recognized this. (2) Correctly conclude that there is a difference between the two means (i.e., correctly reject the null hypothesis of no difference in favor of the alternative hypothesis [H_1 or H_a] that there is a difference, in which case the mean of the treated group would fall in the area labeled rejection region or further to the right. This implies that the second mean arose from a population with a different underlying mean than the population that gave rise to the first mean and the experimenter correctly recognized this. (3) Incorrectly conclude that there is a difference between the two means, when in fact there is not a difference (i.e., incorrectly reject the null hypothesis in favor of the alternative hypothesis when, in fact, the null hypothesis should not be rejected), in which case the value of the second mean happened to fall into the rejection, or alpha region, but actually arose from the same population as the first mean. This is known as a type I error, and its probability of occurrence is based on the alpha error level set by the experimenter (i.e., how much chance is one willing to take of saying that there is a difference when in fact there is not?). This will determine the size or area of the rejection region. A type I error implies that the second mean arose from a population with the same mean as the population that gave rise to the first mean, but the experimenter failed to recognize this because the second mean fell so far out in the tail of the distributor, as shown. (4) Incorrectly conclude that there is no difference between two means when, in fact, there is a difference (i.e., incorrectly accept, or fail to reject, the null hypothesis when it is false). In this case, the second mean falls somewhere in the beta region, thus leading the experimenter to believe that the second mean came from the same population that gave rise to the first. This is known as a type II error, and its probability of occurrence is based on where the experimenter sets the power ($1 -$ the beta error level) of a test. Power will determine the size of the beta area on the graph and is usually heavily dependent on sample size. A type II error implies that the second mean arose from a population with a different mean than the population that gave rise to the first mean, but that the experimenter failed to recognize this because the second mean fell somewhat close to the first mean, as shown (i.e., in the beta region).

Sample Size

The estimation of sample size requires considerable statistical skill as well as knowledge of the underlying basic assumptions being made by the investigator. It involves some guesswork, and the resulting calculation may not always yield the correct sample size needed to answer a specific question. This occurs when the investigator's assumptions do not hold true for the sample that is actually enrolled in the study. Sample size should always be calculated during the development of the clinical investigative protocol.

Sample size is most frequently calculated via computer programs, but the investigator and the statistician must still be able to make various assumptions that they think are likely to be met during the study. For chi-square tests (discussed later), the investigator needs to know the outcome of interest (which should be specifically defined), an estimate of the magnitude of effect (i.e., how much difference can one expect between, for example, a control group and a treated group), the desired type I error level (usually .05), and the type II (beta error) level (i.e., 1-power). With these pieces of information, the calculations are relatively straightforward and can be ascertained from tables or using appropriate computer programs. To calculate a sample size needed for a parametric test, such as the *t* test, one must also estimate the variance in the variable of interest. The variance estimate may come from published data or from a pilot study that was designed to preliminarily assess the question under consideration.

Because many sample size calculations result in the requirement of an unrealistic number of patients, the statistician is often asked to find ways to decrease the number of patients needed. Sample size may be decreased by increasing the acceptable type I error level, increasing the acceptable type II error level by increasing the size of difference to detect a statistically significant difference (which should also be clinically significant), and by choosing an outcome variable with a smaller amount of variance. The most common ways to do this include improving the precision of the measurements of the outcome variable, training investiga-

Table 8–8

Outcome of Study

		ACCEPT H_0	REJECT H_0
True situation	H_0	Correct	Type I error
	H_a	Type II error	Correct

tors, using better equipment, and repeatedly measuring the outcome.

Post Hoc Power Analysis

In the event that an investigation yields nonsignificant differences, the concern is that the investigator has committed a type II error. The options to address this situation include calculation of the size of the difference one could detect as statistically significant with sufficient power (e.g., 80 percent) given the sample size and variance obtained in the study (minimum detectable difference). Three other options include calculation of the power of the study to find the actual (observed) difference between groups statistically significant, calculation of the power of the study to find clinically meaningful differences, and calculation of the sample size that would be necessary to find the observed difference statistically significant.

Minimum Detectable Difference

The first option is used frequently and requires further explanation. Minimum detectable difference calculations estimate the amount of difference between groups that the investigator would be able to detect given the size of the sample and the variance. If the minimum detectable difference is much larger than would be considered clinically significant, the investigator could conclude that the investigation did not include a sufficient number of patients to detect a clinically meaningful difference as statistically significant. If the minimum detectable difference is smaller than the difference that is considered clinically significant, the test was adequately powered and the investigator may conclude that in fact there is no difference between the samples.

Confidence Intervals (Limits) on Statistical Tests of Inference

CIs (described earlier) are frequently calculated when one conducts a statistical hypothesis test. They may be calculated for the *t* test, chi-square test, analysis of variance, regression, and most other tests of inference. A 95 percent CI is a range of values wherein the experimenter thinks that there is a 95 percent probability that the true underlying (unknown) mean (or difference in means) lies. The most frequently reported CI is at the 95 percent level. The confidence limits are related to the *P* value. If one calculates the CI of a test that compares two means or difference in means, and zero is within in the range of 95 percent CI, then the statistical test (*P* value) should not be significant because there is some probability that the true difference between the two means is zero.

Statistical Versus Clinical Versus Biologic Significance

An important concept that is frequently overlooked is that a statistically significant difference may not necessarily indicate clinical significance. Particularly if the sample size is large, many tests may result in a statistically significant finding when in fact there is a relatively small degree of clinically significant difference between the two groups. Biologic significance as compared with statistical significance has come into the forefront with the testing of the new immune response modifiers (biologic agents). For example, the sought-after effect of a drug to reduce the number of CD4-positive cells may in fact be significant yet produce no clinical effect. The solution to this is to include not only measures of surrogate (e.g., laboratory) markers of efficacy but also outcomes that allow for the interpretation of the clinical significance of such a biologic effect.

One-Sample Tests

Statistical hypothesis testing may be completed on studies involving one or more groups. The most frequent approach to analyzing data from a clinical investigation that involves only one group is to compare that group with a known population or expected value.

Binomial Test of Proportions

Perhaps the most frequently used test for comparing one sample to a known population is the binomial test. This test asks the question, "What is the probability of x number of successes in N independent trials, given that the probability of success on any one trial is y?" In other words, what is the probability of a fair coin producing 7 heads in 10 flips of the coin given that the probability of a "success" (heads) is 0.5 on each toss. The binomial test yields an exact probability (*P* value) for the 7 successes as well as the probability of obtaining results even more extreme (i.e., 8 of 10, 9 of 10, and 10 of 10 heads). The binomial test has limited applicability in describing the statistical probability that a therapy is beneficial because the odds of success are typically not known. For example, one may ask, "What is the probability of 50 patients with JRA treated with methotrexate experiencing improvement by some index or measure?" The problem is that one is typically unsure of the exact probability of a success in one independent trial. In some situations, the probability of success is arbitrarily given the value of .5 (i.e., 50 percent chance) to either confirm or fail to confirm that level of probability of success.

Goodness-of-Fit Chi-Square Test

The *goodness-of-fit* chi-square test is related to Pearson's chi-square test (discussed later), in which observed proportions are compared with expected values. The goodness-of-fit chi-square test can be used to test the significance of a single proportion or a theoretical model, such as the mode of inheritance of a gene. A reference population is often used to obtain the expected values. Suppose the known frequency of an allele that is thought to produce risk for polyarticular JRA is known to be 2 in 100 in the general population (ignore population stratification for this example). However, the observed frequency in a sample of patients with polyarticular JRA is 10 in 100. Is this much deviation from the expected significant? One calculates how well the observed frequencies fit the model from the general population with the formula: the sum of (observed − expected)^2 ÷ expected values. Therefore, $(10 - 2)^2 \div 2$ (for those with the allele) + $(90 - 98)^2 \div 98$ (for those without the allele) for a sum of about 33. A chi-square table is consulted (as described in greater detail later), and the value of 33 is found to be highly statistically significant.

One-Sample *t* Test

When a statistical inference is desired on a single mean, the *one-sample t test* may be used. The test is similar to the student *t test* for comparing two means, described later. Suppose one wishes to determine whether the mean height of 9- to 10-year-old females with systemic lupus erythematosus is significantly less than that of the general population of 9- to 10-year-old females. One would set up the *critical ratio* for *t* as

$$t = \bar{x} - \mu_o/(s - \sqrt{n})$$

where $\bar{x}$ is the mean of the sample of patients with systemic lupus erythematosus, μ_o is the general population mean, s is the sample S.D., and n is the sample size. One then consults a t table list of critical values and determines whether t is significant at some predetermined level in consideration of the degrees of freedom or independence (which here is n − 1).

Two-Sample Tests

The two-sample test to be used is determined by the level of the data, and certain other assumptions, as defined later.

Chi-Square Test With One Degree of Freedom

For categorical (nominal) data and ordinal data with very few ranks, the most frequently used hypothesis test is the Pearson chi-square (X^2) test. This nonparametric statistical test of inference is for assessing the association between the two variables. It is most commonly performed on contingency tables such as a 2 × 2 cross-tabulation, which has 1 degree of freedom (1df). The numbers in the cells represent counts (frequencies), and *each cell must be independent of all other cells* (i.e., an individual patient can contribute only once to the entire table). Thus, to observe the association between HLA-DR8 and oligoarticular JRA, a 2 × 2 table can be constructed with HLA-DR8 positive or negative as the column headings and oligoarticular JRA present or absent (i.e., control subjects) as the row headings (Table 8–9). The chi-square statistic is based on how much difference there is between "observed" and "expected" frequencies. The null hypothesis is that there is a random distribution of outcome in each "exposure"

Table 8–9

Example of the Calculation of Chi-Square With 1 Degree of Freedom

		HLA – DR 8		ROW TOTALS OF OBSERVED VALUES
		Present	**Absent**	
OLIGOARTICULAR JRA	**Present**	*cell a* observed = 42 expected = 15	*cell b* observed = 46 expected = 73	88
	Absent (Controls)	*cell c* observed = 41 expected = 68	*cell d* observed = 369 expected = 342	410
	COLUMN TOTALS OF OBSERVED VALUES	83	415	N = 498

Expected value in a cell is the row total × column total divided by the total N (i.e., r_ic_i/N)
Expected value in cell a = (83 × 88) / 498 ≅ 15
Expected value in cell b = (88 × 415) / 498 ≅ 73
Expected value in cell c = (83 × 410) / 498 ≅ 68
Expected value in cell d = (410 × 415) / 498 ≅ 342

$$X^2 = \frac{(42-15)^2}{15} + \frac{(46-73)^2}{73} + \frac{(41-68)^2}{68} + \frac{(369-342)^2}{342} = 71$$

A chi-square value of 71 is significant at the .000001 level.
The odds ratio (i.e., ad/bc) = 8.2.

Adapted from Nepom BS, Malhortra U, Schwarz DA, et al: HLA and T cell receptor polymorphisms in pauciarticular-onset juvenile rheumatoid arthritis. Arthritis Rheum 34: 1260–1267, Copyright © 1991 Wiley-Liss, Inc. Reprinted by permission of Wiley-Liss, Inc., a subsidiary of John Wiley & Sons, Inc.

group—that is, the columns are independent of the rows. Expected values are calculated from row and column totals. Thus, in Table 8–9, the expected value in cells a, b, c, and d are 15, 73, 68, and 342, respectively.

The next step is to find the differences between each of the observed and expected values, square it to eliminate the negative sign, and divide by the expected value. To obtain the chi-square statistic, one sums the results from each cell.

$$X^2 = \Sigma \frac{(O_{ij} - E_{ij})^2}{E_{ij}}$$

A short-cut formula for calculating the chi-square with 1df is

$$X^2 = \frac{(ad - bc)^2 N}{(a + b)(c + d)(a + c)(b + d)}$$

Significance of the resulting chi-square statistic is determined from a table of critical values. There are several useful points to remember about the interpretation of the statistic.

For chi-square with 1df (i.e., 2 × 2 tables), the statistic becomes significant at the .05 level if the value is *3.841* or greater, and the larger the chi-square value, the more significant it is. Most tables of critical values report 2-tailed probabilities. Divide the *P* value by 2 for the 1-tailed probability. Chi-square analysis with greater than 1df (i.e., tables larger than 2 × 2) requires larger values to be significant.

Continuity Correction of Yates. When the total N for a 2 × 2 chi-square table is less than about 40, the Yates continuity correction is used to compensate for deviations from the theoretical (smooth) probability distribution. The resulting chi-square value is smaller and the resulting statistical inference will be more conservative. The technique involves subtracting 1/2 from the absolute value of each $O_{ij} - E_{ij}$. Mathematically, this is stated as follows:

$$X^2 = \Sigma \frac{(|O_{ij} - E_{ij}| - 1/2)^2}{E_{ij}}$$

$$\frac{(|ad - bc| - N/2)^2}{(a + b)(c + d)(a + c)(b + d)}$$

Fisher's Exact Test. *Fisher's exact test* is used as a replacement for the chi-square test when the expected frequency of one or more cells is less than 5. This test is commonly used in studies in which one or more events are rare.

McNemar's Test. The chi-square test assumes independence of the cells, as noted earlier. However, experimental designs exist for observing categorical outcomes more than once in the same patient. McNemar's test (also known as the paired or matched chi-square) provides a way of testing the hypotheses in such designs. McNemar's chi-square statistic can be calculated with the following formula:

$$X^2_{McNemar} = \frac{(b - c)^2}{b + c}$$

or, with the continuity correction,

$$X2c_{McNemar} = \frac{(|b - c| - 1)^2}{b + c}$$

An example is shown in Table 8–10. Two different concentrations of an analgesic lotion are given to 51 patients with arthritis. The null hypothesis is that the proportion of patients that receive relief from analgesic lotion 1 is the same as that from lotion 2. The results show that the null hypothesis cannot be rejected according to the McNemar's test.

Mantel-Haenszel Chi-Square Test. This procedure is known as a stratified chi-square test and is frequently used to detect confounding variables. The procedure involves breaking the contingency table into various strata and then calculating an overall relative risk in which the results from each stratum are weighted by the sample size of the stratum.

Common Errors With Chi-Square Tests. Perhaps because of its frequent use, the chi-square test is often employed or interpreted inappropriately. Some of the more common mistakes include unnecessary conversion of continuous or ordinal level data to categorical data in order to use the chi-square test, nonindependence of the cells in the table (exception is when McNemar's chi-square test is being used), use of the chi-square rather than Fisher's exact test when expected cell frequencies fall below 5, and confusion of statistical significance by chi-square values with clinical or biologic importance.

Student's *t* Test

What the chi-square test is to categorical data, the *t* test is to continuous data. This test is used for comparing

Table 8–10

Example of the McNemar Chi-Square Test

- Fifty-one patients with arthritis pain in both hands are treated with two different lotions containing different concentrations of an analgesic lotion. One lotion is placed on the left hand and the other on the right hand of each patient. Each patient rates each hand as experiencing pain *relief* or *no relief*.
- Null hypothesis. The same proportion of patients receive relief from lotion 1 and lotion 2.

	LOTION 1	
LOTION 2	Relief	No relief
Relief	11	6
No relief	10	24

$X^2c_{McNemar}$ (i.e., McNemar chi-square with the Yates correction) = $(|6 - 10| - 1)^2/6 + 10 = 0.562$.

Interpret from regular X^2 table with 1 degree of freedom.
0.562 is less than 3.841, therefore do not reject the null hypothesis.

two sample means from either independent or matched samples. That is, is the difference between $\bar{x}_t - \bar{x}c$ statistically different, where $\bar{x}_t$ is the mean of the treated group and $\bar{x}c$ is the mean of the control group? This difference must be standardized, just as was done in the case of the standard normal variable procedure earlier, so that one set of *t* tables of critical values can be used. In the case of independent samples, the numerator of the *t* statistic is the difference in means and the denominator is the standard error of the difference. This is calculated as

$$\sqrt{s^2_p(1/n_t + 1/n_c)}$$

where s^2_p is the *pooled variance*, n_t is the *sample size of the treated group*, and n_c is the *sample size of the control group*: the degrees of freedom are calculated as $n_t + n_c - 2$, and a table of critical *t* values, either for 1-tailed or 2-tailed tests (depending on the hypothesis being tested), is consulted to determine whether the *t* statistic is significant.

The matched *t* test is more efficient (i.e., more powerful) than the independent test. The computer calculates the difference (retaining the sign) for each matched pair (i.e., $d_i = x_{1i} - x_{2i}$ where i represents each of *n* successive pairs). The mean difference ($\bar{d}$) and the estimated standard error of the difference ($s_d/\sqrt{n}$) are calculated. The null hypothesis ($\delta = 0$) is tested by: t paired $= \bar{d}/(s_d/\sqrt{n})$. The degrees of freedom is equal to $n - 1$, where *n* is the number of pairs. A table of critical *t* values is consulted to determine whether the test statistic is significant.

Nonparametric *t* Tests

The *t* tests described earlier are parametric tests. That is, they make assumptions about the underlying distributions, including normality and equality of variances between groups. The *t* test is a very *robust* test; it is still valid even when these assumptions are substantially violated. Modern data-analysis computer software programs provide relevant statistics and tests of underlying assumptions when one conducts a parametric test, and the resulting displays may warn the investigator that the results of the test may not be valid. If the violations are severe, the investigator can transform the data using, for example, either natural logarithms (described earlier) or nonparametric tests. Nonparametric tests ignore the magnitude of differences between values taken on by the variables and work with ranks. No assumptions are made about the distribution of the data. In the case of the *t* test, either the *Mann-Whitney U test* is used for independent data or the *Wilcoxon Signed Rank test* is used for paired data.

K Sample Tests

Clinical investigations involving more than two samples (groups) require that modifications be made to the analysis plan to accommodate the need for multiple comparisons.

Chi-Square With More Than One Degree of Freedom

When analyzing categorical data, there may be more than two categories for one or both variables (i.e., the table may be larger than 2 × 2). However, if the chi-square test statistic is found to be significant in a table larger than 2 × 2, it is frequently difficult to determine *which* proportions were different. One must then attempt to either collapse the number of cells in the table or break the table up into several smaller tables. This may require adjustment of the resulting *P* values because of multiple comparisons. The degrees of freedom of contingency tables larger than 2 × 2 are equal to the number of rows minus 1 plus the number of columns minus 1. For example, a 2 × 3 table has (2 − 1 + 3 − 1), or 3, degrees of freedom.

Analysis of Variance

One-Way Analysis of Variance (ANOVA)

The use of repeated *t* tests to detect differences among more than two means is considered unacceptable because the resulting *P* value does not accurately describe the chance one has taken of committing a type I error. The one-way ANOVA is used for the purpose of comparing greater than two sample means. Simply stated, ANOVA divides the total variance among all subjects into two portions, the amount of variance due to the difference between the groups of subjects, and the amount of variance due to differences within each group: The ratio of the amount *between* and the amount *within* each group is known as the *F ratio*. The corresponding test of significance is known as the *F test*. If statistical significance is achieved, the investigator must go one step further. The significance may have arisen because just two means were different from one another, or perhaps all the means were different from one another. To determine exactly which means were different, tests must accommodate the fact that multiple comparisons are being made. One thus applies a *multiple comparison*. Commonly used multiple comparison tests include *Tukey's Honest Significant Difference test*, the *Newman-Keuls test*, *Scheffé's Multiple Contrasts test*, and if one wishes to make multiple comparisons to only one (control) group, *Dunnett's test*.

Multi-Way ANOVA

ANOVA procedures have an additional capability that can increase the efficiency of analyses when one wishes to compare two or more independent variables on one dependent variable simultaneously. Suppose one wished to test the effects of methotrexate and a physical therapy (PT) program on the disease status of a group of patients with polyarticular JRA. One could carry out two separate studies and conduct *t* tests for treatment effects on the methotrexate-treated patients and the PT-treated patients and compare each with placebo or no PT. This approach requires substantial numbers of patients to meet sample-size requirements for each study. However, a *two-way ANOVA factorial design* could make much more efficient use of the available subjects and provide information about the *interaction* (effect modification) between methotrexate and PT. In this situation, patients could be randomized to both treatments, yielding four groups (methotrexate alone, PT alone, both methotrexate and PT, and neither treatment). In addition to providing information about the effect of each treatment alone (i.e., the two *main effects*), a two-way ANOVA factorial design examines the effect of the interaction between the two treatments. ANOVA techniques can be extended to three-way, four-way, and beyond, provided the sample size is large enough.

Nonparametric ANOVA

ANOVA procedures discussed to this point are parametric tests and, as such, make various assumptions about the underlying distribution. If these assumptions are substantially violated, the nonparametric equivalent of ANOVA, the Kruskal-Wallis test, can be used. This test is subject to the same sample-size limitations as the chi-square test. If the sample size in any group is less than five, one must use Fisher's exact test and exact probabilities, as described earlier.

Correlation and Regression

One of the most important measures of statistical correlation is the *Pearson product-moment correlation*. This statistic is appropriate for estimating the relationship between two variables, x and y, both of which are measured along a continuous scale. Correlation is a two-way model that does not require assumptions of causality. The correlation (r) can vary between −1 and +1. The magnitude of the correlation demonstrates the strength of the relationship between the two variables. The larger the absolute variable of the correlation, the more strongly associated are "x" and "y." In the extreme, where $r = \pm 1.0$, all the data values will fall perfectly on a straight line. As r approaches zero, the data demonstrate greater scatter about a best-fit line for their relationship. The sign of the correlation indicates the direction of the relationship. A positive sign means that the two variables are directly related (i.e., both tend to increase or decrease together). A negative sign for r indicates that the two variables are inversely related (i.e., the value of one of the variables tends to decrease as the other increases).

Correlation assumes that the joint distribution of x and y is bivariate normal. That is, y is normally distributed at all values of x, and vice versa. If this assumption is violated substantially, the nonparametric *Spearman rank correlation*, which yields a *Spearman's rho* (r_s), is used. Because Spearman rank correlation deals with ranks, it can be used with continuous variables that violate assumptions and for ordinal data.

Regression is a one-way model in which predictor or explanatory independent (x) variables are thought to affect the (y) dependent outcome variables, but not vice versa. In simple regression models (i.e., models that include only a single predictor), as well as in multiple regression models, the direction of the effects must be pre-specified. The simple linear regression equation is $y = a + bx$ where a is the intercept and b is the coefficient. Thus, by using various values of x in the equation, the predicted value of y for a given x can be determined. Simple regression models serve as the building blocks for the larger, more complex, and more realistic models. These include polynomial regression models and structural equation models.

Multiple Linear Regression

The technique whereby a multitude of independent variables (x_1, x_2, x_3, etc.) can be simultaneously investigated for their influence on a linear related dependent variable (y) is known as *multiple linear regression*. The method models the dependent variable as a linear function of all the (k) independent variables. That is,

$$y = a + b_1x_1 + b_2x_2 + b_3x_3 \ldots b_kx_k$$

It is particularly helpful in evaluating extraneous variables as possible confounders of the linear relationship between two continuous variables. In other words, linear regression permits the investigator to assess the separate *unconfounded effects* of several independent variables on a single dependent variable. The x_i's can be continuous or categorical variables. The b_i's are the regression coefficients. Each b_i is "corrected" simultaneously for the linear relationship between its associated x_i and all the other x_i's, as well as for the linear relationship between the other x_i's and y. An overall r^2 value is calculated for the model. It represents the percentage of the total variance of y accounted for by the linear relationship with all the x_i's. A common mistake is to refer to multiple linear regression as a multivariate technique. Technically, it is not because it deals with multiple independent rather than multiple dependent variables.

Multiple Logistic Regression

Multiple logistic regression is distinguished from multiple linear regression in that the outcome (dependent) variable is dichotomous (diseased or not diseased). Its aim is the same as that for all model-building techniques: to derive the best-fitting, most parsimonious (smallest or most efficient), and biologically reasonable model to describe the relationship between an outcome (dependent variable) and a set of predictors (independent variables). Here, the independent variables are called *covariates*. (Multiple logistic regression is not technically a multivariate technique—it deals with only one dependent variable.) Importantly, in multiple logistic regression, the predictor variables may be of any data level (categorical, ordinal, or continuous). A major use of this technique is to examine a series of predictor variables to determine those that best predict a certain outcome. A pediatric rheumatology example of the use of this technique can be found in the paper by Ruperto and associates,[26] in which predictor variables measurable during the very early stages of JRA (e.g., number of active joints during the first 6 months of illness, ESR) were tested to determine what their relative predictive ability was for either a favorable or less favorable outcome (i.e., a dichotomous, dependent variable) at least 5 years later. An excellent reference guide to this technique is provided by Hosmer and Lemeshow.[55]

Analysis of Covariance (ANCOVA)

The analysis of covariance (ANCOVA) combines the principles of ANOVA and regression. A chief advantage of this technique is that, unlike ANOVA, the independent variables can be of any data level. ANCOVA is often used to adjust for initial (baseline) differences between or among groups. That is, one of its chief purposes is to eliminate systematic bias. For example, suppose two groups of patients had unequal numbers of swollen joints at baseline (even though the study may have been randomized). The initial number of swollen joints is then used as the *covariate*. ANCOVA would adjust the post-treatment means of the groups to what they would have been if all groups had started out equally on the covariate.

The other purpose of ANCOVA is to reduce the within-group (or error) variances, thus making the test more efficient (powerful). For example, suppose a clinical trial investigates the effect on the ESR of a biologic agent and an active comparator. Subjects are randomized to receive one or the other, and the change in the ESR is observed. Within each treatment group, there is considerable variation of the ESR reflecting individual differences among patients in the degree of active inflammation. In other words, the ESR and active inflammation are covarying (covariates). If one could statistically remove this part of the within-group variability by allowing the degree of inflammation to be the covariate in the analysis, a smaller error term would result, and the test would gain power. ANCOVA provides a method to do this. In summary, ANCOVA provides a method for adjusting for differences at baseline between groups and reduces the amount of variation within groups due to covariates, thus increasing power and capability to detect differences.

Survival Analysis

Survival (life table) analysis was developed primarily for the study of how long a particular cohort of subjects survives. The term *survival data* is now used in a broader sense for data that involves time to a certain event, such as time to failure of a drug or time before remission.[55] There are two basic types of life table analysis: The fixed-interval (*actuarial*) model and the *Kaplan-Meier survival analysis*. The latter is used much more frequently in medicine than the former. In actuarial analysis, the lengths of each interval shown on the x-axis are all equal (e.g., 1 year). This is the technique used by life insurance companies to estimate the probability of a person surviving to a certain age. In the Kaplan-Meier approach, the end of an interval is demarcated by an event. The horizontal components of the lines are not equal as they are in the actuarial technique. An example of the actuarial method in pediatric rheumatology can be found in a study by Giannini and colleagues[61] of the time to occurrence of eye disease among patients with certain major histocompatibility complex alleles. An example of the Kaplan-Meier approach can be found in the study by Lovell and associates,[46] in which *time to failure* in subjects given placebo was compared with *time to failure* in those taking etanercept. Methods exist for comparing the difference of the life table graphs; the most frequently used is the generalized Wilcoxon test. Figure 8–7 is a graphic representation of a comparison between the characteristic lines of actuarial and Kaplan-Meier analysis. An outstanding reference for survival analysis techniques is that of Lee.[56]

Measures of Agreement Among and Within Raters

It is often necessary to express in statistical terms how well various raters agree with one another (*inter-rater*

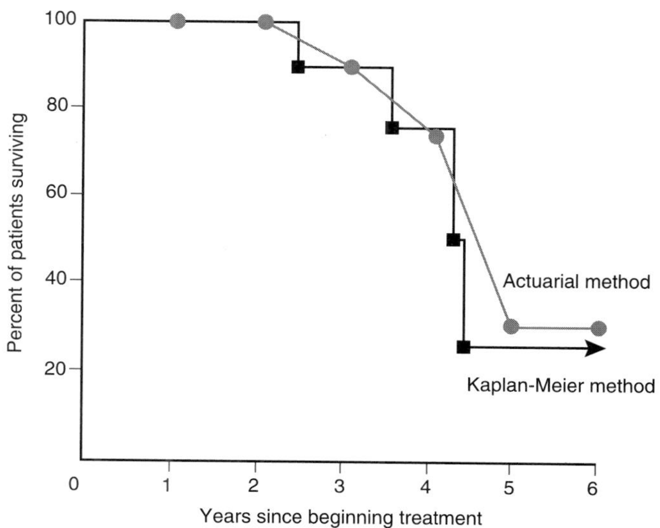

Figure 8–7. Comparison of Kaplan-Meier and actuarial survival curves showing a theoretical example of the percentage of patients surviving after 0 to 6 years of treatment. (Modified from Kramer MS: Clinical Epidemiology and Biostatistics: A Primer for Clinical Investigators and Decision-Makers. Berlin-Heidelberg-New York, Springer-Verlag, 1988, p 246, © 1988 Springer-Verlag.)

agreement) or with themselves (*intra-rater agreement*). Lack of agreement, either among or within raters, indicates that the values for the measure are unreliable. Of course, this has dire consequences for the interpretation of the results and for statistical interpretation. Various tests exist for expressing the degree of agreement between and within raters.

The most frequently used test to express rater agreement when the outcome is dichotomous is the *kappa test ratio* (known also as Cohen's kappa, κ). Table 8–11 shows a conventional 2 × 2 table in which the results of the agreement between two different raters of a variable (e.g., joint space narrowing on radiograph) is judged to be either positive or negative. The κ statistic is given by (observed agreement − agreement expected by chance) ÷ (maximum possible agreement − agreement expected by chance). κ scores range from −1, indicating perfect disagreement, to +1, indicating perfect agreement. A score of 0 indicates the agreement expected by chance. κ scores are often expressed as percentages, with less than 20 percent considered negligible agreement, 20 percent to 40 percent considered minimal, 40 percent to 60 percent considered fair, 60 percent to 80 percent considered good, and over 80 percent considered excellent agreement.[52]

Three or more categories (i.e., ordinal data) require the use of the more complex *weighted kappa test. Kendall's W,* or *coefficient of concordance,* can also be used. W values range from 0, which indicates poor agreement, to +1, indicating perfect agreement among all raters. W cannot be negative because not all the raters can disagree completely when there are more than two.

Multivariate Analyses

This section provides a basic concept of multivariate statistics and an overview of the more popular and increasingly used multivariate tests. Interested readers are referred to the text by Stevens[57] for in-depth discussions of the concepts and tests presented here.

Multivariate statistics are appropriate when the experimental design simultaneously investigates two dependent variables (DVs)—for example, bone mineral density and bone mineral content during a trial of calcium supplementation in prepubescent girls with polyarticular JRA. Testing of the two DVs in the calcium-supplementation and no-supplementation groups by, say, the *t* test is not appropriate because the tests are not independent of one another. That is, the two DVs are highly correlated with each other (and if one is known, the other can be guessed). Furthermore, just as the interaction among independent variables in a factorial ANOVA provides new information, so too does the use of multivariate tests that consider more than one DV simultaneously. Multivariate techniques may use nominal, ordinal, or continuous data.

Hotelling's T^2 Test

Just as the *t* test is used when one wishes to compare one DV in two different groups, Hotelling's T^2 test is used when there are two groups with multiple DVs. The process involves the comparisons of, for example, the *vectors of the means* in the treated and in the control group: A *centroid* for the groups is calculated, which is the point at which the mean values of the two DVs intersect for the control group when they are plotted on an x-y graph. The S.D. and the amount of correlation between the variables are used to calculate whether the T^2 statistic is significant. Multivariate significance implies that there is a linear combination of the dependent variables that is significantly separating the groups. However, significance from the T^2 statistic may arise from one or more of the DVs under consideration. Discriminant function analysis (described later) is used to determine which variables are contributing the most to the significant finding.

Table 8–11

Standard 2 × 2 Table Comparing the Test Results Reported by Two Raters

		RATER NO. 1		
		Positive	Negative	TOTAL
	Positive	a	b	a + b
RATER NO. 2	Negative	c	d	c + d
	TOTAL	a + c	b + d	a + b + c + d

Interpretation of the cells is as follows:
a = positive/positive rater agreement
b = negative/positive rater agreement
c = positive/negative rater agreement
d = negative/negative rater agreement

Formulas are as follows:
a + d = observed agreement (A_o)
$a + b + c + d$ = maximum possible agreement (N)
$(a + d)/(a + b + c + d)$ = overall percent agreement
$[(a + b)(a + c)]/(a + b + c + d)$ = cell *a* agreement expected by chance
$[(c + d)(b + d)]/(a + b + c + d)$ = cell *d* agreement expected by chance
cell *a* agreement expected by chance + cell *d* agreement expected by chance = total agreement expected by chance (A_c)
$(A_o - A_c)/(N - A_c)$ = kappa

Multivariate Analysis of Variance (MANOVA)

Just as ANOVA was used for the comparison of the means of more than two means, so too is MANOVA (rather than Hotelling's T^2) used in situations where there are more than two groups and multiple DVs. Its use instead of separate univariate ANOVA is related to accounting for intercorrelations among the DVs. Vectors of means are calculated and the centroid for each group is compared with the grand centroid (similar to the variance within, versus variance between, groups tested in univariate ANOVA). Similarly, the within-group variability has to be computed for each of the dependent variables. There are numerous ways to calculate the significance of MANOVA, the most common of which is Wilk's lambda. As with Hotelling's T^2, significance can arise from one or several of the variables, and discriminant function analysis is needed to sort it out.

Discriminant Function Analysis

In situations where many DVs exist, statistically significant differences among the groups can arise from the effect of one, several, or all of the variables. Discriminant function analysis identifies the variables that are most important in accounting for the observed differences. In addition, discriminant function analysis allows the determination of the groups that differ more in some DVs than in others. The process derives an equation (function) that best discriminates between the groups. The equation is similar to a regression equation and is the first variable multiplied by its weight, plus the second variable multiplied by its weight, and so on. In this case, rather than predicting a value of a DV as in regression, one is predicting group membership. Again, as in stepwise regression, computer programs can add and subtract variables from the equation (based on significance of Wilk's lambda test) until the combination that best discriminates the groups is arrived at.

Factor Analysis

Factor analysis is used for data exploration to reveal patterns of interrelationships among variables that are not readily apparent, for confirmation of hypotheses, and for reducing the number of variables to a manageable level. In situations involving many different observations concerning the same patient or groups of patients, factor analysis can be used to determine if it is possible that some of these observations are a result of just a few underlying factors. That is, the correlation among many DVs may be explained by some underlying factor(s). For example, the fact that a young boy is experiencing swollen joints, a rash, intermittent fevers, and a drop in hemoglobin with an increase in white blood cell count is a result of underlying factors. He is experiencing the onset of systemic JRA, and pathologic processes are taking place in his hematopoietic system. When groups of patients are studied, the symptoms will "load" on the underlying factors differentially. *Factor loading* is expressed in a *factor loading matrix,* in which each row of the matrix is a variable and each column is a factor. Such a matrix examines how highly each variable correlates with, or loads on, each factor. Each variable may load onto one or more variables. Next, one must decide which factors are most important to keep and which can be discarded as not contributing enough to the explanation of the variables. This is done by calculating an *eigenvalue,* which is the amount of variance in the data explained by a particular factor. The procedure to this point is called *principle component analysis.* Additional steps in factor analysis include rotation of axes to determine which are *general factors* (most variables load significantly on it) and which are *bipolar factors* (some variables load positively and some load negatively on it). *Factorial complexity* is determined by observing how many variables load significantly on two or more factors.

Multivariate Analysis of Covariance (MANCOVA)

This procedure is an extension of univariate ANCOVA in which group means at follow-up are adjusted for differences at baseline and within-group variance is reduced by removing variation due to covariates. The objective of MANCOVA is to determine whether several groups differ on a set of DVs after the follow-up means have been adjusted for any initial differences on the covariates at baseline.

Canonical Correlation

This multivariate procedure, an extension of multiple regression, is used to examine the nature of the association or interrelation between two sets of variables. Canonical correlation breaks down the complex association into additive pieces to determine the number and nature of independent relationships existing between two sets of variables.

Sample Size for Multivariate Tests

A rule of thumb is that there should be at least 10 subjects for each DV investigated in the study. A study in which the subject:variable ratio is smaller is likely to be unreliable.

JUDGING THE QUALITY OF A REPORT OF A CLINICAL INVESTIGATION

The most helpful and up-to-date series of guides to the reader of clinical reports has appeared in the *Journal of the American Medical Association* in recent years.[2–21] This *Users' Guides to the Medical Literature* series provides logical checklists of questions for a reader attempting to weigh the evidence from many different types of clinical studies. In brief, each *Guide* asks three basic questions:

- Are the results of the study valid?
- What were the results?
- Will the results help me in caring for my patients?

Practical examples from everyday clinical situations are then used to illustrate how one determines the answer and eventually weighs the evidence from the report. Because not all epidemiologic studies deal with patients, judging the quality of an epidemiologic investigation requires an approach that is similar to but separate from judging clinical investigations. The suggestions offered by Walker[62] provide a compact guide to reporting results of an epidemiologic study and can be used for judging a report.

Judging the Evidence From a Clinical Trial and the CONSORT Statement

Although the *Users' Guides* just cited contain information for judging clinical trials, more detailed guides are available. Chalmers and colleagues[63] provided a complete guide to the assessment of clinical trials that was used for many years. It remains as one of the most comprehensive reviews of the topic. In the 1980s, the *New England Journal of Medicine* recommended that contributing authors follow the suggestions of DerSimonian and coworkers[64] when preparing reports of clinical trials. In 1995, a group of medical journal editors, clinical epidemiologists, and statisticians developed a consensus statement about how randomized controlled trials should be reported—the *Consolidated Standards of Reporting Trials*, or *CONSORT*, statement.[65] This statement is now endorsed by the *Journal of the American Medical Association*[66] and is incorporated into the *Journal's* "Instructions to Authors." The statement contains a checklist of 21 items that deal chiefly with methods, results, and discussion. It identifies key pieces of information necessary to evaluate the internal and external validity of a report. A flow diagram is also recommended (using a two-group parallel design randomized controlled trial as an example) that provides a graphic display of allocation and status of patients throughout the trial. Some modification of the statement's recommendations is usually necessary because of differences in study design. Overall, however, it provides an outstanding template on which to formulate or judge the report of a clinical trial.

References

1. Evidence-Based Medicine Working Group: Evidence-based medicine: a new approach to teaching the practice of medicine. JAMA 268: 2420–2425, 1992.

1a. Brunner HI, Giannini EH: Evidence-based medicine in pediatric rheumatology [Review]. Clin Exp Rheum 18: 407–414, 2000.

2. Guyatt GH, Rennie D: Users' Guides to the Medical Literature. JAMA 270: 2096–2097, 1993.
3. Oxman AD, Sackett DL, Guyatt GH, for the Evidence-Based Medicine Working Group: Users' Guides to the Medical Literature. I: How to get started. JAMA 270: 2093–2098, 1993.
4. Guyatt GH, Sackett DL, Cook DJ, for the Evidence-Based Medicine Working Group: Users' Guides to the Medical Literature. II: How to use an article about therapy or prevention. A: Are the results of the study valid? JAMA 270: 2598–2601, 1993.
5. Guyatt GH, Sackett DL, Cook DJ, for the Evidence-Based Medicine Working Group: Users' Guides to the Medical Literature. II: How to use an article about therapy or prevention. B: What were the results and will they help me in caring for my patients? JAMA 271: 59–63, 1994.
6. Jaeschke R, Guyatt GH, Sackett DL, for the Evidence-Based Medicine Working Group: Users' Guides to the Medical Literature. III: How to use an article about a diagnostic test. A: Are the results of the study valid? JAMA 271: 389–391, 1994.
7. Jaeschke R, Guyatt GH, Sackett DL, for the Evidence-Based Medicine Working Group: Users' Guides to the Medical Literature. III: How to use an article about a diagnostic test. B: What are the results and will they help me in caring for my patients? JAMA 271: 703–707, 1994.
8. Levine M, Walter S, Lee H, for the Evidence-Based Medicine Working Group: Users' Guides to the Medical Literature. IV: How to use an article about harm. JAMA 271: 1615–1619, 1994.
9. Laupacis A, Wells G, Richardson WS, Tugwell P, for the Evidence-Based Medicine Working Group: Users' Guides to the Medical Literature. V: How to use an article about prognosis. JAMA 272: 234–237, 1994.
10. Oxman AD, Cook DJ, Guyatt GH, for the Evidence-Based Medicine Working Group: Users' Guides to the Medical Literature. VI: How to use an overview. JAMA 272: 1367–1371, 1994.
11. Richardson WS, Detsky AS, for the Evidence-Based Medicine Working Group: Users' Guides to the Medical Literature. VII: How to use a clinical decision analysis. A: Are the results of the study valid? JAMA 273: 1292–1295, 1995.
12. Richardson WS, Detsky AS, for the Evidence-Based Medicine Working Group: Users' Guides to the Medical Literature. VII: How to use a clinical decision analysis. B: What are the results and will they help me in caring for my patients? JAMA 273: 1610–1613, 1995.
13. Hayward RSA, Wilson MC, Tunis SR, for the Evidence-Based Medicine Working Group: Users' Guides to the Medical Literature. VIII: How to use clinical practice guidelines. A: Are the recommendations valid? JAMA 274: 570–574, 1995.
14. Wilson MC, Hayward RSA, Tunis SR, for the Evidence-Based Medicine Working Group: Users' Guides to the Medical Literature. VIII: How to use clinical practice guidelines. B: What are the recommendations and will they help you in caring for your patients? JAMA 274: 1630–1632, 1995.
15. Guyatt GH, Sackett DL, Sinclair JC, for the Evidence-Based Medicine Working Group: Users' Guides to the Medical Literature. IX: A method for grading healthcare recommendations. JAMA 274: 1800–1804, 1995.
16. Naylor CD, Guyatt GH, for the Evidence-Based Medicine Working Group: Users' Guides to the Medical Literature. X: How to use an article reporting variations in the outcomes of health services. JAMA 275: 554–558, 1996.
17. Naylor CD, Guyatt GH, for the Evidence-Based Medicine Working Group: Users' Guides to the Medical Literature. XI: How to use an article about a clinical utilization review. JAMA 275: 1435–1439, 1996.
18. Guyatt GH, Naylor CD, Juniper E, for the Evidence-Based Medicine Working Group: Users' Guides to the Medical Literature. XII: How to use articles about health-related quality of life. JAMA 277: 1232–1237, 1997.
19. Drummond MF, Richardson WS, O'Brien BJ, for the Evidence-Based Medicine Working Group: Users' Guides to the Medical Literature. XIII: How to use an article on economic analysis of clinical practice. A: Are the results of the study valid? JAMA 277: 1552–1557, 1997.
20. O'Brien BJ, Heyland D, Richardson WS, for the Evidence-Based Medicine Working Group: Users' Guides to the Medical Literature. XIII: How to use an article on economic analysis of clinical practice. B: What are the results and will they help me in caring for my patients? JAMA 277: 1802–1806, 1997.
21. Dans AL, Dans LF, Guyatt GH, for the Evidence-Based Medicine Working Group: Users' Guides to the Medical Literature. XIV: How to decide on the applicability of clinical trial results to your patient. JAMA 279: 545–549, 1998.
22. Moses LE: Statistics in practice. Statistical concepts fundamental to investigations. N Engl J Med 312: 890–897, 1985.
23. Hill AB: The environment and disease: association or causation. Proc R Soc Med 58: 295–300, 1965.
24. Inman RD, Johnston ME, Hodge M, et al: Postdysenteric reactive arthritis. A clinical and immunogenetic study following an outbreak of salmonellosis. Arthritis Rheum 31: 1377–1383, 1988.
25. Ruperto N, Levinson JE, Ravelli A, et al: Long-term health outcomes and quality of life in American and Italian inception cohorts of patients with juvenile rheumatoid arthritis. I: Outcome status. J Rheumatol 24: 945–951, 1997.
26. Ruperto N, Levinson JE, Ravelli A, et al: Long-term health out-

comes and quality of life in American and Italian inception cohorts of patients with juvenile rheumatoid arthritis. II: Early predictors of outcome. J Rheumatol 24: 952–958, 1997.
27. Andersson Gäre B, Fasth A: The natural history of juvenile chronic arthritis: a population based cohort study. II: Outcome. J Rheumatol 22: 308–319, 1995.
28. Ansell BM: Prognosis in juvenile chronic polyarthritis. Clin Rheum Dis 2: 397–412, 1976.
29. Kwoh CK, Simms RW, Anderson LG, et al: Guidelines for the management of rheumatoid arthritis. Arthritis Rheum 39: 713–722, 1996.
30. Giannini EH, Cawkwell CD: Drug treatment in children with juvenile rheumatoid arthritis—past, present, and future. Pediatr Clin North Am 42: 1099–1125, 1995.
31. Food and Drug Administration: Guidance for industry: clinical development programs for drugs, devices, and biological products for the treatment of rheumatoid arthritis. U.S. Government Printing Office, 1999. www.fda/gov/cder/1208fne.htm.
32. U.S. DHSS PF: Guidance for Industry: clinical development programs for drugs, devices, and biological products for the treatment of rheumatoid arthritis (RA). U.S. Government Printing Office, 1998.
33. Food and Drug Administration: Guidance for industry: structure and content of clinical study reports. U.S. Government Printing Office, 1996 www.fda.gov/cder/guidance/index.htm
34. Food and Drug Administration: Guidance for industry: E6 Good clinical practice: consolidated guidance. U.S. Government Printing Office, 1996 www.fda.gov/cder/guidance/index.htm.
35. Food and Drug Administration: Guidance for industry. E8: general considerations for clinical trials. U.S. Government Printing Office, 1999 www.fda.gov/cder/guidance/index.htm.
36. Food and Drug Administration: Guidance for industry. E9: Statistical principles for clinical trials. U.S. Government Printing Office, 1999 www.fda.gov/cder/guidance/index.htm.
37. Weiner DL, Yuh L: Bioavailability studies. *In* Buncher CR, Tsay J-Y (eds): Statistics in the Pharmaceutical Industry. New York, Marcel Dekker, 1994, pp 215–245.
38. Lovell DJ, Giannini EH, Whitmore JB, et al: Safety and efficacy of tumor necrosis factor receptor p75 Fc fusion protein (TNFR: Fc;Enbrel) in polyarticular juvenile rheumatoid arthritis. Arthritis Rheum 41(Suppl): S130, 1998.
39. Giannini EH: Can non-fundable trials be conducted anyway? The case for open, randomized, actively-controlled trials in rheumatology. Ann Rheum Dis 57: 128–130, 1998.
40. Shaikov AV, Maximov AA, Speransky AI, et al: Repetitive use of pulse therapy with methylprednisolone and cyclophosphamide in addition to oral methotrexate in children with systemic juvenile rheumatoid arthritis—preliminary results of a longterm study. J Rheumatol 19: 612–616, 1992.
41. Giannini EH: The N of 1 trials design in the rheumatic diseases. Arthritis Care Res 1: 109–115, 1998.
41a. Temple R, Ellenberg SS: Placebo-controlled trials and active-control trials in the evaluation of new treatments. Part 1: Ethical and scientific issues. Ann Intern Med 133: 455–463, 2000.
42. Fortin PR, Stucki G, Katz JN: Measuring relevant change: an emerging challenge in rheumatologic clinical trials. Arthritis Rheum 38: 1027–1030, 1995.
43. Felson DT, Anderson JJ, Boers M, et al: American College of Rheumatology preliminary definition of improvement in rheumatoid arthritis. Arthritis Rheum 38: 727–735, 1995.
44. Giannini EH, Ruperto N, Ravelli A, et al: Preliminary definition of improvement in juvenile arthritis. Arthritis Rheum 40: 1202–1209, 1997.
45. Ruperto N, Ravelli A, Falcini F, et al: Performance of the preliminary definition of improvement in juvenile chronic arthritis patients treated with methotrexate. Ann Rheum Dis 57: 38–41, 1998.
46. Lovell DJ, Giannini EH, Reiff A, et al: Etanercept in children with polyarticular juvenile rheumatoid arthritis. N Engl J Med 342: 763–769, 2000.
47. Ruperto N, Ravelli A, Falcini F, et al: Responsiveness of outcome measures in juvenile chronic arthritis. Rheumatology 38: 176–180, 1999.
48. Pinals RS, Masi AT, Larsen RA: Preliminary criteria for clinical remission in rheumatoid arthritis. Arthritis Rheum 24: 1308–1315, 1981.
49. Larsen A, Dale K, Eek M: Radiographic evaluation of rheumatoid arthritis and related conditions by standard reference films. Acta Radiol [Diagn] (Stockh) 18: 481–491, 1977.
50. Sharp JT, Young DY, Bluhm GB, et al: How many joints in the hands and wrists should be included in a score of radiologic abnormalities used to assess rheumatoid arthritis? Arthritis Rheum 28: 1326–1335, 1985.
50a. Ware JE Jr, Sherbourne CD: The MOS 36-item short-form health survey (SF-36). I. Conceptual framework and item selection. Med Care 30: 473–483, 1992.
51. Mantel N, Haenszel W: Statistical aspects of the analysis of data from retrospective studies of disease. J Natl Cancer Inst 22: 719–748, 1959.
52. Jekel JF, Elmore JG, Katz DL: Epidemiology, Biostatistics, and Preventative Medicine, 1st ed. Philadelphia, WB Saunders, 1996.
53. Huck SW, Cormier WH: Reading Statistics and Research, 2nd ed. Baltimore, HarperCollins College Publishers, 1996.
54. Knapp RG, Miller MC III: Clinical Epidemiology and Biostatistics. Malvern, PA, Harwal, 1992.
55. Hosmer DW, Lemeshow S: Applied Logistic Regression. New York, John Wiley & Sons, 1989.
56. Lee ET: Statistical Methods for Survival Data Analysis, 2nd ed. New York, John Wiley & Sons, 1999.
57. Stevens J: Applied Multivariate Statistics for the Social Sciences, 3rd ed. Mahwah, NJ, Lawrence Erlbaum, 1996.
58. Brophy JM, Joseph L: Placing trials in context using Bayesian analysis: GUSTO revisited by Reverend Bayes. JAMA 273: 871–875, 1995.
59. Brown GW: *P* values. Am J Dis Child 144: 493–495, 1990.
60. Rothman KJ: No adjustments are needed for multiple comparisons. Epidemiology 1: 43–46, 1990.
61. Giannini EH, Malagon C, Van Kerckhove C, et al: Actuarial analysis of iridocyclitis risk in HLA characterized early-onset pauciarticular JRA (EOPA-JRA) patients. J Rheumatol 19(Suppl 33): 118, 1992.
62. Walker AM: Reporting the results of epidemiologic studies. Am J Pub Health 76: 556–558, 1986.
63. Chalmers TC, Smith HS Jr, Blackburn B, et al: A method for assessing the quality of a randomized control trial. Controlled Clin Trials 2: 31–49, 1981.
64. DerSimonian R, Charette LJ, McPeek B, Mosteller F: Reporting on methods in clinical trials. N Engl J Med 306: 1332–1337, 1982.
65. Standards of Reporting Trials Group: A proposal for structured reporting of randomized controlled trials. JAMA 272: 1926–1931, 1994.
66. Rennie D: How to report randomized controlled trials—the CONSORT statement. JAMA 276: 649, 1996.

9

Assessment of Health Status, Function, and Outcome

Ciarán M. Duffy and Daniel J. Lovell

The rheumatic diseases of childhood influence many if not all aspects of the child's life—not only physical but also social,[1] emotional,[2] intellectual, and economic.[3] Indeed, childhood rheumatic disease affects not only the child but also the entire family.[4] Conversely, the family's status and functioning can significantly affect the outcome of the child's illness.[4] This chapter deals with the methods used and tools developed to quantitatively assess this web of influence.

BACKGROUND

Many interests and influences have led to the current popularity of measuring "quality of life" (QOL). This term was originally developed by sociologists to try to determine the effect of material affluence on people's lives. This sociologic approach was developed in the United States during World War II. The concept broadened so that it eventually included education, social welfare, economics, and industrial growth.[5] This broad societal approach was also incorporated into questionnaires that were developed to assess the status of an individual within this broad framework of concern.

Many of these areas of concern or domains, although important to an individual, are well outside the influence of disease and healthcare interventions. It is for this reason that other terminology to describe QOL was developed. Various authors have used terms such as health-related quality of life (HRQL), life satisfaction, self-esteem, well-being, general health, functional status, and life adjustment to describe the aspects of QOL that relate to the overall global health status of human beings.[5] Considerable confusion remains about the actual terminology and definitions in this field.

For the purpose of this chapter, *functional status* is defined as the ability of an individual to perform daily activities. Discussion of QOL will be restricted to HRQL. However, both functional status and HRQL are complex concepts that contain numerous subcomponents. There are differences of opinion among the experts as to what constitutes HRQL. Various tools have been developed to measure HRQL. These tools are further subdivided into generic and disease-specific HRQL measures. Generic HRQL measures are those that purport to be broadly equal across types and severity of disease, across different medical treatments or health interventions, and across different demographic or cultural subgroups. They are designed to capture aspects of health and disease that cross broad diagnostic categories and social and demographic subgroups. Disease-specific HRQL measures are those designed to assess specific disease diagnostic groups for specific diseases or patient populations, often with the goal of becoming more responsive to changes in individual subject disease status or in treatment.

Recent decades have seen the development and validation of a variety of tools to measure functional status and generic and disease-specific HRQL. These tools were first developed for application to adult rheumatology, but more recently specific tools have been developed for use in childhood-onset rheumatic diseases.

Why Measure Quality of Life?

QOL measurements have been used for a wide variety of purposes. One of the earliest and, at the time, one of the strongest motivations for measuring HRQL was to allow comparisons of health gains or efficiency of health-related interventions across broad population groups so as to be able to compare health gains achieved in treating different patient groups. This information has been used in measurement of health outcomes in a variety of health-related systems of care to assist in prioritizing allocations of limited healthcare resources.[5–7] In the field of rheumatology, HRQL has gained wide popularity because it has been shown to measure outcomes that are of direct interest and importance to patients, to effectively measure patient status, to predict patient outcome, and to be a reliable and effective measure of treatment impact.[8–11]

This already complex field is further complicated by the fact that a number of terms and measurement techniques have been imported from the field of questionnaire development and are foreign to and certainly not easily understood by healthcare personnel. The most important concepts and terms are included in Table 9–1 and are described in the following discussion.

Table 9–1
Glossary of Terms Commonly Used in Quality of Life Literature

Term	Definition
Ceiling effect	Situation in which the highest score on an instrument does not represent the best status a subject can have; patients with the highest score can still experience more improvement
Construct validity	Degree to which an instrument correlates with other measures based on a priori predictions of the degree of correlation
Content validity	Extent to which items in the instrument comprehensively assess the domain of interest
Convergent validity	Correlation of instrument scores to accepted but not gold-standard parameters measuring the same domain
Criterion validity	Comparison of results on an instrument as a gold standard; such a gold standard does not exist for QOL
Discriminant instrument	Designed to most effectively differentiate groups of people
Domain or dimension	Area of behavior or experience that is being measured
Evaluative instrument	Designed to most effectively detect change in the status of a person over time
Face validity	Estimation of whether an instrument appears to be measuring what it is intended to measure (does it look reasonable?); seldom quantitated
Floor effects	Situation in which the lowest possible score on an instrument does not represent the worst status a subject can have; patients with the worst score can still deteriorate further
Generalizability	Extent to which an instrument can yield accurate and reliable results when used in circumstances or subjects different from those in which it was originally validated—for example, can be used in varying socioeconomic, ethnic, geographic disease types, or disease severity
Model	A theoretical framework of what is being measured and how the instrument should perform
Patient preference instrument	Instrument designed so that individuals select those parameters on the instrument that are the most important to them
Predictive validity	Extent to which a score on an instrument at one point predicts patient outcome at a later time
Reliability	Extent to which a measuring procedure yields the same results on repeated trials if all the conditions remain unchanged
Sensitivity to change	Extent to which scores on an instrument given at different times in the same subject(s) will change if there is a true change in the status of the subject(s)
Surrogate or proxy reporter	Someone who answers on behalf of another and reports what the surrogate thinks the subject would answer (e.g., parent reporting for a child)

QOL, quality of life.

Hierarchy of Outcomes

Critical to understanding this area is having a clear vision of the hierarchy of outcomes and outcome measures. The first level of outcome assessment is the measurement of disease activity. This is the aspect of outcome assessment that has been the traditional focus of trials in rheumatology. Disease activity measures include those parameters most familiar to clinicians—for example, joint counts, morning stiffness, erythrocyte sedimentation rate. The major drawback to measures in this area is that they are not really what the patient is interested in. However, measures of disease activity are still widely used in clinical trials because inhibition of the disease process or activity is essential to effective therapeutic intervention—especially pharmacologic intervention. At this time, measurement of disease activity is a necessary but insufficient approach to measuring patient outcome. Furthermore, when the performance characteristics of the traditional disease activity measures used in rheumatology were scientifically assessed, many were found to be unreliable, redundant, insensitive to change, or not correlated with long-term patient outcome.[9]

The next level up the hierarchy is measurement of *functional status.* The focus here is on measuring the ability of the person to perform physical activities of daily life—for example, dressing, walking, climbing stairs, and self-care. Obviously, these functions are relevant to the patient. Several instruments have been developed and validated to quantitate functional status in patients with childhood arthritis. These instruments are discussed in greater detail later in this chapter.

The next level in the measurement hierarchy is represented by *QOL tools.* Although some authors have made distinctions between QOL and health status, many others use these terms interchangeably. They may not have separate meanings.[11] In general, QOL is the more commonly used term. Measures at this level are in accordance with the World Health Organization (WHO) view that health is a state of physical, mental, and social well-being.[12] Disease-specific HRQL measures, such as the Health Assessment Questionnaire (HAQ) or the Arthritis Impact Measurement Scale (AIMS), were developed to incorporate the broad WHO concept of health but specifically address areas that are affected by rheumatic disease. For example, the HAQ includes questions addressing mortality, functional status, physical discomfort, psychological discomfort, treatment side effects, and economic impact.[9] Major advances have been made in the development and validation of disease-specific HRQL tools for juvenile arthritis.

PROCESS OF TOOL OR INSTRUMENT DEVELOPMENT

The development and validation process for functional assessment or QOL tools or instruments has been well established, but for most healthcare providers the terminology and statistical approaches are unfamiliar. Certainly, it is clear that the development of a new functional assessment or QOL tool is labor intensive, requires sequential studies, needs input from a wide range of persons, and requires frequent revisions of the original tool prior to completion. For example, over 20 iterations were required in the development of the HAQ. The development process for two of the functional assessment tools validated for children with juvenile arthritis required 3 to 5 years for each questionnaire.[13–16] Given the broader scope of content, QOL tools in childhood arthritis have taken at least as long.[17, 18] In fact, some are still at some stage of validation.[19] The process of developing and validating health measurement questionnaires has been described in textbooks,[20, 21] and several articles thoroughly describe the steps used for tools specifically focused on children with rheumatic diseases.[17, 22]

The five steps involved in this process are determining what the questionnaire is going to measure and in whom, devising the potential items, selecting the items, assessing reliability, and assessing validity.[20]

Step 1: Determining What the Questionnaire Is Going to Measure and in Whom

Is the questionnaire focused on functional status or the broader HRQL? What disease or diseases will be assessed? A key question to answer at this point is: Is there truly a need to develop a new questionnaire?

There are hundreds of validated questionnaires, and review of the literature may well reveal one that will serve the purpose. Researchers tend to magnify the deficiencies of existing measures and significantly underestimate the effort required to develop an adequate new measure.[20] There are several compendia of measuring scales.[23–25] If one or more existent scales are found, these scales need to be evaluated.

The first assessment involves evaluation of face and content validity. *Face validity* merely refers to the subjective assessment of whether the instrument is assessing the desired qualities (i.e., does it look like it might work?). *Content validity* is an assessment of whether the instrument samples all the important domains. Usually, these forms of validity are assessed by a group of experts and are rarely quantified. Published studies of the reliability and validity of the existent tools should be reviewed. *Reliability* refers to the ability of a tool to measure reproducibly. Do the results obtained with the tool change or remain the same when appropriate? *Validity* refers to whether the test is measuring what was intended. Specific steps in assessing reliability and validity are discussed later (see "Step 4: Assessing Reliability" and "Step 5: Assessing Validity"). If the conclusion is that no existent questionnaires are satisfactory, much work awaits the brave souls who choose to develop a new tool.

Step 2: Devising the Potential Items

Devising the potential items is a critical step because no questionnaire is stronger than the individual items included in its makeup.

New items generally come from four sources: theory, research, expert opinion, and clinical observation.[20] *Theory* refers to the general framework driving the questionnaire development (e.g., what domains are going to be measured? Is the tool going to be defined to be primarily a discriminant or an evaluative instrument?). These types of overarching theoretical concepts determine the types of items generated. *Research* can refer to investigating existent tools and including or adapting items from them, or new research performed especially to generate new items. This form of research often involves the use of experts in the field to generate lists of potential items. For example, children with a rheumatic disease, parents, and healthcare professionals have been asked to generate the items for several of the functional assessment and HRQL tools used in pediatric rheumatology. There are no hard and fast rules governing the use of these various approaches to item generation. Most instruments have been developed with a combination of these approaches. It is generally better to involve a variety of persons to avoid skewing the questions. The number of items generated usually greatly exceeds the eventual number included in the final form of the instrument.

Step 3: Selecting the Items

This process, one hopes, results in a small subset of the questions generated in step 2 that contains enough questions to cover adequately the domain or domains under investigation (content validity) but is not so long as to be difficult to complete. First, questions that are ambiguous or difficult to understand are eliminated. Questions should not require reading skills above those of a 12-year-old.[20] Usually, the items are tested on a group of subjects similar to the proposed target audience to identify questions that are confusing, are ambiguous, contain jargon, or are double-barreled (contain two questions in one, e.g., "Do you feel tired and depressed?"). Subjects are asked to read each item and indicate whether they understand it, but they are not asked to actually respond to the item.

The instrument developer can additionally ask the individual to explain what they think the item is asking—the *probe technique*. Generally, the remaining items are administered to a group of subjects. Items that are answered uniformly positive or negative by a large proportion of the group are eliminated. Internal consistency of the items relates to the fact that each item is actually measuring some aspect of the domain in question (i.e., the responses on the individual items should be moderately correlated to each other and each item should correlate with the total score on the instrument—*homogeneity of the items*).[20] If a scale has multiple dimensions or domains within the same scale, the measurement of homogeneity is more complex because individual items need to be more highly correlated with the other items in the particular dimension in question than with the other dimensions in the scale. A statistical technique commonly used in evaluating multidimensional scales is factor analysis.[25]

Step 4: Assessing Reliability

Reliability refers to measurements that are reproducible and consistent. In scales that utilize one person to observe and rate the performance of another, intraobserver and interobserver reliability need to be determined. *Intraobserver reliability* is the ability of an observer to generate similar results at different times if the status of the subject does not change. *Interobserver reliability* refers to the ability of different individuals to agree with each other when independently assessing a subject at one point in time. When the subject is self-administering the instrument (or a surrogate is reporting), test–retest comparability is assessed. The subject (or surrogate) is asked to complete the instrument at two different points in time. The time between tests needs to be long enough that the subject is not likely to remember prior answers but not so long that the subject's true status changes. Usually, 1 to 2 weeks is allowed to elapse between tests in evaluations of rheumatic disease instruments.

Step 5: Assessing Validity

Validity refers to the fact that the scale is actually measuring what we want it to. For example, is the scale truly measuring "sex appeal"? Obviously, determining validity is a more difficult task if the quality to be measured is as complex and somewhat abstract as sex appeal or HRQL. One way to look at validity testing is to assess the "3 Cs"—content, criterion, and construct validity.[20, 24, 25] *Content validity* refers to how well an instrument measures across the entire range of possible states of the subjects in question. For example, can an instrument effectively measure patients with very mild or very severe arthritis as well as those with moderate arthritis? Or, stated another way, if an instrument indicates that a subject has severe arthritis, how accurately does it track with other aspects of severe arthritis?

Criterion validity refers to the correlation of the new scale with one that is widely accepted—a "gold standard."[20] In actuality, no such gold standard exists for HRQL instruments in pediatric rheumatology.[17, 18, 26] In adult rheumatology, widely used and respected tools such as the HAQ or AIMS represent such a gold standard or are at least very close. Commonly, developers choose aspects of the disease that are, if not golden, very high-quality silver—for example, "need for joint replacement surgery" as an indicator of significant joint damage. *Concurrent validity* is a measure of how tightly the new instrument results correlate with the need for joint replacement surgery at one point in time. *Predictive validity* measures how well the new instrument correlates with the need for joint replacement surgery at a later point in time. Concurrent and predictive validity are estimates of construct validity. *Construct validity* is a measure of how well the new instrument correlates with other measures based on a priori predictions of the degree of such correlations. For example, physical dimensions of an instrument should correlate better with measures of disease activity than a psychosocial dimension would.

The rest of this chapter describes the various tools available in pediatric rheumatology.

AVAILABLE INSTRUMENTS

Background

There is an increasing need to incorporate estimates of physical, social, and mental functioning into health assessment, especially in the assessment of chronic diseases.[27] For this reason, emphasis has been placed on the development of "clinimetric" indices,[28] some of which provide an all-encompassing measure of QOL.[29] QOL includes both health status and functional status. Furthermore, QOL measurement should attempt to incorporate some aspect of the patients' own perception of what aspects of their life significantly affect them and to what extent this is influenced by their disease.[30]

Measurement instruments of this type may be generic or disease-specific, with the latter having greater applicability for clinical trials because of greater sensitivity in the detection of important clinical change (responsiveness[29]). The most widely used rheumatic disease–specific measurement instruments for adults with rheumatoid arthritis include the AIMS,[31] the HAQ,[32] and the McMaster-Toronto arthritis patient preference questionnaire (MACTAR)[33] (Table 9–2). These instruments have been demonstrated to be reliable, valid, and responsive in a variety of conditions[34–39] and are now considered to be required for inclusion in clinical trials.[40] The MACTAR allows patients to preferentially select items that have a direct effect on them and thus individualizes the instrument for the patient, resulting in enhanced responsiveness. This approach has been shown to be particularly useful in clinical trials.[41]

The ideal instrument should be practical and easy to use, should be capable of completion by the parents or child within a short time, should measure physical function (and, as suggested by Singsen, should also measure psychological function and social function, including school, family, and behavioral issues), and should include a measurement of pain.[42] Other important qualities of the ideal instrument for measuring QOL in childhood arthritis are shown in Table 9–3.

None of the instruments used meets all of the criteria. However, each instrument has unique characteristics that make it distinct; thus, each one may have different indications for use. Each one is discussed with an emphasis on its development, its measurement

Table 9–2

Instruments Developed for Adults With Rheumatoid Arthritis

Arthritis Impact Measurement Scales (AIMS)
Health Assessment Questionnare (HAQ)
McMaster-Toronto Arthritis (MACTAR) Patient Preference Questionnaire
McMaster Health Index Questionnaire (MHIQ)

Table 9–3

Required Properties of the Ideal Instrument for Juvenile Arthritis

Reliability
Validity
Responsiveness (sensitivity to change)
Discriminative ability
Easy to use and score
Applicable to a wide age range and to a heterogeneous population
Measures physical function comprehensively
Measures quality of life (including psychosocial functioning) comprehensively

properties, and the settings in which it might be used. For a more complete description of these instruments, the reader is referred to reviews.[18, 26]

Although instruments have been developed for diseases other than inflammatory arthritides in adults, few such instruments have been developed for application in children. Those that have been developed specifically for children, and adult instruments that have shown utility in children, are also discussed in brief.

Instruments Available for Use in Juvenile Arthritis

Disease-specific measures include the Childhood Arthritis Impact Measurement Scales (CHAIMS),[43] the Childhood Health Assessment Questionnaire (CHAQ),[14] the Juvenile Arthritis Functional Assessment Report (JAFAR),[15] the Juvenile Arthritis Self-report Index (JASI),[44] the Juvenile Arthritis Quality of Life Questionnaire (JAQQ),[17] and the Childhood Arthritis Health Profile (CAHP)[19] (Table 9–4), all of which were designed for use in juvenile arthritis.

Childhood Arthritis Impact Measurement Scales

The CHAIMS was the first disease-specific measure developed for juvenile rheumatoid arthritis (JRA).[43] This was a modification of the AIMS.[31] Seventy-seven patients with JRA were studied. Several scales could not be administered to the parents of children under 6 years of age because the items did not apply. The overall measurement properties of the instrument, however, were not good except for the pain dimension, which showed good reliability and convergent validity. Face and content validity were not discussed and responsiveness was not tested in this study. Unfortunately, this is the only study published on the evaluation of this instrument, which has not enjoyed widespread use.

Table 9–4

Instruments Developed for Juvenile Arthritis

Childhood Arthritis Impact Measurement Scales (CHAIMS)
Childhood Health Assessment Questionnaire (CHAQ)
Juvenile Arthritis Functional Assessment Scale (JAFAS) and Report (JAFAR)
Juvenile Arthritis Self-report Index (JASI)
Juvenile Arthritis Quality of Life Questionnaire (JAQQ)
Childhood Arthritis Health Profile (CAHP)

Childhood Health Assessment Questionnaire

The CHAQ, which was derived from the adult HAQ,[32] was published in 1994.[14] It comprises two indices, Disability and Discomfort. The Disability Index assesses function in eight areas—dressing and grooming, arising, eating, walking, hygiene, reach, grip, and activities—distributed among a total of 30 items. In each functional area, at least one question is relevant to children of all ages. Each question is rated on a four-point scale of difficulty in performance, scored from 0 to 3. The question with the highest score determines the score for that functional area. If aids or devices are used or assistance is required, the minimum score for that functional area is 2. The Disability Index is calculated as the mean of the eight functional areas. Discomfort is determined by the presence of pain measured by a 100-mm visual analogue scale (VAS), extrapolated to a score of 0 to 3. In addition, a 100-mm VAS measures patient/parent global assessment of arthritis.

In the original validation study,[14] the CHAQ was completed by the parents in all cases and by children 8 years of age and older in a mean of 10 minutes. Mean scores for parents and children were not significantly different from one another and were highly correlated, suggesting that parents can reliably report for their children. Mean scores for patients with JRA were 0.84 for the Disability Index (range, 0 to 2.9) and 0.82 for the Discomfort Index (range, 0 to 2.8). With the Disability Index, excellent test–retest reliability was established. Convergent validity was also good, with excellent correlations with Steinbrocker's functional class, active joint count, disease activity index, and degree of morning stiffness. Responsiveness was also established.[45]

Andersson Gare and colleagues demonstrated excellent reliability, convergent validity, and discriminant validity for a Swedish translation of the CHAQ for both indices in a large cohort of patients with JRA and juvenile spondyloarthritides (JSpA).[46] It was also proved to be a useful instrument for outcome evaluation in longitudinal studies.[47, 48] The CHAQ has also been used in a variety of settings and translated into a number of different languages while maintaining excellent reliability, validity, and parent–child correlations.[49–53] In addition to testing in JRA and JSpA, it has also been evaluated in juvenile dermatomyositis (JDM), in which it was shown to have excellent responsiveness in an open study of 20 children with JDM after the introduction of glucocorticoids.[56] Although the CHAQ does not measure psychosocial function in its present form, an earlier version showed reasonable measurement properties in this domain[57]; however, this has not been maintained in the version in current use.

The CHAQ has excellent reliability and validity and good discriminative properties; thus, it has good predictive qualities and is of value for longitudinal studies. Preliminary data suggest that it is responsive, although this needs to be clearly established in a controlled trial before the CHAQ can be considered the definitive instrument for efficacy or effectiveness trials. It does not attempt to measure overall health or QOL, and in the evaluation of children this is an important deficiency. However, it can be administered to children of all ages, in several languages, and thus is of great potential use in the clinical setting for the long-term follow-up of children with JRA, JSpA, JDM, and probably other childhood rheumatic diseases.

Juvenile Arthritis Functional Assessment Scale and Report

The Juvenile Arthritis Functional Assessment Scale (JAFAS),[58] published in 1989, preceded the publication of the JAFAR, which appeared in 1991.[13] The JAFAS is an observer-based scale, whereas the JAFAR is a patient- or parent-completed report. Items for both instruments were derived from the AIMS, the HAQ, and the McMaster Health Index Questionnaire.[59]

The JAFAS requires standardized simple equipment and can be administered in about 10 minutes by a health professional who times the child's performance on 10 physical tasks. Good reliability and convergent validity have been demonstrated. Responsiveness has not been assessed. The major limitation of the JAFAS is the requirement of a trained observer and standardized equipment.

The JAFAR comprises one dimension and contains 23 items that assess ability to perform physical tasks in children older than 7 years on a three-point scale scored from 0 to 2; thus, the score range is 0 to 46, with the lower score indicating better function. Two separate versions are available, one for the child (JAFAR-C) and one for the parents (JAFAR-P). The original study included 72 patients and parents of children with JRA. The mean scores in JRA patients for the JAFAR-C and JAFAR-P were 4.39 and 4.38, respectively; although close to the normal range, these scores were significantly different from those of controls. Reliability was good for both versions. Construct validity was good, with predictable correlations among JAFAR-C, JAFAR-P, JAFAS, and pain. Convergent validity was also good, with moderate correlations with disease activity index and active joint counts.

Similar measurement properties were found in an English study, in which both versions of the JAFAR were highly correlated with one another and with active joint count, pain, Steinbrocker class, and stiffness score, but not with measures of psychologic dysfunction.[60] A Dutch translation of the JAFAR also showed good measurement properties, although the CHAQ did slightly better than the JAFAR in this particular study.[52] Sensitivity to change or responsiveness was established in a trial by Giannini and associates[61] in their randomized, blinded-withdrawal study of intravenous immunoglobulin in polyarticular JRA. An effect size of 0.5 was demonstrated for the JAFAR; this was similar to but no better than those for the active joint count and overall articular severity score.

The JAFAR has excellent reliability and validity. Although data from a small controlled trial suggest that it is responsive, further work is needed in larger trials to clearly establish the JAFAR's responsiveness and to determine its true value for use in efficacy or effectiveness trials. Its greatest drawback is the fact that it cannot be administered to children under 7 years of age, which prohibits its use in children with early-onset JRA. Nonetheless, the JAFAR is a practical instrument that is of great use in the clinical setting and in the longitudinal follow-up of a majority of children with chronic arthritis.

Juvenile Arthritis Self-Report Index

The JASI was developed with a specific focus on physical activity in children over 8 years of age with JRA. Its emphasis is on responsiveness and it is aimed, primarily, at rehabilitation interventions. Through a detailed process[62]—which involved patients, parents, teachers, therapists, and pediatric rheumatologists—an instrument with 100 items, distributed in five categories of physical function (self-care, domestic, mobility, school, and extracurricular), was developed. Score range is from 0 to 100, with higher scores indicating better function. A seven-point Likert scale of difficulty in performing tasks was included. In a secondary component, the JASI Part II, patients identify up to five tasks that are most problematic, and these tasks are evaluated on sequential follow-up. This maneuver, derived from the MACTAR, makes this component of the JASI potentially more responsive and patient-specific.

In a subsequent study, the JASI was shown to have good measurement properties.[22] It was completed for the most part by the patients in a mean time of 49.8 minutes (including 10 minutes of instruction). Mean JASI Part I score for the group was 78.2 (range, 20–100), suggesting overall excellent function. Despite this, there was a reasonable spread of scores, suggesting that the JASI has discriminative ability. Reliability was demonstrated with excellent intraclass correlations. Construct validity was established by demonstration of predicted correlations with other measurements. In a subsample of patients, level of agreement was good between JASI scores and observation of performance of tasks by a therapist. The JASI Part II was also reliable, but less so. Because potentially stable subjects were selected for study, the opportunity to demonstrate change was substantially reduced and the rate of change was not compared with that in other measures.

The JASI was developed meticulously, resulting in excellent reliability and validity. Data for the JASI Part II suggest that it is responsive, although further data are needed to clearly establish this. Its greatest drawback is the fact that it cannot be administered to children under 8 years of age, which prohibits its use in children with early-onset JRA. Also, because it is comprehensive, it takes a long time to complete, which may make it less attractive for clinical use. Nonetheless, the JASI is a comprehensive instrument with excellent measurement properties whose greatest value is probably as a research tool for longitudinal studies.

Juvenile Arthritis Quality of Life Questionnaire

A summary of the development of the JAQQ was published in 1997.[17] Principles of instrument development similar to those for the JASI were followed.[62] The parents of 91 patients with JRA and JSpA were interviewed to generate items for the JAQQ. For subjects 9 years of age and older, parents and children were interviewed separately, a process that showed a very high level of agreement between patients and parents over a wide array of perceived difficulties.[63] Additional items on psychosocial function were obtained from the Child Behavior Checklist of Achenbach and Edelbrook.[64] Generated items were subsequently reduced to 85 by application of scores assigned by patients, parents, and a panel of experts. The panel then categorized items into four dimensions (gross motor function, fine motor function, psychosocial function, and general symptoms), each with approximately equal numbers of items. A seven-point Likert scale of frequency of difficulty with the particular item in question was used.

In a manner similar to that invoked for the JASI Part II and derived from the MACTAR, identification of items specific to individual patients is emphasized. In the JAQQ, respondents are asked to identify up to five items in each dimension with which they are having difficulty; they may also volunteer their own items for each dimension. Each item is scored from 1 to 7, based on how often the particular item is a problem for the child, with 7 indicating worst function. If an item is deemed inappropriate or unsuitable for the child, a score of 0 is assigned for that item. The mean score for the highest-scoring five items is computed as the Dimension Score; the Total JAQQ Score is computed as the mean across the four dimensions, still with a score range from 1 to 7. Change scores are computed from one administration to the next.

The JAQQ was pretested in 30 patients with JRA and JSpA, mean age 8.23 years (range, 1.66 to 18.33). It was administered without difficulty on two separate occasions a mean of 5 weeks apart. It took 20 minutes on initial completion and 5 minutes on subsequent completions. Construct validity was demonstrated by correlations that agreed with a priori predictions, being moderate for most dimensions with measures of disease activity and excellent with pain. Correlations for the psychosocial dimension were less, as predicted, being best with pain. Responsiveness was demonstrated by correlations of change scores, which were moderate with the sum of joint severity score and physician global assessment of change, and excellent with pain. Responsiveness was also demonstrated by the ability of the JAQQ to discriminate among patients according to physician global assessment of change.

After this pretest, the item number was reduced to 74—gross motor function (17 items), fine motor function (16 items), psychosocial function (22 items), and general symptoms (19 items). A pain dimension was added as a supplement to the JAQQ, which included a 100-mm VAS, a five-point Likert scale, and for children under 10 years of age, a five-point happy face/sad face model.[65] Face and content validity of this version were confirmed by 20 pediatric rheumatologists and therapists. Construct validity and responsiveness of this version were established in a follow-up study, which included 62 patients with JRA and JSpA.[66] Responsiveness was further established in 49 patients before and after institution of new drug therapy, a mean of 8 weeks apart.[67] In this study, effect sizes were better for the JAQQ than for other measures. In a further study that included 120 patients with JRA and JSpA, who were entered immediately after beginning a new treatment, responsiveness of the JAQQ was shown to be maintained over time, with an effect size for the JAQQ of 0.71 a mean of 6 months later, compared with 0.26 for active joint count.[68] This series of studies, published in abstract form, clearly suggests superior responsiveness for the JAQQ.

The JAQQ has been developed as a detailed measurement, resulting in excellent validity and responsiveness. Importantly, it measures overall health or QOL, it can be administered to children of all ages and disease-onset types in a reasonable period of time with minimal assistance, and it can also be scored quickly by hand; this makes it practical for use in the clinical setting. Perhaps its biggest drawback is that for each child, an essentially different instrument is completed because of the JAQQ's unique scoring system; this may make comparison between groups difficult, and thus its discriminative ability may be compromised. This drawback needs further study. Nonetheless, the JAQQ has excellent responsiveness; it may be the best instrument for clinical trials.

Childhood Arthritis Health Profile

Tucker and her group in Boston developed the CAHP,[19] which to date has been published only in abstract form. This instrument was developed to capture the broad range of health states in children with JRA, including physical and psychosocial function. It is a parent report that is self-administered, consisting of three modules (generic health status measures, JRA-specific health status measures, and patient characteristics). The initial report focused on the development, validity, and reliability of the functional scales—both JRA-specific and generic. Items for inclusion were generated from 80 parents of children with JRA, aged 5 to 15 years. Three functional scales—gross motor function, fine motor function, and role activities (play, family, friends)—were determined for the JRA-specific scales. Internal reliability was demonstrated by good interitem correlations within scales and minimal item scale variation. Correlation coefficients among the JRA-specific scales ranged from 0.84 to 0.97; correlation coefficients with the generic functioning scales were 0.73, demonstrating validity of these scales and further suggesting that the JRA-specific scales provide information beyond that of the generic functioning scales.

In a follow-up report, also published in abstract form,[69] the JRA-specific scales were compared with clinician-rated disease severity and activity. Significant differences were apparent across disease severity and activity for gross motor

Table 9–5

Comparative Properties of Instruments Developed for Juvenile Arthritis

	CHAIMS	CHAQ	JAFAR	JASI	JAQQ	CAHP
Reliability	Weak	Strong	Strong	Strong	NA	Moderate
Validity	Weak	Strong	Strong	Strong	Strong	Moderate
Responsiveness	No	Weak	Weak	Moderate	Very strong	NA
Discriminative ability	Weak	Moderate	Moderate	Strong	Weak	Moderate
Applicable to a wide age range	No	Very strong	No	No	Very strong	Moderate
Applicable to a heterogeneous population	Weak	Very strong	Strong	No	Very strong	NA
Measures physical function	Weak	Moderate	Moderate	Strong	Strong	Strong
Measures quality of life	No	No	No	No	Strong	Strong
Measures pain	No	Moderate	Moderate	No	Strong	No
Tested widely	No	Strong	Moderate	No	No	No
Easy to use	No	Strong	Strong	No	Strong	No

CHAIMS, Childhood Arthritis Impact Measurement Scales; CHAQ, Childhood Health Assessment Questionnaire; JAFAR, Juvenile Arthritis Functional Assessment Report; JASI, Juvenile Arthritis Self-report Index; JAQQ, Juvenile Arthritis Quality of Life Questionnaire; CAHP, Childhood Arthritis Health Profile.

No, property absent; weak, property present but weak; moderate, property present and moderately strong; strong, property present and strong; very strong, property present and very strong.

function, fine motor function, usual role activities affected by JRA, and school functioning. This study confirms the discriminative ability of the CAHP.

The CAHP is a promising instrument, but too few data have been published to determine its usefulness. Because of its comprehensiveness and complexity, it is unlikely to be of practical use in the clinical setting. Nonetheless, because of its discriminative ability, it will likely have a role as a research tool for longitudinal studies. Further data on this instrument are forthcoming.

Instruments Available for Use in Rheumatic Diseases Other Than Juvenile Arthritis

As already mentioned, the CHAQ has been used and demonstrated to have good measurement properties, including responsiveness in JDM.[56] The Childhood Myositis Assessment Scale (CMAS) has been developed to measure muscle strength and endurance in children with JDM.[70] The CMAS has been shown how to have outstanding intraobserver and interobserver reliability. A modification of the Fibromyalgia Impact Questionnaire (FIQ)[71] has been used in adolescents with some success, but few data are available on how to modify this instrument for such use.[72]

A range of instruments are available for other rheumatic diseases in adults, such as the Systemic Lupus Erythematosus Disease Activity Index (SLEDAI), Systemic Lupus International Collaborating Clinics (SLICC), and British Isles Lupus Assessment Group (BILAG) for SLE, but none of these has been adapted specifically for use in children (see Chapter 18).

CONCLUSIONS

We have outlined the essential properties of any instrument for application in children with rheumatic diseases and have discussed the various instruments now available. We have focused predominantly on the six outcome measures that have been developed for JRA. The properties of these various instruments are compared in Table 9–5. It is clear that they differ significantly from one another and have been developed with different objectives in mind; thus, each has unique qualities. Four measures—the CHAIMS, CHAQ, JAFAR, and JASI—specifically focus on physical function, whereas the others—the JAQQ and the CAHP—attempt to measure overall health and QOL in addition to physical function.

The CHAIMS has been less well studied, and its measurement properties are not good; thus, it is unlikely to have a continuing role. The CHAQ and JAFAR have excellent measurement properties and have received the most widespread use. They are simple to use and can be completed quickly. Although they are of value as research tools, their greatest value is probably in the clinical setting. The CHAQ, by virtue of the fact that it applies to all age groups, has a distinct advantage over the JAFAR. The JASI has excellent measurement properties. Because it is comprehensive and takes considerable time to complete, it is probably better used as a research tool rather than a clinical tool. The JAQQ is also comprehensive, although it can be completed more quickly than the JASI. It can be administered to all age groups and is highly responsive; thus, its most appropriate role is in clinical trials, for which it was specifically designed. The CAHP also has excellent measurement properties, particularly in its discriminative ability. It is comprehensive and cannot be completed quickly; thus, its role will most likely be as a research tool for longitudinal studies.

This has been a very exciting and active area of research in recent years. Work is still ongoing, however, and the emphasis over the next few years should be on comparative studies between these various instruments to clearly establish the role of each.

References

1. Ross CK, Lavigne JV, Hayford JR, et al: Psychological factors affecting reported pain in juvenile rheumatoid arthritis. J Ped Psychol 18: 561, 1989.

2. Miller JJ: Psychosocial factors related to rheumatic diseases in childhood. J Rheumatol 20: 1, 1993.
3. Allaire SH, DeNardo BS, Szer IS, et al: The economic impacts of juvenile chronic arthritis. J Rheumatol 19: 1952, 1992.
4. Timko C, Baumgartner M, Moos RH, et al: Parental risk and resistance factors among children with juvenile rheumatic disease: a four-year predictive study. J Behav Med 16: 571, 1993.
5. Carr AJ, Thompson PW, Kirwan FR: Quality of life measures. Br J Rheumatol 35: 275, 1996.
6. Bell MJ, Bombardier C, Tugwell P: Measurement of functional status, quality of life, and utility in rheumatoid arthritis. Arthritis Rheum 33: 591, 1990.
7. Kaplan RM, Coons SJ, Anderson JP: Quality of life and policy analysis in arthritis. Arthritis Care Res 5: 173–183, 1992.
8. Tugwell P, Bombardier C, Buchanan WW, et al: Methotrexate in rheumatoid arthritis. Impact on quality of life assessed by traditional standard-item and individualized patient preference health status questionnaires. Arch Intern Med 150: 59–62, 1990.
9. Fries JF: Toward an understanding of patient outcome measurement. Arthritis Rheum 26: 697, 1983.
10. Ward MM: Clinical measures in rheumatoid arthritis—which ones are most useful in assessing patients? J Rheumatol 21: 17, 1993.
11. Duffy CM, Arsenault L: The juvenile arthritis quality of life questionnaire—a responsive index for chronic childhood arthritis. Arthritis Rheum 35(Suppl): S222, 1992.
12. World Health Organization: The First Ten Years of the World Health Organization. Geneva, WHO, 1958.
13. Howe S, Levinson J, Shear E, et al: Development of a disability measurement tool for juvenile rheumatoid arthritis—the Juvenile Arthritis Functional Assessment Report for children and their parents. Arthritis Rheum 34: 873, 1991.
14. Singh G, Athreya BH, Fries JF, et al: Measurement of health status in children with juvenile rheumatoid arthritis. Arthritis Rheum 37: 1761, 1994.
15. Lovell DJ: Newer functional outcome measurements in Juvenile Rheumatoid Arthritis: a progress report. J Rheumatol 19(Suppl 33): 28, 1992.
16. Graham TB, Lovell DJ: Outcome in pediatric rheumatic disease. Curr Opin Rheum 9: 434, 1997.
17. Duffy CM, Arsenault L, Watanabe Duffy KN, et al: The Juvenile Arthritis Quality of Life Questionnaire—development of a new responsive index for juvenile rheumatoid arthritis and juvenile spondyloarthritides. J Rheumatol 24: 738, 1997.
18. Duffy CM, Watanabe Duffy KN: Health assessment in the rheumatic diseases of childhood. Curr Opin Rheumatol 9: 440, 1997.
19. Tucker LB, De Nardo BA, Abetz LN, et al: The Childhood Arthritis Health Profile (CAHP): validity and reliability of the condition specific scales. Arthritis Rheum 38: S183, 1995.
20. Streiner DK, Norman GR: Health Measurement Scales—A Practical Guide to Their Development and Use. Oxford, England, Oxford University Press, 1989.
21. Kirshner B, Guyatt G: A methodologic framework for assessing health indices. J Chron Dis 38: 27, 1985.
22. Wright VF, Longo Kimber J, Law M, et al: The Juvenile Arthritis Functional Status Index (JASI): a validation study. J Rheumatol 23: 1066, 1996.
23. Orvaschel H, Walsh G: The Assessment of Adaptive Functioning in Children: A Review of Existing Measures Suitable for Epidemiological and Clinical Services Research. Rockville, MD, National Institutes of Mental Health, 1984.
24. McDowell I, Newell C: Measuring Health—A Guide to Rating Scales and Questionnaires. Oxford, England, Oxford University Press, 1987.
25. Normal GR, Streiner DL: PDQ Statistics. Toronto, BC Decker, 1986.
26. Murray KJ, Passo MH: Functional measures in children with rheumatic diseases. Pediatr Clin North Am 42: 1127, 1995.
27. Brook RH, Appel FA: Quality of care assessment: choosing a model for peer review. N Engl J Med 288: 1323, 1973.
28. Feinstein AR, Josephy BR, Wells CK: Scientific and clinical problems in indexes of functional disability. Ann Intern Med 105: 413, 1986.
29. Guyatt GH, Veldhuyzen Van Zanten SJO, Feeny DH, Patrick DL: Measuring quality of life in clinical trials: a taxonomy and review. Can Med Assoc J 140: 1441, 1989.
30. Gill TM, Feinstein AR: A critical appraisal of the quality of quality of life measurements. JAMA 272: 619, 1994.
31. Meenan RF, Gertman PM, Mason JH: Measuring health status in arthritis: the Arthritis Impact Measurement Scales. Arthritis Rheum 23: 146, 1980.
32. Fries JF, Spitz P, Kraines RG, et al: Measurement of patient outcome in arthritis. Arthritis Rheum 23: 137, 1980.
33. Tugwell P, Bombardier C, Buchanan WW, et al: The MACTAR patient preference questionnaire—an individualized functional priority approach for assessing improvement in clinical trials in rheumatoid arthritis. J Rheumatol 14: 446, 1987.
34. Meenan RF, Gertman PM, Mason JH, et al: The Arthritis Impact Measurement Scales. Further investigations of a health status measure. Arthritis Rheum 25: 1048, 1982.
35. Potts MK, Brandt K: Evidence of the validity of the Arthritis Impact Measurement Scales. Arthritis Rheum 30: 93, 1987.
36. Duffy CM, Watanabe Duffy KN, Gladman DD, et al: Utility of the Arthritis Impact Measurement Scales for patients with psoriatic arthritis. J Rheumatol 19: 1727, 1992.
37. Anderson JJ, Firschein HE, Meenan RF: Sensitivity of a health status measure to short-term clinical changes in arthritis. Arthritis Rheum 32: 844, 1989.
38. Fries JF, Spitz PW, Young DY: The dimensions of health outcomes: the Health Assessment Questionnaire, disability and pain scales. J Rheumatol 9: 789, 1982.
39. Pincus T, Callaghan LF, Brooks RH, et al: Self-report questionnaire scores in rheumatoid arthritis compared with traditional physical, radiographic and laboratory measures. Ann Intern Med 110: 259, 1989.
40. Felson DT, Anderson JJ, Boers M, et al: The American College of Rheumatology core set of disease activity measures for rheumatoid arthritis clinical trials. Arthritis Rheum 36: 729, 1993.
41. Tugwell P, Bombardier C, Buchanan WW, et al: Methotrexate in rheumatoid arthritis patients. Impact on quality of life: assessed by traditional standard-item and individualized patient preference health status questionnaires. Arch Intern Med 150: 59, 1990.
42. Singsen BH: Health status (arthritis impact) in children with chronic rheumatic diseases. Current measurement issues and an approach to instrument design. Arthritis Care Res 4: 87, 1991.
43. Coulton CJ, Zborowsky E, Lipton J, et al: Assessment of the reliability and validity of the Arthritis Impact Measurement Scales for children with juvenile arthritis. Arthritis Rheum 30: 819, 1987.
44. Wright VF, Law M, Crombie V, et al: Development of a self-report functional status index for juvenile rheumatoid arthritis. J Rheumatol 21: 536, 1994.
45. Singh G, Brown B, Athreya B: Functional status in juvenile rheumatoid arthritis: sensitivity to change of the Childhood Health Assessment Questionnaire. Arthritis Rheum 34: S81, 1991.
46. Andersson Gare B, Fasth A, Wiklund I: Measurement of functional status in juvenile chronic arthritis: evaluation of a Swedish version of the Childhood Health Assessment Questionnaire. Clin Exp Rheumatol 11: 569, 1993.
47. Andersson Gare B, Fasth A: The natural history of juvenile chronic arthritis: a population based cohort study. II: outcome. J Rheumatol 22: 308, 1995.
48. Ruperto N, Ravelli A, Levison JE, et al: Long term health outcomes and quality of life in American and Italian inception cohorts of patients with juvenile rheumatoid arthritis. II: early predictors of outcome. J Rheumatol 24: 952, 1997.
49. Doherty E, Yanni G, Conroy RM, et al: A comparison of child and parent ratings of disability and pain in juvenile chronic arthritis. J Rheumatol 20: 1563, 1993.
50. Len C, Goldenberg J, Bosi Ferraz M, et al: Crosscultural reliability of the Childhood Health Assessment Questionnaire. J Rheumatol 21: 2349, 1994.
51. Fantini F, Corvaglia G, Bergomi P, et al: Validation of the Italian version of the Stanford Childhood Health Assessment Questionnaire for measuring functional status for children with chronic arthritis. Clin Exp Rheumatol 13: 785, 1995.
52. Van der Net J, Prakken ABJ, Helders PJM, et al: Correlates of disablement in polyarticular juvenile chronic arthritis—a cross sectional study. Br J Rheumatol 35: 91, 1996.
53. Goycochea-Robles MV, Garduno-Espinosa J, Vilchis-Guizar E, et al: Validation of a Spanish version of the Childhood Health Assessment Questionnaire. J Rheumatol 24: 2242, 1997.

54. Arguedas O, Andersson Gare B, Fasth A, et al: Development of a Costa Rican version of the Childhood Health Assessment Questionnaire. J Rheumatol 24: 2233, 1997.
55. Flato B, Soskaar D, Vinje O, et al: Measuring disability in early juvenile arthritis: evaluation of a Norwegian version of the Childhood Health Assessment Questionnaire. J Rheumatol 25: 1851, 1998.
56. Feldman BM, Ayling-Campos A, Luy L, et al: Measuring disability in juvenile dermatomyositis: validity of the Childhood Health Assessment Questionnaire. J Rheumatol 22: 326, 1995.
57. Billings AG, Moos RF, Miller JJ, et al: Psychosocial adaptation in juvenile rheumatic disease. A controlled evaluation. Health Psychol 6: 343, 1987.
58. Lovell DJ, Howe S, Shear S, et al: Development of a disability measurement tool for juvenile rheumatoid arthritis. Arthritis Rheum 32: 1390, 1989.
59. Chambers LW, MacDonald LA, Tugwell P, et al: The McMaster Health Index Questionnaire as a measure of the quality of life for patients with rheumatoid disease. J Rheumatol 9: 780, 1982.
60. Baildam EM, Holt PJL, Conway SC, et al: The association between physical function and psychological problems in children with juvenile chronic arthritis. Br J Rheumatol 34: 470, 1995.
61. Giannini EH, Lovell DJ, Silverman ED, for the Pediatric Rheumatology Collaborative Study Group: Intravenous immunoglobulin in the treatment of polyarticular juvenile rheumatoid arthritis: a phase I/II study. J Rheumatol 23: 919, 1996.
62. Kirshner B, Guyatt G: A methodologic framework for assessing health indices. J Chronic Dis 38: 27, 1985.
63. Duffy CM, Arsenault L, Watanabe Duffy KN: Level of agreement between parents and children in rating dysfunction in juvenile rheumatoid arthritis and juvenile spondyloarthritides. J Rheumatol 20: 2134, 1993.
64. Achenbach TM, Edelbrook C: Manual for the Child Behavior Checklist and Revised Child Behavior profile. Burlington, VT, Queen City, 1983.
65. Maunuksela EL, Olkkala KT, Korpela R: Measurement of pain in children with self-reporting and behavioural assessment. Clin Pharmacol Ther 42: 137, 1987.
66. Duffy CM, Arsenault L, Watanabe Duffy KN, et al: Validity and sensitivity to change of the Juvenile Arthritis Quality of Life Questionnaire (JAQQ) [Abstract]. Arthritis Rheum 36(Suppl): S144, 1993.
67. Duffy CM, Arsenault L, Watanabe Duffy KN, et al: Relative sensitivity to change of the Juvenile Arthritis Quality of Life Questionnaire following a new treatment. Arthritis Rheum 37(Suppl): S196, 1994.
68. Duffy CM, Arsenault L, Watanabe Duffy KN, et al: Relative sensitivity to change of the Juvenile Arthritis Quality of Life Questionnaire on sequential follow up. Arthritis Rheum 38(Suppl): S178, 1995.
69. Tucker LB, De Nardo BA, Schaller JG: The Childhood Arthritis Health Profile: Correlation of juvenile-rheumatoid arthritis specific scales with disease severity and activity. Arthritis Rheum 39(Suppl): S57, 1996.
70. Lovell DJ, Giannini EH, Rider L, et al: Validation and rater reliability of the Childhood Myositis Assessment Scale (CMAS). Arthritis Rheum 38(Suppl): S183, 1995.
71. Burckhardt CS, Clark SR, Bennett RM: Fibromyalgia and quality of life. Comparative analysis. J Rheumatol 20: 59–62, 1993.
72. Schanberg LE, Keefe FJ, Lefebvre JD, et al: Pain coping strategies in children with juvenile primary fibromyalgia syndrome: correlation with pain, physical function, and psychological distress. Arthritis Care Res 9: 89, 1996.

10

A General Approach to Management of Children With Rheumatic Diseases

Balu H. Athreya

Patient Profile—*MM is a 15-year-old girl with sudden onset of polyarticular arthritis. She has 2 to 3 hours of morning stiffness. She feels tired all the time. She has been a star basketball player for the school. The stiffness and pain are interfering with her sports. On examination she has arthritis involving small and large joints. There is a knee flexion contracture of 15 degrees bilaterally. She is anemic, with a hemoglobin of 9 g/dl (90 g/L), and has rheumatoid factor in her serum.*

She is stiff and unable to move from class to class or to climb stairs in the morning. She refuses to adhere to the treatment regimen. She forgets to take her medicines and does not follow through with home therapy.

MM's mother is a single parent who works full time. She is unable to communicate with her daughter and help her follow the treatment program. They depend on public transportation and are unable to attend regularly the therapy program. The interaction during the clinic visit suggests a long-standing parent-child conflict.

There are three components to this clinical description—the *disease*, the *illness*, and the *predicaments*.[1]

The *disease* is rheumatoid factor (RF)–positive juvenile rheumatoid arthritis (JRA), and the treatment of this disease is well described in Chapter 12.

The *illness* is characterized in this patient by pain and stiffness. There is prolonged morning stiffness. There are flexion contractures of the knee joints. She is tired all the time. These are all manifestations of the disease. Another child may have more pain and less stiffness. Treating the primary disease should lessen these symptoms. In addition, MM will need physical therapy. The patient and her mother will have to make adaptations in their daily routine. These require changes in family attitude based on acceptance. The illness behavior is characterized in this patient by refusal to adhere to a treatment program—probably driven by lack of knowledge, anger, frustration, and the usual adolescent rebellion.

MM's *predicaments* are personal and social. She happens to be the only child of a working single parent from a poor socioeconomic group. As we subsequently learned, this girl was the mother figure in this family. The mother was not capable of taking care of herself and was dependent on the daughter. Now the mother had to take a more responsible role, which she found difficult. This put a greater burden on the girl, who saw her dreams for the future coming apart. This attractive, athletic girl had all her hopes shattered. She could not play for her school team. She was angry!

The girl and her mother need continuing support and counseling to deal with the illness, the illness behavior, and their special predicament. We cannot change their predicament. But we can help them seek help and support. We can help them change their attitudes so that they can carry on with their lives in spite of the disease.

Thus, the management of rheumatic diseases involves several components (Table 10–1). This chapter is an overview of principles involved in the care of children with chronic illness, with special emphasis on

Table 10–1

Components of Management of Children With Rheumatic Diseases

1. Medical and surgical management
2. Family-centered, community-based, coordinated care (school, outreach)
3. Psychosocial management (social services, mental health services, financial)
4. Musculoskeletal rehabilitation (PT/OT/orthopedics)
5. Well-child care issues (growth and development, nutrition, immunization, anticipatory guidance)
6. Continuity of care
7. Cost-effective care

OT, occupational therapy; PT, physical therapy.

the rheumatic diseases. Rheumatic diseases are chronic; most are characterized by an unpredictable course, with periods of exacerbation and remission. They are multisystem diseases requiring consultations from medical and surgical specialists. Many of these disorders cause muscle weakness and joint contractures with functional disabilities. Therefore, children with rheumatic diseases often require physical and occupational therapy services.

There are multiple dimensions to the effects of chronic illness on the child and on the members of the family.[2] Several studies have established the impact of chronic illness, specifically rheumatic diseases, on psychosocial development,[2, 3] family,[4] school life,[5, 6] and family finances.[7, 8] Studies focusing on rheumatic diseases have shown that children with arthritis generally function well as adults. Many of them complete college, may raise children, and work full time.[9, 10] However, they also may have physical and psychosocial impairments.[10] Earlier studies suggesting greater psychosocial problems in children with JRA[11] have not been completely substantiated in more recent reports.[12] All of the psychosocial and physical problems assume greater importance when the children reach adolescence or when they grow up to be adults with continuing disease activity.[13] For all of these reasons, a program of care for children with rheumatic diseases should be comprehensive: family-centered, community-based, coordinated, and cost-effective.[14]

Accurate diagnosis is the first step. Rheumatic diseases may be acute and explosive in onset or evolve over a period of months and years. Only one organ system may be affected, or several systems may be involved, mimicking several other inflammatory and noninflammatory diseases. We may not be able to place an accurate diagnostic label at first and still may have to manage life-threatening complications and functional disabilities. Great skill and patience are required to support the families to manage their problems in the face of uncertainties in diagnosis and prognosis. Therein reside the challenges and pleasures of rheumatology.

Expertise should be the cornerstone of the care of children with rheumatic diseases. Therefore, comprehensive treatment centers should be based in tertiary-care academic centers. The treatment team (Fig. 10–1) should consist of a pediatric rheumatologist, a nurse specialist, physical and occupational therapists, and a social worker, all working with the child's primary care physician. Consultations with an orthopedic surgeon, ophthalmologist, psychologist, nutritionist, and dentist should be available when required. The child and the family should be the central focus of the team.

The primary physician's role should include care of intercurrent illness, immunizations, anticipatory guidance on developmental issues, and working with community resources such as the school system. The pediatric rheumatology team should provide detailed guidelines and directions for the management of specific problems based on their expertise and experience.

Three essential steps are required to help the families and the primary physician to function effectively:

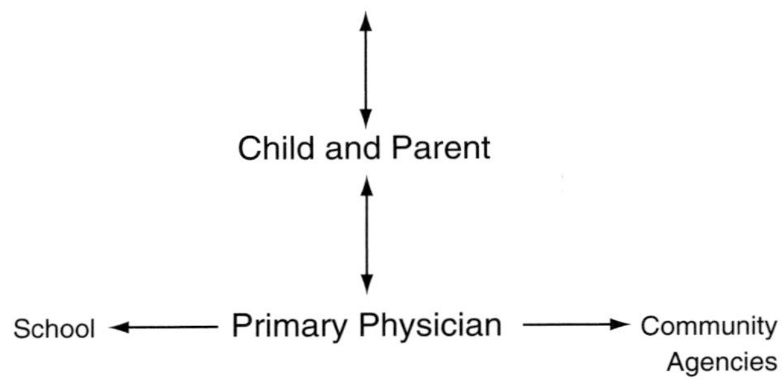

Figure 10–1. Team care.

1. Education of the family
2. Effective two-way communication between the primary physician and the specialists
3. Availability of one contact person in the rheumatology team

In 1975, a report from England that was based on interviews of families of children with chronic problems concluded that families need a *single* person they can call with any questions.[15] A specially trained nurse has fulfilled this function effectively in many pediatric rheumatology centers.[16]

No cure is available for most of the rheumatic diseases. Fortunately, most of these diseases can be controlled with the available newer drugs. Spontaneous remissions do occur. Newer developments in pharmacology and biotechnology have opened up new approaches to the control of inflammation and the modulation of immune responses. Permanent cure and prevention may be realized in the new millennium. Until then, goals of treatment should include control of inflammation and maintenance of function (Table 10–2).

It is important to remember that it is not adequate to plan for control of the disease alone. We have to plan for the whole child and for the future.

Table 10–2

Objectives of the Treatment of Rheumatic Diseases*

Immediate	Control inflammation Relieve pain and discomfort Prevent deformities Preserve function
Long-term	Minimize side effects of the disease and treatment Promote normal growth and development Minimize impact of chronic illness on family Educate the child and family Rehabilitation

*See Chapter 12, under Treatment.

CHILD- AND FAMILY-CENTERED, COMMUNITY-BASED, COORDINATED CARE

Hobbs and Perrin,[2] in their landmark study, documented that the needs of children with chronic illness and disabilities are nonspecific and generic for the most part. In addition to medical management of each disease, these children need to live at home, attend school like other children, and be able to access special services such as physical, occupational, and speech therapy in their own communities. Their families need support for transportation, childcare, and care of siblings. Some families may need mental health services and financial counseling.

These services are difficult to access even in a metropolitan area and are unavailable in remote rural areas. In the United States, the American Academy of Pediatrics, the Surgeon General's Office, and the Bureau of Maternal and Child Health met with parents of children with chronic diseases or disabilities and members of their healthcare teams to explore the needs of children with chronic illness and disabilities. As a result, Doctor C. Everett Koop, then Surgeon General, encouraged the development of a system of family-centered, community-based, coordinated care to improve the lives of these children and their families.[17] The following steps were recognized as important in implementing this approach[14]:

1. Recognizing the pivotal role of the child and the family in the planning of care
2. Developing resources in the community where these children live
3. Recognizing parents and professionals as equals in a partnership of care
4. Empowering the family with information by education and support
5. Encouraging pediatricians to assume a greater role in case coordination, become knowledgeable about available local resources, and work with community agencies
6. Increasing communication among disciplines and from patients to health professionals
7. Breaking barriers to the development of such a system

EDUCATION

Children with rheumatic diseases and their parents require education and counseling on several issues. These are discussed in detail in several publications (Appendix 10–1). The mode of teaching has to vary to suit the needs and skills of parents. Language barriers, cultural backgrounds, and literacy issues have to be kept in mind before such programs are organized.

Education about the disease, medications, adverse effects of medications, and therapy programs has to take place both individually by the pediatric rheumatologist and in groups as part of parent support groups. Information required by parents varies with the time that has passed since diagnosis. It also depends on the developmental needs of the child. Therefore, education must be individualized. Information is easily available on the Internet. However, families need help to receive information from reliable sources such as the Arthritis Foundation (*www.arthritis.org*), and they need assistance with interpretation of the information they gather. Parents and patients in the United States are encouraged to attend educational sessions organized by the American Juvenile Arthritis Organization (AJAO) for patients, siblings, and parents as part of annual regional and national meetings.

COUNSELING

A trusting relationship is the most important requirement for effective counseling. To be trusted, one has to be trustworthy. Open, honest communication with the child and the parent is one major component of this relationship. One has to listen carefully before offering advice.

Collecting information about the child's illness, the child's behavior, and family dynamics may require many visits and observations. One has to listen to what they *say* and observe what they *do*. Nonverbal cues have to be attended to. While treating the impact of the disease on the child and the attendant weaknesses in the family, we have to be on the lookout for their strengths. The strength may be in the extended family, an interested schoolteacher, or a loving grandparent. We have to know the strengths because we can build only on their strengths and find ways to compensate for their weaknesses. Some families grow in strength in the presence of adversity. Factors that contribute to successful coping should be supported and encouraged.

Children with physical disabilities and deformities and children who look different because of a rash or steroid therapy are bound to feel different and self-conscious. Physical disability and fluctuation in disease activity may make it difficult for the children to participate in social and family activities. Emphasis on what they *can* do and planning activities in which they can participate should help their sense of self-worth and morale. There should be alternative plans and backup arrangements. Involvement of the siblings and other children in helping the disabled child during activities should help create a successful experience for everyone.

ADHERENCE (COMPLIANCE)

Children with chronic illness soon become tired of taking medicines day after day with no end in sight. They often ask why they have to do mindless exercises that do not appear to help them anyway. Therefore, compliance with medication and therapy programs becomes a major issue for children with chronic diseases.[18] The word *compliance* implies that the physician

Table 10–3

Factors Affecting Compliance in Treatment of Children

Compliance Is Increased By

Agreement among patient, family, and treatment team with respect to goals of treatment
Understanding the disease and the treatment approach
Setting and resetting short-term achievable goals
Frequent positive reinforcement

Compliance Is Decreased By

Poor understanding of the disease and the treatment approach
Conflict between patient and healthcare providers with respect to treatment goals
Setting treatment goals that are unachievable or too long-term
Complexity or awkwardness of medication regimens
Adverse side effects of drugs
Remission and flareup of disease

gives orders and the patient obeys. But the ideal situation is an informed patient who chooses to follow the treatment prescribed by a trusted physician after being convinced of the benefits and made aware of the consequences of not following the treatment. In other words, the patient chooses to adhere to the prescribed program. In pediatrics, we have to consider the child, the parent, and the caretaker to make sure the treatment plan is followed. Patient and parent education and incorporation of the needs of the family members in planning the care are essential to ensure that the patient adheres to the plan (Table 10–3). Listening to the specific needs of the child and the family and incorporating them into the plan—even if these needs are irrelevant—and designing a plan that accounts for the stresses and strengths of the family and their cultural values increases the likelihood of the plan being followed.

SIBLING ISSUES

Stress related to living with chronic illness affects every member of the family, including siblings. The role of siblings and their impact on developmental needs of the patient may vary with the age and cognitive level of siblings, their perception of the child with chronic illness, parental attitudes, and the demands placed on unaffected siblings.[19, 20] The gamut of feelings ranges from guilt (that siblings are responsible for the sick child in some magical way) to fear of catching the illness and embarrassment.[21]

Siblings may resent the extra time and attention given to the affected child and perceived favoritism in matters of discipline. Realistically, parents may not be able to provide adequate time to satisfy the developmental needs of the siblings. This is a particular problem for the single parent.

In one study that explored the feelings of siblings of children with chronic illness (which included children with JRA, ankylosing spondylitis, systemic lupus erythematosus [SLE], and scleroderma), some children had no problem revealing the illness of their brother or sister to others.[20] Their reasons included "to explain the need for obvious treatment schedules or if an unforeseen problem develops." Some children preferred not to reveal for fear that the ill child would be teased. Depending on the parental demands, some siblings had an important role in the medical treatment of the affected child (such as reminding about medications and helping with therapy); others were protected from this role. Others took a more protective role in the school and outside of the home.

Disease severity, parental functioning, family stress, and family support systems are some of the determinants of the effects of chronic illness on siblings. In spite of ambivalent feelings, siblings of children with arthritis function well in life.[22] With the proper approach, they become a great source of extra support, both at home and at school. It is important to evaluate the needs of siblings in caring for children with chronic illness and help support their needs. Some ideas to reduce the negative impact on siblings are given in Table 10–4.

SCHOOL ISSUES

Rheumatic diseases in general do not affect the ability of the child to learn and think. Children with arthritis can and should attend school except in special circumstances. *School is the child's job.* However, the school system must often institute several adaptations to the standardized schedule.[5, 6] In the United States, children with chronic illness and disabilities *must* be educated in the "least restrictive environment." *Individualized education plans* (IEPs) have to be formulated at the parent's request, and there are strong "due process" requirements.[23] Depending on the medical condition and the disability, one or more of the "related school services" listed in Table 10–5 may have to be provided for children with special healthcare needs to ensure proper educational opportunities.[6, 24]

Special school services are important components of community-based services. They provide physical adaptations in schools for handicapped access, elevators, classes on the same floor, and a duplicate set of books. Transportation, school counseling, nutrition, adaptive physical education, and homebound instruction are some of the other services that may be needed.[5, 24]

Table 10–4

Approaches to Siblings of Children With Chronic Illness

Include siblings in clinic visits
Talk with siblings and explore their needs
Determine the perception of the siblings on the impact of the illness on family members
Help them deal with their friends' questions
Encourage and enlist sibling participation in developing care plans
Conduct sibling group discussions at local and national support groups

Table 10–5

Related School Services Needed by Chronically Ill Children

School health services	Support therapies
Administration of medications	Physical therapy
Implementation of medical procedures	Occupational therapy
Emergency preparations	Speech and language therapy
Schedule modifications	Counseling services
Modified physical education	School
Transportation	Career
Building accessibility	Personal
Toileting/lifting assistance	

Data from Walker DK, Jacobs FH: Chronically ill children in schools. *In* Hobbs N, Perrin J (eds): The Constant Shadow: Issues in Chronic Childhood Illness in America. San Francisco, Jossey-Bass, 1984.

Modified with permission from Walker DK: Care of chronically ill children in schools. Pediatr Clin North Am 31: 221, 1984.

A number of common concerns expressed by children and parents, as well as suggested solutions, are given in Table 10–6. The nurse can provide an individualized checklist to parents (Appendix 10–2); this list can be shared with the school nurse or teacher. School nurses are some of the best advocates for children with disabilities and special needs. Well-informed school nurses can work with teachers and physical education instructors and make appropriate modifications within the school. Therefore, communication between the tertiary center staff (particularly the nurse) and the school nurses is essential. In addition, special educational programs for school nurses are very useful in our experience. Finally, if the child is considering post–high school vocational training or college, early planning is essential. *This should start at the beginning of secondary school at the very latest.* One of our successful "graduates" wrote a checklist in preparation for her entry into college (Table 10–7).

TRANSITION

Transition to adult care is a process that should start in pediatric rheumatology centers when the child reaches the adolescent age group.[13, 25] Preparation of these children requires attention to functional vocational evaluation and training, independent living skills, and self-advocacy.

Growing up through adolescence into young adult life is a major task for any child. This becomes a challenge for children with chronic illness and their parents.[13] Adolescents with chronic diseases have to be encouraged to take control of their disease management gradually. This requires preparation of the family and the child before adolescence. Both the physicians and the parents have to let go of the child in a sensitive and gradual way. The parent has to trust, and the child has to prove that he or she can be trusted to take care of ongoing management and needs. Adolescent support groups with professional leadership may be helpful. Some of the subjects that should be addressed, both in individual sessions and in group discussions,

Table 10–6

Common School Concerns for Students With Rheumatic Diseases

DIFFICULTY	STRATEGIES
Climbing stairs or walking long distances	• Request elevator permit • Schedule classes to decrease walking and climbing • Request extra time getting from class to class • Use a wheelchair if needed
Inactivity, stiffness due to prolonged sitting	• Change position every 20 min • Sit at the side/back of the room to allow walking around without disturbing class • Ask to be assigned jobs that permit walking (collect papers)
Carrying books/cafeteria tray	• Keep two sets of books: one in appropriate class, one at home • Have a buddy help carry books • Get a backpack/shoulder bag for books • Determine cafeteria assistance plan (helper, reserved seat, wheeled cart)
Getting up from desk	• Request an easel-top desk or special chair
Handwriting (slow, messy, painful)	• Use "fat" pen/pencil, crayons • Use a felt-tip pen • Stretch hands every 10 min • Use a tape recorder for note taking • Photocopy classmate's notes • Use a computer for reports • Request an alternative to timed tests (oral test, extra time, computer) • Educate teacher—messy writing may be unavoidable at times
Shoulder movement and dressing	• Wear loose-fitting clothing • Wear clothes with Velcro closures • Get adaptive equipment from occupational therapist
Reaching locker	• Modify locker or request alternative storage place • Use two lockers with key locks instead of dials
Raising hand	• Devise alternative signaling method

From Raising a Child with Arthritis—A Parent's Guide 1998. Atlanta, Arthritis Foundation, 1998. ©1998. Reprinted with permission of the Arthritis Foundation 1330 W. Peachtree St., Atlanta, GA 30309. For more information please call the Arthritis Foundation's Information Line at 1.800.283.7800 or log on to www.arthritis.org

Table 10–7

Rheumatic Diseases and Planning for College

1. Visit the college before choosing in order to evaluate the walking distance between buildings, stairs, elevators, and general accessibility.
2. Know the different climate changes, i.e., if you are better in the summer you may want to pick a campus with a warm climate. Also, climate changes can cause flare-ups or increased stiffness.
3. It is always good to get to know a local doctor in your college area or health service before troubles occur so he or she knows your past history and can help you right away if there are any problems.
4. If you have the chance to pick your own schedule during your first year, make sure you give yourself enough time to get from one class to another, i.e., if you have to walk to buildings from one end of campus to the other.
5. Also *try not to overburden yourself* with classes and too many credit hours—there will always be bad days, so expect them.
6. If you are not a morning person or if you are a night owl, schedule your classes in the afternoon.
7. And always—no matter how "bad" the food is—eat as regularly as possible—breakfast, lunch, and dinner. It helps in the long run, even if your stomach does not think so at the time.
8. Take extra medicine with you at the start of school and give yourself time to find out where the nearest pharmacy is.

are preparing for college, sexuality, alcohol and drugs, and vocational planning.

FINANCIAL ISSUES

Children with chronic illness account for a large proportion of healthcare expenditures in the United States.[8, 26] For instance, families of children with rheumatic diseases may have to spend hundreds to thousands of unreimbursed dollars out of pocket per year.[4, 7] This does not even include time lost from work. In the current competitive environment, children with chronic illness and disabilities are particularly vulnerable. The high cost that goes with chronic illness, and the pressures to cut costs, may make it difficult to provide adequate and appropriate care for children with chronic illness and disabilities.[26] In the United States, families have to be educated about various types of coverage and how to work with Health Maintenance Organizations (HMOs) and insurance companies. They have to learn about child welfare systems and social security benefits. They have to learn to work with their school systems. Parents have to be advocates for their children and learn both their rights and responsibilities and those of their children.[23] Both parents and physicians have to work through the political process to bring about changes in financing of medical care that will ensure access to appropriate services for all children with disabilities.[27]

A special program developed by the AJAO teaches several skills to parents so that they can become advocates for their children. In this program, a parent and a health professional who works with the child learn to list items of care essential for that specific child and learn strategies to achieve those goals.

UNCONVENTIONAL REMEDIES

When scientific medicine truthfully acknowledges its ignorance about the etiology of rheumatic diseases and the lack of permanent cure, it is easy for parents to believe those who promise miracles. This is also the age of alternative medicine.[28] There are pressures from well-meaning friends and relatives to try unproven remedies widely advertised in newspapers and on the Internet. Southwood and colleagues[29] reported that 70 percent of patients with juvenile arthritis had used unconventional remedies. Even when patients do not discuss it, we can assume that most of them have tried or are trying one or more remedies. It is better to keep an open and noncritical relationship with patients and their family members so that they feel comfortable talking about it. It is important for pediatric rheumatologists to be aware of the currently available alternative remedies so they can provide proper guidance when patients ask about such methods. This is an opportunity to educate parents on the conduct of scientific studies and to explain to them the difference between controlled trials and testimonials. It is better to let them try some remedies that are innocuous, caution about some potentially dangerous treatments (megavitamins), and refuse to be part of certain other approaches (bee-sting therapy). It is always wise to allow room for parents to come back without losing face and feeling humiliated.

PHYSICAL AND OCCUPATIONAL THERAPY

Physical and occupational therapy programs are vital to the management of rheumatic diseases in children. A variety of modalities and treatment approaches are used without adequate proof of their efficacy.[30] For example, it is not known whether a resting splint to prevent dysfunctional positioning of the wrist during sleep is better than a functional splint during activities to prevent misalignment of the wrist joint. Consequently, there are differences of opinion as to what modality to use and how aggressive one should be. A 1996 survey of pediatric rheumatology centers from the United States, United Kingdom, and Canada developed a consensus on the need for early intervention and a team approach to therapy. However, there were differences in the timing of physiotherapy exercises, monitoring of joint range of motion (ROM), and treatment of acutely inflamed joints.[30] This study and a workshop conducted in Germany led to the following principles, about which most centers agree:

- Use heat or cold, depending on preference
- Stretch individual joints
- Use traction or prone lying for hip flexion contracture
- Re-educate for improvement of posture and gait
- Use resting splints for wrist

Needs for therapy services may vary with the specific rheumatic disease, whether disabilities are acute or chronic. For minor problems and prevention of contracture, standard exercises to maintain ROM can be taught to parents by the pediatric rheumatologist and the nurses (Figs. 10–2 to 10–11). Usual indications for referral to therapists are listed in Table 10–8.

Most minor problems can be handled at home with standard exercises. However, such management requires adherence to a routine that is often hard to achieve or maintain. When more aggressive therapy is required, an outpatient program is indicated with two or three sessions a week. Even with this frequency, carryover into the daily routine is essential to maintain the benefits. Occasionally, children require intensive inpatient rehabilitation, which is becoming increasingly difficult to finance in the United States. Fortunately, the need for such inpatient rehabilitation is becoming less frequent thanks to better medical management. Children whose disability is serious enough to interfere with attendance at a regular school may be able to receive school-based therapy that follows an IEP.

The overall goals of rehabilitation are to maximize function, to prevent deformities, and to help the child achieve developmental milestones—physical, psychosocial, emotional, educational, and vocational. The concept is to help the child and family lead *as normal a life as possible*. Goals have to be set in collaboration with the parents and the child. One has to account for the needs of the family, their strengths and weaknesses, their economic and human resources, their coping styles, and their cultural values. The child's developmental level and interests also have to be acknowledged.

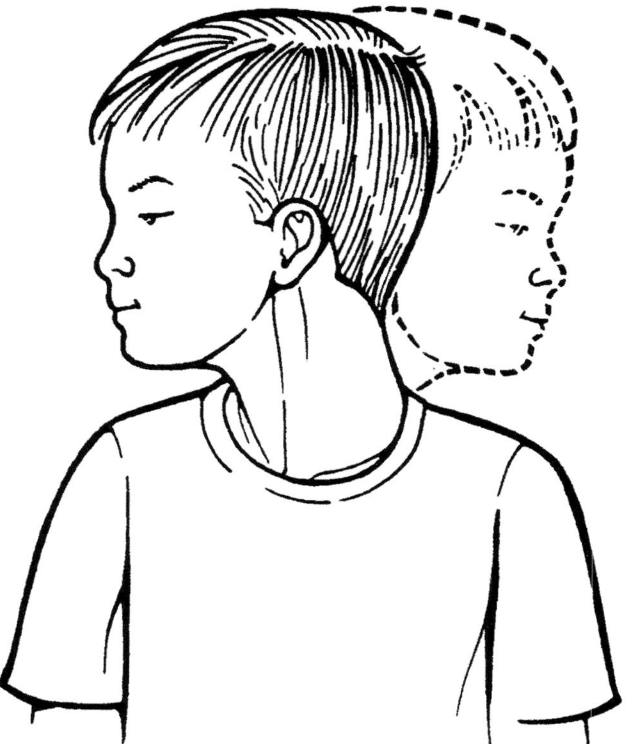

Figure 10–2. Neck. Turn the head toward one shoulder and then the other. Repeat two to three times on each side. (From Raising a Child with Arthritis—A Parent's Guide 1998. Atlanta, Arthritis Foundation, 1998. ©1998. Reprinted with permission of the Arthritis Foundation 1330 W. Peachtree St., Atlanta, GA 30309. For more information please call the Arthritis Foundation's Information Line at 1.800.283.7800 or log on to www.arthritis.org)

Table 10–8

Indications for Referral to Therapists

Involvement of multiple joints
Severe pain or stiffness of joints and muscles
Established contracture, limitation in activities of daily living (even single area)
Preoperative management
Postoperative management
Rapidly progressive disease
Prescription for assistive devices (e.g., crutches, wheelchair)
Failure to respond to standard exercise
Parent-child conflict resulting in poor compliance with therapy

The initial step is a thorough evaluation. This should include collecting information on fatigue, morning stiffness, the patient's and parents' perception of pain, level of endurance, and independence in activities of daily living (ADL) including mobility. The child's ability to participate in school, sports, and recreation should be meticulously evaluated.

The joints are then examined to assess the specific joints involved, activity of the disease, pain, severity of involvement, and active and passive ROM. Several instruments are now available to document pain, ROM, and function, which should be completed before and periodically through therapy to measure progress.[31] It is also important to observe the child's posture, gait, and deficits in ROM during activity; compensatory movements; and adaptive skills.

Essential components of treatment should include rest, management of fatigue and pain, posture and positioning, therapeutic exercises, and improving ADL.[32–34] Conditioning exercises and sports activities are discussed later.

Rest

It is preferable for children with arthritis to be as active as possible. General bed rest is rarely prescribed except for children with severe arthritis or myositis and for children with systemic disease associated with myocarditis or pericarditis. We allow children to set their own limits based on pain and endurance; we suggest that, if necessary, they allow themselves a rest period during the day, usually immediately after school.

Localized rest to an acutely inflamed joint is provided with a splint or a bivalved cast. If a splint or cast is applied, the limb should be taken out once or twice a day and ROM exercises or isometric exercises should be performed.

Fatigue

Fatigue is a common problem for children with rheumatic diseases. It is a particular complaint for children

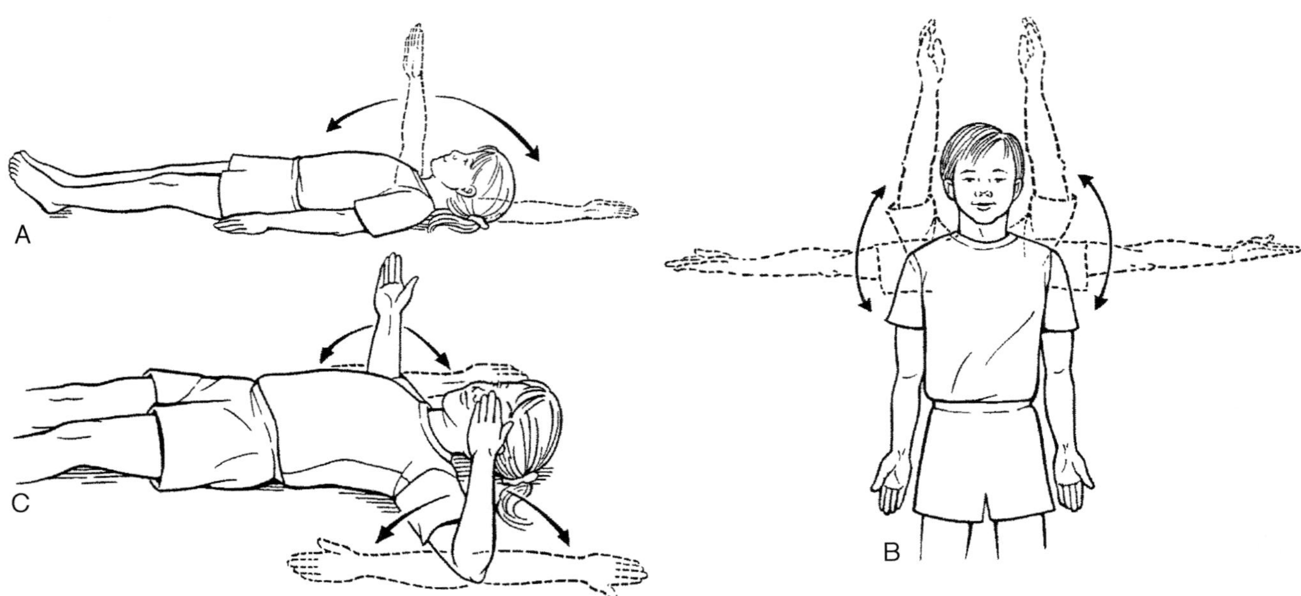

Figure 10–3. *A,* **Shoulder.** Lie on the floor with both arms at your sides. Raise one arm over the head, keeping the elbow straight, until the back of the hand reaches the floor. Return the arm slowly to the side. Repeat this exercise with the other arm. Repeat, alternating arms, two to three times. *B,* **Shoulder abduction.** Start with the arms down at the sides with palms facing out. Raise the arms out to the sides and up until palms touch, keeping elbows straight. Hold briefly, then return arms to the sides. Repeat two to three times. *C,* **Shoulder rotation.** Lying down, place arms straight out from the shoulder, palms toward ceiling; bend at the elbow with the fingers pointing toward ceiling; roll arms forward so the hands point straight down toward feet (internal rotation); roll arms backward so the hands point toward the head (external rotation). Repeat two to three times. (A–C, From Raising a Child with Arthritis—A Parent's Guide 1998. Atlanta, Arthritis Foundation, 1998. ©1998. Reprinted with permission of the Arthritis Foundation 1330 W. Peachtree St., Atlanta, GA 30309. For more information please call the Arthritis Foundation's Information Line at 1.800.283.7800 or log on to www.arthritis.org)

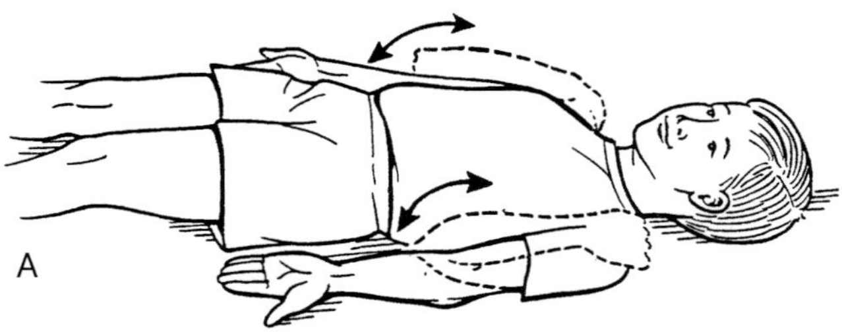

Figure 10–4. **Elbow.** *A,* Lie on floor with both arms at sides, palms facing the ceiling. Bring hands to shoulders by bending elbows. Return hands to the floor by straightening elbows. *B,* Bend elbows and hold them close to the sides of the body with forearms parallel to the floor and palms down; slowly turn forearms so palms face ceiling; hold to the count of three and turn arms so palms face the floor again. (A and B, From Raising a Child with Arthritis—A Parent's Guide 1998. Atlanta, Arthritis Foundation, 1998. ©1998. Reprinted with permission of the Arthritis Foundation 1330 W. Peachtree St., Atlanta, GA 30309. For more information please call the Arthritis Foundation's Information Line at 1.800.283.7800 or log on to www.arthritis.org)

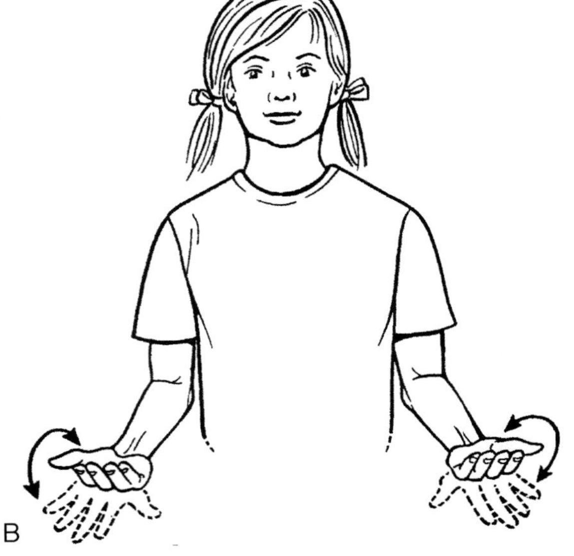

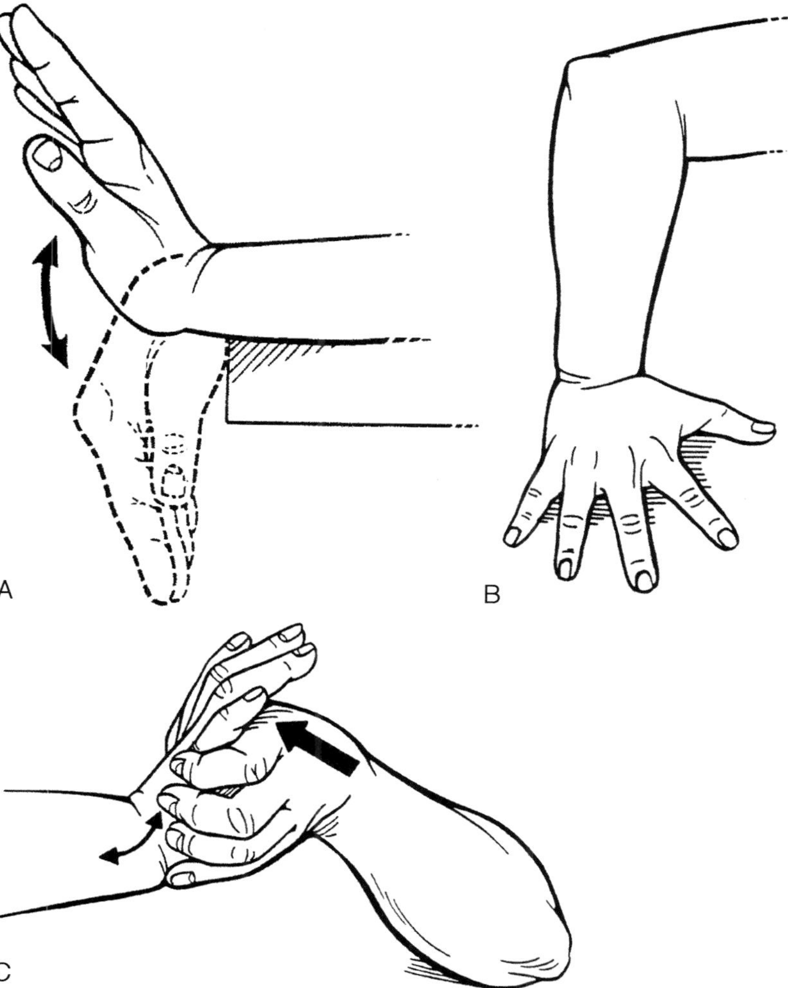

Figure 10–5. Wrist. *A,* With the forearm resting firmly on a table top and the hand hanging over the edge of the table, bend the wrist up as far as possible. Hold. Bend the wrist down as far as possible. Hold. Repeat two to three times. *B,* Place the hand on a table or other flat surface. Raise elbow toward ceiling until wrinkles appear at the wrist. *C,* Grasp the hand with the opposite hand. Put the palms together, with fingers around the opposite hand. Push the hand backward, stretching the wrist. Hold. Repeat two to three times. (A–C, From Raising a Child with Arthritis—A Parent's Guide 1998. Atlanta, Arthritis Foundation, 1998. ©1998. Reprinted with permission of the Arthritis Foundation 1330 W. Peachtree St., Atlanta, GA 30309. For more information please call the Arthritis Foundation's Information Line at 1.800.283.7800 or log on to www.arthritis.org)

with systemic diseases, anemia, and myocarditis. A defined period of rest during the middle of the day is ideal, although it is not always practical. Treatment of the systemic disease and anemia often corrects the fatigue. Children with functional disorders and chronic pain syndromes complain of fatigue that interferes with school attendance and participation in sports. This is often associated with nonrestorative sleep. Pharmacologic and behavioral approaches are needed to help promote sleep and thereby relieve fatigue. Fatigue out of proportion to disease activity deserves close scrutiny to differentiate between medical and psychological causes.

Pain

Pain is a major component of many of the inflammatory musculoskeletal conditions.[35] Children with chronic arthritis often do not complain of pain because they become used to living with a certain level of constant pain. In addition to control of inflammation and use of analgesics, other modalities such as biofeedback and transcutaneous electrical nerve stimulation (TENS) may have to be tried, depending on the clinical diagnosis, acuteness or chronicity of pain, the child's developmental status, various effects of the pain on function, and psychosocial issues.

Pain due to an acutely inflamed joint is treated with joint aspiration, intra-articular injection with glucocorticoid, if appropriate, and use of nonsteroidal anti-inflammatory drugs. In addition, the joint can be placed in a resting splint for a few days until the inflammation subsides. The splint should be removed two or three times a day and the joint moved through ROM actively or passively to avoid atrophy of muscles and joint stiffness.

Children with *myositis* and pain need to rest and be allowed to move to their tolerance. An active exercise program should not be started until pain and tenderness subside.

Pain out of proportion to swelling of the joint needs careful evaluation to rule out other diagnoses such as leukemia. In patients with JRA or SLE, severe pain or sudden onset of pain in one joint may indicate septic arthritis.

Pain after activity is not uncommon in children with rheumatic diseases. Standard treatment is rest and ice,

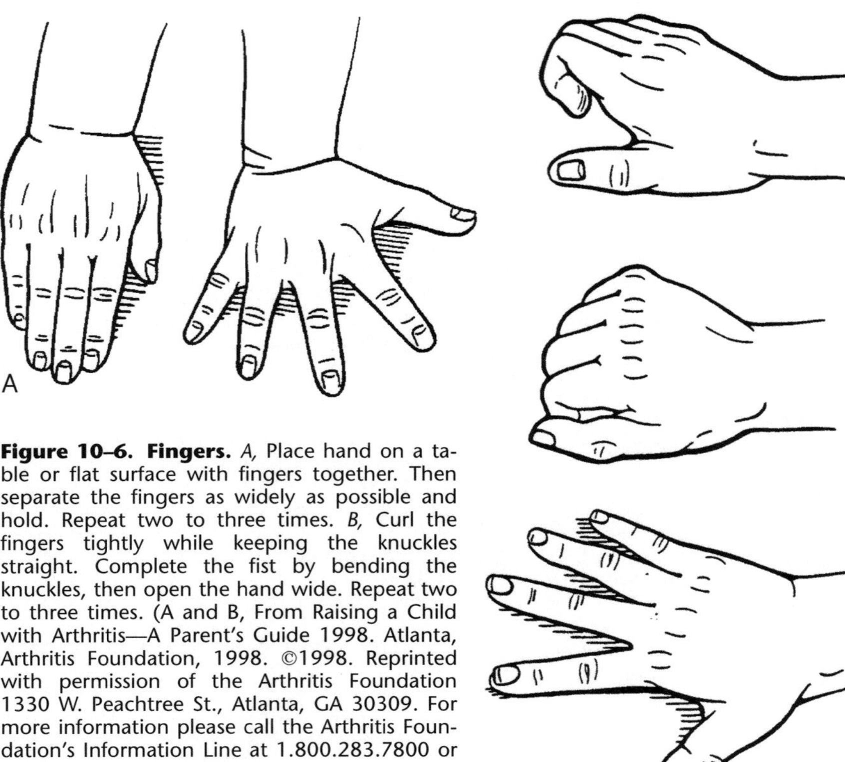

Figure 10–6. Fingers. *A,* Place hand on a table or flat surface with fingers together. Then separate the fingers as widely as possible and hold. Repeat two to three times. *B,* Curl the fingers tightly while keeping the knuckles straight. Complete the fist by bending the knuckles, then open the hand wide. Repeat two to three times. (A and B, From Raising a Child with Arthritis—A Parent's Guide 1998. Atlanta, Arthritis Foundation, 1998. ©1998. Reprinted with permission of the Arthritis Foundation 1330 W. Peachtree St., Atlanta, GA 30309. For more information please call the Arthritis Foundation's Information Line at 1.800.283.7800 or log on to www.arthritis.org)

and an occasional analgesic. We encourage children to be as active as possible and to set their own limits. Our guideline is that if the joint pain after activity lasts more than 45 to 60 minutes, the activity level or duration should be decreased.

Chronic Pain

Secondary morbidity in chronic illness is to a large extent unexplored territory. It is also important to remember that chronic pain, whether organic in origin or unexplained, can lead to depression, and, conversely, occult depression can present itself as chronic pain.[36]

Children with rheumatic diseases may also experience cycles of intense and intractable pain not amenable to a pharmacologic approach. Some of them experience secondary fibromyalgia with such classic features as tender points and lack of sleep. This pattern affects their emotional stability and function and leads to a vicious circle. In these children, a cognitive-behavioral approach may be indicated.[37] Other techniques such as TENS, visual imagery, relaxation, and management of time and stress may be helpful.

Approaches to pain control in regional pain, overuse, and pain amplification syndromes is discussed in appropriate chapters. It is important to remember that

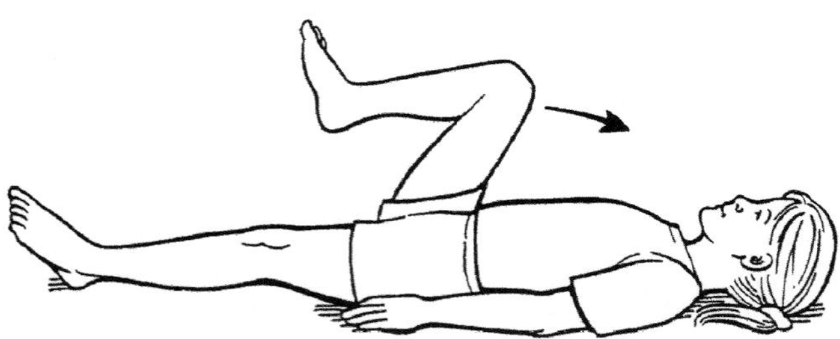

Figure 10–7. Hip and knee. Lying on the back, bend one knee toward the chest, then lower the knee. Repeat with the other knee, two to three times each leg. (From Raising a Child with Arthritis—A Parent's Guide 1998. Atlanta, Arthritis Foundation, 1998. ©1998. Reprinted with permission of the Arthritis Foundation 1330 W. Peachtree St., Atlanta, GA 30309. For more information please call the Arthritis Foundation's Information Line at 1.800.283.7800 or log on to www.arthritis.org)

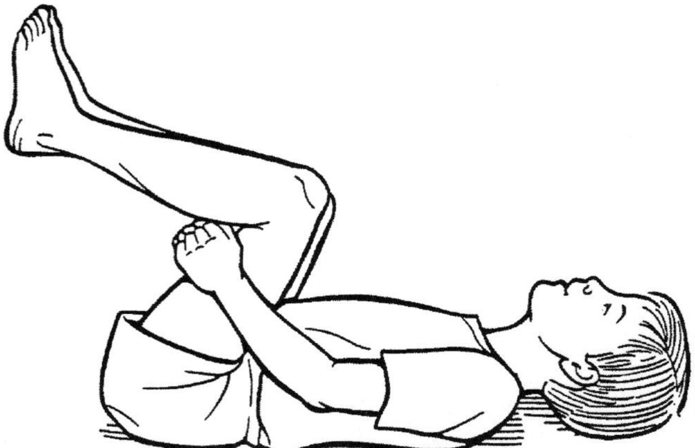

Figure 10–8. Back. Lie on the back with knees bent. Keep the back flat against the floor. Raise both bent knees toward the chest. Place hands behind thighs and pull toward the chest. Lower legs to original position. (From Raising a Child with Arthritis—A Parent's Guide 1998. Atlanta, Arthritis Foundation, 1998. ©1998. Reprinted with permission of the Arthritis Foundation 1330 W. Peachtree St., Atlanta, GA 30309. For more information please call the Arthritis Foundation's Information Line at 1.800.283.7800 or log on to www.arthritis.org)

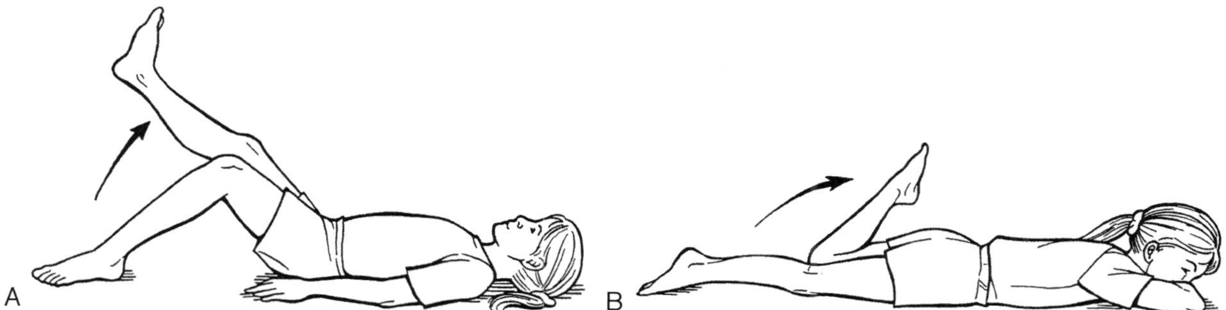

Figure 10–9. *A,* **Thigh.** Lie on the back with one leg bent at the knee and one leg straight. Raise the straight leg, keeping the knee as straight as possible. Keep the small of the back on the floor. Lower the leg and repeat with other leg. *B,* **Knee.** Lying on the stomach, bend one knee, bringing the heel toward the buttocks. Then lower the leg and repeat with the other knee. Repeat two to three times with each leg. (A and B, From Raising a Child with Arthritis—A Parent's Guide 1998. Atlanta, Arthritis Foundation, 1998. ©1998. Reprinted with permission of the Arthritis Foundation 1330 W. Peachtree St., Atlanta, GA 30309. For more information please call the Arthritis Foundation's Information Line at 1.800.283.7800 or log on to www.arthritis.org)

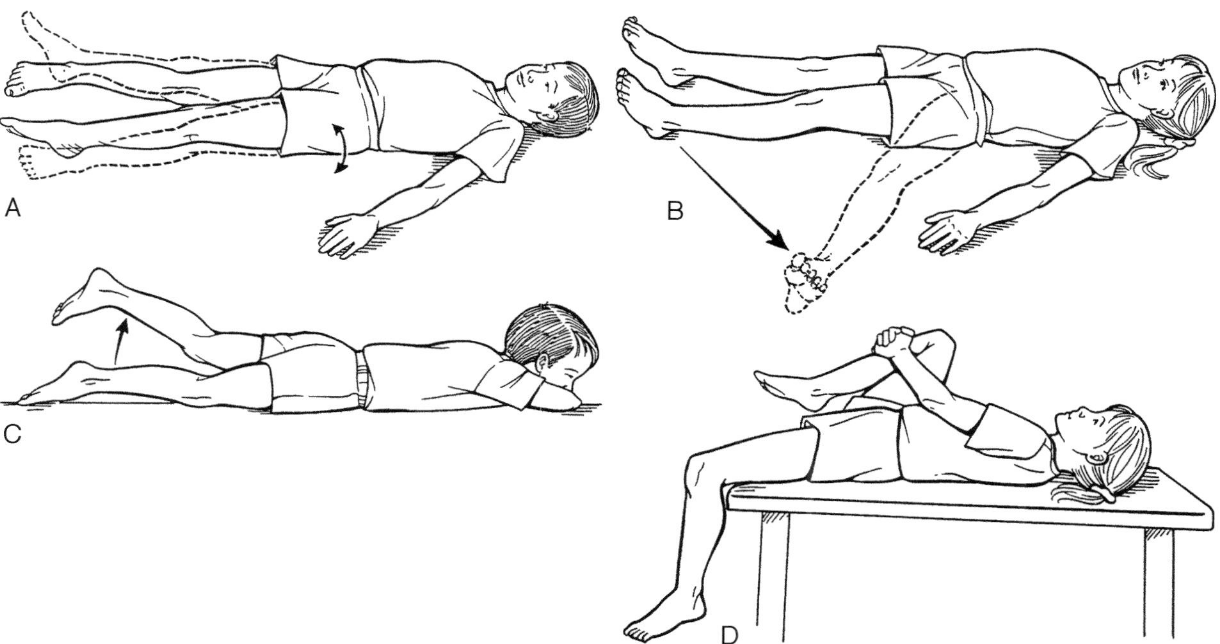

Figure 10–10. Hip. *A,* Lie flat on the back with legs straight, about 6 inches apart. Roll the legs in and out, keeping the knees straight. Repeat two to three times. *B,* Lie flat on the floor with the legs straight, about 6 inches apart. Slide one leg out to the side and return. Repeat with the other leg. Repeat two to three times with each leg. *C,* Lying on the stomach, lift one leg. Try to keep the knee straight. Then lower the leg and repeat with the other leg. Repeat two to three times with each leg. *D,* Lying on a table with knees bent over the edge, bring one knee up to the chest. At the same time, keep the other thigh flat on the table. Hold for a count of 10. Lower the leg. Repeat with the other leg. (A–D, From Raising a Child with Arthritis—A Parent's Guide 1998. Atlanta, Arthritis Foundation, 1998. ©1998. Reprinted with permission of the Arthritis Foundation 1330 W. Peachtree St., Atlanta, GA 30309. For more information please call the Arthritis Foundation's Information Line at 1.800.283.7800 or log on to www.arthritis.org)

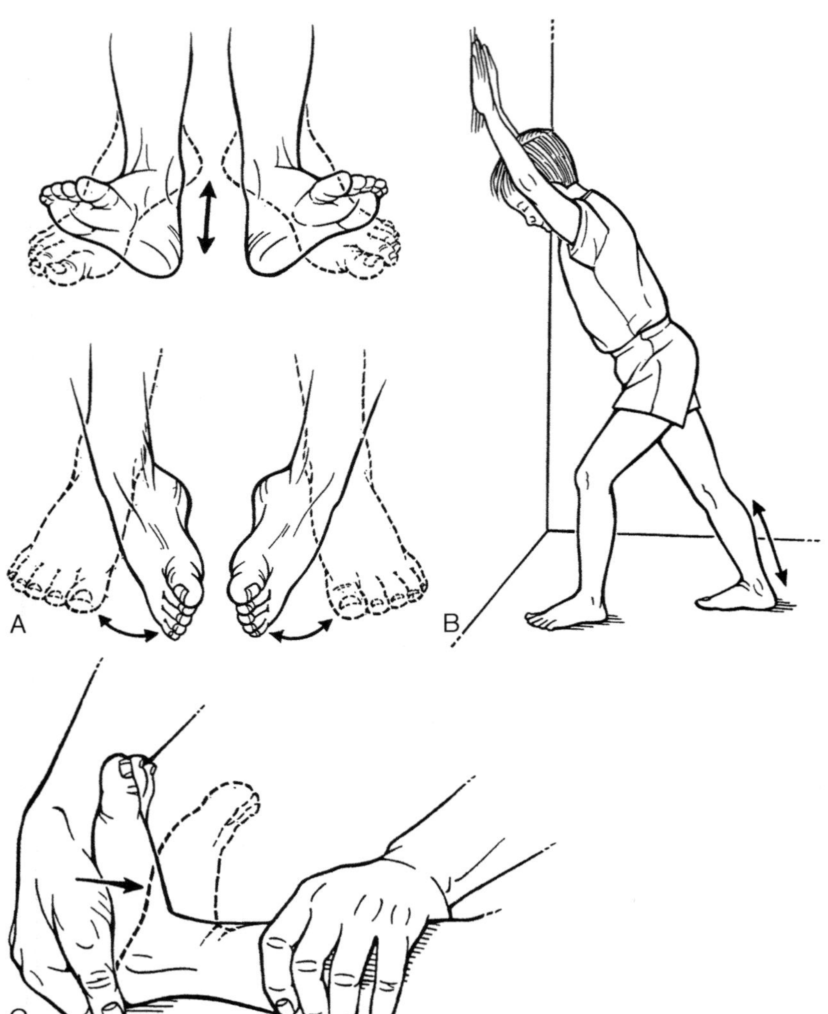

Figure 10–11. *A,* **Ankle.** Sit in a chair with the feet on the floor. First, keeping the heels down, lift the toes up as high as possible. Then, keeping the front of the feet on the floor, lift the heels up as high as possible. Finally, turn the soles of both feet toward each other, then turn them away from each other. Repeat each movement two to three times. *B,* **Lower leg (calf).** Standing an arm's length away from the wall, place both hands on the wall, above the head. Place one leg straight back, keeping the foot flat on the floor and the knee straight; the forward leg should be bent at the knee. Hold until a pull is felt in the back of the straight leg and count slowly to 10. Repeat two to three times with each leg. *C,* **Lower leg.** With your child lying on her back with her legs straight, place your hand under her heel. Grasp her foot and lean the lower part of your arm against the sole of her foot. Bend her foot toward the knee, but don't use too much pressure. With the other hand, grasp the leg between the ankle and knee to steady the leg. Hold for a count of 10 or 15. Repeat with the other leg. (A–C, From Raising a Child with Arthritis—A Parent's Guide 1998. Atlanta, Arthritis Foundation, 1998. ©1998. Reprinted with permission of the Arthritis Foundation 1330 W. Peachtree St., Atlanta, GA 30309. For more information please call the Arthritis Foundation's Information Line at 1.800.283.7800 or log on to www.arthritis.org)

emotions, cultural factors, and family dynamics play a major part in pain perception. Therefore, exclusively medical management of pain in these syndromes is unlikely to be successful. This is particularly true in reflex neurovascular dystrophy.[35, 38]

For all of these reasons, it is important to obtain a complete developmental and psychosocial history in children with chronic pain, particularly in children in whom repeated examinations and laboratory results are negative.

Children with chronic pain present a management challenge because of the psychodynamics and the time needed to care for them. Referral to a pain clinic, psychologist, or psychiatrist is sometimes needed.

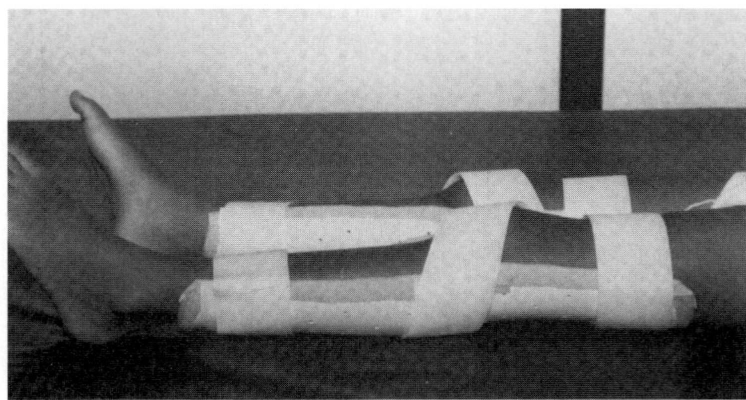

Figure 10–12. Lower-extremity resting splint. This posterior shell is worn during the hours of sleep to rest the knees in extension. (From Scull SA, Dow MB, Athreya BH: Physical and occupational therapy for children with rheumatic diseases. Pediatr Clin North Am 33: 1067, 1986.)

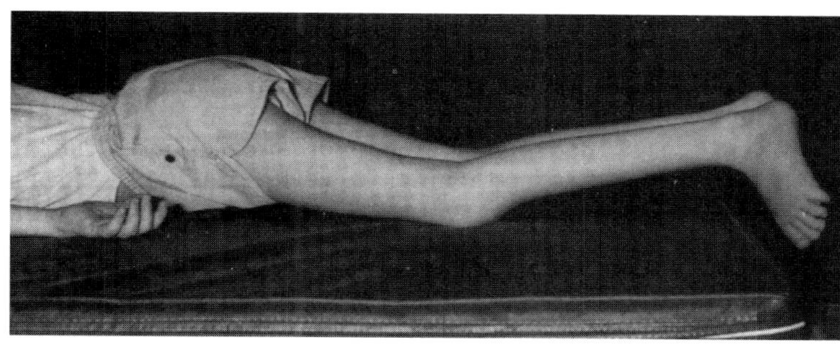

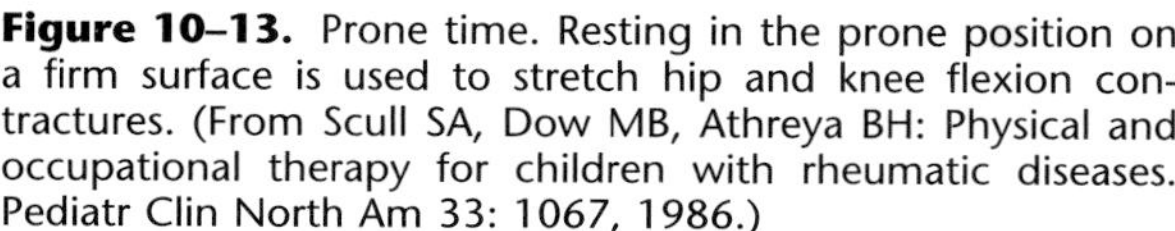

Figure 10–13. Prone time. Resting in the prone position on a firm surface is used to stretch hip and knee flexion contractures. (From Scull SA, Dow MB, Athreya BH: Physical and occupational therapy for children with rheumatic diseases. Pediatr Clin North Am 33: 1067, 1986.)

Posture/Positioning

Children with arthritis assume a number of dysfunctional postures unconsciously as their bodies adapt to the pain and limitation of ROM. It is important to remind them to sit with a straight back and shoulders braced. This is particularly important for children with spondyloarthropathies. Attention should be given to the school chair to ensure that good posture is maintained. The position for reading books or work on the computer should provide for good neck and wrist positions. Children with cervical spine involvement should sleep with a single pillow or very soft pillow. Resting knee or wrist splints may be indicated for use at night to prevent poor positioning of these joints during sleep (Fig. 10–12). Lying prone at least 20 minutes a day may help prevent hip flexion contractures (Fig. 10–13).

Therapeutic Exercises

Therapeutic exercises serve several functions.[32–34, 39] They may be aimed at improving ROM of joints, strengthening muscles, or promoting conditioning and endurance.[39] There are several types of exercises.[34, 40] In active exercises, the patient is asked to move the joint. These are useful to stretch and strengthen muscles (e.g., touching toes to stretch hamstrings—Fig. 10–14). Passive exercises (active-assistive) are performed by the therapist and are useful when there is a flare of arthritis, when a joint has lost motion, and in young children. Resistive exercises are used to strengthen muscles. For example, resistance is applied as the joint moves through its range.

Stretching exercises such as those for the treatment of tight heel cords or hip flexion contracture are done preferably by the therapist.

Strengthening exercises may be isometric or isotonic. When the muscle is contracted without permitting joint motion, it is called *isometric*. Quadriceps setting for an acutely inflamed joint is an isometric exercise. *Isotonic* exercises performed against gravity along with ROM and resistive exercises are useful to strengthen muscles. A child should master ROM exercises and muscle strengthening exercises before proceeding onto endurance/conditioning exercises and sports activities (Fig. 10–15).

Exercises should be done every day, either in the morning or in the evening, for at least 20 to 30 minutes. This routine may be difficult to accomplish, particularly in the morning in a family in which both parents work and there are other children. It is best for the child to take a warm bath before performing exercises. The parents and the child (particularly the adolescent) should be educated on the importance and the techniques of performing home therapy exercises. The therapist should demonstrate the exercise and let the parents practice under supervision. A written description with figures (see Figs. 10–2 to 10–11) is useful.

Exercises should be age-appropriate and accommodate the family's daily schedule. Young children are easily bored with exercises, and insistence by parents on a rigid routine may lead to parent-child conflicts.

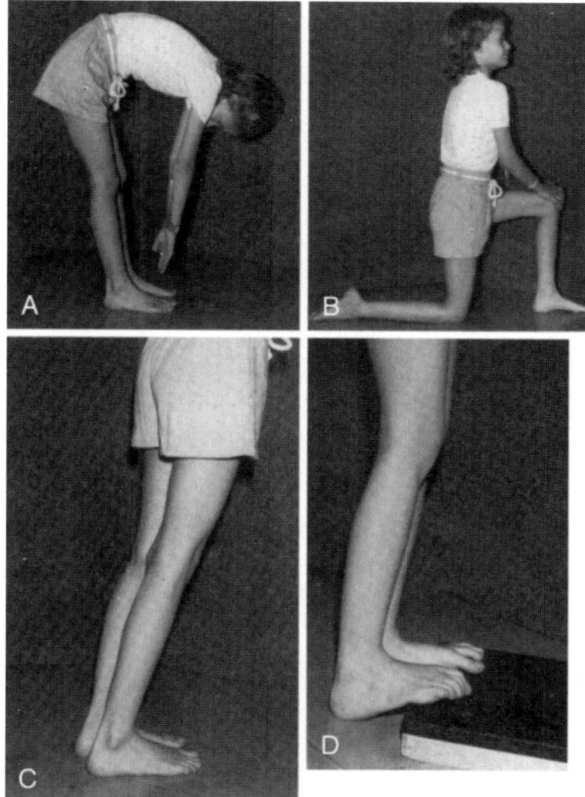

Figure 10–14. Lower-extremity stretching exercises. Active exercises to stretch hamstrings *(A)*, iliopsoas *(B)*, and heel cords *(C* and *D)*. (From Scull SA, Dow MB, Athreya BH: Physical and occupational therapy for children with rheumatic diseases. Pediatr Clin North Am 33: 1067, 1986.)

Table 10–9

Play Exercises by Age Group: A Guide for Parents

AGES 6 MO–3 YR

Playing in warm water with toys moves all joints and helps pain
Toys that pull apart (pop beads)—to strengthen hands and arms
Tickle bottoms of feet—to bend knees and hips
Put plastic ring over ankle and leg and take it off
Pushing and catching a balloon or soft beach ball—to strengthen arms
Kicking a balloon or soft beach ball—to bend knees and strengthen legs
Squeeze and roll clay—to strengthen hand and bend wrist
Tricycle or toys to scoot—to strengthen leg muscles and move the joints of the legs

AGES 4–8 YR

Warm bath and playing with toys in the water—to move all joints and help pain
Pieces of elastic to pull into funny shapes; *Theraband* is a thin elastic sheet that you can draw on and pull into funny shapes; available from a PT or dental supply house—to strengthen arms and hands
Any crafts the child likes—usually strengthen and move joints of arms and hands
Clay to squeeze and roll—to strengthen hand and bend wrist
Tricycle or bicycle—to move leg in many positions
Swimming classes—total body exercise

AGES 9–13 YR

Swimming—total body exercise
Crafts—usually strengthens and moves joints of arm and hands
Bicycling—gives leg joints movements and strengthens leg muscles
School activities (including gym)—total body movement.* Ask your doctor if your child should not play "contact" sports or do headstands. (Although children with JRA are usually encouraged to take part in gym to their tolerance, there may be times when it is not advisable, or your physician may suggest avoiding specific gym activities; please check this out with your physician)
Hitting and catching softballs or volleyballs—arm strength
Ballet—total body movement

AGES 13 YR AND OVER

By this age, the teenager should be helping to plan the exercise activities; the parents, teen, and staff can talk together about what the teen likes to do and what joints need extra moving

PT, physical therapist.
Adapted from Giesecke LL, Athreya BH, Doughty RA: Home Care Guide on Juvenile Rheumatoid Arthritis (for Parents). Atlantic City, NJ, Children's Seashore House, 1985; and Scull SA, Dow MB, Athreya BH: Physical and occupational therapy for children with rheumatic diseases. Pediatr Clin North Am 33: 1060, 1986.

Therefore, it may be easier to incorporate these exercises into games, recreational activities, and play (Table 10–9).

Activities of Daily Living

ADL include tasks in self-care, dressing, feeding, and hygiene. Age-appropriate independence in these activities may be difficult for children with arthritis. For children who have difficulties such as turning doorknobs or opening jars, simple and more efficient techniques to perform these activities and other joint protection techniques must be taught. For more severe conditions, adaptive devices may be needed (Fig. 10–16). In certain situations, modifications to the home may be necessary, particularly for children in wheelchairs.

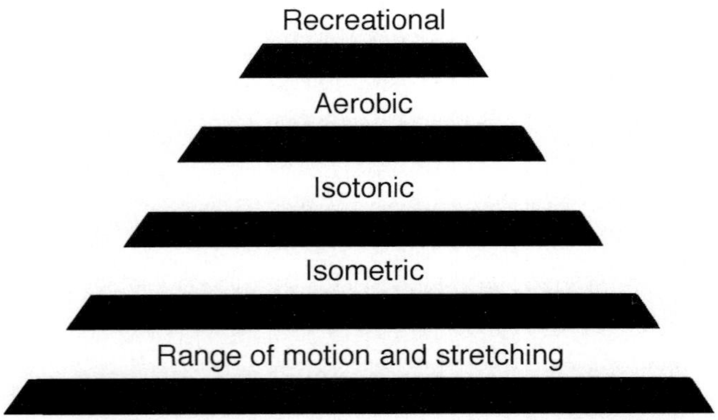

Recreational
Aerobic
Isotonic
Isometric
Range of motion and stretching

Children with arthritis should begin with range-of-motion exercises. They may progress upward on the pyramid as their disease regresses or is controlled medically.

Figure 10–15. Pyramid of graded progress in an exercise program. (From Hicks JE: Exercise in patients with inflammatory arthritis. Rheum Dis Clin North Am 16: 857, 1990.)

Sports and Exercise

Children with rheumatic diseases fatigue easily and have reduced cardiopulmonary reserve.[41] Several factors limit the exercise capacity of these children, including the severity of involvement of joints and muscles, involvement of the cardiovascular or the respiratory system, and anemia. In addition, psychological factors[42] and parental concerns may add to the lowered physical fitness of these children.[43]

Involving children in age-appropriate games and play activities is an ideal way to maintain ROM of joints, increase muscle strength, improve conditioning, and boost self-esteem. Better compliance is an added bonus. Various age-appropriate activities are listed in Table 10–9. Young children can ride in their Hot-Wheels or bicycle (Fig. 10–17). By adjusting the height of the seat and making sure they do not slide up and down, one can improve ROM of the knee to gain increased flexion or extension. By reversing the handle, one can increase extension of the wrist (Fig. 10–18).

School-aged children should be encouraged to participate in physical education classes to their tolerance. Adaptive gym classes and allowing children to set

Table 10–10

Sport Selection for Patients With Arthritis*

Recommended: *Most individuals with arthritis can participate safely*		
Badminton	Darts	Swimming
Billiards	Fishing	Table Tennis
Croquet	Horseshoes	Walking/hiking
Cycling	Shuffleboard	Wiffle ball
Self-Limiting: *Reasonable activities in which students may try to participate to the best of their ability; the risk:benefit ratio should be evaluated for each individual*		
Baseball (not pitcher/ catcher)	Cross-country skiing	Ice skating
Basketball	Dance	Roller skating
Canoeing	Golf	Rowing
Cheerleading	Horseback riding (supervised)	Softball
Tennis		
Contraindicated: *Sports for which the risk of joint damage outweighs the benefits*		
Ballet (en pointe)	Gymnastics	Track
Bowling	Hockey	Trampoline
Boxing	Lacrosse	Tumbling
Diving (if C-spine involved)	Martial arts	Volleyball
Downhill skiing	Skateboarding	Weightlifting
Football	Soccer	Wrestling
	Speed skating	

**Note*—These general guidelines should assist in planning sporting activities for the student with arthritis. However, specific recommendations for each child should be developed jointly with the pediatric rheumatologist or physical therapist because children with rheumatic disease exhibit a wide range of disabilities.

Adapted by permission from B. Goldberg, 1995, *Sports and Exercise for Children with Chronic Health Conditions.* (Champaign, IL: Human Kinetics Publishers), 141.

their limits should encourage participation. However, activities that involve weight-bearing or stress on affected joints, such as headstands, somersaults, chin-ups, and handstands, should be avoided. The trampoline is usually contraindicated. Contact sports and activities that generate torsional forces on involved joints (e.g., downhill skiing) should be avoided in children with severe arthritis. In general, cycling and swimming are safe and beneficial for most children with arthritis. A guideline for recommended sports activities is given in Table 10–10.

Therapeutic Modalities

Heat, cold, splinting, bracing (orthotics), and water exercises are some of the modalities used in the treatment of rheumatic diseases.

Heat and Cold

Both intra-articular temperature and blood flow are increased in inflamed joints. Consequently, the metabolism of articular tissues is altered.[44] However, studies on the value of heat and cold in altering the intra-articular temperature and blood flow and in relief of symptoms have yielded inconclusive results. Based on an extensive review of the literature, Karen Hayes[45] came to the following conclusions:

> Both heat and cold appear to be effective in managing pain, stiffness, and limitation of ROM. Heat may be more effective for joint motion and cold more effective for pain reduction. Therefore, a patient with acute disease may benefit with cold as well as with heat; patients with chronic disease may benefit with heat. Preference of the patient may be the best determinant of modality used.

Deep or superficial heat can be used. A warm tub bath or shower in the morning helps reduce stiffness. A heated pool (88° to 92°F; 31° to 33°C) is ideal for therapeutic exercises,[46] but one has to be careful about vasodilatation and hypotension. Children with moderate to severe anemia often do not tolerate warm pools. Moist packs may be useful to relieve muscle spasm. Deep heat in the form of paraffin baths may be beneficial, particularly for the small joints of the hand. Deep heat application, such as diathermy or ultrasound, is not usually recommended for children because of potential damage to the cartilage. Cold packs and ice packs are ideal for acute swelling and pain and for postexercise pain.

Splints

Splints, braces, and orthotic devices are used for a variety of purposes. These include support for acutely inflamed joints (resting splints), maintenance of joints in functional positions during activity (dynamic splints) (Fig. 10–19), stretching contracted joints (corrective splints), and provision of shock absorption (shoe insert). Splints may be made from a variety of compounds such as plaster of Paris, polypropylene, Aquaplast, or fiberglass. Materials to be used depend on the purpose, need for repeated adjustments, and cost.

Resting Splints. Resting splints are used to rest acutely inflamed joints. A joint is maintained in a functional position in the splint for most of the day. The splint is removed once or twice a day to exercise the muscles and move the joint through its ROM, if possible. Resting splints are often used to maintain position and prevent deformities at the wrists, knees, and ankles. The most commonly used splints are wrist splints (Fig. 10–20) to maintain the wrist in a functional position during the night, and knee splints (see Fig. 10–12) to prevent knee-flexion contractures. If a knee-flexion contracture is greater than 20 degrees, it may be necessary to use serial casting (corrective splint) or dynamic splinting. Although cervical collars may not be totally efficacious to prevent motion at the atlantoaxial joint, we often suggest that children with cervical spine involvement use a firm collar during car rides.

Functional Splints. Functional splints are designed to support joints during ADL and to reduce stress. For example, a molded ankle-foot orthosis (AFO) may be used to maintain the stretch of the Achilles tendon during weight bearing. A shoe insert may be used

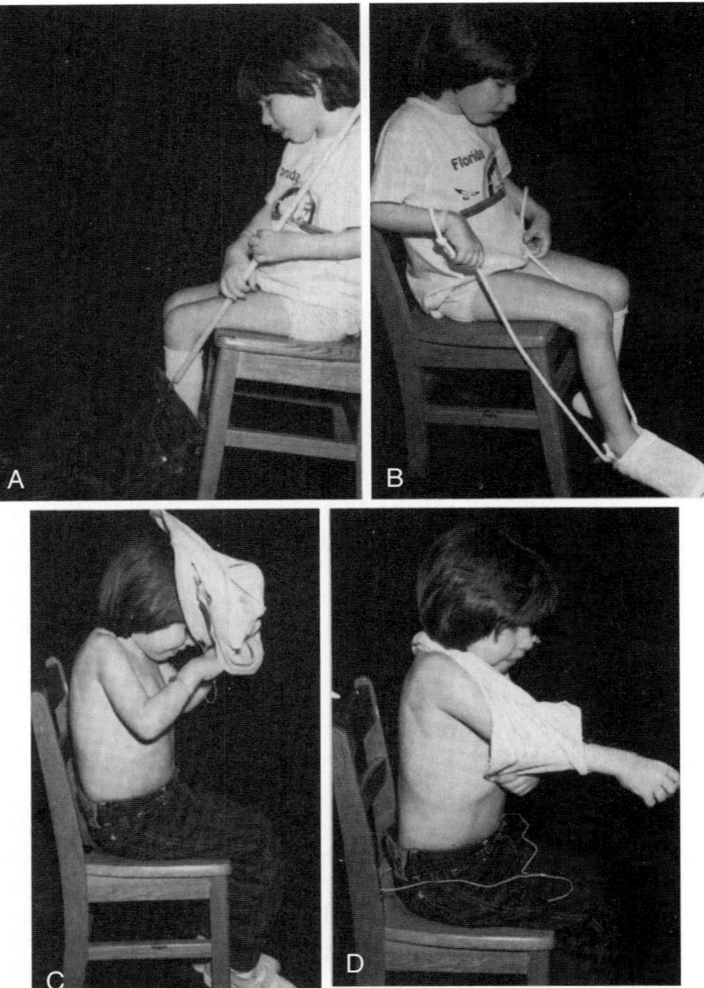

Figure 10–16. Dressing aids. *A,* Dressing stick. *B,* Sock aid. *C* and *D,* Coat hanger "hoops" are used to train this child for independence. (From Scull SA, Dow MB, Athreya BH: Physical and occupational therapy for children with rheumatic diseases. Pediatr Clin North Am 33: 1067, 1986.)

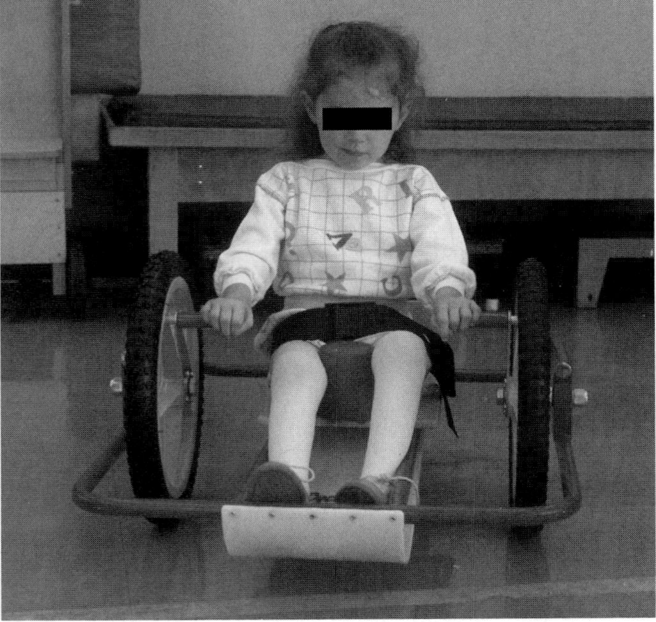

Figure 10–17. Child in Hot-Wheels: Seat or pedal can be adjusted to increase flexion or extension at the knee.

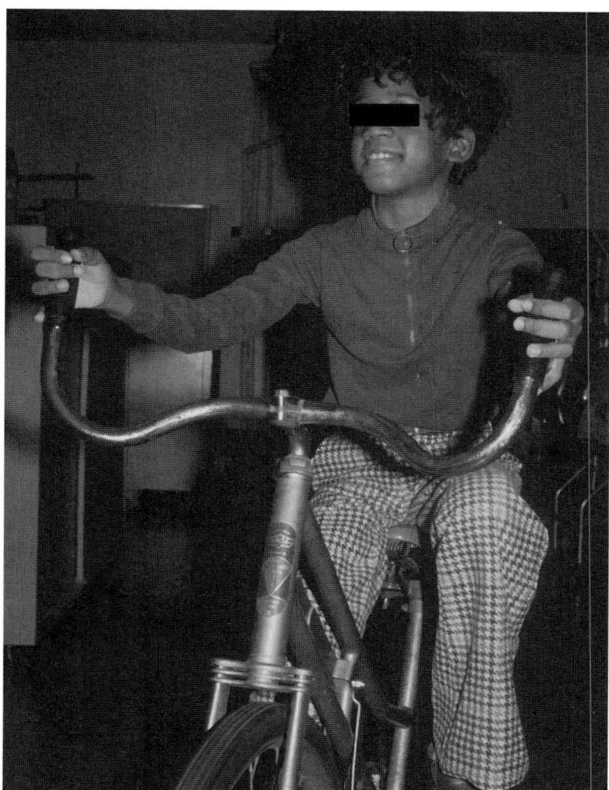

Figure 10–18. Handle-bar reversed, forcing wrist joints into extension.

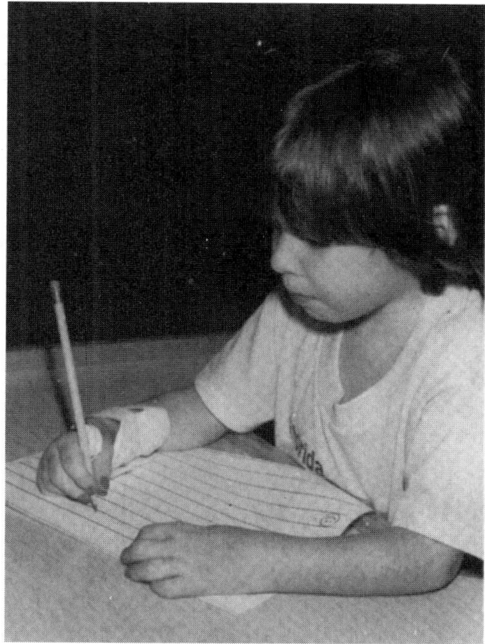

Figure 10–19. Wrist support splint. (From Scull SA, Dow MB, Athreya BH: Physical and occupational therapy for children with rheumatic diseases. Pediatr Clin North Am 33: 1067, 1986.)

to decrease pain during weight bearing. Some splints produce a constant stretch to the muscles during walking and upper-extremity function (dynamic splints) (Fig. 10–21). Biomechanical orthotics are small, custom-made devices such as shoe inserts designed to correct the alignment or to relieve pain.

Water Exercises

Therapy in water (pool or whirlpool) is one of the best and most acceptable forms of therapy for children with arthritis.[46, 47] The buoyancy of water facilitates weight bearing. Water can also be used to provide resistance to muscle movement. Children can walk in water up to their chest to reduce load on their hips. A heated pool may be useful to reduce stiffness. Finally, swimming itself is a great exercise, both for ROM and for aerobic conditioning. Water therapy is ideal for children with severe morning stiffness and for postoperative rehabilitation.

Shoe Modification

Citing their detailed analysis of feet in JRA, Truckenbrodt and associates[48] defined eight major deformities (Table 10–11). The most common are pes planovalgus due to involvement of subtalar joints, pes cavus due to inflammation of the intertarsal joints, and pseudocavus due to inflammation of the upper ankle joint and the talonavicular joint. Soft, comfortable footwear with good arch support, such as sneakers, is recommended for most common problems. Cushioning with a foam insole may reduce force of impact. For children with metatarsal pain, metatarsal bars or rocker-bottom soles may help with push-off.

Postsurgical Therapy

The therapist should be involved from the beginning when surgery is planned. Therapists are in a position to recommend the goals of surgery because they have

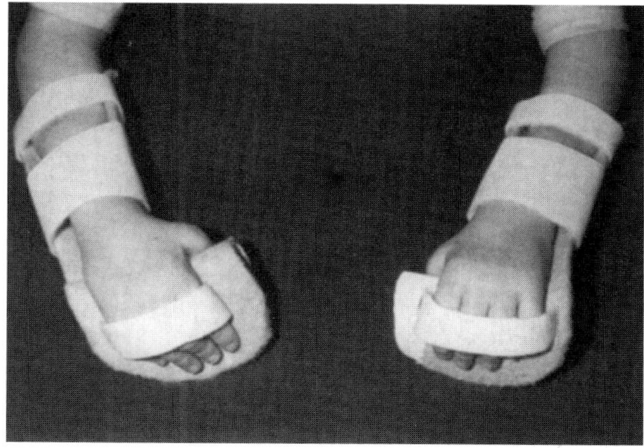

Figure 10–20. Wrist cock-up splint—a resting splint for wrist and fingers. (From Scull SA, Dow MB, Athreya BH: Physical and occupation therapy for children with rheumatic diseases. Pediatr Clin North Am 33: 1067, 1986.)

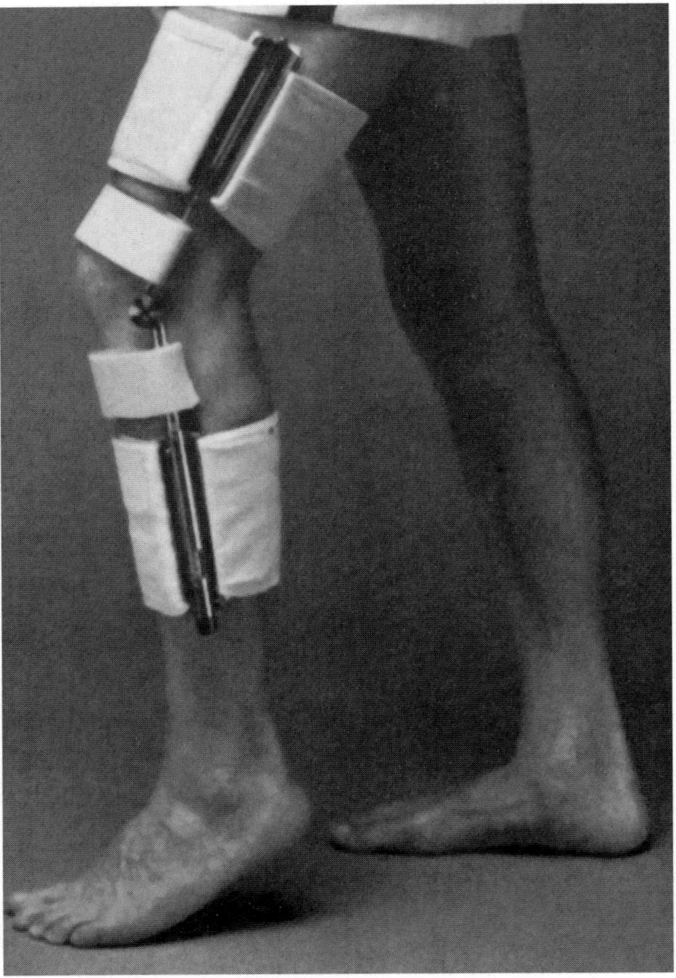

Figure 10–21. Dynamic splint.

worked with the child and the child's personality and have reviewed the disability and its current functional limitations. Children should be taught to exercise thoroughly the muscles they will be asked to use increasingly after surgery. Early mobilization is essential to prevent loss of motion. Positioning and splinting or a passive ROM machine may have to be used to maintain newly acquired motion. Postoperative therapy may include active and passive ROM, water therapy, and gradual increase in weight bearing.[34, 49]

General strategies to manage various problems encountered in patients with rheumatic diseases are given in Table 10–12.

Table 10–11

Most Frequent Deviations of the Foot in Juvenile Chronic Arthritis; Various Combinations Are Possible

Pes planovalgus
Pes cavus
Heelfoot (pseudocavus)
Hallux flexus/rigidus
Hallux valgus
Forefoot adduction
Claw toes
Hammer toes

From Truckenbrodt H, Hafner R, von Altenbockum C: Functional joint analysis of the foot in juvenile chronic arthritis. Clin Exp Rheumatol 12(Suppl 10): 591, 1994.

Table 10–12

Strategies for Managing Various Problems Associated With Rheumatic Diseases

Morning stiffness	Sleep in a sleeping bag Early-morning shower Pool therapy
Decreased range of motion	Therapeutic exercises Active Active-assistive (passive) Resistive Aerobic
Position	Posture Splint Brace
Stretch	Splints Braces
Muscle weakness	Strengthening exercises Active Faradic electrical stimulation
Limitation of activities of daily living	Functional training Adaptive devices
Painful feet	Shoe inserts Functional orthoses
Leg-length differences	Heel or shoe lift

Courtesy of S. Bowyer, MD.

GROWTH AND NUTRITION

Abnormalities of growth and nutrition have been well documented in children with JRA,[50–54] although similar studies are not available for children with SLE and other rheumatic diseases.

Growth retardation is common in children with rheumatic diseases (except in those with oligoarticular JRA). Growth retardation is associated with active disease, particularly in young children.[50] Steroid therapy is well known to accentuate this problem, even at low doses.[52] Even children with polyarticular JRA who have not undergone steroid therapy tend to be smaller.[53] In some of these children, the growth delay, if not severe, normalizes once the disease is controlled, provided there are no secondary problems such as the use of glucocorticoids. One of the major reasons for growth retardation is poor nutrition or undernutrition.

A variety of factors contribute to the nutritional problems in children with JRA.[55] These include poor appetite due to the activity of the disease or secondary to the inflammatory drugs used to treat JRA; mechanical feeding difficulties related to temporomandibular joint function, retrognathia, or dental problems; unprescribed dietary alterations; and fad diets.

Growth retardation, obesity, and protein-energy malnutrition are common problems among children with rheumatic diseases. Patients with chronic diseases often try fad diets. Parents and patients are greatly interested in learning about good nutrition. Therefore, more attention should be paid to educate children and their families on proper nutrition.

Ideally, all children should be followed closely, with documentation of height and weight at every visit or at least three to four times a year. A simple nutritional scoring device has been developed with good sensitivity and specificity.[56] This should be used to screen and refer patients to a nutritionist as needed. However, the services of a nutritionist are not always available. Nurses should discuss family issues, and families often confide in nurses. Therefore, nurses may be in an ideal position to administer nutritional screening tests, provide recommendations for adequate nutrition and vitamin and calcium supplementation, and refer to a nutritionist if needed.[57, 58]

CALCIUM AND BONE

In addition to nutritional screening for protein-energy malnutrition, some children on chronic glucocorticoid therapy may need advice on correction or prevention of osteopenia. Studies have documented that inadequate bone mineralization is almost universal in children with JRA, even if they are not taking glucocorticoids.[59, 60] This problem is accentuated by poor nutrition, lack of physical activity, and glucocorticoid therapy.

Control of disease activity is the most important step in ameliorating this process. Reversal of protein-calorie malnutrition with adequate diet and supplementation with vitamin D (400 units/day) and calcium (1.2 g/day) are essential to prevent osteopenia. Phosphonate compounds may have to be used in children with severe osteopenia and pathologic fractures, although experience with these agents in children is limited.[61] Where available, use of deflazacort for long-term therapy may be less deleterious for bone mineralization.[62]

GROWTH AND GROWTH HORMONE THERAPY

Generalized growth retardation may be associated with JRA,[50, 51, 63] SLE, dermatomyositis, and systemic sclerosis secondary to the disease or its treatment. On occasion, the initial manifestation of SLE may be growth retardation. Patients with JRA and SLE have been treated with human growth hormone,[64, 65] although the exact mechanism of growth retardation in these diseases has not been well understood. Although serum growth hormone levels were not deficient when measured on a single sample of serum, measurement of pulsatile secretion of growth hormone confirmed a low 24-hour secretion.[66] Serum levels of insulin-like growth factor binding protein-3 (IGF-BP3) have been found to be low,[67, 68] and treatment with human growth hormone (hGH) has been shown to increase growth velocity in some children. This increase is often associated with correction of IGF-1 and IGF-BP3.[67, 68]

There are several concerns with the use of hGH in children. Use of recombinant hGH in other conditions has been associated with malignancy, increased growth of pigmented nevi, and scoliosis.[69] A 1998 report describes reactivation of lupus nephritis in a 15-year-old boy with SLE on hGH therapy.[70] Finally, treatment with hGH is very expensive. For these reasons, hGH therapy is not recommended for the treatment of short stature associated with rheumatic diseases. This is an area for preventive medicine in rheumatology; with more adequate control of inflammation and better nutritional advice, growth retardation can perhaps be minimized, if not prevented.

IMMUNIZATION

There are two major questions related to immunization and rheumatic diseases: (1) Is there any relationship between immunization and onset or exacerbation of these diseases? (2) What are the recommendations for children with rheumatic diseases who are taking various medications?

Several reports suggest that immunization may precipitate an arthritic or vasculitic disorder. In one study from England on a large population of children immunized with measles-mumps-rubella (MMR) vaccine, the incidence of joint complaints increased during a 6-week period after immunization, compared with a control group. However, objective arthritis was rare and not persistent.[71] Acute joint symptoms and arthritis are common after rubella vaccination, particularly in young women.[72] Although earlier studies in adolescents suggested that chronic arthritis can occur after rubella vaccination,[73] a larger study did not substantiate this finding.[74] There are reports of systemic vasculitis following hepatitis B[75] and influenza[76] immunizations.

In the only available study on the relationship between influenza immunization and arthritis in children, Malleson and colleagues[77] did not find exacerbation of arthritis associated with influenza virus vaccination. In the same study, they documented that antibody responses were satisfactory even in children on prednisone.

At present, it appears that the benefits of immunization far outweigh any risk of exacerbation of the disease in most situations (see Chapter 12). We encourage the family to keep the regular schedule of immunizations while cautioning them about the possibility of a flareup. There are, however, a *few exceptions*:

- Active disease: Children with severe, active disease should not receive any immunization.
- Children on immunosuppressive therapy and glucocorticoid therapy should *not* receive any live virus vaccine. Recommendations made by the Committee on Infectious Diseases of the American Academy of Pediatrics should be followed for these children.[78]
- Children on intravenous immunoglobulin should

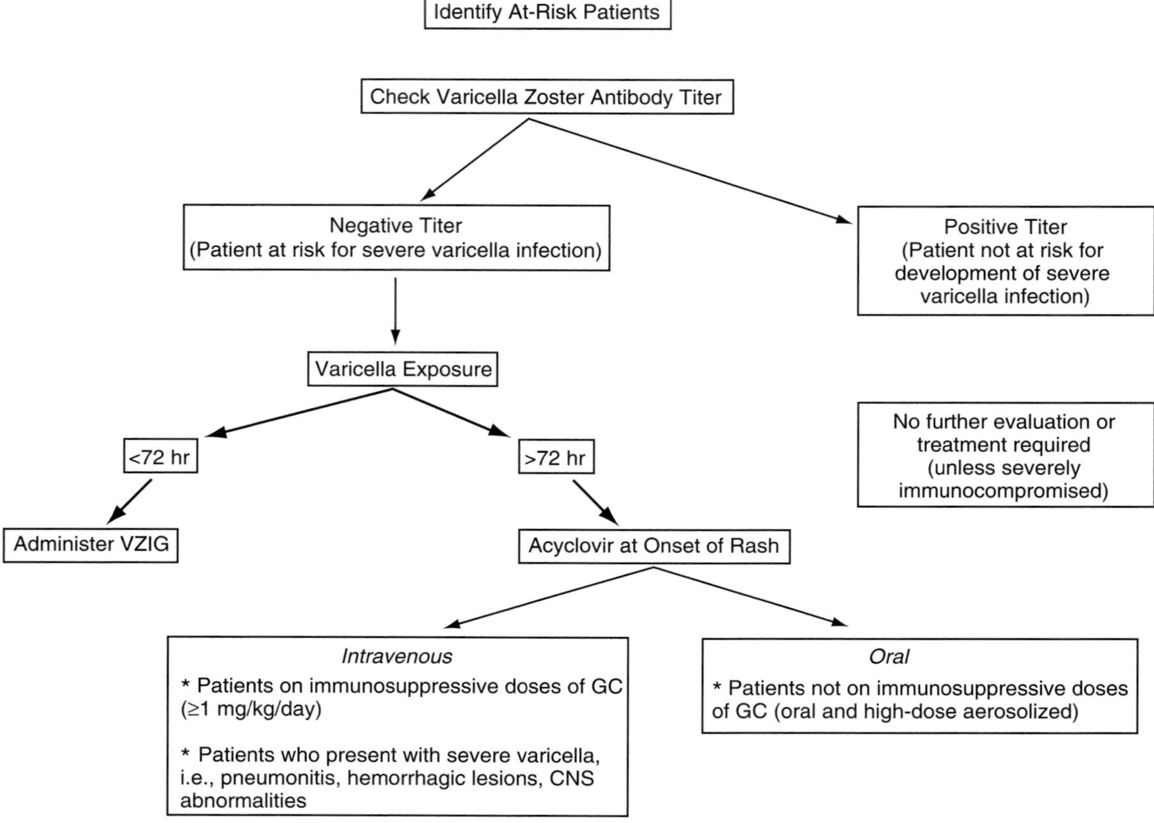

Figure 10–22. Proposed algorithm for the management of varicella infection. GC, glucocorticoid (prednisone). (Reproduced by permission of Pediatrics in Review. From Spahn JD, Kamada AK: Special considerations in the use of glucocorticoids in children. Reproduced by permission of Pediatrics in Review, volume 16, page 270, copyright 1995.)

wait for at least 3 months after the last dose before any immunization in order to ensure an adequate immune response.[79]

- The potential for Reye's syndrome in children treated with salicylates in association with varicella or influenza has been widely discussed.[80] One current strategy for managing varicella exposure in children is outlined in Figure 10–22. Routine use of varicella vaccine will change these recommendations. Varicella vaccination is generally contraindicated in children taking glucocorticoids in doses of 2 mg/kg/day equivalent.[78] For children on smaller doses, the risk:benefit ratio has to be assessed. It is ideal to wait at least 2 weeks after discontinuation of glucocorticoid therapy before immunization with live virus vaccines. Salicylate should not be used for at least 6 weeks after varicella vaccine administration.
- Children on chronic salicylate therapy and all children with SLE, dermatomyositis with significant muscle weakness, systemic scleroderma with cardiopulmonary or renal disease, and systemic vasculitides may benefit from yearly influenza virus vaccination. Early concerns that influenza immunization may cause a flareup of arthritis are probably not justified.[77] Recent studies also indicate that patients on glucocorticoids and immunosuppressives respond to influenza vaccine[77, 81] and pneumococcal vaccines[82] with adequate antibody titers. However, such immunization should not give rise to a false sense of security because immunity is not guaranteed.
- Children with SLE and splenic hypofunction should receive pneumococcal vaccine.[82, 83]

References

1. Taylor DC: The components of sickness: disease, illness and predicaments. Lancet 2: 1008, 1979.
2. Hobbs N, Perrin JM: Issues in the Care of Children With Chronic Illness: A Source Book on Problems, Services and Policies. San Francisco, Josey-Bass, 1985.
3. Pless IB, Power C, Peckham CS: Long term psychosocial sequelae of chronic physical disorders in childhood. Pediatrics 91: 1131, 1993.
4. McCormick MC, Stemmler MM, Athreya BH: The impact of childhood rheumatic diseases on the family. Arthritis Rheum 29: 872, 1986.
5. Lovell DA, Athreya BH, Emery HM, et al: School attendance and patterns, special services and special needs in pediatric patients with rheumatic diseases. Arthritis Care Res 3: 196, 1990.
6. Walker DK: Care of chronically ill children in schools. Pediatr Clin North Am 31: 221, 1984.
7. Allaire SA, DeNardo BS, Szer IS, et al: The economic impact of juvenile rheumatoid arthritis. J Rheumatol 19: 952, 1992.
8. Newacheck PW, Taylor WR: Childhood chronic illness: prevalence, severity and impact. Am J Public Health 82: 364, 1992.
9. Miller JJ: Psychosocial factors related to rheumatic diseases in childhood. J Rheumatol 20(Suppl 38): 1, 1993.
10. Peterson LS, Mason T, Nelson AM: Psychosocial outcomes and health status of adults who have had juvenile rheumatoid

arthritis—a controlled, population-based study. Arthritis Rheum 40: 2235, 1997.
11. McAnarney ER, Pless IB, Satterwhite B, et al: Psychological problems of children with chronic juvenile arthritis. Pediatrics 53: 523, 1974.
12. Frank RG, Hagglund KJ, Schopp LH, et al: Disease and family contributors to adaptation in juvenile rheumatoid arthritis and juvenile diabetes. Arthritis Care Res 11: 166, 1998.
13. Rettig P, Athreya BH: Leaving home—preparing the adolescent with arthritis for coping with independence and the adult rheumatology world. *In* Isenberg D, Miller JJ (eds): Adolescent Rheumatology. London, Martin Dunitz, 1998.
14. Brewer EJ, McPherson M, Magrab P, et al: Family-centered, community-based, coordinated care for children with special healthcare needs. Pediatrics 83: 1055, 1989.
15. Mervyn FA: "They get this training but they don't know how you feel." Horsham, England, National Fund for Research into Crippling Diseases, 1975.
16. Athreya BH: Regionalized arthritis resources. Arthritis Rheum 20(Suppl): 604, 1977.
17. Koop CE: Surgeon-General's Report: Children With Special Healthcare Needs—Campaign '87—Commitment to Family-Centered, Coordinated Care for Children With Special Health Care Needs. Washington, D.C., U.S. Department of Health and Human Services, Government Printing Office, 1987.
18. Rapoff MA, Lindsley CB, Christophersen ER: Parent perception of problems experienced by their children in complying with treatments for juvenile rheumatoid arthritis. Arch Phys Med Rehabil 66: 427, 1985.
19. Swartz DR: Dealing with chronic illness in childhood. Pediatr Rev 6: 67, 1984.
20. Gallo AM, Breitmayer BJ, Knafl KA, et al: Stigma in childhood chronic illness: a well sibling perspective. Pediatr Nurs 17: 21, 1991.
21. Birenbaum A: On managing a courtesy stigma. J Health Soc Behav 11: 196, 1970.
22. Daniels D, Miller JJ, Billings AG, et al: Psychosocial functioning of siblings of children with rheumatic disease. J Pediatr 109: 379, 1986.
23. Cassidy JT, Lindsley CB: Legal rights of children with musculoskeletal disabilities. Bull Rheum Dis 45: 1, 1996.
24. Spencer CH, Fife RZ, Rabinovich E: The school experience of children with arthritis: coping in the 1990's and transition into adulthood. Pediatr Clin North Am 42: 1285, 1995.
25. White PH: Success on the road to adulthood: issues and hurdles for adolescents with disabilities. Rheum Dis Clin North Am 23: 697, 1997.
26. Neff JM, Anderson G: Protecting children with chronic illness in a competitive marketplace. JAMA 274: 1866, 1995.
27. American Academy of Pediatrics: Committee on Children with Disabilities: managed care and children with special health care needs. A subject review. Pediatrics 102: 657, 1998.
28. Jonas WB: Alternative medicine—learning from the past, examining the present, advancing to the future. JAMA 280: 1616, 1998.
29. Southwood TR, Malleson PN, Roberts-Thomson P, et al: Unconventional remedies used for patients with juvenile arthritis. Pediatrics 85: 150, 1990.
30. Hackett J, Johnson B, Parkin A, et al: Physiotherapy and occupational therapy for juvenile chronic arthritis: custom and practice in five centers in the UK, USA, and Canada. Br J Rheumatol 35: 695, 1996.
31. Murray KJ, Passo MH: Functional measures in children with rheumatic diseases. Pediatr Clin North Am 42: 1127, 1995.
32. Scull SA, Dow MB, Athreya BH: Physical and occupational therapy for children with rheumatic diseases. Pediatr Clin North Am 33: 1053, 1986.
33. Emery HM, Bowyer SL: Physical modalities of therapy in pediatric rheumatic diseases. Rheum Dis Clin North Am 17: 1001, 1991.
34. Hicks JE, Nichols JJ, Swezey RL: Handbook of Rehabilitative Rheumatology. Atlanta, American Rheumatism Association (ACR), 1988.
35. Varni JW, Bernstein BH: Evaluation and management of pain in children with rheumatic diseases. Rheum Dis Clin North Am 17: 985, 1991.
36. McGrath PJ, Unruh AM: Pain in children and adolescents. New York, Elsevier Amsterdam, 1987, pp 289–316.
37. Walco GA, Varni JW, Ilowite NT: Cognitive-behavioral management in children with juvenile rheumatoid arthritis. Pediatrics 89: 1075, 1992.
38. Sherry DD, Weisman R: Psychological aspects of childhood reflex neurovascular dystrophy. Pediatrics 81: 572, 1988.
39. Rhodes VJ: Physical therapy management of patients with juvenile rheumatoid arthritis. Phys Ther 71: 910, 1991.
40. Basmajian JV: Therapeutic Exercises, 4th ed. Baltimore, Williams & Wilkins, 1984, pp 303–308.
41. Giannini MJ, Potas EJ: Aerobic capacity in juvenile arthritis patients and healthy children. Arthritis Care Res 4: 131, 1991.
42. Malleson PN, Bennett SM, MacKinnon M, et al: Physical fitness and its relationship to other indices of health status in children with chronic arthritis. J Rheumatol 23: 1059, 1996.
43. Klepper SE, Darbee J, Effgen SK, et al: Physical fitness levels in children with polyarticular juvenile rheumatoid arthritis. Arthritis Care Res 5: 93, 1992.
44. Castor CW, Yaron M: Connective tissue activation. VIII: the effects of temperature studied in vitro. Arch Phys Med Rehabil 57: 5, 1976.
45. Hayes KW: Heat and cold in the management of rheumatoid arthritis. Arthritis Care Res 6: 156, 1993.
46. McNeal RL: Aquatic therapy for patients with rheumatic diseases. Rheum Dis Clin North Am 16: 915, 1990.
47. Campion MR: Hydrotherapy in Pediatrics, 2nd ed. Oxford, Butterworth-Heinemann, 1991.
48. Truckenbrodt H, Hafner R, von Altenbockum C: Functional joint analysis of the foot in juvenile chronic arthritis. Clin Exp Rheumatol 12(Suppl 10): S91, 1994.
49. Swann M: The surgery of juvenile chronic arthritis: an overview. Clin Orthop 259: 70, 1990.
50. Ansell BM, Bywaters EGL: Growth in Still's diseases. Ann Rheum Dis 15: 295, 1956.
51. Laaksonen AL: A prognostic study of juvenile rheumatoid arthritis: analysis of 544 cases. Acta Paediatr Scand 166(Suppl): 49, 1966.
52. Bacon MC, Raiten DJ, Craft N, et al: Nutritional status and its relationship to growth among children with juvenile rheumatoid arthritis. Arthritis Care Res 2:14, 1989.
53. Bernstein BH, Stobie D, Singsen BH, et al: Growth retardation in juvenile rheumatoid arthritis (JRA). Arthritis Rheum 20(Suppl): 212, 1977.
54. Henderson CJ, Lovell DJ: Assessment of protein-energy malnutrition in children and adolescents with juvenile rheumatoid arthritis. Arthritis Care Res 2: 108, 1989.
55. Henderson CJ, Lovell DJ: Nutritional aspects of JRA. Rheum Dis Clin North Am 17: 403, 1991.
56. Henderson CJ, Lovell DJ, Gregg D: A nutritional screening test for use in children and adolescents with juvenile rheumatoid arthritis. J Rheumatol 19: 1276, 1992.
57. Purdy K, Dwyer JT, Holland M, et al: You are what you eat: healthy food choices, nutrition and the child with juvenile rheumatoid arthritis. Pediatr Nurs 22: 391, 1996.
58. Garceau AO, Dwyer HT, Holland T: A practical approach to nutrition in the patient with juvenile rheumatoid arthritis. Clin Nutr 8: 55, 1989.
59. Pepmueller PH, Cassidy JT, Allen SH, et al: Bone mineralization and bone mineral metabolism in children with juvenile rheumatoid arthritis. Arthritis Rheum 39: 746, 1996.
60. Cassidy JT, Hillman LS: Abnormality in skeletal growth in children with juvenile rheumatoid arthritis. Rheum Dis Clin North Am 23: 499, 1997.
61. Bianchi ML, Cimaz R, Baldare M, et al: Efficacy and safety of alendronate for the treatment of osteoporosis in diffuse connective tissue diseases in children: a prospective multicenter study. Arthritis Rheum 43: 1960, 2000.
62. Loftus J, Allen R, Hesp R, et al: Randomized double-blind trial of deflazacort versus prednisone in juvenile chronic (or rheumatoid) arthritis: a relatively bone-sparing effect of deflazacort. Pediatrics 88: 428, 1991.
63. White PA: Growth abnormalities in children with juvenile rheumatoid arthritis. Clin Orthop 259: 46, 1990.
64. Davies UM, Rooney M, Preece MA, et al: Treatment of growth retardation in juvenile chronic arthritis with recombinant growth hormone. J Rheumatol 21: 153, 1994.

65. Rooney M, Davies UM, Reeve J, et al: Bone mineral content and bone mineral metabolism: changes after growth hormone treatment in juvenile chronic arthritis. J Rheumatol 27: 1073, 2000.
66. Hopp RJ, Degan J, Corley K, et al: Evaluation of growth hormone secretion in children with juvenile rheumatoid arthritis and short stature. Neb Med J 80: 52, 1995.
67. Touati G, Prieur A-M, Ruiz JC, et al: Beneficial effects of one-year growth hormone administration to children with juvenile chronic arthritis on chronic steroid therapy. I: effects on growth velocity and body composition. J Clin Endocrinol Metab 83: 403, 1998.
68. Davies UM, Jones J, Reeve J, et al: Juvenile rheumatoid arthritis: effects of disease activity and recombinant human growth hormone on insulin-like growth factor 1, insulin-like growth factor binding proteins 1 and 3, and osteocalcin. Arthritis Rheum 40: 332, 1997.
69. Allen DB: Safety of human growth hormone therapy: current topics. J Pediatr 128: S8, 1996.
70. Yap HK, Murugesan B, Lee BW: Subclinical activation of lupus nephritis by recombinant human growth hormone. Pediatr Nephrol 12: 133, 1998.
71. Benjamin CM, Chew GC, Silman AJ: Joint and limb symptoms in children after immunization with measles, mumps and rubella vaccine. BMJ 304: 1075, 1992.
72. Institute of Medicine: Adverse effects of pertussis and rubella vaccines. *In* Howson CP, Howe CJ, Fineberg HV (eds): A report of the Committee to Review the Adverse Consequences of Pertussis and Rubella Vaccines. Washington, DC, National Academy Press, 1991.
73. Tingle AJ, Allen M, Petty RE, et al: Rubella-associated arthritis 1. Comparative study of joint manifestations associated with natural rubella infection and RA-27/3 rubella immunization. Ann Rheum Dis 45: 110, 1986.
74. Ray P, Black S, Shinefield H, et al: Risk of chronic arthropathy among women after rubella vaccination. JAMA 278: 551, 1997.
75. Castrasana-Isla CJ, Herrera-Martinez G, Vega-Molina J: Erythema nodosum and Takayasu's arteritis after immunization with plasma derived hepatitis B vaccine. J Rheumatol 20: 1417, 1993.
76. Mader R, Narendran A, Lewtas J, et al: Systemic vasculitis following influenza vaccination—report of 3 cases and literature review. J Rheumatol 20: 1429, 1993.
77. Malleson PN, Tekano J, Scheiefle D, et al: Influenza immunization in children with chronic arthritis: a prospective study. J Rheumatol 20: 1769, 1993.
78. Report of the Committee on Infectious Diseases, 24th ed. Elk Grove Village, IL, American Academy of Pediatrics, 1997, pp 50–58.
79. Rowley AH, Shulman ST: Current therapy for acute Kawasaki syndrome. J Pediatr 118: 987, 1991.
80. Hurwitz ES, Barrett MJ, Bregman D, et al: Public Health Service study of Reye's syndrome and medications. Report of the main study. JAMA 257: 1905, 1987.
81. Lucy Park C, Frank AL, Sullivan M, et al: Influenza vaccination of children during acute asthma exacerbation and concurrent prednisone therapy. Pediatrics 98: 196, 1996.
82. Battafarano DF, Battafarano NJ, Larsen L, et al: Antigen-specific antibody responses in lupus patients following immunization. Arthritis Rheum 41: 1828, 1998.
83. Lipnick R, Karsh J, Stahl NI, et al: Pneumococcal immunization in patients with systemic lupus erythematosus treated with immunosuppressives. J Rheumatol 12: 1118, 1985.

Appendix 10–1 Resources for Further Information on Rheumatic Diseases for Patients and Parents

1. American Juvenile Arthritis Organization
   Resource Catalog (1998)—Arthritis Foundation
   1330 W. Peachtree Street, Atlanta, GA 30309 U.S.A.
   http://www.arthritis.org/ajao
2. Lupus Foundation of America Inc.
   1300 Piccard Drive, Suite 200
   Rockville, MD 20850 U.S.A.
3. Scleroderma Foundation
   83 Newbury Street
   Danvers, MA 01923 U.S.A.
4. Spondylitis Association of America
   14827 Ventura Boulevard, Suite 119
   PO Box 5872
   Sherman Oaks, CA 91403 U.S.A.
5. Family Village—A great website for information on all chronic diseases and rare syndromes. Gives information for resources in England also *http://www.familyvillage.wisc.edu.*
6. National Center for Youth with Disabilities
   University of Minnesota
   PO Box 721
   420 Delaware Street S.E.
   Minneapolis, MN 55455 U.S.A.
7. On TRAC—Taking Responsibility for Adolescent/Adult Care
   British Columbia's Children's Hospital
   Room 2, D20
   4480 Oak Street
   Vancouver, BC V6H 3V4 Canada

MONOGRAPHS/BOOKS

1. Raising a Child with Arthritis—A Parent's Guide. Atlanta, Arthritis Foundation, 1998.
2. Tucker LB, Denardo BA, Stebulis JA, Schaller JG: Your Child with Arthritis—A Family Guide for Caregiving. Baltimore, The John's Hopkins University Press, 1996.

Appendix 10–2 Example of a School Communication Form

PEDIATRIC RHEUMATOLOGY PROGRAM

____
(Date)

________________________________ ________________
(Student's Name) (Date of Birth)

__________ is followed by Rheumatology for __________. This chronic disease is characterized by joint swelling, pain and stiffness and fatigue. In addition, this student has __________. We recommend the following services be provided by the school:

- ❑ Modified physical education to include:
  - ❑ Activities to tolerance, allow student to set own limits
  - ❑ No contact sports
  - ❑ Swimming is encouraged
  - ❑ No repeated stress or pounding to affected joints
  - ❑ No weight bearing on wrists and arms, such as handstands, cartwheels, rings
- ❑ Adaptive physical education
- ❑ Two (2) sets of books
- ❑ Use of elevators if available
- ❑ Extra time between classes
- ❑ Provision for locker on each floor if applicable
- ❑ Modified assignments to include use of tape recorder
- ❑ Computer
- ❑ Extended time lines for completion of assignments and tests
- ❑ Use of oral tests
- ❑ No timed tests
- ❑ No grades for handwriting
- ❑ Door-to-door transportation
- ❑ Physical and Occupational Therapist evaluations to plan for accessibility and adaptation needs in school environment (as needed and on a quarterly basis)
- ❑ We request that home instruction be implemented if more than two (2) consecutive school days are missed.
- ❑ IEP that includes all of the above and ongoing OT and PT
- ❑ Other: ________________________________

We are enclosing a booklet for teachers. Attached please find a list of common school problems and solutions experienced by students with arthritis. Thank you in advance for your assistance and cooperation regarding this student.

Sincerely,

____________________ ____________________
Attending Rheumatologist Rheumatology Nurse Specialist

IEP, Individualized education plan; OT, occupational therapy; PT, physical therapy.

Chronic Arthritis

2

11

The Juvenile Idiopathic Arthritides

Ross E. Petty and James T. Cassidy

Chronic arthritis in childhood is a complex area of study and investigation, not least because of inconsistencies of definition and terminology. In order to avoid confusion in the discussions in this section of the book, it is necessary to understand this problem and its potential solutions.

The place of childhood arthritis in classifications has been problematic for decades. The heterogeneity of these diseases was discussed by Diamant-Berger[1] and Still,[2] who recognized that many children with chronic arthritis had a disease that was quite unlike adult rheumatoid arthritis; however, subsequent workers have differed as to whether childhood arthritis should be grouped with adult rheumatoid arthritis or with the spondyloarthropathies.[3]

In the 1970s, two sets of criteria were proposed to classify chronic arthritis in childhood independent of classifications used for adult patients: those developed and tested by a committee of the American College of Rheumatology (ACR)[4] and those of the European League Against Rheumatism (EULAR).[5] A third classification has been proposed by the Pediatric Task Force of the International League of Associations for Rheumatology (ILAR)[6,7] to overcome difficulties in the universal application of either the ACR or the EULAR criteria. These three classifications are compared in Table 11–1. All three classifications have many characteristics in common, as shown in Table 11–2.

COMPARISON OF THE ACR, EULAR, AND ILAR CRITERIA

ACR Criteria for Classification of Juvenile Rheumatoid Arthritis

The ACR criteria define arthritis, the age limit, and the duration of disease necessary for a diagnosis. They also recognize three types of onset (pauciarticular, polyarticular, and systemic). These criteria indicate the need to exclude other diseases, including the seronegative spondyloarthropathies (juvenile ankylosing spondylitis and related diseases). The requirement that age at onset of arthritis be less than 16 years is a criterion based more on practice patterns in the United States than on age-related biologic variation in disease. Furthermore, although persistent objective arthritis in one or more joints for 6 weeks is sufficient for diagnosis, duration of at least 6 months is required before the onset type can be certain (unless characteristic systemic features are present).

The type of onset of juvenile rheumatoid arthritis (JRA) is defined by a constellation of clinical signs present during the first 6 months of illness.[4] Pauciarticular JRA is defined as arthritis in four or fewer joints. Monarthritis (arthritis in a single joint) is a subtype of this onset group. Polyarticular JRA is defined as arthritis in five or more joints during the first 6 months of disease. In the determination of the onset type, each joint is counted separately, except for the joints of the cervical spine, carpus, and tarsus, each of which is counted as one joint.[4] Systemic-onset JRA is characterized by a daily (quotidian) fever spiking to greater than 39°C for at least 2 weeks in association with arthritis of one or more joints. Most children with systemic-onset JRA also have a characteristic rash and many have other evidence of extra-articular involvement such as lymphadenopathy, hepatosplenomegaly, and pericarditis.

The ACR criteria have been widely used and have been tested and revised.[8,9] They are easy to apply, but many children with diseases such as psoriatic arthritis or early ankylosing spondylitis would also meet the criteria for pauciarticular or polyarticular JRA. Herein lies one of the problems in applying the criteria: the necessity to exclude other diseases for which there are no validated diagnostic or classification criteria. Thus, valid exclusion of patients with juvenile ankylosing spondylitis and juvenile psoriatic arthritis, in the absence of compatible criteria for those disorders in childhood, makes strict application of the ACR criteria difficult if not impossible.

EULAR Criteria for Classification of Juvenile Chronic Arthritis

In 1977, a EULAR conference on the Care of Rheumatic Children in Oslo proposed the term *juvenile chronic*

Table 11–1

Comparison of Classifications of Childhood Arthritis

ACR[4]	EULAR[5]	ILAR[6, 7]
Juvenile rheumatoid arthritis	Juvenile chronic arthritis	Juvenile idiopathic arthritis
Systemic	Systemic	Systemic
Polyarticular	Polyarticular JCA	Polyarticular RF-negative
	Juvenile rheumatoid arthritis	Polyarticular RF-positive
Pauciarticular	Pauciarticular	Oligoarticular
		Persistent
		Extended
	Juvenile psoriatic arthritis	Psoriatic arthritis
	Juvenile ankylosing spondylitis	Enthesitis-related arthritis
		Other arthritis

ACR, American College of Rheumatology; EULAR, European League Against Rheumatism; ILAR, International League of Associations for Rheumatology; RF, rheumatoid factor.

arthritis (JCA) for the heterogeneous group of disorders that present as juvenile arthritis (see Table 11–2).[5] The onset types of JCA were distinguished as pauciarticular, polyarticular, and systemic (defined as they are by the ACR criteria). The diagnosis of JCA requires that the arthritis begin before 16 years of age, that it last for at least 3 months, and that other diseases be excluded: infectious arthritis, specific nonrheumatologic abnormalities such as familial Mediterranean fever, sarcoidosis, hematologic disorders and neoplastic disease, the other major connective tissue diseases, vasculitis, rheumatic fever, systemic lupus erythematosus, and the postinfectious arthropathies. Included within the term JCA are the types of arthritis defined as JRA by the ACR criteria, together with juvenile ankylosing spondylitis, psoriatic arthropathy, and arthropathies associated with inflammatory bowel disease.

In the EULAR classification, the term *juvenile rheumatoid arthritis* is reserved for children with arthritis and rheumatoid factor (RF) seropositivity, although no definition of RF seropositivity is provided. The only substantial differences between the ACR and the EULAR criteria are (1) the inclusion of juvenile ankylosing spondylitis, psoriatic arthritis, and the arthritis of inflammatory bowel disease and (2) the restriction of the term *juvenile rheumatoid arthritis*. For the student of pediatric rheumatology, however, the differences in nomenclature require care in interpreting the literature because the terms JRA and JCA are often incorrectly used interchangeably. This dilemma has been the subject of several publications.[10–13]

As with the ACR criteria, imprecision is introduced because of the absence of criteria for juvenile ankylosing spondylitis and psoriatic arthritis. The EULAR criteria have frequently been used with slight (but important) modifications in studies and publications, further contributing to imprecision.

ILAR Criteria for Classification of the Juvenile Idiopathic Arthritides

In 1993, the Pediatric Standing Committee of ILAR established a taskforce to develop a classification of the idiopathic arthritides of childhood. The ILAR classification[6] and its revision[7] were proposed by an international group of pediatric rheumatologists with the aim of achieving as much homogeneity within categories as possible in order to facilitate communication and clinical research (and thereby enhance patient care). It

Table 11–2

Characteristics of the ACR, EULAR, and ILAR Classifications of Childhood Arthritis

CHARACTERISTIC	ACR	EULAR	ILAR
Basis of classification	Clinical Onset and course	Clinical and serologic (RF) Onset only	Clinical and serologic (RF) Onset and course
Onset types	Three	Six	Seven
Course subtypes	Nine	None	Two
Age at onset of arthritis	≤16 yr	≤16 yr	≤16 yr
Duration of arthritis	≥6 wk	≥3 mo	≥6 wk
Includes "JAS"	No	Yes	Yes
Includes "JPsA"	No	Yes	Yes
Includes "IBD"	No	Yes	Yes
Includes reactive arthritis	No	No	No
Exclusion of other diseases	Yes	Yes	Yes

ACR, American College of Rheumatology; EULAR, European League Against Rheumatism; IBD, inflammatory bowel disease; ILAR, International League of Associations for Rheumatology; JAS, juvenile ankylosing spondylitis; JPsA, juvenile psoriatic arthritis; RF, rheumatoid factor.

was intended not that the classification would encompass all juvenile arthropathies but that there should be no overlap among the categories. Seven categories were proposed:

- Systemic arthritis
- Oligoarthritis (which may be either persistent or extended)
- Polyarthritis with negative results on testing for RF
- Polyarthritis with positive results on testing for RF
- Psoriatic arthritis
- Enthesitis-related arthritis
- Other arthritis (see Table 11–1)

The categories are further defined with exclusions that attempt to enhance homogeneity by identifying patients with a family history of psoriasis or a human leukocyte antigen B27 (HLA-B27)–related disorder.

Systemic arthritis refers to children with arthritis of any number of joints together with a documented typical quotidian fever of at least 2 weeks' duration and one or more of the following:

- Typical rash
- Generalized lymphadenopathy
- Enlargement of liver or spleen
- Serositis

The classification implies but does not stipulate that the presence of psoriasis or a family history of psoriasis excludes a patient from this category.

Oligoarthritis is defined as arthritis affecting four or fewer joints during the first 6 months of disease. Children with psoriasis or a family history of psoriasis or HLA-B27–associated disease are excluded from this category, as are those with RF or systemic arthritis and the HLA-B27–positive boy with onset of arthritis after 8 years of age. If the number of affected joints never exceeds four, the term *persistent oligoarthritis* is used. If, after the initial 6 months of disease, the total number of affected joints exceeds four, the term *extended oligoarthritis* is used.

Polyarthritis is defined as arthritis affecting more than four joints during the first 6 months of disease. Patients with systemic arthritis are excluded. *Polyarthritis–rheumatoid factor negative* is used to categorize polyarthritis when there is no detectable RF. *Polyarthritis–rheumatoid factor positive* is used when (1) five or more joints are affected during the first 6 months of disease and (2) RF is detected on at least two occasions at least 3 months apart with a standard method in a laboratory with an accepted standard.

Psoriatic arthritis is defined as arthritis and psoriasis or as arthritis and at least two of the following:

- Dactylitis
- Nail abnormalities (pitting or onycholysis)
- Family history of psoriasis confirmed by a dermatologist in at least one first-degree relative.

The presence of systemic arthritis or RF would exclude a patient from this category.

Enthesitis-related arthritis is defined as (1) arthritis and enthesitis or (2) arthritis *or* enthesitis plus two of the following:

- Sacroiliac joint tenderness, inflammatory spinal pain, or both
- HLA-B27
- Family history in first- or second-degree relative of medically confirmed HLA-B27–associated disease
- Acute anterior uveitis
- Onset of arthritis in a boy after the age of 8 years

Patients with psoriasis or a family history of psoriasis confirmed by a dermatologist in a first- or second-degree relative would exclude a patient from this category.

The category *other arthritis* includes conditions that, for whatever reason, either do not meet the criteria for any other category or meet the criteria for more than one category.

The ILAR classification has a number of advantages. These criteria were proposed by a group of experts who represented pediatric rheumatologic practice in the United States, the United Kingdom, France, Canada, Australia, South Africa, Argentina, Mexico, and China, thereby including all of the regional leagues of the ILAR. By avoiding both the terms *rheumatoid* and *chronic*, it was hoped that the ILAR classification criteria would meet with approval on both sides of the Atlantic, where these particular terms carry pejorative emotional as well as medical meanings. They overcome the problem of defining excluded diseases, a difficulty with both the ACR and the EULAR criteria, by including and clearly defining categories for psoriatic arthritis and enthesitis-related arthritis. The ILAR classification appears to have gained acceptance in some (but not all) parts of the world. These criteria still require validation, and in a process that is intended to be ongoing will almost certainly be modified as new evidence from HLA and other studies becomes available.

THE SPONDYLOARTHROPATHY CONCEPT

In pediatric rheumatology, the term *spondyloarthropathy* refers to four disorders that share the tendency to include arthritis and enthesitis and to be associated with the HLA antigen B27. They are

- Juvenile ankylosing spondylitis
- The axial arthropathies of juvenile psoriatic arthritis
- The arthritides of inflammatory bowel disease
- The reactive forms of arthritis (including Reiter's syndrome)

Although there are several reasons to consider these disorders as a group, there are also many distinguishing features among them, and within each of the four disorders there is considerable heterogeneity. The ILAR classification, therefore, has avoided the term *spondyloarthropathy* altogether and has recognized relatively discrete entities: enthesitis-related arthritis (which would include most if not all children now considered to have ankylosing spondylitis) and psoriatic arthritis. The reactive arthritides are not included in the ILAR classification because, for the most part, they have

Table 11–3

Comparative Frequencies of Types of Childhood Arthritis

DIAGNOSTIC CATEGORY	N	%
JRA* Systemic	578	11.2
Polyarticular	1206	23.3
Pauciarticular	2291	44.4
JPsA†	269	5.2
JAS	127	2.5
Undifferentiated spondyloarthropathy	535	10.4
Reiter's syndrome	50	<1
Arthritis with IBD	106	2.1
Total	5162	

IBD, inflammatory bowel disease; JAS, juvenile ankylosing spondylitis; JPsA, juvenile psoriatic arthritis; JRA, juvenile rheumatoid arthritis.
*Includes JRA (ACR criteria) and JCA (EULAR criteria).
†Vancouver criteria (14).
Data derived from references 15–17.

known causes and are not, therefore, truly idiopathic. Arthritis with inflammatory bowel disease is not separately categorized but is recognized as a descriptor in the enthesitis-related arthritis category.

CHRONIC ARTHRITIS IN CHILDHOOD

It has been difficult to ascertain the population frequencies (incidence, prevalence) of the various types of childhood arthritis because of the use of differing classification criteria and the relative rarity of each category. Three national registries have provided important information regarding relative frequencies of the various forms of childhood arthritis, although there is no certainty that comparable criteria are being consistently used. Data from the three registries are summarized in Table 11–3. JRA (ACR criteria) is most common, and within that category, pauciarticular disease is most frequent. The spondyloarthropathies are much less common, although the differences in frequency suggest that different criteria are being used to make this diagnosis[15–17] and that there are differences in HLA-B27 frequencies in various ethnic and geographic groups. Unfortunately, similar data are not available from much of the world.

TERMINOLOGY

In this edition, the terminology of the ACR criteria is retained for reasons that are both traditional and practical. Until such time as the ILAR classification (or a revision of the current criteria) is validated and widely used, it seemed prudent to use terminology with which most pediatric rheumatologists are familiar. From a practical standpoint, it is not possible to accurately reevaluate all of the literature about JRA or JCA in light of the ILAR classification. Because the literature has yet to embrace the ILAR criteria, writing this edition only in the context of the ILAR criteria would have invited confusion and misinterpretation of currently available data about childhood arthritis. Throughout the book, every attempt has been made to ensure that the terms JCA and JRA are used as they are defined and to reflect accurately the cited publications. In the future, the practice of pediatric rheumatology will undoubtedly reflect the demonstrated utility and validity of the proposed ILAR classification scheme, and we can hope that scientific advances in our knowledge of etiology and pathogenesis will significantly decrease the "idiopathic" categories.

References

1. Diamant-Berger M-S: Du Rhumatisme Noueux (Polyarthrite deformante) Chez les Enfants. Paris, Lecrosnier et Babe, 1891. (Reprinted by Editions Louis Parente, Paris, 1988.)
2. Still GF: On a form of chronic joint disease in children. Med Chirurg Trans 80: 47, 1897. (Reprinted in Am J Dis Child 132: 195, 1978.)
3. Wright V, Moll JM: Seronegative Polyarthritis. Amsterdam, North Holland, 1976.
4. Brewer EJ Jr, Bass J, Baum J, et al: Current proposed revision of JRA criteria. Arthritis Rheum 20(Suppl): 195, 1977.
5. European League Against Rheumatism: EULAR Bulletin No. 4: Nomenclature and Classification of Arthritis in Children. Basel, National Zeitung AG, 1977.
6. Fink CW, and the Task Force for Classification Criteria: Proposal for the development of classification criteria for idiopathic arthritides of childhood. J Rheumatol 22: 1566, 1995.
7. Petty RE, Southwood TR, Baum J, et al: Revision of the proposed classification criteria for juvenile idiopathic arthritis: Durban 1997. J Rheumatol 25: 1991, 1998.
8. Brewer EJ Jr, Bass JC, Cassidy JT, et al, for the JRA Criteria Subcommittee: Criteria for classification of juvenile rheumatoid arthritis. Bull Rheum Dis 25: 712, 1972.
9. Cassidy JT, Levinson JE, Bass JC, et al: A study of classification criteria for a diagnosis of juvenile rheumatoid arthritis. Arthritis Rheum 29: 274, 1986.
10. Childhood arthritis: the name game [Editorial]. Br J Rheumatol 32: 421, 1993.
11. Holt PJL: The classification of juvenile chronic arthritis. Clin Exp Rheumatol 8: 331, 1990.
12. Huppertz H-I: Viewpoint: time for change in pediatric rheumatology. Rheumatol Int 13: 37, 1993.
13. Cassidy JT: What's in a name? Nomenclature of juvenile arthritis. A North American view. J Rheumatol 20(Suppl 40): 4, 1993.
14. Southwood TR, Petty RE, Malleson PN, et al: Psoriatic arthritis in children. Arthritis Rheum 32: 1007, 1989.
15. Malleson PN, Fung MY, Rosenberg AM, for the Canadian Pediatric Rheumatology Association: The incidence of pediatric rheumatic diseases: results from the Canadian Pediatric Rheumatology Association Disease Registry. J Rheumatol 23: 1981, 1996.
16. Bowyer S, Roettcher P, and the Members of the Pediatric Rheumatology Database Research Group. Pediatric Rheumatology clinic populations in the US: results of a 3-year survey. J Rheumatol 23: 1968, 1996.
17. Symmons DPM, Jones M, Osborne J, et al: Pediatric rheumatology in the UK: data from the British Pediatric Rheumatology Group National Diagnostic Register. J Rheumatol 23: 1975, 1993.

12

Juvenile Rheumatoid Arthritis

James T. Cassidy and Ross E. Petty

Juvenile rheumatoid arthritis (JRA), one of the most common rheumatic diseases of childhood, is also one of the more frequent chronic illnesses of children and an important cause of short- and long-term disability. Although it has been customary to refer to JRA as one disease, it is almost certainly three or more diseases, each of which may have the same or different causes or a closely related series of host responses. It is characterized predominantly by idiopathic peripheral arthritis (Fig. 12–1) with an immunoinflammatory pathogenesis, possibly activated by contact with an external antigen or antigens. At least two of the principal phenotypes (oligoarthritis and polyarthritis) occur in children with specific, but dauntingly complex, immunogenetic predispositions.

HISTORICAL REVIEW

The idea that inflammatory polyarthritis occurred in childhood was first suggested in 1864 by Cornil,[1] who described a 29-year-old woman who had had chronic inflammatory arthritis since the age of 12. Diamant-Berger[2] reviewed the subject in 1890 and included 35 previously published cases and three of his own. He commented on the acute onset of disease, predominant involvement of large joints, a course characterized by exacerbations and remissions, frequent disturbances of normal growth, and a generally good prognosis.

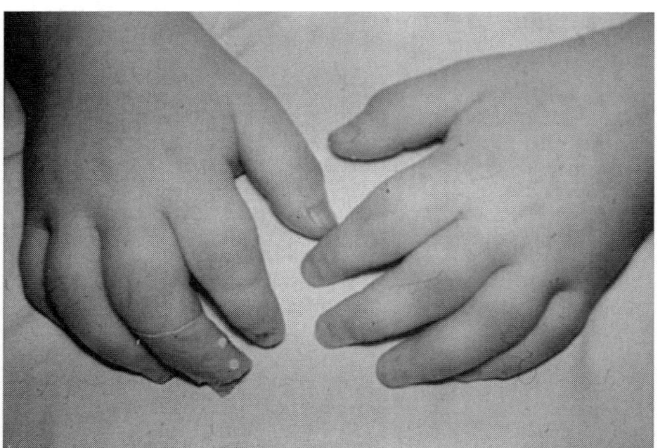

Figure 12–1. The joints of the wrists and hands of a 2½-year-old boy with systemic-onset juvenile rheumatoid arthritis (JRA) are swollen, warm, and painful. The proximal and distal interphalangeal joints are erythematous. There are flexion contractures of the fingers.

Still[3] presented the classic description of chronic childhood arthritis in 1897 while he was a medical registrar at the Hospital for Sick Children, Great Ormond Street, London. He pointed out that the disease almost always began before the second dentition, was more frequent in girls, and was usually of insidious onset. An acute onset of disease in 12 patients who had lymphadenopathy, splenomegaly, and fever was described in detail. Serositis characterized by pleuritis and pericarditis was common. The rash of JRA was not noted. Still observed that there was often no articular pain and that children exhibited a marked tendency to early contracture and muscle atrophy. The cervical spine was affected in the majority of cases, often during the early stages of the disease. On the basis of the disease's marked differences in children and adults, Still suggested that childhood arthritis might have a different etiology from rheumatoid arthritis or might include more than one disease. This classic description is an outstanding example of bedside observation.[4] Today, the acute systemic onset of JRA is still sometimes called *Still's disease*.

In 1901, Hirschsprung[5] confirmed Still's observations that a chronic articular disease was associated with lymphadenopathy and splenomegaly in young children; he also noted the occurrence of hepatomegaly. In 1939, Atkinson[6] published a review of 118 cases of Still's disease, 86 of whom were patients with severe arthritis, lymphadenopathy, and splenomegaly. In the excellent review of Edstrom,[7] only 3 of 65 children with chronic arthritis had marked lymphadenopathy and splenomegaly, and Bille[8] found no examples of "Still's disease" among his 65 patients with chronic childhood arthritis.

Few other large series were published before the 1950s. Those that are well documented include studies by Colver,[9] Holzmuller,[10] Coss and Boots,[11] Pickard,[12] and Lockie and Norcross.[13] Monographs on the subject were published by Wissler in 1942[14] and Francon in 1946.[15] French authors, such as Francon, have often used the term *syndrome de Chauffard-Still* for children with chronic arthritis, lymphadenopathy, and splenomegaly. Coss and Boots[11] thought that Still's disease was not an independent clinical entity and that the term *juvenile rheumatoid arthritis* should be used to refer to all cases of idiopathic inflammatory arthritis. Dawson[16] supported this view but stressed that significant differences between children and adults were evidenced by the severity and frequency of the systemic symptoms and by interference with normal growth and development. Many early authors stressed that JRA could begin as a type of monarthritis that most frequently affected the knee and could persist in one joint for the duration of the illness or for several years before other joints were involved.[7, 8, 10, 12]

Until Colver published the first follow-up examinations of JRA in 1937,[9] the prognosis in this disease was considered to be poor.[17, 18] Extended periods of observation of patients with onset in childhood led some early authors to conclude that severe destruction of cartilage occurred in many children and that ankylosis would supervene in most.[19, 20] Subsequent studies showed that, although the mortality rate was in the range of 7 to 9 percent,[12, 13] recovery was complete in the majority of children.[7, 12, 13] In Edstrom's study,[7] 87 percent of patients seen early in the course of their disease experienced good functional recovery; even 65 percent of those reviewed after the first or second year of disease had a good prognosis. However, only 39 percent of children seen later than 2 years after onset returned to normal function. A long, uninterrupted period of active disease was significantly associated with a poor prognosis; only 6 percent of children whose disease became quiescent within the first 4 years developed severe disability.

Sury identified 151 patients from 1920 to 1948 who had a chronic form of arthritis with onset before the age of 15 years.[21] Thirty-nine percent of referred patients and 19 percent of the children from Copenhagen were severely disabled. The peak age at onset in 100 girls was between 2 and 4 years of age. In 8 of 51 boys, onset was during the first year of life. Of 41 patients whose disease began with monarthritis, 23 had persistent disease in that one joint for at least the first year. On necropsy, 12 children had verrucous endocarditis.

DEFINITION AND CLASSIFICATION

The classification criteria and terminology of the American College of Rheumatology (ACR)[22] are retained in this chapter for purposes of clarity and consistency. Although new criteria for the idiopathic arthritides of childhood have recently been proposed,[23, 23a, 23b] almost all of the published data are based on either the European League Against Rheumatism (EULAR)[24] or the ACR[22] criteria. There is no worldwide agreement on the use of diagnostic terms for JRA or on classification.[25, 26] The reader is referred to Chapter 11 for a discussion and comparison of criteria.[27–31] In any case, early diagnosis of JRA is facilitated by recognition of the three major types of presentation: oligoarthritis (60 percent), polyarthritis (30 percent), and systemic disease (10 percent) (Table 12–1). These are defined by a constellation of clinical signs and symptoms during the first 6 months of illness.[22–24, 32]

EPIDEMIOLOGY

JRA is not a rare disease, but the true frequency of its occurrence is not known (see Chapter 1). In historical reviews, 2.7 to 5.2 percent of all patients with rheumatoid arthritis (RA) experienced onset before 15 years of age.[33–35] JRA has been described in all races and geographic areas, although its incidence and prevalence vary considerably throughout the world,[36, 37] which partly reflects the ethnicity and environment of the population under study.[37a, 37b] The immunogenetic susceptibility to JRA is most obvious in children who have an oligoarticular onset, especially young girls (<6 years of age). The possibility of interaction of environmental triggers is most clearly evident in systemic-onset JRA, with studies supporting seasonal variation in incidence.[38–40, 40a]

Oen and Cheang[36] published a meticulous review of the epidemiology of childhood arthritis. Considered as confounding variables were the diagnostic criteria employed, disease exclusions, source of the data (population, clinic, practitioner, health survey), geographic origin, race, and years of observation. No significant differences were found for diagnostic criteria or duration of the study. However, prevalence was higher for population-based studies and for data from North America, whereas clinic-based studies were more homogeneous in results.

Incidence

The incidence of JRA based on the ACR criteria[22] has varied from 2 to 20 per 100,000 population (Table 12–2).[35–37, 41–60] A clinic survey in the state of Michigan from 1960 to 1970 found a minimal incidence of 9.2 per 100,000 children at risk per year.[42] Estimates in Finland range from 6 to 8 per 100,000 in Laaksonen's study[35] to 18.2 per 100,000 (95 percent confidence interval [CI], 10.8 to 28.7) in the study of Kunnamo and colleagues.[45] In Norway,[57] the incidence was 22.6 per 100,000 (oligoarticular disease, 11.8; and systemic onset, 0.8). However, 42 percent of these children were human leukocyte antigen (HLA)-B27 positive. Data from the Mayo

Table 12–1

Characteristics of JRA by Type of Onset

	POLYARTHRITIS	OLIGOARTHRITIS (PAUCIARTICULAR DISEASE)	SYSTEMIC DISEASE
Frequency of cases	30%	60%	10%
Number of joints involved	≥5	≤4	Variable
Age at onset	Throughout childhood; peak at 1–3 yr	Early childhood; peak at 1–2 yr	Throughout childhood; no peak
Sex ratio (F:M)	3:1	5:1	1:1
Systemic involvement	Moderate involvement	Not present	Prominent
Occurrence of chronic uveitis	5%	20%	Rare
Frequency of seropositivity			
Rheumatoid factors	10% (increases with age)	Rare	Rare
Antinuclear antibodies	40–50%	75–85%*	10%
Prognosis	Guarded to moderately good	Excellent except for eyesight	Moderate to poor

*In girls with uveitis.

Table 12–2

Studies of Incidence and Prevalence of Chronic Childhood Arthritis

AUTHORS	REF.	ORIGIN	YEAR	DIAGNOSTIC CRITERIA	INCIDENCE (100,000/yr)	PREVALENCE (per 100,000)
Group 1						
Towner et al.	43	USA	1983	EULAR, ACR	10.8–13.9	83.7–113.4
Peterson et al.	54	USA	1996	ACR	11.7	86.1–94
Mielants et al.	48	Belgium	1993	EULAR	—	167
Gare	37	Sweden	1994	EULAR	10.9	86.3
Manners et al.	51	Australia	1996	EULAR	—	400
Kaipiainsen-Sepparnen et al.	52	Finland	1996	ACR	14	—
Ozen et al.	56	Turkey	1998	EULAR	—	64
Kiessling et al.	59	Germany	1998	EULAR	3.5	20
Group II						
Gewanter et al.	44	USA	1983	ACR	—	16–43
Kunnamo et al.	45	Finland	1986	ACR	18.2	—
Prieur et al.	46	France	1987	EULAR	1.3–1.9	8–10
Arguedas et al.	58	Costa Rica	1998	EULAR	6.8	31.4
Group III						
Laaksonen	35	Finland	1966	English	6–8	75–100
Bywaters	41	UK	1968	English	—	60–70
Sullivan et al.	42	USA	1975	ACR	9.2	65
Rosenberg et al.	47	Canada	1990	ACR	5–8	39.7
Denardo et al.	49	USA	1994	ACR	4	—
Oen et al.	40	Canada	1995	ACR	5	32
Malleson et al.	50	Canada	1996	ACR	8	40
Symmonds et al.	53	UK	1996	EULAR	10	—
Fujikowa et al.	55	Japan	1997	ACR	0.83	—
Moe et al.	57	Norway	1998	EULAR	22.6	148.1

ACR, American College of Rheumatology; EULAR, European League Against Rheumatism.
Group I: Predominantly population-based; Group II: Surveys of medical practitioners; Group III: Clinic-based.

Clinic in Minnesota reported an incidence of 13.9 per 100,000 (95 percent CI, 9.9 to 18.8).[43] A more recent study from the same center indicated that the frequency of JRA has been decreasing in recent decades from 15 per 100,000 for 1960 to 1969 to 7.8 per 100,000 for 1980 to 1993,[54] Seasonal variation was also apparent in this investigation,[54] in Sweden[37] and in Manitoba.[39, 40] This trend, however, was not confirmed in a larger study from Canada.[39]

Prevalence

Prevalence based on the ACR criteria[22] has varied from 16 to 150 per 100,000 (see Table 12–2).[36, 60] Bywaters[41] found the prevalence of "Still's disease" in English school children to be approximately 65 per 100,000. In the Tecumseh Community Health Survey of 2000 children between 6 and 15 years of age,[61] 10 percent complained of joint pain, just under 10 percent related a history of previous joint swelling, and 5 percent had morning stiffness, although only 2 children were found to have JRA on examination, a prevalence close to that estimated by Bywaters.[41] The 10-year weighted cumulative prevalence in Michigan was 46 for girls and 19 for boys.[42] The prevalence was 86.3 per 100,000 in the Swedish study[37, 62] and 83.7 to 113.4 per 100,000 (95 percent CI, 69.1 to 196.3) in Minnesota.[43] In Norway,[57] the point prevalence was 148.1 per 100,000. As a number of studies suggest, these figures undoubtedly represent minima.[46, 62] The survey by Manners and associates[51] in Australia of 12-year-old school children reported a prevalence of 400 per 100,000 based on an examination of each child included in the survey. Clearly, rheumatic symptoms, past or present, are not uncommon in children and far exceed the estimated prevalence of "JRA" when objective criteria are used and an examination is performed by an experienced pediatric rheumatologist. Two national health surveys in the United States and one in Canada estimated the prevalence of JRA at 220,[63] 121,[64] and 1300[65] per 100,000 at risk.

Age at Onset

JRA is arbitrarily defined as arthritis beginning before the age of 16 years.[22, 66, 67] Although onset before 6 months of age is distinctly unusual, the age at onset is often quite young, with the highest frequency occurring between 1 and 3 years of age.[7, 11, 13, 21, 35, 42, 68–72] This age distribution is most evident in girls with oligoarthritis, and less so in those with polyarticular onset. Systemic onset has no increased frequency at any particular age.

The distribution of ages at onset of arthritis in 300 children in whom the definition of JRA conformed to that of the ACR is shown in Figure 12–2.[42] The peak age at onset was between 1 and 3 years of age for the total group and for girls, but for boys this relationship was much less impressive. As shown in Figures 12–3, 12–4, and 12–5,[42] the early peak was largely accounted for by girls with oligoarticular and polyarticular

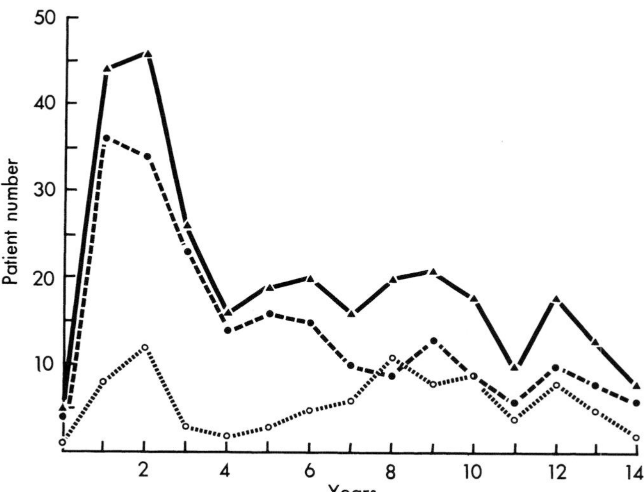

Figure 12–2. Age at onset of JRA in 300 children: total group (-▲-), girls (-●-), and boys (-○-). For the total group and for girls, a large peak is observed at 1 to 2 years. A bimodal distribution with peaks at 2 years and at 8 to 10 years suggests heterogeneity of arthritis in boys. (From Sullivan DB, Cassidy JT, Petty RE: Pathogenic implications of age of onset in juvenile rheumatoid arthritis. Arthritis Rheum 18: 251, 1975.)

JRA. Figure 12–4 shows a second, somewhat broader peak centered at 9 years of age. The contributions of boys and girls to this peak were approximately equal. The relatively high proportion of boys in the second peak raised the question of whether this group represented in part another disease, such as occult juvenile ankylosing spondylitis (JAS).[73] Whatever the correct interpretation, the heterogeneity in distribution of age at onset of different types of JRA points to the probability that this disorder includes a number of fairly distinct entities.

Sex Ratio

Twice as many girls as boys develop JRA.[42, 74] Girls with an oligoarticular onset outnumber boys by a ratio

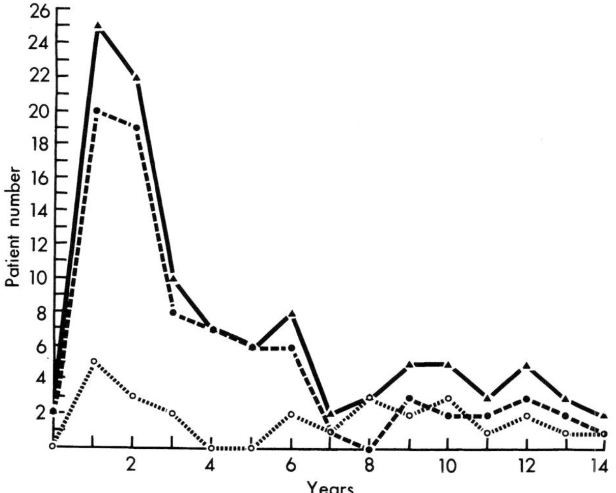

Figure 12–3. Age at onset of oligoarticular JRA: total group (-▲-), girls (-●-), boys (-○-). (From Sullivan DB, Cassidy JT, Petty RE: Pathogenic implications of age of onset in juvenile rheumatoid arthritis. Arthritis Rheum 18: 251, 1975.)

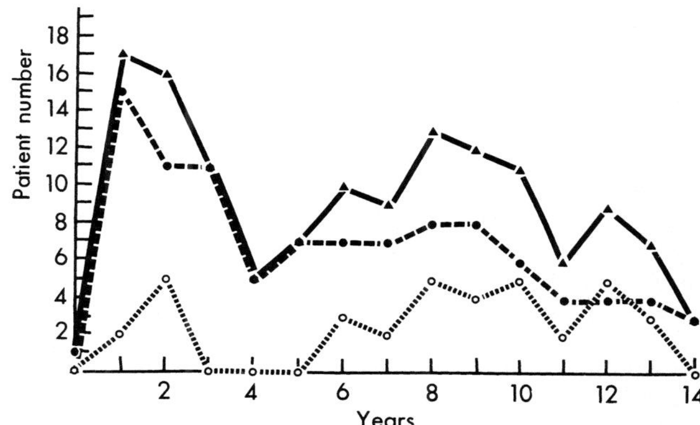

Figure 12–4. Age at onset of polyarticular JRA: total group (-▲-), girls (-●-), boys (-○-). (From Sullivan DB, Cassidy JT, Petty RE: Pathogenic implications of age of onset in juvenile rheumatoid arthritis. Arthritis Rheum 18: 251, 1975.)

of 3:1. In children with uveitis, the ratio of girls to boys is even higher—5:1 to 6.6:1.[75–77] Among children with polyarticular onset, girls outnumber boys in a ratio of 2.8:1. In striking contrast, systemic onset occurs with equal frequency in boys and girls. These differences in sex ratios suggest either that there are three (or more) different diseases included under the designation of JRA or that disease expression is modified by sex chromosome–determined factors.

Geographic and Racial Distribution

The incidence and prevalence data outlined previously were derived primarily from North American or European white populations. There are few comparable data for children of other geographic or racial groups.[78–80] Nonetheless, suggestions of racial disparity in frequency exist.[36, 81, 82] The observations by Hanson and colleagues,[83] and our own, suggest that in North America there are proportionately fewer black than white children with JRA. The impression that this discrepancy may be a reflection of referral differences is negated in part by the higher frequency of black children with systemic lupus erythematosus (SLE) and juvenile dermatomyositis in relation to white children with SLE and juvenile dermatomyositis in the same clinics. Some reports suggest that JRA and RA are less frequent in African than in European populations; in Nigerian Africans, however, the proportion of all pa-

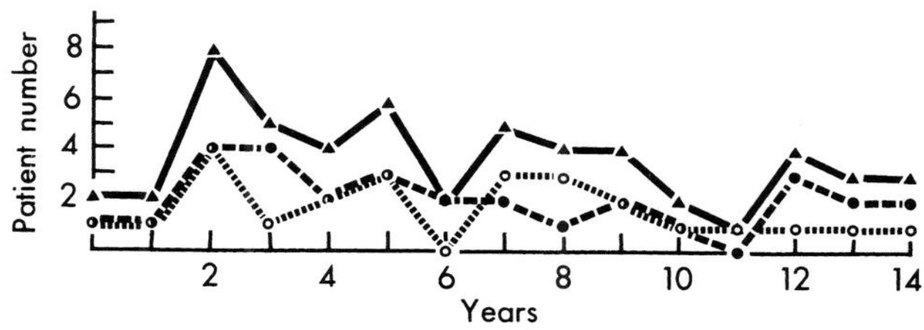

Figure 12–5. Age at onset of systemic JRA: total group (-▲-), girls (-●-), boys (-○-). (From Sullivan DB, Cassidy JT, Petty RE: Pathogenic implications of age of onset in juvenile rheumatoid arthritis. Arthritis Rheum 18: 251, 1975.)

tients with onset of chronic inflammatory arthritis in childhood may be somewhat higher.[78]

Oligoarticular onset is the least frequent type encountered in Africa and in black children in North America. JRA may be less common in North Americans of Chinese ancestry than in North American whites.[79] An analysis of white and North American aboriginal children in the same rheumatology clinic in Canada suggests that, although JRA occurs in aboriginal children, its frequency is not higher than that for the white population, whereas HLA-B27–associated arthritis is appreciably more frequent in the aboriginal group.[84] However, Oen and colleagues[85] noted a high yearly incidence of JRA (23.6 per 100,000), in addition to a high frequency of seronegative spondyloarthropathies, in Inuit children of northern Canada. The data reported by Boyer and associates[86] suggest that the incidence of rheumatoid factor (RF)-seropositive polyarthritis is increased in southeast Alaskan Indian children. The numbers of patients in these studies are small, however, and conclusions with respect to actual incidence and prevalence of chronic arthritis in aboriginal North American children are tentative.

ETIOLOGY AND PATHOGENESIS

As indicated previously, JRA is not a single disease. These children represent a heterogeneity of phenotypes with at least three primary modes of onset. Two observations are paramount in considering the pathogenesis and etiology of JRA.[87] First, it is an *autoimmune disease*. T-cell abnormalities and the pathologic characteristics of the chronic synovitis suggest a possible cell-mediated pathogenesis.[87, 88] Multiple autoantibodies, immune complexes, and complement activation indicate potential humoral abnormalities. Second, JRA is most assuredly a *complex genetic trait* (oligogenic or polygenic).[89] The various forms of JRA display nonmendelian inheritance, and interactions of multiple genes are likely important in these diseases. Many of the putative genetic predispositions are within the major histocompatibility complex (MHC) region on chromosome 6; however, non-MHC genes undoubtedly play a role in some of the syndromes.

Although there are undoubtedly genetic predispositions, and putative environmental triggers, any theory of pathogenesis of JRA must account for a number of factors, including the clinical heterogeneity of the disease; the higher prevalence in girls, especially for oligoarticular disease with uveitis; the rather narrow peak ages at onset, especially for oligoarthritis; the absence of a peak age at onset for systemic disease; and the widespread immunologic perturbations. There may be multiple etiologic events, or JRA may result from a single pathogenic vector with diverse clinical patterns evolving from interactions with the host. It may be postulated that an infectious agent, infecting a child at a point of vulnerability—defined by age, intercurrent illness, prior antigenic experience, immunologic maturity, or immunogenetic predisposition—results in a permanent infection, which emerges as a clinical disorder. It is necessary to consider differing sets of conditions for development of each onset type and course subtype. Possible causes include aberrant immunologic regulation, psychological stress, trauma, hormonal abnormalities, and infection.

Immunologic Factors

A number of observations contribute to the hypothesis that the immune system is intimately involved in the pathogenesis of JRA. First, there is abundant evidence of altered immunity, abnormal immunoregulation, and cytokine production.[87, 90–92, 92a–92c] Second, there is an association between specific immunodeficiencies and rheumatic diseases, including JRA (see Chapter 35). Third, there is a close relationship between immune reactivity and inflammation, the hallmark of arthritis (see Chapter 5). Whether JRA is principally an immunogenetically determined disorder or an antigen-driven immunologic response is uncertain. One study alleged that breast feeding has a protective effect on the development of JRA,[93] especially in oligoarticular disease; however, a strong relationship was not confirmed in another investigation.[94]

Immune Complexes

Complement activation and consumption probably play a role in perpetuation of the inflammatory reaction and in determining specificity of response.[95, 96] Levels of circulating immune complexes (ICs) in JRA parallel activity of the disease and systemic features.[88, 97, 98, 98a] The pro-inflammatory activity of circulating ICs appears to be related to their size.[99] Complement activation is also reflected in levels of fragment Bb of the alternative pathway and C4d, which correlate with circulating ICs and clinical activity of the disease.[100, 100a] The circulating complexes consistently contain immunoglobulin (Ig) M RFs[101–103] even though most of these children are seronegative by conventional RF testing. They are positive, however, for hidden RFs detected by acid gel filtration of their sera.[104, 105] Levels of these tightly bound RFs correlate with activity of the disease, particularly in children with polyarthritis.[106] The pro-inflammatory potential of such ICs may be enhanced because of their resistance to normal complement-mediated degradation because of this interaction with RFs.[107–109] The ICs identified in synovial fluid also vary in size, composition, ability to activate complement, and potential for induction of cytokine secretion.[88, 99, 110]

T Lymphocytes

Recent speculations on the pathogenesis of JRA have centered on the possibility that there is a disordered T_H1/T_H2 interaction (see Chapters 4 and 5).[111, 112, 112a] T_H1 cells, or inflammatory CD4+ T cells, predominantly secrete interleukin-2 (IL-2), IL-3, interferon-γ (IFN-γ), granulocyte colony-stimulating factor (GM-CSF), tumor necrosis factor α (TNF-α), and TNF-β, and activate macrophages. T_H2 cells secrete IL-3, IL-4, IL-5, IL-6, and IL-10, GM-CSF and TNF-α, which effect activation and differentiation of B cells. Murray and colleagues[113] studied synovial T-cell infiltrates in 17 children (12 polyarticular, 5 oligoarticular) and found that the level of T-cell activation (CD3+ IL-2R+) was significantly higher in oligoarthritis (especially for CD8 cells) and that the CD4:CD8 ratio was lower. In a subsequent report,[114] the immunohistologic patterns of expression of synovial T_H1 and T_H2 cells was studied and increased secretion of IL-4 was noted. Ozen and colleagues[56] observed a marked T_H1 response in synovial fluid mononuclear cells in four of five children with JRA by immunofluorescent identification of intracellular cytokines by flow cytometric analysis (increased IFN-γ in addition to IL-4). Co-culture with heat-shock protein (HSP) 60 produced only a slight increase in IFN-γ products in the one synovial fluid sample tested.

Gattorno and colleagues[115] investigated the pattern of cytokine production in T-cell clones from synovial fluid mononuclear cells in five children with oligoarthritis. Large amounts of IFN-γ were produced with a predominant T_H/T_H0 pattern. Raziuddin and coworkers found a mixed T_H-cell response in stimulated peripheral blood mononuclear cells in systemic-onset disease.[116] Synovial fluid T cells appear to be similar in type and responsiveness to those in peripheral blood in some studies,[117, 118] but in others CD4+ T cells were decreased in synovial fluid but increased in synovial tissue.[119, 120] In most instances, T cells from the synovial fluid or membrane had increased expression of activation markers.[117, 118, 121–123, 123a]

Peripheral Blood Mononuclear Cells

The results of studies of T-lymphocyte phenotypes in the peripheral blood have been inconsistent and are difficult to interpret because of absence or inadequacy of control data. In general, studies of T-cell responses to mitogens such as phytohemagglutinin or concanavalin A indicate that proliferation is normal in children with inactive or oligoarticular disease but diminished in those with active disease.[124–127] Aberrations in suppressor T-lymphocyte function may be instrumental in the immunopathogenesis of JRA and permit overproduction of autoantibodies.[119, 124, 128–134] Some studies of peripheral blood lymphocytes have shown normal ratios of CD4 (helper/inducer) to CD8 (suppressor/cytotoxic) T cells.[118, 135] However, Morimoto and coworkers[124] found decreased CD4 and increased CD8 cells, an apparent result of antibody to CD4+ T cells that was present in the sera of patients with active JRA. Others have also found increased CD8+ T cells in children with systemic- and polyarticular-onset JRA,[136, 136a] whereas others noted decreased CD8+ T cells, particularly in systemic-onset disease.[137, 138] In contrast, B-cell numbers are increased in these children.[134, 135] Similar discrepancies have been observed in the frequencies of markers of T-cell activation: Tac or IL-2 receptor expression was found to be normal,[118, 139] HLA-DR antigens normal[139, 140] or increased,[135] and very-late-activation antigen (VLA)-1 increased only in children with active disease.[139] Although many of these studies suggest a global T-cell regulatory defect, their results may have been influenced by therapy. Massa and colleagues[141] found that treatment with methotrexate led to a decrease in CD4−, CD8− and γ/δ T-cell numbers in children with JRA.

Cytokine Profiles

Investigations of the cytokine network in children with JRA are often contradictory and incomplete, making interpretation of pathogenic mechanisms difficult. Differing results are undoubtedly related to the assay methods employed, stage and activity of the disease, treatment, identification of onset type and course subtype, and whether plasma, serum, or synovial fluid was analyzed. Therefore, only the more definitive and positive results are summarized in this section. Three excellent reviews have been published (see also Chapter 5).[92, 142, 143]

Systemic-Onset Disease. Abnormal expression of the three primary inflammatory cytokines (IL-6, IL-1, and TNF-α) is characteristic of this onset type. De Benedetti and Martini[142] have questioned whether systemic JRA is an IL-6–mediated disease. Evidence to support that hypothesis is imposing. IL-6 is markedly elevated in concentration in the vascular compartment[144–148] and in synovial fluid.[144–146] Its level is increased just before each febrile spike and correlates with the systemic activity of the disease, arthritis, and increase in acute-phase reactants.[144, 146, 149] The abnormalities in regulation of IL-6 are also putatively responsible for the impoverishment of linear growth, thrombocytosis, and microcytic anemia.[144–146, 150, 151] Complexes of IL-6 with its soluble receptor, sIL-6R, prolong the activity of the cytokine and thereby potentiate its effects.[146, 150] De Benedetti and colleagues[92, 152] have suggested that polymorphism of the IL-6 gene may affect IL-6 gene expression and contribute to cytokine dysregulation. IL-6 likely induces an increase in the concentration of IL-1Ra, which is also coincident with the febrile peak.[146–149] Soluble IL-2R is increased in concentration; its level correlates with the activity of the disease.[148, 153–155] IL-7 levels are also increased.[156] Finally, there are marked increases in sTNFαRp55 in the vascular compartment and lesser elevations of sTNFαRp75 in the blood and synovial fluid.[148]

Polyarthritis. Studies in polyarticular children have not always distinguished between RF-seronegative and RF-seropositive disease. In general, sIL-2R is moderately increased in the vascular compartment[148, 150, 153–155] and synovial fluid,[155] and its level correlates with the activity of the arthritis. IL-1α is increased in the blood[155] and IL-1β in the synovial fluid.[155] The soluble TNFαRp55 is increased in both,[148, 157] but the ratio of sTNF/TNF-α may be low.[157a]

Oligoarthritis. The cytokine pattern in children with oligoarticular disease of early onset is similar to that in polyarthritis. Soluble IL-2R is increased in the blood, and its level correlates with activity of the clinical disease.[148, 153] IL-1β is increased in the blood, along with TNF-α.[148] The soluble TNFαRp55 is also increased in the blood.[148]

T-Cell Receptor Polymorphism

Abnormalities of assembly and interactions of the trimolecular complex (consisting of putative antigen and genes controlling selection of T-cell receptor [TCR] peptide chains and HLA specificities) are of increasing importance in considering the immunopathogenesis of JRA.[158] Oligoclonal selection of the TCR beta chain has been demonstrated in JRA, a finding that is more characteristic of synovial fluid and tissues than of peripheral blood.[159, 160] Maksymowych and associates[161] confirmed a high frequency of the TCR allele TCR-Vβ6.1 among HLA-DQA*0101-positive children. A subsequent report identified this TCR null allele as a risk factor for a polyarticular course in children with early-onset oligoarticular disease positive for DQA1*0101.[162] This association was not confirmed in a study from Norway,[163] nor did Nepom and coworkers[164] identify TCR polymorphism in their studies of oligoarticular-onset JRA. In the report of Thompson and colleagues,[160] TCR-Vβ8 was clonally expanded in children with polyarticular disease and TCR-Vβ20 was increased in those with oligoarthritis.

Autoantibodies

B-lymphocyte numbers are normal to increased in children with JRA, depending on onset type, but their mitogen responsiveness may be impaired.[135, 165] Immunoglobulin levels tend be high,[166] at least partly reflecting the nonspecific inflammatory response. Antibody levels to specific viruses are also increased.[167] Antibody responses to new T-cell–dependent antigens such as bacteriophage OX 174 may be defective.[168]

Autoantibodies to nuclear, immunoglobulin, and other antigens are common in sera of children with JRA.[169] Among these autoimmune phenomena are antibodies to histones[170–177]; antineutrophil cytoplasmic antibodies[178, 179, 179a]; antiperinuclear, antikeratin, and anti-RA 33 antibodies[180, 180a]; and anticardiolipin antibodies.[174, 181, 181a] Antibodies to high-mobility group (HMG) proteins are increased in JRA to a defined epitope on HMG-17, and in oligoarticular disease to an HMG-2 protein.[182, 182a] Autoantibodies to types I, II, and IV collagen have been demonstrated in some studies.[183, 184] Immunity to cartilage link protein has been found.[185] IgA antigliadin antibodies have been described.[186] These autoantibodies may more likely be epiphenomena than direct participants in pathogenesis, except for complications such as vasculitis, in which ICs participate in vascular inflammation.

Psychological Factors

It is well documented that psychological stress is particularly common in families of children with JRA.[187, 188] It has not been possible, however, to be certain whether the psychosocial disturbances preceded or followed the development of arthritis. Current research indicates that psychological factors inherent in the family and child affect their adaptation to chronic illness but are unlikely to have played any role in the causation of the disease. Studies from The Netherlands demonstrate that JRA is associated with dysregulation of the autonomic nervous system, which leads to lack of an appropriate response of the child's immune system to stimuli.[189, 190]

Physical Trauma

JRA has been reported by parents to follow minor physical trauma to an extremity. Such trauma may serve as a localizing factor, or it may simply call attention to an already inflamed and weakened joint. Benign hypermobility and the rare syndrome of congenital insensitivity to pain are both associated with trauma and may predispose to joint inflammation. The fact that certain joints (e.g., the knee in oligoarticular JRA) are most frequently affected could be interpreted to suggest that trauma associated with weight bearing in the young child is a factor in initiating chronic inflammation. There are many contradictions to these suggestions, however, and the precise role of trauma remains unknown.

Hormonal Factors

In a study by Khalkhali-Ellis and colleagues,[191] androgen levels in children with JRA and in aged-matched controls were similar for progesterone and dehydroepiandrosterone (DHEA). In prepubertal JRA patients, 17-beta estradiol was undetectable, however, and concentration of the sulfated conjugate of DHEA was significantly less than in controls. Testosterone was lower in the synovial fluid than in matched serum; patients with the lowest synovial fluid levels were those with disease of the longest duration. Thus, the low androgen levels in children with JRA may contribute to pathogenesis because androgens exert a protective effect against cartilage degradation.[192]

A number of studies have identified an interesting association between elevated serum prolactin levels and JRA as well as SLE (see Chapter 18). Levels were elevated in children with JRA and were associated with antinuclear antigen (ANA) seropositivity.[193] Modest hyperprolactinemia was also identified in prepubertal girls who were ANA-seropositive and had oligoarthritis.[194, 194a] The prolactin concentration correlated with levels of IL-6 and with a chronic course of the disease.

Infection

That infections can cause arthritis in children is not in doubt. Arthritis following viral infections is probably common, although it is usually self-limited.[195] The possible role of infection in causing JRA[196] is supported by the finding that chronic arthritis is especially common in children who have impaired defense mechanisms and overt forms of immunodeficiency such as selective IgA deficiency, hypogammaglobulinemia, or deficiency of the C2 complement component (see Chapter 35).

There is considerable evidence that viral infections do not cause just transient arthritis but are associated with human autoimmune disease.[197] Persistent rubella virus infection has been demonstrated in children with JRA.[198, 199] In the study by Chantler and coworkers,[198] virus was isolated from peripheral blood or synovial fluid mononuclear cells in 0 of 16 controls and in 7 of 19 children with chronic rheumatic diseases (i.e., from 2 of 2 with polyarticular-, 2 of 6 with oligoarticular-, and 1 of 5 with systemic-onset JRA, and from 2 of 6 with JAS). Although this study provided the strongest support for an etiologic relationship between rubella virus and chronic childhood arthritis, it has not been confirmed in other centers.[200, 201]

Postvaccination arthritis has been described after measles-mumps-rubella (MMR) vaccination, and chronic arthropathy has been documented in one study (predominantly in females[202]) but not in another.[201] HLA-DR associations with rubella vaccine arthritis have been demonstrated.[203] Arthritis has developed after routine vaccinations,[203a] and RA has resulted following hepatitis B vaccination.[203b, 203c] Arthritis in children has also been linked to perinatal infection with the influenza virus A2H2N2.[204, 205] This unique epidemiologic study demonstrated the possibility of delayed expression of disease resulting from a presumed intrauterine or neonatal viral infection, not unlike the long-term effects that have been documented with intrauterine rubella infection. A somewhat tenuous link between chronic arthritis and parvovirus B19 has also been noted.[206–208] Remission following viral infections has been described.[208a, 208b]

Mycoplasma, β-hemolytic streptococcus, and enteric organisms (*Salmonella, Shigella, Campylobacter,* and *Yersinia*) are all known to cause reactive arthritis (see Chapter 33), but not JRA. The role (if any) of chlamydial infection has been raised.[209] The observation that children with oligoarticular arthritis and uveitis frequently have antibodies to bacterial peptidoglycan supports the possibility of a causative role for bacterial infection in this disease.[210] The cyclical pattern of incidence of JRA documented from 1979 to 1992 in Manitoba by Oen and colleagues[40] correlated with the occurrence of infections to *Mycoplasma pneumoniae*. Humoral and cellular immune responses to highly conserved bacterial HSPs are present in children with JRA.[211–217] HSPs have been demonstrated in the serum and synovial fluid of children with JRA.[217–219] Van Eden and colleagues[220] postulated that reactive T cells are part of the normal immune repertoire for TCR V-gene products; self-HSPs and bacterial HSPs may trigger this response.[221–223] In 13 of 15 children with oligoarthritis, T-lymphocyte proliferative responses to HSP 60 were detected an average of 12 weeks before remission of the inflammatory disease.[217, 218] These investigators hypothesized that induction of tolerance to specific T-cell epitopes of HSP 60 by nasal administration may be a promising route of immunotherapy for childhood arthritis.[224] Albani and associates[216, 225] demonstrated immune responses to the dnaJ HSP from *Escherichia coli,* especially in children with polyarticular disease. This protein has five amino acids that are homologous with those in the binding groove of DRB1 that in itself is increased in frequency in children with polyarticular JRA. Thus, molecular mimicry may play a role in the pathogenesis of JRA.[226–228]

GENETIC BACKGROUND

Familial Juvenile Rheumatoid Arthritis

Familial JRA is rare, and multigeneration cases are seldom recognized. Although JRA rarely occurs in affected siblings, data on HLA segregation underscore a hereditary basis to the immunopathogenesis of the disease.[229, 230] Within any one family, JRA tends to have the same type of onset, even having the same complication of uveitis.[231] An examination of time of onset of arthritis in families in which two or more children were affected indicated that the interval between onset of arthritis in each pair of siblings varied from 7 months to 11 years. In no instance was disease onset simultaneous, although in most cases the ages at onset were similar.

The development of JRA in twins has been extensively studied.[230, 232–235] A concordance rate of 44 percent has been reported in identical twins and a rate of 4 percent in dizygotic twins.[236] Ansell and colleagues[234, 237] indicated that two of five pairs of identical twins were concordant for arthritis; in one pair of twin boys, however, diagnosis of ankylosing spondylitis was made later. Six nonidentical twins were discordant for disease. Studies by Clemens and associates[238, 239] in over 3000 children with juvenile chronic arthritis (JCA) documented a remarkable concordance between siblings for onset of disease, clinical manifestations, and disease course (Table 12–3). Nine of 11 sibling pairs who were concordant for type of onset shared two DR antigens; the other two pairs shared one HLA-DR antigen.[239] A multicenter study reconfirmed these findings in 71 sibling pairs, 94 percent of whom were white, in which both (or in three families, three siblings) had JRA.[230] The mean interval between onset of disease in the siblings was 4.4 years (S.D., 4.2). More than three quarters were concordant for onset type, and 79 percent were concordant for disease course. Among seven sets of twins, the interval between disease onset was shorter (3.3 months), and all were concordant for onset type (six oligoarthritis, one polyarthritis) and course subtype. Uveitis occurred in 16 sibling pairs but was concordant in only 3 pairs.

One further association bears attention: the occurrence of JRA and adult RA in the same family. Documentation of this event is scant, and it must be concluded that JRA and RA

Table 12–3

Sibling Studies in Children With Oligoarticular JCA

CHARACTERISTIC	NUMBER CONCORDANT (12 SIBLING PAIRS)
Sex	9
Age at onset (within 3 yr)	11
Type of onset: Oligoarthritis	10
Polyarthritis	1
Course of disease: Oligoarthritis	9
Polyarthritis	2
ANA test: Both positive	7
Both negative	3
Chronic uveitis: Both affected	4
Neither affected	5

Adapted from Clemens LE, Albert E, Ansell BM: Sibling pairs affected by chronic arthritis of childhood: evidence for a genetic predisposition. J Rheumatol 12: 108, 1985.

uncommonly occur in the same family, which is consistent with their differences in HLA associations. Rossen and colleagues,[240] however, studied four families with multiple cases of RA and JRA and concluded from histocompatibility data that susceptibility to arthritis was influenced by a dominant allele with variable penetrance and expressivity. An increased frequency of autoantibodies has been documented in first-degree relatives of children with chronic arthritis.[241]

Human Leukocyte Antigen Relationships

Although JRA has rarely been documented in siblings or in children whose first-degree relatives have another rheumatic disease, over 50 studies of histocompatibility antigens point clearly to the role of HLA genetic polymorphisms predisposing to these diseases.[89, 229, 236, 242–252, 253–267, 267a–267c] These investigations also provide evidence of fundamental distinctions between adult RA and JRA.[268, 269] It had been hoped that HLA specificities might aid in the reclassification of children with chronic arthritis,[262, 270] but this remains an unfulfilled aspiration. Only recently has it been confirmed that risk and protective effects of these immunogenetic profiles are age related for each onset type and a number of course subtypes: These complex interactions and age- and sex-specific windows of susceptibility and protection are examined in detail in the provocative paper by Murray and colleagues.[271] Figure 12–6 shows population details for class I and II genes from this study of 680 patients with JRA (oligoarticular 55 percent, polyarticular 27 percent, systemic 18 percent), and 254 ethnically matched unrelated controls. An increased frequency of certain class III MHC genes may contribute to susceptibility in some populations[272] but not in others.[256, 273, 274]

Associations With Class I Antigens

An increased frequency of A2, B27, and B35 has been documented in children with JRA.[272, 275–278] A2 is associated predominantly with early-onset oligoarticular disease in girls.[271] An increase in B27 in early studies was possibly related to inclusion of children with JAS (the recently proposed *enthesitis-related arthritis*).[279–281] Later investigations document inconsistent increases in the frequency of this antigen in subgroups of children with JRA.[278, 282] However, B27 may confer an age-related risk to oligoarticular JRA in boys (50 percent risk at 7.3 years; 80 percent risk at 11.9 years) (see Fig. 12–6*B*).[271]

Associations With Class II Antigens

Class II genetic associations are more numerous and complex in relation to specific onset types and course subtypes than are the few documented class I specificities.[236] These associations are most obvious in children with early-onset oligoarthritis and in RF-seropositive polyarthritis. They are more heterogeneous and inconclusive in RF-seronegative polyarthritis and systemic disease. Terminology has changed over the years for many of these specificities. Figure 12–7 (from a paper by Nepom and Glass[283]) partially clarifies this transition from serologically defined specificities to oligonucleotide-defined alleles. Most studies address specificities that are more frequent; however, Dw2 and Dw7 are decreased in children with chronic arthritis.[253] Interpretation of data on class II associations are incomplete and still evolving with recognition of clinical onset types and course subtypes of disease, better techniques to assess association and linkage in ethnically and geographically homogeneous populations, sibships[253a] and parental groups, and the age and sex variations in risk and protective effects.

Oligoarthritis

DR8, DR5, DR6, DPB1*0201, and certain DQ alleles are more frequent in children with early-onset oligoarthritis[271, 272, 278, 284] and in oligoarticular JRA, with relative risks in the range of 2 to 13.[244–246, 254, 272, 278, 285, 286] Although these associations suggest multiple gene effects, extended HLA haplotypes dependent on linkage disequilibrium are probably not responsible for the spectrum of the associations. The transmission disequilibrium test was used by Moroldo and colleagues[278] to examine linkage and association in 101 white families with a child who had oligoarthritis. DR8 and DR5 (as well as A2, B27, and B35) had significantly higher frequencies of transmission to the affected child. DR4 and DR7 were found less often. These data suggest that these numerous HLA associations partly reflect linkage between the HLA genetic region in children with JRA and a population stratification effect. However, age and sex influenced these effects. An association with DR6 has been reported in a few studies.[287] Using restriction fragment length polymorphisms, Morling and colleagues[285] found that children with oligoarticular JRA had increases in the frequencies of DRB1*08; DRB3*01/02/03 (DRw52); DQA1*0401 and 0501; DQB1*0301; DPA1*0201; and DPB1*02 compared

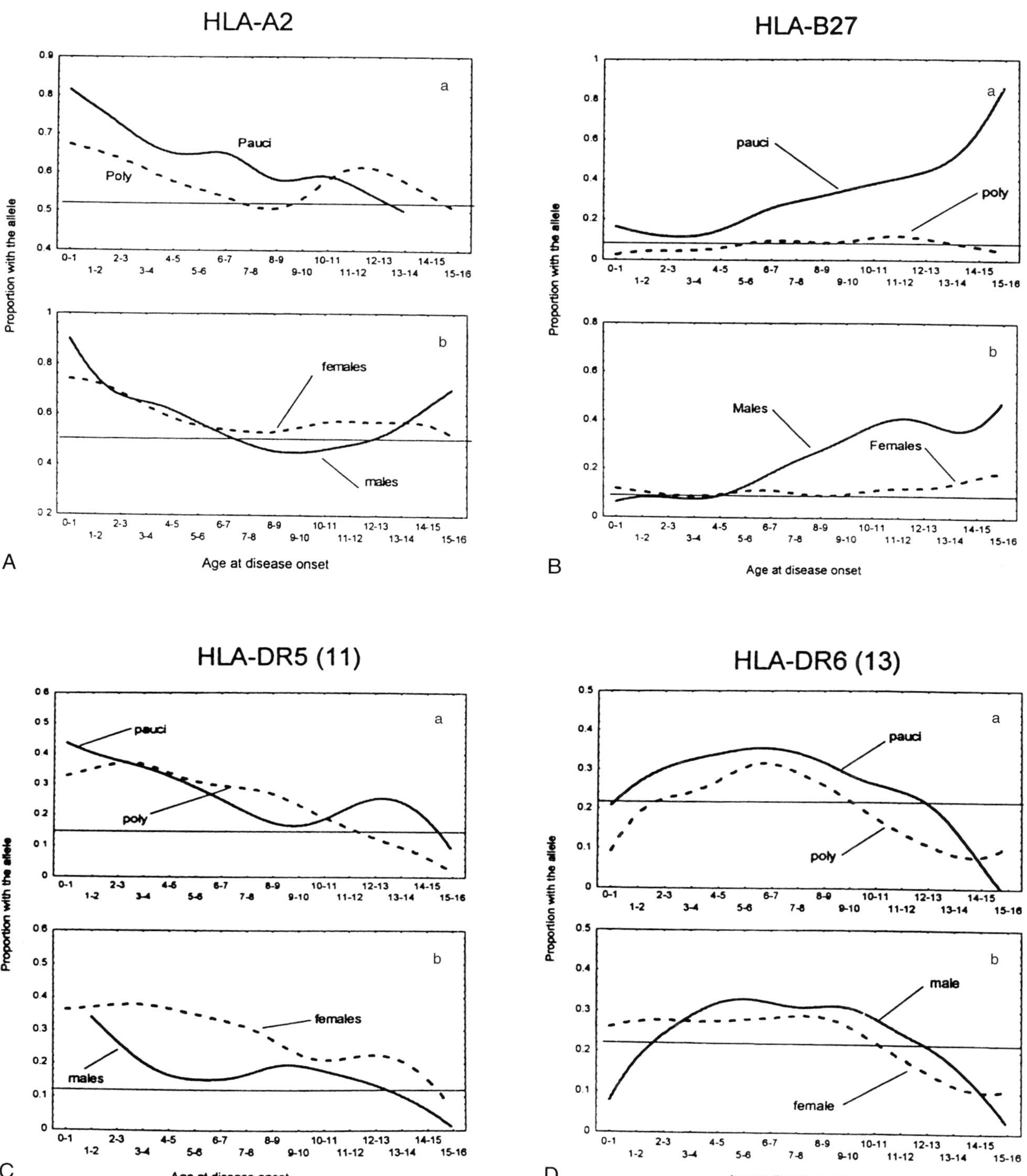

Figure 12–6. *A*, Proportion of the study population, **a**, by disease-onset type, and **b**, by sex, in each age-at-onset category with the human leukocyte antigen (HLA) A2 allele. *Horizontal line* shows the frequency of the allele in the control group. *B*, Proportion of the study population, **a**, by disease-onset type, and **b**, by gender, in each age-at-onset category with the HLA-B27 allele. *Horizontal line* shows the frequency of the allele in the control group. *C*, Proportion of the study population, **a**, by disease-onset type, and **b**, by gender, in each age-at-onset category with the HLA-DR5 (11) allele. *Horizontal line* shows the frequency of the allele in the control group. *D*, Proportion of the study population, **a**, by disease-onset type, and **b**, by gender, in each age-at-onset category with the HLA-DR6 (13) allele. *Horizontal line* shows the frequency of the allele in the control group.

Illustration continued on following page

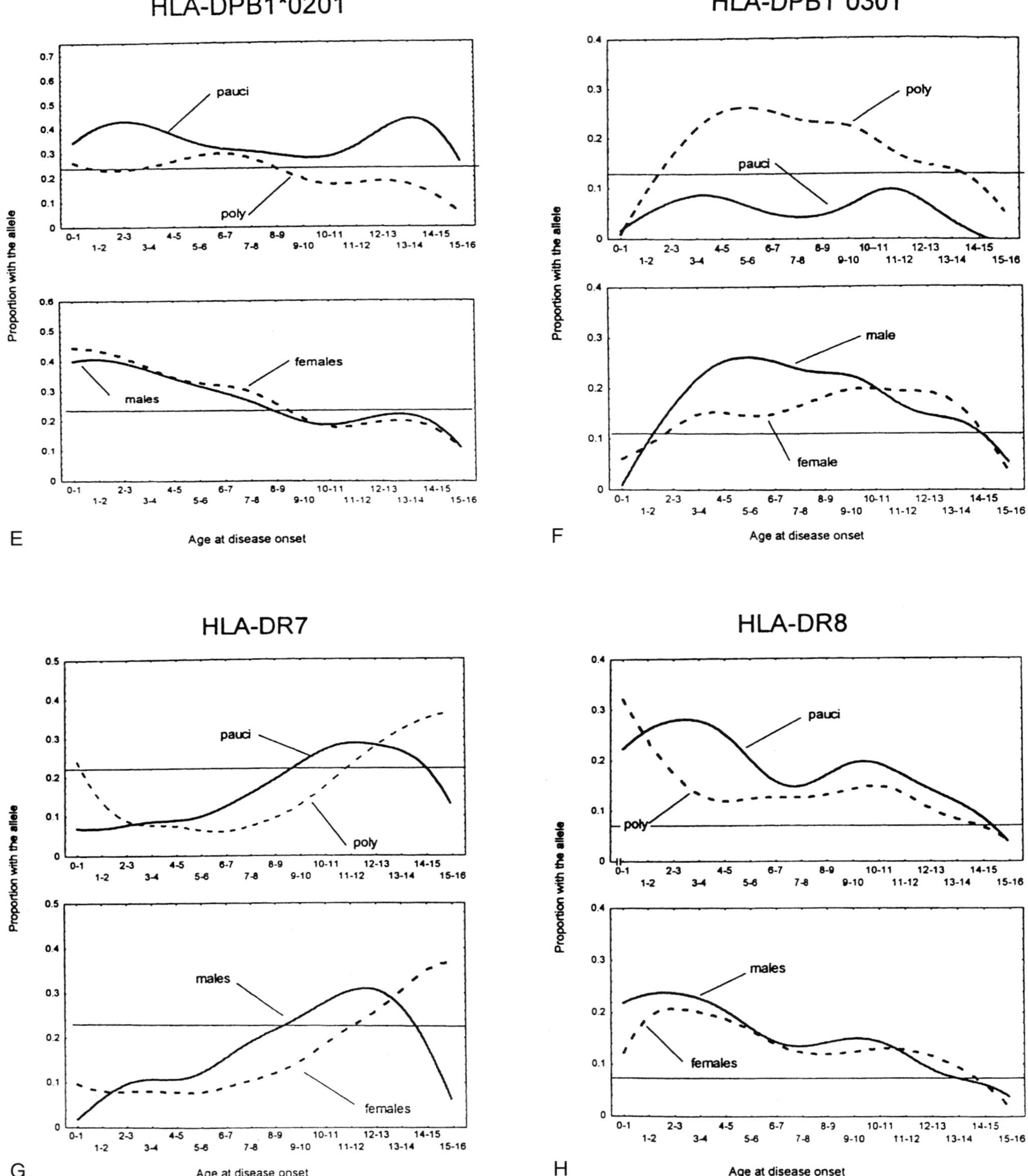

Figure 12–6 *(Continued). E,* Proportion of the study population, **a**, by disease-onset type, and **b**, by gender, in each age-at-onset category with the HLA-DPB1*0201 allele. *Horizontal line* shows the frequency of the allele in the control group. *F,* Proportion of the study population, **a**, by disease-onset type, and **b**, by gender, in each age-at-onset category with the HLA-DPB1*0301 allele. *Horizontal line* shows the frequency of the allele in the control group. *G,* Proportion of the study population, **a**, by disease-onset type, and **b**, by gender, in each age-at-onset category with the HLA-DR7 allele. *Horizontal line* shows the frequency of the allele in the control group. *H,* Proportion of the study population, **a**, by disease-onset type, and **b**, by gender, in each age-at-onset category with the HLA-DR8 allele. *Horizontal line* shows the frequency of the allele in the control group.

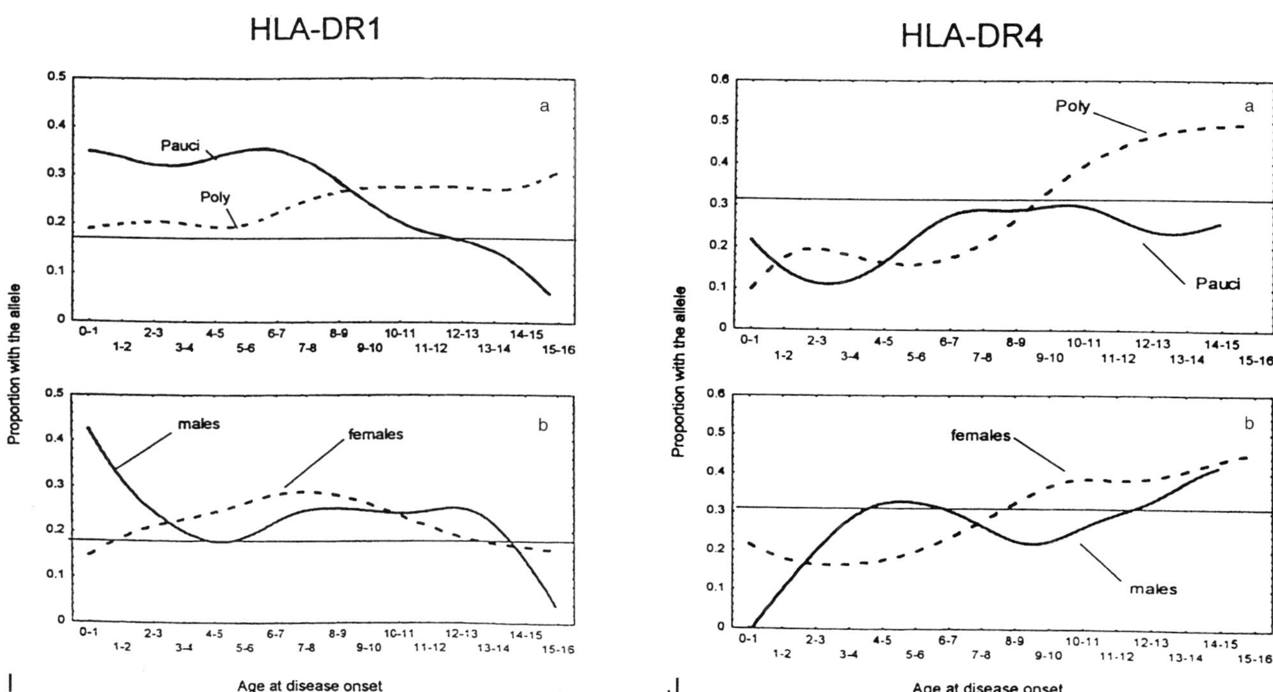

Figure 12–6 *(Continued). I,* Proportion of the study population, **a**, by disease-onset type, and **b**, by gender, in each age-at-onset category with the HLA-DR1 allele. *Horizontal line* shows the frequency of the allele in the control group. *J,* Proportion of the study population, **a**, by disease-onset type, and **b**, by gender, in each age-at-onset category with the HLA-DR4 allele. *Horizontal line* shows the frequency of the allele in the control group. Pauci = pauciarticular; poly = polyarticular. *(A–J,* From Murray KJ, Moroldo MB, Donnelly P, et al: Age-specific effects of juvenile rheumatoid arthritis-associated HLA alleles. Arthritis Rheum 42: 1843–1853, Copyright © 1999. Wiley-Liss, Inc. Reprinted by permission of Wiley-Liss, Inc., a subsidiary of John Wiley & Sons, Inc.)

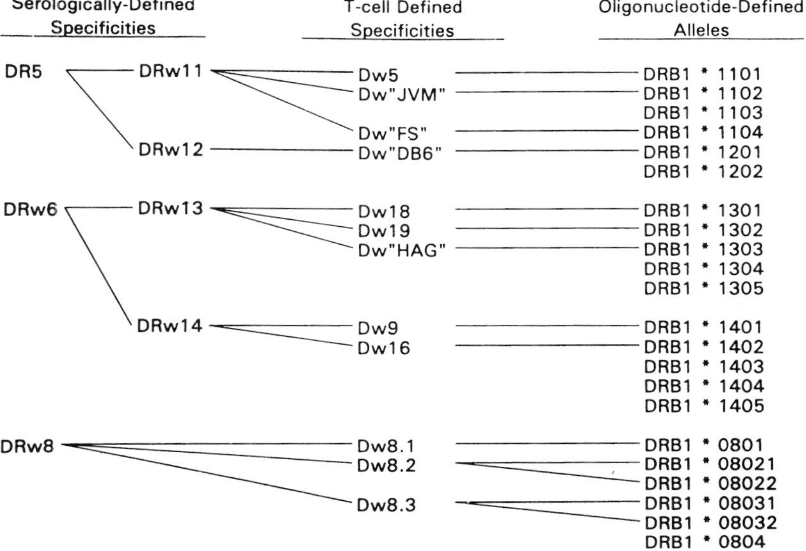

Figure 12–7. Examination of identification of specific HLA alleles. Several examples within HLA-DR gene families demonstrate the improvement of HLA typing methodology; serologically defined "public specificities" like HLA-DR5, which was further divided by serology into HLA-DRw11 and HLA-DRw12; the often more discriminatory T cell–defined specificities like HLA-Dw5 and HLA-DW "JVM"; and the most recent use of allele-specific oligonucleotide probes, which take advantage of DNA sequence separation to distinguish individual alleles. (From Nepom BS, Glass DN: Juvenile rheumatoid arthritis and HLA: report of the Park City III workshop. J Rheumatol Suppl 33: 70–74, 1992.)

with healthy controls. Both subtypes of DR5 (DR11 and DR12) and DR8 (DRB1*0801) contributed to susceptibility to early-onset oligoarticular disease.[288] DR11, DR12, and DR8 haplotypes share similar DQA1 alleles: DQA1*0401, *0501, and *0601.[289, 290] These three DQ alleles have a common motif in exon 2 at the 42 to 53 positions that was present in 86 percent of children with JCA but in only 36 percent of controls.[289, 291] Haas and colleagues[290] demonstrated that distinct differences in the DQA1 promoter are strongly associated with susceptibility to early-onset disease. Nepom and associates[164] identified a 13-nucleotide region of sequence identity in the first hypervariable region of DR5, DR6, and DR8 alleles that is a possible "shared epitope" that could be important in antigen recognition.

DR1 and DR4 are less frequently present in young girls with persistent oligoarticular JRA and ANA seropositivity and may be protective in the very young (see Fig. 12–6*J*). DR1 is a risk factor for extended oligoarthritis as well as for polyarthritis in older children.[89] It is in linkage dysequilibrium with DQA*0101, which was associated in one study with progressive erosive disease in children with early-onset oligoarticular JRA and was negatively associated with the presence of uveitis.[292] This DQA gene, although not present in all children with the disease, may be critically important in the development of this onset type.[293] It is also a binding site for the 45-kD DEK proto-oncogene[294] along with A2 (0201).[295] Anti-DEK antibodies are characteristic of oligoarticular-onset disease (78 percent positive), especially in children who are ANA seropositive and have a history of uveitis, and may negate the regulatory function of the gene,[296] or may simply be a reflection of autoimmunity.[296a] One study associated ANA seropositivity in early-onset disease with DQB1*0603.[297]

Oligoarticular JRA is also associated with DP2 (DPB1*0201),[248, 258, 298] which is present in 64 percent of patients compared with 25 percent of controls. It has been suggested that this DP allele increases the risk conferred by DR alleles but is not sufficient in itself to increase susceptibility to oligoarticular JRA.[277] A number of studies have discussed interaction between alleles at different loci in producing susceptibility to disease.[285, 291] Interaction between class I and class II genes has led to the hypothesis that at least two genetic loci are involved in the predisposition to oligoarthritis, which have been named *JRA 1* and *JRA 2*.[89, 249, 278, 292, 299, 300] A third locus, *JRA 3*, has been postulated for a DP gene.

Polyarthritis

In contrast with the correlations already discussed, HLA-Dw4, DR1, and DR4 are risk factors for polyarticular onset.[162, 238, 244, 249, 251, 252, 254, 271, 301] DR1 (DQA1*0101) is also a risk factor for polyarthritis in older children and is associated with TCR-BV6S1 null alleles.[162] The strong association between RF-seropositive polyarthritis and DR4-related susceptibility alleles and their shared epitope parallels that in RF-seropositive RA in adults. White children with RF-seropositive polyarthritis have a high frequency of two copies of alleles of DR4, particularly for the combinations of Dw4 (DRB1*0401) and Dw14 (DRB1*0404).[252, 301] Data from a study of Canadian First Nation children with RF-seropositive polyarticular JRA indicated that DRB1*0901 may be a risk factor in that population, whereas DRB1*08 alleles were possibly protective.[302] Inconsistent HLA typing has been found in RF-seronegative polyarthritis. Dw4 is only slightly increased in frequency,[248] but there are increases in the frequencies of DR8, DR5 (as in oligoarticular JRA), DR1 (as in RF-seronegative adult RA), and DP3.[253, 261, 273, 303]

Systemic-Onset Disease

Studies of class II associations with systemic-onset JRA have yielded inconsistent results; DR5, DR8, Dw7, and possibly DR4,[236] as well as DPB1 polymorphism,[284] have been reported to be more frequent in certain populations, but this is not consistently confirmed. One study found no association between DR4 and severe arthritis in children with systemic-onset JRA.[304]

Interactions With Nonhuman Leukocyte Antigen Genes

A number of non-HLA genes, either on chromosome 6 or on other chromosomes, may be important in either a predisposition to JRA or its pathogenesis.[305] A weak association with TAP2B, a polymorphism in a member of the adenosine triphosphate–binding cassette superfamily, is present for early-onset disease.[306] TAP1B may function as an additive susceptibility factor.[307] Interaction with other non-HLA genes is also possible, such as IL-1A2, a variant of the IL-1α gene, in early-onset oligoarthritis.[308] The gene for the cytokine IL-1α, or a gene for which its polymorphism is a marker, may contribute risk for early-onset disease and uveitis.[308, 309] One study suggested that homozygosity of the B allele of the LMP2 proteosome subunit may increase susceptibility to a putative subtype of JRA that is associated with B27.[310]

Associations With Other Autoimmune Diseases and Chromosomal Abnormalities

There may also be an association of the various types of onset of JRA with genetic and chromosomal abnormalities[311] and other autoimmune diseases (see Chapters 36 and 37, and Appendix). Most frequently reported is *insulin-dependent diabetes mellitus*.[312, 313] In a referral diabetic clinic population of 200 children, 6 had polyarticular JRA and 1 had probable early JAS.[312] Four of the children also had autoimmune thyroiditis.[313a] We have also observed a number of children with JRA and either thyroiditis or diabetes mellitus. A syndrome that includes flexion contractures, short stature, and skin changes may complicate diabetes mellitus, the so-called Rosenbloom syndrome, and should not be confused with inflammatory joint disease (see Chapter 36).[314, 315] Myasthenia gravis has been reported in four children with chronic arthritis.[316]

Other non-HLA genetic associations have been suggested that might increase a predisposition to JRA. Among these are *selective IgA deficiency*[317] (see Chapter 35) and the *velocardiofacial syndrome*.[318] One child with arthritis and deletion of the short arm of chromosome 18 was IgA deficient.[319] The phenotypic profile of the chromosome translocation in the velocardiofacial syndrome—del (22q11.2)—includes chronic destructive arthritis, normal numbers of T lymphocytes, and normal or elevated serum immunoglobulins.[320, 321] No children had the complete DiGeorge syndrome. Sullivan and associates[318] suggested that T-cell immunodeficiency in a subgroup of patients with this syndrome permits polyarthritis to develop. *Turner's syndrome* has also been identified in a number of patients with JRA.[321a] In a study of this association,[322] 18 of approximately 500 children with JRA were found to have Turner's syndrome. Polyarticular disease was present in 7 who had progressive seronegative arthritis and a 45 XO genotype. It is not entirely clear whether the arthropathy of *Down syndrome* differs from idiopathic JRA.[311, 323] In children whom we have seen with Down syndrome and arthritis, the joint disease has been indistinguishable from polyarticular JRA. In some of these children, the arthritis is more like that associated with psoriasis, and the latter is seemingly increased in frequency in trisomy 21. Polyarthritis has been reported in a child with partial trisomy 5q, monosomy 2p.[311]

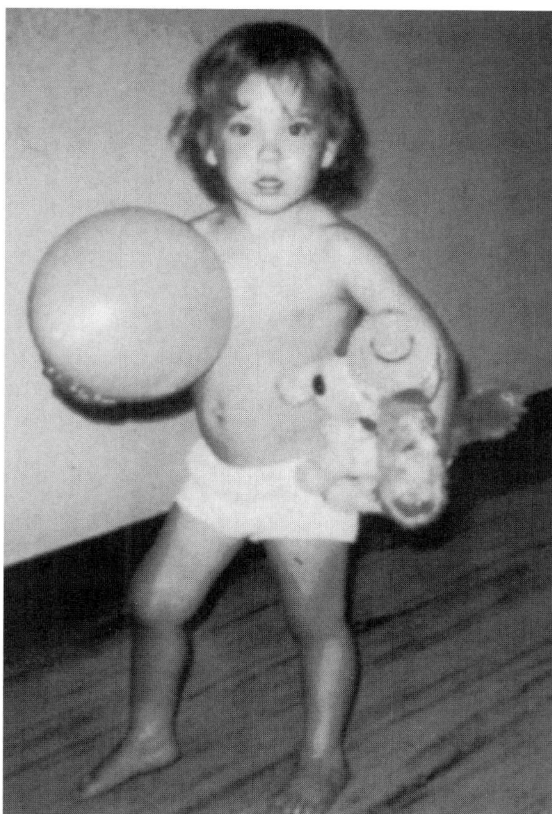

Figure 12–8. Oligoarticular JRA causing swelling and flexion contracture of the right knee of 1 year's duration in this 3-year-old girl. The combination of overgrowth of the right leg and flexion contracture of the right knee has resulted in a circumduction gait and toe-walking. The child has never expressed pain and seems unconcerned about her limp and disability.

TYPES OF ONSET

The relative frequencies of the three onset types of JRA have varied considerably in published series and reflect the same biases that confound estimates of incidence and prevalence. In general, oligoarthritis is most frequent at 56 to 60 percent, polyarthritis is next at 25 to 28 percent, and systemic disease is least common (10 to 12 percent in white populations).[36]

Oligoarticular Onset

In at least 60 percent of children with JRA, the first 6 months of disease is characterized by low-grade inflammation in four or fewer joints (see Table 12–1) (Fig. 12–8). This onset type corresponds to pauciarticular onset of the ACR[22] and EULAR criteria[24] or to oligoarthritis of the International League of Associations of Rheumatology (ILAR) classification.[23] These children are not systemically ill, and except for chronic uveitis, extra-articular manifestations are distinctly unusual. Oligoarthritis in a child is predominantly a disease of the lower extremities. The knees are most commonly involved, followed by the ankles and elbows.[324] The hips are almost always spared. The other joints demonstrate no definite pattern of involvement, and although it is our impression that wrists and small joints of the hands or feet are seldom affected in oligoarticular JRA at onset, others disagree.[325] In at least half of the children, only a single joint is affected (monarticular onset), usually the knee.[326–328] Uveitis may be present at onset of the disease, eventually affects up to 20 percent of children, and is usually asymptomatic.

Diagnosis

The differential diagnosis depends on a number of factors, including the onset type and pattern of joint involvement, the duration of disease at the time the child is evaluated, and the sex and age of the child. In some instances, oligoarticular JRA is a diagnosis of exclusion.[329, 330] In a child with monarthritis of recent onset (i.e., seen within 72 hours of onset), the differential diagnosis must include septic arthritis, trauma (including nonaccidental trauma resulting in a hemarthrosis), and hematologic disease (including hemophilia, leukemia, and malignancy) (Table 12–4).[331] If the monarthritis is long-standing, sepsis (except for tuberculosis), trauma, and malignancy are very unlikely. A painful joint effusion of short duration may be caused by trauma or, rarely in children, may be associated with an internal structural abnormality such as a discoid meniscus[332] or osteochondritis dissecans (see Chapter 16). The monarthritis of hemophilia results from bleeding into a major joint, which is often initiated by even

Table 12–4

Monarticular JRA: Differential Diagnosis

Acute Onset of Monarthritis

- Early rheumatic disease
  - Oligoarticular JRA
  - Seronegative spondyloarthropathy
- Arthritis related to infection
  - Septic arthritis
  - Reactive arthritis
- Malignancy
  - Leukemia
  - Neuroblastoma
- Hemophilia

Chronic Monarthritis

- Oligoarticular JRA
- Juvenile ankylosing spondylitis
- Juvenile psoriatic arthritis
- Villonodular synovitis
- Sarcoidosis

minor trauma. Recurrent involvement has been described in occult celiac disease.[333, 334] Rare causes of chronic monarthritis, such as tuberculosis, sarcoidosis, and villonodular synovitis, should also be considered. A migrating monarthritis, sometimes associated with fever and a rash, has been described in children of Assyrian ancestry.[335] The various forms of idiopathic osteolysis may mimic arthritis of a limited number of joints (e.g., wrists) at onset (see Chapter 37). A patient is occasionally encountered in whom arthritis has resulted from administration of a drug such as isotretinoin[336, 337] or antithyroid medication.[338, 339]

JRA is by far the most common cause of chronic oligoarthritis, especially in girls younger than 6 years. Psoriatic arthritis, which affects large and small joints in an asymmetric pattern, is also a possibility at this age (see Chapter 14). JAS is a more likely cause of a monarthritis or oligoarthritis of the lower extremities with onset in the older child or adolescent.[340] A diagnosis of oligoarticular JRA or psoriatic arthritis may be substantiated by the demonstration of asymptomatic anterior uveitis by slit-lamp examination, although sarcoidosis also rarely presents in this way. ANA seropositivity supports the diagnosis of JRA or psoriatic arthritis but may also be found in some healthy children[341] and in some children with noninflammatory musculoskeletal pain.[342] Lyme disease may present as an oligoarthritis (see Chapter 32).

In the child with oligoarticular JRA, the affected joint is swollen and often warm but usually not very painful, tender, or red. The child is not systemically ill. If a joint is acutely painful and erythematous, or if the child is febrile, septic arthritis is more likely the correct diagnosis.[343, 344] Immediate joint aspiration is always indicated in such a patient to exclude septic arthritis or osteomyelitis. Synovial biopsy with a Parker-Pearson needle or by arthroscopy is useful in children with monarthritis in whom granulomatous disease is suspected.[121, 326, 345] Culture and microscopic examination of synovial tissue may be more rewarding in the case of tuberculosis than culture of the fluid only. A negative purified protein derivative (PPD) skin test virtually excludes the diagnosis of active tuberculosis. Biopsy should not be performed simply to confirm a diagnosis of JRA.

Arthritis of the hip joint is rare at the onset of oligoarticular JRA. In our experience of 145 children with oligoarthritis seen early in their course, only 1 girl had initial involvement of the hip. Onset of apparent arthritis in the hip in a very young child should be considered first to be a septic process or a congenital dislocation.[346] In the older child, osteonecrosis of the femoral head (Legg-Calvé-Perthes disease) is a diagnostic consideration. In the adolescent age group, a slipped capital femoral epiphysis may initially mimic JRA. In older boys, JAS may present as unilateral or bilateral hip disease (see Chapter 13). In children with transient synovitis of the hip,[347, 348] pain may be severe, but the process is self-limited, lasting no more than 1 to a few weeks; the results of all laboratory and radiologic studies are normal (see Chapter 13).

Course of the Disease and Prognosis

The course of oligoarticular JRA is variable (Table 12–5). Some children pursue an oligoarticular course and

Table 12–5

JRA: Onset Types and Course Subtypes

ONSET TYPE	COURSE SUBTYPE	PROFILE	OUTCOME
Oligoarthritis (122) ≤4 Joints Lower extremities	ANA seropositive (66)	Female Young age Chronic uveitis	Excellent (except eyes)
	RF seropositive (8)	Polyarthritis Erosions Unremitting	Poor
	HLA-B27–positive (9)	Male Older age	Good
	Seronegative (38)		Good

ANA, antinuclear antibody; HLA, human leukocyte antigen; RF, rheumatoid factor.

From Cassidy JT, Levinson JE, Bass JC, et al: A study of classification criteria for a diagnosis of juvenile rheumatoid arthritis. Arthritis Rheum 29: 274–281, 1986.

go into remission, although flares of disease may occur many years later. In a second group, there is a progressive increase in the number of affected joints, so that by a year or 2 after onset, they have a polyarticular pattern of disease (extended oligoarthritis). The child with oligoarthritis fares best from the standpoint of joint disease but worst from the risk of uveitis. Because of the limited extent of the joint involvement, serious functional disability is uncommon. Fixed flexion contractures may persist, however, or osteoarthritis of a weight-bearing joint may eventually develop late in the course of the disease after clinical remission (Fig. 12–9). However, in the Cincinnati series, 41 percent of patients with oligoarticular onset still had active arthritis 10 years later.[349]

Arthritis in these children remains monarticular or oligoarticular, in general, especially if the knee or knees are the only joints involved at onset, or if disease develops in a few more joints (≤4) than were affected initially (Tables 12–6 and 12–7). After the first 6 months, approximately 5 to 10 percent experience a course of multiple joint disease not unlike that of the child with polyarthritis (extended oligoarthritis).[54, 350, 351] This phenomenon is recognized in the ACR criteria[22] by a specified course subtype, and in the ILAR criteria[23] by the fact that the category of oligoarthritis is subdivided into persistent and extended groups.[350, 351] The majority of these children, however, have fewer cumulative joints involved than the child who has had a typical onset of polyarthritis. A number of these children behave more like those in the RF-negative polyarticular-onset group.[22] A few are RF seropositive and have a guarded outcome similar to patients with the RF-seropositive polyarticular form.[22, 352] We have not observed a child with established oligoarthritis who developed manifestations of acute systemic disease, such as a rheumatoid rash or an intermittent fever. In this regard, it is important in a discussion of prognosis to exclude from this group children with a typical systemic onset who have involvement of only one or a few joints.

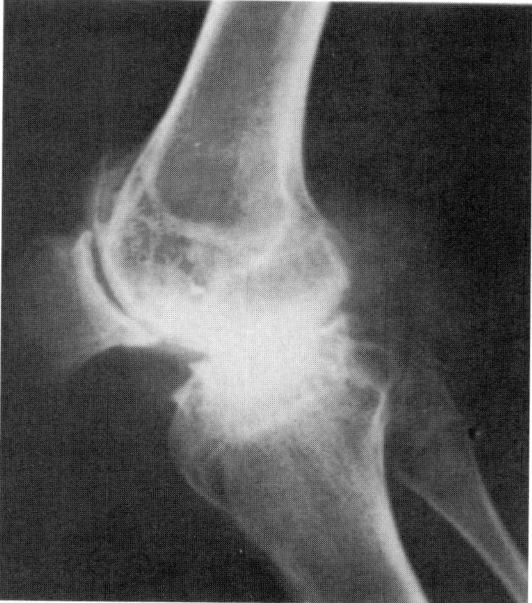

Figure 12–9. Severe degenerative arthritis in a 20-year-old woman who has had monarthritis of the left knee since the age of 3 years. Note the large, square patella and osteophytes.

Table 12–6

Course of Oligoarticular JRA in 40 Children

	CLINICAL COURSE		
	Monarthritis	**Oligoarthritis**	**Polyarthritis**
Number of patients	9	19	12
Years of oligoarthritis preceding further joint disease			
Range	3–8	½–9	½–5
Median	5	3	1
Remission (%)	20	15	20
Bone erosions (%)	—	20	60
Functional capacity (%)			
I, II	100	70	40
III, IV	—	30	60

Modified from Cassidy JT, Brody GL, Martel W: Monarticular juvenile rheumatoid arthritis. J Pediatr 70: 847, 1967.

Polyarticular Onset

Polyarticular JRA is defined as the presence of arthritis in five or more joints during the first 6 months of disease (see Table 12–1) (Fig. 12–10).[67] Disease in children with this type of onset is classified as polyarticular onset by the ACR criteria,[22] as RF-negative polyarticular onset by the EULAR criteria, or if RF-positive as JRA,[24] and as RF-negative or RF-positive polyarthritis by the ILAR classification.[23] Onset may be acute but is more often insidious, with progressive involvement of additional joints. The arthritis may be remittent or indolent, tends to be symmetric, and usually involves the large joints of the knees, wrists, elbows, and ankles. The cervical spine and temporomandibular joints are often involved in polyarticular JRA. Small-joint disease of the hands or feet may occur early or late in the course of the disease.[353] The interphalangeal joint of the thumb, the second and third metacarpophalangeal (MCP) joints, and the proximal interphalangeal (PIP) joints are most commonly involved; the other MCP and PIP joints are less frequently involved. The distal interphalangeal (DIP) joints are affected in 10 to 45 percent of children in association with involvement of the other small joints. The joints are swollen and warm but are not usually erythematous. Often, the digits exhibit soft tissue swelling between the joints as much as around them. Boutonnière deformities (PIP joint flexion and DIP hyperextension) and flexion contractures are more common than swan-neck deformities (PIP joint hyperextension and DIP flexion).[354]

An important subgroup of children with polyarticular JRA, predominantly girls, includes those who have onset late in childhood or adolescence and are RF

Table 12–7

Sequential Pattern of Joint Involvement in 40 Children With Oligoarticular Onset of JRA

SITE OF ARTHRITIS	INITIAL ARTICULAR DISEASE	PERSISTENT MONARTICULAR DISEASE	OLIGOARTICULAR DISEASE	
			Initial	Subsequent
Knee	30	9	12	11
Ankle	4	0	3	12
Wrist	2	0	0	1
Hip	2	0	2	1
Elbow	1	0	1	1
Proximal interphalangeal joint	1	0	1	1
Cervical spine	0	0	0	1

Modified from Cassidy JT, Brody GL, Martel W: Monarticular juvenile rheumatoid arthritis. J Pediatr 70: 847, 1967.

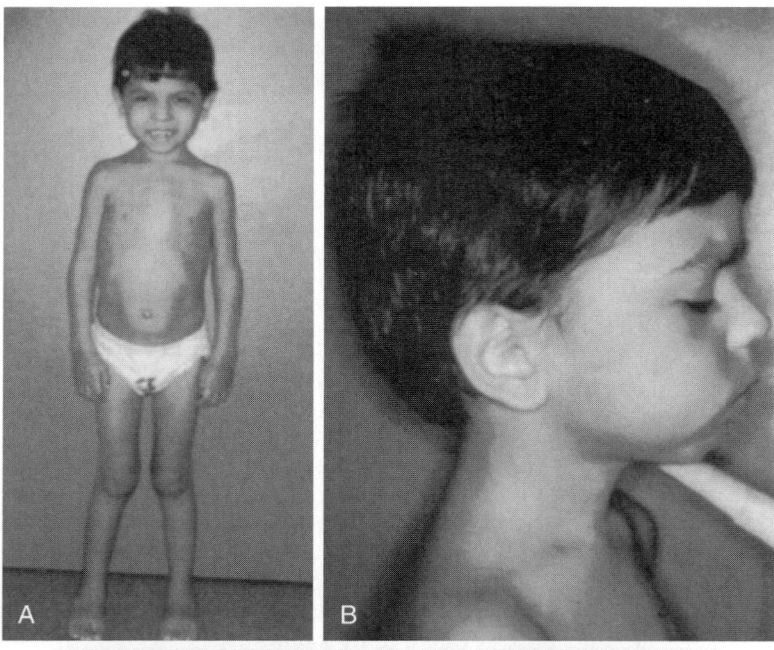

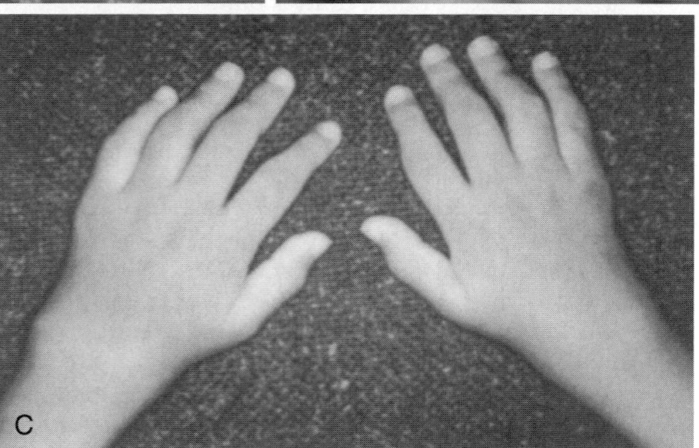

Figure 12–10. The symmetric arthritis in large and small joints of the 6-year-old boy shown here is characteristic of polyarticular JRA. *A*, Flexion contractures at the elbows, hips, and knees and a slight valgus deformity at the knees. The wrists and proximal interphalangeal joints are held in flexion. *B*, The lack of hyperextension of the cervical spine. A cervical collar is required for support. *C*, Symmetric polyarthritis affecting the metacarpophalangeal, proximal interphalangeal, and radiocarpal joints.

seropositive. These patients often develop a pattern of involvement more like that of adult RA, with rheumatoid nodules, early onset of erosive synovitis, and a chronic course persisting well into adulthood. In children with RF-seronegative polyarthritis, there is less tendency for the disease to encompass a large number of joints, to be symmetric, to involve the small joints of the hands or feet, or to be associated with rheumatoid nodules.

Systemic manifestations in children with polyarthritis include low-grade fever and slight to moderate hepatosplenomegaly or lymphadenopathy. Small pericardial effusions may be detected on echocardiographs, but clinically evident pericarditis or pleuritis is infrequent. Chronic uveitis develops less frequently than in early-onset oligoarticular disease.

Ansell[324] found that the knees, wrists, and ankles were most commonly affected in children with polyarticular JCA and that the arthritis was usually symmetric. Approximately 20 percent of children had MCP joint disease, and a similar number, but not necessarily the same children, had PIP joint involvement. Approximately one fourth had involvement of the DIP joints. Joints of the second and third fingers were most commonly affected. Tenosynovitis of the dorsal flexor tendon sheaths of the hands occurred in one sixth of the patients and in one or more of the other flexor tendons in one fifth. Involvement of a PIP joint or flexor tendon sheath was particularly common in children younger than 5 years. Arthritis of the metatarsophalangeal or PIP joints of the feet was also common.

Diagnosis

The differential diagnosis of polyarthritis is considerably different from that of oligoarthritis (Table 12–8). Septic polyarthritis is unusual (see Chapter 31), although arthritis caused by *Neisseria gonorrhoeae* may have an early migratory polyarticular phase, and infectious arthritis in children may involve more than one joint. Lyme disease may be polyarticular, but it can usually be differentiated from polyarticular JRA by its intermittent pattern of activity and the accompanying cutaneous, neurologic, and cardiac abnormalities.[355]

The onset of polyarthritis in a preadolescent or adolescent girl should suggest the possible diagnosis of SLE. The arthritis of SLE may mimic that of JRA,[356] and without serologic studies the correct diagnosis may be difficult or impossible to make until the later occurrence of one of the more characteristic clinical hallmarks of SLE: butterfly rash, alopecia, nephritis, central nervous system disease, Raynaud's phenomenon, leukopenia, hemolytic anemia. Any of these clinical findings, or the presence of an active urinary sediment in a child with polyarthritis, strongly suggests the diagnosis of SLE. This diagnosis would be supported by the presence of anti-dsDNA antibodies or hypocomplementemia.[357] Ragsdale and colleagues[358] presented the course of 10 children who developed SLE after an initial diagnosis of JRA. In all cases, anti-dsDNA antibodies were detectable before the development of clinical disease characteristic of SLE. Raynaud's phenomenon in the child with arthritis should always include a differential diagnosis such as scleroderma, SLE, or mixed connective tissue disease; in our experience, Raynaud's phenomenon has not been associated with JRA. Although anemia is common in severe JRA, it is not Coombs' positive and the presence of hemolytic anemia would support the diagnosis of another connective tissue disease, usually SLE.

The differential diagnosis of polyarthritis also includes the spondyloarthropathies. Children with JAS usually have large joint oligoarthropathy of the lower extremities at onset rather than disease of the axial skeleton and may have polyarthritis.[359] Transient pain in the lower back or buttock may be an early sign.[340] The diagnosis of JAS should be considered particularly in a boy older than 10 years with a family history of ankylosing spondylitis or another of the spondyloarthropathies. The presence of enthesitis in a child with polyarthritis makes the probability of a diagnosis of JAS much more likely (see Chapter 13).[360, 361] RF and ANA are invariably absent in children with JAS; on the other hand, the HLA-B27 antigen is present in more than 92 percent of these children, compared with 6 to 8 percent in the general North American white population.[362] A firm diagnosis of JAS may not be possible at onset of peripheral arthritis and depends ultimately on demonstration of characteristic radiologic features in the sacroiliac joints. Occult inflammatory bowel disease may present as, or be complicated by, polyarthritis that is usually more transient than that of JRA. Whipple's disease may cause peripheral arthritis in children but is very rare.

Dermatomyositis or scleroderma occasionally presents with arthritis. The associated features of these illnesses generally lead quickly to a correct diagnosis. Dermatomyositis is almost invariably associated with the characteristic skin rash, and isolated polymyositis is rare. Scleroderma, on the other hand, may begin insidiously, and subtle subcutaneous calcifications may be misinterpreted as rheumatoid nodules.

Malignant infiltration of bone or synovium may mimic polyarthritis, although in most instances the lesion is in juxta-articular bone rather than in the joint.[363, 364] Sometimes, however, joint effusions occur in children with malignancies.[365] Nonarticular bone pain

Table 12–8

Polyarticular JRA: Differential Diagnosis

- Seronegative spondyloarthropathy
  - Juvenile ankylosing spondylitis
  - Juvenile psoriatic arthritis
  - Arthritides of inflammatory bowel disease
- Systemic lupus erythematosus
- Polyarthritis related to infection
  - Lyme disease
  - Reactive arthritis
- Other
  - Sarcoidosis
  - Familial hypertrophic synovitis syndromes
  - Mucopolysaccharidoses

or tenderness, back pain with rest or activity, and severe constitutional symptoms may be warning clues.[331] In addition to the systemic manifestations of malignancy, many children with hematologic malignancies have moderate to severe anemia or elevation of the erythrocyte sedimentation rate (ESR) that is out of keeping with other features of their disease. The leukocyte count or platelet count may be low or normal, whereas in children with JRA, these laboratory measurements usually are increased.[366] The serum level of lactic dehydrogenase is often very high.[367] Radiographs of affected joints may suggest one of these disorders; however, the correct diagnosis in some children may be delayed for 3 to 6 months. Examination of the bone marrow is usually diagnostic (e.g., leukemia, neuroblastoma). Arthritis as a manifestation of malignancy becomes increasingly uncommon during late adolescence as red marrow ceases to occupy the metaphyses of the long bones.

Sickle cell anemia in the very young child causes a dactylitis (hand-foot syndrome) that may mimic true arthritis, and in other children it causes microinfarcts that give rise to periostitis and periarthritis.[368] Occasionally, the hypermobility syndrome or one of the Ehlers-Danlos syndromes may present as arthritis (see Chapter 16).[369] Swelling, pain, and temperature and color changes associated with reflex sympathetic dystrophy are usually unilateral and are readily differentiated from signs of JRA (see Chapter 17). Rarely, a child with a mucopolysaccharidosis, particularly Morquio's or Scheie's syndrome, may have joint stiffness or bony enlargement suggesting polyarthritis (see Chapter 37). Children with immunodeficiencies, especially selective IgA deficiency and hypogammaglobulinemia, may have an arthritis that mimics JRA (see Chapter 35).

Jacobs and associates[370] and Athreya and coworkers[371] described children with *familial hypertrophic synovitis* who developed characteristic flexion contractures of the finger joints during the first few months of life. A bent thumb, the first diagnostic sign of this disorder, was often noted soon after birth. Symmetric effusions affected the large joints. Progressive but minimal limitation of motion of the joints developed with age. There was usually no pain or systemic manifestation of fever or inflammation. Autosomal dominant inheritance was suggested in some families. Hypertrophic villi with giant cells but no other inflammatory infiltrates were present on histologic examination of the synovium. Synovial lining cells were hyperplastic, but vascular endothelial proliferation was not prominent. Radiographs demonstrated flattening of the proximal ossification centers of the femurs. *Familial arthritis and camptodactyly* has also been described,[372] which is associated in some cases with pericarditis.[373, 374] We have seen two children who had an isolated joint contracture resembling JRA in whom the eventual diagnosis was *myositis ossificans progressiva* (see Chapter 20). This diagnosis was not evident in either child until later in the course, when typical ossifications in muscle were observed radiographically. *Familial osteochondritis dissecans* may mimic polyarticular JRA.[375]

The generalized soft tissue puffiness of the dorsa of the hands and feet in disorders such as *lymphedema praecox, Noonan's syndrome,* and *Turner's syndrome* may mimic swelling caused by a combination of small joint effusions and tenosynovitis in children with polyarticular JRA.[322, 376] The absence of other evidence of inflammation in these disorders should readily differentiate such conditions from polyarticular JRA. Other rare causes of diagnostic confusion include Poncet's disease (see Chapter 31)[377] and the Torg syndrome.[378]

Course of the Disease and Prognosis

The child most at risk for an unsatisfactory outcome is the one who has been referred late after onset or has a relatively late age at onset and long duration of disease, early involvement of the small joints of the hands and feet, rapid appearance of erosions, unremitting inflammatory activity, RF seropositivity, and subcutaneous nodules (Tables 12–9 and 12–10).[22] These children have the greatest number of joints involved, often 20 or more, and eventual disability is largely related to the extent of articular involvement.[379] Widespread symmetric involvement of the PIP and MCP joints of the hands or feet is characteristically associated in polyarthritis with a more guarded outlook than disease that is confined to the large joints. This is the so-called adult pattern of JRA, and it is related to development of RF seropositivity. Hip disease occurs in approximately one half of the children and almost always is accompanied by persistent inflammatory disease.[380–382] Unfortunately, it often leads inexorably to destruction or abnormal development of the femoral heads and acetabula. This type of severe hip disease is a major cause of disability in JRA, and hip involvement is justifiably interpreted as a poor prognostic sign. Limitation of range of articular motion often develops early and is related to synovial proliferation, effusion, or muscle spasm. Later on, it may result from contractures of soft tissues, joint destruction, or ankylosis.[383] Remission is unlikely if arthritis has persisted longer than 7 years. Onset of puberty has no relation to activity of the disease or likelihood of a remission. In the Cincinnati series, 45 percent of the patients still had active arthritis 10 years after onset.[349]

Systemic Onset

Ten percent of children have onset of JRA with severe systemic involvement that may precede development of overt arthritis by weeks, months, or rarely years (see Table 12–1) (Fig. 12–11). The longest interval between

Table 12–9

Association of Rheumatoid Factor in Children With JRA

Rheumatoid factor as detected by latex fixation or sheep cell agglutination tests is most frequent in children with:
- Polyarticular disease
- Older age at onset
- Older presenting age
- Rheumatoid nodules
- Bone erosions
- Poorer functional class
- HLA-Dw4 (DRB1*0401) and -Dw14 (DRB1*0404)

HLA, human leukocyte antigen.

Table 12–10

JRA: Onset Types and Course Subtypes

ONSET TYPE	COURSE SUBTYPE	PROFILE	OUTCOME
Polyarthritis (78) ≥5 Joints Upper and lower extremities	RF seropositive (16)	Female Older age Hand/wrist Erosions Nodules Unremitting	Poor
	ANA seropositive (38)	Female Younger age	Good
	Seronegative (24)		Variable

ANA, antinuclear antibody; RF, rheumatoid factor.

From Cassidy JT, Levinson JE, Bass JC, et al: A study of classification criteria for a diagnosis of juvenile rheumatoid arthritis. Arthritis Rheum 29: 274–281, 1986.

onset of systemic signs and appearance of arthritis in our patients was approximately 10 years! The presence of arthritis must be confirmed, however, before a diagnosis of JRA can be considered definite.

The designation of systemic onset is used in all three of the classification systems—ACR,[22] EULAR,[24] and ILAR.[23] The diagnostic hallmark of this onset type is a high spiking fever.[384] The temperature rises to 39°C or higher on a daily or twice-daily basis, with a rapid return to baseline or below the baseline (Fig. 12–12).

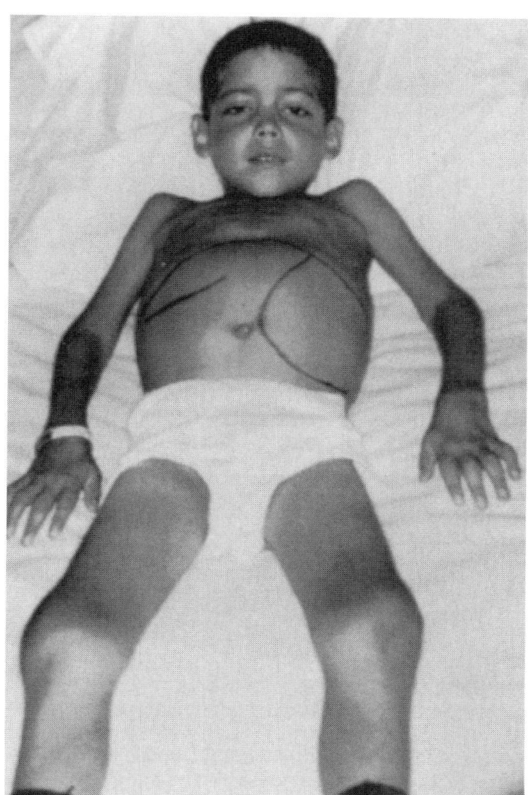

Figure 12–11. This 8-year-old boy experienced onset of systemic JRA at the age of 4 years. There is symmetric large and small joint arthritis. Note the axillary lymphadenopathy and marked hepatosplenomegaly.

This quotidian pattern is highly suggestive of the diagnosis of JRA, although very early in the course of the disease the classic quotidian fever may not be apparent, and the pattern may be indistinguishable from that of sepsis. The fever may occur at any time of the day but is characteristically present in the late afternoon to evening in conjunction with the rash. The temperature may be subnormal in the morning. Chills are frequent at the time of the fever, but rigor is rare. These children are often quite ill while febrile but surprisingly well during the rest of the day. Hyperpyrexia, a temperature higher than 40.5°C, is a rare but serious complication of an acute systemic onset.

The intermittent fever is almost always accompanied by a classic rash that consists of discrete, erythematous macules 2 to 5 mm in size (Fig. 12–13).[385, 386] This rheumatoid rash is usually described as being salmon pink,

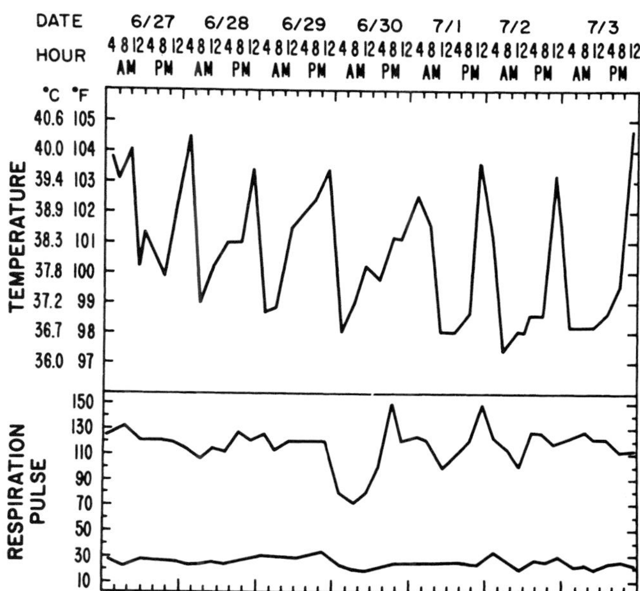

Figure 12–12. Intermittent fever of systemic-onset JRA in a 3-year-old girl. The fever spikes usually occurred daily in the late evening to early morning (quotidian pattern), returned to normal or below normal, and were accompanied by severe malaise, tachycardia, and rash.

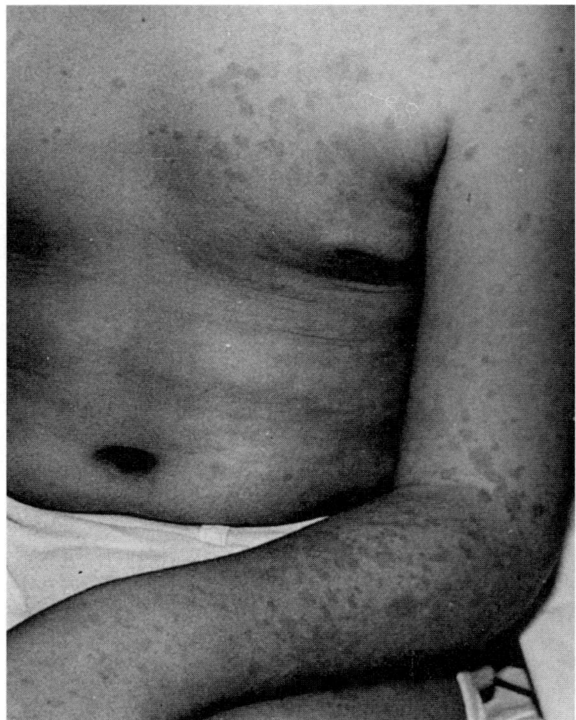

Figure 12–13. Typical rash of systemic-onset JRA in a 3-year-old boy. The rash is salmon-colored, macular, and nonpruritic. Individual lesions are transient, occur in crops over the trunk and extremities, and may occur in a linear distribution (Koebner's phenomenon) after minor trauma such as a scratch.

but very early in the disease it may be more erythematous, although never purpuric. It most commonly occurs on the trunk and proximal extremities but may develop on the face, palms, or soles. The macules are often surrounded by a zone of pallor, and larger lesions develop central clearing. The rash tends to be migratory and is strikingly evanescent in any one area: Individual lesions disappear within a few hours and leave no residua. The rash may be much more persistent in children who are systemically very ill, and it may reappear with each systemic exacerbation. Individual lesions may be elicited by rubbing or scratching the skin (the *Koebner phenomenon* or *isomorphic response*) or by a hot bath or psychological stress. The rash is occasionally pruritic,[387] particularly in the older patient.

In addition to the characteristic fever and rash, children with systemic-onset JRA have other visceral involvement, including hepatosplenomegaly, lymphadenopathy, pericarditis, or other evidence of serositis. Hepatosplenomegaly and generalized lymphadenopathy can be prominent and occur in most children with active systemic disease.

Diagnosis

The differential diagnosis of a child suspected of having systemic-onset JRA may be difficult, especially at onset or early in the course of the disease, when the child may have a high spiking fever and evidence of systemic inflammation but no arthritis and no specific sign or symptom that allows a definitive diagnosis.[388] In such children, the possibilities of malignancy, inflammatory bowel disease, vasculitis such as polyarteritis nodosa, or other connective tissue diseases such as SLE should be considered (Table 12–11). Children with systemic-onset disease may be thought to have an acute infectious disease or septicemia. Infectious mononucleosis and other viral illnesses may mimic systemic-onset JRA, but for the most part the arthropathies secondary to viral infections are transient. Documenting the presence of arthritis or a rheumatoid rash helps to establish a diagnosis of JRA. Laboratory tests are of little value in diagnosis. In many instances, the diagnosis of systemic-onset JRA is one of exclusion until a full complement of characteristic abnormalities has been observed, a process that may take several months or possibly years. Many unusual entities such as neonatal-onset multisystem inflammatory disease (NOMID) or chronic inflammatory neurologic and articular syndrome (CINCA) need to be excluded (see Chapter 24).[389–392]

Fever in children with infectious diseases is of the septic type. It is more hectic, spikes less predictably, and usually does not repetitively return to the baseline each day as does the fever of JRA, and the child remains ill even during a relatively afebrile interval. A sustained or remittent fever is characteristic of acute rheumatic fever and should respond dramatically to salicylates. Although many children with systemic JRA have isolated pericarditis, a pericardial effusion with evidence of endocarditis such as a diastolic murmur suggests a diagnosis of rheumatic fever or bacterial endocarditis. Onset of rheumatic fever in the developed countries of the world generally occurs in children between the ages of 5 and 15 years (see Chapter 34). The arthritis is characteristically acute and painful, migratory, and asymmetric, involving the peripheral joints without sequelae. The initial episode usually lasts no longer than 6 weeks but may persist for as long as 3 months. Evidence of a prior infection with β-hemolytic group A streptococci is present; however, the antistreptolysin O titer may be chronically increased to a moderate degree in one third of children with JRA as a manifestation of inflammation rather than evi-

Table 12–11

Systemic-Onset JRA: Differential Diagnosis of Fever of Unknown Origin

- Infection
- Inflammatory bowel disease
- Malignancy
- Connective tissue diseases
  - Systemic lupus erythematosus
  - Juvenile dermatomyositis
  - Vasculitis (polyarteritis nodosa)
- Castleman's disease
- Familial Mediterranean fever
- Hyper IgD syndrome

IgD, immunoglobulin D.

dence of recent streptococcal infection.[393] In acute rheumatic fever, a two-tube rise or fall in antistreptolysin O titer should be documented.

Adult-Onset Still's Disease. Adult-onset Still's disease was first reported in 1942.[394] It may present in either sex as fever of unknown origin. Hallmarks of adult-onset Still's disease are similar to those of childhood-onset disease.[395–404, 404a] Bywaters[395] described 14 young women with characteristic features of Still's disease, including fever, rash, polyarthritis, and an elevated ESR. In a National Institutes of Health study, all of the patients were men, and half were actually experiencing an exacerbation of arthritis after a long remission of systemic disease that began in childhood.[396] The clinical picture of adult-onset Still's disease often suggests a systemic infection, and in some patients a viral etiology has been implicated.[403] If investigations for infectious, hematologic, or neoplastic causes are unrewarding, diagnostic suspicion often focuses on a connective tissue disease. Characteristic radiographic changes (e.g., pericapitate involvement) have been described.[404, 405]

Course of the Disease and Prognosis

The acute manifestations of the systemic-onset form of JRA are variable in duration and last from weeks to months. Systemic features such as fever, rash, and pericarditis tend to subside during the initial months to years of the disease (2 to 5 years) but may recur in conjunction with exacerbations of the arthritis.[22, 406] About half of the children with systemic onset eventually recover almost completely, often after a pattern of oligoarticular disease for a variable period (Table 12–12). The other half continue to show progressive involvement of more and more joints and moderate to severe functional disability in some studies[22, 407, 407a] but not in others.[408] The eventual functional outcome in these children depends more on the number of joints involved and on continuing activity than on the nature of the systemic disease.[408a] The persistence of systemic symptoms without arthritis is unusual and is seldom a cause of permanent disability. However, in the Cincinnati series, 48 percent of children with systemic onset still had active arthritis 10 years later.[349]

The *macrophage activation syndrome* (MAS), or reactive hematophagocytic lymphohistiocytosis, is a rare but acute complication that is most common in boys and is associated with serious morbidity and sometimes death (Table 12–13).[409] It may also occur in disorders of infectious and neoplastic origin, and a few cases have also been described in adult-onset Still's disease.[410] It is characterized by the rapid development of hepatic failure with encephalopathy, purpura, bruising, and mucosal bleeding sometimes associated with renal failure with hematuria and proteinuria.[411, 412] Persistent fever, lymphadenopathy and hepatosplenomegaly, leukopenia, anemia, thrombocytopenia, and elevated liver enzyme concentrations are present. The ESR is paradoxically low in association with hypofibrinogenemia induced by consumptive coagulopathy and disseminated intravascular coagulation. The prothrombin time and the partial thromboplastin time are prolonged, and blood levels of the vitamin K–dependent clotting factors are low. Fibrin degradation products are present in the serum. Cytokines derived from macrophages and T cells are very high, in particular levels of IFN-γ and TNF-α along with a number of other cytokines, the so-called cytokine storm.[142] Subclinical coagulation abnormalities characterized by prolonged prothrombin and partial thromboplastin times, and increased fibrin degradation products, fibrinopeptide A, and factor VIII–related antigen, have been reported to be common in systemic-onset JRA but not in polyarticular disease.[413, 414] Active systemic disease is also associated with elevated levels of fibrin D-dimer[415] and soluble adhesion molecules.[416] These markers of fibrin degradation correlated with severe disease, fever, and leukocytosis, and serial levels fell with continuing clinical response to disease-modifying agents. Acquired factor VIII inhibitor has been described in some children.[417]

The etiology of this disorder is unknown, but in some children it is associated with an abrupt change in medications. This has often been related to the introduction of treatment with a gold compound, nonsteroidal anti-inflammatory drug (NSAID), sulfasalazine, or other agents such as hydroxychloroquine and D-penicillamine.[418–420] In other cases, the MAS may occur spontaneously[421] or be related to the incidental presence of a viral infection.[422] The MAS in children with JRA obviously reflects a variety of underlying pathogenic mechanisms and environmental triggers.

In one of the original reports of the syndrome, 7 children were described by Silverman and associates,[412] and the supposition was offered that the onset had been triggered by the

Table 12–12

JRA: Onset Types and Course Subtypes

ONSET TYPE	COURSE SUBTYPE	PROFILE	OUTCOME
Systemic disease (51) Variable number of joints and location	Oligoarthritis (30)		Good
	Polyarthritis (21)	Erosions	Poor

From Cassidy JT, Levinson JE, Bass JC, et al: A study of classification criteria for a diagnosis of juvenile rheumatoid arthritis. Arthritis Rheum 29: 274–281, 1986. Copyright © 1986 Wiley-Liss, Inc. Reprinted by permission of Wiley-Liss, Inc., a subsidiary of John Wiley & Sons, Inc.

Table 12–13

Systemic-Onset JRA: Macrophage Activation Syndrome

Acutely ill with bruising, purpura, mucosal bleeding
- ↑ Nodes, liver, spleen
- ↓ Blood cell counts, ESR
- ↑ AST, ALT, PT, PTT, fibrin-split products
- ↓ Fibrinogen, clotting factors

Bone marrow: active phagocytosis by macrophages and histiocytes
Treatment: IV glucocorticoid, cyclosporin

ALT, alanine aminotransferase; AST, aspartate aminotransferase; ESR, erythrocyte sedimentation rate; IV, intravenous, PT, prothrombin time; PTT, partial thromboplastin time.

use of NSAIDs. Jacobs and colleagues[418] reported 4 patients who died after a second gold injection with disseminated intravascular coagulation, jaundice, and other systemic involvement. Scott and colleagues[413] described 2 children with systemic onset who developed fulminant purpura and peripheral gangrene. Smith and coworkers[423] described the presence of microthrombi and endothelial proliferation in skin biopsy specimens from 10 patients with the disorder. They postulated that continuing damage to endothelial cells and the resulting vasculitis induced disseminated intravascular coagulation. Prieur and Stephan[424] studied 44 published cases and suggested that activated macrophages release proteinases that trigger the plasminogen-plasmin cascade. MAS has also been described in children with rheumatic diseases who have been recipients of autologous stem cell transplantation and subsequently experienced overwhelming viremia.

MAS must be treated vigorously and rapidly because of the extreme morbidity and high fatality rate. One approach has been to use intravenous methylprednisolone pulse therapy,[411, 412] although some cases have been glucocorticoid resistant.[425, 426] Mouy and associates[427] described the use of cyclosporine in five children with this disorder, with rapid resolution of their illness over the course of a few days.

CLINICAL MANIFESTATIONS

Constitutional Signs and Symptoms

Morning stiffness and gelling after inactivity are common manifestations of inflammatory joint disease. They are infrequently vocalized by the young child but frequently reported by parents as morning slowness or stiffness. Anorexia, weight loss, and growth failure occur in many children, especially those with systemic onset. Significant fatigue is rarely a feature of oligoarthritis but is a common symptom in children with polyarticular or systemic disease, especially at onset and during periods of poor disease control. It may be expressed as an increased sleep requirement, lack of energy, or increased irritability. Night pain may interrupt sleep and contribute to fatigue. Sleep fragmentation may also exacerbate pain as well as fatigue in these children.[428]

Pain

The child with JRA may not complain of pain at rest,[429–432] but active or passive motion of a joint elicits pain, particularly at the extremes of the range of motion. Pain is usually described as aching or stretching and is of mild to moderate severity. In contrast, children with pain-amplification syndromes almost always describe pain as extremely severe (see Chapter 17).[432a] Pain elicited by pressure or tenderness is usually maximal at the joint line or over hypertrophied, inflamed synovium. Bone pain or tenderness is not characteristic of JRA, and its presence should alert the examiner to the possibility of a malignancy involving bone.

The manner in which a child communicates discomfort or dysfunction varies according to developmental age. The child may express increased irritability or the joints may be tender on examination or painful in motion. In the young child, there may be no complaints of pain, although it is not clear that the child is not experiencing pain.[429–432] Young children with JRA, however, may alter the manner in which the affected joint is used, assume a posture of guarding the joints, or entirely refuse to use a limb in order to avoid pain. Their expression of pain is thereby physical rather than vocal. In such circumstances, parents report that the child does not appear to be in pain but that he or she limps or reverts to more infantile patterns of movement.

The relation of cognitive stage to expression of pain is not certain. Some studies detected no age-related differences in reporting of pain.[433, 434] In others, younger children with limited joint disease complained of the most severe pain,[435] and in still others, older children reported more pain.[429, 431, 432, 436, 437] This was related, it was suggested, to their concern about the significance and consequences of the disease.[437]

A considerable debate continues about pain perception in children with arthritis.[432, 438] Two studies concluded that children with JRA perceived less pain than their adult counterparts, although in both, the evaluation instruments were not ideal.[429, 436] One investigation reported that these children had lower pain thresholds than healthy children.[439] In another study, Sherry and associates[440] stated that only 14 percent of children with JRA (mostly oligoarticular type) studied in an outpatient setting indicated that they had no pain. In a more recent report, all 57 children with chronic arthritis, aged 7 to 17 years, reported the presence of pain, usually described as aching.[433] No differences were found with respect to type of onset of arthritis, sex, age, or disease duration. There was often an overall lack of association between the child's psychosocial functioning and reports of the nature or intensity of the pain.[433, 441] Pain may be an important component of functional disability. It may limit school attendance, physical activity, and social interactions.[442]

In some studies, the child's report of pain intensity correlated with the physician's estimate of disease activity or severity,[441] but in others no correlation was found.[433, 436] In a study by Ilowite and colleagues,[443] pain as assessed by a pediatric pain questionnaire was compared with the results of thermography of affected joints. Correlations between the visual analogue scores determined by parents and those by physicians were significant ($P < .01$ and $< .05$, respectively). However, correlation between the children's scores and thermography was not significant ($P > .05$). The authors interpreted these findings to indicate that relationships among the multifactorial aspects of the subjective pain response in joint inflammation were far from direct. Severity of JRA accounted for only a relatively small percentage of the variance among factors that influence the subjective pain response.[435]

Both acute and chronic pain in children are often underappreciated and therefore undertreated.[433, 441] Children may not complain of pain per se because of their level of cognitive development, and pain might better be evaluated by a child's responses to physical examination of the joints than simply by inquiring about the presence of pain. Measurement of pain in children is facilitated by the use of instruments such as the Pediatric Pain Questionnaire[444] or a visual analogue scale.[445] Using a visual analogue scale, Varni and colleagues[444] confirmed that reports of pain by children as young as 5 years correlated well with reports made by parents and physicians. It therefore seems reasonable to conclude that children with JRA experience as much pain as adults when that pain is accurately evaluated in relation to developmental stages.

A study of children with JRA[431] indicates that many often report pain as a major symptom that affects their daily activities. The pain was modestly correlated with long disease duration, older age, and variables related to demographic scales. Disease status and measurable psychological variables accounted for a modest amount of variance in pain scores. The results suggested that factors that were contributing to pain in children with JRA were quite different from those that had been identified in adults with RA. Another study[446] examined psychological variables in children with JRA and identified three psychological measures in the children and family that significantly affected functioning: Greater emotional distress in the child and in the mother, and a lower level of family harmony, all correlated with a higher degree of reported pain in the child.

Characteristics of Joint Inflammation

The arthritic joint exhibits the cardinal signs of inflammation: swelling, erythema, heat, pain, and loss of function (see Fig. 12–1). Swelling of a joint may result from periarticular soft tissue edema, from intra-articular effusion, or from hypertrophy of the synovial membrane. In JRA, effusion and hypertrophy of the synovial membrane are common, whereas in arthritis accompanying diseases such as Henoch-Schönlein purpura, periarticular swelling is more prominent. Involved joints are often warm but usually not erythematous. In contrast, the joint may be erythematous in septic arthritis or acute rheumatic fever and in some of the other reactive arthritides.

Distribution of Affected Joints

Any joint can be affected by JRA, but large joints are most frequently involved. Small joints of the hands and feet may also be affected, particularly in polyarticular-onset JRA. The examiner's attention must also be directed to the temporomandibular joint and to the cervical, thoracic, and lumbosacral spine. The sternoclavicular, acromioclavicular, and manubriosternal joints are infrequently affected. Cricoarytenoid arthritis is unusual in JRA but may be responsible for acute airway obstruction.[447–450] Inflammation of the synovial joints of the middle ear, the incudomalleal and incudostapedial articulations, is rarely detected clinically. Tympanometric studies, however, have indicated that subclinical disease may be present in almost two thirds of children with JRA.[451]

Disease in the apophyseal joints of the cervical spine occurs at onset in approximately 2 percent of children with JRA[324] and may present as a torticollis.[452] Approximately 60 percent of patients eventually develop involvement of this area of the axial skeleton.[453–455] The characteristic initial complaints are stiffness and pain at the back of the neck; rapid loss of extension and rotation may result. Unilateral apophyseal joint disease may result in asymmetry of neck extension. Subluxation of the atlantoaxial joints may occur early, rendering the child at risk for injury in an accident or with attempted intubation prior to general anesthesia. Cervical spine ankylosis carries much the same risks. It may be a major problem for the anesthetist because of difficulty in obtaining adequate neck extension and the necessity to use nasotracheal rather than orotracheal intubation, or an anesthetic technique of employing a laryngeal mask. Involvement of the thoracolumbar apophyseal joints is generally not appreciated clinically. However, scoliosis, possibly reflecting asymmetric apophyseal joint inflammation, was more frequent in one early study by as much as 30 times.[456, 457] It is our impression that scoliosis is now much less frequent. Minimal reactive sclerosis of the sacroiliac joints may occur in a few children with JRA (<5 percent) and should be distinguished from the more pronounced disease observed in JAS.[359, 383] The sacroiliac joints may eventually fuse in JRA, particularly in children who have been bedridden.[383]

Small outpouchings of synovium are not uncommon in JRA and are particularly evident at the extensor hood of the PIP joints and around the wrist or ankle. Large synovial cysts are an unusual complication. These may appear in the popliteal space (Baker's cyst) (Fig. 12–14) and dissect into the calf.[458–460] Occasionally,

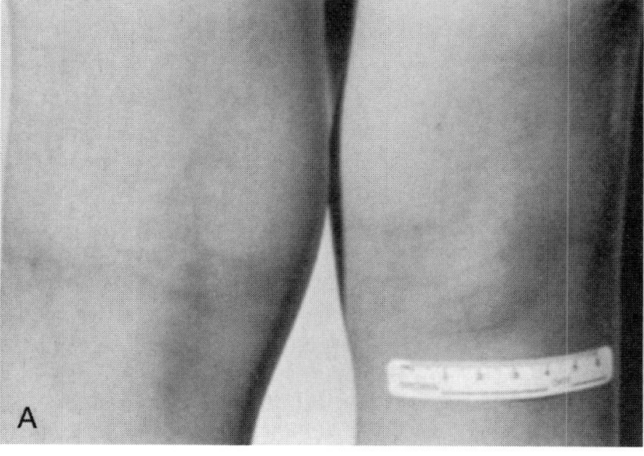

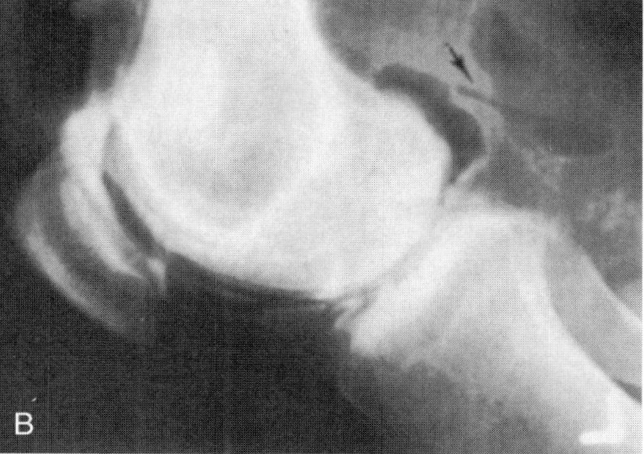

Figure 12–14. *A*, Popliteal cyst (Baker's cyst) in a young girl with oligoarticular JRA. The cyst was associated with pain at the back of the knee, was somewhat tender, and transilluminated. Aspiration yielded clear yellow fluid of low inflammatory activity. *B*, An arthrogram of a popliteal fossa cyst shows the contrast medium outlining the communication (*arrow*) between the synovial space and this dissecting cyst in an 18-year-old boy who has had JRA since the age of 9 years.

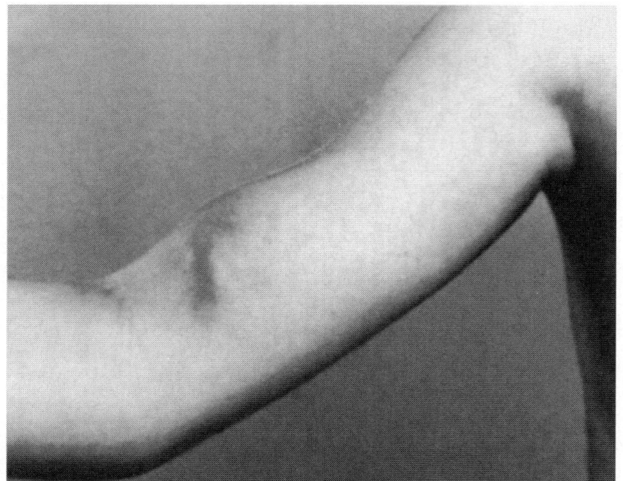

Figure 12–15. Brachial synovial cyst. A 6-year-old girl experienced this dissecting cyst of her right arm as the first manifestation of JRA. Later, bilateral effusions developed in both knees.

popliteal cysts rupture into adjacent calf muscles. This event is characterized by sudden sharp pain and swelling in the calf, followed by crescentic ecchymoses about the malleoli. A normal child may occasionally develop a transient popliteal cyst.[461] Less commonly, synovial cysts occur in the antecubital area or anterior to the shoulder.[462] Synovial cysts may be the initial or sole presentation of JRA and, when unilateral, may be misinterpreted as a tumor or as deep venous thrombosis (Fig. 12–15). Ultrasound imaging, magnetic resonance imaging, or arthrography aid in correct diagnosis.

Tenosynovitis

Tenosynovitis is more common in JRA than is usually appreciated, but it is generally not a striking or isolated clinical complaint. The most common sites of tenosynovitis are the extensor tendon sheaths on the dorsum of the hand, the extensor sheaths over the dorsum of the foot, and those of the posterior tibial tendon and the peroneus longus and brevis tendons around the ankle. Loss of extension of the fingers may result from stenosing synovitis of the flexor tendon sheaths and may be responsible, in part, for a claw-hand deformity.[463] Clinically recognized carpal tunnel syndrome is uncommon in children with involvement of the wrists. Tenosynovitis of the superior oblique tendon of the eye may cause pain on upward gaze, sometimes with diplopia, the *Brown syndrome*.[287, 464, 465]

EXTRA-ARTICULAR MANIFESTATIONS OF DISEASE

The frequency with which extra-articular complications occur during the course of JRA emphasizes the systemic nature of this disease (Table 12–14).[466] It should also serve to remind us that, on occasion, therapy induces systemic complications that may in themselves contribute significantly to morbidity.

Abnormalities of General Growth and Development

Abnormalities of growth and development are frequent complications of JRA or its treatment. Linear growth is retarded during periods of active systemic disease.[467, 468, 468a] Accelerated growth may occur with suppression of the active disease by therapy or during a remission. It is unusual, however, for a child who has suffered prolonged arrest or slowing of growth to return to the previous growth channel. Puberty and the appearance of secondary sexual characteristics are often delayed. Levels of growth hormone and insulin-like growth factors I and II are often normal in children with JRA but may be reduced.[469] Insulin-like growth factor I was low in the study of Davies and colleagues,[469] and in the investigation of De Benedetti and coworkers, inversely correlated with IL-6 levels in systemic disease.[151]

Many early studies commented on the general arrest of development, retardation of linear growth, asymmetry of development, or persistence of infantile proportions.[3, 11] In a study of 119 children, Ansell and Bywaters[467] found that long duration of active disease was associated with reduction of

Table 12–14

Estimated Frequency of Extra-Articular Manifestations in JRA by Onset Type

	POLYARTICULAR (%)	OLIGOARTICULAR (%)	SYSTEMIC (%)
Fever	30	0	100
Rheumatoid rash	2	0	95
Rheumatoid nodules	10	0	5
Hepatosplenomegaly	10	0	85
Lymphadenopathy	5	0	70
Chronic uveitis	5	20	1
Pericarditis	5	0	35
Pleuritis	1	0	20
Abdominal pain	1	0	10

linear growth even in children who had not received glucocorticoid drugs. During remission, height returned to normal in 2 to 3 years if premature epiphyseal fusion had not occurred. Stunting was severe only in children with long-standing, active disease. Similar findings were reported in the extensive prognostic investigation by Laaksonen[35] of 544 children with JRA. In a sequential study of height in 31 children with JRA,[468] about half were below the 3rd percentile for age and sex at the 5- to 7.5-year follow-up interval. However, 3 of 9 children were below the 3rd percentile at onset of disease. Undetected disease of some duration might have accounted for this finding.

In a study of 56 children between the ages of 4 and 18 years who had JRA for more than 1 year, Bacon and White[470] found that mean height for age was below the 35th percentile for children with polyarticular and systemic JRA. Mean weight for age and weight per height were significantly diminished in those with polyarticular disease. In a study of adults who had had JRA, Lovell[471] documented growth retardation (height <5th percentile) in 50 percent of children with systemic onset, 11 percent of those with oligoarticular onset, and 16 percent of those with polyarticular onset. Glucocorticoid therapy could only partly explain these observations.

Glucocorticoid medications also result in measurable growth retardation or may intensify that initiated by the disease.[472, 473] Growth retardation is evident in children treated with prednisone in a dose estimated to be equal to or greater than 5 mg/M^2/day for 6 months or more.[474] Laaksonen and colleagues,[475] however, found that glucocorticoids in this dose range did not produce growth retardation when used for short periods.

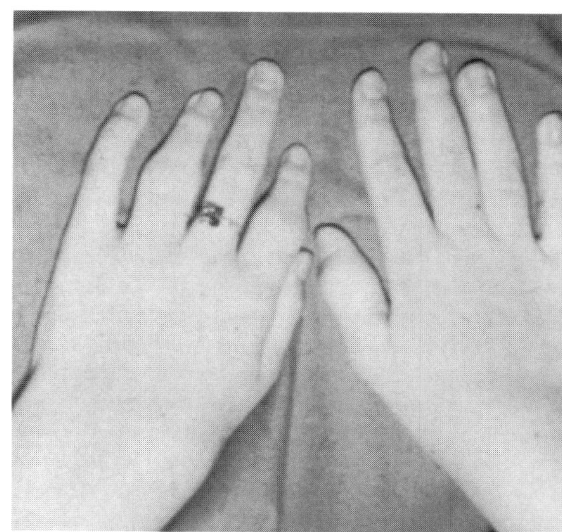

Figure 12–16. Arthritis of the second and fourth proximal interphalangeal joints on the left hand, associated with brachydactyly of those fingers.

Localized Growth Disturbances

Localized growth disturbances result from destruction of a growth center, accelerated development of ossification centers of the long bones of an inflamed joint, or premature fusion of the physis. Brachydactyly of the digits develops from premature closure of the epiphyseal growth plates. During early active disease, development of the ossification centers is accelerated, apparently related to the hyperemia of inflammation. The ultimate result may be either overgrowth of the affected limb or premature fusion of the involved epiphyses, resulting in diminished length.[70, 72, 383] This latter phenomenon may be widespread and symmetric, resulting in small hands and feet, or it may be isolated, as in the example of brachydactyly illustrated in Figure 12–16.

Arthritis of the lower limb, especially of the knee, frequently causes accelerated growth and epiphyseal maturation. If this occurs in one knee only, a discrepancy of leg lengths occurs.[383, 476, 477] Only rarely does premature epiphyseal fusion result in shortening of the affected leg. Although accurate clinical measurement of leg length is difficult,[478] a good estimate can be obtained by (1) measuring the distance from the superior anterior iliac spine to the medial malleolus in the supine position, (2) estimating leg lengths with the child in a supine position by comparison of malleolar symmetry, or (3) using a set of boards of calibrated thickness to determine which is required to level the iliac crests when the child is standing. A difference of greater than 0.5 cm is probably significant, and differences of 5 cm or more occasionally occur. Inability to completely extend both knees makes these measurements invalid, however, and under these circumstances, visual comparison of the heights of the equally flexed knees in a supine position gives some indication of the presence of a leg-length inequality. Apparent leg-length inequality may also result from pelvic rotation and scoliosis. As the child grows, inequalities of minimal to moderate degree may disappear, but they persist in up to two thirds of these children.

Whether the long-term result is shortening or lengthening of the affected limb appears to depend considerably on the age of the child or, more precisely, the degree of maturation of the skeleton at the time of the inflammatory insult. If the child is very young and the potential for growth considerable, the affected limb tends to grow longer. If the disease occurs shortly before the physis would be expected to fuse, shortening of the affected limb is more likely.[467, 479]

Micrognathia is a striking example of localized growth retardation (Fig. 12–17). Marked alterations of facial morphology (bird-face deformity) may result.[480–482] In a Swedish survey of 70 children with active JCA, 56 percent had symptoms (crepitus, pain, difficulty opening the mouth) and 41 percent had radiographic evidence of temporomandibular joint pathology attributable to arthritis.[483] In 1 patient, the disease began in a temporomandibular joint. Another study corroborated the frequency (50 percent) of temporomandibular joint abnormalities and alterations in mandibular growth in JRA.[484] Extreme micrognathia is most likely if arthritis begins before 4 years of age.

The mandible ossifies by intramembranous bone production. Its growth is affected by a number of factors, two of which contribute to mandibular growth abnormalities:

Pain in a temporomandibular joint may inhibit normal masseter muscle development, which in turn retards mandib-

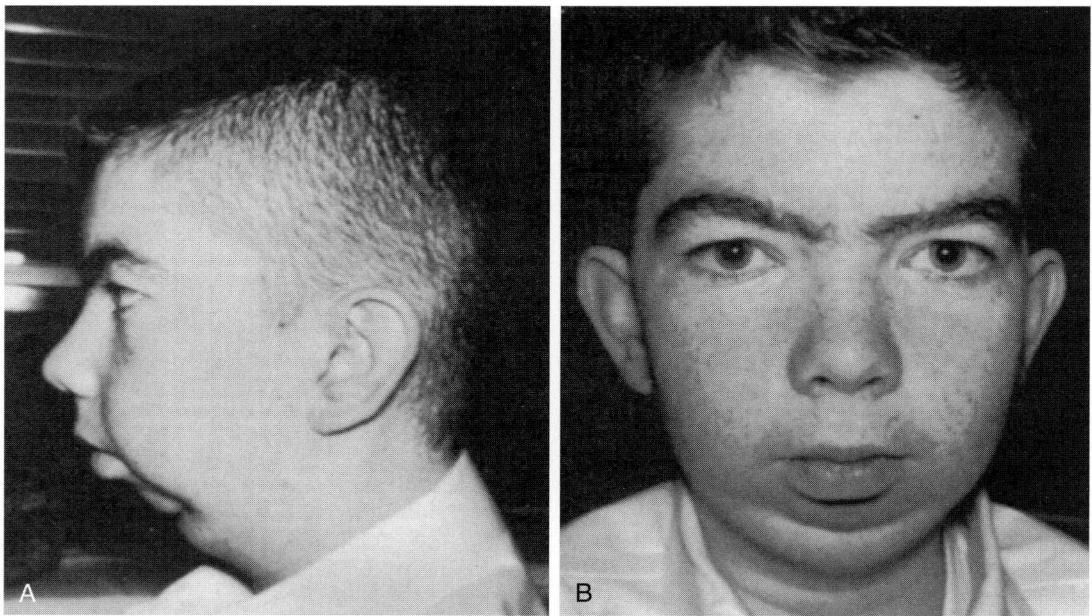

Figure 12–17. *A*, JRA began in this young man at the age of 2 years and has pursued an unremitting polyarticular course. Disease of both temporomandibular joints has caused micrognathia and retrognathia, with an anterior open underbite. *B*, Frontal view of the same patient.

ular bone development, resulting in a shortened mandibular ramus and body.

Destruction of the condyle of the mandible causes further diminution of overall mandibular height.

In some children, overgrowth of the condyle may contribute to temporomandibular joint dysfunction.[485] An association of micrognathia and arthritis of the apophyseal joints of the cervical spine per se has been asserted in a number of studies,[486–492] but this observation may not be valid. Although the stereotypical mandibular abnormality associated with JRA is bilateral micrognathia with an anterior open overbite, unilateral temporomandibular joint disease is much more common than bilateral disease. It is characterized by mandibular asymmetry; deviation to the affected side on opening the jaw; difficulty in palpating the affected mandibular condyle; and pain, tenderness, or crepitus of one or both temporomandibular joints (Fig. 12–18).[493, 494] In many instances, temporomandibular joint arthritis appears to be asymptomatic, although some children report a preference to chew on the unaffected side, experience pain with maximal opening of the mouth, or are aware of clicking or other sounds accompanying movement of the joint. Little is understood about the effect of JRA on dental caries or periodontal disease.[495]

Osteopenia

Osteopenia has emerged as a potentially major determinant of functional outcome in young adults who have had JRA.[496–501] Children with chronic arthritis develop a diminished bone mass compared with normal children and thereby are at increased risk for fractures

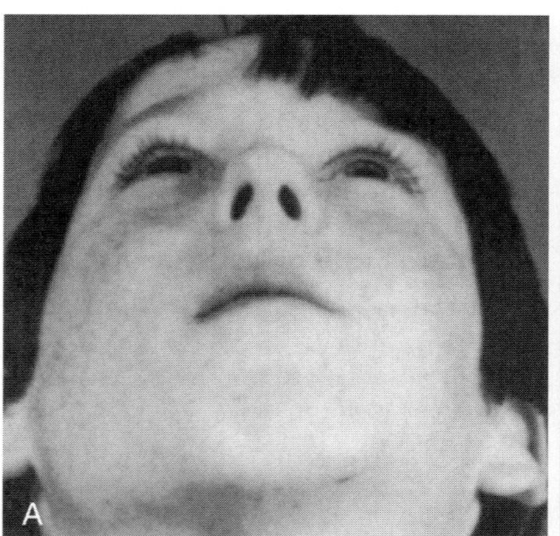

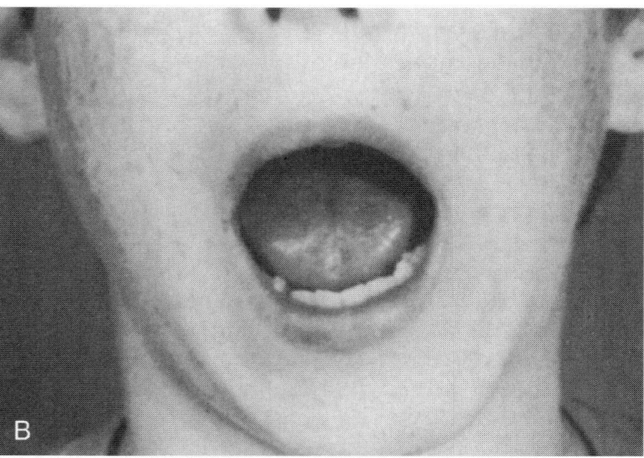

Figure 12–18. *A*, Unilateral temporomandibular joint disease on the left has resulted in underdevelopment of the left side of the mandible and face. *B*, Asymmetry of opening of the mouth in the same patient, caused by left-sided temporomandibular joint disease. The mandible moves toward the affected side when the mouth is open.

in adulthood and for earlier onset of osteoporosis, although only a few studies specific to that hypothesis are currently available.[502, 502a, 502b] An important determinant of future fracture risk is the peak bone mass achieved by the end of skeletal maturation, which is nearly complete by the late years of adolescence.[503]

Although bone mineral density may be decreased at all sites in children with JRA,[504] the appendicular skeleton is predominantly affected.[499] Failure to develop adequate bone mineralization is virtually universal in children with JRA and is predominantly characterized by inadequate bone formation for age, low bone turnover,[505, 506] and depressed formation instead of increased bone resorption. A failure to undergo the normal increase in bone mass during puberty is common in children with JRA, in whom bone formation must exceed resorption for skeletal growth, and markedly decreases their potential to achieve an adequate peak skeletal mass. Thus, onset of accelerated skeletal maturation with puberty is a critical period of potential medical intervention. Conversely, therapeutic maneuvers later during adolescence offer less promise of reversal of inadequate bone mineralization.

One aspect of this problem is the nutritional status of the child. Many children with chronic diseases are poorly nourished; this is no less true for children with chronic arthritis. Protein–energy malnutrition has been estimated to occur in 10 to 50 percent of children with JRA.[507, 508] Some anthropometric measurements indicate that subcutaneous fat in these children is normal or increased.[509, 510] However, malnutrition in these patients is indicated by diminished arm muscle circumference and low serum levels of the short-half-life proteins, retinol-binding protein and prealbumin. These findings are consistent with the fact that when malnutrition is complicated by inflammation, weight loss tends to come from lean body mass such as skeletal muscle rather than from fat.[511]

Children with active JRA are often anorectic, and in one study, their dietary intake was only three quarters of the recommended dietary allowance for age.[512] A number of factors contribute to decreased food intake. Inflammatory mediators such as IL-1 and TNF-α are increased in children with JRA and have been shown to cause anorexia.[513] Anorexia occurs in children with liver disease, a potential complication of systemic-onset JRA. Gastritis associated with anti-inflammatory medications contributes further to a poor appetite. Occasionally, temporomandibular joint pain inhibits adequate food consumption.

Organ-Specific Extra-Articular Manifestations

Skin and Subcutaneous Tissue

Nodules

Rheumatoid nodules occur in 5 to 10 percent of children with JRA, almost always confined to those with polyarthritis (Fig. 12–19).[514–516] Nodules are most frequently below the olecranon, but they also occur at other pressure points, on the digital flexor tendon sheaths, Achilles tendons, and occiput, as well as on the bridge of the nose in a child who wears glasses.

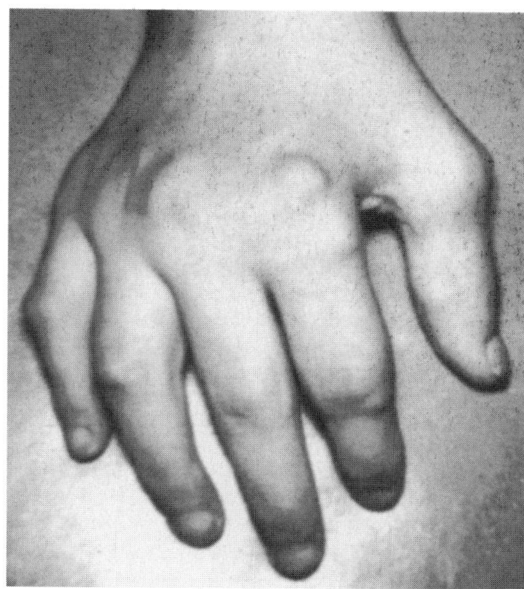

Figure 12–19. Multiple rheumatoid nodules over the metacarpophalangeal (MCP) and proximal interphalangeal joints were a constant feature of polyarticular JRA in this girl. They appeared over joints, pressure points, and tendon sheaths. Note also the radial deviation of the second and third MCP joints, the ulnar deviation of the radiocarpal joint, and the loss of extension of the interphalangeal joint of the thumb.

Typical rheumatoid nodules are firm or hard, usually mobile, and nontender. The overlying skin may be erythematous. They may be solitary or multiple, may change in size over time, and may persist for months to years. They are almost always associated with RF seropositivity and in this respect are generally regarded as a poor prognostic sign. Rheumatoid nodules must be distinguished from those of rheumatic fever and the so-called benign rheumatoid nodules that are not associated with objective arthritis (Table 12–15).

Benign rheumatoid nodules or *pseudorheumatoid nodules* occur as isolated abnormalities in otherwise healthy children (Fig. 12–20).[517–522] They are painless, may be single or multiple, and sometimes become quite large (>5 cm). They occur espe-

Table 12–15

Nodules in Children With Rheumatic Diseases

Rheumatoid nodules	Polyarticular JRA
Benign rheumatoid nodules	No associated disease
Deep granuloma annulare	No associated disease
Rheumatic fever nodules	Acute rheumatic fever
Extensor sheath nodules	Scleroderma
Calcinotic nodules	Scleroderma Dermatomyositis
Erythema nodosum	Postinfectious
Superficial aneurysms	Polyarteritis nodosa

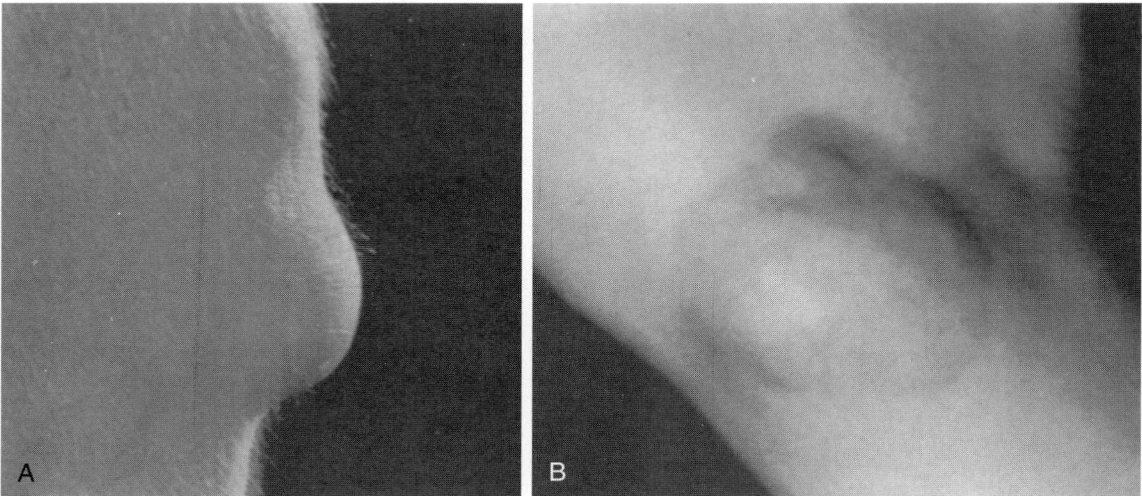

Figure 12–20. *A,* A large benign rheumatoid nodule overlies the tibial tubercle in this young boy. *B,* The lesion of granuloma annulare is histologically indistinguishable from the benign rheumatoid nodule shown in *A.* (*B,* Courtesy of Dr. J. Prendiville).

cially over bony prominences such as the anterior tibia or scalp and are characterized by spontaneous regression and recurrence. They frequently recur after surgical excision. In a very few patients, arthritis may develop at an older age.[521] RF and ANA are absent. Histologically, they resemble the nodules of adult RA. *Subcutaneous granuloma annulare,* a relatively common disease in children, may be histologically indistinguishable from either rheumatoid or pseudorheumatoid nodules.[523] Its clinical appearance, location (shins, dorsum of the foot), umbilicated appearance, and the absence of other disease confirm the diagnosis. Other diseases such as *multicentric reticulohistiocytosis* are associated with subcutaneous nodules (see Chapter 36).[524]

Skin Involvement

The classic rheumatoid rash of systemic-onset JRA has already been described. A second cutaneous change, occurring particularly in children with polyarticular JRA affecting the small joints of the hands, is a dark discoloration of the skin over the PIP joints.[525] The presence of this finding may reflect disease chronicity. In children with tender joints, retention keratosis may simulate a pigmented lesion. The presence of psoriasis or typical nail pitting should suggest the diagnosis of juvenile psoriatic arthritis rather than JRA (see Chapter 14).

Lymphedema

Asymmetric lymphedema of the subcutaneous tissues of one or more extremities has been documented in several children with JRA.[526–528] The swelling is usually painless and may be somewhat pitting (Fig. 12–21). The cause is unknown except for its relationship to inflammation, but it does not seem to be related to local obstruction caused by joint swelling. The course is chronic but may improve over several years. Treatment includes the use of pressure "stockings" or "gloves."

Vasculitis

Rheumatoid vasculitis is rare and occurs most often in the older child with RF-positive polyarthritis (Table 12–16) (Fig. 12–22). This devastating, widespread, small to medium-sized vessel involvement must be distinguished from benign digital vasculitis (Fig. 12–23), which is more frequent, and may occasionally be associated with vascular calcification that is apparent

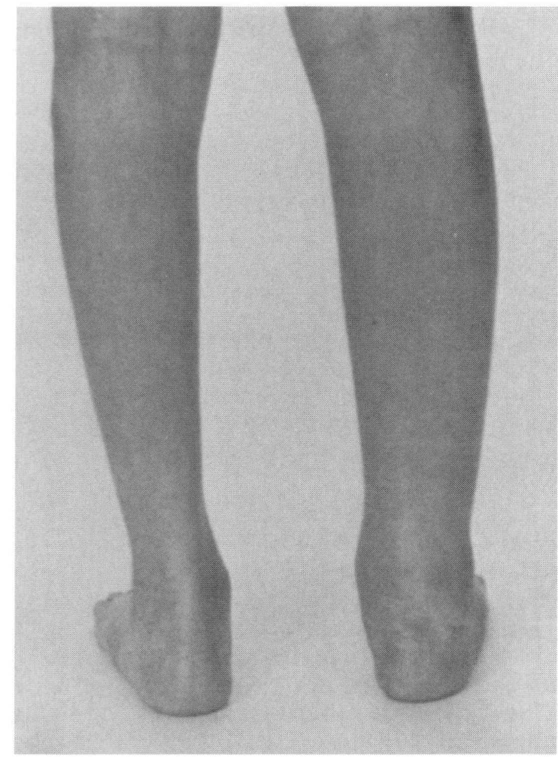

Figure 12–21. Lymphedema of the leg in a 10-year-old girl with long-standing oligoarticular JRA. Edema extended to mid-thigh.

Table 12–16

Clinical Features of Rheumatoid Vasculitis

Fever
Peripheral neuropathy
Cutaneous ulcers
Digital arteritis
Raynaud's phenomenon
Gastrointestinal hemorrhage
Mesenteric thrombosis
Myocardial infarction
Nephritis

on radiographs along the course of the digital arteries.[529, 530, 583]

Pityriasis lichenoides et varioliformis acuta (PLEVA or Mucha-Habermann disease) has been recorded in a few children with JRA,[531, 532] scleroderma,[531] Takayasu's arteritis,[533] polyarteritis nodosa,[532] Wegener's granulomatosis,[534] and other vasculitides[532, 535] (see Chapters 28 through 30). These are rare occurrences, however, and may be entirely coincidental.

Muscle Disease

Atrophy and weakness of muscles around inflamed joints is characteristic of JRA and is often accompanied by a shortening of the muscles and tendons that gives rise to flexion contractures. A nonspecific myositis may account for some of the associated fatigue and muscle weakness. It does not have a characteristic distribution, and histopathologic studies are sparse. Data from adults with RA suggest that it is characterized by perivasculitis and lymphocytic infiltrates (lymphorrhages). Serum levels of muscle enzymes are not increased. Rarely, a large, tender erythematous area of epidermal and dermal inflammation and myositis develops as part of acute systemic disease. A few children with systemic disease and widespread, prolonged, active arthritis develop profound and progressive muscle atrophy, which is most severe and persistent if it occurs before 3 years of age.[477] Isaac's syndrome (neuromyotonia) has been described in a young girl with systemic-onset JRA.[536]

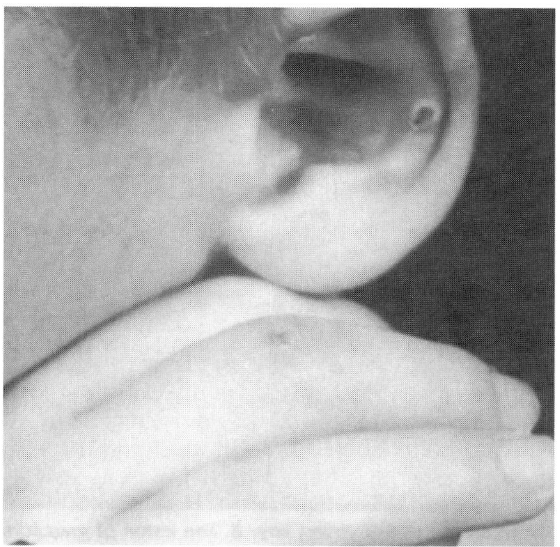

Figure 12–22. Systemic necrotizing vasculitis in a 6-year-old boy with systemic JRA. He developed widespread cutaneous and visceral vasculitis that led to his death 1 year after onset of disease.

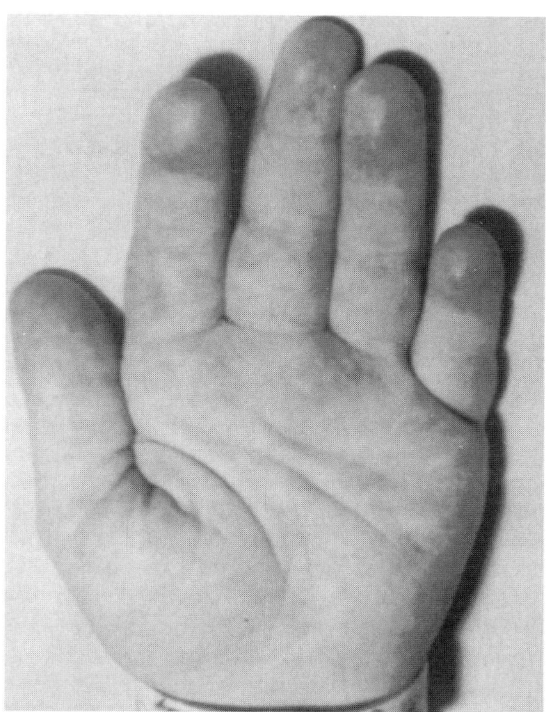

Figure 12–23. Punctate erythema of the palms and finger pads was the sole manifestation of benign perivasculitis in this 5-year-old girl with JRA. The lesions were not raised or tender, and they disappeared after treatment with nonsteroidal anti-inflammatory drugs.

Cardiac Disease

Pericarditis

The overall prevalence of pericardial involvement in JRA is estimated at 3 to 9 percent.[537, 538] Pericarditis and pericardial effusions occur almost exclusively in systemic-onset disease (Fig. 12–24).[538, 539–544] Pericarditis tends to occur in the older child, but it is not related to sex, age at onset, or severity of joint disease.[539] It may precede development of arthritis or occur at any time during the course of the disease, usually accompanied by a systemic exacerbation. Episodes generally persist for 1 to 8 weeks. Most pericardial effusions are asymptomatic, although some children have dyspnea or precordial pain that may be referred to the back, shoulder, or neck. Examination may document diminished heart sounds, tachycardia, cardiomegaly, and a pericardial friction rub, usually at the left lower sternal border (Table 12–17).[542] In many cases, pericardial effusions develop insidiously, are not accompanied by ob-

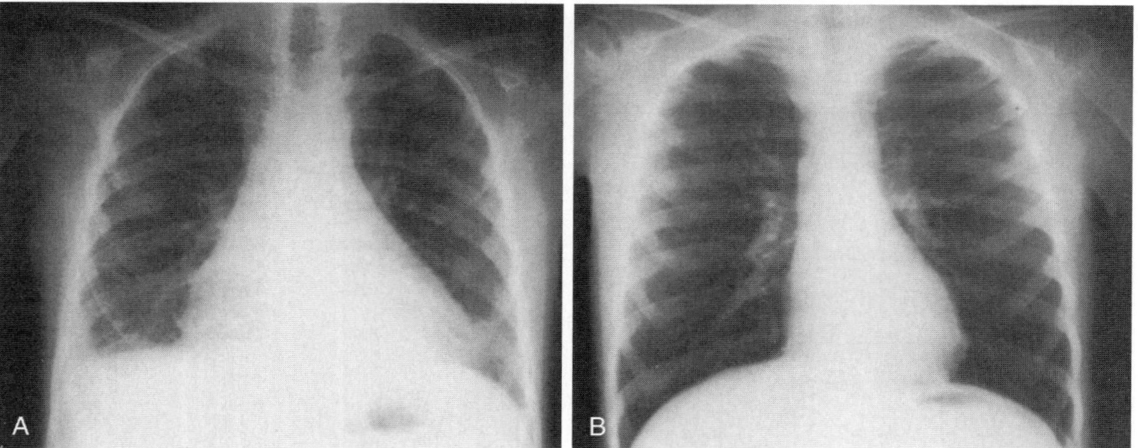

Figure 12–24. *A,* A chest radiograph shows an acute pericardial effusion in a 9-year-old girl with systemic-onset JRA at 3 years of age. The effusion was accompanied by precordial discomfort, dyspnea, and fever and lasted for 1 month. *B,* A chest radiograph taken 1 month later shows resolution of the effusion and pleural reaction.

vious cardiomegaly or electrocardiographic changes, and escape recognition except by echocardiography.[540, 543] In a study from Los Angeles,[543] an effusion or pericardial thickening was present in 36 percent of patients; 81 percent of children who had active systemic manifestations at the time of the study had abnormal echocardiographic findings (low voltage, ST segment elevation, diffuse T-wave inversion). In more than half, pericarditis would not have been diagnosed without echocardiography.

Tamponade is rare[537, 538, 541, 544–547] and is characterized by venous distention, hepatomegaly, and peripheral edema. Pulsus paradoxus (wherein the pulse volume and systolic blood pressure decrease during deep inspiration) can be demonstrated. An enlarged cardiac silhouette is present on chest radiograph, and pericardial fluid is confirmed by echocardiography. Chronic constrictive pericarditis is very rare[541, 545, 546, 548] and is characterized by pulsus paradoxus, a small heart, venous distention, ascites, and peripheral edema. In general, children with pericarditis do not fare worse than others in outcome; this complication should not necessarily be regarded as a poor prognostic sign, although pericarditis is frequently present in children with JRA who die.[539, 542]

Table 12–17

Manifestations of Pericarditis in Children With JRA

Symptoms:	Precordial pain	38%
	Dyspnea	20
Signs:	Tachycardia	83
	Friction rub	67
	Tachypnea	60
Investigations:		
Radiography: Cardiomegaly		71
Electrocardiography:		
ST segment elevation		31
T wave abnormality		71
Echocardiography: Effusion		>90

Modified from Brewer E Jr: Juvenile rheumatoid arthritis—cardiac involvement. Arthritis Rheum 20(Suppl): 231, 1977.

Myocarditis

Myocarditis is much less common than pericarditis and may result in cardiomegaly and congestive heart failure.[418, 549, 549a] In 3 children reported by Miller and French,[549] failure occurred in the absence of overt pericardial effusions in children with severe active systemic disease. At necropsy, diffuse myocardial changes typical of congestive cardiomyopathy were present in 1 child. Goldenberg and colleagues[538] reported 4 children with perimyocarditis and 2 with myocarditis in a retrospective study of 172 children with JRA.

Endocarditis

Valvular disease, seemingly unrelated to other causes, has been documented in more than 10 children with JRA (Table 12–18).[542, 544, 550–556] Eight had aortic insufficiency, and 2 had mitral insufficiency. Sudden deterioration in cardiac function may occur: Valve replacement was necessary in some of these patients.

Pleuropulmonary Disease

Parenchymal pulmonary disease is rare, but diffuse interstitial fibrosis occurs in a small number of children[557–560] and may precede other evidence of JRA.[561–563] Athreya and colleagues[559] noted interstitial disease in 8 of 191 children with JRA, all of whom had a systemic onset. Another report detailed pathologic findings in a child who died of pulmonary fibrosis.[557] Pulmonary function studies in 16 children with JRA documented abnormalities in 10 of them.[561] In some children, these may be the result of respiratory muscle weakness.[564, 564a] Pleural effusions may occur with carditis or may be

Table 12–18

Children With JRA and Valvular Heart Disease

AUTHOR (REF.)	SEX	ARTHRITIS: Age at Onset (Years)	ARTHRITIS: Type of Onset*	RF	VALVULAR DISEASE: Type	VALVULAR DISEASE: Age at Onset (Years)	TREATMENT	OUTCOME
Brewer[542]	—	—	O	—	MI	After 11 mo of arthritis	—	—
	—	—	—	—	MI	After long-standing disease	—	—
Leak et al[551]	F	9.5	P	Pos	AI	12	Prosthesis, chlorambucil	Good
	F	10	P	Pos	AI	16	Prosthesis	Good
	F	8	P	Pos	AI	15	—	Died
	F	8	P	Pos	AI	18	None	Stable
Svantesson et al[544]	—	—	—	—	AI	—	—	—
Kramer et al[552]	F	2	S	—	AI	27	Prosthesis	Good
Hull et al[553]	F	0.6	O	—	AI	8	Chlorambucil	Improved
Delgado et al[554]	F	1.5	O	Pos	AI	9.7	Prosthesis	Good

*Type of onset: P = polyarthritis, O = oligoarthritis, S = systemic disease
AI, aortic insufficiency; MI, mitral insufficiency; RF, rheumatoid factor
Modified from Delgado EA, Petty RE, Malleson PN, et al: Aortic valve insufficiency and coronary artery narrowing in a child with polyarticular juvenile rheumatoid arthritis. J Rheumatol 15: 144, 1988.

asymptomatic and be detected only as incidental findings on chest radiographs. One child we observed had idiopathic pulmonary hemosiderosis as the first sign of JRA; another was described with primary pulmonary hypertension.[565] Pulmonary rheumatoid nodules as described in adult RA are rare in childhood.

Gastrointestinal Tract

Except for symptoms induced by medications,[565a] gastrointestinal (GI) tract disease is rarely described in children with JRA. Intestinal pseudo-obstruction[566] has been noted, and we have observed this complication in one 4-year-old girl with systemic-onset JRA. Peritonitis has been documented in two children.[567] Mast cell–associated gastritis was described in three children with RF-seronegative arthritis, although it was not certain whether the gastritis was directly associated with the arthritis or reflected treatment with NSAIDs.[568] In children with major GI tract disease, the possibilities of inflammatory bowel disease,[569] celiac disease,[333, 570, 571] or cystic fibrosis[572]—all of which may be associated with arthritis that resembles JRA—should be considered. Sjögren's syndrome is uncommonly identified in children with JRA but occasionally complicates RF-positive polyarthritis (see Chapter 23).[573, 574]

Lymphadenopathy and Splenomegaly

Enlargements of lymph nodes and spleen may occur alone or together and are characteristic of systemic-onset JRA. Marked symmetric lymphadenopathy is particularly common in the anterior cervical, axillary, and inguinal areas and may suggest the diagnosis of lymphoma. Mesenteric lymphadenopathy may cause abdominal pain or distention and lead to an erroneous diagnosis of an acute surgical abdomen.

Splenomegaly is common in systemic-onset disease and is generally most prominent within the first years after onset (Table 12–19). The degree of splenomegaly may be extreme (see Fig. 12–11), but it is uncommonly associated with Felty's syndrome (splenic neutropenia).[575, 576] However, we have treated an 11-year-old girl with polyarticular JRA, nodules, and RF seropositivity who had splenomegaly and marked neutropenia that responded to treatment with glucocorticoids. Functional hyposplenia (as in SLE) has not been reported in JRA.

Hepatic Disease

Hepatomegaly is less common than splenomegaly and occurs almost exclusively in children with systemic-onset disease. Moderate to marked enlargement of the liver is often associated with only mild derangement of functional studies and relatively nonspecific histopathologic changes.[577] This type of liver disease is most evident at onset and generally diminishes with time. Chronic liver disease does not occur. Massive enlargement of the liver is usually accompanied by abdominal distention and pain. Progressive hepatomegaly is characteristic of secondary amyloidosis. Unexplained acute yellow atrophy has been recorded.[578] Occasionally, a fatty liver is associated with glucocorticoid administration. Hepatitis (transaminasemia) related to NSAID therapy may occur (see Chapter 7). A rare, and apparently benign, transient elevation of serum alkaline phosphatase has been noted in several children with

Table 12–19

Splenomegaly in Children With Juvenile Rheumatoid Arthritis

Systemic-onset JRA	85%
Felty's syndrome	Rare, in polyarticular disease
Amyloidosis	Rare, in severe, prolonged disease
Hemophagocytic syndrome	Uncommon, in systemic disease

JRA.[579, 580] This abnormality presumably does not result from hepatotoxicity, although it may be confused with it. Reye's syndrome occasionally occurred in children treated with aspirin.[581] Intercurrent infection with varicella or influenza appears to precipitate this serious complication (see Chapter 7).

Neurologic Disease

Involvement of the central nervous system during the course of JRA is usually related to complicating factors such as metabolic derangement, salicylate toxicity, high fever, embolism, and other systemic disease.[582–584] In some children, central nervous system disease has been so overwhelming as to suggest a primary relationship with JRA.[585, 586] These reports may have represented unrecognized instances of Reye's syndrome. Cerebral and cutaneous vasculitis has been described in one child with RF-seropositive JRA.[587]

Renal Disease

Urinary tract abnormalities may occur as a complication of JRA or as toxic effects secondary to treatment.[588–590] Intermittent hematuria or proteinuria is an occasional finding in some children, but it should be noted that low-grade proteinuria and hematuria occasionally occur in normal children.[591] Microscopic hematuria and low-grade proteinuria may reflect the effects of medications, including NSAIDs, gold, or D-penicillamine. Abnormal urinary findings also raise the possibility that the child has vasculitis[592] or intravascular coagulation,[593] a disease such as SLE, or rarely amyloidosis.[594] Renal papillary necrosis has been described in a number of children and is thought to be partly related to NSAID use (see Chapter 7). Hypercalciuria has been identified as an additional cause of hematuria in some children.[595] Retroperitoneal fibrosis has been reported as a cause of renal failure and obstructive uropathy.[596]

In Anttila's study of 165 children with JRA,[588, 589] transient microscopic hematuria was observed in 23 percent, leukocyturia in 25 percent, and low-grade proteinuria in 42 percent. Recurrent or persistent hematuria (4 percent), leukocyturia (6 percent), and proteinuria (2 percent) were uncommon. Hematuria and leukocyturia were more frequent during the initial observation period. Proteinuria was associated with the presence of extra-articular disease, prolonged duration of active disease, and amyloidosis (40 percent of the children who died). Renal biopsy was performed in 35 percent of these children and showed minimal glomerular changes in 22 percent and tubular atrophy in 13 percent. Chronic pyelonephritis was a common finding at necropsy. Interstitial nephritis and gold-induced nephrotic syndrome were rare.

More recent studies of renal dysfunction in children with JRA suggest that abnormalities of tubular function are common.[597] Although the frequency of proteinuria (2.3 percent), hemoglobinuria (3.5 percent), erythrocyturia (4.1 percent), and leukocyturia (5.3 percent) were low in a study of 176 children with chronic arthritis, urinary β_2-microglobulin or *N*-acetyl-beta-glucosaminidase levels were elevated in 38.5 percent. Increased excretion of these proteins was associated with active polyarticular disease and was most frequent in children receiving slow-acting antirheumatic drugs or two or more NSAIDs. It is not clear whether these changes represent the effects of the disease or drug-related toxicity. It is our experience that when persistent urinary sediment changes are observed, they are most frequently related to medications (NSAIDs, gold), papillary necrosis, pyelonephritis, or the evolution of JRA into SLE.

Chronic Uveitis

One of the most devastating complications of JRA is chronic nongranulomatous uveitis.[21, 75, 598–600] It is predominantly a chronic, anterior, nongranulomatous inflammation affecting the iris and ciliary body—an iridocyclitis (Fig. 12–25). The posterior uveal tract, the choroid, is rarely affected clinically (Fig. 12–26). Papillitis has been reported in 3 patients,[75, 76, 601] and macular edema and degeneration have been described in 1 or 2 others.[602] Less common ocular complications include scleritis, episcleritis, and keratoconjunctivitis sicca. In Kanski's study,[603] only 3 of 131 children with chronic uveitis developed keratoconjunctivitis sicca.

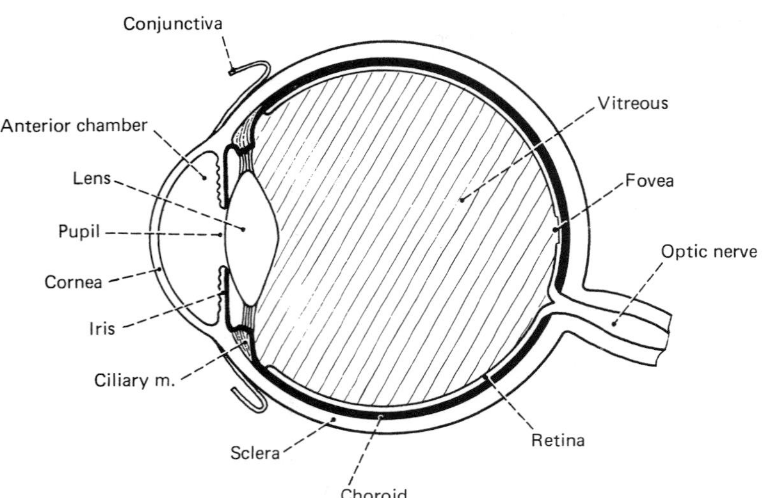

Figure 12–25. Schematic view of a sagittal section of the eye. Chronic anterior uveitis (iridocyclitis) involves the iris and ciliary muscle primarily, but secondary effects occur in the cornea, anterior chamber, lens, vitreous, and (rarely) retina.

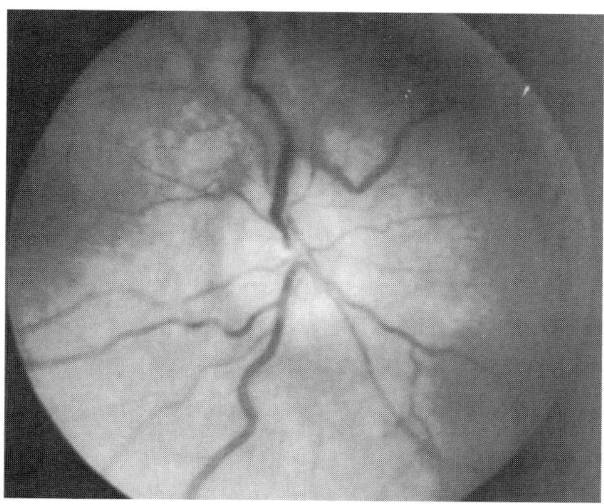

Figure 12–26. Retinal edema and hyperemia in the left eye, representing posterior uveitis in a 6-year-old girl with a 1-year history of JRA. She had minimal blurring of vision. Anterior uveitis and synechiae were also present.

Ohm[604] first described chronic uveitis and band keratopathy in a child with arthritis in 1910. The association of ocular disease and JRA was confirmed by several authors.[605–607] In Sury's patients,[21] chronic uveitis was found in 15 percent of the total, and two thirds of these patients had band keratopathy. The majority of his patients had an insidious onset of uveitis with little or no early disturbance of vision; diagnosis was often delayed until slit-lamp examination.

Epidemiology

Chronic uveitis is especially likely in young girls with oligoarthritis of early age at onset who are ANA seropositive (Table 12–20).[75, 76, 286, 598, 600, 608–616] On average, uveitis is found in 15 to 20 percent of children with oligoarticular JRA[326, 327, 617] and in about 5 percent of those with polyarticular-onset disease. Uveitis is rare in children with systemic-onset disease.[600, 602, 608, 618, 619]

Table 12–20

Characteristics of Children With JRA and Chronic Uveitis in Reported Series

	OVERALL	RANGE
Male:female	1:4.4	1:3 to 1:7.5
Age at onset of arthritis (yr)	4	2 to 5
Onset type (%)		
Oligoarticular	82	63 to 95
Polyarticular	18	7 to 37
Systemic	<1	0 to 6

From Petty RE: Current knowledge of the etiology and pathogenesis of chronic uveitis accompanying juvenile rheumatoid arthritis. Rheum Dis Clin North Am 13: 19, 1987.

The frequency of uveitis has varied considerably in reported series:

Laaksonen, 5.5 percent[35]
Minnesota, 4 percent[43]
Sweden, 10 percent[62]
Finland, 16 percent[45]
Turkey, 7 percent[620]
Greece, 12.5 percent[288]
Norway, 14 percent[57]

JRA with uveitis has been reported in whites, African-Americans, Hispanic Americans,[621] black and Indian South African children,[80] and Polynesians from New Zealand.[622] We have observed this complication in North American aboriginal children.

Etiology and Pathogenesis

The pathogenesis of chronic uveitis and the basis of its association with JRA are not known.[623] A hypothetical approach to understanding the pathogenesis of the disease is shown in Figure 12–27. Children with uveitis and JRA have a higher frequency of immunity to solu-

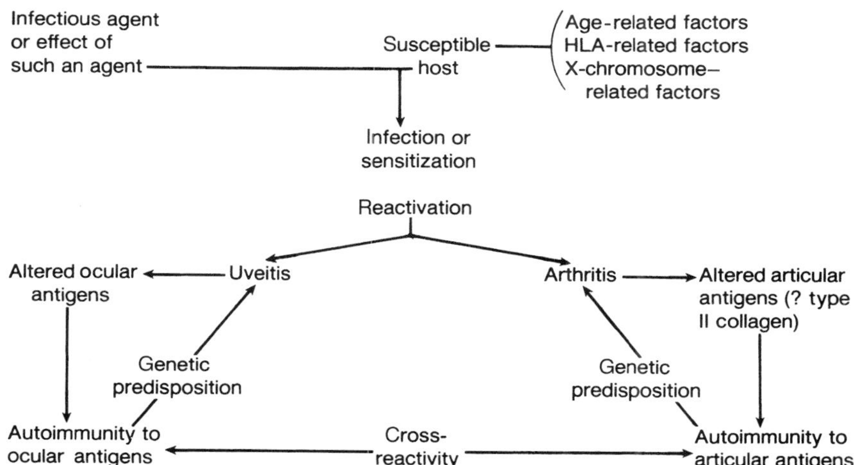

Figure 12–27. Hypothetical approach to the pathogenesis of chronic uveitis in children with chronic joint inflammation. (From Petty RE: Current knowledge of the etiology and pathogenesis of chronic uveitis accompanying juvenile rheumatoid arthritis. Rheum Dis Clin North Am 13: 19, 1987.)

ble retinal antigen (S antigen)[276, 624, 625] and to a low-molecular-weight iris antigen[626, 627] than children with arthritis alone. It is not clear whether immunity to these ocular antigens is pathogenic or merely reflects the inflammatory process.

Genetic Background

The most frequent alleles associated with early-onset oligoarthritis, ANA seropositivity, and uveitis are A2, DR5 (DRB1*1104), DR1 (DRB1*0101), DP2 (DPB1*0201), DQ1 (DQA1*0501), DR6, and DRw52.[286, 628, 629] Malagon and coworkers[286, 629] compared 72 children with early-onset oligoarticular arthritis and uveitis with 77 children with early-onset oligoarticular arthritis but no uveitis. They found that DR5 correlated with the presence of uveitis and DR1 correlated with its absence. The presence of DR8 had no association with uveitis but was increased in all children with oligoarthritis compared with controls. In the study by Melin-Aldana and colleagues,[630] DR5 (DRB1*1104) was significantly associated with an increased risk of uveitis along with DQA1*0501 and DQB1*0301, with which it was in linkage disequilibrium. A2 was significantly associated with anti-DEK antibodies, which occurred in 97 percent of children with uveitis.[293]

Clinical Manifestations

The onset of chronic uveitis is usually insidious and often entirely asymptomatic, although up to one half of the children have some symptoms attributable to the uveitis (pain, redness, headache, photophobia, change in vision) later in the course of their disease (Table 12–21). Uveitis is detected in less than 10 percent of patients before the onset of arthritis,[603] usually in the course of a routine ophthalmic examination. In almost half of all patients with uveitis, it presents just before, at the time arthritis is diagnosed, or shortly thereafter.[75, 603, 615] Most children develop uveitis within 5 to 7 years of onset of arthritis, although the risk is never entirely absent[75, 77, 609, 631] (Fig. 12–28). The disease is bilateral in approximately 70 to 80 percent of children.[75, 598, 614] Patients with unilateral disease are unlikely to develop bilateral involvement after the first year of disease; however, there are exceptions, and unilateral uveitis may persist for many years in a few children before the other eye is involved.

The early detection of chronic uveitis requires slit-lamp biomicroscopy, which should be performed at the time of diagnosis in every child with JRA and repeated at prescribed intervals during the first few years of the disease. The frequency of ophthalmic examinations is influenced by the level of risk of uveitis (Table 12–22). We recommend that slit-lamp examinations be performed every 3 months for the first 2 years in children in the high-risk group (early age at onset, oligoarthritis, female sex, ANA seropositivity) and every 4 to 6 months thereafter for a period of 7 years at a minimum (Table 12–23). In children with polyarticular disease, slit-lamp examinations should be done initially at 4- to 6-month intervals. In children who have a systemic onset, examinations once a year after the first year are probably sufficient. Any child who has had uveitis should be considered at high risk, even if it has remitted, and continued surveillance is mandatory.

The earliest signs of uveitis on slit-lamp examination are the presence of inflammatory cells and increased protein concentration ("flare") in the aqueous humor of the anterior chamber of the eye (Fig. 12–29). Deposition of inflammatory cells on the inner surface of the

Table 12–22

Factors Determining the Risk of Uveitis in Children With JRA

FACTOR	LOW RISK	HIGH RISK
Sex	Male	Female
Age at onset of arthritis	>6 yr	<6 yr
Type of onset of arthritis	Systemic	Oligoarticular
Duration of arthritis	>4 yr	<4 yr
ANA	Absent	Present
RF	Present	Absent

ANA, antinuclear antibody; RF, rheumatoid factor.

Table 12–21

Ocular Signs and Symptoms in Children With Chronic Uveitis and Arthritis

CHARACTERISTIC	MEAN	RANGE
Bilateral uveitis (%)	64	25–89
Symptoms (%)		
Ocular pain and/or redness		0–25
Change in vision		0–20
Photophobia		0–8
Headache		0–6
None	65	51–97

From Petty RE: Current knowledge of the etiology and pathogenesis of chronic uveitis accompanying juvenile rheumatoid arthritis. Rheum Dis Clin North Am 13: 19, 1987.

Table 12–23

Frequency of Ocular Examinations in Children With JRA

In a child who has never had uveitis:
Oligoarticular onset
  At initial visit and every 3 mo for 2 yr, then every 4 to 6 mo for 7 yr, then once a yr
Polyarticular onset
  At initial visit and every 4 to 6 mo for 5 yr, then once a yr
Systemic onset
  At initial visit, then once a yr

In a child who has had uveitis:
With inactive ocular disease
  Every 3 mo
With active ocular disease
  As indicated by response to therapy

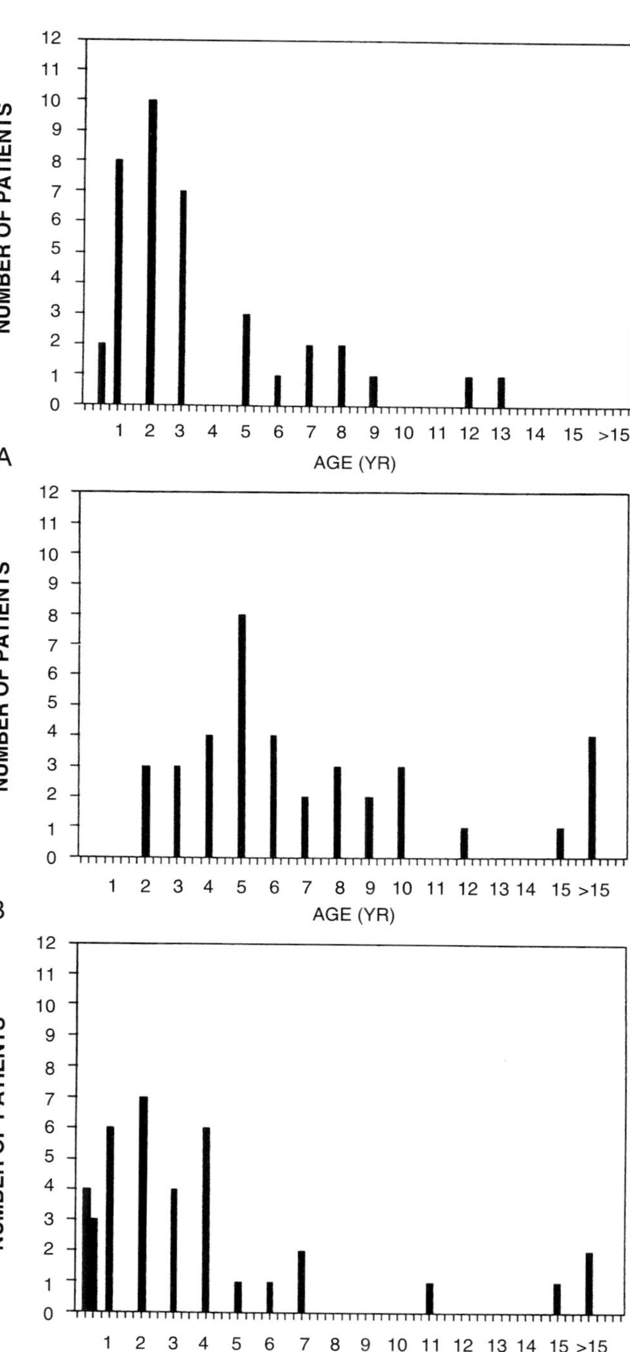

Figure 12–28. These graphs show the temporal relationships between arthritis and uveitis in children with JRA. *A,* The distribution of age at onset of arthritis in a series of 38 children who developed uveitis. *B,* The distribution of age at onset of uveitis in the same children. Note that in four patients, uveitis began after their 15th birthday: at 15½, 18, 31, and 39 years of age. *C,* Interval between the onset of arthritis and the diagnosis of uveitis in these patients. Note that for 1 patient the interval was 29 years, and for another, 34 years.

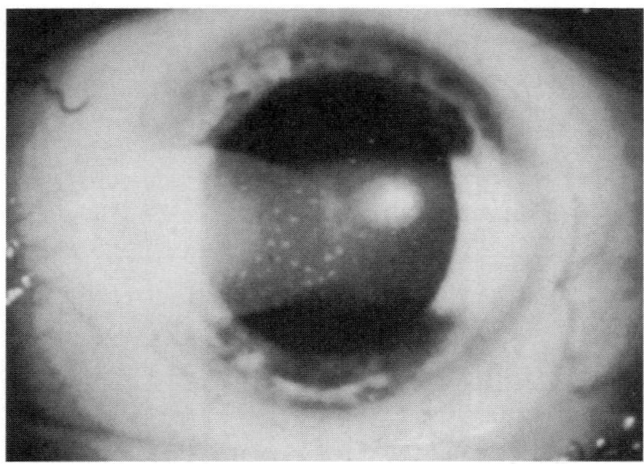

Figure 12–29. A slit-lamp examination shows "flare" in the fluid of the anterior chamber (caused by increased protein content) and keratic precipitates on the posterior surface of the cornea, representing small collections of inflammatory cells. (Courtesy of Dr. H. J. Kaplan.)

cornea (keratopunctate deposits or keratic precipitates) may develop later. Posterior synechiae between the iris and the anterior surface of the lens result in an irregular or poorly reactive pupil (Table 12–24) (Fig. 12–30). This abnormality may be the first obvious clue to the presence of uveitis on ophthalmoscopic examination, but it is unfortunately often a sign of disease of considerable duration or severity.

Band keratopathy occurs late (Fig. 12–31). Secondary cataracts are also common, but glaucoma and phthisis bulbi are rare late manifestations of uveitis. These complications are still occasionally encountered in some children with chronic uveitis in spite of vigorous and carefully monitored ophthalmic treatment, but such complications are less frequent now. Band keratopathy and cataracts occurred in 42 to 58 percent of patients in reported series, and glaucoma occurred in 19 to 22 percent.[619, 623, 632]

Pathology

Reports of the histopathology of uveitis are few. Descriptions of extremely severe, long-standing disease that led to blindness do not necessarily illuminate the pathogenic process.[633] Reported changes include increased iris vascularity[634] with scanty lymphocyte and plasma-cell infiltrates.[634, 635] Plasma cells containing IgM have been described in one patient.[636] Patients in whom granulomatous changes were present may have had sarcoidosis rather than JRA.[637, 638] Immunoglobulin levels were increased in the aqueous humor of children with JRA and uveitis.[639, 640] Studies of the vitreous showed an increased IgG concentration, activated C3c, and increased C1q binding, suggesting the presence of ICs.[641] Kaplan and associates[642] found that 90 percent of vitreous lymphocytes in one adult with uveitis and "juvenile" RA were B lymphocytes.

Table 12–24

Frequency of Complications of Chronic Uveitis in Reported Series

COMPLICATION	MEAN (%)	RANGE
Synechiae	62	37–75
Band keratopathy	37	11–56
Cataract	40	6–75
Glaucoma	18	8–25
Phthisis bulbi	9	0–14

From Petty RE: Current knowledge of the etiology and pathogenesis of chronic uveitis accompanying juvenile rheumatoid arthritis. Rheum Dis Clin North Am 13: 19, 1987.

Differential Diagnosis

Uveitis and arthritis occur together in a number of diseases with high frequency.[619, 643] Uveitis also occurs in children without evidence of joint involvement as an isolated disorder.[644] Inflammation of the anterior uveal tract is found in Kawasaki disease,[645] complicates JAS,[359] and is observed in children with psoriatic arthritis,[613, 646] arthropathy of inflammatory bowel disease,[647–649] and Reiter's syndrome.[650, 651] Uveitis also occurs in NOMID,[652–655] sarcoidosis,[637, 638, 656, 657] Blau's syndrome,[658, 659] Vogt-Koyanagi-Harada syndrome, and Behçet's disease.[619] Posterior uveitis is rare and should suggest the diagnosis of sarcoidosis rather than JRA.

Laboratory Examination

The most common laboratory abnormality associated with chronic uveitis is ANA seropositivity. ANAs are usually present in low titer (<1:640) and for the most part are of unknown specificity.[76, 603, 660–662] When tissue sections were used as substrate, ANAs were found with significantly higher frequency (65 to 88 percent) in children with oligoarticular JRA and uveitis than in those with oligoarticular JRA alone.[660, 661] Neuteboom and coworkers[663] found ANAs in 55 percent of children with uveitis and chronic arthritis with HEp-2 cells sub-

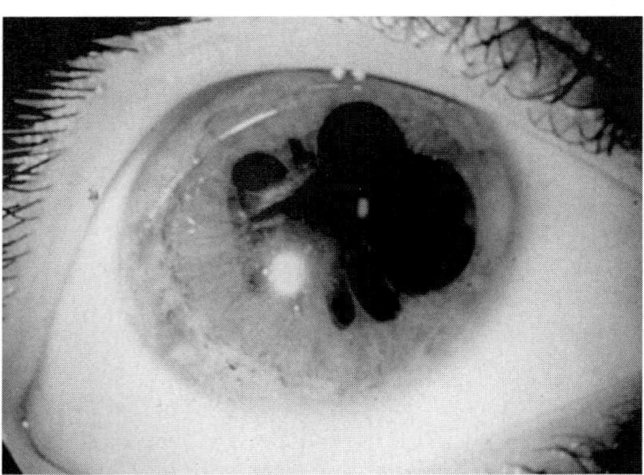

Figure 12–30. Left eye of a 7-year-old boy shows an irregular pupil that resulted from adhesions of the iris to the anterior surface of the lens.

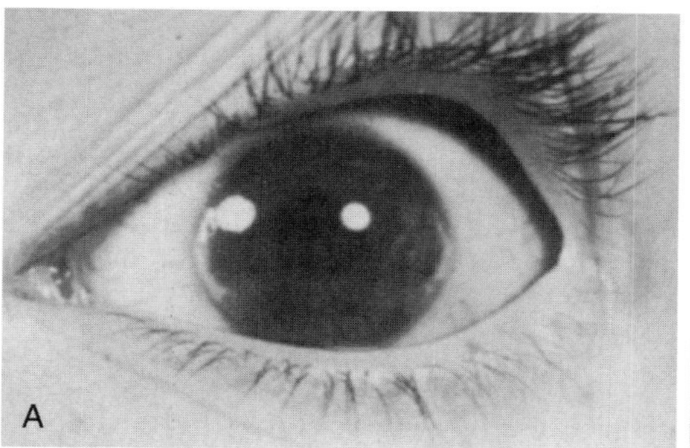

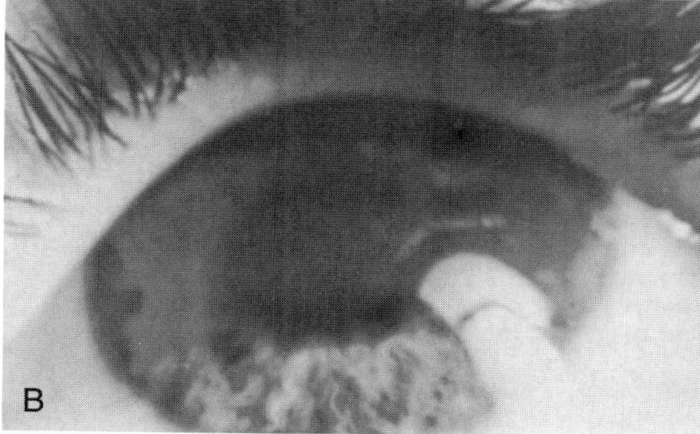

Figure 12–31. *A,* Early band keratopathy is noted as a semilunar band just inside the limbus medially and laterally. It does not extend across the pupil. *B,* The semiopaque band extends across the midplane of the cornea in this example of more advanced band keratopathy. It is fenestrated and does not extend to the limbus.

strate, but in only 32 percent when rat liver was used. They detected antibody to dsDNA in 3 of 22 and anti-SS-A in 1 of 22 children with uveitis. Using HeLa cells as a source of nuclear material, they also demonstrated reactivity of sera from children with arthritis and uveitis to a 15-kD antigen by Western blotting. With rare exceptions, antibodies to RNA or DNA in children with JRA and uveitis have not been detected.[357, 664] Reactivity to histones has been associated with oligoarticular disease and uveitis.[173, 175] Massa and colleagues[665] reported that ANA-seropositive patients had significantly elevated IgG antibodies to nucleosomes H3 and H4, to DNA-free subparticles, and to H3H4-DNA, but that these antibodies were generally not associated with uveitis.

Management

The treatment of chronic uveitis should be supervised by an ophthalmologist who is experienced in management of this complication.[666] The initial approach consists of glucocorticoid eye drops (dexamethasone or methylprednisolone) with or without a mydriatic to dilate the pupil and help prevent posterior synechiae. A short-acting mydriatic drug is preferred, given if possible once a day in the evening, so that pupillary dilatation does not interfere with school work and reading. Some data suggest that NSAIDs may be of some benefit.[667–669] Although this effect is not a major one, it should be considered when NSAID treatment of arthritis is altered.

In unresponsive disease, glucocorticoid drops may be given hourly during waking hours, with glucocorticoid ointment placed in the conjunctival sac at bedtime. Chylack[76] reported that 36 percent of children did not respond to topical glucocorticoids after 6 months of intensive therapy and therefore required systemic administration of the drug (Table 12–25). In a few instances, subtenon injections of glucocorticoid may be required. It may be advisable in more serious cases to employ supplemental oral prednisone in low dosage (e.g., 2 to 4 mg/day). Some children may require larger amounts of oral glucocorticoid; single daily or alternate-day therapy may be useful in these patients.[603] On rare occasions, we have used high-dose intravenous methylprednisolone (30 mg/kg) with benefit. Although the slit-lamp examination may return to normal soon after treatment is initiated, it is not advisable to discontinue steroids at that time because of the frequent reappearance of signs of inflammation. Long-term ophthalmic glucocorticoid administration may lead to the development of Cushing's syndrome. Methotrexate may be an effective mode of therapy in children with severe uveitis in whom all other forms of treatment have failed.[670, 671]

Chlorambucil,[672, 673] cyclosporin,[674] and plasmapheresis[675] may be useful in some cases of idiopathic uveitis, but their role in the uveitis of JRA is not clarified. Cyclosporin was given to 14 children with chronic uveitis refractory to glucocorticoids for a mean duration of 21 months.[676] Visual acuity was improved or did not deteriorate further in 92 percent of eyes, and results of the ophthalmic examination were improved in 76 percent. In a follow-up study, the same investigators studied the use of mycophenolate mofetil to treat 9 cyclosporin nonresponders.[677] Eight eyes improved in visual acuity; by ophthalmoscopy score, 5 were unchanged and 2 eyes worsened. Refractory uveitis has also been treated with intravenous immunoglobulin (IVIG).[678] Smiley[609] noted that neither adrenocorticotrophic hormone nor azathioprine had proved efficacious in controlling ocular inflammation. Gold salts and D-penicillamine are ineffective.

Band keratopathy has been treated with topical chelation and by lasers. Cataracts seldom interfere significantly with vision, but they may require surgical removal. The management of complicated uveitis and glaucoma remains unsatis-

Table 12–25

Therapeutic Response to Glucocorticoids and Mydriatics in Children With Uveitis and JRA

RESPONSE	(%)
Rapid response (<3 mo)	45
Slow response (3–6 mo)	13
No response (>6 mo)	36
Uncertain	6

Modified from Chylack LT Jr: The ocular manifestations of juvenile rheumatoid arthritis. Arthritis Rheum 20(Suppl): 217, 1977.

factory, but results of lensectomy or vitrectomy for complicated cataract are improved.[598] The subject of cataract surgery in children with JRA and uveitis is thoroughly reviewed by Hooper and coworkers.[679] It is their recommendation that cataract surgery be performed only in the absence of vitreous opacities, hypotony, or cyclitic membrane formation; that the anterior chamber be free of inflammatory cells; and that combining anterior segment surgery with a pars plana vitrectomy is the safest approach. Perioperative glucocorticoids are recommended. The timing of cataract extraction challenges the judgment of the ophthalmologist in weighing the danger of operation on an inflamed eye against the risk of amblyopia. Operative complications are minimized with microsurgery and cryoextraction.

Course of the Disease and Prognosis

Smiley[609] emphasized that the course of chronic uveitis is rarely less than 2 years and often as long as 17 or 18 years. Our experience and that of others,[600] however, indicates that some children have much shorter courses. The activity of the uveitis does not parallel that of the arthritis,[75, 77, 608, 609, 632, 680] and may occur for the first time after the arthritis is in remission. Visual loss may occur because of complications of the uveitis or as a result of amblyopia related to suppression of visual images from a cataract. Although prognosis for sight in chronic uveitis has been improving, visual outcome still remains far less than satisfactory, with estimates of blindness (<20/400 OU) as high as 15 to 30 percent.[75, 609, 614] It has been suggested that the frequency and severity of uveitis may actually be decreasing.[613, 615, 616, 681, 682] Whether this represents intrinsically less severe disease (a "benign" form of uveitis), earlier treatment, or more aggressive therapy is not certain.

The prognosis for uveitis is worse in children in whom the onset of uveitis occurs before diagnosis of arthritis or shortly thereafter.[598, 612, 615] It is also worse in those with an initial severe inflammatory response,[612] chronicity of inflammation,[286] or ANA seronegativity.[615] Kanski's review[598] of the Taplow experience confirmed that visual prognosis was good in 25 percent and fair in 50 percent of studied patients. The remaining 25 percent developed visual impairment from cataract or glaucoma. The visual outcomes of patients in six series are summarized in Table 12–26.

In the early Ann Arbor series, 3 children (8 percent) completely recovered from their uveitis and 55 percent retained normal vision.[75] However, 16 percent of the children were blind in one or both eyes. During the course of the disease, even minimal symptoms were associated with moderate to advanced ocular disease. Twenty-five children had protracted or recurrent ocular inflammation. A series of patients from the same center 10 years later[612] described an improved prognosis. Visual outcome was worse if uveitis was present at the time of diagnosis of arthritis and in children with persistently active disease. In the Taplow series, however, Kanski noted that 8 of 26 eyes with continuously active uveitis for more than 10 years remained unaffected by secondary complications and retained normal visual acuity.[603] Cabral and colleagues,[613] in 49 patients (82 affected eyes), reported that only 15 affected eyes had corrected visual acuity of 20/40 or worse, at an average of 9.4 years after onset of uveitis, and 8 had corrected visual acuity of 20/200 or worse. This study confirmed the correlations between a poor visual prognosis and the presence of uveitis at diagnosis of arthritis, complications (e.g., synechiae), and persistent disease activity.

PATHOLOGY

The histopathologic features of JRA are similar to those described in RA.[20, 683–685] In synovial biopsy specimens, there is villous hypertrophy and hyperplasia of the synovial lining layer (Fig. 12–32). The subsynovial tissues are hyperemic and edematous. Vascular endothelial hyperplasia is often prominent, along with infiltration by lymphocytes and plasma cells. There is a selective accumulation in the synovium of activated T cells, which are clustered around antigen-presenting dendritic cells. Fibrin may be layered onto the superficial surface of the synovium or incorporated within it. An exuberant inflammatory process eventually results in progressive erosion and destruction of articular cartilage, and later of contiguous bone with pannus formation. We have not observed rheumatoid nodules and necrotizing vasculitis in synovial tissue from chil-

Table 12–26
Visual Outcome of Uveitis in Children With JRA

SERIES	CHYLACK[76, 608]	SMILEY ET AL.[609]	CASSIDY ET AL.[75]	WOLF ET AL.[612]	KANSKI[598]	MALAGON ET AL.[286]	CABRAL ET AL.[1221]	DANA ET AL.[614]	CHALOM ET AL.[615]	KOTANIEMI ET AL.[600]
Year of publication	1975	1976	1977	1987	1990	1992	1994	1997	1997	1999
Frequency (%)	17.2		10.3		20				9.3	14
Number of patients	36	61	38	51	315	72	49	43	74	16
Number of affected eyes	72		67	89			82	76		24
Mean follow-up (yr)	14	10	4.8	12.7	7.3		9.4	12.2		6.8
Normal vision (%) ≥20/160	79	34	55	61	25	69	85	75	89	81
Visual loss (%) ≤20/200	22	66	45	39	25	31	15	25	11	19
Blind (%) ≤20/400										
Unilateral		13	5	24			8		0	6
Bilateral		16	11	5			2		0	0

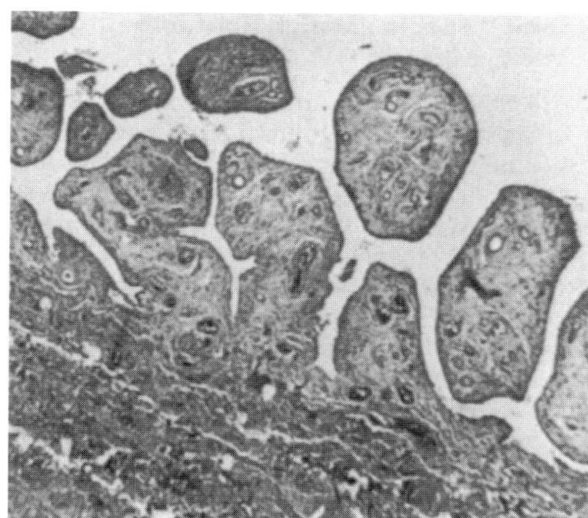

Figure 12–32. Photomicrograph of synovial tissue from the knee of a young boy with oligoarticular JRA shows villous hyperplasia and hypertrophy, edema, proliferation of new blood vessels, and infiltration by mononuclear cells.

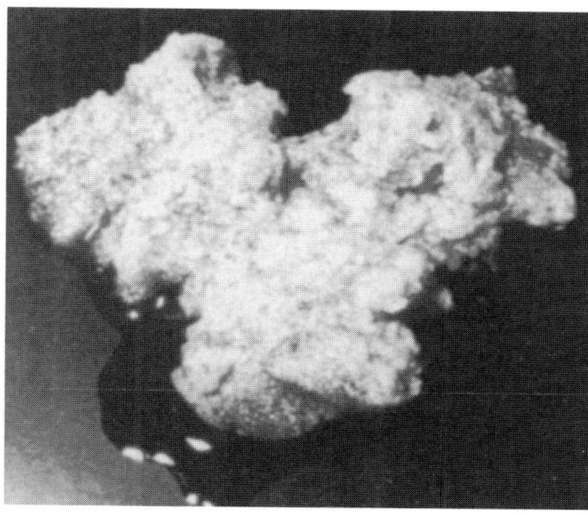

Figure 12–33. Rice bodies from the knee of a 15-year-old boy with persistent arthritis of knees and ankle.

dren with JRA. Oligoarthritis and polyarthritis cannot be distinguished on the basis of their synovial histopathology.[326, 686]

In RA, the primary infiltrating cell is the T lymphocyte, which may be distributed diffusely throughout the synovium or form nodules or germinal centers.[687] CD4+ helper-inducer T cells and CD8+ suppressor-cytotoxic T cells may be visible. In addition, macrophages and dendritic cells abound in mature synovitis. In late disease, B lymphocytes and plasma cells producing RF can be demonstrated. Multinucleated giant cells and mast cells are also present. Hypertrophy of synovial lining cells, fibroblasts, and blood vessels leads to the development of papillary fronds that may reach 2.5 cm × 0.2 cm in size. Extension of the inflammatory granulation tissue or pannus that spreads from the synovium and invades the cartilage and bone results in osteolysis, which is visible radiographically as erosion and subchondral cyst formation. Erosions occur preferentially in the "bare" areas of the joint where bone is not covered by articular cartilage (see Chapter 2). They are irregular but sharply defined. Dissolution of the cartilage (chondrolysis) results from enzymatic digestion by neutral proteases, cathepsin, and collagenase from cells of the pannus. ICs may also contribute to chondrolysis.[688] Metaplasia of the granulation tissue may result in formation of new cartilage, bone, or fibrous tissue, resulting in ankylosis.[687] End-stage disease is characterized by deformity, subluxation, and fibrous or bony ankylosis.

Joint destruction usually occurs much later in the course of JRA than in adult disease, and permanent joint damage is absent in many children with JRA even after years of chronic inflammation. (Newer studies with magnetic resonance imaging are likely to change our impression of the extent of joint damage in early disease.) The greater thickness of juvenile cartilage may offer some protection in this regard. The hyaline cartilage of the hip is destroyed in progressive stages during the course of severe JRA, and during healing it may be replaced by a fibrocartilaginous layer.[689] Rice bodies consist primarily of amorphous fibrous material, fibrin, and small amounts of collagen (Fig. 12–33).[690–692] Viable cells are incorporated within this matrix and appear more normal than the synovial cells of the inflammatory foci. The majority of these cells resemble type B synovial lining cells, although a few type A cells are also visible. Residual blood vessels in some of these bodies attest to their former attachment to the synovial membrane.

The rash of JRA is one of the most characteristic clinical hallmarks of the disease. It is characterized by minimal perivascular infiltration of mononuclear cells around capillaries and venules in the subdermal tissues.[385] A neutrophilic perivasculitis resembling that of the rash of rheumatic fever may accompany the more flagrant lesions.

Subcutaneous nodules may be histopathologically typical of rheumatoid nodules (Fig. 12–34) or they may have a looser connective tissue framework resembling that of the nodules of rheumatic fever.[514, 693] Classic rheumatoid nodules consist of three distinct zones: a central area of necrosis and granulation tissue surrounded by a radially arranged palisade of connective tissue cells that, in turn, is enveloped by chronic inflammatory cells. In JRA, the central area of fibrinoid necrosis and the epithelioid palisades may be absent or less structured.

The serosal lining surfaces of the pleural, pericardial, and peritoneal cavities of the body may exhibit nonspecific fibrous serositis that is characterized clinically by

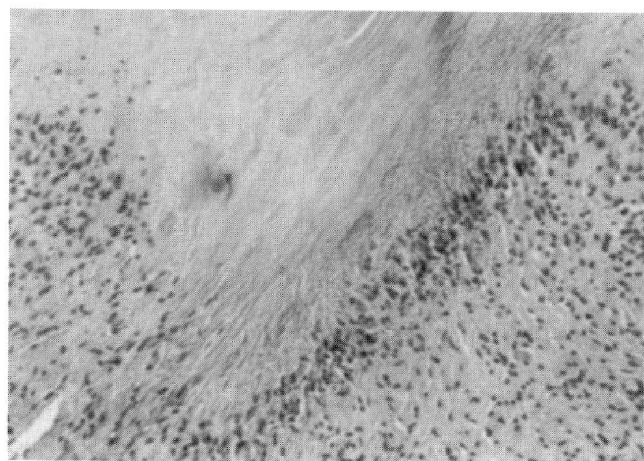

Figure 12–34. Photomicrograph of a rheumatoid nodule shows a central area of fibrinoid necrosis surrounded by a palisade of epithelioid cells and peripheral fibroblastic proliferation.

effusion and pain. Enlargement of the lymph nodes is related to a nonspecific follicular hyperplasia that in rare instances may closely resemble lymphoma. Hepatic abnormalities are characterized by a nonspecific collection of periportal inflammatory cells and hyperplasia of Kupffer's cells.

LABORATORY EXAMINATION

Although the laboratory may provide support for a diagnosis of JRA, that diagnosis is essentially clinical: no laboratory test or combination of studies can confirm the diagnosis of JRA. The laboratory can be used to provide evidence of inflammation, to support the clinical diagnosis of JRA, to monitor toxicity of therapy, and, as a research tool, to understand better the pathogenesis of the disease.

Blood Indices

Hematologic abnormalities reflect, in a general way, the extent of the inflammatory disease. Children with oligoarthritis seldom exhibit any hematologic aberrations beyond that of mild anemia (Table 12–27). Those with moderately extensive joint disease usually have a normocytic hypochromic anemia. The anemia may be moderately severe, with a hemoglobin in the range of 7 to 10 g/dl (70 to 100 g/L) in children with systemic onset.[694, 695] Although the anemia in JRA is attributable to chronic disease (low serum iron, low total iron-binding capacity, adequate hemosiderin stores),[694, 696] iron deficiency may also play a role.[696a] Plasma iron transport and iron available for erythropoiesis are reduced in systemic disease.[697] More severe anemia may respond to recombinant erythropoietin in combination with intravenous iron therapy.[697, 698] Serum ferritin is elevated in children with active JRA and correlates closely with systemic activity[699, 700]; in that sense, such elevations do not reflect iron stores but a response as an acute-phase reactant. Erythroid aplasia has been reported[701, 702]; hypoplastic crises in some instances may represent a virus-associated hemophagocytic syndrome[703–705] or the MAS.[409]

Leukocytosis is common in children with active disease, and leukocyte counts are strikingly high (30,000 to 50,000/mm^3; 30 to 50 $\times$ 10^9/L) in children with systemic-onset JRA. Polymorphonuclear leukocytes predominate. The platelet count may rise dramatically in severe systemic or polyarticular involvement; in disease of long standing, thrombocytosis may signal an exacerbation. Thrombocytopenia is rare[706] and may indicate an evolution of the disease into SLE.[358]

Erythrocyte Sedimentation Rate and C-Reactive Protein

The ESR is a useful measure of active disease at onset and during follow-up of a child with JRA, especially in polyarticular or systemic onset.[707] It is occasionally helpful in monitoring therapeutic efficacy of a medication program, although the ESR does not necessarily correlate with the articular response to medications.[708] The C-reactive protein may be a more reliable monitor of the inflammatory response; at least it is less often increased in a child in whom no clinical inflammatory disease can be found.[708, 709]

Serum Immunoglobulins

Increases in the serum levels of the immunoglobulins are correlated with activity of the disease and reflect the acute phase response.[166, 684, 710–713] Extreme hypergammaglobulinemia is present in the sickest children and returns toward normal with clinical improvement (Table 12–28). Viral antibody titers may also be increased in JRA,[714] but antibodies to rubella and rubeola viruses are usually similar to those of appropriate control groups or are associated with a polyclonal increase in immunoglobulin concentrations.[167, 715, 716]

Thirty-seven percent of 200 children with JRA had hypergammaglobulinemia, defined as a level of 1.96 S.D. or higher from normal, in at least one immunoglobulin class.[166, 713] The

Table 12–27

Laboratory Abnormalities in JRA

ABNORMALITY	POLYARTHRITIS	OLIGOARTHRITIS	SYSTEMIC ONSET
Anemia	+	−	+ +
Leukopenia	−	−	−
Thrombocytopenia	−	−	−
Leukocytosis	+	−	+ + +
Thrombocytosis	+	−	+ +
Antinuclear antibodies	+	+ +	−
Anti-dsDNA antibodies	−	−	−
Rheumatoid factors	+	−	−
Antistreptococcal antibodies	+	−	+
Hypocomplementemia	−	−	−
Elevated hepatic enzyme levels	+	−	+ +
Elevated muscle enzyme levels	−	−	−
Abnormal urinalysis	+	−	+

− = absent; + = minimal; + + = moderate; + + + = severe.

Table 12–28

Clinical Correlations of Increased Serum Immunoglobulin (Ig) Levels in Children With JRA

Highest Ig levels occur in children with:
  Polyarticular disease
  Systemic disease
  Poor functional class
IgM is increased more than IgG or IgA
IgM increase correlates with presence of rheumatoid factor and rheumatoid nodules
Elevations of IgM and IgG are greater in boys than in girls
Degree of elevation of IgA correlates with the presence of active disease and erosions

lowest values were found in children with oligoarthritis, including those who had uveitis. In general, persistent hypergammaglobulinemia was an important hallmark of a deteriorating clinical course and poor therapeutic response. Although increases in IgG concentrations were characteristic of early disease, IgA levels appeared to be associated with the extent of articular and systemic disease and might be a more sensitive indicator of the immunoinflammatory process. Selective IgA deficiency occurred in 4 percent of the children. In addition, abnormally low levels of IgA were more frequent than in normal controls (Fig. 12–35). No relation of immunoglobulin concentrations to age at onset or duration of disease was found. IgA and IgM levels correlated with the type of onset and sex (see Table 12–28).

In contrast, another study found normal levels of immunoglobulins in 86 to 94 percent of children with JRA.[717] Significantly increased concentrations of IgG, IgA, and complement factor C4 were found in children with active disease, whereas elevated IgM levels were characteristic of the disease itself. Studies by the same authors indicated that serum antibody levels to enteric bacteria (*E. coli* 055 and 086, common antigen, *Shigella* polyvalent antigen) were normal in JRA.[718] Only IgA antibodies were found in higher titers in these children. No abnormalities of immunoglobulin allotypes

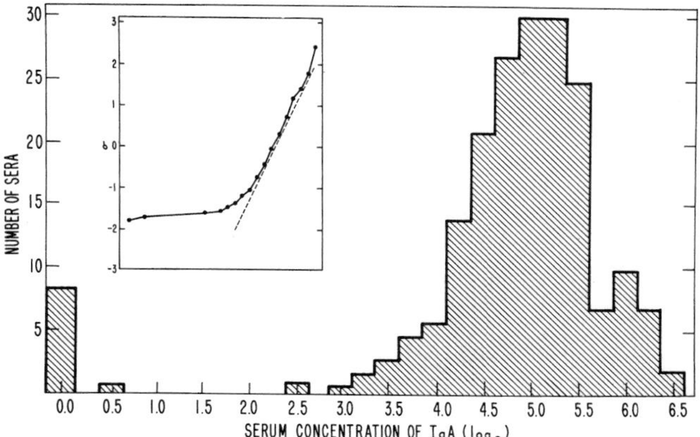

Figure 12–35. Relative frequency distributions of serum concentrations of immunoglobulin A (IgA) in children with JRA plotted as natural logarithms against the number of sera. Cumulative distributions on a normal probability scale are shown in the insert; the dotted lines are computed from ± 1.96 S.D. of the data (95% confidence limits). (From Cassidy JT, Petty RE, Sullivan DB: Abnormalities in the distribution of serum immunoglobulin concentrations in juvenile rheumatoid arthritis. J Clin Invest 52: 1931, 1973.)

have been reported.[719] Marked increases in low-molecular-weight IgM have been described, presumably reflecting a perturbation of intracellular assembly of subunits.[720]

Rheumatoid Factors

The latex fixation and sensitized sheep cell agglutination tests for the detection of classic IgM anti-IgG RFs are positive in a variable percentage of children with JRA, depending on the age of the population under study and onset type.[393, 707, 721–728] Early studies on RFs are summarized in Table 12–29. In the U.S. Pediatric Rheumatic Disease Registry,[729] 20 of 686 children (3 percent) with a polyarticular onset in JRA were RF

Table 12–29

Rheumatoid Factors in Children With JRA

			CORRELATIONS WITH RHEUMATOID FACTOR SEROPOSITIVITY								
AUTHOR/NO. OF CHILDREN	TEST USED	PERCENTAGE POSITIVE	Sex	Age	Late Onset	Long Duration	Type of Onset	Functional Capacity	Stage	Activity	Nodules
Bywaters et al.[721]	DAT	13	–		+	–				–	+ + +
142		45									
Toumbis et al.[722]	SCAT	40		+ +	–		–		–	–	–
45	LFT	13									
Sievers et al.[393]	SCAT	23		+ + +	+	–			–		
200	LFT	31									
Laaksonen[35]	SCAT	11	+		+ + +		+	+ + +	+ + +		
439	LFT	29	(F)								
Cassidy and Valkenburg[723]	HEAT	14	–	+	+ +	–					+ + +
	LFT	19									
110											
Hanson et al.[724]	SCAT	15	+		+ + +	–					+ + +
110	LFT	23	(F)								
Petty et al.[707]	LFT	13	+	+ +	+ +	–	+				
200			(F)								

DAT, differential agglutination test; HEAT, human erythrocyte agglutination test; LFT, latex fixation test; SCAT, sheep cell agglutination test; –, no correlation; +, correlated.

Modified from Petty RE, Cassidy JT, Sullivan DB: Serologic studies in juvenile rheumatoid arthritis. A review. Arthritis Rheum 20 (Suppl): 260, 1977.

Table 12–30

Utility of Rheumatoid Factor as a Diagnostic Test

	JUVENILE RHEUMATOID ARTHRITIS	
RHEUMATOID FACTOR	Present	Absent
Present	5	6
Absent	100	326

Sensitivity = 5/105 (4.8%); specificity = 326/332 (98%).

Modified from Eichenfield AH, Athreya BH, Doughty RA, et al: Utility of rheumatoid factor in the diagnosis of juvenile rheumatoid arthritis. Pediatrics 78: 480, 1986.

positive. In a study by Oen and colleagues[730] in Canadian First Nations children, the high frequency of RF-positive polyarticular disease (42 percent) was undoubtedly related to the high prevalence of HLA-DRB1 antigens bearing the RA shared epitope. RFs are unusual in a child younger than 7 years and are seldom helpful diagnostically at onset of disease. The diagnostic importance of RF seropositivity in a child with possible JRA is mitigated by the frequent occurrence of abnormal titers in the other connective tissue diseases of childhood, especially in SLE. In a study of the diagnostic utility of RF serology in children,[728] RF tests were as likely to be positive in children with diseases other than JRA as in those with JRA (Table 12–30). As a diagnostic aid, therefore, tests for RFs are of little utility.

However, children with high titers of RFs likely represent a subgroup distinct from the larger number of children with seronegative disease. The evidence for this hypothesis is not unequivocal because studies often identify the seropositive group in retrospect. RFs are more common in children with later age of onset of arthritis and in those who are older, have subcutaneous rheumatoid nodules or articular erosions, or are in a poor functional class (Tables 12–31 and 12–32).[723] The percentage of children with RF seropositivity also rises progressively as the age of onset or the duration of disease of the cohort group under study increases (see Table 12–29). These observations suggest that RFs might be a result rather than a determining event in children who go on to develop unremitting, disabling disease during the early adult years.

Many studies have demonstrated other types of antiglobulins in the sera of children with JRA or have reported more sensitive and specific tests for RFs.[96, 102, 104, 731–742, 742a] The majority of children with seronegative JRA can be shown to have IgG anti-IgG antibodies as demonstrated by immunosorbent techniques.[731, 734–736, 740] Pepsin agglutinators of the IgG class are found more often in children with JRA than are classic RFs.[732] Miller and colleagues[736] employed five different immunosorbents to search for occult antiglobulins. Antiglobulins detected by binding to sepharose-linked globulin followed by acid elution were found in 8 normal children and in 52 children with JRA. Only 4 children with JRA had significantly elevated levels. These authors concluded that the presence of these antiglobulins per se was not diagnostically helpful in distinguishing children with JRA.

In the studies of Moore and associates,[96, 102, 104, 251, 737–739, 741] 68 to 75 percent of children with JRA were shown to have "hidden RFs," defined as IgM 19S antiglobulins detected by acid elution of IgM-containing fractions of serum from a gel filtration column. Hidden RFs were found in 59 percent of children with JRA who lacked classic RFs by using a complement-dependent hemolytic assay, and their presence correlated well with disease activity. Not only were hidden RFs more frequent in children with JRA, but they were also of higher titer than in healthy children or other disease control groups. Titers correlated with activity of the disease and did not differ significantly between polyarticular and oligoarticular disease. Hidden RFs could be inhibited more readily by the use of human IgG than IgG of animal origin, although the detection system continued to be a hemolytic assay employing rabbit IgG. These studies have focused on North American and European patients. In a survey of 43 children from Turkey,[743] 19S IgM hidden RFs were found in 56 percent (46 percent oligoarthritis, 64 percent polyarthritis, 80 percent systemic onset). The latex fixation test was positive in only 1 patient who had polyarticular disease. Hidden RFs were present in lower percentages in India[744, 745] and Greece.[746]

Antinuclear Antibodies

Tests for ANAs are more useful than those for RF in the diagnosis of JRA.[707, 747, 748] Early studies of ANAs are summarized in Table 12–33. Standardized serum dilution titers are usually low to moderate (≤1:256).

Table 12–31

Relation of Rheumatoid Factor Positivity and Age in Children With JRA

	AGE AT STUDY		AGE AT ONSET		DURATION OF DISEASE	
YEARS	No.	Positive (%)	No.	Positive (%)	No.	Positive (%)
0–4	7	0	42	12	49	18
5–9	29	7	37	16	35	20
10–14	32	25	31	42	15	27
15–19	18	22	—	—	5	20
20–24	14	36	—	—	4	50
25+	10	50	—	—	2	50

Modified from Cassidy JT, Valkenburg HA: A five year prospective study of rheumatoid factor tests in juvenile rheumatoid arthritis. Arthritis Rheum 10: 83, 1967.

Table 12–32

Relation of Functional Capacity to Rheumatoid Factor Positivity in JRA

	CAPACITY	NUMBER	MEDIAN AGE	MEDIAN DURATION	POSITIVE RF TEST	
					Number	%
I	No limitation	19	14	4	1	5
II	Minimal	38	12	4	7	18
III	Moderate	34	14	6	12	35
IV	Severe	19	16	6	4	21

Modified from Cassidy JT, Valkenburg HA: A five year prospective study of rheumatoid factor tests in juvenile rheumatoid arthritis. Arthritis Rheum 10: 83, 1967.

Most ANAs are of the IgG class, although antibodies of the IgM and IgA classes are found. The frequency of ANAs is highest in girls who are younger at onset of arthritis and lowest in older boys and in children with systemic disease (Table 12–34).[74, 660, 661, 727, 732, 747, 749–757] ANAs reach their highest prevalence (65 to 85 percent) in children who have oligoarthritis and uveitis.[288, 660, 661, 757] Thus, determination of ANA seropositivity is supportive of the diagnosis of JRA and important in identification of children most at risk for chronic uveitis. Studies have demonstrated persistent ANA seropositivity in a small but significant group of children with musculoskeletal complaints in whom no autoimmune or rheumatic disease was found.[341, 342] Care must therefore be exercised in interpreting the significance of a positive ANA test in children who do not have objective evidence of arthritis.[748, 758–760]

At present, tests for ANAs are most often performed on HEp-2 cells. The frequency of ANA seropositivity in children with JRA is increased using this substrate compared with mouse liver, as is background positivity in normal children.[753, 754, 756, 761] The most common patterns are homogeneous and speckled. In addition, a pattern of nuclear fluorescence of mitotic figures has been described in children with oligoarthritis and chronic uveitis.[756]

The antigenic specificities of ANAs have not been identified.[762] Evaluation of specificities by Western blot with HEp-2 cell nuclei demonstrated extensive heterogeneity of reactivity.[171, 763] Antibodies to core histones are common. The appearance of antibody to dsDNA during the course of JRA should be recognized as a warning of a transition to SLE. In a study of 77 children, the frequency of positive results for antibodies to defined nuclear antigens (Sm, RNP, DNA, RNA, RAP, SS-A, and SS-B) was only 13 percent.[751] However, the authors noted a small group of girls with polyarthritis and late onset of disease who had an increased frequency of RFs or antibodies to the RAP antigen. These studies suggested that these patients might be infected with the Epstein-Barr virus (which is associated with anti-RAP) and that this virus might play a role in the pathogenesis of JRA. In another study, granulocyte-specific ANAs of the IgG class were found in all children with uveitis but in none with acute systemic-onset JRA, and they also tended to correlate with the number of affected joints.[752] Half of the granulocyte-specific ANAs were capable of fixing complement and correlated with active disease.[764]

Table 12–33

Antinuclear Antibodies in Children With JRA

STUDY (REF.)	SUBSTRATE	NO. STUDIED	SERUM DILUTION	POSITIVE (%)		CORRELATION
				JRA	Normal	
Petty et al.[660]	Mouse liver	200	Undiluted	38	2	Young age Female Oligoarthritis or polyarthritis Chronic uveitis
Schaller et al.[661]	Rat liver	JRA with chronic iridocyclitis: 58	1:10	88	0	Iridocyclitis
		JRA without iridocyclitis: 133		30		
Rudnicki et al.[727]	Mouse liver	85		24		
Alspaugh and Miller[751]	Mouse kidney	77		57		
Permin et al.[752]	Rat liver; WBC	100		66		
Patel et al.[753]	HEp-2 cells	217		60		
Rosenberg et al.[754]	HEp-2 cells	61		62		
McCune et al.[756]	HEp-2 cells	207	1:40	53	6	Chronic uveitis

Table 12–34

Associations of ANA in Children With JRA

ANA positivity in children with RA is associated with
Oligoarticular and, to a lesser extent, polyarticular onset
Female sex
Young age at onset
Presence of chronic uveitis
Absence of bone erosions

ANA, antinuclear antibodies.

Serum Complement and Immune Complexes

The third component of complement (C3) is often elevated in the sera of children with active JRA, acting as an acute phase protein.[765] The activated form of the molecule C3 (C3d) may be increased as well.[763, 766, 767] Increased levels of C3c and C3d were found in 7 of 10 children with systemic JRA, 16 of 29 with active polyarthritis, and 7 of 20 with active oligoarthritis.[763] Activation products were found in only 2 of 20 children with inactive joint disease. This observation indicates that the pathogenesis of JRA may include complement-mediated tissue damage. ICs are present in the sera of some children with systemic onset of disease and polyarthritis.[96–98, 768] In one study, ICs were detected by C1q binding in 22 percent of children with JRA, most often in those who were RF seropositive.[97, 768a] On the basis of these studies, it was suggested that children with a systemic onset might have a relative defect in antibody-forming capacity or in macrophage function that results in decreased clearance of circulating ICs.

Plasma Lipids

Dyslipoproteinemia occurs de novo in children with JRA, separate from the effects of glucocorticoids.[769, 770] Tselepis and colleagues[771] reported that 14 patients with active arthritis had lower plasma cholesterol and high-density lipoprotein cholesterol levels and higher triglycerides than both comparable children with another disease and controls. In addition, these investigators found that plasma platelet activating factor acetylhydrolase activity was also decreased in parallel with the activity of the disease. These low levels of platelet activating factor acetylhydrolase activity may have resulted in a loss of anti-inflammatory activity in these patients because platelet activating factor is a lipid mediator of inflammation.

Synovial Fluid Analysis

Synovial fluid in JRA is usually a group II or inflammatory fluid (see Appendix); however, the level of the leukocyte count does not always correlate with the degree of clinical activity (Table 12–35).[326] Very low counts, such as 600 cells/mm^3 (0.6 $\times$ 10^9/L), have been observed in fluid from joints clinically involved by intensely active and symptomatic disease. Conversely, counts in the range of septic arthritis, such as 100,000 cells/mm^3 (100 $\times$ 10^9/L), have been described in children with otherwise classic JRA.[772, 773] The principal cellular constituents are polymorphonuclear neutrophils and mononuclear cells including lymphoid dendritic cells.[774] Synovial fluid levels of glucose may be low in JRA, as in adult RA. Synovial fluid complement levels are not as uniformly depressed in JRA as in adult disease.[775–777] Rynes and colleagues[776] found intra-articular activation of the classical complement pathway, but not the alternative pathway, in some children with JRA. Complement activation products, however, were not detected in the joint fluid of children with oligoarticular JRA in the study by Miller and associates.[767] Complexes of IgG, IgG RF, and complement components along with hidden RF have been described in both synovial tissue and eluates.[777–779] The concentration of glycosaminoglycans in synovial fluid (hyaluronic acid and chondroitin sulfates) is decreased in children with JRA compared with normal controls, accounting for the low viscosity of inflamed synovial fluid.[780]

RADIOLOGIC EXAMINATION

Investigative Techniques

Technical advances in imaging techniques since about 1990 have contributed considerably to the radiologic investigation of the child with JRA.[781] Radiologic abnormalities in JRA have been reviewed by Reed and Wilmot.[782] Although plain film radiography is still the mainstay of imaging techniques, computed tomography, high-resolution ultrasonography, radionuclide imaging, and magnetic resonance imaging (MRI) have

Table 12–35

Synovial Fluid Analysis in Children With Oligoarticular JRA

Gross characteristics	Yellow, clear to opalescent
Total white cell count (mm^3)	
Range	150–41,600
Median	10,000
Average	11,400
Polymorphonuclear neutrophils (%)	
Range	18–88
Median	52
Average	56
Mucin clot test (%)	
Excellent	20
Good	20
Fair	15
Poor	45

Modified from Cassidy JT, Brody GL, Martel W: Monarticular juvenile rheumatoid arthritis. J Pediatr 70: 867, 1967.

begun to contribute considerably to our knowledge of early articular changes in JRA.

A radiograph is the best initial investigation in most situations. The only exceptions to this rule are radiographs of the lumbosacral spine and the sacroiliac joints: Unless the indications are very specific, the information gained may not justify the amount of radiation administered. In any event, care should be taken to minimize radiation exposure and maximize information obtained by consultation with a pediatric radiologist. Ultrasonography is often the best way of identifying intra-articular fluid, particularly in joints such as the hip and shoulder, where fluid may be difficult to demonstrate clinically (Fig. 12–36).[783, 783a] Ultrasound studies of the wrist may help delineate joint effusion from tenosynovitis or a ganglion cyst.[784] Computed tomography can demonstrate otherwise poorly defined lesions in the sacroiliac joints, temporomandibular joints, or feet, but otherwise is of limited value in the study of JRA. Thermography is not widely available,

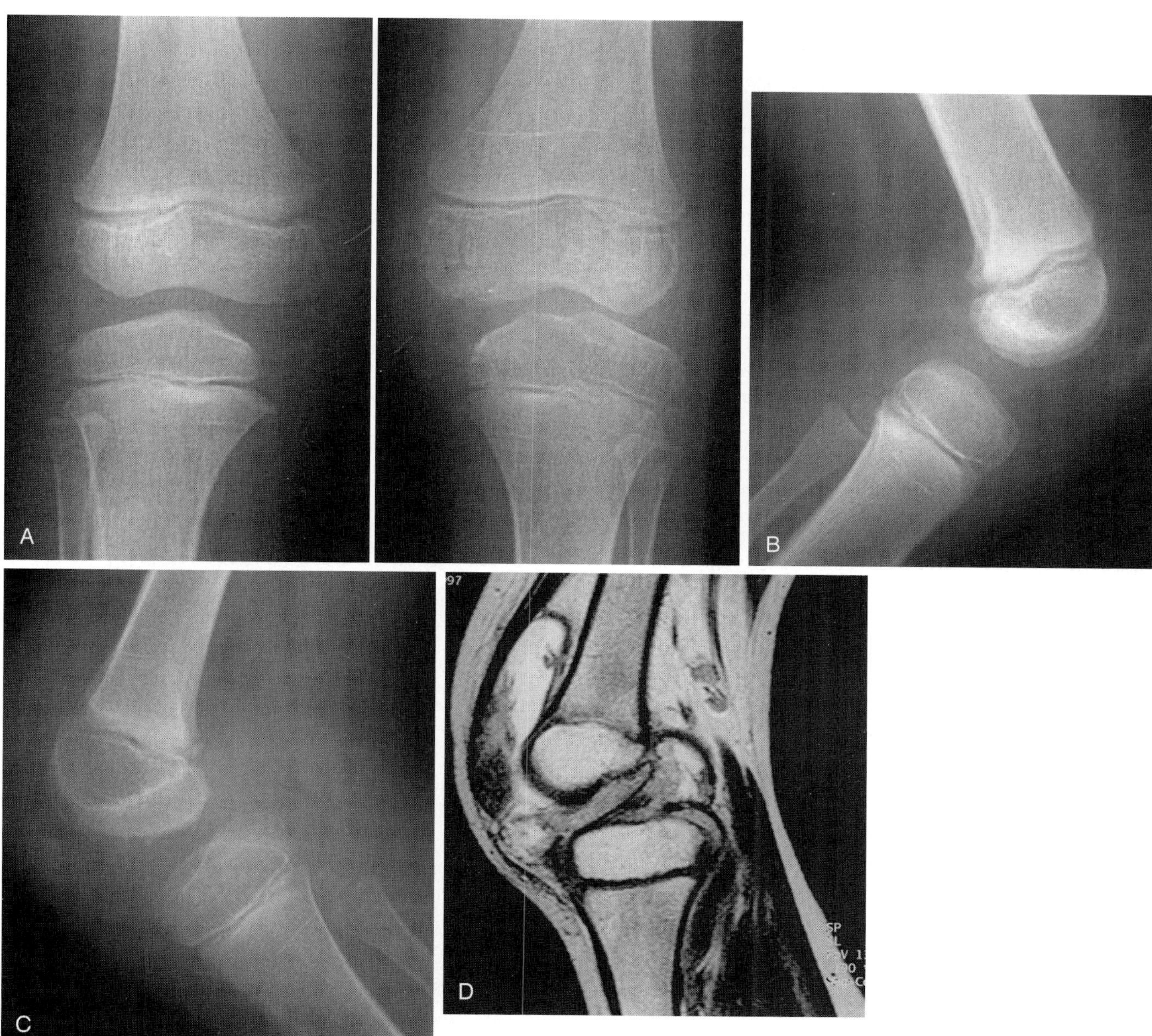

Figure 12–36. *A–C,* These are anteroposterior and lateral films of the knees of a 3-year-old girl who developed monarthritis of the left knee at the age of 2 years with an initial flexion contracture of 32 degrees. There is marked joint space narrowing and regional osteoporosis of the left knee, and epiphyseal enlargement. *D,* Post-gadolinium MRI sagittal studies of the left knee. There is a large joint effusion with marked inflammatory synovial hypertrophy demonstrated by enhancement of the pannus throughout all compartments of the joint. There is also thinning and irregularity of the articular cartilage involving the femur, tibia, and patella. There is almost bone-on-bone apposition of the femorotibial articulation. Asymmetric enlargements of the epiphyses of the left knee are visible, with relative hypoplasia of the menisci.

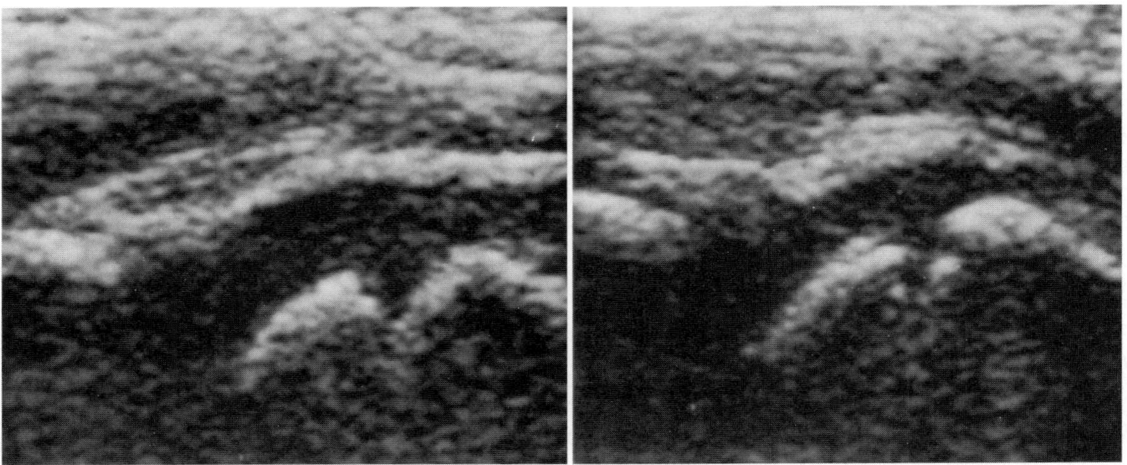

Figure 12–37. Ultrasound of the hip joints of a child with an effusion in one hip (left) indicated by displacement of the capsule away from the femoral heads. The image on the right is normal. (Courtesy of Drs. R. Cairns and D. Stringer.)

although it can document the extent and degree of joint inflammation by registering heat output.[785]

The role of arthrography in the investigation of a child with JRA has been supplanted to some extent by MRI, but arthrography can be helpful in demonstrating popliteal cysts and loose bodies.[786] Radionuclide imaging, particularly with ^{99m}Tc, is a sensitive but less specific investigative tool. The blood-flow phase illustrates vascular integrity; the blood-pool phase evaluates the homeostasis of inflow versus outflow; the bone-uptake phase demonstrates lesions characterized by a decrease or increase in retention of isotope. Unlike other imaging techniques, radionuclide scans demonstrate hemodynamics and metabolic activity in bone or joint at the time the study is being performed. Radionuclide scans therefore provide early evidence of joint inflammation with increased uptake of the isotope on both sides of the joint. They do not necessarily differentiate JRA from septic arthritis or other joint diseases.

MRI has the potential to illuminate our understanding of intra-articular pathology in a way that no other imaging technique can (Fig. 12–37).[783a, 787] It is now possible to identify abnormalities of noncalcified tissues long before they evolve into lesions that cause the bony changes detectable by plain radiography.[787–790] The diagnostic and therapeutic implications of the information gained by these techniques, especially MRI, are enormous.[786, 791, 792] Intravenous gadolinium is taken up by synovial tissue and can be used in conjunction with MRI to differentiate actively inflamed synovium from synovial fluid.[786, 791] MRI may prove especially valuable in permitting an early, accurate diagnosis of many of the rare and unusual causes of monarthritis.[793]

Overview

Early radiographic changes reflect inflammation; they include periarticular soft tissue swelling and (sometimes) widening of the joint space caused by increased intra-articular fluid or synovial hypertrophy. Juxta-articular osteoporosis and growth-arrest lines are common early abnormalities.[782] Generalized osteoporosis may also be significant, especially in the postpubertal girl with polyarticular JRA.[499] Periosteal new bone apposition occurs most commonly in the short tubular bones of the phalanges, metacarpals, and metatarsals (Fig. 12–38) but occasionally involves the long bones as well.[70, 72, 383, 794–796] Widening of the midportions of the phalanges from periosteal new bone apposition is a characteristic feature of polyarthritis.

Later radiologic changes include joint-space narrowing, marginal erosions, subluxation, and ankylosis.[794] Thinning of cartilage is difficult to assess radio-

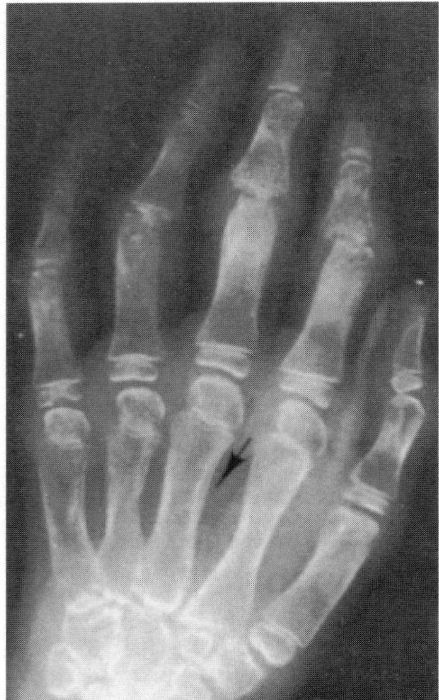

Figure 12–38. Severe polyarticular JRA in an 8-year-old girl. Demineralization is widespread, and there is damage to the proximal epiphyses of the middle phalanges and soft tissue swelling around the PIP joints. Periosteal new bone apposition (*arrow*) is present on the metacarpals.

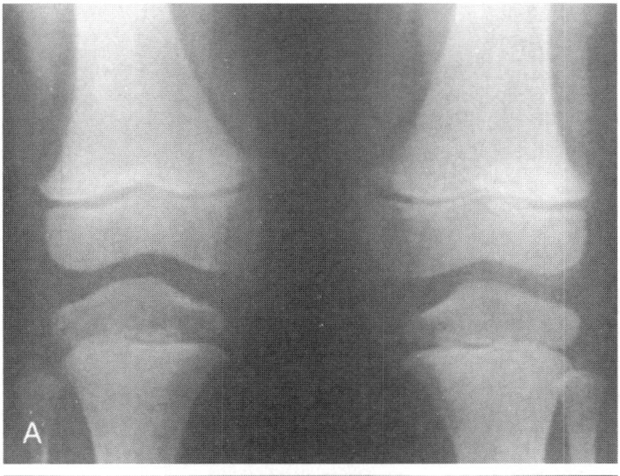

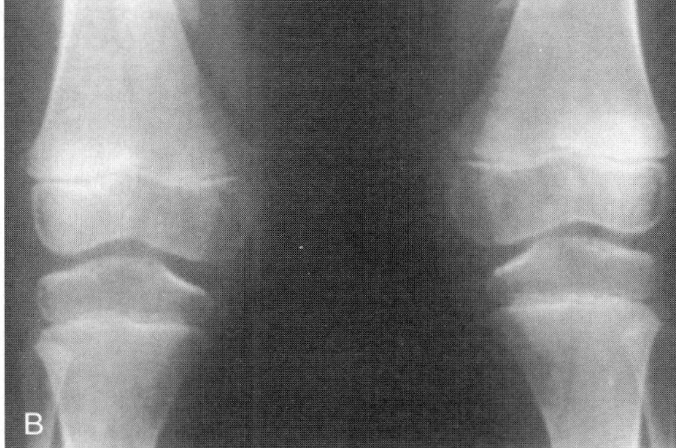

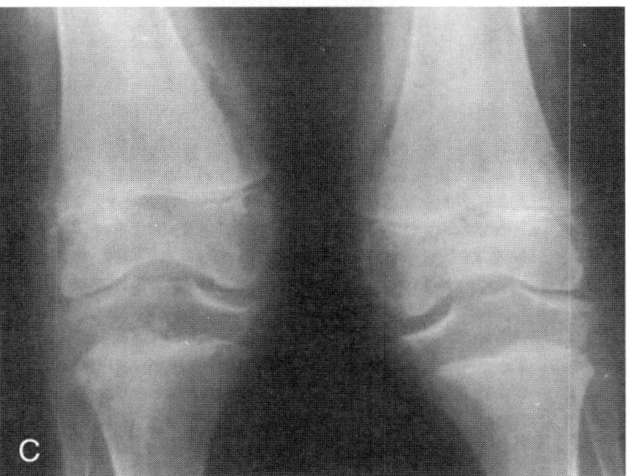

Figure 12–39. These radiographs illustrate the 5-year progression of osteoporosis, joint-space narrowing, and degenerative changes in the knees of a girl with oligoarticular JRA. *A*, In this radiograph, taken 2 years after onset of disease, there is only minimal epiphyseal advancement and osteoporosis. *B*, After 4 years of disease, there is increased prominence of the trabecular pattern secondary to osteoporosis, narrowing of the joint spaces, and remodeling of the normal contours of the articular surfaces. *C*, After 5 years of disease, there is marked narrowing of joint spaces and flattening of the tibial plateaus. Degenerative changes include squaring of the femoral condyles, the development of osteophytes at the medial margin of the tibial plateaus, and the development of subchondral cysts in the femoral epiphyses.

graphically and is often called joint-space narrowing. In fact, it is the layer of noncalcified cartilage overlying bone, not the joint space, that is narrowed. Such a change is best evaluated in joints of the lower extremity if the radiograph is taken with the patient standing (Fig. 12–39). Erosions are often not generally demonstrable by plain radiographs before 2 years of active disease, even in a child with polyarthritis. Indeed, in some children with limited joint disease, erosions may not be visible even after 1 or 2 decades of constant effusion and swelling of a joint. However, in one long-term study of children with JRA,[797] erosive changes of the small joints of the hands and feet were present at 5 years in 67 of 70 children with RF-seropositive disease.

Subluxation involves large as well as small joints. Of the large joints, subluxation is most common in the wrist, hip, and shoulder. Subluxation of the tibiotalar, hip, shoulder, elbow, and other joints may also occur. Bony ankylosis occurs earlier in children than in adults and is particularly pronounced in the carpal and tarsal joints and in the cervical spine. Ankylosis can be confirmed by computed tomography. Aseptic necrosis of the femoral head, humeral epiphysis, or tibial plateau is not common in children with JRA, even in those treated with high-dose glucocorticoids for long periods,[798] although early series reported osteonecrosis more frequently.[799] Some studies frequently report fractures related to JRA or severe generalized osteoporosis.[794, 800–802] They are particularly common in children who have had severe disease and undergone long periods of immobilization or steroid therapy. The supracondylar area of the femur is a characteristic site of a fracture that follows manipulation for contracture of the knee. Microfractures of the growth plates may be related to abnormal mechanical stress in JRA. The normally balanced muscle forces about joints are altered by severe joint deformities, erosion, and subluxation as well as by inflammation of the periarticular connective tissues. Abnormal compression forces on the growth plates result.

Localized growth disturbances are among the most remarkable skeletal changes in JRA. Epiphyseal ossification centers are advanced in development within weeks of onset of the disease.[803–805] This finding is most obvious when the disease is asymmetric (Fig. 12–40). Radial atrophy (overtubulation) often accompanies linear overgrowth of the long bones. Even if arthritis is confined to the knee, growth of the pelvis on the same side may be stunted, and coxa valga may be present.

Sequential radiologic changes have been examined in relation to the type of onset of the disease (Table 12–36).[794] Early findings of soft tissue swelling or osteoporosis were detected in 45 percent of children with polyarthritis or systemic-onset disease and in 75 percent of those with oligoarthritis. Periosteal new bone formation and striking metaphyseal rarefaction were found only in children with polyarthritis and systemic-onset disease (Fig. 12–41). Metaphyseal bands related to focal osteoporosis and hyperemia of the zone of ossification of the epiphyseal plate were common. Periosteal new bone formation occurred adjacent to involved joints but not in children with monarthritis or oligoarthritis in spite of a subsequent polyarticular course in some of these patients.

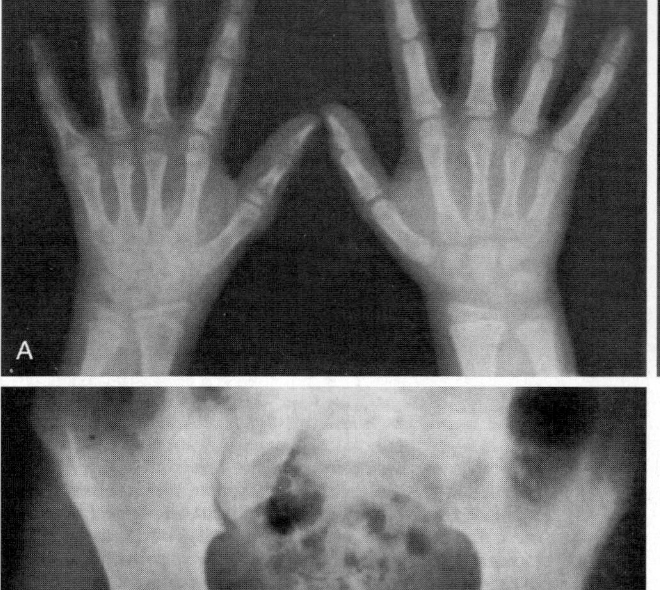

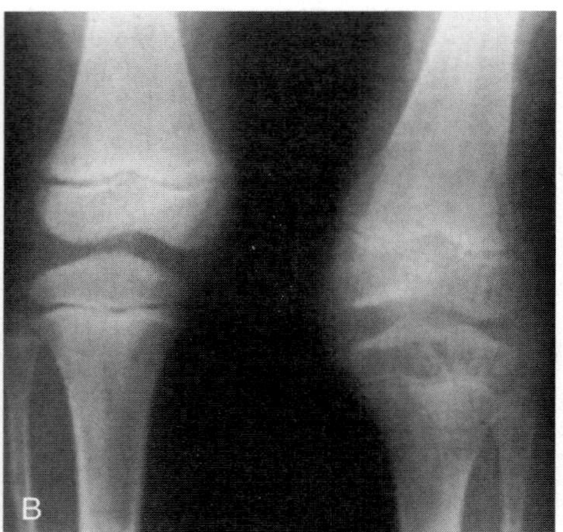

Figure 12–40. These radiographs illustrate localized growth disturbances in children with JRA. *A*, Arthritis persisted for 7 years in the left wrist of this 9-year-old girl, causing osteoporosis and acceleration of maturation of growth centers, resulting in a small hand. *B*, Monarthritis of the left knee has persisted for 8 years in this 14-year-old girl, causing osteoporosis, epiphyseal advancement and enlargement, discrepancy in leg length (left leg longer than right leg), and radial atrophy of the long bones. *C*, Pelvis of the patient described in *B* shows regional demineralization and miniaturization of the left side of the pelvis. Arthritis has not been present in the hip, and these changes are secondary to the effects of inflammatory disease of the left knee.

Advanced radiologic changes were also related to the type of onset of disease (Fig. 12–42). Destruction of cartilage and bone was marked in children with polyarticular- or systemic-onset disease and was less frequent and usually less severe even in those with oligoarthritis who subsequently developed polyarthritis. Bony ankylosis was a late change. Large joint subluxation, especially at the hip, was particularly characteristic. Fractures of the epiphyses and vertebral compression fractures occurred only in children with severe, longstanding disease. The increased frequency of these findings in children with systemic disease was probably related to extended use of glucocorticoid drugs in this group because fractures were rare in children in whom these agents had not

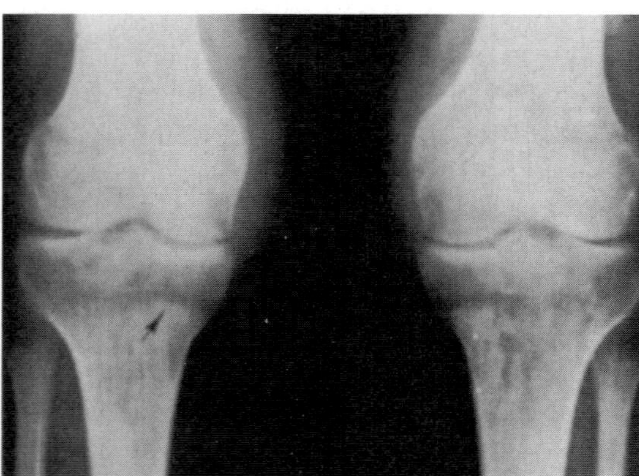

Figure 12–41. Zones of metaphyseal rarefaction in both tibias (*arrow*). These abnormalities are not specific for JRA and are later replaced by growth arrest lines.

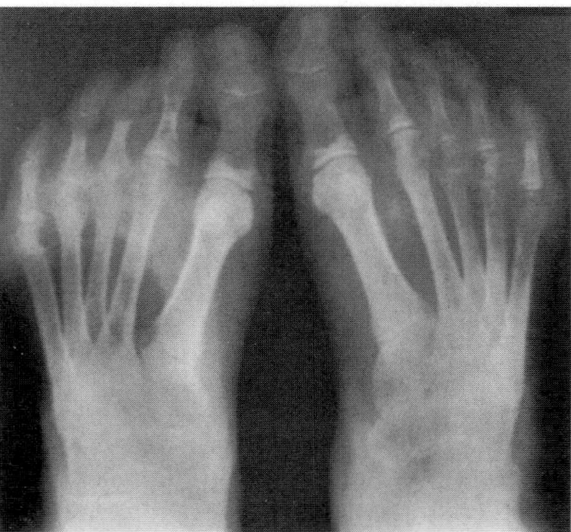

Figure 12–42. Severe symmetric erosions of the heads of the second through fifth metatarsals. The poorly corticated lesions are prominent on the inferomedial aspects of the bones.

Table 12–36

Clinicoradiologic Correlations in Children With JRA

	TYPE OF ONSET		
	Polyarthritis (%)	Oligoarthritis (%)	Systemic Disease (%)
Early changes			
Soft tissue swelling or osteoporosis	45	75	45
Periosteal new bone apposition	30	—	50
Metaphyseal rarefaction	5	—	5
Advanced changes			
Cartilage destruction	55	25	50
Bone destruction	35	25	20
Bony ankylosis	25	5	15
Large-joint subluxation	15	5	20
Epiphyseal fractures	5	—	40
Vertebral compression	20	—	25
Growth abnormalities			
Long bones: under- or overgrowth	30	50	15
Brachydactyly	20	5	30
Micrognathia	15	5	40
Accelerated epiphyseal maturation	5	35	20
Spondylitis			
Cervical	35	10	20
Atlantoaxial subluxation	15	—	5
Dorsolumbar	5	—	5
Sacroiliac	5	5	—

Modified from Cassidy JT, Martel W: Juvenile rheumatoid arthritis: clinicoradiologic correlations. Arthritis Rheum 20(Suppl): 207, 1977.

been used. Fractures were not observed in children who had oligoarthritis.

Growth abnormalities were particularly evident in children with monarticular or oligoarticular disease. Longitudinal overgrowth was the rule, although affected bones were generally smaller in diameter than normal. Brachydactyly and micrognathia occurred predominantly in children with systemic disease and in those with early age at onset; it occurred to a lesser extent in those with polyarthritis. Accelerated epiphyseal maturation during active disease was sometimes associated with future stunting of full growth of the affected bones. Spondylitis typical of JRA was noted in all regions of the axial skeleton. Abnormalities of the upper segments of the cervical spine were the most characteristic change, and a few children had arthritis of the cervical spine at onset of disease. Atlantoaxial subluxation and disease of the thoracolumbar spine did not develop in children with monarthritis, even of long duration. Dwarfing or remodeling of the dorsolumbar vertebral bodies, probably attributable to arthritis of the apophyseal joints of that region, occurred in a few patients. Characteristic sacroiliac arthritis, both with and without coincident cervical disease, was present in four children but was distinguishable from that of JAS.

Changes in Specific Joints

Spine

Characteristic radiologic abnormalities of the axial skeleton occur in JRA.[383, 806] The predominant changes are in the apophyseal joints of the upper cervical segments. Bony fusion is frequent, often observed first at the C2-C3 level (Fig. 12–43). Fusion of adjacent spinous processes may also be present. A single lateral film of the cervical spine may not be sufficient to determine the presence of ankylosis in this location. The distance between spinous processes in flexion and in extension should be compared to confirm that fusion has occurred.

Atlantoaxial subluxation is also common (Fig. 12–44). The upper limit of the atlanto-odontoid distance in children is approximately 4 mm, measured at the bottom of the arch of C1 on a lateral film taken in flexion with a 40-inch tube to film distance.[807] There is normally a small amount of displacement between the bodies of C2 and C3 in the young child (2 to 12 years of age); this change should not be misinterpreted as early subluxation. Instability of the atlantoaxial joint may lead to impingement on the cord and brain stem (Fig. 12–45). There may also be cephalad encroachment of the odontoid into the foramen magnum.

Locke and colleagues[807] studied the atlanto-odontoid distance in 200 normal children aged 3 to 15 years. If the measurement was greater than 4 mm in the neutral position, an atlantoaxial subluxation was usually confirmed. Age and sex were not significant factors in evaluating these measurements. Other signs of atlantoaxial subluxation were increased tissue density anterior to the cervical spine, flexion greater than 10 degrees between the atlas and the axis, compensatory curve of the lower cervical spine, and narrowing of the atlantovertebral foramen.

Narrowing of an intervertebral disk associated with atrophy or maldevelopment of adjacent vertebral bodies probably reflects fusion of the adjacent apophyseal joint(s) even though it may not be well delineated radiologically.[383] Vertebral bodies at areas of fusion fail to grow normally and are smaller and narrower than contiguous vertebral bodies (an altered ratio of height to width). The corresponding intervertebral spaces are reduced, and the disk is sometimes calcified. Verte-

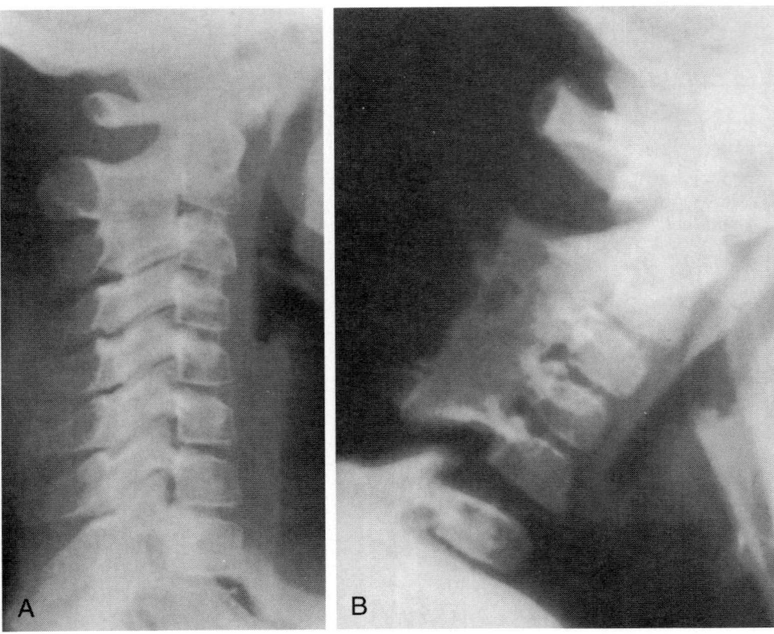

Figure 12–43. *A*, Fusion of the spinous processes of the second and third cervical vertebrae in a teenage girl with early onset of JRA. *B*, More extensive fusion of spinous processes resulting in a severe pseudoarticulation and accompanied by destructive changes at the C5–C6 junction. There were no neurologic signs.

bral compression fractures are sometimes apparent, especially in children who have been treated with glucocorticoids (Fig. 12–46), and are most common in the thoracolumbar vertebrae.[383, 550, 802] Scoliosis of the thoracolumbar spine is more common in children with JRA than in healthy children.[456, 457]

Sacroiliac Joints

Sacroiliac arthritis in JRA is not characterized by the degree of reactive sclerosis that occurs in JAS (Fig. 12–47).[383, 808] In long-standing disease, however, there may be subchondral sclerosis and secondary cartilage space narrowing. Late fusion may occur in children with severe disease who have been in a wheelchair or at bed rest for long periods of time.[383]

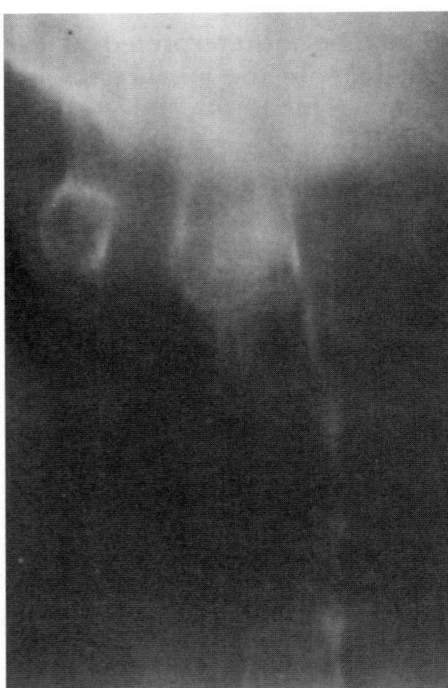

Figure 12–44. A lateral tomogram of the atlantoaxial joint shows approximately 8 mm of separation between the anterior surface of the odontoid and the posterior surface of the atlas.

Temporomandibular Joint

The temporomandibular joint is usually evaluated by Panorex views and, if necessary, tomography or (more recently) MRI.[809] Flattening or even complete dissolution of the mandibular condyle may occur (Fig. 12–48).[494, 794] Mandibular asymmetry with undergrowth on the affected side may be present if the disease predominantly affects one temporomandibular joint.[493, 810]

Shoulder

The shoulder is involved in fewer than 8 percent of children with JRA at onset,[324] although perhaps one third eventually develop disease in this joint.[811, 812] Children with oligoarthritis rarely have shoulder disease, but in those with polyarticular or systemic-onset disease, the frequency of involvement rises to 50 and 80 percent, respectively, and is almost always bilateral.[812] Loss of range of motion is most marked in internal rotation and is accompanied by marked atrophy and weakness of the rotator cuff.[812] Dabrowski and associates[811] described erosions, cysts, and enlargement and flattening of the medial side of the humeral head. Superior subluxation of the shoulder and avascular necrosis may result. Disease of the acromioclavicular joint is uncommon.[811]

Elbow, Wrist, and Hand

Erosions, subluxations, and enlargement of the radial head may occur. Subluxation at the radiocarpal joint is

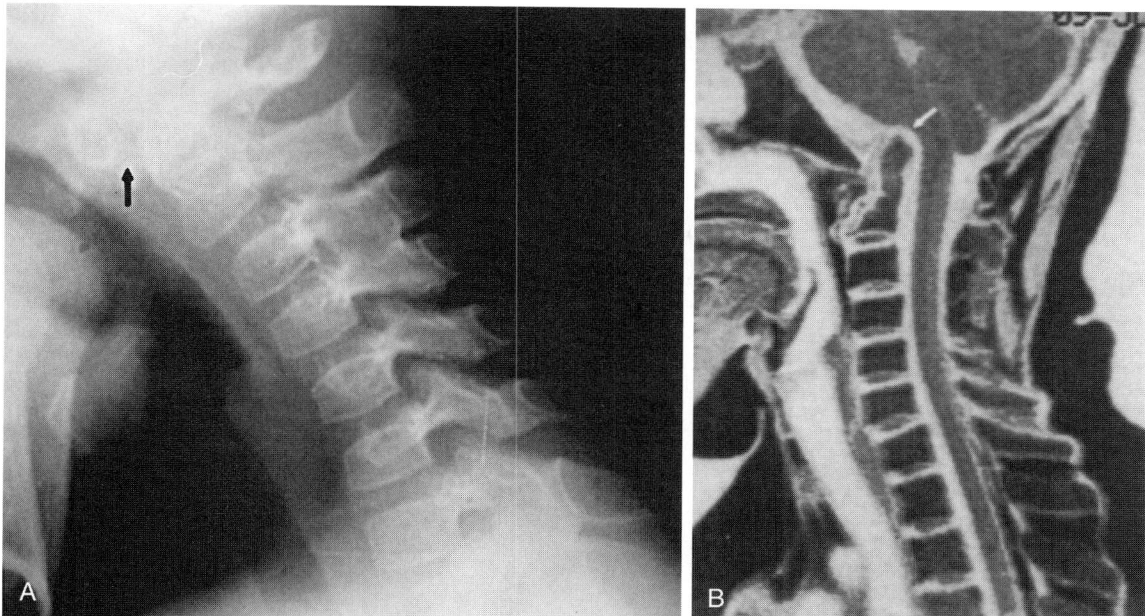

Figure 12–45. *A*, Lateral spine of 12-year-old girl with systemic onset of JRA at the age of 11 years with atlantoaxial subluxation *(arrow)* and fusion of C3–C4. *B*, Magnetic resonance image of the cervical spine at age 26 years. Note the impingement of the odontoid on the upper cervical cord *(arrow)*. (*B*, Courtesy of Dr. J. W. McCune.)

a characteristic radiologic abnormality, particularly in the child with long-standing wrist disease. Reduced carpal length is a consistent finding.[813] Bony ankylosis of the carpal bones is another characteristic change (Fig. 12–49), and similar changes may occur in the MCP joints. In the wrist, there may be disproportionate shortening of the ulna, with the result that the radius compensates by becoming bowed. Pronounced ulnar subluxation of the wrist is characteristic.

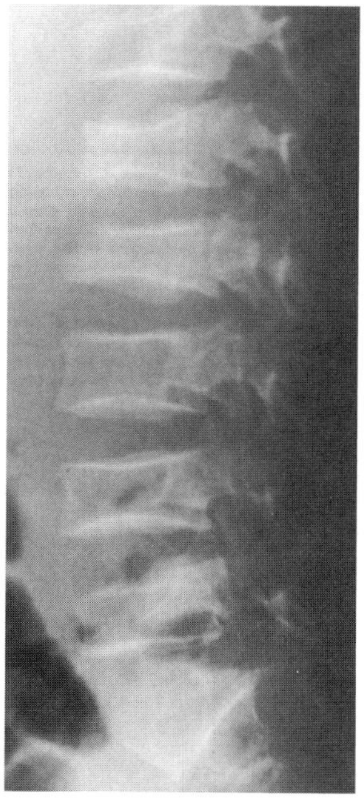

Figure 12–46. Radiograph of the lumbar vertebrae of a 12-year-old girl with severe debilitating JRA requiring glucocorticoid therapy shows numerous areas of vertebral compression.

A radiographic picture of marked bony overgrowth and enlargement of the epiphyses may also be apparent at the interphalangeal joints. Failure of growth of small tubular bones results in brachydactyly. This condition is occasionally but not always related to premature epiphyseal fusion, especially when selective stunting of one or two bones occurs. A common site for this finding is the fourth metacarpal bone. Asymmetric fusion may occur when only a portion of the epiphyseal plate is affected, resulting in abnormal angulation of the joint. Radial deviation at the MCP joints is more characteristic than ulnar drift. In severe, late, uncontrolled disease, bony destruction in the hand may be extensive (Fig. 12–50).[814]

Hip Joint

Subluxation of the hip is best demonstrated on a weight-bearing anteroposterior radiograph to confirm upward and lateral displacement of the femoral head (Fig. 12–51). Ultrasonography may demonstrate increased intra-articular fluid or synovial hypertrophy, particularly between the femoral head and the medial margin of the acetabulum. Protrusio acetabuli may also develop (Fig. 12–52). This complication is sometimes rapidly progressive.[815] Osteonecrosis of the femoral head is not as frequent in JRA as in SLE, but if suspected, this condition should be evaluated by a radionuclide scan or MRI.[816, 817]

Kobayakawa and coworkers[799] reported a high frequency of necrosis of the femoral head. Of 206 children hospitalized

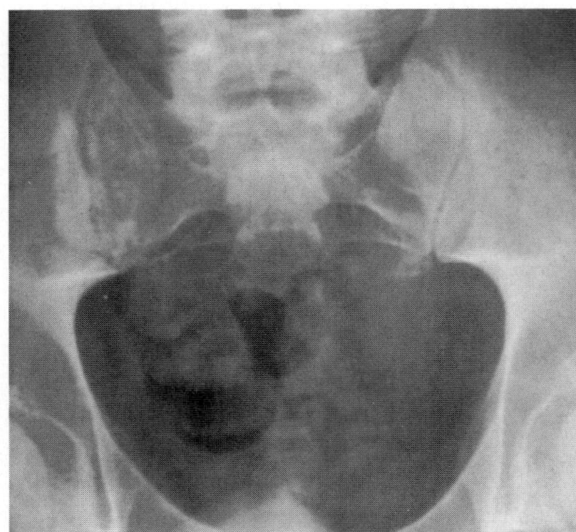

Figure 12–47. Minimal disease of the right sacroiliac joint is present in this 14-year-old boy with polyarticular JRA. Minimal irregularity in the inferior portion of the sacroiliac joint may be difficult to differentiate from the effects of overlying bowel gas shadows.

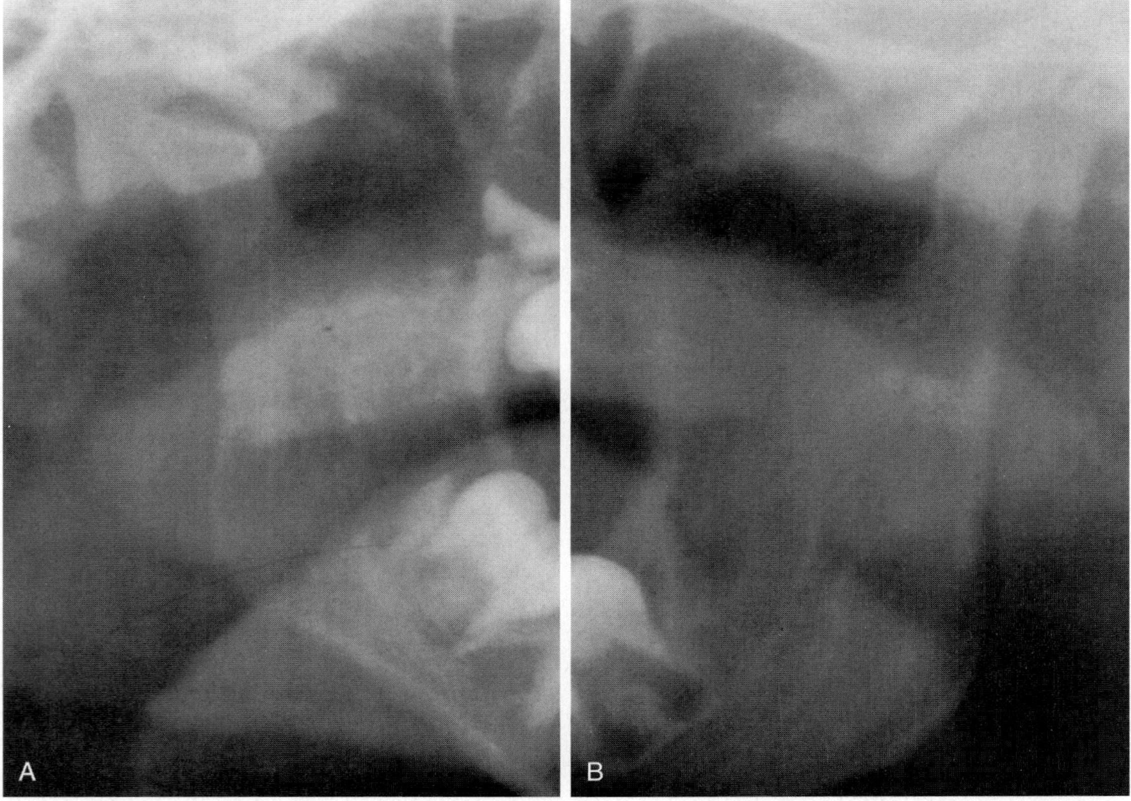

Figure 12–48. *A,* The left mandibular condyle is eroded and flattened and the ramus of the mandible is shortened. *B,* The normal right side of the same patient is shown for comparison. (*A* and *B,* Courtesy of Dr. B. Blasberg.)

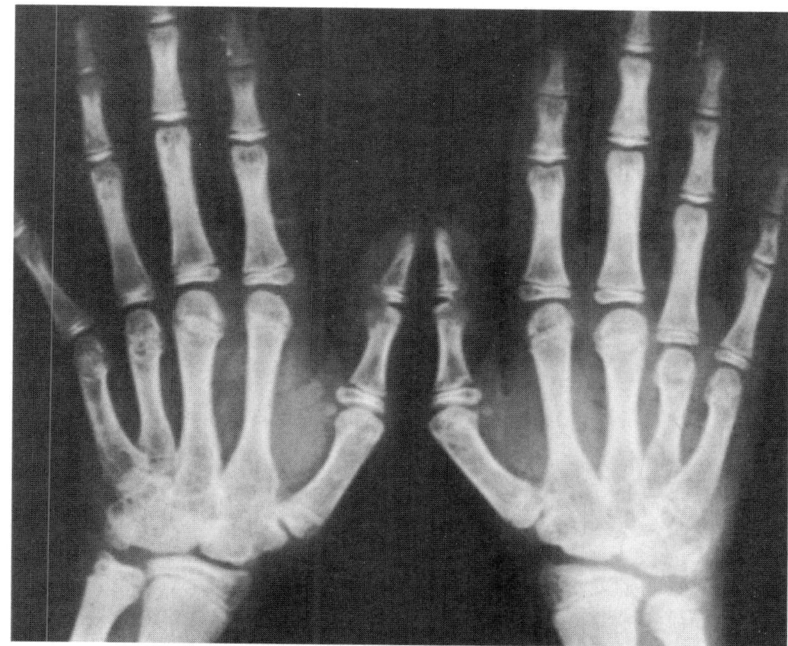

Figure 12–49. Extensive ankylosis of the carpal and metacarpal joints in a 12-year-old girl 2 years after onset of polyarticular JRA. The entire carpus is ankylosed, and there are fusions between the carpals and the second and third metacarpals as well. There is also undergrowth of the fourth right metacarpal and disruption of the radiocarpal relationship.

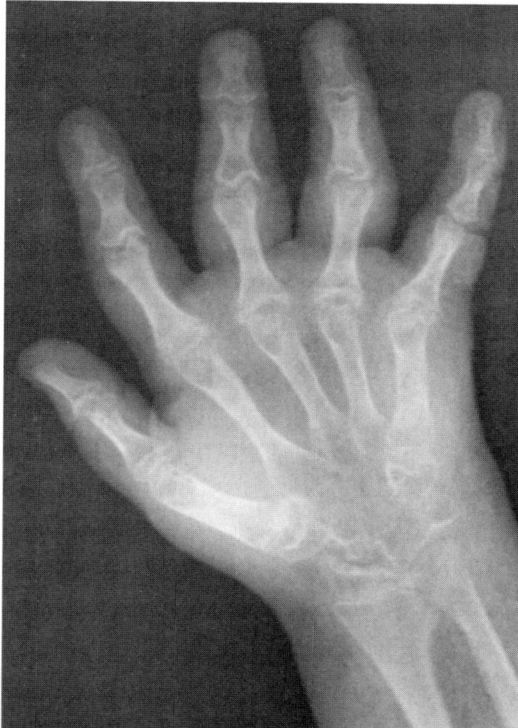

Figure 12–50. Radiograph of the hand of a 15-year-old girl taken shortly before her death. Severe polyarthritis was present, with marked bony overgrowth and enlargement of the epiphyses. Erosions and destruction of the small joints were evident, with invagination of the abutting bones. The distal interphalangeal joints were also involved, and partial ankylosis of the carpus was present.

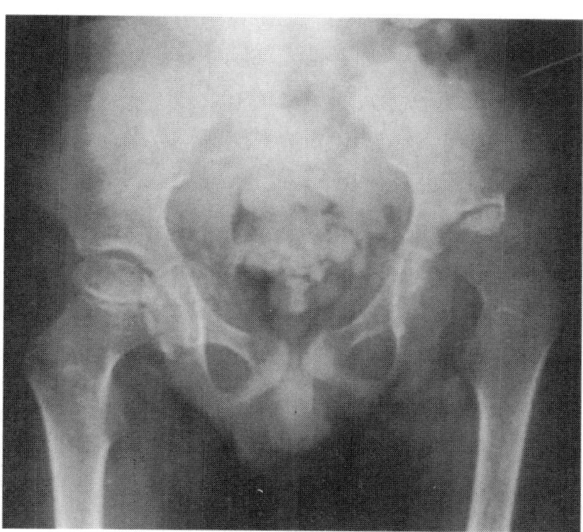

Figure 12–51. Marked subluxation of the left hip of a 5-year-old boy with onset of severe, unremitting JRA at the age of 1½ years. The femoral neck is osteoporotic, and there is the appearance of aseptic necrosis of the femoral head, which is subluxed laterally and superiorly out of a shallow, poorly formed acetabulum.

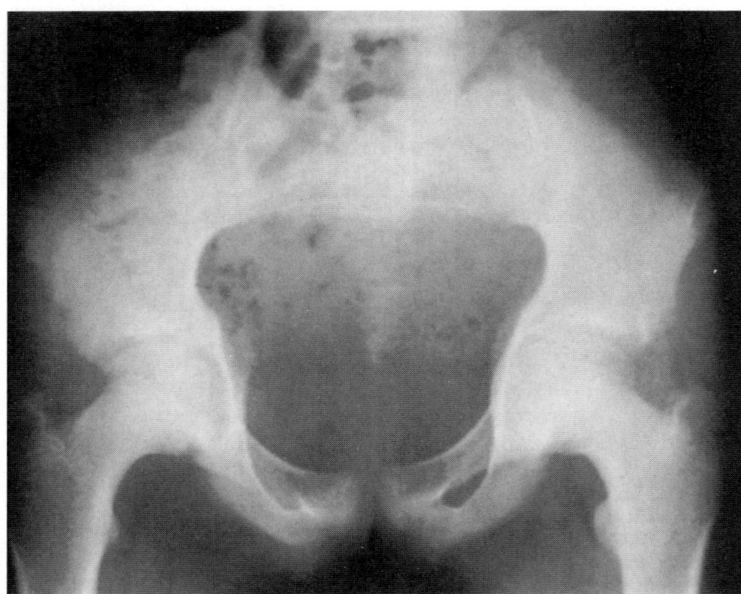

Figure 12–52. Protrusio acetabuli of the left hip in a girl with long-standing JRA. Pain in the hip was accompanied by marked reduction in range of motion, although at the time the overall disease activity was minimal.

for treatment of JCA, 36 (17.5 percent) had pain or restricted hip motion. Definite radiographic evidence of avascular necrosis of the femoral head (condensation, fragmentation, resorption, and flattening of the epiphysis) was found in 10 hips in 6 children, and signs suggestive of this diagnosis were found in a further 20 hips in 13 children. A sclerotic rim at the base of the femoral neck (suggesting earlier ischemia) was also noted.[799, 818] A more recent study demonstrated a low frequency of osteonecrosis.[798]

Knee

Rosberg and Laine[819] noted that the medial femoral condyle tended to enlarge more than the lateral condyle in children with arthritis of the knee. Progression of the radiographic changes of the knee are documented in Figure 12–39. Overgrowth of the patella may be marked in long-standing disease (see Fig. 12–9). Erosion and enlargement of the intercondylar notch of the femur occur. These changes have also been reported as characteristic of hemophilia and tuberculosis. Popliteal fossa cysts are best demonstrated by ultrasound imaging.[820] Children with monarthritis in whom the diagnosis is uncertain should undergo MRI in order to evaluate other causes of persistent joint swelling.[793]

Ankle, Subtalar Joints, and Foot

Loss of "joint space" is frequent in long-standing arthritis of the ankle or subtalar joints. Aseptic necrosis of the dome of the talus may also occur. Intertarsal joint narrowing and fusion occur in JRA but are more characteristic of seronegative spondyloarthritis (tarsitis).[821] Erosive disease (see Fig. 12–42) and localized growth disturbances (Fig. 12–53) are typical of severe polyarticular disease. MRI is particularly useful in the identification of the extent of inflammation of the ankle joint and may confirm the presence of synovitis at a multiplicity of sites: tibia–talar, subtalar, and talonavicular joints, and peroneal and posterior tibial tendon sheaths.[822]

TREATMENT

Approach to Management

The rheumatic diseases grouped under the term JRA cannot yet be cured; fortunately, spontaneous remissions occur in many children, and in the interim, disease control is hopefully achievable. The aims of treatment are, therefore, to control pain and preserve range of motion, muscle strength, and function; to manage systemic complications; and to facilitate normal nutrition, growth, and physical and psychological development (see Chapter 10) (Table 12–37).[430, 823–827] Although the major focus of medical therapy is on the arthritis,

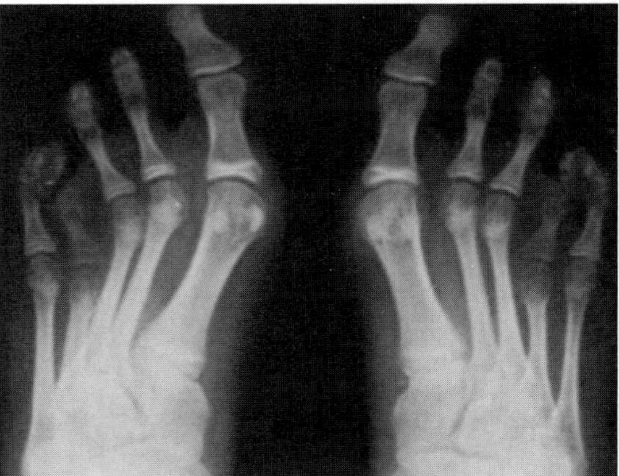

Figure 12–53. Brachydactyly of the fourth metatarsal bones and juxta-articular osteoporosis of the fourth metatarsophalangeal joint in a child with JRA affecting those joints.

Table 12–37

Objectives of the Treatment of JRA

Immediate
- Relieve discomfort
- Preserve function
- Prevent deformities
- Control inflammation

Long-term
- Minimize side effects of disease and treatment
- Promote normal growth and development
- Rehabilitate
- Educate

other extra-articular complications of the disease (e.g., uveitis, serositis, growth retardation, and osteopenia) may require intervention. The treatment program should be family centered, community based, and well coordinated.[828, 829] An ideal approach involves a multidisciplinary team that consists of a pediatric rheumatologist, nurse clinician, social worker, physical therapist, occupational therapist, and psychologist (Table 12–38). Consultation with a physiatrist, psychiatrist, orthopedic surgeon, dentist, or nutritionist is sought when indicated. Regular ophthalmic consultation is mandatory.

Because JRA is characterized by chronic and recurrent inflammation of the joints and varying systemic manifestations, the child and family must often accept the need for long-term treatment and surveillance. Patient and family education and incorporation of the family's needs into the management program are essential in order to facilitate optimal compliance and therapeutic benefit (Table 12–39).[830, 831] Most children with chronic arthritis require elements of pharmacologic, physical, and psychosocial approaches (Table 12–40). A priority in the management of the child with JRA is to foster normal psychological and social development and participation in peer-group activities. Attendance at school is strongly encouraged; only rarely is home instruction justified.[832] The child should also remain in the physical education program at school if at all possible, if not as a participant then as an involved member of the class assigned to other activities; alternatively, the child should be enrolled in adaptive physical education. Children should largely determine their own level of activity. Inappropriate restriction of recess time or peer-group association can be harmful both physically and psychologically.

Table 12–38

The Treatment Team

Child
Family

Pediatric Rheumatologist

Physical Therapist
Occupational Therapist
Nurse
Social Worker
Psychologist
Ophthalmologist
Dentist
Nutritionist
Orthopedic Surgeon

Table 12–39

Factors Affecting Compliance in Treatment of Children With JRA

Compliance is increased by
- Agreement among patient, family, and treatment team with respect to goals of treatment
- Understanding the disease and the treatment approach
- Setting and resetting short-term achievable goals
- Frequent positive reinforcement

Compliance is decreased by
- Poor understanding of the disease and the treatment approach
- Conflict between patient and health care providers with respect to treatment goals
- Setting treatment goals that are unachievable or too long-term
- Complexity or awkwardness of medication regimens
- Adverse side effects of drugs
- Remission and flare of disease

The traditional approach to the pharmacologic treatment of children with JRA is to begin with the safest, simplest, and most conservative measures.[833, 833a] If this approach proves inadequate, other therapeutic modalities are promptly selected in an orderly progression. Thus, NSAIDs are the mainstay of initial treatment. Two developments, however, have fundamentally altered the current approach to treatment beyond that point: Intra-articular glucocorticoids have proved effective in treating limited joint disease; and low-dose methotrexate has substantially changed the approach to early treatment options. New therapeutic modalities such as etanercept promise even further improvements in the risk:benefit ratio. Thus, the traditional "pyramid" of management is in the process of being dismantled, inverted, or otherwise changed to reflect these advances in therapy.[834, 835] Although combination therapy is attractive in a child with severe disease in whom more limited pharmacologic regimens have failed, adequate clinical studies of effectiveness and safety are generally lacking (Fig. 12–54).[836–840]

It is not usually possible at onset of the disease to predict which child will recover and who might go on to have unremitting disease with lingering disability or enter adulthood with serious functional impairment.[841–843] Therefore, the initial therapeutic approach must be vigorous in all children. Furthermore, therapeutic strategies must recognize the three types of on-

Table 12–40

Psychosocial and Educational Management of Children With JRA

- Understand the patient's and parents' goals
- Understand the psychological effect of fluctuations in disease activity
- Undertake early realistic career planning
- Emphasize the benefit of regular school participation
- Facilitate normal peer group interaction

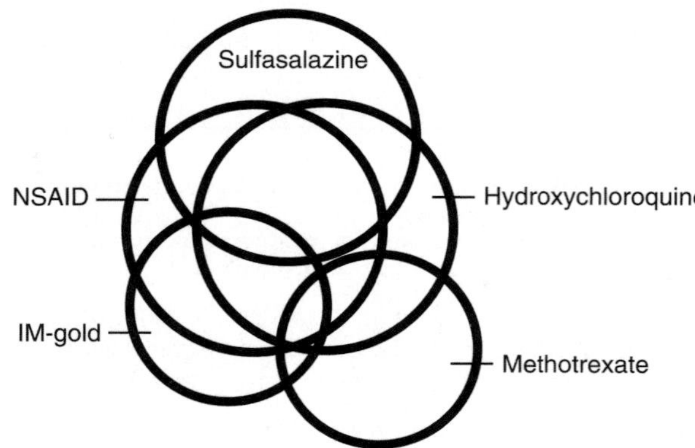

Figure 12–54. Venn diagram illustrates potential combinations of therapeutic modalities. IM, intramuscular; NSAID, nonsteroidal anti-inflammatory drug.

set: oligoarthritis, polyarthritis, and systemic disease (Fig. 12–55). Evolution of the course subtypes and recognition of prognostic indicators will lead to modifications of the program in keeping with the response of the child. Evidence of improvement is based on a review of the clinical course, repeated physical examinations, charting of the articular severity index and global responses, and laboratory estimates of inflammation.[843a, 843b] It is undoubtedly true that a number of these evaluations are redundant.[844, 845] Therapy with an NSAID should be continued for at least 6 months after all evidence of active disease has disappeared. Methotrexate therapy should be continued for a year or longer in the same circumstances. In children, potentially toxic regimens such as prolonged steroid use and immunosuppressive drugs should be employed only in uncontrolled or life-threatening disease.

It is almost impossible to be confident of the therapeutic risk:benefit ratio for many of the medical regimens used for treating a child with chronic arthritis. Experimental data and clinical observation confirm the efficacy of NSAIDs, methotrexate, or glucocorticoids. It is not as certain that other medications such as hydroxychloroquine, sulfasalazine, D-penicillamine, IVIG, or cyclosporin confer statistically and clinically significant benefit. Toxicity is often a foremost concern in the long-term use of steroids or immunosuppressive agents such as azathioprine or cyclophosphamide. Because of the relative lack of scientific guidance by appropriately designed studies, undertaken in adequate numbers of children with appropriate control of confounding factors such as type of onset and course of the disease, the experience and judgment of the pediatric rheumatologist often become the most important principles of guidance for the therapy of a child.

Basic Medical Program

In most children, one of the NSAIDs is the basic approach to therapy (Table 12–41) (see Chapter 7).[846] All of these drugs have antipyretic, analgesic, and anti-inflammatory actions, and—for those that have been approved for use in children—a record of long-term safety. Most current drugs inhibit the activity of cyclo-

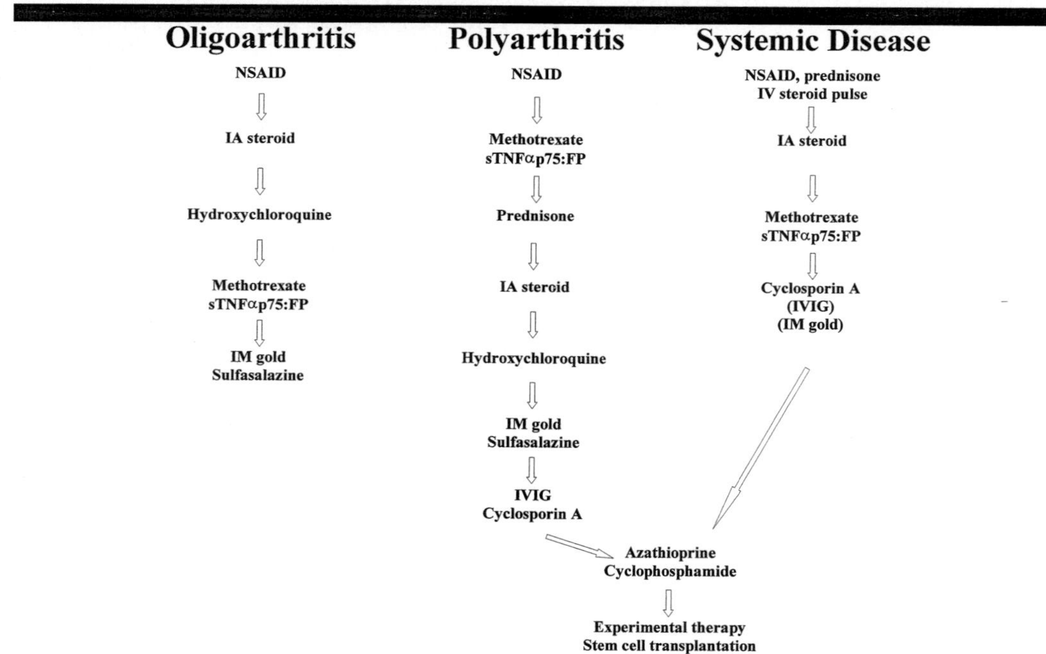

Figure 12–55. Potential sequential therapeutic steps according to onset/course types and clinical response. IA, intra-articular; IM, intramuscular; IV, intravenous; IVIG, intravenous immunoglobulin; NSAID, nonsteroidal anti-inflammatory drug; TNF, tumor necrosis factor.

Table 12–41
Nonsteroidal Anti-Inflammatory Drugs Used in JRA

DRUG	DOSE (mg/kg/d)	MAXIMUM (mg/d)	ADMINISTRATION (ORAL)
Aspirin	75–90	4800	t.i.d. or q.i.d.
Naproxen	15–20	750	b.i.d.
Tolmetin	25–30	1600	t.i.d.
Ibuprofen	35–45	2400	q.i.d.
Indomethacin	1–2	150	t.i.d. or q.i.d.
Diclofenac	2–3	150	q.i.d.
Sulindac	4–6	300	b.i.d. or t.i.d.
Piroxicam	0.3–0.6	20	q.d.

oxygenases 1 and 2 and therefore have the potential to induce GI irritation.[847, 848] The new selective cyclooxygenase 2 (Cox-2) inhibitors have just become generally available but have not been evaluated in children.[849]

Nonsteroidal Anti-Inflammatory Drugs

Only a few of the NSAIDs have been approved in the United States for use in children (e.g., naproxen, tolmetin, and ibuprofen).[850] Results of trials of several other NSAIDs indicate that they are as effective as but no more effective than salicylates, naproxen, or tolmetin. The clinical trials of NSAIDs by the Pediatric Rheumatology Collaborative Study Group (PRCSG) led to the conclusion that approximately 65 percent of children who were going to respond did so by 4 weeks of therapy; however, some children were late responders: A 100-percent level of response was not obtained before 12 weeks in 72 of the 127 children who experienced a favorable outcome.[851] Clinical response to a NSAID is variable and relatively unpredictable. A child may not respond to one drug, or eventually lose an initial response, and yet respond to another drug. In such cases, it is logical to select an NSAID from a different chemical class than was first used (salicylic, propionic, indoleacetic, pyrrolealkaonic, *N*-phenylanthranilic acids, or oxicams) (see Chapter 7).

Naproxen is effective in management of joint inflammation in a dose of 15 to 20 mg/kg/day given with food.[852–856] It need be given only twice daily, and it is available as a suspension (125 mg/5 ml), a definite advantage in the treatment of the young child. Naproxen is usually well tolerated, although mild epigastric discomfort is occasionally encountered. Cutaneous pseudoporphyria, a side effect of this drug and occasionally of other NSAIDs, is characterized by a bullous eruption on the face, hands, and other sun-exposed areas, often leaving an irregular shallow scar (see Chapter 7).[857–861]

Ibuprofen is a relatively mild anti-inflammatory agent. It is usually well tolerated and may have a role in treatment of minimal to moderate disease.[862, 863] Tablets are prescribed in a dose of approximately 35 mg/kg/day, divided into four doses given with food. The suspension (100 mg/5 ml) consists of both the S and the R enantiomers and is not absorbed as well as the tablets. It should therefore be given at a dose of approximately 45 mg/kg/day divided into four doses.[864]

Tolmetin in a dose of 25 to 30 mg/kg/day, given in three divided doses with food, is effective as an anti-inflammatory drug.[856, 865, 866] We have observed severe gastric erosion, however, including perforation in three patients who were taking tolmetin. Diclofenac must be given in four doses, but it may be useful in children who are unable to tolerate other NSAIDs because of gastric side effects.[856, 867, 868] Sulindac is an inactive prodrug that is converted in vivo to the active sulfide and therefore theoretically offers little exposure to the GI mucosa.[869] It has also been suggested that it is less nephrotoxic than other NSAIDs,[870, 871] although this has not always been confirmed.[872] Celecoxib and rofecoxib, the first of a new class of Cox-2 inhibitors, have been introduced for treatment of arthritis in adults. These drugs are reputedly less likely than traditional NSAIDs to cause gastric irritation such as peptic ulcer disease.[848]

Other NSAIDs have specific indications, although their use in childhood has often not been officially approved. Indomethacin, in a dose of 1 to 2 mg/kg/day to a maximum of 125 mg/day, is useful in treating the fever and pericarditis of systemic-onset JRA.[873, 874] The fever of systemic onset often responds poorly to the usual NSAIDs, even in high doses.[873] In many children, it responds only to prednisone or alternatively to indomethacin. Indomethacin is a potent anti-inflammatory drug, but it frequently causes headache or epigastric pain. It has been of particular value in the older child, but its overall use has been limited, perhaps inappropriately, by occasional serious side effects and early reports of masked infections and sudden deaths.[875, 876] Piroxicam needs to be given only once a day, and it may be particularly useful in the older child or adolescent in whom compliance with taking prescribed medication is a problem.[877–879]

Aspirin

The role of aspirin as the drug of choice in initial management has been supplanted by the newer NSAIDs. The reasons for this are related more to convenience of administration and relative freedom from side effects than to superior efficacy. Aspirin likely resulted in more frequent transaminasemia than the newer NSAIDs.[880–882] Nonetheless, considering its long and extensive use, aspirin has a remarkable record of effectiveness in suppressing fever and other aspects of inflammation and a proven record of long-term safety.[883] Its epitaph has not yet been carved in stone, and because of its low cost, aspirin will probably continue to be a part of the pediatric rheumatologist's anti-inflammatory armamentarium, if not at the forefront of the battle.

Aspirin is started at 75 to 90 mg/kg/day in four doses given with food to minimize gastric irritation and to ensure therapeutic blood levels.[884–886] Lower doses per kilogram may be indicated in children weighing more than 25 kg. The therapeutic serum salicylate level is 20 to 25 mg/dl (1.45 to 1.8 mmol/L), usually measured 2 hours after the morning dose. It may be difficult to reach therapeutic levels in children with acute systemic disease, but increasing the dose beyond 130 mg/kg often results in salicylism. If high doses are required initially, they should be reduced gradually to maintenance levels as the systemic manifestations of the disease subside. Awakening the child at night to administer aspirin is not necessary, because the serum half-life of salicylate is prolonged once therapeutic levels have been achieved. Aspirin should not be chewed, because it may cause gingival inflammation and erosions of the biting surfaces of the teeth.[887, 888] An adequate trial of aspirin should last at least 6 weeks. The fever of systemic onset may not respond to aspirin before 3 to 4 weeks of treatment.

Salicylate toxicity is discussed in Chapter 7. However, two side effects deserve special mention here because they require specific management strategies. The potential association of Reye's syndrome with varicella or influenza infection and aspirin administration has been emphasized by epidemiologic data and in the United States by directives from the Centers for Disease Control and the Food and Drug Administration.[581, 889–893] Use of the varicella vaccine will improve safety of medication use in children with JRA. Acyclovir should be employed in immunocompromised children who develop the disease. Zoster–immune globulin should also be used in children with JRA within 96 hours of known intimate exposure to varicella.

In the child exposed to influenza, the situation is more complex. Because influenza is difficult to identify clinically, all drugs except glucocorticoids should be discontinued in any child with vomiting or diarrhea until GI symptoms have ceased. All children with JRA should be immunized yearly for the currently recommended strains of influenza as an added precaution. Such immunization should not give rise to a false sense of security, however, because immunity is not guaranteed. Early concerns[894] that influenza immunization might cause a flare of arthritis seem to be unjustified.[895, 896]

Aspirin and other NSAIDs are associated with interstitial nephritis and renal papillary necrosis. A few children with JRA may develop analgesic nephropathy when taking aspirin alone.[897, 898] Azotemia and hypertension do not occur in children with NSAID nephropathy per se, but the NSAID should be discontinued or the dose reduced if renal involvement is suspected. It is estimated that this complication may occur in approximately 1 percent of children with JRA who receive NSAID therapy.

Analgesics. Although it is not an anti-inflammatory drug, acetaminophen given two to three times a day may be useful for control of pain or fever in the systemically ill child with JRA. This drug should not be used for long-term basic management of the disease because, when used with an NSAID, it may contribute to interstitial nephritis. Ketorolac has profound analgesic effects but less prominent anti-inflammatory effects. Its principal use is in the short-term management of pain. Although controversial, the use of opioids (oxycodone) for severe rheumatic pain should be considered in special circumstances, especially for short-term indications.[899]

Recent studies[435, 900, 900a] examined psychological approaches to treatment for children with JRA who had higher levels of associated pain. The treatment protocol included relaxation training, electromyography, and biofeedback for the child, and training in the use of behavioral techniques for managing daily physical therapy and school attendance for the mothers. The results have provided modest support for the use of psychological interventions in children whose pain significantly affected the activities of daily living.

Methotrexate

Methotrexate, because of its relatively rapid onset of action and acceptable toxicity, can justifiably be considered as the initial second-line agent in many children.[901–906] The advantages of this medication are efficacy at relatively low doses, oral administration, and apparent lack of oncogenicity or production of sterility.[349, 905, 907, 908] Three to 6 months is considered an adequate therapeutic trial. Principal toxicities are directed at the bone marrow, liver, and lung (see Chapter 7). Cirrhosis of the liver is not an expected toxic effect in children on weekly therapy.[909–912] Malnutrition, viral hepatitis, diabetes mellitus, obesity, or alcohol consumption increase the risk. In this respect, the guidelines recommended by the ACR should be observed.[913] Routine liver biopsies are not indicated. Methotrexate-induced pneumonitis has been reported rarely in children (Fig. 12–56).[914–917] Accelerated nodulosis is equally uncommon.[360, 907, 915, 918] Because some NSAIDs may interfere with the protein-binding and excretion of methotrexate, their dosage should be kept constant during treatment.[919] Folic acid, 1 mg/day, is given during treatment with no diminution in effectiveness.[920, 920a] Monthly monitoring for toxicity includes a complete blood count, white blood cell differential and platelet counts, and measurement of serum levels of liver enzymes. Later bimonthly studies are adequate.

The drug is given as a single weekly dose on an empty stomach with clear liquids 60 minutes before breakfast.[921] The injectable preparation (25 mg/ml) can be used orally in children in order to prescribe the correct amount. The minimum oral starting dose is 10 mg/M^2 weekly ($\geq$0.3 mg/kg). If questions concerning adequate absorption arise,[922] an initial assessment of the serum concentration of the drug at 1 hour should be considered, with adjustment based on its level ($\geq 6 \times 10^{-7}$ M).[923, 924] The drug should be administered subcutaneously if clinical response is inadequate, oral administration is associated with nausea, vomiting, or an increase in hepatic enzymes, or a higher dose range (0.65 to 1.0 mg/kg, with a maximum dose of approximately 30 mg/week) is chosen for a trial of effectiveness.[925–927] Intramuscular administration is effective but not necessary.[927]

Clinical improvement of arthritis and relatively low toxicity have been reported in a number of studies (Table 12–42).[901–904, 908, 923, 925, 928–935] Assessments included number of swollen joints, morning stiffness, systemic features of the disease, mean daily dose of glucocorticoid, erythrocyte sedimentation rate, and C-reactive protein concentration. Reviews by Wallace and colleagues[932] and others[905, 928, 936, 937] suggest that virtually all children respond to methotrexate and that approximately one half achieve a remission. The poorest response rate is associated with systemic-onset disease, the best with oligoarthritis.[938] Methotrexate is discontinued if no objective response is documented in the initial trial or if toxicity develops.

The double-blind random trial of methotrexate by the

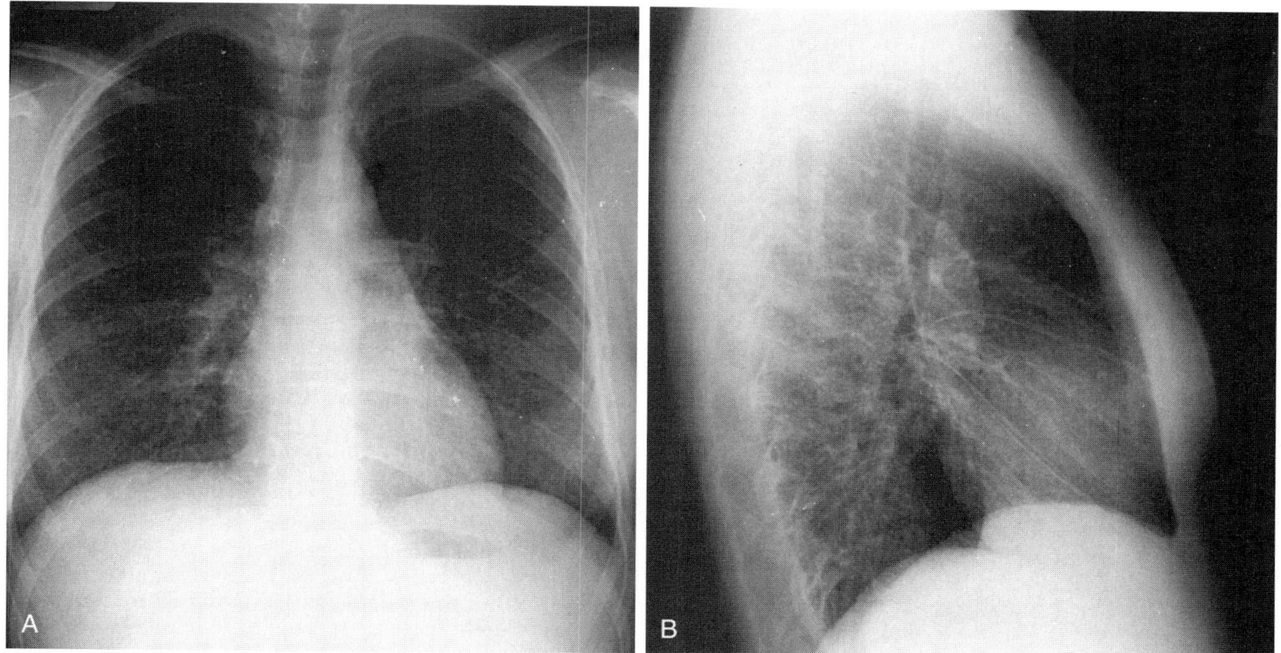

Figure 12–56. Posteroanterior and lateral radiographs of the chest of a 13½-year-old girl who developed polyarticular JRA in the summer of 1997. In December of that year, low-dose methotrexate was started at 7.5 mg once a week. These films were obtained in May 1998. They show a diffuse, fine, fibronodular, interstitial infiltrate throughout the lower two-thirds of the parenchyma. At that time, she was asymptomatic and there were no abnormalities on examination of the chest. Pulmonary function tests revealed a mild restrictive pattern with an initial diffusing capacity of the lungs for carbon monoxide of 79 percent of predicted. High-resolution computed tomographic examination confirmed the presence of bilateral, linear, and reticular nodular interstitial infiltrates. The methotrexate was stopped and, over the course of the next year, the radiographic appearance gradually returned toward normal along with pulmonary function.

Table 12–42

Studies of Efficacy and Toxicity of Methotrexate in Treatment of JRA

	SERIES											
	Truckenbrodt & Hafner[901]	Wallace et al[923]	Speckmaier et al[902]	Rose et al[928]	Halle & Prieur[903]	Lepore & Pennesi[929]	Graham et al[930]	Giannini et al[904]*	Giannini et al[904]*	Wallace et al[932]	Ravelli et al[934]	Huang[935]
Year	1986	1989	1989	1990	1991	1992	1992	1992	1992	1993	1995	1996
Study design	R			R			R	C	C			
Patients *(n)*	19	23	12	29	30	14	62	40	46	49	29	26
Male/female	7/12			14/15			8/54	11/29	13/33			9/19
Type of onset *(n)*												
Polyarthritis	3	10	0	13	13	9	62			24	10	20
Oligoarthritis	4	4	0	1	7	3	0			16	0	0
Systemic	12	9	12	15	10	2	0	11	9	9	19	6
Dose												
mg/M²/wk	4–17		2.5–10	5–15			10–20	5	10		7.5–11	10–15
mg/kg/wk		0.11–0.6			0.4–0.8	0.3–0.5				0.11–1.1		
Treatment duration (mo)												
Mean	10.5	19.2	6	18.5		12	13.4	6	6		6	3
Range	4–10	6–52		8–39	6–30		19–65			12–18		6–72
Outcome												
Improvement (%)	53	91	33	48–83	50			63	72	45	50	73
Toxicity (%)	6	10	1	3	12		10	13	8			23
Drug stopped	0			0	1		0	1	2			1

C, double-blind, placebo-controlled; R, retrospective.
*Giannini et al[904] includes two studies.

Table 12–43

Results of Discontinuation of Methotrexate in JRA

	MONTHS TO CONTROL (x ± SD)	MONTHS FROM CONTROL TO DISCONTINUATION OF MTX (x ± SD)	RELAPSE (%)	MONTHS TO RELAPSE (x & RANGE)	REMISSION (%)
SA	25±14	6±5	50	10 (4–16)	50
PA	17±15	8±15	53	9 (1–36)	47
OA	9±5	7±3	50	16 (6–24)	50
Total	16±4	7±4	52	11 (1–36)	48

SA, systemic-onset arthritis; PA, polyarticular arthritis; OA, oligoarticular arthritis.

Adapted from Gottlieb BS, Keenan GF, Lu T, et al: Discontinuation of methotrexate treatment in juvenile rheumatoid arthritis. Adapted by permission of Pediatrics vol 100: page 996, table 3, copyright 1997.

PRCSG included two doses of 5 mg/M²/week and 10 mg/M²/week along with a placebo control group.[904] Statistical improvement in articular severity was observed with a mean of 26 for the placebo group and 63 for the 10-mg group. Recalculating these data by the newer Pavia criteria for response[845, 939, 940] (three or more of any six core variables improved by at least 30 percent, with up to one variable worse) indicated that 72 percent of children improved with methotrexate versus 44 percent of the placebo group.[931, 941] The drug was discontinued in 2 of 45 patients (hematuria, persistent transaminasemia). One placebo patient developed severe GI irritation.

A report of Wallace and coworkers[923] included 23 children with seropositive polyarthritis who were treated with doses of methotrexate that ranged from 0.1 to 0.6 mg/kg/week. Twenty-one improved significantly, and a remission was noted in 2 children. It was possible to reduce the dose of glucocorticoids in 6 of 9 children. The average time to clinical response was approximately 3.3 months (range, 1 to 8 months). It was not possible to identify clinical involvement that would predict improvement. A study by Harel and associates[942] found that carpal length as a measure of cartilage loss was significantly improved in 11 of the 17 children who responded to 2.5 years of therapy, in which all of the nonresponders had a deterioration of carpal length. Ravelli and colleagues[943] provided further evidence of the effectiveness of methotrexate in that there was radiologic improvement or a slowing of deterioration of carpal length in children who had responded during a 2-year period of administration. Carpal length was significantly shorter in nonresponders. A younger age at onset and being a male correlated with a higher risk of poorer radiologic outcome.

It is somewhat difficult to be sure whether to categorize methotrexate as an anti-inflammatory drug or a remittent drug. Methotrexate therapy should be continued even after a sustained remission of the disease is achieved.[938, 944] Early withdrawal has resulted in an exacerbation of the arthritis, and reinstitution of the drug did not always result in a satisfactory clinical response. However, in children who have entered a remission, it is necessary to discontinue methotrexate at some time. The question is *when*.[941] A study by Ravelli and coworkers[944] indicated that one third of children had a relapse after discontinuation of the drug. The child most at risk was the one who had had a oligoarticular onset with a subsequent polyarticular course.[944a]

A study by Gottlieb and colleagues[938] has strengthened the conclusion that methotrexate is a remittive agent. Approximately 50 percent of children in all onset groups who developed a relapse approximately 11 months after withdrawal of the drug (Table 12–43). Only 50 percent regained control of the disease an average of 15 months after reinstitution of therapy. The most convincing evidence of the disease-modifying nature of methotrexate was the long period of time after withdrawal before relapse (range, 1.5 to 36 months). The authors identified younger age of onset (<5 years) as indicating a more likely chance of relapse. Perhaps therapy with methotrexate should be prolonged for many months, even years, after a remission has been achieved. One might also consider a different mode of withdrawal, such as decreasing administration to every 2 weeks for a period of time, before discontinuation.

Advanced Therapy

The slow-acting antirheumatic drugs (SAARDs), or disease-modifying antirheumatic drugs, consist of the antimalarials, injectable and oral gold compounds, sulfasalazine, and D-penicillamine (Table 12–44). Much of the data regarding therapeutic efficacy of these drugs has been inferred from uncontrolled studies.[945, 946] The fact that their beneficial effects are not observed for several weeks to months, coupled with the unpredictable, relapsing, remitting course of JRA, makes evaluation of this group of medications difficult. When the toxicity of many of the members of this group is ac-

Table 12–44

Slow-Acting Antirheumatic Drugs Used in JRA

DRUG	DOSE	ADMINISTRATION
Hydroxychloroquine	6 mg/kg/d (maximum 400 mg/d)	Oral q.d. or b.i.d. with food
Sulfasalazine	50 mg/kg/d (maximum 2 g/d)	Oral b.i.d. with food
Aurothiomalate	1 mg/kg/wk (maximum 50 mg/wk)	IM q 1–4 wk
Auranofin	0.1–0.2 mg/kg/d (maximum 9 mg/d)	Oral q.d. or b.i.d. with food
Penicillamine	5–10 mg/kg/d (maximum 750 mg/d)	Oral q.d. or b.i.d. 2 hr before meals

Table 12–45

Disease Outcome in Children With JRA Treated With Slow-Acting Antirheumatic Drugs

DRUG (NO. OF PATIENTS)	IMPROVEMENT (%)	REMISSION (%)
Antimalarial drugs (242)	40	27
Gold (340)	47	16
Penicillamine (467)	64	2
Sulfasalazine (28)	61	4

Modified from Grondin C, Malleson P, Petty RE: Slow acting anti-rheumatic drugs in chronic arthritis in childhood. Semin Arthritis Rheum 18: 38, 1988.

counted for, enthusiasm for their use must be somewhat restrained. Until recently, however, these agents were the mainstay of second-line therapy in children with polyarticular JRA in whom NSAIDs had produced no response.[840] Methotrexate now rivals—and in many clinics has replaced—the SAARDs in this capacity.[937] On the other hand, SAARDs can be added to the medical program for children who have an incomplete response to a combination of NSAID and methotrexate during an initial trial period.[908] *Introduction of newer approaches to therapy, such as TNF-α blockade, will undoubtedly lead to changes in therapeutic recommendations.*

Choice among the SAARDs is influenced by the severity of disease for which they are prescribed and by the efficacy (Table 12–45), rapidity of response, and toxicity (Table 12–46) of each drug. Hydroxychloroquine is often our initial choice because it is somewhat more rapid in effect than other drugs and its toxicity is minimal. However, it is not an especially potent agent and is therefore most often used in an adjunctive capacity. Gold and D-penicillamine are widely thought to be more potent in their antiarthritic effect, but they require a period of 3 to 6 months before efficacy can be evaluated, and they have considerable toxicity. Sulfasalazine may act more quickly than gold or D-penicillamine, is possibly less toxic (but not necessarily so), and is especially useful in children with seronegative spondyloarthropathies. All members of this group of drugs can be used with NSAIDs or glucocorticoids. Combination therapy with, for example, gold and hydroxychloroquine is not contraindicated, but there is little evidence to support the practice, and a wider spectrum of toxicity would be anticipated. Children with systemic-onset JRA may be at much greater risk for toxic reactions from any of the SAARDs, and sometimes even NSAIDs, than children with the other types of onset.[412, 418–420, 424] The most serious of these is MAS with the acute onset of neutropenia and diffuse intravascular coagulation.

Hydroxychloroquine

Hydroxychloroquine is a useful adjunctive agent for treatment of the older child with JRA (Tables 12–47 and 12–48).[419, 945, 947–950] The therapeutic effect of hydroxychloroquine in JRA is usually subtle and is rarely evident before 2 to 3 months of therapy. If no improvement is demonstrated after treatment for 6 months, it should be discontinued. Hydroxychloroquine is almost never used alone but is added to an NSAID regimen in a dose of 5 to 6 mg/kg/day.[947] The medication is available only in 200-mg tablets, and it is often not possible to achieve the exact dose per day. An alternative schedule involves calculating the weekly dose and then distributing the correct number of tablets during the week. The drug should be taken with food because it can be an irritant to the GI tract. An ophthalmic examination, including testing of color vision and visual fields, is usually performed before therapy is started and every 6 months thereafter.[951, 952]

Generally, the drug has not been recommended in children younger than 4 years, and occasionally younger than 7 years of age, because of their inability to discern colors adequately for testing on grids or visual fields. Although retinal

Table 12–46

Toxicity of the Slow-Acting Antirheumatic Drugs Used in Treatment of JRA

TOXICITY	ANTIMALARIAL DRUGS	GOLD SALTS	PENICILLAMINE	SULFASALAZINE
No. of patients	242	340	467	28
Toxicity (%)	24	41	23	37
Toxicity requiring drug discontinuation	7	21	9	10
Type of toxicity				
Bone marrow	10	35	16	23
Kidney	28	20	21	0
Skin	8	20	16	23
GI	3	—	20	31
Mouth	—	5	3	8
Miscellaneous	51	20	24	15

Modified from Grondin C, Malleson P, Petty RE: Slow acting anti-rheumatic drugs in chronic arthritis in childhood. Semin Arthritis Rheum 18: 38, 1988.

Table 12–47

Design of Trials of Antimalarial Drugs in JRA

SERIES (REF.)	STUDY DESIGN	OTHER DRUGS USED
1. Stillman[948]	Retrospective	
2. Kvien et al.[949]	Open, comparative, randomized	Penicillamine, gold compounds a. 4 treated during systemic phase b. 15 treated after systemic phase
3. Manners and Ansell[419]	Retrospective	Penicillamine
4. Brewer et al.[950]	Prospective, randomized, double-blind, placebo	
5. Grondin et al.[945]	Retrospective	

Modified from Grondin C, Malleson P, Petty RE: Slow acting anti-rheumatic drugs in chronic arthritis in childhood. Semin Arthritis Rheum 18: 38, 1988.

toxicity is very rare,[951, 952] hydroxychloroquine should be discontinued at the first suspicion of retinopathy because the effects of this drug are cumulative.[953] Chloroquine is less frequently used than hydroxychloroquine and probably has greater ocular toxicity.[954–957] Stillman[948] noted that 3 of 125 children treated with antimalarial drugs developed nonprogressive retinopathy (macular degeneration) that was attributable to the medication. Two of the children had taken chloroquine as well as hydroxychloroquine. Corneal deposition of drug may also occur and is usually accepted as an indication for lowering the dose of the drug rather than discontinuing it.

The therapeutic effect of hydroxychloroquine has not been conclusively proved in randomized, double-blind studies. In a number of therapeutic trials involving approximately 240 children,[945] clinical improvement occurred in 15 to 75 percent and remission in 45 percent of patients. Toxicity occurred in up to 60 percent of the children and required discontinuation of the medication in 10 percent. (This high level of toxicity does not reflect our current experience.) An extensive double-blind trial by the PRCSG compared hydroxychloroquine to D-penicillamine or an NSAID. [950] In this trial, 162 children with severe, poorly controlled arthritis were observed over 12 months. Eighty-eight percent of the children completed 6 months of the trial, and 76 percent completed 12 months. At that time, the three evaluation groups included 43 (hydroxychloroquine), 46 (D-penicillamine), and 34 (NSAID). Although no unequivocal therapeutic advantages could be attributed to hydroxychloroquine or D-penicillamine compared with placebo, it was difficult to explain why children on placebo did so well because failure of a therapeutic trial with an NSAID was an entry criterion. The authors noted that 60 percent of the hydroxychloroquine group, 46 percent of those on D-penicillamine, and 39 percent of the children on placebo demonstrated clinical improvement at 12 months of therapy.[958] However, improvement of pain on motion was noted in the hydroxychloroquine group more often than in children treated only with placebo. Late benefit was unlikely to be documented if a favorable response had not occurred by 6 months. No subgroup of children could be identified who were likely to respond to either drug.[959] Hydroxychloroquine may also be beneficial in amelioration of the dyslipoproteinemia that occurs in JRA and secondary to glucocorticoid treatment.[960]

Table 12–48

Results of Trials of Antimalarial Drugs in JRA

SERIES*	1	2	3a	3b	4	5
Patients (no.)	125	25	4	15	57	19
Male/female	—	10/15	—	—	—	5/14
Type of onset (no.)						
Polyarthritis	57	12	0	0	—	7
Oligoarthritis	52	13	0	0	—	9
Systemic disease	16	0	4	15	—	0
Dose (mg/kg/wk)	7.7	5	4–7	4–7	6	5–6
Duration of treatment						
Mean (yr)	—	0.96	2.4	2.4	1.0	1.16
Range	0.06–5.3	—	—	—	—	0.17–2.33
Outcome						
Improvement (%)	32	20	75	47	74	16
Remission (%)	45	44	0	0	0	5
Toxicity						
Total (%)	15	8	0	7	61	11
Drug stopped (%)	10	0	0	7	4	0

*See Table 12–47 for series 1 through 5.

Modified from Grondin C, Malleson P, Petty RE: Slow acting anti-rheumatic drugs in chronic arthritis in childhood. Semin Arthritis Rheum 18: 38, 1988.

Parenteral Gold Compounds

Parenteral gold compounds (sodium aurothiomalate and aurothioglucose) are indicated in children with polyarthritis in whom a program of NSAIDs has failed and whose disease is extensive or progressing.[961–970] Gold treatment should be initiated earlier, rather than later, in children with rapidly progressing RF-seropositive polyarthritis in whom methotrexate therapy has failed. The basic anti-inflammatory regimen of NSAIDs is continued during administration of gold compounds. Before gold therapy is started, it should be determined that the child's hematologic, renal, and hepatic functions are normal (complete blood count, urinalysis, blood urea nitrogen and creatinine concentrations, and serum levels of liver enzymes). A 5-mg intramuscular test dose is given initially, and weekly doses thereafter are gradually increased to a level of approximately 0.75 to 1 mg/kg/week (maximum, 50 mg/week).[971] If objective, satisfactory improvement or a remission is achieved in 6 months, therapy is maintained at the same dose with injections every 2 weeks for approximately 3 months, then every 3 weeks for 3 months. If signs of improvement have continued during this interval, the gold injections may be decreased to every 4 weeks thereafter, with periodic adjustments based on growth and body weight.

Before each administration, the child should be assessed for any associated toxicity, such as stomatitis, dermatitis, pruritus, depression of any of the cellular elements of the blood, hematuria, or proteinuria. A decrease in the leukocyte count below 3500/mm^3 (3.5 $\times$ 10^9/L), a fall in the absolute neutrophil count of 50 percent or more, or development of thrombocytopenia or eosinophilia, hematuria, or clinical symptoms or signs of gold toxicity are indications for at least a temporary interruption of therapy.[972] Therapy may be cautiously resumed at a lower dose after the symptoms or signs of toxicity disappear. Contraindications to reinstitution of gold therapy are severe leukopenia or neutropenia, proteinuria, exfoliative dermatitis, significant oral ulcerations, or consumptive coagulopathy. In our experience, the most common toxicities are hematuria and dermatitis.

It is estimated that approximately 25 percent of children receiving intramuscular gold undergo serious toxicity and are unable to complete a course of treatment; 25 percent do not improve objectively while receiving the initial course; and the remaining 50 percent develop substantial relief or complete remission and should continue receiving gold for a longer period of time. We are reluctant to discontinue use of gold in children who have had a satisfactory response. There is no convincing evidence of long-term cumulative toxicity, at least in adult RA. Perhaps, after many years of remission, the medication may be cautiously discontinued. Relapses, if they occur, are generally delayed by 3 to 4 months after cessation of therapy. Gold toxicity may be immunogenetically related.[973, 974]

Intramuscular gold has been used to treat children with arthritis for 50 years.[11, 68, 961–965, 967–970] Many of the reported clinical studies are summarized in Tables 12–49 and 12–50.[419, 945, 949, 961, 963–965, 967–969] Most trials demonstrated that 40 to 70 percent of patients improved after treatment. None of these studies was prospective, placebo-controlled, or blinded; six were retrospective,[419, 945, 963–965, 967] and four were open comparisons with D-penicillamine or other anti-inflammatory drugs.[949, 961, 968, 969] Toxicity occurred in 20 to 50 percent of patients and was severe enough to necessitate cessation of therapy in 7 to 30 percent of those affected. In general, the serum concentration of a gold compound has not correlated with the clinical response. In one study,[966] levels were monitored in 66 children with JRA who were treated with gold sodium thiomalate. The results indicated that the dose of the gold compound should be approximately 0.7 mg/kg or 20 mg/M^2 to achieve a peak serum level of approximately 500 to 600 μg/dl. The maximum single dose should never exceed 27 mg/M^2.[15]

Brewer and associates[967] reported a trial of 6 months of gold therapy in 51 children. The dosage was 1 mg/kg/week for 20 weeks and then 1 mg/kg every 2 to 4 weeks for years. Of these children, 63 percent experienced a decrease in severity of the arthritis. In general, children who had the most favorable response had more severe joint involvement; duration of disease and onset type were not related to a beneficial response. Five children developed toxicity (fever, nephrotic syndrome, progressive anemia, hematuria, psychological disturbance) before the 6-month period was completed. Eight children experienced toxicity (dermatitis, nausea, headache, mild anemia, swelling at the injection site,

Table 12–49

Design of Trials of Intramuscular Gold Compounds in JRA

SERIES (REF.)	STUDY DESIGN	OTHER DRUGS USED
1. Sairanen and Laaksonen[962]	Open, comparative	Sulfasalazine, chloroquine, phenylbutazone
2. Hicks et al.[963]	Retrospective	
3. Debendetti et al.[964]	Retrospective	
4. Levinson et al.[965]	Retrospective	
5. Brewer et al.[967]	Retrospective	
6. Ansell et al.[968]	Open, comparative, randomized	Penicillamine
7. Ansell and Hall[969]	Open, comparative, randomized	Penicillamine
8. Kvien et al.[970]	Open, comparative, randomized	Penicillamine, antimalarials used previously
9. Manners and Ansell[419]	Retrospective	a. 24 treated during systemic phase b. 24 treated after systemic phase
10. Grondin et al.[945]	Retrospective	

Modified from Grondin C, Malleson P, Petty RE: Slow acting anti-rheumatic drugs in chronic arthritis in childhood. Semin Arthritis Rheum 18: 38, 1988.

Table 12–50

Results of Trials of Intramuscular Gold Compounds in JRA

SERIES*	1	2	3	4	5	6	7	8	9a	9b	10
Patients (no.)	54	40	14	52	63	10	24	39	24	24	28
Male/female	22/32	12/28	6/8	—	20/43	—	9/15	11/28	—	—	5/23
Type of onset (no.)											
Polyarthritis	—	—	5	—	20	10	—	17	—	—	20
Oligoarrthritis	—	—	3	—	14	—	—	22	—	—	5
Systemic disease	—	30	6	—	29	—	—	0	24	24	3
Dose (mg/kg/wk)	—	1	1	1	—	—	—	0.7	—	—	1
Duration of treatment											
Mean (yr)	—	1.75	2.75	—	0.5	—	—	0.96	1.8	3.8	1.95
Range	0.25–3.0	—	0.23–7.6	0.5–1.0	—	1.0–3.0	—	—	—	—	0.08–8.0
Outcome											
Improvement (%)	78	52	43	32	49	70	50	46	0	42	18
Remission (%)	4	18	57	41	0	10	13	13	8	0	29
Toxicity											
Total (%)	50	48	43	52	21	20	—	23	—	—	43
Drug stopped (%)	30	20	7	—	8	20	17	13	58	25	25

*See Table 12–49 for series 1 through 10.
Modified from Grondin C, Malleson P, Petty RE: Slow acting anti-rheumatic drugs in chronic arthritis in childhood. Semin Arthritis Rheum 18: 38, 1988.

occult blood in the stool) after 6 months. During treatment, only 1 child showed radiologic evidence of disease progression. There was no placebo group.

Levinson and coworkers[965] conducted a trial of gold therapy in 44 children. There was improvement in arthritic and systemic manifestations in 73 percent. Gold failed to produce a response in the remaining children. In a therapeutic study by Manners and Ansell,[419] 48 children with systemic-onset disease had no improvement of the systemic features of the disease and only 10 of the 24 children with unremitting polyarthritis achieved objective benefit. However, 14 children developed potentially life-threatening toxicities that included disseminated intravascular coagulation and cholestatic jaundice (comparable to the macrophage activation syndrome).

The oral gold compound auranofin, or triethylsphosphine gold, was first used for the treatment of JRA in 1983[975] and was subsequently evaluated in a number of studies,[976–980] including a 6-month, double-blind, parallel, randomized, placebo-controlled trial in more than 200 children.[980] Most investigations suggested, and this controlled study conclusively demonstrated, that the effect of auranofin was modest at best and was probably not significantly better than placebo. The safety of this oral gold compound at a starting dose of 0.1 to 0.2 mg/kg/day (maximum 9 mg/day) was documented in the initial study.[975] Steady-state serum levels were reached in 10 to 12 weeks of therapy. Toxicity was relatively mild and occurred in 9 children: diarrhea in 6, abdominal pain in 6, rash in 3, pruritus in 2, and nausea in 1. Toxicity and efficacy did not seem to correlate with the serum level or an increase in the daily dose.

Sulfasalazine

Sulfasalazine has been reported to have modest efficacy in some children with chronic arthritis, and it has the advantage of a more rapid onset of anti-inflammatory action than occurs with the other SAARDs.[981–984, 984a] This drug should not be used in children with known hypersensitivity to sulfa drugs or salicylate, impaired renal or hepatic function, or specific contraindications such as porphyria or glucose-6-phosphate dehydrogenase deficiency. Severe side effects (fever, rash, elevation of serum levels of liver enzymes, and the macrophage activation syndrome) have been reported in children with systemic-onset disease.[981, 985, 986] Sulfasalazine is started at a dose of 500 mg/day given with food. This dose is increased by 500 mg/day every week until a dose of 50 mg/kg/day (maximum of 2000 mg) is reached. Enteric-coated sulfasalazine may be preferable in order to reduce dyspepsia. Monitoring for toxicity includes measurement of hemoglobin, differential leukocyte count, platelet count, and serum levels of liver enzymes every 4 weeks initially and then every 3 months (see Chapter 7). Benefit is usually apparent within 4 to 8 weeks of initiating therapy.

There are only a few published studies on the effectiveness and safety of sulfasalazine in children. Ansell and colleagues[981] noted that good responses to sulfasalazine in a dose of 40 mg/kg/day were most likely in HLA-B27–positive boys who were older than 9 years at onset of arthritis. (This group corresponds to those children who would probably develop ankylosing spondylitis later in life.) Grondin and associates[945] reported that 4 of 12 children had a significant improvement in their arthritis, 1 entered remission, but 2 developed toxicity. In a 24-week study from the Netherlands, 35 children with polyarticular or oligoarticular disease received sulfasalazine and 34 were given a placebo.[983] Those on sulfasalazine had a significant improvement in joint counts and laboratory indices. Ten children (almost one third) developed serious toxicity and were removed from the study. Adverse reactions tended to occur early in treatment and resolved with stopping the medication.

D-Penicillamine

D-Penicillamine is rarely used in the treatment of children with JRA since recognition of the superior effectiveness of methotrexate and publication of the PRCSG's study in which neither D-penicillamine nor

Table 12–51

Design of Trials of D-Penicillamine in JRA

SERIES (REF.)	STUDY DESIGN	OTHER DRUGS
1. Schairer and Stoeber[988]	Retrospective	
2. Schairer and Stoeber[988]	Open, comparative, randomized	Gold compounds
3. Ansell et al.[968]	Open, comparative, randomized	Gold compounds
4. Ansell and Hall[969]	Open, comparative, randomized	Gold compounds
5. Ansell and Hall[969]	Open	Gold compounds
6. Kvien et al.[970]	Open, comparative, randomized	Gold compounds, antimalarials used previously
7. Prieur et al.[989]	Multicenter, double-blind, placebo	
8. Manners and Ansell[419]	Retrospective	a. 11 treated during systemic phase b. 27 treated after systemic phase
9. Brewer et al.[950]	Prospective, randomized, double-blind, placebo	Hydroxychloroqine
10. Grondin et al.[945]	Retrospective	

Modified from Grondin C, Malleson P, Petty RE: Slow acting anti-rheumatic drugs in chronic arthritis in childhood. Semin Arthritis Rheum 18: 38, 1988.

hydroxychloroquine was shown to be superior to placebo.[950] Indications for the use of D-penicillamine are the same as those for intramuscular gold. The dose is approximately 10 mg/kg/day (maximum of 750 mg/day). This level is achieved in three increments at intervals of 8 to 12 weeks each. The drug must be taken on an empty stomach to prevent heavy metals in food from chelating with it and rendering it ineffective. A complete blood count and urinalysis are performed once a week until the maximum dose is achieved, after which monitoring at monthly intervals is sufficient. Toxicity of D-penicillamine is fully discussed in Chapter 7. Of particular concern is the possible induction of a lupus-like syndrome,[987] dermatitis, thrombocytopenia, and proteinuria. D-Penicillamine toxicity is not necessarily dose-dependent and may be related to the presence of HLA-Dw33 (HLA-DR3)[973] and the C4 null allele.[974]

Studies of the efficacy and toxicity of D-penicillamine in treating childhood arthritis are summarized in Tables 12–51 and 12–52.[419, 945, 950, 968–970, 988, 989] Three studies were retrospective,[419, 945, 988] four were open randomized comparisons of gold and D-penicillamine,[949, 967–969] and two were double-blind, placebo-controlled trials.[950, 989] Therapeutic benefit was comparable to that of intramuscular gold, and toxicity was similar or slightly increased. Improvement was documented in 10 to 75 percent of children and remission in 20 percent. Toxicity occurred in 10 to 55 percent, with discontinuation of the drug being necessary in at least 65 percent. In a double-blind study by Prieur and colleagues,[989] there was no observed difference in the rate of remission of children treated with D-penicillamine or placebo. The withdrawal rate for lack of efficacy was about 35 percent, and 18 percent of patients experienced adverse reactions. The most significant toxicities were renal, cutaneous, GI, or bone marrow suppression; these included drug-induced lupus, dermatitis resembling pemphigus, polymyositis, Goodpasture's syndrome, and myasthenia gravis.

Glucocorticoid Drugs

Glucocorticoid medications are indicated in the management of children with JRA for uncontrolled or life-

Table 12–52

Results of Trials of D-Penicillamine in JRA

SERIES*	1	2	3	4	5	6	7	8a	8b	9	10
Patients (no.)	235	29	10	26	26	38	38	11	27	54	11
Male/female	—	—	—	10/16	—	8/30	11/27	—	—	—	3/8
Type of onset (no.)											
Polyarthritis	—	—	10	—	—	16	15	0	0	—	7
Oligoarthritis	—	—	—	—	—	21	7	0	0	—	3
Systemic disease	0	0	—	—	—	1	16	11	27	—	1
Dose (mg/kg/d)	10–30	—	—	15–30	15–30	10	10	—	—	10	4.4–21
Duration of treatment											
Mean (yr)	—	—	—	3.0	3.0	0.96	0.5	0.7	3.3	1.0	1.5
Range	0.1–4.0	—	1.0–3.0	—	—	—	—	—	—	—	0.3–3.3
Outcome											
Improvement (%)	74	66	90	61	53	32	—	0	60	67	9
Remission (%)	0	0	10	8	0	11	18	0	0	0	0
Toxicity											
Total (%)	12	10	10	—	—	40	32	—	—	54	36
Drug stopped (%)	5	10	—	19	42	18	5	64	19	4	18

*See Table 12–51 for series 1 through 10.

Modified from Grondin C, Malleson P, Petty RE: Slow acting anti-rheumatic drugs in chronic arthritis in childhood. Semin Arthritis Rheum 18: 38, 1988.

threatening systemic disease, in treatment of chronic uveitis as local ophthalmic drops or injections, and as intra-articular agents. Systemic glucocorticoids should be instituted only with a well-considered therapeutic plan and a clear set of clinical objectives.[990, 991] Disease control may not be possible except at a cost of unacceptable glucocorticoid toxicity, and some disease activity may have to be accepted in exchange for less drug toxicity. Systemic glucocorticoid therapy, even in high doses, probably does not limit the duration of active disease, prevent extra-articular complications, or alter the eventual outcome of the disease.[475, 992, 993] Given orally or intravenously, these agents are more suited to management of systemic rather than articular disease.

Although the use of glucocorticoid drugs alone to suppress joint inflammation is to be discouraged, low-dose or alternate-day prednisone is of benefit in children with severe polyarthritis who are unresponsive to other therapeutic programs.[994] Low-dose prednisone (i.e., 0.1 to 0.2 mg/kg) can be used as a "bridging" agent in the initial treatment of the moderately to severely affected child who is started at the same time on other, slower acting anti-inflammatory drugs.

For severe uncontrolled systemic manifestations of JRA with marked disability, prednisone is often prescribed as a single daily morning dose of 0.25 to 1.0 mg/kg/day (maximum 40 mg) or in divided doses in more severe disease. After satisfactory control of the systemic manifestations is achieved, or when it is obvious that acceptable control is not attainable, prednisone should be gradually decreased if at all possible as advanced therapy is introduced.

Prolonged use of systemic glucocorticoids leads to iatrogenic Cushing's syndrome, growth suppression, fractures, cataracts, and increased susceptibility to overwhelming infection (see Chapter 7).[995] In spite of these unavoidable toxicities, systemic glucocorticoids are important and effective agents for the treatment of some of the most serious manifestations of JRA. Growth retardation commonly occurs in children who receive long-term steroids, even in doses comparable to physiologic replacement (prednisone 3 to 5 mg/M^2/day or 0.075 to 0.125 mg/kg/day).[474] This effect (among others) is related to blunting of growth hormone release, interference with collagen synthesis and delayed skeletal maturation, and negative effects on insulin-like growth factor reactivity. Effects of glucocorticoids on growth and bone mineralization may be ameliorated by the use of deflazacort.[996, 997]

It is important that the child and family be aware of the signs and symptoms of glucocorticoid toxicity and understand that the drug must not be discontinued abruptly under any circumstances because of the risk of precipitating an adrenal crisis. Vomiting or diarrhea in a child who is receiving steroids requires parenteral glucocorticoid in an equivalent dose (see Chapter 7). Children on systemic glucocorticoids should wear an identification bracelet or necklace indicating their name, diagnosis, and the fact that they are on a steroid. This precaution facilitates emergency intravenous steroid administration in the presence of serious trauma or stress. Supplemental steroid is also necessary before and during surgical anesthesia. Although a number of choices exist for the specific drug to be used in these circumstances, one preference is dexamethasone for intramuscular administration before the operation and the use of intravenous hydrocortisone during the procedure.

It often becomes difficult to reduce the dose of a glucocorticoid because of a child's adaptation to chronic steroid excess. "Steroid pseudorheumatism" may complicate even slow withdrawal of the drug, particularly at lower dose levels.[475, 998] This syndrome is characterized by increased stiffness, joint pain, fever, irritability, and malaise with each reduction of dose. It can be minimized if reductions are 1 mg or less in the lower dosage ranges and not more often than every 1 to 2 weeks.

Steroid Pulse Therapy

Intravenous pulse glucocorticoid therapy offers an alternative approach to serious, unresponsive disease: The effect is immediate, and it is hoped that long-term toxicity is decreased.[999, 1000–1002] Methylprednisolone is the drug of choice in a dose of 10 to 30/mg/kg per pulse. Protocols consist of single pulses spaced a month apart, three pulses given sequentially 3 days each month, or three pulses administered on alternate days each month. Pulse therapy is not without potentially serious toxicities and should always be given in a short-stay clinic with cardiovascular monitoring during the infusion and for a time thereafter, with careful attention to electrolyte and fluid balance and to the potential for cardiac arrhythmia or acute hypertension.[1003] In a study by Adebajo and Hall,[1002] 18 patients with systemic-onset disease in whom conventional therapies had failed were treated with intravenous methylprednisolone with good results and no adverse effects. Only 1 month after the first dose, 10 patients were free of systemic symptoms and 8 had experienced an improvement in joint count. Three patients eventually entered a full remission.

Intra-Articular Glucocorticoids

Depot preparations of glucocorticoid drugs may be injected directly into the joint.[1004–1007] The role of this therapeutic approach is changing, but at present it is clearly indicated (1) in the management of oligoarticular JRA that has not responded to an appropriate program of NSAIDs or (2) as an aid to physical therapy of an inflamed contracted joint. Intra-articular glucocorticoid therapy should be considered in the child with polyarticular JRA with one or several target joints that have not responded to NSAIDs and slow-acting anti-inflammatory drugs. Intra-articular injections, however, should be given for only a limited number of times (e.g., three times in a single joint during a 6-month period). Triamcinolone hexacetonide is the drug of choice at a dose of 20 to 40 mg for large joints.[1008] With the use of topical anesthesia (lidocaine 2.5 percent/prilocaine 2.5 percent cream—EMLA) and then local infiltration with lidocaine, most children older than 7 years can cooperate with the procedure. Younger children, or those in whom a hip joint or several joints are being injected, require conscious sedation (midazolam) or general anesthesia. As in any such procedure, aseptic technique must be followed.

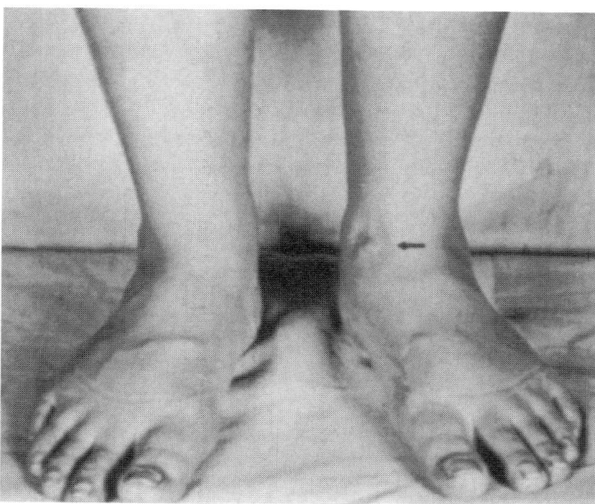

Figure 12–57. Subcutaneous atrophy shown 10 months after intra-articular injection of triamcinolone acetonide tertiary-butylacetate.

The efficacy and safety of intra-articular steroid administration has been studied by a number of authors.[986, 1004–1008, 1008a, 1009] Almost all patients experience a beneficial response; in 60 percent, the response persists for at least 6 months, and in 45 percent, there is no evidence of inflammation in the injected joint for at least 1 year.[1004, 1006] Side effects are uncommon, although two deserve special mention. The risk of subcutaneous atrophy at the site of injection (Fig. 12–57)[1010, 1011] can be avoided or minimized by careful prevention of leakage of the depot preparation around the needle track. Furthermore, intra-articular or periarticular calcification occurs in approximately 15 percent of treated patients.[1006, 1009, 1012] It is seldom symptomatic or clinically detectable but is readily apparent on radiographs (Fig. 12–58). Systemic side effects are rare, although a beneficial "overflow" effect may occur in uninjected joints. We have twice observed prolonged depression after intra-articular injection of triamcinolone hexacetonide. Intra-articular septa, demonstrable by ultrasonography, may impede free distribution of injected glucocorticoid within the joint and prevent a complete therapeutic response.[1013]

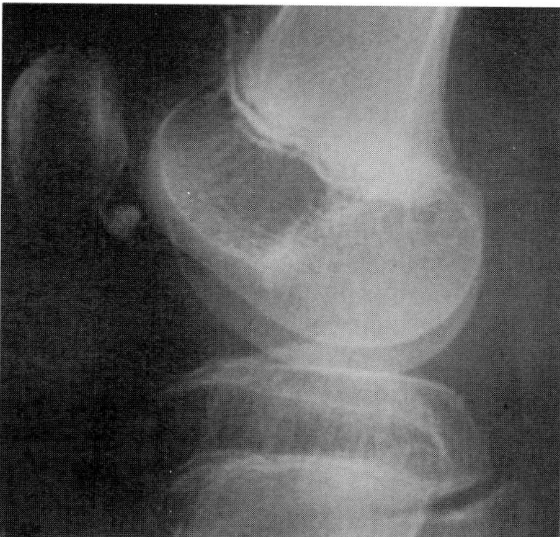

Figure 12–58. An area of subcutaneous calcification occurring 1 year after intra-articular injection of triamcinolone hexacetonide. The calcific deposit was not symptomatic and was not detectable clinically. (Courtesy of Dr. R. Cairns.)

In a study from Israel by Padeh and Passwell,[1011] the efficacy and safety of intra-articular triamcinolone hexacetonide was examined in 70 children with arthritis who had received 300 injections. Excellent benefit was achieved in 246 of 300 joints (82 percent) for longer than 6 months. Discontinuation of other medications was possible in 61 percent of these patients. In 115 of 141 children (82 percent) with oligoarthritis, a complete remission or correction of joint contracture developed in 55 joints. Eleven patients with popliteal cysts and 12 with tenosynovitis experienced satisfactory resolution of the abnormality. Three patients developed subcutaneous atrophy that eventually resolved. Two had a transient postinjection flare of joint pain and increased swelling. None of 20 examined by radiography developed periarticular calcifications. In a retrospective series by Sherry and colleagues,[1014] repeated intra-articular steroid injections were compared with traditional therapy as management for unilateral knee arthritis. Fewer leg-length and thigh-circumference discrepancies developed with steroid use.

Intravenous Immunoglobulin

IVIG for the treatment of JRA and other rheumatic diseases has received considerable attention, but results of clinical trials are inconsistent.[1015, 1016] A controlled randomized trial of IVIG by the PRCSG in children with systemic-onset disease indicated that the drug had little benefit compared with placebo.[1017] However, the results were considered inconclusive because of the small sample size. In an additional trial in children with polyarticular disease,[1018] 1.5 to 2.0 g/kg of IVIG was given twice a month for the first 2 months and then monthly for up to 6 months thereafter, with a maximum dose of 100 g. Responders were randomized at 4 months to continuation of the IVIG or placebo: 19 of the children responded during this open phase of the study. Ten children who were continued on IVIG were able to complete that phase of the study with benefit; however, only 4 of those randomized to placebo maintained their previous level of clinical response. There were no adverse effects. The authors concluded that approximately 75 percent of the children with polyarticular JRA would benefit from IVIG.

An early study of IVIG was reported by Groothoff and van Leeuwen.[1019] Silverman and associates[1020] noted good short-term effects on the systemic manifestations of children with systemic-onset JRA and less consistent improvement in joint disease. In a follow-up study,[1021] 27 children with systemic-onset JRA were treated with monthly IVIG for 4 to 54 months. By 6 months, 20 patients had a significant decrease in the number of days with fever or a marked decrease (>50 percent) in the number of actively inflamed joints. At a mean of 37.6 months' follow-up, 11 of the initial responder patients were in remission, 3 had improved but had chronically active disease, and 6 were nonresponsive. Of the initial 5 nonresponders, 1 developed an incomplete response to IVIG. Prieur and colleagues[1022] studied the use of IVIG treatment in 13 children with systemic-onset and in 3 with polyarticular disease. The rash was improved in 4 of the 10 patients with systemic-onset disease, fever in 6, and lymphadenopathy and splenomegaly in 3. Joint disease was not consistently affected in the short or long term, and progression of systemic features (pericarditis, polyarthritis) or side effects of the IVIG (purpura, urticaria) required further treatment with prednisone or other drugs. Eleven patients received at least 17, and as many as 52, monthly infusions.

Cytotoxic and Immunosuppressive Drugs

Clinical experience with cytotoxic drugs in JRA is largely anecdotal or uncontrolled. Use of the immunosuppressive and cytotoxic drugs should be reserved for children with life-threatening complications, major steroid toxicity, or severe progressive erosive arthritis.[1023, 1024] A number of medications have been studied for this purpose including the purine analogues 6-mercaptopurine and azathioprine[1023, 1025] and the alkylating agents cyclophosphamide[836, 837, 839] and chloroambucil.[836, 1026, 1027] Successful therapy for amyloidosis in children with JRA usually required the use of chlorambucil.[1026, 1028–1031] In one study at 15 years' follow-up,[1032] 68 percent of children with chronic arthritis complicated by amyloidosis who had been treated with chlorambucil (0.08–0.15 mg/kg/day) were alive; the mortality rate in the untreated group was 100 percent. Complications of chlorambucil therapy include sterility and an increased risk of malignancies.[1033, 1034] Trials of leflunomide, an inhibitor of pyrimidine synthesis, have not been published for children but have been encouraging in adults with RA.[1035–1037]

Cyclosporin

Few studies of cyclosporin in the treatment of chronic arthritis in children have been reported.[1038–1040] It is given in an oral dose of 3 to 5 mg/kg/day as two divided doses exactly 12 hours apart. Blood-pressure determinations should be performed at home twice a day for 2 weeks and then evaluated periodically along with urinalyses and estimates of renal function.[1041–1043] There may also be a small long-term risk of lymphoma (recently disputed).[1044] Ostensen and coworkers[1039] gave the drug to 14 children in a dose of 4 to 15 mg/kg/day for 6 to 20 months. Three of the 11 were able to undergo glucocorticoid dose reduction; 4 developed acute exacerbations of disease while on the drug. Serum creatinine concentration increased in 11, hypertrichosis occurred in 14, and hypertension developed in 1 child. Anemia occurred in 9, and the drug was discontinued in 3. The role of this drug in treatment of arthritis in children is uncertain, but it likely is important in treating the macrophage activation syndrome accompanying systemic-onset disease.[409, 427]

Tumor Necrosis Factor Inhibition

Although a number of experimental approaches to severe adult RA have been evaluated in therapeutic trials in recent decades, few have been employed in children without further demonstration of efficacy and safety. However, more recent approaches considered for children include soluble TNF-α receptor p75 fusion protein (etanercept)[1045–1050] and monoclonal antibody to TNF-α (infliximab).[1051–1057, 1057a]

In a clinical trial,[1045] etanercept in a dose of 0.4 mg/kg subcutaneously twice a week was given to 69 children with polyarticular-course JRA that had been refractory or intolerant to methotrexate (22 systemic, 7 oligoarticular, and 40 polyarticular onsets). Ages ranged from 5 to 17 years, with a median duration of 5.5 years. At 3 months, 51 patients (74 percent) met standardized clinical response criteria (≥30 percent improvement in three of six core set criteria and ≥30 percent worsening in not more than one of six criteria and a minimum of two active joints). The responders were then randomized to continued administration of TNFR:Fc or placebo (in addition to a baseline NSAID or low-dose prednisone) for an additional 4 months. There was a clinically and statistically impressive improvement in 19 of 25 children who had been continued on etanercept, and a disease flare in 20 of 26 children in the placebo group ($P = .007$). The median time to a disease flare in the children on etanercept was at least 116 days compared with 28 days in the placebo group. Each component of the JRA core set criteria worsened in the arm that received placebo and remained stable or improved in the arm that continued on etanercept. The data suggested the possibility of a higher flare rate among those patients with a higher baseline ESR. Of patients who demonstrated a clinical response at 90 days, those remaining on etanercept improved from month 3 through month 7, whereas those who received placebo did not have any improvement. The drug was well tolerated with only mild to moderate upper respiratory infections or injection-site reactions.

Studies have not been performed to assess the effects of continued etanercept therapy in patients who do not respond within 3 months of initiating therapy or develop a relapse on the drug, or its effectiveness if used without concomitant methotrexate. There are undoubtedly children who are only partially, or not responsive to TNF-α blockade, especially those with systemic-onset disease. Toxicities are also unclarified on long-term administration. Demyelinating disease and pancytopenia have been described in a drug warning from the company. Other biologics that interfere with TNF-α (infliximab) are becoming available and may prove useful in selected children.

Autologous Stem Cell Transplantation

Bone marrow transplantation has been initiated as experimental treatment for severe autoimmune diseases unresponsive to conventional therapy.[1058, 1059] Autologous stem cell transplantation (ASCT) is being evaluated currently in a small number of children with JRA.[1060–1063, 1064a, 1064b] In one clinical protocol,[1064] bone marrow harvest was followed by T-cell depletion and a conditioning regime (antithymocyte globulin, cyclophosphamide, total body radiation). ASCT has been undertaken in children with polyarticular (1 patient) and systemic-onset (4 patients) arthritis who had progressive, unremitting disease. At final evaluation, 3 patients were in drug-free remission and 1 had mild oligoarthritis. Although follow-up has been short and patient numbers limited, the authors judged these results to be encouraging. More recently, a number of deaths from post-transplantation viral infections have been reported in greater than 30 children who have been transplanted.

Biologic Response Modifiers

A number of immune modulators have been tried therapeutically in children with JRA (see Chapter 7). Transfer factor, after an initial encouraging report, did not prove effective.[1065] Other immunoregulatory drugs such as levamisole were too toxic.[1066] Thymopentin, the active pentapeptide of thymopoietin, was given intravenously to 10 children with systemic-onset JRA and into the joint in 3 children with oligoarthritis.[1067] There was no effect on joint disease, but fever was controlled and the size of lymph nodes, liver, and spleen was decreased. The ratio of CD4 to CD8 T cells returned toward normal. There did not appear to be any toxicity.

Recombinant IFN-γ has been used experimentally.[1068] In one study,[1069] it was given to children (6 systemic onset, 3 polyarthritis, 1 oligoarthritis) in whom other therapies had failed after a long duration of disease of 5 to 11 years. Eight patients had significant improvement and 7 entered remission. Two with systemic onset had no response, and 4 relapsed with exacerbations. One child developed a severe infection. Plasmapheresis has been recommended for severe disease[1070] and may be particularly indicated if high levels of circulating immune complexes are demonstrated. Lymphapheresis and total lymphoid radiation have not been adequately studied in controlled series of patients with JRA.[1071] Tolerance induction by oral administration of type II collagen is currently under review as a therapeutic agent.[1072, 1073] Induction of tolerance to epitopes of HSP 60 as potential therapy for childhood arthritis has been reviewed under "Infection," earlier in this chapter.

Growth Hormone

The best approach to the treatment of growth failure and short stature in JRA is uncertain.[1074] Most children have normal baseline and stimulated blood levels of growth hormone[472, 473, 1075, 1076, 1076a, 1076b] and insulin-like growth factors I and II,[469, 1076, 1077] but not all.[469, 1078, 1079] Growth hormone has been used with varying success, although early studies may not have used sufficient doses.[469, 472, 1075, 1078, 1080]

Davies and colleagues[469] treated 28 children who were growth impaired with one of two regimens of growth hormone, 12 IU/M^2 or 24 IU/M^2 per week. All patients showed adequate baseline secretion of growth hormone. Although almost all children had an increase in height during 1 year of treatment, those on the higher dose of growth hormone grew better. Investigations indicate that daily growth hormone in a weekly dose of 0.3 mg/kg initiates a return to normal growth rates for 1 to 2 years.[1081] However, glucocorticoid in a prednisone-equivalent dose of greater than 0.35 mg/kg/day interferes with growth hormone responsiveness.[1081, 1082] In the study by Touati and associates,[1079] recombinant growth hormone in a dose of 1.4 IU/kg/week partially counteracted the adverse effects of glucocorticoids on linear growth velocity and lean body mass. In children with rheumatic diseases, the immunostimulatory effects of growth hormone lead to the theoretical possibility of interference with immunosuppression.[1083] In one study,[1084, 1085] growth hormone slightly increased allograft rejection rates. Growth hormone may also increase cytochrome P-450 activity[1086] and thereby alter clearance of specific drugs (glucocorticoids, sex steroids, anticonvulsants, cyclosporine).

Nutrition

The child's overall nutrition, development, and growth are important aspects of the long-term management of JRA.[507, 1087] Growth retardation and impaired bone mineralization almost invariably occur during periods of active disease and are exacerbated by glucocorticoid administration, anorexia, or inanition. Nutrition and vitamin supplementation (vitamin D and folic acid) are often indicated. Assessment of nutritional status should be a component of every patient's evaluation.[1088, 1089] Henderson and Lovell[1090] suggested the use of a four-parameter test to screen for protein–energy malnutrition. The presence of any two of the following abnormalities indicates the need for a detailed nutritional assessment:

- Weight below 5th percentile
- Weight-for-height index below 80th percentile
- Arm circumference below 5th percentile
- Serum albumin less than 2.8 mg/dl (28 g/L)

Management of malnutrition is often difficult in the systemically ill, anorectic child. Nocturnal nasogastric feeding occasionally is necessary to maintain adequate nutrition in such a child.[471]

Additional clinical research is required to document therapeutic modalities to prevent and manage osteopenia during periods of active disease.[499] In a controlled study of 70 pairs of identical twins, Johnston and coworkers[1091] demonstrated that normal children on an average American diet could increase their bone mass over a 3-year period with dietary calcium supplementation. Future studies of bone mineral content and bone metabolism should more completely elucidate the mechanisms of decreased bone turnover in children with JRA; determine whether dietary interventions such as calcium or vitamin D supplementation,[1092–1094] intensive exercise programs,[1095–1097] or use of medications such as alendronate[1098, 1099] or growth hormone[1099a, 1099b] might improve outcomes; or whether better suppression of the underlying inflammatory disease is ultimately required.

Physical and Occupational Therapy

The objectives of physical therapy and occupational therapy are to minimize pain, maintain and restore function, and prevent deformity and disability (Table 12–53).[1100–1103] These aspects of treatment are critically important in the child's total management program. In many children, a rest period after returning from school in the afternoon and increased time for sleep at night are advisable. Most children, however, determine

Table 12–53

Treatment in JRA: Physical Measures

Relief of pain
Heat/cold
Maintenance of joint function
Splints
ROM exercises (active/passive)
Posture/prone-lying exercises
Adequate rest/adequate exercise
Balanced physical activity
Selected peer sports (tricycle, swimming)

ROM, range of motion.

their own levels of activity. Only rarely have we found that either pushing them beyond their present capabilities or unduly restricting daily activities is profitable. Normal play must be encouraged, and the family must realize how vital this is to the growing child in terms of peer group interactions and physical fitness, including achieving and maintaining a desirable level of musculoskeletal and cardiopulmonary conditioning.[1104–1106, 1106a] It is important, however, to avoid specific activities that cause overtiring or increased joint pain. Undesirable play is that which places excessive stress on affected joints. Tricycle or bicycle riding and swimming are almost always helpful and do not add undue loading to the joints. Swimming has the added advantage of providing active range of motion and muscle strengthening without weight bearing. Although activities such as bicycling and swimming are excellent ways of maintaining muscle strength and range of motion, they are not a substitute for a well-designed active and passive therapy program: The child tends to function within the current range rather than regain lost range of motion.

Skilled physical and occupational therapists are able to assess the time and intensity of a therapy program that the child can tolerate.[1107] Daily physical therapy performed at home should seldom exceed 30 minutes twice a day (and should often be much shorter). The child's age and temperament, the duration of morning stiffness, and the presence of systemic disease must all be considered in designing a physical therapy program. If possible, adaptive play and games are designed to achieve the desired results. The child and parents should agree on realistic goals. It is sometimes difficult for the parent to carry out a home physical therapy program and maintain a healthy parent-child relationship. In such circumstances, twice-weekly visits to a physical therapist may be a better plan than daily home therapy by the parent. In some children, it is desirable to institute intensive physical and occupational therapy programs for 1 to 3 weeks once or twice a year in order to prevent loss of function.

During periods of active inflammation, joint pain and stiffness are reduced by appropriate warming. A hot bath in the morning and application of heat prior to physical therapy reduce stiffness and pain and maximize function. In children with a great deal of muscle spasm, ice may be more beneficial than heat but is often not preferred. Passive stretching is usually needed to regain lost range of motion. Active exercise is required to rebuild muscle strength. Atrophy of the extensor muscles begins early, and active exercise must be instituted during the initial phases of the disease to maintain the strength of these muscle groups.

Cock-up splints for the wrists (Fig. 12–59), ring splints for the fingers (Fig. 12–60), and orthoplast posterior resting splints for the knees may be used to prevent malpositioning or for the long-term correction of deformity. The maintenance of normal range of motion or reduction of minimal contractures often requires gentle stretching and the use of resting splints. A cervical collar with a plastic insert should be worn by children with cervical spine disease during automobile travel (Fig. 12–61). Malpositioning and neck discomfort may be minimized by the use of a soft collar while studying and a desk with a tilt top on which the child can do homework. At night, a small pillow under the neck, rather than under the head, is an effective way to reduce neck discomfort. Dynamic splints are helpful for certain joint contractures (elbow and knee) (Fig. 12–62). For severe contractures—especially of the wrist, elbow, or knee—serial casting with active exercises every 2 days when the cast is removed may be more effective. If stretching or casting is too forceful or is improperly performed, subluxation of the knee or wrist or even fracture of osteoporotic bone can occur.

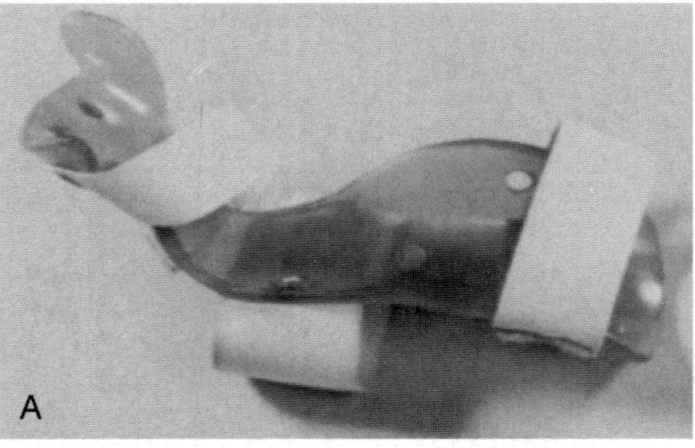

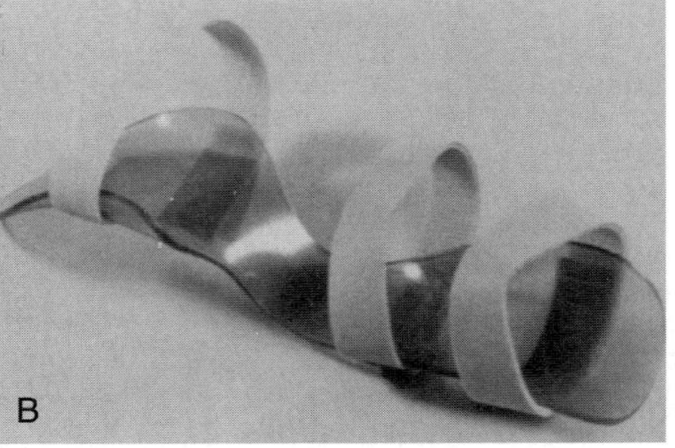

Figure 12–59. *A*, Traditional wrist cock-up splint for maintaining extension at the wrist while the child is at rest. In designing such a splint, one must ensure that the carpus is protected from subluxing forces and that the radiocarpal joint is in neither ulnar nor radial deviation. *B*, A platform splint that simultaneously maintains positioning of the wrist, metacarpophalangeal joints, and proximal interphalangeal joints.

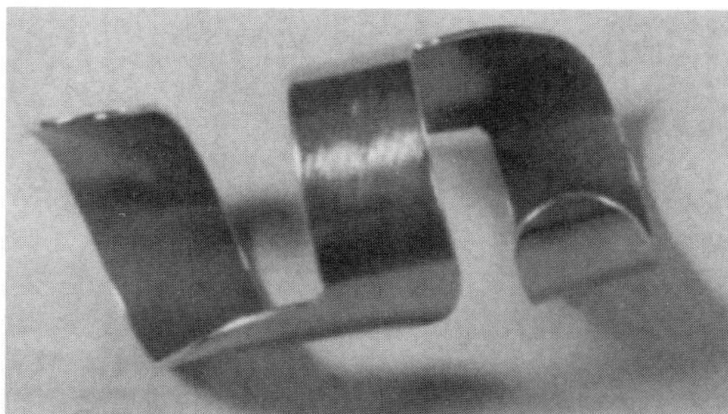

Figure 12–60. Ring splint to prevent or treat flexion contractures while preventing hyperextension of the proximal interphalangeal joint.

Appropriate footwear is essential in the child with arthritis of the joints of the ankle and foot.[1108] Shoes should be lightweight but provide firm lateral support. In children with a leg-length discrepancy, a heel lift or an addition to the bottom of the shoe of the shorter leg should be used, depending on the depth needed. In general, the total compensation should be somewhat less than the leg-length discrepancy. In children with pain or inflammation of the metatarsophalangeal joints or excessive pronation or supination, a custom-fitted hard insole that slips into the shoe provides considerable comfort and improvement of the gait. Hip flexion contractures can be difficult to treat. Prone lying for a significant period of time (at least 1 hour/day) helps to reduce the degree of contracture. A study has analyzed gait alterations in children with chronic arthritis.[1109]

Orthopedic Surgery

At present, orthopedic surgery has a limited but important role in management of JRA in young children.[1110–1113] In the older child, however, surgical approaches to joint contractures, dislocations, or joint replacement become important components of therapy, and the orthopedic surgeon plays an important role at this stage.[1113–1115] Approaches to some problems such as limb overgrowth have not been completely clarified.[1116] In some reports, surgical epiphyseal arrest was judged to be necessary in approximately one third of patients.[479, 1117]

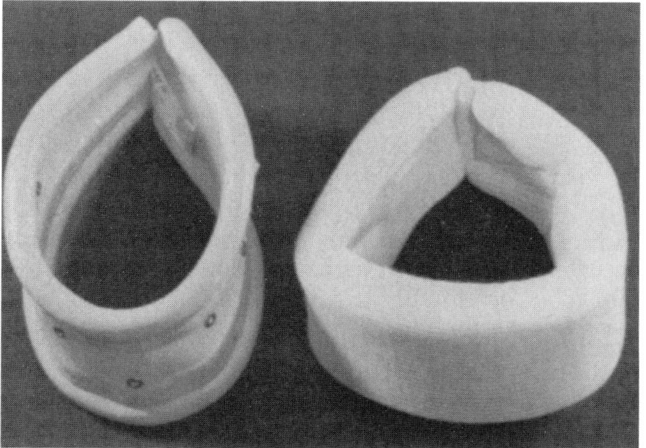

Figure 12–61. Firm and soft collars for helping to maintain the position of the head in a child with cervical spine disease.

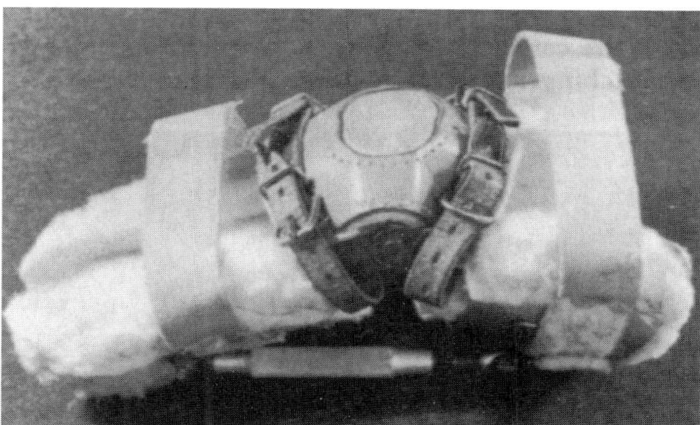

Figure 12–62. Turnbuckle extension splint for treatment of flexion contracture at the knee. The knee cage keeps the knee joint in as much extension as is comfortable. The turnbuckle is gradually adjusted to increase the extension force.

Synovectomy

The long-term outcome of children with JRA and joint disease is not altered by prophylactic synovectomy. Synovectomy, however, may be useful in some children for relief of mechanical impairment of joint motion related to joint pain or synovial hypertrophy.[1110, 1111, 1118–1125] Care must be taken to prevent a postsurgical contracture, and the use of a continuous-motion apparatus has been recommended for this purpose, especially in the young child. Arthroscopic surgery greatly reduces the morbidity associated with synovectomy.[1126–1128]

Soft Tissue Surgery

Soft tissue releases, posterior capsulotomy, and tendon lengthening occasionally are useful in a child with a severe contracture of the knee or hip.[1124, 1129] In other instances, balanced traction is necessary to expedite the treatment of a knee contracture, although this is often difficult to maintain in the young child. Tenosynovectomy may be indicated to reduce the risk of tendon rupture over the dorsum of the wrist or for adhesive flexor tenosynovitis and trigger finger, which sometimes occurs in children who are RF seropositive.

Reconstructive Surgery

Reconstructive surgery has become important in the older patient with marked disability.[1114, 1130] Total joint prostheses, particularly for the hip[382, 818, 832, 1131–1142] or knee,[1138, 1143, 1144, 1144a] have proved to be of great benefit

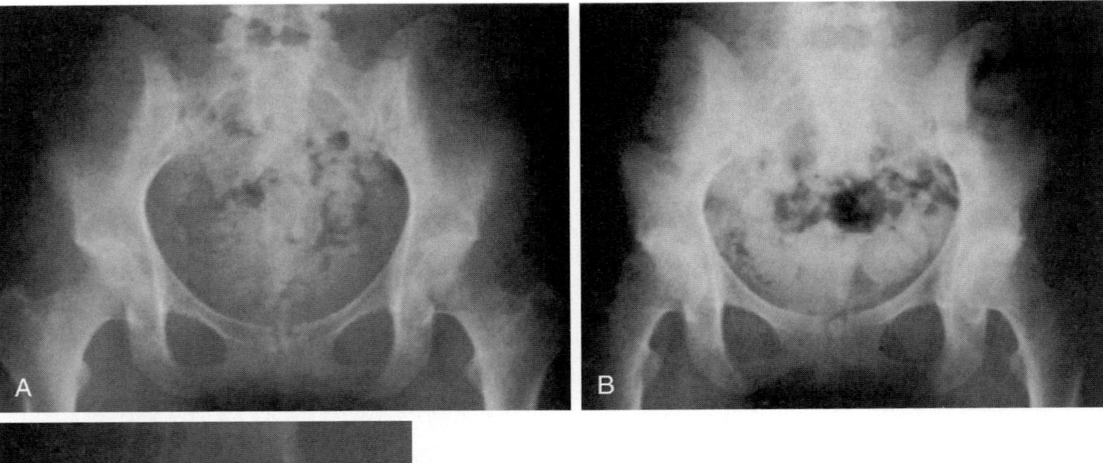

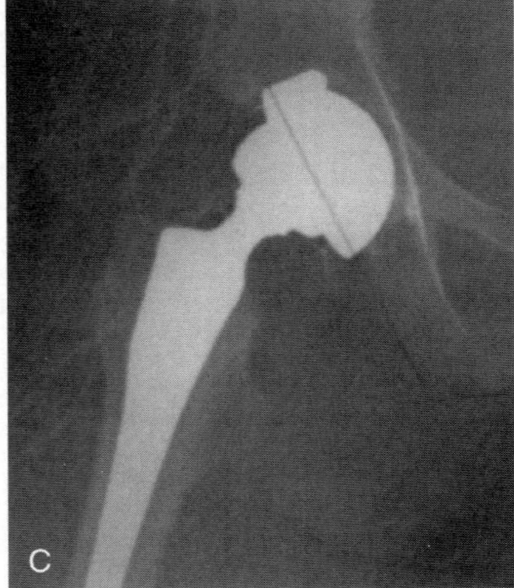

Figure 12–63. *A*, Radiograph of the hips of a 21-year-old woman in whom polyarticular JRA began at the age of 13 years. There is marked narrowing of the joint space with preservation of the contour of the femoral heads. *B*, Radiograph of the same patient 1 year later. Deformity and erosion of the femoral heads are evident. *C*, Radiograph of the total joint replacement in the same patient.

(Fig. 12–63). Generally, surgery is best put off until bone growth has ceased.[1110, 1111, 1130] Other special considerations include the status of the other lower extremity joints, activity of the rheumatic disease in general, currently unresolved questions concerning wear and longevity of the prosthesis, and possible lack of adequate motivation for rehabilitation in some patients. Many children with polyarthritis are further incapacitated either before or after lower extremity surgery because of difficulty with crutch walking from increased use of the hands or wrists, flexion contractures of the elbows, or involvement of the shoulder joints.[811, 1145] Preservation of muscle function in anticipation of surgical intervention requires a rehabilitation program over many years devoted to maintaining as nearly normal muscle strength as possible.

Singsen and associates[1132] studied the course of 29 total hip prostheses in 14 children with JRA and in 2 with JAS. The ages of these children were 12 to 18 years; the median duration of the hip disease was 7 years. Uncontrolled pain was the primary indication for replacement in 5 and severe functional disability in 24 patients. Postoperative range of motion and freedom from pain were improved uniformly. Crowe and coworkers[1133] reported on 22 hip arthroplasties in 15 patients, 14 to 26 years of age, followed for an average of 10 years before surgery. After surgery, the majority of these patients could walk unassisted and experienced marked improvement in self-image. Flexion deformities decreased, and the average arc of flexion–extension increased. Pain was significantly relieved in all but 1 child. Gudmundsson and coworkers[1137] reviewed their experience with 29 total hip replacements in 16 patients with JRA who were between 13 and 26 years of age at the time of surgery. At an average of 64 months after surgery, 20 hips were pain-free and 7 had slight pain on movement. Range and ambulation were improved. Children with temporomandibular joint disease may require reconstructive surgery of the mandibular condyle because of facial pain. Those with micrognathia may profit cosmetically from a combined orthodontic and surgical approach.[1146, 1147]

Counseling the Family

It is of signal importance that the child and the parents be educated about the present state of knowledge of JRA, its outcome, and therapy.[1148–1153] The family must share in coordination of disease management, which should be community based.[1149, 1154] An optimistic attitude must be maintained. Counseling should be initiated by the physician at the time of the first visit and reinforced and continued at follow-up by the team. Educational efforts are repeated as needed during the subsequent clinical course, especially in an effort to increase compliance.[1155, 1156] We have found it useful to ask parents to write down the problems encountered between visits and to bring this list to their appointments.

In management of the child with JRA, the first priority concomitant with initial efforts to control the activity of the disease is to foster normal psychologic and social development.[1157–1161] Attendance at school is an integral part of this program.[1162–1167] Home instruction is rarely indicated; most pediatricians sense that physically disabled students do better in regular schools.[1168, 1169] Some families of children with JRA have had psychologically important disruptions such as divorce, separation, death, or adoption, and they often display severe emotional disturbances.[1170–1177] More recent studies from North America indicate that families with children with chronic illnesses are much more functional.[1178, 1179]

It is important to emphasize that coordinated care of the child with chronic disease requires a team effort. This concept presents problems for newly established clinical services because of the number of personnel who need to be involved in an ideal program in addition to the child, the family, the school, and the community agencies. One study found that in most children with chronic arthritis, basic care was either divided or duplicated and many aspects of a total supportive program were neglected.[1180] These authors and others found that a pattern of division, duplication, and neglect was typical of the fragmented care of the majority of children with a chronic disease.

LONG-TERM OUTCOME

The course of JRA is especially unpredictable at onset of disease. Nonetheless, certain generalizations can be made because the type of onset is associated to some extent with the future unfolding of the disease and its manifestations (see Tables 12–5, 12–10, and 12–12).[22, 35, 37, 83, 1181–1184, 1184a, 1184b] After the pattern of the disease is well established, the course tends to be more predictable and repetitive. After this initial observation period of variable duration, it is usually possible to begin to estimate prognosis and therapeutic response, on which changes in the management program can be based. It is impossible to predict the eventual disease outcome in any individual child with JRA.[1185] Furthermore, "outcome" is a complex concept that can be measured in a number of ways. The classification of functional capacity may be used to estimate physical function, although it has not been specifically validated for children (Table 12–54).

Table 12–54

Classification of Functional Status in JRA

STATUS	DEFINITION*
I	Completely able to perform usual activities of daily living (self-care, vocational, and avocational)
II	Able to perform usual self-care and vocational activities, but limited in avocational activities
III	Able to perform usual self-care activities, but limited in vocational and avocational activities
IV	Limited in ability to perform usual self-care, vocational and avocational activites

*Usual self-care activities include dressing, feeding, bathing, grooming, and toileting. Avocational (recreational and/or leisure) and vocational (work school, homemaking) activities are patient-desired and age- and sex-specific.

From Hochberg MC, Chang RW, Dwosh I, et al: The American College of rheumatology 1991 revised criteria for the classification of global functional status in rheumatoid arthritis. Arthritis Rheum 35: 498, 1992.

Functional Disability and Psychosocial Outcome

It has been estimated that, historically, 70 to 90 percent of children with JRA have a satisfactory outcome without serious disability.[488, 1181, 1185–1190] A small percentage (perhaps 5 percent) have a recurrence of arthritis as adults.[396, 1191–1194] Approximately 10 to 17 percent of children with JRA enter adulthood with moderate to severe functional disabilities.[349, 1194a, 1194b] Delay in referral and initiation of an acceptable therapeutic program are associated with a poorer functional outcome (Table 12–55). Sequential measurements of health status on standardized instruments of assessment have proved valuable for judging a child's functional adaptations (see Chapter 9).[1195]

Hill and coworkers[1193] studied 53 adults for an average of 14.5 years after JRA had been diagnosed. Two thirds of this group had mild to moderate disease, good sexual adjustment, and average educational achievement, employment history, and adjustment to life. One third, however, had severe disease, and many had progressive disability. Continued inflammatory activity of the arthritis, rather than severity of residual disability or deformity, seemed to be the chief factor that prevented adjustment as an adult. Laaksonen[35] reported that the disease had resolved completely in 30 percent of her patients at the time of reassessment (an average of 16 years from the onset of disease). There was minimal to moderate disability in 40 percent and severe incapacitation in 30 percent. Complete recovery was most common when the total duration of active arthritis was 7 years or less, as it was in 51 percent of the group, and least common when duration was 8 to 16 years, as it was in 10 percent. Even systemic-onset disease may lead to few functional impairments in

Table 12–55

Relation Between Functional Capacity and Interval Between Onset and Referral

	FUNCTIONAL CAPACITY*				
YEARS	I	II	III	IV	TOTAL
1	10	23	4	2	39
2	11	34	18	2	65
3	6	12	11	2	31
4	3	10	12	7	32
5+	2	9	13	9	33

*Steinbrocker classification.

Table 12–56

Functional Outcome 15 Years After Onset in 225 Children With Juvenile Chronic Arthritis: Taplow Experience

	NUMBER IN GROUP	PERCENTAGE IN GROUP	
		Normal	Limited
Education (≤16 yr of age)	30	77	23
Employment	150	90	10
Marriage (♀ only)	45	80	20

Modified from Ansell BM, Wood PHN: Prognosis in juvenile chronic polyarthritis. Clin Rheum Dis 2: 397, 1976.

adulthood,[408] comparable with the outcome in children with polyarticular disease.[379]

Irrespective of the type of onset or pattern of the course of the disease, 83 percent of the children who were followed for 15 years at Taplow were able to work, attend school, or be self-sufficient (Tables 12–56 and 12–57).[488] In general, active synovitis tended to diminish as the years passed, although by 1 year after onset, the total number of joints involved was slightly greater than at 3 months. At 5 years, there was considerable improvement in all groups, especially in the wrists, knees, and ankles. Shoulders and hips, however, showed a slightly increased frequency of involvement at that time. Many joints had only limitation of motion and no objective hallmarks of active disease, such as soft tissue swelling or effusion. Small joint disease of the hands and feet increased only slightly in frequency with continuing observation. An important observation from this study was how rapidly joint deformity and disability could occur. This was particularly true for subluxation of the wrists, varus and valgus deformities of the feet, and flexion contractures at the knees and hips.

These observations underscore the urgency of efforts to maintain range of motion and functional positioning while at rest in the overall management of the child's disease. Cervical spine disease was the presenting complaint in only 2 percent of patients. Two children had persistent torticollis. At the 1-year follow-up, however, 10 percent had limitation of cervical spine motion; at the 15-year follow-up, 20 percent had limited neck motion. Limitation of motion in the thoracic and lumbar spine tended to occur relatively later and was the result of vertebral fractures, scoliosis, or an unsuspected diagnosis of JAS. The temporomandibular joint was abnormal in fewer than one sixth of these children. The jaw did not achieve full adult development in one fifth of the patients, which correlated closely with evidence of cervical spine disease in this study.

The data of Wallace and Levinson[349] (compiled in 1991) showed poorer long-term results (Table 12–58).[35, 349, 488, 1187, 1188, 1191, 1193] At 15 to 20 years of follow-up, 17 percent of patients were in Steinbrocker functional capacity III to IV and 45 percent still had active disease. A study by Ruperto and colleagues[842] evaluated long-term outcome in a group of 227 patients followed in Cincinnati and in Pavia. This study evaluated the effect on outcome of specific demographic, clinical, and immunologic variables that were present during the first 6 months of the illness. The mean duration of disease at assessment was 15 years (range, 15.3 to 36.1 years). The best predictor of greater long-term disability was the initial articular severity score. Early hand involvement was also a strong predictor of disability and poorer overall well-being. ANA seropositivity was associated with less disability. This study found that quality-of-life scores were much more difficult to forecast because of the multiple domains that were functioning in this type of outcome. An extension of this study[841] involving many of the same patients indicated that long-term outcome, based on quality-of-life scales and health-assessment questionnaires, was favorable in most patients with JRA 5 years or more after onset of symptoms.

In a study from the United Kingdom,[1196] the functional and psychologic outcome of 43 patients with polyarticular disease, with a mean duration of 19.7 years and a mean age of 26.7 years was assessed. The female:male ratio was 3:1. Severe disability was present in 8 percent of the patients with systemic-onset disease, 34 percent of those who were RF seronegative, 38 percent of those who were RF seropositive, and 86 percent of children who had extended oligoarthritis—related primarily to ocular disease. The RF-seropositive and extended oligoarticular groups, however, were also the most disabled in terms of continuing active disease (85 and 71 percent, respectively). Clinical depression was

Table 12–57

Prognosis in Children With Juvenile Chronic Arthritis: 15-Year Follow-Up at Taplow

	NUMBER OF CHILDREN	LIMITATION (%)			DEAD (%)
		None—Slight	Severe	Very Severe	
Duration of disease before referral					
<1 yr	95	84	6	0	7
>1 yr	148	63	24	5	7
Age at onset					
<6 yr	103	62	24	5	9
≥11 yr	71	83	11	1	4
Type of onset					
Systemic	79	57	25	4	14
Polyarticular	151	71	22	4	3
Oligoarticular	62	89	8	2	2
Initial functional status					
Very severe	87	52	30	9	9
None or slight	97	93	4	0	3

Modified from Ansell BM, Wood PHN: Prognosis in juvenile chronic polyarthritis. Clin Rheum Dis 2: 397, 1976.

Table 12–58

Functional Outcome of JRA

AUTHOR	YR FOLLOW-UP (mean)	CLASSES III AND IV (%)
Laaksonen (1966)[35]	≥16	48
Jeremy et al (1968)[1191]	5–20 (18)	24
Ansell and Wood (1976)[488]	≥15	23
Hill et al (1976)[1193]	(14.5)	33
Hanson et al (1977)[1187]	5–25 (10)	28
Stoeber (1981)[1188]	10–22 (15)	41
Wallace and Levinson (1991)[349]	15–20	17

Data from Wallace CA, Levenson JE: Juvenile rheumatoid arthritis: outcome and treatment for the 1990s. Rheum Dis Clin North Am 17: 891, 1991.

diagnosed in 21 percent. Despite these negative observations, 66 percent of these patients were employed and 38 percent judged that their arthritis had no effect on their ability to form interpersonal relationships.

More recently, investigators have attempted to avoid the confounding factors of referral-based and clinic follow-up by primarily basing their outcome studies on population surveys. Some have also taken the approach recommended by the World Health Organization in 1980 to examine functional adaptation in relation to impairment (based on organ disease), disability (related to personal quality of life), and handicap (related to society's perception of the functioning ability of the individual).[1197]

A study by Peterson and colleagues[1177] from the Mayo Clinic evaluated the physical and psychosocial impact of JRA in a population-based cohort of adults who had had the disease during childhood. Controls were age- and sex-matched. Forty-four patients were included (73 percent oligoarticular-onset, 16 percent polyarticular-onset, 11 percent systemic-onset disease). Average follow-up was 24.7 years. The patients with JRA had greater disability, more bodily pain, increased fatigue, poorer health perception, and decreased physical functioning along with lower rates of employment and lower levels of exercise compared with the control group. On the other hand, their level of educational achievement, annual income, health insurance status, and rate of pregnancy and childbirth were similar to those of controls. This study concluded that adults who had had JRA experienced long-term physical and psychosocial impairment that have been often ignored in the evaluation of functional outcome. Persistent pain has been repeatedly observed by us and others,[1197a] and may have a neurologic basis (see Chapter 3, Spinal Cord).

Another study from Norway by Flato and colleagues[1198] included 53 patients with JRA and 19 with juvenile spondyloarthropathy. Forty-three (60 percent) of the 72 patients were in a remission at the time of the study, and 60 percent reported no disability. This study and a subsequent report[1199] supported the conclusion that long-term outcome was more favorable than previously reported, perhaps related to less bias of admission to the study and by the early use of more aggressive therapeutic regimens. This group of investigators had previously indicated that poor psychosocial functioning in 22 percent of the patients on follow-up was associated with premorbid psychosocial dysfunction, chronic family difficulties, and major life events.[1199] They also confirmed that approximately 19 percent of the patients were still suffering from chronic pain without evidence of active arthritis.[1198] It is also our impression that a chronic pain syndrome may persist in these patients well after their JRA has remitted.

A number of investigations of adaptation to chronic illnesses in children have been completed recently.[1178, 1179, 1200, 1200a, 1200b] Studies of adaptation have been limited by assumptions that disease groups of chronic illnesses are homogeneous and that comprehensive adaptation models involve both risk and resistant factors within the child and family. In one study, 107 children with JRA, 114 with insulin-dependent diabetes mellitus, and 88 healthy controls were evaluated every 6 months for 2 years. Differences were observed between mothers and fathers with regard to dependent variables of depression, anxiety, somatization, strain at work, days of work loss due to child's illness, and extent to which the illness interfered with leisure time in the family. Married mothers missed more work than fathers but demonstrated less overall functional impairment. Single mothers did not differ from married mothers or fathers. The dependent variables—particularly those related to depression, anxiety, and strain at work—decreased for all parents during the 2 years of observation. Premorbid diagnostic groups were associated with maternal depression and paternal distress in passive coping. Parental depression and distress were associated with the child's behavior in the illness, complaints of pain, and ability to deal with anger and disappointment. Anger level and anger expression styles were highly associated with depression.[1201] Angry children who turned their anger inward were most likely to report depression. The child's functioning did not appear to be related to the clinical diagnostic group. Trajectories within the child's and family's adaptations could be identified independent of the diagnostic groups.[1179] This and other studies[1202] have concluded that interventions to ameliorate parental distress would certainly have beneficial effects on child behavior and parental reactions to that behavior and the chronic illness.

Transition of the child to young-adult identification, vocational planning, and eventually a place in adult life has been the subject of a number of current projects. Excellent summaries are contained in publications by Spencer and colleagues,[1203] Chamberlain and Rooney,[1204] and White.[1205–1207]

Death

In early studies of JRA, the death rate was 2 to 4 percent.[1208, 1209] The disease-associated death rate is now perhaps less than 1 percent in Europe and less than 0.5 percent in North America. The majority of the deaths associated with JRA in Europe were related to amyloidosis, and in the United States deaths occurred in children with systemic onset of disease and, in many cases, were related to infection. Infections were associated in the early studies with glucocorticoid therapy and are currently less often fatal.

Amyloidosis refers to the tissue deposition of the fibrillar protein amyloid[1210] and is discussed in Chapter 36. *Secondary amyloidosis* occurs as a complication of chronic inflammatory conditions such as arthritis or infection and in diseases such as familial Mediterranean fever. It is characterized by proteinuria and the nephrotic syndrome, diarrhea, hepatosplenomegaly, or unexplained anemia in a child with profound hypergammaglobulinemia. Amyloidosis may be preceded by marked elevations of C-reactive protein, an acute phase reactant that is similar in structure to serum amyloid A (SAA) protein.[1211] SAA protein responds as an acute-phase reactant and is increased in concentration in children with active

Table 12–59

Death in Patients With JRA: University of Michigan, 1960 to 1980

SEX	AGE AT ONSET (yr)	AGE AT DEATH (yr)	DURATION OF DISEASE	TYPE OF ONSET	ACTIVITY OF DISEASE	FUNCTIONAL CAPACITY	BONE EROSIONS	RHEUMATOID NODULES	RHEUMATOID FACTOR	ANTINUCLEAR ANTIBODY	CAUSE OF DEATH
F	6	13	7	Systemic	+++	IV	++	++	++	ND	Febrile illness, dehydration
M	8	12	4	Systemic	++	IV	–	++	+	++++	Chronic pulmonary disease
F	2	16	14	Systemic	++	IV	++	–	++++	–	Medication error (adrenal insufficiency)
M	2	22	20	Systemic	+++	IV	++	–	–	ND	Congestive heart failure, pneumonitis
M	2	11	9	Systemic	+++	IV	+	–	+++	–	Chronic pulmonary disease, pneumonitis
F	13	27	14	Systemic	++	III	+	++	+++	++++	Anesthetic accident
F	3	7	4	Systemic	++++	III	–	–	–	ND	Congestive heart failure
M	7	32	19	Systemic	–	III	++	–	–	–	Acute myocardial infarction
F	5	6	1	Systemic	++	III	–	–	–	–	Cardiopulmonary failure

ND, no data.

disease. Although no HLA associations have been confirmed in children who experience amyloidosis,[1212] a genetic marker for amyloid P component has been identified in one study by restriction fragment length polymorphism.[1213] Secondary amyloidosis as a complication of JRA is exceedingly rare in North America but occurred in approximately 5 to 7 percent of children with chronic arthritis in certain areas of the world, particularly England, Scandinavia, Poland, and Germany.[1214, 1215] Amyloidosis is diagnosed by examination of tissue sections stained by Congo red dye. Under the polarizing microscope, the deposits assume a green color that is virtually pathognomonic. Rectal submucosa is the most frequently recommended biopsy site; renal biopsy may be hazardous because of an increased tendency toward bleeding. Radionuclide imaging using radioiodinated autologous serum amyloid P is a noninvasive technique for diagnosis and monitoring of amyloidosis.[1216, 1217]

The major causes of death in 46 children followed by Bywaters at Taplow[1218, 1219] were renal failure (which in half of the children was associated with amyloidosis) and infections. At the 15-year evaluation, excess mortality was identified in girls who had onset arthritis early in life. After 15 years of arthritis, the frequency of amyloidosis had risen to 7.4 percent among children with arthritis in the United Kingdom.[1215] It was rarely observed as early as 1 year after onset of the arthritis but could develop as late as 23 years after onset, most commonly in children with systemic disease. Spontaneous remissions occurred. Even in Europe, amyloidosis as a complication of chronic arthritis appears to be on the decline, with a decreasing number of deaths[1026, 1027, 1220]; however, a recent series from Turkey reported a 10 percent frequency.[620]

Table 12–59 describes characteristics of nine children with JRA who died in our Ann Arbor series up to 1980. Almost all of these deaths occurred late during the course of disease and in children who had systemic-onset disease. One death resulted from an acute myocardial infarction in a young man who had been treated with glucocorticoid drugs for many years.

PERSPECTIVE

In spite of new insights into causation and considerable advances in treatment, JRA remains an important cause of chronic pain and disability in childhood. Particularly when considering heroic pharmacologic therapy, one should remember that the disease is often self-limited, albeit after years of activity, and is seldom fatal. On the other hand, undue delay in instituting advanced treatment that may be effective can result in irretrievable damage to joints and other organs and impaired skeletal maturation. The art of medicine is at least as important as its science in guiding the pediatric rheumatologist's planning of a therapeutic approach to a chronic illness such as JRA. An important factor working in favor of the program of management is the child's unceasing potential for growth. To a large extent, it is this intrinsic endowment for future physical and psychological development that enables so much to be accomplished in the vast majority of children with JRA. Even so, much work remains in clarifying the nature and management of these diseases and their complications.

References

1. Cornil MV: Memoire sur les coincidences pathologiques du rhumatisme articulaire chronique. C R Mem Soc Biol (Paris) 4: 3, 1864.
2. Diamant-Berger MS: Du Rhumatisme Noueux (Polyarthrite Deformante) Chez Les Enfants. Paris, Lecrosnier et Babe, 1891.
3. Still GF: On a form of chronic joint disease in children. Med Chir Trans 80: 47, 1897.
4. Keen JH: George Frederic Still—registrar, Great Ormond Street Children's Hospital. Br J Rheumatol 37: 1247, 1998.
5. Hirschsprung H: Multipel, kronisk, infektios Ledsygdom I Barnealderen. Hospitalstid 421, 1901.
6. Atkinson FRB: Still's disease. Br J Child Dis 36: 100, 1939.
7. Edstrom G: Rheumatoid arthritis in children. Acta Paediatr Scand 34: 334, 1947.
8. Bille BSV: Kronisk polyartrit hos barn och dess guldbehandling. Nord Med 37: 307, 1948.
9. Colver T: The prognosis in rheumatoid arthritis in childhood. Arch Dis Child 12: 253, 1937.
10. Holzmuller G: Beitrag zur Frage der Pathogenese und Therapie der primar-chronischen Gelenkerkrankungen im Kindesalter. Ztschr F Rheumaforsch 5: 57, 1942.
11. Coss JA, Boots RH: Juvenile rheumatoid arthritis. J Pediatr 29: 143, 1946.
12. Pickard NS: Rheumatoid arthritis in children. A clinical study. Arch Intern Med 80: 771, 1947.
13. Lockie LM, Norcross BM: Juvenile rheumatoid arthritis. Pediatrics 2: 694, 1948.
14. Wissler H: Der Rheumatismus im Kindesalter. Teil 2: Die chronische Polyartritis des Kindes. Der Rheumatismus Bd 24. Steinkopff, Dresden und Leipzig 152, 1942.
15. Francon F: Conferences Cliniques De Rhumatologie Pratique. Conference Proceeding, 1946. Publication #386, Paris, France.
16. Dawson MH: Rheumatoid arthritis in children (Still's disease). *In* Palmer WW (ed): Nelson Loose-Leaf Medicine. New York, T Nelson & Sons, 1946, p 626.
17. Spitzy H: Ueber das Vorkommen multipier chronischer deformierende Glenkentzundungen im Kindesalter. Jahrb Kinderheilk 49: 286, 1899.
18. Chevallier P: La maladie de Chaufffard-Still et les syndromes voisins. Rev Med Paris 47: 77, 1930.
19. Sundt H: Om arthritis deformans i Barnealderen. Med Rev 38: 145, 1921.
20. Portis RB: Pathology of chronic arthritis of children (Still's disease). Am J Dis Child 55: 1000, 1938.
21. Sury B: Rheumatoid Arthritis in Children. A Clinical Study. Copenhagen, Munksgaard, 1952.
22. Cassidy JT, Levinson JE, Bass JC, et al: A study of classification criteria for a diagnosis of juvenile rheumatoid arthritis. Arthritis Rheum 29: 274–281, 1986.
23. Petty RE, Southwood TR, Baum J, et al: Revision of the proposed classification criteria for juvenile idiopathic arthritis: Durban, 1997. J Rheumatol 25: 1991–1994, 1998.

23a. Foeldvari, I, Bidde M: Validation of the proposed ILAR classification criteria for juvenile idiopathic arthritis. International League of Associations for Rheumatology. J Rheumatol 27: 1069–1072, 2000.

23b. Ramsey SE, Bolaria RK, Cabral DA, et al: Comparison of criteria for the classification of childhood arthritis. J Rheumatol 27: 1283–1286, 2000.

24. European League Against Rheumatism (EULAR): Nomenclature and Classification of Arthritis in Children. Bulletin 4. Basel, Nathional Zeitung AG, 1977.
25. Cassidy JT: What's in a name? Nomenclature of juvenile arthritis. A North American view. J Rheumatol Suppl 40: 4–8, 1993.
26. Cassidy JT: The classification and nomenclature of idiopathic peripheral arthritis in children. *In* Isenberg DA, Tucker LB (eds): Controversies in Rheumatology. London, Martin Dunetz, 1997, pp 117–126.
27. Fries JF, Hochberg MC, Medsger TA Jr, et al: Criteria for rheumatic disease. Different types and different functions. The American College of Rheumatology Diagnostic and Therapeutic Criteria Committee. Arthritis Rheum 37: 454–462, 1994.
28. Hanson V: From Still's disease and JRA to JCPA, JCA, and

JA: medical progress or biased ascertainment? J Rheumatol 9: 819–820, 1982.
29. Prieur AM, Petty RE: Definitions and classifications of chronic arthritis in children. Baillieres Clin Paediatr 1: 695, 1993.
30. Southwood TR, Woo P: Childhood arthritis: the name game. Br J Rheumatol 32: 421–423, 1993.
31. Prieur AM: What's in a name? Nomenclature of juvenile arthritis. A European view. J Rheumatol Suppl 40: 9–11, 1993.
32. Fink CW: Proposal for the development of classification criteria for idiopathic arthritides of childhood. J Rheumatol 22: 1566–1569, 1995.
33. Barkin RE: Clinical course of juvenile rheumatoid arthritis. Bull Rheum Dis 3: 19, 1952.
34. Norcross BM: Juvenile rheumatoid arthritis. Minn Med 42: 1760, 1959.
35. Laaksonen AL: A prognostic study of juvenile rheumatoid arthritis. Analysis of 544 Cases. Acta Paediatr Scand Suppl 1966, pp 1–163.
36. Oen KG, Cheang M: Epidemiology of chronic arthritis in childhood. Semin Arthritis Rheum 26: 575–591, 1996.
37. Gare BA: Juvenile Chronic Arthritis. A Population Based Study on Epidemiology, Natural History and Outcome. Goteborg, Sweden, University of Goteborg, 1994.
37a. Gare BA: Juvenile arthritis—who gets it, where and when? A review of current data on incidence and prevalence. Clin Exp Rheumatol 17:367–374, 1999.
37b. Nielsen HE, Dorup J, Herlin T, et al: Epidemiology of juvenile chronic arthritis: risk dependent on sibship, parental income, and housing. J Rheumatol 26: 1600–1605, 1999.
38. Lindsley CB: Seasonal variation in systemic onset juvenile rheumatoid arthritis. Arthritis Rheum 30: 838–839, 1987.
39. Feldman BM, Birdi N, Boone JE, et al: Seasonal onset of systemic-onset juvenile rheumatoid arthritis. J Pediatr 129: 513–518, 1996.
40. Oen K, Fast M, Postl B: Epidemiology of juvenile rheumatoid arthritis in Manitoba, Canada, 1975–92: cycles in incidence. J Rheumatol 22: 745–750, 1995.
40a. Uziel Y, Pomeranz A, Brik R, et al: Seasonal variation in systemic onset juvenile rheumatoid arthritis in Israel. J Rheumatol 26: 1187–1189, 1999.
41. Bywaters EG: Diagnostic criteria for Still's disease (juvenile RA). *In* Bennett PH, Wood PHN (eds): Population Studies of the Rheumatic Diseases. Amsterdam, Excerpta Medica, 1968, p 235.
42. Sullivan DB, Cassidy JT, Petty RE: Pathogenic implications of age of onset in juvenile rheumatoid arthritis. Arthritis Rheum 18: 251–255, 1975.
43. Towner SR, Michet CJ Jr, O'Fallon WM, et al: The epidemiology of juvenile arthritis in Rochester, Minnesota 1960–1979. Arthritis Rheum 26: 1208–1213, 1983.
44. Gewanter HL, Roghmann KJ, Baum J: The prevalence of juvenile arthritis. Arthritis Rheum 26: 599–603, 1983.
45. Kunnamo I, Kallio P, Pelkonen P: Incidence of arthritis in urban Finnish children. A prospective study. Arthritis Rheum 29: 1232–1238, 1986.
46. Prieur AM, Le Gall E, Karman F, et al: Epidemiologic survey of juvenile chronic arthritis in France. Comparison of data obtained from two different regions. Clin Exp Rheumatol 5: 217–223, 1987.
47. Rosenberg AM: Analysis of a pediatric rheumatology clinic population. J Rheumatol 17: 827–830, 1990.
48. Mielants H, Veys EM, Maertens M, et al: Prevalence of inflammatory rheumatic diseases in an adolescent urban student population, age 12 to 18, in Belgium. Clin Exp Rheumatol 11: 563–567, 1993.
49. Denardo BA, Tucker LB, Miller LC, et al: Demography of a regional pediatric rheumatology patient population. Affiliated Children's Arthritis Centers of New England. J Rheumatol 21: 1553–1561, 1994.
50. Malleson PN, Fung MY, Rosenberg AM: The incidence of pediatric rheumatic diseases: results from the Canadian Pediatric Rheumatology Association Disease Registry. J Rheumatol 23: 1981–1987, 1996.
51. Manners PJ, Diepeveen DA: Prevalence of juvenile chronic arthritis in a population of 12-year-old children in urban Australia. Pediatrics 98: 84–90, 1996.
52. Kaipiainen-Seppanen O, Savolainen A: Incidence of chronic juvenile rheumatic diseases in Finland during 1980–1990. Clin Exp Rheumatol 14: 441–444, 1996.
53. Symmons DP, Jones M, Osborne J, et al: Pediatric rheumatology in the United Kingdom: data from the British Pediatric Rheumatology Group National Diagnostic Register. J Rheumatol 23: 1975–1980, 1996.
54. Peterson LS, Mason T, Nelson AM, et al: Juvenile rheumatoid arthritis in Rochester, Minnesota 1960–1993. Is the epidemiology changing? Arthritis Rheum 39: 1385–1390, 1996.
55. Fujikawa S, Okuni M: A nationwide surveillance study of rheumatic diseases among Japanese children. Acta Paediatr Jpn 39: 242–244, 1997.
56. Ozen S, Karaaslan Y, Ozdemir O, et al: Prevalence of juvenile chronic arthritis and familial Mediterranean fever in Turkey: a field study. J Rheumatol 25: 2445–2449, 1998.
57. Moe N, Rygg M: Epidemiology of juvenile chronic arthritis in northern Norway: a ten-year retrospective study. Clin Exp Rheumatol 16: 99–101, 1998.
58. Arguedas O, Fasth A, Andersson-Gare B, et al: Juvenile chronic arthritis in urban San Jose, Costa Rica: a 2 year prospective study. J Rheumatol 25: 1844–1850, 1998.
59. Kiessling U, Doring E, Listing J, et al: Incidence and prevalence of juvenile chronic arthritis in East Berlin 1980–88. J Rheumatol 25: 1837–1843, 1998.
60. Gare BA: Epidemiology. Baillieres Clin Rheumatol 12: 191–208, 1998.
61. Mikkelson WM, Dodge HJ, Duff IF, et al: Clinical and serological estimates of the prevalence of rheumatoid arthritis in the population of Tecumseh, Michigan 1959–60. *In* Kellgren J (ed): The Epidemiology of Chronic Rheumatism. Philadelphia, FA Davis, 1963, p 239.
62. Gare BA, Fasth A, Andersson J, et al: Incidence and prevalence of juvenile chronic arthritis: a population survey. Ann Rheum Dis 46: 277–281, 1987.
63. Bonham GS: Prevalence of chronic skin and musculoskeletal conditions. United States—1976. Vital Health Stat [10]: i–57, 1978.
64. Newacheck PW, Halfon N, Budetti PP: Prevalence of activity limiting chronic conditions among children based on household interviews. J Chronic Dis 39: 63–71, 1986.
65. Lee P, Helewa A, Smythe HA, et al: Epidemiology of musculoskeletal disorders (complaints) and related disability in Canada. J Rheumatol 12: 1169–1173, 1985.
66. Brewer EJ, Bass JC, Cassidy JT: Criteria for the classification of juvenile rheumatoid arthritis. Bull Rheum Dis 23: 712–719, 1972.
67. Brewer EJ Jr, Bass J, Baum J, et al: Current proposed revision of JRA Criteria. JRA Criteria Subcommittee of the Diagnostic and Therapeutic Criteria Committee of the American Rheumatism Section of The Arthritis Foundation. Arthritis Rheum 20: 195–199, 1977.
68. Edstrom G: Rheumatoid arthritis and Still's disease in children. A survey of 161 cases. Arthritis Rheum 1: 497, 1958.
69. Ansell BM: Heberden Oration, 1977. Chronic arthritis in childhood. Ann Rheum Dis 37: 107–120, 1978.
70. Sairanen E: On rheumatoid arthritis in children. A clinicoroentgenological study. Acta Rheum Scand(Suppl)2: 1, 1958.
71. Schesinger BE, Forsyth CC, White RH: Observations on the clinical course and treatment of one hundred cases of Still's disease. Arch Dis Child 36: 65, 1961.
72. Grokoest AW, Snyder AL, Schlaeger R: Juvenile Rheumatoid Arthritis. Boston, Little, Brown, 1962.
73. Schaller JG: Juvenile rheumatoid arthritis: Series 1. Arthritis Rheum 20: 165–170, 1977.
74. Aaron S, Fraser PA, Jackson JM, et al: Sex ratio and sibship size in juvenile rheumatoid arthritis kindreds. Arthritis Rheum 28: 753–758, 1985.
75. Cassidy JT, Sullivan DB, Petty RE: Clinical patterns of chronic iridocyclitis in children with juvenile rheumatoid arthritis. Arthritis Rheum 20: 224–227, 1977.
76. Chylack LT Jr: The ocular manifestations of juvenile rheumatoid arthritis. Arthritis Rheum 20(Suppl): 217–223, 1977.
77. Schaller J, Kupfer C, Wedgwood RJ: Iridocyclitis in juvenile rheumatoid arthritis. Pediatrics 44: 92–100, 1969.

78. Greenwood BM: Polyarthritis in Western Nigeria. II. Still's disease. Ann Rheum Dis 28: 617–623, 1969.
79. Hill RH: Juvenile arthritis in various racial groups in British Columbia. Arthritis Rheum 20: 162, 1977.
80. Haffejee IE, Raga J, Coovadia HM: Juvenile chronic arthritis in black and Indian South African children. S Afr Med J 65: 510–514, 1984.
81. Graham TB, Glass DN: Juvenile rheumatoid arthritis: ethnic differences in diagnostic types. J Rheumatol 24: 1677–1679, 1997.
82. Schwartz MM, Simpson P, Kerr KL, et al: Juvenile rheumatoid arthritis in African Americans. J Rheumatol 24: 1826–1829, 1997.
83. Hanson V, Kornreich HK, Bernstein B, et al: Three subtypes of juvenile rheumatoid arthritis (correlations of age at onset, sex, and serologic factors). Arthritis Rheum Suppl 20: 184, 1977.
84. Rosenberg AM, Petty RE, Oen KG, et al: Rheumatic diseases in Western Canadian Indian children. J Rheumatol 9: 589–592, 1982.
85. Oen K, Postl B, Chalmers IM, et al: Rheumatic diseases in an Inuit population. Arthritis Rheum 29: 65–74, 1986.
86. Boyer GS, Lanier AP, Templin DW, et al: Spondyloarthropathy and rheumatoid arthritis in Alaskan Yupik Eskimos. J Rheumatol 17: 489–496, 1990.
87. Lang BA, Shore A: A review of current concepts on the pathogenesis of juvenile rheumatoid arthritis. J Rheumatol Suppl 21: 1–15, 1990.
88. Jarvis JN: Pathogenesis and mechanisms of inflammation in the childhood rheumatic diseases. Curr Opin Rheumatol 10: 459–467, 1998.
89. Glass DN, Giannini EH: JRA as a complex genetic trait. Arthritis Rheum 42: 2261–2268, 1999.
90. Lipnick RN, Tsokos GC: Immune abnormalities in the pathogenesis of juvenile rheumatoid arthritis. Clin Exp Rheumatol 8: 177–186, 1990.
91. Lipnick RN, Tsokos GC, Magilavy DB: Immune abnormalities in the pathogenesis of juvenile rheumatoid arthritis. Rheum Dis Clin North Am 17: 843–857, 1991.
92. De Benedetti F, Ravelli A, Martini A: Cytokines in juvenile rheumatoid arthritis. Curr Opin Rheumatol 9: 428–433, 1997.
92a. Moore TL: Immunopathogenesis of juvenile rheumatoid arthritis. Curr Opin Rheumatol 11: 377–383, 1999.
92b. Maeno N, Takei S, Imanaka H, et al: Increased circulating vascular endothelial growth factor is correlated with disease activity in polyarticular juvenile rheumatoid arthritis. J Rheumatol 26: 2244–2248, 1999.
92c. De Benedetti F, Vivarelli M, Pignatti P, et al: Circulating levels of soluble E-selectin, P-selectin and intercellular adhesion molecule-1 in patients with juvenile idiopathic arthritis. J Rheumatol 27: 2246–2250, 2000.
93. Mason T, Rabinovich CE, Fredrickson DD, et al: Breast feeding and the development of juvenile rheumatoid arthritis. J Rheumatol 22: 1166–1170, 1995.
94. Rosenberg AM: Evaluation of associations between breast feeding and subsequent development of juvenile rheumatoid arthritis. J Rheumatol 23: 1080–1082, 1996.
95. Pachman LM, Baldwin SM: Assays of complement in polyarticular juvenile rheumatoid arthritis. Arthritis Rheum 20: 467–470, 1977.
96. Moore TL, Dorner RW: Separation and characterization of complement-fixing immune complexes in juvenile rheumatoid arthritis patients. Rheumatol Int 6: 49–52, 1986.
97. Rossen RD, Brewer EJ, Person DA, et al: Circulating immune complexes and antinuclear antibodies in juvenile rheumatoid arthritis. Arthritis Rheum 20: 1485–1490, 1977.
98. Moran H, Ansell BM, Mowbray JF, et al: Antigen-antibody complexes in the serum of patients with juvenile chronic arthritis. Arch Dis Child 54: 120–122, 1979.
98a. Khalkhali-Ellis Z, Bulla GA, Schlesinger LS, et al: C1q-containing immune complexes purified from sera of juvenile rheumatoid arthritis patients mediate IL-8 production by human synoviocytes: role of C1q receptors. J Immunol 163: 4612–4620, 1999.
99. Jarvis JN, Diebold MM, Chadwell MK, et al: Composition and biological behaviour of immune complexes isolated from synovial fluid of patients with juvenile rheumatoid arthritis (JRA). Clin Exp Immunol 100: 514–518, 1995.
100. Jarvis JN, Taylor H, Iobidze M, et al: Complement activation and immune complexes in children with polyarticular juvenile rheumatoid arthritis: a longitudinal study. J Rheumatol 21: 1124–1127, 1994.
100a. Aggarwal A, Bhardwaj A, Alam S, et al: Evidence for activation of the alternate complement pathway in patients with juvenile rheumatoid arthritis. Rheumatology (Oxford) 39: 189–192, 2000.
101. Moore TL, Sheridan PW, Zuckner J, et al: Separation and characterization of immune complexes containing 19S IgM rheumatoid factor-IgG in juvenile arthritis. Arthritis Rheum 26: 165–169, 1983.
102. Moore TL, Osborn TG, Dorner RW: 19S IgM rheumatoid factor-7S IgG rheumatoid factor immune complexes isolated in sera of patients with juvenile rheumatoid arthritis. Pediatr Res 20: 977–981, 1986.
103. Jarvis JN, Iobidze M, Taylor H, et al: A comparison of immunoglobulin G–containing high-molecular-weight complexes isolated from children with juvenile rheumatoid arthritis and congenital human immunodeficiency virus infection. Pediatr Res 34: 781–784, 1993.
104. Moore T, Dorner RW, Zuckner J: Hidden rheumatoid factor in seronegative juvenile rheumatoid arthritis. Ann Rheum Dis 33: 255–257, 1974.
105. Moore TL, Dorner RW, Osborn TG, et al: Hidden 19S IgM rheumatoid factors. Semin Arthritis Rheum 18: 72–75, 1988.
106. Jarvis JN, Pousak T, Krenz M: Detection of IgM rheumatoid factors by enzyme-linked immunosorbent assay in children with juvenile rheumatoid arthritis: correlation with articular disease and laboratory abnormalities. Pediatrics 90: 945–949, 1992.
107. Mitchell WS, Naama JK, Veitch J, et al: IgM-RF prevents complement–mediated inhibition of immune precipitation. Immunology 52: 445–448, 1984.
108. Doekes G, Schouten J, Cats A, et al: Reduction of the complement activation capacity of soluble IgG aggregates and immune complexes by IgM-rheumatoid factor. Immunology 55: 555–564, 1985.
109. Jarvis JN, Lockman JC, Levine RP: IgM rheumatoid factor and the inhibition of covalent binding of C4b to IgG in immune complexes. Clin Exp Rheumatol 11: 135–141, 1993.
110. Jarvis JN, Wang W, Moore HT, et al: In vitro induction of proinflammatory cytokine secretion by juvenile rheumatoid arthritis synovial fluid immune complexes. Arthritis Rheum 40: 2039–2046, 1997.
111. Woo P: The cytokine network in juvenile chronic arthritis. Ann Med 29: 145–147, 1997.
112. Woo P: Cytokines in juvenile chronic arthritis. Baillieres Clin Rheumatol 12: 219–228, 1998.
112a. Harjacek M, Diaz-Cano S, Alman BA, et al: Prominent expression of mRNA for proinflammatory cytokines in synovium in patients with juvenile rheumatoid arthritis or chronic Lyme arthritis. J Rheumatol 27: 497–503, 2000.
113. Murray KJ, Luyrink L, Grom AA, et al: Immunohistological characteristics of T cell infiltrates in different forms of childhood onset chronic arthritis. J Rheumatol 23: 2116–2124, 1996.
114. Murray KJ, Grom AA, Thompson SD, et al: Contrasting cytokine profiles in the synovium of different forms of juvenile rheumatoid arthritis and juvenile spondyloarthropathy: prominence of interleukin 4 in restricted disease. J Rheumatol 25: 1388–1398, 1998.
115. Gattorno M, Facchetti P, Ghiotto F, et al: Synovial fluid T cell clones from oligoarticular juvenile arthritis patients display a prevalent Th1/Th0–type pattern of cytokine secretion irrespective of immunophenotype. Clin Exp Immunol 109: 4–11, 1997.
116. Raziuddin S, Bahabri S, Al-Dalaan A, et al: A mixed Th1/Th2 cell cytokine response predominates in systemic onset juvenile rheumatoid arthritis: immunoregulatory IL-10 function. Clin Immunol Immunopathol 86: 192–198, 1998.
117. De Maria A, Malnati M, Moretta A, et al: CD3+4–8–WT31–(T cell receptor gamma+) cells and other unusual phenotypes are frequently detected among spontaneously interleukin 2–responsive T lymphocytes present in the joint fluid in juvenile

rheumatoid arthritis. A clonal analysis. Eur J Immunol 17: 1815–1819, 1987.
118. Bergroth V, Konttinen YT, Pelkonen P, et al: Synovial fluid lymphocytes in different subtypes of juvenile rheumatoid arthritis. Arthritis Rheum 31: 780–783, 1988.
119. Thoen J, Forre O, Waalen K, et al: Phenotypes of T lymphocytes from peripheral blood and synovial fluid of patients with rheumatoid arthritis and juvenile rheumatoid arthritis. Evidence in favour of normal helper and suppressor functions of T lymphocytes from patients with juvenile rheumatoid arthritis. Scand J Rheumatol 16: 247–256, 1987.
120. Agosti E, Radillo O, Narchi G, et al: Immunological patterns in monoarticular juvenile rheumatoid arthritis. Clin Exp Rheumatol 6: 319–324, 1988.
121. Konttinen YT, Bergroth V, Kunnamo I, et al: The value of biopsy in patients with monarticular juvenile rheumatoid arthritis of recent onset. Arthritis Rheum 29: 47–53, 1986.
122. Silverman ED, Isacovics B, Petsche D, et al: Synovial fluid cells in juvenile arthritis: evidence of selective T cell migration to inflamed tissue. Clin Exp Immunol 91: 90–95, 1993.
123. Kutukculer N, Caglayan S, Aydogdu F: Study of pro-inflammatory (TNF-alpha, IL-1alpha, IL-6) and T-cell–derived (IL-2, IL-4) cytokines in plasma and synovial fluid of patients with juvenile chronic arthritis: correlations with clinical and laboratory parameters. Clin Rheumatol 17: 288–292, 1998.
123a. Wedderburn LR, Robinson N, Patel A, et al: Selective recruitment of polarized T cells expressing CCR5 and CXCR3 to the inflamed joints of children with juvenile idiopathic arthritis. Arthritis Rheum 43: 765–774, 2000.
124. Morimoto C, Reinherz EL, Borel Y, et al: Autoantibody to an immunoregulatory inducer population in patients with juvenile rheumatoid arthritis. J Clin Invest 67: 753–761, 1981.
125. Astrup LB, Morling N, Ryder LP, et al: Concanavalin-A-activated suppressor cells in patients with juvenile rheumatoid arthritis. Scand J Immunol 16: 361–367, 1982.
126. Ellsworth JE, Stein LD, Thebert PJ, et al: Abnormalities of lymphokine generation in children with juvenile rheumatoid arthritis. Pediatr Res 16: 221A, 1982.
127. Abrahamsen TG, Froland SS, Natvig JB: In vitro mitogen stimulation of synovial fluid lymphocytes from rheumatoid arthritis and juvenile rheumatoid arthritis patients: dissociation between the response to antigens and polyclonal mitogens. Scand J Immunol 7: 81–90, 1978.
128. Strelkauskas AJ, Callery RT, McDowell J, et al: Direct evidence for loss of human suppressor cells during active autoimmune disease. Proc Natl Acad Sci U S A 75: 5150–5154, 1978.
129. Barron KS, Lewis DE, Brewer EJ, et al: Cytotoxic anti-T cell antibodies in children with juvenile rheumatoid arthritis. Arthritis Rheum 27: 1272–1280, 1984.
130. Williams RC Jr, Froelich CJ, Kilpatrick K, et al: T gamma subset specificity of lymphocyte reactive factors in juvenile rheumatoid arthritis and systemic lupus erythematosus sera. Arthritis Rheum 24: 585–591, 1981.
131. Oen K, Wilkins JA, Krzekotowska D: OKT4:OKT8 ratios of circulating T cells and in vitro suppressor cell function of patients with juvenile rheumatoid arthritis (JRA). J Rheumatol 12: 321–327, 1985.
132. Murata H, Yata J: Defect of suppressor cell induction in patients with juvenile rheumatoid arthritis. Asian Pac J Allergy Immunol 4: 95–99, 1986.
133. Alpert SD, Turek PJ, Foung SK, et al: Human monoclonal anti-T cell antibody from a patient with juvenile rheumatoid arthritis. J Immunol 138: 104–108, 1987.
134. Tsokos GC, Mavridis A, Inghirami G, et al: Cellular immunity in patients with systemic juvenile rheumatoid arthritis. Clin Immunol Immunopathol 42: 86–92, 1987.
135. Tsokos GC, Inghirami G, Pillemer SR, et al: Immunoregulatory aberrations in patients with polyarticular juvenile rheumatoid arthritis. Clin Immunol Immunopathol 47: 62–74, 1988.
136. Alarcon-Riquelme ME, Vazquez-Mellado J, Gomez-Cordillo M, et al: Immunoregulatory defects in juvenile rheumatoid arthritis. Comparison between patients with the systemic or polyarticular forms. J Rheumatol 15: 1547–1550, 1988.
136a. Wedderburn LR, Maini MK, Patel A, et al: Molecular fingerprinting reveals non-overlapping T cell oligoclonality between an inflamed site and peripheral blood. Int Immunol 11: 535–543, 1999.
137. Oen K: Defects in pokeweed mitogen (PWM) induced immunoglobulin (Ig) synthesis by lymphocytes of patients with juvenile rheumatoid arthritis. J Rheumatol 12: 728–734, 1985.
138. Doublog JH, Chattoppadhyay C, Forre O, et al: Con A-induced suppressor cell activity and T-lymphocyte subpopulations in peripheral blood lymphocytes of patients with rheumatoid arthritis and juvenile rheumatoid arthritis. Scand J Immunol 13: 367–373, 1981.
139. Odum N, Morling N, Platz P, et al: Increased prevalence of late stage T cell activation antigen (VLA-1) in active juvenile chronic arthritis. Ann Rheum Dis 46: 846–852, 1987.
140. Forre O, Thoen J, Dobloug JH, et al: Detection of T-lymphocyte subpopulation in the peripheral blood and the synovium of patients with rheumatoid arthritis and juvenile rheumatoid arthritis using monoclonal antibodies. Scand J Immunol 15: 221–226, 1982.
141. Massa M, De Benedetti F, Robbioni P, et al: Association of methotrexate treatment with a decrease of double negative (CD4–CD8–) and gamma/delta T cell levels in patients with juvenile rheumatoid arthritis. J Rheumatol 20: 1944–1948, 1993.
142. De Benedetti F, Martini A: Is systemic juvenile rheumatoid arthritis an interleukin 6 mediated disease? J Rheumatol 25: 203–207, 1998.
143. Mangge H, Schauenstein K: Cytokines in juvenile rheumatoid arthritis (JRA). Cytokine 10: 471–480, 1998.
144. De Benedetti F, Massa M, Robbioni P, et al: Correlation of serum interleukin-6 levels with joint involvement and thrombocytosis in systemic juvenile rheumatoid arthritis. Arthritis Rheum 34: 1158–1163, 1991.
145. Lepore L, Pennesi M, Saletta S, et al: Study of IL-2, IL-6, TNF alpha, IFN gamma and beta in the serum and synovial fluid of patients with juvenile chronic arthritis. Clin Exp Rheumatol 12: 561–565, 1994.
146. Rooney M, David J, Symons J, et al: Inflammatory cytokine responses in juvenile chronic arthritis. Br J Rheumatol 34: 454–460, 1995.
147. De Benedetti F, Pignatti P, Massa M, et al: Circulating levels of interleukin 1 beta and of interleukin 1 receptor antagonist in systemic juvenile chronic arthritis. Clin Exp Rheumatol 13: 779–784, 1995.
148. Mangge H, Kenzian H, Gallistl S, et al: Serum cytokines in juvenile rheumatoid arthritis. Correlation with conventional inflammation parameters and clinical subtypes. Arthritis Rheum 38: 211–220, 1995.
149. Prieur AM, Kaufmann MT, Griscelli C, et al: Specific interleukin-1 inhibitor in serum and urine of children with systemic juvenile chronic arthritis. Lancet 2: 1240–1242, 1987.
150. De Benedetti F, Massa M, Pignatti P, et al: Serum soluble interleukin 6 (IL-6) receptor and IL-6/soluble IL-6 receptor complex in systemic juvenile rheumatoid arthritis. J Clin Invest 93: 2114–2119, 1994.
151. De Benedetti F, Alonzi T, Moretta A, et al: Interleukin 6 causes growth impairment in transgenic mice through a decrease in insulin-like growth factor-I. A model for stunted growth in children with chronic inflammation. J Clin Invest 99: 643–650, 1997.
152. Fishman D, Faulds G, Jeffery R, et al: The effect of novel polymorphisms in the interleukin-6 (IL-6) gene on IL-6 transcription and plasma IL-6 levels, and an association with systemic-onset juvenile chronic arthritis. J Clin Invest 102: 1369–1376, 1998.
153. Silverman ED, Laxer RM, Nelson DL, et al: Soluble interleukin-2 receptor in juvenile rheumatoid arthritis. J Rheumatol 18: 1398–1402, 1991.
154. Lipnick RN, Sfikakis PP, Klipple GL, et al: Elevated soluble CD8 antigen and soluble interleukin-2 receptors in the sera of patients with juvenile rheumatoid arthritis. Clin Immunol Immunopathol 68: 64–67, 1993.
155. Madson KL, Moore TL, Lawrence JM III, et al: Cytokine levels in serum and synovial fluid of patients with juvenile rheumatoid arthritis. J Rheumatol 21: 2359–2363, 1994.
156. De Benedetti F, Massa M, Pignatti P, et al: Elevated circulating interleukin-7 levels in patients with systemic juvenile rheumatoid arthritis. J Rheumatol 22: 1581–1585, 1995.

157. Gattorno M, Picco P, Buoncompagni A, et al: Serum p55 and p75 tumour necrosis factor receptors as markers of disease activity in juvenile chronic arthritis. Ann Rheum Dis 55: 243–247, 1996.
157a. Rooney M, Varsani H, Martin K, et al: Tumour necrosis factor alpha and its soluble receptors in juvenile chronic arthritis. Rheumatology (Oxford) 39: 432–438, 2000.
158. Grom AA, Giannini EH, Glass DN: Juvenile rheumatoid arthritis and the trimolecular complex (HLA, T cell receptor, and antigen). Differences from rheumatoid arthritis. Arthritis Rheum 37: 601–607, 1994.
159. Sioud M, Kjeldsen-Kragh J, Suleyman S, et al: Limited heterogeneity of T cell receptor variable region gene usage in juvenile rheumatoid arthritis synovial T cells. Eur J Immunol 22: 2413–2418, 1992.
160. Thompson SD, Murray KJ, Grom AA, et al: Comparative sequence analysis of the human T cell receptor beta chain in juvenile rheumatoid arthritis and juvenile spondylarthropathies: evidence for antigenic selection of T cells in the synovium. Arthritis Rheum 41: 482–497, 1998.
161. Maksymowych WP, Gabriel CA, Luyrink L, et al: Polymorphism in a T-cell receptor variable gene is associated with susceptibility to a juvenile rheumatoid arthritis subset. Immunogenetics 35: 257–262, 1992.
162. Grom AA, von Knorre C, Murray KJ, et al: T-cell receptor BV6S1 null alleles and HLA-DR1 haplotypes in polyarticular outcome juvenile rheumatoid arthritis. Hum Immunol 45: 152–156, 1996.
163. Ploski R, Hansen T, Forre O: Lack of association with T-cell receptor TCRBV6S1*2 allele in HLA-DQA1*0101–positive Norwegian juvenile chronic arthritis patients. Immunogenetics 38: 444–445, 1993.
164. Nepom BS, Malhotra U, Schwarz DA, et al: HLA and T cell receptor polymorphisms in pauciarticular-onset juvenile rheumatoid arthritis. Arthritis Rheum 34: 1260–1267, 1991.
165. Oen K, Krzekotowska D: In vitro immunoglobulin production by lymphocytes of patients with juvenile rheumatoid arthritis: effects of Staphylococcus aureus Cowan I stimulation and monocyte depletion. J Rheumatol 15: 1539–1546, 1988.
166. Cassidy JT, Petty RE, Sullivan DB: Abnormalities in the distribution of serum immunoglobulin concentrations in juvenile rheumatoid arthritis. J Clin Invest 52: 1931–1936, 1973.
167. Cassidy JT, Shillis JL, Brandon FB, et al: Viral antibody titers to rubella and rubeola in juvenile rheumatoid arthritis. Pediatrics 54: 239–244, 1974.
168. Ilowite NT, Wedgwood RJ, Rose LM, et al: Impaired in vivo and in vitro antibody responses to bacteriophage phi X 174 in juvenile rheumatoid arthritis. J Rheumatol 14: 957–963, 1987.
169. Leak AM: Autoantibody profile in juvenile chronic arthritis. Ann Rheum Dis 47: 178–182, 1988.
170. Pauls JD, Silverman E, Laxer RM, et al: Antibodies to histones H1 and H5 in sera of patients with juvenile rheumatoid arthritis. Arthritis Rheum 32: 877–883, 1989.
171. Malleson P, Petty RE, Fung M, et al: Reactivity of antinuclear antibodies with histones and other antigens in juvenile rheumatoid arthritis. Arthritis Rheum 32: 919–923, 1989.
172. Monestier M, Losman JA, Fasy TM, et al: Antihistone antibodies in antinuclear antibody-positive juvenile arthritis. Arthritis Rheum 33: 1836–1841, 1990.
173. Leak AM, Woo P: Juvenile chronic arthritis, chronic iridocyclitis, and reactivity to histones. Ann Rheum Dis 50: 653–657, 1991.
174. Malleson PN, Fung MY, Petty RE, et al: Autoantibodies in chronic arthritis of childhood: relations with each other and with histocompatibility antigens. Ann Rheum Dis 51: 1301–1306, 1992.
175. Leak AM, Tuaillon N, Muller S, et al: Study of antibodies to histones and histone synthetic peptides in pauciarticular juvenile chronic arthritis. Br J Rheumatol 32: 426–431, 1993.
176. Stemmer C, Tuaillon N, Prieur AM, et al: Mapping of B-cell epitopes recognized by antibodies to histones in subsets of juvenile chronic arthritis. Clin Immunol Immunopathol 76: 82–89, 1995.
177. Kageura H: Activation of dorsal development by contact between the cortical dorsal determinant and the equatorial core cytoplasm in eggs of Xenopus laevis. Development 124: 1543–1551, 1997.
178. Speckmaier M, Rother E, Terreri T, et al: Prevalence of antineutrophil cytoplasmic antibodies (ANCA) in juvenile chronic arthritis. Clin Exp Rheumatol 14: 211–216, 1996.
179. Mulder L, van Rossum M, Horst G, et al: Antineutrophil cytoplasmic antibodies in juvenile chronic arthritis. J Rheumatol 24: 568–575, 1997.
179a. Bakkaloglu A, Ozen S, Saatci U, et al: Antineutrophil cytoplasmic antibodies in juvenile chronic arthritis. Clin Rheumatol 18: 304–307, 1999.
180. Gabay C, Prieur AM, Meyer O: Occurrence of antiperinuclear, antikeratin, and anti-RA 33 antibodies in juvenile chronic arthritis. Ann Rheum Dis 52: 785–789, 1993.
180a. Serra CR, Rodrigues SH, Sztajnbok FR, et al: Antiperinuclear factor and antibodies to the stratum corneum of rat esophagus in juvenile idiopathic arthritis. J Pediatr 134: 507–509, 1999.
181. Gattorno M, Buoncompagni A, Molinari AC, et al: Antiphospholipid antibodies in paediatric systemic lupus erythematosus, juvenile chronic arthritis and overlap syndromes: SLE patients with both lupus anticoagulant and high-titre anticardiolipin antibodies are at risk for clinical manifestations related to the antiphospholipid syndrome. Br J Rheumatol 34: 873–881, 1995.
181a. Serra CR, Rodrigues SH, Silva NP, et al: Clinical significance of anticardiolipin antibodies in juvenile idiopathic arthritis. Clin Exp Rheumatol 17: 375–380, 1999.
182. Jung F, Neuer G, Bautz FA: Antibodies against a peptide sequence located in the linker region of the HMG-1/2 box domains in sera from patients with juvenile rheumatoid arthritis. Arthritis Rheum 40: 1803–1809, 1997.
182a. Rosenberg AM, Cordeiro DM: Relationship between sex and antibodies to high mobility group proteins 1 and 2 in juvenile idiopathic arthritis. J Rheumatol 27: 2489–2493, 2000.
183. Rosenberg AM, Hunt DW, Petty RE: Antibodies to native type I collagen in childhood rheumatic diseases. J Rheumatol 11: 421–424, 1984.
184. Petty RE, Hunt DW, Rosenberg AM: Antibodies to type IV collagen in rheumatic diseases. J Rheumatol 13: 246–253, 1986.
185. Guerassimov A, Duffy C, Zhang Y, et al: Immunity to cartilage link protein in patients with juvenile rheumatoid arthritis. J Rheumatol 24: 959–964, 1997.
186. Pellegrini G, Scotta MS, Soardo S, et al: Elevated IgA antigliadin antibodies in juvenile chronic arthritis. Clin Exp Rheumatol 9: 653–656, 1991.
187. Henoch MJ, Batson JW, Baum J: Psychosocial factors in juvenile rheumatoid arthritis. Arthritis Rheum 21: 229–233, 1978.
188. Vandvik IH, Hoyeraal HM, Fagertun H: Chronic family difficulties and stressful life events in recent onset juvenile arthritis. J Rheumatol 16: 1088–1092, 1989.
189. Kuis W, Jong-de Vos VS, Sinnema G, et al: The autonomic nervous system and the immune system in juvenile rheumatoid arthritis. Brain Behav Immun 10: 387–398, 1996.
190. Kuis W, Kavelaars A, Prakken BJ, et al: Dialogue between the brain and the immune system in juvenile chronic arthritis. Rev Rhum Engl Ed 64: 146S–148S, 1997.
191. Khalkhali-Ellis Z, Moore TL, Hendrix MJ: Reduced levels of testosterone and dehydroepiandrosterone sulphate in the serum and synovial fluid of juvenile rheumatoid arthritis patients correlates with disease severity. Clin Exp Rheumatol 16: 753–756, 1998.
192. Da Silva JA, Larbre JP, Spector TD, et al: Protective effect of androgens against inflammation induced cartilage degradation in male rodents. Ann Rheum Dis 52: 285–291, 1993.
193. McMurray RW, Allen SH, Pepmueller PH, et al: Elevated serum prolactin levels in children with juvenile rheumatoid arthritis and antinuclear antibody seropositivity. J Rheumatol 22: 1577–1580, 1995.
194. Picco P, Gattorno M, Buoncompagni A, et al: Prolactin and interleukin 6 in prepubertal girls with juvenile chronic arthritis. J Rheumatol 25: 347–351, 1998.
194a. Picco P, Gattorno M, Buoncompagni A, et al: Interactions between prolactin and the proinflammatory cytokine network in juvenile chronic arthritis. Ann N Y Acad Sci 876: 262–265, 1999.

195. Petty RE, Tingle AJ: Arthritis and viral infection. J Pediatr 113: 948–949, 1988.
196. Pugh MT, Southwood TR, Gaston JS: The role of infection in juvenile chronic arthritis. Br J Rheumatol 32: 838–844, 1993.
197. Vaughan JH: Viruses and autoimmune disease [editorial]. J Rheumatol 23: 1831–1833, 1996.
198. Chantler JK, Tingle AJ, Petty RE: Persistent rubella virus infection associated with chronic arthritis in children. N Engl J Med 313: 1117–1123, 1985.
199. Smith CA, Petty RE, Tingle AJ: Rubella virus and arthritis. Rheum Dis Clin North Am 13: 265–274, 1987.
200. Phillips PE, Dougherty RM: Detection of rubella virus using polymerase chain reaction after vaccination and in arthritis. Arthritis Rheum Suppl 33:S134, 1990.
201. Frenkel LM, Nielsen K, Garakian A, et al: A search for persistent rubella virus infection in persons with chronic symptoms after rubella and rubella immunization and in patients with juvenile rheumatoid arthritis. Clin Infect Dis 22: 287–294, 1996.
202. Weibel RE, Benor DE: Chronic arthropathy and musculoskeletal symptoms associated with rubella vaccines. A review of 124 claims submitted to the National Vaccine Injury Compensation Program. Arthritis Rheum 39: 1529–1534, 1996.
203. Mitchell LA, Tingle AJ, MacWilliam L, et al: HLA-DR class II associations with rubella vaccine-induced joint manifestations. J Infect Dis 177: 5–12, 1998.
203a. Maillefert JF, Tonolli-Serabian I, Cherasse A, et al: Arthritis following combined vaccine against diphtheria, poliomyelitis, and tetanus toxoid. Clin Exp Rheumatol 18: 255–256, 2000.
203b. Pope JE, Stevens A, Howson W, et al: The development of rheumatoid arthritis after recombinant hepatitis B vaccination. J Rheumatol 25: 1687–1693, 1998.
203c. Maillefert JF, Sibilia J, Toussirot E, et al: Rheumatic disorders developed after hepatitis B vaccination. Rheumatology (Oxford) 38: 978–983, 1999.
204. Pritchard MH, Matthews N, Munro J: Antibodies to influenza A in a cluster of children with juvenile chronic arthritis. Br J Rheumatol 27: 176–180, 1988.
205. Pritchard MH, Munro J: Successful treatment of juvenile chronic arthritis with a specific antiviral agent. Br J Rheumatol 28: 521–524, 1989.
206. Schwarz TF, Roggendorf M, Suschke H, et al: Human parvovirus B19 infection and juvenile chronic polyarthritis. Infection 15: 264–265, 1987.
207. Nocton JJ, Miller LC, Tucker LB, et al: Human parvovirus B19–associated arthritis in children. J Pediatr 122: 186–190, 1993.
208. Soderlund M, von Essen R, Haapasaari J, et al: Persistence of parvovirus B19 DNA in synovial membranes of young patients with and without chronic arthropathy. Lancet 349: 1063–1065, 1997.
208a. Saulsbury FT: Remission of juvenile rheumatoid arthritis with varicella infection. J Rheumatol 26:1606–1608, 1999.
208b. Bateman HE, Kirou KA, Paget SA, et al: Remission of juvenile rheumatoid arthritis after infection with parvovirus B19. J Rheumatol 26: 2482–2484, 1999.
209. Maximov AA, Shaikov AV, Lovell DJ, et al: Chlamydial associated syndrome of arthritis and eye involvement in young children. J Rheumatol 19: 1794–1797, 1992.
210. Burgos-Vargas R, Howard A, Ansell BM: Antibodies to peptidoglycan in juvenile onset ankylosing spondylitis and pauciarticular onset juvenile arthritis associated with chronic iridocyclitis. J Rheumatol 13: 760–762, 1986.
211. de Graeff-Meeder ER, van der Zee R, Rijkers GT, et al: Recognition of human 60 kD heat shock protein by mononuclear cells from patients with juvenile chronic arthritis. Lancet 337: 1368–1372, 1991.
212. Boog CJ, de Graeff-Meeder ER, Lucassen MA, et al: Two monoclonal antibodies generated against human hsp60 show reactivity with synovial membranes of patients with juvenile chronic arthritis. J Exp Med 175: 1805–1810, 1992.
213. de Graeff-Meeder ER, Rijkers GT, Voorhorst-Ogink MM, et al: Antibodies to human HSP60 in patients with juvenile chronic arthritis, diabetes mellitus, and cystic fibrosis. Pediatr Res 34: 424–428, 1993.
214. de Graeff-Meeder ER, van Eden W, Rijkers GT, et al: Heat-shock proteins and juvenile chronic arthritis. Clin Exp Rheumatol 11(Suppl)9:S25–S28, 1993.
215. Life P, Hassell A, Williams K, et al: Responses to gram negative enteric bacterial antigens by synovial T cells from patients with juvenile chronic arthritis: recognition of heat shock protein HSP60. J Rheumatol 20: 1388–1396, 1993.
216. Albani S, Ravelli A, Massa M, et al: Immune responses to the *Escherichia coli* dnaJ heat shock protein in juvenile rheumatoid arthritis and their correlation with disease activity. J Pediatr 124: 561–565, 1994.
217. Prakken AB, van Hoeij MJ, Kuis W, et al: T-cell reactivity to human HSP60 in oligo-articular juvenile chronic arthritis is associated with a favorable prognosis and the generation of regulatory cytokines in the inflamed joint. Immunol Lett 57: 139–142, 1997.
218. Prakken AB, van Eden W, Rijkers GT, et al: Autoreactivity to human heat-shock protein 60 predicts disease remission in oligoarticular juvenile rheumatoid arthritis. Arthritis Rheum 39: 1826–1832, 1996.
219. Conroy SE, Tucker L, Latchman DS, et al: Incidence of anti Hsp 90 and 70 antibodies in children with SLE, juvenile dermatomyositis and juvenile chronic arthritis. Clin Exp Rheumatol 14: 99–104, 1996.
220. van Eden W, Anderton SM, van der Zee R, et al: (Altered) self peptides and the regulation of self reactivity in the peripheral T cell pool. Immunol Rev 149: 55–73, 1996.
221. van der Zee R, Anderton SM, Prakken AB, et al: T cell responses to conserved bacterial heat-shock-protein epitopes induce resistance in experimental autoimmunity. Semin Immunol 10: 35–41, 1998.
222. van Eden W, van der Zee R, Paul AG, et al: Do heat shock proteins control the balance of T-cell regulation in inflammatory diseases? Immunol Today 19: 303–307, 1998.
223. van Eden W, van der Zee R, Taams LS, et al: Heat-shock protein T-cell epitopes trigger a spreading regulatory control in a diversified arthritogenic T-cell response. Immunol Rev 164: 169–174, 1998.
224. Prakken B, Wauben M, van Kooten P, et al: Nasal administration of arthritis-related T cell epitopes of heat shock protein 60 as a promising way for immunotherapy in chronic arthritis. Biotherapy 10: 205–211, 1998.
225. Albani S, Keystone EC, Nelson JL, et al: Positive selection in autoimmunity: abnormal immune responses to a bacterial dnaJ antigenic determinant in patients with early rheumatoid arthritis. Nat Med 1: 448–452, 1995.
226. Danieli MG, Markovits D, Gabrielli A, et al: Juvenile rheumatoid arthritis patients manifest immune reactivity to the mycobacterial 65–kDa heat shock protein, to its 180–188 peptide, and to a partially homologous peptide of the proteoglycan link protein. Clin Immunol Immunopathol 64: 121–128, 1992.
227. Nuallain EM, Monaghan H, Reen DJ: Antibody response of restricted isotype to heat shock proteins in juvenile chronic arthritis. Scand J Immunol 38: 83–88, 1993.
228. Albani S: Infection and molecular mimicry in autoimmune diseases of childhood. Clin Exp Rheumatol 12(Suppl)10:S35–S41, 1994.
229. Howard JF, Sigsbee A, Glass DN: HLA genetics and inherited predisposition to JRA. J Rheumatol 12: 7–12, 1985.
230. Moroldo MB, Tague BL, Shear ES, et al: Juvenile rheumatoid arthritis in affected sibpairs. Arthritis Rheum 40: 1962–1966, 1997.
231. Rosenberg AM, Petty RE: Similar patterns of juvenile rheumatoid arthritis within families. Arthritis Rheum 23: 951–953, 1980.
232. Baum J, Fink C: Juvenile rheumatoid arthritis in monozygotic twins: a case report and review of the literature. Arthritis Rheum 11: 33–36, 1968.
233. Kapusta MA, Metrakos JD, Pinsky L, et al: Juvenile rheumatoid arthritis in a mother and her identical twin sons. Arthritis Rheum 12: 411–413, 1969.
234. Ansell BM, Bywaters EG, Lawrence JS: Familial aggregation and twin studies in Still's disease. Juvenile chronic polyarthritis. Rheumatology 2: 37–61, 1969.
235. Husby G, Williams RC Jr, Tung KS, et al: Immunologic studies in identical twins concordant for juvenile rheumatoid arthritis

but discordant for monoclonal gammopathy and amyloidosis. J Lab Clin Med 111: 307–314, 1988.
236. Nepom B: The immunogenetics of juvenile rheumatoid arthritis. Rheum Dis Clin North Am 17: 825–842, 1991.
237. Ansell BM, Bywaters EGL, Lawrence JS: A family study in Still's disease. Ann Rheum Dis 21: 243, 1962.
238. Clemens LE, Albert E, Ansell BM: HLA studies in IgM rheumatoid-factor-positive arthritis of childhood. Ann Rheum Dis 42: 431–434, 1983.
239. Clemens LE, Albert E, Ansell BM: Sibling pairs affected by chronic arthritis of childhood: evidence for a genetic predisposition. J Rheumatol 12: 108–113, 1985.
240. Rossen RD, Brewer EJ, Sharp RM, et al: Familial rheumatoid arthritis: linkage of HLA to disease susceptibility locus in four families where proband presented with juvenile rheumatoid arthritis. J Clin Invest 65: 629–642, 1980.
241. Southwood TR, Roberts-Thomson PJ, Ahern MJ, et al: Autoantibodies in patients with juvenile chronic arthritis and their immediate family relatives. Ann Rheum Dis 49: 968–972, 1990.
242. Hall A, Ansell BM, James DCO, et al: HL-A antigens in juvenile chronic polyarthritis (Still's disease). Ann Rheum Dis Suppl 34: 36, 1975.
243. Gershwin ME, Opelz G, Terasaki PI, et al: Frequency of HLA-Dw3 in juvenile rheumatoid arthritis. Tissue Antigens 10: 330–336, 1977.
244. Stastny P, Fink CW: Different HLA-D associations in adult and juvenile rheumatoid arthritis. J Clin Invest 63: 124–130, 1979.
245. Glass D, Litvin D, Wallace K, et al: Early-onset pauciarticular juvenile rheumatoid arthritis associated with human leukocyte antigen-DRw5, iritis, and antinuclear antibody. J Clin Invest 66: 426–429, 1980.
246. Suciu-Foca N, Godfrey M, Jacobs J, et al: Increased frequency of DRw5 in pauciarticular juvenile rheumatoid arthritis. *In* Terasaki P (ed): Histocompatibility Testing 1980. Los Angeles, University of California Press, 1980, p 953.
247. Glass DN, Litvin DA: Heterogeneity of HLA associations in systemic onset juvenile rheumatoid arthritis. Arthritis Rheum 23: 796–799, 1980.
248. Morling N, Hellesen C, Jakobsen BK, et al: HLA-A, B, C, D, DR antigens and primed lymphocyte typing (PLT) defined DP-antigens in juvenile chronic arthritis. Tissue Antigens 17: 433–441, 1981.
249. Forre O, Dobloug JH, Hoyeraal HM, et al: HLA antigens in juvenile arthritis. Genetic basis for the different subtypes. Arthritis Rheum 26: 35–38, 1983.
250. Ansell BM, Albert ED: Juvenile chronic arthritis, pauciarticular type. *In* Albert ED, Baur MR, Mayr WR (eds): Histocompatibility Testing, 1984. New York, Springer-Verlag, 1984, p 368.
251. Moore TL, Oldfather JW, Osborn TG, et al: HLA antigens in black and white patients with juvenile arthritis: associations with rheumatoid factor, hidden rheumatoid factor, antinuclear antibodies, and immune complex levels. J Rheumatol 11: 188–196, 1984.
252. Nepom BS, Nepom GT, Mickelson E, et al: Specific HLA-DR4–associated histocompatibility molecules characterize patients with seropositive juvenile rheumatoid arthritis. J Clin Invest 74: 287–291, 1984.
253. Morling N, Friis J, Heilmann C, et al: HLA antigen frequencies in juvenile chronic arthritis. Scand J Rheumatol 14: 209–216, 1985.
253a. Prahalad S, Ryna MH, Shear ES, et al: Juvenile rheumatoid arthritis: linkage to HLA demonstrated by allele sharing in affected sibpairs. Arthritis Rheum 43: 2335–2338, 2000.
254. Sher MR, Schultz JS, Ragsdale CG, et al: HLA-DR and MT associations with the clinical and serologic manifestations of pauciarticular onset juvenile rheumatoid arthritis. J Rheumatol 12: 114–118, 1985.
255. Miller ML, Aaron S, Jackson J, et al: HLA gene frequencies in children and adults with systemic onset juvenile rheumatoid arthritis. Arthritis Rheum 28: 146–150, 1985.
256. Brautbar C, Mukamel M, Yaron M, et al: Immunogenetics of juvenile chronic arthritis in Israel. J Rheumatol 13: 1072–1075, 1986.
257. Manners PJ, Dawkins RL, McCluskey J, et al: An immunogenetic study of juvenile chronic arthritis. Aust Paediatr J 22: 317–321, 1986.
258. Hoffman RW, Shaw S, Francis LC, et al: HLA-DP antigens in patients with pauciarticular juvenile rheumatoid arthritis. Arthritis Rheum 29: 1057–1062, 1986.
259. Nepom BS, Palmer J, Kim SJ, et al: Specific genomic markers for the HLA-DQ subregion discriminate between DR4+ insulin-dependent diabetes mellitus and DR4+ seropositive juvenile rheumatoid arthritis. J Exp Med 164: 345–350, 1986.
260. Stastny P: HLA and the role of T cells in the predisposition to disease. Rheum Dis Clin North Am 13: 1–6, 1987.
261. Fernandez-Vina MA, Fink CW, Stastny P: HLA antigens in juvenile arthritis. Pauciarticular and polyarticular juvenile arthritis are immunogenetically distinct. Arthritis Rheum 33: 1787–1794, 1990.
262. De Inocencio J, Giannini EH, Glass DN: Can genetic markers contribute to the classification of juvenile rheumatoid arthritis? J Rheumatol Suppl 40: 12–18, 1993.
263. Haas JP, Nevinny-Stickel C, Schoenwald U, et al: Susceptible and protective major histocompatibility complex class II alleles in early-onset pauciarticular juvenile chronic arthritis. Hum Immunol 41: 225–233, 1994.
264. Fernandez-Vina M, Fink CW, Stastny P: HLA associations in juvenile arthritis. Clin Exp Rheumatol 12: 205–214, 1994.
265. Fink CW, Fernandez-Vina M, Stastny P: Clinical and genetic evidence that juvenile arthritis is not a single disease. Pediatr Clin North Am 42: 1155–1169, 1995.
266. Fink CW, Fernandez-Vina M: The genetics of juvenile rheumatoid arthritis. Bull Rheum Dis 44: 5–8, 1995.
267. Ploski R: Immunogenetic polymorphism and disease mechanisms in juvenile chronic arthritis. Rev Rhum Engl Ed 64: 127S–130S, 1997.
267a. Pratsidou-Gertsi P, Kanakoudi-Tsakalidou F, Spyropoulou M, et al: Nationwide collaborative study of HLA class II associations with distinct types of juvenile chronic arthritis (JCA) in Greece. Eur J Immunogenet 26: 299–310, 1999.
267b. Sanjeevi CB, Miller EN, Dabadghao P, et al: Polymorphism at NRAMP1 and D2S1471 loci associated with juvenile rheumatoid arthritis. Arthritis Rheum 43: 1397–1404, 2000.
267c. Thomas E, Barrett JH, Donn RP, et al: Subtyping of juvenile idiopathic arthritis using latent class analysis. British Paediatric Rheumatology Group. Arthritis Rheum 43: 1496–1503, 2000.
268. Jacobs JC, Berdon WE, Johnston AD: HLA-B27–associated spondyloarthritis and enthesopathy in childhood: clinical, pathologic, and radiographic observations in 58 patients. J Pediatr 100: 521–528, 1982.
269. Sheerin KA, Giannini EH, Brewer EJ Jr, et al: HLA-B27–associated arthropathy in childhood: long-term clinical and diagnostic outcome. Arthritis Rheum 31: 1165–1170, 1988.
270. Suciu-Foca N, Jacobs J, Godfrey M, et al: HLA-DR5 in juvenile rheumatoid arthritis confined to few joints [letter]. Lancet 2: 40, 1980.
271. Murray KJ, Moroldo MB, Donnelly P, et al: Age-specific effects of juvenile rheumatoid arthritis-associated HLA alleles. Arthritis Rheum 42: 1843–1853, 1999.
272. Hall PJ, Burman SJ, Laurent MR, et al: Genetic susceptibility to early onset pauciarticular juvenile chronic arthritis: a study of HLA and complement markers in 158 British patients. Ann Rheum Dis 45: 464–474, 1986.
273. Arnaiz-Villena A, Gomez-Reino JJ, Gamir ML, et al: DR, C4, and Bf allotypes in juvenile rheumatoid arthritis. Arthritis Rheum 27: 1281–1285, 1984.
274. Vicario JL, Martinez-Laso J, Gomez-Reino JJ, et al: Both HLA class II and class III DNA polymorphisms are linked to juvenile rheumatoid arthritis susceptibility. Clin Immunol Immunopathol 56: 22–28, 1990.
275. Oen K, Petty RE, Schroeder ML: An association between HLA-A2 and juvenile rheumatoid arthritis in girls. J Rheumatol 9: 916–920, 1982.
276. Petty RE, Hunt DW, Rollins DF, et al: Immunity to soluble retinal antigen in patients with uveitis accompanying juvenile rheumatoid arthritis. Arthritis Rheum 30: 287–293, 1987.
277. Paul C, Schoenwald U, Truckenbrodt H, et al: HLA-DP/DR interaction in early onset pauciarticular juvenile chronic arthritis. Immunogenetics 37: 442–448, 1993.
278. Moroldo MB, Donnelly P, Saunders J, et al: Transmission disequilibrium as a test of linkage and association between HLA

alleles and pauciarticular-onset juvenile rheumatoid arthritis. Arthritis Rheum 41: 1620–1624, 1998.
279. Rachelefsky GS, Terasaki PI, Katz R, et al: Increased prevalence of W27 in juvenile rheumatoid arthritis. N Engl J Med 290: 892–893, 1974.
280. Schaller JG, Ochs HD, Thomas ED, et al: Histocompatibility antigens in childhood-onset arthritis. J Pediatr 88: 926–930, 1976.
281. Prieur AM: HLA B27 associated chronic arthritis in children: review of 65 cases. Scand J Rheumatol Suppl 66: 51–56, 1987.
282. Wordsworth P: Genes in the spondyloarthropathies. Rheum Dis Clin North Am 24: 845–863, 1998.
283. Nepom BS, Glass DN: Juvenile rheumatoid arthritis and HLA: report of the Park City III workshop. J Rheumatol Suppl 33: 70–74, 1992.
284. Paul C, Yao Z, Nevinny-Stickel C, et al: Immunogenetics of juvenile chronic arthritis. I. HLA interaction between A2, DR5/8–DR/DQ, and DPB1*0201 is a general feature of all subsets of early onset pauciarticular juvenile chronic arthritis. II. DPB1 polymorphism plays a role in systemic juvenile chronic arthritis. Tissue Antigens 45: 280–283, 1995.
285. Morling N, Friis J, Fugger L, et al: DNA polymorphism of HLA class II genes in pauciarticular juvenile rheumatoid arthritis. Tissue Antigens 38: 16–23, 1991.
286. Malagon C, Van Kerckhove C, Giannini EH, et al: The iridocyclitis of early onset pauciarticular juvenile rheumatoid arthritis: outcome in immunogenetically characterized patients. J Rheumatol 19: 160–163, 1992.
287. Moore AT, Morin JD: Bilateral acquired inflammatory Brown's syndrome. J Pediatr Ophthalmol Strabismus 22: 26–30, 1985.
288. Dracou C, Constantinidou N, Constantopoulos A: Juvenile chronic arthritis profile in Greek children. Acta Paediatr Jpn 40: 558–563, 1998.
289. Haas JP, Andreas A, Rutkowski B, et al: A model for the role of HLA-DQ molecules in the pathogenesis of juvenile chronic arthritis. Rheumatol Int 11: 191–197, 1991.
290. Haas JP, Kimura A, Truckenbrodt H, et al: Early-onset pauciarticular juvenile chronic arthritis is associated with a mutation in the Y-box of the HLA-DQA1 promoter. Tissue Antigens 45: 317–321, 1995.
291. Scholz S, Albert ED: Immunogenetic aspects of juvenile chronic arthritis. Clin Exp Rheumatol 11(Suppl)9:S37–S41, 1993.
292. Van Kerckhove C, Luyrink L, Taylor J, et al: HLA-DQA1*0101 haplotypes and disease outcome in early onset pauciarticular juvenile rheumatoid arthritis. J Rheumatol 18: 874–879, 1991.
293. Murray KJ, Szer W, Grom AA, et al: Antibodies to the 45 kDa DEK nuclear antigen in pauciarticular onset juvenile rheumatoid arthritis and iridocyclitis: selective association with MHC gene. J Rheumatol 24: 560–567, 1997.
294. Adams BS, Tan HMD: Allele-specific DQA1 promotor binding by DEK. A putative autoantigen in juvenile rheumatoid arthritis. Arthritis Rheum 41:S188, 1998.
295. Forero L, Zwirner NW, Fink CW, et al: Juvenile arthritis, HLA-A2 and binding of DEK oncogene-peptides. Hum Immunol 59: 443–450, 1998.
296. Szer IS, Sierakowska H, Szer W: A novel autoantibody to the putative oncoprotein DEK in pauciarticular onset juvenile rheumatoid arthritis. J Rheumatol 21: 2136–2142, 1994.
296a. Dong X, Wang J, Kabir FN, et al: Autoantibodies to DEK oncoprotein in human inflammatory disease. Arthritis Rheum 43: 85–93, 2000.
297. Donn RP, Thomson W, Pepper L, et al: Antinuclear antibodies in early onset pauciarticular juvenile chronic arthritis (JCA) are associated with HLA-DQB1*0603: a possible JCA-associated human leucocyte antigen haplotype. Br J Rheumatol 34: 461–465, 1995.
298. Begovich AB, Bugawan TL, Nepom BS, et al: A specific HLA-DP beta allele is associated with pauciarticular juvenile rheumatoid arthritis but not adult rheumatoid arthritis. Proc Natl Acad Sci U S A 86: 9489–9493, 1989.
299. Albert ED, Scholz S: Juvenile arthritis: genetic update. Baillieres Clin Rheumatol 12: 209–218, 1998.
300. Feichtlbauer P, Gomolka M, Brunnler G, et al: HLA region microsatellite polymorphisms in juvenile arthritis. Tissue Antigens 52: 220–229, 1998.
301. Vehe RK, Begovich AB, Nepom BS: HLA susceptibility genes in rheumatoid factor positive juvenile rheumatoid arthritis. J Rheumatol Suppl 26: 11–15, 1990.
302. Oen K, El Gabalawy HS, Canvin JM, et al: HLA associations of seropositive rheumatoid arthritis in a Cree and Ojibway population. J Rheumatol 25: 2319–2323, 1998.
303. Gao X, Fernandez-Vina M, Olsen NJ, et al: HLA-DPB1*0301 is a major risk factor for rheumatoid factor-negative adult rheumatoid arthritis. Arthritis Rheum 34: 1310–1312, 1991.
304. Desaymard C, Kaplan C, Fournier C, et al: Major histocompatibility complex markers and disease heterogeneity in one hundred eight patients with systemic onset juvenile chronic arthritis. Rev Rhum Engl Ed 63: 9–16, 1996.
305. Ploski R, Forre O: Non-HLA genes and susceptibility to juvenile chronic arthritis. Clin Exp Rheumatol 12(Suppl)10:S15–S17, 1994.
306. Donn RP, Davies EJ, Holt PL, et al: Increased frequency of TAP2B in early onset pauciarticular juvenile chronic arthritis. Ann Rheum Dis 53: 261–264, 1994.
307. Ploski R, Undlien DE, Vinje O, et al: Polymorphism of human major histocompatibility complex-encoded transporter associated with antigen processing (TAP) genes and susceptibility to juvenile rheumatoid arthritis. Hum Immunol 39: 54–60, 1994.
308. Ploski R, McDowell TL, Symons JA, et al: Interaction between HLA-DR and HLA-DP, and between HLA and interleukin 1 alpha in juvenile rheumatoid arthritis indicates heterogeneity of pathogenic mechanisms of the disease. Hum Immunol 42: 343–347, 1995.
309. McDowell TL, Symons JA, Ploski R, et al: A genetic association between juvenile rheumatoid arthritis and a novel interleukin-1 alpha polymorphism. Arthritis Rheum 38: 221–228, 1995.
310. Pryhuber KG, Murray KJ, Donnelly P, et al: Polymorphism in the LMP2 gene influences disease susceptibility and severity in HLA-B27 associated juvenile rheumatoid arthritis. J Rheumatol 23: 747–752, 1996.
311. Ihnat DH, McIlvain-Simpson G, Conard K, et al: Inflammatory arthropathies in children with chromosomal abnormalities. J Rheumatol 20: 742–746, 1993.
312. Rudolf MC, Genel M, Tamborlane WV Jr, et al: Juvenile rheumatoid arthritis in children with diabetes mellitus. J Pediatr 99: 519–524, 1981.
313. Daugbjerg PS, Pedersen FK: Arthritis in a 15–year-old boy with juvenile diabetes mellitus. Dan Med Bull 31: 346–347, 1984.
313a. Mihailova D, Grigorova R, Vassileva B, et al: Autoimmune thyroid disorders in juvenile chronic arthritis and systemic lupus erythematosus. Adv Exp Med Biol 455: 55–60, 1999.
314. Rosenbloom AL, Silverstein JH, Lezotte DC, et al: Limited joint mobility in childhood diabetes mellitus indicates increased risk for microvascular disease. N Engl J Med 305: 191–194, 1981.
315. Sherry DD, Rothstein RR, Petty RE: Joint contractures preceding insulin-dependent diabetes mellitus. Arthritis Rheum 25: 1362–1364, 1982.
316. Glass JB, Sher PK, Lennon VA, et al: The association of pauciarticular juvenile arthritis and myasthenia gravis. Am J Dis Child 145: 1176–1180, 1991.
317. Cassidy JT, Petty RE, Sullivan DB: Occurrence of selective IgA deficiency in children with juvenile rheumatoid arthritis. Arthritis Rheum 20: 181–183, 1977.
318. Sullivan KE, McDonald-McGinn DM, Driscoll DA, et al: Juvenile rheumatoid arthritis-like polyarthritis in chromosome 22q11.2 deletion syndrome (DiGeorge anomalad/velocardiofacial syndrome/conotruncal anomaly face syndrome). Arthritis Rheum 40: 430–436, 1997.
319. Petty RE, Malleson P, Kalousek DK: Chronic arthritis in two children with partial deletion of chromosome 18. J Rheumatol 14: 586–587, 1987.
320. Verloes A, Curry C, Jamar M, et al: Juvenile rheumatoid arthritis and del(22q11) syndrome: a non-random association. J Med Genet 35: 943–947, 1998.
321. Zori RT, Boyar FZ, Williams WN, et al: Prevalence of 22q11 region deletions in patients with velopharyngeal insufficiency. Am J Med Genet 77: 8–11, 1998.
321a. Wihlborg CE, Babyn PS, Schneider R: The association between Turner's syndrome and juvenile rheumatoid arthritis. Pediatr Radiol 29:676–681, 1999.

322. Zulian F, Schumacher HR, Calore A, et al: Juvenile arthritis in Turner's syndrome: a multicenter study. Clin Exp Rheumatol 16: 489–494, 1998.
323. Olson JC, Bender JC, Levinson JE, et al: Arthropathy of Down syndrome. Pediatrics 86: 931–936, 1990.
324. Ansell BM: Joint manifestations in children with juvenile chronic polyarthritis. Arthritis Rheum 20: 204–206, 1977.
325. Sharma S, Sherry DD: Joint distribution at presentation in children with pauciarticular arthritis. J Pediatr 134: 642–643, 1999.
326. Cassidy JT, Brody GL, Martel W: Monarticular juvenile rheumatoid arthritis. J Pediatr 70: 867–875, 1967.
327. Bywaters EGL, Ansell BM: Monoarticular arthritis in children. Ann Rheum Dis 24: 116, 1965.
328. Schaller J, Wedgwood RJ: Pauciarticular juvenile rheumatoid arthritis. Arthritis Rheum 12: 330, 1969.
329. Brewer EJ Jr: Pitfalls in the diagnosis of juvenile rheumatoid arthritis. Pediatr Clin North Am 33: 1015–1032, 1986.
330. Cassidy JT: Miscellaneous conditions associated with arthritis in children. Pediatr Clin North Am 33: 1033–1052, 1986.
331. Cabral DA, Tucker LB: Malignancies in children who initially present with rheumatic complaints. J Pediatr 134: 53–57, 1999.
332. Rush PJ, Shore A, Wilmot D, et al: Discoid meniscus presenting as juvenile rheumatoid arthritis. J Rheumatol 13: 1173–1177, 1986.
333. Lepore L, Martelossi S, Pennesi M, et al: Prevalence of celiac disease in patients with juvenile chronic arthritis. J Pediatr 129: 311–313, 1996.
334. Falcini F, Ferrari R, Simonini G, et al: Recurrent monoarthritis in an 11-year-old boy with occult coeliac disease. Successful and stable remission after gluten-free diet. Clin Exp Rheumatol 17: 509–511, 1999.
335. Miller JJ III, Emery HM: Migrating monopredominant arthritis in children of Assyrian ancestry. J Rheumatol 23: 178–180, 1996.
336. Dubourg G, Koeger AC, Huchet B, et al: Acute monoarthritis in a patient under isotretinoin. Rev Rhum Engl Ed 63: 228–229, 1996.
337. De Francesco V, Stinco G, Campanella M: Acute arthritis during isotretinoin treatment for acne conglobata. Dermatology 194: 195, 1997.
338. Bajaj S, Bell MJ, Shumak S, et al: Antithyroid arthritis syndrome. J Rheumatol 25: 1235–1239, 1998.
339. Mathieu E, Fain O, Sitbon M, et al: Systemic adverse effect of antithyroid drugs. Clin Rheumatol 18: 66–68, 1999.
340. Burgos-Vargas R, Vazquez-Mellado J: The early clinical recognition of juvenile-onset ankylosing spondylitis and its differentiation from juvenile rheumatoid arthritis. Arthritis Rheum 38: 835–844, 1995.
341. Allen RC, Dewez P, Stuart L, et al: Antinuclear antibodies using HEp-2 cells in normal children and in children with common infections. J Paediatr Child Health 27: 39–42, 1991.
342. Cabral DA, Petty RE, Fung M, et al: Persistent antinuclear antibodies in children without identifiable inflammatory rheumatic or autoimmune disease. Pediatrics 89: 441–444, 1992.
343. Fink CW, Dich VQ, Howard J Jr, et al: Infections of bones and joints in children. Arthritis Rheum 20: 578–583, 1977.
344. Kornreich HK, Bernstein BH, Key KK, et al: The rheumatic presentation of osteomyelitis. Arthritis Rheum 22: 631, 1979.
345. Jacobs JC, Phillips PE, Johnston AD: Needle biopsy of the synovium of children. Pediatrics 57: 696–701, 1976.
346. Cooperman DR, Emery H, Keller C: Factors relating to hip joint arthritis following three childhood diseases—juvenile rheumatoid arthritis, Perthes disease, and postreduction avascular necrosis in congenital hip dislocation. J Pediatr Orthop 6: 706–712, 1986.
347. Hellstrom B: The diagnosis and course of rheumatoid arthritis and benign aseptic arthritis in children. Acta Paediatr Scand 50: 529, 1961.
348. Jacobs BW: Synovitis of the hip in children and its significance. Pediatrics 47: 558–566, 1971.
349. Wallace CA, Levinson JE: Juvenile rheumatoid arthritis: outcome and treatment for the 1990s. Rheum Dis Clin North Am 17: 891–905, 1991.
350. Ramsey SE, Bolaria RK, Cabral DA, et al: Comparison of proposed ILAR and existing classification systems for childhood arthritis. Arthritis Rheum 40:S47, 1998.
351. Cassidy JT: Comparison of the ILAR and ACR classification criteria for oligoarthritis in children. Arthritis Rheum 42: S180, 1999.
352. Sailer M, Cabral D, Petty RE, et al: Rheumatoid factor positive, oligoarticular onset juvenile rheumatoid arthritis. J Rheumatol 24: 586–588, 1997.
353. Naidu SH, Ostrov BE, Pellegrini VD Jr: Isolated digital swelling as the initial presentation of juvenile rheumatoid arthritis. J Hand Surg [Am] 22: 653–657, 1997.
354. Chaplin D, Pulkki T, Saarimaa A, et al: Wrist and finger deformities in juvenile rheumatoid arthritis. Acta Rheumatol Scand 15: 206–223, 1969.
355. Sood SK: Lyme disease. Pediatr Infect Dis J 18: 913–925, 1999.
356. Martini A, Ravelli A, Viola S, et al: Systemic lupus erythematosus with Jaccoud's arthropathy mimicking juvenile rheumatoid arthritis. Arthritis Rheum 30: 1062–1064, 1987.
357. Cassidy JT, Walker SE, Soderstrom SJ, et al: Diagnostic significance of antibody to native deoxyribonucleic acid in children with juvenile rheumatoid arthritis and other connective tissue diseases. J Pediatr 93: 416–420, 1978.
358. Ragsdale CG, Petty RE, Cassidy JT, et al: The clinical progression of apparent juvenile rheumatoid arthritis to systemic lupus erythematosus. J Rheumatol 7: 50–55, 1980.
359. Ladd JR, Cassidy JT, Martel W: Juvenile ankylosing spondylitis. Arthritis Rheum 14: 579–590, 1971.
360. Rosenberg AM, Petty RE: A syndrome of seronegative enthesopathy and arthropathy in children. Arthritis Rheum 25: 1041–1047, 1982.
361. Cabral DA, Oen KG, Petty RE: SEA syndrome revisited: a longterm followup of children with a syndrome of seronegative enthesopathy and arthropathy. J Rheumatol 19: 1282–1285, 1992.
362. Friis J, Morling N, Pedersen FK, et al: HLA-B27 in juvenile chronic arthritis. J Rheumatol 12: 119–122, 1985.
363. Yaw KM: Pediatric bone tumors. Semin Surg Oncol 16: 173–183, 1999.
364. Bolling WS, Beauchamp CP: Presentation and evaluation of bone tumors. Instr Course Lect 48: 607–612, 1999.
365. Schaller J: Arthritis as a presenting manifestation of malignancy in children. J Pediatr 81: 793–797, 1972.
366. Fink CW, Windmiller J, Sartain P: Arthritis as the presenting feature of childhood leukemia. Arthritis Rheum 15: 347–349, 1972.
367. Wallendal M, Stork L, Hollister JR: The discriminating value of serum lactate dehydrogenase levels in children with malignant neoplasms presenting as joint pain. Arch Pediatr Adolesc Med 150: 70–73, 1996.
368. Weinberg AG, Currarino G: Sickle cell dactylitis: histopathologic observations. Am J Clin Pathol 58: 518–523, 1972.
369. Gedalia A, Person DA, Brewer EJ Jr, et al: Hypermobility of the joints in juvenile episodic arthritis/arthralgia. J Pediatr 107: 873–876, 1985.
370. Jacobs JC, Downey JA: Juvenile rheumatoid arthritis. *In* Downey JA, Low NL (eds): The Child with Disabling Illness. Philadelphia, WB Saunders, 1974, p 5.
371. Athreya BH, Schumacher HR: Pathologic features of a familial arthropathy associated with congenital flexion contractures of fingers. Arthritis Rheum 21: 429–437, 1978.
372. Malleson P, Schaller JG, Dega F, et al: Familial arthritis and camptodactyly. Arthritis Rheum 24: 1199–1204, 1981.
373. Bulutlar G, Yazici H, Ozdogan H, et al: A familial syndrome of pericarditis, arthritis, camptodactyly, and coxa vara. Arthritis Rheum 29: 436–438, 1986.
374. Laxer RM, Cameron BJ, Chaisson D, et al: The camptodactyly-arthropathy-pericarditis syndrome: case report and literature review. Arthritis Rheum 29: 439–444, 1986.
375. Robinson RP, Franck WA, Carey EJ, et al: Familial polyarticular osteochondritis dissecans masquerading as juvenile rheumatoid arthritis. J Rheumatol 5: 190–194, 1978.
376. Balestrazzi P, Ferraccioli GF, Ambanelli U, et al: Juvenile rheumatoid arthritis in Turner's syndrome. Clin Exp Rheumatol 4: 61–62, 1986.
377. Pugh MT, Southwood TR: [Tuberculous rheumatism, Poncet disease: a sterile controversy? (editorial)]. Rev Rhum Ed Fr 60: 855–860, 1993.

378. Eisenstein DM, Poznanski AK, Pachman LM: Torg osteolysis syndrome. Am J Med Genet 80: 207–212, 1998.
379. van der Net J, Prakken AB, Helders PJ, et al: Correlates of disablement in polyarticular juvenile chronic arthritis—a cross-sectional study. Br J Rheumatol 35: 91–100, 1996.
380. Isdale IC: Hip disease in juvenile rheumatoid arthritis. Ann Rheum Dis 29: 603–608, 1970.
381. Rombouts JJ, Rombouts-Lindemans C: Involvement of the hip in juvenile rheumatoid arthritis. A radiological study with special reference to growth disturbances. Acta Rheumatol Scand 17: 248–267, 1971.
382. Blane CE, Ragsdale CG, Hensinger RN: Late effects of JRA on the hip. J Pediatr Orthop 7: 677–680, 1987.
383. Martel W, Holt JF, Cassidy JT: Roentgenologic manifestations of juvenile rheumatoid arthritis. AJR 88: 400, 1962.
384. McMinn FJ, Bywaters EGL: Differences between the fever of Still's disease and that of rheumatic fever. Ann Rheum Dis 18: 293, 1959.
385. Isdale IC, Bywaters EGL: The rash of rheumatoid arthritis and Still's disease. Q J Med 25: 377, 1956.
386. Ansell BA, Rudge S, Schaller JG: A Colour Atlas of Paediatric Rheumatology. Aylesbury, UK, Wolfe, 1991.
387. Schaller J, Wedgwood RJ: Pruritus associated with the rash of juvenile rheumatoid arthritis. Pediatrics 45: 296–298, 1970.
388. Miller LC, Sisson BA, Tucker LB, et al: Prolonged fevers of unknown origin in children: patterns of presentation and outcome. J Pediatr 129: 419–423, 1996.
389. Prieur AM, Griscelli C, Lampert F, et al: A chronic, infantile, neurological, cutaneous and articular (CINCA) syndrome. A specific entity analysed in 30 patients. Scand J Rheumatol Suppl 66: 57–68, 1987.
390. Torbiak RP, Dent PB, Cockshott WP: NOMID—a neonatal syndrome of multisystem inflammation. Skeletal Radiol 18: 359–364, 1989.
391. De Cunto CL, Liberatore DI, San Roman JL, et al: Infantile-onset multisystem inflammatory disease: a differential diagnosis of systemic juvenile rheumatoid arthritis. J Pediatr 130: 551–556, 1997.
392. Hashkes PJ, Lovell DJ: Recognition of infantile-onset multisystem inflammatory disease as a unique entity. J Pediatr 130: 513–515, 1997.
393. Sievers K, Ahvonen P: Serological patterns in juvenile rheumatoid arthritis. Rheumatism 19: 88, 1963.
394. Pindborg S: Et tilfaelde af Still's sygdom. Ugeskr Laeger 104: 1417, 1942.
395. Bywaters EG: Still's disease in the adult. Ann Rheum Dis 30: 121–133, 1971.
396. Aptekar RG, Decker JL, Bujak JS, et al: Adult onset juvenile rheumatoid arthritis. Arthritis Rheum 16: 715–718, 1973.
397. Elkon KB, Hughes GR, Bywaters EG, et al: Adult-onset Still's disease. Twenty-year followup and further studies of patients with active disease. Arthritis Rheum 25: 647–654, 1982.
398. Wouters JM, van Rijswijk MH, van de Putte LB: Adult onset Still's disease in the elderly: a report of two cases. J Rheumatol 12: 791–793, 1985.
399. Wouters JM, Reekers P, van de Putte LB: Adult-onset Still's disease. Disease course and HLA associations. Arthritis Rheum 29: 415–418, 1986.
400. Wouters JM, van de Putte LB: Adult-onset Still's disease; clinical and laboratory features, treatment and progress of 45 cases. Q J Med 61: 1055–1065, 1986.
401. Cush JJ, Medsger TA Jr, Christy WC, et al: Adult-onset Still's disease. Clinical course and outcome. Arthritis Rheum 30: 186–194, 1987.
402. Reginato AJ, Schumacher HR Jr, Baker DG, et al: Adult onset Still's disease: experience in 23 patients and literature review with emphasis on organ failure. Semin Arthritis Rheum 17: 39–57, 1987.
403. Roberts-Thomson PJ, Southwood TR, Moore BW, et al: Adult onset Still's disease or coxsackie polyarthritis? Aust N Z J Med 16: 509–511, 1986.
404. Bjorkengren AG, Pathria MN, Sartoris DJ, et al: Carpal alterations in adult-onset Still disease, juvenile chronic arthritis, and adult-onset rheumatoid arthritis: comparative study. Radiology 165: 545–548, 1987.
404a. Lin SJ, Chao HC, Yan DC: Different articular outcomes of Still's disease in Chinese children and adults. Clin Rheumatol 19: 127–130, 2000.
405. Medsger TA Jr, Christy WC: Carpal arthritis with ankylosis in late onset Still's disease. Arthritis Rheum 19: 232–242, 1976.
406. Prieur AM, Ansell BM, Bardfeld R, et al: Is onset type evaluated during the first 3 months of disease satisfactory for defining the sub-groups of juvenile chronic arthritis? A EULAR Cooperative Study (1983–1986). Clin Exp Rheumatol 8: 321–325, 1990.
407. Schneider R, Lang BA, Reilly BJ, et al: Prognostic indicators of joint destruction in systemic-onset juvenile rheumatoid arthritis. J Pediatr 120: 200–205, 1992.
407a. Lin SJ, Huang JL, Chao HC, et al: A follow-up study of systemic-onset juvenile rheumatoid arthritis in children. Taiwan Erh Ko I Hsueh Hui Tsa Chih 40: 176–181, 1999.
408. van der Net J, Kuis W, Prakken AB, et al: Correlates of disablement in systemic onset juvenile chronic arthritis. A cross sectional study. Scand J Rheumatol 26: 188–196, 1997.
408a. Lomater C, Gerloni V, Gattinara M, et al: Systemic onset juvenile idiopathic arthritis: a retrospective study of 80 consecutive patients followed for 10 years. J Rheumatol 27:491–496, 2000.
409. Grom AA, Passo M: Macrophage activation syndrome in systemic juvenile rheumatoid arthritis. J Pediatr 129: 630–632, 1996.
410. Aellen P, Raccaud O, Waldburger M, et al: [Still's disease in adults with disseminated intravascular coagulation]. Schweiz Rundsch Med Prax 80: 376–378, 1991.
411. Hadchouel M, Prieur AM, Griscelli C: Acute hemorrhagic, hepatic, and neurologic manifestations in juvenile rheumatoid arthritis: possible relationship to drugs or infection. J Pediatr 106: 561–566, 1985.
412. Silverman ED, Miller JJ III, Bernstein B, et al: Consumption coagulopathy associated with systemic juvenile rheumatoid arthritis. J Pediatr 103: 872–876, 1983.
413. Scott JP, Gerber P, Maryjowski MC, et al: Evidence for intravascular coagulation in systemic onset, but not polyarticular, juvenile rheumatoid arthritis. Arthritis Rheum 28: 256–261, 1985.
414. Gallistl S, Mangge H, Neuwirth G, et al: Activation of the haemostatic system in children with juvenile rheumatoid arthritis correlates with disease activity. Thromb Res 92: 267–272, 1998.
415. Bloom BJ, Tucker LB, Miller LC, et al: Fibrin D-dimer as a marker of disease activity in systemic onset juvenile rheumatoid arthritis. J Rheumatol 25: 1620–1625, 1998.
416. Bloom BJ, Miller LC, Tucker LB, et al: Soluble adhesion molecules in juvenile rheumatoid arthritis. J Rheumatol 26: 2044–2048, 1999.
417. De Inocencio J, Lovell DJ, Gabriel CA: Acquired factor VIII inhibitor in juvenile rheumatoid arthritis. Pediatrics 94: 550–553, 1994.
418. Jacobs JC, Gorin LJ, Hanissian AS, et al: Consumption coagulopathy after gold therapy for JRA. J Pediatr 105: 674–675, 1984.
419. Manners PJ, Ansell BM: Slow-acting antirheumatic drug use in systemic onset juvenile chronic arthritis. Pediatrics 77: 99–103, 1986.
420. Barash J, Cooper M, Tauber Z: Hepatic, cutaneous and hematologic manifestations in juvenile chronic arthritis. Clin Exp Rheumatol 9: 541–543, 1991.
421. Bray VJ, Singleton JD: Disseminated intravascular coagulation in Still's disease. Semin Arthritis Rheum 24: 222–229, 1994.
422. Coffernils M, Soupart A, Pradier O, et al: Hyperferritinemia in adult onset Still's disease and the hemophagocytic syndrome. J Rheumatol 19: 1425–1427, 1992.
423. Smith KJ, Skelton HG, Yeager J, et al: Cutaneous histopathologic, immunohistochemical, and clinical manifestations in patients with hemophagocytic syndrome. Military Medical Consortium for Applied Retroviral Research (MMCARR). Arch Dermatol 128: 193–200, 1992.
424. Prieur AM, Stephan JL: [Macrophage activation syndrome in rheumatic diseases in children]. Rev Rhum Ed Fr 61: 447–451, 1994.
425. Stephan JL, Zeller J, Hubert P, et al: Macrophage activation syndrome and rheumatic disease in childhood: a report of four new cases. Clin Exp Rheumatol 11: 451–456, 1993.

426. Fishman D, Rooney M, Woo P: Successful management of reactive haemophagocytic syndrome in systemic-onset juvenile chronic arthritis [letter]. Br J Rheumatol 34: 888, 1995.
427. Mouy R, Stephan JL, Pillet P, et al: Efficacy of cyclosporine A in the treatment of macrophage activation syndrome in juvenile arthritis: report of five cases. J Pediatr 129: 750–754, 1996.
428. Zamir G, Press J, Tal A, et al: Sleep fragmentation in children with juvenile rheumatoid arthritis. J Rheumatol 25: 1191–1197, 1998.
429. Laaksonen AL, Laine V: A comparative study of joint pain in adult and juvenile rheumatoid arthritis. Ann Rheum Dis 20: 386, 1961.
430. Brewer EJ, Giannini EH, Person DA: Juvenile Rheumatoid Arthritis, 2nd ed. Philadelphia, WB Saunders, 1982.
431. Hagglund KJ, Schopp LM, Alberts KR, et al: Predicting pain among children with juvenile rheumatoid arthritis. Arthritis Care Res 8: 36–42, 1995.
432. Kuis W, Heijnen CJ, Hogeweg JA, et al: How painful is juvenile chronic arthritis? Arch Dis Child 77: 451–453, 1997.
432a. Schikler KN: Is it juvenile rheumatoid arthritis or fibromyalgia? Med Clin North Am 84: 967–982, 2000.
433. Vandvik IH, Eckblad G: Relationship between pain, disease severity and psychosocial function in patients with juvenile chronic arthritis (JCA). Scand J Rheumatol 19: 295–302, 1990.
434. Ross DM, Ross SA: Childhood pain: the school-aged child's viewpoint. Pain 20: 179–191, 1984.
435. Walco GA, Varni JW, Ilowite NT: Cognitive-behavioral pain management in children with juvenile rheumatoid arthritis. Pediatrics 89: 1075–1079, 1992.
436. Scott PJ, Ansell BM, Huskisson EC: Measurement of pain in juvenile chronic polyarthritis. Ann Rheum Dis 36: 186–187, 1977.
437. Beales JG, Keen JH, Holt PJ: The child's perception of the disease and the experience of pain in juvenile chronic arthritis. J Rheumatol 10: 61–65, 1983.
438. Kuis W, Heijnen CJ, Sinnema G, et al: Pain in childhood rheumatic arthritis. Baillieres Clin Rheumatol 12: 229–244, 1998.
439. Thastum M, Zachariae R, Scholer M, et al: Cold pressor pain: comparing responses of juvenile arthritis patients and their parents. Scand J Rheumatol 26: 272–279, 1997.
440. Sherry DD, Bohnsack J, Salmonson K, et al: Painless juvenile rheumatoid arthritis. J Pediatr 116: 921–923, 1990.
441. Thompson KL, Varni JW, Hanson V: Comprehensive assessment of pain in juvenile rheumatoid arthritis: an empirical model. J Pediatr Psychol 12: 241–255, 1987.
442. Lovell DJ, Athreya B, Emery HM, et al: School attendance and pattern: special services and special needs in pediatric patients with rheumatic diseases. Arthritis Care Res 3: 196, 1990.
443. Ilowite NT, Walco GA, Pochaczevsky R: Assessment of pain in patients with juvenile rheumatoid arthritis: relation between pain intensity and degree of joint inflammation. Ann Rheum Dis 51: 343–346, 1992.
444. Varni JW, Thompson KL, Hanson V: The Varni/Thompson Pediatric Pain Questionnaire. I. Chronic musculoskeletal pain in juvenile rheumatoid arthritis. Pain 28: 27–38, 1987.
445. McGrath PA, Seifert CE, Speechley KN, et al: A new analogue scale for assessing children's pain: an initial validation study. Pain 64: 435–443, 1996.
446. Ross CK, Lavigne JV, Hayford JR, et al: Psychological factors affecting reported pain in juvenile rheumatoid arthritis. J Pediatr Psychol 18: 561–573, 1993.
447. Jacobs JC, Hui RM: Cricoarytenoid arthritis and airway obstruction in juvenile rheumatoid arthritis. Pediatrics 59: 292–294, 1977.
448. Malleson P, Riding K, Petty R: Stridor due to cricoarytenoid arthritis in pauciarticular onset juvenile rheumatoid arthritis. J Rheumatol 13: 952–953, 1986.
449. Goldhagen JL: Cricoarytenoiditis as a cause of acute airway obstruction in children. Ann Emerg Med 17: 532–533, 1988.
450. Bertolani MF, Bergamini BM, Marotti F, et al: Cricoarytenoid arthritis as an early sign of juvenile chronic arthritis. Clin Exp Rheumatol 15: 115–116, 1997.
451. Siamopoulou-Mavridou A, Asimakopoulos D, Mavridis A, et al: Middle ear function in patients with juvenile chronic arthritis. Ann Rheum Dis 49: 620–623, 1990.
452. Uziel Y, Rathaus V, Pomeranz A, et al: Torticollis as the sole initial presenting sign of systemic onset juvenile rheumatoid arthritis. J Rheumatol 25: 166–168, 1998.
453. Grancher M: Du rhumatisme cervical chez l'enfant. Bull Med (Paris) 2: 283, 1988.
454. Barkin RE, Stillman JS, Potter TA: The spondylitis of juvenile rheumatoid arthritis. N Engl J Med 253: 1107, 1955.
455. Ziff M, Contreras V, McEven C: Spondylitis in postpubertal patients with rheumatoid arthritis of juvenile onset. Ann Rheum Dis 15: 40, 1956.
456. Rombouts JJ, Rombouts-Lindemans C: Scoliosis in juvenile rheumatoid arthritis. J Bone Joint Surg 56B: 478–483, 1974.
457. Ross AC, Edgar MA, Swann M, et al: Scoliosis in juvenile chronic arthritis. J Bone Joint Surg [Br] 69: 175–178, 1987.
458. Baldassare AR, Auclair RJ, Carls GL, et al: Dissecting popliteal cyst in a child with juvenile rheumatoid arthritis. J Rheumatol 4: 186–188, 1977.
459. Bamzai A, Krieger M, Kretschmer RR: Synovial cysts in juvenile rheumatoid arthritis. Ann Rheum Dis 37: 101–103, 1978.
460. Rennebohm RM, Towbin RB, Crowe WE, et al: Popliteal cysts in juvenile rheumatoid arthritis. Am J Roentgenol 140: 123–125, 1983.
461. Dinham JM: Popliteal cysts in children. The case against surgery. J Bone Joint Surg [Br] 57: 69–71, 1975.
462. Bloom BJ, Tucker LB, Miller LC, et al: Bicipital synovial cysts in juvenile rheumatoid arthritis: clinical description and sonographic correlation. J Rheumatol 22: 1953–1955, 1995.
463. Ansell BM, Bywaters EGL: Finger contractures due to tendon lesions as a mode of presentation of rheumatoid arthritis. Ann Rheum Dis 12: 283, 1953.
464. Wang FM, Wertenbaker C, Behrens MM, et al: Acquired Brown's syndrome in children with juvenile rheumatoid arthritis. Ophthalmology 91: 23–26, 1984.
465. Kaufman LD, Sibony PA, Anand AK, et al: Superior oblique tenosynovitis (Brown's syndrome) as a manifestation of adult Still's disease. J Rheumatol 14: 625–627, 1987.
466. Sury B, Vesterdal E: Extra-articular lesions in juvenile rheumatoid arthritis. A survey based upon a study of 151 cases. Acta Rheumatol Scand 14: 309–316, 1968.
467. Ansell BM, Bywaters EGL: Growth in Still's disease. Ann Rheum Dis 15: 295, 1956.
468. Bernstein BH, Stobie D, Singsen BH, et al: Growth retardation in juvenile rheumatoid arthritis (JRA). Arthritis Rheum 20: 212–216, 1977.
468a. Saha MT, Verronen P, Laippala P, et al: Growth of prepubertal children with juvenile chronic arthritis. Acta Paediatr 88: 724–728, 1999.
469. Davies UM, Jones J, Reeve J, et al: Juvenile rheumatoid arthritis. Effects of disease activity and recombinant human growth hormone on insulin-like growth factor 1, insulin-like growth factor binding proteins 1 and 3, and osteocalcin. Arthritis Rheum 40: 332–340, 1997.
470. Bacon MC, White P: A new approach to the assessment of growth in JRA. Arthritis Rheum 30:S132, 1987.
471. Lovell DJ, White PH: Growth and nutrition in juvenile rheumatoid arthritis. *In* Woo P, White PH, Ansell BM (eds): Paediatric Rheumatology Update. Oxford, Oxford University Press, 1990.
472. Ward DJ, Hartog M, Ansell BM: Corticosteroid-induced dwarfism in Still's disease treated with human growth hormone. Clinical and metabolic effects including hydroxyproline excretion in two cases. Ann Rheum Dis 25: 416–421, 1966.
473. Sturge RA, Beardwell C, Hartog M, et al: Cortisol and growth hormone secretion in relation to linear growth: patients with Still's disease on different therapeutic regimens. Br Med J 3: 547–551, 1970.
474. Allen DB, Julius JR, Breen TJ, et al: Treatment of glucocorticoid-induced growth suppression with growth hormone. National Cooperative Growth Study. J Clin Endocrinol Metab 83: 2824–2829, 1998.
475. Laaksonen AL, Sunell JE, Westeren H, et al: Adrenocortical function in children with juvenile rheumatoid arthritis and other connective tissue disorders. Scand J Rheumatol 3: 137–142, 1974.
476. Bunger C, Bulow J, Tondevold E, et al: Microcirculation of the juvenile knee in chronic arthritis. Clin Orthop 204: 294–302, 1986.

477. Vostrejs M, Hollister JR: Muscle atrophy and leg length discrepancies in pauciarticular juvenile rheumatoid arthritis. Am J Dis Child 142: 343–345, 1988.
478. Woerman AL, Bender-Macleod SA: Leg length discrepancy assessment: accuracy and precision of five clinical methods of evaluation. J Orthop Sports Phys Ther 5: 230, 1984.
479. Simon S, Whiffen J, Shapiro F: Leg-length discrepancies in monoarticular and pauciarticular juvenile rheumatoid arthritis. J Bone Joint Surg [Am] 63: 209–215, 1981.
480. Pearson MH, Ronning O: Lesions of the mandibular condyle in juvenile chronic arthritis. Br J Orthod 23: 49–56, 1996.
481. Hanna VE, Rider SF, Moore TL, et al: Effects of systemic onset juvenile rheumatoid arthritis on facial morphology and temporomandibular joint form and function. J Rheumatol 23: 155–158, 1996.
482. Mericle PM, Wilson VK, Moore TL, et al: Effects of polyarticular and pauciarticular onset juvenile rheumatoid arthritis on facial and mandibular growth. J Rheumatol 23: 159–165, 1996.
483. Olson L, Eckerdal O, Hallonsten AL, et al: Craniomandibular function in juvenile chronic arthritis. A clinical and radiographic study. Swed Dent J 15: 71–83, 1991.
484. Ronchezel MV, Hilario MO, Goldenberg J, et al: Temporomandibular joint and mandibular growth alterations in patients with juvenile rheumatoid arthritis. J Rheumatol 22: 1956–1961, 1995.
485. Avrahami E, Segal R, Solomon A, et al: Direct coronal high resolution computed tomography of the temporomandibular joints in patients with rheumatoid arthritis. J Rheumatol 16: 298–301, 1989.
486. Sairanen E: On the etiology of growth disturbance of the mandible in juvenile rheumatoid arthritis. Acta Rheumatol Scand 16: 136–143, 1970.
487. Ogus H: Rheumatoid arthritis of the temporomandibular joint. Br J Oral Surg 12: 275–284, 1975.
488. Ansell BM, Wood PHN: Prognosis in juvenile chronic polyarthritis. Clin Rheum Dis 2: 397, 1976.
489. Bjork A, Skieller V: Contrasting mandibular growth and facial development in long face syndrome, juvenile rheumatoid polyarthritis, and mandibulofacial dysostosis. J Craniofac Genet Dev Biol Suppl 1: 127–138, 1985.
490. Ganik R, Williams FA: Diagnosis and management of juvenile rheumatoid arthritis with TMJ involvement. Cranio 4: 254–262, 1986.
491. Stabrun AE: Mandibular morphology and position in juvenile rheumatoid arthritis. A study on postero-anterior radiographs. Eur J Orthod 7: 288–298, 1985.
492. Stabrun AE, Larheim TA, Rosler M, et al: Impaired mandibular function and its possible effect on mandibular growth in juvenile rheumatoid arthritis. Eur J Orthod 9: 43–50, 1987.
493. Blasberg B, Lowe AA, Petty RE, et al: Temporomandibular joint disease in children with juvenile rheumatoid arthritis. Arthritis Rheum 30:S27, 1987.
494. Marini I, Vecchiet F, Spiazzi L, et al: Stomatognathic function in juvenile rheumatoid arthritis and in developmental openbite subjects. ASDC J Dent Child 66: 30–35, 1999.
495. Walton AG, Welbury RR, Foster HE, et al: Juvenile chronic arthritis: a dental review. Oral Dis 5: 68–75, 1999.
496. Hillman L, Cassidy JT, Johnson L, et al: Vitamin D metabolism and bone mineralization in children with juvenile rheumatoid arthritis. J Pediatr 124: 910–916, 1994.
497. Woo PM: Growth retardation and osteoporosis in juvenile chronic arthritis. Clin Exp Rheumatol 12(Suppl)10:S87–S90, 1994.
498. Cassidy JT, Langman CB, Allen SH, et al: Bone mineral metabolism in children with juvenile rheumatoid arthritis. Pediatr Clin North Am 42: 1017–1033, 1995.
499. Cassidy JT, Hillman LS: Abnormalities in skeletal growth in children with juvenile rheumatoid arthritis. Rheum Dis Clin North Am 23: 499–522, 1997.
500. Henderson CJ, Cawkwell GD, Specker BL, et al: Predictors of total body bone mineral density in non-corticosteroid-treated prepubertal children with juvenile rheumatoid arthritis. Arthritis Rheum 40: 1967–1975, 1997.
501. Kotaniemi A, Savolainen A, Kroger H, et al: Development of bone mineral density at the lumbar spine and femoral neck in juvenile chronic arthritis—a prospective one year followup study. J Rheumatol 25: 2450–2455, 1998.
502. Zak M, Hassager C, Lovell DJ, et al: Assessment of bone mineral density in adults with a history of juvenile chronic arthritis: a cross-sectional long-term followup study. Arthritis Rheum 42: 790–798, 1999.
502a. Henderson CJ, Specker BL, Sierra RI, et al: Total-body bone mineral content in non-corticosteroid-treated postpubertal females with juvenile rheumatoid arthritis: frequency of osteopenia and contributing factors. Arthritis Rheum 43: 531–540, 2000.
502b. Haugen M, Lien G, Flato B, et al: Young adults with juvenile arthritis in remission attain normal peak bone mass at the lumbar spine and forearm. Arthritis Rheum 43: 1504–1510, 2000.
503. Cassidy JT: Osteopenia and osteoporosis in children. Clin Exp Rheumatol 17: 245–250, 1999.
504. Kotaniemi A: Growth retardation and bone loss as determinants of axial osteopenia in juvenile chronic arthritis. Scand J Rheumatol 26: 14–18, 1997.
505. Falcini F, Ermini M, Bagnoli F: Bone turnover is reduced in children with juvenile rheumatoid arthritis. J Endocrinol Invest 21: 31–36, 1998.
506. Pereira RM, Falco V, Corrente JE, et al: Abnormalities in the biochemical markers of bone turnover in children with juvenile chronic arthritis. Clin Exp Rheumatol 17: 251–255, 1999.
507. Johansson U, Portinsson S, Akesson A, et al: Nutritional status in girls with juvenile chronic arthritis. Hum Nutr Clin Nutr 40: 57–67, 1986.
508. Lovell DJ, Gregg D, Heubi J, et al: Nutritional status in juvenile rheumatoid arthritis: an interim report. Arthritis Rheum 29: 567, 1986.
509. Warady BD, McCammon SP, Lindsley CB: Anthropometric assessment of patients with juvenile rheumatoid arthritis. Top Clin Nutr 4: 7, 1989.
510. Henderson CJ, Lovell DJ: Assessment of protein-energy malnutrition in children and adolescents with juvenile rheumatoid arthritis. Arthritis Care Res 2: 108–113, 1989.
511. Kremer JM: Nutrition and rheumatic diseases. *In* Ruddy S, Harris ED Jr, Sledge CB (eds): Kelley's Textbook of Rheumatology, 6th ed. Philadelphia, WB Saunders, 2000, pp 713–727.
512. Miller ML, Chacko JA, Young EA: Dietary deficiencies in children with juvenile rheumatoid arthritis. Arthritis Care Res 2: 22–24, 1989.
513. Tracey KJ, Wei H, Manogue KR, et al: Cachectin/tumor necrosis factor induces cachexia, anemia, and inflammation. J Exp Med 167: 1211–1227, 1988.
514. Bywaters EGL, Glynn LE, Zeldis A: Subcutaneous nodules of Still's disease. Ann Rheum Dis 17: 278, 1958.
515. Bywaters EG, Cardoe N: Multiple nodules in juvenile chronic polyarthritis. Ann Rheum Dis 31: 421, 1972.
516. Kaye BR, Kaye RL, Bobrove A: Rheumatoid nodules. Review of the spectrum of associated conditions and proposal of a new classification, with a report of four seronegative cases. Am J Med 76: 279–292, 1984.
517. Beatty EC: Rheumatic-like nodules occurring in nonrheumatic children. Arch Pathol 68: 154, 1959.
518. Taranta A: Occurrence of rheumatic-like subcutaneous nodules without evidence of joint or heart disease. N Engl J Med 226: 13, 1962.
519. Altman RS, Caffrey PR: Isolated subcutaneous rheumatic nodules. Pediatrics 34: 869, 1964.
520. Burrington JD: "Pseudorheumatoid" nodules in children: report of 10 cases. Pediatrics 45: 473–478, 1970.
521. Simons FE, Schaller JG: Benign rheumatoid nodules. Pediatrics 56: 29–33, 1975.
522. Schaller JG: Benign rheumatoid nodules. Arthritis Rheum Suppl 20: 277, 1977.
523. Mesara BW, Brody GL, Oberman HA: "Pseudorheumatoid" subcutaneous nodules. Am J Clin Pathol 45: 684–691, 1966.
524. Havill S, Duffill M, Rademaker M: Multicentric reticulohistiocytosis in a child. Australas J Dermatol 40: 44–46, 1999.
525. Gedalia A, Gewanter H, Baum J: Dark skin discoloration of finger joints in juvenile arthritis. J Rheumatol 16: 797–799, 1989.
526. Athreya BH, Ostrov BE, Eichenfield AH, et al: Lymphedema

associated with juvenile rheumatoid arthritis. J Rheumatol 16: 1338–1340, 1989.
527. Bardare M, Falcini F, Hertzberger-ten Cate R, et al: Idiopathic limb edema in children with chronic arthritis: a multicenter report of 12 cases. J Rheumatol 24: 384–388, 1997.
528. Schmit P, Prieur AM, Brunelle F: Juvenile rheumatoid arthritis and lymphoedema: lymphangiographic aspects. Pediatr Radiol 29: 364–366, 1999.
529. Forsyth CC: Calcification of the digital arteries in a child with rheumatoid arthritis. Arch Dis Child 35: 296, 1960.
530. Reid MM, Fannin TF: Extensive vascular calcification in association with juvenile rheumatoid arthritis and amyloidosis. Arch Dis Child 43: 607–610, 1968.
531. Ellsworth JE, Cassidy JT, Ragsdale CG, et al: Mucha-Habermann disease in children—the association with rheumatic diseases. J Rheumatol 9: 319–324, 1982.
532. Person DA, He XH, Brewer EJ: Vasculitis in children with juvenile rheumatoid arthritis. J Rheumatol 13: 219, 1986.
533. Hall S, Nelson AM: Takayasu's arteritis and juvenile rheumatoid arthritis. J Rheumatol 13: 431–433, 1986.
534. Wedderburn LR, Kwan JT, Thompson PW, et al: Juvenile chronic arthritis and Wegener's granulomatosis. Br J Rheumatol 31: 121–123, 1992.
535. Cullen B, Mongey AB, Molony J: Juvenile chronic arthritis associated with systemic vasculitis. Ir Med J 79: 72–74, 1986.
536. Le Gars L, Clerc D, Cariou D, et al: Systemic juvenile rheumatoid arthritis and associated Isaacs' syndrome. J Rheumatol 24: 178–180, 1997.
537. Alukal MK, Costello PB, Green FA: Cardiac tamponade in systemic juvenile rheumatoid arthritis requiring emergency pericardiectomy. J Rheumatol 11: 222–225, 1984.
538. Goldenberg J, Ferraz MB, Pessoa AP, et al: Symptomatic cardiac involvement in juvenile rheumatoid arthritis. Int J Cardiol 34: 57–62, 1992.
539. Lietman PS, Bywaters EGL: Pericarditis in juvenile rheumatoid arthritis. Pediatrics 32: 855, 1963.
540. Bernstein B, Takahashi M, Hanson V: Cardiac involvement in juvenile rheumatoid arthritis. J Pediatr 85: 313–317, 1974.
541. Scharf J, Levy J, Benderly A, et al: Pericardial tamponade in juvenile rheumatoid arthritis. Arthritis Rheum 19: 760–762, 1976.
542. Brewer E Jr: Juvenile rheumatoid arthritis—cardiac involvement. Arthritis Rheum 20: 231–236, 1977.
543. Bernstein B: Pericarditis in juvenile rheumatoid arthritis. Arthritis Rheum Suppl 20: 241, 1977.
544. Svantesson H, Bjorkhem G, Elborgh R: Cardiac involvement in juvenile rheumatoid arthritis. A follow-up study. Acta Paediatr Scand 72: 345–350, 1983.
545. Majeed HA, Kvasnicka J: Juvenile rheumatoid arthritis with cardiac tamponade. Ann Rheum Dis 37: 273–276, 1978.
546. Yancey CL, Doughty RA, Cohlan BA, et al: Pericarditis and cardiac tamponade in juvenile rheumatoid arthritis. Pediatrics 68: 369–373, 1981.
547. Goldenberg J, Pessoa AP, Roizenblatt S, et al: Cardiac tamponade in juvenile chronic arthritis: report of two cases and review of publications. Ann Rheum Dis 49: 549–553, 1990.
548. Bauer-Vinassac D, Chapsal J, Duboc D, et al: [Aortic insufficiency and rapidly developing constrictive pericarditis in rheumatoid polyarthritis of juvenile onset. Apropos of a case and review of the literature]. Ann Med Interne (Paris) 138: 141–142, 1987.
549. Miller JJ III, French JW: Myocarditis in juvenile rheumatoid arthritis. Am J Dis Child 131: 205–209, 1977.
549a. Oguz D, Ocal B, Ertan U, et al: Left ventricular diastolic functions in juvenile rheumatoid arthritis. Pediatr Cardiol 21: 374–377, 2000.
550. Martel W, Cassidy JT, Brody GL, et al: Spinal cord lesions in juvenile rheumatoid arthritis. J Can Assoc Radiol 20: 32–36, 1969.
551. Leak AM, Millar-Craig MW, Ansell BM: Aortic regurgitation in seropositive juvenile arthritis. Ann Rheum Dis 40: 229–234, 1981.
552. Kramer PH, Imboden JB Jr, Waldman FM, et al: Severe aortic insufficiency in juvenile chronic arthritis. Am J Med 74: 1088–1091, 1983.
553. Hull RG, Hall MA, Prasad AN: Aortic incompetence in pauciarticular juvenile chronic arthritis. Arch Dis Child 61: 409–410, 1986.
554. Delgado EA, Petty RE, Malleson PN, et al: Aortic valve insufficiency and coronary artery narrowing in a child with polyarticular juvenile rheumatoid arthritis. J Rheumatol 15: 144–147, 1988.
555. Karademir S, Oner A, Atalay S, et al: Mitral and aortic insufficiency in polyarticular juvenile rheumatoid arthritis. Acta Paediatr 85: 380, 1996.
556. Trehan A, Singh S, Ambalavanan N, et al: Valvular heart disease: rheumatic or rheumatoid? Indian Pediatr 34: 641–644, 1997.
557. Brinkman GL, Chaikof L: Rheumatoid lung disease. Am Rev Respir Dis 80: 732, 1959.
558. Jordan JD, Snyder CH: Rheumatoid disease of the lung and cor pulmonale. Observations in a child. Am J Dis Child 108: 174, 1964.
559. Athreya BH, Doughty RA, Bookspan M, et al: Pulmonary manifestations of juvenile rheumatoid arthritis. A report of eight cases and review. Clin Chest Med 1: 361–374, 1980.
560. Lovell D, Lindsley C, Langston C: Lymphoid interstitial pneumonia in juvenile rheumatoid arthritis. J Pediatr 105: 947–950, 1984.
561. Wagener JS, Taussig LM, DeBenedetti C, et al: Pulmonary function in juvenile rheumatoid arthritis. J Pediatr 99: 108–110, 1981.
562. Uziel Y, Hen B, Cordoba M, et al: Lymphocytic interstitial pneumonitis preceding polyarticular juvenile rheumatoid arthritis. Clin Exp Rheumatol 16: 617–619, 1998.
563. Noyes BE, Albers GM, deMello DE, et al: Early onset of pulmonary parenchymal disease associated with juvenile rheumatoid arthritis. Pediatr Pulmonol 24: 444–446, 1997.
564. Braidy JF, Poulson JM: Diaphragmatic weakness and myositis associated with systemic juvenile rheumatoid arthritis. Can Med Assoc J 130: 47–49, 1984.
564a. Knook LM, De Kleer IM, Van der Ent CK, et al: Lung function abnormalities and respiratory muscle weakness in children with juvenile chronic arthritis. Eur Respir J 14: 529–533, 1999.
565. Padeh S, Laxer RM, Silver MM, et al: Primary pulmonary hypertension in a patient with systemic-onset juvenile arthritis. Arthritis Rheum 34: 1575–1579, 1991.
565a. Len C, Hilario MO, Kawakami E, et al: Gastroduodenal lesions in children with juvenile rheumatoid arthritis. Hepatogastroenterology 46: 991–996, 1999.
566. Snape WJ Jr: Pseudo-obstruction and other obstructive disorders. Clin Gastroenterol 11: 593–608, 1982.
567. Bhettay E, Thomson AJ: Peritonitis in juvenile chronic arthritis. A report of 2 cases. S Afr Med J 68: 605–606, 1985.
568. Lindsley CB, Miner PB Jr: Seronegative juvenile rheumatoid arthritis and mast cell-associated gastritis. Arthritis Rheum 34: 106–109, 1991.
569. Lindsley C, Schaller JG: Arthritis associated with inflammatory bowel disease in children. J Pediatr 84: 16, 1974.
570. Parke AL, Fagan EA, Chadwick VS, et al: Coeliac disease and rheumatoid arthritis. Ann Rheum Dis 43: 378–380, 1984.
571. George EK, Hertzberger-ten Cate R, van Suijlekom-Smit LW, et al: Juvenile chronic arthritis and coeliac disease in The Netherlands. Clin Exp Rheumatol 14: 571–575, 1996.
572. Rush PJ, Shore A, Coblentz C, et al: The musculoskeletal manifestations of cystic fibrosis. Semin Arthritis Rheum 15: 213–225, 1986.
573. Jackson J, Anderson L, Schur PH, et al: Sjögren's syndrome in juvenile rheumatoid arthritis. Arthritis Rheum 16: 122, 1973.
574. McLaughlin WS: Sjögren's syndrome and juvenile rheumatoid arthritis. Proc Br Soc Dent Maxillofac Radiol 1: 17–21, 1986.
575. Rosenberg AM, Mitchell DM, Card RT: Felty's syndrome in a child. J Rheumatol 11: 835–837, 1984.
576. Toomey K, Hepburn B: Felty syndrome in juvenile arthritis. J Pediatr 106: 254–255, 1985.
577. Schaller J, Beckwith B, Wedgwood RJ: Hepatic involvement in juvenile rheumatoid arthritis. J Pediatr 77: 203–210, 1970.
578. Boone JE: Hepatic disease and mortality in juvenile rheumatoid arthritis. Arthritis Rheum Suppl 20: 257, 1977.
579. Jacobs JC: JRA and hyperphosphataemia. J Pediatr 107: 828–829, 1985.

580. Lockitch G, Pudek MR, Halstead AC: Isolated elevation of serum alkaline phosphatase. J Pediatr 105: 773–775, 1984.
581. Rennebohm RM, Heubi JE, Daugherty CC, et al: Reye syndrome in children receiving salicylate therapy for connective tissue disease. J Pediatr 107: 877–880, 1985.
582. Russell AS: Cerebral complications in juvenile rheumatoid arthritis. Can Med Assoc J 108: 19, 1973.
583. Lang H, Anttila R, Svekus A, et al: EEG findings in juvenile rheumatoid arthritis and other connective tissue diseases in children. Acta Paediatr Scand 63: 373–380, 1974.
584. Sievers K, Nissila M, Sievers UM: Cerebral vasculitis visualized by angiography in juvenile rheumatoid arthritis simulating brain tumor. Acta Rheumatol Scand 14: 222–232, 1968.
585. Jan JE, Hill RH, Low MD: Cerebral complications in juvenile rheumatoid arthritis. Can Med Assoc J 107: 623–625, 1972.
586. Calabro JJ: Other extraarticular manifestations of juvenile rheumatoid arthritis. Arthritis Rheum 20: 237–240, 1977.
587. Gururaj AK, Chand RP, Chuah SP: Cerebral infarction in juvenile rheumatoid arthritis. Clin Neurol Neurosurg 90: 261–263, 1988.
588. Anttila R, Laaksonen AL: Renal disease in juvenile rheumatoid arthritis. Acta Rheumatol Scand 15: 99–111, 1969.
589. Anttila R: Renal involvement in juvenile rheumatoid arthritis. A clinical and histopathological study. Acta Paediatr Scand Suppl 227: 3–73, 1972.
590. Mertens JC, Huizinga TW, Hagen EC, et al: Extracapillary glomerulonephritis in a patient with juvenile chronic arthritis. J Rheumatol 23: 1633–1635, 1996.
591. Dodge WF, West EF, Smith EH, et al: Proteinuria and hematuria in schoolchildren: epidemiology and early natural history. J Pediatr 88: 327–347, 1976.
592. Dhib M, Prieur AM, Courville S, et al: Crescentic glomerulonephritis in juvenile chronic arthritis. J Rheumatol 23: 1636–1640, 1996.
593. von Kemp K, Dehaen F, Huybrechts M, et al: Hematuria as presenting sign in Wissler-Fanconi syndrome. J Rheumatol 14: 145–146, 1987.
594. Levy M, Prieur AM, Gubler MC, et al: Renal involvement in juvenile chronic arthritis: clinical and pathologic features. Am J Kidney Dis 9: 138–146, 1987.
595. Stapleton FB, Hanissian AS, Miller LA: Hypercalciuria in children with juvenile rheumatoid arthritis: association with hematuria. J Pediatr 107: 235–239, 1985.
596. Tsai TC, Chang PY, Chen BF, et al: Retroperitoneal fibrosis and juvenile rheumatoid arthritis. Pediatr Nephrol 10: 208–209, 1996.
597. Malleson PN, Lockitch G, Mackinnon M, et al: Renal disease in chronic arthritis of childhood. A study of urinary N-acetyl-beta-glucosaminidase and beta 2–microglobulin excretion. Arthritis Rheum 33: 1560–1566, 1990.
598. Kanski JJ: Juvenile arthritis and uveitis. Surv Ophthalmol 34: 253–267, 1990.
599. Chanteau S, Glaziou P, Plichart C, et al: Wuchereria bancrofti filariasis in French Polynesia: age-specific patterns of microfilaremia, circulating antigen, and specific IgG and IgG4 responses according to transmission level. Int J Parasitol 25: 81–85, 1995.
600. Kotaniemi K, Kaipiainen-Seppanen O, Savolainen A, et al: A population-based study on uveitis in juvenile rheumatoid arthritis. Clin Exp Rheumatol 17: 119–122, 1999.
601. Chadwick AJ, Rosen ES: Papillitis and Still's disease. Am J Ophthalmol 65: 784–787, 1968.
602. Jose DG, Good RA: Iridocyclitis and pauciarticular juvenile rheumatoid arthritis. J Pediatr 78: 910–911, 1971.
603. Kanski JJ: Anterior uveitis in juvenile rheumatoid arthritis. Arch Ophthalmol 95: 1794–1797, 1977.
604. Ohm J: Bandformige Hornhauttrubung bei einem neunjhrigen Madchen und ihre Behandlung mit subkonjunktivalen Jodkalium-einspritzungen. Klin Monatsbl Augenheilkd 48: 243, 1910.
605. Friedlander A: 2 Tilfaelde af kronisk septisk Polyartritis i Barnealderen med Ojenkomplikationer. Ugeskr Laeger 95: 1190, 1933.
606. Holm E: Iridocyclitis and ribbon-like keratitis in cases of infantile polyarthritis (Still's disease). Trans Ophthalmol Soc U K 55: 478, 1935.
607. Blegvad O: Iridocyclitis and disease of the joints in children. Acta Ophthalmol (Copenh) 19: 219, 1941.
608. Chylack LT Jr, Bienfang DC, Bellows AR, et al: Ocular manifestations of juvenile rheumatoid arthritis. Am J Ophthalmol 79: 1026–1033, 1975.
609. Smiley WK: The eye in juvenile chronic polyarthritis. Clin Rheum Dis 2: 413, 1976.
610. Schaller JG: Iridocyclitis. Arthritis Rheum Suppl 20: 227, 1977.
611. Rosenberg AM: Uveitis associated with juvenile rheumatoid arthritis. Semin Arthritis Rheum 16: 158–173, 1987.
612. Wolf MD, Lichter PR, Ragsdale CG: Prognostic factors in the uveitis of juvenile rheumatoid arthritis. Ophthalmology 94: 1242–1248, 1987.
613. Cabral DA, Petty RE, Malleson PN: Visual prognosis in children with chronic uveitis and arthritis. Arthritis Rheum 35:S229, 1992.
614. Dana MR, Merayo-Lloves J, Schaumberg DA, et al: Visual outcomes prognosticators in juvenile rheumatoid arthritis-associated uveitis. Ophthalmology 104: 236–244, 1997.
615. Chalom EC, Goldsmith DP, Koehler MA, et al: Prevalence and outcome of uveitis in a regional cohort of patients with juvenile rheumatoid arthritis. J Rheumatol 24: 2031–2034, 1997.
616. Malleson P: Prevalence and outcome of uveitis in a regional cohort of patients with juvenile rheumatoid arthritis. J Rheumatol 25: 1242, 1998.
617. Cassidy JT, Martel W: Monarticular juvenile rheumatoid arthritis. Arthritis Rheum 7: 298, 1964.
618. Key SN III, Kimura SJ: Iridocyclitis associated with juvenile rheumatoid arthritis. Am J Ophthalmol 80: 425–429, 1975.
619. Kanski JJ, Shun-Shin GA: Systemic uveitis syndromes in childhood: an analysis of 340 cases. Ophthalmology 91: 1247–1252, 1984.
620. Ozdogan H, Kasapcopur O, Dede H, et al: Juvenile chronic arthritis in a Turkish population. Clin Exp Rheumatol 9: 431–435, 1991.
621. Spalter HF: The visual prognosis in juvenile rheumatoid arthritis. Trans Am Ophthalmol Soc 73: 554–570, 1976.
622. McGill NW, Gow PJ: Juvenile rheumatoid arthritis in Auckland: a long term follow-up study with particular reference to uveitis. Aust N Z J Med 17: 305–308, 1987.
623. Petty RE: Current knowledge of the etiology and pathogenesis of chronic uveitis accompanying juvenile rheumatoid arthritis. Rheum Dis Clin North Am 13: 19–36, 1987.
624. Petty RE, Hunt DW: Immunity to ocular and collagen antigens in childhood arthritis and uveitis. Int Arch Allergy Appl Immunol 89: 31–37, 1989.
625. Gupta D, Singh VK, Rajasingh J, et al: Cellular immune responses of patients with juvenile chronic arthritis to retinal antigens and their synthetic peptides. Immunol Res 15: 74–83, 1996.
626. Uchiyama RC, Osborn TG, Moore TL: Antibodies to iris and retina detected in sera from patients with juvenile rheumatoid arthritis with iridocyclitis by indirect immunofluorescence studies on human eye tissue. J Rheumatol 16: 1074–1078, 1989.
627. Hunt DW, Petty RE, Millar F: Iris protein antibodies in serum of patients with juvenile rheumatoid arthritis and uveitis. Int Arch Allergy Immunol 100: 314–318, 1993.
628. Ploski R, Vinje O, Ronningen KS, et al: HLA class II alleles and heterogeneity of juvenile rheumatoid arthritis. DRB1*0101 may define a novel subset of the disease. Arthritis Rheum 36: 465–472, 1993.
629. Giannini EH, Malagon CN, Van Kerckhove C, et al: Longitudinal analysis of HLA associated risks for iridocyclitis in juvenile rheumatoid arthritis. J Rheumatol 18: 1394–1397, 1991.
630. Melin-Aldana H, Giannini EH, Taylor J, et al: Human leukocyte antigen-DRB1*1104 in the chronic iridocyclitis of pauciarticular juvenile rheumatoid arthritis. J Pediatr 121: 56–60, 1992.
631. Akduman L, Kaplan HJ, Tychsen L: Prevalence of uveitis in an outpatient juvenile arthritis clinic: onset of uveitis more than a decade after onset of arthritis. J Ophthalmic Nurs Technol 16: 177–182, 1997.
632. Rosenberg AM, Oen KG: The relationship between ocular and articular disease activity in children with juvenile rheumatoid arthritis and associated uveitis. Arthritis Rheum 29: 797–800, 1986.

633. Sabates R, Smith T, Apple D: Ocular histopathology in juvenile rheumatoid arthritis. Ann Ophthalmol 11: 733–737, 1979.
634. Chylack LT Jr, Dueker DK, Pihlaja DJ: Ocular manifestations of juvenile rheumatoid arthritis: pathology, fluorescein iris angiography, and patient care patterns. *In* Miller JJ III (ed): Juvenile Rheumatoid Arthritis. Littleton, MA, PSG, 1978, p 149.
635. Merriam JC, Chylack LT Jr, Albert DM: Early-onset pauciarticular juvenile rheumatoid arthritis. A histopathologic study. Arch Ophthalmol 101: 1085–1092, 1983.
636. Godfrey WA, Lindsley CB, Cuppage FE: Localization of IgM in plasma cells in the iris of a patient with iridocyclitis and juvenile rheumatoid arthritis. Arthritis Rheum 24: 1195–1198, 1981.
637. Hollwich F, Damaske E: [Eye symptoms in Still's disease]. Med Monatsschr 22: 109–114, 1968.
638. Hinzpeter EN, Naumann G, Bartelheimer HK: Ocular histopathology in Still's disease. Ophthalmol Res 2: 16, 1971.
639. Rahi AH, Kanski JJ, Fielder A: Immunoglobulins and antinuclear antibodies in aqueous humour from patients with juvenile "rheumatoid" arthritis (Still's disease). Trans Ophthalmol Soc U K 97: 217–222, 1977.
640. Kanski JJ: Clinical and immunological study of anterior uveitis in juvenile chronic polyarthritis. Trans Ophthalmol Soc U K 96: 123–130, 1976.
641. Person DA, Leatherwood CM, Brewer EJ, et al: Immunology of the vitreous in juvenile rheumatoid arthritis. Arthritis Rheum 24: 591, 1981.
642. Kaplan HJ, Aaberg TM, Keller RH: Recurrent clinical uveitis. Cell surface markers on vitreous lymphocytes. Arch Ophthalmol 100: 585–587, 1982.
643. Kanski JJ: Care of children with anterior uveitis. Trans Ophthalmol Soc U K 101 (Pt 3): 387–390, 1981.
644. Perkins ES: Pattern of uveitis in children. Br J Ophthalmol 50: 169–185, 1966.
645. Ohno S, Miyajima T, Higuchi M, et al: Ocular manifestations of Kawasaki's disease (mucocutaneous lymph node syndrome). Am J Ophthalmol 93: 713–717, 1982.
646. Shore A, Ansell BM: Juvenile psoriatic arthritis—an analysis of 60 cases. J Pediatr 100: 529–535, 1982.
647. Lindsley CB, Schaller JG: Arthritis associated with inflammatory bowel disease in children. J Pediatr 84: 16, 1974.
648. Passo M, Brandt K, Fitzgerald J: Arthritis associated with inflammatory bowel disease in children: relationship between arthritis and activity of the inflammatory bowel disease. Arthritis Rheum 22: 645, 1979.
649. Rankin GB, Watts HD, Melnyk CS, et al: National Cooperative Crohn's Disease Study: extraintestinal manifestations and perianal complications. Gastroenterology 77: 914–920, 1979.
650. Davies NE, Haverty JR, Boatwright M: Reiter's disease associated with shigellosis. South Med J 62: 1011–1014, 1969.
651. Iveson JM, Nanda BS, Hancock JA, et al: Reiter's disease in three boys. Ann Rheum Dis 34: 364–368, 1975.
652. Ansell MB, Bywaters EG, Elderkin FM: Familial arthropathy with rash, uveitis and mental retardation. Proc R Soc Med 68: 584–585, 1975.
653. Prieur AM, Griscelli C: Arthropathy with rash, chronic meningitis, eye lesions, and mental retardation. J Pediatr 99: 79–83, 1981.
654. Kaufman RA, Lovell DJ: Infantile-onset multisystem inflammatory disease: radiologic findings. Radiology 160: 741–746, 1986.
655. Yarom A, Rennebohm RM, Levinson JE: Infantile multisystem inflammatory disease: a specific syndrome? J Pediatr 106: 390–396, 1985.
656. Lindsley CB, Godfrey WA: Childhood sarcoidosis manifesting as juvenile rheumatoid arthritis. Pediatrics 76: 765–768, 1985.
657. Hoover DL, Khan JA, Giangiacomo J: Pediatric ocular sarcoidosis. Surv Ophthalmol 30: 215–228, 1986.
658. Blau EB: Familial granulomatous arthritis, iritis, and rash. J Pediatr 107: 689–693, 1985.
659. Pastores GM, Michels VV, Stickler GB, et al: Autosomal dominant granulomatous arthritis, uveitis, skin rash, and synovial cysts. J Pediatr 117: 403–408, 1990.
660. Petty RE, Cassidy JT, Sullivan DB: Clinical correlates of antinuclear antibodies in juvenile rheumatoid arthritis. J Pediatr 83: 386–389, 1973.
661. Schaller JG, Johnson GD, Holborow EJ, et al: The association of antinuclear antibodies with the chronic iridocyclitis of juvenile rheumatoid arthritis (Still's disease). Arthritis Rheum 17: 409–416, 1974.
662. Rosenberg AM, Romanchuk KG: Antinuclear antibodies in arthritic and nonarthritic children with uveitis. J Rheumatol 17: 60–61, 1990.
663. Neuteboom GH, Hertzberger-ten Cate R, de Jong J, et al: Antibodies to a 15 kD nuclear antigen in patients with juvenile chronic arthritis and uveitis. Invest Ophthalmol Vis Sci 33: 1657–1660, 1992.
664. Epstein WV, Tan M, Easterbrook M: Serum antibody to double-stranded RNA and DNA in patients with idiopathic and secondary uveitis. N Engl J Med 285: 1502–1506, 1971.
665. Massa M, De Benedetti F, Pignatti P, et al: Lack of temporal association of iridocyclitis with IgG reactivities to core histones and nucleosome subparticles in pauciarticular juvenile chronic arthritis. Br J Rheumatol 34: 507–511, 1995.
666. Nguyen QD, Foster CS: Saving the vision of children with juvenile rheumatoid arthritis-associated uveitis. JAMA 280: 1133–1134, 1998.
667. Olson NY, Lindsley CB, Godfrey WA: Treatment of chronic childhood iridocyclitis with nonsteroidal anti-inflammatory drugs. J Allerg Clin Immunol 79: 220, 1981.
668. March WF, Coniglione TC: Ibuprofen in the treatment of uveitis. Ann Ophthalmol 17: 103–104, 1985.
669. Dunne JA, Jacobs N, Morrison A, et al: Efficacy in anterior uveitis of two known steroids and topical tolmetin. Br J Ophthalmol 69: 120–125, 1985.
670. Weiss AH, Wallace CA, Sherry DD: Methotrexate for resistant chronic uveitis in children with juvenile rheumatoid arthritis. J Pediatr 133: 266–268, 1998.
671. Shetty AK, Zganjar BE, Ellis GS Jr, et al: Low-dose methotrexate in the treatment of severe juvenile rheumatoid arthritis and sarcoid iritis. J Pediatr Ophthalmol Strabismus 36: 125–128, 1999.
672. Mehra R, Moore TL, Catalano D, et al: Chlorambucil in the treatment of iridocyclitis in juvenile rheumatoid arthritis. J Rheumatol 8: 141–144, 1981.
673. Palmer RG, Kanski JJ, Ansell BM: Chlorambucil in the treatment of intractable uveitis associated with juvenile chronic arthritis. J Rheumatol 12: 967–970, 1985.
674. Nussenblatt RB, Palestine AG, Chan CC: Cyclosporin A therapy in the treatment of intraocular inflammatory disease resistant to systemic corticosteroids and cytotoxic agents. Am J Ophthalmol 96: 275–282, 1983.
675. Wizemann AJ, Wizemann V: Therapeutic effects of short-term plasma exchange in endogenous uveitis. Am J Ophthalmol 97: 565–572, 1984.
676. Kilmartin DJ, Forrester JV, Dick AD: Cyclosporin A therapy in refractory non-infectious childhood uveitis. Br J Ophthalmol 82: 737–742, 1998.
677. Kilmartin DJ, Forrester JV, Dick AD: Rescue therapy with mycophenolate mofetil in refractory uveitis. Lancet 352: 35–36, 1998.
678. Rosenbaum JT, George RK, Gordon C: The treatment of refractory uveitis with intravenous immunoglobulin. Am J Ophthalmol 127: 545–549, 1999.
679. Hooper PL, Rao NA, Smith RE: Cataract extraction in uveitis patients. Surv Ophthalmol 35: 120–144, 1990.
680. Cimaz RG, Fink CW: The articular prognosis of pauciarticular onset juvenile arthritis is not influenced by the presence of uveitis. J Rheumatol 23: 357–359, 1996.
681. Sherry DD, Mellins ED, Wedgwood RJ: Decreasing severity of chronic uveitis in children with pauciarticular arthritis. Am J Dis Child 145: 1026–1028, 1991.
682. Gori S, Broglia AM, Ravelli A, et al: Frequency and complications of chronic iridocyclitis in ANA-positive pauciarticular juvenile chronic arthritis. Int Ophthalmol 18: 225–228, 1994.
683. Bywaters EG: Pathologic aspects of juvenile chronic polyarthritis. Arthritis Rheum 20: 271–276, 1977.
684. Houba V, Bardfeld R: Serum immunoglobulins in juvenile rheumatoid arthritis. Ann Rheum Dis 28: 55–57, 1969.
685. Wynne-Roberts CR, Anderson CH, Turano AM, et al: Light- and electron-microscopic findings of juvenile rheumatoid ar-

thritis synovium: comparison with normal juvenile synovium. Semin Arthritis Rheum 7: 287–302, 1978.
686. Fletcher MR, Scott JT: Chronic monarticular synovitis. Diagnostic and prognostic features. Ann Rheum Dis 34: 171–176, 1975.
687. Harris ED Jr: Rheumatoid Arthritis. Philadelphia, WB Saunders, 1997.
688. Cooke TDV: The interaction and local disease manifestations of immune complexes in articular collagenous tissue. *In* Maroudas A, Holborow EJ (eds): Studies in Joint Disease. London, Pittman, 1980, p 158.
689. Bernstein B, Forrester D, Singsen B, et al: Hip joint restoration in juvenile rheumatoid arthritis. Arthritis Rheum 20: 1099–1104, 1977.
690. Berg E, Wainwright R, Barton B, et al: On the nature of rheumatoid rice bodies: an immunologic, histochemical, and electron microscope study. Arthritis Rheum 20: 1343–1349, 1977.
691. Wynne-Roberts CR, Cassidy JT: Juvenile rheumatoid arthritis with rice bodies: light and electron microscopic studies. Ann Rheum Dis 38: 8–13, 1979.
692. Chung C, Coley BD, Martin LC: Rice bodies in juvenile rheumatoid arthritis. AJR Am J Roentgenol 170: 698–700, 1998.
693. Bennett GA, Zeller JW, Bauer W: Subcutaneous nodules of rheumatoid arthritis and rheumatic fever. A pathologic study. Arch Pathol 30: 70, 1970.
694. Harvey AR, Pippard MJ, Ansell BM: Microcytic anaemia in juvenile chronic arthritis. Scand J Rheumatol 16: 53–59, 1987.
695. Prouse PJ, Harvey AR, Bonner B, et al: Anaemia in juvenile chronic arthritis: serum inhibition of normal erythropoiesis in vitro. Ann Rheum Dis 46: 127–134, 1987.
696. Kirel B, Yetgin S, Saatci U, et al: Anaemia in juvenile chronic arthritis. Clin Rheumatol 15: 236–241, 1996.
696a. Kivivuori SM, Pelkonen P, Ylijoki H, et al: Elevated serum transferrin receptor concentration in children with juvenile chronic arthritis as evidence of iron deficiency. Rheumatology (Oxford) 39: 193–197, 2000.
697. Cazzola M, Ponchio L, De Benedetti F, et al: Defective iron supply for erythropoiesis and adequate endogenous erythropoietin production in the anemia associated with systemic-onset juvenile chronic arthritis. Blood 87: 4824–4830, 1996.
698. Fantini F, Gattinara M, Gerloni V, et al: Severe anemia associated with active systemic-onset juvenile rheumatoid arthritis successfully treated with recombinant human erythropoietin: a pilot study [letter]. Arthritis Rheum 35: 724–726, 1992.
699. Craft AW, Eastham EJ, Bell JI, et al: Serum ferritin in juvenile chronic polyarthritis. Ann Rheum Dis 36: 271–273, 1977.
700. Pelkonen P, Swanljung K, Siimes MA: Ferritinemia as an indicator of systemic disease activity in children with systemic juvenile rheumatoid arthritis. Acta Paediatr Scand 75: 64–68, 1986.
701. Rubin RN, Walker BK, Ballas SK, et al: Erythroid aplasia in juvenile rheumatoid arthritis. Am J Dis Child 132: 760–762, 1978.
702. Ewer AK, Darbyshire PJ, Southwood TR: Systemic-onset juvenile chronic arthritis and bone marrow hypoplasia. Br J Rheumatol 32: 78–80, 1993.
703. Heaton DC, Moller PW: Still's disease associated with Coxsackie infection and haemophagocytic syndrome. Ann Rheum Dis 44: 341–344, 1985.
704. Morris JA, Adamson AR, Holt PJ, et al: Still's disease and the virus-associated haemophagocytic syndrome. Ann Rheum Dis 44: 349–353, 1985.
705. Prieur AM, Fischer A, Griscelli C: Still's disease and haemophagocytic syndrome [letter]. Ann Rheum Dis 44: 806, 1985.
706. Sherry DD, Kredich DW: Transient thrombocytopenia in systemic onset juvenile rheumatoid arthritis. Pediatrics 76: 600–603, 1985.
707. Petty RE, Cassidy JT, Sullivan DB: Serologic studies in juvenile rheumatoid arthritis: a review. Arthritis Rheum 20: 260–267, 1977.
708. Giannini EH, Brewer EJ: Poor correlation between the erythrocyte sedimentation rate and clinical activity in juvenile rheumatoid arthritis. Clin Rheumatol 6: 197–201, 1987.
709. Hussein A, Stein J, Ehrich JH: C-reactive protein in the assessment of disease activity in juvenile rheumatoid arthritis and juvenile spondyloarthritis. Scand J Rheumatol 16: 101–105, 1987.
710. Salmi TT, Schmidt E, Laaksonen AL, et al: Levels of serum immunoglobulins in juvenile rheumatoid arthritis. Ann Clin Res 5: 395–397, 1973.
711. Goel KM, Logan RW, Barnard WP, et al: Serum immunoglobulin and beta 1C-beta 1A globulin concentrations in juvenile rheumatoid arthritis. Ann Rheum Dis 33: 35–38, 1974.
712. Hoyeraal HM, Mellbye OJ: Humoral immunity in juvenile rheumatoid arthritis. Ann Rheum Dis 33: 248–254, 1974.
713. Cassidy JT: Clinical correlations of serum immunoglobulin concentrations in juvenile chronic arthritis. *In* Munthe E (ed): The Care of Rheumatic Children. Basel, EULAR, 1978, p 141.
714. Ogra PL, Chiba Y, Ogra SS, et al: Rubella-virus infection in juvenile rheumatoid arthritis. Lancet 1: 1157–1161, 1975.
715. Linnemann CC Jr, Levinson JE, Buncher CR, et al: Rubella antibody levels in juvenile rheumatoid arthritis. Ann Rheum Dis 34: 354–358, 1975.
716. Schnitzer TJ, Ansell BM, Hawkins GT, et al: Significance of rubella virus infection in juvenile chronic polyarthritis. Ann Rheum Dis 36: 468–470, 1977.
717. Gutowska-Grzegorczyk G, Baum J: Serum immunoglobulin and complement interrelationships in juvenile rheumatoid arthritis. J Rheumatol 4: 179–185, 1977.
718. Gutowska-Grzegorczyk G, Baum J: Antibody levels to enteric bacteria in juvenile rheumatoid arthritis. Arthritis Rheum 20: 779–784, 1977.
719. Hall PJ, de Lange GG, Ansell BM: Immunoglobulin allotypes in families with pauciarticular-onset juvenile chronic arthritis. Tissue Antigens 25: 212–215, 1985.
720. Roberts-Thomson PJ, Shepherd K, Southwood TR, et al: Low molecular weight IgM in juvenile chronic arthritis. Arch Dis Child 63: 1453–1456, 1988.
721. Bywaters EGL, Carter ME, Scott FET: Differential agglutination titre (D.A.T.) in juvenile rheumatoid arthritis. Ann Rheum Dis 18: 225, 1959.
722. Toumbis A, Franklin EC, McEwen C, et al: Clinical and serologic observations in patients with juvenile rheumatoid arthritis and their relatives. J Pediatr 62: 463, 1963.
723. Cassidy JT, Valkenburg HA: A five year prospective study of rheumatoid factor tests in juvenile rheumatoid arthritis. Arthritis Rheum 10: 83–90, 1967.
724. Hanson V, Drexler E, Kornreich H: The relationship of rheumatoid factor to age of onset in juvenile rheumatoid arthritis. Arthritis Rheum 12: 82–86, 1969.
725. Bluestone R, Goldberg LS, Katz RM, et al: Juvenile rheumatoid arthritis—a serologic survey of 200 consecutive patients. J Pediatr 77: 98–102, 1970.
726. Bianco NE, Panush RS, Stillman JS, et al: Immunologic studies of juvenile rheumatoid arthritis. Arthritis Rheum 14: 685–696, 1971.
727. Rudnicki RD, Ruderman M, Scull E, et al: Clinical features and serologic abnormalities in juvenile rheumatoid arthritis. Arthritis Rheum 17: 1007–1015, 1974.
728. Eichenfield AH, Athreya BH, Doughty RA, et al: Utility of rheumatoid factor in the diagnosis of juvenile rheumatoid arthritis. Pediatrics 78: 480–484, 1986.
729. Bowyer S, Roettcher P: Pediatric rheumatology clinic populations in the United States: results of a 3 year survey. Pediatric Rheumatology Database Research Group. J Rheumatol 23: 1968–1974, 1996.
730. Oen K, Schroeder M, Jacobson K, et al: Juvenile rheumatoid arthritis in a Canadian First Nations (aboriginal) population: onset subtypes and HLA associations. J Rheumatol 25: 783–790, 1998.
731. Torrigiani G, Ansell BM, Chown EE, et al: Raised IgG antiglobulin factors in Still's disease. Ann Rheum Dis 28: 424–427, 1969.
732. Munthe E: Anti-IgG and antinuclear antibodies in juvenile rheumatoid arthritis. Scand J Rheumatol 1: 161–170, 1972.
733. Prieur AM, Bach JF, Griscelli C, et al: Rheumatoid rosette in juvenile rheumatoid arthritis. Arch Dis Child 49: 438–442, 1974.
734. Florin-Christensen A, Arana RM, Morteo OG, et al: IgG, IgA, IgM, and IgD antiglobulins in juvenile rheumatoid arthritis. Ann Rheum Dis 33: 32–34, 1974.
735. Schur PH, Bianco NE, Panush RS: Antigammaglobulins in

normal individuals and in patients with adult and juvenile rheumatoid arthritis and osteoarthritis. Rheumatology 6: 156–166, 1975.
736. Miller JJ III, Olds-Arroyo L, Akasaka T: Antiglobulins in juvenile rheumatoid arthritis. Arthritis Rheum 20: 729–735, 1977.
737. Moore TL, Dorner RW: 19S IgM Forssman-type heterophile antibodies in juvenile rheumatoid arthritis. Arthritis Rheum 23: 1262–1267, 1980.
738. Emancipator K, Moore TL, Dorner RW, et al: Hidden and classical 19S IgM rheumatoid factor in a juvenile rheumatoid arthritis patient. J Rheumatol 12: 372–375, 1985.
739. Speiser JC, Moore TL, Weiss TD, et al: Hidden 19S IgM rheumatoid factor in adults with juvenile rheumatoid arthritis onset. Ann Rheum Dis 44: 294–298, 1985.
740. Schlump U, Howard A, Ansell BM: IgG-anti-IgG antibodies in juvenile chronic arthritis. Scand J Rheumatol 14: 65–68, 1985.
741. Moore TL, el-Najdawi E, Dorner RW: IgM rheumatoid factor plaque-forming cells in juvenile rheumatoid arthritis. Arthritis Rheum 30: 335–338, 1987.
742. Magsaam J, Ferjencik P, Tempels M, et al: A new method for the detection of hidden IgM rheumatoid factor in patients with juvenile rheumatoid arthritis. J Rheumatol 14: 964–967, 1987.
742a. Bharadwaj A, Aggarwal A, Misra R: Clinical relevance of IgA rheumatoid factor (RF) in children with juvenile rheumatoid arthritis. Rheumatol Int 19: 47–49, 1999.
743. Ince A, Akhter IM, Moore TL, et al: Hidden 19S IgM rheumatoid factors in Turkish patients with juvenile rheumatoid arthritis. J Rheumatol 25: 190–192, 1999.
744. Aggarwal A, Misra R: Juvenile chronic arthritis in India: is it different from that seen in Western countries? Rheumatol Int 14: 53–56, 1994.
745. Danda D, Naveed M, Misra R: Detection of IgM hidden rheumatoid factor in juvenile rheumatoid arthritis: a novel approach using high performance liquid chromatography. J Indian Rheum Assoc 2(Suppl): 80–84, 1994.
746. Siamopoulou-Mavridou A, Mavridis AK, Terzoglou C, et al: Autoantibodies in Greek juvenile chronic arthritis patients. Clin Exp Rheumatol 9: 647–652, 1991.
747. Haynes DC, Gershwin ME, Robbins DL, et al: Autoantibody profiles in juvenile arthritis. J Rheumatol 13: 358–363, 1986.
748. Malleson PN, Sailer M, Mackinnon MJ: Usefulness of antinuclear antibody testing to screen for rheumatic diseases. Arch Dis Child 77: 299–304, 1997.
749. Kornreich HK, Drexler E, Hanson V: Antinuclear factors in childhood rheumatic diseases. J Pediatr 69: 1039–1045, 1966.
750. Miller JJ, Henrich VL, Brandstrup NE: Sex difference in incidence of antinuclear factors in juvenile rheumatoid arthritis. Pediatrics 38: 916–918, 1966.
751. Alspaugh MA, Miller JJ: A study of specificities of antinuclear antibodies in juvenile rheumatoid arthritis. J Pediatr 90: 391–395, 1977.
752. Permin H, Horbov S, Wiik A, et al: Antinuclear antibodies in juvenile chronic arthritis. Acta Paediatr Scand 67: 181–185, 1978.
753. Patel NJ, Osborn TG, Moore TL: Antinuclear antibodies in juvenile arthritis using the HEp-2 cell substrate. Arthritis Rheum 26:S57, 1983.
754. Rosenberg AM, Cordeiro DM, Knaus RP: Studies on the specificity of antinuclear antibodies in juvenile rheumatoid arthritis. Arthritis Rheum 26:S57, 1983.
755. Osborne TG, Moore TL: Speckled pattern antinuclear antibodies in juvenile rheumatoid arthritis. Arthritis Rheum 28:S56, 1985.
756. McCune WJ, Wise PT, Cassidy JT: A comparison of antibody tests in children with juvenile rheumatoid arthritis. J Rheumatol 13: 980, 1986.
757. Leak AM, Ansell BM, Burman SJ: Antinuclear antibody studies in juvenile chronic arthritis. Arch Dis Child 61: 168–172, 1986.
758. Deane PM, Liard G, Siegel DM, et al: The outcome of children referred to a pediatric rheumatology clinic with a positive antinuclear antibody test but without an autoimmune disease. Pediatrics 95: 892–895, 1995.
759. Craig WY, Ledue TB, Johnson AM, et al: The distribution of antinuclear antibody titers in "normal" children and adults. J Rheumatol 26: 914–919, 1999.
760. Rosenberg AM, Semchuk KM, McDuffie HH, et al: Prevalence of antinuclear antibodies in a rural population. J Toxicol Environ Health 57: 225–236, 1999.
761. Arroyave CM, Giambrone MJ, Rich KC, et al: The frequency of antinuclear antibody (ANA) in children by use of mouse kidney (MK) and human epithelial cells (HEp-2) as substrates. J Allergy Clin Immunol 82: 741–744, 1988.
762. Southwood TR, Malleson PN: Antinuclear antibodies and juvenile chronic arthritis (JCA): search for a specific autoantibody associated with JCA. Ann Rheum Dis 50: 595–598, 1991.
763. Miller JJ III, Hsu YP, Moss R, et al: The immunologic and clinical associations of the split products of C3 in plasma in juvenile rheumatoid arthritis. Arthritis Rheum 22: 502–507, 1979.
764. Hoyeraal HM: Granulocyte reactive antinuclear factors in juvenile rheumatoid arthritis. Scand J Rheumatol 5: 84–90, 1976.
765. Hoyeraal HM, Mellbye OJ: High levels of serum complement factors in juvenile rheumatoid arthritis. Ann Rheum Dis 33: 243–247, 1974.
766. Miller JJ III, Olds LC, Silverman ED, et al: Different patterns of C3 and C4 activation in the varied types of juvenile arthritis. Pediatr Res 20: 1332–1337, 1986.
767. Miller JJ III, Olds LC, Huene DB: Complement activation products and factors influencing phagocyte migration in synovial fluids from children with chronic arthritis. Clin Exp Rheumatol 4: 53–56, 1986.
768. Miller JJ III, Osborne CL, Hsu YP: Clq binding in serum in juvenile rheumatoid arthritis. J Rheumatol 7: 665–670, 1980.
768a. Bhardwaj A, Aggarwal A, Agarwal V, et al: Role of IgM and IgA rheumatoid factors in complement activation in patients with juvenile rheumatoid arthritis. Indian J Med Res 111: 103–109, 2000.
769. Iiowite NT, Samuel P, Beseler L, et al: Dyslipoproteinemia in juvenile rheumatoid arthritis. J Pediatr 114: 823–826, 1989.
770. Bakkaloglu A, Kirel B, Ozen S, et al: Plasma lipids and lipoproteins in juvenile chronic arthritis. Clin Rheumatol 15: 341–345, 1996.
771. Tselepis AD, Elisaf M, Besis S, et al: Association of the inflammatory state in active juvenile rheumatoid arthritis with hypo-high-density lipoproteinemia and reduced lipoprotein-associated platelet-activating factor acetylhydrolase activity. Arthritis Rheum 42: 373–383, 1999.
772. Zuckner J, Baldassare AR, Chang F, et al: High synovial fluid leukocyte counts of noninfectious etiology. Arthritis Rheum Suppl 20: 270, 1977.
773. Baldassare AR, Chang F, Zuckner J: Markedly raised synovial fluid leucocyte counts not associated with infectious arthritis in children. Ann Rheum Dis 37: 404–409, 1978.
774. Harding B, Knight SC: The distribution of dendritic cells in the synovial fluids of patients with arthritis. Clin Exp Immunol 63: 594–600, 1986.
775. Hedberg H: The total complement activity of synovial fluid in juvenile forms of arthritis. Acta Rheumatol Scand 17: 279–285, 1971.
776. Rynes RI, Ruddy S, Spragg J, et al: Intraarticular activation of the complement system in patients with juvenile rheumatoid arthritis. Arthritis Rheum 19: 161–168, 1976.
777. Mollnes TE, Paus A: Complement activation in synovial fluid and tissue from patients with juvenile rheumatoid arthritis. Arthritis Rheum 29: 1359–1364, 1986.
778. Munthe E: Complexes of IgG and IgG rheumatoid factor in synovial tissues of juvenile rheumatoid arthritis. Scand J Rheumatol 1: 153–160, 1972.
779. Martin CL, Pachman LM: Synovial fluid in seronegative juvenile rheumatoid arthritis: studies of immunoglobulins, complements, and alpha 2–macroglobulin. Arthritis Rheum 23: 1256–1261, 1980.
780. Spelling PF, Heise N, Toledo OM: Glycosaminoglycans in the synovial fluids of patients with juvenile rheumatoid arthritis. Clin Exp Rheumatol 9: 195–199, 1991.
781. Poznanski AK: Radiological approaches to pediatric joint disease. J Rheumatol Suppl 33: 78–93, 1992.
782. Reed MH, Wilmot DM: The radiology of juvenile rheumatoid arthritis. A review of the English language literature. J Rheumatol Suppl 31: 2–22, 1991.

783. Fedrizzi MS, Ronchezel MV, Hilario MO, et al: Ultrasonography in the early diagnosis of hip joint involvement in juvenile rheumatoid arthritis. J Rheumatol 24: 1820–1825, 1997.
783a. Lamer S, Sebag GH: MRI and ultrasound in children with juvenile chronic arthritis. Eur J Radiol 33: 85–93, 2000.
784. Goldenstein C, McCauley R, Troy M, et al: Ultrasonography in the evaluation of wrist swelling in children. J Rheumatol 16: 1079–1087, 1989.
785. Viitanen SM, Laaksonen AL: Thermography in juvenile rheumatoid arthritis. Acta Rheumatol Scand 16: 91–98, 1970.
786. Herve-Somma CM, Sebag GH, Prieur AM, et al: Juvenile rheumatoid arthritis of the knee: MR evaluation with Gd-DOTA. Radiology 182: 93–98, 1992.
787. Senac MO Jr, Deutsch D, Bernstein BH, et al: MR imaging in juvenile rheumatoid arthritis. Am J Roentgenol 150: 873–878, 1988.
788. Yulish BS, Lieberman JM, Newman AJ, et al: Juvenile rheumatoid arthritis: assessment with MR imaging. Radiology 165: 149–152, 1987.
789. Verbruggen LA, Shahabpour M, Van Roy P, et al: Magnetic resonance imaging of articular destruction in juvenile rheumatoid arthritis. Arthritis Rheum 33: 1426–1430, 1990.
790. Ruhoy MK, Tucker L, McCauley RG: Hypertrophic bursopathy of the subacromial-subdeltoid bursa in juvenile rheumatoid arthritis: sonographic appearance. Pediatr Radiol 26: 353–355, 1996.
791. Murray JG, Ridley NT, Mitchell N, et al: Juvenile chronic arthritis of the hip: value of contrast-enhanced MR imaging. Clin Radiol 51: 99–102, 1996.
792. Graham TB, Blebea JS, Gylys-Morin V, et al: Magnetic resonance imaging in juvenile rheumatoid arthritis. Semin Arthritis Rheum 27: 161–168, 1997.
793. Ramsey SE, Cairns RA, Cabral DA, et al: Knee magnetic resonance imaging in childhood chronic monarthritis. J Rheumatol 26: 2238–2243, 1999.
794. Cassidy JT, Martel W: Juvenile rheumatoid arthritis: clinicoradiologic correlations. Arthritis Rheum 20: 207–211, 1977.
795. Ansell BM, Kent PA: Radiological changes in juvenile chronic polyarthritis. Skeletal Radiol 1: 129, 1977.
796. Pettersson H, Rydholm U: Radiologic classification of joint destruction in juvenile chronic arthritis. Acta Radiol [Diagn] (Stockh) 26: 719–722, 1985.
797. Williams RA, Ansell BM: Radiological findings in seropositive juvenile chronic arthritis (juvenile rheumatoid arthritis) with particular reference to progression. Ann Rheum Dis 44: 685–693, 1985.
798. Lang BA, Schneider R, Reilly BJ, et al: Radiologic features of systemic onset juvenile rheumatoid arthritis. J Rheumatol 22: 168–173, 1995.
799. Kobayakawa M, Rydholm U, Wingstrand H, et al: Femoral head necrosis in juvenile chronic arthritis. Acta Orthop Scand 60: 164–169, 1989.
800. Badley BWD, Ansell BM: Fractures in Still's disease. Ann Rheum Dis 19: 135, 1960.
801. Elsasser U, Wilkins B, Hesp R, et al: Bone rarefaction and crush fractures in juvenile chronic arthritis. Arch Dis Child 57: 377–380, 1982.
802. Varonos S, Ansell BM, Reeve J: Vertebral collapse in juvenile chronic arthritis: its relationship with glucocorticoid therapy. Calcif Tissue Int 41: 75–78, 1987.
803. Brattstrom M: Asymmetry of ossification and rate of growth of long bones in children with unilateral juvenile gonarthritis. Acta Rheumatol Scand 9: 102, 1963.
804. Brattstrom M, Sundberg J: Juvenile rheumatoid gonarthritis. I. Clinical and roentgenological study. Acta Rheumatol Scand 11: 266–278, 1965.
805. Sundberg J, Brattstrom M: Juvenile rheumatoid gonarthritis. II. Disturbance of ossification and growth. Acta Rheumatol Scand 11: 279–290, 1965.
806. Hensinger RN, DeVito PD, Ragsdale CG: Changes in the cervical spine in juvenile rheumatoid arthritis. J Bone Joint Surg [Am] 68: 189–198, 1986.
807. Locke GR, Gardner JI, Van Epps EF: Atlas-dens interval (ADI) in children: a survey based on 200 normal cervical spines. Am J Roentgenol Radium Ther Nucl Med 97: 135–140, 1966.
808. Hall MA, Burgos VR, Ansell BM: Sacroiliitis in juvenile chronic arthritis. A 10–year follow-up. Clin Exp Rheumatol 5(Suppl 1): S65–S67, 1987.
809. Kuseler A, Pedersen TK, Herlin T, et al: Contrast enhanced magnetic resonance imaging as a method to diagnose early inflammatory changes in the temporomandibular joint in children with juvenile chronic arthritis. J Rheumatol 25: 1406–1412, 1998.
810. Pedersen TK, Herlin T, Melsen B: Non-surgical treatment of the unilateral affection of the temporomandibular joint in children with juvenile chronic arthritis. Clin Exp Rheumatol 11(Suppl 9):S79, 1993.
811. Dabrowski W, Fonseka N, Ansell BM, et al: Shoulder problems in juvenile chronic polyarthritis. Scand J Rheumatol 8: 49–53, 1979.
812. Libby AK, Sherry DD, Dudgeon BJ: Shoulder limitation in juvenile rheumatoid arthritis. Arch Phys Med Rehabil 72: 382–384, 1991.
813. Poznanski AK, Hernandez RJ, Guire KE, et al: Carpal length in children—a useful measurement in the diagnosis of rheumatoid arthritis and some congenital malformation syndromes. Radiology 129: 661–668, 1978.
814. Belt EA, Kaarela K, Kauppi MJ, et al: Assessment of mutilans-like hand deformities in chronic inflammatory joint diseases. A radiographic study of 52 patients. Ann Rheum Dis 58: 250–252, 1999.
815. Hughes RA, Tempos K, Ansell BM: A review of the diagnoses of hip pain presentation in the adolescent. Br J Rheumatol 27: 450–453, 1988.
816. Gabriel H, Fitzgerald SW, Myers MT, et al: MR imaging of hip disorders. Radiographics 14: 763–781, 1994.
817. Fantini F, Corradi A, Gerloni V, et al: The natural history of hip involvement in juvenile rheumatoid arthritis: a radiological and magnetic resonance imaging follow-up study. Rev Rhum Engl Ed 64: 173S–178S, 1997.
818. Patriquin HB, Camerlain M, Trias A: Late sequelae of juvenile rheumatoid arthritis of the hip: a follow-up study into adulthood. Pediatr Radiol 14: 151–157, 1984.
819. Rosberg G, Laine V: Natural history of radiological changes of knee joint in juvenile rheumatoid arthritis. Acta Paediatr Scand 56: 671–675, 1967.
820. Cellerini M, Salti S, Trapani S, et al: Correlation between clinical and ultrasound assessment of the knee in children with mono-articular or pauci-articular juvenile rheumatoid arthritis. Pediatr Radiol 29: 117–123, 1999.
821. Garcia-Morteo O, Gusis SE, Somma LF, et al: Tarsal ankylosis in juvenile and adult onset rheumatoid arthritis. J Rheumatol 15: 298–300, 1988.
822. Remedios D, Martin K, Kaplan G, et al: Juvenile chronic arthritis: diagnosis and management of tibio-talar and sub-talar disease. Br J Rheumatol 36: 1214–1217, 1997.
823. Ansell BM: Treatment of juvenile chronic arthritis. Clin Rheum Dis 1: 443, 1975.
824. Levinson JE: The ideal program for juvenile arthritis. Arthritis Rheum 20: 607–610, 1977.
825. Orozco-Alcala JJ, Baum J: Treatment of juvenile rheumatoid arthritis—a world survey. J Rheumatol 1: 187–189, 1974.
826. Malleson PN: Management of childhood arthritis. Part 1: Acute arthritis. Arch Dis Child 76: 460–462, 1997.
827. Malleson PN: Management of childhood arthritis. Part 2: Chronic arthritis. Arch Dis Child 76: 541–544, 1997.
828. Hobbs N, Perrin JM (eds): Issues in the Care of Children With Chronic Illness. A Source Book on Problems, Services, and Policies. San Francisco, Jossey-Bass, 1985.
829. Hobbs N, Perrin JM, Ireys HT: Chronically Ill Children and Their Families. Problems, Prospects, and Proposals From the Vanderbilt Study. San Francisco, Jossey-Bass, 1985.
830. Rapoff MA, Purviance MR, Lindsley CB: Educational and behavioral strategies for improving medication compliance in juvenile rheumatoid arthritis. Arch Phys Med Rehabil 69: 439–441, 1988.
831. Andre M, Hedengren E, Hagelberg S, et al: Perceived ability to manage juvenile chronic arthritis among adolescents and parents: development of a questionnaire to assess medical issues, exercise, pain, and social support. Arthritis Care Res 12: 229–237, 1999.

832. Chmell MJ, Scott RD, Thomas WH, et al: Total hip arthroplasty with cement for juvenile rheumatoid arthritis. Results at a minimum of ten years in patients less than thirty years old. J Bone Joint Surg [Am] 79: 44–52, 1997.
833. Cron RQ, Sharma S, Sherry DD: Current Treatment by United States and Canadian Pediatric Rheumatologists. J Rheumatol 26: 2036–2038, 1999.
833a. Cassidy JT: Medical management of children with juvenile rheumatoid arthritis. Drugs 58: 831–850, 1999.
834. Levinson JE, Wallace CA: Dismantling the pyramid. J Rheumatol Suppl 33: 6–10, 1992.
835. Kuis W, Wulffraat NM, Prakken AB: New therapeutic strategies in juvenile chronic arthritis. Neth J Med 53: 134–136, 1998.
836. Shaikov AV, Maximov AA, Speransky AI, et al: Repetitive use of pulse therapy with methylprednisolone and cyclophosphamide in addition to oral methotrexate in children with systemic juvenile rheumatoid arthritis—preliminary results of a long-term study. J Rheumatol 19: 612–616, 1992.
837. Lehman TJ: Aggressive therapy for childhood rheumatic diseases. When are immunosuppressives appropriate? Arthritis Rheum 36: 71–74, 1993.
838. Schaller JG: Therapy for childhood rheumatic diseases. Have we been doing enough? Arthritis Rheum 36: 65–70, 1993.
839. Wallace CA, Sherry DD: Trial of intravenous pulse cyclophosphamide and methylprednisolone in the treatment of severe systemic-onset juvenile rheumatoid arthritis. Arthritis Rheum 40: 1852–1855, 1997.
840. Wallace CA: On beyond methotrexate treatment of severe juvenile rheumatoid arthritis. Clin Exp Rheumatol 17: 499–504, 1999.
841. Ruperto N, Levinson JE, Ravelli A, et al: Long-term health outcomes and quality of life in American and Italian inception cohorts of patients with juvenile rheumatoid arthritis. I. Outcome status. J Rheumatol 24: 945–951, 1997.
842. Ruperto N, Ravelli A, Levinson JE, et al: Long-term health outcomes and quality of life in American and Italian inception cohorts of patients with juvenile rheumatoid arthritis. II. Early predictors of outcome. J Rheumatol 24: 952–958, 1997.
843. Petty RE: Prognosis in children with rheumatic diseases: justification for consideration of new therapies. Rheumatology (Oxford) 38: 739–742, 1999.
843a. Ruperto N, Ravelli A, Migliavacca D, et al: Responsiveness of clinical measures in children with oligoarticular juvenile chronic arthritis. J Rheumatol 26: 1827–1830, 1999.
843b. Feldman BM, Grundland B, McCullough L, et al: Distinction of quality of life, health related quality of life, and health status in children referred for rheumatologic care. J Rheumatol 27: 226–233, 2000.
844. Cassidy JT, Johnson JC, Hewett JE, et al: The clinical utility of measures of disease severity in children with juvenile rheumatoid arthritis (JRA). Clin Exp Rheumatol 12:S122, 1994.
845. Ruperto N, Ravelli A, Falcini F, et al: Responsiveness of outcome measures in juvenile chronic arthritis. Italian Pediatric Rheumatology Study Group. Rheumatology (Oxford) 38: 176–180, 1999.
846. Lindsley CB: Uses of nonsteroidal anti-inflammatory drugs in pediatrics. Am J Dis Child 147: 229–236, 1993.
847. Keenan GF, Giannini EH, Athreya BH: Clinically significant gastropathy associated with nonsteroidal antiinflammatory drug use in children with juvenile rheumatoid arthritis. J Rheumatol 22: 1149–1151, 1995.
848. Cryer B, Feldman M: Cyclooxygenase-1 and cyclooxygenase-2 selectivity of widely used nonsteroidal anti-inflammatory drugs. Am J Med 104: 413–421, 1998.
849. Golden BD, Abramson SB: Selective cyclooxygenase-2 inhibitors. Rheum Dis Clin North Am 25: 359–378, 1999.
850. Giannini EH, Lovell DJ, Hepburn B: FDA draft guidelines for the clinical evaluation of antiinflammatory and antirheumatic drugs in children. Executive summary. Arthritis Rheum 38: 715–718, 1995.
851. Lovell DJ, Giannini EH, Brewer EJ Jr: Time course of response to nonsteroidal antiinflammatory drugs in juvenile rheumatoid arthritis. Arthritis Rheum 27: 1433–1437, 1984.
852. Makela AL: Naproxen in the treatment of juvenile rheumatoid arthritis. Metabolism, safety and efficacy. Scand J Rheumatol 6: 193–205, 1977.
853. Moran H, Hanna DB, Ansell BM, et al: Naproxen in juvenile chronic polyarthritis. Ann Rheum Dis 38: 152–154, 1979.
854. Nicholls A, Hazleman B, Todd RM, et al: Long-term evaluation of naproxen suspension in juvenile chronic arthritis. Curr Med Res Opin 8: 204–207, 1982.
855. Laxer RM, Silverman ED, St-Cyr C, et al: A six-month open safety assessment of a naproxen suspension formulation in the therapy of juvenile rheumatoid arthritis. Clin Ther 10: 381–387, 1988.
856. Leak AM, Richter MR, Clemens LE, et al: A crossover study of naproxen, diclofenac and tolmetin in seronegative juvenile chronic arthritis. Clin Exp Rheumatol 6: 157–160, 1988.
857. Levy ML, Barron KS, Eichenfield A, et al: Naproxen-induced pseudoporphyria: a distinctive photodermatitis. J Pediatr 117: 660–664, 1990.
858. Allen R, Rogers M, Humphrey I: Naproxen induced pseudoporphyria in juvenile chronic arthritis. J Rheumatol 18: 893–896, 1991.
859. Lang BA, Finlayson LA: Naproxen-induced pseudoporphyria in patients with juvenile rheumatoid arthritis. J Pediatr 124: 639–642, 1994.
860. Wallace CA, Farrow D, Sherry DD: Increased risk of facial scars in children taking nonsteroidal antiinflammatory drugs. J Pediatr 125: 819–822, 1994.
861. Girschick HJ, Hamm H, Ganser G, et al: Naproxen-induced pseudoporphyria: appearance of new skin lesions after discontinuation of treatment. Scand J Rheumatol 24: 108–111, 1995.
862. Steans A, Manners PJ, Robinson IG: A multicentre, long-term evaluation of the safety and efficacy of ibuprofen syrup in children with juvenile chronic arthritis. Br J Clin Pract 44: 172–175, 1990.
863. Giannini EH, Brewer EJ, Miller ML, et al: Ibuprofen suspension in the treatment of juvenile rheumatoid arthritis. Pediatric Rheumatology Collaborative Study Group. J Pediatr 117: 645–652, 1990.
864. Makela AL, Lempiainen M, Ylijoki H: Ibuprofen levels in serum and synovial fluid. Scand J Rheumatol Suppl 39: 15–17, 1981.
865. Levinson JE, Baum J, Brewer E Jr, et al: Comparison of tolmetin sodium and aspirin in the treatment of juvenile rheumatoid arthritis. J Pediatr 91: 799–804, 1977.
866. Gewanter HL, Baum J: The use of tolmetin sodium in systemic onset juvenile rheumatoid arthritis. Arthritis Rheum 24: 1316–1319, 1981.
867. Todd PA, Sorkin EM: Diclofenac sodium. A reappraisal of its pharmacodynamic and pharmacokinetic properties, and therapeutic efficacy. Drugs 35: 244–285, 1988.
868. Minisola G, Dardano B, Calderazzo L, et al: [Clinical efficacy of sodium diclofenac in chronic juvenile polyarthritis]. Pediatr Med Chir 12: 169–173, 1990.
869. Bhettay E: Double-blind study of sulindac and aspirin in juvenile chronic arthritis. S Afr Med J 70: 724–726, 1986.
870. Ciabattoni G, Cinotti GA, Pierucci A, et al: Effects of sulindac and ibuprofen in patients with chronic glomerular disease. Evidence for the dependence of renal function on prostacyclin. N Engl J Med 310: 279–283, 1984.
871. Whelton A, Hamilton CW: Nonsteroidal anti-inflammatory drugs: effects on kidney function. J Clin Pharmacol 31: 588–598, 1991.
872. Brater DC, Anderson S, Baird B, et al: Effects of ibuprofen, naproxen, and sulindac on prostaglandins in men. Kidney Int 27: 66–73, 1985.
873. Brewer EJ Jr: A comparative evaluation of indomethacin, acetaminophen and placebo as antipyretic agents in children. Arthritis Rheum 11: 645–651, 1968.
874. Sherry DD, Patterson MW, Petty RE: The use of indomethacin in the treatment of pericarditis in childhood. J Pediatr 100: 995–998, 1982.
875. Jacobs JS: Sudden death in arthritic children receiving large doses of indomethacin. JAMA 199: 932–934, 1967.
876. Balduck N, Otten J, Verbruggen L, et al: Sudden death of a child with juvenile chronic arthritis, probably due to indomethacin [letter]. Eur J Pediatr 146: 620, 1987.
877. Williams PL, Ansell BM, Bell A, et al: Multicentre study of piroxicam versus naproxen in juvenile chronic arthritis, with

special reference to problem areas in clinical trials of nonsteroidal anti-inflammatory drugs in childhood. Br J Rheumatol 25: 67–71, 1986.

878. Garcia-Morteo O, Maldonado-Cocco JA, Cuttica R, et al: Piroxicam in juvenile rheumatoid arthritis. Eur J Rheumatol Inflamm 8: 49–53, 1987.
879. Makela AL, Olkkola KT, Mattila MJ: Steady state pharmacokinetics of piroxicam in children with rheumatic diseases. Eur J Clin Pharmacol 41: 79–81, 1991.
880. Athreya BH, Moser G, Cecil HS, et al: Aspirin-induced hepatotoxicity in juvenile rheumatoid arthritis. A prospective study. Arthritis Rheum 18: 347–352, 1975.
881. Miller JJ III, Weissman DB: Correlations between transaminase concentrations and serum salicylate concentration in juvenile rheumatoid arthritis. Arthritis Rheum 19: 115–118, 1976.
882. Bernstein BH, Singsen BH, King KK, et al: Aspirin-induced hepatotoxicity and its effect on juvenile rheumatoid arthritis. Am J Dis Child 131: 659–663, 1977.
883. Rumack B (ed): Aspirin and acetaminophen. Pediatrics (Suppl) 26: 867–946, 1978.
884. Pachman LM, Olufs R, Procknal JA, et al: Pharmacokinetic monitoring of salicylate therapy in children with juvenile rheumatoid arthritis. Arthritis Rheum 22: 826–831, 1979.
885. Poe TE, Mutchie KD, Saunders GH, et al: Total and free salicylate concentrations in juvenile rheumatoid arthritis. J Rheumatol 7: 717–723, 1980.
886. Kvien TK, Olsson B, Hoyeraal HM: Acetylsalicylic acid and juvenile rheumatoid arthritis. Effect of dosage interval on the serum salicylic acid level. Acta Paediatr Scand 74: 755–759, 1985.
887. Weaver AL, Sullivan RE, Kramer WS: Iatrogenic tooth erosions in juvenile rheumatoid arthritis patients. Clin Res 30: 810A, 1982.
888. Tanchyk AP: Prevention of tooth erosion from salicylate therapy in juvenile rheumatoid arthritis. Gen Dent 34: 479–480, 1986.
889. Ulshen MH, Grand RJ, Crain JD, et al: Hepatoxicity with encephalopathy associated with aspirin therapy in rheumatoid arthritis. J Pediatr 93: 1034–1037, 1978.
890. Remington PL, Shabino CL, McGee H, et al: Reye syndrome and juvenile rheumatoid arthritis in Michigan. Am J Dis Child 139: 870–872, 1985.
891. Kauffman RE, Roberts RJ: Aspirin use and Reye syndrome. Pediatrics 79: 1049–1050, 1987.
892. Arrowsmith JB, Kennedy DL, Kuritsky JN, et al: National patterns of aspirin use and Reye syndrome reporting, United States, 1980 to 1985. Pediatrics 79: 858–863, 1987.
893. Hurwitz ES, Barrett MJ, Bregman D, et al: Public Health Service study of Reye's syndrome and medications. Report of the main study. JAMA 257: 1905–1911, 1987.
894. Olson NY, Lindsley CB: Influenza immunization in children with chronic arthritis [letter]. J Rheumatol 21: 1581–1582, 1994.
895. Malleson PN, Tekano JL, Scheifele DW, et al: Influenza immunization in children with chronic arthritis: a prospective study. J Rheumatol 20: 1769–1773, 1993.
896. Prieur AM: Vaccination and rheumatic diseases. Rev Rhum Engl Ed 64: 158S–160S, 1997.
897. Wortmann DW, Kelsch RC, Kuhns L, et al: Renal papillary necrosis in juvenile rheumatoid arthritis. J Pediatr 97: 37–40, 1980.
898. Allen RC, Petty RE, Lirenman DS, et al: Renal papillary necrosis in children with chronic arthritis. Am J Dis Child 140: 20–22, 1986.
899. Ytterberg SR, Mahowald ML, Woods SR: Codeine and oxycodone use in patients with chronic rheumatic disease pain. Arthritis Rheum 41: 1603–1612, 1998.
900. Lovell DJ, Walco GA: Pain associated with juvenile rheumatoid arthritis. Pediatr Clin North Am 36: 1015–1027, 1989.

900a. Schangberg LE, Sandstrom MJ: Causes of pain in children with arthritis. Rheum Dis Clin North Am 25: 31–53, vi, 1999.

901. Truckenbrodt H, Hafner R: Methotrexate therapy in juvenile rheumatoid arthritis: a retrospective study. Arthritis Rheum 29: 801–807, 1986.
902. Speckmaier M, Findeisen J, Woo P, et al: Low-dose methotrexate in systemic onset juvenile chronic arthritis. Clin Exp Rheumatol 7: 647–650, 1989.
903. Halle F, Prieur AM: Evaluation of methotrexate in the treatment of juvenile chronic arthritis according to the subtype. Clin Exp Rheumatol 9: 297–302, 1991.
904. Giannini EH, Brewer EJ, Kuzmina N, et al: Methotrexate in resistant juvenile rheumatoid arthritis. Results of the U.S.A.-U.S.S.R. double-blind, placebo-controlled trial. The Pediatric Rheumatology Collaborative Study Group and The Cooperative Children's Study Group. N Engl J Med 326: 1043–1049, 1992.
905. Lovell DJ: Ten years of experience with methotrexate. Past, present and future. Rev Rhum Engl Ed 64: 186S–188S, 1997.
906. Singsen BH, Goldbach-Mansky R: Methotrexate in the treatment of juvenile rheumatoid arthritis and other pediatric rheumatoid and nonrheumatic disorders. Rheum Dis Clin North Am 23: 811–840, 1997.
907. Giannini EH, Cassidy JT, Brewer EJ, et al: Comparative efficacy and safety of advanced drug therapy in children with juvenile rheumatoid arthritis. Semin Arthritis Rheum 23: 34–46, 1993.
908. Wallace CA: The use of methotrexate in childhood rheumatic diseases. Arthritis Rheum 41: 381–391, 1998.
909. Martini A, Ravelli A, Viola S, et al: Methotrexate hepatotoxic effects in children with juvenile rheumatoid arthritis [letter]. J Pediatr 119: 333–334, 1991.
910. Kugathasan S, Newman AJ, Dahms BB, et al: Liver biopsy findings in patients with juvenile rheumatoid arthritis receiving long-term, weekly methotrexate therapy. J Pediatr 128: 149–151, 1996.
911. Hashkes PJ, Balistreri WF, Bove KE, et al: The long-term effect of methotrexate therapy on the liver in patients with juvenile rheumatoid arthritis. Arthritis Rheum 40: 2226–2234, 1997.
912. Hashkes PJ, Balistreri WF, Bove KE, et al: The relationship of hepatotoxic risk factors and liver histology in methotrexate therapy for juvenile rheumatoid arthritis. J Pediatr 134: 47–52, 1999.
913. Kremer JM, Alarcon GS, Lightfoot RW Jr, et al: Methotrexate for rheumatoid arthritis. Suggested guidelines for monitoring liver toxicity. American College of Rheumatology. Arthritis Rheum 37: 316–328, 1994.
914. Searles G, McKendry RJ: Methotrexate pneumonitis in rheumatoid arthritis: potential risk factors. Four case reports and a review of the literature. J Rheumatol 14: 1164–1171, 1987.
915. Falcini F, Taccetti G, Ermini M, et al: Methotrexate-associated appearance and rapid progression of rheumatoid nodules in systemic-onset juvenile rheumatoid arthritis. Arthritis Rheum 40: 175–178, 1997.
916. Cron RQ, Sherry DD, Wallace CA: Methotrexate-induced hypersensitivity pneumonitis in a child with juvenile rheumatoid arthritis. J Pediatr 132: 901–902, 1998.
917. Camiciottoli G, Trapani S, Castellani W, et al: Effect on lung function of methotrexate and non-steroid anti-inflammatory drugs in children with juvenile rheumatoid arthritis. Rheumatol Int 18: 11–16, 1998.
918. Muzaffer MA, Schneider R, Cameron BJ, et al: Accelerated nodulosis during methotrexate therapy for juvenile rheumatoid arthritis. J Pediatr 128: 698–700, 1996.
919. Wallace CA, Smith AL, Sherry DD: Pilot investigation of naproxen/methotrexate interaction in patients with juvenile rheumatoid arthritis. J Rheumatol 20: 1764–1768, 1993.
920. Hunt PG, Rose CD, McIlvain-Simpson G, et al: The effects of daily intake of folic acid on the efficacy of methotrexate therapy in children with juvenile rheumatoid arthritis. A controlled study. J Rheumatol 24: 2230–2232, 1997.

920a. Ravelli A, Migliavacca D, Viola S, et al: Efficacy of folinic acid in reducing methotrexate toxicity in juvenile idiopathic arthritis. Clin Exp Rheumatol 17: 625–627, 1999.

921. Dupuis LL, Koren G, Silverman ED, et al: Influence of food on the bioavailability of oral methotrexate in children. J Rheumatol 22: 1570–1573, 1995.
922. Albertioni F, Flato B, Seideman P, et al: Methotrexate in juvenile rheumatoid arthritis. Evidence of age dependent pharmacokinetics. Eur J Clin Pharmacol 47: 507–511, 1995.
923. Wallace CA, Bleyer WA, Sherry DD, et al: Toxicity and serum levels of methotrexate in children with juvenile rheumatoid arthritis. Arthritis Rheum 32: 677–681, 1989.
924. Wallace CA, Sherry DD: A practical approach to avoidance of methotrexate toxicity. J Rheumatol 22: 1009–1012, 1995.

925. Wallace CA, Sherry DD: Preliminary report of higher dose methotrexate treatment in juvenile rheumatoid arthritis. J Rheumatol 19: 1604–1607, 1992.
926. Reiff A, Shaham B, Wood BP, et al: High dose methotrexate in the treatment of refractory juvenile rheumatoid arthritis. Clin Exp Rheumatol 13: 113–118, 1995.
927. Ravelli A, Gerloni V, Corona F, et al: Oral versus intramuscular methotrexate in juvenile chronic arthritis. Italian Pediatric Rheumatology Study Group. Clin Exp Rheumatol 16: 181–183, 1998.
928. Rose CD, Singsen BH, Eichenfield AH, et al: Safety and efficacy of methotrexate therapy for juvenile rheumatoid arthritis. J Pediatr 117: 653–659, 1990.
929. Lepore L, Pennesi M: [Treatment with low-dose methotrexate in intractable juvenile chronic arthritis]. Pediatr Med Chir 14: 509–512, 1992.
930. Graham LD, Myones BL, Rivas-Chacon RF, et al: Morbidity associated with long-term methotrexate therapy in juvenile rheumatoid arthritis. J Pediatr 120: 468–473, 1992.
931. Moroldo MB, Giannini EH: Estimates of the discriminant ability of definitions of improvement for juvenile rheumatoid arthritis. J Rheumatol 25: 986–989, 1998.
932. Wallace CA, Sherry DD, Mellins ED, et al: Predicting remission in juvenile rheumatoid arthritis with methotrexate treatment. J Rheumatol 20: 118–122, 1993.
933. Ravelli A, Ramenghi B, Di Fuccia G, et al: Factors associated with response to methotrexate in systemic-onset juvenile chronic arthritis. Acta Paediatr 83: 428–432, 1994.
934. Ravelli A, Viola S, Ramenghi B, et al: Evaluation of response to methotrexate by a functional index in juvenile chronic arthritis. Clin Rheumatol 14: 322–326, 1995.
935. Huang JL: Methotrexate in the treatment of children with chronic arthritis—long-term observations of efficacy and safety. Br J Clin Pract 50: 311–314, 1996.
936. Giannini EH, Cassidy JT: Methotrexate in juvenile rheumatoid arthritis. Do the benefits outweigh the risks? Drug Saf 9: 325–339, 1993.
937. Giannini EH, Cawkwell GD: Drug treatment in children with juvenile rheumatoid arthritis. Past, present, and future. Pediatr Clin North Am 42: 1099–1125, 1995.
938. Gottlieb BS, Keenan GF, Lu T, et al: Discontinuation of methotrexate treatment in juvenile rheumatoid arthritis. Pediatrics 100: 994–997, 1997.
939. Giannini EH, Ruperto N, Ravelli A, et al: Preliminary definition of improvement in juvenile arthritis. Arthritis Rheum 40: 1202–1209, 1997.
940. Ruperto N, Ravelli A, Falcini F, et al: Performance of the preliminary definition of improvement in juvenile chronic arthritis patients treated with methotrexate. Italian Pediatric Rheumatology Study Group. Ann Rheum Dis 57: 38–41, 1998.
941. Cassidy JT: Outcomes research in the therapeutic use of methotrexate in children with chronic peripheral arthritis [editorial]. J Pediatr 133: 179–180, 1998.
942. Harel L, Wagner-Weiner L, Poznanski AK, et al: Effects of methotrexate on radiologic progression in juvenile rheumatoid arthritis. Arthritis Rheum 36: 1370–1374, 1993.
943. Ravelli A, Viola S, Ramenghi B, et al: Radiologic progression in patients with juvenile chronic arthritis treated with methotrexate. J Pediatr 133: 262–265, 1998.
944. Ravelli A, Viola S, Ramenghi B, et al: Frequency of relapse after discontinuation of methotrexate therapy for clinical remission in juvenile rheumatoid arthritis. J Rheumatol 22: 1574–1576, 1995.
944a. Ravelli A, Viola S, Migliavacca D, et al: The extended oligoarticular subtype is the best predictor of methotrexate efficacy in juvenile idiopathic arthritis. J Pediatr 135: 316–320, 1999.
945. Grondin C, Malleson P, Petty RE: Slow-acting antirheumatic drugs in chronic arthritis of childhood. Semin Arthritis Rheum 18: 38–47, 1988.
946. Rosenberg AM: Treatment of juvenile rheumatoid arthritis: approach to patients who fail standard therapy. J Rheumatol 23: 1652–1656, 1996.
947. Laaksonen AL, Koskiahde V, Juva K: Dosage of antimalarial drugs for children with juvenile rheumatoid arthritis and systemic lupus erythematosus. A clinical study with determination of serum concentrations of chloroquine and hydroxychloroquine. Scand J Rheumatol 3: 103–108, 1974.
948. Stillman JS: Antimalarials in the treatment of juvenile rheumatoid arthritis. *In* Moore TD (ed): Arthritis in Childhood. Columbus, Ohio, Ross Laboratories, 1981, p 125.
949. Kvien TK, Hoyeraal HM, Sandstad B: Slow acting antirheumatic drugs in patients with juvenile rheumatoid arthritis—evaluated in a randomized, parallel 50-week clinical trial. J Rheumatol 12: 533–539, 1985.
950. Brewer EJ, Giannini EH, Kuzmina N, et al: Penicillamine and hydroxychloroquine in the treatment of severe juvenile rheumatoid arthritis. Results of the U.S.A.-U.S.S.R. double-blind placebo-controlled trial. N Engl J Med 314: 1269–1276, 1986.
951. Rynes RI: Ophthalmologic considerations in using antimalarials in the United States. Lupus 5(Suppl 1): S73–S74, 1996.
952. Rynes RI: Antimalarial drugs in the treatment of rheumatological diseases. Br J Rheumatol 36: 799–805, 1997.
953. Sassaman FW, Cassidy JT, Alpern M, et al: Electroretinography in patients with connective tissue diseases treated with hydroxychloroquine. Am J Ophthalmol 70: 515–523, 1970.
954. Bernstein HN: Ocular safety of hydroxychloroquine. Ann Ophthalmol 23: 292–296, 1991.
955. Houpt JB: A rheumatologist's verdict on the safety of chloroquine versus hydroxychloroquine. Liability in off-label prescribing. J Rheumatol 26: 1864–1866, 1999.
956. Easterbrook M: An opthalmological view on the efficacy and safety of chloroquine versus hydroxychloroquine. J Rheumatol 26: 1866–1868, 1999.
957. Esdaile JM: More thoughts about antimalarials: should one prescribe chloroquine? J Rheumatol 26: 1868, 1999.
958. Van Kerckhove C, Giannini EH, Lovell DJ: Temporal patterns of response to D-penicillamine, hydroxychloroquine, and placebo in juvenile rheumatoid arthritis patients. Arthritis Rheum 31: 1252–1258, 1988.
959. Giannini EH, Brewer EJ, Kuzmina N, et al: Characteristics of responders and nonresponders to slow-acting antirheumatic drugs in juvenile rheumatoid arthritis. Arthritis Rheum 31: 15–20, 1988.
960. Wallace DJ, Metzger AL, Stecher VJ, et al: Cholesterol-lowering effect of hydroxychloroquine in patients with rheumatic disease: reversal of deleterious effects of steroids on lipids. Am J Med 89: 322–326, 1990.
961. Sairanen E, Laaksonen AL: The toxicity of gold therapy in children suffering from rheumatoid arthritis. Ann Paediatr Fenn 8: 105, 1962.
962. Sairanen E, Laaksonen AL: The results of gold therapy in juvenile rheumatoid arthritis. Ann Paediatr Fenn 10: 274, 1963.
963. Hicks RM, Hanson V, Kornreich HK: The use of gold in the treatment of juvenile rheumatoid arthritis. Arthritis Rheum 13: 323, 1970.
964. Debendetti C, Tretbar H, Corrigan JJ Jr: Gold therapy in juvenile rheumatoid arthritis. Ariz Med 33: 373–376, 1976.
965. Levinson JE, Balz GP, Bondi S: Gold therapy. Arthritis Rheum 20: 531–535, 1977.
966. Makela AL, Peltola O, Makela P: Gold serum levels in children with juvenile rheumatoid arthritis. Scand J Rheumatol 7: 161–165, 1978.
967. Brewer EJ Jr, Giannini EH, Barkley E: Gold therapy in the management of juvenile rheumatoid arthritis. Arthritis Rheum 23: 404–411, 1980.
968. Ansell BM, Hall MA, Ribero S: A comparative study of gold and penacillamine in seropositive juvenile chronic arthritis (juvenile rheumatoid arthritis). Ann Rheum Dis 40: 522, 1981.
969. Ansell BM, Hall MA: Penicillamine in chronic arthritis of childhood. J Rheumatol Suppl 7: 112–115, 1981.
970. Kvien TK, Hoyeraal HM, Sandstad B: Gold sodium thiomalate and D-penicillamine. A controlled, comparative study in patients with pauciarticular and polyarticular juvenile rheumatoid arthritis. Scand J Rheumatol 14: 346–354, 1985.
971. The Research Subcommittee of the Empire Rheumatism Council: Gold therapy in rheumatoid arthritis. Final report of a multicentre controlled trial. Ann Rheum Dis 20: 315–333, 1961.
972. Aaron S, Davis P, Percy J: Neutropenia occurring during the course of chrysotherapy: a review of 25 cases. J Rheumatol 12: 897–899, 1985.

973. Wooley PH, Griffin J, Panayi GS, et al: HLA-DR antigens and toxic reaction to sodium aurothiomalate and D-penicillamine in patients with rheumatoid arthritis. N Engl J Med 303: 300–302, 1980.
974. Clarkson RW, Sanders PA, Grennan DM: Complement C4 null alleles as a marker of gold or D-penicillamine toxicity in the treatment of rheumatoid arthritis. Br J Rheumatol 31: 53–54, 1992.
975. Brewer EJ Jr, Giannini EH, Person DA: Early experiences with auranofin in juvenile rheumatoid arthritis. Am J Med 75: 152–156, 1983.
976. Giannini EH, Brewer EJ Jr, Person DA: Auranofin in the treatment of juvenile rheumatoid arthritis. J Pediatr 102: 138–141, 1983.
977. Giannini EH, Brewer EJ, Person DA, et al: Longterm auranofin therapy in patients with juvenile rheumatoid arthritis. J Rheumatol 13: 768–770, 1986.
978. Kvien TK, Hoyeraal HM, Sandstad B, et al: Auranofin therapy in juvenile rheumatoid arthritis: a 48–week phase II study. Scand J Rheumatol Suppl 63: 79–83, 1986.
979. Brewer EJ, Giannini EH: Oral gold (auranofin) in juvenile rheumatoid arthritis—results of the double-blind, placebo controlled trial. Arthritis Rheum 30:S31, 1987.
980. Giannini EH, Brewer EJ Jr, Kuzmina N, et al: Auranofin in the treatment of juvenile rheumatoid arthritis. Results of the USA-USSR double-blind, placebo-controlled trial. The USA Pediatric Rheumatology Collaborative Study Group. The USSR Cooperative Children's Study Group. Arthritis Rheum 33: 466–476, 1990.
981. Ansell BM, Hall MA, Loftus JK, et al: A multicentre pilot study of sulphasalazine in juvenile chronic arthritis. Clin Exp Rheumatol 9: 201–203, 1991.
982. Imundo LF, Jacobs JC: Sulfasalazine therapy for juvenile rheumatoid arthritis. J Rheumatol 23: 360–366, 1996.
983. van Rossum MA, Fiselier TJ, Franssen MJ, et al: Sulfasalazine in the treatment of juvenile chronic arthritis: a randomized, double-blind, placebo-controlled, multicenter study. Dutch Juvenile Chronic Arthritis Study Group. Arthritis Rheum 41: 808–816, 1998.
984. Huang JL, Chen LC: Sulphasalazine in the treatment of children with chronic arthritis. Clin Rheumatol 17: 359–363, 1998.
984a. Varbanova BB, Dyankov ED: Sulphasalazine. An alternative drug for second-line treatment of juvenile chronic arthritis. Adv Exp Med Biol 455: 331–336, 1999.
985. Ozdogan H, Turunc M, Deringol B, et al: Sulphasalazine in the treatment of juvenile rheumatoid arthritis: a preliminary open trial. J Rheumatol 13: 124–125, 1986.
986. Hertzberger-ten Cate R, Cats A: Toxicity of sulfasalazine in systemic juvenile chronic arthritis. Clin Exp Rheumatol 9: 85–88, 1991.
987. Enzenauer RJ, West SG, Rubin RL: D-Penicillamine–induced lupus erythematosus. Arthritis Rheum 33: 1582–1585, 1990.
988. Schairer H, Stoeber E: Long-term follow-up of 235 cases of juvenile rheumatoid arthritis treated with D-penicillamine. *In* Munthe E (ed): Penicillamine Research in Rheumatoid Disease. Oslo, Fabricius and Sonner, 1977, pp 279–281.
989. Prieur AM, Piussan C, Manigne P, et al: Evaluation of D-penicillamine in juvenile chronic arthritis. A double-blind, multicenter study. Arthritis Rheum 28: 376–382, 1985.
990. Prieur AM: The place of corticosteroid therapy in juvenile chronic arthritis in 1992. J Rheumatol Suppl 37: 32–34, 1993.
991. Southwood TR: Report from a symposium on corticosteroid therapy in juvenile chronic arthritis. Clin Exp Rheumatol 11: 91–94, 1993.
992. Schaller JG: Corticosteroids in juvenile rheumatoid arthritis. Arthritis Rheum 20: 537–543, 1977.
993. Stoeber E: Juvenile chronic polyarthritis and Still's syndrome. Doc Geigy 1: 1–20, 1977.
994. Ansell BM, Bywaters EG: Alternate-day corticosteroid therapy in juvenile chronic polyarthritis. J Rheumatol 1: 176–186, 1974.
995. Axelrod L: Glucocorticoid therapy. Medicine (Baltimore) 55: 39–65, 1976.
996. Loftus J, Allen R, Hesp R, et al: Randomized, double-blind trial of deflazacort versus prednisone in juvenile chronic (or rheumatoid) arthritis: a relatively bone-sparing effect of deflazacort. Pediatrics 88: 428–436, 1991.
997. Falcini F, Trapani S, Ermini M, et al: Deflazacort in pediatric rheumatic diseases needs a frequent follow-up of bone densitometry [letter]. Pediatrics 95: 318, 1995.
998. Slocumb CH: Relative cortisone deficiency simulating exacerbation of arthritis. Bull Rheum Dis 3: 21, 1952.
999. Miller JJ III: Prolonged use of large intravenous steroid pulses in the rheumatic diseases of children. Pediatrics 65: 989–994, 1980.
1000. Oppermann J, Mobius D: Therapeutical and immunological effects of methylprednisolone pulse therapy in comparison with intravenous immunoglobulin. Treatment in patients with juvenile chronic arthritis. Acta Univ Carol [Med] (Praha) 40: 117–121, 1994.
1001. Picco P, Gattorno M, Buoncompagni A, et al: 6–Methylprednisolone 'mini-pulses': a new modality of glucocorticoid treatment in systemic onset juvenile chronic arthritis. Scand J Rheumatol 25: 24–27, 1996.
1002. Adebajo AO, Hall MA: The use of intravenous pulsed Methylprednisolone in the treatment of systemic-onset juvenile chronic arthritis. Br J Rheumatol 37: 1240–1242, 1998.
1003. Klein-Gitelman MS, Pachman LM: Intravenous corticosteroids: adverse reactions are more variable than expected in children. J Rheumatol 25: 1995–2002, 1998.
1004. Allen RC, Gross KR, Laxer RM, et al: Intraarticular triamcinolone hexacetonide in the management of chronic arthritis in children. Arthritis Rheum 29: 997–1001, 1986.
1005. Earley A, Cuttica RJ, McCullough C, et al: Triamcinolone into the knee joint in juvenile chronic arthritis. Clin Exp Rheumatol 6: 153–155, 1988.
1006. Sparling M, Malleson P, Wood B, et al: Radiographic followup of joints injected with triamcinolone hexacetonide for the management of childhood arthritis. Arthritis Rheum 33: 821–826, 1990.
1007. Dent PB, Walker N: Intra-articular corticosteroids in the treatment of juvenile rheumatoid arthritis. Curr Opin Rheumatol 10: 475–480, 1998.
1008. Bird HA, Ring EF, Bacon PA: A thermographic and clinical comparison of three intra-articular steroid preparations in rheumatoid arthritis. Ann Rheum Dis 38: 36–39, 1979.
1008a. Yang MH, Lee WI, Chen LC, et al: Intraarticular triamcinolone hexacetonide injection in children with chronic arthritis: a survey of clinical practice. Taiwan Erh Ko I hsueh Hui Tsa Chih 40: 182–185, 1999.
1009. Huppertz HI, Tschammler A, Horwitz AE, Schwab KO: Intraarticular corticosteroids for chronic arthritis in children: efficacy and effects on cartilage growth. J Pediatr 127: 317–321, 1995.
1010. Cassidy JT, Bole GG: Cutaneous atrophy secondary to intraarticular corticosteroid administration. Ann Intern Med 65: 1008–1018, 1966.
1011. Padeh S, Passwell JH: Intraarticular corticosteroid injection in the management of children with chronic arthritis. Arthritis Rheum 41: 1210–1214, 1998.
1012. Gilsanz V, Bernstein BH: Joint calcification following intraarticular corticosteroid therapy. Radiology 151: 647–649, 1984.
1013. Hertzberger-ten Cate R, Jung I, Bos CF: Septa within the suprapatellar region blocking intra-articular steroids in pauciarticular juvenile chronic arthritis. Clin Exp Rheumatol 10: 93–94, 1992.
1014. Sherry DD, Stein LD, Reed AM, et al: Prevention of leg length discrepancy in young children with pauciarticular juvenile rheumatoid arthritis by treatment with intraarticular steroids. Arthritis Rheum 42: 2330–2334, 1999.
1015. Stein LD, Roifman CM: Intravenous immunoglobulin therapy. Bull Rheum Dis 44: 3–5, 1995.
1016. Prieur AM: Intravenous immunoglobulins in Still's disease: still controversial, still unproven. J Rheumatol 23: 797–800, 1996.
1017. Silverman ED, Cawkwell GD, Lovell DJ, et al: Intravenous immunoglobulin in the treatment of systemic juvenile rheumatoid arthritis: a randomized placebo controlled trial. Pediatric Rheumatology Collaborative Study Group. J Rheumatol 21: 2353–2358, 1994.
1018. Giannini EH, Lovell DJ, Silverman ED, et al: Intravenous immunoglobulin in the treatment of polyarticular juvenile rheu-

matoid arthritis: a phase I/II study. Pediatric Rheumatology Collaborative Study Group. J Rheumatol 23: 919–924, 1996.
1019. Groothoff JW, van Leeuwen EF: High dose intravenous gammaglobulin in chronic systemic juvenile arthritis. Br Med J (Clin Res Ed) 296: 1362–1363, 1988.
1020. Silverman ED, Laxer RM, Greenwald M, et al: Intravenous gamma globulin therapy in systemic juvenile rheumatoid arthritis. Arthritis Rheum 33: 1015–1022, 1990.
1021. Uziel Y, Laxer RM, Schneider R, et al: Intravenous immunoglobulin therapy in systemic onset juvenile rheumatoid arthritis: a followup study. J Rheumatol 23: 910–918, 1996.
1022. Prieur AM, Adleff A, Debre M, et al: High dose immunoglobulin therapy in severe juvenile chronic arthritis: long-term follow-up in 16 patients. Clin Exp Rheumatol 8: 603–608, 1990.
1023. Savolainen HA, Kautiainen H, Isomaki H, et al: Azathioprine in patients with juvenile chronic arthritis: a longterm followup study. J Rheumatol 24: 2444–2450, 1997.
1024. Laxer RM: Long-term toxicity of immune suppression in juvenile rheumatic diseases. Rheumatology (Oxford) 38: 743–746, 1999.
1025. Kvien TK, Hoyeraal HM, Sandstad B: Azathioprine versus placebo in patients with juvenile rheumatoid arthritis: a single center double blind comparative study. J Rheumatol 13: 118–123, 1986.
1025a. Lin YT, Yang YH, Tsai MJ, et al: Long-term effects of azathioprine therapy for juvenile rheumatoid arthritis. J Formos Med Assoc 99: 330–335, 2000.
1026. Savolainen HA, Isomaki HA: Decrease in the number of deaths from secondary amyloidosis in patients with juvenile rheumatoid arthritis. J Rheumatol 20: 1201–1203, 1993.
1027. Ansell BM: Chlorambucil therapy in juvenile chronic arthritis (juvenile idiopathic arthritis). J Rheumatol 26: 765–766, 1999.
1028. Ansell BM, Eghtedari A, Bywaters EG: Chlorambucil in the management of juvenile chronic polyarthritis complicated by amyloidosis. Ann Rheum Dis 30: 331, 1971.
1029. Deschenes G, Prieur AM, Hayem F, et al: Renal amyloidosis in juvenile chronic arthritis: evolution after chlorambucil treatment. Pediatr Nephrol 4: 463–469, 1990.
1030. Rostropowicz-Denisiewicz K: Some remarks on management of juvenile chronic arthritis complicated by amyloidosis. Acta Univ Carol [Med] (Praha) 40: 91–94, 1994.
1031. Savolainen HA: Chlorambucil in severe juvenile chronic arthritis: longterm followup with special reference to amyloidosis. J Rheumatol 26: 898–903, 1999.
1032. David J: Amyloidosis in juvenile chronic arthritis. Clin Exp Rheumatol 9: 73–78, 1991.
1033. Prieur AM, Balafrej M, Griscelli C, et al: [Results and long-term risks of immuno-suppressive treatment in chronic juvenile arthritis. Apropos of 40 cases]. Rev Rhum Mal Osteoartic 46: 85–90, 1979.
1034. Buriot D, Prieur AM, Lebranchu Y, et al: [Acute leukemia in 3 children with chronic juvenile arthritis treated with chlorambucil]. Arch Fr Pediatr 36: 592–598, 1979.
1035. Rozman B: Clinical experience with leflunomide in rheumatoid arthritis. Leflunomide Investigators' Group. J Rheumatol Suppl 53: 27–32, 1998.
1036. Weaver A, Caldwell J, Olsen N: Treatment of active rheumatoid arthritis with leflunomide compared to placebo or methotrexate. Arthritis Rheum 41:S131, 1998.
1037. Weinblatt ME, Kremer JM, Coblyn JS, et al: Pharmacokinetics, safety, and efficacy of combination treatment with methotrexate and leflunomide in patients with active rheumatoid arthritis. Arthritis Rheum 42: 1322–1328, 1999.
1038. Bjerkhoel F, Forre O: Cyclosporin treatment of a patient with severe systemic juvenile rheumatoid arthritis. Scand J Rheumatol 17: 483–486, 1988.
1039. Ostensen M, Hoyeraal HM, Kass E: Tolerance of cyclosporine A in children with refractory juvenile rheumatoid arthritis. J Rheumatol 15: 1536–1538, 1988.
1040. Reiff A, Rawlings DJ, Shaham B, et al: Preliminary evidence for cyclosporin A as an alternative in the treatment of recalcitrant juvenile rheumatoid arthritis and juvenile dermatomyositis. J Rheumatol 24: 2436–2443, 1997.
1041. Myers BD, Ross J, Newton L, et al: Cyclosporine-associated chronic nephropathy. N Engl J Med 311: 699–705, 1984.
1042. Rogers AJ, Yoshimura N, Kerman RH, et al: Immunopharmacodynamic evaluation of cyclosporine-treated renal allograft recipients. Transplantation 38: 657–664, 1984.
1043. Palestine AG, Austin HA III, Balow JE, et al: Renal histopathologic alterations in patients treated with cyclosporine for uveitis. N Engl J Med 314: 1293–1298, 1986.
1044. van den Borne BE, Landewe RB, Houkes I, et al: No increased risk of malignancies and mortality in cyclosporin A-treated patients with rheumatoid arthritis. Arthritis Rheum 41: 1930–1937, 1998.
1045. Lovell DJ, Giannini EH, Reiff A, et al: Etanercept in children with polyarticular juvenile rheumatoid arthritis. Pediatric Rheumatology Collaborative Study Group. N Engl J Med 342: 763–769, 2000.
1046. Keystone EC: The role of tumor necrosis factor antagonism in clinical practice. J Rheumatol 26(Suppl)57: 22–28, 1999.
1047. Moreland LW: Inhibitors of tumor necrosis factor for rheumatoid arthritis. J Rheumatol 26(Suppl 57): 7–15, 1999.
1048. Moreland LW, Schiff MH, Baumgartner SW, et al: Etanercept therapy in rheumatoid arthritis. A randomized, controlled trial. Ann Intern Med 130: 478–486, 1999.
1049. Weinblatt ME, Kremer JM, Bankhurst AD, et al: A trial of etanercept, a recombinant tumor necrosis factor receptor: Fc fusion protein, in patients with rheumatoid arthritis receiving methotrexate. N Engl J Med 340: 253–259, 1999.
1050. Kietz D, Pepmueller PH, Moore TL: Clinical response to etanercept in polyarticular course JRA. J Rheumatol 28: 360–362, 2001.
1051. Elliott MJ, Maini RN, Feldmann M, et al: Randomised double-blind comparison of chimeric monoclonal antibody to tumour necrosis factor alpha (cA2) versus placebo in rheumatoid arthritis. Lancet 344: 1105–1110, 1994.
1052. Elliott MJ, Maini RN, Feldmann M, et al: Repeated therapy with monoclonal antibody to tumour necrosis factor alpha (cA2) in patients with rheumatoid arthritis. Lancet 344: 1125–1127, 1994.
1053. Maini RN, Elliott M, Brennan FM, et al: Targeting TNF alpha for the therapy of rheumatoid arthritis. Clin Exp Rheumatol 12(Suppl 11): S63–S66, 1994.
1054. Elliott MJ, Woo P, Charles P, et al: Suppression of fever and the acute-phase response in a patient with juvenile chronic arthritis treated with monoclonal antibody to tumour necrosis factor-alpha (cA2). Br J Rheumatol 36: 589–593, 1997.
1055. Maini RN, Breedveld FC, Kalden JR, et al: Therapeutic efficacy of multiple intravenous infusions of anti-tumor necrosis factor alpha monoclonal antibody combined with low-dose weekly methotrexate in rheumatoid arthritis. Arthritis Rheum 41: 1552–1563, 1998.
1056. Choy EH, Kingsley GH, Panayi GS: Monoclonal antibody therapy in rheumatoid arthritis. Br J Rheumatol 37: 484–490, 1998.
1057. Rau R, Sander O, den Broeder A, et al: Long-term efficacy and tolerability of multiple I.V. doses of a fully human anti-TNF-antibody D2E7 in patients with rheumatoid arthritis. Arthritis Rheum 41:S55, 1998.
1057a. Pisetsky DS: Tumor necrosis factor blockers in rheumatoid arthritis. N Engl J Med 342: 810–811, 2000.
1058. Messner RP: The potential of bone marrow stem cell transplantation in the treatment of autoimmune diseases [editorial]. J Rheumatol 24: 819–821, 1997.
1059. Tyndall A, Gratwohl A: Bone marrow transplantation in the treatment of autoimmune diseases. Br J Rheumatol 36: 1–3, 1997.
1060. Wulffraat NM, Vlieger A, Brinkman JP, et al: Autologous stem cell transplantation (ASCT) in refractory polyarticular and systemic JCA. Arthritis Rheum 41:S129, 1998.
1061. Quartier P, Prieur AM, Fischer A: Haemopoietic stem-cell transplantation for juvenile chronic arthritis. Lancet 353: 1885–1886, 1999.
1062. Kuis W, Wulffraat NM, Petty RE: Autologous stem cell transplantation: an alternative for refractory juvenile chronic arthritis. Rheumatology (Oxford) 38: 737–738, 1999.
1063. Wulffraat NM, Kuis W: Autologous stem cell transplantation: a possible treatment for refractory juvenile chronic arthritis? Rheumatology (Oxford) 38: 764–766, 1999.
1064. Wulffraat NM, Kuis W, Petty R: Addendum: proposed guide-

lines for autologous stem cell transplantation in juvenile chronic arthritis. Paediatric Rheumatology Workshop. Rheumatology (Oxford) 38: 777–778, 1999.

1064a. Vossen JM, Brinkman DM, Bakker B, et al: Rationale for high-dose cyclophosphamide and medium-dose total body irradiation in the conditioning of children with progressive systemic and polyarticular juvenile chronic arthritis before autologous stem cell transplantation. Rheumatology (Oxford) 38: 762–763, 1999.

1064b. Tyndall A, Millikan S: Bone marrow transplantation. Baillieres Best Pract Res Clin Rheumatol 13: 719–735, 1999.

1065. Hoyeraal HM, Froland SS, Salvesen CF, et al: No effect of transfer factor in juvenile rheumatoid arthritis by double-blind trial. Ann Rheum Dis 37: 175–179, 1978.

1066. Prieur AM, Buriot D, Lefur JM, et al: Possible toxicity of levamisole in children with rheumatoid arthritis. J Pediatr 93: 304–305, 1978.

1067. Bardare M, Corona F, Ogliari MT, et al: Thymopentin in the treatment of juvenile chronic arthritis. Clin Exp Rheumatol 8: 89–93, 1990.

1068. Pernice W, Schuchmann L, Dippell J, et al: Therapy for systemic juvenile rheumatoid arthritis with gamma-interferon: a pilot study of nine patients. Arthritis Rheum 32: 643–646, 1989.

1069. Coto C, Varela G, Hernandez V, et al: Use of recombinant interferon gamma in pediatric patients with advanced juvenile chronic arthritis. Biotherapy 11: 15–20, 1998.

1070. Lepore L, Agosti E, Pitacco F, et al: [Therapy with plasmapheresis and lymphoplasmapheresis combined with immunosuppressive agents in 2 cases of intractable juvenile rheumatoid arthritis]. Pediatr Med Chir 9: 321–324, 1987.

1071. Field EH, Strober S, Hoppe RT, et al: Sustained improvement of intractable rheumatoid arthritis after total lymphoid irradiation. Arthritis Rheum 26: 937–946, 1983.

1072. Barnett ML, Combitchi D, Trentham DE: A pilot trial of oral type II collagen in the treatment of juvenile rheumatoid arthritis. Arthritis Rheum 39: 623–628, 1996.

1073. McKown KM, Carbone LD, Kaplan SB, et al: Lack of efficacy of oral bovine type II collagen added to existing therapy in rheumatoid arthritis. Arthritis Rheum 42: 1204–1208, 1999.

1074. Allen DB, Blizzard RM, Rosenfeld RG: The use—and misuse—of growth hormone. Contemp Pediatr 12: 45–50, 53, 1995.

1075. Butenandt O: Rheumatoid arthritis and growth retardation in children: treatment with human growth hormone. Eur J Pediatr 130: 15–28, 1979.

1076. Allen R, Jimenez M, Cowell C: Physiologic growth hormone secretion and somatomedin levels in juvenile rheumatoid arthritis. Arthritis Rheum Suppl 31:S118, 1988.

1076a. Chikanaza IC: Neuroendocrine immune features of pediatric inflammatory rheumatic diseases. Ann N Y Acad Sci 876: 71–80, 1999.

1076b. Tsatsoulis A, Simaopoulou A, Petsoukis C, et al: Study of growth hormone secretion and action in growth-retarded children with juvenile chronic arthritis (JCA). Growth Horm IGF Res 9: 143–149, 1999.

1077. Bennett AE, Silverman ED, Miller JJ III, et al: Insulin-like growth factors I and II in children with systemic onset juvenile arthritis. J Rheumatol 15: 655–658, 1988.

1078. Hopp RJ, Degan J, Corley K, et al: Evaluation of growth hormone secretion in children with juvenile rheumatoid arthritis and short stature. Nebr Med J 80: 52–57, 1995.

1079. Touati G, Prieur AM, Ruiz JC, et al: Beneficial effects of one-year growth hormone administration to children with juvenile chronic arthritis on chronic steroid therapy. I. Effects on growth velocity and body composition. J Clin Endocrinol Metab 83: 403–409, 1998.

1080. Svantesson H: Treatment of growth failure with human growth hormone in patients with juvenile chronic arthritis. A pilot study. Clin Exp Rheumatol 9(Suppl 6): 47–50, 1991.

1081. Allen DB, Goldberg BD: Stimulation of collagen synthesis and linear growth by growth hormone in glucocorticoid-treated children. Pediatrics 89: 416–421, 1992.

1082. Simon D, Touati G, Prieur AM, et al: Growth hormone treatment of short stature and metabolic dysfunction in juvenile chronic arthritis. Acta Paediatr Suppl 88: 100–105, 1999.

1083. Manfredi R, Tumietto F, Azzaroli L, et al: Growth hormone (GH) and the immune system: impaired phagocytic function in children with idiopathic GH deficiency is corrected by treatment with biosynthetic GH. J Pediatr Endocrinol 7: 245–251, 1994.

1084. Broyer M, Guest G, Crosnier H, et al: Recombinant growth hormone in children after renal transplantation. Societe Francaise de Nephrologie Pediatrique. Lancet 343: 539–540, 1994.

1085. Crosnier H, Guest G, Souberbielle JC, et al: [Treatment with recombinant human growth hormone (rhGH) in children with chronic kidney failure or renal transplantation]. Arch Pediatr 1: 716–722, 1994.

1086. Cheung NW, Liddle C, Coverdale S, et al: Growth hormone treatment increases cytochrome P450–mediated antipyrine clearance in man. J Clin Endocrinol Metab 81: 1999–2001, 1996.

1087. Mortensen AL, Allen JR, Allen RC: Nutritional assessment of children with juvenile chronic arthritis. J Paediatr Child Health 26: 335–338, 1990.

1088. Henderson CJ, Lovell DJ, Specker BL, et al: Physical activity in children with juvenile rheumatoid arthritis: quantification and evaluation. Arthritis Care Res 8: 114–119, 1995.

1089. Knops N, Wulffraat N, Lodder S, et al: Resting energy expenditure and nutritional status in children with juvenile rheumatoid arthritis. J Rheumatol 26: 2039–2043, 1999.

1090. Henderson CJ, Lovell DJ: Nutritional aspects of juvenile rheumatoid arthritis. Rheum Dis Clin North Am 17: 403–413, 1991.

1091. Johnston CC Jr, Miller JZ, Slemenda CW, et al: Calcium supplementation and increases in bone mineral density in children. N Engl J Med 327: 82–87, 1992.

1092. Chan GM: Dietary calcium and bone mineral status of children and adolescents. Am J Dis Child 145: 631–634, 1991.

1093. Chanetsa F, Hillman L, Cassidy JT: Fractional calcium absorption in children with juvenile rheumatoid arthritis supplemented with vitamin D. J Rheumatol 27(Suppl 58): 94, 1999.

1094. Hillman LS, Chanetsa F, Popescu M, et al: Calcium and vitamin D supplementation in children with JRA. Arthritis Rheum 42: 1999.

1095. Als OS, Gotfredsen A, Riis BJ, et al: Are disease duration and degree of functional impairment determinants of bone loss in rheumatoid arthritis? Ann Rheum Dis 44: 406–411, 1985.

1096. Hopp R, Degan J, Gallagher JC, et al: Estimation of bone mineral density in children with juvenile rheumatoid arthritis. J Rheumatol 18: 1235–1239, 1991.

1097. Kotaniemi A, Savolainen A, Kroger H, et al: Weight-bearing physical activity, calcium intake, systemic glucocorticoids, chronic inflammation, and body constitution as determinants of lumbar and femoral bone mineral in juvenile chronic arthritis. Scand J Rheumatol 28: 19–26, 1999.

1098. Falcini F, Trapani S, Ermini M, et al: Intravenous administration of alendronate counteracts the in vivo effects of glucocorticoids on bone remodeling. Calcif Tissue Int 58: 166–169, 1996.

1099. Bianchi ML, Cimaz R, Bardare M, et al: Efficacy and safety of alendronate for the treatment of osteoporosis in diffuse connective tissue diseases in children: a prospective multicenter study. Arthritis Rheum 43: 1960–1966, 2000.

1099a. Rooney M, Davies UM, Reeve J, et al: Bone mineral content and bone mineral metabolism: Changes after growth hormone treatment in juvenile chronic arthritis. J Rheumatol 27: 1073–1081, 2000.

1099b. Touati G, Ruiz JC, Porquet D, et al: Effects on bone metabolism of one year recombinant human growth hormone administration to children with juvenile chronic arthritis undergoing chronic steroid therapy. J Rheumatol 27: 1287–1293, 2000.

1100. Donovan WH: Physical measures in the treatment of juvenile rheumatoid arthritis. Arthritis Rheum 20: 553–557, 1977.

1101. Scull SA, Dow MB, Athreya BH: Physical and occupational therapy for children with rheumatic diseases. Pediatr Clin North Am 33: 1053–1077, 1986.

1102. Emery HM, Kucinski J: Management of Juvenile Rheumatoid Arthritis. A Handbook for Occupational and Physical Therapists. Chicago, LaRabida Children's Hospital and Research Center, 1987.

1103. Fan JS, Wessel J, Ellsworth J: The relationship between strength and function in females with juvenile rheumatoid arthritis. J Rheumatol 25: 1399–1405, 1998.

1104. Singsen BH: Physical fitness in children with juvenile rheuma-

toid arthritis and other chronic pediatric illnesses. Pediatr Clin North Am 42: 1035–1050, 1995.
1105. Malleson PN, Bennett SM, Mackinnon M, et al: Physical fitness and its relationship to other indices of health status in children with chronic arthritis. J Rheumatol 23: 1059–1065, 1996.
1106. Wessel J, Kaup C, Fan J: Isometric strength measurements in children with arthritis: reliability and relation to function. Arthritis Care Res 12: 238–246, 1999.
1106a. Klepper SE: Effects of an eight-week physical conditioning program on disease signs and symptoms in children with chronic arthritis. Arthritis Care Res 12: 52–60, 1999.
1107. Hackett J, Johnson B, Parkin A, et al: Physiotherapy and occupational therapy for juvenile chronic arthritis: custom and practice in five centres in the UK, USA and Canada. Br J Rheumatol 35: 695–699, 1996.
1108. Lechner DE, McCarthy CF, Holden MK: Gait deviations in patients with juvenile rheumatoid arthritis. Phys Ther 67: 1335–1341, 1987.
1109. Frigo C, Bardare M, Corona F, et al: Gait alterations in patients with juvenile chronic arthritis: a computerized analysis. J Orthop Rheumatol 9: 82–90, 1996.
1110. Arden GP, Ansell BM (eds): Surgical Management of Juvenile Chronic Polyarthritis. London, Academic Press, 1978.
1111. Arden GP: Surgical treatment of juvenile rheumatoid arthritis. Ann Chir Gynaecol Suppl 198: 103–109, 1985.
1112. Greene WB: Surgical alternatives for adolescents with severe arthritis. Bull Rheum Dis 43: 3–5, 1994.
1113. Pahle JA: Orthopaedic management of juvenile chronic arthritis (JCA). Z Rheumatol 55: 376–387, 1996.
1114. Swann M: The surgery of juvenile chronic arthritis. An overview. Clin Orthop 259: 70–75, 1990.
1115. Hamalainen M: Surgical treatment of juvenile rheumatoid arthritis. Clin Exp Rheumatol 12(Suppl 10): S107–S112, 1994.
1116. Price CT: Are we there yet? Management of limb-length inequality. J Pediatr Orthop 16: 141–143, 1996.
1117. Rydholm U, Brattstrom H, Bylander B, et al: Stapling of the knee in juvenile chronic arthritis. J Pediatr Orthop 7: 63–68, 1987.
1118. Fink CW, Baum J, Paradies LH, et al: Synovectomy in juvenile rheumatoid arthritis. Ann Rheum Dis 28: 612–616, 1969.
1119. Eyring EJ, Longert A, Bass JC: Synovectomy in juvenile rheumatoid arthritis. Indications and short-term results. J Bone Joint Surg [Am] 53: 638–651, 1971.
1120. Granberry WM, Brewer EJ Jr: Results of synovectomy in children with rheumatoid arthritis. Clin Orthop 101: 120–126, 1974.
1121. Granberry WM: Synovectomy in juvenile rheumatoid arthritis. Arthritis Rheum 20: 561–564, 1977.
1122. Jacobsen ST, Levinson JE, Crawford AH: Late results of synovectomy in juvenile rheumatoid arthritis. J Bone Joint Surg [Am] 67: 8–15, 1985.
1123. Rydholm U, Elborgh R, Ranstam J, et al: Synovectomy of the knee in juvenile chronic arthritis. A retrospective, consecutive follow-up study. J Bone Joint Surg [Br] 68: 223–228, 1986.
1124. Swann M, Ansell BM: Soft-tissue release of the hips in children with juvenile chronic arthritis. J Bone Joint Surg [Br] 68: 404–408, 1986.
1125. Kvien TK, Pahle JA, Hoyeraal HM, et al: Comparison of synovectomy and no synovectomy in patients with juvenile rheumatoid arthritis. A 24–month controlled study. Scand J Rheumatol 16: 81–91, 1987.
1126. Rydholm U: Arthroscopy of the knee in juvenile chronic arthritis. Scand J Rheumatol 15: 109–112, 1986.
1127. Paus A, Pahle JA: The value of arthroscopy in the diagnosis and treatment of patients with juvenile rheumatoid arthritis. Ann Chir Gynaecol 75: 168–171, 1986.
1128. Gattinara M, Lomater C, Paresce E, et al: Arthroscopic synovectomy of the knee joint in the treatment of patients with juvenile chronic arthritis. Acta Univ Carol [Med] (Praha) 40: 113–115, 1994.
1129. Rydholm U, Brattstrom H, Lidgren L: Soft tissue release for knee flexion contracture in juvenile chronic arthritis. J Pediatr Orthop 6: 448–451, 1986.
1130. Sledge CB: Joint replacement surgery in juvenile rheumatoid arthritis. Arthritis Rheum 20: 567–572, 1977.
1131. Arden GP, Ansell BM, Hunter MJ: Total hip replacement in juvenile chronic polyarthritis and ankylosing spondylitis. Clin Orthop 84: 130–136, 1972.
1132. Singsen BH, Isaacson AS, Bernstein BH, et al: Total hip replacement in children with arthritis. Arthritis Rheum 21: 401–406, 1978.
1133. Crowe W, Hausleman C, Shear S, et al: Total hip arthroplasty in children with juvenile rheumatoid arthritis. Arthritis Rheum 22: 602, 1979.
1134. Colville J, Raunio P: Total hip replacement in juvenile rheumatoid arthritis. Analysis of 59 hips. Acta Orthop Scand 50: 197–203, 1979.
1135. Lachiewicz PF, McCaskill B, Inglis A, et al: Total hip arthroplasty in juvenile rheumatoid arthritis. Two to eleven-year results. J Bone Joint Surg [Am] 68: 502–508, 1986.
1136. Ruddlesdin C, Ansell BM, Arden GP, et al: Total hip replacement in children with juvenile chronic arthritis. J Bone Joint Surg [Br] 68: 218–222, 1986.
1137. Gudmundsson GH, Harving S, Pilgaard S: The Charnley total hip arthroplasty in juvenile rheumatoid arthritis patients. Orthopedics 12: 385–388, 1989.
1138. Hamalainen M: Surgical treatment of the hip and knee joint in juvenile rheumatoid arthritis. Ryumachi 33: 473, 1993.
1139. McCullough CJ: Surgical management of the hip in juvenile chronic arthritis. Br J Rheumatol 33: 178–183, 1994.
1140. Lehtimaki MY, Lehto MU, Kautiainen H, et al: Survivorship of the Charnley total hip arthroplasty in juvenile chronic arthritis. A follow-up of 186 cases for 22 years. J Bone Joint Surg [Br] 79: 792–795, 1997.
1141. Lehtimaki MY, Kautiainen H, Hamalainen MM, et al: Hip involvement in seropositive rheumatoid arthritis. Survivorship analysis with a 15-year follow-up. Scand J Rheumatol 27: 406–409, 1998.
1142. Haber D, Goodman SB: Total hip arthroplasty in juvenile chronic arthritis: a consecutive series. J Arthroplasty 13: 259–265, 1998.
1143. Rydholm U, Boegard T, Lidgren L: Total knee replacement in juvenile chronic arthritis. Scand J Rheumatol 14: 329–335, 1985.
1144. Carmichael E, Chaplin DM: Total knee arthroplasty in juvenile rheumatoid arthritis. A seven-year follow-up study. Clin Orthop 210: 192–200, 1986.
1144a. Lyback CO, Belt EA, Hamalainen MM, et al: Survivorship of AGC knee replacement in juvenile chronic arthritis: 13-year follow-up of 77 knees. J Arthroplasty 15: 166–170, 2000.
1145. Harrison SH: Wrist and hand problems and their management. *In* Arden GP, Ansell BM (eds): Surgical Management of Juvenile Chronic Arthritis. London, Academic Press, 1978, p 161.
1146. Guyuron B: Facial deformity of juvenile rheumatoid arthritis. Plast Reconstr Surg 81: 948–951, 1988.
1147. Myall RW, West RA, Horwitz H, et al: Jaw deformity caused by juvenile rheumatoid arthritis and its correction. Arthritis Rheum 31: 1305–1310, 1988.
1148. Arthritis Foundation: We Can: A Guide for Parents of Children with Arthritis. Atlanta, Arthritis Foundation, 1985.
1149. Athreya BH, McCormick MC: Impact of chronic illness on families. Rheum Dis Clin North Am 13: 123–131, 1987.
1150. Meenan RF: Health status assessment in pediatric rheumatology. Rheum Dis Clin North Am 13: 133–140, 1987.
1151. Brewer EJ Jr, Angel KC: Parenting a Child With Arthritis. Los Angeles, Lowell House, 1992.
1152. Barlow J, Shaw KL, Southwood TR: Do psychosocial interventions have a role to play in paediatric rheumatology? Br J Rheumatol 37: 573–578, 1998.
1153. Tucker LB, Denardo BA, Stebulis JA, et al: Your Child With Arthritis. A Family Guide for Caregiving. Baltimore, Johns Hopkins Press, 1999.
1154. Surgeon General's Report: Children with Special Health Care Needs. Commitment to: Family-centered, Community-based, Coordinated Care. Rockville, MD, U.S. Department of Health and Human Services, 1987.
1155. Rapoff MA, Lindsley CB, Christophersen ER: Parent perceptions of problems experienced by their children in complying with treatments for juvenile rheumatoid arthritis. Arch Phys Med Rehabil 66: 427–429, 1985.
1156. Kroll T, Barlow JH, Shaw K: Treatment adherence in juvenile rheumatoid arthritis—a review. Scand J Rheumatol 28: 10–18, 1999.

1157. Cleveland SE, Reitman EE, Brewer EJ Jr: Psychological factors in juvenile rheumatoid arthritis. Arthritis Rheum 8: 1152–1158, 1965.
1158. Morse J: Aspiration and achievement. A study of one hundred patients with juvenile rheumatoid arthritis. Rehabil Lit 33: 290–303, 1972.
1159. King K, Hanson V: Psychosocial aspects of juvenile rheumatoid arthritis. Pediatr Clin North Am 33: 1221–1237, 1986.
1160. Keltikangas-Jarvinen L: Body-image disturbances ensuing from juvenile rheumatoid arthritis, a preliminary study. Percept Mot Skills 64: 984, 1987.
1161. Ungerer JA, Horgan B, Chaitow J, et al: Psychosocial functioning in children and young adults with juvenile arthritis. Pediatrics 81: 195–202, 1988.
1162. Whitehouse R, Shope J, Kulik CL: Psychosocial functioning in children and young adults with juvenile rheumatoid arthritis. Arthritis Rheum 25:S11, 1982.
1163. Whitehouse R, Shope JT, Graham-Tomasi G, et al: Educational needs of school personnel working with children with juvenile rheumatoid arthritis. Arthritis Rheum 26:S84, 1983.
1164. Spencer CH, Zanga J, Passo M, et al: The child with arthritis in the school setting. Pediatr Clin North Am 33: 1251–1264, 1986.
1165. White PH, McPherson M, Levinson JE: Community programs for children with rheumatic diseases. Pediatr Clin North Am 33: 1239–1249, 1986.
1166. Taylor J, Passo MH, Champion VL: School problems and teacher responsibilities in juvenile rheumatoid arthritis. J Sch Health 57: 186–190, 1987.
1167. Cassidy JT, Lindsley CB: Legal rights of children with musculoskeletal disabilities. Bull Rheum Dis 45: 1–5, 1996.
1168. Cope C, Anderson E: Special Units in Disabled Schools. Studies in Education. London, Institute of Education, University of London, 1977.
1169. Sturge C, Garralda ME, Boissin M, et al: School attendance and juvenile chronic arthritis. Br J Rheumatol 36: 1218–1223, 1997.
1170. McAnarney ER, Pless IB, Satterwhite B, et al: Psychological problems of children with chronic juvenile arthritis. Pediatrics 53: 523–528, 1974.
1171. Weil-Halpern F, Rapoport D, Hatt A, et al: La polyarthrite chronique de l'enfant dans la structure hospitalière. Etude psychosociologique. La consultation. Ann Pediatr 22: 499, 1975.
1172. Mozziconacci P: Pour une "prise en charge psychologique" des polyarthrites juvéniles. Ann Pediatr 23: 415, 1976.
1173. Weil-Halpern F, Rapoport D, Hatt A, et al: La polyarthrite chronique juvénile dans la structure hospitalière. Etude psy-cho-sociologique. L'hospitalisation. Ann Pediatr 23: 420, 1976.
1174. Hatt A, Weil-Halpern F, Rapoport D, et al: La polyarthrite chronique juvénile dans la structure hospitalière. Etude psychologique des enfants atteints. Ann Pediatr 23: 429, 1976.
1175. Rapoport D, Hatt A, Weil-Halpern F, et al: La polyarthrite chronique juvénile dans la structure hospitalière. IV. Etude psychologique des enfants atteints. Ann Pediatr 23: 437, 1976.
1176. Tursz A: La polyarthrite chronique juvenile dans la structure hospitaliere. V. Scolarite, vie sociale et familiale. Ann Pediatr 23: 442, 1976.
1177. Peterson LS, Mason T, Nelson AM, et al: Psychosocial outcomes and health status of adults who have had juvenile rheumatoid arthritis: a controlled, population-based study. Arthritis Rheum 40: 2235–2240, 1997.
1178. Frank RG, Hagglund KJ, Schopp LH, et al: Disease and family contributors to adaptation in juvenile rheumatoid arthritis and juvenile diabetes. Arthritis Care Res 11: 166–176, 1998.
1179. Frank RG, Thayer JF, Hagglund KJ, et al: Trajectories of adaptation in pediatric chronic illness: the importance of the individual. J Consult Clin Psychol 66: 521–532, 1998.
1180. Pless IB, Satterwhite B, Van Vechten D: Division, duplication and neglect: patterns of care for children with chronic disorders. Child Care Health Dev 4: 9–19, 1978.
1181. Ansell BM, Bywaters EGL: Prognosis in Still's disease. Bull Rheum Dis 9: 189, 1959.
1182. Allen RC, Ansell BM: Juvenile chronic arthritis—clinical subgroups with particular relationship to adult patterns of disease. Postgrad Med J 62: 821–826, 1986.
1183. Gare BA, Fasth A: The natural history of juvenile chronic arthritis: a population based cohort study. I. Onset and disease process. J Rheumatol 22: 295–307, 1995.
1184. Gare BA, Fasth A: The natural history of juvenile chronic arthritis: a population based cohort study. II. Outcome. J Rheumatol 22: 308–319, 1995.
1184a. Ansell BM: Prognosis in juvenile arthritis. Adv Exp Med Biol 455: 27–33, 1999.
1184b. Minden K, Kiessling U, Listing J, et al: Prognosis of patients with juvenile chronic arthritis and juvenile spondyloarthropathy. J Rheumatol 27: 2256–2263, 2000.
1185. Dequeker J, Mardjuadi A: Prognostic factors in juvenile chronic arthritis. J Rheumatol 9: 909–915, 1982.
1186. Goel KM, Shanks RA: Follow-up study of 100 cases of juvenile rheumatoid arthritis. Ann Rheum Dis 33: 25–31, 1974.
1187. Hanson V, Kornreich H, Bernstein B, et al: Prognosis of juvenile rheumatoid arthritis. Arthritis Rheum 20: 279–284, 1977.
1188. Stoeber E: Prognosis in juvenile chronic arthritis. Follow-up of 433 chronic rheumatic children. Eur J Pediatr 135: 225–228, 1981.
1189. Michels H, Hafner R, Morhart R, et al: Five year follow-up of a prospective cohort of juvenile chronic arthritis with recent onset. Clin Rheumatol 6(Suppl 2): 87–92, 1987.
1190. Billings AG, Moos RH, Miller JJ III, et al: Psychosocial adaptation in juvenile rheumatic disease: a controlled evaluation. Health Psychol 6: 343–359, 1987.
1191. Jeremy R, Schaller J, Arkless R, et al: Juvenile rheumatoid arthritis persisting into adulthood. Am J Med 45: 419–434, 1968.
1192. Ansell BM: Still's disease followed into adult life. Proc R Soc Med 62: 912, 1969.
1193. Hill RH, Herstein A, Walters K: Juvenile rheumatoid arthritis: follow-up into adulthood—medical, sexual and social status. Can Med Assoc J 114: 790–796, 1976.
1194. FitzGerald O, Bresnihan B: Juvenile chronic arthritis: spectrum of disease in an adult rheumatology department. Ir J Med Sci 155: 266–271, 1986.
1194a. Zak M, Pedersen FK: Juvenile chronic arthritis into adulthood: a long-term follow-up study. Rheumatology (Oxford) 39: 198–204, 2000.
1194b. Cuesta IA, Kerr K, Simpson P, et al: Subspecialty referrals for pauciarticular juvenile rheumatoid arthritis. Arch Pediatr Adolesc Med 154: 122–125, 2000.
1195. Burgos-Vargas R: Assessment of quality of life in children with rheumatic disease. J Rheumatol 26: 1432–1435, 1999.
1196. David J, Cooper C, Hickey L, et al: The functional and psychological outcomes of juvenile chronic arthritis in young adulthood. Br J Rheumatol 33: 876–881, 1994.
1197. Hutchison T: The classification of disability. Arch Dis Child 73: 91–93, 1995.
1197a. Rapoff MA, Lindsley CB: The pain puzzle: a visual and conceptual metaphor for understanding and treating pain in pediatric rheumatic disese. J Rheumatol 27(Suppl 58): 29–33, 2000.
1198. Flato B, Aasland A, Vinje O, et al: Outcome and predictive factors in juvenile rheumatoid arthritis and juvenile spondyloarthropathy. J Rheumatol 25: 366–375, 1998.
1199. Aasland A, Flato B, Vandvik IH: Psychosocial outcome in juvenile chronic arthritis: a nine-year follow-up. Clin Exp Rheumatol 15: 561–568, 1997.
1200. Carter BD, Kronenberger WG, Edwards JF, et al: Psychological symptoms in chronic fatigue and juvenile rheumatoid arthritis. Pediatrics 103: 975–979, 1999.
1200a. Huygen AC, Kuis W, Sinnema G: Psychological, behavioural, and social adjustment in children and adolescents with juvenile chronic arthritis. Ann Rheum Dis 59: 276–282, 2000.
1200b. Noll RB, Kozlowski K, Gerhardt C, et al: Social, emotional, and behavioral functioning of children with juvenile rheumatoid arthritis. Arthritis Rheum 43: 1387–1396, 2000.
1201. Hagglund KJ, Clay DL, Frank RG, et al: Assessing anger expression in children and adolescents. J Pediatr Psychol 19: 291–304, 1994.
1202. Cassidy JT, Johnson JC, Hewett JE, et al: Parental distress in families of children with juvenile rheumatoid arthritis. Arthritis Rheum 37:S405, 1994.
1203. Spencer CH, Fife RZ, Rabinovich CE: The school experience of children with arthritis. Coping in the 1990s and transition into adulthood. Pediatr Clin North Am 42: 1285–1298, 1995.

1204. Chamberlain MA, Rooney CM: Young adults with arthritis: meeting their transitional needs. Br J Rheumatol 35: 84–90, 1996.
1205. White PH: Future expectations: adolescents with rheumatic diseases and their transition into adulthood. Br J Rheumatol 35: 80–83, 1996.
1206. White PH: Resilience in children with disabilities—transition to adulthood. J Rheumatol 23: 960–962, 1996.
1207. White PH: Success on the road to adulthood. Issues and hurdles for adolescents with disabilities. Rheum Dis Clin North Am 23: 697–707, 1997.
1208. Baum J, Gutowska G: Death in juvenile rheumatoid arthritis. Arthritis Rheum Suppl 20: 253, 1977.
1209. Bernstein B: Death in juvenile rheumatoid arthritis. Arthritis Rheum Suppl 20: 256, 1977.
1210. Woo P: Amyloidosis in pediatric rheumatic diseases. J Rheumatol Suppl 35: 10–16, 1992.
1211. Gwyther M, Schwarz H, Howard A, et al: C-reactive protein in juvenile chronic arthritis: an indicator of disease activity and possibly amyloidosis. Ann Rheum Dis 41: 259–262, 1982.
1212. Burman SJ, Hall PJ, Bedford PA, et al: HLA antigen frequencies among patients with juvenile chronic arthritis and amyloidosis: a brief report. Clin Exp Rheumatol 4: 261–263, 1986.
1213. Woo P, O'Brien J, Robson M, et al: A genetic marker for systemic amyloidosis in juvenile arthritis. Lancet 2: 767–769, 1987.
1214. Calabro JJ: Amyloidosis and juvenile rheumatoid arthritis. J Pediatr 75: 521, 1969.
1215. Schnitzer TJ, Ansell BM: Amyloidosis in juvenile chronic polyarthritis. Arthritis Rheum 20: 245–252, 1977.
1216. Hawkins PN, Myers MJ, Lavender JP, et al: Diagnostic radionuclide imaging of amyloid: biological targeting by circulating human serum amyloid P component. Lancet 1: 1413–1418, 1988.
1217. Hawkins PN, Richardson S, Vigushin DM, et al: Serum amyloid P component scintigraphy and turnover studies for diagnosis and quantitative monitoring of AA amyloidosis in juvenile rheumatoid arthritis. Arthritis Rheum 36: 842–851, 1993.
1218. Bywaters EGL: Deaths in juvenile chronic polyarthritis. Arthritis Rheum Suppl 20: 256, 1977.
1219. Arden GP: Sepsis in juvenile chronic polyarthritis. *In* Arden GP, Ansell BM (eds): Surgical Management of Juvenile Chronic Polyarthritis. London, Academic Press, 1978, p 225.
1220. David J, Vouyiouka O, Ansell BM, et al: Amyloidosis in juvenile chronic arthritis: a morbidity and mortality study. Clin Exp Rheumatol 11: 85–90, 1993.
1221. Cabral DA, Petty RE, Malleson PN, et al: Visual prognosis in children with chronic anterior uveitis and arthritis. J Rheumatol 21: 2370–2375, 1994.

13

Juvenile Ankylosing Spondylitis

Ross E. Petty and James T. Cassidy

SPONDYLOARTHROPATHY

Definition and Classification

The term *spondyloarthropathy* is used traditionally to refer to a group of rheumatic diseases that affect the joints of the axial skeleton (as well as peripheral joints) and that differ from juvenile rheumatoid arthritis (JRA) in many ways. Wright and Moll[1] introduced the term *spondarthritis* to include ankylosing spondylitis (AS), psoriatic arthritis, Reiter's disease, ulcerative colitis, Crohn's disease, juvenile chronic arthritis, Whipple's disease, Behçet's syndrome, reactive arthritis, and acute anterior uveitis. They noted that patients with these conditions lacked rheumatoid factor (RF) and subcutaneous nodules but had inflammatory peripheral arthritis; many had radiologic sacroiliac arthritis with or without AS. They also observed a tendency toward a familial aggregation of such diseases. It is the familiality of these disorders, based on the presence of the histocompatibility antigen (HLA)-B27, that currently unites the somewhat smaller group included under the title *seronegative spondyloarthritis*: AS, the arthritides of inflammatory bowel disease (IBD), reactive arthritis including Reiter's syndrome, and psoriatic arthritis.

There are several reasons for grouping these disorders together under the heading of spondyloarthropathy:

- Inflammation of the joints of the axial skeleton (spine and sacroiliac joints) and of entheses is a clinical feature frequently exhibited by members of this group of diseases that is seldom observed in the other chronic arthritides such as JRA.
- Relatives of children with juvenile ankylosing spondylitis (JAS) commonly have AS, psoriatic arthritis, IBD, or less commonly, Reiter's syndrome. This genetic influence is related to the high frequency of HLA-B27 in patients with spondyloarthritis.
- A number of extra-articular features are shared by several diseases in this group. Iritis, usually acute, occurs in all members of the group. The cutaneous manifestations of psoriasis and Reiter's syndrome may be indistinguishable.
- RFs are absent, and other autoantibodies are infrequent.

Thus, although individual members of the spondyloarthropathy group differ from each other, they share characteristics that distinguish them from the disease complex of JRA and other connective tissue diseases (Table 13–1). However, this grouping does not recognize the heterogeneity within each of the four disease categories, particularly psoriatic arthritis and the arthritides of IBD. Thus, only some of the patients with psoriasis and arthritis have involvement of the axial joints, and most children with arthritis related to IBD have peripheral arthritis rather than spinal involvement.

In the system of classification of juvenile idiopathic arthritides proposed by the International League of

Table 13–1

Overlapping Characteristics of the Spondyloarthropathies

	ENTHESITIS	AXIAL ARTHRITIS	PERIPHERAL ARTHRITIS	B27-POSITIVE	ANA-POSITIVE	RF-POSITIVE	SYSTEMIC DISEASE: Iritis	Skin	MM	GI
JAS	+ + +	+ + +	+ + +	+ + +	−	−	+	−	−	−
JPsA	+	+ +	+ + +	+	+ +	−	+	+ + +	−	−
IBD	+	+ +	+ + +	+ +	−	−	+	+	+	+ + + +
RS	+ +	+	+ + +	+ + +	−	−	+	+	+	+ + +

ANA, antinuclear antibodies; GI, gastrointestinal tract; IBD, inflammatory bowel disease; JAS, juvenile ankylosing spondylitis; JPsA, juvenile psoriatic arthritis; MM, mucous membranes; RF, rheumatoid factor; RS, Reiter's syndrome.

−, absent; +, <25%; + +, 25–50%; + + +, 50–75%; + + + +, 75% or more.

Table 13–2

SEA Syndrome: Classification Criteria

Onset of musculoskeletal symptoms before age 17 yr
Absence of rheumatoid factors and antinuclear antibodies
Presence of enthesitis
Presence of arthralgia or arthritis

SEA, seronegativity, enthesitis, arthritis.

From Rosenberg AM, Petty RE: A syndrome of seronegative enthesopathy and arthropathy in children. Arthritis Rheum 25: 1041, Copyright © 1982 Wiley-Liss, Inc. Reprinted by permission of Wiley-Liss, Inc., a subsidiary of John Wiley & Sons, Inc.

Associations for Rheumatology (ILAR),[2, 3] the dilemma of classification of these diseases is dealt with by recognizing enthesitis-related arthritis (ERA) and juvenile psoriatic arthritis as separate categories. Within the ERA category, attention is given to arthritis related to IBD. Reactive arthritis is not included within the juvenile idiopathic arthritides because these disorders are known to be caused by immune reactions to specific infections. (See Chapter 11 for further discussion of the subject of classification of childhood arthritis.)

In addition to the extra-articular signs and symptoms in Table 13–1, recognition of the syndrome of seronegativity, enthesitis, and arthritis (SEA syndrome),[4] which is an early manifestation of many patients with a spondyloarthropathy, assists in the identification of affected children—in many, if not most, of whom sacroiliac arthritis, particularly JAS, will eventually develop.

Seronegativity, Enthesitis, and Arthritis (SEA Syndrome)

Many children with SEA syndrome have some of the characteristics of JAS but lack the sacroiliac joint changes needed to confirm a diagnosis by accepted criteria (New York criteria).[5] In 1982, a group of 39 such children, representing approximately 20 percent of a pediatric rheumatic disease clinic population, were described as having the SEA syndrome (Table 13–2).[4] These children were seronegative (lacked RFs and antinuclear antibodies [ANAs]), had enthesitis (usually around the heel or knee), and had arthritis of a few joints, particularly the large and small joints of the lower extremities. Table 13–3 is a comparison of children with the SEA syndrome and those with JRA or JAS.

Entheses—the sites of attachment of ligament, tendon, fascia, or capsule to bone—are characteristic sites of inflammation in the spondyloarthropathies. Although the presence of exquisite, well-localized tenderness at characteristic entheses strongly suggests spondyloarthropathy, it must be noted that enthesitis occurs occasionally in JRA and even in systemic lupus erythematosus; such findings could also be confused with other noninflammatory conditions such as Osgood-Schlatter disease and Sever's disease. The ultimate diagnosis in a child with idiopathic SEA syndrome cannot be evident until development of the full clinical spectrum of disease over the course of time. The disorder remits in some children, and they will presumably never develop a diagnosable seronegative spondyloarthropathy. Others progress to JRA or systemic lupus erythematosus. It seems probable, however, that most will be diagnosed as having JAS (Fig. 13–1).

Of the 39 children with SEA syndrome in the original report, 8 had bilateral sacroiliitis consistent with a diagnosis of JAS; 2 each had IBD and reactive arthritis; and 1 had Reiter's syndrome.[4] The remaining 26 children had idiopathic SEA syndrome—no other rheumatic disease being identified. The striking similarities of this group of patients and those with JAS with regard to age, sex, mean number of affected joints, and family history of arthritis and back symptoms suggested that the SEA syndrome might be an early or mild form of JAS. The high frequency of HLA-B27 in both groups further supported this possibility.

A follow-up study of 36 of these children a mean of 11 years after onset indicated that they experienced a varied course.[6] Twelve of the 23 patients (52 percent) who did not have a definite spondyloarthropathy at the time of the original report now had definite or possible spondyloarthropathy. The presence of HLA-B27 (62 percent, $P < .004$) and arthritis (as opposed to arthralgia, $P < .05$) and the onset of disease after the age of 5 years ($P < .01$) correlated with the evolution of idiopathic SEA syndrome to an identifiable spondyloarthropathy. Overall, 64 percent had definite or possible spondyloarthropathy, 10 percent JRA, 13 percent noninflammatory diseases, and 5 percent continuing idiopathic SEA syndrome.

Burgos-Vargas and Clark[7] described a group of Mexican children with the SEA syndrome who developed an inexora-

Table 13–3

Comparison of JRA, JAS, and SEA Syndrome

	JRA	JAS	SEA
Male:female ratio	1:4	7:1	9:1
Average age at onset (yr)	5	>10	10
Average number of joints	9 (may be many)	6 (rarely many)	5 (rarely many)
Family history of arthritis (%)	30	65	65
Back signs (%)	2	100	45
ANA positive (%)	30–80	0	0
RF positive (%)	15	0	0
HLA-B27 positive (%)	15	90	72

JRA, juvenile rheumatoid arthritis; JAS, juvenile ankylosing spondylitis; SEA, syndome of seronegativity, enthesitis, and arthritis; ANA, antinuclear antibodies; RF, rheumatoid factor.

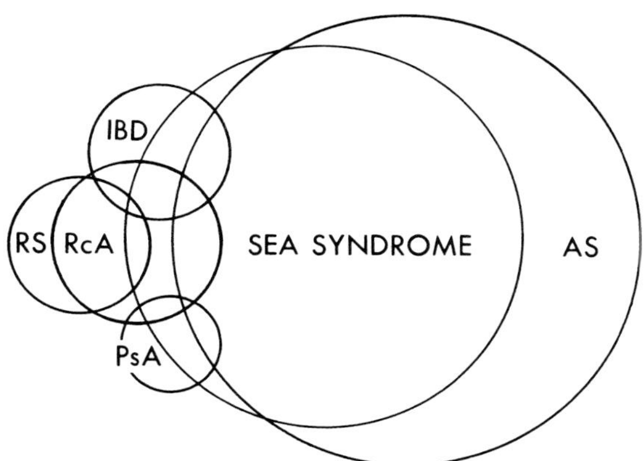

Figure 13–1. Diagnostic considerations in children with the SEA (seronegativity, enthesitis, arthritis) syndrome. AS, ankylosing spondylitis; IBD, inflammatory bowel disease; PsA, psoriatic arthritis; RcA, reactive arthritis; RS, Reiter's syndrome.

ble course of progressive axial disease and sacroiliac arthritis. Within 5 years of onset, 75 percent had definite JAS. This is in contrast with the aforementioned report of Cabral and colleagues,[6] in which clinical progression was more varied and remissions were more frequent. A definite diagnosis in these latter children was often achieved only with a follow-up of approximately 10 years.

Jacobs and associates[8] studied 58 patients selected on the basis of the presence of HLA-B27 who were seen in the pediatric rheumatology clinic for a mean of 5 years. Two thirds were boys, and most had onset of symptoms after 9 years of age, none had RF, and only 7 had ANAs (8.6 percent). Altogether, 51 of 58 had disease that satisfied the American College of Rheumatology (ACR) criteria for a diagnosis of JRA,[9] 1 had Reiter's syndrome, and 6 had episodic arthritis and enthesitis. In all, 75 percent of the children with HLA-B27 had enthesitis and many had other features of one of the spondyloarthropathies, although definitive diagnostic outcomes were not presented.

Sheerin and associates[10] followed 36 of 85 children with arthropathy and HLA-B27 positivity for a mean of approximately 9 years. Although only 2 of these children met the New York criteria for AS, 27 of the 36 (75 percent) fulfilled the authors' criteria for JAS. Five of their patients (24 percent) had enthesitis at onset, and at follow-up 22 patients (61 percent) had enthesitis or a history compatible with enthesitis. A group of 26 children with atypical spondyloarthropathy who fulfilled diagnostic criteria for the SEA syndrome or one of the HLA-B27 syndromes were followed by Hussein and colleagues[11] in an effort to define common characteristics among these various diseases. No diagnostic outcome at follow-up was described in this study, although the proposed criteria tested favorably.

JUVENILE ANKYLOSING SPONDYLITIS

Definition and Classification

JAS is a chronic inflammatory arthritis of the peripheral and axial skeletons, frequently accompanied by enthesitis, characterized by RF or ANA seronegativity, and having a genetic basis. *Arthritis of the sacroiliac joints, which eventually develops in all patients with JAS, may take years or even decades to become apparent.* For the purpose of this discussion, radiologic evidence of inflammation of the sacroiliac joints is required for a definitive diagnosis of JAS.

A number of attempts to develop criteria for the classification or diagnosis of AS have been published.[2, 3, 5, 12, 13] The New York criteria define adult AS (Table 13–4).[5] The more inclusive criteria of Amor and coworkers[12] (Table 13–5) and the European Spondylarthropathy Study Group (ESSG)[13] (Table 13–6) describe spondyloarthropathy, a much broader category. In the ILAR classification[2, 3] (Table 13–7), the category ERA best describes what is currently called JAS. These criteria have not yet been formally compared with the definition used in this chapter or with the New York criteria for AS.

Epidemiology

Incidence and Prevalence

JAS is less frequently recognized in childhood than is JRA, partly because it may be difficult to differentiate early JAS from JRA and partly because it has only relatively recently been recognized that JAS is probably almost as common as JRA in some geographic areas. Striking differences in the frequency of JAS in different racial and ethnic groups reflect differences in the frequency of the HLA-B27 antigen. Increasing awareness of the possibility of the occurrence of AS-like diseases in childhood and their clinical and laboratory differentiation from other chronic arthritides of childhood will probably result in an increase in the proportion of children with chronic arthritis in this category.

The relative frequencies of JAS derived from data accumulated in the national pediatric rheumatic diseases registries of Canada,[14] the United States,[15] and the United Kingdom,[16] and from studies in Finland[17]

Table 13–4

New York Criteria for a Diagnosis of Ankylosing Spondylitis (AS)

Clinical Criteria

1. Limitation of lumbar spine motion in all three planes
2. Pain or history of pain at the dorsolumbar junction or lumbar spine
3. Limitation of chest expansion to 2.5 cm or less at the level of the 4th intercostal space

Definite AS

Grade 3–4 bilateral sacroiliac arthritis on radiograph with at least 1 clinical criterion, *or*
Grade 3–4 unilateral or grade 2 bilateral sacroiliac arthritis on radiograph with criterion 1 or criteria 2 and 3

Probable AS

Grade 3–4 bilateral sacroiliac arthritis on radiograph without clinical criteria

From Bennett PH, Wood PHN: Population Studies of the Rheumatic Diseases. New York, Excerpta Medica, 1968, p 456.

Table 13–5

Amor Criteria for Classification of Spondyloarthropathies

CRITERION	POINTS
Clinical	
Lumbar or thoracic night pain or stiffness	1
Asymmetric oligoarthritis	2
Buttock pain alternating in site or	1
triggered by pelvic movement	2
Sausage digit	2
Enthesopathy	2
Iritis	2
Nonspecific urethritis or cervicitis within 1 mo before onset	1
Diarrhea within 1 mo before onset	1
Psoriasis, balanitis, or chronic enterocolitis	2
Radiologic	
Sacroiliitis (≥ stage 2 if bilateral; ≥ stage 3 if unilateral)	3
Genetic	
Presence of HLA-B27, family history of pelvospondylitis, Reiter's disease, psoriasis, uveitis, or chronic enterocolitis	2
Therapeutic	
Amelioration of pain within 48 hr of treatment with nonsteroidal anti-inflammatory drug	2

A definite diagnosis of spondyloarthropathy is confirmed if 6 or more points are present (sensitivity, 91.9%; specificity, 97.9%)

From Amor B, Dougados M, Mijiyawa M: Critères de classification des spondylarthropathies. Rev Rhum Mal Osteoartic 57: 85, © 1990. Wiley-Liss, Inc. Reprinted by permission of Wiley-Liss, Inc., a subsidiary of John Wiley & Sons, Inc.

and Sweden,[18] are presented in Table 13–8. JAS accounted for 1 to 7 percent of children with chronic arthritis in these studies.

Estimates of the prevalence of AS in adults also range widely among ethnic and racial groups. Using modified New York criteria, including radiographic evidence of sacroiliac arthritis, Carter and coworkers[19] determined a prevalence of 129 per 100,000 (0.13 percent) in an American population of Northern European extraction. This number undoubtedly represents a minimum estimate. A follow-up study of the same population confirmed that the incidence of AS was not changing.[20] On the basis of the prevalence of HLA-B27 and the frequency of sacroiliac arthritis in the B27-positive population, the prevalence of AS has been estimated at 0.86 to 1 percent,[21, 22] highest in B27-positive persons.[21] Although this estimate includes asymptomatic persons, it also excludes the 8 percent of the AS population who do not have B27, and it may be a more accurate reflection of the prevalence of the entire spectrum of AS, whereas the estimate of Carter and colleagues more accurately represents patients with clinically and radiologically evident disease.

Table 13–6

Classification Criteria of the European Spondylarthropathy Study Group (ESSG)

Inflammatory spinal pain
or
Synovitis (asymmetric or predominantly in lower limbs)
plus
One of the following:
- Positive family history
- Psoriasis
- Inflammatory bowel disease
- Urethritis, cervicitis, or diarrhea within 1 mo before arthritis
- Buttock pain alternating between right and left gluteal areas
- Enthesopathy
- Sacroiliitis

From Dougados M, van der Linden S, Juhlin R, et al: The European Spondylarthropathy Study Group preliminary criteria for the classification of spondylarthropathy. Arthritis Rheum 34: 1218, 1991.

Table 13–7

Enthesitis-Related Arthritis (ILAR Classification)

Definition

Arthritis and enthesitis
or
Arthritis or enthesitis with at least two of:
- Sacroiliac joint tenderness and/or inflammatory spinal pain
- Presence of HLA-B27
- Family history in at least one first- or second-degree relative of medically confirmed HLA-B27–associated disease
- Anterior uveitis that is usually associated with pain, redness, or photophobia
- Onset of arthritis in a boy after 8 yr of age

Exclusions

- Psoriasis confirmed by a dermatologist in at least one first- or second-degree relative
- Presence of systemic arthritis

ILAR, International League of Associations for Rheumatology.
From Petty RE, Southwood TR, Baum J, et al: Revision of the proposed classification criteria for juvenile idiopathic arthritis: Durban, 1997. J Rheumatol 25: 1991, 1998.

Few data are specifically related to geographic and racial differences in the incidence of JAS. The low incidence of AS in North American blacks[23] and in Japanese,[24] and a high frequency in the Haida Indians of Pacific Canada,[25] reflect, in part, the frequency of B27 in these populations. Other factors may be significant, however, because this antigen occurs in only 50 percent of American blacks with AS[26] and in only 65 to 90 percent of Japanese with AS.[23]

It is not entirely clear that JAS and AS are the same diseases, although they are undoubtedly closely related. The proportion of adults with AS who developed an onset of disease in childhood ranges from 8.6 percent[13] to 11 percent.[27] The prevalence of JAS could thus be extrapolated to be from 11 to 86 per 100,000 children (0.01 to 0.08 percent). If this admittedly rough estimate is near the mark, the prevalence of JAS is close to or may exceed that of JRA! This possibility is startling when one considers the relative infrequency with which the disease is recognized in childhood. Ladd and colleagues[28] reported 15 patients with onset of JAS (New York criteria) before age 17 years, seen over a 10-year period, during which 208 children with JRA were registered in the same clinic, a ratio of approximately 1:14.

Age at Onset

JAS usually has its onset in late childhood or adolescence, although instances of onset in younger children

Table 13–8

Relative Frequencies of Juvenile Rheumatoid Arthritis (JRA), Juvenile Ankylosing Spondylitis (JAS), and the Spondyloarthropathies (SpA)

	JRA*	JAS	SpA
United Kingdom[16]	1483 (79%)	37 (2%)	348 (19%)
United States[15]	2071 (71%)	75 (3%)	757 (26%)
Canada[14]	521 (61%)	65 (7%)†	274 (32%)
Finland[17]	114 (99%)	1 (1%)	—
Sweden[18]	216 (96%)	2 (1%)	7 (3%)

*Equivalent to the American College of Rheumatology definition.
†Includes 15 children with definite and 50 with probable JAS.

have been recorded.[29, 30] The age distribution appears to be homogeneous and presumably is continuous with that described in adult populations, suggesting that, at least on this basis, the disease as seen in adults is the same as that in children.[28, 31, 32]

Sex Ratio

JAS has a much higher frequency in boys than in girls: of 247 children with this disorder, 216 were boys, a ratio of 7 boys to 1 girl.[28, 31–37] This disproportionate representation of boys may not accurately represent the actual occurrence of the disease in girls. The strong correlation between JAS and HLA-B27 and the equal distribution of this antigen in males and females suggest that JAS could be as common in girls as in boys. Furthermore, in radiographic surveys of adult blood donors with B27, sacroiliac joint arthritis was as common in women as in men.[38] In a large questionnaire survey of members of the National Ankylosing Spondylitis Society in the United Kingdom, the male:female ratio was 2.7:1.[27] Manifestations in the female may be less severe,[39] and women with AS may have more peripheral and less axial disease.[40] It is possible that these observations contribute to the relative infrequency of the diagnosis in women.

Etiology and Pathogenesis

There is no known cause of JAS. The clinical, genetic, and epidemiologic similarities of JAS and diseases such as Reiter's syndrome and reactive arthritis, in which bacterial enteric or genitourinary tract infections are known to play a triggering role, suggest an infectious etiology, although none has been proved. Although no bacteria can be isolated from the joint, a local response to antigen is supported by antibody and cellular immune studies.[41] The strong association with HLA-B27 suggests that a genetically determined mechanism is central to pathogenesis.[21] HLA-B27 itself may be involved in pathogenesis or merely serve as a marker gene. Inflammation of the gastrointestinal tract may be related in AS to this association with HLA antigens[42] as well as cellular immunity to cartilage proteoglycans.[43]

Molecular mimicry, in which there is an immune response to an amino acid sequence that is shared by certain B27 molecules and some *Klebsiella* species, has been suggested as a pathogenic mechanism. Reports[44] of an association between B27 and gastrointestinal isolation of *Klebsiella* species in adults with AS suggest a role for these organisms, but these studies remain largely unconfirmed.[45] The reactivity of synovial fluid lymphocytes to microbial antigens has been shown to correlate with the specificity of extra-articular bacterial isolates in adult patients with chronic arthritis.[46] A modulatory effect of the surface expression of the B27 molecule on the invasive capability of arthritogenic bacteria, such as *Yersinia enterocolitica* and *Salmonella enteritidis*, has been demonstrated in murine cells[47, 48] but not in human fibroblasts or lymphocytes.[49, 50] Some investigators have found that, although bacterial invasion of B27 expressing cells is normal, killing of the organisms in such cells is impaired, with the result that infective organisms persist within the host.[51] The B27 transgenic rat is an important animal model for studying these relationships.[52, 53] The observations of Mielants and associates[54, 55] support a pathogenic relationship between AS and JAS and inflammation of the gut.

Genetic Background

There is often a striking familial occurrence of AS and related diseases in adults and children. Ansell and colleagues[56] noted that 6 of 12 monozygotic twin pairs concordant for arthritis were HLA-B27 positive, which made the diagnosis of JAS likely (if not certain) in these children. Family studies have indicated that AS is inherited as an autosomal dominant trait with penetrance of about 20 percent.[57] Although the risk of development of AS in a B27-positive person is not precisely known, epidemiologic studies in adults suggest that AS occurs 10 to 20 times more frequently in relatives of patients with AS and 50 to 80 times more frequently in their siblings.[58, 59] The general risk that a B27-heterozygous parent with AS will have a male child with the disease is approximately 5 to 10 percent (20 percent if the child is B27 positive; close to zero if the child is B27 negative).[59] The risk of having a female child with JAS is lower.

The studies of Brewerton and colleagues[58] and Schlosstein

Table 13–9

Genetic Associations With Ankylosing Spondylitis (AS) or Juvenile Ankylosing Spondylitis (JAS)

GENE	ASSOCIATION	REFERENCE(S)
HLA-B27	↑ in AS, JAS	58, 60, 28, 31–37
HLA-A2	↑ in AS, JAS	67, 68
HLA-A28	↑ in B27-positive AS	69, 70
HLA-B60	↑ in AS	71, 72
HLA-DRB1*08	↑ in Mexican children with JAS	75
LMP-2A	↑ in Mexicans with AS, JAS, and iritis	76
LMP-2 b/b	↑ in JAS	77

and colleagues[60] (and subsequently many others) indicated that B27 was strongly associated with AS in adults. The association between JAS and the B27 antigen is as strong in children as in adults. Of 247 children with JAS, B27 was present in 91 percent.[28, 31–37] One study demonstrated restriction fragment length polymorphisms of B27 that had striking associations with AS.[61] There are now at least 12 known subtypes of B27[62]; all except 1 are associated with AS. Specifically, no specific associations with B27 subtypes have been identified by oligonucleotide probes B*2701-2706.[63] In the Gambian population of Africa, a unique subtype, B2703, has been shown not to be associated with AS.[64] The possibility that homozygosity for B27 was responsible for the juvenile onset of AS was not supported by data in one small study.[65]

Although HLA-B27 has the strongest genetic association with AS and contributes the greatest share (15 to 60 percent) of the attributable genetic risk,[57, 66] other genetic factors undoubtedly play a role. Thus, B27-positive persons with a family history of AS have a tenfold greater risk of AS than that of B27-positive persons with no family history of AS.[59] There is also an increase in HLA-A2, an association that is shared with other chronic arthritides of childhood.[67] Woodrow[68] has used meta-analysis to calculate a relative risk of spondylitis of 1.72 in A2-positive patients. Reports of an increased frequency of HLA-A28 in B27-positive patients with AS suggest that this antigen also may contribute to disease susceptibility.[69, 70] HLA-B60 is increased in adults with AS independent of the presence of B27.[71, 72] The reported increased frequency of Cw1 and Cw2[73, 74] probably reflects a linkage disequilibrium with HLA-B27. In contrast with JRA, there are few known class II associations with JAS. A higher frequency of HLA DRB1*08 (44.9 percent) was reported in a Mexican population with JAS than in a control population (25.4 percent)[75] (Table 13–9).

Other genetic indicators have also been studied in JAS. Maksymowych and colleagues[76] reported that the LMP2A allele frequency in patients with adult- and juvenile-onset AS with uveitis was twice that in those without this complication (odds ratio, 2.51). Ploski and colleagues[77] reported an increase of B*4001, DRB1*08, and DPB1*0301 and the LMP2 b/b phenotype in patients with JAS compared with B27-positive controls or adults with AS. These differences between JAS and adult AS require further investigation to determine the relationship between the disease in the two age ranges.

Clinical Manifestations

The initial manifestations of JAS usually include arthritis of one or more peripheral joints, usually in the lower extremities, together with enthesitis at one or more sites around the knee or foot. Systemic signs are usually minimal, but there may be low-grade fever. Symptoms related to the back are usually absent at disease onset but become evident during the disease course in most adolescents.

Arthritis

The presenting joint symptoms that have been recorded in the largest reported series of children with JAS are summarized in Table 13–10. The initial musculoskeletal symptoms are often difficult for the child to localize and include pain in the buttocks, groin, thighs, or heels, or around the shoulders. The vague quality and localization of this pain and its frequent spontaneous disappearance early in the disease are recurring sources of delay and confusion in diagnosis.

In distinction to AS in adults, JAS in children seldom causes symptoms of involvement of the axial skeleton

Table 13–10

Musculoskeletal Signs and Symptoms in Juvenile Ankylosing Spondylitis (JAS)

Clinical Evidence of Joint Involvement at Onset*	
(Arthritis, painful limitation of range of motion)	
Proximal limb joints	35%
Distal limb joints	44%
Upper limb joints	16%
Lower limb joints	82%
Axial skeleton joints	24%
Joint Involvement During Disease Course*	
No peripheral joints affected	3%
1–4 peripheral joints affected	43%
More than 4 peripheral joints affected	54%
Lumbosacral spine affected†	90%
Sacroiliac joint involvement†	95%
Enthesitis	
Around the knee†	80%
Around the ankle and foot†	90%
Muscle Pain, Wasting†	50%

Note: Clinical or radiographic evidence of involvement of the sacroiliac joints, and particularly the lumbosacral spine, may not be evident until adulthood.

*Data from published studies.

†Estimate.

at onset; only 24 percent of reported children have pain, stiffness, or limitation of motion of the lumbosacral spine or sacroiliac joints at presentation. In contrast, peripheral joint symptoms occur at onset in 82 percent (see Table 13–10). With the exception of one report in which hip disease was frequent at onset,[78] distal joints are affected more commonly than are proximal joints. All reports agree that at onset, disease of the lower-extremity joints is much more characteristic (82 percent) than involvement of the upper extremities (16 percent).

In most instances, the number of joints involved is limited (four or fewer), although approximately 25 percent of children experience a polyarticular onset. Shoulders are not uncommonly affected, and even the temporomandibular joint may become involved. The least commonly affected joints are the small joints of the hands. Pain at costosternal and sternoclavicular joints and the sternomanubrium, often in conjunction with tenderness over the proximal clavicle, may be associated with significant impairment of chest expansion. In the series of Schaller and associates,[32] five of seven patients had decreased chest expansion. Aside from the number and distribution of the affected joints, there is nothing clinically to distinguish the peripheral joint disease of JAS from that of JRA. Burgos-Vargas and colleagues[79] have pointed out that there is a subgroup of children with typical adult-type onset of disease. Whether this presentation represents a distinct entity or merely an extreme end of the spectrum of clinical characteristics at onset is not certain.[80]

Enthesitis

The presence of enthesitis is the most helpful feature in differentiating JAS from JRA.[81] Enthesitis is a characteristic early manifestation of JAS and occurs with greater frequency in JAS than in adult-onset AS. Inflammation at these sites frequently produces severe pain and resultant disability, which may be the child's most important complaints.

The most common sites of enthesitis are the same as those described in the SEA syndrome.

Iritis

The iritis of JAS is characterized by a red, painful, photophobic eye. It is usually unilateral, frequently recurs, and generally leaves no ocular residua. It rarely precedes the onset of musculoskeletal complaints. Acute iritis occurs in 20 percent of adults with AS, particularly in those with peripheral joint involvement, but may be less common in JAS. In the series of Ladd and colleagues,[28] 1 of 15 patients experienced acute iritis; in the series of Schaller and associates,[33] 2 of 20 patients developed this complication. However, Hafner[34] recorded acute iritis in 14 percent of 71 patients with JAS, and Ansell[30] noted acute iritis in 27 percent of a group of 77 patients. These higher figures may reflect a longer follow-up period in the latter two studies.

Cardiopulmonary Disease

None of 36 consecutive patients with JAS followed for a mean of 4.3 years had symptoms related to the cardiovascular system, and only 1 had a murmur of aortic regurgitation.[82] Echocardiographs documented no structural abnormalities, and electrocardiography revealed no conduction defects, but color Doppler assessment showed mild mitral regurgitation in 2 patients and mild aortic regurgitation in 3 patients. Systolic ventricular function was impaired in 1 patient. Although cardiovascular disease is uncommon in JAS, it can occasionally be severe, and marked aortic insufficiency, sometimes with aortic dilatation, has been reported in at least 7 patients with JAS,[83–89] in 1 patient with sacroiliac arthritis and regional enteritis,[30] and in 1 patient with juvenile Reiter's syndrome.[90] The apparently low frequency of such complications in JAS may reflect the fact that follow-up has been of much shorter duration than in adults, in whom cardiac disease develops in approximately 5 percent of patients an average of 15 years after onset of spondylitis.[91] A study in adults with AS using transesophageal echocardiography demonstrated aortic root abnormalities and valve disease in 82 percent of patients compared with 27 percent of controls. Valve thickening was demonstrable as nodularity of the aortic cusps and basal thickening of the anterior mitral valve leaflet, creating the characteristic subaortic bump. Aortic valve regurgitation was present in almost half of the patients.[92]

Few data relating to pleuropulmonary disease in JAS are available. In a study of 18 children aged 8 to 17 years who fulfilled the Amor criteria[12] for the diagnosis of spondyloarthropathies, abnormalities of pulmonary function were detected in 33 percent.[93] All patients had normal-appearing chest radiographs at baseline and at 2-year follow-up. No patient had symptoms attributable to the respiratory system, and all had normal chest expansion. Nonetheless, 6 patients (33 percent) had abnormalities on pulmonary function tests. The most common abnormality was reduction in the forced vital capacity (22 percent). Occasionally, increased functional residual capacity (11 percent) and residual volume (5 percent) were observed. These restrictive patterns were more common than diffusion defects, and diffusing capacity of the lungs for carbon monoxide was reduced in only 11 percent. Small airways disease was not present.

In adults, although diminished chest expansion and resultant decreased vital capacity are not infrequent, clinically detected parenchymal pulmonary disease is rare. In the review by Rosenow and associates,[94] 1.3 percent of 2080 adults with AS had radiographic evidence of pleuropulmonary disease, that is, apical pleural thickening. High-resolution computed tomography (CT) in 26 adults with AS demonstrated a much higher frequency of pulmonary parenchymal abnormalities (69 percent) than was demonstrated by plain radiograph (15 percent).[95] These included interstitial lung disease in 4 patients, bronchiectasis in 6, paraseptal emphysema in 3, and tracheal dilatation and apical fibrosis in 2 each. Cor pulmonale can develop secondary to kyphoscoliosis and decreased chest wall movement characteristic of advanced spondylitis but has not been reported in children or adolescents.

Nervous System

Central nervous system disease rarely occurs in JAS. Atlantoaxial subluxation leading to severe cervico-occipital pain has been reported in one boy with JAS,[96] and we have seen this complication in two other boys with the SEA syndrome.[97] The cauda equina syndrome, caused by bony impingement on the cauda equina and characterized by weakness of the sphincters of bowel and bladder, saddle anesthesia, and leg weakness, occurs in adults with AS[98] but has not been reported in JAS.

Renal Disease

Renal abnormalities in JAS are rare. Renal papillary necrosis, thought to be secondary to nonsteroidal anti-inflammatory drugs (NSAIDs), has been reported.[99] Immunoglobulin A (IgA) nephropathy, occasionally with uveitis,[100] has also been noted among 115 adults with AS or other seronegative spondyloarthropathies.[101] Most such patients have elevated serum IgA concentrations; some have hypertension and impaired renal function.

Amyloidosis is extremely rare in the rheumatic diseases of childhood, particularly in North America. However, Ansell[30] documented amyloidosis in 3.8 percent of 77 patients with JAS in the United Kingdom seen before 1980; she noted its association with severe peripheral arthropathy and persistently elevated erythrocyte sedimentation rate (ESR).

Pathology

Studies of the pathology of JAS have not been reported, but it is probable that changes are similar to those of adult AS. It is generally stated that the synovitis is much milder and the degree of cartilage erosion in peripheral joints much less in AS than in adult rheumatoid arthritis (RA).[102] The synovitis itself is otherwise virtually indistinguishable from that of RA, although there may be relatively more polymorphonuclear leukocytes. Cells of the synovial membrane express tumor necrosis factor (TNF)-α, TNF-β, and TNF receptors similar to those of children with JRA.[103] Enthesitis, said by Ball[104] to be the hallmark of AS, is characterized by nonspecific inflammation. Granulation tissue, infiltrated with lymphocytes and plasma cells and causing localized osteitis, replaces the bony and cartilaginous attachment of the ligament or tendon. Healing of this lesion gives rise to a bony spur. When this process occurs at the insertion of the plantar fascia into the calcaneus, it produces a calcaneal spur; when it occurs at the attachment of the outer fibers of the annulus fibrosus to the anterolateral aspects of the rim of the vertebral body, it gives rise to a syndesmophyte.

The characteristic pathologic changes in the apophyseal joints and the sacroiliac joints are enchondral and capsular ossification. The earliest lesion in the sacroiliac joints is subchondral inflammation leading to the formation of granulation tissue with few inflammatory cells. The surfaces of the sacroiliac joints are little affected, and pannus is not present.[105] Enchondral ossification on the iliac side of the joint accounts for the radiographic appearance of erosions. Ball comments, "As a rule, it seems that in any synovial joint in ankylosing spondylitis the outcome represents a balance of erosive synovitis and capsular and/or ligamentous ossification. In joints of low mobility the ossific process tends to be the dominant feature."[106]

Diagnosis

The onset of JAS may be insidious and characterized by intermittent musculoskeletal pain or objective inflammation of joints, particularly those of the lower extremities. In other patients, oligoarthritis may have an abrupt onset. A complete physical examination should be an integral part of any rheumatologic evaluation; in children with JAS, it may provide important diagnostic information indicating the presence of a complication such as iritis or cardiovascular disease. Furthermore, cutaneous, mucous membrane, gastrointestinal, or genitourinary abnormalities may influence the examiner to consider an alternative diagnosis from among the other members of the spondyloarthropathy group.[107]

Criteria for the diagnosis of AS in adults (see Tables 13–4 through 13–6) are not applicable to the younger age group for a number of reasons: data for some of the physical measurements have not been published for children, or if reported (back range)[108] have not yet been validated in a population of children with JAS. Furthermore, the limitations of spine and chest motion may reflect disease duration and are therefore of little help in facilitating early diagnosis.[109] The fact that peripheral joint disease usually precedes axial involvement by years in many children precludes an early diagnosis by criteria in which abnormalities in axial motion or radiologic changes are essential diagnostic features. Reasons for these differences between adults and children—whether they have an immunologic, genetic, biochemical, or structural basis—are not understood.[110, 111]

There remains a clear need for the development and standardization of diagnostic criteria for JAS. In one such study,[112] 2958 consecutive children with various forms of childhood arthritis (including 324 definite spondyloarthropathies and 334 possible spondyloarthropathies) and 2300 control subjects were evaluated with the adult AS criteria of Amor and coworkers[12] and the ESSG (see Tables 13–5 and 13–6).[13] Children with JAS were identified by the Amor criteria with a sensitivity of 73.5 percent and specificity of 97.6 percent; and by the ESSG criteria with a sensitivity of 78.7 percent and specificity of 92.2 percent. Proposals for the reclassification of the juvenile idiopathic arthritides include the category ERA.[3, 4] This category recognizes those patients considered to have JAS or SEA syndrome. The ILAR criteria are less inclusive than either the Amor or the ESSG criteria, which also include children with psoriatic arthritis and the arthritis of IBD.

Musculoskeletal Examination

The diagnosis of JAS depends on careful clinical observations, often over several years. The musculoskeletal examination can be divided into three parts: (1) examination of the entheses, (2) examination of the peripheral joints, and (3) examination of the joints of the axial skeleton, including those of the pelvis, spine, and chest.

Entheses

A careful history and a thorough but gentle palpation of entheses may reveal evidence of past or present inflammation. Enthesitis is often remarkably discrete and painful. A diagnosis of JAS is strongly supported by marked tenderness on the patella at the 2, 6, and 10 o'clock positions, at the tibial tuberosity, at the attachment of the Achilles tendon or plantar fascia to the calcaneus, at the attachment of the plantar fascia to the base of the fifth metatarsal, and at the heads of the metatarsals (Fig. 13–2).

Tenderness is less commonly demonstrable at the greater trochanters of the femurs, superior anterior iliac spines, pubic symphysis, and ischial tuberosities, and seldom demonstrable at entheses of the upper extremities. Symptoms of pain or tenderness at the origin of the adductor longus near the symphysis pubis[113] and at the costochondral junctions, although infrequent, also support the diagnosis of JAS. Careful observation of stance and gait may indicate that the child stands or moves so as to avoid pressure on inflamed entheses.

Peripheral Joints

The peripheral arthropathy of JAS may be indistinguishable from that of JRA or other spondyloarthropathies, although the number and distribution of affected joints provide helpful clues to the differentiation of these diseases. The arthritis of JAS is often asymmetric and involves the lower extremities. Isolated hip joint disease may be the presenting feature of JAS[114] but would be highly unlikely in a child with JRA. Although involvement of one or both knees is characteristic of both oligoarticular JRA and JAS, the child's sex and age at onset are useful distinguishing features. Small joints of the toes are seldom affected in JRA but are commonly involved in JAS. Thus, for example, the

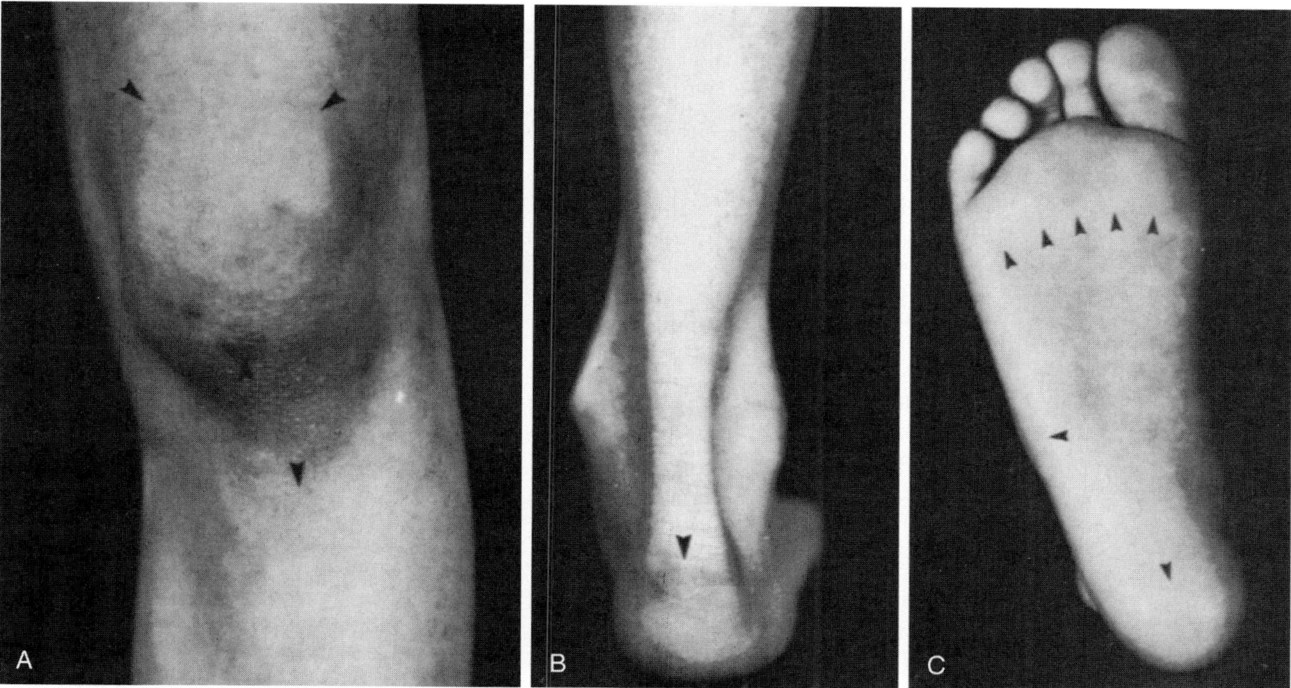

Figure 13–2. *A, Arrows* indicate the most common sites of tenderness associated with enthesitis at the insertions of the quadriceps muscles into the patella and the attachments of the patellar ligament to the patella and tibial tuberosity. *B, Arrow* indicates the site of enthesitic tenderness at the insertion of the Achilles tendon into the calcaneus. *C, Arrows* indicate the most common sites of tenderness associated with enthesitis at the insertion of the plantar fascia into the calcaneus, base of the fifth metatarsal, and heads of the first through fifth metatarsals. Swelling in this area is best visualized by having the child lie prone on the examining table with the feet over the edge. (*B* and *C,* From Petty RE, Malleson P: Spondyloarthropathies of childhood. Pediatr Clin North Am 33: 1079, 1986.)

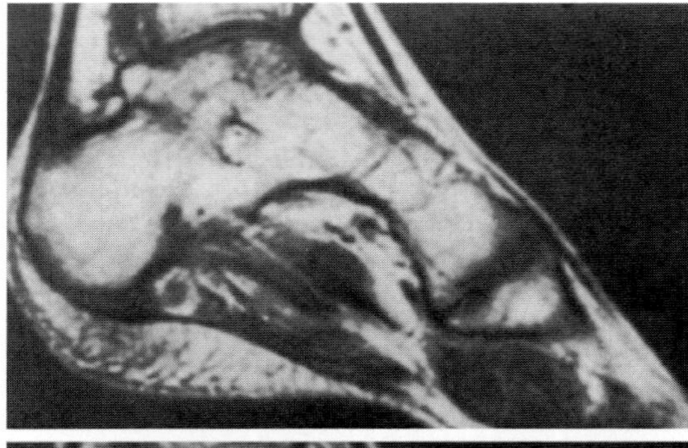

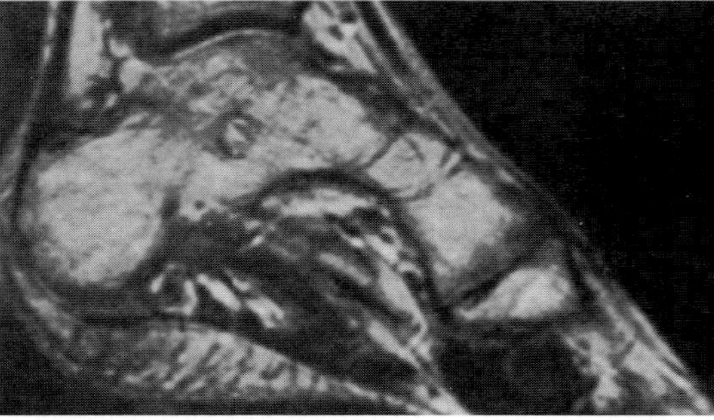

Figure 13–3. Magnetic resonance images of bony ankylosis on T1 (top) and hyperintensive signals coming from the synovial sheath and bursae on T2 (bottom). (From Burgos-Vargas R, Granados-Arriola J: Ankylosing spondylitis and related diseases in the Mexican mestizo. Spine: State of the Art Reviews 44: 665, 1990.)

presence of arthritis in the metatarsophalangeal joint of the first toe, the ankle, and the knee—particularly in a boy over the age of 8 years—strongly suggests a diagnosis of JAS. In contrast, symmetric disease of the small joints of the hands or polyarticular disease, particularly in a girl, is more likely to be the result of JRA.

A highly characteristic intertarsal joint inflammation (tarsitis) occurs in many children with JAS (Fig. 13–3). Such children have pain, tenderness, and restriction of movement in the midfoot, which, in the presence of disease of the first metatarsophalangeal joint, often results in a characteristic deformity of the foot. Burgos-Vargas and associates[115] concluded that a diagnosis of JAS could be confirmed or strongly suspected shortly after onset of disease in children who displayed enthesopathy, midtarsal foot involvement, sparing of the hands, and progressive onset of lumbosacral disease.

Axial Skeleton

Examination of the joints of the axial skeleton is central to the diagnosis of JAS. In patients with sacroiliac joint inflammation, pain may be elicited by direct pressure over one or both sacroiliac joints, compression of the pelvis, or distraction of the sacroiliac joints (Patrick's test). Examination of the back should first be directed at detecting asymmetry in the standing position. Abnormalities in contour, such as loss of the normal lumbar lordosis or thoracic kyphosis, are best observed while the child is standing upright. The contour of the back on full forward flexion may demonstrate loss of the normal smooth curve in the lower part of the thoracolumbar spine (Fig. 13–4), or there may be restriction of hyperextension, signifying early axial disease. The rigid spine of long-standing AS is rare in children.

Although observations of abnormalities of the contour of the back are often more informative than actual numerical measurements, sequential measurement of thoracolumbar spinal mobility is useful in documenting progression of disease. The modified Schober test[116, 117] provides one such index (Fig. 13–5). With the child standing with the feet together, a line joining the dimples of Venus is used as a surface landmark for the lumbosacral junction. A mark is made 5 cm below (point A) and 10 cm above (point B) the lumbosacral junction. With the patient in maximal forward flexion and with the knees straight, the increase in distance between points A and B is used as an indicator of lumbosacral spine mobility. Normal values plus or minus 1 S.D. are shown in Figure 13–6.[108] Care should be exercised in the interpretation of this measurement because there are clearly large normal variations at each age and the data have not been adequately validated in children with musculoskeletal disease. In general, however, a modified Schober measurement of less than 6 cm (i.e., an increase from 15 cm to less than 21 cm) should be regarded as abnormal. Measurement of the distance from fingertips to floor on maximal forward flexion is often used to quantitate spinal motion but is poorly reproducible and does not correlate with the Schober measurement. Furthermore, finger-to-floor distance reflects hip as well as back flexion.

Pain at the costosternal and costovertebral joints may be elicited by firm palpation. Sternomanubrial

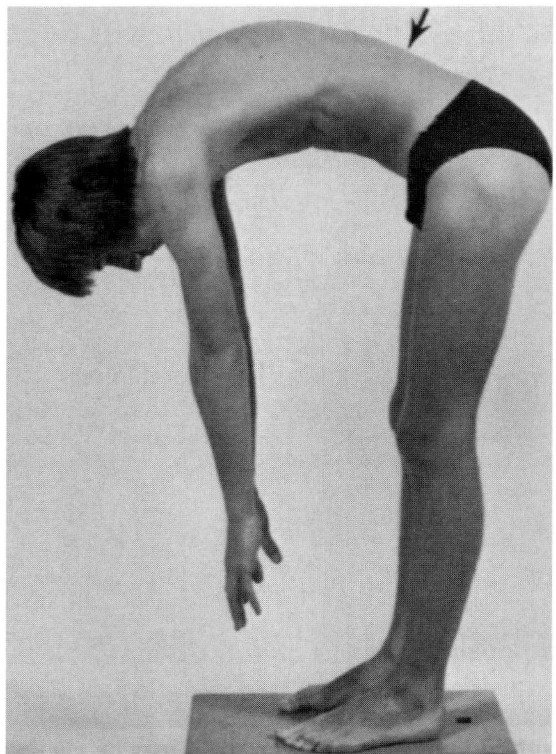

Figure 13–4. A 15-year-old boy shown in the position of maximal forward flexion. Note the flattened back (*arrow*). Radiographs demonstrated bilateral sacroiliac arthritis but no abnormality of the lumbosacral spine.

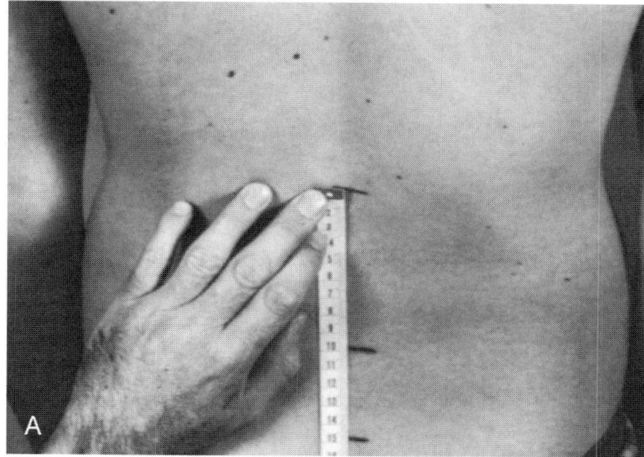

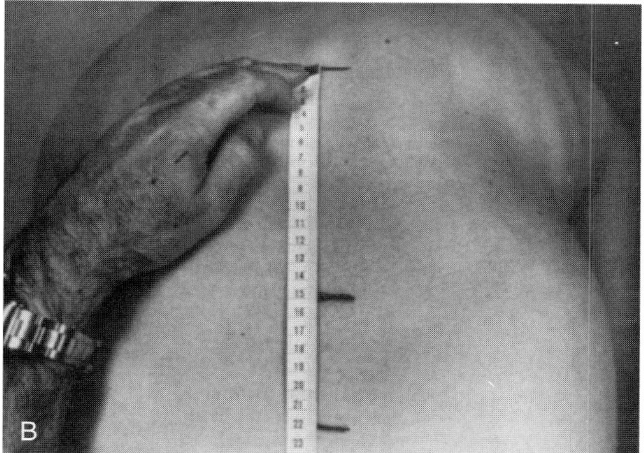

Figure 13–5. Shober's test. *A,* Measurement 10 cm above and 5 cm below the lumbosacral junction (the dimples of Venus) in the upright position. *B,* Measurement of the distance between the upper and the lower marks when the child is bending forward.

tenderness sometimes occurs, but sternoclavicular pain is more common. Thoracic joint disease may be reflected in limitation of chest expansion. Normal thoracic excursion varies a great deal, and normal age- and sex-adjusted ranges have not been established. However, in a specific child, sequential measurement of thoracic motion may be very useful in detecting progressive loss of range. In the adolescent, any thoracic excursion of less than 5 cm (maximum expiration to maximum inspiration, measured at the 4th intercostal space) should be regarded with caution. Even in the absence of chest wall symptoms, chest expansion in children with JAS may be restricted to 1 or 2 cm.

Differential Diagnosis

At onset, JAS may mimic other inflammatory arthropathies such as oligoarticular JRA, mechanical causes of back or lower extremity pain, or (very occasionally) infection or malignancy. It is the combination of arthritis, enthesitis, and axial skeletal involvement that points to a spondyloarthropathy; the absence of cutaneous, gastrointestinal, or genitourinary tract disease further narrows the diagnosis to JAS. In most instances, however, children with spondyloarthropathies lack sacroiliac and back symptoms at onset of disease and differentiation of JAS from JRA and other disorders of the entheses, back, and sacroiliac joints may be difficult.

Arthritis of the cervical spine is infrequent in JAS and, when present, mimics that in children with polyarticular JRA. Thoracolumbar pain may reflect Scheuermann's disease as well as arthritis. Lumbar and lumbosacral spine pain have a myriad of causes, including spondylolysis, spondylolisthesis, osteoid osteoma, osteomyelitis, diskitis, and (rarely) lumbar disk herniation. Trauma may cause chronic pain in the sacrum and coccyx.

Sacroiliac joint tenderness occurs in many patients with JAS, but septic sacroiliac joint disease, osteomyelitis, and familial Mediterranean fever[118] also cause pain in and around these joints. Ewing's sarcoma of the ilium may present as sacroiliac joint pain.

Pain that mimics enthesitis may result from a number of causes, including excessive running or jogging. Usually, the pain of traumatic enthesopathy is less severe and more diffuse than that caused by inflammation. Osteochondrosis of the tibial tuberosity (Osgood-Schlatter disease), of the inferior pole of the patella (Sinding-Larsen-Johansson syndrome), or the apophysis of the calcaneus (Sever's disease) may mimic inflammatory enthesitis in those sites. The coexistence of enthesitis at multiple sites usually eliminates these disorders from consideration. The absence of HLA-B27 positivity also assists in differentiating these disorders from the inflammatory enthesitis of JAS.[119] Pressure over bony prominences, including entheses, may produce pain in children with leukemia or bone tumors. In most instances, however, the pain resulting from such infiltrative diseases is less discrete and more severe than that of inflammatory enthesitis, frequently awakening the child from sleep.

Laboratory Examination

There are few distinguishing laboratory features in children with JAS. Anemia is usually mild in JAS and characteristic of the anemia of chronic inflammation. White blood cell counts are usually normal or moderately elevated, with normal differential counts. Indices of inflammation are frequently abnormal. The platelet count and the ESR are often elevated and may remain so for years. Very high values for the ESR (>100 mm) occasionally occur in JAS but should also alert the physician to the possibility of occult IBD. Conversely, a normal ESR may accompany clinically active disease. Elevated immunoglobulin levels reflect inflammation, and selective deficiency of IgA has been reported.[120, 121] High levels of IgA and C4[122, 123] and of circulating immune complexes[124] in adults with AS suggest an immunoreactive state.

Characteristically, RFs are absent in children with JAS. ANAs do not occur in children with JAS more commonly than in the healthy population. Antiphospholipid antibodies have been demonstrated in 29 percent of adults with AS,[125] but children with JAS have

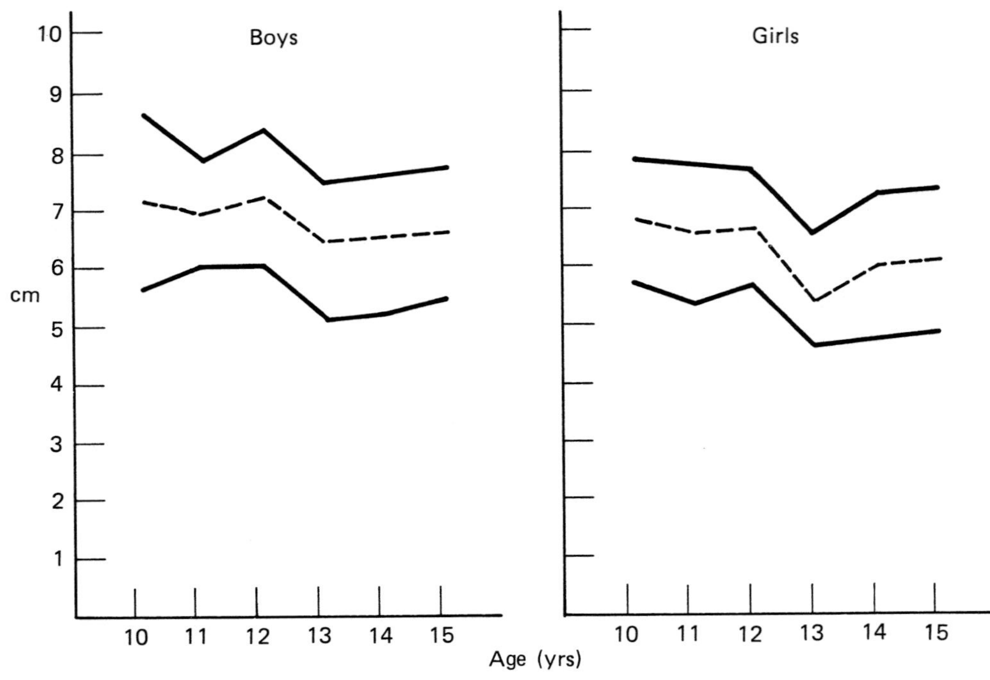

Figure 13–6. Normal values for modified Schober's test: mean ± S.D. (Adapted from Moran HM, Hall MA, Barr A, et al: Spinal mobility in the adolescent. Br J Rheumatol Rehab 18: 181, 1979. © 1979, British Society for Rheumatology. Formerly Rheumatol Rehab.)

not been studied. Although there are no reports of systematic studies of other autoantibodies in JAS, experience suggests that they are not detectable.

HLA-B27 is present in 90 percent of children with JAS; it does not constitute a diagnostic test but rather *an indicator of risk*. The diagnosis of JAS rests on clinical characteristics, and the use of HLA typing for diagnosis may lead to misdiagnosis, although HLA typing is important as a criterion to classify patients.

There are no specific studies of synovial fluid from children with JAS, but the changes are probably similar to those in adults with AS, in which the differential white blood cell count includes more neutrophils and fewer lymphocytes than in RA.[126] It has been reported that the predominant large mononuclear cell in synovial fluid in RA is lymphocyte derived, whereas that in AS is of macrophage origin.[127] Macrophages containing degenerated neutrophils are more common in synovial fluid of patients with AS and related diseases such as Reiter's syndrome than in RA.[128] Descriptions of the synovial fluid are otherwise similar to those in RA except that the complement level is usually normal[129] or increased.[30]

Radiologic Examination

Sacroiliac Joints

Radiographic demonstration of bilateral sacroiliac arthritis is necessary to establish the unequivocal diagnosis of JAS using the New York criteria,[5] although the classic radiographic changes of bilateral sacroiliac disease may not occur for several years after the onset of disease and are not requirements for a diagnosis of ERA by the ILAR criteria.[2, 3] The use of radiographic criteria poses a dilemma when applied to JAS, not only because of the late development of sacroiliac joint changes in this disease but also because interpretation of sacroiliac joint radiographs in children and adolescents is difficult, even for the experienced radiologist. Nonetheless, characteristic radiographic changes in the sacroiliac joints, peripheral joints, and entheses aid in diagnosis and confirm the clinical diagnostic impression (Table 13–11).[130, 131]

Table 13–11

Radiologic Characteristics of Juvenile Ankylosing Spondylitis (JAS)

Sacroiliitis (Bilateral)

Diffuse osteoporosis of the pelvis
Blurring of subchondral margins
Erosions (iliac side first)
Reactive sclerosis
Joint space narrowing
Fusion (late)

Enthesitis (e.g., at Calcaneus, tibial tuberosity)

Soft tissue swelling
Erosions or spur formation at insertions

Peripheral Joints

Soft tissue swelling
Accelerated ossification and epiphyseal overgrowth
Periostitis
Joint-space narrowing, erosions
Ankylosis

Vertebral Column

Vertebral epiphysitis with anterior vertebral squaring
Anterior ligament calcification
"Bamboo spine"

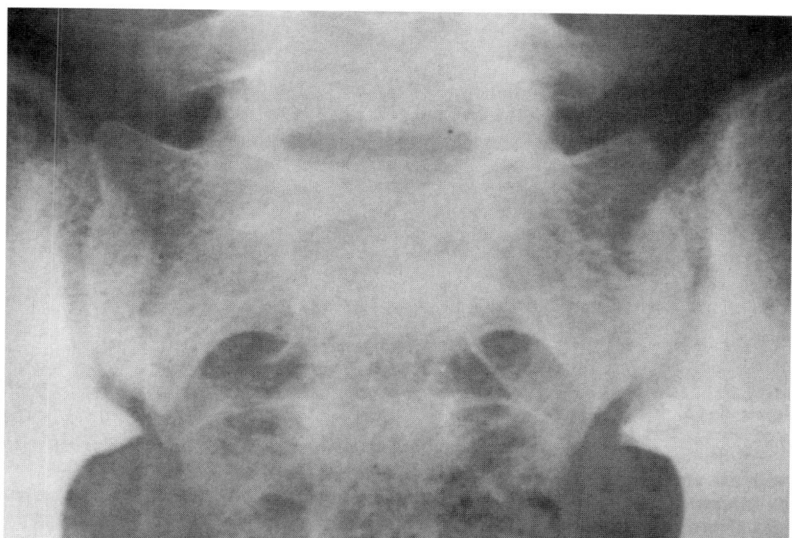

Figure 13–7. Juvenile ankylosing spondylitis. Early radiographic changes (angulated view). There is moderate reactive sclerosis of both sacroiliac joints with widening, irregularity, and haziness of the subchondral bone margins in this 11-year-old boy at onset of disease. (From Ladd JR, Cassidy JT, Martel W: Juvenile ankylosing spondylitis. Arthritis Rheum 14: 579, 1971.)

Radiographic techniques used to evaluate sacroiliac joints vary from institution to institution. A single anteroposterior view of the pelvis may provide an adequate screening examination of the sacroiliac joints and minimizes radiation exposure, although posteroanterior, stereoscopic, angulated (30 degree), or oblique views are preferred by some pediatric radiologists for definitive evaluation. Figures 13–7 through 13–9 provide examples of the abnormalities demonstrable on plain radiographs. Ansell[30] noted that the mean interval from onset of symptoms to radiographic evidence of sacroiliac arthritis was 6.5 years (range, 1 to 15 years). In the report by Ladd and colleagues,[28] sacroiliac joint arthritis was consistently the first radiographic abnormality of the axial skeleton and diagnostic findings were confirmed at the onset of low back symptoms in the majority of children when technically adequate views of the sacroiliac joints were obtained. A systematic search for widening or narrowing of the sacroiliac joints, sclerosis on the iliac or sacral sides of the joints, and fusion of the sacroiliac joints is required to maximize the yield from this investigation.

The apparent widening of the sacroiliac joint is the result of erosions of the subchondral border occurring particularly in the inferior synovial portion of the joint (see Fig. 13–7). The lesion may appear initially as haziness of the bony margins, followed by dissolution of the subchondral bone plate that results in a punched-out appearance. Although these changes may be unilateral initially, they eventually become bilateral and symmetric. An osteoblastic reaction occurring on both sides of the joint results in increased density or reactive sclerosis (see Fig. 13–8). Late changes may include fusion of the sacroiliac joints and regional osteoporosis (see Fig. 13–9).

The sacroiliac joint has some unique anatomic characteristics, an understanding of which assists in the interpretation of certain radiologic features. The sacral side of the joint is covered by hyaline cartilage, whereas the iliac side is pro-

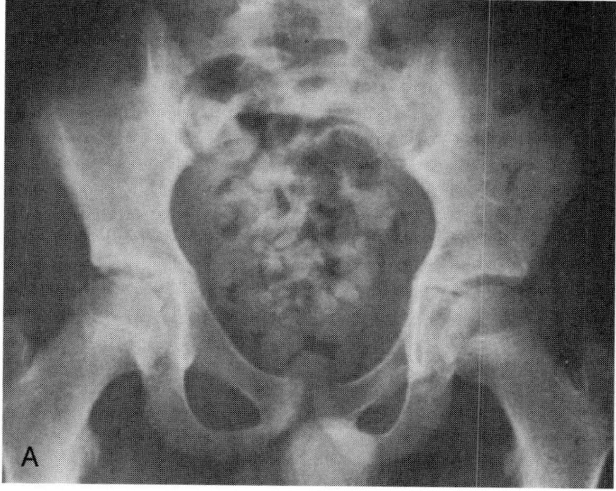

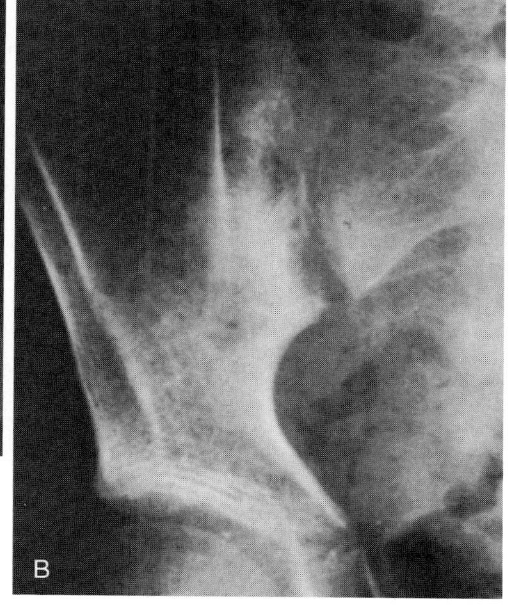

Figure 13–8. Juvenile ankylosing spondylitis. Moderately advanced radiographic changes. *A,* The widening, erosions, and reactive sclerosis are marked on this anteroposterior view of the pelvis. *B,* Oblique view of right sacroiliac joint demonstrates the same changes in more detail.

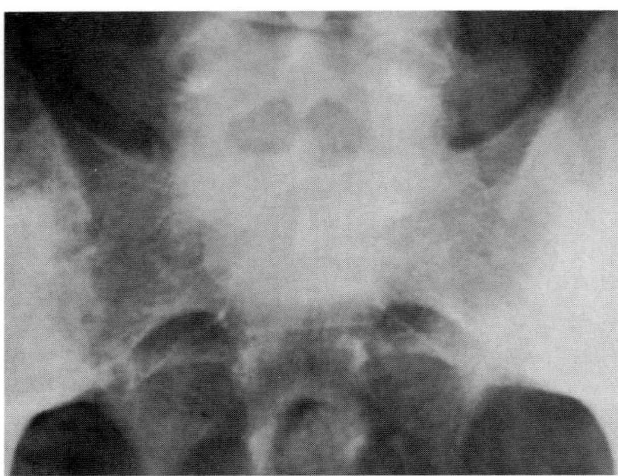

Figure 13–9. Juvenile ankylosing spondylitis. Advanced radiographic changes (angulated view). This film was obtained 14 years after onset of clinical disease in the patient shown in Figure 13–7. The sacroiliac joints are virtually fused, especially on the left, but there is still marked bilateral reactive sclerosis and erosions on the right. (From Ladd JR, Cassidy JT, Martel W: Juvenile ankylosing spondylitis. Arthritis Rheum 14: 579, 1971.)

tected only by a thin layer of fibrocartilage. This difference may account for the higher frequency of abnormalities on the iliac side of the joints. Only the lower one third to one half of the sacroiliac joint is diarthrodial and enclosed in a synovial membrane; the upper portion is a fibrous synostosis.[132]

CT is a considerable advance over plain radiography for demonstrating abnormalities in the sacroiliac joints. In a study of 40 adults with sacroiliac disease, conventional radiography yielded abnormal results in 10 but CT documented abnormalities in 30 patients. CT was particularly useful in the early stages of the disease.[133] Tomograms at three levels through the synovial portion of the joint are sufficient to demonstrate all but the smallest erosions (Fig. 13–10). A CT technique described by Oudjhane and colleagues[134] may even be more efficient at demonstrating erosions and sclerosis of the sacroiliac joints.

Magnetic resonance imaging (MRI) identifies early changes in both the sacroiliac joints and the spine and may prove to be the most sensitive indicator of inflammation of these joints. In a large study, dynamic MRI was used to evaluate the sacroiliac joints of 100 children under the age of 16 years with probable spondyloarthropathies (ESSG criteria) and 30 control children.[135] Dynamic MRI was capable of demonstrating early sacroiliac joint inflammation in many patients in whom other studies were unrevealing, particularly in children with acute disease. The authors, however, point out that this investigation should not be used in every child with back pain (because of cost) but that knowledge of the involvement of the sacroiliac joints could influence the choice of anti-inflammatory therapy.

Scintigraphic study of the sacroiliac joint is of limited value in the growing child or adolescent, unless there are distinct unilateral abnormalities. Sufficient experience in the interpretation of radionuclide scans in this age group is required before interpretation of bone scans can be relied on, and even then the yield is limited. Increased uptake in one sacroiliac joint can result not only from inflammation or infection but from asymmetric weight-bearing caused by arthritis in a lower-extremity joint or from enthesitis around the foot.

For purposes of documenting abnormalities of the sacroiliac joints in children and adolescents with suspected JAS, it is our practice to begin with a plain anteroposterior radiograph of the pelvis. Unless erosions are clearly demonstrable, we then obtain a CT examination. If uncertainty remains, we think that MRI is the most appropriate investigation unless the changes are clearly unilateral, in which case a scintigraphic study may be of help. From the viewpoint of classification, only plain radiographs are used; the application of newer techniques to diagnostic and classification clearly requires study.

Spine

Radiologic changes in the lumbosacral spine are less frequent and occur much later than abnormalities in

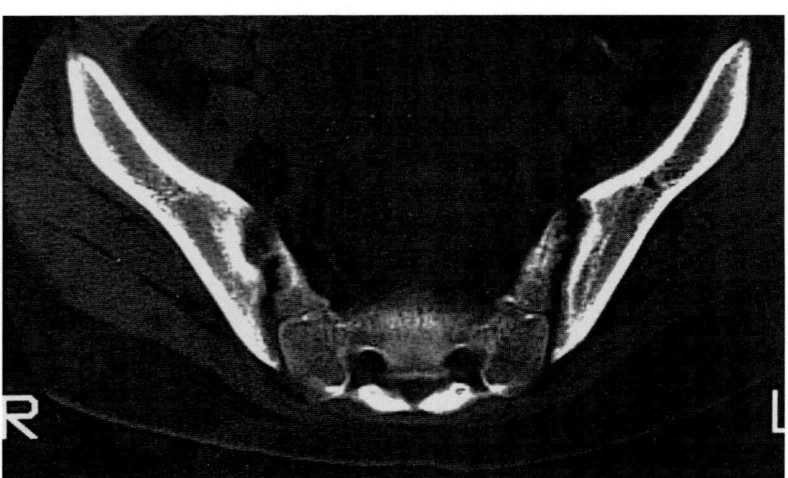

Figure 13–10. Coronal computed tomography scan of the sacroiliac joints in a child with ankylosing spondylitis. The image demonstrates bilateral sclerosis and erosions on the iliac sides of the sacroiliac joints, worse on the right than on the left.

the sacroiliac joint.[28] Periostitis with deposition of new bone along the anterior margin of the vertebral border results first in the "shining corner" and then in flattening of the normally slightly concave anterior margin of the vertebral body (Fig. 13–11). Syndesmophyte formation (Fig. 13–12), the hallmark of advanced disease in adults, is rare in children and adolescents but develops during the adult years in some patients with juvenile-onset disease. Periostitis at the iliac crests or the inferior pubic rami, or erosion at the symphysis pubis, is uncommon in children.

Arthritis affecting the cervical spine is less commonly symptomatic than that of the lumbosacral spine but may cause severe damage. This is documented by the MRI study shown in Figure 13–13C.

Entheses

Radiographic evaluation of entheses around the calcaneus and rarely the patella may show subtle changes in soft tissue density. Loss of the distinct margins of the Achilles tendon at its insertion, together with effacement of the triangular fat shadow, may be an early sign of inflammation at this site. Erosion of the bone at the insertion of the Achilles tendon or spur formation at that site is readily evaluated by a lateral radiograph of the calcaneus (Fig. 13–14). Azouz and Duffy[131] have described changes in the bone marrow subjacent to an inflamed enthesis in children with JAS.

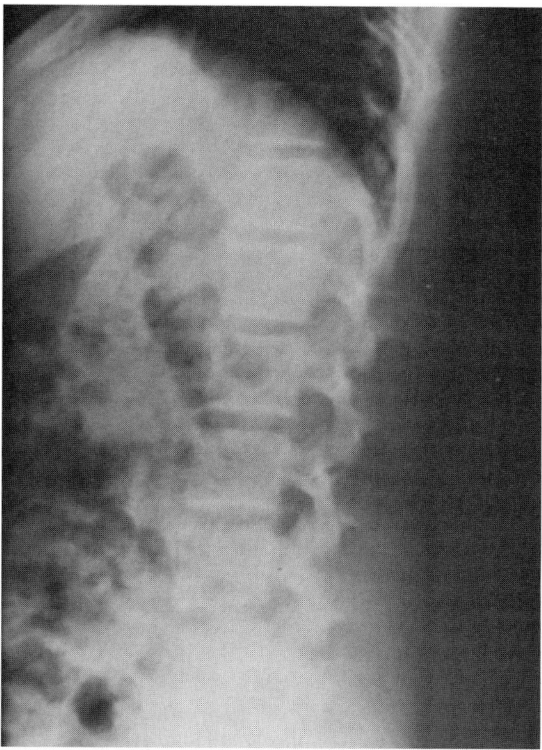

Figure 13–11. Lateral spine film shows marked straightening of the lumbar spine in early juvenile ankylosing spondylitis.

Peripheral Joints

Radiographic changes of peripheral joints are characterized by juxta-articular osteoporosis and joint space narrowing, especially at the hips, knees, and ankle joints. Erosions such as those that develop in children with JRA are exceptional. A characteristic ring osteophyte may be evident in the femur (Fig. 13–15). Ankylosis may occur but is not common in childhood, except at the intertarsal joints.

Treatment

General Management

Children with JAS have frequently had undiagnosed symptoms for months or years or have been diagnosed as having JRA or other disorders. The counsel of a team of health professionals—including physical and occupational therapists, nurses, social workers, and physicians—helps provide necessary education and care. Explanation of the correct diagnosis, its chronicity, possible complications, and the need for long-term medication, physical therapy, and medical follow-up facilitates compliance with therapeutic recommendations. In the older adolescent, realistic career goals must be discussed with the occupational therapist, who can advise the patient about ways of minimizing work-related stress to the low back and joints of the lower extremities. The child should be encouraged to participate as fully as possible in age-appropriate social and recreational activities. The relatively good long-term prognosis should be emphasized, particularly in the adolescent, who may regard the diagnosis of JAS as the end of recreational, social, educational, and career goals.

Management should be individualized according to the patient's specific problems. If widespread severe joint inflammation is the overwhelming problem, systemic anti-inflammatory medications (including NSAIDs, glucocorticoids, and sulfasalazine) are appropriate. If the joint disease is localized, it may be more useful to use NSAIDs and intra-articular triamcinolone hexacetonide in particularly problematic joints. Enthesitis, particularly around the foot, is unlikely to respond to systemic anti-inflammatory drugs alone; the use of custom-made orthotics often provides dramatic relief of calcaneal or metatarsal enthesitis. In all patients, exercise and maintenance of good posture to minimize loss of range of motion in the spine and its articulations are recommended. A firm mattress and thin pillow are important adjuncts to the program. Smoking should be strongly discouraged because of its demonstrated effect on range of motion of the spine and chest and adverse effects on pulmonary function[136] as well as its other detrimental effects on the lungs.

Anti-Inflammatory Medications

NSAIDs form the basis of the pharmacologic management of JAS. Although there are no reported trials of

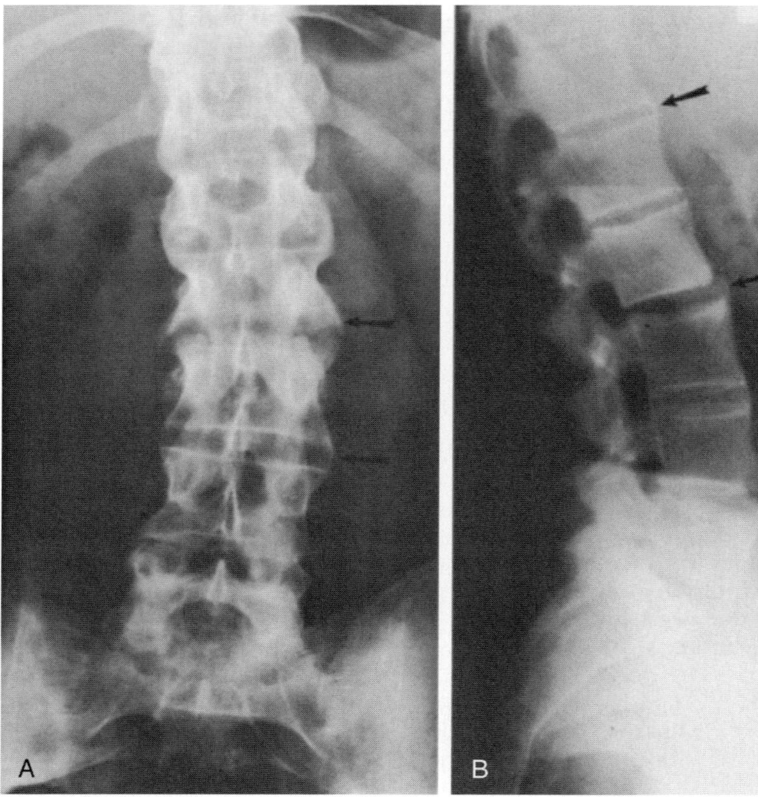

Figure 13–12. Radiographs of the lumbar spine. *A,* Syndesmophytes (*arrows*). *B,* Calcification of the anulus fibrosus (*arrows*) and anterior squaring. The bamboo-like appearance of the spine indicates long-standing juvenile ankylosing spondylitis and is a rare finding in childhood. These films were obtained from a 36-year-old man with onset of disease at the age of 14 years. (*A* and *B,* From Ladd JR, Cassidy JT, Martel W: Juvenile ankylosing spondylitis. Arthritis Rheum 14: 579, 1971.)

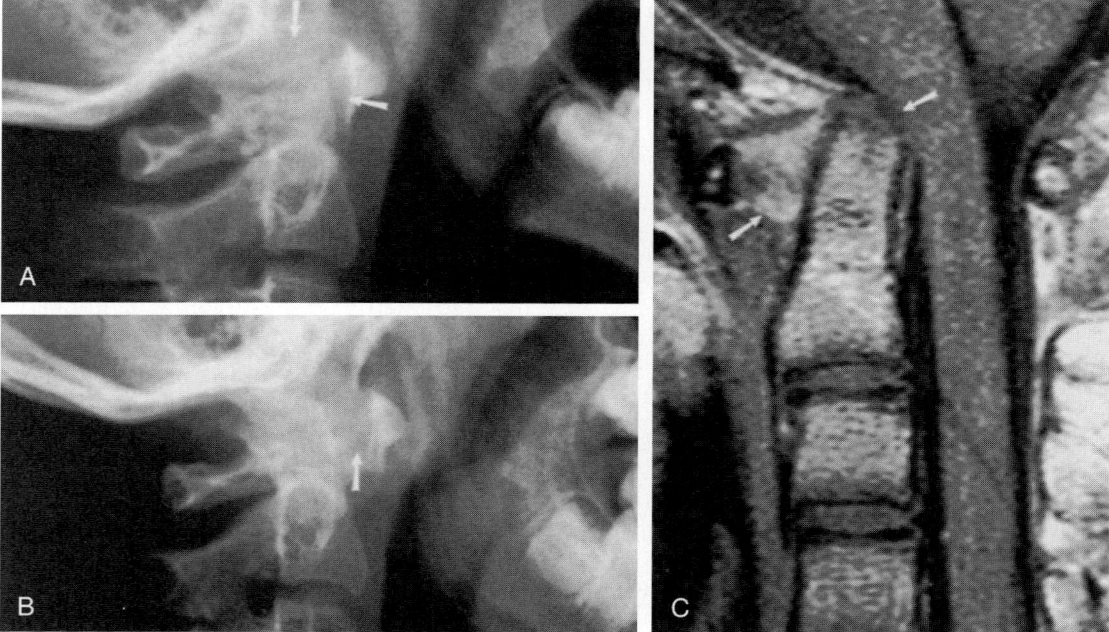

Figure 13–13. Close-up views of radiographs of the upper cervical spine in a child with juvenile ankylosing spondylitis. *A,* Extension view identifies the upper limit of the odontoid process of C2 (*arrow*) and the posteroinferior margin of the anterior arch of C1 (*arrow*). *B,* Flexion view documents a widened atlantoaxial space (*arrow*) confirming the presence of subluxation. *C,* Magnetic resonance image (T2-weighted) delineates an inflammatory mass in the space between the C1 anterior arch and the odontoid process (*lower arrow*) and indentation of the odontoid on the lower medulla/upper cervical cord (*upper arrow*).

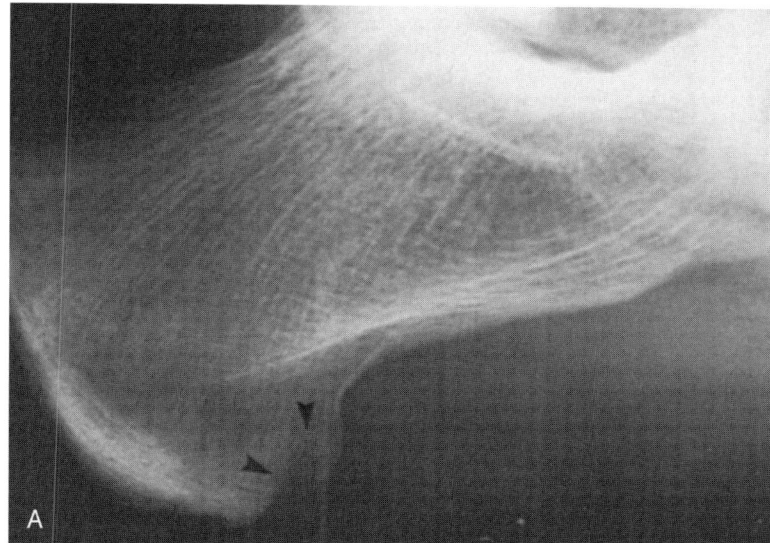

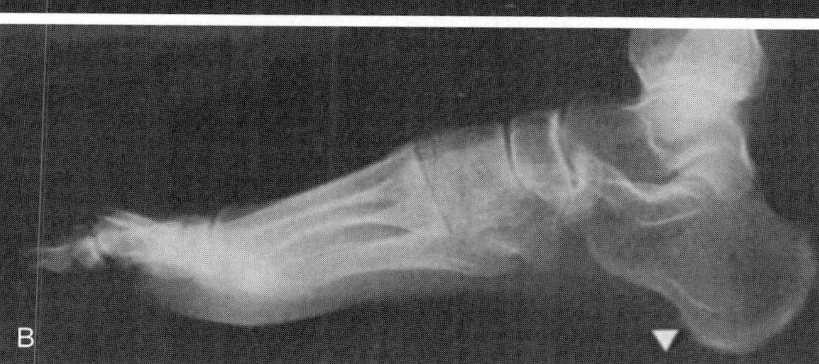

Figure 13–14. Lateral radiographs of the calcaneus show erosions at the site of insertion of the plantar fascia into the calcaneus (*A, arrowheads*) and spur formation at the insertion of the plantar fascia into the calcaneus (*B, arrowhead*). (*A,* From Petty RE, Malleson P: Spondyloarthropathies of childhood. Pediatr Clin North Am 33: 1079, 1986.)

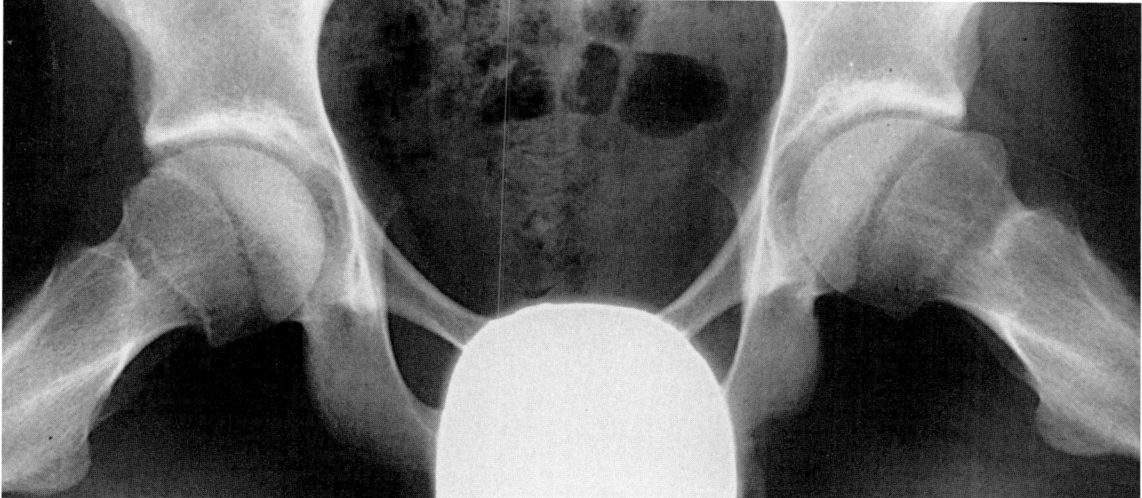

Figure 13–15. Radiograph of the hips of an adolescent boy with ankylosing spondylitis demonstrates bilateral rim osteophytes at the junction of the femoral head and neck.

NSAIDs in JAS, it is our clinical impression that these patients respond best to naproxen, tolmetin, or indomethacin. Because of lower toxicity, we recommend the use of naproxen (15 mg/kg/day) or tolmetin (25 to 30 mg/kg/day) before using indomethacin (1 to 2 mg/kg/day). Although indomethacin is often effective, toxicity is common and the drug must be prescribed and monitored carefully, beginning with low doses. Headache, epigastric pain, and inability to pay attention in school occur in 20 to 30 percent of children taking this drug and frequently necessitate cessation of its use.

Sulfasalazine has gained currency in the treatment of JAS, based largely on experience in adults,[137–143] although no prospective, randomized, placebo-controlled trials have been reported. In an open multicenter study, children with HLA-B27–positive late-onset oligoarthritis responded well to sulfasalazine.[144] This specific group of patients appeared to be those who responded best in other small trials as well.[145, 146] The response rate to sulfasalazine was as high in patients with the juvenile spondyloarthropathies as in those with JRA, but the duration of response was found to be shorter in those with the spondyloarthropathies.[147] The doses used in these studies ranged from 40 to 50 mg/kg/day. The beneficial effects are usually not evident for several weeks to 3 months after initiating treatment. Toxicity to bone marrow and liver must be monitored closely.

Glucocorticoids have a place in the management of the severely ill patient with JAS given orally or intravenously,[148] as topical agents in the management of acute iritis, and administered intra-articularly in children with limited, but severe, joint disease.[149, 150] The use of CT to guide injection of 40 mg of triamcinolone hexacetonide into the sacroiliac joints was reported in 30 adults with AS.[151] The injections were considered effective as judged both clinically and by dynamic MRI. Local injections of glucocorticoids at sites of enthesitis may occasionally be useful, particularly at the plantar fascia–calcaneal junction, taking care to avoid direct injection into tendon or extravasation into subcutaneous tissue.

There is little reported experience with other second agents. In general, gold and D-penicillamine are not recommended. Hydroxychloroquine and methotrexate are sometimes used, but there are no reports of their efficacy in children. In an open study of adults with AS who had not responded to NSAIDs and sulfasalazine, modest benefit was demonstrated with the use of methotrexate in a dose of 7.5 to 15 mg/wk.[152] There are no reports of the use of immunosuppressive drugs in children or adults with AS. In a single patient treated with azathioprine, severe pancytopenia developed because of an accompanying and presumably coincidental mutation of the thiopurine methyltransferase gene.[153]

Physical and Occupational Therapy

Physical therapy should be aimed at preventing loss of range of motion and poor functional positioning in the spine and chest, as well as stabilizing or regaining lost range in peripheral joints. Attention to posture and daily active range-of-motion exercises for the back and deep-breathing exercises for the chest help preserve range. Some young patients with JAS breathe predominantly with the diaphragm and have to be retaught to use the intercostal muscles. Strengthening of abdominal and back muscles should be undertaken cautiously. Swimming is an ideal form of physical activity that can be encouraged to augment these specific exercises.

Painful enthesitis in the feet may be dramatically relieved by the use of custom-made orthotics, fitted to support the fat cushion under the heel and to take pressure off the plantar aspects of the heel and metatarsophalangeal joints. If the Achilles enthesis alone is involved, the use of a slightly higher heel may help to reduce the stress at this site. Therapeutic ultrasonography and transcutaneous nerve stimulation are sometimes useful in the management of pain caused by enthesitis around the foot. Enthesitis may be quite resistant to therapy and be the most functionally limiting aspect of the disease.

Surgery

Orthopedic surgery has a limited role in the management of childhood JAS. Later in life, joint reconstruction and replacement are invaluable contributions to function and quality of life in the patient with severely damaged joints. The outcome of total hip replacement surgery in young adults followed for up to 30 years indicates that the probability that both components of the Charnley low-friction arthroplasty will survive 10 years is 91 percent; it was 70 percent at the 20-year follow-up.[154] Bony ankylosis as a result of exuberant overgrowth of bone around the prosthesis has been reported after hip joint replacement as an almost unique complication related to this disease.[30]

Course of the Disease and Prognosis

The early course of JAS is often remitting and may be mild. Often, it is only in retrospect that the musculoskeletal complaints are recognized as harbingers of JAS. Almost half of these children have four or fewer joints affected during the entire course of the disease; even in those in whom this number is exceeded, it is uncommon cumulatively to have more than six or seven inflamed joints. It should be noted that with few exceptions, children with JAS eventually develop peripheral joint disease, if they do not have it at onset. Lower-extremity predominance remains the rule throughout the disease, with hips, knees, and ankles and feet much more commonly affected than upper-extremity joints. Enthesitis may increase in frequency during the course of the disease.[155]

Long-term follow-up is essential to the care of the child with JAS. Subtle losses in range of motion of the thorax or back should be detected as early as possible.

Ansell[30] noted that limitation of range of motion of the spine was not detected until 11 to 33 years after onset of symptoms. A similar delay was also reported in the series of Ladd and coworkers.[28] From more recent experience, it is our impression, however, that limitation of range of back motion may occur much earlier. In the study of Burgos-Vargas and colleagues,[7] all patients had decreased back mobility by 5 years.

Accurate data on the outcome of children with JAS are very limited, and long-term outcome studies are badly needed. Outcome measures for adults with AS have been proposed[156] and could be evaluated in patients with JAS. At least during the years of childhood and adolescence, the functional outcome is probably good.[157] In one study,[158] however, outcome in JAS was worse than in AS. The persistence of peripheral joint disease may be more common in children than in adults, and persistent hip disease, in particular, is associated with a poor functional outcome.[155, 159] Acute iritis seldom leaves significant residua, even when it is recurrent, but uncommonly can be severe. Aortitis is rare but if present could contribute to late morbidity and mortality.

References

1. Wright V, Moll JM: Seronegative Polyarthritis. Amsterdam, The Netherlands, North Holland, 1976.
2. Fink CW and the Task Force for Classification Criteria: Proposal for the development of classification criteria for idiopathic arthritides of childhood. J Rheumatol 22: 1566, 1995.
3. Petty RE, Southwood TR, Baum J, et al: Revision of the proposed classification criteria for juvenile idiopathic arthritis: Durban, 1997. J Rheumatol 25: 1991, 1998.
4. Rosenberg AM, Petty RE: A syndrome of seronegative enthesopathy and arthropathy in children. Arthritis Rheum 25: 1041, 1982.
5. Bennett PH, Wood PHN: Population Studies of the Rheumatic Diseases. New York, Excerpta Medica, 1968, p 456.
6. Cabral DA, Oen KG, Petty RE: SEA syndrome revisited: a long-term follow-up of children with a syndrome of seronegative enthesopathy and arthropathy. J Rheumatol 19: 1282, 1992.
7. Burgos-Vargas R, Clark P: Axial involvement in the seronegative enthesopathy and arthropathy syndrome and its progression to ankylosing spondylitis. J Rheumatol 16: 192, 1989.
8. Jacobs JC, Beardon WE, Johnston AD: HLA-B27–associated spondyloarthritis and enthesopathy in childhood: clinical, pathologic and radiographic observations in 58 patients. J Pediatr 100: 521, 1983.
9. Cassidy JT, Levinson JE, Bass JC, et al: A study of classification criteria for a diagnosis of juvenile rheumatoid arthritis. Arthritis Rheum 29: 274, 1986.
10. Sheerin KA, Giannini EH, Brewer EJ, et al: HLA-B27–associated arthropathy in childhood: long-term clinical and diagnostic outcome. Arthritis Rheum 31: 1165, 1988.
11. Hussein A, Abdul-Khaliq H, van der Hardt H: Atypical spondyloarthritis in children: proposed diagnostic criteria. Eur J Pediatr 148: 513, 1989.
12. Amor B, Dougados M, Mijiyawa M: Critères de classification des spondylarthropathies. Rev Rhum Mal Osteoartic 57: 85, 1990.
13. Dougados M, van der Linden, S, Juhlin R, et al: The European Spondylarthropathy Study Group preliminary criteria for the classification of spondylarthropathy. Arthritis Rheum 34: 1218, 1991.
14. Malleson PN, Fung Y, Rosenberg AM, et al: The incidence of pediatric rheumatic diseases: results from the Canadian Pediatric Rheumatology Association Disease Registry. J Rheumatol 23: 1981, 1996.
15. Bowyer S, Roettcher P: Pediatric rheumatology clinic populations in the United States: results of a 3 year survey. J Rheumatol 23: 1968, 1986.
16. Symmons DPM, Jones M, Osborne J, et al: Pediatric rheumatology in the United Kingdom: data from the British Pediatric Rheumatology Group National Diagnostic Register. J Rheumatol 23: 1975, 1986.
17. Kaipiainen-Seppanen O, Savvolainen A: Incidence of chronic juvenile rheumatic diseases in Finland during 1980–1990. Clin Exp Rheumatol 14: 441, 1996.
18. Andersson-Gare B, Fasth A, Andersson J, et al: Incidence and prevalence of juvenile chronic arthritis: a population survey. Ann Rheum Dis 46: 277, 1987.
19. Carter ET, McKenna CH, Brian DD, et al: Epidemiology of ankylosing spondylitis in Rochester, Minnesota, 1935–1973. Arthritis Rheum 22: 365, 1979.
20. Carbone LD, Cooper C, Michet CJ, et al: Ankylosing spondylitis in Rochester, Minnesota, 1935–1989. Is the epidemiology changing? Arthritis Rheum 35: 1476, 1992.
21. Calin A: The epidemiology of ankylosing spondylitis: a clinician's point of view. *In* Lawrence RC, Shulman LE (eds): Epidemiology of the Rheumatic Diseases. New York, Gower, 1984, p 51.
22. Braun J, Bollow M, Remlinger G, et al: Prevalence of spondyloarthropathies in HLA-B27 positive and negative blood donors. Arthritis Rheum 41: 58, 1998.
23. Baum J, Ziff M: The rarity of ankylosing spondylitis in the black race. Arthritis Rheum 14: 12, 1971.
24. Sonozaki H, Seki H, Chang S, et al: Human lymphocyte antigen HL-A27 in Japanese patients with ankylosing spondylitis. Tissue Antigens 5: 131, 1975.
25. Gofton JP, Robinson HS, Trueman GE: Ankylosing spondylitis in a Canadian Indian population. Ann Rheum Dis 25: 525, 1966.
26. Good AE, Kawanishi H, Schultz JS: HLA B27 in blacks with ankylosing spondylitis or Reiter's disease. N Engl J Med 294: 166, 1976.
27. Gomez KS, Raza K, Jones SD, et al: Juvenile onset ankylosing spondylitis—more girls than we thought? J Rheumatol 24: 735, 1997
28. Ladd JR, Cassidy JT, Martel W: Juvenile ankylosing spondylitis. Arthritis Rheum 14: 579, 1971.
29. Edstrom G, Thune S, Wittbom-Cigen G: Juvenile ankylosing spondylitis. Acta Rheumatol Scand 6: 161, 1960.
30. Ansell BM: Juvenile spondylitis and related disorders. *In* Moll JMH (ed): Ankylosing Spondylitis. Edinburgh, Churchill Livingstone, 1980, p 120.
31. Bywaters EGL: Ankylosing spondylitis in childhood. Clin Rheum Dis 2: 387, 1976.
32. Schaller J, Bitnun S, Wedgwood RJ: Ankylosing spondylitis with childhood onset. J Pediatr 74: 505, 1969.
33. Schaller J: Ankylosing spondylitis of childhood onset. Arthritis Rheum 20(Suppl): 398, 1977.
34. Hafner R: Die juvenile Spondarthritis. Retrospektive Untersuchung an 71 Patienten. Monatsschr Kinderheilkd 135: 41, 1987.
35. Veys EM, Coigne E, Mielants H, et al: HLA and juvenile rheumatoid polyarthritis. Tissue Antigens 8: 62, 1976.
36. Sturrock RD, Dick HM, Henderson N, et al: Association of HLA 27 in juvenile rheumatoid arthritis and ankylosing spondylitis. J Rheumatol 1: 269, 1974.
37. Edmonds J, Morris RI, Metzger AL, et al: Follow-up study of juvenile chronic polyarthritis with particular reference to histocompatibility antigen W. 27. Ann Rheum Dis 33: 289, 1974.
38. Calin A, Fries JF: Striking prevalence of ankylosing spondylitis in "healthy" w27 positive males and females. A controlled study. N Engl J Med 293: 835, 1975.
39. Masi AT: HLA-B27 and other host interactions in spondyloarthropathy syndromes. J Rheumatol 5: 359, 1978.
40. Resnick D, Dwopsh IL, Goergen TG, et al: Clinical and radiographic abnormalities in ankylosing spondylitis: a comparison of men and women. Radiography 119: 293, 1976.
41. Keat A: Infections and the immunopathogenesis of seronegative spondyloarthropathies. Curr Opin Rheumatol 4: 494, 1992.
42. Mielants H, Veys EM, Joos R, et al: HLA antigens in seronegative spondyloarthropathies. Reactive arthritis and arthritis in ankylosing spondylitis: relation to gut inflammation. J Rheumatol 14: 466, 1987.

43. Jobanputra P, Choy EHS, Kingsley GH, et al: Cellular immunity to cartilage proteoglycans: relevance to the pathogenesis of ankylosing spondylitis. Ann Rheum Dis 51: 959, 1992.
44. Geczy AF, Seger K, Bashir HV, et al: The role of *Klebsiella* in the pathogenesis of ankylosing spondylitis: II. Evidence for a specific B27-associated marker on the lymphocytes of patients with ankylosing spondylitis. J Clin lab Immunol 3: 23, 1980.
45. Cameron FH, Russell PJ, Easter JF, et al: Failure of *Klebsiella pneumoniae* antibodies to cross-react with peripheral blood mononuclear cells from patients with ankylosing spondylitis. Arthritis Rheum 30: 300, 1987.
46. Ford DK, Da Roza DM, Schultzer M: Lymphocytes from the site of disease but not blood lymphocytes indicate the cause of arthritis. Ann Rheum Dis 44: 701, 1985.
47. Kapasi K, Inman RD: HLA-B27 expression modulates gram-negative bacterial invasion into transfected L cells. J Immunol 148: 3554, 1992.
48. Kapasi K, Inman RD: ME 1 epitope of HLA B27 confers class I mediated modulation of gram-negative bacterial invasion. J Immunol 153: 833, 1994.
49. Ortiz-Alvarez O, Yu D, Petty RE, Finlay BB: HLA-B27 does not affect invasion of arthritogenic bacteria into human cells. J Rheumatol 25: 1765, 1998.
50. Huppertz H-I, Heesemann J: Invasion and persistence of Salmonella in human fibroblasts positive or negative for endogenous HLA B27. Ann Rheum Dis 56: 671, 1997.
51. Granfors K: Host-microbe interaction in HLA-B27 associated diseases. Ann Med 29: 153, 1997.
52. Taurog J: Immunology, genetics and animal models of the spondyloarthropathies. Curr Opin Rheumatol 2: 586, 1990.
53. Breban M, Hammer RE, Richardson JA, Taurog JD: Transfer of the inflammatory disease of HLA-B27 transgenic rats by bone marrow engraftment. J Exp Med 178: 1607, 1993.
54. Mielants H, Veys EM, Goemaere S, et al: A prospective study of patients with spondyloarthropathy with special reference to HLA-B27 and to gut histology. J Rheumatol 20: 1353, 1993.
55. Mielants H, Veys EM, Cuvelier C, et al: The evolution of spondyloarthropathies in relation to gut histology: III. Relation between gut and joint. J Rheumatol 22: 2279, 1995.
56. Ansell BM, Bywaters EGL, Lawrence JS: Familial aggregation and twin studies in Still's disease. Juvenile chronic polyarthritis. Rheumatology 2: 37, 1969.
57. Rubin LA, Amos CI, Wade JA, et al: Investigating the genetic basis for ankylosing spondylitis. Arthritis Rheum 37: 1212, 1994.
58. Brewerton DA, Caffrey M, Hart FD: Ankylosing spondylitis and HL-A 27. Lancet 1: 194, 1973.
59. Van der Linden SM, Valkenburg HA, deJongh BM, et al: The risk of developing ankylosing spondylitis in HLA-B27 positive individuals. A comparison of relative of spondylitis patients with the general population. Arthritis Rheum 27: 241, 1984.
60. Schlosstein L, Terasaki PI, Bluestone R, et al: High association of an HL-A antigen, W27, with ankylosing spondylitis. N Engl J Med 288: 704, 1973.
61. McDaniel DO, Barger DO, Reveille JD, et al: Analysis of restriction fragment length polymorphisms in rheumatic diseases. Rheum Dis Clin North Am 13: 353, 1987.
62. Khan, MA: Spondyloarthropathies. Curr Opin Rheumatol 10: 279, 1998
63. MacLean L: HLA-B27 subtypes: implications for the spondyloarthropathies. Ann Rheum Dis 51: 929, 1992.
64. Hill AVS, Allsopp CEM, Kwiatkowski D, et al: HLA class I typing by PCR: HLA B27 and an African B27 subtype. Lancet 337: 640, 1991.
65. Kvien TK, Moller P, Dale K: Juvenile ankylosing spondylitis and HLA B27 homozygosity. Scand J Rheumatol 14: 47, 1985.
66. Brown MA, Kennedy LG, MacGregor AJ, et al: Susceptibility to ankylosing spondylitis in twins: the role of genes, HLA, and the environment. Arthritis Rheum 40: 1823, 1997.
67. Oen K, Petty RE, Schroeder M-L: An association between HLA-A2 and juvenile rheumatoid arthritis in girls. J Rheumatol 9: 916, 1982.
68. Woodrow JC: Genetics. *In* Moll JMH (ed): Ankylosing Spondylitis. Edinburgh, Churchill Livingstone, 1980, p 26.
69. Arnett FH Jr, Schacter BZ, Hochberg MC, et al: HLA-A28 in patients with B27-associated rheumatic diseases. Arthritis Rheum 20: 106, 1977.
70. Calin A, Porta J, Payne R: HLA-A28 in B27 positive controls and patients with ankylosing spondylitis. Arthritis Rheum 20: 1428, 1977.
71. Robinson WP, van der Linden SM, Khan MA, et al: HLA-Bw60 increases susceptibility to ankylosing spondylitis in HLA-B27 + patients. Arthritis Rheum 32: 1135, 1989.
72. Brown MA, Pile KD, Kennedy LG, et al: HLA class I associations of ankylosing spondylitis in the white population in the United Kingdom. Ann Rheum Dis 55: 268, 1996.
73. Truog P, Steiger U, Contu I, et al: Ankylosing spondylitis (AS): a population and family study using HL-A serology and MLR. *In* Kissmeyer-Nielsen F (ed): Histocompatibility Testing. Copenhagen, Munksgaard, 1975, p 788.
74. Van den Berg-Loonen EM, Dekker-Saeys BJ, Meuwissen SGM, et al: Histocompatibility antigens and other genetic markers in ankylosing spondylitis and inflammatory bowel diseases. J Immunogenet 4: 167, 1977.
75. Maksymowych WP, Gorodezky C, Olivo A, et al: HLA-DRB1*08 influences the development of disease in Mexican Mestizo with spondyloarthropathy. J Rheumatol 24: 904–907, 1997.
76. Maksymowych WP, Jhangri GS, Gorodezky C, et al: The LMP2 polymorphism is associated with susceptibility to acute anterior uveitis in HLA-B27 positive juvenile and adult Mexican subjects with ankylosing spondylitis. Ann Rheum Dis 56: 488, 1997.
77. Ploski R, Flato B, Vinje O, et al: Association to HLA-DRB1*08, HLA-DPB1*0301 and homozygosity for an HLA-linked proteasome gene in juvenile ankylosing spondylitis. Hum Immunol 44: 88, 1995.
78. Kleinman P, Rivelis M, Schneider R, et al: Juvenile ankylosing spondylitis. Pediatr Radiol 125: 775, 1977.
79. Burgos-Vargas R, Vazquez-Mellado J, Cassis N, et al: Genuine ankylosing spondylitis in children: a case-control study of patients with early definite disease according to adult onset criteria. J Rheumatol 23: 2140, 1996.
80. Petty RE: Is ankylosing spondylitis in childhood a distinct entity? J Rheumatol 23: 2013, 1996.
81. Niepel GA, Sit'aj S: Enthesopathy. Clin Rheum Dis 5: 857, 1979.
82. Stamato T, Laxer RM, de Freitas C, et al: Prevalence of cardiac manifestations of juvenile ankylosing spondylitis. Am J Cardiol 75: 744, 1995.
83. Stewart SL, Robbins DL, Castles JJ: Acute fulminant aortic and mitral insufficiency in ankylosing spondylitis. N Engl J Med 299: 1448, 1978.
84. Reid GD, Patterson MWH, Patterson AC, et al: Aortic insufficiency in association with juvenile ankylosing spondylitis. J Pediatr 95: 78, 1979.
85. Kean WF, Anastassiades TP, Ford PM: Aortic incompetence in HLA B27-positive juvenile arthritis. Ann Rheum Dis 39: 294, 1980.
86. Gore JE, Vizcarrondo FE, Rieffel CN: Juvenile ankylosing spondylitis and aortic regurgitation: a case presentation. Pediatrics 68: 423, 1981.
87. Pelkonen P, Byring R, Pesonen I, et al: Rapidly progressive aortic incompetence in juvenile ankylosing spondylitis: a case report. Arthritis Rheum 27: 698, 1984.
88. Kim TH, Jung SS, Sohn SJ, et al: Aneurysmal dilatation of ascending aorta and aortic insufficiency in juvenile spondylarthropathy. Scand J Rheumatol 26: 218, 1997.
89. Simpson J, Borzy MS, Silberbach GM: Aortic regurgitation at diagnosis of HLA-B27 associated spondyloarthropathy. J Rheumatol 22: 332, 1995.
90. Hubscher O, Graci Y, Susini J: Aortic insufficiency in Reiter's syndrome of juvenile onset. J Rheumatol 11: 94, 1984.
91. Toone E, Johnson WL: The clinical and pathological cardiac manifestations of rheumatoid spondylitis. Va Med 95: 132, 1968.
92. Roldan CA, Chavez J, Wiest PW, et al: Aortic root disease and valve disease associated with ankylosing spondylitis. J Am Coll Cardiol 32: 1397, 1998.
93. Camiciottoli G, Trapani S, Ermini M, et al: Pulmonary function in children affected by juvenile spondyloarthropathy. J Rheumatol 26: 1382, 1999.
94. Rosenow EC, Strimlan CV, Muhm JR, et al: Pleuropulmonary manifestations of ankylosing spondylitis. Mayo Clin Proc 52: 641, 1977.
95. Fenlon HM, Casserly I, Sant SM, Breatnach E: Plain radiographs

and thoracic high-resolution CT in patients with ankylosing spondylitis. AJR 168: 1067, 1997.
96. Reid GD, Hill RH: Atlantoaxial subluxation in juvenile ankylosing spondylitis. J Pediatr 93: 531, 1978.
97. Foster HE, Cairns RA, Burnell RH, et al: Atlantoaxial subluxation in children with seronegative enthesopathy and arthropathy syndrome: 2 case reports and a review of the literature. J Rheumatol 22: 548, 1995.
98. Bartleson JD, Cohen MD, Harrington TM, et al: Cauda equina syndrome secondary to long-standing ankylosing spondylitis. Ann Neurol 14: 662, 1983.
99. Allen RC, Petty RE, Lirenman DS, et al: Renal papillary necrosis in children with chronic arthritis treated with non-steroidal anti-inflammatory drugs. Am J Dis Child 140: 20, 1986.
100. Mustonen J: IgA glomerulonephritis and associated diseases. Ann Clin Res 16: 161, 1984.
101. Bruneau C, Villiaumey JH, Avouac B, et al: Seronegative spondyloarthropathies and IgA glomerulonephritis: a report of four cases and a review of the literature. Semin Arthritis Rheum 15: 179, 1986.
102. Julkunen H: Synovial inflammatory cell reaction in chronic arthritis. Acta Rheumatol Scand 12: 188, 1966.
103. Grom AA, Murray KJ, Luyrink L, et al: Patterns of expression of tumor necrosis factor α, tumor necrosis factor β, and their receptors in synovia of patients with juvenile rheumatoid arthritis and juvenile spondyloarthropathy. Arthritis Rheum 39: 1703, 1996.
104. Ball J: Enthesopathy of rheumatoid and ankylosing spondylitis. Ann Rheum Dis 30: 213, 1971.
105. Shichikawa K, Tsujimoto M, Nishioka J, et al: Histopathology of early sacroiliitis and enthesitis in ankylosing spondylitis. Adv Inflammat Res 9: 15, 1985.
106. Ball J: Pathology and pathogenesis. *In* Moll JMH (ed): Ankylosing Spondylitis. Edinburgh, Churchill Livingstone, 1980, p 96.
107. Turner PG, Green JH, Galasko CSB: Back pain in childhood. Spine 8: 812, 1989.
108. Moran HM, Hall MA, Barr A, et al: Spinal mobility in the adolescent. Rheumatol Rehab 18: 181, 1979.
109. The HSG, Steven MM, van der Linden S, et al: Evaluation of diagnostic criteria for ankylosing spondylitis: a comparison of the Rome, New York and modified New York criteria in patients with a positive clinical history screening test for ankylosing spondylitis. Br J Rheumatol 24: 242, 1985.
110. Petty RE, Malleson P: Spondyloarthropathies of childhood. Pediatr Clin North Am 33: 1079, 1986.
111. Burgos-Vargas R, Petty RE: Juvenile ankylosing spondylitis. Rheum Dis Clin North Am 18: 123, 1992.
112. Prieur A-M, Listrat M, Dougados M, Amor B: Critères de classification des spondylarthropathies chez les enfants. Arch Fr Pediatr 50: 379, 1993.
113. Olivieri I, Barbieri P, Geiningnam G, et al: Isolated juvenile onset HLA-B27 associated peripheral enthesitis. J Rheumatol 17: 567, 1990.
114. Bowyer S: Hip contracture as the presenting sign in children with HLA-B27 arthritis. J Rheumatol 1995;22: 165.
115. Burgos-Vargas R, Naranjo A, Castillo J, et al: Ankylosing spondylitis in the Mexican mestizo: patterns of disease according to age at onset. J Rheumatol 16: 186, 1989.
116. Macrae IF, Wright V: Measurement of back movement. Ann Rheum Dis 28: 584, 1969.
117. Moll JMH, Wright V: Normal range of spinal mobility: an objective clinical study. Ann Rheum Dis 30: 381, 1971.
118. Lehman TJA, Hanson V, Kornreich H, et al: HLA-B-27 negative sacroiliitis: a manifestation of familial Mediterranean fever in childhood. Pediatrics 61: 423, 1978.
119. Sherry DD, Petty RE, Tredwell S, et al: Histocompatibility antigens in Osgood-Schlatter's disease. J Pediatr Orthop 5: 302, 1985.
120. Barkely DO, Hohermuth HJ, Howard A, et al: IgA deficiency in juvenile chronic polyarthritis. J Rheumatol 6: 219, 1979.
121. Cassidy JT: Selective IgA deficiency and chronic arthritis in children. *In* Moore TD (ed): Arthritis in Childhood. Report of the Eightieth Ross Conference in Pediatric Research. Columbus, OH, Ross Laboratories, 1981, p 82.
122. Kinsella TD, Espinoza L, Vasey FB: Serum complement and immunoglobulin levels in sporadic and familial ankylosing spondylitis. J Rheumatol 2: 308, 1975.
123. Cowling P, Ebringer R, Ebringer A: Association of inflammation and raised serum IgA in ankylosing spondylitis. Ann Rheum Dis 39: 545, 1980.
124. Corrigall V, Panayi GS, Unger A, et al: Detection of immune complexes in serum of patients with ankylosing spondylitis. Ann Rheum Dis 37: 159, 1978.
125. Juanola X, Mateo L, Domenech P, et al: Prevalence of antiphospholipid antibodies in patients with ankylosing spondylitis. J Rheumatol 22: 1891, 1995.
126. Kendall MJ, Farr M, Meynell MJ, et al: Synovial fluid in ankylosing spondylitis. Ann Rheum Dis 32: 487, 1973.
127. Traycoff RB, Pascal E, Schumacher HR Jr: Mononuclear cells in human synovial fluid. Identification of lymphoblasts in rheumatoid arthritis. Arthritis Rheum 19: 743, 1976.
128. Spriggs AJ, Boddington MM, Mowat AG: Joint fluid cytology in Reiter's disease. Ann Rheum Dis 37: 557, 1978.
129. Bunch TW, Hunder GG, McDuffie FC, et al: Synovial fluid complement determination as a diagnostic aid in inflammatory joint disease. Mayo Clin Proc 49: 715, 1974.
130. Riley MJ, Ansell BM, Bywaters EGL: Radiological manifestations of ankylosing spondylitis according to age at onset. Ann Rheum Dis 30: 138, 1971.
131. Azouz EM, Duffy CM: Juvenile spondyloarthropathies: clinical manifestations and medical imaging. Skel Radiol 24: 399, 1995.
132. Bellamy N, Park W, Rooney PS: What do we know about the sacroiliac joint? Semin Arthritis Rheum 12: 282, 1983.
133. Geijer M, Sihlbom H, Gothlin JH, Nordborg E: The role of CT in the diagnosis of sacro-iliitis. Acta Radiol 39: 265, 1998.
134. Oudjhane K, Azouz EM, Hughes S, Paquin JD: Computed tomography of the sacroiliac joints in children. Can Assoc Radiol J 44: 313, 1993.
135. Bollow M, Biedermann T, Kannenberg J, et al: Use of dynamic magnetic resonance imaging to detect sacroiliitis in HLA B-27 positive and negative children with juvenile arthritides. J Rheumatol 25: 556, 1998.
136. Averns HL, Oxtoby J, Taylor HG, et al: Smoking and outcome in ankylosing spondylitis. Scand J Rheumatol 25: 138, 1996.
137. Dougados M, Boumier P, Amor B: Sulphasalazine in ankylosing spondylitis: a double-blind, controlled study in 60 patients. Br Med J 293: 911, 1986.
138. Dougados M, Maetzel A, Mijiyawa M, et al: Evaluation of sulphasalazine in the treatment of spondyloarthropathies. Ann Rheum Dis 51: 955, 1992.
139. Feltelius N, Hallgren R: Sulphasalazine in ankylosing spondylitis. Ann Rheum Dis 45: 396, 1986.
140. Nissila M, Lehtinen K, Leirisalo-Repo M, et al: Sulphasalazine in the treatment of ankylosing spondylitis. A twenty-six-week placebo-controlled clinical trial. Arthritis Rheum 31: 1111, 1988.
141. Davis MJ, Sawes PT, Beswick E, et al: Sulphasalazine therapy in ankylosing spondylitis: its effects on disease activity, immunoglobulin A, and the complex immunoglobulin A-alpha$_1$-antitrypsin. Br J Rheumatol 28: 410, 1989.
142. Fraser SM, Sturrock RD: Evaluation of sulphasalazine in ankylosing spondylitis—an interventional study. Br J Rheumatol 29: 37, 1990.
143. Corkill MM, Jobanputra P, Gibson T, et al: A controlled trial of sulphasalazine treatment of chronic ankylosing spondylitis: failure to demonstrate clinical effect. Br J Rheumatol 29: 41, 1990.
144. Ansell BM, Hall MA, Loftus JK, et al: A multicentre pilot study of sulphasalazine in juvenile chronic arthritis. Clin Exp Rheumatol 9: 201, 1991.
145. Suschke HJ: Die therapie der juvenilen chronischen arthritis mit sulfasalzin. Z Rheumatol 46: 83, 1987.
146. Joss R, Veys EM, Mielants H, et al: Sulfasalazine treatment in juvenile chronic arthritis: an open study. J Rheumatol 18: 880, 1991.
147. Huang JL, Chen LC: Sulphasalazine in the treatment of children with chronic arthritis. Clin Rheumatol 17: 359–363, 1998.
148. Miller JJ: Prolonged use of large intravenous steroid pulses in the rheumatic diseases of children. Pediatrics 65: 989, 1980.
149. Allen RC, Gross KR, Laxer RM, et al: Intraarticular triamcinolone hexacetonide in the management of chronic arthritis in children. Arthritis Rheum 29: 997, 1986.

150. Huppertz H-I, Tschammler A, Horwitz AE, Schwab O: Intra-articular corticosteroids for chronic arthritis in children: efficacy and effects on cartilage and growth. J Pediatr 127: 317, 1995.
151. Braun J, Bollow M, Seyrekbasan F, et al: Computed tomography guided corticosteroid injection of the sacroiliac joint in patients with spondyloarthropathy with sacroiliitis: clinical outcome and followup by dynamic magnetic resonance imaging. Arthritis Rheum 39: 659, 1996.
152. Creemers MCW, Franssen JAM, van de Putte LBA, et al: Methotrexate in severe ankylosing spondylitis: an open study. J Rheumatol 22: 1104, 1995.
153. Leipold G, Schutz, Haas JP, Oellerich M: Azathioprine-induced severe pancytopenia due to a homozygous two-point mutation of the thiopurine methyltransferase gene in a patient with juvenile HLA-B27–associated spondylarthritis. Arthritis Rheum 40: 1896, 1997.
154. Sochart DH, Porter ML: Long-term results of total hip replacement in young patients who had ankylosing spondylitis. Eighteen to thirty-year results with survivorship analysis. J Bone Joint Surg Am 79: 1181, 1997.
155. Burgos-Vargas R, Vazquez-Mellado J: Cohort study comparing juvenile ankylosing spondylitis (JAS) and juvenile rheumatoid arthritis (JRA). J Rheumatol 19(Suppl 33): 118, 1992.
156. van der Heijde D, Bellamy N, Calin A, et al: Preliminary core sets for endpoints in ankylosing spondylitis. Arthritis Rheum 24: 2225, 1997.
157. Calin A, Elswood J: The natural history of juvenile-onset ankylosing spondylitis: as 24-year retrospective case-control study. Br J Rheumatol 27: 91, 1988.
158. Garcia-Morteo O, Maldonado-Cocco JA, Suarez-Almazor ME, et al: Ankylosing spondylitis of juvenile onset: comparison with adult onset disease. Scand J Rheumatol 12: 246, 1983.
159. Marks SH, Barnett M, Calin A: A case-control study of juvenile- and adult-onset ankylosing spondylitis. J Rheumatol 9: 739, 1982.

14

Psoriatic Arthritis

Taunton R. Southwood

DEFINITION AND CLASSIFICATION

The diagnosis of juvenile psoriatic arthritis (JPsA) is straightforward if arthritis begins before 16 years of age and psoriasis is present at the same time. However, the onset of arthritis and psoriasis may not be simultaneous, as is highlighted in a traditional definition of the disease: an inflammatory arthritis beginning before the age of 16 years, associated with psoriasis, either preceding the onset of psoriasis or occurring within the subsequent 15 years.[1] More recent attempts to formulate criteria for the diagnosis and classification of psoriatic arthritis include the "Vancouver criteria"[2] and an international consensus proposal of classification criteria for juvenile idiopathic arthritis[3] (Table 14–1). An important feature of both sets of criteria is the recognition of a diagnosis of JPsA in a child with arthritis who has yet to develop the rash of psoriasis. This entity, also known as *psoriatic arthritis sine psoriasis*, has also been recognized in adults.[4] A follow-up study of children with probable psoriatic arthritis defined by the Vancouver criteria found that definite psoriatic arthritis had occurred in approximately half of the children after a mean of 2.1 years.[5]

Key clinical elements of the classification criteria for JPsA include arthritis, psoriasis, a family history of psoriasis, dactylitis, and nail pitting. Arthritis is defined as swelling within a joint or limitation in range of joint movement with joint pain or tenderness that persists for more than 6 weeks, is observed by a physician, and is not due to primarily mechanical disorders. Dactylitis can be distinguished from arthritis if swelling of one or more digits extends beyond the joint margins. It represents the combined effects of arthritis and tenosynovitis. Psoriasis, and a positive family history of psoriasis in a first-degree relative (parent or sibling), requires that the skin rash be diagnosed with certainty as psoriasis. Such strict definitions may be difficult to use in clinical situations but help improve communication and attempts at understanding the etiology and pathogenesis of the disease.[6]

There is an apparent disparity between psoriatic arthritis observed during the childhood years and the disease that begins during adulthood,[7] which appears to be part of the spectrum of spondyloarthropathies,[8–10] with a proposed "common thread" being the presence of enthesitis.[11] In contrast, JPsA shares few of the characteristics of the spondyloarthropathies, such as sacroiliac disease, enthesitis, acute uveitis, or an association with human leukocyte antigen (HLA)-B27. At onset, JPsA is similar to the asymmetric oligoarticular disease described by Moll and Wright[12] (Table 14–2). The arbitrary time point of 16 years used to differentiate childhood from adult disease may have little biologic or pathologic relevance. For this reason, information about adult psoriatic arthritis is considered in the following discussions of the epidemiology, pathology, clinical features, and treatment of psoriatic arthritis in children.

EPIDEMIOLOGY

Incidence and Prevalence

Psoriasis affects 1 to 3 percent of the general population,[13] and as many as 20 to 30 percent of patients are reported to have an associated arthritis.[14–16] In the pediatric population, the frequency of psoriasis is lower (about 0.5 percent of the population younger than 16 years of age[17]); the proportion with arthritis may also be lower. These figures must be viewed with

Table 14–1

Criteria for Diagnosis and Classification of Juvenile Psoriatic Arthritis

ILAR CRITERIA (DURBAN, 1997)[3]	VANCOUVER CRITERIA (1989)[2]
Arthritis and psoriasis, or Arthritis and at least two of: Dactylitis Nail pitting or onycholysis Family history of psoriasis in a first-degree relative Excluding: Presence of rheumatoid factor Presence of another form of juvenile idiopathic arthritis	Definite juvenile psoriatic arthritis: Arthritis with typical psoriatic rash, or Arthritis with three of the following minor criteria: Nail pitting or onycholysis Family history of psoriasis (first- or second-degree relative) Psoriasis-like rash Dactylitis Probable juvenile psoriatic arthritis: arthritis with two of four minor criteria

ILAR, International League of Associations for Rheumatology.

Table 14–2

Classification of Psoriatic Arthritis

ONSET TYPE	CHARACTERISTICS	PERCENT
Monarticular or asymmetric oligoarthritis	Dactylitis, often becomes polyarticular	70
Symmetric polyarthritis	Polyarticular, large and small joints	15
Predominant distal interphalangeal joint	Accompanying nail disease	5
Spondylitis	Peripheral arthritis with sacroiliac joint disease	5
Arthritis mutilans	Severely deforming, often with sacroiliac joint disease and ankylosis	5

caution, however, because at least half of the children with psoriatic arthritis develop joint inflammation before the onset of psoriasis.

Published studies suggest that JPsA accounts for 2 to 15 percent of all children with chronic arthritis.[18–20] Several recent surveys of arthritis in children that used similar diagnostic criteria have confirmed that JPsA accounts for approximately 7 percent of all cases of chronic childhood arthritis (Table 14–3).[18–21] Estimates of the incidence have suggested that 2.3 to 3 per 100,000 children develop psoriatic arthritis every year, with a prevalence of 10 to 15 per 100,000.[2, 21] The ethnic associations of psoriatic arthritis have only rarely been studied, but a multicenter survey in the United States found that over 90 percent of patients with definite psoriatic arthritis were white, 5 percent were Hispanic, and 2.5 percent were African-American.[18] Psoriatic arthritis has also been reported in Chinese, Indians, and Malaysians living in Singapore.[24]

Age at Onset and Sex Ratio

In the pediatric population, the age at onset of psoriatic arthritis appears to be bimodally distributed.[2] A first peak occurs during the preschool years (mainly in girls), and a second occurs during mid to late childhood, centering around 10 years of age. Unlike adult psoriatic arthritis, psoriasis begins after the arthritis in the majority of children, and simultaneous onset is found in less than 10 percent (Table 14–4).[1, 2, 19, 21a–c] This may explain the earlier age of diagnosis of probable psoriatic arthritis (7.4 ± 4.5 years) compared with definite psoriatic arthritis (10 ± 4.9 years) noted in an American survey.[18] It is uncommon for the disease to begin before 1 year of age. The youngest child with psoriatic arthritis in the author's personal experience was 4 months old when arthritis in a knee and dactylitis of a toe were noted, in the absence of other features of psoriasis except for a maternal history of psoriasis. JPsA is somewhat more frequent in girls than boys (see Table 14–4), and in one survey girls accounted for 60 percent of 128 cases of JPsA.[20] The incidence of arthritis in adults who have psoriasis is 3.5 per 100,000 men and 3.4 per 100,000 women.[24]

ETIOLOGY AND PATHOGENESIS

At present, the cause of JPsA is unknown. Satisfactory theories of the etiology and pathogenesis of JPsA should explain not only the link between psoriasis and arthritis but also how a predisposition to psoriasis might lead to arthritis and even the peculiarly asymmetric large and small joint involvement in the disease.

Environmental Triggers

There have been few reports of psoriatic arthritis precipitated by physical trauma.[25, 26] Other environmental triggers, such as bacterial infections, have also been implicated. The onset of psoriasis in children may be preceded by streptococcal upper respiratory tract infection and, less commonly, skin infection.[27, 28] Laboratory studies in children with psoriatic arthritis have demonstrated synovial fluid T-cell responses to streptococci (Bhayani H, Black A, Southwood T, unpublished observations, 1998).[29, 30]

Viral infections have also been implicated in the disease, and JPsA may follow viral infections such as chickenpox.[1] However, a wider study of the epidemiology of childhood arthritis found no correlations between the onset of JPsA and coincident infections with mycoplasma, respiratory syncytial virus, adenovirus, influenza A and B, parainfluenza, rubella, cytomegalovirus, or herpes simplex.[31]

Pathogenesis

There is increasing evidence that psoriatic arthritis is mediated by activated CD8-positive T cells. These cells

Table 14–3

Epidemiology of Juvenile Psoriatic Arthritis

AUTHOR	TOTAL	JPsA (%)	ONSET AGE (yr)	F:M RATIO	INCIDENCE (per 100,000)
Gare and Fasth, 1992[21]	213	2.8	11.5	1.0	0.3
Bowyer et al, 1996[18]	1568	5.5	8.7	1.3	
Malleson et al, 1996[19]	861	7.0	10.1	1.6	0.23
Symmons et al, 1996[20]	1831	7.0	10.1	1.6	

JPsA, juvenile psoriatic arthritis; Total, number of patients surveyed.

Table 14–4

Juvenile Psoriatic Arthritis: Summary of Reported Series

	LAMBERT ET AL[21a]	CALABRO[21b]	SILLS[22]	SHORE AND ANSELL[1]	WESOLOWSKA[21c]	SOUTHWOOD ET AL[2]	TOTAL
Patients (n)	43	12	24	60	21	35	195
Male:female ratio	11:32	5:7	7:17	35:25	13:8	24:11	0.95:1
Age at onset (yr)							
Joint disease	9.3	NA	10	11	NA	6.7	6.7–11.0
Skin disease	10.4	12	11	8.8	NA	12.6	8.8–12.6
Disease sequence							
Psoriasis first (%)	40	67	33	42	33	43	33–67
Arthritis first (%)	53	33	58	43	62	48	33–62
Simultaneous onset (%)	7	0	9	15	5	10	5–15
Oligo-onset (≤4 joints) (%)	55	42	58	73	86	94	42–94
Poly-onset (≥5 joints) (%)	45	58	42	27	14	6	6–58
DIP joints affected (%)	21	50	62	42	10	29	10–62
Sacroiliac arthritis (%)	28	17	29	47*	100*	11	11–100
Nail changes (%)	70	92	83	77	86	51	51–92
Uveitis (%)	9	0	13	8	14	17	0–17

DIP, distal interphalangeal; NA, not available.
*Only selected patients had pelvic radiographs.

invade the epidermis in psoriatic skin lesions induced by the Koebner response, and long-lived CD8-positive clones have been recovered from psoriatic skin biopsies.[32, 33] Synovial fluid CD8-positive T cell numbers are increased in patients with psoriatic arthritis compared with other forms of arthritis,[34] although in the synovium itself the ratio of CD4 to CD8-positive T cells is variable.[35] Patients with psoriatic arthritis who are infected with human immunodeficiency virus often undergo a flare in the arthritis activity when CD4-positive T cell numbers are low.[36]

Cytokines appear to be important in the pathogenesis of psoriatic arthritis.[37, 38] Interleukin (IL)-2 has been demonstrated in the synovium of patients with psoriatic arthritis but not rheumatoid arthritis.[39] The proinflammatory cytokines tumor necrosis factor (TNF)-α, IL-1β, and IL-8, as well as TNF-α and IL-2 receptors, have been detected in psoriatic arthritis synovial fluid.[40] It is interesting that IL-4 and IL-10, cytokines associated with downregulation of the immune response, have been detected more frequently in the synovium of children whose arthritis remains oligoarticular, compared with those who follow a more aggressive disease course that evolves from oligoarthritis to polyarthritis, a pattern similar to that in psoriatic arthritis.[41]

Psoriasis can be induced in scid/scid mice by minor histocompatibility mismatched naive CD4-positive T cells.[42] Expression of alpha 2, alpha 5, or beta 1 integrin subunits by murine suprabasal keratinocytes is also associated with histopathologic changes characteristic of human psoriasis.[43] In a mouse model of psoriasis in which bone morphogenic protein 6 is overexpressed, overproduction of bone pro-osteoblastic cytokines leads to the periostitis and enthesitis typical of psoriatic arthritis.[44]

GENETIC BACKGROUND

There is convincing clinical evidence of a strong genetic component to psoriasis and psoriatic arthritis.[45] A concordance of 55 to 70 percent is documented for psoriasis and psoriatic arthritis in monozygotic twins.[46] A family history of psoriasis in first- or second-degree relatives was recorded in 40 to 63 percent of children with psoriatic arthritis, compared with 21 percent of children with other forms of chronic arthritis.[2] However, differing genetic susceptibilities may underlie psoriasis and psoriatic arthritis. Genomic DNA extracted from 395 probands with psoriasis provided strong evidence for a susceptibility gene on chromosome 6p, close to the HLA region, which was inherited paternally.[47] However, in probands with psoriatic arthritis, the investigators found that this linkage was less evident and there was no paternal effect. There appear to be ethnic differences in the occurrence of psoriatic arthritis in adults. In an Asian population of multiple ethnicity, psoriatic arthritis was significantly more common in patients of Indian extraction, compared with Chinese and Malaysians.[24]

Given the probable importance of synovial CD8-positive T cells in the pathology of psoriatic arthritis, it might be expected that major histocompatibility complex class I molecules are important in this disease; indeed, adult psoriatic arthritis has been associated with HLA-B13, B17, B19, B39, and Cw6.[48] It has been suggested that various HLA markers are associated with peripheral joint disease progression in psoriatic arthritis. In one study, B22 appeared to be "protective," whereas B39 and DQw3 were associated with progressive disease.[49] The presence of HLA-B27 in patients with psoriatic arthritis is associated with spinal inflammation and sacroiliitis.[50] None of these associations has been convincingly demonstrated in JPsA, although the number of children investigated has been comparatively small. Childhood disease appears to be linked to the major histocompatibility complex class II molecules DR1 and DR6 5, and it has been suggested that the haplotype HLA-DRB1*01, -DQA1*0101, -DQB1*05 predisposes to the disease (Thomson et al, submitted). DRB1*04, DQA1*03, and DQB1*03 appear to be "pro-

Table 14–5

Joints Affected in Juvenile Psoriatic Arthritis

Joint	SHORE AND ANSELL[1] Initial (%)	SHORE AND ANSELL[1] Cumulative (%)	SOUTHWOOD ET AL[2] Initial (%)	SOUTHWOOD ET AL[2] Cumulative (%)
Knee	53	77	57	89
Finger	28	40	17	60
Toe	25	45	20	46
Ankle	21	63	14	63
Wrist	11	62	11	23
Elbow	10	43	0	20
Hindfoot	8	38	6	23
MCP	8	53	—	—
DIP finger	8	42	—	—
MTP	7	33	—	—
Cervical spine	7	32	3	17
Lower spine	—	—	0	11
Sacroiliac joints	—	—	0	11
Hip	5	38	11	23
Sternoclavicular	0	15	—	—
Temporomandibular	—	—	0	34
Shoulder	—	—	0	9

DIP, distal interphalangeal; MCP, metacarpophalangeal; MTP, metatarsophalangeal.

tective" alleles, which are found in significantly fewer patients than expected in the normal population. Childhood psoriatic arthritis differs from other forms of childhood arthritis in that it is not associated with A2 or DR8.[5]

It is important to note that genes other than those coding the HLA system have been implicated in the pathogenesis of psoriatic arthritis. Immunologic heavy-chain gene polymorphisms and T cell–receptor polymorphisms have been associated with psoriatic arthritis.[51, 52] A mutation of the proinflammatory cytokine TNF-α promotor was present in 32 percent of patients with psoriatic arthritis, compared with only 7 percent of controls.[53] The functional implications of this mutation have yet to be determined.

CLINICAL MANIFESTATIONS

Clinical Patterns

JPsA usually begins with inflammation of only a few joints during the first 6 months of the disease, initially making its differentiation from oligoarticular juvenile rheumatoid arthritis (JRA) difficult. Less commonly, children with psoriatic arthritis have symmetric polyarthritis at disease onset. It has been suggested that, in adults, psoriatic arthritis is less painful than other forms of arthritis,[54] and the uncomplaining younger child often presents with an apparently painless limp. Most older children, however, have symptoms of joint stiffness and pain, particularly on awakening.

The course of the disease is usually characterized by an increase in the number of affected joints. Occasionally, the reverse pattern is observed, that is, an initial polyarthritis resolves with the exception of one or two persistently inflamed joints. There appear to be several clinical patterns of JPsA that are similar to those in adult psoriatic arthritis (see Table 14–2). A scattered asymmetric polyarthritis is the most common long-term manifestation of psoriatic arthritis in both children and adults. Longitudinal follow-up studies have suggested that the most clinically useful subgrouping is (1) patients who develop axial disease who are likely to be HLA-B27–positive and (2) those with peripheral joint disease who are likely to be HLA-B27–negative.[50]

Arthritis

The most commonly affected joint is the knee, but JPsA also has a particular predilection for the small joints of the hands and feet (Table 14–5).[2, 5] A predominantly asymmetric large and small joint arthritis is typical. Swelling of a single small joint, especially in a toe (Fig. 14–1), is highly suggestive of psoriatic arthritis because isolated small joint disease is uncommon in other forms of chronic arthritis. Distal interphalangeal (DIP) joint involvement occurred in 29 percent of children in one series,[2] and dactylitis (defined as swelling of a digital joint and periarticular tissues extending beyond the joint margin, often giving a typical "sausage digit" appearance) occurred in 49 percent (Fig. 14–1).[2] The presence of dactylitis implies underlying tendinitis, and tendon nodules have been described in 14 percent of children. The limb girdle joints (glenohumeral and hip), and cervical spine are relatively spared in psoriatic arthritis compared with other juvenile arthritides. Sacroiliitis occurs in a minority of patients.[5]

Enthesitis

Enthesitis, inflammation of the entheses (the sites of insertion into bone of tendon, ligament, or joint cap-

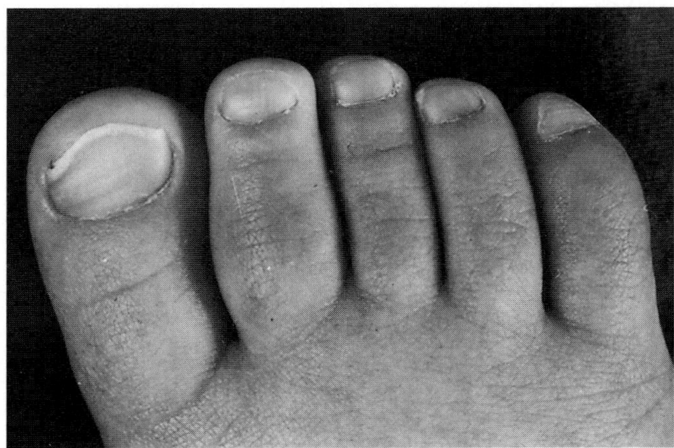

Figure 14–1. Dactylitis in a child with psoriatic arthritis. The second and fifth toes are diffusely swollen. (From Petty RE, Malleson P: Spondyloarthropathies of childhood. Pediatr Clin North Am 33: 1079, 1986.)

sule), has been proposed as an important unifying clinicopathologic feature in adult psoriatic arthritis.[11] Patients have been described in whom isolated enthesitis occurs in association with psoriasis.[55] In JPsA, however, clinical evidence of enthesitis is unusual and correlates more closely with the disease that predisposes to ankylosing spondylitis (i.e., enthesitis-related arthritis—see Chapter 13).

Extra-Articular Manifestations

Skin Disease

The typical rash of psoriasis in children is characterized by well-demarcated, erythematous, scaly lesions occurring over the extensor surfaces of the elbows and forearms, knees, and interphalangeal joints. This form of psoriatic skin lesion, psoriasis vulgaris, occurs in over 80 percent of children who have the skin rash of psoriatic arthritis. Less common presentations include guttate psoriasis, inverse (flexural) psoriasis, pustular psoriasis, and the generalized forms (von Zumbusch and erythrodermic generalized psoriasis). In small children, the rash may not be obvious; a careful search of the hairline behind the ears, navel, and groin may be revealing (Fig. 14–2). Auspitz's sign, a small pinpoint area of bleeding found on removing a psoriatic skin scale, perhaps reflects the underlying predisposition to angiogenesis.[56]

A number of disorders enter into the differential diagnoses, including atopic eczema and contact dermatitis, drug eruptions, tinea corporis, and less commonly in children, pityriasis rosea, lichen planus, discoid lupus, and mycosis fungoides.[57, 58] The onset of the skin manifestations of the disease is rarely coincident with the onset of the joint disease. In most adult studies, the rash of psoriasis appears to precede the onset of arthritis, but in children the ratio is evenly divided (see Table 14–4). Approximately 25 percent of children with JPsA sine psoriasis develop a typical psoriatic rash within 2 years.[5]

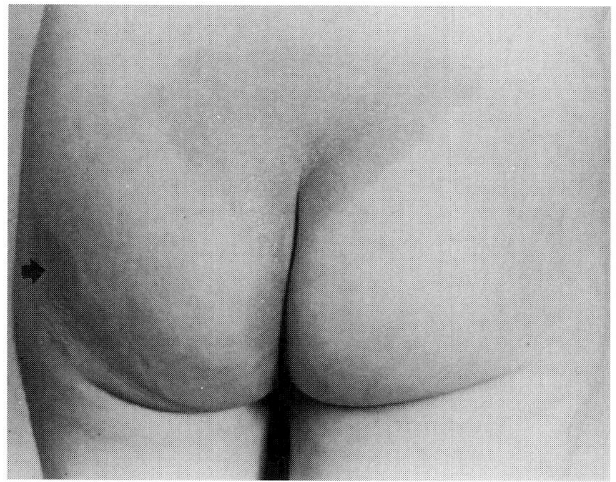

Figure 14–2. This scaly pink rash over the sacrum and in the gluteal crease was initially treated as "diaper" dermatitis. The isolated patch on the left buttock suggested the diagnosis of psoriasis (*arrow*).

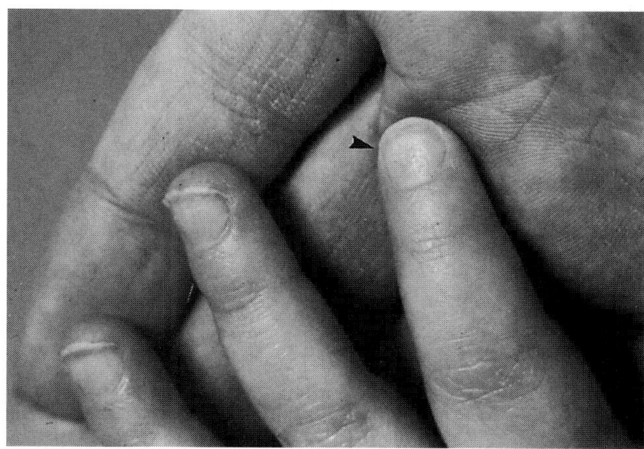

Figure 14–3. The nail of the index finger has multiple pits (*arrowhead*) characteristic of psoriasis. The digit is also swollen, suggesting dactylitis. (From Petty RE, Malleson P: Spondyloarthropathies of childhood. Pediatr Clin North Am 33: 1079, 1986.)

Nail Changes

There are several forms of nail involvement in psoriasis. The most common is nail pitting (found in about one third of patients), and the least common is the complete nail dystrophy of onycholysis. Nail pits are typically small (0.5 to 1 mm diameter), round, shallow, and dimple-like, most easily seen on the fingernails as a disruption to the normal reflection of light from the nail surface (Fig. 14–3). Horizontal, but not longitudinal, nail ridging is also associated with psoriasis. The association of nail dystrophy and DIP joint arthritis is not as common in children as in adults.[59] Typical nail pitting may occur in normal persons, in children with fungal infections of the nail, those with eczema, and in children who bite their nails. There is a close anatomic relationship between the DIP joints and the nail beds, and it is possible that subclinical enthesitis may explain the presence of nail dystrophy.[11] An alternative explanation is that abnormal angiogenesis leads to altered nail bed blood supply. Although nailfold capillaries usually appear normal on magnified inspection,[60] nailfold video capillaroscopy has demonstrated morphologic abnormalities.[60a]

Uveitis

The ocular inflammation that may accompany JPsA, anterior uveitis, is usually asymptomatic. Rarely, older patients may complain of reduced visual acuity and photophobia. Young children may appear to squint in bright light. The acute symptomatic anterior uveitis observed in 5 to 10 percent of adult patients[60b] is rare in childhood disease. All children with JPsA should undergo regular slit-lamp examination of the anterior chamber by an experienced ophthalmologist at least every 6 months. Signs of anterior uveitis apparent on slit-lamp biomicroscopy include protein flare and increased cells in the anterior chamber, similar to the signs in anterior uveitis accompanying oligoarticular

JRA. Patients with long-standing uveitis may have an irregular pupil with posterior synechiae, band keratopathy, cataract formation, and even blindness. In the younger patient, chronic anterior uveitis occurs with a frequency similar to that in oligoarticular JRA (approximately 20 percent of patients) and is associated with antinuclear antibodies.[2] There is a suggestion[60c] that the chronic anterior uveitis associated with psoriatic arthritis is relatively resistant to treatment with topical glucocorticoids, although this has not been tested formally.

Other Systemic Manifestations

It is uncommon for children with psoriatic arthritis to have fever, but patients with significant arthritis may have all of the constitutional features of a chronic inflammatory disease such as anorexia, anemia, and poor growth. Amyloidosis has been reported.[1] Rarely, features of colitis, mucositis, and urethritis occur in adults with psoriatic arthritis. The *SAPHO* syndrome (synovitis, acne, pustulosis, hyperostosis, and osteitis) and *CRMO* (chronic recurrent multifocal osteomyelitis) have been postulated to be part of the same spectrum of disease as psoriatic arthritis.[61] Reported cardiac manifestations include aortic incompetence and mitral valve prolapse.[62] Upper limb lymphedema is a rare complication of psoriatic arthritis in adults.[63]

PATHOLOGY

Little is known about specific histopathologic changes in children with psoriatic arthritis. The inflammatory synovial infiltrate is indistinguishable by light microscopy from that of other forms of chronic arthritis.[64] Synovial histology of 14 children with long-standing psoriatic arthritis demonstrated hyperemia and an inflammatory round cell infiltrate.[1] There are no other systematic studies of the histopathology of the synovium in children with psoriatic arthritis; most information is gleaned from the study of adults with the disease.

The histopathology of inflamed synovium and lesional skin is typified by marked angiogenesis. In the skin, this may be explained by increased production of IL-8 by keratinocytes, a cytokine with proangiogenic properties.[65] Distinctive capillary hyperemia and neovascularity, with tortuous and bushy vessels, have been demonstrated by knee arthroscopy in patients with early psoriatic arthritis.[56] At the cellular level, these changes are reflected by endothelial cell hypertrophy, dilated rough endoplasmic reticulum, thickened arteriolar basement membranes, and increased deposition of perivascular collagen.[66] Endothelial cell expression of adhesion molecules such as CD54, which interact with CD11a/CD18 expressed on the surface of T cells, has been demonstrated in affected skin and synovium.[67] The vascular changes are likely to contribute to the inflammatory process by attracting T cells to the synovial compartment. Cutaneous lymphocyte antigen and its receptor E-selectin are expressed in both skin and joint.[68, 69] T cells expressing cutaneous antigen, however, appear to migrate preferentially to the skin only, not the joint.[70] In three patients with psoriatic arthritis, T cells expressing the chemokine receptor CCR5 were present in greater numbers in synovial fluid than in peripheral blood, although this finding does not appear to discriminate among the various forms of inflammatory arthritis.[71] Evidence of selective T cell traffic between the affected skin and inflamed joint is equivocal.

LABORATORY EXAMINATION

No laboratory tests are pathognomonic for JPsA. Most patients have elevated acute-phase reactants (erythrocyte sedimentation rate, C-reactive protein), the anemia of chronic disease, and thrombocytosis, as do adults with the disease.[72] However, approximately one third of patients have no laboratory evidence of an acute-phase response, which occasionally misleads the clinician into excluding the diagnosis of arthritis. Antinuclear antibodies are found in 30 to 60 percent of all children with psoriatic arthritis. Although the antigenic specificities of the antinuclear antibodies are unknown, antihistone antibodies have been reported.[2] Rheumatoid factor is not present.

RADIOLOGIC EXAMINATION

Plain radiographic features of psoriatic arthritis generally follow a sequence of changes similar to those of other forms of childhood arthritis.[73–75] In early arthritis, particularly within the first few weeks of the disease, soft tissue swelling around the joint (with or without joint effusion) is the only abnormality. Periarticular osteoporosis may occur within a few months of the onset of joint swelling, and periosteal new bone formation is common in digits affected by dactylitis (Fig. 14–4). The presence of periostitis due to enthesitis may contribute to the "pencil in cup" appearance of the DIP joint found in adults with the disease.[76] Such an appearance cannot be explained by synovitis alone because the joint itself contains only a vestigial amount of synovium.[11] Instead, there may be a central erosion surrounded by joint capsular calcification at the sites of the flexor and extensor digitorum entheses. Joint-space narrowing, indicating significant cartilage loss, and erosive disease of bone are usually late features of psoriatic arthritis (Fig. 14–5). Bone remodeling may eventually occur, secondary to persistent periostitis, altered epiphyseal growth, and osteoporosis. Sacroiliac erosions are uncommon, and the osteolysis typical of adult psoriatic arthritis is rare in children. Other imaging techniques (including magnetic resonance imaging, nuclear scans with technetium-99m–labeled immunoglobulin, and ultrasonography) have been used to demonstrate the presence of enthesitis.[77, 78]

TREATMENT

Unfortunately, because no controlled trials have tested the efficacy and safety of medication in children with

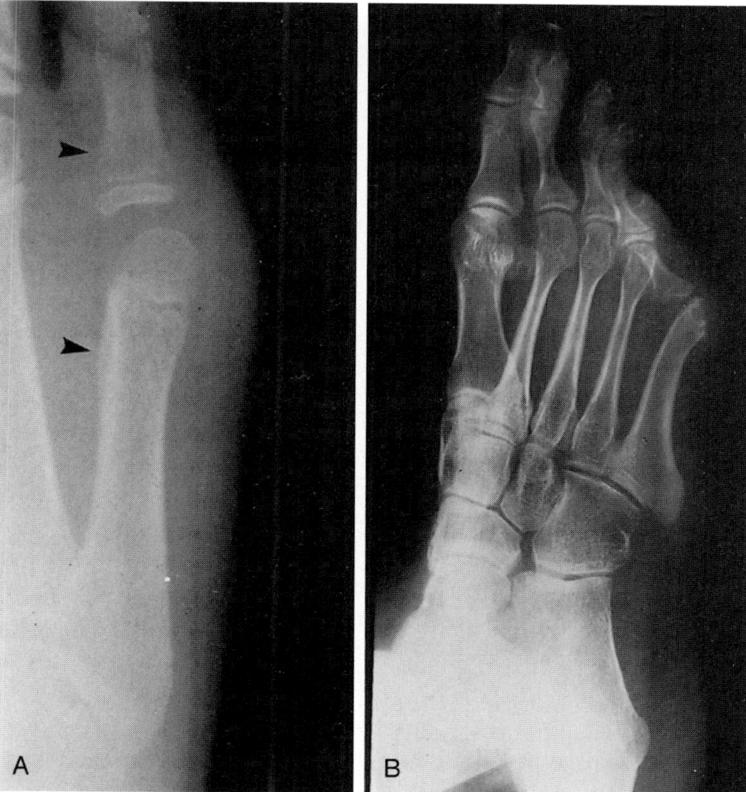

Figure 14–4. *A*, Radiograph shows periostitis of the fifth metatarsal and proximal phalanx of a 14-year-old boy with psoriatic arthritis of recent onset (*arrowheads*). *B*, Radiograph of the foot of a 12-year-old girl with psoriatic arthritis of several years' duration. There is marked erosion of the head of the fifth metatarsal and the base of the proximal phalanx with dislocation of the joint. The other joints are relatively normal. (*A*, from Petty RE, Malleson P: Spondyloarthropathies of childhood. Pediatr Clin North Am 33: 1079, 1986.)

JPsA, the treatment approach is based on studies of other forms of arthritis in children and studies of adults with psoriatic arthritis. Many experienced clinicians use a combination of nonsteroidal anti-inflammatory drugs (NSAIDs) and intra-articular long-acting glucocorticoids (e.g., triamcinolone hexacetonide) for the initial treatment of oligoarthritis, adding methotrexate at the first evidence of progression to polyarticular disease. Naproxen (10 to 20 mg/kg/day in two divided doses) or ibuprofen (30 to 60 mg/kg/day in three or

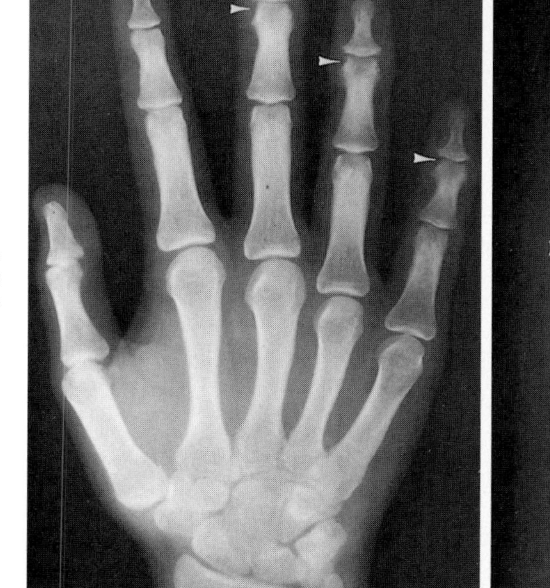

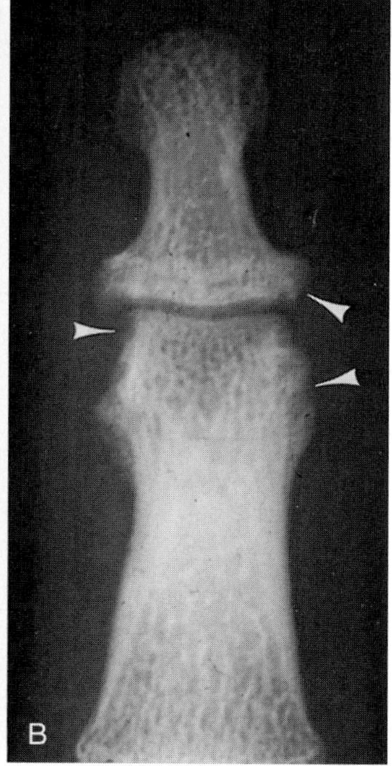

Figure 14–5. *A*, Psoriatic arthropathy affecting the distal interphalangeal joints of the third to fifth fingers (*arrowheads*). *B*, Magnified view of the distal interphalangeal joint of the third finger.

four doses per day) is most commonly used, especially in younger children. Other NSAIDs, such as piroxicam (0.5 mg/kg/day in a single dose) or indomethacin (up to 2.5 mg/kg/day), have been used successfully in the symptomatic treatment of psoriatic arthritis in children. All NSAIDs are taken with or just after food; gastric irritation can be further relieved with misoprostol or an H_2 blocker such as ranitidine. Patients with JPsA do not appear to have more drug side effects than children with other forms of arthritis.

Intra-articular triamcinolone hexacetonide (1 mg/kg per large joint, 0.5 mg/kg for small joints) is effective in treating the oligoarthritic phase of psoriatic arthritis, but its efficacy in polyarticular disease is less clear. Intra-articular glucocorticoids do not appear to be effective for treating dactylitis or tenosynovitis, particularly after the underlying bone has become thickened by periosteal reaction. There is some anecdotal evidence that the response to repeated joint injections diminishes over time, perhaps as the degree of joint destruction becomes more severe.

Methotrexate is the most frequently used slow-acting antirheumatic drug to treat psoriatic arthritis in children and adults,[79–88] occasionally in combination with oral glucocorticoids.[79] Methotrexate treatment is usually initiated at a dose of 0.5 mg/kg by mouth once a week given at least an hour before eating. If the patient is able to tolerate this dose but the drug is ineffective, the dose may be gradually increased to a maximum of 1 mg/kg/week. Common side effects include nausea, abdominal pain, and mood change. Changing from oral to subcutaneous administration may improve efficacy and reduce side effects. It is possible that the early use of methotrexate may reduce the rate of progression of the disease and even the risk of polyarthritic evolution. Methotrexate may also help to control the rash of psoriasis.

In several studies, including a 12-month prospective, randomized, controlled trial of psoriatic arthritis treatment in adults, cyclosporin appeared to be as effective as methotrexate for the control of the disease.[89–93] However, long-term administration of cyclosporin has been associated with hypertension, and a life-table analysis has suggested that methotrexate is likely to be better tolerated.[93] Hypertension is rare in most children treated with cyclosporin for arthritis, although they may develop raised creatinine levels.

As yet, there are only anecdotal reports of the use of biologic agents such as soluble TNF-α receptor in the treatment of JPsA. A wide variety of conventional and unconventional drugs have been used to treat psoriatic arthritis in adults, including sulfasalazine,[94–96] gold,[97–100] azathioprine,[101] chloroquine,[102] etretinate,[103] fish oil,[104–106] vitamin D_3,[107] bromocriptine,[108] and photochemotherapy.[109–111] A few reports of surgical approaches to psoriatic arthritis have been published.[112–114] Children with psoriatic arthritis have successfully undergone total hip replacement. The role of disease education is important in managing psoriatic arthritis in young people.[115]

The skin rash of psoriasis usually responds to a combination of moisturizing emollients to prevent fissuring, keratolytics for descaling the skin (e.g., 5% salicylic acid emollient), coal tar preparations, antihistamines to prevent pruritus, and topical glucocorticoid creams.[57]

COURSE OF THE DISEASE AND PROGNOSIS

Psoriatic arthritis has a relatively poor outlook compared with other oligoarticular forms of chronic arthritis in childhood. In a study of 63 children with psoriatic arthritis who had been monitored for over 5 years, 70 percent continued to have active arthritis and one third of these had limited vocational and avocational activities.[5] Ten percent of patients reported by Shore and Ansell[1] were severely incapacitated by their disease. A study of the prognosis of adult psoriatic arthritis has suggested that patients who were HLA-B27–positive and had axial disease were more likely to develop erosions than those who had peripheral joint involvement only.[50] Deaths in JPsA secondary to amyloidosis have been reported.[1] The influence of methotrexate and more aggressive therapeutic approaches on the prognosis of psoriatic arthritis in children has yet to be assessed.

References

1. Shore A, Ansell BM: Juvenile psoriatic arthritis—an analysis of 60 cases. J Pediatr 100: 529, 1982.
2. Southwood TR, Petty RE, Malleson PN, et al: Psoriatic arthritis in children. Arthritis Rheum 32: 1007, 1989.
3. Petty RE, Southwood TR, Baum J, et al: Revision of the proposed classification criteria for juvenile idiopathic arthritis: Durban 1997. J Rheumatol 25: 10, 1998.
4. Barth WF: Psoriatic arthritis sine psoriasis. *In* Klippel JH, Dieppe P (eds): Rheumatology. London, Mosby, 1994, pp 34.1–34.3.
5. Roberton DM, Cabral DA, Malleson PN, Petty RE: Juvenile psoriatic arthritis: follow-up and evaluation of diagnostic criteria. J Rheumatol 23: 1, 166, 1996.
6. Petty RE, Southwood TR: Classification of childhood arthritis: divide and conquer. J Rheumatol 25:1991, 1998.
7. Scarpa R: Juvenile psoriatic arthritis: a new clinical entity? J Rheumatol 23: 408, 1996.
8. Moll JMH, Wright V: Psoriatic arthritis. Semin Arthritis Rheum 3: 55, 1973.
9. Dougados M, van der Linden S, Juhlin R, et al: The European Spondylarthropathy Study Group preliminary criteria for the classification of spondylarthropathy. Arthritis Rheum 34: 1218, 1991.
10. Thomson GTD, Inman RD: Diagnostic conundra in the spondyloarthropathies: towards a base for revised nosology. J Rheumatol 17: 426, 1990.
11. McGonagle D, Conaghan PG, Emery P: Psoriatic arthritis. Arthritis Rheum 42: 1080, 1999.
12. Moll JM, Wright V: Psoriatic arthritis. Semin Arthritis Rheum 3: 55, 1973.
13. Christophers E, Mrowietz U: Psoriasis. *In* Freedberg IM, Eisen AZ, Wolff K, et al (eds): Fitzpatrick's Dermatology in General Medicine, 5th ed. New York, McGraw-Hill, 1999, pp 495–521.
14. Baker H: Epidemiological aspects of psoriasis. Br J Dermatol 78: 249, 1966.
15. Barii-Druko V, Dobri I, Pai A, et al: Frequency of psoriatic arthritis in general population and among psoriatics in department of dermatology. Acta Dermatol Venereol 74(Suppl 186): 107, 1994.
16. Green L, Meyers OL, Gordon W, Briggs B: Arthritis in psoriasis. Ann Rheum Dis 40: 366, 1981.

17. Church R: The prospect of psoriasis. Br J Dermatol 70: 139, 1958.
18. Bowyer S, Roettcher P, members of the Pediatric Rheumatology Database Research Group: Pediatric rheumatology clinic populations in the United States: results of a 3 year survey. J Rheumatol 23: 1968, 1996.
19. Malleson PN, Fung MY, Rosenberg AM: The incidence of pediatric rheumatic diseases: results from the Canadian Pediatric Rheumatology Association Disease Registry. J Rheumatol 23: 1981, 1996.
20. Symmons DPM, Jones M, Osborne J, et al: Pediatric rheumatology in the United Kingdom: data from the British Paediatric Rheumatology Group National Diagnostic Register. J Rheumatol 23: 1975, 1996.
21. Gare BA, Fasth A: Epidemiology of juvenile chronic arthritis in southwestern Sweden: a 5-year prospective population study. Pediatrics 90: 950, 1992.
21a. Lambert JR, Ansell BM, Stephenson E, et al: Psoriatic arthritis in childhood. Clin Rheum Dis 2: 339, 1976.
21b. Calabro JJ: Psoriatic arthritis in children. Arthritis Rheum 20(Suppl): 415, 1977.
21c. Wesolowska H: Clinical course of psoriatic arthropathy in children. Mater Med Pol 55: 185, 1985.
22. Sills EL: Psoriatic arthritis in childhood. Johns Hopkins Med J 146: 49, 1980.
23. Thumboo J, Tham SN, Tay YK, et al: Patterns of psoriatic arthritis in Orientals. J Rheumatol 24: 1949, 1997.
24. Harrison BJ, Silman AJ, Barrett EM, et al: Presence of psoriasis does not influence the presentation or short-term outcome of patients with early inflammatory polyarthritis. J Rheumatol 24: 1744, 1997.
25. Langevitz P, Buskila D, Gladman DD: Psoriatic arthritis precipitated by physical trauma. J Rheumatol 17: 695, 1990.
26. Punzi L, Pianon M, Bertazzolo N, et al: Clinical laboratory and immunogenetic aspects of post-traumatic psoriatic arthritis: a study of 25 patients. Clin Exp Rheumatol 16: 277, 1998.
27. Telfer NR, Chalmers RJ, Whale K, Colman G: The role of streptococcal infection in the initiation of guttate psoriasis. Arch Dermatol 128: 39, 1992.
28. Vasey FB, Deitz C, Fenske NA, et al: Possible involvement of group A streptococci in the pathogenesis of psoriatic arthritis. J Rheumatol 9: 719, 1982.
29. Rantakokko K, Rimpiläninen M, Uksila J, et al: Antibodies to streptococcal cell wall in psoriatic arthritis and cutaneous psoriasis. Clin Exp Rheumatol 15: 399, 1997.
30. Grilington FM, Skinner MA, Birchall NM, Tan PLI: $\gamma\delta$ + T cells from patients with psoriatic and rheumatoid arthritis respond to streptococcal antigen. J Rheumatol 20:983, 1993.
31. Oen K, Fast M, Postl B: Epidemiology of juvenile rheumatoid arthritis in Manitoba, Canada, 1975–1992: cycles in incidence. J Rheumatol 22:745, 1995.
32. Paukkonnen K, Naukkarinen A, Horstmanheimo M: The development of manifest psoriatic lesions is linked with the invasion of CD8+ T cells and CD11c+ macrophages into the epidermis. Arch Dermatol Res 284: 375, 1992.
33. Chang JC, Smith LR, Froning KJ, et al: Persistence of T cell clones in psoriatic lesions. Arch Dermatol 133: 703, 1997.
34. Costello P, Bresnihan B, O'Farrelly C, Fitzgerald O: Predominance of CD8+ T lymphocytes in psoriatic arthritis. J Rheumatol 26: 1117, 1999.
35. Konig A, Krenn V, Gillitzer R, et al: Inflammatory infiltrate and interleukin-8 expression in the synovium of psoriatic arthritis—an immunohistochemical and mRNA analysis. Rheumatol Int 17: 159, 1997.
36. Vasey FB, Seleznick MJ, Fenske NA, Espinoza LR: New signposts on the road to understanding psoriatic arthritis. J Rheumatol 16: 1405, 1989.
37. Ritchlin C, Hass-Smith SA, Hicks D, et al: Patterns of cytokine production in psoriatic synovium. J Rheumatol 25: 1544, 1998.
38. Gottlieb SL, Gilleaudeau P, Johnson R, et al: Response of psoriasis to a lymphocyte-selective toxin (DAB389IL-2) suggests a primary immune but not keratinocyte, pathogenic basis. Nat Med 1: 442, 1995.
39. Wong WM, Howell WM, Coy SD, et al: Interleukin-2 is found in the synovium of psoriatic arthritis and spondyloarthritis, not in rheumatoid arthritis. Scand J Rheumatol 25: 239, 1996.
40. Partsch G, Wagner E, Leeb BF, et al: Upregulation of cytokine receptors sTNF-R55, sTNF-R75, and sIL-2R in psoriatic arthritis synovial fluid. J Rheumatol 25: 105, 1998.
41. Murray KJ, Grom AA, Thompson SD, et al: Contrasting cytokine profiles in the synovium of different forms of juvenile rheumatoid arthritis and juvenile spondyloarthropathy: prominence of interleukin 4 in restricted disease. J Rheumatol 25: 1388, 1998.
42. Carroll JM, Romero MR, Watt FM: Suprabasal integrin expression in the epidermis of transgenic mice results in developmental defects and a phenotype resembling psoriasis. Cell 83: 957, 1995.
43. Schön MP, Detmar M, Parker CM: Murine psoriasis-like disorder induced by naïve CD4+ T cells. Nat Med 3:183, 1997.
44. Blessing M, Schirmacher P, Kaiser S: Overexpression of bone morphogenic protein-6 (BMP-6) in the epidermis of transgenic mice: inhibition or stimulation of proliferation depending on the pattern of transgene expression and formation of psoriatic lesions. J Cell Biol 135: 227, 1996.
45. Tomfohrde J, Silverman A, Barnes R, et al: Gene for familial psoriasis susceptibility mapped to the distal end of human chromosome 17q. Science 264: 1141, 1994.
46. Eldar JT, Henseler T, Christophers E, et al: Of genes and antigens. The genetics of psoriasis. J Invest Dermatol 103(Suppl): 150S, 1994.
47. Burden AD, Javed S, Bailey M, et al: Genetics of psoriasis: paternal inheritance and a locus on chromosome 6p. J Invest Dermatol 110: 958, 1998.
48. Gladman DD, Anhorn KA, Schachter RK, Mervart H: HLA antigens in psoriatic arthritis. J Rheumatol 13: 586, 1986.
49. Gladman DD, Farewell VT, Kopciuk A, Cook RJ: HLA markers and progression in psoriatic arthritis. J Rheumatol 25: 730, 1998.
50. Marsal S, Armadens-Gil L, Martinez M, et al: Clinical radiographic and HLA associations as markers for different patterns of psoriatic arthritis. Rheumatology 38: 332, 1999.
51. Sakkas LI, Marchesoni A, Kerr LA, et al: Immunoglobulin heavy chain gene polymorphism in Italian patients with psoriasis and psoriatic arthritis. Br J Rheumatol 30: 449, 1991.
52. Sakkas LI, Loqueman N, Bird H, et al: HLA class II and T cell receptor gene polymorphisms in psoriatic arthritis and psoriasis. J Rheumatol 17: 1487, 1990.
53. Hohler R, Kruger A, Schneider PM, et al: A TNF-alpha promoter polymorphism is associated with juvenile onset psoriasis and psoriatic arthritis. J Invest Dermatol 109: 562, 1997.
54. Buskila D, Langevitz P, Gladman DD, et al: Patients with rheumatoid arthritis are more tender than those with psoriatic arthritis. J Rheumatol 19: 1115, 1992.
55. Salvarani C, Cantini F, Olivieri I, et al: Isolated peripheral enthesitis and/or dactylitis: a subset of psoriatic arthritis. J Rheumatol 24: 1106, 1997.
56. Reece RJ, Canete JD, Parsons WJ, et al: Distinct vascular patterns of early synovitis in psoriatic, reactive and rheumatoid arthritis. Arthritis Rheum 42, 1481, 1999.
57. Griffiths C, Kirby B: Psoriasis management within primary care. Prescriber 10: 47, 1999.
58. Abel EA, DiCocco LM, Orenberg EK, et al: Drugs in exacerbation of psoriasis. J Am Acad Dermatol 15: 1007, 1986.
59. Eastmond CJ, Wright V: The nail dystrophy of psoriatic arthritis. Ann Rheum Dis 38: 226, 1979.
60. Hafner R, Michels H: Psoriatic arthritis in children. Curr Opin Rheumatol 8: 467, 1996.
60a. Bhushan M, Moore T, Herrick AL, Griffiths CE: Nailfold capillary microscopy in psoriasis. Br J Dermatol 142: 1171, 2000.
60b. Paiva ES, Macaluso DC, Edwards A, Rosenbaum JT: Characterization of uveitis in patients with psoriatic arthritis. Ann Rheum Dis 59: 67, 2000.
60c. Cabral DA, Petty RE, Malleson PN, et al: Visual prognosis in children with chronic anterior uveitis and arthritis. J Rheumatol 21: 2370, 1994.
61. Laxer RM, Shore AD, Manson D, et al: Chronic recurrent multifocal osteomyelitis and psoriasis—a report of a new association and review of related disorders. Semin Arthritis Rheum 17: 260, 1988.
62. Pines A, Ehrenfeld M, Fisman EZ, et al: Mitral valve prolapse in psoriatic arthritis. Arch Intern Med 146: 1371, 1986.

63. Mulherin DM, FitzGerald O, Bresnihan B: Lymphedema of the upper limb in patients with psoriatic arthritis. Semin Arthritis Rheum 22: 350, 1993.
64. Murray KJ, Lorie L, Grom AA, et al: Immunohistological characteristics of T cell infiltrates in different forms of childhood onset chronic arthritis. J Rheumatol 23: 2116, 1996.
65. Nickoloff BJ, Mitra RS, Sailer D, et al: Aberrant production of interleukin-8 and thrombospondin-1 by psoriatic keratinocytes mediates angiogenesis. Am J Pathol 144: 137, 1994.
66. Espinoza LR, Vasey FB, Espinoza CG, et al: Vascular changes in psoriatic synovium. A light and electron microscope study. Arthritis Rheum 25: 677, 1982.
67. Dunky A, Neumuller J, Menzel J: Interactions of lymphocytes from patients with psoriatic arthritis or healthy controls and cultured endothelial cells. Clin Immunol Immunopathol 85: 297, 1997.
68. Jones SM, Dixey J, Hall ND, McHugh NJ: Expression of the cutaneous lymphocyte antigen and its counter-receptor E-selectin in the skin and joints of patients with psoriatic arthritis. Br J Rheumatol 36: 748, 1997.
69. Veale D, Yanni G, Rogers S, et al: Reduced synovial membrane macrophage numbers, ELAM-1 expression, and lining layer hyperplasia in psoriatic arthritis as compared with rheumatoid arthritis. Arthritis Rheum 36: 893, 1993.
70. Pitzalis C, Cauli A, Pipitone N, et al: Cutaneous lymphocyte antigen-positive T lymphocytes preferentially migrate to the skin but not to the joint in psoriatic arthritis. Arthritis Rheum 39: 137, 1996.
71. Mack M, Bruhl H, Gruber R, et al: Predominance of mononuclear cells expressing the chemokine receptor CCR5 in synovial effusions of patients with different forms of arthritis. Arthritis Rheum 42: 981, 1999.
72. Khan MA, Kammer GM: Laboratory findings and pathology in psoriatic arthritis. *In* Gerber LH, Espinoza LR (eds): Psoriatic Arthritis. Orlando, FL, Grune & Stratton, 1985, p 109.
73. Gladman DD, Stafford-Brady F, Chang CH, et al: Clinical and radiological progression in psoriatic arthritis. J Rheumatol 17: 809, 1990.
74. Macchioni P, Boiardi L, Cremonesi T, et al: The relationship between serum-soluble interleukin-2 receptor and radiological evolution in psoriatic arthritis patients. Rheum Int 18: 1, 27, 1998.
75. Jenkinson T, Armas J, Evison G, et al: The cervical spine of psoriatic arthritis: a clinical and radiological study. Br J Rheumatol 33: 255, 1994.
76. Fournie B, Granel J, Bonnet M, et al: Incidence of signs explaining psoriatic rheumatism in radiological involvement of the fingers and toes. Rev Rhum 59: 1777, 1992.
77. Lehtinen A, Traavisainen M, Leirisalo-Repo M: Sonographic analysis of enthesopathy in the lower extremities of patients with spondyloarthropathy. Clin Exp Rheumatol 12: 143, 1994.
78. Stoeger A, Mur E, Penz-Schneeweiss D, et al: Technetium-99m human immunoglobulin scintigraphy in psoriatic arthropathy: first results. Eur J Nucl Med 21: 342, 1994.
79. Bjorksten B, Back OL: Methotrexate and prednisolone treatment of a child with psoriatic arthritis. Acta Paediatr Scand 64: 664, 1975.
80. Abu-Shakra M, Gladman DD, Thorne JC, et al: Long-term methotrexate therapy in psoriatic arthritis: clinical and radiological outcome. J Rheumatol 22: 241, 1995.
81. Black RL, O'Brien WM, Van Scott EJ, et al: Methotrexate therapy in psoriatic arthritis. Double blind study on 21 patients. JAMA 189: 743, 1964.
82. Cuellar ML, Espinoza LR: Methotrexate use in psoriasis and psoriatic arthritis. Rheum Dis Clin North Am 23:797, 1997.
83. Espinoza LR, Zakkraoni L, Espinoza CG, et al: Psoriatic arthritis clinical response and side effects of methotrexate therapy. J Rheumatol 19: 872, 1992.
84. Falk ES, Vandbakk Ø: Prevalence of psoriatic arthritis clinical response and side effects of methotrexate therapy. Acta Dermatol Venereol 73(Suppl): 6, 1993.
85. Roenigk HH, Fowler-Bergfeld W, Curtis GH: Methotrexate for psoriasis in weekly oral doses. Arch Dermatol 99: 86, 1969.
86. Spadaro A, Taccari E, Sensi F, et al: Soluble interleukin-2 receptor and interleukin-6 levels: evaluation during cyclosporin A and methotrexate treatment in psoriatic arthritis. Clin Rheumatol 17: 83, 1998.
87. Wilkens RF, Williams HJ, Ward JR, et al: Randomized, double-blind, placebo controlled trial of low-dose pulse methotrexate in psoriatic arthritis. Arthritis Rheum 27: 376, 1984.
88. Zacharias H, Zacharias E: Methotrexate treatment of psoriatic arthritis. Acta Dermatol Venereol 67: 270, 1987.
89. Ellis CN, Fradin MS, Messana JM, et al: Cyclosporin for plaque-type psoriasis. Results of a multidose, double-blind trial. N Engl J Med 324: 277, 1991.
90. Gupta AK, Matteson EI, Ellis CN, et al: Cyclosporin in the treatment of psoriatic arthritis. Arch Dermatol 125: 507, 1989.
91. Macchioni P, Boiardi L, Meliconi R, et al: Serum chemokines in patients with psoriatic arthritis treated with cyclosporin A. J Rheumatol 25: 320, 1998.
92. Olivieri I, Salvarani C, Cantini F, et al: Therapy with cyclosporin in psoriatic arthritis. Semin Arthritis Rheum 27: 36, 1997.
93. Spadaro A, Taccari E, Mohtadi B, et al: Life-table analysis of cyclosporin A treatment in psoriatic arthritis: comparison with other disease-modifying antirheumatic drugs. Clin Exp Rheumatol 15: 609, 1997.
94. Farr M, Kitas GD, Waterhouse L, et al: Sulphasalazine in psoriatic arthritis: a double blind placebo-controlled study. Br J Rheumatol 29: 46, 1990.
95. Fraser SM, Hopkins R, Hunter JA, et al: Sulphasalazine in the management of psoriatic arthritis. Br J Rheumatol 32: 923, 1993.
96. Rahman PA, Gladman DD: Sulphasalazine in psoriatic arthritis. J Rheumatol 22: 1601, 1995.
97. Carrett S, Calin A: Evaluation of auranofin in psoriatic arthritis: a double blind placebo controlled trial. Arthritis Rheum 32: 158, 1989.
98. Dowart BB, Gall EP, Schumacher HR, Krauser RE: Chrysotherapy in psoriatic arthritis: efficacy and toxicity compared to rheumatoid arthritis. Arthritis Rheum 21: 513, 1978.
99. Mader R, Gladman DD, Long J, et al: Injectable gold for the treatment of psoriatic arthritis—long term follow-up. Clin Invest Med 18: 139, 1995.
100. Palit J, Hill J, Capell HA, et al: A multicentre double-blind comparison of auranofin, intramuscular gold thiomalate and placebo in patients with psoriatic arthritis. Br J Rheumatol 29: 280, 1990.
101. Levy JJ, Paulus HE, Barnett EV, et al: A double blind controlled evaluation of azathioprine treatment in rheumatoid arthritis and psoriatic arthritis. Arthritis Rheum 15: 116, 1972.
102. Gladman DD, Blake R, Brubacher B, Farewell VT: Chloroquine therapy in psoriatic arthritis. J Rheumatol 19: 1724, 1992.
103. Klinkhoff AV, Gertner E, Chalmers A, et al: Pilot study of etretinate in psoriatic arthritis. J Rheumatol 16: 789–791, 1989.
104. Gupta AK, Ellis CN, Telliner DC, et al: Double blind, placebo controlled study to evaluate the efficacy of fish oil and low dose UVB in the treatment of psoriasis. Br J Dermatol 120: 801, 1989.
105. Veale DJ, Torley HI, Richards IM, et al: A double-blind placebo controlled trial of efamol marine on skin and joint symptoms of psoriatic arthritis. Br J Rheumatol 33: 954, 1994.
106. Peloso P, Gladman DD: Fish oils in the treatment of psoriatic arthritis: an open study. Arthritis Rheum 35(Suppl 9): S225, 1992.
107. Huckins D, Felson DT, Holick M: Treatment of psoriatic arthritis with oral 1,25-dihydroxyvitamin D3: a pilot study. Arthritis Rheum 33: 1723, 1990.
108. Buskila D, Sukenik S, Holcberg G, Horowitz J: Improvement of psoriatic arthritis in a patient treated with bromocriptine for hyperprolactinemia. J Rheumatol 18: 611–612, 1991.
109. de Misa RF, Azafia JM, Harto A, et al: Psoriatic arthritis: one year of treatment with extracorporeal photochemotherapy. J Am Acad Dermatol 30: 1037, 1994.
110. Parish JA, Fitzpatrick TB, Tanenbaum L, Pathak MA: Photochemotherapy of psoriasis with oral methoxsalen and longwave ultraviolet light. N Engl J Med 291: 1207, 1974.
111. Perlman SG, Gerber LH, Roberts M, et al: Photochemotherapy and psoriatic arthritis. A prospective study. Ann Intern Med 91: 717, 1979.

112. Hicken GJ, Kitaoka HB, Valente RM: Foot and ankle surgery in patients with psoriasis. Clin Orthop Rel Res 300: 204, 1994.
113. Peterson AW, Shepherd LH: Fascia lata interpositional arthroplasty in the treatment of temporomandibular joint ankylosis caused by psoriatic arthritis. Int J Oral Maxillofac Surg 21: 137, 1992.
114. Zangger P, Gladman DD, Bogoch ER: Musculoskeletal surgery in psoriatic arthritis. J Rheumatol 25: 4, 725, 1998.
115. Lubrano E, Helliwell P, Parsons W, et al: Patient education in psoriatic arthritis: a cross sectional study on knowledge by a validated self-administered questionnaire. J Rheumatol 25: 1560, 1998.

15

Arthropathies of Inflammatory Bowel Disease

Ross E. Petty and James T. Cassidy

DEFINITION AND CLASSIFICATION

The arthropathies of inflammatory bowel disease (IBD) may be defined as any noninfectious arthritis occurring before or during the course of either regional enteritis (RE; Crohn's disease) or ulcerative colitis (UC). Arthritis is probably the most common extraintestinal complication of these disorders. There are two patterns of joint inflammation: peripheral polyarthritis and, less commonly, involvement of the sacroiliac (SI) joints.

EPIDEMIOLOGY

Incidence and Prevalence

Arthropathy has been reported in 7 to 21 percent of children with IBD[1–5] (Table 15–1). Passo and colleagues[5] found arthritis in 9 percent of the 44 children with UC and in 15.5 percent of 58 children with RE. Arthralgia was much more common, occurring in 32 percent of those with UC and 22 percent of those with RE.[5] Differentiation of UC from RE is not always easy, and differences in the reported frequencies of arthritis in each may reflect differences in the accuracy of diagnosis in these types of IBD.[2, 3] Other children have myalgia, skeletal pain associated with glucocorticoid-induced osteopenia, or secondary hypertrophic osteoarthropathy without objective arthritis.

Age at Onset and Sex Ratio

In their study of 136 patients with onset of IBD before the age of 20 years, Lindsley and Schaller[4] concluded that age at onset of IBD in patients with arthritis did not differ significantly from that in children without arthritis. The ratios of boys to girls in those with and without peripheral arthritis were almost identical, although the 5 children who developed spondylitis were boys.

ETIOLOGY AND PATHOGENESIS

The causes of both IBD and the accompanying arthritis are obscure. The possible roles of gastrointestinal (GI) infections or allergic reactions to foods absorbed across an inflamed mucosa remain speculative. The SI arthritis probably shares its etiology with that of ankylosing spondylitis, and the studies of enteric species and immunity to them may be relevant.[6] The peripheral arthropathy may involve entirely different immunoinflammatory mechanisms (immune complexes) and is

Table 15–1
Arthritis in Inflammatory Bowel Disease in Children

AUTHOR	DISEASE	NO. OF PATIENTS	NO. WITH ARTHRITIS	% WITH ARTHRITIS
Farmer & Michener, 1979[1]	RE	522	39	7
Hamilton et al, 1979[2]	RE	58	11	19
Burbige et al, 1975[3]	RE	58	6	10
Lindsley & Schaller, 1974[4]	RE	50	5	10
Passo et al, 1986[5]	RE	58	9	15
Lindsley & Schaller, 1974[4]	UC	86	18	21
Hamilton et al, 1979[2]	UC	87	8	9
Passo et al, 1986[5]	UC	44	4	9

RE, regional enteritis; UC, ulcerative colitis.

clinically more closely related to the activity of the intestinal disease.

GENETIC BACKGROUND

There is a pronounced tendency for familial clustering of UC and RE. Hamilton and associates[2] reported that approximately 15 percent of children with UC and 8 percent of those with RE had first-degree relatives with IBD. Both diseases are more common in children of Jewish descent, who composed 21 percent of the IBD population, compared with 2 percent of the general population in one study.[2] Published reports support the view that genes of the major histocompatibility complex are important in determining susceptibility to UC in particular,[7] but inherited predispositions are undoubtedly polygenic. In Japanese[8] and Jewish patients,[9] but not in other ethnic groups, human leukocyte antigen (HLA)–DRB1*1502 (DR2) is increased in frequency. It is estimated that SI arthritis is at least 30 times more common in patients with IBD than in the general population,[10] a fact that reflects the high frequency of HLA-B27 in such patients. The peripheral polyarthritis accompanying IBD has no known HLA association.

CLINICAL MANIFESTATIONS

Arthritis and Enthesitis

Two distinct patterns of joint disease occur. The more common pattern of arthritis in patients with IBD is inflammation affecting peripheral joints. Lindsley and Schaller[4] noted that in 11 of 18 children, four or fewer joints were affected at onset or during the course of the illness; in 5 children, five to nine joints were affected; in only 2 children were more than 10 joints affected. (In these last 2 patients, small joints of the hand were involved.) Lower extremity joints, especially ankles and knees, were most frequently affected,[3–5] although upper extremity joints, occasionally also including small joints of the hand and the temporomandibular joints, may be involved. Episodes of acute peripheral arthritis are usually brief, lasting 1 or 2 weeks (occasionally longer), and tend to recur.[5] In some children, arthritis may last for several months, particularly if the GI disease is active. Rarely, joint inflammation persists for months, although permanent functional loss or joint damage is unusual. Whereas the SI arthritis bears little relation to the activity of the gut disease, the peripheral arthritis reflects the activity and course of the GI inflammation. A clinical flare-up in a child's arthritis is suggestive of poor control of the underlying IBD.

SI arthritis, which may be asymptomatic but often is characterized by pain and stiffness in the lower back, buttocks, or thighs, is a much less common complication of IBD than is polyarthritis. It is sometimes accompanied by enthesitis identical to that occurring in other forms of spondyloarthritis. SI arthritis may also be associated with chronic symmetric oligoarthritis predominantly affecting the joints of the lower limbs. In the study of Passo and colleagues,[5] no patient had spondyloarthritis.

Hypertrophic osteoarthropathy is an occasionally very painful musculoskeletal complication of IBD.[11] The pain occurs symmetrically in the limbs (rather than the joints) and may be accompanied by increased sweating and purple discoloration of the affected limbs.

Extra-Articular Manifestations of Disease

Gastrointestinal Disease

Cramping abdominal pain, often with localized or generalized tenderness, anorexia, and diarrhea, sometimes occurring at night, is characteristic of IBD. Differentiation of UC and RE on the basis of GI symptoms alone is unreliable, although bloody diarrhea is highly suggestive of UC, whereas perianal skin tags and fistulae are typical of RE (Table 15–2).

GI tract symptoms usually precede joint disease by months or years, although occasionally both systems are affected simultaneously or joint symptoms precede intestinal disease. In the latter case, arthritis resembles that of juvenile rheumatoid arthritis, juvenile ankylosing spondylitis, or the syndrome of seronegativity enthesopathy and arthropathy, with a course punctuated by intermittent abdominal pain that may be ascribed to the effects of anti-inflammatory drugs. Low-grade diarrhea, anemia, unexplained fever, weight loss, growth retardation out of proportion to the extent and activity of the joint disease, or a family history of IBD should alert the physician to the possibility of occult IBD. Mucocutaneous lesions (erythema nodosum, aphthous stomatitis, pyoderma gangrenosum) seem to be

Table 15–2

Gastrointestinal and Other Systemic Disease in Children With Inflammatory Bowel Diseases

SYMPTOM OR SIGN	ULCERATIVE COLITIS	REGIONAL ENTERITIS
Diarrhea	+ + + +	+ +
Hematochezia	+ +	+
Abdominal pain	+ +	+ + +
Weight loss	+ +	+ + + +
Fever	+	+ + +
Vomiting	+	+ +
Perianal disease	+	+ + +
Finger clubbing	+	+ +
Erythema nodosum	+	+
Oral lesions	+	+
Uveitis	(+)	(+)
Pyoderma gangrenosum	(+)	(+)

(+), rare; +, <25%; + +, 25%–50%; + + +, 50%–75%; + + + +, 75% or more.

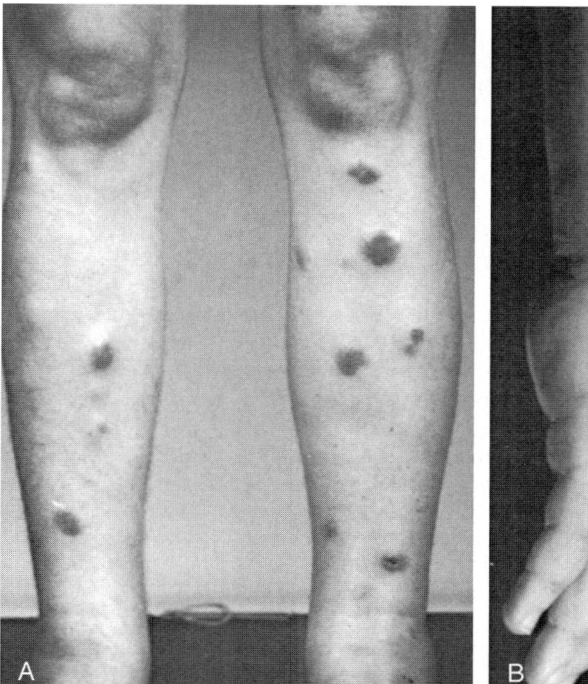

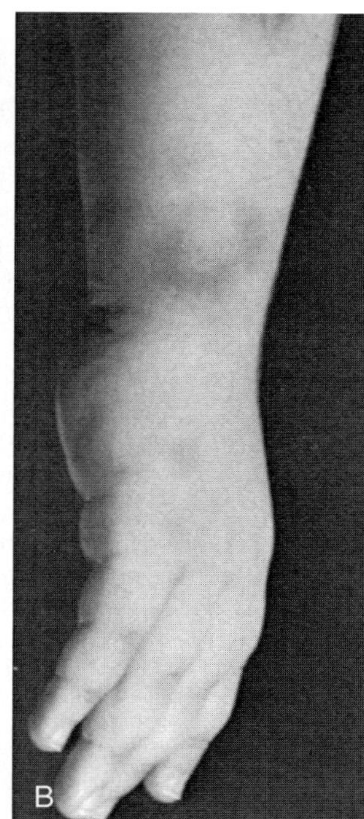

Figure 15–1. Erythema nodosum. *A*, This young girl had tender, circumscribed purple-red nodules on the shins. *B*, Lesions on the forearm of a child.

more common in children who have arthritis (especially peripheral arthritis) as a complication of IBD, although this association is not supported by some clinical studies.[5]

Although there are no clear-cut correlations between the extent of GI inflammation and arthritis, most reports support the view that there is a higher frequency of arthritis in children with extensive, as opposed to segmental, bowel disease.[1, 2, 5] Patients with arthritis usually have active gut disease, although the onset of arthritis is not necessarily related to obvious flare-ups in the GI tract inflammation.

Cutaneous Disease

Erythema Nodosum

The lesions of erythema nodosum (nodular panniculitis) occur most commonly in the subcutaneous fat of the pretibial region (Fig. 15–1) as erythematous, painful, slightly elevated lesions, 1 to 2 cm in diameter, erupting in groups and reappearing in new areas after several days. The nodules tend to persist for several weeks and recur in crops for several months. As they heal, they frequently leave pigmented areas that persist for many months. Articular pain and synovitis accompany each exacerbation in approximately two thirds of instances. Although erythema nodosum may occur as a distinct, isolated clinical syndrome, it is commonly associated with systemic illness of diverse causes, including IBD.[12, 13]

Pyoderma Gangrenosum

The lesions of pyoderma gangrenosum may occur alone or in concert with IBD (Fig. 15–2). They often arise after minor trauma, may be single or multiple, and usually begin as a pustule that breaks down and rapidly enlarges to form a painful, chronic, deep, undermined ulcer with a red, raised border. They have rarely been reported in children, and in adults the lesions occur with IBD, rheumatoid arthritis, or other diseases.[14] A single report of pyoderma gangrenosum in a 2-year-old boy with joint effusions but without IBD was associated with enhanced leukocyte mobility.[15] There have been no other reports of this phenomenon.

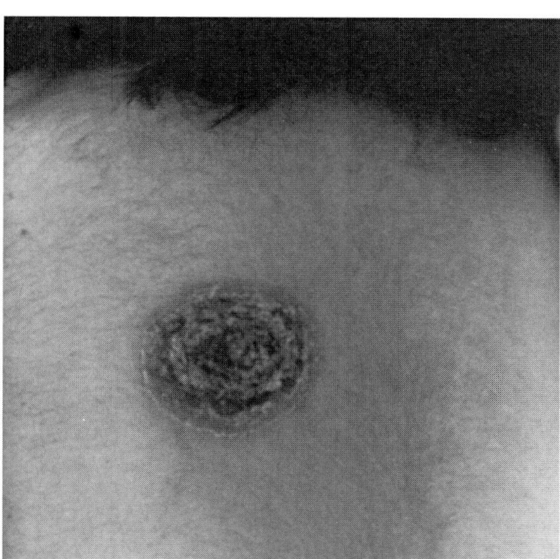

Figure 15–2. Pyoderma gangrenosum on the upper back of a child. These lesions begin as nodules but progress to ulcers with considerable loss of subcutaneous tissue.

Vasculitis

Vasculitis of several types has been reported in patients with IBD and arthritis. Involvement of large vessels was found in at least two studies.[16, 17] Takayasu's arteritis in patients with RE was first described in 1970[18] and has been reported in several other adults and in a 15-year-old boy,[19] as well as in a young adult with UC and juvenile ankylosing spondylitis.[20] It seems unlikely that coincidence could account for the simultaneous occurrence of these rare diseases, but data are insufficient to allow certainty about its significance. A syndrome of cutaneous vasculitis, glomerulonephritis, and circulating immune complexes was reported in two adults with IBD and spondyloarthritis (one with juvenile-onset colitis).[21] Immunoglobulin (Ig) A nephropathy has been described in ankylosing spondylitis and in at least three patients with IBD.[22, 23] Cutaneous vasculitis was noted as the presenting feature in a 14-year-old girl with RE.[24]

Uveitis

Lyons and Rosenbaum[25] compared the characteristics of uveitis in 17 adults with IBD and 89 patients with spondyloarthritis. Twelve of the 15 patients with uveitis and IBD had RE, and 82 percent were female. Uveitis accompanying IBD was usually bilateral, posterior, and of insidious onset and chronic duration. The frequency of HLA-B27 was half that in the spondyloarthritis group. Episcleritis, scleritis, and glaucoma were more common among patients with IBD. At least in adults, the uveitis associated with IBD was frequently complicated by cataract (35 percent), glaucoma (24 percent), cystoid macular edema (24 percent), or posterior synechiae (29 percent).[25] There are no reported studies of uveitis in children with IBD and arthritis.

PATHOLOGY

The histopathology of the synovitis of IBD is nonspecific, with proliferation of lining cells and infiltration of the synovium with lymphocytes, plasma cells, and histiocytes.[26] Granulomatous synovitis occasionally occurs.[27] For a discussion of the histopathology of IBD, the reader is referred to current textbooks of gastroenterology.

DIAGNOSIS AND LABORATORY EXAMINATION

Making the diagnosis of arthritis associated with IBD rests on recognition of the significance of this association and on a high level of clinical suspicion. A diagnosis of IBD should be suspected in any child with arthritis accompanied by lower abdominal pain, hematochezia, unexplained weight loss, anemia, or fever. This suspicion would be supported by laboratory evidence of inflammation (high erythrocyte sedimentation rate and other acute-phase reactants, low serum albumin), and negative results for rheumatoid factor and antinuclear antibody tests. Antibodies to neutrophil cytoplasmic antigens (pANCA) are frequently present in the sera of children with IBD. Tests for antineutrophil cytoplasmic antibody (ANCA) were positive in 73 percent of children with UC and 14 percent of those with RE.[28] In spite of the association of this autoantibody with systemic vasculitis, vasculitis does not appear to be more frequent in ANCA-positive patients with IBD.[29]

Synovial fluid analyses of children with IBD have not been reported, although in adults counts of synovial fluid white blood cells have ranged from 5000 to 15,000/mm^3 (5 to 15 $\times$ 10^9/L), with a predominance of neutrophils. Synovial fluid protein, glucose, and hemolytic complement levels have been normal.[30] Occult GI blood loss can be verified by repeated stool guaiac examinations.

RADIOLOGIC EXAMINATION

Radiographs of peripheral joints document only soft tissue thickening and joint effusions. SI arthritis, when it occurs, is not clearly distinguishable from that associated with juvenile ankylosing spondylitis. Spur formation, the result of enthesitis, is sometimes identified at the insertion of the plantar fascia into the calcaneus. Periostitis may be demonstrable by radiographs or radionuclide scanning (Fig. 15–3). Burbige and coworkers[3] noted erosive lesions secondary to granulomatous synovitis in one child.

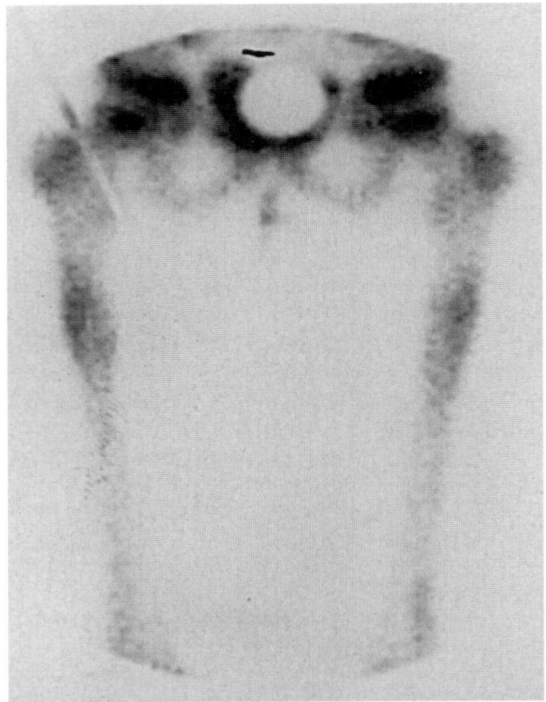

Figure 15–3. Bone scan documents increased uptake in the sacroiliac joints and along the femoral shafts, representing sacroiliac joint arthritis and periostitis in a 14-year-old girl with ulcerative colitis.

TREATMENT

Successful management of the peripheral arthritis depends on effective treatment of the GI tract disease: Control of the primary disease usually results in remission of the peripheral arthritis. Colectomy in UC may be followed by a striking remission in peripheral joint symptoms, although colectomy for the control of peripheral joint arthritis alone is certainly not indicated. Peripheral arthritis may be managed with nonsteroidal anti-inflammatory agents, but there is increasing evidence that these drugs can exacerbate IBD.[31] Selective cyclo-oxygenase-2 inhibitors may be important in this situation. Early use of sulfasalazine or glucocorticoids may provide the best management of the arthropathy of IBD directly by way of its beneficial effect on the GI inflammation, although no therapeutic trials have been published. For persistent arthritis in one or two joints, intra-articular triamcinolone hexacetonide should be considered. The peripheral joint arthritis is usually of quite short duration, and physical therapy is usually not necessary.

The HLA-B27–associated spondylitis of IBD is much more likely than the peripheral arthritis to persist and progress without remission, independent of the activity of the GI disease, and unaffected by procedures such as colectomy. It is therefore much more difficult to manage in the long term. Sulfasalazine is the drug of choice in a dose of 50 mg/kg/day to a maximum of 2.5 g/day. A physical therapy program with range-of-motion exercises to maintain back and chest motion (as for juvenile ankylosing spondylitis) may help to prevent or slow the effects of the disease. Custom-made orthotics may be useful to minimize pain secondary to enthesitis around the foot. Vasculitis accompanying IBD should be treated with systemic glucocorticoids. Topical glucocorticoids are used to treat uveitis.

COURSE OF THE DISEASE AND PROGNOSIS

The outcome of the GI disease is the most important determinant of overall prognosis in the child with IBD and arthritis.[1] Prognosis of the peripheral joint disease is usually excellent, although axial skeleton disease may progress independent of the course of the GI inflammation. Permanent changes in the spine and hips are frequent in this group of children. Poor nutrition and accompanying growth retardation may be major problems.

References

1. Farmer RG, Michener WM: Prognosis of Crohn's disease with onset in childhood or adolescence. Dig Dis Sci 24: 752, 1979.
2. Hamilton JR, Bruce MD, Abdourhaman M, et al: Inflammatory bowel disease in children and adolescents. Adv Pediatr 26: 311, 1979.
3. Burbige EJ, Shi-Shung H, Bayless TM: Clinical manifestations of Crohn's disease in children and adolescents. Pediatrics 55: 866, 1975.
4. Lindsley C, Schaller JG: Arthritis associated with inflammatory bowel disease in children. J Pediatr 84: 16, 1974.
5. Passo MH, Fitzgerald JF, Brandt KD: Arthritis associated with inflammatory bowel disease in children. Relationship of joint disease to activity and severity of bowel lesion. Dig Dis Sci 31: 492, 1986.
6. Keat A: Infections and the immunopathogenesis of seronegative spondyloarthropathies. Curr Opin Rheumatol 4: 494, 1992.
7. Satsangi J, Jewell DP, Bell JI: The genetics of inflammatory bowel disease. Gut 40: 572, 1997.
8. Futami S, Aoyama N, Honsako Y, et al: HLA-DRB1*1502 alleles, subtype of DR15 is associated with susceptibility to ulcerative colitis and its progression. Dig Dis Sci 40: 814, 1995.
9. Toyoda H, Wang S-J, Yang H, et al: Distinct association of HLA class II genes with inflammatory bowel disease. Gastroenterology 104: 741, 1993.
10. Brewerton DA, James DCO: The histocompatibility antigen HLA-27 and disease. Semin Arthritis Rheum 4: 191, 1975.
11. Neale G, Kelsall AR, Doyte FH: Crohn's disease and diffuse symmetrical periostitis. Gut 9: 383, 1968.
12. Lorber J: The changing etiology of erythema nodosum in children. Arch Dis Child 33: 137, 1958.
13. Winkelmann RK, Forstrom L: New observations in the histopathology of erythema nodosum. J Invest Dermatol 65: 441, 1975.
14. Hurwitz S: Clinical Pediatric Dermatology, 2nd ed. Philadelphia, WB Saunders, 1993, p 684.
15. Jacobs JC, Goetzl EJ: "Streaking leukocyte factor," arthritis and pyoderma gangrenosum. Pediatrics 56: 570, 1975.
16. Yassinger S, Adelman R, Cantor D: Association of inflammatory bowel disease and large vascular lesions. Gastroenterology 71: 844, 1976.
17. Gormally S, Bourke W, Kierse B, et al: Isolated cerebral thromboembolism and Crohn disease. Eur J Pediatr 154: 815, 1995.
18. Soloway M, Loir TW, Linton DW: Takayasu's arteritis: report of a case with unusual findings. Am J Cardiol 25: 258, 1970.
19. Hilário MOE, Terreri MTRA, Prismich G, et al: Association of ankylosing spondylitis, Crohn's disease and Takayasu's arteritis in a child. Clin Exp Rheumatol 16: 92, 1998.
20. Aoyagi S, Akashi H, Kawara T, et al: Aortic root replacement for Takayasu arteritis associated with ulcerative colitis and ankylosing spondylitis—report of a case. Jpn Circ J 62: 64, 1998.
21. Peeters AJ, van den Wall BAW, Daha MR, Breeveld FC: Inflammatory bowel disease and ankylosing spondylitis was associated with cutaneous vasculitis, glomerulonephritis and circulating IgA immune complexes. Ann Rheum Dis 49: 638, 1990.
22. Dard S, Kenouch S, Mery JP, et al: A new association: ankylosing spondylitis (AS) and Berger disease (BD). Kidney Int 24: 129, 1983.
23. McCallum D, Smith L, Harley F, et al: IgA nephropathy and thin basement membrane disease in association with Crohn disease. Pediatr Nephrol 11: 637, 1997.
24. Kay MH, Wyllie R: Cutaneous vasculitis as the initial manifestation of Crohn's disease in a pediatric patient. Am J Gastroenterol 93: 1014, 1998.
25. Lyons JL, Rosenbaum JT: Uveitis associated with inflammatory bowel disease compared with uveitis associated with spondyloarthropathy. Arch Ophthalmol 115: 61, 1997.
26. Ansell BM, Wigley RAD: Arthritis manifestations in regional enteritis. Ann Rheum Dis 23: 64, 1964.
27. Lindstrom H, Wramsby H, Ostberg G: Granulomatous arthritis in Crohn's disease. Gut 13: 257, 1972.
28. Olives JP, Breton A, Hugot JP, et al: Antineutrophil cytoplasmic antibodies in children with inflammatory bowel disease: prevalence and diagnostic value. J Pediatr Gastrol Nutr 25: 142, 1997.
29. Rosa C, Esposito C, Caglioti A, et al: Does the presence of ANCA in patients with ulcerative colitis necessarily imply renal involvement? Nephrol Dial Transplant 11: 2426, 1996.
30. Bunch TW, Hunder GG, McDuffie FC, et al: Synovial fluid complement determination as a diagnostic aid in inflammatory joint disease. Mayo Clin Proc 49: 715, 1974.
31. Evans JMM, McMahon AD, Murray FE, et al: Non-steroidal anti-inflammatory drugs are associated with emergency admission to hospital for colitis due to inflammatory bowel disease. Gut 40: 619, 1997.

16

Nonrheumatic Musculoskeletal Pain

David D. Sherry and Peter N. Malleson

Musculoskeletal pain of noninflammatory origin is a common cause of morbidity in childhood. Noninflammatory causes of pain are much more common than rheumatic ones, and their identification and differentiation from other causes of musculoskeletal pain such as infection or malignancy are essential in order to institute appropriate therapy and to avoid unnecessary investigations.

PAIN ASSOCIATED WITH HYPERMOBILITY

Generalized Hypermobility

The term *benign hypermobility syndrome* is applied to those children with musculoskeletal pain associated with generalized hypermobility of the joints (or "double-jointedness") without any associated congenital syndrome or abnormality of connective tissue, such as Marfan or Ehlers-Danlos syndrome.[1–3] Some of the more common syndromes associated with hypermobility are listed in Table 16–1; many of these conditions may be far from benign. The criteria for hypermobility have evolved over the years, and currently most authors use either the nine-point Beighton scale or the modified criteria of Carter and Wilkinson (Table 16–2).[4, 5] Estimates of the frequency of hypermobility range from 8 to 20 percent in white populations; Chinese and West Africans have a much higher prevalence of hypermobility.[4, 6–9] Girls are affected about twice as often as boys. A family history of hypermobility is common.

Hypermobility is often associated with intermittent nocturnal pains that may occur after certain activities. Children aged 3 to 10 years are mostly affected, as the prevalence of hypermobility decreases with age.[7–11] Rarely is such a child dysfunctional. Mild joint effusions may be observed. Reassurance is the initial treatment of hypermobility. Supportive footwear is helpful for many. Some children will benefit from an evening dose of acetaminophen or a nonsteroidal anti-inflammatory agent. A very few children will require a change of activity, although it is important that the alteration of activity not be interpreted by the family or child as a recommendation to stop participating in physical activities. Older, more severely affected children may be helped by formal physical therapy.[12]

Although generally innocuous, there are several less benign associations with hypermobility. In infants, delayed development of major motor skills may lead to unnecessary anxiety and physiotherapy.[13, 14] Joint pain, if not identified as related to hypermobility, may also lead to unnecessary laboratory investigations and treatments in a mistaken belief that the pains are rheumatic in origin.[15] A benign bleeding tendency has been reported in children with hypermobile thumbs.[16] In both children and adults, soft tissue rheumatism, including diffuse idiopathic musculoskeletal pain and fibromyalgia, is more common in hypermobile patients.[17, 18]

Although hypermobility may enable a child to be a good gymnast, injuries may be more frequent in hypermobile athletes[19–21] as well as in individuals undergoing strenuous training, including military recruits.[22] Temporomandibular joint dysfunction may be a consequence of hypermobility.[23–25] Proprioception of the knee, reported to be diminished in hypermobile females, may lead to poor biomechanical loading and microtrauma.[26]

Patients with chondromalacia patellae (anterior knee pain) are more likely to be hypermobile than are control patients.[27] Back pain is also more common in hypermobile patients, especially if their activities involve a lot of sitting or standing; individuals whose activities require frequently changing positions experienced less back pain.[27, 28] Premature osteoarthritis has been suggested as a consequence of hypermobility, but the evidence is not convincing.[29] One study showed no difference in bone density between those with and those without hypermobility.[30]

Children who "crack their knuckles" are frequently hypermobile. Parents are often concerned that this activity might lead to joint damage, but it is probably not a cause of later osteoarthritis.[31]

Fortunately, children with benign hypermobility syndrome are not at an increased risk for aortic dilatation or mitral valve prolapse.[30, 32, 33] A number of children do not fulfill criteria for generalized hypermobil-

Table 16–1

Selected Conditions Associated With Hypermobility

Marfan Syndrome
Tall and thin
Arm span greater than height
Lower ratio of upper-body segment to lower-body segment (long legs); normal ratio is 0.85 in whites and 0.92 in blacks
Arachnodactyly
Pectus excavatum or carinatum
Kyphoscoliosis
Dislocation of the lens of the eye
Aortic root dilatation
Heart murmurs, midsystolic click
Hernias
Autosomal dominant disorder due to mutations of fibrillin gene on chromosome 15
Homocystinuria
Marfanoid habitus
Major risk of thrombotic events
Autosomal recessive disorder usually associated with cystathionine β–synthase deficiency due to mutations of gene on long arm of chromosome 21
Stickler's Syndrome
Marfanoid habitus
Typical facial appearance: malar hypoplasia, depressed nasal bridge, epicanthal folds, micrognathia
Cleft palate (Pierre Robin sequence)
Severe myopia (may lead to retinal detachment)
Sensorineural hearing loss
Mitral valve prolapse
Autosomal dominant disorder due to mutations of type II collagen gene on chromosome 12
Ehlers-Danlos Syndromes
Skin abnormalities: thin, hyperelastic, cigarette paper scars, easy bruising
Dislocation of joints
Rarely, artery aneurysms; hollow organ rupture
Heterogeneous conditions; at least nine types with different inheritance patterns
Osteogenesis Imperfecta
Blue sclerae
Fragile bones with multiple fractures and deformities
Short stature
Spinal deformity
Different types; usually autosomal dominant inheritance
Involves abnormalities of type I collagen
Williams' Syndrome
Short stature
Characteristic elfin facial appearance
Hoarse voice
Friendly and loquacious
Developmental delay
Supravalvular stenosis
Occasionally hypercalcemia
Initially hypermobile but later become hypomobile without pain
Sporadic and inherited cases due to deletion of elastin allele on chromosome 7
Down Syndrome (Trisomy 21)
Hypotonia
Developmental delay
Characteristic facial appearance; epicanthal folds
Short stature
Endocardial cushion defects
Broad hands with simian creases
Brushfield (depigmented) spots of the iris
Usually inherited in a sporadic fashion

For further details about these conditions, the reader is referred to Chapter 37, Smith's Recognizable Patterns of Human Malformation,[157] and McKusick's Heritable Disorders of Connective Tissue.[158]

ity, being hypermobile in only a few joints. They too can develop pain, probably as a consequence of the imbalance between the hypermobile and the less mobile joints.

Table 16–2

Criteria for Hypermobility

Modified Criteria of Carter and Wilkinson
Three of five are required to establish a diagnosis of hypermobility
Touch thumb to volar forearm
Hyperextend metacarpophalangeal joints so fingers parallel forearm
>10° hyperextension of elbows
>10° hyperextension of knees
Touch palms to floor with knees straight
Beighton Scale
≥ 6 points defines hypermobility
Touch thumb to volar forearm (one point each for right and left)
Extend 5th metacarpophalangeal joint to 90° (one point each for right and left)
>10° hyperextension of elbow (one point each for right and left)
>10° hyperextension of knee (one point each for right and left)
Touch palms to floor with knees straight (one point)
Other noncriteria features of many children with hypermobility
Put heel behind head
Excessive internal rotation to hip
Excessive ankle dorsiflexion
Excessive eversion of the foot
Passively touch elbows behind the back

Pes Planus

The flexible flat foot is normal in very young children. Most infants have no longitudinal arch, and the development of this arch is part of normal growth.[34] In children, the arch may exist when they are toe-standing or lying but may disappear on weight bearing. Usually, flexible flat feet are not a cause of significant discomfort. A patient with flat feet and hindfoot valgus is shown in Figure 16–1.

The occasional adolescent with a short Achilles tendon and hypermobile flat foot may have pain from excessive weight bearing on the talar head.[35] This defect is rare, however, being present in only 25 of 3619 male soldiers.[36] Treatment is controversial. Wenger and associates[37] reported a prospective randomized trial of 98 children with flat feet receiving no treatment or treated with corrective orthopedic shoes, a Helfet heel-cup, or a custom-molded plastic insert. There was sig-

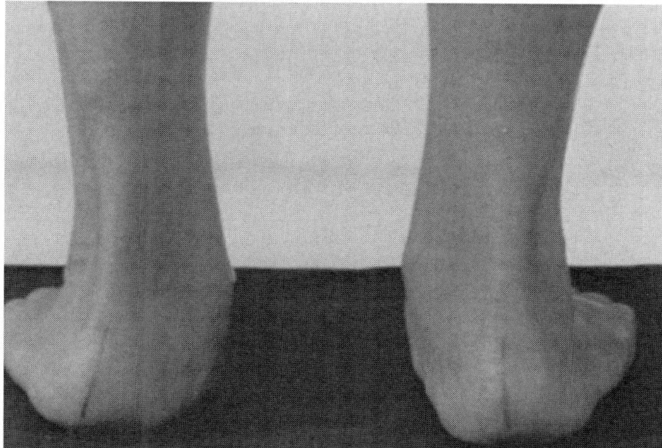

Figure 16–1. Pes planus with left hindfoot valgus. (Courtesy of Dr. G. Kuchta.)

nificant improvement in most children irrespective of treatment group. Orthotic devices that involve only the hindfoot do not reduce the mediolateral ground forces in adults with pes planus.[38] Mosca recommends aggressive heel cord stretching and adjusting of the shoes; if that fails, then a soft foot orthosis may be tried.[35] Surgery is indicated only in the most extreme cases in skeletally mature adolescents.[35, 39]

Pes planus (and pes cavus) in the athlete may be associated with overuse injury more commonly than in those with a normal-appearing arch.[40] Interestingly, neither pes planus nor pes cavus (which can also be a cause of foot discomfort) has been shown to be a significant predictor of injury in army recruits,[41] and one study reports fewer stress fractures in those with low arches.[42] No therapeutic studies in these populations are available.

In contrast to the mobile flat foot, a rigid flat foot is always pathologic. It may result from tarsal coalition, in which a bone or cartilaginous bridge is present between tarsal bones, usually the talus and the calcaneus or the navicular and the calcaneus (Fig. 16–2). As the bridge ossifies, motion is restricted and pain may result; 25 percent of children with tarsal coalition have symptoms.[43] Computed tomography will usually show the defect, and surgical intervention is required if conservative management fails.

Genu Recurvatum

Genu recurvatum, like pes planus, may be part of a generalized hypermobility syndrome or may occur as an isolated phenomenon. Symptomatic genu recurvatum occurs most commonly in adolescent girls and is associated with popliteal pain and an increased incidence of anterior cruciate ligament injury.[22, 44] Symptoms are worse with standing or walking and are relieved by rest. Athletes may have particular difficulty.[22]

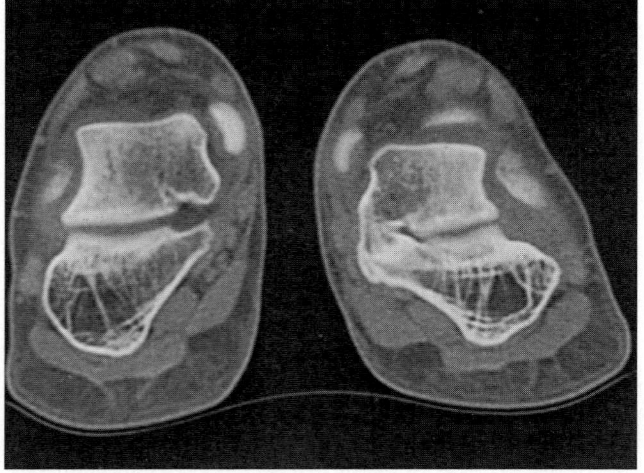

Figure 16–2. This computed tomography scan illustrates the bony bridge between the calcaneus and talus on the right side. The left hindfoot is normal. This feature may not be detectable on plain radiographs. (Courtesy of Dr. R. Cairns.)

Treatment includes correction of biomechanical faults by use of orthotics; improving knee proprioception and muscle control, especially quadriceps strength, as well as gait; and maintaining good knee alignment during functional activities.[44]

Recurrent Patellar Dislocation

As part of the hypermobility syndrome or as an isolated phenomenon, the patella may dislocate laterally. This is accompanied by a sensation of giving way with sudden pain and the inability to straighten the leg. The knee is held in a position of about 25 degrees of flexion. It may be associated with a congenital abnormality of the patella (unifaceted or bipartite patella), of the femoral condyles (shallow intercondylar groove), or of the patellar ligament (lateral attachment). Repeated episodes of dislocation lead to premature degeneration of the articular cartilage of the patellofemoral joint. The patellar apprehension sign suggests the diagnosis: contraction of the quadriceps muscle when the examiner attempts to displace the patella laterally. Femoral anteversion, patella alta, and an increased Q-angle are also commonly found. Treatment consists of short-arc active and resistive exercises to strengthen the musculature around the knee joint, especially the vastus medialis, to centralize the patella. If these interventions fail, surgical realignment of the extensor system may be indicated.[45]

Hypomobility

Although not studied in a formal fashion, it is our impression that a few children with slightly limited joint mobility (either as part of an underlying syndrome or as one end of the normal spectrum of joint mobility) may also present with arthralgias. It is not uncommon for children with back and lower extremity arthralgias to have tight hamstring, quadriceps, and calf muscles.[46] Bowyer reported that four of five children with hip contractures due to an underlying spondyloarthropathy experienced hip pain.[47] We have seen several children with a variety of individually relatively uncommon disorders, including hypothyroidism and hyalinosis,[48] who seemed to be in pain because of very stiff joints (Table 16–3). Two sisters with familial fibrosing serositis[49] developed multiple joint pain and contractures. Most children with marked stiffness due to conditions such as arthrogryposis, Williams' syndrome, and cerebral palsy do not complain of arthralgias, so careful evaluation for underlying disorders is indicated.

PAIN SYNDROMES RELATED TO OVERUSE

Patellofemoral Pain

Pain in the anterior aspect of the knee, originating in the patellofemoral joint, is quite common (Table 16–

Table 16–3

Selected Conditions Associated With Hypomobility or Joint Contractures

Diabetes mellitus (diabetic cheiroarthropathy)
  Tightening of skin and soft tissues of fingers
  Short stature
Scleroderma and scleroderma-like conditions
Mucopolysaccharidoses and mucolipidoses with dysostosis multiplex
  Autosomal recessive inheritance except in Hunter's syndrome, which is X-linked
Hyalinosis
Familial fibrosing serositis
  Progressive contractures of fingers and toes
  Fibrosing pleuritis and constrictive pericarditis
  Probably autosomal recessive inheritance
Camptodactyly syndromes (several familial conditions including Blau's syndrome)
Flexion contractures of fingers
Beals' contractural arachnodactyly syndrome
  Marfanoid features
  Crumpled ears
  Cardiac abnormalities unusual
  Linked to fibrillin-like gene on chromosome 5 (autosomal dominant inheritance)
Winchester's syndrome
  Multicentric osteolysis particularly of fingers starting in infancy
  Autosomal recessive inheritance

For further details about the inherited conditions listed here, the reader is referred to Chapter 37, Smith's Recognizable Patterns of Human Malformation,[157] and McKusick's Heritable Disorders of Connective Tissue.[158]

4).[50, 51] It is characterized by pain and tenderness in the region of the medial patellar facet and crepitation on movement of the joint. There are several possible causes of this disorder.[52–56] If the syndrome is accompanied by fissuring and fibrillation of the posterior surface of the patella, the term *chondromalacia patellae* is used. It is most common in teenage girls. There is insidious development of retropatellar knee pain. Pain occurs at first with activity that stresses the quadriceps, such as deep knee bends, climbing or descending stairs, or running, and is lessened by rest. Pain recurs with prolonged sitting with the knee flexed and can be relieved by extension of the leg. On physical examination, knee flexion may be accompanied by patellar crepitus. Pain may be reproduced by compression of the patella and by palpation along its inferomedial edge. Pain may also be elicited if the upward movement of the patella is restrained when the quadriceps muscle is contracted. A small effusion may be present. Findings on standard radiographs and laboratory investigations are normal. Arthroscopy may reveal ridging and strands of degenerating cartilage on the retropatellar surface.

Patellofemoral pain syndromes can be chronic and difficult to treat. Activities that provoke pain should be avoided. Strengthening of the muscles around the knee, especially the vastus medialis muscle, may help prevent progression of the problem. A knee strap or elastic support may provide some relief. Correction of pronated feet by custom-fitted orthoses and weight reduction in the overweight teenager may help. Surgical procedures, including shaving off the patellar irregularities, are of questionable benefit.

Plica Syndromes

The medial and lateral plicae arise from synovial bands that separate the compartments of the knee during development. These folds do not usually cause symptoms; however, some experts believe that if they become thickened, they may cause pain in the knee (Table 16–5).[57]

The *mediopatellar plica syndrome* is the more common and causes pain with flexion of the knee; erosion of cartilage may eventually occur. There is often an area of tenderness over the superomedial border of the femoral condyle and locking or snapping during movement of the joint. Diagnosis is made by arthroscopy; if necessary, resection can be performed at the same time.

Stress Fractures and Physeal and Apophyseal Injuries

Stress injuries occur when bones, physes, or apophyses (sites of growth cartilage where tendons insert) are damaged by their exposure to repetitive, nonviolent loads. The onset of pain and localized weakness due to reflex inhibition are usually insidious, occurring in an athletic adolescent who is doing a repetitive activity such as long-distance running. Physical examination reveals localized bone tenderness with reproduction of pain on resisted movement. Early radiographs may be normal or show only soft tissue swelling. Later radiographs demonstrate callus formation (Fig. 16–3), physeal widening, or apophyseal fragmentation. There is significant overlap between these conditions and the osteochondroses (see later text and Table 16–6).

Table 16–4

Patellofemoral Pain Syndromes

Age at onset	Adolescent to young adulthood
Sex ratio	Girls > boys
Symptoms	Insidious onset of exertional knee pain, difficulty descending stairs and walking downhill, need to sit with legs straight ("theater sign")
Signs	Patellar tenderness on compression; quadriceps weakness; inhibition sign; small joint effusion

Table 16–5

Mediopatellar Plica Syndrome

Age at onset	Adolescence
Symptoms	Medial knee pain, intermittent aching increased with activity or motion, giving way on weight bearing, locking
Signs	Medial palpable band, snapping on motion
Arthroscopy	Fibrous band with hemorrhage and inflammation identified

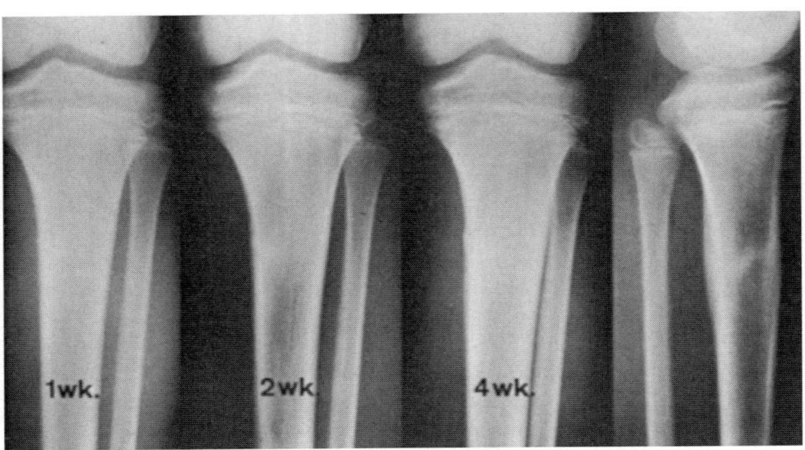

Figure 16–3. Serial radiographs document the evolution of a stress fracture in a 10-year-old girl who was the hopscotch champion of her block. Two weeks after the onset of leg pain, the fracture line is evident. After 4 weeks, the fracture callus is seen. (Courtesy of Dr. Robert N. Hensinger.)

Lower Limb Conditions

The classic stress fracture is the march fracture of the metatarsals seen in members of the military. The most common site of a stress fracture in children, however, is the proximal third of the tibia, with metatarsal fractures being uncommon (see Fig. 16–3).

Pelvic Apophysitis

Pain may occur where abdominal and hip muscles insert into the pelvis. Particular conditions involve the insertion of the sartorius into the anterior superior iliac spine, the insertion of the rectus femoris into the anterior inferior iliac spine, the insertion of the ilio-

Table 16–6

The Osteochondroses

AREA AFFECTED	EPONYM	MECHANISM
Upper Extremity		
Basal phalanges	Thiemann	Trauma
Second metacarpal head	Mauclaire	Trauma
Lunate	Kienböck	Osteonecrosis
Carpal navicular	Prieser	Trauma
Distal ulna	Burns	Trauma
Capitellum of humerus	Panner	Trauma? Avascular necrosis
Head of humerus	Hass	Trauma
Lower Extremity		
Second metatarsal head	Freiberg	Osteonecrosis
Fifth metatarsal base	Iselin	Trauma
Tarsal navicular	Köhler	Normal variation
Talus	Diaz	Trauma
Calcaneal apophysis	Sever	Normal variation
Distal tibia	Liffert-Arkin	Trauma
Tibial tubercle	Osgood-Schlatter	Trauma
Proximal tibia	Blount	Trauma
Intercondylar spines	Caffey	?
Primary patellar center	Köhler	?
Secondary patellar center	Sinding-Larsen-Johansson	Repeated trauma
Greater trochanter	Mandl	?
Femoral epiphysis	Legg-Calvé-Perthes	Osteonecrosis
Femoral epiphysis	Meyer's dysplasia	Normal variation
Axial Skeleton		
Vertebral body	Calvé	?
Disk	Schmorl	?
Vertebral epiphysis	Scheuermann	Repeated trauma
Iliac crest	Buchman	?
Symphysis pubis	Pierson	?
Ischiopubic synchondrosis	Van Neck	Normal variant
Ischial apophysis	Milch	?

Adapted from Brower AC: The osteochondroses. Orthop Clin North Am 14: 99, 1983; Resnick D: The osteochondroses. *In* Resnick D, Niwayama G (eds): Diagnosis of Bone and Joint Disorders. Philadelphia, WB Saunders, 1981, p 2874; and other sources.

Table 16–7

Osgood-Schlatter Disease

Age at onset	Athletic adolescents
Sex ratio	Boys > girls
Symptoms	Pain over the tibial tubercle exacerbated by exercise, unable to kneel because of pain
Signs	Tenderness and swelling over the attachment of the infrapatellar tendon
Investigations	Radiograph shows soft tissue swelling, enlarged and sometimes fragmented tubercle

psoas into the lesser trochanter, and the insertion of the abdominal musculature into the iliac crest apophysis.[58] These conditions are associated with a dull pain in the general area of the hip on activity and may therefore be confused with intra-articular hip disease. The occurrence of pain on resisted contractions of involved muscles, in which the hip joint itself is not allowed to move, is indicative that the pain is not due to intrinsic hip disease.

Osgood-Schlatter Disease

Osgood-Schlatter disease[59, 60] is an osteochondrosis caused by repeated trauma to the tibial tuberosity. Essentially it is a microavulsion fracture resulting when the infrapatellar tendon pulls out from the tibial tuberosity.[61] It commonly occurs in athletic adolescents (Table 16–7).[62] There is a complaint of pain over the tibial tubercle that is exacerbated by exercise or kneeling. On examination, tenderness and, often, swelling of the tibial tubercle and patellar tendon insertion are present. Radiographs, which should be obtained to exclude other conditions, may show soft tissue swelling and an enlarged and fragmented tubercle (Fig. 16–4). It is normal, however, for the tibial tubercle to appear irregular in adolescence, and it may be difficult to differentiate normal development from disease. Ultrasonography can help in identifying the lesion.[63] Laboratory studies reveal no evidence of chronic inflammation. Rest or use of a basketball knee protector is usually sufficient treatment. The outcome is usually very good.[64]

Sinding-Larsen-Johansson Disease

Sinding-Larsen-Johansson disease is an osteochondrosis caused by repeated trauma to the inferior pole (secondary ossification center) of the patella (Fig. 16–5); essentially it is an avulsion fracture resulting when the infrapatellar tendon pulls out from the patella.[65, 66] It may be confused with Osgood-Schlatter disease or infrapatellar tendinitis, in which pain at the inferior pole of the patella may also occur. Treatment consists of rest or reduction in physical activities that involve the legs; most cases resolve within 3 to 12 months.

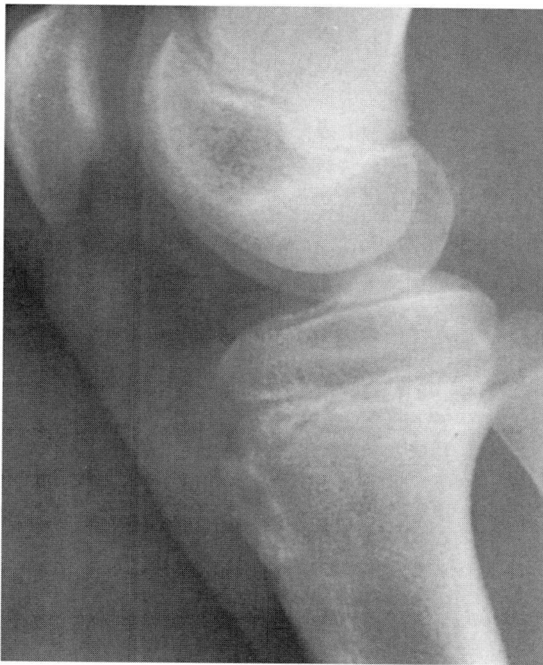

Figure 16–4. Radiograph of the knee of a boy with Osgood-Schlatter disease. In addition to fragmentation of the apophysis, the soft tissues overlying the tibial tubercle are thickened. (Courtesy of Dr. R. Cairns.)

Sever's Disease

Sever's disease is a common cause of heel pain, usually occurring in physically active individuals in early adolescence. The etiology is uncertain. Liberson and colleagues[67] suggested that radiographic findings of a dense calcaneal apophysis are normal, occurring as commonly in control subjects as in subjects with heel pain, but that radiographic lucencies or fragmentation

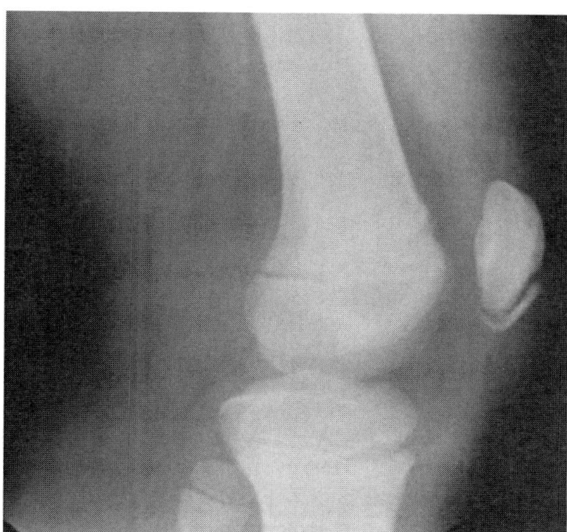

Figure 16–5. Radiograph of the knee of a boy with Sinding-Larsen-Johansson disease. The lower pole of the patella has been separated from the patella.

changes are more commonly associated with pain. Based on radiographic changes, computed tomographic scans, and histologic examinations, these authors hypothesized that the cause of Sever's disease is a process of remodeling of the calcaneal apophysis secondary to repetitive stresses of traction from the Achilles tendon and plantar fascia, and impact from weight bearing. This remodeling process is usually a normal subclinical event but becomes symptomatic when it becomes excessive.

Upper Limb Conditions

Upper limb stress injuries occur less commonly than lower limb conditions.

Shoulder pain on active and resisted movement is associated with widening of the proximal humeral physis and occurs in children in sports such as baseball pitching that involve repetitive overarm movements *(Little League shoulder)*.[68] These overarm movements can also be associated with pain at the elbow due to an apophyseal injury to the medial epicondyle (golfer's elbow). A similar injury is *tennis elbow*, in which the pain is due to apophysitis of the lateral epicondyle at the insertion of the common wrist extensors. These elbow syndromes can be helped by the use of a "tennis elbow strap," which is applied fairly tightly around the forearm just distal to the tender site. It is believed to help diminish the pain by altering the apparent origin of the extensor and flexor muscles. Glucocorticoid injections into the site of maximal tenderness are often required if the symptoms persist for more than a few weeks.

Little Leaguer elbow is another stress injury in which there is a painful fragmentation of the capitellum of the distal humerus. Its pathogenesis and its relation to Panner's osteochondrosis are unclear. *Panner's disease* usually affects boys under 10 years of age and is not associated with obvious repetitive trauma. The whole ossific nucleus becomes flattened and fragmented, but the condition resolves with no long-term sequelae. Traumatic damage to the capitellum is probably due to compressive forces between the radial head and the capitellum. It occurs in older children and is more likely to be associated with joint loose bodies, and there may be persistent elbow abnormalities despite surgical intervention.[69] Injuries to the olecranon occurring in young elite gymnasts have also been described.[70]

Soft Tissue Stress Injuries

Repetitive trauma can cause soft tissue injuries in addition to bony lesions. Tenosynovitis is relatively common, particularly in the athletic adolescent and in relatively inactive children who, without proper preparation, overengage in an activity (the "weekend warrior").

Shin Splints

The term *shin splints* is applied to a pain syndrome in the posteromedial aspect of the lower half of the shin, usually in older adolescents. It is associated with running, jogging, or walking, is worse with the activity, and is relieved by rest.[71] It is due to periostitis at the insertion of the soleus muscle.[72] The diagnosis is confirmed by the demonstration of tenderness at the posteromedial border of the distal tibia. Stress fractures can mimic shin splints. Rarely, an anterior compartment syndrome resulting from hemorrhage or edema, accompanied by ischemic changes in the foot, is confused with shin splints. Shin splints are best prevented by adequate stretching and strengthening and avoidance of jogging or walking on hard surfaces. Treatment is symptomatic with rest, stretching, ice, anti-inflammatory drugs, close attention to shoes, and a graduated rehabilitation program.[71, 72] Orthotics may help patients with pronated feet or excessive subtalar motion.

Tenosynovitis

Although tenosynovitis commonly accompanies rheumatic disease, it can also occur as a result of unaccustomed repetitive movement, especially around the ankle (Achilles tenosynovitis, anterior tibial tenosynovitis) or at the wrists, or as stenosing tenosynovitis of the abductor pollicis longus or extensor pollicis brevis *(de Quervain's disease)*. Treatment requires rest, with splinting if needed, and possibly injection of glucocorticoid into the tendon sheath.

For a complete discussion of these and other overuse syndromes, the reader is referred to the work of Sheon and coworkers.[73]

OSTEOCHONDROSES

As indicated earlier, there is a great deal of commonality between many of the stress-related injuries and the osteochondroses, and dividing the discussion into individual conditions is somewhat arbitrary. Some members of this heterogeneous group of disorders are described under "Apophyseal Injuries"; others, of particular significance to pediatric rheumatologists, are discussed briefly in the following sections. Some of the conditions commonly considered to be osteochondroses are probably variants of normal ossification, some are probably due to stress injury, and others may be due to avascular necrosis without any obvious precipitating trauma, perhaps occurring because of some inherent predisposition to vascular insufficiency. This uncertainty of the etiology has led to confusion and contradictory nomenclature and classification.

Brower defined osteochondrosis as "a condition in which the primary or secondary ossification centre in the growing child undergoes aseptic necrosis with gradual resorption of dead bone and replacement by reparative osseous tissue."[74] Resnick uses a somewhat broader definition: any of "a group of disorders that share certain features: predilection for the immature skeleton; involvement of an epiphysis, apophysis, or epiphysioid bone; and a radiographic picture that is dominated by fragmentation, collapse, sclerosis, and frequently, reossification with reconstitution of the osseous contour."[75] From a clinical point of view, osteochondroses might be defined as idiopathic, acquired, localized disorders of cartilage and bone, often characterized by localized pain.

The osteochondroses usually affect a single site but may be bilateral; they are characteristically observed in children between the ages of 3 and 12 years and are much more common in boys than in girls. In large part, these disorders have been defined by their radiologic appearance, although, as already discussed, it is now clear that some of these findings are normal variants. In Table 16–6, the osteochondroses are listed according to the site affected and the putative etiology is indicated.

Legg-Calvé-Perthes Disease

Legg-Calvé-Perthes disease was independently and simultaneously described by Legg,[76] Calvé,[77] and Perthes.[78] It is an idiopathic *avascular necrosis* of the femoral head occurring in children between about the ages of 5 and 10 years. It is about four times more common in boys than girls and affects both hips in 10 to 15 percent of cases. There is an increased incidence in family members of an index case; Asians and whites are more frequently affected than are Native Australians, Native Americans, and blacks, and it occurs more frequently in urban than in rural areas.[79] It has been noted that children with Legg-Calvé-Perthes disease have delayed skeletal maturation and reduced height.[80]

The etiology of Legg-Calvé-Perthes disease is unknown, but it is generally accepted that the condition occurs in individuals whose vascular supply to the femoral head is particularly vulnerable to interruption. There is evidence that children in the Legg-Calvé-Perthes age range have a less extensive anastomotic vascular network to the femoral epiphysis than at other ages, and that boys have a less complete network than girls. It has recently been suggested that the factor V Leiden gene, responsible for resistance to protein C activation and therefore associated with an increased risk of thrombosis, is found more commonly in individuals with Legg-Calvé-Perthes disease.[81]

Affected children present with a limp and varying degrees of hip pain. Radiographs taken shortly after the onset of symptoms are often normal, but later radiographs show a progression through four stages: (1) an initial stage, at which there may be a small ossific nucleus, widening of the joint space, irregularity of the physis, and a subchondral radiolucent area; (2) a fragmentation stage, at which the bony epiphysis begins to fragment and there are patchy areas of increased radiolucency and radiodensity; (3) a reossification stage, at which normal bone density returns, radiodensities develop in previously radiolucent areas, and abnormalities of the shape of the femoral head and neck appear; and (4) the healed stage, at which the bone density is normal but the head is left with residual deformities. These changes may take several years to complete. Bone scans and magnetic resonance imaging studies have a greater sensitivity for the detection of early disease than do plain radiographs (Fig. 16–6).

The prognosis of Legg-Calvé-Perthes disease is dependent on how extensively involved the epiphyseal head is. The greater the extent of the necrosis, the more likely the femoral head is to become widened and flattened and uncontainable within the acetabulum. These changes predispose the individual to decreased range of movement at the hip and later changes of osteoarthritis. The aim of all forms of treatment for this condition is to maintain the femoral head well covered within the acetabulum, so as to minimize the deformity of the head. There is considerable uncertainty about the benefits of different surgical procedures compared with nonsurgical interventions such as splints[82, 83] A study by Lahdes-Vasama and associates[83] demonstrated that femoral heads with less than 50 percent involvement have a significantly better radiographic outcome than that in those with greater than 50 percent involvement, and that hips treated by femoral varus osteotomies did only a little better than those treated with containment splints. The more severely affected hips may benefit from operative intervention. Overall, two thirds of hips had a good long-term radiographic outcome.

Scheuermann's Disease

Scheuermann's disease (juvenile kyphosis) may be considered to be an osteochondrosis caused by repeated trauma to the ring apophysis of the vertebral body, although there is no consistency of its definition. It is most common in girls between 13 and 17 years of age who present with pain in the midthoracic or lumbar spine, or it can be painless but causes a round shoulder appearance and dorsal kyphosis. Radiographically, it is associated with anterior wedging of one to three adjacent vertebral bodies by at least 5 degrees each.[84] The kyphosis is thoracic in 75 percent of patients and thoracolumbar in most of the rest, except for the rare child with disease limited to the lumbar spine.[85] A prominent fixed dorsal kyphosis with a compensatory increase in the lumbar lordosis is characteristic. Tightness of the pectoral and hamstring muscles has been noted.[86] A standing lateral radiograph of the spine reveals anterior vertebral wedging, irregularity of vertebral end plates (Schmorl's nodes), increased anteroposterior diameter of the affected vertebral bodies, and increased dorsal kyphosis (Fig. 16–7). Treatment consists of simple analgesia and, occasionally, the use of a back brace to prevent flexion. The process is self-limited and the outcome is usually very good.

Köhler's Disease

Köhler's disease is an osteochondrosis of the tarsal navicular bone. It tends to affect children between 4

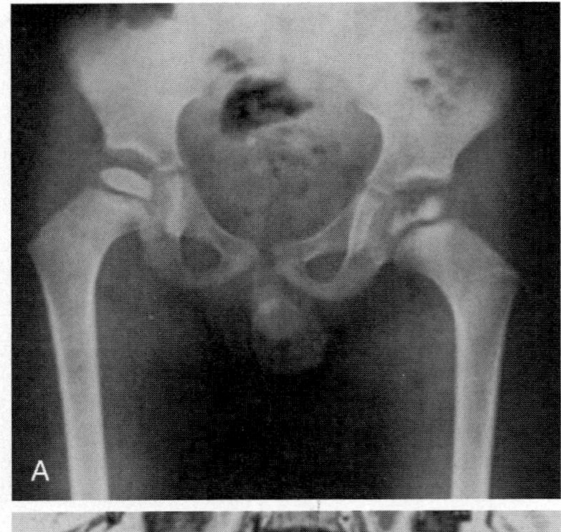

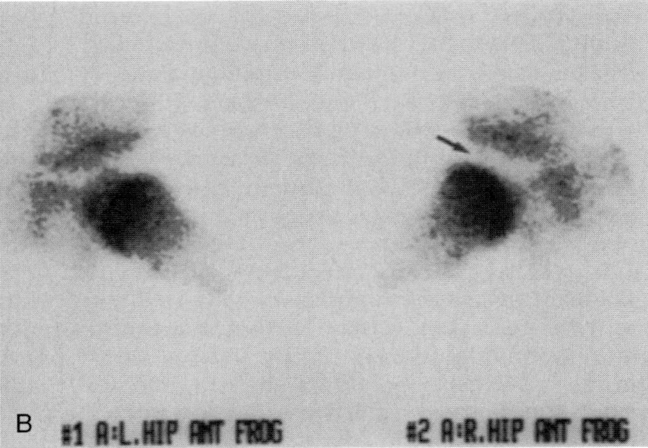

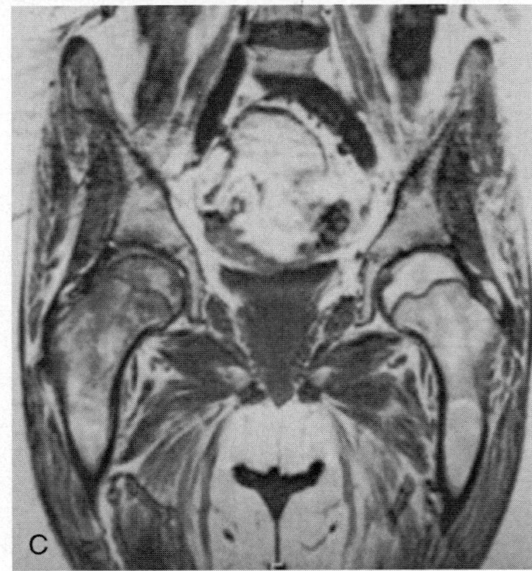

Figure 16–6. Progression of Legg-Calvé-Perthes disease. *A,* On the right side, the capital femoral epiphysis is flattened and sclerotic; on the left, it is fragmented. The femoral metaphyses are widened, especially on the left side. *B,* Technetium-99m bone scan of another patient shows absence of uptake of the isotope in the right capital femoral epiphysis *(arrow),* but normal uptake in the left side. *C,* Magnetic resonance image of aseptic necrosis of the right femoral head, thought to be related to prolonged glucocorticoid intake, in a boy with dermatomyositis. The entire femoral head and the marrow in the metaphysis are abnormal. (*A* and *C,* courtesy of Dr. R. Cairns; *B,* courtesy of Dr. H. Nadel.)

and 9 years of age who present with onset of insidious foot pain and a limp. The affected child characteristically bears weight on the lateral aspect of the foot.[87] Some authorities consider the radiographic findings of navicular narrowing, increased density, and sometimes fragmentation to be a variant of normal ossification (Fig. 16–8). There is no evidence that treatment affects outcome, which appears to be almost always associated with complete recovery; any persistent or late-onset foot complaints are usually due to other unrelated pathology.[88]

Freiberg's Disease

Freiberg's disease is an osteochondrosis of the second metatarsal head occurring most frequently in adolescent girls. Other metatarsal heads are occasionally affected. It causes localized pain on weight bearing, sometimes with swelling in the region of the second metatarsal head. This condition has usually been ascribed to trauma.[89] A retrospective study of 31 patients, however, elicited a history of trauma in only 15 percent, and pedobarographic studies failed to show abnormal high pressure at the affected metatarsal head.[90] This study noted that in 85 percent of cases, the affected metatarsal was the longest in the foot, and that this might, in some poorly explained way, predispose the metatarsal head to vascular insufficiency and infarction. Radiographs reveal increased density or flattening of the affected metatarsal head (Fig. 16–9). Treatment is usually supportive with shoe inserts to reduce weight bearing on the metatarsal heads, and rest (casting may be necessary for pain control).[39] The outcome is usually good.

Thiemann's Disease

Thiemann's disease is an osteochondrosis caused by osteonecrosis of the phalangeal epiphyses, possibly secondary to trauma. Thiemann's disease is characterized by progressive, painless enlargement during adolescence of the epiphysis of the proximal interphalangeal joints of the hands and the interphalangeal joints of the first toes.[91, 92] Flexion contractures of the large joints also occur. Radiologically, there is irregularity of the epiphyses of the digits. Results of tests for acute phase reactants are normal. Disability is minimal. The condition may be familial.[93–95]

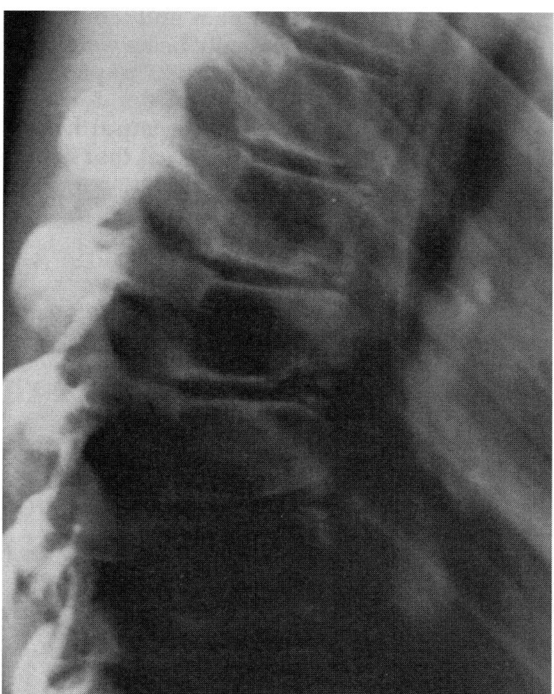

Figure 16–7. This lateral radiograph of the spine illustrates the abnormalities of the anterior margins of the vertebral bodies characteristic of Scheuermann's disease, resulting in anterior wedging. (Courtesy of Dr. R. Cairns.)

TRAUMA-INDUCED CONDITIONS

Some of the apophyseal stress injuries described earlier may be more severe and be associated with avulsion injuries. In these situations, surgical intervention may be required. This section does not attempt to cover all the types of musculoskeletal conditions caused by trauma, rather focusing on conditions that are more likely to come to the attention of the pediatric rheumatologist. For more detailed information, the reader is referred to the *Oxford Textbook of Sports Medicine*[96] or a standard orthopedic textbook.

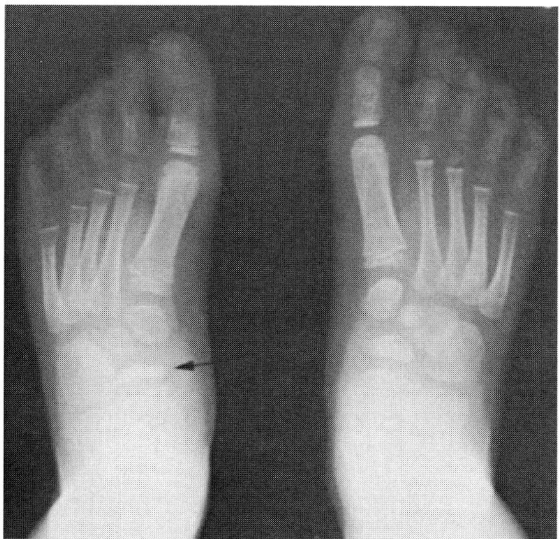

Figure 16–8. Köhler's disease. The tarsal navicular on the left *(arrow)* is sclerotic. (Courtesy of Dr. R. Cairns.)

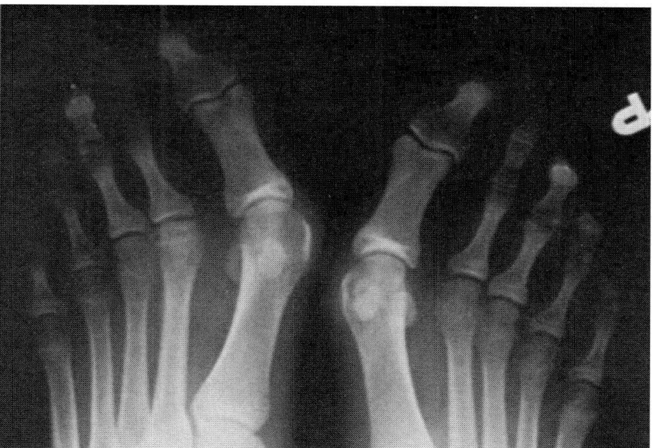

Figure 16–9. Freiberg's disease affecting the left second metatarsal head. (Courtesy of Dr. R. Cairns.)

Osteochondritis Dissecans

Osteochondritis dissecans is a condition in which there is partial or complete separation of articular cartilage with or without involvement of the subchondral bone. It is related to trauma, but is more frequently due to repeated microtrauma and overuse than to a single traumatic episode.[97] Bilateral lesions are common (approximately 20 percent). Occasional familial cases suggest that a genetic predisposition to vascular insufficiency of the subchondral bone may be of etiologic importance. Although the condition is usually recognized by plain radiography, because of the appearance of a subchondral fracture, the use of magnetic resonance imaging has led to an increased recognition that pure cartilaginous separation can occur, when radiographs may appear normal (Fig. 16–10). The inner aspect of the distal femoral medial condyle is the most commonly affected area (Fig. 16–11); however, osteochondritis dissecans of the dome of the talus (Fig. 16–12), the capitellum, or the patella also occurs fairly commonly.

Osteochondritis dissecans is characterized by activity-related pain, sometimes with recurrent bland effusions. If there has been complete separation of a fragment, there may be joint locking. Magnetic resonance imaging may become the method of choice for staging the lesion. Intact cartilage, contrast enhancement of the lesion, and absence of osseous "cystic" defects are designated stage 1. Treatment can be conservative (non–weight bearing for a few weeks), avoiding the need for arthroscopy. A cartilage defect with or without complete separation of the fragment, fluid around an undetached fragment, an osseous "cystic" lesion, or a dislodged fragment are stage 2 findings, probably requiring arthroscopy and surgical intervention. Persis-

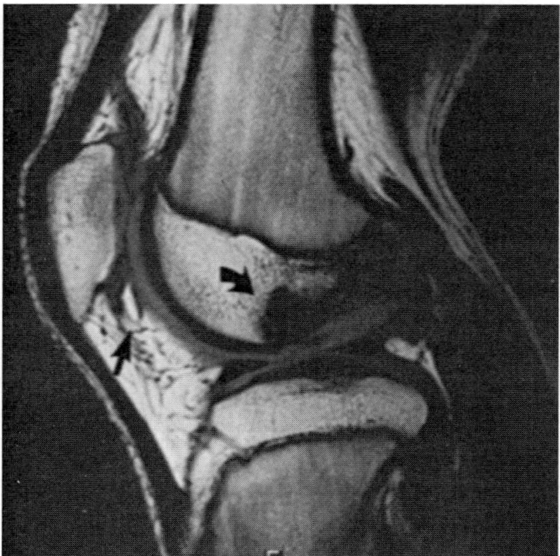

Figure 16–10. In this magnetic resonance image, the area from which the osteochondral fragment has arisen is seen as a black area in the posterior part of the articular surface of the femur *(curved arrow)*. The loose fragment of cartilage is indicated by the *straight arrow*. (Courtesy of Dr. R. Cairns.)

tence of symptoms despite non–weight bearing in individuals with stage 1 findings also usually requires arthroscopic investigation. Surgical interventions include trying to relocate the fragments by various fixation methods, and removing the loose bodies. Patients with open physes have an excellent prognosis, whereas older subjects with closed physes are at much greater risk of developing secondary osteoarthritic changes.

Traumatic Arthritis

Joint swelling associated with trauma occurs in older school-aged children and adolescents. An effusion arising immediately after an injury is more likely to be associated with intra-articular hemorrhage, fracture, or joint derangement than swelling that develops over several hours. A history of injury is often elicited in children with juvenile rheumatoid arthritis because a minor injury brings a swollen joint to parental attention. Trauma, especially minor trauma, is not an explanation for joint swelling in a young child, and internal joint derangements (meniscal tears) are very rare. Juvenile rheumatoid arthritis is far more common than traumatic arthritis in the very young. Transient joint swelling can result, however, from patellar subluxation or from repetitive trauma associated with overuse syndromes or structurally abnormal joints in older children.

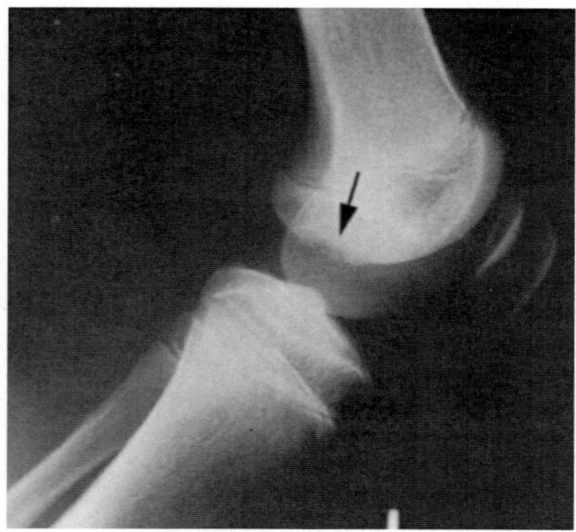

Figure 16–11. Osteochondritis dissecans is evident in the posterior aspect of the medial femoral condyle *(arrow)*. The loose fragment of cartilage and bone is not evident. (Courtesy of Dr. R. Cairns.)

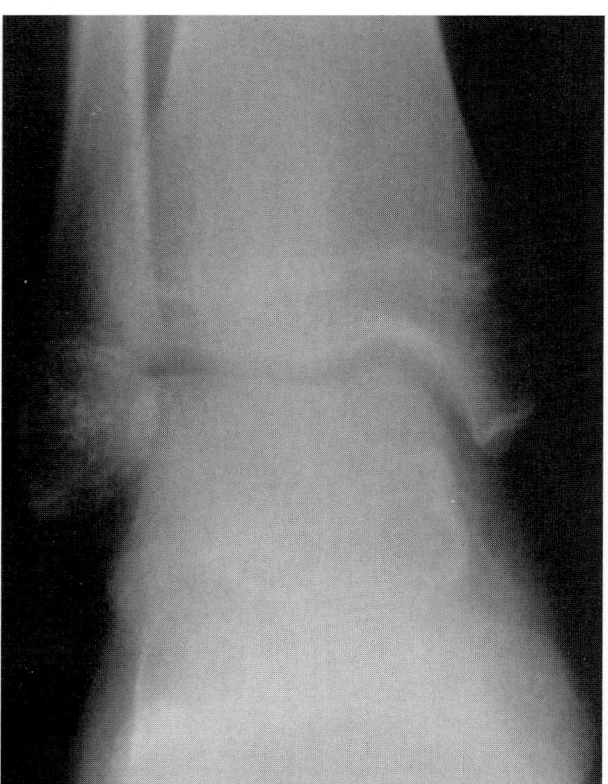

Figure 16–12. Osteochondritis dissecans is seen on the medial side of the dome of the talus.

Slipped Capital Femoral Epiphysis

Although slipped capital femoral epiphysis (SCFE) and acute chondrolysis of the hip are discussed here, their actual relationship to trauma is unclear, and there is often no significant history of trauma elicited, although it seems probable that abnormal mechanical loading contributes to their occurrence. In SCFE, there is onset of limp and pain in the affected hip. In the case of a subacute or a chronic-on-subacute slip, the onset of symptoms is insidious. Occasionally after a moderate injury, an acute slip can develop, resulting in pain and inability to walk. Radiographs are usually diagnostic, assuming a good lateral (axial) view of the hip is obtained, showing a posterior and downward slip of the femoral head on the neck due to a separation through the growth plate between the zones of hypertrophic and calcified cartilage. If a diagnosis is made, the child should be given crutches and made non–weight bearing until he or she can be seen urgently by the orthopedic surgeon. The condition most commonly affects overweight boys in early to mid-adolescence.

Generally the slip is classified as mild if it is less than one third the diameter of the femoral head and severe if the slip is greater than this amount. More recently, new classification schemes have been described that are probably of more prognostic utility than the traditional ones.[98] It has also been suggested that decreased radionuclide uptake on bone scans by the physis of the greater trochanter on the affected side, and later its premature closure on radiographs, is a predictive sign for the development of acute chondrolysis.[99] Bilateral slipped epiphyses are common (approximately 33 percent).[100] Treatment is by fixation, usually with a single central screw. Acute chondrolysis is a complication of both treated and untreated SCFE and occurs in about 6 percent of cases; avascular necrosis occurs in about 5 percent of cases.[101]

Acute Chondrolysis of the Hip

Acute chondrolysis of the hip is an unusual condition in which there is hip pain and limitation of movement in association with radiographic evidence of progressive loss of articular cartilage. It can occur as an apparently idiopathic event or secondary to other hip pathology, particularly SCFE or Legg-Calvé-Perthes disease. Idiopathic chondrolysis usually occurs in adolescents and may be more frequent in black girls.[101] Although the potential for severe disability is significant, many children have minimal symptoms on long-term follow-up, and radiographs can show apparent restoration of joint cartilage, often with lateral overgrowth of the femoral head and lateral acetabular osteophyte formation.[102] In those children with persistent symptoms, there is progressive loss of joint space and eventual ankylosis. It has been suggested that idiopathic chondrolysis may be due to synovitis of the hip, perhaps from a spondyloarthropathy[101, 103]; however, other studies have failed to show histologic evidence of significant synovial inflammation.[102] Chondrolysis associated with a SCFE appears to have a better long-term prognosis than idiopathic chondrolysis.[98]

Nonaccidental Injury

An abused infant or child is sometimes suspected of having a rheumatic disease because of the refusal to walk or bear weight, the presence of a joint effusion, or the presence of skin lesions that are thought to be vasculitic in origin. These children may be misdiagnosed as having juvenile rheumatoid arthritis if a proper history is not obtained. Beating a child over the hands and knuckles results in brawny induration of the dorsal surfaces of the hands as well as thickened, dense round bones and bone chips on radiographs. Physical abuse should be considered in the child who has a history of repeated visits to the emergency department because of poorly explained trauma, the occurrence of allegedly spontaneous bruises, or hemarthrosis without an underlying bleeding disorder. Radiographic demonstration of multiple fractures and periosteal new bone formation is characteristic. The syndrome termed *Munchausen's syndrome by proxy* is a bizarre form of child abuse induced by the parent in order to bring the child to medical attention, usually to meet the pathologic psychological needs of the mother.

There is the rare child with ecchymoses and deep bruising due to Henoch-Schönlein purpura who is thought to have been abused.[104] Awareness of this will save the child and family much suffering.

Frostbite Arthropathy

Frostbite is a cold-induced necrosis of the superficial tissues due to freezing. The acral or exposed areas, including the fingers, toes, nose, and ears, are predominantly affected. Immediately after exposure, the diagnosis of frostbite can be made by the characteristic appearance of swollen red fingers or toes. The history of cold exposure should be obvious, although the parents may not have been aware of the increased susceptibility of the very young child to cold injury. Vasomotor changes suggesting Raynaud's phenomenon may persist for months. In the growing child, frostbite produces a characteristic stunting of growth of the small bones and acro-osteolysis (Fig. 16–13).[105–107] Secondary symptoms of osteoarthritis may develop in early adulthood.

Pernio (Chilblains)

Pernio is due to a prior cold injury, not as severe as frostbite, that generally occurs in cold, damp climates or after exposure to cold water or snow. Pernio presents as burning pain, with associated red to purple, swollen papules (or even blisters) on exposed fingers or toes.[108] It can recur within a few minutes of cold reexposure. A history of wet cold exposure and typical skin changes establish the diagnosis. If the condition is severe, treatment with nifedipine may be beneficial.

Congenital Indifference to Pain

In the rare syndromes of congenital indifference to pain, affected children develop swollen but painless joints associated with induration or necrosis of the toes and fingers (Fig. 16–14).[109] Children with this condition, which may be an autosomal recessive trait, also frequently have anhydrosis, self-mutilating behaviors, and mental retardation. This *Charcot* type of arthropathy results in severely damaged, unstable joints that may eventually require arthrodesis to maintain some

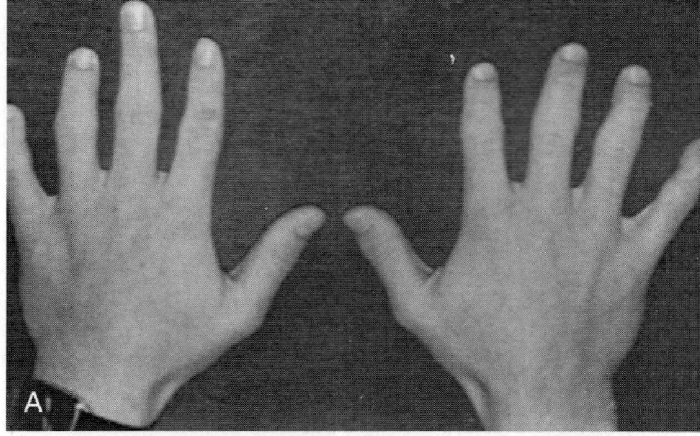

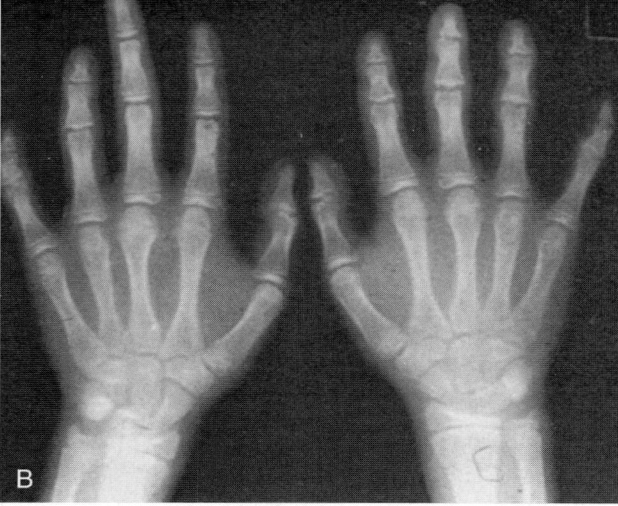

Figure 16–13. The effects of frostbite: Necrosis of the distal epiphyses of all digits except the thumbs and left second and third fingers has resulted in growth failure.

degree of function. One study suggested that substance P nerve fibers may be absent in this condition, confirming the importance of substance P in nociception within normal diarthrodial joints.[110] In three unrelated children with this condition, different abnormalities of the tyrosine kinase receptor gene for nerve growth factor have been found, indicating that abnormalities of this gene may be responsible for this condition.[111]

PAIN SYNDROMES AFFECTING THE BACK, CHEST, OR NECK

Noninflammatory disorders of the back, chest, or neck are important causes of chronic or recurrent pain in children. Pain can arise from a wide variety of causes, including congenital, developmental, or acquired defects as well as from nonmusculoskeletal diseases. In a study from Norway, 75 percent of schoolchildren had body pain and 25 percent reported pain several days a week.[112]

Back pain in the general pediatric population is very frequent in first world countries. A study from Denmark reported that at least 50 percent of teenagers had one episode of back pain[113]; a frequency of 74 percent was reported from Switzerland[114] and 44 percent from Iceland[115] (where 21 percent had weekly back pain). The prevalence is even higher in athletes[116, 117] but surprisingly is only 32 percent in those with idiopathic scoliosis.[118] Volinn reviewed the literature and concluded that low back pain was two- to fourfold higher in Swedish, German, and Belgium populations than in southern Chinese, Indonesian, Nigerian, and Filipino farmers.[119] In contrast, back pain is a relatively infrequent reason for referral to a pediatric orthopedic surgeon,[120] accounting for 2 percent of referrals. In those children seen by an orthopedic surgeon because of low back pain, no specific cause could be found in almost half; Scheuermann's disease was present in 15 percent, spondylolysis in 13 percent, infection in 8 percent, disk prolapse in 6 percent, and tumor in 6 percent.[120] A common cause of back pain in very young children is diskitis (see Chapter 31).

Chest pain is also a fairly frequent complaint in the pediatric population. Rowe and coworkers[121] reported that 6 of 1000 emergency department visits in a children's hospital were for chest pain. Chest pain occurred with equal frequency in boys and girls. Of 366 patients, 28 percent were diagnosed with chest wall pain; only 1 percent (5 of 336) had cardiac causes (Table 16–8).

Spondylolysis and Spondylolisthesis

Spondylolysis is a defect in the pars interarticularis, most commonly of the fifth lumbar vertebra (L5). In one study of 185 children with spondylolysis, 193 defects were detected, 1 at L2, 6 at L3, 16 at L4, 168 at L5, and 2 at L6.[122] The affected vertebra may slip anteriorly, giving rise to *spondylolisthesis*. Spondylolysis occurs in 6 percent of the population and frequently is asymptomatic.[123, 124] It is uncommon before the age of 5 years and is usually seen in the older adolescent. Spondylolysis is generally due to a stress or fatigue fracture of

Table 16–8

Causes of Chest Pain in Children Presenting to an Emergency Department

CATEGORY	%	CONDITIONS INCLUDED
Chest wall	28	Costochondritis, Tietze's syndrome, musculoskeletal pain, breast tenderness
Lung/pleura	19	Asthma, infection, embolism, pleurisy, pneumothorax
Trauma	15	Contusion, abrasion
Psychogenic	5	Depression, anxiety, conversion disorder, hyperventilation
Other	21	Esophagitis, gastritis, upper respiratory tract infection, constipation, cardiac causes
Unknown	12	Chest pain of undetermined cause

Adapted and reprinted from, by permission of the publisher, Rowe BH, Dulberg CS, Peterson RG, et al: Characteristics of children presenting with chest pain to a pediatric emergency department. Can Med Assoc J 143: 388, 1990.

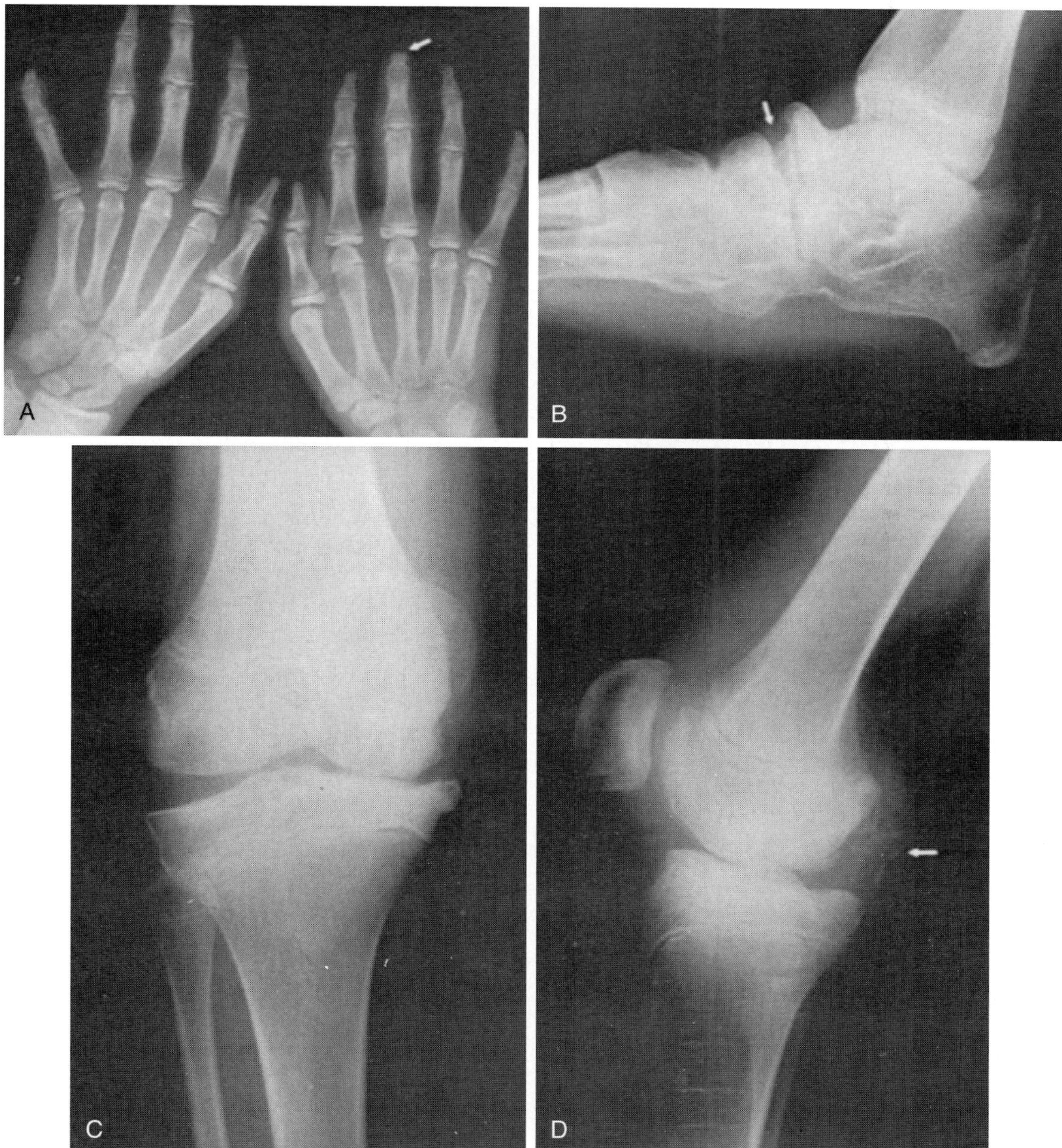

Figure 16–14. Radiographs of the effects of congenital indifference to pain. *A,* This child has lost the tips of several fingers *(arrow). B,* Hypertrophic and destructive changes are visible in the calcaneus, talus, and midfoot *(arrow). C* and *D,* There is marked loss of the medial compartment space and calcifications typical of Charcot's arthropathy. Clinically, the knees were warm and contained large effusions *(arrow* in *D).*

the pars interarticularis, but there may be a genetic component, since it is more common in first-order relatives.[124] Either condition can give rise to low back pain that may occur with activity and radiate down the posterior thigh. Occasionally, pain can be elicited by palpation of the involved vertebra, and a defect may be noted if a slip has occurred. Results of the neurologic examination are normal but there may be tightness and spasm of the hamstring muscles. Having the child hyperextend the back and lift a leg exacerbates the pain.[125] The diagnosis is usually clear from oblique and lateral radiographs (Fig 16–15), although bone scintigraphy may be needed in selected cases.[125] Treatment is usually conservative, with rest, analgesics, and a back corset or bracing to limit extension.[122–124] Continuation in sports is allowable.[126] The outcome is excellent for most patients; approximately 3 percent of patients with spondylolysis develop spondylolisthesis.

Intervertebral Disk Herniation

Disk herniation is rare in childhood, with estimates of the incidence in the Japanese population ranging from

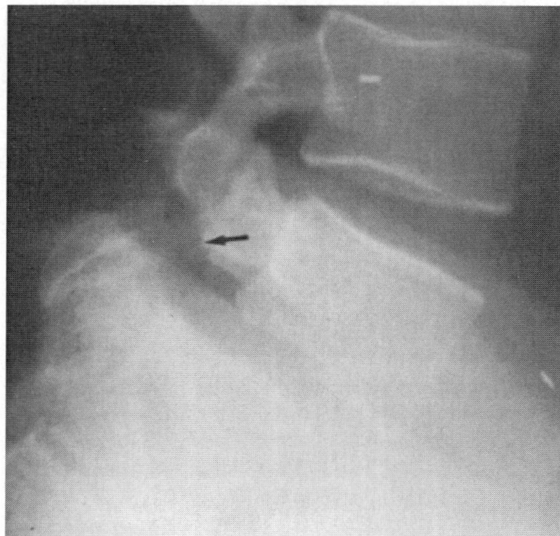

Figure 16–15. Spondylolysis affecting the pars interarticularis of L5 *(arrow)* is visible in this oblique view radiograph of the lumbar spine of a child with low back pain. The posterior elements on the oblique view form the "Scotty dog," and the pars interarticularis appears as the dog's neck. There is also spondylolisthesis with an anterior slip of L5 on S1.

1.69 per 100,000 in the 10- to 12-year-old age group, to 3.15 per 100,000 in the 13- to 15-year-old age group, and 9.63 per 100,000 in high school students aged 16 to 18 years.[127] These estimates are similar to those for the adult population in the United States.[128] Disk herniation accounted for 6 percent of 61 children younger than 16 years of age who were seen in an orthopedics clinic because of low back pain.[120] Boys may be slightly more frequently affected than girls.[129–131] The vast majority of herniated disks are at L4-5 and L5-S1. The onset of pain is usually insidious with stiffness of the lower lumbar spine with or without radicular pain down the leg (which can be the presenting complaint in some patients). Coughing, sneezing, and bending may aggravate the pain. Examination reveals limitation of forward bending and straight-leg raising and, in 25 percent, weakness of the plantar flexors. Plain radiographs are seldom helpful, although the disk space is narrowed in 20 percent of patients and there may be a slight posterior calcification if there is a slipped apophysis; diagnosis is evident on magnetic resonance images or computed tomography scans. Conservative treatment with rest, analgesics, and physical therapy is successful in up to 80 percent of cases.[123] The long-term success of surgery in adolescents is quite good.[131] (See also the discussion of diskitis in Chapter 31.)

Slipping Rib Syndrome

The slipping rib syndrome is produced by trauma to the costal cartilages of the eighth to tenth ribs.[132] These cartilages attach to each other by fibrous tissue rather than to the sternum. Interruption of this fibrous tissue by trauma permits a rib to impinge on the adjacent rib, causing a click and sharp pain under the ribs. The symptoms may be precipitated in a number of ways, including forward flexion, deep breathing, and the raising of the ipsilateral arm. The physician can reproduce the symptoms by hooking fingers under the inferior margins of the affected ribs and pulling anteriorly. Treatment consists of injection of local anesthetic or surgical excision of the subluxating cartilaginous rib tip.[133]

Costochondritis

Costochondritis, characterized by anterior chest wall pain that is reproduced by palpation of one or more of the costal cartilages, has been reported to be quite common in adolescents, constituting the reason for 4 percent of outpatient visits to one adolescent clinic.[134] It may result from trauma or idiopathic inflammation.[135] One or, occasionally, two or more costochondral junctions (usually the second or third) are painful and tender. The associated pain is usually acute and stabbing, often related to position or deep breathing. The syndrome can be self-limited or chronic and intermittent, lasting from a few months to a few years. Local anesthetic injections and anti-inflammatory medication may provide symptomatic relief.

The term *Tietze's syndrome* is usually applied to a costochondritis in which, in addition to pain and tenderness of one or more costal cartilages, there is swelling overlying the affected costal cartilage.

Torticollis

Torticollis, or wryneck, can accompany juvenile rheumatoid arthritis as a manifestation of cervical spine disease, develop due to a neurologic abnormality, or be caused by an idiopathic shortening of a sternocleidomastoid muscle. Squints, if uncorrected surgically, may lead to a head tilt that can become permanent, with asymmetry of the facial structures. Acute torticollis is transient if associated with trauma or cervical adenitis. The phenothiazine group of drugs and psychogenic disorders may also cause torticollis.[136] Intensive physiotherapy[137] and botulinum toxin[138] should be administered before consideration of surgical release.

Neuralgic Amyotrophy

Neuralgic amyotrophy (brachial plexus neuropathy) presents as an acute onset of pain in a shoulder, followed by localized muscle wasting, but not by restricted range of motion.[139–143] It can be unilateral or bilateral and may follow a vaccination or infection. Some cases are familial.[139, 140] It tends to occur in the older child. Recovery requires many months of intensive physical therapy. Brachial neuritis follows a similar pattern but is accompanied by paralysis of the affected part. In a similar fashion, lumbosacral plexus neuropathy can occur, leading to leg pain and paralysis.[144] Characteristic electromyographic findings of damage to both the nerve roots and the peripheral nerves usually confirm the diagnosis.

OTHER MISCELLANEOUS CONDITIONS

Growing Pains

The term *growing pains* has significant positive and negative connotations. The positive aspect is that most parents accept it as a benign condition. Frequently, an immediate family member or family friend had been diagnosed with growing pains that resolved without sequelae. The negative aspect is that this diagnosis has been too frequently applied to children who actually have a serious rheumatic or malignant disease. The term is a misnomer, since growth itself is not associated with the etiology of the pain. We prefer the term *benign nocturnal pains of childhood*; however, no generally accepted alternative term exists.[145–147] The term should be restricted to identify a fairly narrow spectrum of complaints (Table 16–9). Children who have unusual symptoms or abnormal findings on examination should not be diagnosed as having growing pains.

Surveys of schoolchildren have indicated that as many as 10 to 20 percent have had growing pains.[145, 147, 148] Most growing pains occur in preschool- to school-aged children. The pain is sometimes crampy, usually localized to the lower extremities, often deep in the thigh, shin, or calf, or behind the knee. Benign pain in the groin, back, or upper extremity is far less frequent. Growing pains may be precipitated by exercise and are usually relieved by massage. They occur in the evening or at night and often interrupt sleep. A few children have pain almost every night. Growing pains are never associated with a limp, and symptoms disappear by morning. Children with such pain have completely normal patterns of activity and normal physical examinations during and after the episode. Results of laboratory studies and radiographs are normal.

The pathophysiology of the pain is unknown. Long experience with such pains in many children, however, has proved that they do not portend serious illness. Successful management of growing pains includes education of the child and family about the benign nature of the problem. Gentle massage with or without analgesics is usually effective. In children with frequent attacks, administration of an evening dose of either acetaminophen or a nonsteroidal anti-inflammatory drug may prove preventive. Passive stretching can also be of benefit.[149]

Table 16–9

Growing Pains (Benign Nocturnal Pains of Childhood)

Age at onset	4 to 12 years
Sex ratio	Probably equal, slightly more girls in some series
Symptoms	Deep aching, cramping pain in thigh or calf, usually in evening or during the night; never present in the morning; bilateral; responds to massage and analgesia
Signs	Physical examination results are normal
Investigations	Laboratory and radiographic studies (if done) have normal results

Erythromelalgia

Erythromelalgia (erythro = red, mel = limb, algia = pain) is a rare condition that presents as episodic burning pain with accompanying erythematous, warm, swollen hands or feet (or both) that is eased by cold and elevation.[150] Affected patients refuse to stop using ice or cold water for their painful extremities. Exercise or heat (even wearing socks) can precipitate an attack.

This condition occurs in three forms: associated with thrombocythemia, primary, and secondary.[151] The most common form is that associated with thrombocythemia, which can occur in isolation or be associated with polycythemia vera or myelofibrosis and is sensitive to treatment with aspirin. Primary erythromelalgia begins in childhood or adolescence and can be familial (autosomal dominant).[152] It affects girls more often than boys. It is almost always symmetric and is resistant to treatment. Secondary erythromelalgia is more common in adults and is associated with an underlying condition other than one associated with a platelet dysfunction and therefore is not aspirin responsive. It usually responds to treatment of the underlying disorder. Additionally, an epidemic form has been reported in southern China due to a poxvirus.[153]

Treatment includes avoidance of exposure to heat, elevation of the extremity, and application of cold during acute attacks. If aspirin is unsuccessful, a host of treatments have been tried, each with a few case reports of benefit, including nifedipine, verapamil, nicardipine, pergolide, bromocriptine, busulfan, propranolol, posterior pituitary extract, epinephrine, biofeedback, hypnosis, sympathectomy, clonazepam, nitroprusside, prostaglandin E_1, amputation, and stereotactic destruction of the ventroposteromedial and centromedian regions of the thalamus.

Restless Legs Syndrome

Restless legs syndrome is a feeling of discomfort in, and an inability to keep from moving, the legs at night after resting or going to bed. It is relieved by activity and, therefore, frequently leads to insomnia. Periodic movements of the limb during sleep are common. These last less than a minute and rarely cause the child to awaken. Restless legs syndrome is more common in older adults but has been reported in children.[154, 155] Reducing caffeine intake is the first therapeutic step. A wide variety of medications, including pramipexole, clonidine, carbidopa/levodopa, and levodopa, have been reported to be helpful.[154, 156]

References

1. Kirk JA, Ansell BM, Bywaters EG: The hypermobility syndrome. Musculoskeletal complaints associated with generalized joint hypermobility. Ann Rheum Dis 26: 419–425, 1967.
2. Jessee EF, Owen DS Jr, Sagar KB: The benign hypermobile joint syndrome. Arthritis Rheum 23: 1053–1056, 1980.
3. Biro F, Gewanter HL, Baum J: The hypermobility syndrome. Pediatrics 72: 701–706, 1983.
4. Carter C, Wilkinson J: Persistent joint laxity and congenital dislocation of the hip. J Bone Joint Surg Br 46: 40–45, 1964.
5. Beighton P, Solomon L, Soskolne C: Articular mobility in an African population. Ann Rheum Dis 32: 413–418, 1973.
6. Gedalia A, Person DA, Brewer EJ Jr, Giannini EH: Hypermobility of the joints in juvenile episodic arthritis/arthralgia. J Pediatr 107: 873–876, 1985.
7. Cheng JC, Chan PS, Hui PW: Joint laxity in children. J Pediatr Orthop 11: 752–756, 1991.
8. Birrell FN, Adebajo AO, Hazleman BL, Silman AJ: High prevalence of joint laxity in West Africans. Br J Rheumatol 33: 56–59, 1994.
9. Mikkelsson M, Salminen JJ, Kautiainen H: Joint hypermobility is not a contributing factor to musculoskeletal pain in pre-adolescents. J Rheumatol 23: 1963–1967, 1996.
10. Gedalia A, Press J: Articular symptoms in hypermobile schoolchildren: a prospective study. J Pediatr 119: 944–946, 1991.
11. El-Garf AK, Mahmoud GA, Mahgoub EH: Hypermobility among Egyptian children: prevalence and features. J Rheumatol 25:1003–1005, 1998.
12. Barton LM, Bird HA: Improving pain by the stabilization of hyperlax joints. J Orthop Rheumatol 9: 46–51, 1996.
13. Benady S, Ivanans T: Hypermobile joints: a benign cause of transitory motor delay in infancy. Clin Pediatr 17: 790,795–796, 1978.
14. Davidovitch M, Tirosh E, Tal Y: The relationship between joint hypermobility and neurodevelopmental attributes in elementary school children. J Child Neurol 9: 417–419, 1994.
15. Lewkonia RM, Ansell BM: Articular hypermobility simulating chronic rheumatic disease. Arch Dis Child 58: 988–992, 1983.
16. Kaplinsky C, Kenet G, Seligsohn U, Rechavi G: Association between hyperflexibility of the thumb and an unexplained bleeding tendency: is it a rule of thumb? Br J Haematol 101: 260–263, 1998.
17. Gedalia A, Press J, Klein M, Buskila D: Joint hypermobility and fibromyalgia in schoolchildren. Ann Rheum Dis 52: 494–496, 1993.
18. Hudson N, Fitzcharles MA, Cohen M, et al: The association of soft-tissue rheumatism and hypermobility. Br J Rheumatol 37: 382–386, 1998.
19. Decoster LC, Vailas JC, Lindsay RH, Williams GR: Prevalence and features of joint hypermobility among adolescent athletes. Arch Pediatr Adolesc Med 151: 989–992, 1997.
20. Klemp P, Stevens JE, Isaacs S: A hypermobility study in ballet dancers. J Rheumatol 11: 692–696, 1984.
21. Everman DB, Robin NH: Hypermobility syndrome. Pediatr Rev 19: 111–117, 1998.
22. Cowan DN, Jones BH, Frykman PN: Lower limb morphology and risk of overuse injury among male infantry trainees. Med Sci Sports Exerc 28: 945–952, 1996.
23. Westling L, Mattiasson A: General joint hypermobility and temporomandibular joint derangement in adolescents. Ann Rheum Dis 51: 87–90, 1992.
24. Harinstein D, Buckingham RB, Braun T, et al: Systemic joint laxity (the hypermobile joint syndrome) is associated with temporomandibular joint dysfunction. Arthritis Rheum 31: 1259–1264, 1988.
25. Adair SM, Hecht C: Association of generalized joint hypermobility with history, signs, and symptoms of temporomandibular joint dysfunction in children. Pediatr Dent 15: 323–326, 1993.
26. Hall MG, Ferrell WR, Sturrock RD, et al: The effect of the hypermobility syndrome on knee joint proprioception. Br J Rheumatol 34: 121–125, 1995.
27. al-Rawi Z, Nessan AH: Joint hypermobility in patients with chondromalacia patellae. Br J Rheumatol 36: 1324–1327, 1997.
28. Larsson LG, Mudholkar GS, Baum J, Srivastava DK: Benefits and liabilities of hypermobility in the back pain disorders of industrial workers. J Intern Med 238: 461–467, 1995.
29. Klemp P: Hypermobility. Ann Rheum Dis 56: 573–575, 1997.
30. Mishra MB, Ryan P, Atkinson P: Extra-articular features of benign joint hypermobility syndrome. Br J Rheumatol 35: 861–866, 1996.
31. Unger DL: Does knuckle cracking lead to arthritis of the fingers? Arthritis Rheum 41: 949–950, 1998.
32. Grahame R, Edwards JC, Pitcher D, et al: A clinical and echocardiographic study of patients with the hypermobility syndrome. Ann Rheum Dis 40: 541–546, 1981.
33. Marks JS, Sharp J, Brear SG, Edwards JD: Normal joint mobility in mitral valve prolapse. Ann Rheum Dis 42: 54–55, 1983.
34. Staheli LT, Chew DE, Corbett M: The longitudinal arch: a survey of eight hundred and eighty-two feet in normal children and adults. J Bone Joint Surg Am 69: 426–428, 1987.
35. Mosca VS: Flexible flatfoot and skewfoot. Instr Course Lect 45: 347–354, 1996.
36. Harris RI, Beath T: Hypermobile flat-foot with short tendo achillis. J Bone Joint Surg Am 30: 116–138, 1948.
37. Wenger DR, Mauldin D, Speck G, et al: Corrective shoes and inserts as treatment for flexible flatfoot in infants and children. J Bone Joint Surg Am 71: 800–810, 1989.
38. Miller CD, Laskowski ER, Suman VJ: Effect of corrective rearfoot orthotic devices on ground reaction forces during ambulation. Mayo Clin Proc 71: 757–762, 1996.
39. Sullivan JA: The child's foot. *In* Morrissy RT, Weinstein SL (eds): Lovell and Winter's Pediatric Orthopaedics. Philadelphia, Lippincott-Raven, 1996, pp 1077–1135.
40. Sneyers CJ, Lysens R, Feys H, Andries R: Influence of malalignment of feet on the plantar pressure pattern in running. Foot Ankle Int 16: 624–632, 1995.
41. Rudzki SJ: Injuries in Australian Army recruits. Part III: The accuracy of a pretraining orthopedic screen in predicting ultimate injury outcome. Mil Med 162: 481–483, 1997.
42. Giladi M, Milgrom C, Stein M, et al: The low arch, a protective factor in stress fractures. Orthop Rev 14: 81–84, 1985.
43. Mosier KM, Asher M: Tarsal coalitions and peroneal spastic flat foot. A review. J Bone Joint Surg Am 66: 976–984, 1984.
44. Loudon JK, Goist HL, Loudon KL: Genu recurvatum syndrome. J Orthop Sports Phys Ther 27: 361–367, 1998.
45. Thabit GD, Micheli LJ: Patellofemoral pain in the pediatric patient. Orthop Clin North Am 23: 567–585, 1992.
46. Tjernstrom B, Rehnberg L: Back pain and arthralgia before and after lengthening: 75 patients questioned after 6 (1–11) years. Acta Orthop Scand 65: 328–332, 1994.
47. Bowyer S: Hip contracture as the presenting sign in children with HLA-B27 arthritis. J Rheumatol 22: 165–167, 1995.
48. Glover MT, Lake BD, Atherton DJ: Infantile systemic hyalinosis: newly recognized disorder of collagen? Pediatrics 87: 228–234, 1991.
49. Verma UN, Misra R, Radhakrisnan S, et al: A syndrome of fibrosing pleuritis, pericarditis, and synovitis with infantile contractures of fingers and toes in 2 sisters: "familial fibrosing serositis." J Rheumatol 22: 2349–2355, 1995.
50. O'Neill DB, Micheli LJ, Warner JP: Patellofemoral stress: a prospective analysis of exercise treatment in adolescents and adults. Am J Sports Med 20: 151, 1992.
51. Yates CK, Grana WA: Patellofemoral pain in children. Clin Orthop 255: 36–43, 1990.
52. Goodfellow J, Hungerford DS, Woods C: Patello-femoral joint mechanics and pathology. 2. Chondromalacia patellae. J Bone Joint Surg Br 58: 291–299, 1976.
53. Insall J: "Chondromalacia patellae": patellar malalignment syndrome. Orthop Clin North Am 10: 117–127, 1979.
54. Outerbridge RE: The etiology of chondromalacia patellae. J Bone Joint Surg Br 43: 752, 1961.
55. Fairbank JC, Pynsent PB, van Poortvliet JA, Phillips H: Mechanical factors in the incidence of knee pain in adolescents and young adults. J Bone Joint Surg Br 66: 685–693, 1984.
56. Radin EL: Chondromalacia of the patella. Bull Rheum Dis 34: 1–6, 1984.
57. Reid GD, Glasgow M, Gordon DA, Wright TA: Pathological plicae of the knee mistaken for arthritis. J Rheumatol 7: 573–576, 1980.

58. Micheli LJ: The traction apophysitises. Clin Sports Med 6: 389–404, 1987.
59. Osgood RB: Lesions of the tibial tubercle occurring during adolescence. Boston Med J 8: 114, 1903.
60. Schlatter C: Verlezungen des schnabelförmigen Forsatzes der oberen Tibiaepiphyse. Beitr Klin Chir 38: 874, 1903.
61. Ogden JA, Southwick WO: Osgood-Schlatter's disease and tibial tuberosity development. Clin Orthop Rel Res 116: 180–189, 1976.
62. Kujala UM, Kvist M, Heinonen O: Osgood-Schlatter's disease in adolescent athletes. Retrospective study of incidence and duration. Am J Sports Med 13: 236–241, 1985.
63. Lanning P, Heikkinen E: Ultrasonic features of the Osgood-Schlatter lesion. J Pediatr Orthop 11: 538–540, 1991.
64. Krause BL, Williams JP, Catterall A: Natural history of Osgood-Schlatter disease. J Pediatr Orthop 10: 65–68, 1990.
65. Medlar RC, Lyne ED: Sinding-Larsen-Johansson disease: its etiology and natural history. J Bone Joint Surg Am 60: 1113–1116, 1978.
66. Gardiner JS, McInerney VK, Avella DG, Valdez NA: Pediatric update: 13. Injuries to the inferior pole of the patella in children. Orthop Rev 19: 643–649, 1990.
67. Liberson A, Lieberson S, Mendes DG, et al: Remodeling of the calcaneus apophysis in the growing child. J Pediatr Orthop Br 4: 74–79, 1995.
68. Barnett LS: Little League shoulder syndrome: proximal humeral epiphyseolysis in adolescent baseball pitchers. A case report. J Bone Joint Surg Am 67: 495–496, 1985.
69. Jawish R, Rigault P, Padovani JP, et al: Osteochondritis dissecans of the humeral capitellum in children. Eur J Pediatr Surg 3: 97–100, 1993.
70. Maffulli N, Chan D, Aldridge MJ: Overuse injuries of the olecranon in young gymnasts. J Bone Joint Surg Br 74: 305–308, 1992.
71. Andrish JT, Bergfeld JA, Walheim J: A prospective study on the management of shin splints. J Bone Joint Surg Am 56: 1697–1700, 1974.
72. Michael RH, Holder LE: The soleus syndrome. A cause of medial tibial stress (shin splints). Am J Sports Med 13: 87–94, 1985.
73. Sheon RP, Moskowitz RW, Goldberg VM: Soft Tissue Rheumatic Pain: Recognition, Management and Prevention. Philadelphia, Lea & Febiger, 1982.
74. Brower AC: The osteochondroses. Orthop Clin North Am 14: 99–117, 1983.
75. Resnick D: The osteochondroses. *In* Resnick D, Niwayama G (eds): Diagnosis of Bone and Joint Disorders. Philadelphia, WB Saunders, 1981, p 2874.
76. Legg AT: An obscure affection of the hip joint. Boston Med Surg J 162: 202, 1910.
77. Calvé J: Sur une forme particulière de coxalgie greffée sur des déformations caractéristiques de l'extremité supérieure du fémur. Rev Chir Orthop 30: 54, 1910.
78. Peltier LF: The Classic: concerning arthritis deformans juvenilis. Professor Georg C. Perthes. Clin Orthop 158: 5–9, 1981.
79. Weinstein SL: Natural history and treatment outcomes of childhood hip disorders. Clin Orthop 344: 227–42, 1997.
80. Eckerwall G, Wingstrand H, Hagglund G, Karlberg J: Growth in 110 children with Legg-Calve-Perthes' disease: a longitudinal infancy childhood puberty growth model study. J Pediatr Orthop B 5: 181–184, 1996.
81. Glueck CJ, Brandt G, Gruppo R, et al: Resistance to activated protein C and Legg-Perthes disease. Clin Orthop 338: 139–152, 1997.
82. Wang L, Bowen JR, Puniak MA, et al: An evaluation of various methods of treatment for Legg-Calve-Perthes disease. Clin Orthop 314: 225–233, 1995.
83. Lahdes-Vasama TT, Marttinen EJ, Merikanto JE: Outcome of Perthes' disease in unselected patients after femoral varus osteotomy and splintage. J Pediatr Orthop B 6: 229–234, 1997.
84. Sorenson KH: Scheuermann's Juvenile Kyphosis. Copenhagen, Munksgaard, 1964.
85. Tachdjian MO: Pediatric Orthopedics. Philadelphia, WB Saunders, 1972.
86. Moe JH, Winter RB, Bradford DS, et al: Juvenile Kyphosis, Scoliosis and Other Spinal Deformities. Philadelphia, WB Saunders, 1978, p 331.
87. Giannestras NJ: Other problems of the forepart of the foot. *In* Giannestras NJ (ed): Foot Disorders. Philadelphia, Lea & Febiger, 1973, p 410.
88. Borges JL, Guille JT, Bowen JR: Kohler's bone disease of the tarsal navicular. J Pediatr Orthop 15: 596–598, 1995.
89. Braddock GTF: Experimental epiphyseal injury and Freiberg's disease. J Bone Joint Surg Br 41: 154, 1959.
90. Stanley D, Betts RP, Rowley DI, Smith TW: Assessment of etiologic factors in the development of Freiberg's disease. J Foot Surg 29: 444–447, 1990.
91. Molloy MG, Hamilton EB: Thiemann's disease. Rheumatol Rehabil 17: 179–180, 1978.
92. Gewanter H, Baum J: Thiemann's disease. J Rheumatol 12: 150–153, 1985.
93. Allison AC, Blumberg BS: Familial osteoarthropathy of the fingers. J Bone Joint Surg Br 40: 538, 1958.
94. Stougaard J: Familial occurrence of osteochondritis dissecans. J Bone Joint Surg Br 46: 542, 1964.
95. Robinson RP, Franck WA, Carey EJ, Goldberg EB: Familial polyarticular osteochondritis dissecans masquerading as juvenile rheumatoid arthritis. J Rheumatol 5: 190–194, 1978.
96. Harries M (ed): Oxford Textbook of Sports Medicine, 2nd ed. New York, Oxford University Press, 1998.
97. Bohndorf K: Osteochondritis (osteochondrosis) dissecans: a review and new MRI classification. Eur Radiol 8: 103–112, 1998.
98. Loder RT: Slipped capital femoral epiphysis in children. Curr Opin Pediatr 7: 95–97, 1995.
99. Mandell GA, Keret D, Harcke HT, Bowen JR: Chondrolysis: detection by bone scintigraphy. J Pediatr Orthop 12: 80–85, 1992.
100. Spero CR, Masciale JP, Tornetta PD, et al: Slipped capital femoral epiphysis in black children: incidence of chondrolysis. J Pediatr Orthop 12: 444–448, 1992.
101. Duncan JW, Nasca R, Schrantz J: Idiopathic chondrolysis of the hip. J Bone Joint Surg Am 61: 1024–1028, 1979.
102. Bleck EE: Idiopathic chondrolysis of the hip. J Bone Joint Surg Am 65: 1266–1275, 1983.
103. Koot MF, Berendsen HA, van der Hoeven H, et al: 3 adolescents with hip pain caused by idiopathic chondrolysis. Ned Tijdschr Geneeskd 137: 86–90, 1993.
104. Brown J, Melinkovich P: Schonlein-Henoch purpura misdiagnosed as suspected child abuse. A case report and literature review. JAMA 256: 617–618, 1986.
105. Carrera GF, Kozin F, McCarty DJ: Arthritis after frostbite injury in children. Arthritis Rheum 22: 1082–1087, 1979.
106. Dreyfuss JR, Glimcher MJ: Epiphyseal injury following frostbite. N Engl J Med 253: 1065, 1955.
107. Brown FE, Spiegel PK, Boyle WEJ: Digital deformity: an effect of frostbite in children. Pediatrics 71: 955–959, 1983.
108. Goette DK: Chilblains (perniosis). J Am Acad Dermatol 23: 257–262, 1990.
109. Nellhaus G: Neurogenic arthropathies (Charcot's joints) in children: description of a case traced to occult spinal dysraphism. Clin Pediatr 14: 647–653, 1975.
110. Derwin KA, Glover RA, Wojtys EM: Nociceptive role of substance-P in the knee joint of a patient with congenital insensitivity to pain. J Pediatr Orthop 14: 258–262, 1994.
111. Indo Y, Tsuruta M, Hayashida Y, et al: Mutations in the TRKA/NGF receptor gene in patients with congenital insensitivity to pain with anhidrosis. Nat Genet 13: 485–488, 1996.
112. Smedbraten BK, Natvig B, Rutle O, Bruusgaard D: Self-reported bodily pain in schoolchildren. Scand J Rheumatol 27: 273–276, 1998.
113. Leboeuf-Yde C, Kyvik KO: At what age does low back pain become a common problem? A study of 29,424 individuals aged 12–41 years. Spine 23: 228–234, 1998.
114. Balague F, Skovron ML, Nordin M, et al: Low back pain in schoolchildren: a study of familial and psychological factors. Spine 20: 1265–1270, 1995.
115. Kristjansdottir G: Prevalence of self-reported back pain in school children: a study of sociodemographic differences. Eur J Pediatr 155: 984–986, 1996.
116. Sward L, Hellstrom M, Jacobsson B, Peterson L: Back pain and radiologic changes in the thoraco-lumbar spine of athletes. Spine 15: 124–129, 1990.
117. Kujala UM, Taimela S, Erkintalo M, et al: Low-back pain in adolescent athletes. Med Sci Sports Exerc 28: 165–170, 1996.

118. Ramirez N, Johnston CE, Browne RH: The prevalence of back pain in children who have idiopathic scoliosis. J Bone Joint Surg Am 79: 364–368, 1997.
119. Volinn E: The epidemiology of low back pain in the rest of the world. A review of surveys in low- and middle-income countries. Spine 22: 1747–1754, 1997.
120. Turner PG, Green JH, Galasko CS: Back pain in childhood. Spine 14: 812–814, 1989.
121. Rowe BH, Dulberg CS, Peterson RG, et al: Characteristics of children presenting with chest pain to a pediatric emergency department. Can Med Assoc J 143: 388–394, 1990.
122. Morita T, Ikata T, Katoh S, Miyake R: Lumbar spondylolysis in children and adolescents. J Bone Joint Surg Br 77: 620–625, 1995.
123. Sponseller PD: Evaluating the child with back pain. Am Fam Physician 54: 1933–1941, 1996.
124. Payne WK 3rd, Ogilvie JW: Back pain in children and adolescents. Pediatr Clin North Am 43: 899–917, 1996.
125. Ralston S, Weir M: Suspecting lumbar spondylolysis in adolescent low back pain. Clin Pediatr 37: 287–293, 1998.
126. Muschik M, Hahnel H, Robinson PN, et al: Competitive sports and the progression of spondylolisthesis. J Pediatr Orthop 16: 364–369, 1996.
127. Matsui H, Terahata N, Tsuji H, et al: Familial predisposition and clustering for juvenile lumbar disc herniation. Spine 17: 1323–1328, 1992.
128. Bruske-Hohlfeld I, Merritt JL, Onofrio BM, et al: Incidence of lumbar disc surgery: a population-based study in Olmsted County, Minnesota, 1950–1979. Spine 15: 31–35, 1990.
129. Nelson CL, Janecki CJ, Gildenberg PL, Sava G: Disk protrusions in the young. Clin Orthop 88: 142–150, 1972.
130. Ishihara H, Matsui H, Hirano N, Tsuji H: Lumbar intervertebral disc herniation in children less than 16 years of age: long-term follow-up study of surgically managed cases. Spine 22: 2044–2049, 1997.
131. Papagelopoulos PJ, Shaughnessy WJ, Ebersold MJ, et al: Long-term outcome of lumbar discectomy in children and adolescents sixteen years of age or younger. J Bone Joint Surg Am 80: 689–698, 1998.
132. Taubman B, Vetter VL: Slipping rib syndrome as a cause of chest pain in children. Clin Pediatr 35: 403–405, 1996.
133. Porter GE: Slipping rib syndrome: an infrequently recognized entity in children. A report of three cases and review of the literature. Pediatrics 76: 810–813, 1985.
134. Brown RT: Costochondritis in adolescents. J Adolesc Health Care 1: 198–201, 1981.
135. Calabro JJ, Marshesano JM: Tietze's syndrome: report of a case with juvenile onset. J Pediatr 68: 985, 1966.
136. Bolthauser E: Differential diagnosis of torticollis in childhood. Schweiz Med Wochenschr 106: 1261, 1976.
137. Smith DL, DeMario MC: Spasmodic torticollis: a case report and review of therapies. J Am Board Fam Pract 9: 435–441, 1996.
138. Lew MF, Adornato BT, Duane DD, et al: Botulinum toxin type B: a double-blind, placebo-controlled, safety and efficacy study in cervical dystonia. Neurology 49: 701–707, 1997.
139. Lane RJ, Dewar JA: Bilateral aneuralgic amyotrophy. Br Med J 1: 895, 1978.
140. Dunn HG, Daube JR, Gomez MR: Heredofamilial brachial plexus neuropathy (hereditary neuralgic amyotrophy with brachial predilection) in childhood. Dev Med Child Neurol 20: 28–46, 1978.
141. Shaywitz BA: Brachial plexus neuropathy in childhood. J Pediatr 86: 913–915, 1975.
142. Bale JF Jr, Thompson JA, Petajan JH, Ziter FA: Childhood brachial plexus neuropathy. J Pediatr 95: 741–742, 1979.
143. Zeharia A, Mukamel M, Frishberg Y, et al: Benign plexus neuropathy in children. J Pediatr 116: 276–278, 1990.
144. van Alfen N, van Engelen BG: Lumbosacral plexus neuropathy: a case report and review of the literature. Clin Neurol Neurosurg 99: 138–141, 1997.
145. Peterson H: Growing pains. Pediatr Clin North Am 33: 1365–1372, 1986.
146. Brady M, Grey M: Growing pains: a myth or a reality. J Pediatr Health Care 3: 219–220, 1989.
147. Oster J, Nielsen A: Growing pains: a clinical investigation of a school population. Acta Paediatr Scand 61: 329–334, 1972.
148. Apley J: One child. *In* Apley J, Ounsted C (eds): One Child. Philadelphia, JB Lippincott, 1982, pp 23–47.
149. Baxter MP, Dulberg C: "Growing pains" in childhood: a proposal for treatment. J Pediatr Orthop 8: 402–406, 1988.
150. Kurzrock R, Cohen PR: Erythromelalgia: review of clinical characteristics and pathophysiology. Am J Med 91: 416–422, 1991.
151. Drenth JP, Michials JJ: Three types of erythromelalgia. Br Med J 301: 454–455, 1990.
152. Finley WH, Lindsey JRJ, Fine JD, et al: Autosomal dominant erythromelalgia. Am J Med Genet 42: 310–315, 1992.
153. Zheng ZM, Zhang JH, Hu JM, et al: Poxviruses isolated from epidemic erythromelalgia in China. Lancet 8580: 296, 1988.
154. Walters AS, Picchietti DL, Ehrenberg BL, Wagner ML: Restless legs syndrome in childhood and adolescence. Pediatr Neurol 11: 241–245, 1994.
155. Walters AS, Hickey K, Maltzman J,: A questionnaire study of 138 patients with restless legs syndrome: The "Night-Walkers" survey. Neurology 46: 92–95, 1996.
156. Lin S-C, Kaplan J, Burger CD, Fredrickson PA: Effect of paramipexole in treatment of resistant restless legs syndrome. Mayo Clin Proc 73: 497–500, 1998.
157. Jones KL: Smith's Recognizable Patterns of Human Malformation, 5th ed. Philadelphia, WB Saunders, 1997.
158. Beighton P: McKusick's Heritable Disorders of Connective Tissue, 5th ed. St. Louis, Mosby, 1993.

17

Idiopathic Musculoskeletal Pain Syndromes

David D. Sherry and Peter N. Malleson

Pediatric rheumatologists care for children with a wide variety of musculoskeletal pains; many of these children do not have an identified inflammatory disease or mechanical derangement to cause the degree of pain and debility manifested. Such children frequently are referred from physician to physician and undergo multiple diagnostic tests and therapeutic trials, all in a vain attempt to ascertain a diagnosis and treatment. The physician who can promptly recognize the underlying syndromes provides a great service to the child and family by halting further medical investigations and initiating specific therapy.

HISTORICAL REVIEW

Chronic musculoskeletal pain in children received virtually no attention until the latter half of the twentieth century. In 1951, Naish and Apley[1] published their work on pediatric limb pains due to nonarthritic causes. There has subsequently been a dearth of studies dealing with this group of children, except for a few epidemiologic reports.[2–6] The largest series of such children presenting to a pediatric rheumatology service was that of 100 children reported in 1991.[7] In 1971, reflex neurovascular dystrophy (complex regional pain syndrome, type I[8]) was described in a child.[9] This disorder has subsequently been the subject of the majority of pediatric reports, most of which deal with very small numbers of subjects.[10–30] The first group of children with fibromyalgia was described in 1985.[31] Since then, many reports on this condition have appeared, again describing very small series.[5, 32–39]

DEFINITION AND CLASSIFICATION

The terms used to describe these conditions are inadequate and can be confusing because many children have features that are shared among different subsets.[7, 40] Authors have separated these children depending on physical features (such as the presence of overt autonomic signs[8] or number of painful points),[31, 41] or location (localized or diffuse).[40] The terminology used is, in one sense, moot because evaluation and treatment are similar between subsets.[42]

In this chapter, we use the terminology proposed by Malleson et al[40] because it is descriptive and acknowledges the fact that the etiology of the pain is unknown (Table 17–1). Discrete subsets exist in each of these groups. Specifically, children who fulfill criteria for fibromyalgia (Table 17–2) are included with those with diffuse idiopathic musculoskeletal pain, and those with complex regional pain syndrome (Table 17–3) are included with those with localized idiopathic musculoskeletal pain. There is a small subset of children with intermittent diffuse or localized idiopathic musculoskeletal pain in whom the criterion for duration is not satisfied, but they are considered because of the recurrent nature of the pain over many months.[42]

EPIDEMIOLOGY

Incidence and Prevalence

Population surveys of schoolchildren confirm that musculoskeletal pain is quite common; back pain is as

Table 17–1

Criteria for Classification of Amplified Pain Syndromes

Diffuse Idiopathic Pain

Criteria for classification require both 1 and 2.

1. Generalized musculoskeletal aching at three or more sites for 3 or more months.
2. Exclusion of diseases that could reasonably explain the symptoms.

Localized Idiopathic Pain

Criteria for classification require all three.

1. Pain localized to one limb persisting
   a. 1 week with medically directed treatment *OR*
   b. 1 month without medically directed treatment
2. Absence of prior trauma that could reasonably explain the symptoms.
3. Exclusion of diseases that could reasonably explain the symptoms.

Data from Malleson PN, Al-Matar M, Petty RE: Idiopathic musculoskeletal pain syndromes in children. J Rheumatol 19: 1786–1789, 1992.

Table 17–2

Classification Criteria for Primary and Concomitant Fibromyalgia (Adults)

For classification purposes, patients will be said to have fibromyalgia if both criteria are satisfied. Widespread pain must have been present for at least 3 months. The presence of a second clinical disorder does not exclude the diagnosis of fibromyalgia.

1. History of Widespread Pain

Definition: Pain is considered widespread when all of the following are present: pain in the left side of the body, pain in the right side of the body, pain above the waist, and pain below the waist. In addition, axial skeletal pain (cervical spine or anterior chest or thoracic spine or low back) must be present. In this definition, shoulder and buttock pain is considered as pain for each involved side. "Low back" pain is considered lower segment pain.

2. Pain in 11 of 18 Tender Point Sites on Digital Palpation

Definition: Pain, on digital palpation, must be present in at least 11 of the following 18 tender point sites:

Occiput: bilateral, at the suboccipital muscle insertions.
Low cervical: bilateral, at the anterior aspects of the intertransverse spaces at C5-C7.
Trapezius: bilateral, at the midpoint of the upper border.
Supraspinatus: bilateral, at origins above the scapula spine near the medial border.
Second rib: bilateral, at the second costochondral junctions, just lateral to the junctions on upper surfaces.
Lateral epicondyle: bilateral, 2 cm distal to the epicondyles.
Gluteal: bilateral, in upper outer quadrants of buttocks in anterior fold of muscle.
Greater trochanter: bilateral, posterior to the trochanteric prominence.
Knees: bilateral, at the medial fat pad proximal to the joint line.

Digital palpation should be performed with an approximate force of 4 kg. For a tender point to be considered "positive," the subject must state that the palpation was painful. "Tender" is not to be considered painful.

Data from Merskey DM, Bogduk N: Classification of Chronic Pain. Descriptions of Chronic Pain Syndromes and Definitions of Pain Terms. Seattle, IASP Press, 1994.

frequent as 20 percent.[3] Limb pain has been reported in 16 percent[4, 6] and fibromyalgia in 6 percent.[5] There are no specific incidence and prevalence data regarding other idiopathic musculoskeletal pain syndromes, but 5 to 8 percent of new patients presenting to North American pediatric rheumatology centers have idiopathic musculoskeletal pain (excluding hypermobility, arthralgia, back pain, and limb pain not yet diagnosed).[43, 44] Although it may be selection bias, many pediatric rheumatologists report that they are diagnosing these syndromes much more commonly in recent years.

Age at Onset

Idiopathic musculoskeletal pain has been described in patients as young as 3 years, but the vast majority of reports involve children in late childhood and adolescence.[7, 10, 12, 19, 31, 40] The mean age is generally 12 or 13 years. Older adolescents may be underrepresented, presumably because they are referred to adult specialists.

Sex Ratio

All large series agree that girls predominate over boys, in a ratio of approximately 4:1.[7, 10, 12, 19, 31, 40] Since women seek medical advice more often than men, there may be a selection bias; however, given the disability involved, this is most likely not a major factor in children.

Geographic and Racial Distribution

There have been no formal investigations regarding the relationship of idiopathic pain syndromes to ethnicity; however, a series from Philadelphia reported a disproportionate number of white patients: 15 of 15.[16] All reports are from developed countries, and comparisons with developing nations, such as that reported in back pain patients,[45] are impossible.

ETIOLOGY AND PATHOGENESIS

The cause (or causes) of the different idiopathic musculoskeletal pain syndromes is unknown. No proper controlled studies exist, especially in children. Childhood disease may differ significantly from that occurring in adults; for example, there is a distinct difference between technetium bone scintigraphy in children and adults with complex regional pain syndrome type I,[16, 46] and children respond much more readily to exercise therapy.[10, 42] Nevertheless, in many children, these syndromes seem to be causally related to injury, illness, or psychological distress, either singly or in combination.

Injury, including surgery, frequently precedes complex regional pain syndrome in adults, and minor in-

Table 17–3

Criteria for Chronic Regional Pain Syndrome

Chronic Regional Pain Syndrome, Type I

1. The presence of an initiating noxious event, or a cause of immobilization.
2. Continuing pain, allodynia, or hyperalgesia with which the pain is disproportionate to any inciting event.
3. Evidence at some time of edema, changes in skin blood flow, or abnormal sudomotor activity in the region of the pain.
4. This diagnosis is excluded by the existence of conditions that would otherwise account for the degree of pain and dysfunction.

Note: Criteria 2–4 must be satisfied.

Chronic Regional Pain Syndrome, Type II

1. The presence of continuing pain, allodynia, or hyperalgesia after a nerve injury, not necessarily limited to the distribution of the injured nerve.
2. Evidence at some time of edema, changes in skin blood flow, or abnormal sudomotor activity in the region of the pain.
3. This diagnosis is excluded by the existence of conditions that would otherwise account for the degree of pain and dysfunction.

Note: All three criteria must be satisfied.

Data from Merskey DM, Bogduk N: Classification of Chronic Pain. Descriptions of Chronic Pain Syndromes and Definitions of Pain Terms. Seattle, IASP Press, 1994.

jury is commonly reported in children. Rarely, more overt trauma may be the inciting event.[20, 22, 47, 48] Minor trauma may play a role in localizing the site of a subsequent idiopathic musculoskeletal pain, and children who are hypermobile may be at increased risk of developing diffuse idiopathic musculoskeletal pain, perhaps due to chronic microtrauma.[36]

Illness such as myocardial infarction has been associated in adults with the complex regional pain syndrome,[49] and arthritis may coexist with idiopathic pain in children.[50] We have also observed idiopathic musculoskeletal pain in children with a variety of illnesses, including cerebral palsy, muscular dystrophy, new-onset diabetes, and leukemia. These associations may or may not be coincidental.

Psychological distress has been a recurring theme in multiple reports of children with idiopathic musculoskeletal pain syndromes, although controlled studies are lacking.[7, 10, 12, 51–54] Clearly some children and their families are overtly psychologically dysfunctional, but whether it is the cause of, the effect of, or unrelated to the development of an idiopathic musculoskeletal pain syndrome is not known. Not all families with a painful, dysfunctional child are inappropriately distressed, however.

The role of hormonal or environmental factors is uncertain. The observation that girls are more frequently affected may reflect the fact that girls have lower pain thresholds, increased levels of hypermobility, and increased frequency of sleep disorders than boys, as well as differences in coping and cultural expectations (in Western countries).[55–57] There is commonly a role model (usually a parent) for either chronic pain or disability. The social history may document multiple recent major life events such as moving, changes in the nuclear family, family illness and deaths, or school stress.[7, 12] Interdependency, or enmeshment, between the patient and the parent (usually the mother) is striking in many families: even when the physician directly addresses the child, the parent will often answer.[7, 12]

The pathophysiology of idiopathic musculoskeletal pain is unknown, but in some children, especially those with localized pain, it seems related to either increased sympathetic nervous system activity or increased alpha-adrenoceptor responsiveness.[58–63] Diffuse pain, especially fibromyalgia, has been extensively studied in adults and a wide variety of hypotheses have been suggested, including abnormal muscle anatomy and physiology, altered sleep pattern, abnormal serotonin metabolism, hypothalamic-pituitary-adrenal axis hypofunction, decreased cerebral blood flow, trauma, and psychological distress. There is no convincing evidence that any of these factors is of primary importance.[64] Two recent studies of a small number of adults with fibromyalgia suggest that they have a deranged sympathetic response to orthostatic stress.[65, 66]

GENETIC BACKGROUND

Idiopathic musculoskeletal pain syndromes have been reported in siblings,[18, 67] parent/child pairs,[32, 51] and even spouses.[33] No genetic studies in children with these syndromes have been reported.

CLINICAL MANIFESTATIONS

Although there are some differences between localized and diffuse idiopathic musculoskeletal pain syndromes, the medical history and physical examination in both are surprisingly consistent. In children with *localized idiopathic musculoskeletal pain,* minor trauma that might not even be clearly recalled is common ("someone must have stepped on my foot"). The pain and consequent disability increase over time regardless of medication. A cast or splint may minimize the pain while it is being worn, but it is our clinical impression that the consequent immobilization is an important factor in perpetuating the pain. Autonomic signs (edema, cyanosis, coolness, or increased perspiration) may be persistent or transient, or not occur at all. Allodynia (pain generated by normally nonpainful stimuli) can be marked ("the breeze of someone walking by hurts") and can lead to significant impairment. This, too, can be transient. Any body part can be involved, and the child may have several areas of pain at presentation. The lower extremity is more commonly involved than the upper, and peripheral body parts are more commonly involved than centrally located areas. Occasionally, only one small area is involved, such as a finger, the nose, or a tooth.[68] Localized pain is usually continuous.

In *diffuse idiopathic musculoskeletal pain,* the onset is usually more gradual and can be quite vague in both location and character. There is an absence of autonomic signs, but affected children complain of poor sleep and depression more often than those with localized pain.[64] These children frequently report a multiplicity of symptoms. Pain is often centrally located, involving the back, chest, abdomen, and head as well as the extremities.

Conversion symptoms are not uncommon.[7] Frequently numbness is reported, but these children can also report paralysis, blindness, or a bizarre (histrionic) gait. Eating disorders can also be present.[26, 69] Even when reporting severe pain, the child often has a markedly incongruent affect, smiling even when reporting severe pain (up to 10 out of 10), and has *la belle indifference* about the pain and dysfunction it causes. A few children demonstrate marked pain behaviors such as crying or screaming with pain. This is more common in those with localized idiopathic musculoskeletal pain. Affected children often seem to be mature for their age, are accomplished in school and in extracurricular activities, and are described by their parents as perfectionistic, empathetic, and pleasers.

Notable points on physical examination include the absence of findings suggesting an underlying disease, normal results of a neurologic examination (paying special attention to sensory tests), and the presence of allodynia. Careful sensory testing, with special attention to dermatomal and peripheral nerve innervation, is required. Allodynia is present if pain is reported

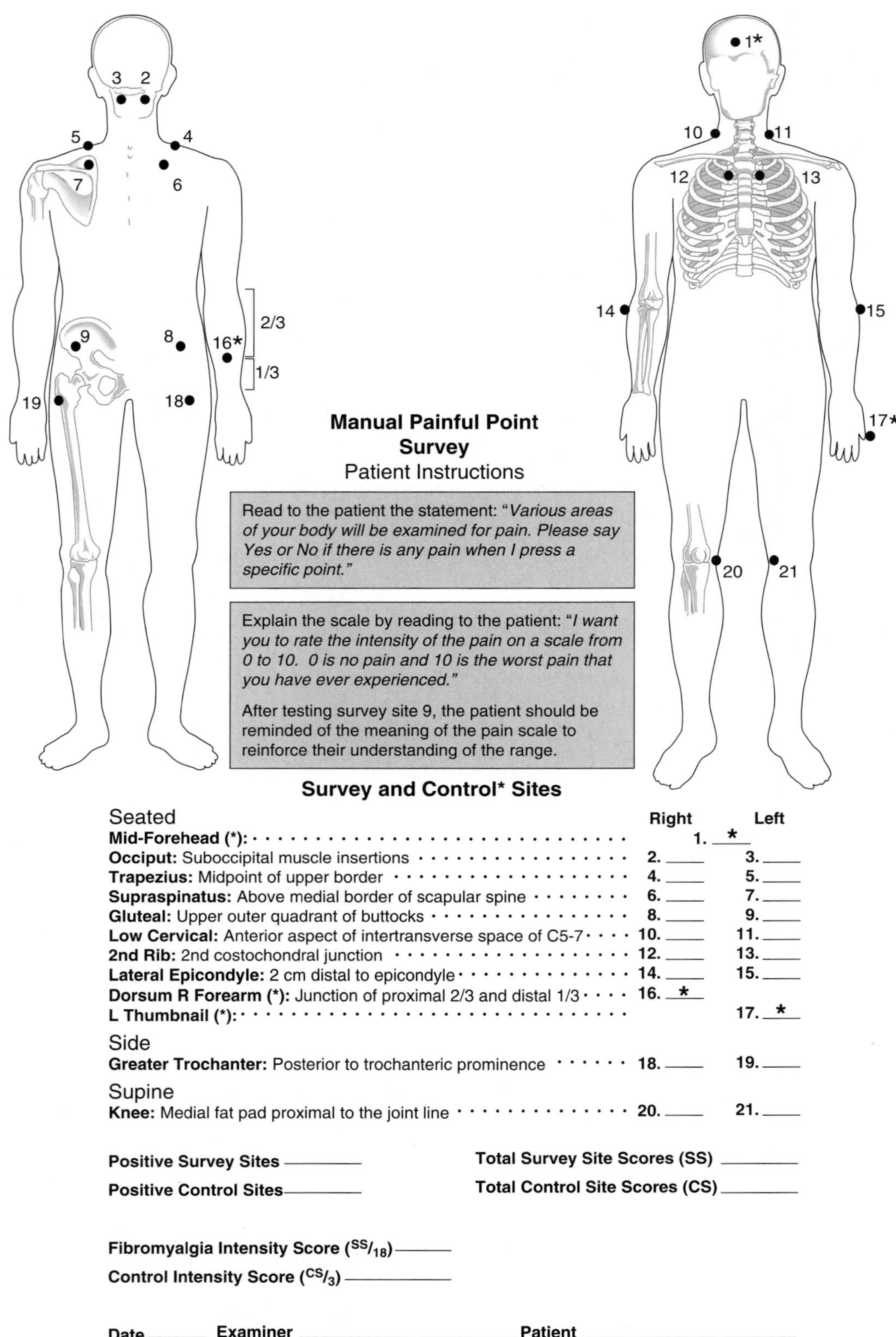

Manual Painful Point Survey

Patient Instructions

Read to the patient the statement: "*Various areas of your body will be examined for pain. Please say Yes or No if there is any pain when I press a specific point.*"

Explain the scale by reading to the patient: "*I want you to rate the intensity of the pain on a scale from 0 to 10. 0 is no pain and 10 is the worst pain that you have ever experienced.*"

After testing survey site 9, the patient should be reminded of the meaning of the pain scale to reinforce their understanding of the range.

Survey and Control* Sites

Seated	Right	Left
Mid-Forehead (*):	1. *	
Occiput: Suboccipital muscle insertions	2. ____	3. ____
Trapezius: Midpoint of upper border	4. ____	5. ____
Supraspinatus: Above medial border of scapular spine	6. ____	7. ____
Gluteal: Upper outer quadrant of buttocks	8. ____	9. ____
Low Cervical: Anterior aspect of intertransverse space of C5-7	10. ____	11. ____
2nd Rib: 2nd costochondral junction	12. ____	13. ____
Lateral Epicondyle: 2 cm distal to epicondyle	14. ____	15. ____
Dorsum R Forearm (*): Junction of proximal 2/3 and distal 1/3	16. *	
L Thumbnail (*):		17. *
Side		
Greater Trochanter: Posterior to trochanteric prominence	18. ____	19. ____
Supine		
Knee: Medial fat pad proximal to the joint line	20. ____	21. ____

Positive Survey Sites ________ **Total Survey Site Scores (SS)** ________

Positive Control Sites ________ **Total Control Site Scores (CS)** ________

Fibromyalgia Intensity Score ($^{SS}/_{18}$) ________

Control Intensity Score ($^{CS}/_{3}$) ________

Date ______ **Examiner** ____________ **Patient** ____________

Figure 17–1. Diagram of painful points in fibromyalgia as defined by the American College of Rheumatology.[41] (From Okifuji A, Turk DC, Sinclair JD, et al: A standardized manual tender point survey: I. Development and determination of a threshold point for the identification of positive tender points in fibromyalgia syndrome. J Rheumatol 24: 377–383, 1997.)

when lightly touching the skin or gently pinching a fold of skin. There can be markedly different borders of allodynia on repeat testing. Signs of autonomic dysfunction, especially coolness and cyanosis, may be present after exercising the limb or may become apparent if the limb is held in a dependent position for a few minutes.

The distribution of painful points is outlined in Table 17–2 and shown in Figure 17–1. Control points such as the forehead, shin, and thumbnail will define how widespread the pain is.[70] We have observed several children who report that their entire body is painful, some even having pain from gentle touching of their hair. It should be noted, however, that a significant number of children with diffuse idiopathic pain do not have tender points, although they are otherwise indistinguishable from those fulfilling criteria for fibromyalgia.

Prolonged back pain in childhood is quite often due to a serious illness and should be carefully investigated.[71] However, there is a subset of children with nonorganic back pain, usually in conjunction with diffuse idiopathic musculoskeletal pain. Distinguishing signs include the axial loading test, distracted straight leg raising, passive rotation test, overreaction, and allodynia (Table 17–4).[72]

PATHOLOGY

There is virtually no information concerning the histopathology of connective or nerve tissues from children with idiopathic musculoskeletal pain syndromes. Three children with complex regional pain syndrome type I had biopsies of skin, muscle, and nerve consistent with ischemic injury.[73] Endothelial swelling, basement membrane thickening and reduplication, and patchy fiber atrophy of muscle were observed.

Table 17–4

Signs of Nonorganic Back Pain

TEST	DESCRIPTION
Axial loading test	A positive test is when back pain is reported while the examiner exerts downward pressure on the top of a standing patient's head. Neck pain may be elicited and is not a positive test.
Distracted straight leg raising	In a positive test, flexion of the hip causes back pain when the patient is supine but not when sitting.
Passive rotation test	A positive test is when the patient reports back pain when passively rotated at the ankles and knees keeping the pelvis, back, and shoulders in the same plane.
Overreaction	Overreaction is defined as excessive wincing, muscle tremors, screaming, or collapsing with pain. "Excessive" is quite subjective and may vary based on age, mental status, cultural influences, or fear.
Allodynia	Report of pain to light touch or a gentle pinch of the skin, usually with a border that varies on repeat testing.

Data from Waddell G, McCulloch JA, Kummel E, Venner RM: Nonorganic physical signs in low-back pain. Spine 5: 117–125, 1980.

DIFFERENTIAL DIAGNOSIS

Exclusion of other painful conditions is necessary before a diagnosis of an idiopathic musculoskeletal pain syndrome can be made (see Table 17–1). Table 17–5 lists disorders that can be confused with idiopathic pain syndromes, many of which are discussed further in other chapters. One condition commonly misdiagnosed as an idiopathic pain syndrome is seronegative enthesopathy arthropathy (SEA syndrome), especially in children with back pain. The most common misdiagnoses for children with an idiopathic pain syndrome are trauma, mechanical pain, or arthritis. Other diagnostic considerations include Fabry's disease, pernio, and neoplasia.

LABORATORY EXAMINATION

Often, the diagnosis of an idiopathic pain syndrome is quite clear and no further investigations are required. If blood and urine tests are obtained, their results are normal. The most common "abnormal" test is a low-titer positive antinuclear antibody titer (1:40), which should be discounted.[74] Two reports describe normal or slightly slowed nerve conduction velocity in patients with complex regional pain syndrome type 1.[17, 23] Any laboratory testing in these children should be done with caution because it may lead to unjustified doubt about the diagnosis, anxiety concerning more serious illnesses, and delay in initiating treatment.

RADIOLOGIC EXAMINATION

Radiographic findings are normal or demonstrate disuse osteoporosis depending on the duration and degree of disability; rarely do children have the spotty osteoporosis that occurs in adults with complex regional pain syndromes.[10] Technetium radionuclide bone scans are probably the most useful study if the diagnosis is in doubt.[16, 24] The most frequent abnormality in childhood idiopathic musculoskeletal pain is decreased uptake in the affected limb. A normal study is good evidence against an underlying bone disease. Magnetic resonance images are normal.

GENERAL ASSESSMENT OF DISEASE ACTIVITY

There are two major independent variables to consider when assessing activity of disease: pain and dysfunction. The report of pain is always valid in these children. Because pain is subjective, the most useful measurement is the self-report, usually on a verbal or visual analogue scale (Fig. 17–2). The quality of pain can be assessed using various instruments.

The amount of reported pain does not directly correlate with the degree of incapacitation, which can vary from almost none to being bedridden. An important observation is that function usually returns before the

Table 17–5

Differential Diagnoses in Children Presenting with Idiopathic Pain Syndromes

DIAGNOSIS	TYPICAL AGE	DISTINGUISHING CHARACTERISTICS
Fabry's disease	Adolescents	Episodic excruciating burning pain in the distal extremities, blue maculopapular hyperkeratotic lesions clustered on the lower trunk and perineum; erythrocyte sedimentation rate is usually elevated
Neoplasia	Any	Episodic or migratory pain or arthritis, generalized malaise, anorexia, and bone pain
Spinal cord tumors	Any	Abnormal neurologic examination, altered gait, or spinal curvature
Erythromelalgia	Adolescents	Pain with erythematous, warm, swollen hands or feet that is eased by cold to the point that patients will refuse to remove ice or cold water from their affected limbs
Pernio (chilblains)	Any	Burning pain, with associated red to purple, swollen, papules on exposed fingers or toes after cold injury
Raynaud's disease	Adolescents	Tricolor change (white, blue, red), associated with tingling, usually not very painful
Hypermobility	Younger	Intermittent nocturnal pains that may occur after certain activities
Restless legs	Adolescents	Nocturnal discomfort in, and an inability to keep from moving, the legs; paresthesias, not pain per se, common and rarely cause awakening
Myofascial pain	Adolescents	Sustained contraction of part of a muscle, especially those about the head, jaw, and upper back; pain well localized and reproduced when that part of the muscle is palpated
Chronic recurrent multifocal osteomyelitis	Any	Specific point tenderness
Chronic compartment syndrome	Adolescents	Severe muscle pain (usually calf) after exercising
Progressive diaphyseal dysplasia	Adolescents	Severe leg pain, fatigue, headaches, weight loss, weakness, and an abnormal, waddling gait; radiographs show cortical thickening and sclerosis of the diaphysis of the long bones
Peripheral mononeuropathy	Adults	Post-traumatic mononeuropathy
Transient migratory osteoporosis	Adolescents	Rapidly developing, painful osteoporosis
Vitamin D deficiency	Adults	Hyperesthetic pain in debilitated patients with multiple reasons to be deficient in vitamin D
Thyroid disease	Any	Widespread musculoskeletal pain with either hypo- or hyperthyroidism with associated symptoms of thyroid dysfunction

pain diminishes. Functional measurements vary depending on the location of the pain and the presence of coexisting conditions such as arthritis or, more commonly, conversion symptoms. Children with both idiopathic musculoskeletal pain and paralysis are extremely dysfunctional.

One study used a visual analogue scale of well-being to compare newly diagnosed children with juvenile rheumatoid arthritis and those with localized idiopathic musculoskeletal pain. This confirmed that the latter group reported significantly worse scores (see Fig. 17–2).[12] It is our impression that these children do, if fact, suffer more than children with other musculoskeletal conditions, which, we speculate, may indicate the degree to which the disorder is a manifestation of psychological distress.

Psychological assessment has been advocated by many authors because, by the time these children are identified, significant psychological dysfunction is almost universally present.[7, 10, 12, 37, 38, 75] Even though it is not necessarily true that these syndromes are psychological in cause, the psychological toll on the child and family is often severe. The degree of psychosocial pathology is highly variable and may range from anxiety or poor coping to borderline personality disturbance, or may involve siblings and other family members.

TREATMENT

The plethora of widely disparate treatments attests to the fact that there are no proven therapies demonstrated by well-controlled therapeutic trials in children with idiopathic musculoskeletal pain.[54] Many reports

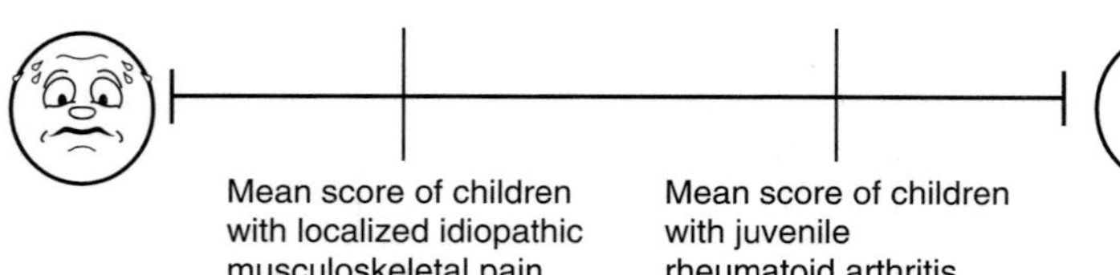

Figure 17–2. Visual analogue scale compares the mean score between children with localized idiopathic musculoskeletal pain and adolescents with newly diagnosed juvenile rheumatoid arthritis. (From Sherry DD, Weisman R: Psychologic aspects of childhood reflex neurovascular dystrophy. Pediatrics 81: 572–578, 1988. Reproduced with permission from Pediatrics, Vol 81, Pages 572–578, 1988.)

describe a single child or a very small group of children. Therefore, anything said about treatment cannot be dogmatic or authoritative.

Treatment should have two goals: restoration of function and relief of pain. Anything less is not satisfactory, although, since pain is subjective and not directly amenable to specific treatment, there are some patients in whom restoration to full function without total pain relief has to be an accepted, albeit less desirable, outcome. Helping the child develop skills to cope with the pain is often effective in relieving the distress and dysfunction caused by the pain, even if the pain persists.

Most reports deal with localized idiopathic musculoskeletal pain, specifically complex regional pain syndrome type I. Of these, most report benefit, in order of success, with exercise therapy, transcutaneous electrical nerve stimulation, and sympathetic blocks.[7, 10–14, 17–20, 23, 25, 27–30] Most authors advocate aggressive exercise therapy aimed at reversing immobility and increasing function. Treatments used less commonly and with variable results include glucocorticoids,[19, 22] tricyclic antidepressants, anticonvulsants, opioids, sympathectomy, biofeedback, behavioral modification, and other forms of psychotherapy.[19, 22, 76, 77] Wilder et al[19] advocated a combination of multiple physical and medical treatments, including sympathetic blocks and sympathectomy, with pain resolution in less than half of their patients. Bernstein et al[10] successfully treated 23 patients with exercise therapy alone and reported long-term follow-up on 20; 12 were without any pain and 5 had occasional discomfort without any physical signs, 2 had moderate discomfort with some swelling, and 1 had a recurrence of neurovascular dystrophy.

There are few reports of treatment of diffuse idiopathic musculoskeletal pain, mainly fibromyalgia, in children. Studies in adults have found combination therapy with education, mild aerobic exercise, a low-dose tricyclic antidepressant, and a nonsteroidal anti-inflammatory agent helpful but not curative.[78] One report of 15 children found cyclobenzaprine to be helpful in 73 percent.[79] However, in a study of 33 children only 3 subjects indicated that they would recommend cyclobenzaprine to other individuals with similar pain.[80] Psychological support has also been advocated.[38, 81]

We have been successful with a team approach for children with both localized and diffuse idiopathic musculoskeletal pain that involves intense exercise therapy directed to the restoration of full function, along with psychological evaluation and therapy (if indicated).[42, 82] The exercise therapy is generally for 5 hours a day, on weekdays, for a mean of 2 weeks. The children are treated one-on-one with the therapist encouraging both speed and quality of movement. Allodynia is treated with desensitization using towel rubs. Children with persistent dysfunctional sleep are given a therapeutic trial of low-dose tricyclic antidepressant medication. Those with clinical depression are usually treated with a serotonin reuptake inhibitor.[83] Analgesics, physical therapy modalities, sympathetic blocks, and steroids are, in our experience, not required. Psychological evaluation is undertaken on all individuals, and most are referred for psychotherapy with family members. Psychological testing is helpful not only in ascertaining whether there are significant family or other environmental stress factors (such as learning disabilities), and whether the child is depressed, but also as a foundation for cognitive-behavioral therapy to teach pain-coping strategies.

COURSE OF THE DISEASE AND PROGNOSIS

No studies of natural history are available, but some children have disease that persists for years. Those with self-limited involvement probably tend not to be evaluated in tertiary centers. There may be many children who have spontaneous remission of illness; 11 of 15 children incidentally diagnosed with fibromyalgia were asymptomatic after 30 months.[35] However, 92 percent of children diagnosed with fibromyalgia in a pediatric rheumatology center still had significant pain 15 to 60 months (mean, 33 months) later.[39]

We have experienced much better short- and long-term outcomes.[82] In general, children with complex regional pain syndrome do better than those without signs of autonomic dysfunction, who, in turn, do better than those with diffuse idiopathic musculoskeletal pain. After a mean of 5 years, 88 percent of the children with autonomic signs were free of pain and fully functional. Most (90 percent) of those without autonomic signs were functional, but only 78 percent were without pain. Initially, 90 percent of the group with diffuse idiopathic musculoskeletal pain were pain free, but this success declined to 50 percent over 5 years. However, 90 percent remained fully active in school or employment. We have not observed a difference in outcome between girls and boys or in younger children compared with older adolescents.

The frequency of relapses is rarely reported but does occur in all forms of idiopathic musculoskeletal pain. The clinical subset of the second episode may be different from the first, even changing between localized and diffuse disease.[7, 40] In our experience, children with relapses are more likely to have significant underlying psychopathology.

In addition to recurrent episodes of idiopathic musculoskeletal pain, children may develop a pain condition involving other organ systems, especially headaches or abdominal pains, and other psychological problems, including conversion disorders (blindness, paralysis), suicide attempts, panic attacks, or eating disorders. Controlled studies have not been done, so it is unclear whether these problems occur at a greater frequency than in the general population.

EVALUATION AND MANAGEMENT OF MUSCULOSKELETAL PAIN

Pain is the subjective expression of an unpleasant sensation associated with actual or perceived tissue dam-

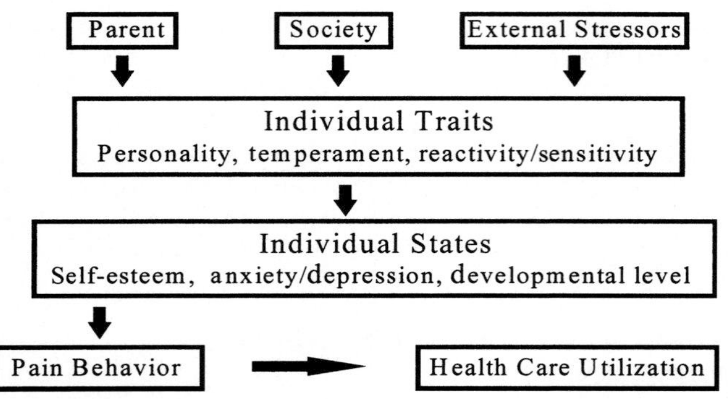

Figure 17–3. Factors influencing pain expression.

age. It is difficult, if not impossible, for an observer to know with any certainty to what extent a child is in pain. Even experienced observers, such as nurses or parents, may differ in their assessments of the degree of pain the child is experiencing. Although parents and children tend to make a similar assessment of the degree of pain, parents may over- or underestimate the child's pain in relation to the child's own self-report. An important premise in the evaluation and management of a child in pain is that the child's report of pain and its severity must be believed. Malingering is exceedingly rare: "Pain is what the patient says it is, and exists when he says it does."[85] Effective management requires that the child feels that he or she is believed.

Many interacting issues determine whether a child's pain disturbs the child's and family's functioning and whether or when medical help is sought (Fig. 17–3). The purpose of the following discussion is to provide a framework for assessment of pain, a logical approach to differential diagnosis, and an initial management of both acute and chronic pain.

Assessment of the Child With Musculoskeletal Pain

History and Physical Examination

In obtaining a history, answers to the following questions should be sought:

- What is the character of the pain?
- Are there any other symptoms?
- Is there a family history of musculoskeletal disease?
- What are the family social, emotional, and educational circumstances?

More detailed questions addressing these four general areas are listed in Table 17–6. In addition to a history of pain-related symptoms, a complete past history and review of systems will help to make certain that the child's overall health is documented. This may be quite time-consuming, but is especially important in children with idiopathic pains, and is the initial step in establishing a trusting relationship with the child and family, who often feel that their concerns have not been considered seriously. The answers elicited by the questions will allow a directed clinical examination, enabling the physician to develop a focused differential diagnosis. The physician can then reasonably determine whether further investigations are indicated. A few key observations to be made during the physical examination are listed in Table 17–7. A list of some of the possible causes of pain categorized by location is provided in Table 17–8.

Table 17–6

History of Musculoskeletal Pain

What Is the Character of the Pain?

Which body parts are painful?
How long has the pain been present?
Is the pain getting better or worse or staying the same?
What makes the pain worse? What makes it better?
Is there diurnal variation in the severity of the pain?
Is the pain present at night? Does it wake the child from sleep?
Does the pain interfere with function? If so, in what way and to what extent?
Is the pain sharp, aching, deep, boring, etc.?
Does the pain radiate or migrate or spread?
Is the painful area tender to touch?
Is the painful area either cold or hot to the touch?
Does the painful part look abnormal?
What is the child's or parent's assessment of the pain severity?

Are There Other Symptoms?

Is there fever?
Is there a rash?
Is there change in gastrointestinal function?
Is there weight loss?
Are there upper or lower respiratory tract symptoms?
Is there muscle weakness?
Is there sleep disturbance?
Is there depression?

Family and Social History

Is there a family history of ankylosing spondylitis, Reiter's syndrome, or inflammatory bowel disease?
Is there a history of severe back pain, heel pain, or acute iritis?
Is there a family history of psoriasis?
Is there a family history of fibromyalgia or other chronic pain condition?
Is there an identifiable stressor in the family, school, or peer group?

Laboratory Examination

It is important to have a clear rationale for undertaking any investigation. In many situations, no testing is

Table 17–7

The Clinical Examination: Several Key Observations

Does the child look well or ill?
Is the child's affect commensurate with the level of child or parental pain assessment?
Is there any joint swelling?
Is there any muscle weakness or atrophy?
Is there any tenderness to palpation? If so, is it over joints, entheses, or muscles?
Is there any evidence of hyperesthesia, allodynia, or skin color changes?
Is there evidence of localized or diffuse neurologic dysfunction?

Table 17–8

Diagnostic Possibilities for Musculoskeletal Pain by Location

Neck
- Idiopathic wry neck (acute self-limited torticollis)
- Intervertebral disk calcification
- Joint subluxation
  - Down syndrome or other skeletal dysplasias
  - Long-standing arthritis
- Diffuse idiopathic pain syndrome

Upper Limb
- General
  - Localized idiopathic pain syndrome
- Shoulder
  - Dislocation
  - Rotator cuff injury (uncommon in children)
  - Impingement syndromes (uncommon in children)
  - Labral tear (probably uncommon in children)
- Elbow
  - "Toddler pulled elbow" (radial head subluxation)
  - Panner's disease
  - Tennis, golf, or Little Leaguer's elbow
- Wrist and hand
  - Arthritis
  - Raynaud's disease
  - Chilblains
  - Erythromelalgia
  - Peripheral neuropathy

Back
- Scheuermann's disease
- Spondylolysis or spondylolisthesis
- Hyperlordosis leading to mechanical strain

Lower Limb
- General
  - Localized idiopathic pain syndrome
- Hip
  - Missed congenital dislocated hip (0–5 yr)
  - Legg-Calvé-Perthes disease (5–10 yr)
  - Slipped capital femoral epiphysis (10–15 yr)
  - Transient synovitis (5–10 yr)
  - Spondyloarthropathy (>10 yr)
- Knee
  - Arthritis
  - Osgood-Schlatter disease
  - Mechanical knee pain (chondromalacia)
  - Discoid meniscus
  - Osteochondritis dissecans
- Ankle and foot
  - Osteochondritis dissecans of talus
  - Sever's disease
  - Köhler's disease
  - Enthesitis of spondyloarthropathy
    - Achilles tendon insertion
    - Plantar fascia insertion
  - Peripheral neuropathy or neuroma
  - Arthritis
  - Stress fracture
  - Erythromelalgia
  - Tarsal coalition

required. A large number of investigations increases the likelihood of false-positive results that may confuse the issue. An evaluation of indices of inflammation (complete blood count, erythrocyte sedimentation rate, or C-reactive protein) is appropriate. It would be dangerous to make a diagnosis of a noninflammatory condition in a child with an abnormal complete blood count or increased acute phase reactants unless the abnormalities could be ascribed to an intercurrent illness. Tests for antinuclear antibodies and rheumatoid factors are of little value in the absence of clinical evidence of inflammatory disease, and false-positive antinuclear antibodies in particular may lead to unnecessary investigations.[86, 87]

Radiologic examinations of symptomatic areas are used to exclude bony changes that might point toward a serious cause of skeletal pain, such as a malignancy or infection. Further imaging studies (computed tomography, magnetic resonance imaging) should be used only to further evaluate abnormalities demonstrated by radiography or bone scintigraphy.

Pain Assessment

Many methods are available to assess pain in children. Because pain is a complex state, influenced by many factors, no single instrument can provide a complete evaluation of pain. Nonetheless, application of one or more of the available instruments will aid in understanding pain in the individual child, and in groups of children with similar diseases.

Physiologic Measures

A number of physiologic measures may be useful to assess pain in very young children or in older children who have limited communication skills. These included heart rate, blood pressure, palmar sweating, transcutaneous oxygen tension, and skin blood flow. Most of these tests have little or no data to support their reliability, validity, sensitivity, specificity, or practicality.[88]

Behavioral Measures

Physicians routinely interpret the child's behavior as an indicator of the severity of pain. However, perhaps because behavioral measurements are integrated into the assessment almost subconsciously, and because of inherent biases about what constitutes appropriate responses to pain, such behavioral assessments may be misleading. Nevertheless, it is important to be able to quantify pain behaviors because they represent important indicators of how a child is dealing with noxious or perceived noxious stimuli. Furthermore, pain behaviors may themselves positively or negatively affect a child's and a family's pain-coping mechanisms, so an ability to measure these behaviors may help the rheumatology team to understand and better manage the child's pain.[89]

A number of different scales of pain behavior have been developed. These include various assessments of crying or other verbal responses, facial expressions, and limb movements.[89] The Children's Hospital of Eastern Ontario Pain Scale (CHEOPS)[90] is a validated and widely used scale. However, this instrument is not sensitive to change in children who have been in pain for several hours, presumably because pain behaviors habituate if the pain persists. In this situation, the

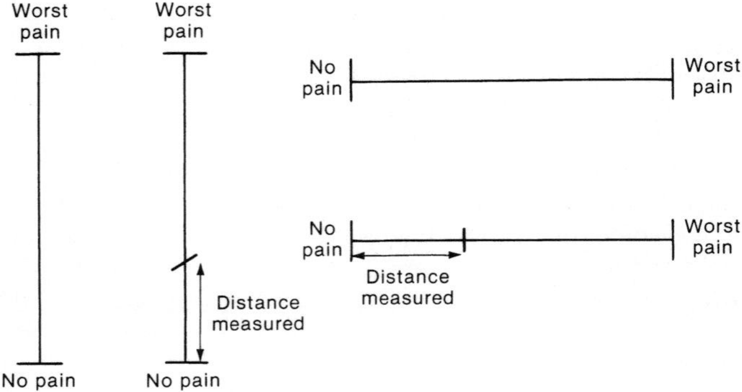

Figure 17–4. Examples of pain scales, ordinarily 10 cm in length. The patient estimates the severity of pain by placing a mark on the line, thus facilitating sequential comparisons and gauging the effect of treatment.

CHEOPS scores are generally low and correlate poorly with self-report measures.[91] Utilizing a standardized observational method with videotapes, Jaworski and colleagues[92] measured pain behaviors in 30 children with juvenile rheumatoid arthritis and concluded that this method was a reliable and valid measure of pain. They also stated that measures of pain behavior might be particularly useful in treatment outcome studies because these behaviors seemed to be relatively independent of depression.

Self-Report Measures

A number of both unidimensional and multidimensional self-report instruments for children were developed during the 1990s.[93]

Unidimensional Pain Measures

The most frequently used simple unidimensional pain scale is the visual analogue scale (VAS). For older children and adults, this is usually a 10-cm horizontal or vertical line anchored by phrases such as "no pain" at one end and "the worst imaginable pain" at the other. The patient puts a mark along the line to represent the level of pain. This mark is measured in millimeters from the "no pain" end to give a value that can be compared over time in a clinical situation, during an intervention trial, or with other individuals in research studies (Fig. 17–4). For younger children, the VAS is usually anchored by a cartoon happy face at one end and a crying face at the other. Variants of the VAS for children include pain thermometers[94] or pain ladders.[95] Other unidimensional scales included Likert scales, in which the pain is rated on a 4-, 5-, or 6-point verbal scale, such as no pain, mild pain, moderate pain, severe pain,[96] or as a number from 1 to 10. A Faces Rating Scale[97] (Fig. 17–5) is a nonverbal nonnumeric Likert scale for younger children.

Multidimensional Pain Measures

Multidimensional instruments are questionnaires that collect information about a number of domains relevant to pain, including pain severity, psychological well-being (anxiety, depression), coping strategies, and self-efficacy. The best known of these in pediatric rheumatology is the Varni/Thompson Pediatric Pain Questionnaire.[98] Other questionnaires are designed to assess pain-coping strategies[99] and competency.[100]

Pain Management

For most of the twentieth century, children's pain was generally ignored and undertreated.[101] Thankfully, since about 1980, there has been a dramatic improvement with the recognition that children *do* have pain, that they can describe it, and that it can be effectively and safely managed.

Management of Acute Pain

Preventing procedural pain is preferable to treating it.[102, 103] The topical application of the eutectic mixture

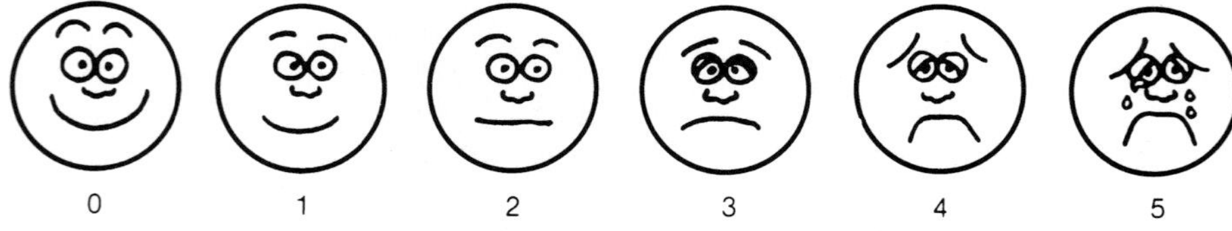

Figure 17–5. Pain assessment in children: faces rating scale. (From Wong D, Whaley L: Clinical Handbook of Pediatric Nursing. 3rd ed. St. Louis, Mosby, 1990.)

Instructions for Faces Rating Scale

1. Explain to the child that each face is for a person who feels happy because he or she feels no pain (hurt, or any word used by the child) or sad because he or she has some or a lot of pain.

   Face 0 = very happy, has no hurt.
   Face 1 = hurts just a little bit.
   Face 2 = hurts a little more.
   Face 3 = hurts even more.
   Face 4 = hurts a whole lot.
   Face 5 = hurts as much as you can imagine, although you don't have to be crying to feel this bad.

2. Have the child choose the face that best describes how he or she feels.

Table 17–9

Drugs for Conscious Sedation

DRUG	DOSAGE AND SCHEDULE
Oral midazolam	0.5 mg/kg in juice 30 min prior to procedure *followed by:*
Intravenous midazolam	0.1–0.2 mg/kg/dose given over 2–3 min repeated ×1 after 5 min if necessary
Intravenous fentanyl	0.5–1.0 μg/kg/dose given over 3–5 min repeated ×1 after 30 min if necessary
Reversal drugs	To be available for urgent use but not to be used routinely
Naloxone	0.1 mg/kg/dose repeated as necessary
Flumazenil	10–25 μg/kg/dose repeated ×2 as necessary

of local anesthetics (EMLA) 1 hour before venipunctures or joint injections minimizes pain associated with these procedures.[104] When a local anesthetic is indicated, addition of 2 ml of sodium bicarbonate to 10 ml of 1 percent lidocaine significantly decreases the stinging sensation associated with injection of the anesthetic drug.[105]

Painful procedures are made more tolerable by careful attention to the environment in which the procedure is performed.[106, 107] Ensuring that the room is quiet; that health care providers approach the child in an unhurried, calm manner; that the child is distracted (by reading or being read to, watching videos, listening to tapes, or playing hand-held computer games) helps the child to cope with pain associated with a procedure. Under most circumstances, the presence of a parent is reassuring to the child and therefore helps to minimize pain.

For younger children undergoing arthrocentesis, conscious sedation with either oral midazolam or a combination of intravenous midazolam and intravenous fentanyl (Table 17–9) is effective in diminishing the pain and anxiety. For young children, or for those requiring injection of multiple joints, however, a brief general course of anesthesia is recommended.

Behavioral techniques and the early and regular use of analgesics are the mainstays of therapy for acute pain that lasts longer than that associated with minor medical procedures.[108] There is convincing evidence that the use of local anesthetics as adjunctive therapy during surgery under general anesthesia can decrease postoperative pain.[109] The routine use of postoperative analgesia, including morphine, has been shown to decrease the time required for convalescence. It is now clear that children can tolerate intravenous morphine well, with a low risk of respiratory depression, and minimal risk of addiction.[110] Most children over 5 years of age are able to use patient-controlled analgesia effectively.[111]

Management of Chronic Pain

The World Health Organization has outlined a progressive therapeutic pain stepladder beginning with simple analgesics.[112] An analgesic with adjunctive therapy is sufficient for most children with rheumatic diseases. Adjunctive therapy includes the behavioral techniques discussed previously as well as various physical modalities (massage, physical therapy, transcutaneous nerve stimulation, acupuncture) or psychological techniques (hypnotherapy, biofeedback).[113] If this approach is insufficient, opioids (usually morphine) are introduced in a stepwise fashion. Children with joint pain resulting from end-stage arthritis require joint replacement to effectively control pain.[114] Occasionally, the nonsteroidal anti-inflammatory drug ketorolac (10 mg 3 to 4 times a day) is of some benefit for older children who are awaiting joint replacement surgery. Ketorolac is approved only for very short-term use.

Pain management in some children requires a cognitive-behavioral approach in a multidisciplinary setting. There are two strands to such treatment.[115] The cognitive strand is aimed at helping children develop more effective coping strategies to deal with pain. The behavioral strand is aimed at decreasing pain behaviors and increasing healthy behaviors. Each of these strands may have several components, depending on the needs of the individual child, as well as the availability and skills of the therapists. The goal of this approach is not to cure the pain, but to help the child and the family discover ways of coping with pain and disability so that they are less disruptive to the child's life.

CONCLUSION

Musculoskeletal pain is common in childhood, and an accurate diagnosis of the cause and a logical and consistent approach to its management are important. A careful history and examination combined with judicious laboratory or radiographic investigations can usually allow a diagnosis to be made. The use of a few simple measures of pain, particularly self-report scales, can help the physician assess how the child and the parent perceive the pain, and thereby enable institution of the most appropriate management. Reassurance, the use of simple analgesics or anti-inflammatory drugs, and physiotherapy are often sufficient. However, some children with chronic pain syndromes need much more complex medical and psychological management strategies involving a multidisciplinary team approach.

References

1. Naish JM, Apley J: "Growing pains": a clinical study of non-arthritic limb pains in children. Arch Dis Child 26: 134–140, 1951.
2. Paice E: Reflex sympathetic dystrophy. Br Med J 310: 1645–1648, 1995.
3. Payne WK 3rd, Ogilvie JW: Back pain in children and adolescents. Pediatr Clin North Am 43: 899–917, 1996.
4. Oster J: Recurrent abdominal pain, headache and limb pains in children and adolescents. Pediatrics 50: 429–436, 1972.
5. Buskila D, Press J, Gedalia A, et al: Assessment of nonarticular tenderness and prevalence of fibromyalgia in children. J Rheumatol 20: 368–370, 1993.

6. Abu-Arafeh I, Russell G: Recurrent limb pain in schoolchildren. Arch Dis Child 74: 336–339, 1996.
7. Sherry DD, McGuire T, Mellins E, et al: Psychosomatic musculoskeletal pain in childhood: clinical and psychological analyses of 100 children. Pediatrics 88: 1093–1099, 1991.
8. Merskey DM, Bogduk N: Classification of Chronic Pain. Descriptions of Chronic Pain Syndromes and Definitions of Pain Terms. Seattle, WA, IASP Press, 1994.
9. Matles AI: Reflex sympathetic dystrophy in a child. A case report. Bull Hosp Joint Dis 32: 193–197, 1971.
10. Bernstein BH, Singsen BH, Kent JT, et al: Reflex neurovascular dystrophy in childhood. J Pediatr 93: 211–215, 1978.
11. Ruggeri SB, Athreya BH, Doughty R, et al: Reflex sympathetic dystrophy in children. Clin Orthop 163: 225–230, 1982.
12. Sherry DD, Weisman R: Psychologic aspects of childhood reflex neurovascular dystrophy. Pediatrics 81: 572–578, 1988.
13. Stilz RJ, Carron H, Sanders DB: Reflex sympathetic dystrophy in a 6-year-old: successful treatment by transcutaneous nerve stimulation. Anesth Analg 56: 438–443, 1977.
14. Silber TJ, Majd M: Reflex sympathetic dystrophy syndrome in children and adolescents. Report of 18 cases and review of the literature. Am J Dis Child 142: 1325–1330, 1988.
15. Kavanagh R, Crisp AJ, Hazelman BL, Coughlan RJ: Reflex sympathetic dystrophy in children. Dystrophic changes are less likely. Br Med J 311: 1503, 1995.
16. Goldsmith DP, Vivino FB, Eichenfield AH, et al: Nuclear imaging and clinical features of childhood reflex neurovascular dystrophy: comparison with adults. Arthritis Rheum 32: 480–485, 1989.
17. Ashwal S, Tomasi L, Neumann M, Schneider S: Reflex sympathetic dystrophy syndrome in children. Pediatr Neurol 4: 38–42, 1988.
18. Rush PJ, Wilmot D, Saunders N, et al: Severe reflex neurovascular dystrophy in childhood. Arthritis Rheum 28: 952–956, 1985.
19. Wilder RT, Berde CB, Wolohan M, et al: Reflex sympathetic dystrophy in children. Clinical characteristics and follow-up of seventy patients. J Bone Joint Surg Am 74: 910–919, 1992.
20. Richlin DM, Carron H, Rowlingson JC, et al: Reflex sympathetic dystrophy: successful treatment by transcutaneous nerve stimulation. J Pediatr 93: 84–86, 1978.
21. Ostrov BE, Eichenfield AH, Goldsmith DP, Schumacher HR: Recurrent reflex sympathetic dystrophy as a manifestation of systemic lupus erythematosus. J Rheumatol 20: 1774–1776, 1993.
22. Kozin F, Haughton V, Ryan L: The reflex sympathetic dystrophy syndrome in a child. J Pediatr 90: 417–419, 1977.
23. Lemahieu RA, Van Laere C, Verbruggen LA: Reflex sympathetic dystrophy: an underreported syndrome in children? Eur J Pediatr 147: 47–50, 1988.
24. Laxer RM, Allen RC, Malleson PN, et al: Technetium 99m-methylene diphosphonate bone scans in children with reflex neurovascular dystrophy. J Pediatr 106: 437–440, 1985.
25. Stanton RP, Malcolm JR, Wesdock KA, Singsen BH: Reflex sympathetic dystrophy in children: an orthopedic perspective. Orthopedics 16: 773–779; discussion 779–780, 1993.
26. Silber TJ: Anorexia nervosa and reflex sympathetic dystrophy syndrome. Psychosomatics 30: 108–111, 1989.
27. Lightman HI, Pochaczevsky R, Aprin H, Ilowite NT: Thermography in childhood reflex sympathetic dystrophy. J Pediatr 111: 551–555, 1987.
28. Kesler RW, Saulsbury FT, Miller LT, Rowlingson JC: Reflex sympathetic dystrophy in children: treatment with transcutaneous electric nerve stimulation. Pediatrics 82: 728–732, 1988.
29. Hood-White R, Gainor J: Reflex sympathetic dystrophy in an 8-year-old: successful treatment by physical therapy. Orthopedics 20: 73–74, 1997.
30. Doolan LA, Brown TC: Reflex sympathetic dystrophy in a child. Anaesth Intens Care 12: 70–72, 1984.
31. Yunus MB, Masi AT: Juvenile primary fibromyalgia syndrome: a clinical study of thirty-three patients and matched normal controls. Arthritis Rheum 28: 138–145, 1985.
32. Buskila D, Neumann L, Hazanov I, Carmi R: Familial aggregation in the fibromyalgia syndrome. Semin Arthritis Rheum 26: 605–611, 1996.
33. Buskila D, Neumann L: Fibromyalgia syndrome (FM) and nonarticular tenderness in relatives of patients with FM. J Rheumatol 24: 941–944, 1997.
34. Buskila D: Fibromyalgia in children: lessons from assessing nonarticular tenderness. J Rheumatol 23: 2017–2019, 1996.
35. Buskila D, Neumann L, Hershman E, et al: Fibromyalgia syndrome in children: an outcome study. J Rheumatol 22: 525–528, 1995.
36. Gedalia A, Press J, Klein M, Buskila D: Joint hypermobility and fibromyalgia in schoolchildren. Ann Rheum Dis 52: 494–496, 1993.
37. Reid GJ, Lang BA, McGrath PJ: Primary juvenile fibromyalgia: psychological adjustment, family functioning, coping, and functional disability. Arthritis Rheum 40: 752–760, 1997.
38. Schanberg LE, Keefe FJ, Lefebvre JC, et al: Pain coping strategies in children with juvenile primary fibromyalgia syndrome: correlation with pain, physical function, and psychological distress. Arthritis Care Res 9: 89–96, 1996.
39. Rabinovich CE, Schanberg LE, Stein LD, Kredich DW: A follow up study of pediatric fibromyalgia patients. Arthritis Rheum 33: S146, 1990.
40. Malleson PN, al-Matar M, Petty RE: Idiopathic musculoskeletal pain syndromes in children. J Rheumatol 19: 1786–1789, 1992.
41. Wolfe F, Smythe HA, Yunus MB, et al: The American College of Rheumatology 1990 criteria for the classification of fibromyalgia: report of the Multicenter Criteria Committee. Arthritis Rheum 33: 160–172, 1990.
42. Sherry DD: Musculoskeletal pain in children. Curr Opin Rheumatol 9: 465–470, 1997.
43. Bowyer S, Roettcher P: Pediatric rheumatology clinic populations in the United States: results of a 3 year survey. Pediatric Rheumatology Database Research Group. J Rheumatol 23: 1968–1974, 1996.
44. Malleson PN, Fung MY, Rosenberg AM: The incidence of pediatric rheumatic diseases: Results from the Canadian Pediatric Rheumatology Association Disease Registry. J Rheumatol 23: 1981–1987, 1996.
45. Volinn E: The epidemiology of low back pain in the rest of the world: a review of surveys in low- and middle-income countries. Spine 22: 1747–1754, 1997.
46. Laxer RM, Shore AD, Manson D, et al: Chronic recurrent multifocal osteomyelitis and psoriasis: a report of a new association and review of related disorders. Semin Arthritis Rheum 17: 260–270, 1988.
47. Wainapel SF: Reflex sympathetic dystrophy following traumatic myelopathy. Pain 18: 345–349, 1984.
48. Gangi A, Dietemann JL, Gasser B, et al: Interstitial laser photocoagulation of osteoid osteomas with use of CT guidance. Radiology 203: 843–848, 1997.
49. Veldman PH, Reynen HM, Arntz IE, Goris RJ: Signs and symptoms of reflex sympathetic dystrophy: prospective study of 829 patients. Lancet 342: 1012–1016, 1993.
50. Sherry DD: Disproportional musculoskeletal pain in children with juvenile rheumatoid arthritis. J Rheumatol 27(Suppl 58): 71, 2000.
51. Balague F, Skovron ML, Nordin M, et al: Low back pain in schoolchildren: a study of familial and psychological factors. Spine 20: 1265–1270, 1995.
52. Lynch ME: Psychological aspects of reflex sympathetic dystrophy: a review of the adult and paediatric literature. Pain 49: 337–347, 1992.
53. Bruehl S, Carlson CR: Predisposing psychological factors in the development of reflex sympathetic dystrophy: a review of the empirical evidence. Clin J Pain 8: 287–299, 1992.
54. White KP, Harth M: An analytical review of 24 controlled clinical trials for fibromyalgia syndrome (FMS). Pain 64: 211–219, 1996.
55. Brazier DK, Venning HE: Conversion disorders in adolescents: a practical approach to rehabilitation. Br J Rheumatol 36: 594–598, 1997.
56. Cicuttini F, Littlejohn GO: Female adolescent rheumatological presentations: the importance of chronic pain syndromes. Aust Paediatr J 25: 21–24, 1989.
57. Prazar G: Conversion reactions in adolescents. Pediatr Rev 8: 279–286, 1987.

58. Price DD, Long S, Huitt C: Sensory testing of pathophysiological mechanisms of pain in patients with reflex sympathetic dystrophy. Pain 49: 163–173, 1992.
59. Arnold JM, Teasell RW, MacLeod AP, et al: Increased venous alpha-adrenoceptor responsiveness in patients with reflex sympathetic dystrophy. Ann Intern Med 118: 619–621, 1993.
60. Chelimsky TC, Low PA, Naessens JM, et al: Value of autonomic testing in reflex sympathetic dystrophy. Mayo Clin Proc 70: 1029–1040, 1995.
61. Cronin KD, Kirsner RL, Fitzroy VP: Diagnosis of reflex sympathetic dysfunction: use of the skin potential response. Anaesthesia 37: 848–852, 1982.
62. Herrick A, el-Hadidy K, Marsh D, Jayson M: Abnormal thermoregulatory responses in patients with reflex sympathetic dystrophy syndrome. J Rheumatol 21: 1319–1324, 1994.
63. Procacci P, Francini F, Maresca M, Zoppi M: Skin potential and EMG changes induced by cutaneous electrical stimulation. II. Subjects with reflex sympathetic dystrophies. Appl Neurophysiol 42: 125–134, 1979.
64. Simms RW: Fibromyalgia syndrome: current concepts in pathophysiology, clinical features, and management. Arthritis Care Res 9: 315–328, 1996.
65. Bou-Holaigah I, Calkins H, Flynn JA, et al: Provocation of hypotension and pain during upright tilt table testing in adults with fibromyalgia. Clin Exp Rheumatol 15: 239–246, 1997.
66. Martinez-Lavin M, Hermosillo AG, Mendoza C, et al: Orthostatic sympathetic derangement in subjects with fibromyalgia. J Rheumatol 24: 714–718, 1997.
67. Erdmann MW, Wynn-Jones CH: "Familial" reflex sympathetic dystrophy syndrome and amputation. Injury 23: 136–138, 1992.
68. Lunter MH, van Albada-Kuiper GA, Heggelman BGF: Reflex sympathetic dystrophy of one finger. Clin Rheumatol 9: 542–544, 1990.
69. Silber TJ: Eating disorders and reflex sympathetic dystrophy syndrome: is there a common pathway? Med Hypotheses 48: 197–200, 1997.
70. Okifuji A, Turk DC, Sinclair JD, et al: A standardized manual tender point survey. I. Development and determination of a threshold point for the identification of positive tender points in fibromyalgia syndrome. J Rheumatol 24: 377–383, 1997.
71. Hollingworth P: Back pain in children. Br J Rheumatol 35: 1022–1028, 1996.
72. Waddell G, McCulloch JA, Kummel E, Venner RM: Nonorganic physical signs in low-back pain. Spine 5: 117–125, 1980.
73. Nickeson R, Brewer E, Person D: Early histologic and radionuclide scan changes in children with reflex sympathetic dystrophy syndrome (RSDS). Arthritis Rheum 28: S72, 1985.
74. Cabral DA, Petty RE, Fung M, Malleson PN: Persistent antinuclear antibodies in children without identifiable inflammatory rheumatic or autoimmune disease. Pediatrics 89: 441–444, 1992.
75. Apley J: One child. *In* Apley J, Ounsted C (eds): One Child. Philadelphia, JB Lippincott, 1982, pp 23–47.
76. Schulman JL: Use of a coping approach in the management of children with conversion reactions. J Am Acad Child Adolesc Psychiatry 27: 785–788, 1988.
77. Alioto JT: Behavioral treatment of reflex sympathetic dystrophy. Psychosomatics 22: 539–540, 1981.
78. Russell IJ: Fibromyalgia syndrome: approaches to management. Bull Rheum Dis 45: 1–4, 1996.
79. Romano TJ: Fibromyalgia in children: diagnosis and treatment. W V Med J 87: 112–114, 1991.
80. Siegel DM, Janeway D, Baum J: Fibromyalgia syndrome in children and adolescents: clinical features at presentation and status at follow-up. Pediatrics 101: 377–382, 1998.
81. Mikkelsson M, Sourander A, Piha J, Salminen JJ: Psychiatric symptoms in preadolescents with musculoskeletal pain and fibromyalgia. Pediatrics 100: 220–227, 1997.
82. Sherry DD: Pain syndromes. *In* Isenberg DA, Miller JJI (eds): Adolescent Rheumatology. London, Marin Duntz Ltd, 1998, pp 197–227.
83. Anonymous: Practice parameters for the assessment and treatment of children and adolescents with depressive disorders. AACAP. J Am Acad Child Adolesc Psychiatry 37(10 Suppl): 63S–83S, 1998.
84. Sherry DD, Wallace CA, Kelley C, et al: Short- and long-term outcomes of children with complex regional pain syndrome type I treated with exercise therapy. Clin J Pain 15: 218–223, 1999.
85. Meinhart NT, McCaffery M: Pain: A Nursing Approach to Assessment and Analysis. New York, Appleton-Century-Crofts, 1983.
86. Eichenfield AH, Athreya BH, Doughty RA, Cebul RD: Utility of rheumatoid factor in the diagnosis of juvenile rheumatoid arthritis. Pediatrics 78: 480–484, 1986.
87. Malleson PN, Sailer M, Mackinnon MJ: Usefulness of antinuclear antibody testing to screen for rheumatic diseases. Arch Dis Child 77: 299–304, 1997.
88. Sweet SD, McGrath PJ: Physiological Measures of Pain. *In* Finley GA, McGrath PJ (eds): Measurement of Pain in Infants and Children. Progress in Pain Research and Management, vol 10. Seattle, IASP Press, 1998, pp 59–81.
89. McGrath PJ: Behavioral Measures of Pain. *In* Finley GA, McGrath PJ (eds): Measurement of Pain in Infants and Children. Progress in Pain Research and Management, vol 10. Seattle, IASP Press, 1998, pp 83–102.
90. McGrath PJ, Johnson G, Goodman JT, et al: CHEOPS: a behavioral scale for rating postoperative pain in children. *In* Fields HL, Dubner R, Cervero F (eds): Advances in Pain Research and Therapy, vol 9. Proceedings of the Fourth World Congress on Pain. New York, Raven, 1985, pp 395–402.
91. Beyer JE, McGrath PJ, Berde CB: Discordance between self-report and behavioral pain measures in children aged 3–7 years after surgery. J Pain Symptom Manage 5: 350–356, 1990.
92. Jaworski TM, Bradley LA, Heck LW, et al: Development of an observation method for assessing pain behaviors in children with juvenile rheumatoid arthritis. Arthritis Rheum 38: 1142–1151, 1995.
93. Champion GD, Goodenough B, von Baeyer CL, Thomas W: Measurement of pain by self-report. *In* Finley GA, McGrath PJ (eds): Measurement of Pain in Infants and Children, Progress in Pain Research and Management, vol 10. Seattle, IASP Press, 1998, pp 123–160.
94. Jay SM, Ozolins M, Elliott CH, Caldwell S: Assessment of children's distress during painful medical procedures. Health Psychol 2: 133–147, 1983.
95. Hester NO, Foster R, Kristensen K: Measurement of pain in children: generalizability and validity of the Pain Ladder and the Poker Chip Tool. *In* Tyler DC, Krane EJ (eds): Pediatric Pain. Advances in Pain Research and Therapy, vol 15. New York, Raven, 1990, pp 79–84.
96. Savedra MC, Tesler MD: Assessing children's and adolescents' pain. Pediatrician 16: 24–29, 1989.
97. Whaley L, Wong DL: Nursing Care of Infants and Children. 3rd ed. St. Louis, CV Mosby, 1987.
98. Varni JW, Thompson KL, Hanson V: The Varni/Thompson Pediatric Pain Questionnaire: I. Chronic musculo-skeletal pain in juvenile rheumatoid arthritis. Pain 28: 27–38, 1987.
99. Varni JW, Waldron SA, Gragg RA, et al: Development of the Waldron/Varni Pediatric Pain Coping Inventory. Pain 67: 141–150, 1996.
100. Harter S: The Perceived Competence Scale for children. Child Dev 53: 87–97, 1982.
101. Schechter NL: The undertreatment of pain in children: an overview. Pediatr Clin North Am 36: 781–794, 1989.
102. Jackson DL, Moore PA, Hargreaves KM: Preoperative nonsteroidal anti-inflammatory medication for the prevention of postoperative dental pain. J Am Dent Assoc 119: 641–647, 1989.
103. Maunuksela E-L: Nonsteroidal anti-inflammatory drugs in pediatric pain management. *In* Schechter NL, Berde CB, Yaster M (eds): Pain in Infants, Children, and Adolescents. Baltimore, Williams & Wilkins, 1993, pp 135–143.
104. Halperin DL, Koren G, Attias D, et al: Topical skin anesthesia for venous, subcutaneous drug reservoir and lumbar punctures in children. Pediatrics 84: 281–284, 1989.
105. McKay W, Morris R, Mushlin P: Sodium bicarbonate attenuates pain on skin infiltration with lidocaine, with or without epinephrine. Anesth Analg 66: 572–574, 1987.
106. Zeltzer LK, Jay SM, Fisher DM: The management of pain associ-

ated with pediatric procedures. Pediatr Clin North Am 36: 941–964, 1989.

107. Gonzalez JC, Routh DK, Saab PG, et al: Effects of parent presence on children's reactions to injections: behavioral, physiological, and subjective aspects. J Pediatr Psychol 14: 449–462, 1989.
108. Sievers TD, Yee JD, Foley ME, et al: Midazolam for conscious sedation during pediatric oncology procedures: safety and recovery parameters. Pediatrics 88: 1172–1179, 1991.
109. Schindler M, Swann M, Crawford M: A comparison of postoperative analgesia provided by wound infiltration or caudal analgesia. Anaesth Int Care 19: 46–49, 1991.
110. Porter J, Jick H: Addiction rare in patients treated with narcotics. N Engl J Med 302: 123, 1980.
111. Gaukroger PB: Patient-controlled analgesia in children. *In* Schechter NL, Berde CB, Yaster M (eds): Pain in Infants, Children, and Adolescents. Baltimore, Williams & Wilkins, 1993, pp 203–211.
112. World Health Organization: Cancer pain relief and palliative care. Geneva, World Health Organization, 1990.
113. Carter B: Holistic/therapeutic nursing care. *In* Child and Infant Pain. London, Chapman & Hall, 1994, pp 89–104.
114. Haber D, Goodman SB: Total hip arthroplasty in juvenile chronic arthritis: a consecutive series. J Arthroplasty 13: 259–265, 1998.
115. Bursch B, Walco GA, Zeltzer L: Clinical assessment and management of chronic pain and pain-associated disability syndrome. Dev Behav Pediatr 19: 45–53, 1998.

Systemic Connective Tissue Diseases

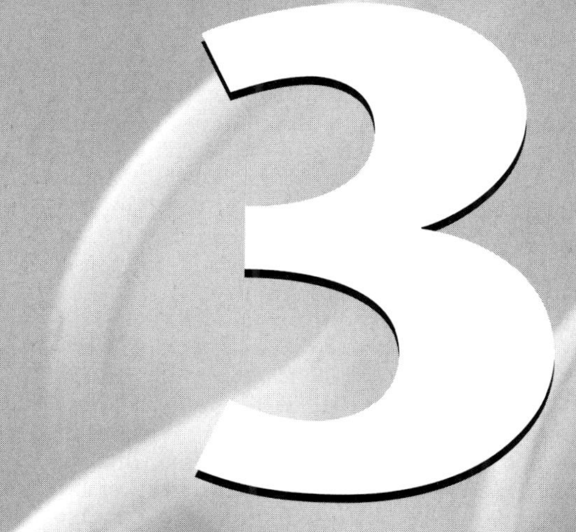

18

Systemic Lupus Erythematosus

Ross E. Petty and James T. Cassidy

Systemic lupus erythematosus (SLE) is an episodic, multisystem, autoimmune disease characterized by widespread inflammation of blood vessels and connective tissues and by the presence of antinuclear antibodies (ANAs), especially antibodies to native (double-stranded) DNA (dsDNA). Its clinical manifestations are extremely variable, and its natural history is unpredictable. Untreated, SLE is often progressive and has a significant fatality rate.

HISTORICAL REVIEW

The word *lupus*, derived from the Latin word for wolf, was originally used in medicine from the 13th to the 19th centuries to describe a dermatitis characterized by recurrent, florid facial ulcerations.[1] The acute and chronic types of the skin disease were first clarified by Kaposi in 1872.[2] In 1895, Osler recognized the systemic nature of this disease, its characteristic exacerbations and remissions, and suggested that "erythema exudativum" was a form of vasculitis.[3] Cardiac involvement was described in detail by Libman and Sacks in 1924,[4] and by Gross in 1940.[5] The clinical features of SLE as recognized today, however, were first delineated by Baehr, Klemperer, and Schifrin in 1935.[6] These authors emphasized that characteristic visceral involvement could occur in the absence of the typical cutaneous lesions.

In 1948, description of the lupus erythematosus (LE) cell by Hargraves, Richmond, and Morton[7] permitted recognition of a broader spectrum of patients with SLE. Not only was the frequency with which the diagnosis was made remarkably increased, but investigation of the mechanism of the formation of LE cells led to an understanding of the autoimmune nature of the disease, that is, the production of circulating antibodies that reacted with nuclear and other self-antigens.

The demonstration of ANAs by the more sensitive technique of indirect immunofluorescence microscopy led to more accurate diagnosis in patients with less typical presentations. Identification of an antibody to dsDNA in the serum and in the pathologic lesions of patients with the disease led to the concept of immune complex disease as an explanation for the pathogenesis of many of the features of SLE. The role of inflammation invoked by soluble immune complexes by way of complement activation was soon demonstrated. Later, altered cell-mediated immunity in active SLE and, more recently, the importance of immunogenetic predispositions have been documented.

The introduction of glucocorticoid drugs for the treatment of connective tissue diseases represented a major advance in the management of SLE. It became possible not only to prolong the lives of severely affected patients and to control acute manifestations of the disease, but also to follow the unfolding course of the illness in successfully treated patients.

DEFINITION AND CLASSIFICATION

The diagnosis of SLE is a clinical one and is supported by specific laboratory abnormalities. Three prominent features suggest the diagnosis:

1. SLE is an *episodic* disease. A history of intermittent symptoms such as arthritis, pleuritis, dermatitis, and nephritis may precede the diagnosis by months or years.
2. SLE is a *multisystem* disease, and children usually present with symptoms and signs of disease affecting more than one organ system.
3. SLE is characterized by the presence of *antinuclear antibodies* (especially those directed to dsDNA) and of other autoantibodies.

Criteria for the Classification of Patients

The most widely used criteria for the classification of SLE are those of the American College of Rheumatology, revised in 1982 (Table 18–1).[8] Although designed as classification criteria, they are widely used for diagnosis as well. In adults, the presence of four criteria has a sensitivity and specificity of 96 percent for the diagnosis of SLE. Evaluations of the 1982 criteria in childhood SLE[9] concluded that they had a sensitivity of 96 percent and a specificity of 100 percent in childhood lupus, as compared with a rheumatic disease control group. Of 103 children with SLE in this study, 99 fulfilled four or more criteria; none of the 101 control subjects did so, and only three of the control subjects fulfilled three criteria.

A 1997 recommendation by the Diagnostic and Therapeutic Criteria Committee of the American College of Rheuma-

Table 18–1

Criteria for the Classification of Systemic Lupus Erythematosus

ACR 1982 CRITERIA*	ACR 1997 CRITERIA†
Malar (butterfly) rash	Malar (butterfly) rash
Discoid-lupus rash	Discoid-lupus rash
Photosensitivity	Photosensitivity
Oral or nasal mucocutaneous ulcerations	Oral or nasal mucocutaneous ulcerations
Nonerosive arthritis	Nonerosive arthritis
Nephritis‡	Nephritis‡
Proteinuria >0.5 g/d	Proteinuria >0.5 g/d
Cellular casts	Cellular casts
Encephalopathy‡	Encephalopathy‡
Seizures	Seizures
Psychosis	Psychosis
Pleuritis or pericarditis	Pleuritis or pericarditis
Cytopenia	Cytopenia
Positive immunoserology‡	Positive immunoserology‡
Antibodies to dsDNA	Antibodies to dsDNA
Antibodies to Sm nuclear antigen	Antibodies to Sm nuclear antigen
Positive LE-cell preparation	
Biologic false positive test for syphilis	Positive finding of antiphospholipid antibodies based on: 1. IgG or IgM anticardiolipin antibodies, *or* 2. Lupus anticoagulant, *or* 3. False positive serologic test for syphilis for at least 6 months, confirmed by *Treponema pallidum* immobilization or fluorescent treponemal antibody absorption test
Positive antinuclear antibody test	Positive antinuclear antibody test

ACR, American College of Rheumatology; LE, lupus erythematosus.
*Adapted from Tan et al.[8]
†Adapted from Hochberg.[10]
‡Any one item satisfies that criterion.

tology[10] modifies the 1982 criteria for positive immunoserology by deleting "positive LE-cell preparation," and changing the criterion "biologic false-positive test for syphilis" to "(1) abnormal serum level of IgG or IgM anticardiolipin antibodies; (2) presence of the lupus anticoagulant demonstrated by a standard method; or (3) a false-positive serologic test for syphilis known to be positive for at least 6 months, and confirmed by negative *Treponema pallidum* immobilization or fluorescent treponemal antibody absorption test." A number of studies have validated the 1982 criteria in adults.[11, 12] The 1997 modification has not yet been validated, and concern about the nonspecificity of the anticardiolipin assay has been raised.[13] An apparent redundancy that has not been addressed is the fact that a positive test for ANA is one criterion, whereas antibodies to dsDNA or to Sm antigen are components of another criterion. Although almost all patients with SLE have ANA, the presence of this antibody has very low specificity for the disease, and since it is almost certain that patients with antibodies to dsDNA or Sm also have ANA, it seems evident that ANA should also be removed as a criterion.

EPIDEMIOLOGY

Incidence and Prevalence

Several large studies in adults with SLE[14–18] have estimated the incidence at 2.0 to 7.6 per 100,000 per year, and the prevalence at 12 to 50 per 100,000. Data in children are few, but, from national registries, it is estimated that the mean annual incidence is 0.36 per 100,000 (CI, 0.23, 0.61) in Canadian children[19] and 0.37[20] to 0.9 per 100,000 per year (CI, 0.10, 0.94)[21] in Finnish children. Using a questionnaire survey of pediatric departments of 1290 hospitals, the frequency of SLE in children in Japan was estimated at 0.47 per 100,000 per year.[22] The estimate in the study of Malleson and colleagues[19] may be the most accurate, since all patients submitted to the registry were evaluated by pediatric rheumatologists. In general, these studies agree with earlier studies from the United States of 0.53[17] and 0.60[18] per 100,000 per year.

Data from pediatric rheumatic disease registries confirm that SLE accounts for less than 1 percent of patients in pediatric rheumatology clinics in the United Kingdom,[23] 1.5 to 3 percent of patients in Canada,[19] and 4.5 percent of patients in the United States.[24] These differences probably reflect many factors, including referral patterns and ethnic diversity. In adults in the United Kingdom, Johnson and colleagues[25] observed a prevalence of SLE in Asians that was three times that in whites; in Afro-Caribbeans, the prevalence was almost six times higher than in whites. Although there are no accurate prevalence data, it has been inferred that there are between 5000 and 10,000 children with SLE in the United States.[26]

Age at Onset

The proportion of all patients with onset of SLE in childhood has been estimated at 15 to 17 percent.[27, 28] This information dates from the 1950s and 1960s, however, and it is likely that the proportion now is even higher. Onset of SLE is rare before 5 years of age and uncommon before adolescence, when it is almost as frequent as in any subsequent decade.

Sex Ratio

Women outnumber men in ratios ranging from 5:1[29] to 10:1[30] in large series of adults with SLE. In childhood, girls are affected 4.5 times more frequently than boys, although the overall ratio varies to some extent with age at onset.[31–34] In one study,[31] the ratio of girls to boys with SLE in the 0- to 9-year-old age range was 4:3; in the 10- to 14-year-old age range, 4:1, and in the 15- to 19-year-old range, 5:1. Three of the youngest patients with SLE were boys, including the youngest child, who had disease onset at the age of 3 years. A similar trend was noted in a study by King and associates[35] in which girls outnumbered boys by 3:1 in the group with onset before 12 years of age and by almost 10:1 in the group with onset after 12 years of age. This difference in sex distribution is not seen in all series, however, and a large study of SLE in children found no difference in the sex ratio of children who were younger or older than 10 years of age at the onset of disease.[26]

Influence of Geography and Race

Systemic lupus erythematosus is recognized worldwide. In studies of 234 children with SLE in the United States in whom racial origin was noted,[31, 35–37] 123 were white, 49 Hispanic American, 52 African-American, and 10 Asian. Although these data suggest a disproportionate representation by children of African-American, Asian, or Hispanic origin, population studies necessary to support this impression have not been reported.[38–42] Nonetheless, surveys suggest a predisposition for SLE among Puerto Rican and nonwhite residents of New York City that is higher than that for non-Hispanic whites.[14] An increased incidence of SLE among Sioux, Crow, Arapaho[43] and southeast Alaskan Indian adults[44] has been noted, but no data relating to children in these groups are available. In the pediatric rheumatology clinic in Vancouver, the proportion of children with SLE whose parents are aboriginal Canadians or from India greatly exceeds their representation in the overall population.[45]

Cook and associates[27] have analyzed the month of onset of symptoms attributable to SLE in 35 children studied in Boston and Cleveland. There was no striking seasonal incidence, although the lupus rash was more likely to be first noted in March or April.

GENETIC BACKGROUND

Family and Twin Studies

There have been numerous studies of genetic factors in patients with SLE, beginning with family studies, in which a higher than expected prevalence of lupus was noted in relatives of patients with the disease. In a case control study, 10 percent of patients with SLE had a first-degree relative with SLE, compared with 1 percent in control patient families.[46] The degree of disease clustering can be expressed as the ratio of the prevalence in families in which there is an affected member to the prevalence of disease within the population as a whole. The risk ratio of affected sibling pairs to population prevalence quantifies sibling-pair familial clustering. This ratio is estimated at 20 in SLE, similar to that seen in diabetes mellitus.[46, 47] Twin studies have shown concordance for SLE in 24 percent of 45 monozygous twin pairs, but only 2 percent of 62 dizygous twin pairs.[48] A connective tissue disease other than SLE occurs in approximately 1 of 10 families of patients with SLE.[49–53] The influence of the sex of the affected parent on inheritance of SLE (imprinting) is a subject of some interest. The transmission of the disease from father to son may mark a specific subset of SLE.[54] A role for genetic imprinting in SLE has not been established, however.

In studies of linkage in SLE, a region of chromosome 1 from 1q31 to 1q42 was identified as an area where a potential disease susceptibility locus was located.[55] This association was found in diverse ethnic groups. The identity of this gene is not yet known.

Histocompatibility Antigens

An explanation of the genetic predisposition to SLE has been sought in the study of antigens of the major histocompatibility complex. HLA-DR2 and HLA-DR3 independently increase the relative risk for development of SLE by two- to threefold in whites.[56] In African-Americans in whom DR3 is infrequent, DR2 and DR7 are associated with SLE. These associations are attributable largely to linkage disequilibrium between DRB1*1501 and DRB5*0101 and DQB1*0602.[57] Class III major histocompatability complex genes (tumor necrosis factor alpha [TNF-α], C4) are probably more important contributors to susceptibility to SLE. Mason and Isenberg[58] state that in white subjects, the haplotype A1;B8;DR3 confers a 10-fold increase in the risk of developing SLE; the presence of two C4A null alleles increases the risk 17-fold.

Although the contribution of specific HLA haplotypes to susceptibility to SLE is modest, there are, nonetheless, strong associations between some HLA genes and specific autoantibodies. These are shown schematically in Figure 18–1. Studies of associations with antigens of the major histocompatability complex and the presence of anti-dsDNA, the serologic hallmark of SLE, have been somewhat conflicting. Griffing and colleagues[59] reported an association between anti-dsDNA and HLA-DR3. Others found associations with DR2[60] or DR7.[61] In one study, 96 percent of patients with high titer antibody to dsDNA had DQB1*0201 (linked to DR3 and DR7), DQB1*0602 (linked to DR2 and DR6), or DQB1*0302 (linked to some DR4 allo-

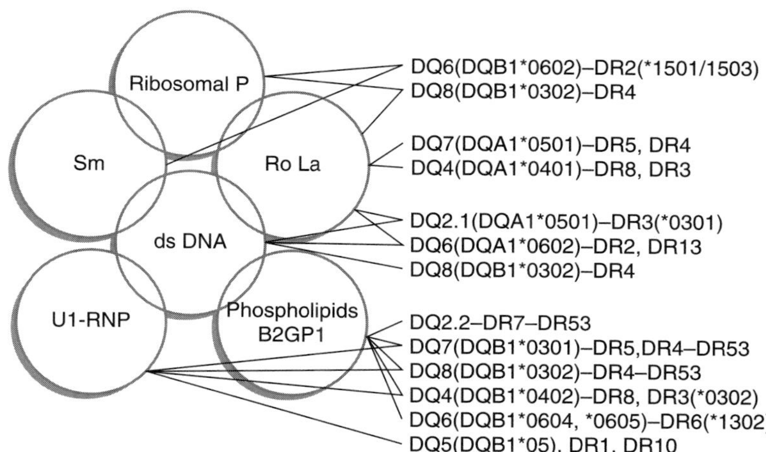

Figure 18–1. This representation illustrates the inter-related human leukocyte antigen (HLA) associations with autoantibody subsets in systemic lupus erythematosus. (From Tan FK, Arnett FC: The genetics of lupus. Curr Opin Rheumatol 10: 399, 1998.)

types).[62] The most important HLA and other genetic associations are summarized in Table 18–2.

Complement Component and Receptor Genes

Deficiencies of C1q, C1r, C1s, C4, and C2 are important but rare genetic causes for lupus-like syndromes.[56] Deficiencies of C1q have been reported in 30 patients with SLE, 80 percent of whom were children at disease onset.[63–65] Absence of C1q, C1r, and C1s is associated with SLE, nephritis, and antibodies to dsDNA, whereas complete absence of C2, C3, and C4 is associated with milder lupus-like syndromes.[63, 66] C4A and possibly C4B null alleles resulting in partial deficiencies have been associated with lupus in several populations.[67] Homozygous C4A deficiency is said to occur in 10 to 15 percent of white lupus patients, although rarely in healthy individuals; partial C4A deficiency occurs in 50 to 80 percent of SLE patients, and in 10 to 20 percent of control subjects.[58] Mutations of the complement regulatory mannose-binding protein have been reported to be increased in patients with SLE.[68] The authors suggest that there may be an additive effect of defective mannose-binding protein and the C4 null allele. Complement deficiencies probably predispose to SLE because of a deficiency of the processing and clearance of immune complexes.

Table 18–2

Genes Associated With Systemic Lupus Erythematosus

Major histocompatibility complex class II
DR2, DR3 in whites
DR2, DR7 in African-Americans
DQ alleles associated with specific autoantibodies
Major histocompatibility complex class III
C2, C3, C4A null, ?C4B
C1q, C1r, C1s
Mannose-binding protein
Tumor necrosis factor-alpha
FcγII, FcγIII

Tumor Necrosis Factor Polymorphisms

The frequency of the TNF-α2 allele is increased in white patients with SLE in the United Kingdom[69] and Sweden,[70] and is part of the HLA-DR3 haplotype that is common in SLE. This allele appears to be increased in white,[71] African-American,[72] and Chinese lupus patients.[73] It has been suggested that individuals who have low levels of TNF-α production may be protected from the development of glomerulonephritis: TNF-α levels are lower in DR2 positive individuals and higher in DR3 and DR4 positive individuals who are more prone to lupus nephritis.[74] Different levels of TNF-α may also explain the discrepant incidences of SLE in West Africans and African Americans, most of whom are of West African descent. An uncommon TNF-α2 allele is common in West Africa and directs high levels of TNF production; absence of this gene in the African-American population results in lower TNF-α production and increased susceptibility to SLE.[75]

Fc Receptor and T-cell Receptor Polymorphisms

There have been conflicting reports of associations of SLE and the isoforms of FcγRI, FcγRII, and FcγRIII, and SLE. An increased frequency of homozygosity for the low affinity FcγRII receptor that binds IgG2 to leukocytes and platelets has been found in one white population,[76] but not in another.[77] The latter study, however, found an increased frequency of the low affinity phenotype in African-Americans with SLE. A single base pair mutation of the FcγRIII gene is also present in increased frequency in patients with SLE.[78]

Early studies suggested that genetically determined differences in the T-cell receptor were associated with SLE, although a recent study discounts this association.[79]

ETIOLOGY AND PATHOGENESIS

Except for drug-induced SLE, the etiology of lupus is unknown. A number of factors may act independently or in concert to trigger onset of the disease: immune dysregulation, hormonal imbalance, and environmental factors including infection, all acting in a genetically predisposed host. The evidence in support of these and other possible etiologies and mechanisms is summarized.

Immune Dysregulation

B Lymphocyte Function

Antibody-mediated mechanisms of disease are operative in many of the clinical manifestations of SLE, such as acute hemolytic anemia, thrombocytopenia, leukopenia, and coagulopathies. In lupus nephritis and vasculitis, antigen-antibody complexes are directly related to the pathologic manifestations of the disease.

B cell numbers are increased in patients with active lupus and are activated to produce increased levels of antibodies, giving rise to hypergammaglobulinemia.[80] The frequency of IgG-secreting B cells in the peripheral blood correlates with disease activity.[81, 82] This may reflect polyclonal B cell activation by an exogenous antigen, antigen-stimulated B cell proliferation, or intrinsic abnormalities of the B cell and its control. CD5+ B cells (B1a B cells) produce IgM antibody of low affinity and may be particularly susceptible to polyclonal activation. They were once believed to be major contributors of autoantibodies, but their role is currently uncertain.

Autoantibodies, such as IgM antibodies to single-stranded and double-stranded DNA (anti-dsDNA), are part of the natural antibody repertoire of normal individuals, but high-affinity IgG anti-dsDNA antibodies are characteristic of SLE. Such antibodies may arise by polyclonal B-cell activation induced by environmental agents such as viruses or bacteria, or may arise by the exposure of the immune system to self DNA-protein complexes in nucleosomes or chromatin. During apoptosis, nuclear and cytoplasmic antigens appear in blebs on the cell membrane. Complexes such as the Ro (SSA) antigen, snRNA, and nucleosomes are presented to the immune system by this mechanism.

In patients with SLE, CD8 T lymphocytes and natural killer cells are defective in their ability to suppress B cell activity and, in fact, may facilitate increased production of autoantibodies.[83] The idiotype–anti-idiotype network that normally functions to modulate antibody production is probably also defective in patients with SLE.[84]

A further contributor to disease pathogenesis is the failure of optimal clearance of immune complexes by the reticuloendothelial system. This represents the effects of a number of factors, including exceeding the capacity of the reticuloendothelial system to remove the high level of complexes generated by autoantibody-antigen interactions, the low level of CR1 complement receptors on cell surfaces,[85] and the presence of low-affinity receptors for IgG2 (FCγRII).[76] Thus B cells produce high levels of antibodies to autoantigens; control of the production of these antibodies is defective and mechanisms that normally eliminate the immune complexes formed by such antibodies are also deficient. These circumstances set the stage for antibody and immune complex-mediated tissue damage.

Immune Complex Mediated Disease

Evidence that immune complexes are important in the pathogenesis of SLE is summarized in Table 18–3. Although immune complexes are often formed in the circulation and deposited in tissues, others are formed in organs in situ. In situ immune complex formation is favored by the affinity of the antigen for the target tissue, such as the basement membrane. This interaction may promote in situ localization of antibodies to dsDNA and the formation of immune complexes, a mechanism that may be of central importance in membranous glomerulonephritis. It has been demonstrated that antigens such as dsDNA bind directly to type IV collagen, a constituent of basement membranes.[86, 87] C1q can bind directly to dsDNA, and therefore complement activation and its consequences might result without participation of autoantibody. Demonstration of properdin in some biopsy specimens is evidence of involvement of the alternative pathway.[88] Complement activation might therefore result either from binding of complement to dsDNA without participation of autoantibody, or from binding of circulating antibody to the tissue-bound dsDNA, and in situ activation of complement. These mechanisms are described in detail elsewhere (see Chapter 5). Alternatively, antibody can bind directly to a cell-surface antigen. This is the case in antierythrocyte and antilymphocyte antibodies that result in hemolytic anemia and lymphocytopenia.

Lupus nephritis is caused by deposition of immune complexes consisting of complement components, immunoglobulins, and nuclear antigens in the glomerular lesions. High titers of antibodies to dsDNA and ribonucleoprotein have been eluted from the renal glomeruli,[89, 90] and have been demonstrated by fluorescence microscopy in the kidney, skin, and central nervous system.

Immunoglobulin antibody complexes of appropriate size activate the complement cascade. As a result, chemotactic factors are generated (C3a, C5a), granulocytes and macrophages are attracted, and inflammation results. A number of factors contribute to immune complex deposition in SLE,

Table 18–3

Evidence of Importance of Immune Complexes in Pathogenesis of Human Systemic Lupus Erythematosus

Spectrum of disease is similar to that of serum sickness, which is known to be immune complex mediated

Complement is activated
- Hypocomplementemia during active disease
- Presence of products of C3 and factor B activation in serum

Immune complexes are demonstrable
- In the serum
- In tissues (renal glomeruli, dermal-epidermal junction, choroid plexus)

including the availability of large amounts of antigen resulting, at least in part, from enhanced apoptosis, the exaggerated autoantibody response, and the diminished clearance of immune complexes by an overburdened or inefficient reticuloendothelial system. Genetic contributions to the failure to eliminate immune complexes effectively include polymorphisms of the FcγRs and the decrease in the complement receptor CR1 on erythrocytes.

Low serum levels of C3 and C4, along with the detection of complement components in immune complexes in the renal glomerulus, indicate that activation of both the classic and alternative pathways is involved in the production of the renal lesions.[91] Activation of the classic complement pathway is initiated by immune complexes, including those containing DNA and anti-dsDNA antibody. C3 and C1q can be demonstrated in the glomerular lesions in the majority of kidney biopsy specimens.

In experimental models of glomerulonephritis, the deposition of immune complexes is influenced by a variety of factors, including filtration pressure, and release of vasoactive amines by IgE-sensitized basophils, in addition to immune complex size, complement fixation, and antibody affinity.[92–96] Undoubtedly, cells of the reticuloendothelial system also play a role in determining the site of deposition of immune complexes. The glomerular mesangium functions normally to clear immune complexes from the vascular compartment and thereby occupies a central pathogenic role in certain types of experimental chronic nephritis.

Deposition of immune complexes in the subendothelial spaces of the choroid plexus may contribute to the clinical manifestations of lupus encephalopathy by interfering with normal cerebrospinal fluid circulation. Immune complexes were demonstrated in the choroid plexus in one 10-year-old girl who died of CNS lupus.[97]

T Lymphocyte Function

Patients with active SLE have a T lymphocytopenia involving, particularly, the CD4+/CD45RA+ subset of T cells that activates CD8+ T cells to suppress hyperactive B cells. T cell abnormalities are summarized in Table 18–4. There is a shift from the T_H0 to the T_H2 cell cytokine phenotype in SLE.[98] As a result, the cytokine profile tends to support B cell activation by interleukin (IL)-10, IL-4, IL-5, and IL-6. (The interactions of cytokines and cells are discussed in detail in Chapter 5.)

Table 18–4

T Lymphocyte Abnormalities in Systemic Lupus Erythematosus (SLE)

- CD4+ T cells
  - Decreased by glucocorticoids
  - Decreased in active SLE
  - Decreased in presence of antilymphocyte antibodies
  - CD4+ subset decreased: CD45 RA+
  - CD4+ subset increased: CD45 RO
- CD8+ T cells
  - Normal or increased in active SLE
- CD3+ double negative (CD4−, CD8−) T cells

Neutrophil Abnormalities

Patients with SLE may be neutropenic, but neutrophil function is usually normal. However, a lupus-like syndrome has been described in some mothers and maternal grandmothers of boys with chronic granulomatous disease, in which bacterial killing by neutrophils is defective.[99–101] There are also several reports of children with chronic granulomatous disease who also have a disease resembling SLE.[102, 103] (See Chapter 35.)

Apoptosis

Apoptosis is receptor-ligand mediated cell death. The Bcl-2 gene product interferes with apoptosis, thereby promoting survival of cells expressing this epitope. Bcl-2 expression is increased in peripheral T lymphocytes from patients with SLE,[104] and its expression correlates with the level of disease activity.[105] Paradoxically, Emlen and colleagues[106] have described increased apoptosis of a mixed population of lymphocytes from patients with SLE in vitro. If this occurs in vivo it could lead to release of nucleosomes that could contain autoantigenic material, thereby enhancing an autoimmune response. The Fas protein is also associated with apoptosis. In SLE, the expression of Fas protein is increased in particular on CD8+ T cells,[107] resulting in increased apoptosis of these cells and lymphocytopenia.[108] Whether mutations of the Fas gene are important in human SLE (as they are in some murine models) is uncertain. A Fas mutation has been described in children with lymphoproliferative disease,[105] but Fas mutations appear to be rare in patients with SLE.[109]

The level of apoptosis could have several implications. Prolongation of the life of cells that are proinflammatory would enhance disease; enhanced apoptosis could result in the exposure of antigen in apoptotic blebs (snRNPs) and nucleosomes (dsDNA, chromatin), thereby stimulating autoantibody formation.

Hormones

Sex hormones do not cause SLE, but they appear to play a role in disease predisposition and, possibly, disease severity or activity. A relative deficiency of androgenic hormones and an increase in estrogenic hormones appears to be characteristic of the patient with SLE, male or female. Studies in children[110] have reported that estrogen levels in children with SLE were normal but that testosterone levels were lower in postpubertal boys and girls with SLE than in normal children or in children with juvenile rheumatoid arthritis (JRA). Children with SLE also had significantly elevated follicle-stimulating hormone, luteinizing hormone, and prolactin.

Other evidence points to an important role of estrogenic hormones in SLE. Thus, lupus occurs primarily in women between menarche and menopause; in childhood and after menopause, the ratio of females to males with the disease is much lower. It has been noted that the activity of SLE is increased in the 2 weeks preceding menstruation,[111] during which time the level of estrogens is increased. Levels of 16α-hydroxyestrone and estriol are increased in women with SLE.[112] Oral contraception and pregnancy have also been alleged to exacerbate SLE, although the data are conflicting. Early studies of the use of oral contraceptives with high levels of estrogen were reportedly associated with increased lupus activity,[113, 114] but more recent reports in which the estrogen dose was much lower failed to show a relationship with disease activity.[115] Increased frequency of flares of SLE during the third trimester of pregnancy or in the post-partum period have been reported in some studies[116] but not in others.[117] In men with SLE, elevated levels of serum 16α-hydroxyestrone[112] and estrone[118] have been demonstrated. A recent study[118a] of 35 males with SLE found no significant differences from controls with respect to serum prolactin, testosterone or estradiol levels. However, gonadotropins (follicle-stimulating hormone, luteinizing hormone) were higher in men with SLE.

Relative deficiency of androgenic hormones may also play a role. Plasma androgens are decreased in SLE in women[119] and men. Males with Klinefelter's syndrome have low levels of testosterone and elevated luteinizing hormone[120] and an increased frequency of SLE.[121–124]

Elevated prolactin levels have been reported in pregnant women[125] and in men with active SLE.[118, 118a] Bromocriptine, which inhibits the secretion of prolactin by the anterior pituitary gland, has been used to suppress activity in these patients and in a few children with SLE.[126]

Environmental Factors

Ultraviolet Irradiation

Ultraviolet B irradiation has multiple effects that are important in the pathogenesis of SLE. Ultraviolet B results in photo-oxidation and degradation of native DNA in the skin, thereby increasing its immunogenicity. It induces apoptosis of keratinocytes.[127] In the process of apoptosis, DNA is degraded to nucleosomes, which are important inducers of ANAs.[128] During apoptosis, apoptotic blebs containing snRNPs such as the 52 kD Ro/SS-A appear on the cell surface, rendering them available as immunogens.[129] Expression by keratinocytes of the intercellular adhesion molecule ICAM-1 is enhanced by ultraviolet B,[130] but suppressed by ultraviolet A.[131] Ultraviolet B increases production of IL-8 and TNF-α in the epidermis,[132] an effect that could increase leukocyte-mediated inflammation. Interestingly, there is evidence that ultraviolet A1 may actually be therapeutic in patients with SLE.[133]

Viral Infection

The role of viruses in the production of the autoimmune abnormalities in SLE is not clear.[134] Tubuloreticular structures that were believed to be viral in origin have not been confirmed as such. Elevated titers of antiviral antibodies[135–139] probably reflect polyclonal B-cell activation rather than specific viral infection. Infection with the Epstein-Barr virus has been considered a possible etiologic candidate in patients with SLE. Epstein-Barr viral DNA was demonstrated in 53 percent of 15 adult SLE patients but in only 21 percent of control subjects in one study[140] and in 100 percent of SLE patients and 72 percent of control subjects in another.[141] The frequency of Epstein-Barr virus detected by polymerase chain reaction studies of peripheral blood leukocytes from 20 children with SLE was no different from the frequency in children with JRA or normal control subjects, however.[142] Studies of immunity to cytomegalovirus and herpes simplex virus I (HSV-I) in adults with SLE indicated that almost 90 percent had antibodies to cytomegalovirus, whereas only 64 percent of patients with rheumatoid arthritis and 43 percent of control subjects were seropositive. The frequency of seropositivity to HSV-1 was the same in patients with SLE or rheumatoid arthritis (80 percent), and only somewhat higher than in the healthy population (59 percent).[143] Although these associations are interesting, studies to date do not prove an etiologic relationship between SLE and any virus. The serologic studies may simply reflect polyclonal B cell activation; the serologic and polymerase chain reaction studies could reflect an effect of SLE on susceptibility to infection with certain viruses, or an effect on their persistence, rather than the cause of SLE.

Drugs and Chemicals

Certain drugs are associated with the induction of a lupus diathesis that differs from idiopathic lupus in being dependent on the presence of the drug. Discontinuation of the offending agent is usually associated with disappearance of the serologic and clinical manifestations of lupus. The etiology and pathogenesis of drug-induced lupus or lupus-like disorders have been recently reviewed.[143a] Drugs implicated in this phenomenon are listed in Table 18–5.[144–151] A review of reported cases documented minocycline-induced lupus in 57 patients with rheumatoid arthritis.[151a] The most common offenders are hydralazine, isoniazid, penicillin, sulfonamides, beta-agonists, and anticonvulsants. Chlorpromazine is associated with a lupus-like syndrome, possibly because it induces apoptosis, thereby leading

Table 18–5

Causes of Drug-Induced Lupus

DEFINITELY ASSOCIATED	POSSIBLY ASSOCIATED
Alpha-methyldopa	Captopril
Chlorpromazine	Carbamazepine
Ethosuximide	L-Canavanine
Hydralazine	Metoprolol
Isoniazid	Minocycline
Phenytoin	Penicillamine
Procainamide	Penicillin
Primidone	Propylthiouracil
Trimethadione	Quinidine
	Sulfonamides

to induction of autoimmunity to nuclear components.[151b]

L-Canavanine, a chemical that is found in alfalfa sprouts and seeds, has been associated with the induction or exacerbation of SLE in a few patients.[152, 153] Furthermore, a diet consisting almost exclusively of alfalfa sprouts and seeds induced reversible SLE in cynomolgus macaque monkeys with high levels of antibody to dsDNA, hypocomplementemia, and diffuse glomerulonephritis.[154] No relationship between use of hair dye and incidence of lupus was found in a recent study.[155]

Other evidence of the role of environmental factors includes the presence of immune complexes in skin biopsy specimens ("lupus band") and lymphocytotoxic antibodies, ANAs, and positive LE-cell preparations among laboratory technicians working with SLE sera.[156] Familial occurrence of SLE has been reported in households where pet dogs had antibodies to dsDNA.[157–159] There have been no recent studies of these questions.

CLINICAL MANIFESTATIONS

Clinical Presentation

Systemic lupus erythematosus ranges from an insidious, chronic illness with a long history of intermittent signs and symptoms to an acute, rapidly fatal disease.[27, 36, 160–166] Constitutional symptoms are very common at onset and during exacerbations (Table 18–6). Intermittent or sustained fever, fatigue, weight loss, and anorexia are manifestations of active disease in most children or may occur as the presenting symptoms. A single system may be affected at onset; however, in most children, multisystem disease is characteristic (Table 18–7).[31] As awareness of the occurrence of SLE in children has increased, early diagnosis has become the rule rather than the exception.

Table 18–6

Clinical Features of Systemic Lupus Erythematosus

Constitutional	Fever, malaise, weight loss
Cutaneous	Butterfly rash, discoid lupus, periungual erythema, photosensitivity, alopecia, mucosal ulcerations
Musculoskeletal	Polyarthralgia and arthritis, tenosynovitis, myopathy, aseptic necrosis
Vascular	Raynaud's phenomenon, livedo reticularis, thrombosis, erythromelalgia, lupus profundus
Cardiac	Pericarditis and effusion, myocarditis, Libman-Sacks endocarditis
Pulmonary	Pleuritis, basilar pneumonitis, atelectasis, hemorrhage
Gastrointestinal	Peritonitis, esophageal dysfunction, colitis
Liver, spleen, nodes	Hepatomegaly, splenomegaly, lymphadenopathy
Neurologic	Organic brain syndrome, seizures, psychosis, chorea, cerebrovascular accident, polyneuritis and peripheral neuropathy, cranial nerve palsies, pseudotumor cerebri
Ocular	Exudates, papilledema, retinopathy
Renal	Glomerulonephritis, nephrotic syndrome, uremia, hypertension

Table 18–7

Manifestations of Systemic Lupus Erythematosus in 58 Children

	PERCENT	
	Initial	Cumulative
Nephritis	84	86
Hypertension	10	28
Arthritis	72	76
Dermatitis	69	76
Malar erythema	51	56
Photosensitivity	16	16
Alopecia	16	20
Oral or nasopharyngeal ulceration	12	16
Raynaud's phenomenon	16	24
Pericarditis	40	47
Pleuritis	31	36
Central nervous system disease	9	31
Hepatomegaly	43	47
Splenomegaly	20	20
Anemia	43	47
Thrombocytopenia	22	27

Modified from Cassidy JT, Sullivan DB, Petty RE, Ragsdale CG: Lupus nephritis and encephalopathy. Prognosis in 58 children. Arthritis Rheum 20(Suppl): 315, Copyright © 1977 Wiley-Liss, Inc. Reprinted by permission of Wiley-Liss, Inc., a subsidiary of John Wiley & Sons, Inc.

Cutaneous Involvement

The rashes of SLE are common at onset and during active disease and are extremely varied in character and distribution. A comprehensive classification and discussion of the cutaneous lesions of SLE can be found in the review by Sontheimer.[167] The classic "butterfly" rash[168] occurs in one third to one half of children at onset of disease,[35, 169] but, although highly suggestive of SLE, it is not pathognomonic (Fig. 18–2). This rash is characteristically symmetric, on both malar eminences, over the bridge of the nose, sometimes on the forehead, but sparing the nasolabial folds. It is usually quite well demarcated and may be slightly raised. Follicular plugging is present, but the lesions do not usually result in scarring. This rash may be precipitated by exposure to sunlight (i.e., it is photosensitive). A similar distribution of erythema occurs in juvenile dermatomyositis, but the lesion is usually less well demarcated. A rare syndrome of telangiectasia in a butterfly-like distribution and membranoproliferative glomerulonephritis may be confused with SLE.[170] As pointed out by Sherwood and colleagues,[170] *Bloom's syndrome*,[171] *Cockayne's syndrome*,[172] and *Rothmund-Thomson syndrome*[173] all have a dermatologic lesion in the butterfly distribution, thereby raising the question of SLE.

A number of other cutaneous manifestations of SLE may occur at onset or during the course of disease. The skin changes in 57 Thai children with SLE are summarized in Table 18–8.[169] Changes such as periungual erythema and livedo reticularis may be underreported in this study, since these abnormalities are

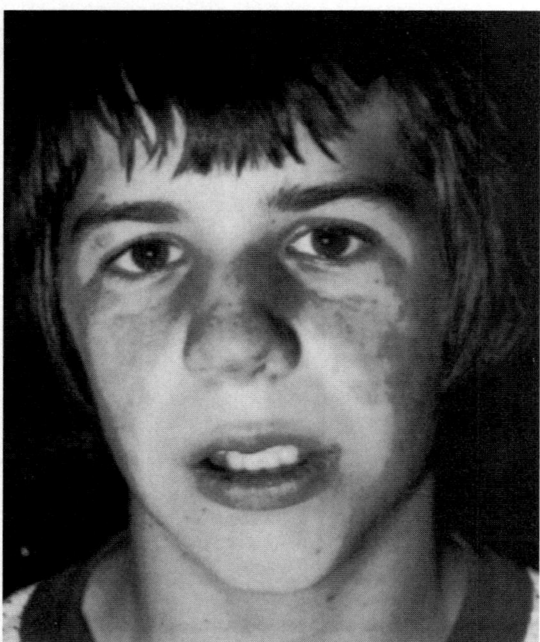

Figure 18–2. Malar erythema of acute SLE. The classic butterfly rash has erupted over both cheeks and spread over the bridge of the nose. It may be punctate and follicular or an erythematous blush. The rash does not leave a scar.

much more readily observed in fair-skinned individuals of European ancestry. Maculopapular rashes as manifestations of vasculitis or perivasculitis may occur anywhere on the body, but particularly on sun-exposed areas (face and upper anterior chest). These lesions are occasionally tender, and angiitic papules on the soles and palms may resemble the Osler nodes and Janeway spots of bacterial endocarditis. Most heal without scarring or pigmentation (Fig. 18–3). Petechiae and purpura may represent perivasculitis or result from thrombocytopenia (Fig. 18–4). Sharply demarcated chronic leg ulcerations may develop around the malleoli (Fig. 18–5), and gangrene may result from severe cutaneous vasculitis or arterial thrombosis associated with the antiphospholipid syndrome. The lesions of subacute cutaneous lupus begin as papules that evolve into annular lesions with raised edges. They are often widespread on trunk, limbs, and face. These lesions may become crusted, hyperpigmented, and atrophic.[174]

Periungual erythema reflects dilatation and tortuosity of the nailfold capillaries, similar to that in dermatomyositis and scleroderma. Nailfold infarcts may also occur (Fig. 18–6). Livedo reticularis occurs, particularly in the lower extremities, reflects active disease, and is associated with the presence of antiphospholipid antibodies.[175]

Discoid lesions in SLE were noted in 19 percent of the patients reported from Thailand,[169] but may be less frequent in children in North America and Europe. Isolated discoid lesions are even less common in children.[176, 177] They most commonly occur on the scalp or limbs in an asymmetric distribution, are sharply demarcated papulosquamous lesions that are often

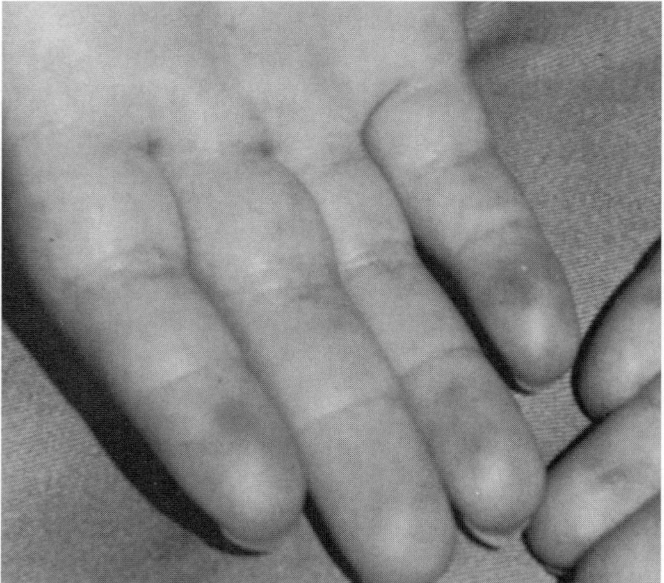

Figure 18–3. Vasculitis seen as punctate erythema of the fingertips of a child with SLE.

Table 18–8

Cutaneous Manifestations of Systemic Lupus Erythematosus in Children

	NUMBER	PERCENT
Skin lesions (all types)	44/57	77
Malar "butterfly" rash	42/57	74
Vasculitis (petechiae, palpable purpura)	22/57	38
Raynaud's phenomenon	4/57	7
Periungual erythema	5/57	9
Periungual gangrene	2/57	4
Nail involvement	2/57	4
Alopecia	18/57	32
Subacute lupus erythematosus	2/57	4
Bullous lupus erythematosus	1/57	2
Discoid lupus erythematosus	11/57	19
Photosensitivity	23/57	40
Urticarial leukocytoclastic vasculitis	1/57	2
Livedo reticularis	1/57	2

Data modified from Wananukul et al.[169]

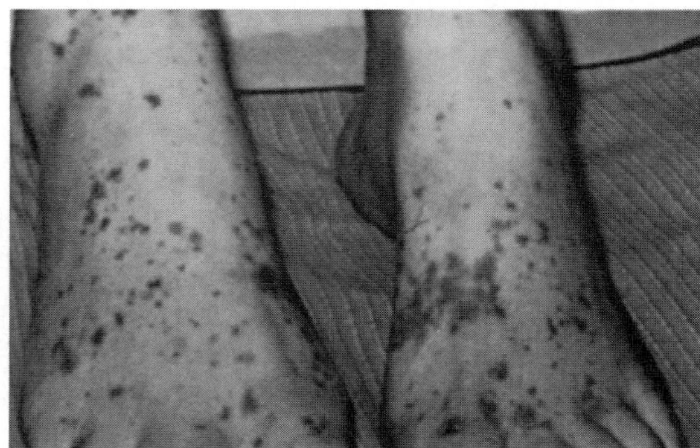

Figure 18–4. Vasculitic purpura in a teenage girl with an acute exacerbation of SLE.

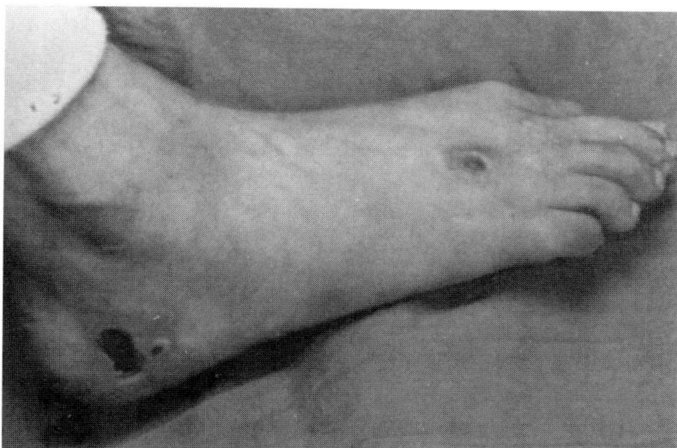

Figure 18–5. Chronic and well-demarcated ulcers of the skin in a child with SLE.

photosensitive, and heal with atrophy, scarring, and alteration of pigmentation (Fig. 18–7). When they occur in the scalp, they may be associated with localized alopecia. Discoid lupus appears to be much more common in black children than in other racial groups.

Alopecia, usually characterized by diffuse thinning of the hair, is associated with active disease. Frontal hair is usually affected initially and becomes brittle and kinky. The initial complaint of the child or parent is that there is excessive hairfall on the pillow, in the hair brush, or after shampooing. Patchy alopecia is less common; total alopecia is very rare. Nail changes, including loss of the nails, occur in up to 15 percent of patients with long-standing disease.[178]

Other infrequent cutaneous complications of SLE include bullae[179–181] and papular mucinosis.[182] Telangiectases occur occasionally. Urticarial lesions can occur at any time. Nodules, either resembling erythema nodosum or rheumatoid nodules, occur in approximately 5 percent of patients and may suggest the presence of an overlap syndrome. Lupus profundus[183] has rarely been described in childhood.[184] Chilblain lupus is a chronic unremitting form of SLE that occurs predominantly in women, although we have observed it in children. It results from cold exposure and possibly hyperviscosity.[185] Persistent warts are common in children with SLE

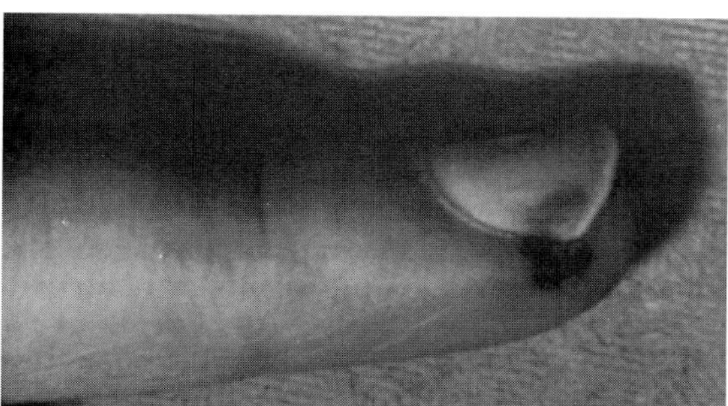

Figure 18–6. Nailfold infarct in a 22-year-old man with SLE for 14 years. Ischemic necrosis of the fingers developed after 2 years of remission from a clinical course punctuated with cardiopulmonary onset, polyarthritis, diffuse proliferative nephritis, and more recently, central nervous system lupus. The digital lesions healed completely in 5 months with prednisone and prazosin therapy.

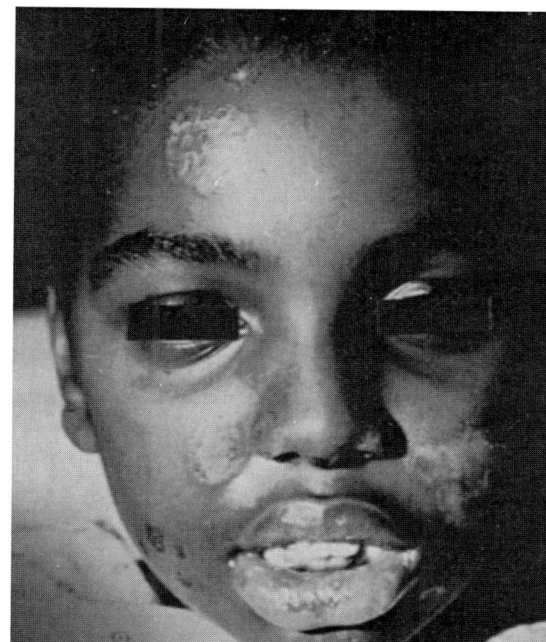

Figure 18–7. Discoid lesions and mucocutaneous disease are present in this teenage boy who had anti-Ro antibody.

and appear to be related both to the disease[186] and to the effects of immunosuppressive treatment.

Mucosal Involvement

The oral mucosa is the site of ulceration in some children with SLE. The classic lesion is a painless, shallow, ragged ulcer on the hard palate. Although this involvement is relatively uncommon, erythema of the hard palate is quite common and suggestive of the diagnosis (Fig. 18–8). Occasionally, ulceration or perforation of the nasal septum is observed. Aphthous stomatitis is perhaps a more frequent but less specific finding, since such changes occur frequently in the otherwise healthy population.

Musculoskeletal Disease

Arthralgia and arthritis affect the majority of children with SLE. The arthritis is characteristically short in duration, lasting 24 to 48 hours, and can be migratory. Joint pain is often severe even though objective findings are minimal. Arthritis commonly involves the small joints of the hands, wrists, elbows, shoulders, knees, and ankles. Tenosynovitis on the dorsum of the hand and wrist commonly accompanies arthritis of the small joints of the hands. In some children, the arthritis is persistent and is characterized by swelling, tenderness, and loss of range of motion. Although the synovitis of SLE may be minimally proliferative, it is only occasionally erosive[187] and usually does not result in permanent deformity. A Jaccoud type of arthritis (reversible subluxation related to tenosynovitis) may be

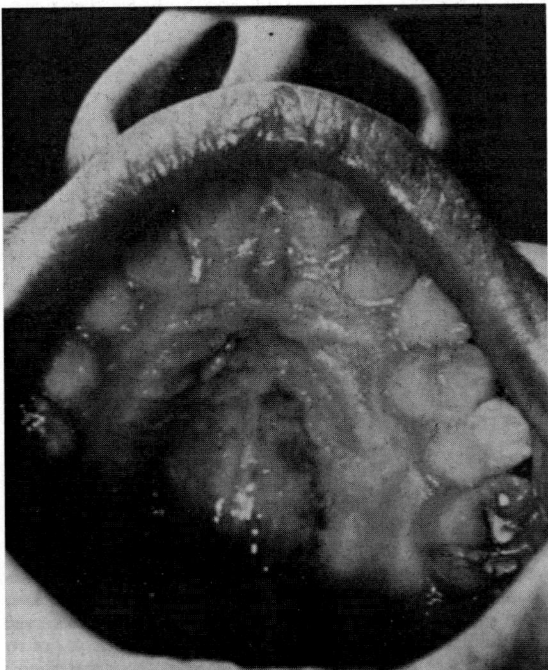

Figure 18–8. Mucocutaneous ulcerations of acute SLE. A shallow, painless, erythematous ulceration with an irregular margin is seen on the hard palate.

associated with the presence of antibodies to U1 ribonucleoprotein (U1RNP).[188]

Myalgia or muscle weakness is characteristic of the acutely ill patient[189] and is most prominent proximally. The occurrence of myositis is often related to the presence of systemic vasculitis and involvement of viscera. Steroid myopathy, in which serum levels of muscle enzymes are normal, must be distinguished later in the disease from a recurrence of myositis, in which enzyme levels are usually elevated. Myasthenia gravis occurs in a small number of patients with SLE, although the significance of the association is uncertain.[190]

Ischemic necrosis of bone is a significant risk in young patients with SLE,[191] especially in those treated for long periods with glucocorticoid drugs.[192–194] It can occur anywhere but is most common in weight-bearing bones, such as the femoral heads and tibial plateaus (Fig. 18–9).

Lupus Nephritis

Lupus nephritis is probably present to some degree in all children with SLE and is a major determinant of the long-term outcome of this disease. Clinically evident nephritis occurs in at least 75 percent of children with lupus[20, 195] and may be more frequent and of greater severity in children than adults.[36] The frequency with which clinically evident renal disease occurs at disease onset is uncertain, and lupus nephritis is usually initially asymptomatic, although a few children develop gross hematuria or edema associated with the nephrotic syndrome. Using data from his own and reported series, Cameron[195] estimated that the most common initial manifestation of nephritis is microscopic hematuria (79 percent), followed by proteinuria, including nephrotic syndrome (55 percent). Decreased glomerular filtration (50 percent) and hypertension (40 percent) were also common, but acute renal failure as a presenting manifestation of renal lupus was rare (1.4 percent). Correlations between clinical disease and renal biopsy abnormalities are summarized in Table 18–9.

Significant renal disease usually develops within 2 years after onset but occasionally appears many years later. Clinical nephritis was recorded 11 years after onset in one child,[27] and 12 years after diagnosis in another.[196] Histologic evidence of renal disease may precede the development of changes in the urinary sediment by months, and routine monitoring of urine for proteinuria and hematuria, as well as assessment of renal function by measurement of creatinine clearance or radionuclide glomerular filtration rates, are essential components of the management of all children from the onset of disease. The expertise of a nephrologist as a member of the team that is providing ongoing care is essential.

Interstitial cystitis occurred early in the course of disease in an 8-year-old girl with SLE and glomerulonephritis. She had not received cyclophosphamide and the disease responded to cyclosporin A.[197]

Central Nervous System Disease

Central nervous system (CNS) disease ranks second only to nephritis as a cause of morbidity and mortality in patients with SLE,[198, 199] occurring in 20 to 40 percent

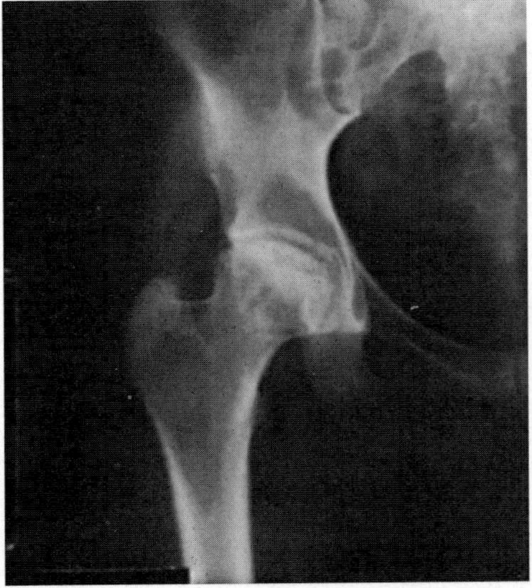

Figure 18–9. Aseptic necrosis of the femoral head in a young woman with SLE who had been treated with prednisone for 11 years. She developed anterior groin pain on weight bearing. The joint space is preserved, but there is mottled increased density and deformity of the femoral head. A semilunar area of separation of the bone is present, indicating osteonecrosis. The patient's symptoms and disability resolved only partially with reduction of prednisone and a trial of no weight bearing.

Table 18–9

Correlations of Histopathologic Characteristics and Clinical State in Lupus Nephritis

TYPE OF RENAL DISEASE	NEPHROTIC SYNDROME	RENAL FAILURE	REMISSION	UREMIC DEATHS
Glomerular				
Mesangial	−	−	+	−
Focal proliferative	±	±	+ +	±
Diffuse proliferative	+ +	+ +	±	+ + +
Membranous	+ + +	+ +	+	+
Extraglomerular				
Interstitial	+	+	±	±
Necrotizing arteritis	±	+	+	±
End-stage	+ +	+ + +	−	+ + +

−, absent; ±, minimal; +, moderate; + +, marked; + + +, very marked.

of affected children.[27, 36, 160, 200–203] Some evidence of CNS involvement is present at disease onset in approximately half of the children and adolescents with lupus, has onset in the first year of disease in 40 percent, or may not appear until many years later.[203] The most common manifestations are listed in Table 18–10.

Neuropsychiatric manifestations appear to be most common and include depression, difficulty concentrating and remembering, and psychosis (including hallucinations and paranoia).[203–206] Depression is particularly common and it may be difficult to differentiate depression caused by concern about the effects of the disease or side-effects of therapy from organic depression. The change in physical appearance caused by glucocorticoid therapy is especially difficult for adolescent patients and alone may lead to major depression and noncompliance with treatment. Emotional lability is common in young patients with SLE, often in the absence of other evidence of CNS disease. An organic brain syndrome characterized by disorientation, memory loss, and progressive intellectual deterioration is a grave development prognostically.[198] It may, of course, be a manifestation of a transient metabolic encephalopathy or be related to malignant hypertension.[207]

Cognitive impairment has been noted in a number of patients with SLE, and it is not uncommon for a child with acute SLE to have increasing difficulty with school and falling academic grades.[208] Silber and colleagues[206] found significant psychometric abnormalities in 21 of 32 children with SLE. Cognitive impairment was present in 52 percent of the children, and an additional 29 percent were considered to be borderline abnormal. A study that compared children with SLE and those with JRA indicated that those with SLE had greater neuropsychologic impairment. Furthermore, a specific deficit in complex problem-solving ability was noted. Long disease duration was found to correlate with lower Intelligence Quotient score.[209]

Headache, a frequent and annoying complaint in patients with SLE, has many causes, and determining the relationship of headache to CNS lupus is often difficult. Most reports note that vascular migraine-like headaches are more frequent in patients with SLE than in control subjects.[210] In a recent questionnaire study of 78 adults with SLE including 10 with CNS involvement and 89 healthy individuals matched for age, sex, and socioeconomic status, however, no difference in the frequency of headache (0–32 percent) was noted.[211] In three girls with cerebral vein thrombosis, unremitting headache was a prominent complaint.[212]

Seizures are occasionally the initial manifestation of lupus. They are usually generalized tonic-clonic in

Table 18–10

Frequencies of Central Nervous System Complications of Systemic Lupus Erythematosus

	STEINLIN ET AL[203] $n = 40$ (%)	PARIKH ET AL[202] $n = 25$ (%)	YANCEY ET AL[199] $n = 16$ (%)
Psychiatric manifestations	48	40	56
Headache	22	64	44
Seizures	20	20	31
Cerebrovascular accidents	15	28	—
Chorea	3	28	—
Peripheral neuropathy	5	—	6
Papilledema	5	—	12
Visual loss	—	8	6
Vertigo	—	4	—
Myelopathy	—	1	—

type, although focal seizures sometimes occur. Cerebrovascular accidents may occur independently or with venous sinus thrombosis or cerebral vein thrombosis,[203, 212] and may be associated with hypertension, antiphospholipid-related thrombosis, or intracranial hemorrhage secondary to thrombocytopenia. Diagnostic tests used in the evaluation of CNS lupus are listed in Table 18–11.

Chorea is an uncommon complication occurring in 4 to 10 percent of children with SLE[31, 32, 36, 199, 213–219] and has developed in only three girls under our observation. It may precede other manifestations of SLE, leading to an incorrect diagnosis of acute rheumatic fever, or it may occur months or years after onset of lupus. It is usually unilateral. A rare manifestation of CNS lupus that resembles Parkinson's disease may be difficult to differentiate from psychosis.[220] One child in a report by Shar and colleagues[220] presented with rigidity, irritability, and mutism leading to an initial diagnosis of psychosis. The second child had progressive bradykinesia and was thought to be depressed. ^{99m}Tc-HmPAO single photon emission computed tomography scanning documented impaired blood flow to the basal ganglia. Both responded to dopamine-agonist drugs. Myelopathy has been rarely reported in children.[221] We have observed transient myelopathy following lumbar puncture in one girl with SLE complicated by a retinal vein thrombosis. It may have been related to an antiphospholipid antibody syndrome.

The results of two recent large studies of neurologic findings in childhood and adolescent onset SLE illustrate the diversity of abnormalities observed. Parikh and colleagues[202] noted neurologic abnormalities in 25 of 108 (23 percent) of a series of patients with onset of SLE before the age of 20 years.[202] Headache occurred in 16 of 25; behavioral changes in 10 of 25 (most commonly depression), hemichorea or chorea in 7, cerebrovascular accident with hemiplegia or diplegia in 7, generalized tonic-clonic seizures in 5, visual loss in 3, and cranial neuropathy in 2. Vertigo and myelopathy each occurred in 1 patient. In a study by Steinlin and coworkers,[203] CNS abnormalities were noted in 40 of 91 patients with onset of SLE before 18 years of age. The gender ratio in patients with CNS involvement was the same as that for the SLE group as a whole. In 47 percent of patients with CNS involvement, it was present at diagnosis; in a further 30 percent, it occurred during the first year of the illness. CNS manifestations in the remaining 23 percent did not occur until up to 7 years after disease onset. The most common manifestations were neuropsychiatric: 11 of 19 patients had frank psychoses, 6 had cognitive impairment or emotional lability, and 2 had severe depression. Psychotic episodes were often multiple and required hospitalization. Severe headache occurred in 9 children; in 5 patients it was present at onset and accompanied by papilledema. Seizures occurred in 8 patients and followed a cerebrovascular accident in 2. Peripheral neuropathy occurred in 2 patients and chorea occurred in 1 patient. Aseptic meningitis was observed in 1 patient and was ascribed to indomethacin. Cranial nerve palsy including facial palsy is rare.[222] Pseudotumor cerebri can develop as a direct complication of active SLE or may be related to inappropriately rapid tapering of the glucocorticoid dose.[223] Narcolepsy (a disorder that is strongly associated with HLA-DR2, DQw1, and is characterized by extreme sleepiness and cataplexy) has been reported in an 18-year-old girl with SLE.[224]

Table 18–11

Evaluation of Central Nervous System Lupus Erythematosus

EXAMINATION	PURPOSE
Cerebrospinal fluid examination	Exclude infection, subarachnoid hemorrhage
Neurocognitive testing	Detection of subtle changes in cognition
Electroencephalography	Provide evidence of diffuse or local abnormality
Computed tomography	Document focal lesion
Magnetic resonance imaging	Characterize focal lesion
Magnetic resonance angiography	Characterize focal lesion
Positron emission tomography	Document abnormal function

Cardiac Involvement

Pericarditis

Pericarditis is the most common cardiac manifestation of SLE, occurring in up to 30 percent of children with acute disease. It may be clinically silent, or it may be represented by precordial pain exacerbated by lying down or deep breathing, and relieved by sitting up and leaning forward. It is often not accompanied by a friction rub or obvious cardiomegaly. Occasionally, lower anterior midline chest pain that is thought to be pleuropericardial in origin may persist for many months or years. Pericardial inflammation leading to constriction[225] or tamponade[226–230] is rare but can be a presenting feature of SLE.[227, 228]

Myocarditis

Myocarditis occurs in approximately 10 to 15 percent of adults with SLE,[231] and in a similar frequency in children.[232] It is characterized clinically by congestive heart failure, cardiomegaly, arrhythmias, and a narrow pulse pressure. The presence of tachycardia in the absence of fever suggests the presence of myocarditis in children with SLE and should prompt electrocardiographic investigation.

Myocardial Infarction

There have been a few instances of myocardial infarction in childhood SLE, usually in older patients with long-standing disease.[233–242] However, the extent of coronary artery disease is probably considerably underestimated and multifactorial in pathogenesis.

Gazarian and colleagues[243] studied children and adolescents with SLE by thallium myocardial perfusion scans, radionuclide angiography with multiple gated acquisition, and resting M-mode and two-dimension echocardiography. None of the patients had a history of ischemic heart disease or electrocardiographic abnormalities. Ventricular wall function was normal, but four children had reversible abnormalities of myocardial perfusion scans indicating deficient myocardial perfusion. One child had a fixed myocardial perfusion defect. Anticardiopin antibodies and elevated plasma lipids were present in many of the children with and without perfusion defects. In this study, duration of glucocorticoid therapy was shorter in the group with perfusion defects, in contrast to the conclusions of studies in adults in which those with the most severe coronary artery disease had highest cumulative dose and longest duration of therapy with prednisone.[244]

Valvulitis

The classic cardiac lesion of SLE, Libman-Sacks endocarditis, is probably less common in children than in adults and is often subclinical. It is characterized by the presence of 1- to 4-mm nodules of fibrinoid necrosis of the supporting collagenous tissues of the valve.[4] The mitral valve is most commonly affected, and the aortic, pulmonic, and tricuspid valves may be involved in descending order of frequency. A clinically significant or changing murmur may or may not be present. Superimposed infectious endocarditis can also occur. Kornreich and Hanson found that the postmortem findings of endocarditis did not correlate well with the presence or absence of heart murmurs during life.[200]

Transesophageal echocardiography in 69 adults with SLE disclosed valvular abnormalities in 61 percent.[245] The most common findings were valvular thickening (51 percent), vegetations (43 percent), regurgitation (25 percent), and stenosis (4 percent). There are reports of valve disease in children with SLE that required surgical replacement of the damaged valve.[245–247] The importance of antiphospholipid antibodies to the development of cardiac valve disease is controversial, although a strong association has been noted in some studies.[248] Similarly, antibodies to SS-A (Ro) and SS-B (La) have been reported to be associated with a higher frequency of valvular disease in children with SLE.[249]

Accelerated Atherosclerosis

Two factors contribute to accelerated atherosclerosis in patients with SLE: long-term administration of glucocorticoid drugs[250] and abnormalities of plasma lipids.[251, 252] In a study of 19 children with SLE, Ilowite and colleagues[251] found dyslipoproteinemia in the majority. The dyslipoproteinemia of active SLE was characterized by elevations of the very low density lipoprotein (VLDL) cholesterol and triglyceride levels and decreases of high density lipoprotein (HDL) cholesterol and apoprotein A-I levels. Glucocorticoid-induced changes included increased total cholesterol, VLDL cholesterol, and triglyceride levels. It has been estimated that approximately 5 percent of adult patients with SLE experience nonfatal myocardial infarctions, and an equal number have fatal infarctions.[233–236, 253–255] However, a much larger percentage develop cardiomyopathy[256] and on angiography 45 percent have been demonstrated to have narrowing of at least one coronary artery.[257] A recent study[257a] measured carotid media–intima thickness by ultrasound in 26 patients with juvenile-onset SLE. Artery thickening was significantly more common in patients with SLE than in controls, and correlated with the presence of nephrotic-range proteinuria.

Pleuropulmonary Disease

Clinical or subclinical pleuropulmonary disease is a frequent manifestation of childhood SLE (Table 18–12). In a study of 22 children with SLE,[45] 17 (77 percent) had respiratory symptoms (cough, chest pain, dyspnea, orthopnea), and radiographic abnormalities were demonstrated in one half. Pleuropulmonary disease may be particularly common in North American Indian children.[45] The most frequently described pleuropulmonary manifestations are pleural effusions and pleuritis,[161, 258] acute and chronic pneumonitis,[259, 260] and pulmonary hemorrhage.[35, 260–263] *Shrinking lung,* the loss of lung volume that is the result of diaphragmatic

Table 18–12

Comparison of Pulmonary Manifestations in Childhood Onset and Adult Onset Systemic Lupus Erythematosus

ABNORMALITY	CHILDHOOD ONSET (%)	ADULT ONSET (%)
Subclinical (abnormal pulmonary function tests only)	60	>50
Pleural effusions	27	>50
Shrinking lungs (diaphragmatic dysfunction)	13	25
Pulmonary infiltrates/atelectasis	13	>50
Acute lupus pneumonitis	9	10
Pneumothorax	9	Occasional
Pleuropulmonary infections	Common	50
Pulmonary hemorrhage	6	<2
Diffuse interstitial disease	Occasional	<5
Pulmonary hypertension	Rare	Occasional

Modified from Delgado EA, Malleson PN, Pirie GE, Petty RE: The pulmonary manifestations of childhood onset systemic lupus erythematosus. Semin Arthritis Rheum 19: 285, 1990.

dysfunction,[264] is less commonly identified, although it may be observed after long-term follow-up as progressive elevation of the level of the diaphragm. Pneumothorax and cavitary nodules have been reported occasionally.[45] A syndrome of reversible hypoxemia has been noted in severely ill adults with SLE without evidence of parenchymal lung involvement.[265] Changes in the quality of the voice (dysphonia or hoarseness) have been noted occasionally in adult patients with SLE,[266, 267] and we have observed two adolescents with persistent hoarseness, which was one of the presenting complaints in one patient.

Pleural effusions are common and may result from inflammatory pleuritis or occasionally be secondary to the nephrotic syndrome. Noninflammatory pleural effusions are usually asymptomatic. Inflammatory pleuritis usually causes unilateral or bilateral pleuritic chest pain that is exacerbated by deep inspiration. Occasionally pleuritic pain is the initial manifestation of the disease. The effusions are usually of small volume and seldom cause respiratory embarrassment, but occasionally very large bilateral pleural effusions occur and may require urgent paracentesis.

Acute lupus pneumonitis consisting of pulmonary infiltrates and atelectasis occurs in 10 to 15 percent of children with SLE.[42, 259, 260] Patients usually have symptoms similar to those who have pulmonary hemorrhage, except that anemia is not a feature, and hemoptysis is absent or minimal. Bibasilar rales may be present, and radiographs reveal basilar infiltrates. Chronic interstitial lung disease characterized by chronic nonproductive cough, recurrent pleuritic chest pain, and dyspnea on exertion has been reported in adults with SLE,[268] but not in children.

Although the overall incidence of pulmonary hemorrhage is estimated at less than 2 percent in a recent large series of adults with SLE,[269] this complication occurred in 6 percent of a series of children with SLE. In another study,[270] pulmonary hemorrhage, sometimes preceded by chest pain and hemoptysis, occurred in seven children and was a major factor in the death of four. A recent case report documented the occurrence of pulmonary hemorrhage as the sole presenting manifestation of lupus in a 13-year-old girl.[271] Intra-alveolar hemorrhage can mimic congestive heart failure and pneumonitis, or it can present with sudden pallor and tachycardia with hemoptysis, although hemoptysis is not always present. A rapidly falling hematocrit with shifting pulmonary infiltrates in a patient with lupus should suggest the diagnosis of pulmonary hemorrhage even in the absence of hemoptysis. Chest radiographs, including computed tomography, demonstrate characteristic changes (Fig. 18–10) Pulmonary hypertension may be present in such patients..

Pneumocystis carinii pneumonia has been documented in three children with SLE, all of whom were receiving glucocorticoids and azathioprine therapy and were mildly lymphopenic.[272] The clinical presentations included cough and dyspnea. Two responded to cotrimoxazole; one died, presumably from the effects of *Pneumocystis* and other concomitant infections.[273] Infection with other opportunistic organisms such as *Nocardia* has also been reported.[274]

The relationship between antiphospholipid antibodies and pulmonary disease has recently been reviewed.[275] The pulmonary disorders that may be associated with antiphospholipid antibodies include pulmonary embolism, pulmonary hypertension, and pulmonary artery thrombosis.

Tests of pulmonary function in patients with SLE often document a moderate to marked functional impairment despite a normal radiologic appearance of the lungs (Table 18–13).[224, 225, 269, 276] Restrictive lung disease and diffusion defects are the most commonly observed abnormalities. Pulmonary function test abnormalities may be present in children with no clinical or radiographic evidence of lung disease. In a study of 15 such children, 40 percent had reduced forced vital capacity and 26 percent had reduced DLCO. These abnormalities increased over time.[277] Unexplained

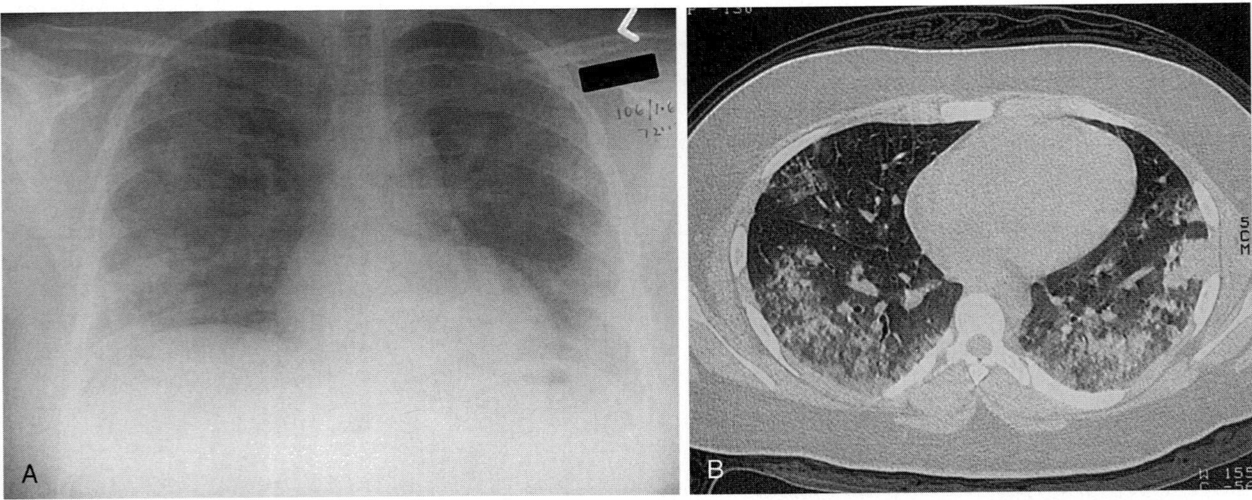

Figure 18–10. Radiograph *(A)* and thin-section computed tomogram *(B)* of the chest of a 14-year-old girl with acute onset of pulmonary hemorrhage and thrombocytopenia as the initial manifestation of SLE showing widespread airspace and interstitial disease. The abnormalities completely resolved after therapy with high-dose prednisone.

Table 18–13

Pulmonary Function in Childhood Onset SLE

STUDY	SUBJECT (*n*)	CLINICAL DISEASE (%)	RADIOGRAPHIC CHANGES (%)	% WITH PULMONARY FUNCTION TEST ABNORMALITY			
				Any	Restrictive	Obstructive	Diffusion
De Jonste et al[259]	8	87	87	87	50	0	100*
Singsen & Platzker[260]	20	†	†	35	35	55	25
Weiss et al[276]	28	?	?	64	61	3	35‡
Delgado et al[45]	13	85	54	62	46	8	67§

*Diffusion measured in 6 children was diminished for surface area, but normal or increased for remaining lung volume.
†Patients with clinical or radiographic evidence of lung disease were excluded from this study.
‡20 patients studied.
§Diffusion abnormal at one time or another in 6 of 9 patients. (Diffusion appropriate for lung size in 4 of the 6.)

dyspnea and cyanosis are present in some patients. If these signs are transient or episodic, subclinical thromboembolic phenomena should be considered.

Disturbances of Coagulation

Antiphospholipid Syndrome

The antiphospholipid syndrome (APLS)[278] is characterized by the presence of antibodies to phospholipids such as cardiolipin, and a number of clinical manifestations shown in Table 18–14.

Based on a study of 667 consecutive patients with SLE, Alarcon-Segovia and coworkers[279] recommended a set of criteria for the classification of APLS. Definite APLS was defined as the presence of a high level of antibody to phospholipid (enzyme-linked immunosorbent assay optical density value for IgG or IgM > 5 SD of the normal mean), plus two or more of the following clinical manifestations: recurrent fetal loss, venous thrombosis, arterial occlusion, leg ulcer, livedo reticularis, hemolytic anemia, or thrombocytopenia. Using such criteria, 10 percent of their patients had APLS.

Table 18–14

Classification Criteria for Antiphospholipid Syndrome

Definite Antiphospholipid Syndrome

Two or more of the following clinical manifestations:
- Recurrent fetal loss
- Venous thrombosis
- Arterial occlusion
- Leg ulcer
- Livedo reticularis
- Hemolytic anemia
- Thrombocytopenia

Plus high level (>5 SD above normal mean) of IgG or IgM antiphospholipid antibody

Probable Antiphospholipid Syndrome

Two or more of the clinical manifestations listed above, and low level (>2, <5 SD above normal mean) of IgG or IgM antiphospholipid antibody

From Alarcon-Segovia D, Perez-Vasquez AR, Villa AR, et al: Preliminary classification criteria for the antiphospholipid syndrome. Semin Arthritis Rheum 21: 275, 1992.

An international consensus statement proposed classification criteria for APLS.[278a] Definite APLS required the presence of one clinical criterion (vascular thrombosis or pregnancy loss) plus one laboratory criterion (presence of β_2 glycoprotein I–dependent anticardiolipin antibodies of medium or high titer, or lupus anticoagulant).

In a retrospective study,[161] 9 percent of 42 children with SLE had one or more episodes of thrombosis, sometimes as the presenting manifestation of the disease. Thrombosis of leg veins was most common, but cerebral artery thrombosis, renal artery thrombosis,[280] and arterial occlusions in other sites have been reported.[281] We have observed such patients in our clinics: one with thrombosis of the retro-orbital plexus and transverse myelitis, a second with thrombosis of the right middle cerebral artery, and a third with thrombosis of the anterior tibial artery. Chorea may also be a manifestation of APLS in childhood.[282] Spontaneous recurrent abortions and cardiovascular crises such as myocardial infarction and valvular lesions[283–285] have been observed in young adults with antiphospholipid antibodies. Menorrhagia in adolescent girls may result from this circulating anticoagulant. Spontaneous bleeding is uncommon, however, and thrombosis is more characteristic.

A number of abnormalities in addition to antiphospholipid antibodies can contribute to intravascular thrombosis in patients with SLE. Elevations of homocysteine levels are associated with arterial thrombotic events in lupus.[286] In adults, acquired protein S deficiency has been identified as an additional risk factor for thrombosis, often in association with antiphospholipid antibodies.[287, 288] Much less commonly, epistaxis, easy bruising, gingival bleeding, or menorrhagia may occur as a result of acquired hypoprothombinemia (factor II deficiency).[289] Such patients also have a lupus anticoagulant, and antibodies to factor II have been demonstrated.[290] The disorder usually responds to glucocorticoids with or without vitamin K and fresh frozen plasma.

Thrombotic Thrombocytopenic Purpura

The combination of thrombocytopenic purpura (TTP) and acute hemolytic anemia (Evans' syndrome) is seen

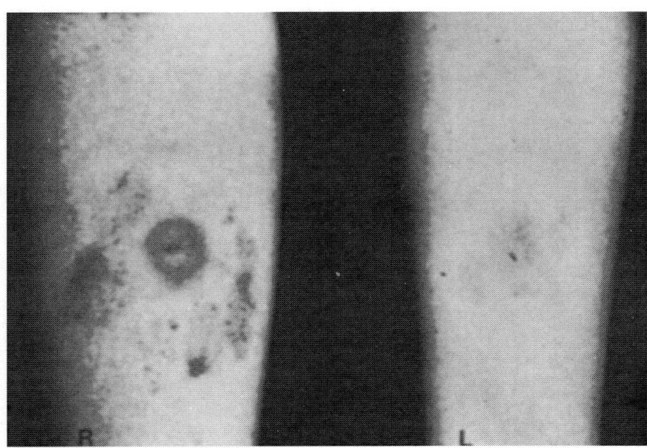

Figure 18–11. Volar surfaces of the forearms of a 10-year-old boy diagnosed as having the Gardner-Diamond syndrome. A large area of inflammatory change and ecchymosis was produced in the right forearm by the subcutaneous injection of "ghosts" prepared from his red blood cell membranes. Except for subcutaneous bleeding, no inflammatory changes were produced in the left arm by injection of a comparable amount of buffer.

in isolation and with SLE.[291, 292] TTP may occur as a hypersensitivity reaction to drugs or recent immunization and may also complicate carcinoma, inflammatory arthritis, and pregnancy. It has been associated with a wide variety of infections. TTP occurs primarily in young women but is similar in many ways to the hemolytic-uremic syndrome seen in children. It has an acute onset and is often fatal. In addition to anemia and purpura, these patients have fever, changing CNS signs, and nephritis.

The primary laboratory abnormalities include leukocytosis, thrombocytopenia, and microangiopathic hemolytic anemia characterized by the presence of bizarre red blood cells, especially helmet cells. The Coombs test is usually negative. Histologically, there is widespread occlusion of arterioles and capillaries by fibrin-containing hyaline thrombi. Punch biopsy of skin can often document these changes.

Although outcome is improving,[292] treatment is often unsuccessful and the course may be brief and fulminant. Glucocorticoids and anticoagulants have been used successfully in some persons, and splenectomy is occasionally performed. Plasmapheresis and blood exchange have been used with some success.[293–295]

Auto-Erythrocyte Sensitization

A syndrome of auto-erythrocyte sensitization, consisting of large inflammatory lesions in the skin in response to minor trauma, was first described by Gardner and Diamond.[296–299] Subcutaneous injection of autologous erythrocyte membranes reproduces the lesions (Fig. 18–11). The syndrome is most often seen in adolescent girls and has been associated with psychiatric disturbances. It has been described in one boy.[299] There is no known relationship of this syndrome to SLE, but its clinical manifestations may mimic SLE.

Vasculitis

The vasculitis of SLE affects small blood vessels, arterioles, and venules, in contrast to polyarteritis, in which there is preferential involvement of the medium-sized arteries.[27, 300] *Lupus crisis* is the sudden development of overwhelming, often fatal, systemic disease resulting from widespread acute vasculitis.

Raynaud's phenomenon, a frequent finding in children with SLE and other diffuse connective tissue diseases, is characterized by sequential color changes in the distal extremities. The initial event is blanching of the distal phalanges, usually related to exposure to cold or emotional upset. This initial phase of digital ischemia is followed by cyanosis caused by anoxia and desaturation. A reactive phase of hyperemia supervenes, accompanied by ischemic pain. To make the diagnosis, the blanching phase and at least one other color phase should be present. Raynaud's phenomenon in SLE is in part vasospastic but is also indicative of structural vascular disease. The skin of the fingers may eventually become atrophic and shiny (sclerodactyly). Vascular necrosis, digital ulceration, and gangrene follow in a minority of affected children (Fig. 18–12). Significant Raynaud's phenomenon should raise the possibility of an overlap syndrome (see Chapter 23). Edema of the lower extremities is usually related to congestive heart failure or nephrotic syndrome rather than to localized vasculitis.

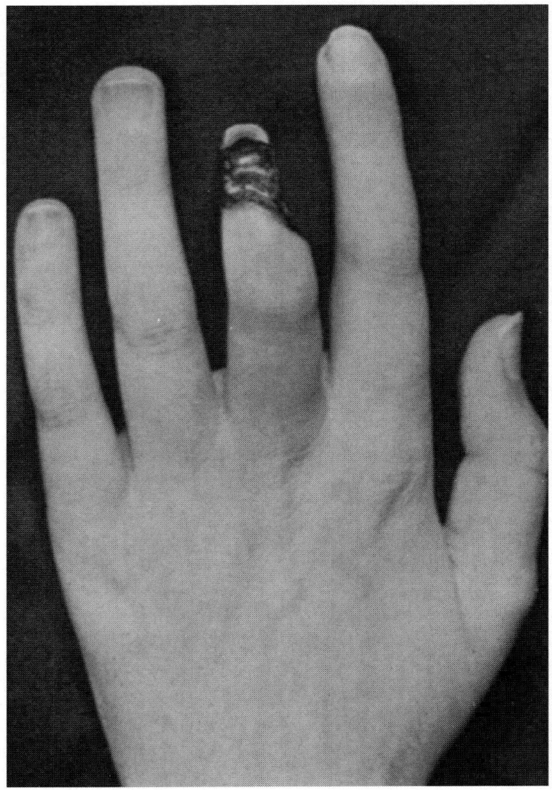

Figure 18–12. Gangrene affecting the distal phalanx of the third finger of a 12-year-old boy with SLE. The distal digit eventually autoamputated.

Ocular Disease

Cotton-wool spots (cytoid bodies) are evidence of retinal vasculitis (Fig. 18–13). They occur singly or in small numbers in a para-arteriolar location in the posterior pole of the retina. They are highly suggestive of the diagnosis of SLE in the absence of other systemic disease such as hypertension, diabetes, or severe anemia, which may cause similar exudative lesions in the nerve cell layer. They have been occasionally reported in children with dermatomyositis, polyarteritis, or scleroderma. Other ocular manifestations include subretinal edema or hemorrhage, occlusion of the central retinal vein, and episcleritis.

Table 18–15

Sjögren's Syndrome

Definition	Keratoconjunctivitis sicca (dry eyes secondary to decreased tear production by lacrimal glands) and xerostomia (dry mouth secondary to decreased saliva production by salivary glands)
Primary Sjögren's syndrome	Not associated with any other disease; rare in childhood
Secondary Sjögren's syndrome	Associated with a connective tissue disease, most often systemic lupus erythematosus or mixed connective tissue; disease uncommon in childhood
Autoantibodies	Anti-Ro(SS-A) (95%) Anti-La(SS-B) (85%)

Sjögren's Syndrome

Keratoconjunctivitis sicca (xerostomia) occurring as part of Sjögren's syndrome is an uncommon complication of childhood SLE. Until 1988, only 11 children had been reported with Sjögren's syndrome accompanying SLE or mixed connective tissue disease (secondary Sjögren's syndrome).[301] It is characterized clinically by a gritty feeling in the eyes, conjunctival injection, and photophobia. Schirmer's test indicates deficient tear flow (< 5 mm wetting of a filter paper strip in 15 minutes), and Rose-Bengal or fluorescein staining of the cornea may demonstrate superficial corneal erosions. Patients with keratoconjunctivitis sicca usually also have inflammation of the salivary glands with a deficiency of saliva resulting in painful or painless unilateral or bilateral parotid gland swelling, difficulty chewing and swallowing, abnormalities of taste, severe dental caries, and halitosis. Demonstration of ectasis of the parotid ducts by sialography[302] or decreased uptake of ^{99m}technetium pertechnetate, or abnormalities on magnetic resonance images[303] support the diagnosis, which is confirmed, if necessary, by biopsy of a minor salivary gland from the lower lip demonstrating periductal lymphocytic infiltrates.[304] Dryness of other mucosal surfaces, including nose, pharynx, and vagina, may occur. Sjögren's syndrome is strongly associated with the presence of antibodies to the extractable nuclear antigens SS-A (Ro) and SS-B (La) (Table 18–15). (See Chapter 23.)

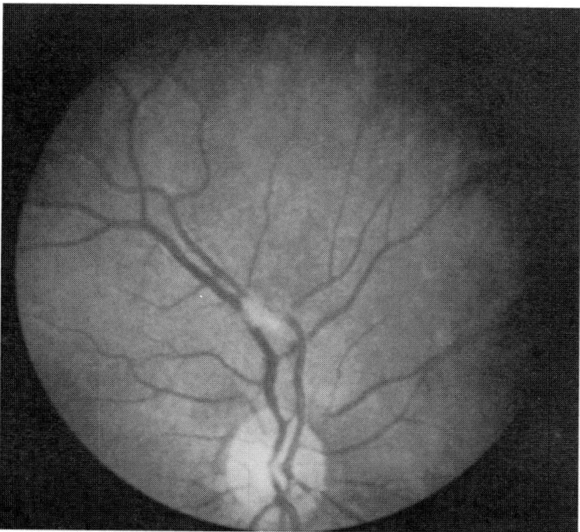

Figure 18–13. An oval white cotton wool spot (CWS) in the posterior retinal pole. A CWS is invariably in a para-arteriolar position and often partially obliterates the adjacent arteriole. CWSs arise from segmental vasculitis within and adjacent to these vessels. The surrounding retina generally shows an edematous sheen. In SLE, one usually finds only a few CWSs. Identical lesions may rarely be seen in other connective tissue diseases. In hypertension, diabetes, or septicemia, numerous CWSs may be present.

Gastrointestinal Manifestations

An association between pancreatitis and SLE has been recorded in a number of children.[305–308] Symptoms include diffuse abdominal pain, nausea, and vomiting. Serum lipase and amylase levels suggest the diagnosis. There is usually a response to glucocorticoids, but the complication is occasionally fatal.[307] Drugs, including glucocorticoids and immunosuppressives, have been implicated in the etiology of pancreatitis, but the evidence for this causality is scant.[307]

Protein-losing enteropathy has been reported in three children and more than 20 adults with SLE.[309] Rare reports of children with SLE and celiac disease,[310] ulcerative colitis,[311] or Crohn's disease[312] probably represent coincidental occurrence of both diseases rather than specific associations.

Hepatic Disease

Hepatomegaly occurs in up to two thirds of children with SLE[36] but is usually of mild degree. In some cases, it may also be a manifestation of fatty infiltration of the liver related in part to glucocorticoid therapy.[313] Jaundice is rare but may result from antibody-mediated hemolysis. Granulomatous hepatitis is rare.[28]

The term *lupoid hepatitis* was first used to describe a disease occurring in young women with hepatitis and systemic, serologic, and occasionally familial evidence of SLE.[314] Its relation to SLE has been controversial[315] and it is now generally agreed that there does not appear to be a true association with SLE.[315–317] Lupoid hepatitis actually comprises a subset of patients with chronic active hepatitis who have hypergammaglobulinemia and autoantibodies, including ANAs, antimitochondrial antibodies, and, in 70 percent, antibodies to smooth muscle, but no antibodies to dsDNA. It is rare in children and must be differentiated from the more common hepatic involvement of SLE.[315] Some cases begin with an episode of acute viral hepatitis. Clinically, these patients develop prolonged jaundice, intermittent fever, and hepatosplenomegaly. Areas of fibrosis, nodular degeneration, and piecemeal necrosis and a striking infiltration of lymphocytes and plasma cells are present in liver biopsy specimens.[315]

Lymphatic Tissue Involvement

Splenomegaly of moderate degree is a feature of active disease. Splenic infarcts or perisplenitis may cause recurrent left upper quadrant pain. Functional asplenia, defined as failure of the spleen to accumulate radiocolloid, is a rare but potentially fatal complication.[318, 319] It is not associated with clinical symptoms, except in the case of overwhelming pneumococcal sepsis. It can be suspected, however, if Howell-Jolly bodies are seen on examination of the peripheral blood smear by interference phase-contrast microscopy, and confirmed by demonstrating failure of splenic uptake of colloid such as ^{99m}technetium-labeled phytate. We have seen two such children, one of whom died of overwhelming pneumococcal sepsis. Spleen scans in 11 other children with active SLE failed to detect any abnormalities. In some instances, the defect is reversible.[319]

About half of the children with SLE have localized or generalized lymphadenopathy. Occasionally, this may be extreme and suggest a diagnosis of lymphoma, a malignancy that rarely has been reported in association with childhood SLE.[320]

Malignancy

In a study of 724 adult patients with SLE who were followed prospectively for 24 years, the overall risk for cancer was not increased over the general population. However, the risk of non-Hodgkin's lymphoma was increased fourfold.[321] An increased frequency of lymphoma was also demonstrated in a Danish study in which increases in lung, liver, and vaginal cancers were also documented.[322] Whether these increased risks are conferred by the disease or by treatment with drugs such as cyclophosphamide is uncertain. In a short-term study of 75 patients with SLE who had received intravenous cyclophosphamide, neoplasia developed in 4.[323]

Autoimmune Endocrinopathies

Autoimmune thyroid disease occurs with increased frequency in children with SLE, and *Hashimoto's thyroiditis* may occasionally herald the onset of the SLE. In one study, 4 of 35 children with SLE had clinically evident hypothyroidism, and a further two had elevated serum T4 concentration but normal levels of thyroid-stimulating hormone. Antithyroglobulin and antimicrosomal antibodies occurred in two thirds of patients with clinical or laboratory evidence of thyroid disease, but antibodies to thyroglobulin and microsomes were present in 30 and 60 percent, respectively, of euthyroid children with SLE.[324] The high frequency of antithyroid autoantibodies in children with SLE is similar to that reported in adults with the disease.[325] No association of SLE with Graves' disease has been reported.

A 15-year-old girl with SLE and symptomatic partial hypoparathyroidism manifested by persistently low levels of parathormone was reported by Gazarian and colleagues.[326] Primary hyperparathyroidism has also been reported in a patient with SLE.[327] One young girl with SLE and juvenile onset diabetes mellitus has been reported,[328] and we have noted the concurrence of the diseases in two patients in our clinics. Pernicious anemia has also been detected in one patient. We have seen one young girl with Addison's disease and SLE, and there have been rare reports of this association in adults.[329] Endocrine gland dysfunction secondary to arterial thrombosis as part of the antiphospholipid syndrome is rare and to our knowledge has not been reported in children.

PATHOLOGY

The basic pathologic lesions of SLE are an immune complex–mediated vasculitis and fibrinoid necrosis, inflammatory cellular infiltrate, and sclerosis of collagen.[330] The characteristic histopathologic lesions of SLE include *hematoxylin bodies* and so-called *onion-skin lesions.* Hematoxylin bodies, which can be found in any organ, are formed by the interaction of antibody to deoxynucleoprotein and degraded nuclear material. They are basophilic structures that, when engulfed by a phagocytic cell, result in the LE cell. In the absence of necrosis, hematoxylin bodies in tissue sections are pathognomonic for SLE. Onion-skin lamination resulting from sclerosis of collagen reflects the effects of arteritis. It is typically seen in the penicilliary arteries of the spleen (Fig. 18–14), and in other organs in association with foci of fibrinoid necrosis.

Vascular endothelial thickening is another characteristic of SLE. Capillaries, venules, and arterioles are

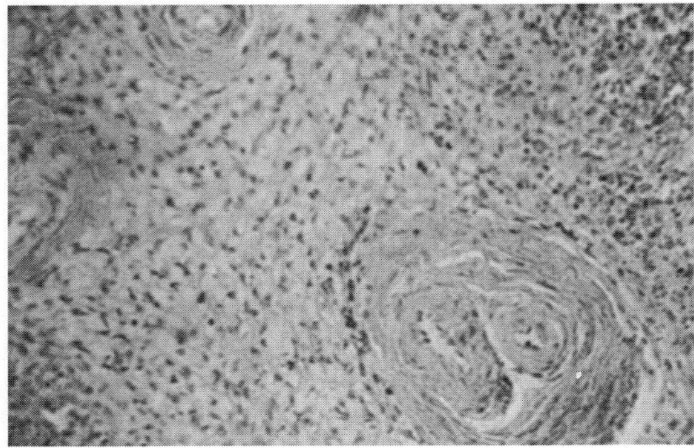

Figure 18–14. Onion-skin lamination of the penicilliary arteries of the spleen illustrating a typical pattern of sclerosis of collagen in SLE. This section was from a young patient who had idiopathic thrombocytopenic purpura and who required a splenectomy. Three years later, she developed the typical manifestations of SLE.

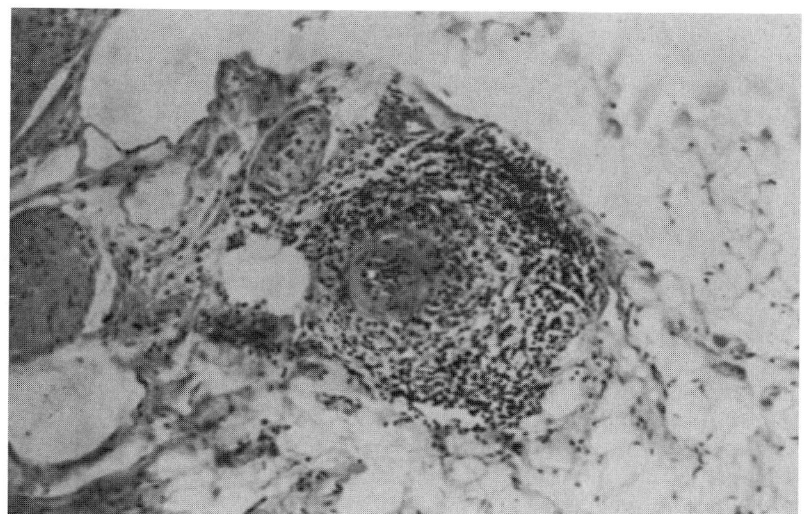

Figure 18–15. Immune complex vasculitis in a patient with SLE. A small artery is the focus of the necrotizing arteritis, with periarterial round cell infiltration and involvement of the adjacent vein.

involved; larger vessels are usually spared. Secondary changes include vascular obstruction and thrombosis, which are uncommon, except in the CNS and mesenteric vessels. In areas of severe inflammation, there may be almost total destruction of the connective tissues combined with cellular necrosis and the deposition of basophilic nuclear debris. These changes are most commonly seen in lymph nodes, heart, and glomeruli, and are attributable to immune complex desposition.

In the most complete histologic study of necropsy findings in children with SLE, Cook and associates[27] noted that the most characteristic microscopic changes were found in the arterioles and consisted of fibrinoid necrosis of the media, proliferation and swelling of the intima, and varying degrees of periarteriolar inflammation (Fig. 18–15). The fibrinoid material is deposited within the interfibrillary ground substance of the connective tissues; nearby connective tissue fibers are irregularly thickened. This pathologic change was first recognized by Klemperer and colleagues[331] and is most often identified in glomeruli and arterioles of the skin, heart, and other parenchymal organs but may be present in necrotic lymph nodes and synovium. It is not distinguishable microscopically from fibrinoid changes of other connective tissue diseases.

Renal Lesions

A wide spectrum of abnormalities, including glomerulonephritis, interstitial nephritis, and necrotizing angiitis, may be seen on studies of renal pathology in SLE. The predominant abnormality, however, is usually one of the types of glomerulonephritis as categorized by the classification of the World Health Organization (WHO) (Table 18–16).[332] Indices of severity and activity can also be applied. The distribution of histologic patterns in 60 patients in the study of Sorof and coworkers[337] is shown in Table 18–17.

Glomerulonephritis

The WHO classification of lupus nephritis (see Table 18–16) recognizes six categories that include at least

Table 18–16

World Health Organization Classification of Lupus Nephritis

Class I	Normal	No detectable disease
Class IIA	Minimal change	Normal LM; mesangial immunoglobulin and complement by IFM; mesangial deposits by EM
Class IIB	Mesangial glomerulitis	IIA plus mesangial hypercellularity (>3 cells per mesangial area or increased mesangial matrix); minimal tubular or interstitial disease
Class III	Focal and segmental proliferation	Focal areas of intra- and extracapillary cellular proliferation, necrosis, karyorrhexis, and leukocyte infiltration in <50% of the glomeruli; subendothelial or mesangial deposits on IFM or EM; focal tubular and intersitial disease
Class IV	Diffuse proliferative glomerulonephritis	Class III changes involving more glomerular surface area and >50% of the glomeruli; IFM and EM show abundant subendothelial deposits; marked interstitial involvement; membranoproliferative variant has prominent mesangial cell proliferation and capillary wall thickening
Class V	Membranous glomerulonephritis	No mesangial, endothelial, or epithelial cellular proliferation; diffusely and uniformly thickened capillary walls; IFM and EM show mesangial and subepithelial deposits; minimal interstitial involvement
Class VI	Glomerular sclerosis	Segmental or extensive sclerosis of glomeruli; fibrous crescents are common

EM, electron microscopy; IFM, immunofluorescence microscopy; LM, light microscopy.

Table 18–17

Relative Frequency of Different Patterns of Renal Histology at Initial and Subsequent Biopsies

WHO CLASS	INITIAL BIOPSY (%)	SECOND BIOPSY (%)	THIRD OR MORE BIOPSY (%)
I	2	0	0
II	23	11	10
III	37	41	40
IV	10	26	10
V	28	22	40

Data from Sorof et al.[337]

two different pathogenic mechanisms. Light, immunofluorescence, and electron microscopic findings are all used to define these categories. WHO class I denotes normal renal histology. Mesangial, focal, and diffuse proliferative glomerulonephritis result from the deposition of immune complexes from the circulation. Membranous glomerulonephritis results, at least in part, from in situ formation of immune complexes. In addition, mixed histologic patterns are common, and changes from one category to another over time are frequent. The relative frequency of each histologic type varies from series to series and reflects, at least in part, the indications used to perform the renal biopsy. However, mesangial and proliferative lesions (classes II, III, and IV) constitute the findings in 90 percent of biopsied patients.[195]

Mesangial nephritis (WHO class II) is the most minimal glomerular lesion seen in lupus nephritis. By light microscopy, glomeruli appear normal (class IIA) or, at most, show a minimal increase in the number of mesangial cells and matrix (class IIB) (Fig. 18–16). The diagnosis depends on the demonstration of mesangial deposition of IgG and C3 by immunofluorescence microscopy (Fig. 18–17). By electron microscopy, electron-dense deposits are noted in the mesangium and along the paramesangial capillary basement membranes. Mesangial disease may progress to focal or diffuse proliferative nephritis.[333, 334] Although children with class II nephritis may have low-grade proteinuria and hematuria, most do not develop renal insufficiency, particularly if the active systemic disease is adequately treated initially, with normalization of serologic abnormalities (Table 18–18).

Focal segmental proliferative glomerulitis (WHO class III) is characterized by mesangial changes, and areas of hypercellularity in fewer than half of the glomeruli in the biopsy specimen (Figs. 18–18 and 18–19). The lesions may be proliferative, necrotizing, or sclerosing, or a combination of these changes. In addition to mesangial changes, the lesions within each glomerulus tend to be located in the peripheral capillary loops, in contrast with the predominant centrilobular distribution in class II lesions or poststreptococcal glomerulonephritis. Segmental proliferation of the glomerular tufts, which is usually accompanied by mesangial proliferation, is also present. Lumpy-bumpy or granular deposits of immunoglobulins and complement components are seen by immunofluorescence microscopy along the basement membranes. By ultrastructural studies, these are subendothelial electron-dense deposits of immune complexes along the capillary basement membrane with accompanying proliferative changes. Less often, a few subepithelial and intramembranous deposits may be found. Focal segmental proliferative nephritis may progress to diffuse disease in from 7[335] to 35 percent of patients.[336] This transition is most likely

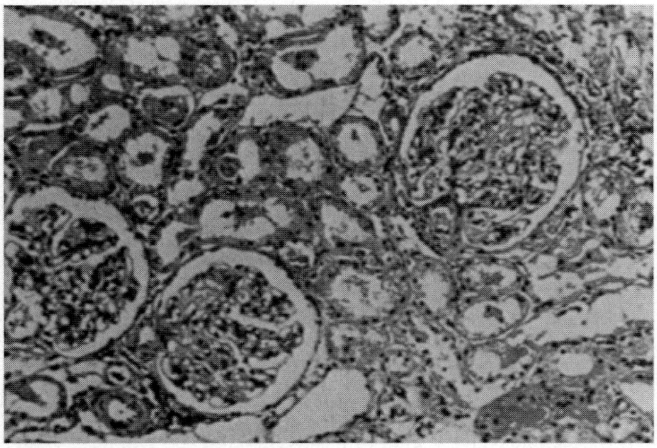

Figure 18–16. Mesangial lupus nephritis. Except for a few lobular areas of hypercellularity, these glomeruli from a renal biopsy of a 12-year-old black girl with acute SLE appear normal.

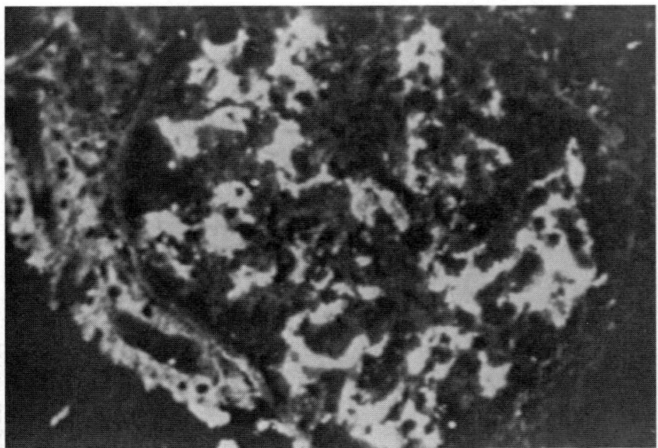

Figure 18–17. Mesangial lupus nephritis. Immunofluorescent section from the patient in Figure 18–16 stained for immunoglobulin G (IgG). Massive deposits of immunoglobulin are identified in the mesangium, in contrast to the paucity of abnormalities identified by light microscopy.

Table 18–18

Mesangial Lupus Nephritis

May be initial immune complex lesion
Usually no clinical features of renal disease, or there may be minimal proteinuria or hematuria
Remission or progression of the nephritis may occur with transition to diffuse or membranous disease

to occur with prolonged, severe, active disease (Table 18–19).

Diffuse proliferative glomerulonephritis (WHO class IV) is characterized by the uniform hypercellularity of more than 50 percent of the glomeruli in the biopsy specimen (Figs. 18–20, 18–21, and 18–22). The severity of the individual glomerular changes is usually more pronounced than in focal disease. Fluorescence microscopy demonstrates the characteristic lumpy-bumpy deposition of immunoglobulin and complement along the peripheral capillary walls, as well as in the mesangium. Interstitial infiltrates and extraglomerular immune complex deposition may also be noted along the tubular basement membranes, within the walls of the peritubular capillaries, or in the interstitium. By electron microscopy, extensive immune deposits occur in the mesangium and subendothelial spaces, and, to a lesser extent, in the subepithelial areas and intramembranously. Ultrastructurally, these electron-dense deposits may exhibit a fingerprint or microtubular appearance, a result of crystallization within the immune complexes (Table 18–20).

Membranous glomerulonephritis (WHO class V) is quite uncommon as an isolated abnormality. The characteristic lesion is deposition of immune complexes along the subepithelial surface of the glomerular basement membrane with obliteration of the foot processes but little cellular proliferation (Figs. 18–23, 18–24). The basement membranes assume a rigid, enlarged, glassy appearance. There may be slight increases in the number of mesangial cells and in the density of the mesangial matrix. Silver or periodic acid-Schiff stains define a spike pattern along the basement membrane related to immune complex deposition on the capillary loops. Fluorescence microscopy shows a granular deposition of IgG and complement along the basement membrane that is usually finer and smaller than the deposits found in diffuse glomerulonephritis. In addition, there may be intra–basement membrane deposits, suggesting that in certain situations immune complexes can traverse the basement membrane from the subendothelial to the subepithelial surfaces (Table 18–21).

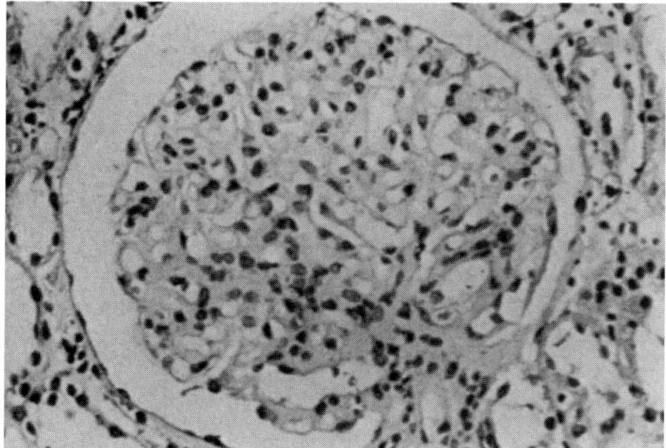

Figure 18–18. Focal proliferative lupus nephritis. A lobular area of hypercellularity and necrosis is seen in an otherwise normal glomerulus. The majority of the glomeruli appeared normal on light microscopy.

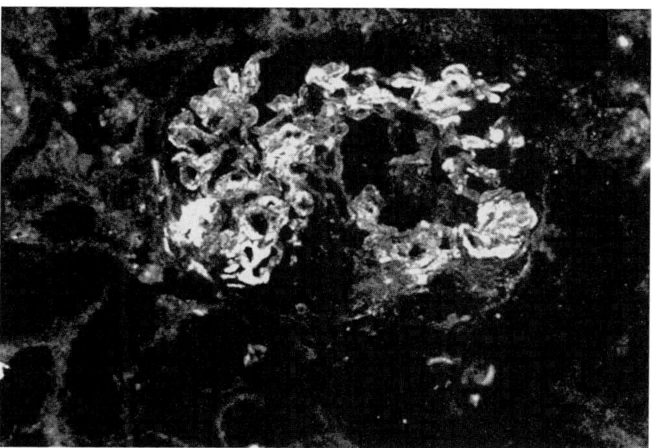

Figure 18–19. Focal proliferative glomerulonephritis demonstrated on direct immunofluorescence microscopy staining for C1q. Some areas of the glomerulus show intense staining, whereas others are entirely normal. (Courtesy of Dr. David Lirenman.)

Glomerular sclerosis (class VI) is actually not a category of the WHO classification but is customarily appended to it to accommodate patients in whom the predominant histologic change is focal segmental glomerular sclerosis. Although extensive sclerosis indicates a poor prognosis, minimal to mild sclerosis may be present in patients who have a stable disease course.[335]

Correlations between glomerular histopathologic changes and clinical features of renal disease are summarized in Table 18–10. Children with mesangial lupus nephritis seldom have clinical evidence of renal disease, although there may be minimal proteinuria and microscopic hematuria. In focal segmental proliferative glomerulitis, there may be proteinuria and mild hematuria, but renal insufficiency is either absent or minimal, and the nephrotic syndrome is distinctly uncommon. Children with diffuse proliferative glomeru-

Table 18–19

Focal Proliferative Lupus Glomerulonephritis

Minimal proteinuria
Microscopic hematuria
Nephrotic syndrome or renal insufficiency in 20%
Responsive to glucocorticoid therapy
Does not usually progress to renal failure

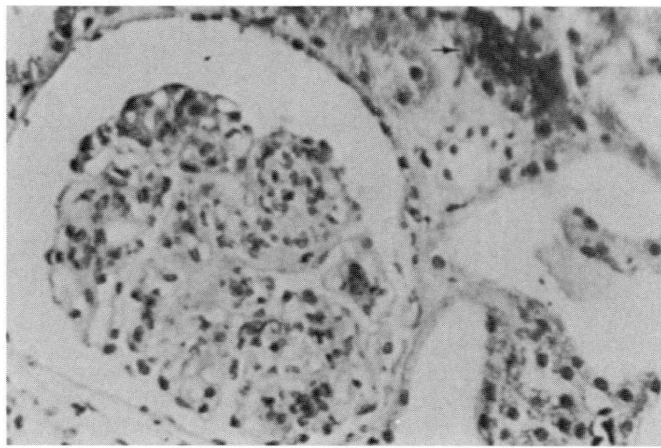

Figure 18–20. Diffuse proliferative lupus glomerulonephritis. All glomeruli in the biopsy core were uniformly involved. Marked hypercellularity, hyaline thrombi, hematoxylin bodies, and areas of necrosis were present. A red blood cell cast *(arrow)* is seen in an adjacent tubule.

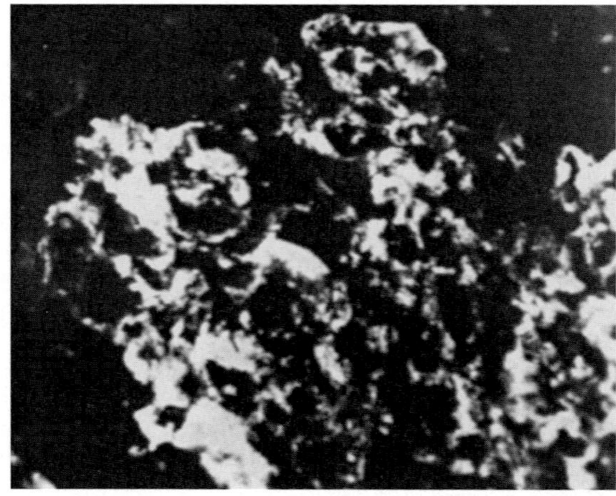

Figure 18–21. Fluorescence microscopy of a renal biopsy section from a young girl who died with central nervous system lupus and nephrotic syndrome. Deposits of IgG are shown in a "lumpy-bumpy" pattern (subendothelial) and a finer granular pattern (epimembranous).

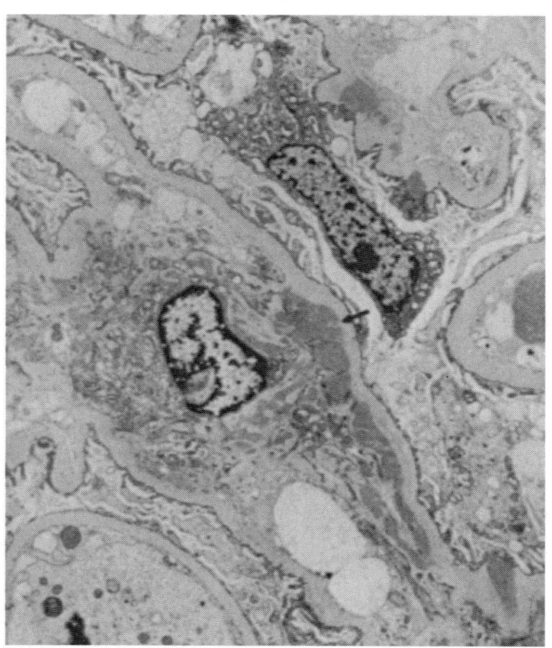

Figure 18–22. Electron microscopy study of a biopsy specimen from a patient with diffuse proliferative glomerulonephritis showing subendothelial and paramesangial immune deposits *(arrow)*.

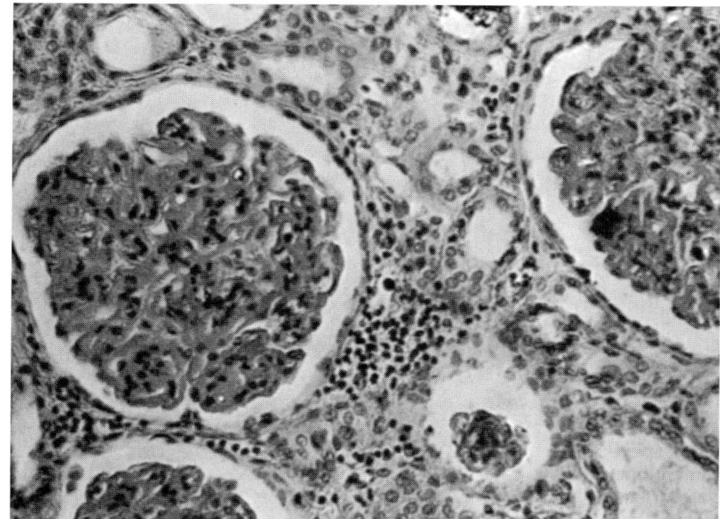

Figure 18–23. Membranous lupus nephritis. This patient was a 17-year-old white girl with nephrotic syndrome and congestive heart failure. She died from arrhythmia. Libman-Sacks endocarditis was found at necropsy (see Fig. 18–27). There was uniform thickening of endothelial walls with a "glassy" refractility on hematoxylin-eosin staining. Minimal hypercellularity was noted, and deposits of inflammatory cells were present in the tubular interstitial tissues.

Table 18–20

Diffuse Proliferative Lupus Glomerulonephritis

Proteinuria and hematuria
Nephrotic syndrome and renal insufficiency in 60%
Limited remission in 50%
Renal failure in some patients, 5–10 years after onset

Table 18–21

Membranous Lupus Glomerulonephritis

Persistent nephrotic syndrome
Hypertension in 30%
Remissions in 30%
Eventual renal insufficiency in majority

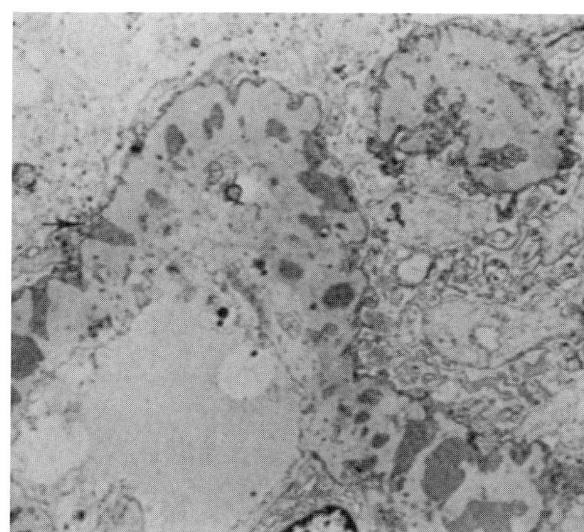

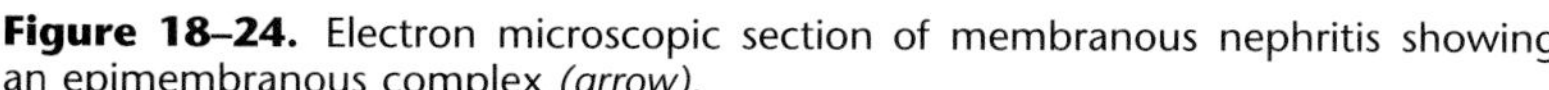

Figure 18–24. Electron microscopic section of membranous nephritis showing an epimembranous complex *(arrow)*.

lonephritis have proteinuria and hematuria in most cases, and, in 60 percent, nephrotic syndrome or renal insufficiency. Children with membranous lupus glomerulonephritis have persistent nephrotic syndrome, and one third have hypertension. The frequency of this lesion may be increasing and was found in 28 percent of initial biopsy samples of children with SLE in one center.[337] Furthermore, the frequency of this histologic pattern at the same center increased from 17 percent prior to 1995 to 64 percent after 1995. Severe glomerular sclerosis represents an end-stage lesion in which the nephrotic syndrome, renal failure, and hypertension are common.

In addition to histologic type, an estimate of the level of inflammatory activity can be made on the basis of the renal biopsy by comparing the number of active lesions to those of chronic disease.[338] Active disease is characterized histologically by the presence of intracapillary cellular proliferation, polymorphonuclear infiltrates, karyorrhexis, epithelial crescents, subendothelial fibrinoid change (wire loops), hyaline, fibrin, or platelet thrombi, interstitial inflammation, and necrotizing vasculitis. Chronicity is marked by segmental, global, mesangial, or vascular sclerosis, glomerular obsolescence, thickening of capillary basement membrane, fibrous adhesions or crescents, and tubulointerstitial scarring (Table 18–22).[339]

Interstitial Nephritis

Approximately half of the children with significant involvement of the glomerulus also have evidence of interstitial nephritis,[340] and the severity of interstitial disease usually correlates with the severity of the glomerular changes. Rarely, severe interstitial nephritis is noted in the absence of glomerular abnormalities. Focal and diffuse infiltration with inflammatory cells, tubular necrosis, and interstitial fibrosis may be observed. Immunoglobulins and complement are deposited along the peritubular capillaries or the tubular basement membrane in a granular pattern. In some patients, tubular acidosis is present.[341] Other patients have interstitial nephritis and isosthenuria as part of Sjögren's syndrome. Analgesic nephropathy as a cause of interstitial inflammation and tubular damage should always be considered in patients with these changes.

Table 18–22

Assessment of Activity and Chronicity in Renal Lupus

INDICATORS OF ACTIVE DISEASE	INDICATORS OF CHRONICITY
Cellular proliferation	Glomerular sclerosis
Necrosis, karyorrhexis	Interstitial fibrosis
Cellular crescents	Fibrous crescents
Wire loops, hyaline thrombi	Tubular atrophy
Leukocytic glomerular infiltration	
Interstitial infiltration	

Necrotizing Angiitis

Some children with lupus nephritis may also demonstrate an immune complex arteriolitis in renal tissues that may be indistinguishable from other forms of necrotizing arteritis. Fibrinoid necrosis, thrombosis, and arteriolar inflammation are usually present. This type of vasculitis may be associated clinically with fulminant renal failure and malignant hypertension or renal venous thromboses.

The role of the renal biopsy in the evaluation of lupus nephritis is controversial.[342] It is seldom needed to make the diagnosis of SLE, but it is indicated in at least three circumstances: (1) in the child with nephrotic syndrome in whom differentiation of diffuse proliferative from membranous glomerulonephritis is important; (2) in one in whom, despite high-dose glucocorticoids, renal function is deteriorating, or there is persistent hematuria or proteinuria or both, to determine whether the renal disease is likely to be responsive to cytotoxic agents (i.e., if there is evidence of activity or chronicity); and (3) as a prerequisite to entry into clinical therapeutic trials.[342]

Extensive glomerular abnormalities have been identified on biopsy of patients who have no clinical evidence of renal disease.[36, 343–346] In two reports of 27 children in whom lupus nephritis was found at necropsy, 6 children had no laboratory or clinical evidence of renal disease during life.[27, 201] Diffuse nephritis without clinically apparent disease may not always portend as poor a prognosis as that for clinically obvious disease.[347–349] Histologic abnormalities change over time in many patients,[337] and sequential biopsy findings have provided some insight into the progression of the renal lesions. However, these studies must be interpreted with caution, since indications for biopsy and the influence of therapy undoubtedly affect the results.[338, 350] In general, however, sequential biopsies in children have demonstrated progression of mesangial or focal proliferative glomerulonephritis to diffuse proliferative glomerulonephritis in months to years.[35, 336, 351–354] Occasionally, progression from diffuse proliferative to membranous disease, or less commonly, from focal proliferative to membranous disease has also been documented.[354, 355] In some studies, improvement was noted in 15 to 20 percent of patients in whom the initial biopsy had shown diffuse proliferative or focal proliferative glomerulonephritis, but membranous disease tended to be worse on subsequent examination.

Skin

The typical cutaneous lesion of acute SLE is liquefaction of the epidermal basilar layer with disruption of the dermal-epidermal junction, edema of the dermis, infiltration of T lymphocytes throughout the epidermis and around blood vessels, and fibrinoid degeneration of the connective tissues (Fig. 18–25). In more chronic lesions, there is epidermal atrophy, hyperkeratosis, follicular plugging, and proliferation of elastic tissues. IgG and C3 can be identified by fluorescence microscopy along the epidermal basement membranes in uninvolved and non–sun-exposed skin as well as in le-

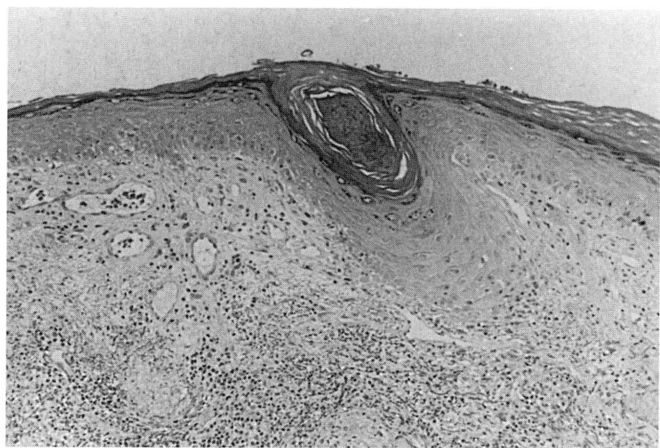

Figure 18–25. Skin biopsy of SLE rash (hematoxylin-eosin, 33×) demonstrating follicular plugging, squamatization, and vacuolation of the basal keratinocytes, thickening of the basement membrane zone, and telangiectasia. There is a small dermal perivascular lymphocytic infiltrate. (Courtesy of Dr. Richard Crawford.)

sional biopsy specimens (Fig. 18–26).[356–359] This finding of the "lupus band" on dermal punch biopsy specimens is not pathognomonic for SLE but may be a useful diagnostic test in difficult cases.

Lungs

The pulmonary histology in acute pulmonary involvement in SLE is nonspecific. A basilar interstitial pneumonitis may lead to atelectasis and basophilic mucinous edema of the alveoli with hyaline membrane formation. There is interstitial infiltration of lymphocytes and other inflammatory cells, alveolar hemorrhage, formation of hyaline membranes, and focal necrosis. Fibrinoid necrosis of arterioles and capillary thrombi may occur, and hematoxylin bodies may be seen.

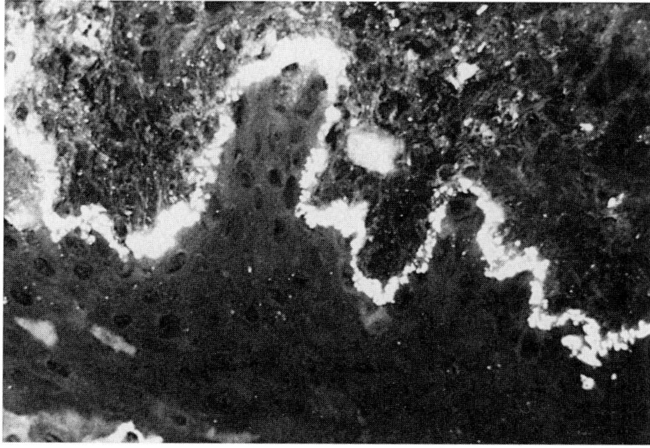

Figure 18–26. This direct immunofluorescence photomicrograph shows granular deposits of IgG along the basement membrane zone ("lupus band") in a biopsy sample of nonaffected skin in a patient with SLE. (Courtesy of Dr. Richard Crawford.)

Heart

All layers of the heart may be involved by the pathologic processes of SLE. Pericarditis consists of focal or diffuse fibrinous deposits or fibrosis. Pericardial fluid contains high numbers of leukocytes, almost all of which are neutrophils.[360] Myocarditis is typified by plasma cell and lymphocyte infiltration of the myocardium, sometimes with fibrosis, especially in steroid-treated patients.[250] The basic lesion of the endocardium consists of nodule formation along the atrial or ventricular surfaces of the valve leaflets, or on the endocardium of the chambers (Fig. 18–27). The Libman-Sacks lesion has been described as having three zones: an outer exudative zone of fibrin containing nuclear debris, including hematoxylin bodies; a middle zone of proliferating fibroblasts; and the inner zone characterized by neovascularization.[361] The mitral valve is most commonly involved.

Central Nervous System

There are no pathognomonic pathologic findings in CNS lupus,[362] and anatomically identifiable lesions do not always account for the neurologic manifestations of the disease.[97] True vasculitis is rare; perivasculitis is more common and may lead to infarction, encephalomalacia, or other focal lesions (Figs. 18–28 and 18–29). Microinfarcts and nonspecific destructive and proliferative arteriolar and capillary lesions occur.[363] Thrombosis as part of the antiphospholipid antibody syndrome may affect small arterioles or venules, although the direct evidence that this is responsible for many of the CNS lesions is unclear. In a study of the brains of patients with chorea (many of whom were children), infarcts, but not arteritis, were found in the basal ganglia.[218] Most patients with chorea and SLE have antiphospholipid antibodies, however.[364]

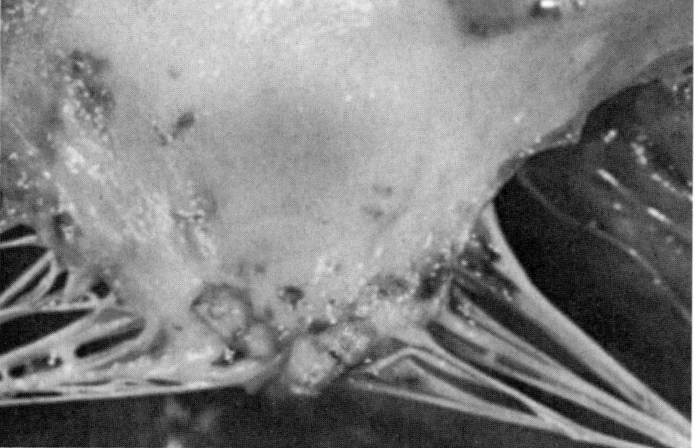

Figure 18–27. Libman-Sacks endocarditis. This patient was a 17-year-old girl with an acute exacerbation of SLE who had cardiac and pulmonary failure. The heart was minimally enlarged. There were a loud systolic murmur and a faint diastolic murmur at the apex. The necropsy examination of the mitral valve leaflets showed many nonbacterial verrucae at the margins.

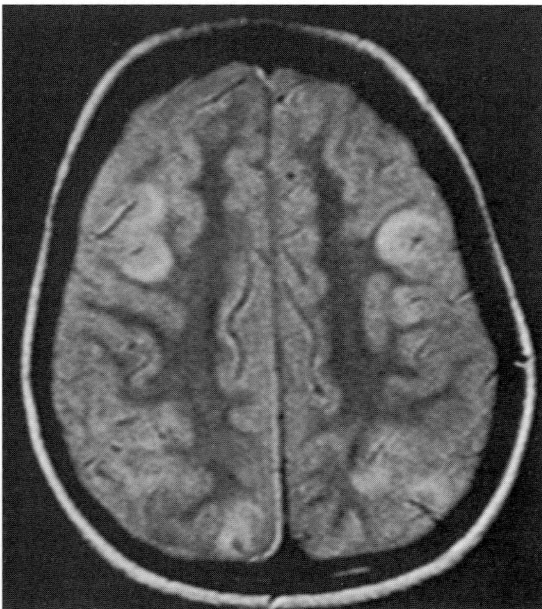

Figure 18–28. Magnetic resonance image of the brain of a 12-year-old girl with SLE who suffered widespread seizures due to central nervous system vasculitis. Pale areas of the deep cortex are observed on the initial study.

Retinal cotton-wool spots (cytoid bodies) represent areas of inflammatory edema and degeneration of the ganglion cells arising from a periarteriolitis within the nerve fiber layer, presumably related to immune complex deposition. In an immunofluorescence microscopy study, immunoglobulin was demonstrated in the vascular layer of the capillaries of the choroid and around the basement membranes of the ciliary processes and bulbar conjunctivae.[365]

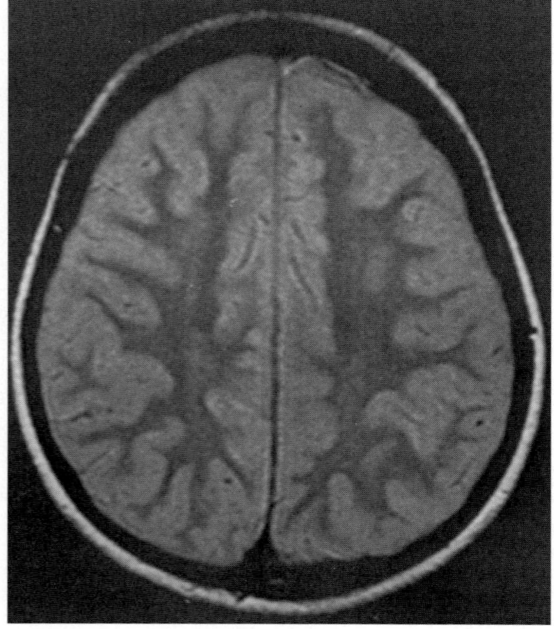

Figure 18–29. The abnormalities seen in Figure 18–28 are no longer demonstrated on a second study 1 month later.

Other Organs

The synovitis in children with SLE is nonspecific and is usually milder in degree than that of JRA. Changes include proliferation of synovial lining cells and microvascular abnormalities, including vasculitis and inflammatory cell infiltration. The myopathy of SLE is not specific and includes necrotizing arteritis, mild interstitial myositis, and vacuolization of muscle fibers.

The walls of the gastrointestinal tract are also sites of focal or diffuse vasculitis. Acute hemorrhage or infarction results from thrombosis of the mesenteric vessels. Mesenteric vasculitis is a rare but serious occurrence in the child with SLE. Hepatic biopsies in 33 adults with SLE and elevated liver enzymes demonstrated steatosis (12 patients), cirrhosis (4), chronic active hepatitis (3), chronic granulomatous hepatitis (3), centrilobular necrosis (3), chronic persistent hepatitis (2), and microabscess (2).[366] More recent studies have noted the presence of multiple fibrin microthrombi, liver infarction, hepatic veno-occlusive disease, and Budd-Chiari syndrome (hepatic vein occlusion with cirrhosis and ascites) related to the presence of antiphospholipid antibodies.[367] Hyperplasia of plasma cells, vasculitis, and the occurrence of hematoxylin bodies characterize lesions of the lymph nodes.

LABORATORY EXAMINATION

Indicators of Inflammation

Most acute-phase indices of inflammation are increased in children with SLE in proportion to the activity of the systemic disease. These include an increased erythrocyte sedimentation rate (ESR), polyclonal hypergammaglobulinemia, and increased serum levels of α_2-globulins.[368–372] C-reactive protein (CRP), an important acute phase protein that is elevated in most inflammatory conditions, is often normal in SLE.[373] However, it is increased in patients with SLE and systemic infection,[374] and in patients with serositis,[375] and arthritis.[376, 377] Serum ferritin is elevated in adult patients with active SLE in contrast to those with rheumatoid arthritis, and correlates with disease activity, but not with the ESR.[378] In at least one study, factor VIII–related antigen (von Willebrand factor) was elevated in approximately half of the children with SLE.[379] The discrepancies among the acute-phase responses may reflect the intricate cytokine abnormalities in SLE, and their influence on the synthesis of specific acute phase proteins. Patients with SLE have low levels of IL-1, the cytokine responsible for the induction of CRP; high ferritin levels may reflect the high IL-6 or TNF-α levels seen in this disease. In some studies, however, correlations between cytokine levels and acute-phase protein levels were inconsistent.[380]

Hematologic Abnormalities

Anemia

Mild or moderate anemia occurs in approximately one half of children with SLE and is usually typical of

Table 18–23

Hematologic Abnormalities in Systemic Lupus Erythematosus

ABNORMALITY	FREQUENCY (%)
Anemia (hematocrit <30%)	50
Acute hemolytic anemia	5
Leukopenia	
<4500 WBC/mm³ (<4.5 × 10⁹/L)	40
<2000 WBC/mm³ (<2 × 10⁹/L)	10
Thrombocytopenia	
<150,000 plts/mm³ (<150 × 10⁹/L)	30
<100,000 plts/mm³ (<100 × 10⁹/L)	5

plts, platelets; WBC, white blood cells.

that which develops in chronic disease (normocytic, hypochromic), with decreased serum iron and normal or slightly reduced iron binding capacity (Table 18–23). In other patients, it reflects autoimmune hemolysis caused by IgG complement-fixing antibodies to erythrocytes that are detected by an antiglobulin (Coombs) test. Occasionally lupus may present with severe hemolytic anemia, but ordinarily the level of hemoglobin is only moderately depressed. Anemia associated with cold agglutinins directed against the I antigen of erythrocyte membranes is also found in some children with SLE. Hemolytic anemia is seldom severe and is rarely fatal. Pernicious anemia has been rarely reported in adults with SLE.[381] Hypersplenism, drug sensitivity, and, rarely, microangiopathy may also contribute to anemia. Drug-induced gastrointestinal tract ulceration occasionally contributes to anemia. The presence of Howell-Jolly bodies indicates the presence of splenic dysfunction and should be looked for regularly (Fig. 18–30).

Leukocytes and Platelets

Leukopenia, particularly lymphocytopenia (<1500 cells/mm³), is a hallmark of acute SLE, although leukocytosis may occur.[35] Severe neutropenia (<1000 neutrophils/mm³; <1 × 10⁹/L) is very uncommon. In contrast, lymphopenia is common, particularly in patients with active disease.[382] In spite of increased production and peripheral destruction of platelets, most children maintain a normal platelet count. In one study, although antiplatelet antibodies were present in 78 percent of patients, only 15 percent were thrombocytopenic.[383] Some children with SLE have clinically important immune thrombocytopenic purpura, usually in association with splenomegaly. Bone marrow examination in these cases confirms an increased number of megakaryocytes with poor platelet budding. Patients with thrombocytopenic purpura and hemolytic anemia (*Evans' syndrome*) may progress to SLE or eventually develop the features of TTP.

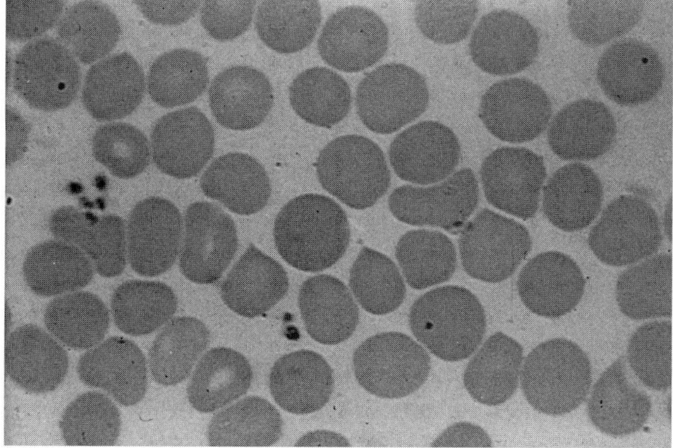

Figure 18–30. Photomicrograph of smear of peripheral blood stained with Wright's stain showing erythrocytes containing small dark Howell-Jolly bodies. (Courtesy of Dr. L. Wadsworth.)

Coagulation Abnormalities

The lupus anticoagulant described in 1952 by Conley and Hartmann was associated with a hemorrhagic disorder that occurred in some patients with SLE.[384] In such patients, the activated partial thromboplastin time and prothrombin time are prolonged. Addition of fresh plasma incompletely corrects the defect. This phenomenon results from the effect of a unique antibody that acts at the junction of the intrinsic and extrinsic coagulation pathways: the conversion of prothrombin to thrombin by thromboplastin is inhibited by interference with the interaction of the prothrombin-activator complex (factors Xa and V, calcium, and phospholipids).[385]

Abnormalities of at least one of nine different tests were demonstrated in 41 percent of patients with SLE, but no individual test (Dilute Russell Viper Venom Time [DRVVT]) detected more than 78 percent of patients with these abnormalities. It is likely, therefore, that a combination of assays is necessary to effectively screen a lupus population for lupus anticoagulant, and in this study, a combination of the DRVVT, APTT, and dilute thromboplastin tissue assay identified all patients with any abnormal test result. A combination of DRVVT and APTT detected 91 percent of those with any abnormal test result.[386] In this study, there were no correlations between abnormal clotting tests and the presence of high titers of anticardiolipin antibodies.

Antinuclear Antibodies

Antinuclear antibodies are present in the sera of almost all children with active SLE (Table 18–24). In fact, the absence of ANAs, particularly in the presence of symptomatic disease, all but excludes the diagnosis of SLE. The titers of ANAs as demonstrated by immunofluorescence microscopy on HEp-2 cells range from low (1:80) in inactive disease, to extremely high (>1:5120) in active disease. There is considerable interpatient variability, and determination of an ANA titer alone is not sufficient to diagnosis SLE or to monitor disease course. The pattern of nuclear immunofluorescence is usually peripheral or homogeneous and suggests the presence of antibodies to dsDNA (Fig. 18–31).

Table 18–24

Characteristic Autoantibodies in Systemic Lupus Erythematosus

ANTINUCLEAR ANTIBODIES	OTHER AUTOANTIBODIES
Anti-dsDNA antibodies	Antierythrocyte antibodies
Anti-DNP antibodies	Antilymphocytotoxic antibodies
Anti-Ro (SS/A) antibodies	Antitissue specific antibodies
Anti-La (SS/B) antibodies	Antiphospholipid antibodies
Anti-Sm antibodies	Rheumatoid factors
Anti-histone antibodies	

The first evidence for the presence of ANAs in SLE was the demonstration of the LE cell (Fig. 18–32).[7] The antibody responsible for this phenomenon is directed to deoxyribonucleoprotein (anti-DNP) or anti-DNA histone. Although the LE-cell test is quite specific for SLE, it can be present in other situations, and its low sensitivity makes it a poor screening test for SLE. For these reasons, and because it is labor-intensive, it has been supplanted by the more sensitive, if less specific, test for ANAs by immunofluorescence.

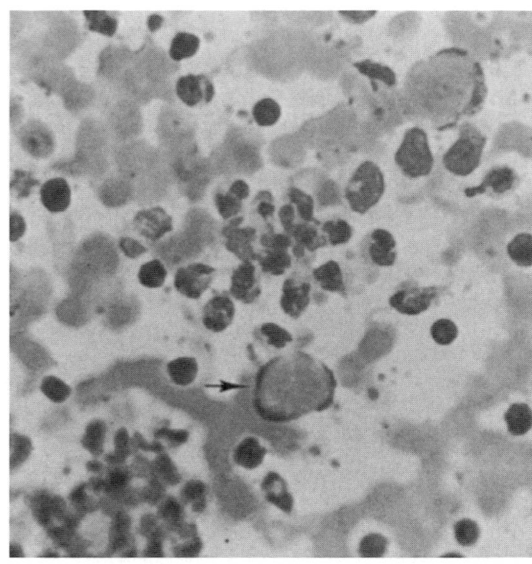

Figure 18–32. Lupus erythematosus cell preparation. The lupus erythematosus cell, a polymorphonuclear leukocyte containing a homogeneous nuclear inclusion, is identified by the *arrow.*

Antibodies to DNA

Antibodies to dsDNA are virtually pathognomonic of SLE, occur in almost all children with active SLE, and are present at particularly high titers in children with active nephritis (Table 18–25).[389–391] They are rarely, if ever, associated with other rheumatic diseases. Antibodies to single-stranded DNA occur in approximately 50 percent of children with SLE but are also present in children with a variety of other rheumatic disorders and infections and are, therefore, of little diagnostic significance. The reader is referred to the excellent recent review of this subject by Hahn.[392]

Antibody to dsDNA is measured by a number of methods, most commonly a radioimmunoassay that uses radiolabeled dsDNA,[387–389] a fluorescence microscopy assay that uses the protozoan *Crithidia luciliae,*[393, 394] or an enzyme-linked immunosorbent assay (ELISA).[395] The radioimmunoassay is sensitive and provides semiquantitative data, but, since the substrate may contain contaminating single-stranded DNA, it may lack specificity. The kinetoplast of *Crithidia luciliae,* on the other hand, consists only of dsDNA, and, although it is less sensitive than radioimmunoassay, assays using this organism are highly specific for the detection of antibodies to dsDNA (Fig. 18–33). ELISAs provide semiquantitative information but, like the radioimmunoassay, may have a higher level of false-positive results. For diagnostic purposes, the *Crithidia* assay is often preferred; for monitoring levels of antibody to dsDNA during the course of therapy, the radioimmunoassay or ELISA is superior. Increased or increasing levels of antibody to dsDNA are often a clue to the development of active renal disease, particularly if accompanied by decreased or decreasing levels of complement.

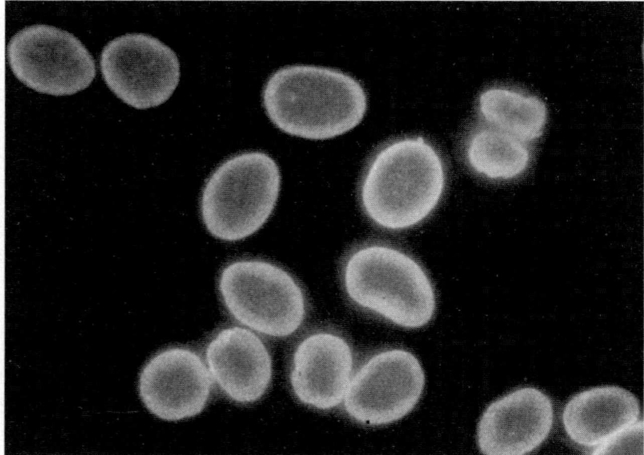

Figure 18–31. Demonstration of antinuclear antibodies (ANA) on HEp 2 cells by indirect immunofluorescence microscopy. The homogeneous pattern of staining is characteristic of SLE. (Courtesy of Kallestad Laboratories, Minneapolis, MN.)

Antibodies to Extractable Nuclear Antigens

Antibodies to the extractable nuclear antigens (Sm, SS-A/Ro, SS-B/La) are strongly associated with SLE, neonatal lupus erythematosus, and Sjögren's syndrome. High titers of anti-RNP are associated with SLE and mixed connective tissue disease. The frequencies of

Table 18–25

Anti-dsDNA Antibodies

Antigenic specificity	Native, double-stranded DNA
Mechanism of action	Forms complement-activating immune complexes that deposit in tissues
Clinical correlations	Highly specific for systemic lupus erythematosus Active glomerulonephritis

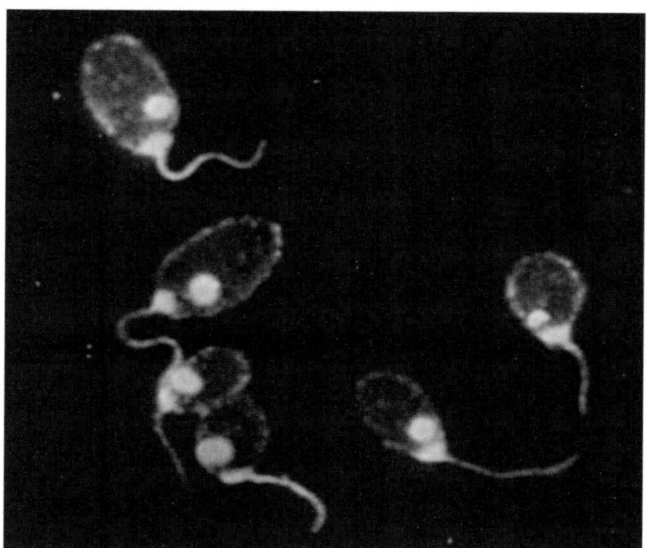

Figure 18–33. Demonstration of antibody to dsDNA using *Crithidia luciliae*. The brightly staining kinetoplast at the base of the flagellum indicates the presence of antibodies to dsDNA, as revealed by indirect immunofluorescence. (Courtesy of Kallestad Laboratories, Minneapolis, MN.)

antibodies to the extractable nuclear antigens are well documented in adults with SLE. In a long-term follow-up of 100 adults with SLE, 39 had anti-Ro, 13 anti-La, and 7 anti-Sm.[396] In a study of 22 children with SLE, anti-Ro was present in 29 percent, anti-La in 10 percent, anti-Sm in 14 percent, and anti-RNP in 19 percent.[45]

Anti-Ro/SS-A. The Ro antigen consists of two polypeptides of 52 kD and 60 kD that are complexed to cytoplasmic RNA Y1, Y3, Y4, and Y5. Most reactive sera recognize the 60 kD moiety. Anti-Ro is most strongly associated with neonatal lupus erythematosus, subacute cutaneous lupus, homozygous C2 and C4 deficiency, interstitial lung disease, skin photosensitivity,[397] and Sjögren's syndrome.[398] These antibodies are also present in about one fourth of patients with typical SLE, particularly in association with active renal disease.[399, 400] Up to 15 percent of normal individuals have low levels of anti-Ro activity.[401] Anti-Ro can be demonstrated by several methods, including immunodiffusion and ELISA (Table 18–26).[402–405]

Patients who have only anti-Ro antibody occasionally have negative findings on tests for ANA by immunofluorescence microscopy on tissue substrates (ANA-negative lupus),[405, 406] although the majority of such patients are positive on HEp-2 cells. We have seen one such patient, a teenaged boy with anti-Ro antibodies, who presented with classic discoid cutaneous lesions, developed CNS disease, and died from cerebromalacia (see Fig. 18–7). Another developed a butterfly rash with anti-Ro antibodies after griseofulvin administration for a presumed cutaneous fungal infection.

Anti-La/SS-B. The La antigen is a 48 kD nuclear phosphoprotein that is complexed to the Y RNAs, as well as to other immature transcripts of RNA polymerase III. Patients with anti-La almost always also have anti-Ro, although the converse is not true. Anti-La is associated with Sjögren's syndrome,[398] and with neonatal lupus.[407] Approximately 5 percent of the normal population have low levels of anti-La detected by ELISA (Table 18–27).

Anti-Sm. The Sm antigen is composed of five small uridine-rich RNAs (U1, U2, U4, U5, and U6) and is associated with a number of polypeptides with which anti-Sm antibodies react.[408] Core Sm proteins B (29 kD), B′ (28 kD), D (16 kD), E (12 kD), F (11 kD), and G (9 kD) have been identified. The polypeptides most often recognized by anti-Sm are B/B′.[408] B′ is found only in human tissues. Antibodies to the Sm antigen complex that are specific for SLE usually occur together with anti-U1 RNP antibodies in CNS disease (Table 18–28),[409, 410] although more recent studies have failed to demonstrate strong associations between anti-Sm and disease characteristics.[411] Anti-Sm antibodies are found in higher frequency in African-Americans than in whites with SLE.[412]

Anti-U1 RNP. Antibodies to a portion of a polypeptide associated with U1 RNA (anti-RNP) are found in low titers in children with SLE, but in high titers are associated with mixed connective tissue disease.[413] They are characterized by a speckled pattern of nuclear fluores-

Table 18–26

Anti-Ro (SS-A) Antibodies

Antigenic specificity	52 and 60 kD peptides complexed to Y1, Y3, Y4, and Y5 RNAs
Mechanism of action	Interferes with RNA translation or transport
Clinical correlations	Neonatal lupus syndromes, especially complete heart block Subacute cutaneous lupus Sjögren's syndrome Renal and pulmonary disease

Table 18–27

Anti-La (SS-B) Antibodies

Antigenic specificity	48 kD nuclear phosphoprotein that is complexed to the Y RNAs
Mechanism of action	Interferes with action of RNA polymerase III
Clinical associations	Neonatal lupus syndromes Sjögren's syndrome Almost always found in association with anti-Ro

Table 18–28

Anti-Sm Antibodies

Antigenic specificity	Uridine rich RNAs U1, U2, U4, U5, and U6 associated with the core Sm peptides B/B′, D, E, F, and G
Mechanism of action	Involved with RNA processing, mRNA synthesis and splicing
Clinical associations	Specific for systemic lupus erythematosus Related to central nervous system disease

Table 18–29

Anti-U1 RNP Antibodies

Antigenic specificities	Polypeptide associated with U1 RNA
Mechanism of action	Interferes with synthesis of RNA
Clinical associations	Low titer: systemic lupus erythematosus High titer: mixed connective tissue disease

cence on tests for ANAs and confirmed by counterimmunoelectrophoresis or ELISA (Table 18–29).

Antihistone Antibodies

Antibodies to histones are present in many children with SLE, but were first detected in drug-induced SLE by Fritzler and Tan.[414] Specificities differ markedly between spontaneous SLE and the various types of drug-induced disease (Table 18–30).[415–417] In procainamide-induced lupus, antibodies react with H2A, H2B, and the H2A-H2B complex. In hydralazine-induced disease, they react primarily with H3 and H4. The finding of antihistone antibodies in the absence of high titers of anti-dsDNA antibodies is highly suggestive of drug-induced SLE. Antibodies to histones are most commonly demonstrated by an enzyme-linked immunoassay.

Other Autoantibodies

Antiphospholipid Antibodies

Most patients with lupus anticoagulant have antibodies to cardiolipin[385] that cross-react with a range of negatively charged phospholipids (Table 18–31).

The reported frequencies of anticardiolipin antibodies in childhood SLE have ranged from 50 percent[418] to 100 percent.[45] A correlation with the presence of CNS disease was observed in one study.[410] A similar antibody species directed against phospholipid is responsible for the false-positive serologic reaction for syphilis seen in this disease.

Antiphospholipid antibodies are not restricted to patients with SLE. They can be detected in a wide variety of neoplastic, infectious, inflammatory, and autoimmune diseases. The reported frequency of anticardiolipin antibodies in childhood SLE was 37 percent in a recent study.[387] In a study of other antiphospholipid antibodies in childhood SLE, a lupus anticoagulant was found in 55 percent and a false-positive serologic test for syphilis in 38 percent.[388]

Table 18–30

Anti-Histone Antibodies

Antigenic specificities	Histone complex (H2A-H2B) H1 > H2B > H2A > H3 > H4
Mechanism of action	? Interferes with nucleosome packaging of DNA
Clinical correlations	Drug-induced lupus; systemic lupus erythematosus

Table 18–31

Anticardiolipin Antibodies

Antigenic specificities	Phospholipids (diphosphatidyl glycerol)
Mechanism of action	Inhibition of prothrombin activator complex (Xa, V, Ca^{2+}, lipid), platelet aggregation, ↓ prostaglandin I_2 release
Clinical correlations	Recurrent thromboses, livedo reticularis, chorea, recurrent fetal loss, cerebrovascular accidents, hypertension

Antiglobulins (Rheumatoid Factors)

Rheumatoid factors are present in approximately 10 to 30 percent of children with SLE, but high titers in children in the presence of a lupus-like disease may suggest the presence of an overlap syndrome. Antibodies to IgA are common in IgA-deficient patients with lupus.[419]

Immune Complexes

Immune complexes are fundamental to the pathogenesis of SLE, and their measurement in the peripheral blood is sometimes useful in patient management, especially if there is uncertainty concerning interpretation of the clinical status, anti-dsDNA titers, or serum complement levels. Methods employing C1q binding,[420] or Raji cells,[421] are the most reliable in SLE. Extensive reviews of the complexity and multiplicity of these assays have been published,[422, 423] and their clinical applicability to the problems of immune complex disease in SLE has been evaluated.[423–425] Abrass and colleagues demonstrated that an abnormal C1q binding was significantly associated with active SLE, including arthritis and nephritis, and correctly predicted a variation in disease activity 82 percent of the time.[426] In this study, detection of serum immune complexes correlated better with disease activity than did the anti-dsDNA or C3 levels, but this has rarely been our experience. Inter-test agreement of immune complex assays is often poor, and correlations with disease subsets or disease activity is variable. For these reasons, immune complex assays are of very limited utility in the diagnosis of management of SLE.[427] Cryoglobulins containing ANA and DNA are sometimes present in active SLE and may be responsible for certain expressions of the disease by intravascular activation of complement or precipitation of the hyperviscosity syndrome (Raynaud's phenomenon, acrocyanosis, purpura, and abdominal pain).

Complement

Determination of the serum complement level is one of the most important laboratory measures of active

SLE.[91, 428, 429] Specific components of the complement sequence, such as C3 and C4, may be assayed, or the total hemolytic complement (CH50) may be titrated by red cell lysis. The CH50 reflects the integrity of the total complement cascade, can be measured for either the classic or alternative pathways of complement activation, and is abnormally low in approximately 90 percent of children with active nephritis. The C3 concentration is depressed less often than the CH50 or C4. A low C4 is a consistent and reliable indicator of active nephritis in SLE if the baseline level is known in a particular patient. A more precise method of determining the state of complement activation is to measure its activation products. Elevations of complement factors Bb and C4d more accurately reflected disease activity than did measurements of C3, C4, or CH50 in one study.[430] Normal or moderately reduced levels of C3 and C4 in a patient with undetectable complement activity as measured by the hemolytic assay suggest a genetically determined deficiency of one of the complement components.[431–435]

Table 18–32

Evaluation of Lupus Nephritis

Urinalysis
Chemical and microscopic; culture if white blood cells present
Measurement of glomerular function
Plasma creatinine, urea nitrogen
Creatinine clearance; 24-hr protein excretion
Radionuclide glomerular filtration rate
Evaluation of disease activity
Serum anti-dsDNA antibody level
Serum complement assay
Renal ultrasonography and biopsy
Light, immunofluorescence, and electron microscopy

Urinalysis and Evaluation of Renal Involvement

Most children with active glomerulonephritis have abnormalities of the urinary sediment that are characteristic of the specific type of renal involvement or have a telescoped urine (a urinary sediment that shows, at one time, the sequential features characteristic of the course of glomerulonephritis). Proteinuria is probably the most common urinary abnormality, but hematuria and red blood cell casts are more important hallmarks of active glomerulitis. The latter are also useful clinical markers in following the course of treatment. Proteinuria is indicative of both glomerular and tubular abnormalities and, like the creatinine clearance, may not be a satisfactory short-term indicator of therapeutic response.

In severe renal disease, the sediment also contains increased numbers of cellular and fatty casts. With the onset of the nephrotic syndrome, doubly refractile oval fat bodies appear and assume the form of Maltese crosses on polarizing microscopy. Profuse proteinuria and a fixed specific gravity (1.010) are characteristic of the chronic phase of lupus nephritis. Broad casts of renal failure are seen at that time, and there may be few cellular elements in the sediment. Other abnormalities may include renal tubular acidosis. Excretion of immunoglobulin and light chains is also increased in nephritis.

Evaluation of the extent and activity of renal involvement in SLE requires the integration of several laboratory features (Table 18–32). The combination of high levels of anti-dsDNA and low levels of complement, especially C4, in the presence of an abnormal urinalysis makes active lupus nephritis a virtual certainty.[428, 436–439] Rarely, a child with seemingly active SLE has a near-normal complement level. (Because serum complement components are increased by inflammatory disease, a previously elevated level may be simply lowered to normal levels by immune complex fixation, rather than being reduced to subnormal levels.) Occasionally, a child with SLE may have hemolytic complement values in the subnormal range for long periods with no other indication of active renal disease. This observation may reflect the catabolic events associated with glucocorticoid therapy, general illness, or uremia that impairs the syntheses of complement components, particularly C3, rather than active disease per se.[440]

In the nephrotic syndrome, serologic markers of active disease, such as anti-dsDNA and even ANAs, may be falsely low because of profuse loss of IgG in the urine. An estimate of glomerular damage may be determined by the size of the proteins that are excreted (selectivity of the proteinuria). As in the idiopathic nephrotic syndrome, more severe disease is characterized by loss of the larger molecules (IgM, α_2-macroglobulin), and an altered ratio of IgG to transferrin.

The role of renal biopsy has been discussed under Necrotizing Angiitis, earlier in this chapter.

Analysis of Inflammatory Fluids

The synovial fluid in SLE is usually a group I noninflammatory fluid with a low white blood cell count ($<2000/mm^3$; $<2 \times 10^9/L$) (see Appendix). The protein content varies from transudative to exudative levels. Synovial fluid complement levels are low, reflecting, in part, the low levels in the blood. The pleural fluid contains increased protein (>3 g/dl), increased white blood cells (2500–5000 with mononuclear cells predominating), glucose levels near those of serum, and decreased C3 and C4. LE cells may be present in the smear.

GENERAL ASSESSMENT

Determination of overall disease activity in a multisystem disease such as SLE is difficult. Attempts to meet this challenge have resulted in the development of a number of disease activity scores. Those most commonly used are the Lupus Activity Index (LAI) (Table

18–33),[441] the SLE Disease Activity Index (SLEDAI) (Table 18–34),[442] the Systemic Lupus Activity Measure (SLAM) (Table 18–35),[443] and the British Isles Lupus Assessment Group (BILAG) Activity Index (Table 18–36).[444] In a recent comparison, the LAI was found to be most reliable, although all four had high validity.[445] SLEDAI has also been evaluated by Hawker and coworkers.[446] In one small study of 11 children and adolescents with SLE, the LAI and SLEDAI were found to compare closely to the physician's global assessment of disease activity.[447] Brunner and colleagues[447a] found SLEDAI, BILAG, and SLAM to be equally sensitive to clinical change in their application to 35 children with SLE.

Attempts have also been made to define a "flare" of disease activity. Sibley and colleagues[448] defined a flare as the exacerbation or development of new signs and symptoms that in the opinion of the attending physician required a change in therapy. Petri and coworkers[441] defined a flare as a change in physician's global assessment of 1 or more on a 3-point scale.

The Systemic Lupus International Collaborating Clinics (SLICC) Damage Index for SLE provides a measure of accumulated organ damage, whether it results from the disease or its treatment, and has been used in children.[449, 449a] Instruments to measure the quality of life in patients with SLE have also been developed and evaluated.[450] These indices have not yet been thoroughly evaluated in children and adolescents.

TREATMENT

Systemic lupus erythematosus is a chronic disease, characterized by remissions and relapses, and is associated with considerable morbidity and significant mortality. Treatment is in itself associated with morbidity, the effects of which may be permanent. The patient and family must cope with a chronic, unpredictable disease that ranges widely in severity. For the physician and other healthcare providers, the challenge is not only to provide the most appropriate pharmacologic care but also to ensure the health of the child in the broadest sense, and to help the child and family cope with the effects of the disease and its treatment. A brief summary of management is outlined in Table 18–37.

General Measures

The importance of general supportive care of the child with SLE cannot be underestimated. Incorporation of the child and parents into the planning of the overall treatment program is best accomplished by informing them in broad terms of the character and treatment of the disease. This is best achieved by a team of healthcare providers who are experienced in the management of children and adolescents with this multisystem disease, including a pediatric rheumatologist, nurse, social worker, and psychologist. It is our practice to seek the consultation of a nephrologist early in the disease course to provide optimal surveillance of the renal complications of the disease. Dermatologists, nutritionists, and other subspecialists, as needed, may become involved in the patient's care. Most children benefit from the continuity provided by surveillance by the same team over the long course of their disease. Although SLE is a serious problem, the steady improvement in long-term outcome justifies a reasonably opti-

Table 18–33

Lupus Activity Index (LAI)

Part I	Physician's global assessment on a visual analogue scale (VAS), from 0 to 5 points		
Part II	Assessment of 4 symptoms (fatigue, rash, joint involvement, serositis) on a VAS from 0 to 3 points		
Part III	Assessment of severity of involvement of 4 organ systems (CNS, renal, pulmonary, hematologic) on a VAS from 0 to 3 points		
Part IV	Assign points for medication used:		
	Prednisone	0–15 mg/d	1 point
		16–39 mg/d	2 points
		>40 mg/d	3 points
	Any immunosuppressive agent	Not used	0 points
		Used	3 points
Part V	Assign points for three laboratory values		
	Proteinuria	1+	1 point
		2+ to 3+	2 points
		4+	3 points
	Anti-dsDNA	0–3 points depending on degree of abnormality	
	C3, C4 or CH50	0–3 points depending on degree of abnormality	
Interpretation			
LAI score is arithmetic mean of the following			
	Part I	Number of points	
	Part II	Mean of 4 point values	
	Part III	Maximum of 4 point values	
	Part IV	Mean of 2 point values	
	Part V	Mean of 3 point values	

Adapted from Petri M, Genovese M, Engle E, Hochberg M: Definition, incidence, and clinical description of flare in systemic lupus erythematosus. A prospective cohort study. Arthritis Rheum 34: 937, © 1991 Wiley-Liss, Inc. Reprinted by permission of Wiley-Liss, Inc., a subsidiary of John Wiley & Sons, Inc.

Table 18–34

Systemic Lupus Erythematosus Disease Activity Index (SLEDAI)

WEIGHT	SCORE	DESCRIPTOR	DEFINITION
8	_____	Seizure	Recent onset. Exclude metabolic, infectious, or drug causes.
8	_____	Psychosis	Altered ability to function in normal activity due to severe disturbance in the perception of reality. Include hallucinations; incoherence; marked loose associations; impoverished thought content; marked illogical thinking; bizarre, disorganized, or catatonic behavior. Exclude uremic and drug causes.
8	_____	Organic brain syndrome	Altered mental function with impaired orientation, memory, or other intellectual function, with rapid onset and fluctuating clinical features. Include clouding of consciousness with reduced capacity to focus, and inability to sustain attention to environment, plus at least two of the following: perceptual disturbance, incoherent speech, insomnia or daytime drowsiness, or increased or decreased psychomotor activity. Exclude metabolic, infectious, or drug causes.
8	_____	Visual disturbance	Retinal changes of SLE. Include cytoid bodies, retinal hemorrhages, serous exudate or hemorrhages in the choroid, or optic neuritis. Exclude hypertensive, infectious, or drug causes.
8	_____	Cranial nerve disorder	New onset of sensory or motor neuropathy involving cranial nerves.
8	_____	Lupus headache	Severe, persistent headache; may be migrainous, but must be nonresponsive to narcotic analgesia.
8	_____	CVA	New onset of cerebrovascular accident(s). Exclude arteriosclerosis.
8	_____	Vasculitis	Ulceration, gangrene, tender finger nodules, periungual infarction, splinter hemorrhages, or biopsy or angiogram proof of vasculitis.
4	_____	Arthritis	More than two joints with pain and signs of inflammation (e.g., tenderness, swelling, or effusion).
4	_____	Myositis	Proximal muscle aching/weakness, associated with elevated creatine kinase/aldolase or electromyogram changes or a biopsy showing myositis.
4	_____	Urinary casts	Heme-granular or red blood cell casts.
4	_____	Hematuria	>5 red blood cells/high power field. Exclude stone, infection, or other cause.
4	_____	Proteinuria	>0.5 g/24 hr. New onset or recent increase of more than 0.5 g/24 hr.
4	_____	Pyuria	>5 white blood cells/high power field. Exclude infection.
2	_____	New rash	New onset or recurrence of inflammatory type rash.
2	_____	Alopecia	New onset or recurrence of abnormal, patchy, or diffuse loss of hair.
2	_____	Mucosal ulcers	New onset or recurrence of oral or nasal ulcerations.
2	_____	Pleurisy	Pleuritic chest pain with pleural rub or effusion, or pleural thickening.
	_____	Pericarditis	Pericardial pain with at least one of the following: rub, effusion, or electrocardiogram or echocardiogram confirmation.
2	_____	Low complement	Decrease in CH_{50}, C3, or C4 below the lower limit of normal for testing laboratory.
2	_____	Increased DNA binding	>25% binding by Farr assay or above normal range for testing laboratory.
1	_____	Fever	>38°C. Exclude infectious cause.
1	_____	Thrombocytopenia	<100,000 platelets/mm^3.
1	_____	Leukopenia	<3000 white blood cells/mm^3. Exclude drug causes.

From Bombardier C, Gladman DD, Urowitz M, et al: Derivation of the SLEDAI. A disease activity index for lupus patients. Arthritis Rheum 35: 630, © 1992 Wiley-Liss, Inc. Reprinted by permission of Wiley-Liss, Inc., a subsidiary of John Wiley & Sons, Inc.

Table 18–35

Systemic Lupus Activity Measure (SLAM)

CATEGORY	MILD	MODERATE	SEVERE
Constitutional			
Weight loss	1		3
Fatigue	1		3
Fever	1		3
Mucocutaneous			
Malar rash or photosensitive rash, or periungual erythema or nailfold infarct	1		
Alopecia	1	2	
Discoid, bullous, or lupus profundus	1	2	3
Cutaneous vasculitis	1	2	3
Ocular			
Cytoid bodies	1		3
Hemorrhages or episcleritis	1		3
Papillitis or pseudotumor cerebri	1		3
Visceral			
Diffuse lymphadenopathy	1	2	
Large liver or spleen	1	2	
Pleural effusion	1	2	3
Pneumonitis	1	2	3
Raynaud's phenomenon	1		
Hypertension	1	2	3
Carditis	1	2	3
Abdominal pain	1	2	3
Neuromuscular			
Stroke	1	2	3
Seizure	1	2	3
Cortical dysfunction	1	2	3
Headache	1	2	3
Myalgia/myositis	1	2	3
Synovitis/tenosynovitis	1	2	3
Laboratory			
Anemia	1	2	3
Leukopenia	1	2	3
Lymphopenia	1	2	3
Thrombocytopenia	1	2	3
Elevated ESR	1	2	3
Elevated serum creatinine	1	2	3
Abnormal urine sediment	1	2	3

Maximum score is 86. For definitions of grade of severity refer to Liang et al.[443]

Modified from Liang MH, Socher SA, Larson MG, Schur PH: Reliability and validity of six systems for the clinical assessment of disease activity in systemic lupus erythematosus. Arthritis Rheum 32: 1107, © 1989 Wiley-Liss, Inc. Reprinted by permission of Wiley-Liss, Inc., a subsidiary of John Wiley & Sons, Inc.

mistic approach to the patient and family and energetic treatment of each exacerbation or complication. It is our opinion that careful attention to all of the details of managing SLE has contributed as much to the improved prognosis as any single therapeutic program or drug.

As with other illnesses in childhood, rigorous restraints on general activity are usually unnecessary and undesirable, not to mention often impossible. Except during periods of severe active disease, regular school attendance should be expected, and communication with and education of concerned teachers and physical education instructors helps ensure the child's optimal participation in school activities. The child should be encouraged to participate in compatible extracurricular activities as the disease permits.

Certain general aspects of treatment are of primary importance. The dangers of exposure to excessive sunlight should be stressed. Sunscreens with sun protection factors greater than 15 that protect against ultraviolet B light[451] should be applied to all exposed skin whenever the child is outside, whether or not it is sunny. Even exposure to fluorescent lights that emit ultraviolet B may be associated with symptoms.[452] A variety of suitable sunscreens is available, some with a water base, which are most appropriate for use on the face, and others that contain alcohol and may be used

Table 18–36

British Isles Lupus Assessment Group (BILAG)

Systems

Nonspecific
Mucocutaneous
Central nervous system
Renal
Musculoskeletal
Cardiovascular and respiratory
Vasculitis
Hematologic

Grading System

A = Intention to treat disease process (not just symptoms) (9 points)
B = Potential problem, mild, or reversible symptoms (4 points)
C = Stable disease (1 point)
D = System unaffected (0 points)

Scoring

A or B in any system denotes active disease. Possible scores range from 0 to 72.

Adapted from Symmons DPM, Coopock JS, Bacon PA, et al: Development and assessment of a computerized index of clinical disease activity in systemic lupus erythematosus. Q J Med 69: 927, 1988. By permission of Oxford University Press.

Table 18–37

Approach to Management of Systemic Lupus Erythematosus

General
- Counseling, education, team approach
- Adequate rest, appropriate nutrition
- Use of sunscreen
- Immunizations, especially antipneumoccocal vaccine
- Prompt management of infection

Nonsteroidal anti-inflammatory drugs
- For musculoskeletal signs and symptoms

Anticoagulation
- If anticardiolipin antibodies are present in significant titers
  - Low-dose aspirin unless thrombosis has occurred
  - Heparin, followed by warfarin if thrombosis has occurred

Hydroxychloroquine
- For cutaneous disease and as an adjunct to glucocorticoids for systemic disease

Glucocorticoids
- Oral prednisone 1–2 mg/kg/d
- IV methylprednisolone initially, and at monthly intervals for maintenance therapy in severe disease

Immunosuppressives
- Azathioprine 1–2 mg/kg/d
- Cyclophosphamide 1–2 mg/kg/d orally; 500–1000 mg/M²/mo (IV)

on other exposed skin. Some are water resistant, but reapplication after bathing or swimming is advisable.

The risk of infection is increased in the child with SLE, and the sequelae of infection may be catastrophic. Prevention of infection by immunization is particularly important in these children, and the recommendations outlined in Chapter 10 should be followed.

A high index of suspicion for infections will facilitate prompt diagnosis and appropriate treatment. Antibiotics should not be used prophylactically and should not be given before appropriate cultures have been obtained. Fever, which may accompany active SLE, should always be considered first to be caused by infection, and cultures of blood, pharynx, and urine should be taken. Functional asplenia[318, 319] makes the child with SLE extremely susceptible to severe, sometimes fatal pneumococcal sepsis. For this reason, children with SLE should be immunized against pneumococci. Basilar pneumonitis should always be initially regarded as bacterial and blood cultures as well as cultures and a Gram stain of sputum should be obtained. Acute CNS disease should also be regarded initially as an effect of infection, and cerebrospinal fluid examinations should be performed.

Laboratory markers of infection may be somewhat blunted by the primary disease. In a child with SLE, elevation of a previously low white blood cell count into the normal range may represent the maximal response to infection. Marked elevations of serum levels of CRP are strongly suggestive of infection in a patient with SLE. The many complications of tuberculosis should be considered in the differential diagnosis. CNS infection with organisms such as *Cryptococcus* may occur.

General Aspects of Pharmacologic Therapy

Specific treatment should be individualized and based on the extent and severity of the disease (see Table 18–37). Four groups of drugs are almost universally used to treat most children and adolescents with lupus at some stage, however.

Nonsteroidal Anti-inflammatory Drugs

The primary role of nonsteroidal anti-inflammatory drugs (NSAIDs) in the management of the child with SLE is to treat musculoskeletal complaints. Myalgia, arthralgia, or arthritis may respond well to anti-inflammatory doses of the NSAIDs. It is our practice to avoid the use of aspirin for this purpose because of the tendency of children with SLE on anti-inflammatory doses of the drug to develop elevations of serum levels of the liver enzymes alanine and aspartic transaminase,[453] and because of the risk of Reye's syndrome. (Low-dose aspirin is not contraindicated, however, and is widely used in children with the antiphospholipid syndrome and SLE.) Occasional reports have linked the use of ibuprofen to the occurrence of aseptic meningitis[454, 455] or other hypersensitivity reactions[456] in patients with SLE. Aseptic meningitis has also been noted following naproxen[457] or tolmetin.[458] Nonetheless, these reports have been very rare, and it seems reasonable to use an NSAID such as naproxen for the management of musculoskeletal pain or inflammation in children with lupus.

Antimalarial Drugs

Antimalarials such as hydroxychloroquine are most often given as an adjunct to therapy with glucocorticoids, rather than as the mainstay of treatment. The role of this medication in the management of SLE has been changing since the studies of the Canadian Hydroxychloroquine Study Group[459, 460] reported that this drug made an important contribution to management of the disease. In a randomized, double-blind, placebo-controlled study of the effect of withdrawing hydroxychloroquine therapy in adults with clinically stable SLE, the frequency and severity of flares of SLE activity were much higher in patients who received the placebo than in those maintained on hydroxychloroquine. In addition, hydroxychloroquine may also have a role in reversing glucocorticoid-induced changes in plasma lipids.[461–463] For both reasons, it is our practice to treat children and adolescents with SLE with hydroxychloroquine (6 mg/kg/day) at the initiation of steroid therapy, and for up to 2 years or more.[464, 465] Because of the possibility that the risk of retinal toxicity from antimalarials is increased in the presence of impaired renal function, children with SLE should be carefully monitored for retinal toxicity related to the drug (see Chapter 7). Children with SLE may be more prone than those with JRA to develop retinal damage.

Glucocorticoids

Without doubt, glucocorticoids constitute the mainstay of pharmacologic therapy for SLE, and almost all children with SLE require oral prednisone or prednisolone, or intravenous methylprednisolone at some stage of the disease. The choice between prednisone and prednisolone is one of personal experience and preference, although some authorities believe that the latter may result in somewhat greater cushingoid effects. High-dose intravenous methylprednisolone is often indicated in children with severe acute disease such as acute hemolytic anemia, CNS disease, and overwhelming systemic disease ("lupus crisis"), or as part of the long-term management of lupus nephritis.

Initial Glucocorticoid Therapy. Initial disease control usually cannot be achieved without daily glucocorticoid administration for a period of several weeks or months, and many children require these drugs for years. Prednisone or prednisolone should be given in a dose sufficient to achieve disease control, often 1 to 2 mg/kg/day (Table 18–38). At least at the initiation of therapy, oral glucocorticoids should be given in three

Table 18–38

Glucocorticoid Therapy for Children With Systemic Lupus Erythematosus

Initiation of Therapy (First 4–6 wk)	
Oral prednisone	15–60 mg/d (0.5–2 mg/kg/d) in at least 2 divided doses (depending on severity and type of organ involvement)
IV methylprednisolone	Indicated for severe disease (active lupus nephritis, hematologic crisis, central nervous system disease) 30 mg/kg/d on 1 to 5 consecutive days
Tapering the Prednisone Dose	
If the dose is 20–60 mg/d	Decrease by 2.5–5.0 mg/wk
If the dose is 10–20 mg/d	Decrease by 1–2.5 mg/wk
If dose <10 mg/d	Decrease by 0.5–1 mg every 2–4 wk

or four divided doses to maximize the anti-inflammatory and immunosuppressive effects. The initial dose of glucocorticoid and the frequency of its administration depend on the severity of the disease and the organ systems affected. The potential benefits of sustained glucocorticoid administration must be balanced against the serious complications that result from this treatment (see Chapter 7).

Low-dose therapy, defined as a dose of prednisone of less than 0.5 mg/kg/day given in divided doses by mouth, is usually sufficient to control fever, dermatitis, arthritis, and serositis within hours to days of starting treatment. Children usually have a dramatically improved sense of well-being and increased energy within days of initiating therapy. Although low-dose glucocorticoids may be sufficient to control hemolytic anemia or thrombocytopenia and reverse abnormalities of the sedimentation rate, anti-dsDNA antibodies, and complement levels, these effects may require several weeks to a few months.

High-dose oral prednisone in the range of 1 to 2 mg/kg/day in divided doses is employed for treatment of acute hemolytic anemia, CNS disease, parenchymal pulmonary disease, and the more severe types of lupus nephritis (Table 18–39).[33, 351, 352, 466, 467] In addition, intravenous methylprednisolone (30 mg/kg/d on 1 or more consecutive days) may be necessary to manage these aspects of the disease, particularly when a rapid response is needed. Hypertension, uremia, and preexisting psychosis are relative contraindications to high steroid doses.

Table 18–39

Approach to Therapy for Lupus Nephritis

Mesangial nephritis	Symptomatic management
Focal nephritis	Prednisone 0.5 mg/kg/d for 2–4 mo, then taper to maintenance level
Diffuse nephritis	Prednisone 1 mg/kg/d for 3–6 mo, then taper to maintenance level Cyclophosphamide 1–2 mg/kg/d, or IV pulse every month for 6 mo, possibly longer
Membranous nephritis	Prednisone 0.5–1 mg/kg/d, possible addition of cyclophosphamide or azathioprine
In all patients, manage hypertension and nephrotic syndrome	

Tapering the Glucocorticoid Dose. After the acute manifestations of the disease are controlled, glucocorticoids should be reduced to the lowest possible level that will maintain the well-being of the child. Tapering from high dose to minimum dose is one of the most challenging aspects of management of the child with SLE. In a justified determination to minimize glucocorticoid toxicity, the physician may be tempted to make an injudiciously rapid dose reduction; too often, the result is a flare of the disease, with a subsequent requirement to increase the dosage by 25 to 50 percent or more. A smooth, gradual tapering of drug dose, with frequent monitoring to make certain that clinical and laboratory measures of disease activity are suppressed, is much more satisfactory. In Table 18–38, average dosage schedules are suggested as guidelines, but these must be individualized as necessary. Ordinarily, the initial glucocorticoid dose is maintained for a period of 3 to 4 weeks. Thereafter, a weekly or biweekly decrease in the daily prednisone dose of approximately 5 mg is appropriate when the child is taking 20 to 60 mg/day. The average reduction every 2 to 4 weeks at daily doses of 10 to 20 mg should be approximately 2.5 mg/day. At doses below 10 mg/day, a biweekly or monthly reduction of the daily dose of not more than 1 mg is appropriate. Consolidation of prednisone administration into a single daily dose, preferably given in the morning, may be successful at levels of 10 mg/day or lower. Alternate-day therapy may risk inadequate disease suppression and, in spite of its obvious advantages with respect to side-effects, has little role in the management of children with acute SLE, although it may be used in children who require low doses (<10 mg/day) to maintain disease control.

No studies in children have been performed comparing these treatment protocols, and the recommendations in the preceding paragraph are based on clinical experience. It is generally agreed that most children with SLE are withdrawn completely from glucocorticoid drugs only with great difficulty during the initial years after diagnosis. Even long-term very low dose maintenance therapy can minimize the tendency toward exacerbations during the protracted course of this disease.

Maintenance Glucocorticoid Therapy. Clinical response, the white blood cell and platelet counts, hemoglobin, serum complement, and levels of anti-dsDNA

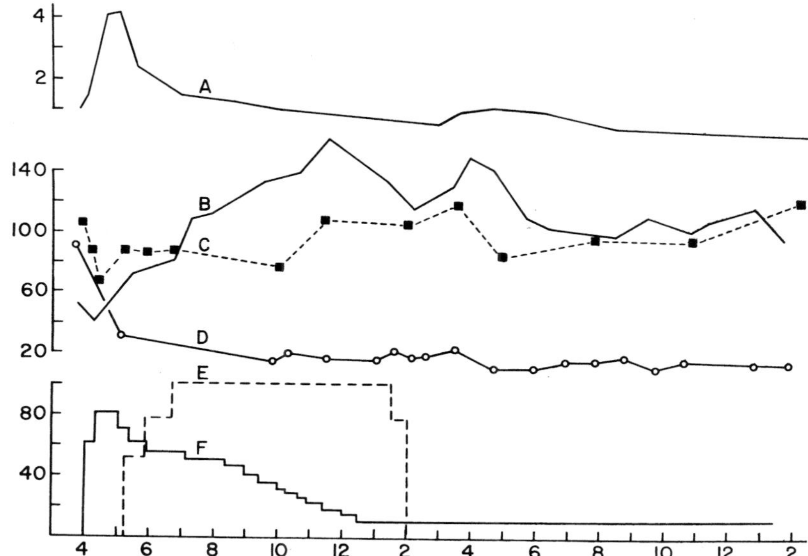

Figure 18–34. The course of a young girl with acute SLE and diffuse proliferative glomerulonephritis is charted in relation to urinary protein values measured in g/24 hours *(A)*; serum hemolytic complement units *(B)*; creatinine clearance in liters/24 hours *(C)*; and anti-DNA antibody expressed as DNA binding in percent *(D)*.

The doses of cyclophosphamide *(E)* and prednisone *(F)* are indicated in mg/day. Gradual resolution of systemic disease was accompanied by a fall in the DNA binding level to a normal value of less than 20 percent and a rise in the serum hemolytic complement level to a normal value above 110 CH_{50} units. Resolution of the acute phase of renal disease was accompanied initially by an increase in urinary protein excretion and a decrease in creatinine clearance. A fall in daily protein excretion and a gradual rise of the creatinine clearance to relatively normal values followed. Initial deterioration in the creatinine clearance rate with glucocorticoid therapy is occasionally observed.

antibodies, together with urinalysis and indices of renal function, are periodically assessed to determine the adequacy of treatment. As long as these parameters are improving, treatment should be maintained. It is our practice not to alter the regimen of glucocorticoid administration, if at all possible, until the serum C3, C4, or CH50 are close to normal, there is no clinically significant hematocytopenia, and the levels of anti-dsDNA have fallen substantially (Fig. 18–34). In many children with proliferative nephritis, treatment with adequate doses of glucocorticoid leads to a return of the urinalysis finding toward normal, although proteinuria and a depressed creatinine clearance are less responsive to therapy. Failure of high-dose prednisone (2 mg/kg/day in divided doses) to result in substantial improvement in clinical, serologic, and urinary abnormalities within 8 weeks should prompt consideration of alternative therapies. The decision to initiate therapy with a cytotoxic drug such as azathioprine or cyclophosphamide is usually influenced by a number of factors, including steroid responsiveness, steroid dependency, and steroid toxicity. A patient who is steroid responsive and dependent at an acceptably low prednisone dose may be best managed without cytotoxic drugs. Side-effects of glucocorticoids are frequently such, however, that institution of another agent is indicated, even if the disease appears to be well controlled.

Immunosuppressive Agents

Most recent pediatric experience has indicated that immunosuppressive agents are often required to control SLE and permit an acceptable quality of life. A meta-analysis of eight studies in adults with SLE that compared the effect of prednisone alone to that of prednisone and azathioprine, or prednisone and cyclophosphamide, demonstrated that an immunosuppressive agent given with prednisone was superior to prednisone alone.[468] Depending to a large extent on the severity of the disease and specific organ involvement, a choice of immunosuppressive agent is made among azathioprine, cyclophosphamide, methotrexate, and cyclosporin A (Table 18–40).

Azathioprine. Azathioprine has probably been used for a longer period of time to treat childhood lupus than any other second-line agent. However, its role is still being defined. It has traditionally been used as the initial second-line agent, largely because of its perceived safety. For children with SLE that is not controlled by acceptable doses of prednisone, addition of azathioprine may be indicated to permit a reduction in steroid dose. Abrupt withdrawal of azathioprine after long-term treatment resulted in an exacerbation of systemic disease in seven of nine patients in one study.[469] The exacerbations were delayed by 3 months and were often refractory to treatment. One patient died during such an exacerbation. Experience in 66 pediatric patients with SLE, 19 of whom were treated with azathioprine, indicated that early treatment with prednisone

Table 18–40

Approach to the Use of Immunosuppressive Drugs in Systemic Lupus Erythematosus

Azathioprine	1–2 mg/kg/d (PO) For patients who are unresponsive to glucocorticoids and hydroxychloroquine, or who develop unacceptable toxicity to these drugs
Cyclophosphamide	1–2 mg/kg/d (PO) For patients with diffuse proliferative glomerulonephritis, or significant CNS disease
	500–1000 mg/M^2 per mo (IV) For patients with life-threatening manifestations, or resistant CNS or renal disease

CNS, central nervous system.

and azathioprine was effective in controlling disease and preserving renal function.[470] It is probable that the appropriate role of azathioprine in childhood SLE is in the management of steroid-resistant or steroid-dependent disease with or without class III or IV nephritis.

Cyclophosphamide. Cyclophosphamide is an important drug for the management of severe aspects of SLE, particularly severe lupus nephritis and CNS disease. Because of its potential toxicity, however, cyclophosphamide is not indicated for minor manifestations of disease and should only be used by experienced clinicians familiar with the anticipated benefits and toxicity of this drug. Cyclophosphamide alone is ineffective[471] and should always be used in conjunction with glucocorticoids where it has been shown to be superior to prednisone alone, especially in severe nephritis.[472] There have been no controlled trials in children, but extensive comparative studies of azathioprine and cyclophosphamide in the management of renal nephritis in adults have been reported by investigators at the U.S. National Institutes of Health.[473, 474] In a comparison of oral prednisone, or prednisone plus either azathioprine, oral cyclophosphamide, intravenous cyclophosphamide, or intravenous cyclophosphamide plus azathioprine, renal function was better in the group receiving oral or intravenous cyclophosphamide than in those receiving azathioprine or prednisone alone. The results of other studies support these conclusions.[475–477] These differences in outcome did not become apparent until 5 to 10 years after treatment was started. The differences in mortality, however, were not impressively different among the treatment groups.[478]

Intravenous pulse cyclophosphamide used in combination with oral prednisone is an effective regimen for the prevention of disease flares and the preservation of renal function in severe disease. A regimen of seven monthly pulses of cyclophosphamide followed by a pulse of cyclophosphamide every 3 months thereafter was found to be optimal.[479] This regimen is also recommended for management of lupus in children and adolescents.[480] The combination of oral prednisone and intravenous pulse cyclophosphamide for the treatment of severe neuropsychiatric lupus in adults and older adolescents was dramatically effective in the majority of patients who had been refractory to other therapy, including glucocorticoids and azathioprine.[481]

Cyclophosphamide is probably the drug of choice among the second-line agents for severe nephritis or CNS disease. Its short- and long-term toxicity limits its prolonged use, however, and in patients who require treatment for longer than 3 years, an alternative should be sought because of the risk of ovarian failure and malignancy. Gonadotropin-releasing hormone (GnRH) and GnRH agonists are currently being investigated for use in preserving gonadal function in patients who require cyclophosphamide therapy.[482]

Methotrexate. Experience with methotrexate to treat childhood SLE is limited.[483–485] In a study of 10 children, the addition of 2.5 to 10 mg of methotrexate per week reduced the requirement for glucocorticoid and permitted cessation of cyclophosphamide in the majority of patients.[474] In contrast, Ravelli and colleagues[485] treated 11 children with methotrexate (12.5–17.0 mg/M^2/week) and prednisone and concluded that although there was initial improvement, methotrexate did not make a major contribution to steroid requirement or disease control. Silverman suggested that methotrexate may have a role in the management of resistant arthritis and skin disease in childhood lupus.[470] The use of intrathecal dexamethasone and methotrexate has been suggested in the treatment of CNS lupus,[486] and benefit from methotrexate has been reported in one patient with interstitial lung disease.[487]

Cyclosporin. An early study showed that cyclosporin in an average daily dose of 5 mg/kg permitted reduction in prednisone dose and better disease control in 8 of 13 children with severe glucocorticoid-dependent or glucocorticoid-resistant SLE in childhood.[488] In an open study of 40 children with class III or IV lupus nephritis and heavy proteinuria, cyclosporin (5 mg/kg/day) was compared with prednisone (2 mg/kg/day) plus cyclophosphamide (2 mg/kg/day). Cyclosporin was as effective as prednisone and cyclophosphamide in reducing proteinuria, allowed significantly greater growth, and was well tolerated.[489] The authors suggested that cyclosporin A could have an important steroid-sparing effect, as reported in adult lupus patients.[490]

Mycophenolate Mofetil. Experience with the use of mycophenolate mofetil in childhood SLE is very limited. Studies of this drug in adults with SLE indicate that, in combination with prednisone, it may be at least as effective as cyclophosphamide.[490a, 490b] The toxicity of this agent at least in the short-term appears to be less than that of cyclophosphamide.

Biological Modulation

Intravenous immunoglobulin (IVIG) has been used to a very limited extent in adults with refractory SLE,[491–493] including those with thrombocytopenia, in whom it evoked a mild but transient improvement in platelet counts.[494, 495] In one small study, IVIG resulted in modest temporary improvement in a measure of disease activity and decline in the titer of anti-dsDNA antibodies.[496] Lafferty and colleagues reported that IVIG was successful in the treatment of the acquired factor VIII inhibitor that had resulted in bleeding.[497] Experience in the use of IVIG to treat manifestations of childhood lupus is largely unreported, and its role should be considered to be very limited at present.

Plasmapheresis may occasionally be of benefit in the child with a severe acute complication such as thrombotic thrombocytopenic purpura,[294] but has not been shown to be beneficial in the treatment of lupus nephritis.[498–500] Whether synchronized plasmapheresis and cyclophosphamide therapy has any significant role in disease management is uncertain.[501] Therapy with monoclonal antibodies directed to CD4[502, 503] or CD5 T-cell antigens[504] may offer some promise, but evidence to date is extremely limited.

Other, essentially experimental, therapies include thalidomide[505] and extracorporeal photochemotherapy.[506] None of these forms of therapy has been evaluated in children. Autologous bone marrow transplantation has been performed in several adolescents with SLE with good short-term effect, but the long-term effectiveness of such therapy is not yet known.[507, 507a]

Management of Specific Aspects of the Disease

Acute Hemolytic Anemia

Acute hemolytic anemia can be a medical emergency requiring the use of high-dose intravenous methylprednisolone (30 mg/kg/day on one or more consecutive days). Some children are unresponsive even to high-dose glucocorticoid therapy. Splenectomy may be necessary in such children, although this procedure may be less efficacious than in the idiopathic form of the disease. For the usual reasons, blood transfusions should be avoided in these patients if not absolutely necessary; in addition, they may be at added risk because of the high frequency of anti-erythrocyte and anti-leukocyte antibodies, and because of the occurrence of anti-IgA antibodies when SLE is associated with selective IgA deficiency.

Antiphospholipid Syndrome

The optimal management of patients with the antiphospholipid syndrome is controversial and depends on the presence of laboratory abnormalities that demonstrate antiphospholipid antibodies or their effects on coagulation, and the history of venous or arterial thrombotic events.[508] In patients who have an antiphospholipid antibody and a platelet count greater than 70,000/mm^3, ($>7 \times 10^9$/L), low-dose aspirin (3 mg/kg/day) is recommended to reduce the risk of vascular occlusion. In patients who have high levels of antibody to cardiolipin, or in whom venous or arterial thrombosis has already occurred, anticoagulation with heparin, followed by warfarin is recommended.[508a]

Central Nervous System Disease

Central nervous system manifestations of SLE usually require high-dose oral or intravenous glucocorticoids once the possibility of infection has been excluded. Thirty-one adults and adolescents with progressing neuropsychiatric SLE as demonstrated by serial imaging studies were treated with intravenous cyclophosphamide (500 mg/M^2). All had received glucocorticoids and one third had received azathioprine or chlorambucil. Improvement was noted in 61 percent and a further 29 percent stabilized after intravenous cyclophosphamide was given.[481] The use of both glucocorticoids and cyclophosphamide in treating CNS lupus in children is supported by another smaller study.[509] Initial therapy in this group of seven children with neuropsychiatric lupus consisted of intravenous methylprednisolone and intravenous cyclophosphamide, followed by intravenous cyclophosphamide every month for at least 3 months, and oral prednisone in a dose of 1 to 2 mg/kg/d. Significant improvement was noted within 1 week of instituting therapy, and all patients recovered except for a residual neurologic deficit in one patient.

Lupus Nephritis

Lupus nephritis almost always requires the use of sustained doses of oral prednisone or prednisolone. The dose and duration of treatment remain controversial, however. Mesangial or focal nephritis may respond to low to moderate doses of prednisone (0.5–1.0 mg/kg/day) given over a period of several months. The efficacy of therapy is judged by a decrease in hematuria, improvement in renal function, and normalization of C3, C4, and CH50, with a fall in the level of anti-dsDNA antibodies. Proteinuria may persist for a lengthy period of time and, if it is the only abnormality, should not prevent tapering the prednisone dose. Diffuse proliferative glomerulonephritis usually requires high-dose prednisone (1–2 mg/kg/day) and, in many cases, the addition of azathioprine (2 mg/kg/day) or cyclophosphamide (2 mg/kg/day). In our experience, cyclophosphamide is the drug of choice in this situation, although if the renal abnormalities are mild, azathioprine may be effective. Management of hypertension with a drug such as nifedipine is essential. If there is not a prompt response to oral cyclophosphamide and prednisone, the addition of intravenous pulse cyclophosphamide and intravenous methylprednisolone is appropriate. Membranous glomerulonephritis is less likely to be responsive to glucocorticoids than is proliferative disease.[510]

The majority of children with SLE do not develop renal insufficiency if they are treated early and maintained in serologic and clinical remission. Systemic exacerbation of the disease or loss of control by inappropriate tapering of medication often leads to a return of the renal abnormalities. Such exacerbations are usually responsive to adequate therapy, and severe renal insufficiency generally does not occur. Some children appear to enter permanent remissions; late in the disease course, gradual deterioration of renal function may again be observed (end-stage renal disease) (Table 18–41) in the absence of serologic deterioration.

Dialysis and transplantation offer final approaches to maintaining life and renal function in patients with end-stage renal disease.[511] Hemodialysis is difficult psychologically for younger children and should be undertaken only in centers with experience in this age group. McCurdy and coworkers[512] reported that renal failure occurred in 22 percent of 71 children with SLE during a 13-year period. Of the 16 patients with renal failure, 2 had successful transplants and were alive and well 2 years later, 4 died of fulminant SLE within 1 month of beginning dialysis, and 10 received chronic dialysis. Of these, 5 died of sepsis. Thus, although dialysis is an important potential intervention in the child with lupus

Table 18–41

End-Stage Lupus Nephritis

Characteristics
Clinically inactive
Normal serum complement, anti-dsDNA
Hypertension
Intermittent sepsis
Management
Minimize glucocorticoids
Antihypertensives
Hemodialysis
Renal transplantation

nephritis, the relatively low long-term success rate should prompt vigorous attempts to prevent progression of renal disease and development of renal failure.

Renal transplantation has offered an alternative long-term approach and has generally been successful.[513] Data from 1982 and 1983 indicate that the 5-year survival rate of all patients who had end-stage renal failure was 80 percent.[514, 515] More recent studies in adult recipients of allografts for end-stage renal failure reported that the graft survival rate at 1 year was 68 percent, and at 5 years was 54 to 60 percent.[516] Graft survival rate at 10 years was 45 percent.[517] Recurrences of the nephritis in the allograft have been noted,[518] but at this stage the disease is usually inactive serologically and permanent remissions occur.[519]

Dyslipoproteinemia

Insufficient attention has been paid to the management of the lipid abnormalities of SLE and prevention of their long-term sequelae. Intermittent monitoring of total cholesterol, very low density cholesterol and triglycerides should alert the physician to the advisability of dietary or pharmacologic intervention. The lipid-lowering effects of hydroxychloroquine should be exploited in achieving this aim.

COURSE OF THE DISEASE AND PROGNOSIS

Systemic lupus erythematosus is characterized by a prolonged course over many years that is punctuated by exacerbations and remissions.[36, 520, 521] The disease may flare at any time, either spontaneously or as a reaction to infection or some other identifiable event. Spontaneous remissions occur. Fever and prominent constitutional symptoms are present at the onset of disease and during exacerbations. In an early study,[31] there was little tendency for involvement of new organ systems during exacerbations except for CNS disease. King and associates[35] found that CNS, cardiac, and renal involvement occurred somewhat more frequently during the course of the disease than at onset.

Morbidity

With the increasing life expectancy of children with SLE, a number of factors that affect the long-term quality of life are assuming increased importance (Table 18–42). These observations are related to previously unappreciated aspects of SLE, complications of drug therapy, especially glucocorticoid and immunosuppressive drugs, and problems with physical and psychological adaptations to a severe chronic illness.

Recurrent infections contribute significantly to the morbidity of children with SLE.[522, 523] In a review of 32 patients with onset of SLE before 16 years of age who had been followed for a period of 10 years (1979–1988),[523] infection occurred in almost two thirds of patients overall, and disseminated infection with *Aspergillus, Candida, Nocardia, Clostridum perfringens*, or *Pseudomonas* contributed to all five deaths. It is not certain whether these infections were primarily related to the longer-term course of the disease in surviving patients or to the therapy, but infections were more common in patients who had received prolonged high-dose glucocorticoid therapy. In contrast to this experience, infection has only occasionally been a serious problem in patients with SLE seen in our clinics. The development of functional asplenia in some children with SLE is a contributing factor to infection with *Streptococcus pneumoniae. Pneumocystis carinii* pneumonitis occurred in one of our patients and *Pseudomonas* osteomyelitis and septic arthritis in another.

Atherosclerotic complications of SLE and its treatment are emerging as an important residual problem of the illness, becoming clinically apparent only after a decade or more of active disease. Whether these developments are related primarily to the lupus per se, to prolonged hyperlipoproteinemia, or the long-term complications of glucocorticoid therapy is not clear. Undoubtedly, all of these factors may contribute to the final prognostic profile.

Mortality

There has been a remarkable improvement in the outcome for patients with SLE during the past three decades (Table 18–43).[35–37, 522–530] Although SLE is a serious, life-threatening disease, an optimistic approach to the care of these children is now justified by current data.

Table 18–42

Morbidity in Childhood Lupus

Renal	Hypertension, dialysis, transplantation
Central nervous system	Organic brain syndrome, seizures, psychosis, neurocognitive dysfunction
Heart	Atherosclerosis, myocardial infarction, cardiomyopathy, valvular disease
Immune	Recurrent infection, functional asplenia, malignancy
Musculoskeletal	Osteopenia, compression fractures, osteonecrosis
Ocular	Cataracts, glaucoma
Endocrine	Diabetes, obesity, growth failure, infertility, fetal wastage

Table 18–43
Survivorship in Children With Systemic Lupus Erythematosus

STUDY (YR)	PATIENTS (n)	PERCENT SURVIVAL 5 yr	10 yr	15 yr
Meislin and Rothfield (1968)[36]	42	42/72*	—	—
Walravens and Chase (1976)[37]	50	—	60–70	—
Garin et al (1976)[353]	49	72	—	—
King et al (1977)[35]	108	78	—	—
Fish et al (1977)[524]	49	—	86	—
Abeles et al (1980)[525]	67	89/100*	—	—
Platt et al (1982)[522]	70	90	85	77
Glidden et al (1983)[527]	55	92	85	—
McCurdy et al (1992)[512]	71	—	28†	
Yang et al (1994)[530]	167‡	91		
Baqi et al (1996)[529]	56§		29	

*% with renal disease/% with no renal disease.
†Life table analysis.
‡All 167 patients had nephritis.
§63% had WHO class III or IV renal histology.

The prognosis for an individual child with SLE, however, is relatively unpredictable. Generalizations about prognosis are especially unreliable during the first 24 months after diagnosis. Estimates can be related to the degree of activity and severity of the systemic disease, the type and progression of nephritis, clinically apparent vasculitis, and the multisystemic character of the disease. The prognosis is poorest in patients with diffuse proliferative nephritis or persistent CNS disease, and is best in those with mesangial disease or focal nephritis.[531–533] Encephalopathy, especially organic brain syndrome and vascular accident have become major factors in survival in some studies.[187, 534]

Sepsis has replaced renal failure as the most common cause of death. This trend is illustrated in Table 18–44. Malignant hypertension, gastrointestinal bleeding and perforation, acute pancreatitis, and pulmonary hemorrhage are other terminal events. Infection may be with common pathogens as well as with opportunistic organisms such as fungi or protozoa. Death from lupus crisis is rare today.

Reports on prognosis before 1968 were based on early experience with glucocorticoids and in general were restricted to children with classic SLE and severe disease.[36, 189] Meislin and Rothfield compared 42 children with 200 adults with SLE seen from 1957 to 1966.[36] Survival at 5 years calculated from the time of diagnosis was 42 percent in children with renal disease, compared with 82 percent in adults, and 72 percent in children without renal disease, compared with 85 percent in adults (see Table 18–44). Comparable studies from other centers published in 1976 and 1977 indicated that children with diffuse proliferative nephritis had a mean 5-year survival of 61 percent[353] to 73 percent.[524] In a later study,[525] the 5-year survival rate in children with renal disease improved to 89 percent, compared with 83 percent in adults, and was 100 percent in children without renal disease, compared with 94 percent in adults.

In the early Los Angeles series,[35] outcome did not appear to be related to the age at onset of disease, but there was an excess mortality in boys: 9 boys (50 percent) died compared with 19 girls (17 percent). Platt and colleagues reviewed 70 children with SLE followed from 1958 to 1981.[522] Survival was 77 percent at 15 years (see Table 18–43). Age at onset and the presence of CNS disease did not affect mortality. Prognosis for life and renal function were poorest after 7 years of follow-up in those with diffuse nephritis.

The relation of mortality to race and gender was evaluated for a 5-year period (1968–1972) using National Center for Health statistics (Table 18–45).[535] The overall mortality rate

Table 18–44
Causes of Death in Children With Systemic Lupus Erythematosus

STUDY (YEAR)	DIED/TOTAL	INFECTION	RENAL	CENTRAL NERVOUS SYSTEM	CARDIAC	OTHER
Meislin and Rothfield 1968[36]	18/42	7	6	2	0	3
Walravens and Chase 1976[37]	12/50	1	4	0	5	3
Garin et al 1976[353]	6/49	2	2	2	0	0
King et al 1977[35]	28/108	8	12	0	0	0
Cassidy et al 1977[31]	11/58*	8	7	1	3	1
Fish et al 1977[524]	7/49	6	0	0	0	0
Abeles et al 1980[525]	10/67	1	3	0	0	6
Platt et al 1982[522]	11/70	9	2	0	1	2
Glidden et al 1983[527]	9/55	3	3	3	0	1

*In some cases, death was attributed to more than one cause.

Table 18–45

Mortality in Childhood Systemic Lupus Erythematosus

AGE (YR)	WHITE MALE	WHITE FEMALE	BLACK MALE	BLACK FEMALE
5–9	0.1	0.4	0.2	0.6
10–14	0.3	1.5	0.8	4.4
15–19	0.9	3.8	1.8	12.9

Data are expressed as mortality rates per 10^6 person-years.

Adapted from Kaslow RA, Masi AT: Age, sex, and race effects on mortality from systemic lupus erythematosus in the United States. Arthritis Rheum 21: 473, © 1978 Wiley-Liss, Inc. Reprinted by permission of Wiley-Liss, Inc., a subsidiary of John Wiley & Sons, Inc.

for females, 6.3 per 10^6 person-years, was four times that for males, 1.6 × 10^6 person-years. Furthermore, black females had a rate of 14.8 compared with 5.2 for white females. Black males and white males were much closer, at 2.2 and 1.5, respectively. These epidemiologic data have been re-evaluated, and the conclusions were again supported.[536] African-Americans, especially young children in this racial group, and Hispanic-American children have a poorer prognosis than white children.[529, 537]

DRUG-INDUCED LUPUS

Serologic or clinical manifestations of lupus develop in some patients taking certain drugs (see Table 18–5). Cutaneous and pleuropericardial disease are most prominent clinical manifestations. CNS disease and lupus nephritis are distinctly uncommon. ANAs usually react with histones,[538, 539] and anti-dsDNA antibody is not usually present. Serum complement levels remain normal. Alarcon-Segovia has divided these reactions into two groups: group I, SLE-like disease related directly to the drug; and group II, disease developing after an allergic reaction to the drug.[540, 541]

The anticonvulsant drugs are the most common cause of drug-induced SLE in childhood.[542, 543] Diphenylhydantoin, mephenytoin, trimethadione, and ethosuximide have been most often incriminated. In the series of Jacobs,[201] 7 of 25 children had a history of seizures, and all had received anticonvulsant drugs before the onset of the symptoms of SLE. Singsen and associates[543] described five children who received ethosuximide, developed SLE with fever, malar rash, and arthritis, and had ANA seropositivity. Pleuropericardial effusions were less commonly observed. Clinical renal disease occurred in seven children and resulted in the deaths of three. Serum ANA titers did not differ significantly from results in 101 asymptomatic patients with seizures. Even after the drug was discontinued, 70 percent of these children remained ANA-positive. It was concluded that asymptomatic children who develop ANA positivity while receiving anticonvulsant drugs should be carefully followed but need not have their medications discontinued.

Patients who develop an SLE-like illness while receiving hydralazine have usually been treated with moderate to high doses of the drug.[544] There has been little relation to the duration of drug therapy[545] or to acetylator phenotype.[546, 547] During drug administration, antihydralazine antibodies were present in some patients, and antibodies to dsDNA were observed with this type of drug hypersensitivity. In some children, the SLE-like disease may not abate when the drug is discontinued.

PERSPECTIVE

Systemic lupus erythematosus is a challenging disease to diagnose and manage. Lupus can assume many guises and should be suspected particularly in older girls or adolescents with systemic illness that includes dermatitis, arthritis, and a myriad of other signs. The course is inevitably prolonged, but the outcome has improved dramatically with the availability of appropriately trained healthcare providers, and the early and judicious use of glucocorticoids, hydroxychloroquine, and second-line agents such as azathioprine and cyclophosphamide. Nonetheless, the disease often remains active throughout adolescence and into adulthood. The transition of the medical care of these young adults from the pediatric to the medical setting is an important part of their ongoing management. A great deal is yet to be learned from the long-term follow-up of patients with childhood onset of SLE.

References

1. Smith CD, Cyr M: The history of lupus erythematosus: From Hippocrates to Osler. Rheum Dis Clin North Am 14: 1, 1988.
2. Kaposi M: New reports on knowledge of lupus erythematosus. Arch Dermatol Syph 4: 36, 1872.
3. Osler W: On the visceral complications of erythema exudativum multiforme. Am J Med 110: 629, 1895.
4. Libman E, Sacks B: A hitherto undescribed form of valvular and mural endocarditis. Arch Intern Med 33: 701, 1924.
5. Gross L: Cardiac lesions in Libman-Sacks disease with a consideration of its relationship to acute diffuse lupus erythematosus. Am J Pathol 16: 375, 1940.
6. Baehr G, Klemperer P, Schifrin A: A diffuse disease of the peripheral circulation usually associated with lupus erythematosus and endocarditis. Trans Assoc Am Phys 50: 139, 1935.
7. Hargraves MM, Richmond H, Morton R: Presentation of two bone marrow elements: The "Tart" cell and the "L.E." cell. Mayo Clin Proc 23: 25, 1948.
8. Tan EM, Cohen AS, Fries JF, et al: The 1982 revised criteria for the classification of systemic lupus erythematosus. Arthritis Rheum 25: 1271, 1982.
9. Ferraz MB, Goldenberg J, Hilario MO, et al: Evaluation of the 1982 ARA lupus criteria data set in pediatric patients. Clin Exp Rheumatol 12: 83, 1994.
10. Hochberg MC: Updating the American College of Rheumatology revised criteria for the classification of systemic lupus erythematosus. Arthritis Rheum 40: 1725, 1997.
11. Trimble RB, Townes AS, Robinson H, et al: Preliminary criteria for the classification of systemic lupus erythematosus. Evaluation in early diagnosed SLE and rheumatoid arthritis. Arthritis Rheum 17: 184, 1974.
12. Passas CM, Wong RL, Peterson M, et al: A comparison of the specificity of the 1971 and 1982 American Rheumatism Association criteria for the classification of systemic lupus erythematosus. Arthritis Rheum 28: 620, 1985.
13. Piette J-C: Updating the American College of Rheumatology criteria for systemic lupus erythematosus: Comments on the letter by Hochberg. Arthritis Rheum 41: 751, 1998.
14. Nobrega FT, Ferguson RH, Kurland LT, et al: Lupus erythematosus in Rochester, Minnesota 1950–65; a preliminary study. *In* Bennett PH, Wood PHN (eds): Population Studies of the Rheumatic Diseases. International Congress Series, No. 148, Excepta Medica Foundation, 1968.
15. Fessel WJ: Systemic lupus erythematosus in the community.

Incidence, prevalence, outcome, and first symptoms; the high prevalence in black women. Arch Intern Med 134: 1027, 1974.
16. Fessel WJ: Epidemiology of systemic lupus erythematosus. Rheum Dis Clin North Am 14: 15, 1988.
17. Hochberg M: The incidence of systemic lupus erythematosus in Baltimore, Maryland, 1970–1977. Arthritis Rheum 28: 80, 1985.
18. Siegel M, Lee ML: The epidemiology of systemic lupus erythematosus. Semin Arthritis Rheum 3: 1, 1973.
19. Malleson PN, Fung MY, Rosenberg AM: The incidence of pediatric rheumatic diseases: Result from the Canadian Pediatric Rheumatology Association Disease Registry. J Rheumatol 23: 1981, 1996.
20. Pelkonen PM, Jalanko HJ, Lantto RR, et al: Incidence of systemic connective tissue diseases in children: A nationwide prospective study in Finland. J Rheumatol 21: 2143, 1994.
21. Kaipiainen-Sappanen O, Savolainen A: Incidence of chronic juvenile rheumatic diseases in Finland during 1980–1990. Clin Exp Rheumatol 14: 441, 1996.
22. Fujikawa S, Okuni M: A nationwide surveillance study of rheumatic diseases among Japanese children. Acta Paediatrica Japonica 39: 242, 1997.
23. Symmons DPM, Jones M, Osborne J, et al: Pediatric Rheumatology in the UK: Data from the British Pediatric Rheumatology Group National Diagnostic Register. J Rheumatol 23: 1975, 1996.
24. Bowyer S, Roettcher P and the members of the Pediatric Rheumatology Database Research Group: Pediatric Rheumatology Clinic populations in the United States: Results of a 3 year survey. J Rheumatol 23: 1968, 1996.
25. Johnson AE, Gordon C, Palmer RG, Bacon PA: The prevalence and incidence of systemic lupus erythematosus in Birmingham, England. Relationship to ethnicity and country of birth. Arthritis Rheum 38: 551, 1995.
26. Lehman TJA, McCurdy DK, Bernstein BH, et al: Systemic lupus erythematosus in the first decade of life. Pediatrics 83: 235, 1989.
27. Cook CD, Wedgwood RJP, Craig JM, et al: Systemic lupus erythematosus. Description of 37 cases in children and a discussion of endocrine therapy in 32 of the cases. Pediatrics 26: 570, 1960.
28. Harvey AM, Shulman LE, Tumulty PH, et al: Systemic lupus erythematosus. A review of the literature and clinical analysis of 138 cases. Medicine (Baltimore) 33: 291, 1954.
29. Lee P, Urowitz MB, Bookman AAM, et al: Systemic lupus erythematosus: A review of 110 cases with reference to nephritis, the nervous system, infections, aseptic necrosis and prognosis. Q J Med 46: 1, 1977.
30. Estes D, Christina CL: The natural history of systemic lupus erythematosus by prospective analysis. Medicine (Baltimore) 50: 85, 1971.
31. Cassidy JT, Sullivan DB, Petty RE, et al: Lupus nephritis and encephalopathy. Prognosis in 58 children. Arthritis Rheum 20 (Suppl): 315, 1977.
32. Norris DG, Colon AR, Stickler GB: Systemic lupus erythematosus in children: The complex problems of diagnosis and treatment encountered in 101 such patients at the Mayo Clinic. Clin Pediatr (Phila) 16: 774, 1977.
33. Hagge WW, Burke EC, Stickler GB: Treatment of systemic lupus erythematosus complicated by nephritis in children. Pediatrics 40: 822, 1967.
34. Celermajer DS, Thorner PS, Baumal R, et al: Sex differences in childhood lupus nephritis. Am J Dis Child 138: 586, 1984.
35. King KK, Kornreich HK, Bernstein BH, et al: The clinical spectrum of systemic lupus erythematosus in childhood. Arthritis Rheum 20(Suppl): 287, 1977.
36. Meislin AG, Rothfield NF: Systemic lupus erythematosus in childhood. Analysis of 42 cases with comparative data on 200 adult cases followed concurrently. Pediatrics 42: 37, 1968.
37. Walravens PA, Chase HP: The prognosis of childhood systemic lupus erythematosus. Am J Dis Child 130: 929, 1976.
38. Kaslow RA: High rate of death caused by systemic lupus erythematosus among U.S. residents of Asian descent. Arthritis Rheum 25: 414, 1982.
39. Feng PH, Boey ML: Systemic lupus erythematosus in Chinese: The Singapore experience. Rheumatol Int 2: 151, 1982.
40. Lee BW, Yap HK, Yip WC, et al: A 10 year review of systemic lupus erythematosus in Singapore children. Aust Paediatr J 23: 163, 1987.
41. Chen JH, Lin CY, Chen WP, et al: Systemic lupus erythematosus in children. Chinese J Microbiol Immunol 20: 23, 1987.
42. Tejani A, Nicastri AD, Chen CK, et al: Lupus nephritis in Black and Hispanic children. Am J Dis Child 137: 481, 1983.
43. Moreton RO, Gershwin MD, Brady C, et al: The incidence of systemic lupus erythematosus in North American Indians. J Rheumatol 3: 186, 1976.
44. Boyer GS, Templin DW, Lanier AP: Rheumatic diseases in Alaskan Indians of the southeast coast: High prevalence of rheumatoid arthritis and systemic lupus erythematosus. J Rheumatol 18: 1477, 1991.
45. Delgado EA, Malleson PN, Pirie GE, Petty RE: The pulmonary manifestations of childhood onset systemic lupus erythematosus. Semin Arthritis Rheum 19: 285, 1990.
46. Hochberg MC: The application of genetic epidemiology to systemic lupus erythematosus. J Rheumatol 14: 867, 1987.
47. Vyse TJ, Todd JA: Genetic analysis of autoimmune disease. Cell 85: 311, 1996.
48. Deapen D, Escalante A, Weinrib L, et al: A revised estimate of twin concordance in systemic lupus erythematosus. Arthritis Rheum 35: 311, 1992.
49. Leonhardt ETG: Family studies in systemic lupus erythematosus. Clin Exp Immunol 2: 743, 1967.
50. Larsen RA: Family studies in systemic lupus erythematosus. J Chronic Dis 25: 187, 1972.
51. DeHoratius RJ, Pillarisetty RP: Antinucleic acid antibodies in systemic lupus erythematosus patients and their families. Incidence and correlation with lymphocytotoxic antibodies. J Clin Invest 56: 1149, 1975.
52. Mitchell AJ, Rusin LHJ, Diaz LA: Circumscribed scleroderma with immunologic evidence of systemic lupus erythematosus. Arch Dermatol 116: 69, 1980.
53. Lippman SM, Arnett FC, Conley CL, et al: Genetic factors predisposing to autoimmune disease. Autoimmune hemolytic anemia, chronic thrombocytopenic purpura, and systemic lupus erythematosus. Am J Med 73: 827, 1982.
54. Lahita RG, Chiorazzi N, Gibofsky A, et al: Familial systemic lupus erythematosus in males. Arthritis Rheum 26: 39, 1983.
55. Tsao BP, Cantor RM, Kalunian KC, et al: Evidence for linkage of a candidate chromosome I region to human systemic lupus erythematosus. J Clin Invest 99: 725, 1997.
56. Tan FK, Arnett FC: The genetics of lupus. Curr Opin Rheumatol 10: 399, 1998.
57. Vyse TJ, and Kotzin BL: Genetic susceptibility to systemic lupus erythematosus. Ann Rev Immunol 16: 261, 1998.
58. Mason LJ, Isenberg DA: Immunopathogenesis of SLE. Baillieres Clin Rheumatol 12: 385, 1998.
59. Griffing WL, Moore SB, Luthra HS, et al: Associations of antibodies to native DNA with HLA-DRw3: A possible major histocompatibility linked human immune response gene. J Exp Med 152: 3195, 1980.
60. Ahearn JM, Provost TT, Dorsch CA, et al: Interrelationships of HLA-DR, MB and MT phenotypes, autoantibody expression and clinical features in systemic lupus erythematosus. Arthritis Rheum 25: 1031, 1982.
61. Schur PH, Meyer I, Garovoy M, Carpenter CD: Associations between systemic lupus erythematosus and the major histocompatibility complex: Clinical and immunologic considerations. Clin Immunol Immunopathol 24: 263, 1982.
62. Khanduja S, Arnett FC, Reveille JD: HLA-DQ beta genes encode an epitope for lupus specific DNA antibodies [abstract]. Clin Res 38: 975A, 1995.
63. Bowness P, Davies KA, Norsworthy PJ, et al: Hereditary C1q deficiency and systemic lupus erythematosus. Q J Med 87: 455, 1994.
64. Slingsby JH, Norsworthy P, Pearce G, et al: Homozygous hereditary C1q deficiency and systemic lupus erythematosus. Arthritis Rheum 39: 663, 1996.
65. Berkel AI, Petry F, Sanal O, et al: Development of systemic lupus erythematosus in a patient with selective complete C1q deficiency. Eur J Pediatr 156: 113, 1997.
66. Walport MJ, Lachmann PJ: Complement deficiencies and abnormalities of the complement system in systemic lupus erythematosus and related disorders. Curr Opin Rheumatol 2: 661, 1990.
67. Arnett FC, Reveille JD: Genetics of systemic lupus erythematosus. Rheum Dis Clin North Am 18: 865, 1992.

68. Davies EJ, Teh LS, Ordi-Ros J, et al: A dysfunctional allele of mannose-binding protein associated with systemic lupus erythematosus in a Spanish population. J Rheumatol 24: 485, 1997.
69. Hajeer AH, Worthington J, Davies EJ, et al: TNF microsatellite a2, b3 and d2 alleles are associated with systemic lupus erythematosus. Tissue Antigens 49: 222, 1997.
70. Sturfelt G, Hellmer G, Trudsson L: TNF microsatellites in systemic lupus erythematosus, a high frequency of the TNFdabc 2–3–1 haplotype in multicase SLE families. Lupus 5: 618, 1996.
71. Wilson AG, Gordon C, di Giovine, FS, et al: A genetic association between systemic lupus erythematosus and tumor necrosis factor alpha. Eur J Immunol 24: 191, 1994.
72. Sullivan KE, Wooten C, Schmeckpeper BJ, et al: A promoter polymorphism of tumor necrosis factor associated with systemic lupus erythematosus in African Americans. Arthritis Rheum 40: 2207, 1997.
73. Lu LY, Ding WZ, Deulofeut R, et al: Molecular analysis of major histocompatibility complex allelic associations with systemic lupus erythematosus. Arthritis Rheum 40: 1138, 1997.
74. Jacob CO, Fronek Z, Lewis GD, et al: Heritable major histocompatibility complex class II-associated differences in production of tumour necrosis factor-α: Relevance to genetic predisposition to systemic lupus erythematosus. Proc Natl Acad Sci U S A 87: 1233, 1990.
75. Wilson AG, Duff GW: Genetics of tumour necrosis factor in systemic lupus erythematosus. Lupus 5: 87, 1996.
76. Duits AJ, Bootsma H, Derksen RHWM, et al: Skewed distribution of IgG Fc receptor IIa (CD32) polymorphism is associated with renal disease in systemic lupus erythematosus patients. Arthritis Rheum 39: 1832, 1995.
77. Salmon JE, Millard S, Schacter LA, et al: FcγRIIA alleles are heritable risk factors for lupus nephritis in African Americans. J Clin Invest 97: 1348, 1995.
78. Wu J, Edberg JC, Redecha PB, et al: A novel polymorphism of FcγIIIa (CD16) alters receptor function and predisposes to autoimmune disease. J Clin Invest 100: 1059, 1997.
79. Huang O, Morris D, Dunckley H, et al: Lack of linkage between antinuclear antibody or clinical features of systemic lupus erythematosus and TCRA/Vb loci in families of subjects with SLE. Lupus 6: 527, 1997.
80. Klinman DM: B-cell abnormalities characteristic of systemic lupus erythematosus. *In* Wallace D, Hahn BH (eds): Dubois' Lupus Erythematosus, 5th ed. Williams & Wilkens. 1997, p 195.
81. Becher TM, Lizzio EF, Mercant LP, et al: Increased multiclonal antibody-forming cell activation in the peripheral blood of patients with SLE. Int Arch All Appl Immunol 66: 293, 1982.
82. Balow JE, Tsokos GC: T and B lymphocyte function in patients with lupus nephritis: Correlation with renal pathology. Clin Nephrol 21: 93, 1984.
83. Linker-Israeli M, Quismorio FP Jr, Horwitz DA: CD8+ lymphocytes from patients with systemic lupus erythematosus sustain, rather than suppress, spontaneous polyclonal IgG production and synergize with CD4+ cells to support antibody synthesis. Arthritis Rheum 33: 1216, 1990.
84. Williams RC Jr, Malone CC, Huffman GR, et al: Active systemic lupus erythematosus is associated with depletion of the natural generic anti-idiotype (anti-F(ab')2 system. J Rheumatol 22: 1074, 1995.
85. Krych M, Atkinson JP, Holers VM: Complement receptors. Curr Opin Immunol 4: 8, 1992.
86. Izui S, Lambert PH, Miescher PA: In vitro demonstration of a particular affinity of glomerular basement membrane and collagen for DNA. A possible basis for a local formation of DNA-anti-DNA complexes in systemic lupus erythematosus. J Exp Med 144: 428, 1976.
87. Gilboa N, Durante D, McIntosh RM: Glomerular deposition of renal tubular epithelial antigen in the patients with systemic lupus erythematosus: Its possible role in lupus nephritis. J Rheumatol 4: 358, 1977.
88. Rothfield N, Ross HA, Minta JO, et al: Glomerular and dermal deposition of properdin in systemic lupus erythematosus. N Engl J Med 287: 681, 1972.
89. Koffler D, Schur PH, Kunkel HG: Immunological studies concerning the nephritis of systemic lupus erythematosus. J Exp Med 126: 607, 1967.
90. Kunkel H: Mechanisms of renal injury in systemic lupus erythematosus. Am J Med 45: 165, 1968.
91. Gewurz H, Pickering RJ, Mergenhagen SE, et al: The complement profile in acute glomerulonephritis, systemic lupus erythematosus and hypocomplementemic chronic glomerulonephritis. Int Arch Allergy Appl Immunol 34: 556, 1968.
92. Gershwin ME, Steinberg AD: Qualitative characteristics of anti-DNA antibodies in lupus nephritis. Arthritis Rheum 17: 947, 1974.
93. Steward MW, Katz FE, West NJ: The role of low affinity antibody in immune complex disease. The quantity of anti-DNA antibodies in NZB/W F1 hybrid mice. Clin Exp Immunol 21: 121, 1975.
94. Winfield JB, Faiferman I, Koffler D: Avidity of anti-DNA antibodies in serum and IgG glomerular eluates from patients with systemic lupus erythematosus. Association of high avidity antinative DNA antibody with glomerulonephritis. J Clin Invest 59: 90, 1977.
95. Leon SA, Green A, Ehrlich GE, et al: Avidity of antibodies in SLE. Relation to severity of renal involvement. Arthritis Rheum 20: 23, 1977.
96. Hale GM, Highton J, Kalmakoff J, et al: Changes in anti-DNA antibody affinity during exacerbations of systemic lupus erythematosus. Scand J Rheumatol 15: 243, 1986.
97. Sher JH, Pertschuk LP: Immunoglobulin G deposits in the choroid plexus of a child with systemic lupus erythematosus. J Pediatr 85: 385, 1974.
98. Viallard JF, Pellegrin JL, Ranchin V, et al: Th1 (IL-2, interferon-gamma (IFN gamma) and Th2 (IL-10, IL-4) cytokine production by peripheral blood mononuclear cells (PBMC) from patients with systemic lupus erythematosus (SLE). Clin Exp Immunol 115: 189, 1999.
99. Schaller J: Illness resembling lupus erythematosus in mothers of boys with chronic granulomatous disease. Ann Intern Med 76: 747, 1972.
100. Finlay AY, Kingston HM, Holt PJA: Chronic granulomatous disease carrier gene dermatosis (CGDCGD). Clin Genet 23: 276, 1983.
101. Barton LL, Johnson CR: Discoid and lupus erythematosus and x-linked chronic granulomatous disease. Pediatr Dermatol 3: 376, 1986.
102. Ortiz-Romero PL, Corell-Almuzara A, Lopez-Estebaranz JL, et al: Lupus-like lesions in a patient with X-linked chronic granulomatous disease and recombinant X chromosome. Dermatology 195: 280, 1997.
103. Schmitt CP, Scharer K, Waldherr R, et al: Glomerulonephritis associated with chronic granulomatous disease and systemic lupus erythematosus. Nephrol Dial Transplant 10: 891, 1995.
104. Aringer M, Wintersberger W, Steiner CW, et al: High levels of bcl-2 protein in circulating T lymphocytes, but not B cells, of patients with systemic lupus erythematosus. Arthritis Rheum 37: 1423, 1994.
105. Rose LM, Latchman DS, Isenberg DA: Apoptosis in peripheral lymphocytes in systemic lupus erythematosus: A review. Brit J Rheumatol 36: 158, 1997.
106. Emlen W, Niebur J, Kadera R: Accelerated apoptosis of lymphocytes from patients with systemic lupus erythematosus. J Immunol 152: 3685, 1994.
107. Mysler E, Bini P, Drappa J, et al: The apoptosis-1/fas protein in human SLE. J Clin Invest 93: 1029, 1994.
108. Elkon KB: Apoptosis in SLE: Too little or too much? Clin Exp Rheumatol 12: 553, 1994.
109. Tsokos GC, Kovacs B, Liossis S-NC: Lymphocytes, cytokines, inflammation and immune trafficking. Curr Opin Rheumatol 9: 380, 1997.
110. Athreya BH, Rafferty JH, Sehgal GS, Lahita RG: Adenohypophyseal and sex hormones in pediatric rheumatic diseases. J Rheumatol 20: 725, 1993.
111. Steinberg AD, Steinberg BJ: Lupus disease activity associated with menstrual cycle. J Rheumatol 12: 816, 1985.
112. Lahita RG, Bradlow HL, Kunkel HG, Fishman J: Increased 16 alpha hydroxylation of estradiol in systemic lupus erythematosus. J Clin Endocrinol Metab 53: 174, 1981.
113. Travers RL, Hughes GRV: Oral contraceptive therapy and systemic lupus erythematosus. J Rheumatol 5: 448, 1978.

114. Jungers P, Dougados M, Pelissier C, et al: Influence of oral contraceptive therapy on the activity of systemic lupus erythematosus. Arthritis Rheum 25: 618, 1982.
115. Julkunen HI: Oral contraceptives in systemic lupus erythematosus. Side effects and influence on the activity of SLE. Scand J Rheumatol 20: 427, 1991.
116. Petri M, Howard D, Repke J: Frequency of lupus flare in pregnancy. The Hopkins Lupus Pregnancy Center experience. Arthritis Rheum 34: 1538, 1991.
117. Lockshin MD: Pregnancy does not cause systemic lupus erythematosus to worsen. Arthritis Rheum 32: 665, 1989.
118. Lavalle C, Loyo E, Paniagua R, et al: Correlation study between prolactin and androgens in male patients with systemic lupus erythematosus. J Rheumatol 14: 268, 1987.
118a. Mok CC, Law CS: Profile of sex hormones in male patients with systemic lupus erythematosus. Lupus 9: 252, 2000.
119. Jungers P, Dougados M, Pélissier C, et al: Influence of oral contraceptive therapy on the activity of systemic lupus erythematosus. Arthritis Rheum 25: 618, 1982.
120. Grumbach MM, Conte FA: Disorders of sex differentiation. *In* Wilson JD, Foster DFW (eds): Williams Textbook of Endocrinology, 8th ed. Philadelphia, WB Saunders, 1992, p 853.
121. Landwirth J, Berger A: Systemic lupus erythematosus and Klinefelter syndrome. Am J Dis Child 126: 851, 1973.
122. Stern R, Fishman J, Brushman H, Kunkel HG: Systemic lupus erythematosus associated with Klinefelter's syndrome. Arthritis Rheum 20: 18, 1977.
123. Fam AG, Izak M, Saiphoo C: Systemic lupus erythematosus and Klinefelter's syndrome. Arthritis Rheum 23: 124, 1980.
124. Sequeira JF, Keser G, Greenstein B, et al: Systemic lupus erythematosus: Sex hormones in male patients. Lupus 3: 315, 1993.
125. Jara-Quezada L, Graef A, Lavalle C: Prolactin and gonadal hormones during pregnancy in systemic lupus erythematosus. J Rheumatol 18: 349, 1991.
126. McMurray RW, Weidensaul D, Allan SH, Walker SE: Efficacy of bromocriptive in an open label therapeutic trial for SLE. J Rheumatol 22: 2084, 1995.
127. Casciola-Rosen L, Rosen A: Ultraviolet light-induced keratinocyte apoptosis: A potential mechanism for the induction of skin lesions and autoantibody production in LE. Lupus 6: 175, 1997.
128. Mohan C, Adams S, Stanik V, Datta SK: Nucleosomes: A major immunogen for pathogenic autoantibody inducing T cells of lupus. J Exp Med 177: 1367, 1993.
129. Rosen A, Casciola-Rosen L, Ahearn J: Novel packages of viral and self-antigens are generated during apoptosis. J Exp Med 179: 1317, 1994.
130. Funk JO, Holler E, Kohlhuber F, et al: Protein kinase C activation is involved in ultraviolet B irradiation-induced endothelial cell ICAM-1 up-regulation and lymphocyte-endothelium interaction in vitro. Scand J Immunol 44: 54, 1996.
131. Treina G, Scaletta C, Fourtanier A, et al: Expression of intercellular adhesion molecule-1 in UVA-irradiated human skin cells in vitro and in vivo. Br J Dermatol 135: 241, 1996.
132. Strickland I, Rhodes LE, Flanagan BF, Friedmann PS: TNF-alpha and IL-8 are upregulated in the epidermis of normal human skin after UVB exposure: Correlation with neutrophil accumulation and E-selectin. J Invest Dermatol 108: 763, 1997.
133. Cohen MR, Isenberg DA: Ultraviolet irradiation in systemic lupus erythematosus: Friend or foe? Br J Rheumatol 35: 1002, 1996.
134. Phillips PE: The role of infectious agents in childhood rheumatic diseases. Models and evidence. Arthritis Rheum 20: 459, 1977.
135. Hollinger FB, Sharp JT, Lidsky MD, et al: Antibodies to viral antigens in systemic lupus erythematosus. Arthritis Rheum 14: 1, 1971.
136. Phillips PE: Raised antibody titres in systemic lupus erythematosus. Lancet 1: 382, 1972.
137. Phillips PE, Christian CL: Virus antibodies in systemic lupus erythematosus and other connective tissue diseases. Ann Rheum Dis 32: 450, 1973.
138. Hurd ER, Dowdle W, Casey H, et al: Virus antibody levels in systemic lupus erythematosus. Arthritis Rheum 15: 267, 1972.
139. Reichlin M, Harley JB: Immune response to the RNA protein particles in systemic lupus erythematosus. Am J Med 85(Suppl 6A): 35, 1988.
140. Incaprere M, Rindi L, Bazzichi A, Garzelli C: Potential role of the Epstein-Barr virus in systemic lupus erythematosus autoimmunity. Clin Exp Rheumatol 16: 289, 1998.
141. James JA, Kaufman KM, Farris AD, et al: An increased prevalence of Epstein-Barr virus infection in young patients suggests a possible etiology for systemic lupus erythematosus. J Clin Invest 100: 3019, 1997.
142. Tsai YT, Chiang BL, Kao YE, Hsieh KH: Detection of Epstein-Barr virus and cytomegalovirus genome in white blood cells from patients with juvenile rheumatoid arthritis and childhood systemic lupus erythematosus. Int Arch All Immunol 106: 235, 1995.
143. Rider JR, Ollier WER, Lock RJ, et al: Human cytomegalovirus infection and systemic lupus erythematosus. Clin Exp Rheumatol 15: 405, 1997.
143a. Rubin RL: Etiology and mechanisms of drug-induced lupus. Curr Opin Rheumatol 11: 357, 1999.
144. Miller JJ III: Drug-induced lupus-like syndromes in children. Arthritis Rheum 20: 308, 1977.
145. Jacobs JC: Drug-induced lupus. JAMA 222: 1557, 1972.
146. Hess EV: Introduction to drug-related lupus. Arthritis Rheum 24: 6, 1981.
147. Hanlon TM, Binkiewixz A, Feingold M, et al: Procainamide HC1-induced lupus syndrome in child with myotonia congenita. Am J Dis Child 113: 491, 1967.
148. Tolaymat A, Levinthal B, Sakarcan A, et al: Systemic lupus erythematosus in a child receiving long-term interferon therapy. J Pediatr 120: 429, 1992.
149. Searles RP, Plymate SR, Troup GM: Familial thioamide-induced lupus syndrome in thyrotoxicosis. J Rheumatol 8: 498, 1981.
150. Vanheula BA, Carswell F: Sulphasalazine-induced systemic lupus erythematosus in a child. Eur J Pediatr 140: 66, 1983.
151. Walshe JM: Penicillamine and the SLE syndrome. J Rheumatol 7: 155, 1981.
151a. Schlienger RG, Bircher AJ, Meier CR: Minocycline-induced lupus. A systematic review. Dermatology 200: 223, 2000.
151b. Hieronymous T, Grotsch P, Blank N, et al: Chlorpromazine induces apoptosis in activated human lymphoblasts: A mechanism supporting the induction of drug-induced lupus erythematosus. Arthritis Rheum 43: 1994, 2000.
152. Prete P: The mechanisms of action of L-canavanine in inducing autoimmune phenomena. Arthritis Rheum 28: 1198, 1985.
153. Manilow MR, Bardana EJ Jr, Goodnight SH: Pancytopenia during ingestion of alfalfa seeds. Lancet I: 615, 1981.
154. Bardana EJ Jr, Manilow MR, Houghton DC, et al: Diet-induced systemic lupus erythematosus in primates. Am J Kidney Dis 1: 345, 1982.
155. Sanchezguerrero J, Karlson EW, Colditz GA, et al: Hair dye use and the risk of developing systemic lupus erythematosus: A cohort study. Arthritis Rheum 39: 657, 1996.
156. Carr RI, Hoffmann AA, Harbeck RJ: Comparison of DNA binding in normal population, general hospital laboratory personnel, and personnel from laboratories studying SLE. J Rheumatol 2: 178, 1975.
157. Beaucher WN, Garman RH, Condemi JJ: Familial lupus erythematosus. Antibodies to DNA in household dogs. N Engl J Med 296: 982, 1977.
158. Lewis RM: Animal model: Canine systemic lupus erythematosus. Am J Pathol 69: 537, 1972.
159. Reinersten JL, Kaslow RA, Klippel JH, et al: An epidemiologic study of households exposed to canine systemic lupus erythematosus. Arthritis Rheum 23: 564, 1980.
160. Coleman WP III, Coleman WP, Derbes VJ, et al: Collagen disease in children. A review of 71 cases. JAMA 237: 1085, 1977.
161. Caeiro F, Michielson FM, Bernstein R, et al: Systemic lupus erythematosus in childhood. Ann Rheum Dis 40: 325, 1981.
162. Schaller J: Lupus in childhood. Clin Rheum Dis 8: 219, 1982.
163. Lee LA, Weston WL: Lupus erythematosus in childhood. Dermatol Clin 4: 151, 1986.
164. Emery H: Clinical aspects of systemic lupus erythematosus in childhood. Pediatr Clin North Am 33: 1177, 1986.
165. Kaufman DB, Laxer RM, Silverman ED, et al: Systemic lupus erythematosus in childhood and adolescence: The problem, epidemiology, incidence, susceptibility, genetics and prognosis. Curr Probl Pediatr 16: 545, 1986.

166. Ansell BM: Perspectives in pediatric systemic lupus erythematosus. J Rheumatol 13: 177, 1987.
167. Sontheimer RD: The lexicon of cutaneous lupus erythematosus: A review and personal perspective on the nomenclature and classification of the cutaneous manifestations of lupus erythematosus. Lupus 6: 84, 1997.
168. Hebra F, Kaposi M: On diseases of the skin including the exanthemata. London: The New Sydenham Society, 1875.
169. Wananukul S, Watana D, Pongprasit P: Cutaneous manifestations of childhood systemic lupus erythematosus. Pediatr Dermatol 15: 342, 1998.
170. Sherwood MC, Pincott JR, Goodwin FJ, Dillon MJ: Dominantly inherited glomerulonephritis and an unusual skin disease. Arch Dis Child 62: 1278, 1997.
171. German J: Bloom's syndrome. Derm Clin 13: 7, 1995.
172. Jung EG: The red face: Photogenodermatoses. Clin Dermatol 11: 275, 1993.
173. Oates RK, Lewis MB, Walker-Smith JA: The Rothmund-Thomson syndrome: Case report of an unusual syndrome. Aust Pediatr J 7: 103, 1971.
174. Sontheimer RD, Provost TT: Cutaneous manifestations of lupus erythematosus. *In* Wallace DJ, Hahn DH (eds): Dubois' Lupus Erythematosus, 4th ed. Philadelphia, Lea & Febiger, 1997.
175. Alarcon-Segovia D, Deleze M, Oria CV, et al: Antiphospholipid antibodies and the antiphospholipid syndrome in systemic lupus erythematosus prospective analysis of 500 consecutive patients. Medicine (Baltimore) 68: 353, 1989.
176. McMullen EA, Armstrong KDB, Bingham EA, Walsh MY: Childhood discoid lupus erythematosus: A report of two cases. Pediatr Dermatol 15: 439, 1992.
177. George PM, Tunnessen WW: Childhood discoid lupus erythematosus. Arch Dermatol 129: 613, 1993.
178. Caputo R, Cappio F, Rigoni C, et al: Pterygium inversum unguis: Report of 19 cases and review of the literature. Arch Dermatol 129: 1307, 1993.
179. Kettler AH, Bean SF, Duffy JO, Gammon R: Systemic lupus erythematosus presenting as a bullous eruption in a child. Arch Dermatol 124: 1083, 1998.
180. Roholt NS, Lapiere JC, Wang JI, et al: Localized linear bullous eruption of systemic lupus erythematosus in a child. Pediatr Dermatol 12: 138, 1995.
181. Shirahama S, Furukawa F, Yagi H, et al: Bullous systemic lupus erythematosus: Detection of antibodies against noncollagenous domain of type VII collagen. J Am Acad Dermatol 38: 844, 1998.
182. Eskreis BD, Bronson DM: Cutaneous mucinosis in a child with systemic lupus erythematosus. Pediatr Dermatol 9: 259, 1992.
183. Peters MS, Su WP: Lupus erythematosus panniculitis. Med Clin North Am 73: 113, 1989.
184. Koransky JS, Esterly NB: Lupus panniculitis (profundus). J Pediatr 98: 241, 1981.
185. Millard LG, Rowell NR: Chilblain lupus erythematosus (Hutchinson). A clinical and laboratory study of 17 patients. Brit J Dermatol 98: 497, 1978.
186. Yell JA, Burge SM: Warts and lupus erythematosus. Lupus 2: 21, 1993.
187. Ragsdale CG, Petty RE, Cassidy JT, et al: The clinical progression of apparent juvenile rheumatoid arthritis to systemic lupus erythematosus. J Rheumatol 7: 50, 1980.
188. Reilly PA, Evison G, McHugh NJ, Maddison PJ: Arthropathy of hands and feet in systemic lupus erythematosus. J Rheumatol 17: 777, 1990.
189. Foote RA, Kimbrough SM, Stevens JC: Lupus myositis. Muscle Nerve 5: 65, 1982.
190. Ciaccio M, Parodi A, Regora A: Myasthenia gravis and lupus erythematosus. Int J Dermatol 28: 317, 1989.
191. Smith FE, Sweet DE, Brunner CM, et al: Avascular necrosis in SLE. An apparent predilection for young patients. Ann Rheum Dis 35: 227, 1976.
192. Griffiths ID, Maini RN, Scott JT: Clinical and radiological features of osteonecrosis in systemic lupus erythematosus. Ann Rheum Dis 38: 413, 1979.
193. Abeles M, Urman JD, Rothfield NF: Aseptic necrosis of bone in systemic lupus erythematosus. Relationship to corticosteroid therapy. Arch Intern Med 138: 750, 1978.
194. Zizic TM, Marcoux C, Hungerford DS, et al: Corticosteroid therapy associated with ischemic necrosis of bone in systemic lupus erythematosus. Am J Med 79: 596, 1985.
195. Cameron JS: Lupus nephritis in childhood and adolescence. Pediatr Nephrol 8: 230, 1994.
196. Reinersten JL, Klippel JH, Johnson AH, et al: Family studies of B lymphocyte alloantigens in systemic lupus erythematosus. J Rheumatol 9: 253, 1982.
197. LaManna A, Polito C, Papale MR, et al: Chronic interstitial cystitis and systemic lupus erythematosus in an 8-year old girl. Pediatr Nephrol 12: 139, 1998.
198. Sergent JS, Lockshin MD, Klempner MS, et al: Central nervous system disease in systemic lupus erythematosus: Therapy and prognosis. Am J Med 58: 644, 1975.
199. Yancey CI, Doughty RA, Athreya BH: Central nervous system involvement in childhood systemic lupus erythematosus. Arthritis Rheum 24: 1389, 1981.
200. Kornreich HK, Hanson V: The rheumatic diseases of childhood. Curr Probl Pediatr 4: 1, 1974.
201. Jacobs JC: Systemic lupus erythematosus in childhood. Report of 35 cases, with discussion of seven apparently induced by anticonvulsant medication, and of prognosis and treatment. Pediatrics 32: 257, 1963.
202. Parikh S, Swaiman KF, Kim Y: Neurologic characteristics of childhood lupus erythematosus. Pediatric Neurology 13: 198, 1995.
203. Steinlin MI, Blaser SI, Gilday DL, et al: Neurologic manifestations of pediatric systemic lupus erythematosus. Pediatric Neurology 13: 191, 1995.
204. Feinglass EJ, Arnett FC, Dorsch CA, et al: Neuropsychiatric manifestations of systemic lupus erythematosus: Diagnosis, clinical spectrum, and relationship to other features of the disease. Medicine (Baltimore) 55: 323, 1976.
205. McCune WJ, Golbus J: Neuropsychiatric lupus. Rheum Dis Clin North Am 14: 149, 1988.
206. Silber TJ, Chatoor I, White PH: Psychiatric manifestations of systemic lupus erythematosus in children and adolescents. A review. Clin Pediatr 23: 331, 1984.
207. Ostrov SG, Quencer RM, Gaylis NB, et al: Cerebral atrophy in systemic lupus erythematosus: Steroid- or disease-induced phenomenon? AJNR 3: 21, 1982.
208. Wyckoff PM, Miller LC, Tucker LB, Schaller JG: Neuropsychological assessment of children and adolescents with systemic lupus erythematosus. Lupus 4: 217, 1995.
209. Papero PH, Bluestein HG, White P, Lipnick RN: Neuropsychologic deficits and anti-neuronal antibodies in pediatric systemic lupus erythematosus. Clin Exp Rheumatol 8: 417, 1990.
210. Isenberg DA, Meyrick-Thomas D, Snaith ML, et al: A study of migraine in systemic lupus erythematosus. Ann Rheum Dis 41: 30, 1982.
211. Sfikakis PP, Mitsikostas DD, Manoussakis MN, et al: Headache in systemic lupus erythematosus: A controlled study. Br J Rheumatol 37: 300, 1995.
212. Uziel Y, Laxer RM, Blaser S, et al: Cerebral vein thrombosis in childhood systemic lupus erythematosus. J Pediatr 126: 722, 1995.
213. Herd JK, Medhi M, Uzendoski DM, et al: Chorea associated with systemic lupus erythematosus: Report of two cases and review of the literature. Pediatrics 61: 308, 1978.
214. Kukla LF, Reddy C, Silkalna G, et al: Systemic lupus erythematosus presenting as chorea. Arch Dis Child 53: 345, 1978.
215. Arisaka O, Obinata K, Sasaki H, et al: Chorea as an initial manifestation of systemic lupus erythematosus. A case report of a 10-year old girl. Clin Pediatr 23: 298, 1984.
216. Bruyn GW, Padberg G: Chorea and systemic lupus erythematosus. A critical review. Eur Neurol 23: 435, 1984.
217. Asherson RA, Derksen RH, Harris EN, et al: Chorea in systemic lupus erythematosus and "lupus-like" disease: Association with antiphospholipid antibodies. Semin Arthritis Rheum 16: 253, 1987.
218. Groothuis JR, Groothuis DR, Mukhopadhyay D, et al: Lupus-associated chorea in childhood. Am J Dis Child 131: 1131, 1977.
219. Zetterstrom R, Berglund G: Systemic lupus erythematosus in childhood. A clinical study. Acta Paediatr Scand 45: 189, 1956.
220. Shar E, Goshen E, Tauber Z, Lahat E: Parkinsonian syndrome complicating systemic lupus erythematosus. Pediatric Neurol 18: 456, 1998.

221. Penn AS, Rowan AJ: Myelopathy in systemic lupus erythematosus. Arch Neurol 18: 337, 1968.
222. Blaustein DA, Blaustein SA: Antinuclear antibody negative systemic lupus erythematosus presenting as bilateral facial paralyses. J Rheumatol 25: 798, 1998.
223. DelGiudice GC, Scher CA, Athreya BH, et al: Pseudotumor cerebri and childhood systemic lupus erythematosus. J Rheumatol 13: 748, 1986.
224. Pablos JL, del Rincon E, Francisco F, Mateo I: Narcolepsy in systemic lupus erythematosus. J Rheumatol 20: 375, 1993.
225. Jacobson EJ, Reza MJ: Constrictive pericarditis in systemic lupus erythematosus. Demonstration of immunoglobulins in the pericardium. Arthritis Rheum 21: 972, 1978.
226. Kahl LE: The spectrum of pericardial tamponade in systemic lupus erythematosus. Arthritis Rheum 35: 1343, 1992.
227. Ehrenfeld M, Asman A, Shpilberg O, Samra Y: Cardiac tamponade as the presenting manifestation of systemic lupus erythematosus. Am J Med 86: 626, 1989.
228. Lerer RJ: Cardiac tamponade as an initial finding in systemic lupus erythematosus. Am J Dis Child 124: 436, 1972.
229. Malcic I, Senecic I, Dasovic A, Radonic M: Incipient pericardial tamponade as the first symptom of systemic lupus erythematosus in 2 children. Reumatizam 42: 19, 1995.
230. Tamura EJ: Cardiac tamponade in a child with systemic lupus erythematosus and IgG2 and IgG4 subclass deficiencies. Eur J Pediatr 157: 475, 1998.
231. Quismorio FP Jr: Cardiac abnormalities in systemic lupus erythematosus. *In* Wallace DJ, Hahn BH (eds): Dubois' Lupus Erythematosus, 5th ed. Baltimore, Williams & Wilkins, 1997, p 653.
232. Oshiro AC, Derbes SJ, Stopa AR, Gedalia A: Anti- Ro/SS-A and anti-La/SS-B antibodies associated with cardiac involvement in childhood systemic lupus erythematosus. Ann Rheum Dis 56: 272, 1997.
233. Ishikawa S, Segar WE, Gilbert EF, et al: Myocardial infarct in a child with systemic lupus erythematosus. Am J Dis Child 132: 696, 1978.
234. Homcy CJ, Liberthson RR, Fallon JT, et al: Ischemic heart disease in systemic lupus erythematosus in the young patient: Report of six cases. Am J Cardiol 49: 478, 1982.
235. Spiera H, Rothenberg RR: Myocardial infarction in four young patients with SLE. J Rheumatol 10: 464, 1983.
236. Haider YS, Roberts WC: Coronary arterial disease in systemic lupus erythematosus; quantification of degrees of narrowing in 22 necropsy patients (21 women) aged 16 to 37 years. Am J Med 70: 775, 1981.
237. Bonfiglio TA, Botti RE, Hagstrom JWC: Coronary arteritis, occlusion, and myocardial infarction due to lupus erythematosus. Am Heart J 83: 153, 1972.
238. Bor I: Myocardial infarction and ischemic heart disease in infants and children: Analysis of 29 cases and review of the literature. Arch Dis Child 44: 268, 1969.
239. Friedman DM, Lazarus HM, Fierman AH: Acute myocardial infarction in pediatric systemic lupus erythematosus. J Pediatr 117: 263, 1990.
240. Schaller JG, Gilliland BG, Ochs HD, et al: Severe systemic lupus erythematosus with nephritis in a boy with deficiency of the fourth component of complement. Arthritis Rheum 20: 1519, 1977.
241. Fearon WF, Cooke JP: Acute myocardial infarction in a young woman with systemic lupus erythematosus. Vasc Med 1: 19, 1996.
242. Miller DJ, Maisch SA, Perez MD, et al: Fatal myocardial infarction in an 8-year-old girl with systemic lupus erythematosus, Raynaud's phenomenon, and secondary antiphospholipid antibody syndrome. J Rheumatol 22: 768, 1995.
243. Gazarian M, Feldman BM, Benson LN, et al: Assessment of myocardial perfusion and function in childhood systemic lupus erythematosus. J Pediatr 132: 109, 1998.
244. Petri M, Perez-Gutthann S, Spence D, Hochberg MC: Risk factors for coronary artery disease in patients with systemic lupus erythematosus. Am J Med 93: 513, 1992.
245. Roldan CA, Shively BK, Crawford MH: An echocardiographic study of valvular heart disease associated with systemic lupus erythematosus. New Engl J Med 335: 1424, 1996.
246. Chauvaud SM, Kalangos A, Berrebi AJ, et al: Systemic lupus erythematosus valvulitis: Mitral valve replacement with a homograft. Ann Thorac Surg 60: 1803, 1995.
247. Morin AM, Boyer AS, Nataf P, Gandjbakhch I: Mitral valve insufficiency caused by systemic lupus erythematosus requiring valve replacement: Three case reports and a review of the literature. Thorac Cardiovasc Surg 44: 314, 1996.
248. Kaplan SD, Chartash EK, Pizzarello RA, Furie RA: Cardiac manifestations of the antiphospholipid syndrome. Am Heart J 124: 1331, 1992.
249. Oshiro AC, Derbes SJ, Stopa AR, Gedalia A: Anti-Ro/SS-A and anti-La/SS-B antibodies associated with cardiac involvement in childhood systemic lupus erythematosus. Ann Rheum Dis 56: 272, 1997.
250. Bulkley BH, Roberts WC: The heart in systemic lupus erythematosus and the changes induced in it by corticosteroid therapy. A study of 36 necropsy patients. Am J Med 58: 243, 1975.
251. Ilowite NT, Samuel P, Ginzler E, et al: Dyslipoproteinemia in pediatric systemic lupus erythematosus. Arthritis Rheum 31: 859, 1988.
252. Smith GW, Hannan SF, Scott PJ, et al: Immune complex-like activity associated with abnormal serum lipoproteins in systemic erythematosus. Clin Exp Immunol 48: 8, 1982.
253. Englund JA, Lucas RV Jr: Cardiac complications in children with systemic lupus erythematosus. Pediatrics 72: 724, 1983.
254. Badui E, Garcia-Rubi D, Robles E, et al: Cardiovascular manifestations in systemic lupus erythematosus. Prospective study of 100 patients. Angiology 36: 431, 1985.
255. Mandell BF: Cardiovascular involvement in systemic lupus erythematosus. Semin Arthritis Rheum 17: 126, 1987.
256. Doherty NE, Siegel RJ: Cardiovascular manifestations of systemic lupus erythematosus. Am Heart J 110: 1257, 1985.
257. Laufer J, Frand M, Milo S: Valve replacement for severe tricuspid regurgitation caused by Libman-Sacks endocarditis. Br Heart J 48: 294, 1982.
257a. Falaschi F, Ravelli A, Martignoni A, et al: Nephrotic-range proteinuria, the major risk factor for early atherosclerosis in juvenile-onset systemic lupus erythematosus. Arthritis Rheum 43: 1405, 2000.
258. Schaller J: Lupus in childhood. Clin Rheum Dis 8: 219, 1982.
259. De Jongste JC, Neyens HJ, Duiveman EJ, et al: Respiratory tract disease in systemic lupus erythematosus. Arch Dis Child 61: 478, 1986.
260. Singsen BH, Platzker CG: Pulmonary involvement in the rheumatic disorders of children. *In* Kendig EL, Chernick V (eds): Disorders of the Respiratory Tract in Children, 4th ed. Philadelphia, WB Saunders, 1983, p 846.
261. Rajani KB, Ashbacher LV, Kinney TR: Pulmonary hemorrhage and systemic lupus erythematosus. J Pediatr 93: 810, 1978.
262. Ramirez RE, Glasier C, Kirks D, et al: Pulmonary hemorrhage associated with systemic lupus erythematosus in children. Radiology 152: 409, 1984.
263. Miller RW, Salcedo JR, Fink RJ, et al: Pulmonary hemorrhage in pediatric patients with systemic lupus erythematosus. J Pediatr 108: 576, 1986.
264. Nadorra RL, Landing BH: Pulmonary lesions in childhood onset systemic lupus erythematosus. Pediatr Pathol 7: 1, 1987.
265. Abramson SG, Dobro J, Eberle MA, et al: Acute reversible hypoxemia in systemic lupus erythematosus. Ann Intern Med 114: 941, 1991.
266. Kraus A, Guerra-Bautista G: Laryngeal involvement as a presenting symptom of systemic lupus erythematosus. Ann Rheum Dis 49: 421, 1990.
267. Teitel AD, MacKenzie CR, Stern R, Paget SA: Laryngeal involvement in systemic lupus erythematosus. Semin Arthritis Rheum 22: 203, 1992.
268. Weinrib L, Sharma OP, Quismorio FP Jr: A long term study of interstitial lung disease in systemic lupus erythematosus. Semin Arthritis Rheum 16: 479, 1990.
269. Schwab EP, Schumacher HR Jr, Freundlich B, Callegari PE: Pulmonary hemorrhage in systemic lupus erythematosus. Semin Arthritis Rheum 23: 8, 1993.
270. Reznik VM, Griswold WR, Lemire JM, Mendoza SA: Pulmonary hemorrhage in children with glomerulonephritis. Pediatr Nephrol 9: 83, 1995.
271. Uziel Y, Laxer RM, Silverman ED: Persistent pulmonary hemor-

rhage as the sole initial clinical manifestation of pediatric systemic lupus erythematosus. Clin Exp Rheumatol 15: 697, 1997.
272. Foster HE, Malleson PN, Petty RE, et al: *Pneumocystis carinii* pneumonia in childhood systemic lupus erythematosus. J Rheumatol 23: 753, 1996.
273. Byard RW, Bourne AJ, Matthews N, et al: Pulmonary strongyloides in a child diagnosed on open lung biopsy. Surgical Pathology 5: 55, 1993.
274. Wang SM, Liu CC, Chen CT, Wu MH: Pulmonary nocardiosis in a child with systemic lupus erythematosus: Report of a case. J Formosan Med Assoc 94: 506, 1995.
275. Asherson RA, Cervera R: Review: Antiphospholipid antibodies and the lung. J Rheumatol 22: 63, 1995.
276. Weiss SG, Wagner-Weiner L, Newcomb RW, et al: Assessment of pulmonary function in childhood systemic lupus erythematosus. Arthritis Rheum 27: S63, 1984.
277. Trapani S, Camiciottoli G, Erminin M, et al: Pulmonary involvement in juvenile systemic lupus erythematosus: A study of lung function in patients asymptomatic for respiratory disease. Lupus 7: 545, 1998.
278. Hughes GRV, Harris EN, Gharavi AE: The anticardiolipin syndrome. J Rheumatol 13: 486, 1986.
278a. Wilson WA, Gharavi AE, Koike T, et al: International consensus statement on preliminary classification criteria for definite antiphospholipid syndrome. Arthritis Rheum 42: 1309, 1999.
279. Alarcon-Segovia D, Perez-Vazauez ME, Villa AR, et al: Preliminary classification criteria for the antiphospholipid syndrome. Semin Arthritis Rheum 21: 275, 1992.
280. Ostuni PA, Lazzarin P, Pengo V, et al: Renal artery thrombosis and hypertension in a 13-year old girl with antiphospholipid syndrome. Ann Rheum Dis 49: 184, 1990.
281. Mechinaud-Lacroix F, Jehan P, Debre MA, et al: Thrombotic manifestations and acute distal ischemia in primary antiphospholipid syndrome in children. Arch Fr Pediatr 40(Suppl 1): 257, 1992.
282. Vlachoyiannopoulos PG, Siamopoulou-Mavridou A: Chorea as a manifestation of the antiphospholipid syndrome. Clin Exp Rheumatol 9: 303, 1991.
283. Asherson RA, Lubbe WF: Cerebral and valve lesions in SLE: Association with antiphospholipid antibodies. J Rheumatol 15: 539, 1988.
284. Lubbe WF, Asherson RA: Intracardiac thrombus in systemic lupus erythematosus associated with lupus anticoagulant. Arthritis Rheum 31: 1453, 1988.
285. Brown JH, Doherty CC, Allen DC, et al: Fatal cardiac failure due to myocardial microthrombi in systemic lupus erythematosus. Br Med J 296: 1505, 1988.
286. Petri M, Roubenoff R, Dallal GE, et al: Plasma homocysteine as a risk factor for atherothrombotic events in systemic lupus erythematosus. Lancet 348: 1120, 1996.
287. Ginsberg JS, Demers C, Brill-Edwards P, et al: Acquired protein S deficiency is associated with antiphospholipid antibodies and increased thrombin generation in patients with systemic lupus erythematosus. Am J Med 98: 379, 1995.
288. Tomas JF, Alberca I, Tabernero MD, et al: Natural anticoagulant protein and antiphospholipid antibodies in systemic lupus erythematosus. J Rheumatol 25: 57, 1998.
289. Eberhard A, Sparling C, Sudbury S, et al: Hypoprothrombinemia in childhood systemic lupus erythematosus. Semin Arthritis Rheum 24: 12, 1994.
290. Fleck RA, Rapaport SI, Roa LVM: Anti-prothrombin antibodies and the lupus anticoagulant. Blood 72: 512, 1988.
291. Gatenby PA, Smith H, Kirwan P, et al: Systemic lupus erythematosus and thrombotic thrombocytopenic purpura. A case report and review of relationship. J Rheumatol 8: 504, 1981.
292. Bell WR, Braine HG, Ness PM, Kickler TS: Improved survival in thrombocytopenic purpura: Hemolytic uremic syndrome. Clinical experience in 108 patients. N Engl J Med 325: 398, 1991.
293. Breckenridge RL Jr, Solberg LA, Pineda AA, et al: Treatment of thrombotic thrombocytopenic purpura with plasma exchange, antiplatelet agents, corticosteroid and plasma infusion. Mayo Clinic experience. J Clin Apheresis 1: 6, 1996.
294. Oen K, Petty RE, Schroeder ML, et al: Thrombotic thrombocytopenic purpura in a girl with systemic lupus erythematosus. J Rheumatol 7: 727, 1980.
295. Rock GA, Shamak KH, Buskard NA, et al: Comparison of plasma exchange with plasma infusion in the treatment of thrombocytopenic purpura. N Engl J Med 325: 393, 1991.
296. Gardner FH, Diamond LK: Autoerythrocyte sensitization: A form of purpura producing painful bruising following autosensitization to red blood cells in certain women. Blood 10: 675, 1995.
297. Ratnoff OD: The psychogenic purpuras: A review of autoerythrocyte sensitization, autosensitization to DNA, "hysterical" and factitial bleeding and the religious stigmata. Semin Hematol 17: 192, 1980.
298. Scott JP, Schiff DW, Githens JH: The autoerythrocyte sensitization syndrome as the primary manifestation of systemic lupus erythematosus. J Pediatr 99: 598, 1981.
299. Kurczynski EM, Cassidy JT, Heyn RM: Autoerythrocyte sensitization in a young boy. Lancet 1: 424, 1973.
300. Ansari A, Larson PH, Bates HD: Vascular manifestations of systemic lupus erythematosus. Angiology 37: 423, 1986.
301. Deprettere AJ, Van Acker KJ, De Clerck LS, et al: Diagnosis of Sjögren's syndrome in children. Am J Dis Child 142: 1185, 1988.
302. Bloch KJ, Buchanan WW, Wohl MJ, Bunim JJ: Sjögren's syndrome. A clinical, pathological, and serological study of sixty-two cases. Medicine (Baltimore) 44: 187, 1965.
303. Spath M, Kruger K, Dresel S, et al: Magnetic resonance imaging of the parotid gland in patients with Sjögren's syndrome. J Rheumatol 18: 1372, 1991.
304. Daniel TE: Labial salivary gland biopsy in Sjögren's syndrome. Arthritis Rheum 27: 147, 1984.
305. Garcia-Consuegra J, Merino R, Alonso A, Goded F: Systemic lupus erythematosus: A case report with unusual manifestations and favourable outcome after plasmapheresis. Eur J Pediatr 151: 581, 1992.
306. Saab S, Corr MP, Weisman MH: Corticosteroids and systemic lupus erythematosus pancreatitis: A case series. J Rheumatol 25: 801, 1998.
307. Kolk A, Horneff G, Wilgenbus KK, et al: Acute lethal necrotising pancreatitis in childhood systemic lupus erythematosus: Possible toxicity of immunosuppressive therapy. Clin Exp Rheumatol 13: 399, 1995.
308. Huang J-L, Huang C-C, Chen C-Y, Hung I-J: Acute pancreatitis: An early manifestation of systemic lupus erythematosus. Pediatr Emerg Care 10: 291, 1994.
309. Molina JF, Brown RF, Gedalia A, Espinoza LR: Protein losing enteropathy as the initial manifestation of childhood systemic lupus erythematosus. J Rheumatol 23: 269, 1996.
310. Mukamel M, Rosenbach Y, Mimount M, Dinari G: Celiac disease associated with systemic lupus erythematosus. Israel J Med Sci 30: 656, 1994.
311. Stevens HP, Ostlere LS, Rustin MH: Systemic lupus erythematosus in association with ulcerative colitis: Related autoimmune diseases. Br J Dermatol 130: 385, 1994.
312. Nagata M, Ogawa Y, Hisano S, Ueda K: Crohn's disease in systemic lupus erythematosus: A case report. Eur J Pediatr 148: 525, 1989.
313. Gibson T, Myers AR: Subclinical liver disease in systemic lupus erythematosus. J Rheumatol 8: 752, 1981.
314. Mackay IR, Taft Li, Cowling DC: Lupoid hepatitis. Lancet 2: 1323, 1956.
315. Hall S, Czaja AJ, Kaufman DK, et al: How lupoid is lupoid hepatitis? J Rheumatol 13: 95, 1986.
316. Maddrey WC: Chronic hepatitis. *In* Zakim D, Boyer TD (eds): Hepatology. A Textbook of Liver Disease, 2nd ed. Philadelphia, WB Saunders, 1990, p 1025.
317. Miller MH, Urowitz MB, Gladman DD: The liver in systemic lupus erythematosus. Q J Med 211: 401, 1984.
318. Dillon AM, Stein HB, English RA: Splenic atrophy in systemic lupus erythematosus. Ann Intern Med 96: 40, 1982.
319. Malleson P, Petty RE, Nadel H, et al: Functional asplenia in childhood onset systemic lupus erythematosus. J Rheumatol 15: 1648, 1988.
320. Efremidis A, Eiser A, Grishman E, Rosenberg V: Hodgkin's lymphoma in an adolescent with SLE. Cancer 53: 142, 1984.
321. Abu-Shakra M, Gladman DD, Urowitz MB: Malignancy in systemic lupus erythematosus. Arthritis Rheum 39: 1050, 1996.
322. Mellemkhaer L, Anderson V, Linet MS, et al: Non-Hodgkin's

lymphoma and other cancers among a cohort of patients with systemic lupus erythematosus. Arthritis Rheum 40: 761, 1997.
323. Martin F, Lauwerys B, Lefebvre C, et al: Side-effects of intravenous cyclophosphamide pulse therapy. Lupus 6: 254, 1997.
324. Eberhard BA, Laxer RM, Eddy AA, Silverman ED: Presence of thyroid abnormalities in children with systemic lupus erythematosus. J Pediatr 119: 277, 1991.
325. Miller FW, Moore GF, Weintraub BD, Steinberg AD: Prevalence of thyroid disease and abnormal thyroid function test results in patients with systemic lupus erythematosus. Arthritis Rheum 30: 1124, 1987.
326. Gazarian M, Laxer RM, Kooh S, Silverman ED: Hypoparathyroidism associated with systemic lupus erythematosus. J Rheumatol 22: 2156, 1995.
327. Benekli M, Savas MC, Erdem Y, et al: Primary hyperparathyroidism in a patient with systemic lupus erythematosus-antiphospholipid syndrome. Nephron 79: 215, 1998.
328. Fruman LS: Diabetes mellitus, islet-cell antibodies and HLA-B8 in a patient with systemic lupus erythematosus. Am J Dis Child 131: 1252, 1977.
329. Koren S, Hanley JG: Adrenal failure in systemic lupus erythematosus. J Rheumatol 24: 1410, 1997.
330. Gardner DL: Systemic lupus erythematosus. *In* Gardner DI (ed): Pathology of the Connective Tissue Diseases, 2nd ed. Baltimore, Williams & Wilkins, 1965, p 144.
331. Klemperer P, Pollack AD, Baehr G: Pathology of disseminated lupus erythematosus. Arch Pathol 32: 569, 1941.
332. Donadio JV Jr: Renal involvement in SLE: The argument for aggressive treatment. *In* Bacon PA, Hadler NM (eds): The Kidney and Rheumatic Disease. Boston, Butterworth Scientific, 1982, p 45.
333. Diamond H: Progression of mesangial and focal to diffuse lupus nephritis. N Engl J Med 291: 693, 1974.
334. Ginzler EM, Nicastri AD, Chen C-K, et al: Progression of mesangial and focal to diffuse lupus nephritis. N Engl J Med 291: 693, 1974.
335. Morel-Maroger L: The course of lupus nephritis: Contribution of serial renal biopsies. *In* Hamburger J (ed): Advances in Nephrology, vol 6. Chicago, Year Book Medical Publishers, 1976, p 79.
336. Zimmerman SW, Jenkins PG, Shelf WD, et al: Progression from minimal or focal to diffuse proliferative lupus nephritis. Lab Invest 32: 665, 1975.
337. Sorof JM, Perez MD, Brewer ED, et al: Increasing incidence of childhood class V lupus nephritis. J Rheumatol 25: 1413, 1998.
338. Balow JE, Austin HA, Muenz LR, et al: Effects of treatment on the evolution of renal abnormalities in lupus nephritis. N Engl J Med 311: 491, 1984.
339. Grande JP, Balow JE: Renal biopsy in lupus nephritis. Lupus 7: 611, 1998.
340. Brentjens FR, Sepulveda M, Baliah T, et al: Interstitial immune complex nephritis in patients with systemic lupus erythematosus. Kidney Int 7: 342, 1975.
341. Fortenberry JD, Kenney RD: Distal renal tubular acidosis as the initial manifestation of systemic lupus erythematosus in an adolescent. J Adolesc Health 12: 148, 1992.
342. Malleson PN: The role of the renal biopsy in childhood onset systemic lupus erythematosus: A viewpoint. Clin Exp Rheumatol 7: 563, 1989.
343. Comerford FR, Cohen AS: The nephropathy of systemic lupus erythematosus: An assessment by clinical, light and electron microscopic criteria. Medicine (Baltimore) 46: 425, 1967.
344. Woolf A, Croker B, Osofsky SG, et al: Nephritis in children and young adults with systemic lupus erythematosus and normal urinary sediment. Pediatrics 64: 678, 1979.
345. Weis LS, Pachman LM, Potter EV, et al: Occult lupus nephropathy: A correlated light, electron and immunofluorescent microscopic study. Histopathology 1: 401, 1977.
346. Mahajan SK, Ordonez NG, Feitelson PJ, et al: Lupus nephropathy without clinical renal involvement. Medicine (Baltimore) 56: 493, 1977.
347. Leehey DJ, Katz AI, Azaran AH, et al: Silent diffuse lupus nephritis: Long-term follow-up. Am J Kidney Dis 2: 188, 1982.
348. Bennett WM, Bardana EJ, Norman DJ, et al: Natural history of "silent" lupus nephritis. Am J Kidney Dis 1: 359, 1982.
349. Magil AB, Ballon HS, Chan V, et al: Diffuse proliferative lupus glomerulonephritis. Determination of prognostic significance of clinical, laboratory and pathologic factors. Medicine (Baltimore) 63: 210, 1984.
350. Stamenkovic I, Favre H, Donath A, et al: Renal biopsy in SLE irrespective of clinical findings: Longterm follow up. Clin Nephrol 26: 109, 1986.
351. Baldwin DS, Lowenstein J, Rothfield NF, et al: The clinical course of the proliferative and membranous forms of lupus nephritis. Ann Intern Med 73: 929, 1970.
352. Baldwin DS, Gluck MC, Lowenstein J, et al: Lupus nephritis. Clinical course as related to morphologic forms and their transitions. Am J Med 62: 12, 1977.
353. Garin EH, Donnelly WH, Fennell RS III, et al: Nephritis in systemic lupus erythematosus in children. J Pediatr 89: 366, 1976.
354. Rush PJ, Baumel R, Shore A, et al: Correlation of renal histology with outcome in children with lupus nephritis. Kidney Int 29: 1066, 1986.
355. Ty A, Fine B: Membranous nephritis in infantile systemic lupus erythematosus associated with chromosomal abnormalities. Clin Nephrol 12: 137, 1979.
356. Schrager MA, Rothfield NF: The lupus band test. Clin Rheum Dis 1: 597, 1975.
357. Grossman J, Schwartz RH, Callerame ML, et al: Systemic lupus erythematosus in a 1-year-old child. Am J Dis Child 129: 123, 1975.
358. Wertheimer D, Barland P: Clinical significance of immune deposits in the skin in SLE. Arthritis Rheum 19: 1249, 1976.
359. Davis BM, Gillian JN: Prognostic significance of subepidermal immune deposits in uninvolved skin of patients with systemic lupus erythematosus: A 10-year longitudinal study. J Invest Dermatol 83: 242, 1984.
360. Mandell BF: Pericardial effusions in patients with systemic lupus erythematosus. Arthritis Rheum 36: 1029, 1993.
361. Shapiro RF, Gamble CN, Wiesner KB, et al: Immunopathogenesis of Libman-Sacks endocarditis. Assessment by light and immunofluorescent microscopy in two cases. Ann Rheum Dis 36: 508, 1977.
362. Johnson RT, Richardson EP: The neurological manifestations of systemic lupus erythematosus. A clinical-pathological study of 24 cases and review of the literature. Medicine (Baltimore) 47: 337, 1968.
363. Hanly JG, Walsh NMG, Sangalang V: Brain pathology in systemic lupus erythematosus. J Rheumatol 19: 732, 1992.
364. Khamashita MA, Gil A, Anciones B, et al: Chorea in systemic lupus erythematosus: Association with antiphospholipid antibodies. Ann Rheum Dis 47: 681, 1988.
365. Aronson AJ, Ordonez NG, Diddie KR, et al: Immune-complex deposition in the eye in systemic lupus erythematosus. Arch Intern Med 139: 1312, 1979.
366. Runyon BA, LaBrecque DR, Anuras S: The spectrum of liver disease in systemic lupus erythematosus: Report of 33 histologically-proved cases and review of the literature. Am J Med 69: 187, 1980.
367. Asherson RA, Khamashta MA, Hughes GRV: The hepatic complications of the antiphospholipid antibodies. Clin Exp Rheumatol 9: 341, 1991.
368. Rothfield NF: Systemic lupus erythematosus. Laboratory studies. Arthritis Rheum 20: 299, 1977.
369. McCarty GA: Update on laboratory studies and relationship to rheumatic and allergic diseases. Ann Allergy 55: 1, 1985.
370. Zein N, Ganuza C, Kushner I: Significance of serum C-reactive protein elevation in patients with systemic lupus erythematosus. Arthritis Rheum 22: 7, 1979.
371. Maury CP, Helve T, Sjöblom C: Serum beta 2-microglobulin, sialic acid, and C-reactive protein in systemic lupus erythematosus. Rheumatol Int 2: 145, 1982.
372. Pepys MB, Lanham JG, DeBeer FC: C-reactive protein in SLE. Clin Rheum Dis 8: 91, 1982.
373. Pereira A, Silva JA, Elkon KB, et al: C-reactive protein levels in systemic lupus erythematosus: A classification criterion? Arthritis Rheum 23: 770, 1980.
374. Morley JJ, Kushner I: Serum C-reactive protein levels in disease. Ann N Y Acad Sci 389: 406, 1982.

375. Ter Borg E, Horst G, Limburg P, et al: C-reactive protein levels during disease exacerbations and infections in systemic lupus erythematosus: A prospective longitudinal study. J Rheumatol 17: 1642, 1990.
376. Moutsopoulos HM, Mavridis AK, Acritidis NC, Avgerinos PC: High C-reactive protein response in lupus polyarthritis. Clin Exp Rheumatol 1: 53, 1983.
377. Spronk PE, terBorg RJ, Kallenberg CG: Patients with systemic lupus erythematosus and Jaccoud's arthropathy: A clinical subset with an increased C-reactive protein response? Ann Rheum Dis 51: 358, 1997.
378. Nishiya K, Hashimoto K: Elevation of serum ferritin levels as a marker for active systemic lupus erythematosus. Clin Exp Rheumatol 15: 39, 1997.
379. Bowyer SL, Ragsdale CG, Sullivan DB: Factor VIII related antigen and childhood rheumatic diseases. J Rheumatol 16: 1093, 1989.
380. Lacki JK, Leszczynski P, Kelemen J, et al: Cytokine concentration in serum of lupus erythematosus patients: The effect on acute phase response. J Med 28: 99, 1997.
381. Costello C, Abdelaal M, Coomes EN: Pernicious anemia and systemic lupus erythematosus in a young woman. J Rheumatol 12: 798, 1985.
382. Rivero SJ, Diaz-Jouanen E, Alarcon-Segovia D: Lymphocytopenia in systemic lupus erythematosus. Arthritis Rheum 21: 295, 1978.
383. Karpatkin S, Strick BS, Karpatkin MB, et al: Cumulative experience in the detection of antiplatelet antibody in 234 patients with idiopathic thrombocytopenic purpura, systemic lupus erythematosus and other clinical disorders. Am J Med 52: 776, 1972.
384. Conley CL, Hartmann RC: A hemorrhagic disorder caused by circulating anticoagulant in patients with disseminated lupus erythematosus. J Clin Invest 31: 621, 1952.
385. Bajaj SP, Rapaport SI, Fierer DS, et al: A mechanism for the hypoprothrombinemia of the acquired hypoprothrombinemia-lupus anticoagulant syndrome. Blood 61: 684, 1983.
386. Johns AS, Chamley L, Ockelford PA, et al: Comparison of tests for the lupus anticoagulant and antiphospholipid antibodies in systemic lupus erythematosus. Clin Exp Rheumatol 12: 523, 1994.
387. Gedalia A, Molina JF, Garcia CO, et al: Anticardiolipin antibodies in childhood rheumatic diseases. Lupus 7: 551, 1998.
388. Seaman DE, Londino AV Jr, Kwok CK, et al: Antiphospholipid antibodies in pediatric systemic lupus erythematosus. Pediatrics 96: 1040, 1995.
389. Lehman TJ, Hanson V, Singsen BH, et al: The role of antibodies directed against double-stranded DNA in the manifestations of systemic lupus erythematosus in childhood. J Pediatr 96: 657, 1980.
390. Morimoto C, Sano H, Abe T, et al: Correlation between clinical activity of systemic lupus erythematosus and the amounts of DNA in DNA/anti-DNA antibody immune complexes. J Immunol 129: 1960, 1982.
391. Miller JJ III, Hsu YP, Osborne CL, et al: Comparison of three assays for anti-DNA with three assays for the measurement of the role of complement in systemic lupus erythematosus in adolescents. J Rheumatol 7: 660, 1980.
392. Hahn BH: Mechanisms of disease: Antibodies to DNA. N Engl J Med 338: 1359, 1998.
393. Crowe W, Kushner I: An immunofluorescent method using *Crithidia luciliae* to detect antibodies to double-stranded DNA. Arthritis Rheum 20: 811, 1977.
394. Deng JS, Rubin RL, Lipscomb MF, et al: Reappraisal of the *Crithidia luciliae* assay for nDNA antibodies: Evidence for histone antibody kinetoplast binding. Am J Clin Pathol 82: 448, 1984.
395. Pisetsky DS, Gonzales TC: The influence of DNA size on the binding of antibodies to DNA in the sera of normal human subjects and patients with systemic lupus erythematosus (SLE). Clin Exp Immunol 116: 354, 1999.
396. Worrall JG, Snaith ML, Batchelor JR, Isenberg DA: SLE: A rheumatological view. Analysis of the clinical features, serology and immunogenetics of 100 SLE patients during long-term follow-up. Q J Med 74: 319, 1990.
397. Reichlin M: Antibodies to ribonuclear proteins in systemic lupus erythematosus. Rheum Dis Clin North Am 20: 29, 1994.
398. Wahren M, Tengner P, Gunnaisson I, et al: RO/SS-A and La/SS-B antibody level variation in patients with Sjögren's and systemic lupus erythematosus. J Autoimmun 11: 29, 1998.
399. Wasicek GA, Reichlin M: Clinical and serological differences between systemic lupus erythematosus patients with antibodies to Ro versus patients with antibodies to Ro and La. J Clin Invest 69: 835, 1982.
400. Wechsler HL, Stavrides A: Systemic lupus erythematosus with anti-Ro antibodies: Clinical, histologic and immunologic findings. J Am Acad Dermatol 6: 73, 1982.
401. Harley JB, Gaither KK: Autoantibodies. Rheum Dis Clin North Am 14: 43, 1988.
402. Meilof JF, Bantjes I, DeJong J, et al: The detection of anti-Ro/SS-S and anti-La/SS-B antibodies. A comparison of counterimmunoelectrophoresis with immunoblot, ELISA, and RNA-precipitation assays. J Immunol Methods 133: 215, 1990.
403. Harmon CE, Deng J, Peebles CL, et al: The importance of tissue substrate in the SS-A (Ro) antigen-antibody system. Arthritis Rheum 27: 166, 1984.
404. Arroyave CM, Giambrone MJ, Rich KC, et al: The frequency of antinuclear antibody in children by use of mouse kidney and human epithelial cells (Hep-2) of substrates. J Allergy Clin Immunol 82: 741, 1988.
405. Maddison PJ, Provost TT, Reichlin M: Serological findings in patients with "ANA-negative" systemic lupus erythematosus. Medicine (Baltimore) 60: 87, 1981.
406. Gillespie JP, Lindsley CB, Linshaw MA, et al: Childhood systemic lupus erythematosus with negative antinuclear antibody test. J Pediatr 98: 578, 1981.
407. Taylor PV, Scott JS, Gerlis LM, et al: Maternal autoantibodies against fetal cardiac antigens in congenital complete heart block. N Engl J Med 315: 667, 1986.
408. Williams DG, Sharpe NG, Wallace G, Latchman DS: A repeated proline-rich sequence in B/B and N is a dominant epitope recognized by human and murine autoantibodies. J Autoimmun 3: 715, 1990.
409. Barada FA Jr, Andrews BS, David JS IV, et al: Antibodies to Sm in patients with systemic lupus erythematosus. Correlations of Sm antibody titers with disease activity and other laboratory parameters. Arthritis Rheum 24: 1236, 1981.
410. Beaufils M, Kouki F, Mignon F, et al: Clinical significance of anti-Sm antibodies in systemic lupus erythematosus. Am J Med 74: 201, 1983.
411. Gulko PS, Reveille JD, Koopman WJ, et al: Survival impact of autoantibodies in systemic lupus erythematosus. J Rheumatol 21: 224, 1994.
412. Arnett FC, Hamilton RG, Roebber MG, et al: Increased frequencies of Sm and nRNP autoantibodies in American blacks compared to whites with systemic lupus erythematosus. J Rheumatol 15: 1773, 1988.
413. Sharp GC, Irvine WS, Tan EM, et al: Mixed connective tissue disease: An apparently distinct rheumatic disease syndrome associated with a specific antibody to an extractable nuclear antigen. Am J Med 52: 148, 1972.
414. Fritzler MJ, Tan EM: Antibodies to histone in drug-induced and idiopathic lupus erythematosus. J Clin Invest 62: 560, 1978.
415. Fritzler MJ, Ryan JP, Kinsella TD: Clinical features of SLE patients with antihistone antibodies. J Rheumatol 9: 46, 1982.
416. Portanova JP, Arndt RE, Tan EM, et al: Anti-histone antibodies in idiopathic and drug-induced lupus recognize distinct intrahistone regions. J Immunol 138: 293, 1987.
417. Rubin RL, Joslin GF, Tan EM: Specificity of antihistone antibodies in systemic lupus erythematosus. Arthritis Rheum 25: 779, 1982.
418. Shergy WJ, Kredich DW, Pisetsky DS: The relationship of anticardiolipin antibodies to disease manifestations in pediatric systemic lupus erythematosus. J Rheumatol 15: 1389, 1988.
419. Petty RE, Palmer NR, Cassidy JT, et al: The association of autoimmune diseases and anti-IgA antibodies in patients with selective IgA deficiency. Clin Exp Immunol 37: 83, 1979.
420. Levinsky RJ, Cameron JS, Soothill JF: Serum immune complexes and disease activity in lupus nephritis. Lancet 1: 564, 1977.
421. Theofilopoulos AN, Wilson CB, Bokisch VA, et al: Binding of soluble immune complexes to human lymphoblastoid cells. II. Use of Raji cells to detect circulating immune complexes in animal and human sera. J Exp Med 140: 1230, 1974.

422. Maini RN, Holborow EJ (eds): Detection and measurement of circulatory soluble antigen-antibody complexes and anti-DNA antibodies. Ann Rheum Dis 36(Suppl 1): 1, 1997.
423. Harbeck RJ, Bardana EJ, Kohler PF, et al: DNA–anti-DNA complexes: Their detection in systemic lupus erythematosus sera. J Clin Invest 52: 789, 1973.
424. Bardana EJ Jr, Harbeck RJ, Hoffman AA, et al: The prognostic and therapeutic implications of DNA–anti-DNA immune complexes in systemic lupus erythematosus. Am J Med 59: 515, 1975.
425. Coppo R, Bosticardo GM, Basolo B, et al: Clinical significance of the detection of circulating immune complexes in lupus nephritis. Nephron 32: 320, 1982.
426. Abrass CK, Nies KM, Louie JS, et al: Correlation and predictive accuracy of circulating immune complexes with disease activity in patients with systemic lupus erythematosus. Arthritis Rheum 23: 273, 1980.
427. Gauthier VJ, Emlen W: Immune complexes in systemic lupus erythematosus. *In* Hahn BH, Wallace DJ (eds): Dubois' Lupus Erythematosus, 5th ed. 1997, p 207.
428. Gewurz H, Pickering RJ, Mergenhagen SE, et al: The complement profile in acute glomerulonephritis, systemic lupus erythematosus and hypocomplementemic chronic glomerulonephritis. Int Arch Allergy Appl Immunol 34: 556, 1968.
429. Singsen BH, Bernstein BH, King KK, et al: Systemic lupus erythematosus in childhood: Correlations between changes in disease activity and serum complement levels. J Pediatr 89: 358, 1976.
430. Buyon JP, Tamerius J, Belmont HM, Abramson SB: Assessment of disease activity and impending flare in patients with systemic lupus erythematosus. Arthritis Rheum 35: 1028, 1992.
431. Agnello V: Complement deficiency states. Medicine (Baltimore) 57: 1, 1978.
432. Atkinson JP: Complement deficiency. Predisposing factor to autoimmune syndromes. Am J Med 85(Suppl 6A): 45, 1988.
433. Osterland CK, Espinoza L, Parker LP, et al: Inherited C2 deficiency and systemic lupus erythematosus: Studies on a family. Ann Intern Med 82: 323, 1975.
434. Gewurz A, Lint TF, Roberts JL, et al: Homozygous C2 deficiency with fulminant lupus erythematosus: Severe nephritis via the alternative complement pathway. Arthritis Rheum 21: 28, 1978.
435. Roberts JL, Schwartz MM, Lewis EJ: Hereditary C2 deficiency and systemic lupus erythematosus associated with severe glomerulonephritis. Clin Exp Immunol 31: 328, 1978.
436. Pincus T, Hughes GRV, Pincus D, et al: Antibodies to DNA in childhood systemic lupus erythematosus. J Pediatr 78: 981, 1971.
437. Hughes GRV, Cohen AS, Christian CL: Anti-DNA activity in systemic lupus erythematosus. A diagnostic and therapeutic guide. Ann Rheum Dis 30: 259, 1971.
438. Adler MK, Baumgarten A, Hecht B, et al: Prognostic significance of DNA-binding capacity patterns in patients with lupus nephritis. Ann Rheum Dis 34: 444, 1975.
439. Garin EH, Donnelly WH, Shulman ST, et al: The significance of serial measurements of serum complement C3 and C4 components and DNA binding capacity in patients with lupus nephritis. Clin Nephrol 12: 148, 1979.
440. Sliwinski AJ, Zvaifler NJ: Decreased synthesis of the third component of complement in hypocomplementemic systemic lupus erythematosus. Clin Exp Immunol 11: 21, 1972.
441. Petri M, Genovese M, Engle E, Hochberg MC: Definition, incidence, and clinical description of flare in systemic lupus erythematosus: A prospective cohort study. Arthritis Rheum 34: 937, 1991.
442. Bombardier C, Gladman DD, Urowitz M, et al: Derivation of the SLEDAI. A disease activity index for lupus patients. Arthritis Rheum 35: 630, 1992.
443. Liang MH, Socher SA, Larson MG, Schur PH: Reliability and validity of six systems for the clinical assessment of disease activity in systemic lupus erythematosus. Arthritis Rheum 32: 1107, 1989.
444. Symmons DPM, Coopock JS, Bacon PA, et al: Development and assessment of a computerized index of clinical disease activity in systemic lupus erythematosus. Q J Med 68: 927, 1988.
445. Petri M, Hellmann D, Hochberg M: Validity and reliability of lupus activity measures in the routine clinic setting. J Rheumatol 19: 53, 1992.
446. Hawker G, Gabriel S, Bombardier C, et al: A reliability study of SLEDAI: A disease activity index for systemic lupus erythematosus. J Rheumatol 20: 657, 1993.
447. Merino R, Mendez S, Garcia-Consuegra, Madero R: Evaluation of two disease activity indices of systemic lupus erythematosus in pediatric patients. Clin Exp Rheumatol 13: 680, 1995.
447a. Brunner HI, Feldman BM, Bombardier C, Silverman ED: Sensitivity of the Systemic Lupus Erythematosus Disease Activity Index, British Isles Lupus Assessment Group Index and Systemic Lupus Activity measure in the evaluation of clinical change in childhood-onset systemic lupus erythematosus. Arthritis Rheum 42: 1354, 1999.
448. Sibley JT, Olszynski WP, Decoteau WE, Sundaram MB: The incidence and prognosis of central nervous system disease in systemic lupus erythematosus. J Rheumatol 19: 47, 1992.
449. Gladman DD, Ginzler E, Goldsmith C, et al: The development and initial validation of the Systemic Lupus International Collaborating Clinics/American College of Rheumatology Damage Index for systemic lupus erythematosus. Arthritis Rheum 39: 363, 1996.
449a. Brunner HI, Silverman ED, Bombardier C, et al: Disease activity and steroids are risk factors for damage, while second line agents are protective in childhood-onset systemic lupus erythematosus. Arthritis Rheum 43(Suppl) S171, 2000.
450. Stoll T, Gordon C, Seifert B, et al: Consistency and validity of patient administered assessment of quality of life by the MOS SF-36. Its association with disease activity and damage in patients with systemic lupus erythematosus. J Rheumatol 24: 1608, 1997.
451. Freeman RG, Knox JM, Owens DW: Cutaneous lesions of lupus erythematosus induced by monochromatic light. Arch Dermatol 100: 677, 1969.
452. Rihner M, McGrath J Jr: Fluorescent light photosensitivity in patients with systemic lupus erythematosus. Arthritis Rheum 35: 949, 1992.
453. Seaman WE, Ishak KG, Plotz PH: Aspirin-induced hepatotoxicity in patients with systemic lupus erythematosus. Ann Intern Med 80: 1, 1974.
454. Samuelson CO, Williams HJ: Ibuprofen-associated aseptic meningitis in systemic lupus erythematosus. West J Med 131: 57, 1979.
455. Jensen S, Glud TK, Bacher T, Ersgaard H: Ibuprofen-induced meningitis in a male with systemic lupus erythematosus. Acta Med Scand 221: 509, 1987.
456. Mandell BF, Raps ED: Severe systemic hypersensitivity reaction of ibuprofen occurring after prolonged therapy. Am J Med 82: 817, 1987.
457. Weksler BB, Lehany AM: Naproxen-induced recurrent aseptic meningitis. DICP 25: 1183, 1991.
458. Ruppert GB, Barth WF: Tolmetin-induced aseptic meningitis. JAMA 245: 67, 1981.
459. The Canadian Hydroxychloroquine Study Group: A randomized study of the effect of withdrawing hydroxychloroquine sulfate in systemic lupus erythematosus. N Engl J Med 324: 150, 1991.
460. Tsakonas E, Joseph L, Esdaile JM, et al: A long-term study of hydroxychloroquine withdrawal on exacerbations of systemic lupus erythematosus. Lupus 7: 80, 1998.
461. Wallace DJ, Metzger AL, Stecher VJ, et al: Cholesterol-lowering effect of hydroxychloroquine in patients with rheumatic disease: Reversal of deleterious effects of steroids on lipids. Am J Med 89: 322, 1990.
462. Hodis HN, Quismorio FP Jr, Wickham E, Blankenhorn DH: The lipid, lipoprotein, and apolipoprotein effects of hydroxychloroquine in patients with systemic lupus erythematosus. J Rheumatol 20: 661, 1993.
463. Petri M: Hydroxychloroquine use in the Baltimore lupus cohort: Effects on lipids, glucose and thrombosis. Lupus 5(Suppl 1): S16, 1996.
464. Laaksonen A-L, Koskiahde V, Juva K: Dosage of antimalarial drugs for children with juvenile rheumatoid arthritis and systemic lupus erythematosus. A clinical study with determination of serum concentration of chloroquine and hydroxychloroquine. Scand J Rheumatol 3: 103, 1974.
465. Rudnicki RD, Gresham GE, Rothfield NF: The efficacy of anti-

malarials in systemic lupus erythematosus. J Rheumatol 2: 323, 1975.
466. Rothfield N, Baldwin D: The clinical course of the proliferative and membranous forms of lupus nephritis. Ann Intern Med 73: 929, 1970.
467. Pollak VE, Pirani CL, Kark RM: Effect of large doses of prednisone on the renal lesions and life span of patients with lupus glomerulonephritis. J Lab Clin Med 57: 495, 1961.
468. Felson DT, Anderson J: Evidence for the superiority of immunosuppressive drugs and prednisone over prednisone alone in lupus nephritis. Results of a pooled analysis. N Engl J Med 311: 1528, 1984.
469. Sharon E, Kaplan D, Diamond HS: Exacerbation of systemic lupus erythematosus after withdrawal of azathioprine therapy. N Engl J Med 288: 122, 1973.
470. Silverman E: What's new in the treatment of pediatric SLE. J Rheumatol 23: 1657, 1996.
471. Fries JF, Sharp GC, McDevitt HO, Holman HR: Cyclophosphamide therapy in systemic lupus erythematosus and polymyositis. Arthritis Rheum 16: 154, 1973.
472. Donadio JV Jr, Holley KE, Ferguson RH, Ilstrup DM: Treatment of diffuse proliferative lupus nephritis with prednisone and combined prednisone and cyclophosphamide. N Engl J Med 299: 1151, 1978.
473. Steinberg AD, Decker JL: A double-blind controlled trial comparing cyclophosphamide, azathioprine and placebo in the treatment of lupus glomerulonephritis. Arthritis Rheum 17: 923, 1974.
474. Steinberg AS, Steinberg SC: Long-term preservation of renal function in patients with lupus nephritis receiving treatment that includes cyclophosphamide versus those treated with prednisone only. Arthritis Rheum 34: 945, 1991.
475. Hahn BH, Kantor OS, Osterland CK: Azathioprine plus prednisone compared with prednisone alone in the treatment of systemic lupus erythematosus. Report of a prospective controlled trial in 24 patients. Ann Intern Med 83: 597, 1975.
476. Barnett EV, Dornfeld L, Lee DB, et al: Longterm survival of lupus nephritis patients treated with azathioprine and prednisone. J Rheumatol 5: 275, 1978.
477. Ginzler E, Sharon E, Diamond H, et al: Long-term maintenance therapy with azathioprine in systemic lupus erythematosus. Arthritis Rheum 18: 27, 1975.
478. Balow JE, Austin HA, Tsokos GC, et al: NIH Conference: Lupus nephritis. 106: 79, 1987.
479. Boumpas DT, Austin HA, Vaughn EM, et al: Controlled trial of pulse methylprednisolone versus two regimens of pulse cyclophosphamide in severe lupus nephritis. Lancet 340: 741, 1992.
480. Lehman TJ: A practical guide to systemic lupus erythematosus. Pediatr Clin North Am 42: 1223, 1995.
481. Neuwelt MC, Lacks S, Kaye BR, et al: Role of intravenous cyclophosphamide in the treatment of severe neuropsychiatric systemic lupus erythematosus. Am J Med 98: 32, 1995.
482. Slater CA, Liang MH, McCune JW, et al: Preserving ovarian function in patients receiving cyclophosphamide. Lupus 8: 3, 1999.
483. Rothenberg RJ, Graziano RM, Grandone JT, et al: The use of methotrexate in steroid-resistant systemic lupus erythematosus. Arthritis Rheum 31: 612, 1988.
484. Abud-Mendoza C, Sturbaum AK, Vazquez-Compean R, Gonzalez-Amaro R: Methotrexate therapy in childhood systemic lupus erythematosus. J Rheumatol 20: 731, 1993.
485. Ravelli A, Ballardini G, Viola S, et al: Methotrexate therapy in refractory pediatric onset systemic lupus erythematosus. J Rheumatol 25: 572, 1998.
486. Valesini G, Priori R, Francia A, et al: Central nervous system involvement in systemic lupus erythematosus: A new therapeutic approach with intrathecal dexamethasone and methotrexate. Springer Semin Immunopathol 16: 313, 1994.
487. Fink SD, Kremer JM: Successful treatment of interstitial lung disease in systemic lupus erythematosus with methotrexate. J Rheumatol 22: 967, 1995.
488. Feuren G, Querin S, Noel LH, et al: Effects of cyclosporine in severe systemic lupus erythematosus. J Pediatr 111: 1063, 1987.
489. Fu LW, Yang LY, Chen WP, Lin CY: Clinical efficacy of cyclosporin A (Neoral) in the treatment of paediatric lupus nephritis with heavy proteinuria. Br J Rheumatol 37: 217, 1998.
490. Caccavo D, Lagana B, Mitterhofer AP, et al: Long-term treatment of systemic lupus erythematosus with cyclosporin A. Arthritis Rheum 40: 27, 1997.
490a. Chan TM, Li FK, Tang CS, et al: Efficacy of mycophenolate mofetil in patients with diffuse proliferative lupus nephritis. N Engl J Med 343: 1156, 2000.
490b. Austin HA, Balow JE: Treatment of lupus nephritis. Semin Nephrol 20: 265, 2000.
491. Akashi K, Magasawa K, Mayumi T, et al: Successful treatment of refractory systemic lupus erythematosus with intravenous immunoglobulins. J Rheumatol 17: 375, 1990.
492. Winder A, Molad Y, Ostfeld I, et al: Treatment of systemic lupus erythematosus by prolonged administration of high dose intravenous immunoglobulin: Report of 2 cases. J Rheumatol 20: 495, 1993.
493. DeVita S, Ferraccioli GF, De Poi E, et al: High dose intravenous immunoglobulin therapy for rheumatic diseases: Clinical relevance and personal experience. Clin Exp Rheumatol 14(Suppl 15): S85, 1996.
494. Cohen MG, Li EK: Limited effects of intravenous IgG in treating systemic lupus erythematosus-associated thrombocytopenia. Arthritis Rheum 34: 787, 1991.
495. terBorg EJ, Kallenberg CGM: Treatment of severe thrombocytopenia in systemic lupus erythematosus with intravenous gammaglobulin. Ann Rheum Dis 51: 1149, 1992.
496. Schroeder JO, Zeuner RA, Euler HH, Loffler H: High dose intravenous immunoglobulins in systemic lupus erythematosus: Clinical and serological results of a pilot study. J Rheumatol 23: 71, 1996.
497. Lafferty TE, Smith JB, Schuster SJ, DeHoratius RJ: Treatment of acquired factor VIII inhibitor using intravenous immunoglobulin in two patients with systemic lupus erythematosus. Arthritis Rheum 40: 775, 1997.
498. Wei N, Klippel JH, Huston DP, et al: Randomised trial of plasma exchange in mild systemic lupus erythematosus. Lancet 1: 17, 1983.
499. Lewis EJ, Hunsicker LG, Lan S-P, et al: A controlled trial of plasmapheresis therapy in severe lupus nephritis. N Engl J Med 326: 1373, 1992.
500. Campion BW: Desperate diseases and plasmapheresis. N Engl J Med 326: 1425, 1992.
501. Hanly JG, Hong C, Zayed E, et al: Immunomodulating effects of synchronised plasmapheresis and intravenous bolus cyclophosphamide in systemic lupus erythematosus. Lupus 4: 457, 1995.
502. Hiepe F, Volk H-D, Apostoloff E, et al: Treatment of severe systemic lupus erythematosus with anti-CD4 monoclonal antibody. Lancet 338: 1529, 1991.
503. Perosa F, Scudeletti M, Imro MA, et al: Anti-CD4 monoclonal antibody (mab) and anti-idiotypic mAb to anti-CD4 in the therapy of autoimmune diseases. Clin Exp Rheumatol 15: 201, 1997.
504. Wacholtz MC, Lipsky PE: Treatment of lupus nephritis with CD5 PLUS, an immunoconjugate of an anti-CD-5 monoclonal antibody and ricin A chain. Arthritis Rheum 35: 837, 1992.
505. Calabrese L, Fleischer AB: Thalidomide: current and potential clinical applications. Am J Med 108: 487, 2000.
506. Knobler RM, Graninger W, Graninger W, et al: Extracorporeal photochemotherapy for the treatment of systemic lupus erythematosus. Arthritis Rheum 35: 319, 1992.
507. Burt RK, Traynor AE, Pope R, et al: Treatment of autoimmune disease by intense immunosuppressive conditioning and autologous hematopoietic stem cell transplantation. Blood 92: 3505, 1998.
507a. Trysberg E, Lindgren I, Tarkowski A: Autologous stem cell transplantation in a case of treatment-resistant central nervous system lupus. Ann Rheum Dis 59: 236, 2000.
508. Lockshin MD: Which patients with antiphospholipid antibody should be treated and how? Rheum Dis Clin North Am 19: 235, 1993.
508a. Wahl DG, Bournameaux H, de Moerloose P, Sarasin FP: Prophylactic antithrombotic therapy for patients with systemic lupus erythematosus with or without antiphospholipid antibodies. Arch Intern Med 160: 2042, 2000.
509. Baca V, Lavalle C, Garcia R, et al: Favorable response to intravenous methylprenisolone and cyclophosphamide in children with severe neuropsychiatric lupus. J Rheumatol 26: 432, 1999.

510. Klein M, Radhakrishnan J, Appel G: Cyclosporine treatment of glomerular diseases. Annu Rev Med 50: 1, 1999.
511. Pollock CA, Ibels LS: Dialysis and transplantation in patients with renal failure due to systemic lupus erythematosus. The Australian and New Zealand experience. Aust N Z J Med 17: 321, 1987.
512. McCurdy DK, Lehman TJA, Bernstein B, et al: Lupus nephritis: Prognostic factors in children. Pediatrics 89: 240, 1992.
513. Jarrett MP, Santhanam S, Del Greco F: The clinical course of end-stage renal disease in systemic lupus erythematosus. Arch Intern Med 143: 1353, 1983.
514. Litsey SE, Noonan JA, O'Connor WN, et al: Maternal connective tissue disease and congenital heart block. Demonstration of immunoglobulin in cardiac tissue. N Engl J Med 312: 98, 1985.
515. Kramer P, Boyer M, Brunner FP, et al: Combined report on regular dialysis and transplantation in Europe XII, 1981. Proc Eur Dial Transplant Assoc 19: 29, 1982.
516. Nossent HC, Swaak TJG, Berden JHM, et al: Systemic lupus erythematosus after renal transplantation: Patient and graft survival and disease activity. Ann Intern Med 114: 183, 1991.
517. Cheigh JS, Kim H, Stenzel KH, et al: Systemic lupus erythematosus in patients with end-stage renal disease: Long-term follow-up on the prognosis of patients and the evolution of lupus activity. Am J Kidney Dis 16: 189, 1990.
518. Kumano K, Sakai T, Mashimo S, et al: A case of recurrent lupus nephritis after renal transplantation. Clin Nephrol 27: 94, 1987.
519. Brown CD, Rao TKS, Maxey RW, et al: Regression of clinical and immunological expression of SLE consequent to the development of uremia. Kidney Int 16: 884, 1979.
520. Estes D, Christian CL: The natural history of systemic lupus erythematosus by prospective analysis. Medicine (Baltimore) 50: 85, 1971.
521. Wedgwood RJ: Prognostic factors in childhood systemic lupus erythematosus. Arthritis Rheum 20: 295, 1977.
522. Platt JL, Burke BA, Fish AJ, et al: Systemic lupus erythematosus in the first two decades of life. Am J Kidney Dis 2: 212, 1982.
523. Lacks S, White P: Morbidity associated with childhood systemic lupus erythematosus. J Rheumatol 17: 941, 1990.
524. Fish AJ, Blau EB, Westberg NG, et al: Systemic lupus erythematosus within the first two decades of life. Am J Med 62: 99, 1977.
525. Abeles M, Urman JD, Weinstein A, et al: SLE in the younger patient: Survival studies. J Rheumatol 7: 515, 1980.
526. Wallace DJ, Podell T, Weiner J, et al: Systemic lupus erythematosus: Survival patterns. Experience with 609 patients. JAMA 245: 934, 1981.
527. Glidden RS, Mantzouranis EC, Borel Y: Systemic lupus erythematosus in childhood: Clinical manifestations and improved survival in fifty-five patients. Clin Immunol Immunopathol 29: 196, 1983.
528. Dumas R: Lupus nephritis. Collaborative study by the French Society of Paediatric Nephrology. Arch Dis Child 60: 126, 1985.
529. Baqi N, Moazami S, Singh A, et al: Lupus nephritis in children: A longitudinal study of prognostic factors and therapy. J Am Soc Nephrol 7: 924, 1998.
530. Yang LY: Lupus nephritis in children: A review of 167 patients. Pediatrics 94: 335, 1994.
531. Rush PJ, Baumal R, Shore A, et al: Correlation of renal histology with outcome in children with lupus nephritis. Kidney Int 29: 1066, 1986.
532. Harisdangkul V, Nilganuwonge S, Rockhold L: Cause of death in systemic lupus erythematosus: A pattern based on age at onset. South Med J 80: 1249, 1987.
533. Austin HA III, Muenz LR, Joyce KM, et al: Prognostic factors in lupus nephritis. Contribution of renal histologic data. Am J Med 75: 382, 1983.
534. Bennahum DA, Messner RP: Recent observations on central nervous system lupus erythematosus. Semin Arthritis Rheum 4: 253, 1975.
535. Kaslow RA, Masi AT: Age, sex and race effects on mortality from systemic lupus erythematosus in the United States. Arthritis Rheum 21: 473, 1978.
536. Gordon MF, Stolley PD, Schinnar R: Trends in recent systemic lupus erythematosus mortality rates. Arthritis Rheum 24: 762, 1981.
537. Tejani A, Nicastri AD, Chen CK, et al: Lupus nephritis in black and Hispanic children. Am J Dis Child 137: 481, 1983.
538. Grossman L, Barland P: Histone reactivity of drug-induced antinuclear antibodies. A comparison of symptomatic and asymptomatic patients. Arthritis Rheum 24: 927, 1981.
539. Fritzler M, Ryan P, Kinsella TD: Clinical features of systemic lupus erythematosus patients with antihistone antibodies. J Rheumatol 9: 46, 1982.
540. Alarcon-Segovia D, Wakim KG, Worthington JW, et al: Clinical and experimental studies on the hydralazine syndrome and its relationship to systemic lupus erythematosus. Medicine (Baltimore) 46: 1, 1967.
541. Alarcon-Segovia D: Drug induced systemic lupus erythematosus and related syndromes. Clin Rheum Dis 1: 573, 1975.
542. Beernink DH, Miller JJ III: Anticonvulsant-induced antinuclear antibodies and lupus-like disease in children. J Pediatr 82: 113, 1973.
543. Singsen BH, Fishman L, Hanson V: Antinuclear antibodies and lupus-like syndromes in children receiving anticonvulsants. Pediatrics 57: 529, 1976.
544. Irias JJ: Hydralazine-induced lupus erythematosus-like syndrome. Am J Dis Child 129: 862, 1975.
545. Hahn BH, Sharp GC, Irvin WS, et al: Immune responses to hydralazine and nuclear antigens in hydralazine-induced lupus erythematosus. Ann Intern Med 76: 365, 1972.
546. Johansson E, Mustakallio KK, Mattila MJ: Polymorphic acetylator phenotype and systemic lupus erythematosus. Acta Med Scand 210: 193, 1981.
547. Baer AN, Woosley RL, Pincus T: Further evidence for the lack of association between acetylator phenotype and systemic lupus erythematosus. Arthritis Rheum 29: 508, 1986.

19

Neonatal Lupus Erythematosus

Earl D. Silverman

Neonatal lupus erythematosus (NLE) is a disease of the developing fetus and neonate defined by characteristic clinical features in the presence of specific maternally derived autoantibodies. The transplacental passage of these autoantibodies is necessary but not sufficient to cause the disease. The specific autoantibodies associated with NLE are directed against a group of small cytoplasmic and nuclear ribonucleoproteins and their associated RNAs, collectively referred to as the RoRNP or Ro particle. The most common clinical manifestations of NLE are cardiac, dermatologic, and hepatic.

ETIOLOGY AND PATHOGENESIS

Maternal autoantibodies directed against the RoRNP or occasionally other autoantigens are required for the development of NLE. However, many mothers with these autoantibodies do not deliver children with NLE. Therefore, other factors, including viral infection, maternal estrogens, and ultraviolet light, may have a role in the development of NLE.[1, 2]

Autoantigens

Anti-Ro and anti-La autoantibodies are directed against the RoRNP.[3, 4] There are at least two Ro proteins, a 60-kD and a 52-kD polypeptide, and a single La protein (48 kD).[3, 5, 6] The Ro and La proteins are closely associated and both are usually found complexed to small RNAs. The Ro and La proteins, rather than their associated RNAs, are the major antigenic targets of the autoantibodies.

La Protein

The La protein is found in association with RNA polymerase III transcripts, which include small viral RNAs, U1RNA, and precursors of both tRNA and 5sRNA.[4, 7–10] La protein has an important role in the production of polymerase III RNA transcripts, can modulate 5′ processing of pre-tRNAs, and therefore is important in controlling transcriptional and post-transcriptional events during the synthesis, maturation, and nuclear export of polymerase III transcripts, including the RNAs to which it binds.[11–14] La exists in at least two forms: one is associated with the Ro protein and the other is independent of Ro.[15] A structural basis for the association of Ro and La proteins has been demonstrated.[16]

Proteins homologous to La exist in many species, including fruit flies (*Drosophila melanogaster*), frogs (*Xenopus laevis*), mosquitoes, and yeast (*Saccharomyces cerevisiae*), demonstrating the importance of La in normal cell function.[17–19] There are species-specific inserts that may be of pathogenic significance in the development of anti-La antibodies and in the pathogenesis of NLE.[20] La is present in numerous nuclear and cytoplasmic complexes, where it acts as a molecular chaperone for polymerase III transcripts, functions as an RNA-folding protein, is important in the very early steps of U6snRNP assembly, and is important during the cell cycle by increasing histone protein production.[21–24]

La binds to, enhances translation of, and alters gene expression of several viral RNAs, including human parainfluenza virus type 3, poliovirus, and human immunodeficiency virus,[25–28] and alters regulation of interferon-inducible protein kinase after viral infection.[29, 30] Infection with poliovirus or adenovirus induces a relocation of La from the nucleus to the cytoplasm and cell surface.[31, 32] The interaction of La with viruses and the subsequent alteration of the cellular distribution of La may permit maternally derived autoantibodies to bind directly to their autoantigen target on the cell surface.

The La protein can shuttle between the nucleus and the cytoplasm, but it is mainly located in the nucleus.[32] During early development in *X. laevis*, there are extremely high levels of La mRNA that progressively and significantly decrease during gestation.[18] This observation may help explain why the developing rather than the adult heart is the target of autoantibodies in NLE. There are three functional La mRNA forms, which are upregulated and downregulated in parallel.[33, 34] In vivo, mRNA for exons 1 and 1′ have been found in endothelial cells and liver cells but not in smooth muscle cells.

Exon 1 resides mostly in the nucleus, whereas exon 1′ La mRNA is mainly in the cytoplasm.[35] Any of the La isoforms may be the target of the immune response in NLE.

Ro Proteins

The function of the Ro proteins has been much more difficult to determine. The 60 kD Ro protein is important in maintaining production of functional 5S rRNA.[36] This function of 60 kD Ro is in association with La, and the two proteins are either complexed together or bind in close proximity to each other.[37] The 52 kD Ro protein is mainly located in the cytoplasm,[38] whereas 60 kD Ro is predominantly found in the nucleus, suggesting that the two Ro antigens likely have different cellular functions. Cell stress in vivo can alter the antigenic configuration and cell surface expression of 52 kD Ro, which would then allow for direct tissue damage by anti-Ro antibodies.[39]

The 52 kD Ro protein has an alternatively spliced form referred to as 52β, whereas the more common protein in adult life is the 52α protein. The 52β form is maximally expressed between 14 and 16 weeks of gestation, a time when the level of 52α expression is at its lowest. In fetal hearts by age 22 to 25 weeks and in adult hearts, the 52β transcript is markedly diminished and 52α is the dominant form. These data suggest that the differential expression of the 52 kD Ro isoforms may be important in the development of heart block because the maximal expression of 52β occurs at the time of cardiac ontogeny, when maternal antibodies begin to cross the placental barrier.[40]

Calreticulin and RoRNP

The most controversial issue regarding RoRNP is its relationship to calreticulin. Some investigators have "demonstrated" that calreticulin is part of RoRNP associated with the hY RNAs, whereas others disagree.[41, 42] Calreticulin was initially described as a calcium-binding protein present in the endoplasmic reticulum. It is present in many animal species, including *Leishmania*,[43] the filarial nematode *Onchocerca volvulus* (specifically the RAL1 protein),[41, 44] *Caenorhabditis elegans*,[45] *D. melanogaster*,[46] and *X. laevis*.[47]

Calreticulin has three structural domains, each with a different function. It is present on the cell membrane of neutrophils and may be shed during cytotoxic T cell activation, which permits calreticulin to be present extracellularly.[48, 49] Although a major function of calreticulin is as a resident calcium-binding protein in the endoplasmic reticulum, it is also found outside of the endoplasmic reticulum in the nuclear envelope, the nucleus, and cytotoxic granules in T cells, and in vesicles of sperm cells.[50, 51] Similar to other autoantigens, stress can increase gene expression of calreticulin.[52, 53] In addition to calcium binding, calreticulin may have a role in (1) regulating T-cell activation,[54] (2) controlling gene transcription including the glucocorticoid receptor,[55–60] (3) modulating integrin-mediated functions,[61–63] (4) inhibiting androgen receptor and retinoic acid receptor transcriptional activities,[59] (5) regulating bone cell function,[60] and (6) processing T-cell receptor alpha and beta proteins and human leukocyte antigen (HLA) proteins.[64–67]

Autoantibodies

In the mid-1980s, it was recognized that NLE in the child was associated with maternal anti-Ro antibodies.[68, 69] Following the discovery that there were two major Ro proteins and the La protein, it became clear that the greatest risk for the development of congenital atrioventricular block (CAVB) was associated with maternal anti–52 kD Ro and anti-La antibodies.[70–76] The risk of NLE was associated with higher mean maternal antibody titers to all three proteins.[71, 77–79] Cutaneous NLE (C-NLE) is associated with higher titers of maternal autoantibodies to these antigens than occur with CAVB.[70–76, 79, 80]

Examination of the fine specificity of the repertoire of maternal anti-La antibodies allowed identification of antibodies directed against a small La polypeptide, named DD, that was found only in the sera of mothers of children with NLE and not in sera from mothers of unaffected children.[71] Although this finding was specific for NLE, it had only a 30 percent sensitivity because many mothers without anti-DD antibodies delivered children with NLE, and anti-DD antibodies were present in only 30 percent of children with NLE.

Similarly, the fine specificity of the anti-Ro antibody response in mothers of children with NLE differs from the anti-Ro response of other women with rheumatic disorders.[81] Differences in the fine specificity of the immune response to the RoRNP may be important in fetal outcome. Further studies are required to determine the "at risk" pregnancies and should examine the response to isoforms of the Ro and La proteins, the relative amount of which can vary during gestation.[33, 40, 82]

Although there still is controversy about whether calreticulin is a part of the RoRNP, autoantibodies directed against calreticulin are present in the sera from patients with autoimmune diseases.[41, 44, 83] Although elevated anti-calreticulin antibody levels have been reported in mothers of children with NLE compared with healthy normal subjects, when the anti-calreticulin response was compared with that of healthy pregnant women, no differences in the mean titer of these autoantibodies could be demonstrated. However, one report found differences in anti-calreticulin antibody titers when compared with normal, healthy control subjects.[84]

The presence of other antigens on the fetal heart or placenta has been suggested to be important in the development, or protection from the development, of CAVB. There is cross-reactivity between a subset of anti-La, but not anti-Ro, antibodies and laminin.[85, 86] Sera from mothers of infants with CAVB may also contain anti-endogenous retrovirus-3 (ERV-3) antibodies. Anti-La, anti-calreticulin, and anti-ERV-3 antibodies can bind to the placenta or placental trophoblast or both.[86–88] Binding of these autoantibodies to placental tissue may alter the quantity and repertoire of these autoantibodies in the fetal circulation and therefore affect binding to the target fetal tissue.[87–89]

Anti-laminin autoantibodies bind to fetal but not adult heart and cardiac tissue, and both ERV-3 and laminin are maximally expressed between 11 and 17 weeks of gestation.[87, 89] Therefore, cardiac laminin, calreticulin, or ERV-3 may be a target for maternal autoantibodies, and direct binding to these fetal cardiac proteins may initiate or potentiate inflammation in the fetal heart.[86, 87, 89]

Antibodies directed against both a p57 recombinant protein and alpha-fodrin have been detected in the sera of mothers of infants with NLE. Anti-p57 antibodies were present in approximately one third of the sera from mothers of children with NLE and were almost always associated with anti-Ro antibodies.[90] Anti–alpha-fodrin antibodies were initially reported to be present in sera from patients with Sjögren's syndrome (SS) but not in the sera from patients with rheumatoid arthritis or systemic lupus erythematosus (SLE).[91] Preliminary data in NLE suggest that maternal anti–120 kD alpha-fodrin antibodies may be an additional serologic marker for the risk of development of NLE.[92]

GENETIC BACKGROUND

HLA-DR and DQ genes are important in the production of anti-Ro and anti-La antibodies. In patients with autoimmune diseases, DR3 was associated with anti-52 kD Ro and anti-La autoantibodies but not anti-60 kD Ro antibodies.[93, 94] This association is present in most but not all ethnic backgrounds and is independent of disease expression.[95–103] High-titer anti-Ro antibodies are associated with the DQw1/DQw2 heterozygote state.[104, 105] In mothers of children with NLE, the HLA antigen profile more closely resembles that which is present in patients with primary SS than that associated with patients with SLE.[77]

It is likely that extended haplotypes are more important than single loci in determining production of anti-Ro and anti-La antibodies. In patients of most ethnic backgrounds, high levels of anti-Ro and anti-La antibodies are associated with all or at least most of DRB1*0301, DQA1*0501, and DQB1*0201 extended haplotype alleles, whereas the DQA1*0501 allele is present in the other patients.[96, 97, 106] Glutamine at position 34 of the DQA1 chain and leucine at position 26 of the DQB1 chain are associated with anti-Ro and anti-La antibodies, although the extended haplotype (in linkage disequilibrium) may have the strongest correlation with this autoantibody response.[107, 108] The genetic control of anti-RoRNP antibodies is further complicated by the demonstration that response to peptides of the 60 kD Ro protein may be under different genetic control and distinct from the HLA associations of the response to the complete 60 kD protein.[109]

In Japanese mothers of children with NLE, the production of both anti-Ro and anti-La antibodies was associated with the extended haplotypes DRB1*1101-DQA1*0501-DQB1*0301 and DRB1*08032-DQA1*0103-DQB1*0601 as well as the individual alleles DRB1*1101, DRB1*08032, and DQB1*0301.[110] All of the anti-Ro and anti-La antibody–positive mothers had DRB1 alleles that shared the same amino acid residues at positions 14 to 31 and 71 of the DRB1 chain and were either homozygous or heterozygous at DQ6, and DQ3 alleles that shared the same amino acid residues at positions 27 to 36 and 71 to 77 of hypervariable regions of the DQB1 chain.[110] Individual manifestations of NLE may also be influenced by maternal HLA, as the maternal DR5 haplotype DRB1*1101-DQA1*0501-DQB1*0301 and individual class II alleles making up this haplotype, including DQA1 alleles with glutamine at position 34 of the first domain, were significantly associated with C-NLE but not CAVB. DQB1*0602 carried on DR2 haplotypes was associated with CAVB but not C-NLE.[111, 112]

Despite the strong association of maternal HLA antigens with NLE, in general there has not been any association of HLA genes in the offspring with the development of NLE, although there have been exceptions.[111–116] One study demonstrated that children with NLE tended to have DRB, DQA, and DQB genes identical to those of their mothers.[117] In addition, one report suggested that DR3 in the fetus might protect against in utero death, whereas another postulated that DR2 in the infant may be protective (although this was associated with maternal DR2).[69, 115]

Multiple genes located outside the MHC locus, including T-cell receptor genes, can influence the onset and progression of autoimmune diseases.[118, 119] The same may be true in NLE.

CLINICAL MANIFESTATIONS OF NEONATAL LUPUS ERYTHEMATOSUS

Cardiac Neonatal Lupus Erythematosus

The most clinically significant manifestations of NLE are cardiac, specifically CAVB. In most cases, the CAVB is isolated, but it may be associated with other cardiac lesions, including endocardial fibroelastosis or patent ductus arteriosus. The first reported case of CAVB associated with maternal autoimmune disease (Mickulisz's syndrome or Sjögren's syndrome) was published around the turn of the last century.[120] However, it was not until the 1950s that it was generally recognized that autoimmune autoantibodies in the mother were associated with NLE. It was another 20 to 30 years until the association with anti-Ro and anti-La antibodies was reported.[70–72, 121–125]

Epidemiology

It is estimated that CAVB occurs in 1 in 14,000 live births, and at least 90 percent of the cases of CAVB are the result of transplacental passage of maternal autoantibodies. This is likely an underestimate of the true incidence of abnormalities of fetal cardiac conduction. Intrauterine deaths are also associated with NLE.[126–131] In most cases, these deaths occurred in fetuses of mothers without a diagnosed autoimmune disease, and the first demonstration of autoantibodies in these mothers occurred during the pregnancy or after delivery of a child with NLE. Our experience suggests that up to 50 percent of pregnancies complicated by fetal CAVB result in intrauterine death and most mothers do not have an autoimmune disease. Therefore, it is likely that CAVB occurs in more than the 1 in 14,000 reported incidence in live births and may be a factor resulting in death of the fetus in 1 in 7000 to 8000 pregnancies carried only to the late second trimester.

Pathology

Although necropsy studies are few, the characteristic pathologic findings in CAVB are an absence or a degeneration of the atrioventricular (AV) node with replacement by fibrosis, calcification, or fatty tissue (Fig. 19–1). The distal conducting system may be normal. The few reports of cases of CAVB not associated with maternal

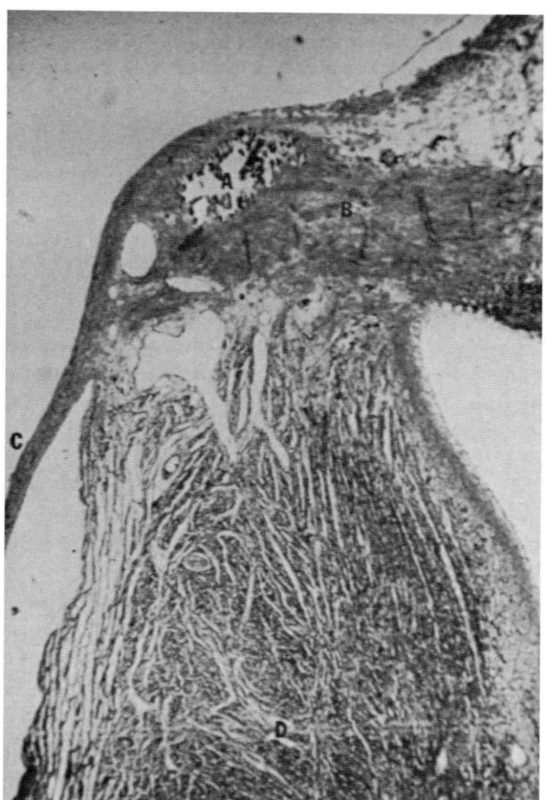

Figure 19–1. Section of ventricular septum from the fetus of a mother with systemic lupus erythematosus. The baby died at birth from nonimmune hydrops secondary to complete congenital heart block. A, Dystrophic calcification in the region of an atrioventricular node; B, dense fibrosis; C, valve leaflet; D, ventricular septum. (Courtesy of Dr. J. Dimmick.)

autoantibodies have demonstrated a normal AV node. Abnormalities also occur in other areas of the heart; therefore, inflammation and scarring may be a more generalized process associated with ventricular endomyocardial fibrosis with complement deposition and an inflammatory cell infiltrate.[122] These latter findings suggest the possibility that the AV node conduction defects may be the result of the susceptibility of the conduction system to inflammatory damage rather than a specific localization of the autoantibodies to this area of the developing heart. It has been proposed that anti-Ro and anti-La antibodies lead to fetal myocarditis, which can result in endocardial fibroelastosis and disruption of the conducting system.[135]

The presence of myocardial inflammation has been substantiated by the demonstration of immunoglobulin G (IgG), complement, and fibrin deposition on the myocardium.[122, 136–139] As the fetus is unable to produce IgG, demonstration of IgG deposits on the myocardium implicates the transplacental passage of maternal immunoglobulin as the likely cause of the pathology. Anti-Ro and anti-La antibodies only rarely cause conduction problems in the mothers of children with NLE, although conduction abnormalities and myocarditis are more common in SLE patients with anti-Ro and anti-La antibodies than in SLE patients without these antibodies.[140]

The most serious intrauterine complication of CAVB is the development of *hydrops fetalis*. Despite early delivery, immediate pacing, and ionotropic therapy, many fetuses or infants with hydrops fetalis will die before delivery or perinatally.[130, 141] A poor outcome is associated with heart rates of less than 55 per minute, a rapid fall in the heart rate, or both.[130]

Treatment

The detection of fetal bradycardia (heart rate less than 120 per minute) requires that the mother be referred for immediate fetal cardiac ultrasonography to confirm the rate and the possible presence of AV block. If isolated AV block is present, the maternal anti-Ro and anti-La antibody status should be determined. Most fetuses will tolerate CAVB if the ventricular rate is greater than 60 per minute. Slower rates and signs of congestive heart failure are associated with poor fetal outcome. To date, however, fetal ventricular pacing has not resulted in a live birth, although pacemakers have been successfully implanted into the fetus.[142, 143] Intrauterine pacemaker therapy still remains a possibility with improving fetoscopy techniques and more experience in preventing infection.[132–134]

The use of direct intraumbilical fetal therapy with digoxin and diuretics followed by treatment of the mother with digoxin has been suggested. However, there are risks associated with this approach to therapy, including infection and the initiation of premature labor. An initial report demonstrated a good response with a live birth in two cases, but in the third the mother developed chorioamnionitis and the fetus died.[144] If intraumbilical therapy is not feasible, then maternal therapy with digoxin and furosemide may be used. If hydrops fetalis persists, then delivery should follow.[145] Some cardiologists have suggested that maternal sympathomimetics can be administered safely and effectively to increase fetal heart rate. In one fetus, isoproterenol given through the umbilical vein resulted in reversal of the hydrops fetalis.[146] Maternal administration of dexamethasone has been used with some success in reversing hydrops fetalis, particularly if it occurs in the late second to early third trimesters.[147] The use of inotropic therapy in the mother may also improve the fetal outcome.

If any or all of these therapies are not successful or not available, a so-called staged approach is advocated. Initially, the mother receives fluorinated glucocorticoids and thyroid-releasing hormone to increase fetal lung development, which is followed 48 hours later by delivery via cesarean section. The delivery is controlled, and intubation, ventilation, and pacemaker insertion or sympathomimetic therapy are available.[148]

If there is good ventricular function, no pleural or pericardial effusions, and a satisfactory cardiac output, direct fetal therapy is not warranted. The current treatment of choice is maternal administration of a fluorinated glucocorticoid such as dexamethasone at a dose of 4 mg/day. This recommendation is based on the successful treatment of CAVB and carditis with dexamethasone. A large series of cases reported that one fetus with third-degree heart block temporarily reverted to second-degree heart block, and one fetus with second-degree heart block reverted to first-degree block. In these cases, the heart rate reverted to the initial rate, but all fetuses were successfully delivered. The three pregnancies with fetuses with hydrops fetalis resulted in permanent reversal of the hydrops after therapy and resulted in live births.[149] Betamethasone can be used instead of dexamethasone.[150]

In the past, it had been suggested that mothers with anti-Ro and anti-La antibodies and a history of delivering a child with CAVB should receive glucocorticoid therapy and undergo plasmapheresis.[151, 152] This aggressive therapy was replaced by the suggestion that glucocorticoid therapy with or without intravenous immunoglobulin should be used prophylactically; there have been case reports of the successful use of this therapy.[135, 153] The risk of recurrence of CAVB is low in subsequent pregnancies, however, and therefore any prophylactic therapy is likely to be "successful." The current recommendation is to monitor pregnancies associated with maternal anti-Ro and anti-La antibodies with serial fetal echocardiograms. Any therapies should be reserved for pregnancies complicated by fetal heart block (of any degree).

Long-Term Cardiac Outcome

The long-term outcome of children with CAVB is guarded. Many children require early pacemaker insertion, and by adolescence most if not all children will require a pacemaker. In a recent extensive review, 14 percent of children died within 3 months of birth; the 3-year survival rate was only 79 percent.[131] Using Kaplan-Meier analysis of more than 100 children with CAVB, we found that all children with CAVB require the insertion of a pacemaker by the age of 15 years. This finding is in agreement with recently published guidelines that all children should have pacemaker insertion before the end of adolescence.[132–134] The decision to insert a permanent pacemaker early after delivery is determined by the ability of the child to tolerate the heart rate: The slower the rate, the more likely that early pacemaker insertion will be necessary.

Cutaneous Neonatal Lupus Erythematosus

The rash of C-NLE was first reported in 1954 in a child born to a mother with an autoimmune disease.[154] It was not until 1981, however, that the association of C-NLE and maternal anti-Ro antibodies was described.[155] Similar to mothers of children with CAVB, mothers of children with C-NLE are usually clinically well despite the presence of circulating anti-Ro or anti-La antibodies or both. It is likely that a skin rash is seen in 25 to 50 percent of children with NLE although it is difficult to determine the true percentage of children born of these mothers who will develop C-NLE, because the rash can be easily missed and spontaneously resolves. The female to male ratio of C-NLE has been reported to be as high as 3:1. The reason for the increased incidence in females may be related to the observation that estrogens enhance surface expression of Ro and La proteins on keratinocyte cells (see section in experimental models).

The photosensitive nature of the skin lesions has led investigators to examine the effect of ultraviolet irradiation on keratinocyte cell surface expression of the components of the RoRNP. The section on experimental models of NLE contains a detailed description of these in vivo and in vitro experiments.

Clinically, the dermatitis more closely resembles the lesions of subacute cutaneous lupus erythematosus (SCLE) than the malar rash of SLE (Figs. 19–2 to 19–4). Of note, most patients with SCLE have anti-Ro antibodies or anti-La antibodies or both, and these antibodies are directed against similar proteins on the RoRNP as the antibodies present in mothers of children with NLE.[81, 156, 157] The rash of C-NLE is rarely in a malar distribution and the lesions are not indurated, whereas follicular plugging or dermal atrophy, typical of discoid lupus erythematosus, is rare.[158] The face and scalp are the most commonly involved areas, but the rash may occur at any site, including the palms and soles. Commonly, it develops around the eyes in a raccoon-like distribution. The rash tends to consist of discrete, round, or elliptical plaques with a fine scale with central clearing and tends to be papulosquamous or characterized by annular erythema. An infant may have either one or both of these typical rashes. In North America, papulosquamous lesions are most commonly described, whereas in Japan, the lesion of annular erythema is more commonly seen.[159]

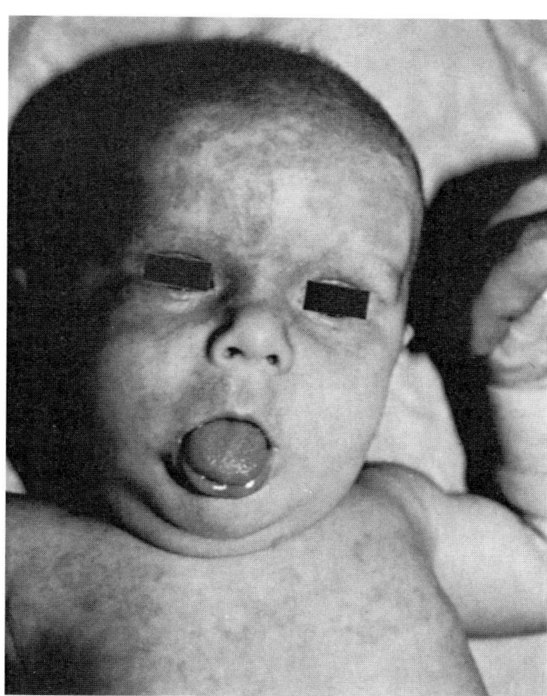

Figure 19–2. Neonatal lupus syndrome. This erythematous rash appeared a day after birth, accompanied by thrombocytopenia and leukopenia. (Courtesy of Drs. D. C. Rada and T. Kestenbaum.)

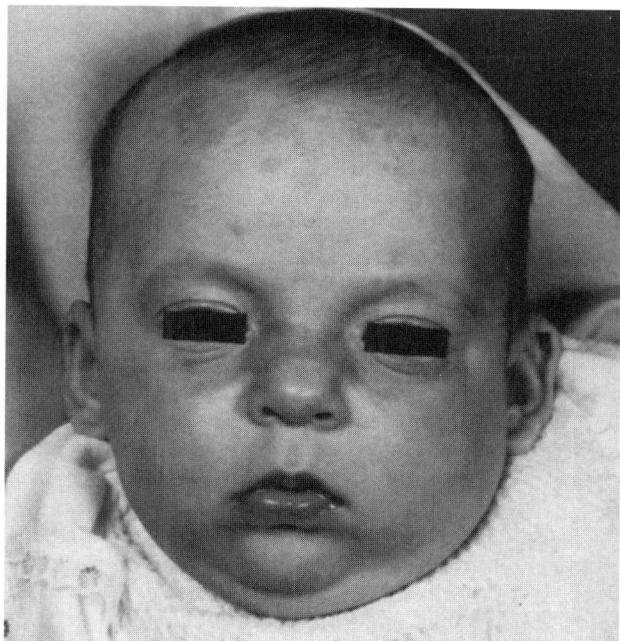

Figure 19–4. Neonatal lupus syndrome. Four-month-old girl with the erythematous rash of neonatal lupus syndrome across the bridge of the nose, lower eyelids, and superior forehead. This baby was born at 33 weeks of gestation with complete congenital heart block. Her mother had high titers of anti-Ro antibody. (From Cassidy JT: Systemic lupus erythematosus, juvenile dermatomyositis, scleroderma, and vasculitis. *In* Kelley WN, Harris ED Jr, Ruddy S, Sledge CB [eds]: Textbook of Rheumatology, 5th ed. Philadelphia, WB Saunders, 1997.)

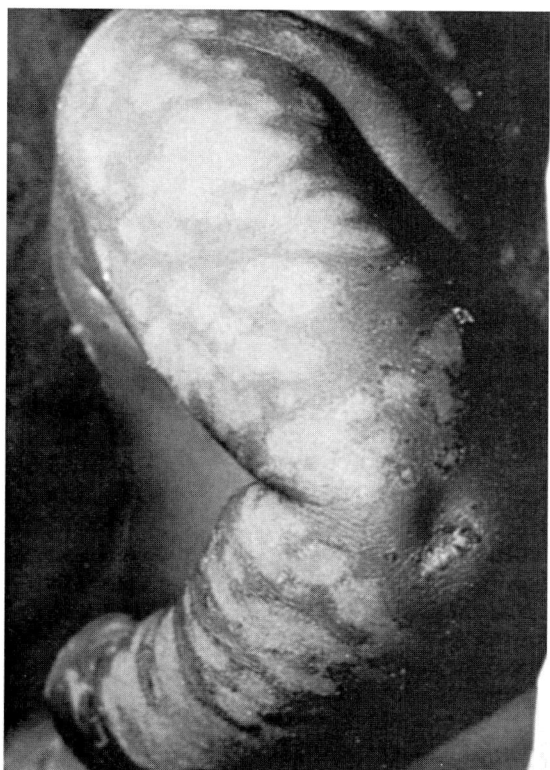

Figure 19–3. A child with neonatal lupus syndrome. The rash on this baby is more discoid in character. (Courtesy of Dr. D. Kredich.)

The dermatitis of C-NLE may be present at birth but more commonly tends to develop postnatally. Usually, it is present by 6 weeks of age, but it may not be recognized until as late as 12 weeks of age. New lesions may appear for several months but rarely develop beyond 6 months of postnatal life, consistent with the disappearance of maternal antibodies from the infant's circulation. The lesions may be induced or exacerbated by sun exposure, but cases of C-NLE that are present at birth, along with the observations that involvement of the soles of the feet and diaper area occur, illustrate that sun exposure is not required for development of the rash. There has been the occasional report of the rash appearing after phototherapy for neonatal jaundice, but this is uncommon.[160]

The lesions of C-NLE are transient and usually resolve without scarring, although some mild epidermal atrophy may result. Cutaneous telangiectasia, beginning at age 6 to 12 months, is seen in approximately 10 percent of affected infants.[158, 161, 162] These cases of telangiectasia may occur in areas that were not initially involved with C-NLE and therefore are not just the result of healing of the initial inflammatory rash.[161] The most common area for telangiectasia is at the temples near the hairline, an area not usually affected by the acute lesions. The telangiectasia tends to be bilateral. It may be the presenting feature of C-NLE, although it is not clear in these instances whether the initial rash was subtle and missed or the telangiectasia occurred de novo without the characteristic earlier rash.[163]

Pathology

Biopsies of the lesions of C-NLE demonstrate the typical abnormal histopathology of SCLE, which includes epidermal basal cell damage, a mild mononuclear cell dermal infiltrate, vacuolation of the basal layer, and epidermal colloid bodies. IgG, IgM, and complement are deposited usually at the dermoepidermal junction.[114, 164, 165]

The vast majority of mothers of infants with C-NLE are anti-Ro antibody positive, often in combination with anti-La antibodies. The percentage of mothers with elevated anti-Ro antibody levels depends on the assay used. A few cases of C-NLE have been reported in association with antibodies to U1RNP in the absence of anti-Ro or anti-La antibody and have included one report of twins discordant for NLE.[166–168] The cutaneous lesions in some of these infants were considered to be atypical in morphologic appearance.[168] We examined one infant with C-NLE who had anti-U1RNP but not anti-Ro or anti-La antibodies when tested by enzyme-linked immunosorbent assay.[169] However, anti-La antibodies were present by immunoblot. It is therefore possible that in some cases of C-NLE the antibodies may be directed to epitopes that cannot be detected by enzyme-linked immunosorbent assay.

Differential Diagnosis

The differential diagnosis of isolated C-NLE includes the other causes of annular and polycyclic lesions as follows[170–176]:

For a polycyclic lesion: urticaria, erythema marginatum, tinea corporis, seborrheic dermatitis, and ichthyosiform genodermatosis

For annular erythema: erythema annulare centrifugum, familial annular erythema, erythema multiforme, infantile epidermodysplastic erythema, infection with *Pityrosporum*, annular erythema of infancy, and erythema gyratum atrophicans

When the rash occurs concomitant with CAVB, the diagnosis is much easier

Treatment

The usual approach to management of C-NLE is reassurance to the parents and continued observation of the child, because the natural history of the skin lesions is spontaneous resolution without scarring; therefore, aggressive treatment is not indicated. However, topical application of a mild glucocorticoid cream may hasten the resolution of the lesions and be used for cosmetic reasons, although it is possible that steroid usage increases the risk of developing telangiectasia. Telangiectasia can be treated with pulse dye laser therapy, although it may also spontaneously improve.[161]

Liver Disease

The first descriptions of hepatic dysfunction in NLE included reports of abnormal levels of liver enzymes and hepatomegaly. Initially, these abnormalities were ascribed to congestive heart failure, intrauterine hydrops fetalis, disseminated intravascular coagulation, or total parenteral nutrition. It was subsequently realized that hepatic involvement occurs in approximately 15 percent of infants with NLE. Liver disease can present as an isolated disorder or in association with C-NLE, CAVB, or any other manifestation of NLE. Usually, there is mild hepatomegaly (with or without splenomegaly) and cholestasis with mildly to moderately elevated transaminases.[177, 178] Hepatitis may be the only manifestation of NLE in a mother with anti-Ro and anti-La autoantibodies.[179] Although a liver biopsy is usually not clinically indicated, histological abnormalities are similar to idiopathic neonatal giant cell hepatitis with mild bile duct obstruction, occasional giant cell transformation, and mild portal fibrosis. It is possible in this regard that idiopathic neonatal hepatitis may be another manifestation of NLE.[177] Liver biopsies should be reserved for infants with clinical evidence of severe dysfunction or with persistent, moderate dysfunction.

Abnormalities of liver function usually resolve, although deaths secondary to hepatic failure before age 6 months have been reported.[180, 181] The only reported case of a repeat biopsy in an infant with abnormalities demonstrated persistence of mild fibrosis but a good long-term outcome.[177] There have not been any instances of late liver failure or cirrhosis developing in children with hepatic involvement from NLE; however, it has been only since about 1980 that hepatic disease has been identified.

Hematologic Disease

Thrombocytopenia is the most common hematologic manifestation, whereas anemia and neutropenia are less frequently seen. Usually, hematologic involvement develops in conjunction with other stigmata of NLE, but thrombocytopenia and anemia have been reported as isolated manifestations of NLE (NLE should therefore be considered in the differential diagnosis of neonatal thrombocytopenia).[182–185] Antiplatelet antibodies have been rarely detected, suggesting that other factors may be responsible for the neonatal thrombocytopenia. The thrombocytopenia may be secondary to anti-Ro or anti-La antibodies, because thrombocytopenia in SLE is associated with these autoantibodies and patients with chronic idiopathic thrombocytopenic purpura may have anti-Ro antibodies.[183, 186–188] There have been isolated reports of aplastic anemia and neonatal thrombosis associated with the transplacental passage of maternal autoantibodies.[185, 189–191]

The thrombocytopenia and other hematologic manifestations tend to resolve over several weeks and, unless there is bleeding, do not require treatment. However, if the condition is severe or life threatening, high-dose glucocorticoids or intravenous immunoglobulin treatment may be necessary.

Other Disease Manifestations

There have been numerous case reports of different diseases of the newborn associated with the transplacental passage of maternal anti-Ro, anti-La, or other autoantibodies as well as unusual clinical manifestations in neonates with classic NLE. When there is a single case report, it is not clear if the illness in the neonate is related to the maternal autoantibodies or just a disease coincidentally occurring in offspring of mothers with autoantibodies. Similarly, when unusual features are seen in patients with definite NLE, it is not yet clear whether the other illness is just coincidental or is the result of maternal autoantibodies.

Multiple neurologic manifestations have been reported. A myelopathy with a gait abnormality and spastic paraparesis has been reported in two cases of infants with C-NLE.[192] The neurologic disease became apparent in one patient at age 1 year and in the other at age 16 months. Although it is possible that there was undiagnosed neonatal thrombocytopenia or vasculitis that resulted in intracerebral hemorrhage or infarction without any other clinical disease, there was no obvious etiology other than the presence of anti-Ro antibodies.[192] Other reported neurologic diseases have included an infant with vasculopathy, a nonspecific marker of an insult to the developing brain, hydrocephalus in two female siblings, and a case of NLE with transient neonatal myasthenia gravis.[193–196] Three children with CAVB have been described with cerebral ultrasonography and color Doppler flow imaging studies that demonstrated evidence of a vasculopathy in the area of the thalamus. The short-term follow-up study of these children revealed no signs of progression or neurologic impairment. The authors suggested that when an infant is seen with clinical signs and symptoms consistent with a vasculopathy in the gangliothalamic region, the children should be examined for other manifestations of NLE and the mothers should be tested for anti-Ro and anti-La antibodies.[194]

Recently, there have been case reports of chondrodysplasia punctata associated with NLE.[197, 198] We have seen a child with C-NLE and radiographic changes in the hip and ankle consistent with this diagnosis. This association requires further investigation.

Individual case reports have included congenital nephrotic syndrome in an infant with NLE[199] and a child with C-NLE and Turner's syndrome.[200]

COURSE OF THE DISEASE AND PROGNOSIS

Children

NLE is a disease caused by maternal autoantibodies and not by the production of these autoantibodies by the fetus or child. The skin, liver, and hematologic complications generally resolve with minimal sequelae, whereas CAVB is permanent. The long-term cardiac outcome of these children is described in the section on CAVB.

It was initially reported that children with NLE may be at a high risk for developing SLE in later life.[201, 202] In our experience, none of a total of more than 100 children with NLE has developed a connective tissue disease; however, most of these children have not been followed for more than 20 years. A report from Japan suggested a less optimistic outcome, as 8 percent of children had persistent or recurrently positive autoantibodies and one met the American College of Rheumatology classification criteria for SLE.[114] The increased risk of autoimmune disease in the offspring may reflect the genetic predisposition of a child born to a mother with an autoimmune disease, as opposed to a direct delayed consequence of having had NLE. The risk of development of an autoimmune disease in the child with NLE is probably not greater than the risk for developing SLE in any other offspring of anti-Ro antibody–positive women with SLE and is likely related to the linkage of HLA class II genes to the production of anti-Ro and anti-La antibodies.[99, 203–207] Parents of these infants should be counseled that the risk of their offspring developing autoimmune diseases is similar to the risk in children of women with SLE.

Mothers

Initially, NLE was the name given to infants born with the characteristic skin or cardiac findings in the presence of maternal connective tissue disease and particularly SLE and SS. Therefore, all mothers of infants with NLE had an autoimmune disease. However, it rapidly became apparent that CAVB and the characteristic rash of C-NLE could be seen in the offspring of mothers who did not have any signs or symptoms of a connective tissue disorder. It was initially surmised that the mothers of children with CAVB would develop a connective tissue disease. We and others found, however, that only a minority of mothers had a connective tissue disease at the time of delivery of their child with CAVB, and at long-term follow-up the majority remained healthy.[76, 208–211]

Because almost all children with NLE are born to mothers with anti-Ro or anti-La antibodies or both,[212] it is important to estimate the risk of delivering a child with NLE from mothers with a known connective tissue disease (in particular SLE) or from mothers who have previously delivered a child with NLE. Large series of pregnancies in women with SLE who had anti-Ro or anti-La antibodies or both have suggested that the risk of delivering a child with NLE varied between 1 and 10 percent.[78, 185, 213, 214] More specifically, in the at-risk group—mothers with anti-Ro or anti-La antibodies—the risk of NLE varied between 2 and 20 percent.[78, 185, 213, 214] We prospectively studied the outcome of 110 pregnancies in anti-Ro and anti-La antibody–positive women and found that the risk of delivering a child with CAVB was less than 3 percent, although there was a 7 percent risk of having a child with C-NLE. Retrospective studies have suggested a recurrence rate for CAVB of between 8 and 25 percent in subsequent pregnancies.[126, 131, 208] Our personal experience of the outcome of pregnancies after the delivery of a child with CAVB suggests that the risk is approximately 10 to 15 percent.

ANIMAL MODELS OF NEONATAL LUPUS ERYTHEMATOSUS

In Vitro Experiments

Culture of isolated neonatal but not adult rabbit cardiac myocytes with sera from anti-Ro or anti-La antibody–positive women led to changes in the repolarization of these cells.[215, 216] Binding of the maternal sera to rabbit tissue was likely the result of the presence of the RoRNP antigen on the surface of fetal hearts.[217, 218] However, unlike that which occurs with keratinocytes, the cellular localization of 48 kD La, 52 kD Ro, or 60 kD Ro in fetal cardiac myocytes is not altered by culture in the presence of either 17β-estradiol or progesterone (see later).[219]

Skin

Irradiation of keratinocytes enhances the expression of Ro, U1RNP, and Sm antigens.[220–222] Estradiol treatment of keratinocytes can induce a marked increase in both mRNA and expression of Ro, U1RNP, and Sm autoantigens.[218, 220, 221, 223] Other factors, including tumor necrosis factor-α and exposure to viruses, upregulate the surface expression of 52 kD Ro and La on keratinocytes.[224] The direct binding of anti-RoRNP antibodies to skin has been demonstrated.[218, 225]

The difference in disease expression in different offspring born to the same mother may be at least partially explained by the demonstration that sera from children with C-NLE can be cytotoxic to keratinocytes from patients with NLE but not to cells obtained from normal individuals. This cytotoxicity was enhanced by ultraviolet B irradiation. These data suggest that keratinocytes from children with C-NLE may have abnormal surface expression of both Ro and La antigens and that ultraviolet irradiation can further increase that expression.[226] These results are consistent with the demonstration that the rash of C-NLE may be present at birth, or photosensitive, and that it does not occur in all infants born to mothers with autoantibodies directed against RoRNP.

Langendorff Experiments

Initial ex vivo experiments examined the effect of anti-Ro– and anti-La–containing sera on conduction in isolated rabbit hearts. The perfusion of isolated Langendorff preparations of adult rabbit hearts with purified IgG from sera containing anti-Ro and anti-La antibodies induced heart block and altered the peak slow inward current.[227] However, sera from women with SLE or SS without a history of delivering a child with NLE also resulted in heart block in the isolated, whole rabbit heart, although the heart block occurred only with perfusion with affinity-purified anti-52 kD antibodies.[228] These observations are not unique to anti-Ro antibody–containing sera, as similar alterations of cardiac conduction have been observed with sera derived from patients with conduction defects associated with Chagas' disease.[229]

Perfusion of Langendorff preparations of human fetal hearts with affinity-purified anti-52 kD Ro derived from mothers of children with CAVB also resulted in the development of complete AV block. At a whole-cell and single-channel level, perfusion experiments with the human heart demonstrated an inhibition of L-type calcium currents.[230] Similarly, when isolated rat hearts were used, 2:1 AV block followed by complete inhibition of AV nodal action potential was demonstrated, and calcium channels were inhibited in isolated cellular preparations.[231] These results suggested that rodents may be an appropriate species for monitoring the fetal effects of maternal anti-Ro and anti-La antibodies.

In Vivo Experiments

Immunization of female BALB/c mice with recombinant RoRNP proteins generates high-titer antibodies that cross the placenta during pregnancy and are associated with varying degrees of AV conduction abnormalities in the pups.[230] However, conduction abnormalities were seen in only a low percentage of the offspring born to these mice, and advanced conduction abnormalities rarely developed.[232]

Apoptosis has been proposed as a mechanism for the observed tissue damage. In human fetal cardiac myocytes, apoptosis results in surface translocation of RoRNP.[233] Therefore, it is possible that apoptosis, a normal event during cardiac development, may result in the binding of maternal anti-RoRNP to the apoptotic cells that cause an inflammatory reaction. The neighboring cells may be damaged as bystanders. Initial binding may be by maternal anti-52 kD Ro antibodies or antibodies to isoforms of the La protein, which are maximally expressed early in gestation, with levels decreasing with gestational age until 25 weeks, when adult levels are achieved.[23] This hypothesis would allow for the selective damage to fetal but not to maternal conducting tissue.

References

1. Smeenk RJ: Immunological aspects of congenital atrioventricular block. Pacing Clin Electrophysiol 20: 2093–2097, 1977.
2. Zhu J: Cytomegalovirus infection induces expression of 60 KD/Ro antigen on human keratinocytes. Lupus 4: 396–406, 1995.
3. Wolin S, Stietz J: The Ro small cytoplasmic ribonucleoproteins:

identification of the antigenic protein and its binding site on the Ro RNAs. Proc Natl Acad Sci U S A 81: 1996–2000, 1984.
4. Lerner MB, Boyle JA, Hardin JA, Steitz JA: Two novel classes of small ribonucleoproteins detected by antibodies associated with lupus erythematosus. Science 211: 400–402, 1981.
5. Ben-Chetrit E, Chan EKL, Sullivan KF, Tan EM: A 52-kD protein is a novel component of the SS-A/Ro antigenic particle. J Exp Med 167: 1560–1571, 1988.
6. Harmon CE, Deng J-S, Peebles CL, Tan EM: The importance of tissue substrate in the SS-A/Ro antigen-antibody system. Arthritis Rheum 27: 166–173, 1984.
7. Hendrick JP, Wolin SL, Rinke J, et al: Ro small cytoplasmic ribonucleoproteins are a subclass of La ribonucleoproteins: further characterization of the Ro and La small ribonucleoproteins from uninfected mammalian cells. Mol Cell Biol 1: 1138–1149, 1981.
8. Rosa MD, Gottlieb E, Lerner MR, Steitz JA: Striking similarities are exhibited by two small Epstein-Barr virus–encoded ribonucleic acids and the adenovirus-associated ribonucleic acids VAI and VAII. Mol Cell Biol 1: 785–796, 1981.
9. Rinke J, Steitz JA: Precursor molecules of both human 5S ribosomal RNA and transfer RNAs are bound by a cellular protein reactive with anti-La lupus antibodies. Cell 29: 149–159, 1982.
10. Madore SJ, Wieben ED, Pederson T: Eukaryotic small ribonucleoproteins: anti-La human autoantibodies react with U1 RNA-protein complexes. J Biol Chem 259: 1929–1933, 1984.
11. Maraia RJ, Kenan DJ, Keene JD: Eukaryotic transcription termination factor La mediates transcript release and facilitates reinitiation by RNA polymerase III. Mol Cell Biol 14: 2147–2158, 1994.
12. Fan H, Goodier JL, Chamberlain JR, et al: 5′ processing of tRNA precursors can be modulated by the human La antigen phosphoprotein. Mol Cell Biol 18: 3201–3211, 1998.
13. Gottlieb E, Steitz JA: The RNA binding protein La influences both the accuracy and the efficiency of RNA polymerase III transcription in vitro. EMBO J 8: 841–850, 1989.
14. Gottlieb E, Steitz JA: Function of the mammalian La protein: evidence for its action in transcription termination by RNA polymerase. EMBO J 8: 851–861, 1989.
15. Deng J-S, Sontheimer RD, Giliam JN: Molecular characteristics of SS-B/La and SS-A/Ro cellular antigens. J Invest Dermatol 84: 86–90, 1985.
16. Dickey WD, van Egmond JE, Hardgrave KL, et al: Presence of anti-La(SS-B) is associated with binding to the 13-kD carboxyl terminus of 60-kD Ro(SS-A) in systemic lupus erythematosus. J Invest Dermatol 100: 412–416, 1993.
17. Pardigon N, Strauss JH: Mosquito homolog of the La autoantigen binds to Sindbis virus RNA. J Virol 70: 1173–1181, 1996.
18. Scherly D, Stutz F, Lin-Marq N, Clarkson SG: La proteins from *Xenopus laevis*. cDNA cloning and developmental expression. J Mol Biol 231: 196–204, 1993.
19. Yoo CJ, Wolin SL: La proteins from *Drosophila melanogaster* and *Saccharomyces cerevisiae*: a yeast homolog of the La autoantigen is dispensable for growth. Mol Cell Biol 14: 5412–5424, 1994.
20. Semsei I, Troster H, Bartsch H, et al: Isolation of rat cDNA clones coding for the autoantigen SS-B/La: detection of species-specific variations. Gene 126: 265–268, 1993.
21. Pannone BK, Xue D, Wolin SL: A role for the yeast La protein in U6 snRNP assembly: evidence that the La protein is a molecular chaperone for RNA polymerase III transcripts. EMBO J 17: 7442–7453, 1998.
22. Rosenblum JS, Pemberton LF, Bonifaci N, Blobel G: Nuclear import and the evolution of a multifunctional RNA-binding protein. J Cell Biol 143: 887–899, 1998.
23. Goodier JL, Fan H, Maraia RJ: A carboxy-terminal basic region controls RNA polymerase III transcription factor activity of human La protein. Mol Cell Biol 17: 5823–5832, 1997.
24. McLaren RS, Caruccio N, Ross J: Human La protein: a stabilizer of histone mRNA. Mol Cell Biol 17: 3028–3036, 1997.
25. De BP, Gupta S, Zhao H, et al: Specific interaction in vitro and in vivo of glyceraldehyde-3-phosphate dehydrogenase and LA protein with cis-acting RNAs of human parainfluenza virus type 3. J Biol Chem 271: 24728–24735, 1996.
26. Craig AW, Svitkin YV, Lee HS, et al: The La autoantigen contains a dimerization domain that is essential for enhancing translation. Mol Cell Biol 17: 163–169, 1997.
27. Chang YN, Kenan DJ, Keene JD, et al: Direct interactions between autoantigen La and human immunodeficiency virus leader RNA. J Virol 68: 7008–7020, 1994.
28. Meerovitch K, Svitkin YV, Lee HS, et al: La autoantigen enhances and corrects aberrant translation of poliovirus RNA in reticulocyte lysate. J Virol 67: 3798–3807, 1993.
29. Huhn P, Pruijn GJ, van Venrooij WJ, Bachmann M: Characterization of the autoantigen La (SS-B) as a dsRNA unwinding enzyme. Nucleic Acids Res 25: 410–416, 1997.
30. Xiao Q, Sharp TV, Jeffrey IW, et al: The La antigen inhibits the activation of the interferon-inducible protein kinase PKR by sequestering and unwinding double-stranded RNA. Nucleic Acids Res 22: 2512–2518, 1994.
31. Peek R, van Venrooij WJ, Simons F, Pruijn G: The SS-A/SS-B autoantigenic complex: localization and assembly. Clin Exp Rheumatol 12: S15–S18, 1994.
32. Shiroki K, Isoyama T, Kuge S, et al: Intracellular redistribution of truncated La protein produced by poliovirus 3Cpro-mediated cleavage. J Virol 73: 2193–2200, 1999.
33. Grolz D, Bachmann M: The nuclear autoantigen La/SS-associated antigen B: one gene, three functional mRNAs. Biochem J 323: 151–158, 1997.
34. Hilker M, Troster H, Grolz D, et al: The autoantigen La/SS-B: analysis of the expression of alternatively spliced La mRNA isoforms. Cell Tissue Res 284: 383–389, 1996.
35. Grolz D, Bachmann M: An altered intracellular distribution of the autoantigen La/SS-B when translated from a La mRNA isoform. Exp Cell Res 234: 329–335, 1997.
36. O'Brien CA, Wolin SL: A possible role for the 60-kD Ro autoantigen in a discard pathway for defective 5S rRNA precursors. Genes Dev 8: 2891–2903, 1994.
37. Shi H, O'Brien CA, Van Horn DJ, Wolin SL: A misfolded form of 5S rRNA is complexed with the Ro and La autoantigens. RNA 2: 769–784, 1996.
38. Pourmand N, Blange I, Ringertz N, Pettersson I: Intracellular localisation of the Ro 52kD auto-antigen in HeLa cells visualised with green fluorescent protein chimeras. Autoimmunity 28: 225–233, 1998.
39. Igarashi T, Itoh Y, Fukunaga Y, Yamamoto M: Stress-induced cell surface expression and antigenic alteration of the Ro/SSA autoantigen. Autoimmunity 22: 33–42, 1995.
40. Buyon JP, Tseng CE, DiDonato F, et al: Cardiac expression of 52β, an alternative transcript of the congenital heart block-associated 52-kd SS-A/Ro autoantigen, is maximal during fetal development. Arthritis Rheum 40: 655–660, 1997.
41. Meilof JF, Van der Lelij A, Rokeach LA, et al: Autoimmunity and filariasis: autoantibodies against cytoplasmic cellular proteins in sera of patients with onchocerciasis. J Immunol 151: 5800–5809, 1993.
42. Lieu TS, Sontheimer RD: A subpopulation of WIL-2 cell calreticulin molecules is associated with RO/SS-A ribonucleoprotein particles. Lupus 6: 40–47, 1997.
43. Joshi M, Pogue GP, Duncan RC, et al: Isolation and characterization of *Leishmania donovani* calreticulin gene and its conservation of the RNA binding activity. Mol Biochem Parasitol 81: 53–64, 1996.
44. Rokeach LA, Haselby JA, Meilof JF, et al: Characterization of the autoantigen calreticulin. J Immunol 147: 3031–3039, 1991.
45. Smith MJ: A *C. elegans* gene encodes a protein homologous to mammalian calreticulin. DNA Seq 2: 235–240, 1992.
46. Smith MJ: Nucleotide sequence of a *Drosophila melanogaster* gene encoding a calreticulin homologue. DNA Seq 3: 247–250, 1992.
47. Treves S, Zorzato F, Pozzan T: Identification of calreticulin isoforms in the central nervous system. Biochem J 287: 579–581, 1992.
48. Dupuis M, Schaerer E, Krause KH, Tschopp J: The calcium-binding protein calreticulin is a major constituent of lytic granules in cytolytic T lymphocytes. J Exp Med 177: 1–7, 1993.
49. Eggleton P, Lieu TS, Zappi EG, et al: Calreticulin is released from activated neutrophils and binds to C1q and mannan-binding protein. Clin Immunol Immunopathol 72: 405–409, 1994.
50. Nash PD, Opas M, Michalak M: Calreticulin: not just another calcium-binding protein. Mol Cell Biochem 135: 71–78, 1994.
51. Baksh S, Spamer C, Heilmann C, Michalak M: Identification

of the Zn2+ binding region in calreticulin. FEBS Lett 376: 53–57, 1995.
52. Nguyen TO, Capra JD, Sontheimer RD: Calreticulin is transcriptionally upregulated by heat shock, calcium and heavy metals. Mol Immunol 33: 379–386, 1996.
53. Waser M, Mesaeli N, Spencer C, Michalak M: Regulation of calreticulin gene expression by calcium. J Cell Biol 138: 547–557, 1997.
54. Burns K, Helgason CD, Bleackley RC, Michalak M: Calreticulin in T-lymphocytes. Identification of calreticulin in T-lymphocytes and demonstration that activation of T cells correlates with increased levels of calreticulin mRNA and protein. J Biol Chem 267: 19039–19042, 1992.
55. Michalak M, Burns K, Andrin C, et al: Endoplasmic reticulum form of calreticulin modulates glucocorticoid-sensitive gene expression. J Biol Chem 271: 29436–29445, 1996.
56. Winrow CJ, Miyata KS, Marcus SL, et al: Calreticulin modulates the in vitro DNA binding but not the in vivo transcriptional activation by peroxisome proliferator-activated receptor/retinoid X receptor heterodimers. Mol Cell Endocrinol 111: 175–179, 1995.
57. Burns K, Duggan B, Atkinson EA, et al: Modulation of gene expression by calreticulin binding to the glucocorticoid receptor. Nature 367: 476–480, 1994.
58. Crossin KL, Tai MH, Krushel LA, et al: Glucocorticoid receptor pathways are involved in the inhibition of astrocyte proliferation. Proc Natl Acad Sci U S A 94: 2687–2692, 1997.
59. Dedhar S, Rennie PS, Shago M, et al: Inhibition of nuclear hormone receptor activity by calreticulin. Nature 367: 480–483, 1994.
60. St-Arnaud R, Prud'homme J, Leung Hagesteijn C, Dedhar S: Constitutive expression of calreticulin in osteoblasts inhibits mineralization. J Cell Biol 131: 1351–1359, 1995.
61. Zhu Q, Zelinka P, White T, Tanzer ML: Calreticulin-integrin bidirectional signaling complex. Biochem Biophys Res Commun 232: 354–358, 1997.
62. Rojiani MV, Finlay BB, Gray V, Dedhar S: In vitro interaction of a polypeptide homologous to human Ro/SS-A antigen (calreticulin) with a highly conserved amino acid sequence in the cytoplasmic domain of integrin alpha subunits. Biochemistry 30: 9859–9866, 1991.
63. Coppolino MG, Woodside MJ, Demaurex N, et al: Calreticulin is essential for integrin-mediated calcium signalling and cell adhesion. Nature 386: 843–847, 1997.
64. Van Leeuwen JEM, Kearse KP: The related molecular chaperones calnexin and calreticulin differentially associate with nascent T cell antigen receptor proteins within the endoplasmic reticulum. J Biol Chem 271: 25345–25349, 1996.
65. Spee P, Neefjes J: TAP-translocated peptides specifically bind proteins in the endoplasmic reticulum, including gp96, protein disulfide isomerase and calreticulin. Eur J Immunol 27: 2441–2449, 1997.
66. Verreck FA, Elferink D, Vermeulen CJ, et al: DR4Dw4/DR53 molecules contain a peptide from the autoantigen calreticulin. Tissue Antigens 45: 270–275, 1995.
67. Max H, Halder T, Kalbus M, et al: A 16mer peptide of the human autoantigen calreticulin is a most prominent HLA-DR4Dw4–associated self-peptide. Hum Immunol 41: 39–45, 1994.
68. Taylor PV, Scott JS, Gerlis LM, et al: Maternal antibodies against fetal cardiac antigens in congenital complete heart block. N Engl J Med 315: 667–672, 1986.
69. Watson RM, Lane AT, Barnett NK, et al: Neonatal lupus erythematosus. A clinical, serological and immunogenetic study with review of the literature. Medicine 63: 362–378, 1984.
70. Buyon JP, E. Ben-Chetrit E, Karp S, et al: Acquired congenital heart block: pattern of maternal antibody response to biochemically defined antigens of the SSA/Ro-SSB/La system in neonatal lupus. J Clin Invest 84: 627–634, 1989.
71. Silverman ED, Buyon J, Laxer RM, et al: Autoantibody response to the Ro/La particle may predict outcome in neonatal lupus erythematosus. Clin Exp Immunol 100: 499–505, 1995.
72. Silverman E, Mamula M, Hardin JA, Laxer R: Importance of the immune response to the Ro/La particle in the development of congenital heart block and neonatal lupus erythematosus. J Rheumatol 18: 120–124, 1991.
73. McCreadie M, Celermajer J, Sholler G, et al: A case control study of congenital heart block: association with maternal antibodies to Ro(SS-A) and La(SS-B). Br J Rheumatol 29: 10–14, 1990.
74. Taylor PV, Taylor KF, Norman A, et al: Prevalence of maternal Ro (SS-A) and La (SS-B) autoantibodies in relation to congenital heart block. Br J Rheumatol 27: 128–132, 1988.
75. Buyon JP, Winchester RJ, Slade SG, et al: Identification of mothers at risk for congenital heart block and other neonatal lupus syndromes in their children. Comparison of enzyme-linked immunosorbent assay and immunoblot for measurement of anti-SS-A/Ro and anti-SS-B/La antibodies. Arthritis Rheum 36: 1263–1273, 1993.
76. Julkunen H, Kurki P, Kaaja R, et al: Isolated congenital heart block. Long-term outcome of mothers and characterization of the immune response to SS-A/Ro and to SS-B/La. Arthritis Rheum 36: 1588–1598, 1993.
77. Julkunen H, Siren MK, Kaaja R, et al: Maternal HLA antigens and antibodies to SS-A/Ro and SS-B/La. Comparison with systemic lupus erythematosus and primary Sjögren's syndrome. Br J Rheumatol 34: 901–907, 1995.
78. Ramsey-Goldman R, Hom D, Deng J-S, et al: Anti-SSA antibodies and fetal outcome in maternal systemic lupus erythematosus. Arthritis Rheum 29: 1269–1273, 1986.
79. Julkunen H, Kaaja R, Siren MK, et al: Immune-mediated congenital heart block (CHB): identifying and counseling patients at risk for having children with CHB. Semin Arthritis Rheum 28: 97–106, 1998.
80. Miyagawa S, Fukumoto T, Hashimoto K, et al: Maternal autoimmune response to recombinant Ro/SSA and La/SSB proteins in Japanese neonatal lupus erythematosus. Autoimmunity 21: 277–282, 1995.
81. Lee LA, Alvarez K, Gross T, et al: The recognition of human 60-kDa Ro ribonucleoprotein particles by antibodies associated with cutaneous lupus and neonatal lupus. J Invest Dermatol 107: 225–228, 1996.
82. Grolz D, Troster H, Semsei I, Bachmann M: Analysis of expression of the gene encoding for the nuclear autoantigen La/SS-B using reporter gene constructs. Biochim Biophys Acta 1396: 278–293, 1998.
83. Rokeach LA, Zimmerman PA, Unnasch TR: Epitopes of the *Onchocerca volvulus* RAL1 antigen, a member of the calreticulin family of proteins, recognized by sera from patients with onchocerciasis. Infect Immun 62: 3696–3704, 1994.
84. Orth T, Dorner T, Meyer Zum Buschenfelde KH, Mayet WJ: Complete congenital heart block is associated with increased autoantibody titers against calreticulin. Eur J Clin Invest 26: 205–215, 1996.
85. Chang SH, Huh MS, Kim HR, et al: Cross-reactivity of antibodies immunoadsorbed to laminin with recombinant human La (SS-B) protein. J Autoimmun 11: 163–167, 1998.
86. Li JM, Horsfall AC, Maini RN: Anti-La (SS-B) but not anti-Ro52 (SS-A) antibodies cross-react with laminin: a role in the pathogenesis of congenital heart block? Clin Exp Immunol 99: 316–324, 1995.
87. Horsfall AC, Li JM, Maini RN: Placental and fetal cardiac laminin are targets for cross-reacting autoantibodies from mothers of children with congenital heart block. J Autoimmun 9: 561–568, 1996.
88. Houen G, Koch C: Human placental calreticulin: Purification, characterization and association with other proteins. Acta Chem Scand 48: 905–911, 1994
89. Li JM, Fan WS, Horsfall AC, et al: The expression of human endogenous retrovirus-3 in fetal cardiac tissue and antibodies in congenital heart block. Clin Exp Immunol 104: 388–393, 1996.
90. Maddison PJ, Lee L, Reichlin M, et al: Anti-p57: a novel association with neonatal lupus. Clin Exp Immunol 99: 42–48, 1995.
91. Haneji N, Nakamura T, Takio K, et al: Identification of alpha-fodrin as a candidate autoantigen in primary Sjögren's syndrome. Science 276: 604–607, 1997.
92. Miyagawa S, Yanagi K, Yoshioka A, et al: Neonatal lupus erythematosus: maternal IgG antibodies bind to a recombinant NH2-terminal fusion protein encoded by human alpha-fodrin cDNA. J Invest Dermatol 111: 1189–1192, 1998.
93. Bell DA, Maddison PJ: Serologic subsets in systemic lupus erythematosus: an examination of autoantibodies in relationship to

clinical features of disease and HLA antigens. Arthritis Rheum 23: 1268–1273, 1980.
94. Ehrfeld H, Hartung K, Renz M, et al: MHC associations of autoantibodies against recombinant Ro and La proteins in systemic lupus erythematosus. Results of a multicenter study. SLE Study Group. Rheumatol Int 12: 169–173, 1992.
95. Fei HM, Kang H, Scharf S, et al: Specific HLA-DQA and HLA-DRB1 alleles confer susceptibility to Sjögren's syndrome and autoantibody production. J Clin Lab Anal 5: 382–391, 1991.
96. Lulli P, Sebastiani GD, Trabace S, et al: HLA antigens in Italian patients with systemic lupus erythematosus: evidence for the association of DQw2 with the autoantibody response to extractable nuclear antigens. Clin Exp Rheumatol 9: 475–479, 1991.
97. Kerttula TO, Collin P, Polvi A, et al: Distinct immunologic features of Finnish Sjögren's syndrome patients with HLA alleles DRB1*0301, DQA1*0501, and DQB1*0201. Alterations in circulating T cell receptor gamma/delta subsets. Arthritis Rheum 39: 1733–1739, 1996.
98. Martin-Villa JM, Martinez-Laso J, Moreno-Pelayo MA, et al: Differential contribution of HLA-DR, DQ, and TAP2 alleles to systemic lupus erythematosus susceptibility in Spanish patients: role of TAP2*01 alleles in Ro autoantibody production. Ann Rheum Dis 57: 214–219, 1998.
99. Miyagawa S, Shinohara K, Nakajima M, et al: Polymorphisms of HLA class II genes and autoimmune responses to Ro/SS-A-La/SS-B among Japanese subjects. Arthritis Rheum 41: 927–934, 1998.
100. Smolen JS, Klippel JH, Penner E, et al: HLA-DR antigens in systemic lupus erythematosus: association with specificity of autoantibody responses to nuclear antigens. Ann Rheum Dis 46: 457–462, 1987.
101. Wilson WA, Scopelitis E, Michalski JP: Association of HLA-DR7 with both antibody to SSA(Ro) and disease susceptibility in blacks with systemic lupus erythematosus. J Rheumatol 11: 653–657, 1984.
102. Miyagawa S, Dohi K, Shima H, Shirai T: HLA antigens in anti-Ro(SS-A)–positive patients with recurrent annular erythema. J Am Acad Dermatol 28: 185–188, 1993.
103. Miyagawa S, Dohi K, Shima H, Shirai T: Absence of HLA-B8 and HLA-DR3 in Japanese patients with Sjögren's syndrome positive for anti-SSA(Ro). J Rheumatol 19: 1922–1924, 1992.
104. Hamilton RG, Harley JB, Bias WB, et al: Two Ro (SS-A) autoantibody responses in systemic lupus erythematosus. Correlation of HLA-DR/DQ specificities with quantitative expression of Ro (SS-A) autoantibody. Arthritis Rheum 31: 496–505, 1988.
105. Fujisaku A, Frank MB, Neas B, et al: HLA-DQ gene complementation and other histocompatibility relationships in man with the anti-Ro/SSA autoantibody response of systemic lupus erythematosus. J Clin Invest 86: 606–611, 1990.
106. Rischmueller M, Lester S, Chen Z, et al: HLA class II phenotype controls diversification of the autoantibody response in primary Sjögren's syndrome (pSS). Clin Exp Immunol 111: 365–371, 1998.
107. Reveille JD, Macleod MJ, Whittington K, Arnett FC: Specific amino acid residues in the second hypervariable region of HLA-DQA1 and DQB1 chain genes promote the Ro (SS-A)/La (SS-B) autoantibody responses. J Immunol 146: 3871–3876, 1991.
108. Skarsvag S, Hansen KE, Moen T, Eggen BM: Distributions of HLA class II alleles in autoantibody subsets among Norwegian patients with systemic lupus erythematosus. Scand J Immunol 42: 564–571, 1995.
109. Scofield RH, Dickey WD, Hardgrave KL, et al: Immunogenetics of epitopes of the carboxyl terminus of the human 60-kD Ro autoantigen. Clin Exp Immunol 99: 256–261, 1995.
110. Miyagawa S, Shinohara K, Kidoguchi K, et al: Neonatal lupus erythematosus: HLA-DR and -DQ distributions are different among the groups of anti-Ro/SSA-positive mothers with different neonatal outcomes. J Invest Dermatol 108: 881–885, 1997.
111. Miyagawa S, Fukumoto T, Hashimoto K, et al: Neonatal lupus erythematosus: haplotypic analysis of HLA class II alleles in child/mother pairs. Arthritis Rheum 40: 982–983, 1997.
112. Miyagawa S, Shinohara K, Kidoguchi K, et al: Neonatal lupus erythematosus: studies on HLA class II genes and autoantibody profiles in Japanese mothers. Autoimmunity 26: 95–101, 1997.
113. Brucato A, Gasparini M, Vignati G, et al: Isolated congenital complete heart block: long-term outcome of children and immunogenetic study. J Rheumatol 22: 541–543, 1995.
114. Kaneko F, Tanji O, Hasegawa T, et al: Neonatal lupus erythematosus in Japan. J Am Acad Dermatol 26: 397–403, 1992.
115. Arnaiz-Villena A, Vazquez-Rodriguez JJ, Vicario JL, et al: Congenital heart block immunogenetics. Evidence of an additional role of HLA class III antigens and independence of Ro autoantibodies. Arthritis Rheum 32: 1421–1426, 1989.
116. Siren MK, Julkunen H, Kaaja R, Koskimies S: Congenital heart block: HLA differences between affected children and healthy siblings in four Finnish families. APMIS 105: 463–468, 1997.
117. Siren MK, Julkunen H, Kaaja R, et al: Role of HLA in congenital heart block: susceptibility alleles in children. Lupus 8: 60–67, 1999.
118. Garchon HJ, Bach JF: The contribution of non-MHC genes to susceptibility to autoimmune diseases. Hum Immunol 32: 1–30, 1991.
119. Frank MB, McArthur R, Harley JB, Fujisaku A: Anti-Ro(SSA) autoantibodies are associated with T cell receptor beta genes in systemic lupus erythematosus patients. J Clin Invest 85: 33–39, 1990.
120. Morquio L: Sur une maladie infantile et familiale caracterisée et la aort subite. Arch Med Enfants 4, 1901.
121. East WR, Lumpkin LR: Systemic lupus erythematosus in the newborn. Minn Med 52: 477–478, 1969.
122. Hogg G: Congenital acute lupus erythematosus associated with subendocardial fibroelastosis. Am J Clin Pathol 28: 648–654, 1957.
123. Taylor PV, Scott JS, Gerlis LM, et al: Connective-tissue disease, antibodies to ribonucleoprotein, and congenital heart block. N Engl J Med 309: 209–212, 1983.
124. Harley JB, Kaine JL, Fox OF, et al: Ro (SS-A) antibody and antigen in a patient with congenital complete heart block. Arthritis Rheum 28: 1321–1325, 1985.
125. Taylor PV, Taylor KF, Norman A, et al: Prevalence of maternal Ro (SS-A) and La (SS-B) autoantibodies in relation to congenital heart block. Br J Rheumatol 27: 128–132, 1988.
126. Julkunen H, Kaaja R, Wallgren E, Teramo K: Isolated congenital heart block: fetal and infant outcome and familial incidence of heart block. Obstet Gynecol 82: 11–16, 1993.
127. Schmidt KG, Ulmer HE, Silverman NH, et al: Perinatal outcome of fetal complete atrioventricular block: a multicenter experience. J Am Coll Cardiol 17: 1360–1366, 1991.
128. Cecconi M, Renzi R, Bettuzzi MG, et al: Congenital isolated complete atrioventricular block: long-term experience with 38 patients. G Ital Cardiol 23: 39–53, 1993.
129. Friedman RA, Moak JP, Garson AJ: Clinical course of idiopathic dilated cardiomyopathy in children. J Am Coll Cardiol 18: 152–156, 1991.
130. Groves AMM, Allan LD, Rosenthal E: Outcome of isolated congenital complete heart block diagnosed in utero. Br Heart J 75: 190–194, 1996.
131. Buyon JP, Hiebert R, Copel J, et al: Autoimmune-associated congenital heart block: demographics, mortality, morbidity and recurrence rates obtained from a national neonatal lupus registry. J Am Coll Cardiol 31: 1658–1666, 1998.
132. Michaelsson M, Riesenfeld T, Jonzon A: Natural history of congenital complete atrioventricular block. Pacing Clin Electrophysiol 20: 2098–2101, 1997.
133. Michaelsson M, Jonzon A, Riesenfeld T: Isolated congenital complete atrioventricular block in adult life: a prospective study. Circulation 92: 442–449, 1995.
134. Friedman RA: Congenital AV block. Pace me now or pace me later? Circulation 92: 283–285, 1995.
135. Herreman G, Sauvaget F, Genereau T, Galezowski N: Congenital atrioventricular block and maternal autoimmune diseases. Ann Med Interne (Paris) 141: 234–238, 1990.
136. Carter JB, Blieden LC, Edwards JE: Congenital heart block. Arch Pathol 97: 51–57, 1974.
137. Hackel DB: Pathology of primary congenital complete heart block. Mod Pathol 1: 114–128, 1988.
138. Ho SY, Fagg N, Anderson RH, et al: Disposition of the atrioventricular conduction tissues in the heart with isomerism of the atrial appendages: its relation to congenital complete heart block. J Am Coll Cardiol 20: 904–910, 1992.

139. Morales B, Hernandez I, Farru O, Chuaqui B: Heart cartilage and disruption of the bundle of His in a case with congenital AV-block and corrected transposition. Pathologe 12: 254–258, 1991.
140. Logar D, Kveder T, Rozman B, Dobovisek J: Possible association between anti-Ro antibodies and myocarditis or cardiac conduction defects in adults with systemic lupus erythematosus. Ann Rheum Dis 49: 627–629, 1990.
141. Groves AM, Allan LD, Rosenthal E: Therapeutic trial of sympathomimetics in three cases of complete heart block in the fetus. Circulation 92: 3394–3396, 1995.
142. Carpenter RJ Jr, Strasburger JF, Garson A Jr, et al: Fetal ventricular pacing for hydrops secondary to complete atrioventricular block. J Am Coll Cardiol 8: 1434–1436, 1986.
143. Walkinshaw SA, Welch CR, McCormack J, Walsh K: In utero pacing for fetal congenital heart block. Fetal Diagn Ther 9: 183–185, 1994.
144. Anandakumar C, Biswas A, Chew SSL, et al: Direct fetal therapy for hydrops secondary to congenital atrioventricular heart block. Obstet Gynecol 87: 835–837, 1996.
145. Harris JP, Alexson CG, Manning JA, Thompson HO: Medical therapy for the hydropic fetus with congenital complete atrioventricular block. Am J Perinatol 10: 217–219, 1993.
146. Lopes LM, Cha SC, Leone C, Zugaib M: Use of sympathomimetic agents in fetal atrioventricular heart block. Arquiv Brasil Cardiol 63: 297–298, 1994.
147. Kiuttu J, Hartikainen AL, Makitalo R, Ruuska P: Congenital heart block with hydrops fetalis treated with high-dose dexamethasone; a case report. Eur J Obstet Gynecol Reprod Biol 42: 155–158, 1991.
148. Deloof E, Devlieger H, Van Hoestenberghe R, et al: Management with a staged approach of the premature hydropic fetus due to complete congenital heart block. Eur J Pediatr 156: 521–523, 1997.
149. Copel JA, Buyon JP, Kleinman CS: Successful in utero therapy of fetal heart block. Am J Obstet Gynecol 173: 1384–1390, 1995.
150. Bierman FZ, Baxi L, Jaffe I, Driscoll J: Fetal hydrops and congenital complete heart block: response to maternal steroid. J Pediatr 1988: 646–648, 1988.
151. Buyon JP, Swersky SH, Fox HE, et al: Intrauterine therapy for presumptive fetal myocarditis with acquired heart block due to systemic lupus erythematosus: experience in a mother with a predominance of SS-B(La) antibodies. Arthritis Rheum 30: 44–49, 1987.
152. Buyon J, Roubey R, Swersky S, et al: Complete congenital heart block: risk of occurrence and therapeutic approach to prevention. J Rheumatol 15: 1104–1108, 1988.
153. Kaaja R, Julkunen H, Ammala P, et al: Congenital heart block: successful prophylactic treatment with intravenous gamma globulin and corticosteroid therapy. Am J Obstet Gynecol 165: 1333–1334, 1991.
154. McCuistion CH, Schoch EP: Possible discoid lupus erythematosus in a newborn infant. Arch Dermatol 70: 782–785, 1954.
155. Franco HL, Weston WL, Peebles C, et al: Autoantibodies directed against sicca syndrome antigens in the neonatal lupus syndrome. J Am Acad Dermatol 4: 67–72, 1981.
156. Deng J-S, Sontheimer RD, Gilliam JN: Relationships between antinuclear antibodies and anti-Ro/SSA antibodies in subacute cutaneous lupus erythematosus. J Am Acad Dermatol 11: 494–499, 1984.
157. Vazquez-Botet M, Rodriguez R, Sanchez JL: Neonatal lupus erythematosus. P R Health Sci J 16: 162–166, 1997.
158. Nitta Y: Lupus erythematosus profundus associated with neonatal lupus erythematosus. Br J Dermatol 136: 112–114, 1997.
159. Miyagawa S, Kitamura W, Yoshioka J, Sakamoto K: Placental transfer of anticytoplasmic antibodies in annular erythema of newborns. Arch Dermatol 117: 569–572, 1981.
160. Gawkrodger DJ, Beveridge GW: Neonatal lupus erythematosus in four successive siblings born to a mother with discoid lupus erythematosus. Br J Dermatol 111: 683–687, 1984.
161. Thornton CM, Eichenfield LF, Shinall EA, et al: Cutaneous telangiectases in neonatal lupus erythematosus. J Am Acad Dermatol 33: 19–25, 1995.
162. Hetem MB, Takada MH, Llorach Velludo MA, Foss NT: Neonatal lupus erythematosus. Int J Dermatol 35: 42–44, 1996.
163. Carrascosa JM, Ribera M, Bielsa I, et al: Cutis marmorata telangiectatica congenita or neonatal lupus? Pediatr Dermatol 13: 230–232, 1996.
164. Lee LA: Neonatal lupus erythematosus. J Invest Dermatol 100: 9S–13S, 1993.
165. Bielsa I, Herrero C, Collado A, et al: Histopathologic findings in cutaneous lupus erythematosus. Arch Dermatol 130: 54–58, 1994.
166. Solomon BA, Laude TA, Shalita AR: Neonatal lupus erythematosus: discordant disease expression of U1RNP-positive antibodies in fraternal twins—is this a subset of neonatal lupus erythematosus or a new distinct syndrome? J Am Acad Dermatol 32: 858–862, 1995.
167. Dugan EM, Tunnessen WW, Honig PJ, Watson RM: U1RNP antibody-positive neonatal lupus. A report of two cases with immunogenetic studies. Arch Dermatol 128: 1490–1494, 1992.
168. Provost TT, Watson R, Gammon WR, et al: The neonatal lupus syndrome associated with U_1RNP (nRNP) antibodies. N Engl J Med 316: 1135–1138, 1987.
169. Sheth AP, Esterly NB, Ratoosh SL, et al: U1RNP positive neonatal lupus erythematosus: association with anti-La antibodies? Br J Dermatol 132: 520–526, 1995.
170. Bouderlique C, Debillon T, Mesnard B, et al: Neonatal lupus presenting as telangiectatic and atrophic lesions. Pediatrie (Bucur) 45: 251–254, 1990.
171. Carrascosa JM, Ribera M, Bielsa I, et al: Cutis marmorata telangiectatica congenita or neonatal lupus? Pediatr Dermatol 13: 230–232, 1996.
172. Giam YC: Cutaneous neonatal lupus erythematosus in Chinese neonates. J Singapore Paediatr Soc 34: 39–43, 1992.
173. Kettler AH, Stone MS, Bruce S, Tschen JA: Annular eruptions of infancy and neonatal lupus erythematosus. Arch Dermatol 123: 298–299, 1987.
174. Lee LA, Weston WL: Cutaneous lupus erythematosus during the neonatal and childhood periods. Lupus 6: 132–138, 1997.
175. Puig L, Moreno A, Alomar A, de Moragas JM: Erythema gyratum atrophicans transiens neonatale: a variant of cutaneous neonatal lupus erythematosus. Pediatr Dermatol 5: 112–116, 1988.
176. Vaughn RY, Guill MA, Cook J: Atrophic plaques in a neonate. Neonatal lupus erythematosus (NLE). Arch Dermatol 128: 683, 686, 1992.
177. Laxer RM, Roberts EA, Gross KR, et al: Liver disease in neonatal lupus erythematosus. J Pediatr 116: 238–242, 1990.
178. Lee LA, Reichlin M, Ruyle SZ, Weston WL: Neonatal lupus liver disease. Lupus 2: 333–338, 1993.
179. Miyagawa S, Dohi K, Yoshioka A, Shirai T: Female predominance of immune response to SSA/Ro antigens and risk of neonatal lupus erythematosus. Br J Dermatol 123: 223–227, 1990.
180. Schoenlebe J, Buyon JP, Zitelli BJ, et al: Neonatal hemochromatosis associated with maternal autoantibodies against Ro/SS-A and La/SS-B ribonucleoproteins. Am J Dis Child 147: 1072–1075, 1993.
181. Rosh JR, Silverman ED, Groisman G, et al: Intrahepatic cholestasis in neonatal lupus erythematosus. J Pediatr Gastroenterol Nutr 17: 310–312, 1993.
182. Fonseca E, Contreras F, Garcia-Frias E, Carrascosa MC: Neonatal lupus erythematosus with multisystem organ involvement preceding cutaneous lesions. Lupus 1: 49–50, 1991.
183. Watson R, Kang JE, May M, et al: Thrombocytopenia in the neonatal lupus syndrome. Arch Dermatol 124: 560–563, 1988.
184. Kleinman D, Katz VL, Kuller JA: Perinatal outcomes in women with systemic lupus erythematosus. J Perinatol 18: 178–182, 1998.
185. Lockshin MD, Bonfa E, Elkon K, Druzin ML: Neonatal lupus risk to newborns of mothers with systemic lupus erythematosus. Arthritis Rheum 31: 697–701, 1988.
186. Kurata Y, Miyagawa S, Kosugi S, et al: High-titer antinuclear antibodies, anti-SSA/Ro antibodies and anti-nuclear RNP antibodies in patients with idiopathic thrombocytopenic purpura. Thromb Haemost 71: 184–187, 1994.
187. Alexander EL, Arnett FC, Provost TT, Stevens MB: Sjögren's syndrome: association of anti-Ro(SS-A) antibodies with vasculitis, hematologic abnormalities, and serologic hyperreactivity. Ann Intern Med 98: 155–159, 1983.

188. Watson RM, Braunstein BL, Watson AJ, et al: Fetal wastage in women with anti-Ro (SSA) antibody. J Rheumatol 13: 90–94, 1986.
189. Wolach B, Choc L, Pomeranz A, et al: Aplastic anemia in neonatal lupus erythematosus. Am J Dis Child 147: 941–944, 1993.
190. Selander B, Cedergren S, Domanski H: A case of severe neonatal lupus erythematosus without cardiac or cutaneous involvement. Acta Paediatr 87: 105–107, 1998.
191. Fonseca E, Contreras F, Garcia-Frias E, Carrascosa MC: Neonatal lupus erythematosus with multisystem organ involvement preceding cutaneous lesions. Lupus 1: 49–50, 1991.
192. Kaye EM, Butler IJ, Conley S: Myelopathy in neonatal and infantile lupus erythematosus. J Neurol Neurosurg Psychiatr 50: 923–926, 1987.
193. Wang HS, Kuo MF, Chang TC: Sonographic lenticulostriate vasculopathy in infants: some associations and a hypothesis. AJNR Am J Neuroradiol 16: 97–102, 1995.
194. Cabanas F, Pellicer A, Valverde E, et al: Central nervous system vasculopathy in neonatal lupus erythematosus. Pediatr Neurol 15: 124–126, 1996.
195. Nakayama FF, Takigawa M, Iwatsuki K, et al: Hydrocephalus in two female siblings with neonatal lupus erythematosus. Arch Dermatol 130: 1210–1212, 1994.
196. Rider LG, Sherry DD, Glass ST: Neonatal lupus erythematosus simulating transient myasthenia gravis at presentation. J Pediatr 118: 417–419, 1991.
197. Elcioglu N, Hall CM: Maternal systemic lupus erythematosus and chondrodysplasia punctata in two sibs: phenocopy or coincidence? J Med Genet 35: 690–694, 1998.
198. Austin-Ward E, Castillo S, Cuchacovich M, et al: Neonatal lupus syndrome: a case with chondrodysplasia punctata and other unusual manifestations. J Med Genet 35: 695–697, 1998.
199. Westenend PJ: Congenital nephrotic syndrome in neonatal lupus syndrome. J Pediatr 126: 851, 1995.
200. Ruas E, Moreno A, Tellechea O, et al: Neonatal lupus erythematosus in an infant with Turner syndrome. Pediatr Dermatol 13: 298–302, 1996.
201. Jackson R, Gulliver M: Neonatal lupus erythematosus progressing into systemic lupus erythematosus. Br J Dermatol 101: 81–86, 1979.
202. Fox RJ, McCuistion CH, Schoch EP: Systemic lupus erythematosus association with previous neonatal lupus erythematosus. Arch Dermatol 115: 340, 1979.
203. Reichlin M, Friday K, Harley JB: Complete congenital heart block followed by anti-Ro/SSA in adult life. Am J Med 84: 339–344, 1988.
204. McCue CM, Manatakas ME, Tingelstad JB, Ruddy S: Congenital heart block in newborns of mothers with connective tissue disease. Circulation 56: 82–90, 1977.
205. Waterworth RF: Systemic lupus erythematosus occurring with congenital complete heart block. N Z Med J 92: 311–312, 1980.
206. Esscher E, Scott JS: Congenital heart block and maternal systemic lupus erythematosus. Br Med J 1: 1235–1238, 1979.
207. Lanham JG, Walport MJ, Hughes GR: Congenital heart block and familial connective tissue disease. J Rheumatol 10: 823–825, 1983.
208. McCune AB, Weston WL, Lee LA: Maternal and fetal outcome in neonatal lupus erythematosus. Ann Intern Med 106: 518–523, 1987.
209. Press J, Uziel Y, Laxer RM, et al: Long-term outcome of mothers of children with complete congenital heart block. Am J Med 100: 328–332, 1996.
210. Waltuck J, Buyon JP: Autoantibody-associated congenital heart block: outcome in mothers and children. Ann Intern Med 120: 544–551, 1994.
211. Brucato A, Franceschini F, Gasparini M, et al: Isolated congenital complete heart block: long-term outcome of mothers, maternal antibody specificity and immunogenetic background. J Rheumatol 22: 533–540, 1995.
212. Knolle P, Mayet W, Lohse AW, et al: Complete congenital heart block in autoimmune hepatitis (SLA-positive). J Hepatol 21: 224–226, 1994.
213. Fu LS, Hwang B, Lee BH: Newborns of Chinese mother with systemic lupus erythematosus (SLE). Acta Paediatr Sinica 33: 341–349, 1992.
214. Leu LY, Lan JL: The influence on pregnancy of anti-SSA/Ro antibodies in systemic lupus erythematosus. Chung Hua Min Kuo Wei Sheng Wu Chi Mien I Hsueh Tsa Chih 25: 12–20, 1992.
215. Alexander EL, Buyon JP, Lane J, et al: Anti-SS-A/Ro SS-B/La antibodies bind to neonatal rabbit cardiac cells and preferentially inhibit in vitro cardiac repolarization. J Autoimmun 2: 463–469, 1989.
216. Alexander E, Buyon JP, Provost TT, Guarnieri T: Anti-Ro/SS-A antibodies in the pathophysiology of congenital heart block in neonatal lupus syndrome, an experimental model. In vitro electrophysiologic and immunocytochemical studies. Arthritis Rheum 35: 176–189, 1992.
217. Deng J-S, Bair LWJ, Shen-Schwarz S, et al: Localization of Ro(SS-A) antigen in the cardiac conduction system. Arthritis Rheum 30: 1232–1238, 1987.
218. Lee LA, Harmon CE, Huff JC, et al: The demonstration of SS-A/Ro antigen in human fetal tissues and in neonatal and adult skin. J Invest Dermatol 85: 143–146, 1985.
219. Tseng CE, Miranda E, Di Donato F, et al: mRNA and protein expression of SSA/Ro and SSB/La in human fetal cardiac myocytes cultured using a novel application of the Langendorff procedure. Pediatr Res 45: 260–269, 1999.
220. Furukawa F, Lyons MB, Lee LA, et al: Estradiol binding to cultured human keratinocytes of antibodies specific for SS-A/Ro and SS-B/La. J Immunol 141: 1480–1488, 1988.
221. Furukawa F, Imamura S, Norris DA: Stimulation of anti-RNP antibody binding to cultured keratinocytes by estradiol. Arch Dermatol Res 283: 258–261, 1991.
222. LeFeber WP, Norris DA, Ryan SR, et al: Ultraviolet light induces binding of antibodies to selected nuclear antigens on cultured keratinocytes. J Clin Invest 74: 1545–1551, 1984.
223. Wang D, Chan EK: 17-Beta-estradiol increases expression of 52-kDa and 60-kDa SS-A/Ro autoantigens in human keratinocytes and breast cancer cell line MCF-7. J Invest Dermatol 107: 610–614, 1996.
224. Dorner T, Chaoui R, Feist E, et al: Significantly increased maternal and fetal IgG autoantibody levels to 52 kD Ro (SS-A) and La(SS-B) in complete congenital heart block. J Autoimmun 8: 675–684, 1995.
225. Lee LA, Weston WL, Krueger GG, et al: An animal model of antibody binding in cutaneous lupus. Arthritis Rheum 29: 782–788, 1986.
226. Yu HS, Chiang LC, Chang CH, et al: The cytotoxic effect of neonatal lupus erythematosus and maternal sera on keratinocyte cultures is complement-dependent and can be augmented by ultraviolet irradiation. Br J Dermatol 135: 297–301, 1996.
227. Garcia S, Nascimento JH, Bonfa E, et al: Cellular mechanism of the conduction abnormalities induced by serum from anti-Ro/SSA-positive patients in rabbit hearts. J Clin Invest 93: 718–724, 1994.
228. Viana VS, Garcia S, Nascimento JH, et al: Induction of in vitro heart block is not restricted to affinity purified anti-52 kDa Ro/SSA antibody from mothers of children with neonatal lupus. Lupus 7: 141–147, 1998.
229. de Oliveira SF, Pedrosa RC, Nascimento JH, et al: Sera from chronic chagasic patients with complex cardiac arrhythmias depress electrogenesis and conduction in isolated rabbit hearts. Circulation 96: 2031–2037, 1997.
230. Boutjdir M, Chen L, Zhang ZH, et al: Arrhythmogenicity of IgG and anti-52-kD SSA/Ro affinity-purified antibodies from mothers of children with congenital heart block. Circ Res 80: 354–362, 1997.
231. Boutjdir M, Chen L, Zhang ZH, et al: Serum and immunoglobulin G from the mother of a child with congenital heart block induce conduction abnormalities and inhibit L-type calcium channels in a rat heart model. Pediatr Res 44: 11–19, 1998.
232. Miranda-Carus ME, Boutjdir M, Tseng CE, et al: Induction of antibodies reactive with SSA/Ro-SSB/La and development of congenital heart block in a murine model. J Immunol 161: 5886–5892, 1998.
233. Miranda ME, Tseng CE, Rashbaum W, et al: Accessibility of SSA/Ro and SSB/La antigens to maternal autoantibodies in apoptotic human fetal cardiac myocytes. J Immunol 161: 5061–5069, 1998.

20

Juvenile Dermatomyositis

James T. Cassidy and Ross E. Petty

Juvenile dermatomyositis (JDM) is a multisystem disease of uncertain etiology that results in nonsuppurative inflammation of striated muscle, skin, and the gastrointestinal tract.[1, 2] It is characterized early in its course by an immune complex vasculitis of varying severity and later by development of calcinosis.

HISTORICAL REVIEW

The clinical presentation of dermatomyositis was described by four different investigators in 1887.[3–6] Unverricht best clarified the cutaneous and muscular manifestations of the disease, introducing the term *dermatomyositis*.[6] That report recognized that the childhood form of the disease was not always fatal, although many of the subsequent reports emphasized a poor prognosis. The clinically distinctive features of JDM were not detailed until some time later.[7–16] Experience with this disease in the presteroid era was reported by Karelitz and Welt (22 children),[7] Scheuermann (47 children),[17] Hecht (5 children),[18] and Selander (22 children).[19] The first full postmortem study that described the classic histopathologic features of the disease in a child was published by Batten in 1912.[20] Pearson[21] recognized the uniqueness of dermatomyositis in children and separated the childhood disease from that occurring in adults in his classification in 1966. Wedgwood and colleagues[8] in 1953 reviewed data on 26 children treated with glucocorticoids, and Cook and colleagues[22] in 1963 reported 15 deaths in 50 children and emphasized again the therapeutic role of these relatively new agents for treatment of this disorder. Sullivan and colleagues[13, 15] in 1972 and 1977 and Rose[14] in 1974 stressed the importance of an adequately high dose and sufficiently long therapeutic course to reverse the previously dismal outlook of childhood dermatomyositis.

DEFINITION AND CLASSIFICATION

In childhood, chronic idiopathic inflammatory myositis is a relatively heterogeneous disorder, although almost all affected children have the characteristic skin and muscle abnormalities of dermatomyositis. JDM differs in a number of respects from the disease as it is observed in adults (Table 20–1). Other types of inflammatory myositis, including polymyositis (muscle inflammation without cutaneous disease)[23–25] and dermatomyositis with other systemic diseases such as malignancy,[26–31] are rare in childhood. Additional considerations include myositis-associated connective tissue diseases,[25, 32–35] such as scleroderma and overlap syndromes, and rare instances in childhood of inclusion body myositis,[25, 36] focal myositis,[37, 38] and eosinophilic myositis.[39]

EPIDEMIOLOGY

Incidence and Prevalence

Rose and Walton[40] estimated the annual incidence of dermatomyositis and polymyositis in Great Britain at 0.4 per 100,000. This is similar to the frequency in the United States of 0.5[41] and 0.55,[42] and to the rate found in studies in Israel of 0.44.[43] In general, 16 to 20 percent of all patients with dermatomyositis have onset in childhood.[41, 44] Estimates of the incidence of JDM are given in Table 20–2.[23, 41, 42, 45–47]

Age at Onset and Sex Ratio

The data of Medsger and coworkers[41] suggest a bimodal distribution of ages at onset of polymyositis and dermatomyositis, with a peak in the 10- to 14-year-old range, and a second, much larger peak in the 45- to 64-year-old age group (Fig. 20–1).[41, 43] Such a distinctly bimodal distribution of ages at onset underlines the clinical heterogeneity of this group of diseases and the uniqueness of the childhood form of the illness. Data from nine series of children with JDM derived from widely divergent geographic areas are illustrated in Figure 20–2. Onset is especially common from the 4th to the 10th year of childhood.[45] The average age at onset is 7 years.[13, 15, 22, 24, 48] For boys the most common age at onset is 6 years, but for girls there appears to be one peak at 6 years and another at 10 years.[45] The disease occurs more frequently in girls than in boys in

Table 20–1
Unique Characteristics of Juvenile Dermatomyositis

Vasculitis is frequent and often severe
Calcinosis is common, especially in the recovery phase
Polymyositis is uncommon
Malignancy is very rare

Table 20–2

Incidence of Juvenile Dermatomyositis

POPULATION	STUDY	INCIDENCE/100,000	SEX RATIO, F:M
United States 1970	Medsger et al.[41]		
0–4 yr		0.06	3:1
5–9 yr		0.37	1:1.3
10–14 yr		0.43	4.7:1
United States 1982	Hanissian et al.[23]	0.32	
PM (n=17)			4.7:1
JDM (n=26)			
United States 1990 (Pennsylvania)	Oddis et al.[42]	0.8 (0.01–1.59)	2.5:1
white female (n=14)		1.1 (0.01–2.19)	2.8:1
white male (n=5)		0.4 (0–1.8)	
black female (n=1)		0.7 (0–1.4)	1:1
black male (n=1)		0.9 (0.01–1.75)	
United Kingdom and Ireland 1995	Symmons et al.[45]		5:1
PM (n=3)			
JDM (n=48)		0.19 (0.14–0.26)	
Finland 1996	Kaipiainen et al.[46]	0.5	
JDM (n=4)			
Japan 1997	Fujikawa et al.[47]	0.16	
PM/JDM			

JDM, juvenile dermatomyositis; PM, polymyositis.

a ratio of 1.4:1 to 2.7:1 or even higher, especially in the group with onset at 10 years of age or older.[23, 32, 45, 46, 49–51] This ratio was reversed in a recent review of the course of JDM in 25 Arab patients.[52] In the pooled data illustrated in Figure 20–2, the female to male ratio was 1.7:1.

Geographic and Racial Distribution

Dermatomyositis is widely distributed throughout the world, although it has been most frequently reported from North American centers. Striking racial differences in the incidence of inflammatory myositis have been described in adults in the United States, with the frequency of the disease in black women in the 55- to 64-year-old group being 10 times that of white women.[41] Such differences are less marked in children, although it has been an impression that JDM occurs more frequently than expected in black children. This belief may reflect referral patterns, but the data of Medsger and colleagues[41] and Oddis and colleagues[42] suggest that it may be a valid observation, at least for girls.

ETIOLOGY AND PATHOGENESIS

The cause of JDM is unknown (Table 20–3).[53–55] Most studies suggest that JDM is autoimmune in pathogenesis and results from an angiopathy. Both cell-mediated immunity to muscle antigens and immune-complex disease may participate in pathogenesis. Response of patient lymphocytes in vitro to allogeneic or autologous muscle extracts has been described in some studies,[56–59] but not all.[60] A cytotoxic effect on muscle monolayers in culture by lymphocytes from children with JDM has been noted,[61–66] but, again, not uniformly.[67] In one study, peripheral blood lymphocytes from four of five children with active disease produced a lympho-

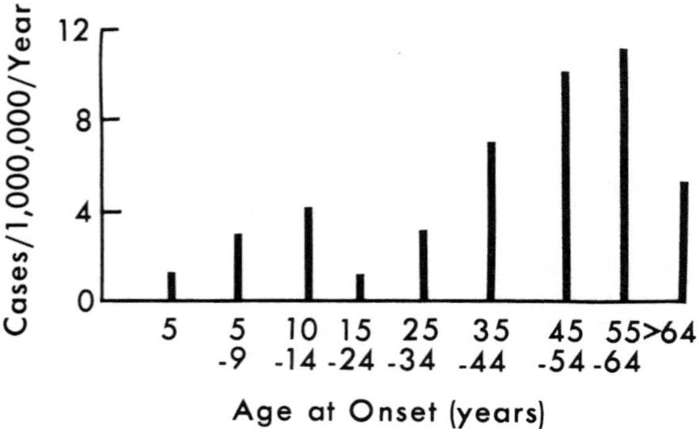

Figure 20–1. Incidence of inflammatory myositis.

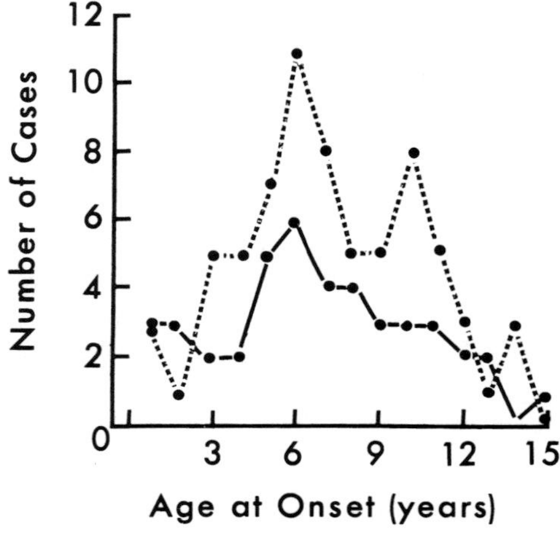

Figure 20–2. Age at onset of dermatomyositis. Girls (●----●); boys (●—●).

Table 20–3

Etiology and Pathogenesis of Juvenile Dermatomyositis (JDM)

POTENTIAL PATHOGENIC MECHANISM	EVIDENCE
Abnormalities of cell-mediated immunity	Patient lymphocytes proliferate in vitro in presence of muscle cells
	Patient lymphocytes are cytotoxic to human fetal or animal myocytes in vitro
	Patient lymphocyte supernatants (lymphokines) are cytotoxic to myocytes in culture
Immune complex disease	Presence of circulating immune complexes in patient sera
	Immunoglobulin and complement deposited in vascular endothelium
Association with immunodeficiency	Occurrence of disease in children with hypogammaglobulinemia, selective IgA deficiency, or C2 complement component deficiency
Relation to infection	Myxovirus-like tubuloreticular structures in endothelial cells in muscle biopsy specimens
	Occurrence of limited myositis in association with influenza
	Increased coxsackie B virus titers in children with JDM (?)
	Increased toxoplasmosis titers in children with JDM (?)
Genetic predisposition	HLA-DRB1*0301 and DQA1*0501

toxin that caused necrosis or impaired protein synthesis in monolayers of human fetal muscle in the presence of homogenates of autologous muscle.[63] Activated T cells undoubtedly are involved in pathogenesis.[67a] Normal muscle cells do not express major histocompatibility class (MHC) class I antigens, but in JDM these antigens are strongly expressed.[68, 69] A recent report suggests that dysregulation of apoptosis in myofibrils, as suggested by the observation of overexpression of bcl-2 protein in muscle specimens from children with this disease, should be considered in pathogenesis.[69a]

An immune-complex–mediated vasculitis may be an important initiating or perpetuating event in JDM.[70–73] Complement activation and immune complex deposition have been demonstrated.[74] Whitaker and Engel[70] identified immunoglobulin (IgG and (IgM) and complement (C3) in vessel walls of skeletal muscle in both childhood and adult dermatomyositis, although the frequency and intensity of deposition were more pronounced in children. Elevated plasma levels of Factor VIII–related antigen, fibrinopeptide A, and C3 provide additional evidence of endothelial cell injury that may be immune-complex induced, although antibodies that are directly stimulatory of or toxic to endothelial cells may also be important.[75]

Reports of both geographic and seasonal clustering of cases support an environmental factor in the causation or triggering of JDM.[45, 52, 76] Onset has often been associated with infections (coxsackie virus, influenza, streptococcus, toxoplasmosis, parvovirus, hepatitis B, borrelia, leishmania).[2, 32] The evidence for the participation of infectious agents is for the most part indirect, however. Although acute muscle inflammation occurs in humans as a result of viral illness, there are no unequivocal data supporting a viral etiology for JDM.[77, 78] Serologic evidence of coxsackievirus B infection was reported in 83 percent of children with early JDM, compared with 25 percent of control subjects,[79, 80] but a search for the presence of viral genome in cells from patients with JDM by the polymerase chain reaction was unsuccessful.[81] Enteroviral titers are similar to those in control groups.[52] Acute transitory myositis may occur after influenza infection.[82–84, 84a] Dermatomyositis has been reported to follow immunizations (e.g., rubella, bacille Calmette-Guérin).[85–89] Relapse with β hemolytic streptococcal disease[32, 90] may be related to molecular mimicry between the streptococcal M5 protein and skeletal muscle myosin and immune responses to homologous peptide regions.[90a, 90b]

Toxoplasma gondii was demonstrated in muscle in one patient with JDM.[91] Antibody titers to Toxoplasma have been found to be elevated in some studies,[92–95] but appropriate environmental controls were lacking. A dermatomyositis-like disease has been described in a few children with agammaglobulinemia in association with echovirus infection[75, 96] and occasionally in patients with selective immunoglobulin A (IgA) deficiency[97] or deficiency of the second component of complement (C2), in whom an inordinate susceptibility to infection might be anticipated[98] (see Chapter 35). Experimental induction of a polymyositis-like syndrome in neonatal animals has also been reported after inoculation with Semliki Forest virus,[99] coxsackievirus,[100, 101] encephalomyocarditis virus,[102] and Ross River virus.[103]

Electron microscopic examination of muscle from children with JDM has demonstrated tubuloreticular structures within endothelial cells that resemble the myxovirus-like particles that have been identified in patients with systemic lupus erythematosus (SLE).[104, 105] This finding, however, may simply reflect degenerative or regenerative alterations in the cytoplasmic constituents of the endothelial cells (Fig. 20–3).[106–108] A study of muscle and peripheral blood mononuclear cells from children with JDM demonstrated the presence of tubuloreticular structures and cylindrical confronting cisternae in all of the six patients studied.[109] The authors concluded that these structures probably represented the effect of interferon-alpha, which could be induced by viral infections in general.

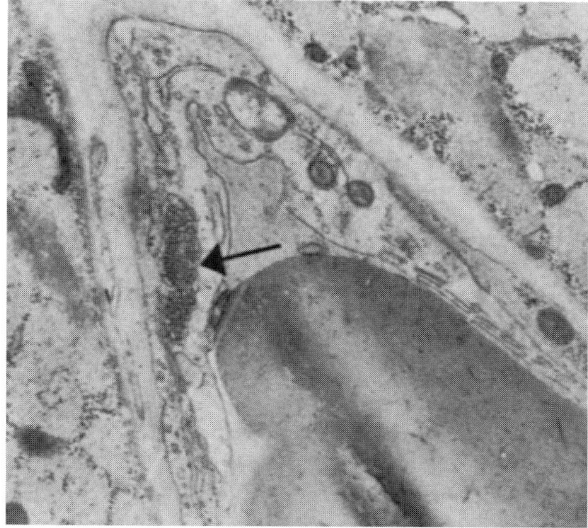

Figure 20–3. Electron microscopy of a proximal muscle biopsy specimen with an abnormal endothelial tubuloreticular structure *(arrow).*

Other reports have confirmed these paramyxovirus-like particles in affected muscle[110, 111] and indicated the possible presence of picornavirus,[112–114] or coxsackie virus.[115, 116]

Experimental myositis can be induced by the injection of muscle homogenates in Freund's adjuvant in guinea pigs,[117] rabbits,[118] and rats.[119] Although this disorder was quite different from JDM, cell-mediated immunity to muscle was noted, and the disease could be transferred by lymphocytes.[120–122] It has not been possible, however, to reproduce in animals the characteristic vasculopathy of JDM.[123, 124]

GENETIC BACKGROUND

Familial Dermatomyositis

JDM is rarely familial, although there are several reports of the occurrence of this disease in more than one family member (Table 20–4).[8, 125–131, 131a] In all instances but one, the disease has been typical dermatomyositis. In the daughter-father pair described by Lewkonia and Buxton,[126] the daughter had typical JDM and the father had polymyositis with positive lupus erythematosus cell preparations. The twin girls reported by Harati and associates[128] developed JDM within 2 weeks of each other after upper respiratory tract infections. There is an increased frequency of autoimmune disease in families of children with JDM.[130]

Human Leukocyte Antigen Relationships

In spite of the infrequency of familial dermatomyositis, there may be an immunogenetic predisposition to this disease marked by the presence of human leukocyte antigens (HLA) B8 and DR3.[132–135] Friedman and colleagues[132, 133] studied HLA antigens in 65 children with JDM seen at five medical centers. B8 was found in 43 percent of these patients (21 percent of control subjects), and DR3 (DRB1*0301) was present in 57 percent (30 percent of control subjects). B8 has been commonly reported to be increased in prevalence among patients with other connective tissue diseases or autoimmune diseases such as SLE, and its increased frequency in JDM is therefore not unexpected. An association with DQA1*0501 in white children with JDM[39, 136] and in other ethnic groups has been published.[137] Class II–associated DM molecules (DMA*0103 and DMB*0102) are also increased in frequency.[137a] A study of Czech children with JDM, however, did not demonstrate an HLA association.[138] A number of distinct HLA associations occur with the myositis-specific antibodies.[139]

Table 20–4

Dermatomyositis in Families

AUTHORS	AGE (yr)	SEX	AFFECTED RELATIVE (AGE)
Lambie and Duff[125]	13	F	Cousin (F, 16 yr)
Lewkonia and Buxton[126]	9	F	Father (25 yr)
Wedgwood et al.[8]	4	F	Identical twin (5 yr)
Harati et al.[128]	12	F	Identical twin (12 yr)
Cassidy et al. (unpublished observations)	9	F	Maternal grandmother (74 yr)
Andrews et al.[131]	2	F	Mother (27 yr)

CLINICAL MANIFESTATIONS

JDM usually presents with a combination of malaise, easy fatigue, muscle weakness, fever, and rash (Table 20–5).[1, 8, 9, 11–15, 138, 140–147] There is great variation in the rapidity of evolution of the clinical manifestations. The disease generally begins with insidious development of progressive muscle weakness and pain, although a more acute onset occurs in approximately one third of children. Symptoms may be present for 2 months or longer before initial diagnosis of the illness.

Constitutional Signs and Symptoms

In most children, the onset of JDM is characterized by fever in the range of 38 to 40°C. These children also complain of ease of fatigue, which probably represents muscle weakness. Malaise, anorexia, and weight loss may occur. Parents of young children with early JDM often report that the child had become irritable and describe alterations in gross motor function or regression of motor milestones.

Musculoskeletal Disease

Muscle weakness at onset is predominantly proximal, and complaints related to weakness of the limb-girdle musculature of the lower extremities are most common. Weakness of the anterior neck flexors and back

Table 20–5

Frequency of Manifestations of Juvenile Dermatomyositis at Onset of the Disease

MANIFESTATION	FREQUENCY (%)
Easy fatigue	80–100
Progressive proximal muscle weakness	16–96
Classic rash	32–84
Fever	50–80
Muscle pain or tenderness	30–80
Lymphadenopathy	50–75
Arthritis	7–38
Hepatomegaly	10–20
Splenomegaly	10–15
Nonspecific rash	10–15
Dyspnea	5–15
Dysphagia	5–9

muscles leads to inability to hold the head upright or maintain a sitting posture. The child may stop walking or be unable to dress or climb stairs. The affected child may also complain of muscle pain or stiffness that is usually only moderate in degree.

Physical examination demonstrates symmetric weakness that is maximal in the proximal muscles: those of the shoulders, hips, and neck flexors, and in the abdominal musculature. Affected muscles are occasionally edematous and indurated and may be tender. Functional muscle examination may demonstrate that the child is unable to rise from a supine position without rolling over, is unable to rise from sitting to standing or to get out of bed without assistance, or is unable to squat or to rise from a squatting position without help; *Gowers' sign* is often present. The child with weakness of the pelvic girdle musculature has difficulty climbing or descending stairs; the *Trendelenburg sign,* if present, indicates weakness of the hip abductors. Later in the disease, or in children with an especially severe course, the distal muscles of the extremities may become involved. Occasionally, the disease is so severe that the child is unable to move at all.

In these severely affected children, who account for approximately 10 percent of those with JDM, pharyngeal, hypopharyngeal, and palatal muscles are affected as well. Difficulty swallowing may be related to this involvement or to esophageal hypomotility.[148] Dysphonia, palatal speech, or regurgitation of liquids through the nose may be early signs of impending difficulties. The threat of aspiration is always present in these children. Although muscle weakness may be impressive, the deep tendon reflexes are usually well preserved,

Sequential musculoskeletal examinations by the same experienced physician or physical therapist should be recorded using a standard scale (Table 20–6).[149, 150] The importance of this examination and its documentation becomes even more critical later during the course of the disease when serum levels of muscle enzymes may be less dependable indicators of disease activity. Selected muscle groups that should always be evaluated are the neck flexors and extensors, shoulder abductors, elbow flexors and extensors, hip flexors, extensors, and abductors, and knee flexors and extensors. Myometry provides a reproducible means of more finely grading changes in muscle strength.

Table 20–6

Scale for Grading Muscle Strength

GRADE	FUNCTION (%)	ACTIVITY LEVEL
0—None	0	No evidence of muscle contractility
1—Trace	15	Evidence of slight contractility; no effective joint motion
2—Poor	25	Full range of motion without gravity
3—Fair	50	Full range of motion against gravity
4—Good	75	Complete range of motion against gravity with some resistance
5—Normal	100	Complete range of motion against gravity with full resistance

Modified from National Foundation: Publication No. 60, 1946.

Some children with JDM have arthralgia or subtle arthritis that is transient and nondeforming, sometimes accompanied by tenosynovitis or flexor nodules. Early development of flexion contractures, particularly at the knees, hips, and shoulders, is common and usually represents the effects of muscle inflammation rather than synovitis. The presence of significant, persistent arthritis in a child with myositis and skin changes of dermatomyositis suggests the possibility of an overlap syndrome such as mixed connective tissue disease. A recent report documented the presence of arthritis in 35 percent of 79 children with JDM, a frequency that is much higher than was previously appreciated.[150a]

Mucocutaneous Disease

In three fourths of the children with JDM, the cutaneous abnormalities are pathognomonic of the disease; in the remainder, a less characteristic rash is present. Occasionally, dermatitis is the first manifestation of the disorder. More often, the cutaneous abnormalities become evident in the first few weeks after the onset of muscle symptoms. The three most typical cutaneous manifestations of early JDM are heliotrope discoloration of the upper eyelids, Gottron's papules, and periungual erythema and capillary loop abnormalities. The classic heliotrope dermatitis occurs over the upper eyelids as a violaceous, reddish purple suffusion often associated with a malar rash that resembles that of SLE in its distribution but is less well demarcated (Fig. 20–4). Edema of the eyelids and face often accompanies this heliotrope dermatitis and may be marked (Fig. 20–5).

The symmetric changes over the extensor surfaces of joints (*Gottron's papules, or collodion patches*) tend to be associated with shiny, erythematous, atrophic, scaly plaques (Fig. 20–6*A* and *B*). These atrophic areas of skin have a bright pink-red appearance. Occasionally, the lesions appear to be thickened and pale early in disease (hence the name "collodion patch"). Gottron's papules are especially common over the proximal interphalangeal joints of the hands and less so over the metacarpophalangeal and distal interphalangeal joints. The skin over the toes is rarely, if ever, affected. The extensor surfaces of the elbows and knees and, less frequently, the malleoli may also be involved. Similar rashes may cover the entire extensor surface of the limbs and can occur on the trunk as well.

Abnormalities of the periungual skin and capillary bed are typical of JDM and are present in 50 to 100 percent of children. The periungual skin is often intensely erythematous, and careful examination with the naked eye or the 40× lens of an ophthalmoscope

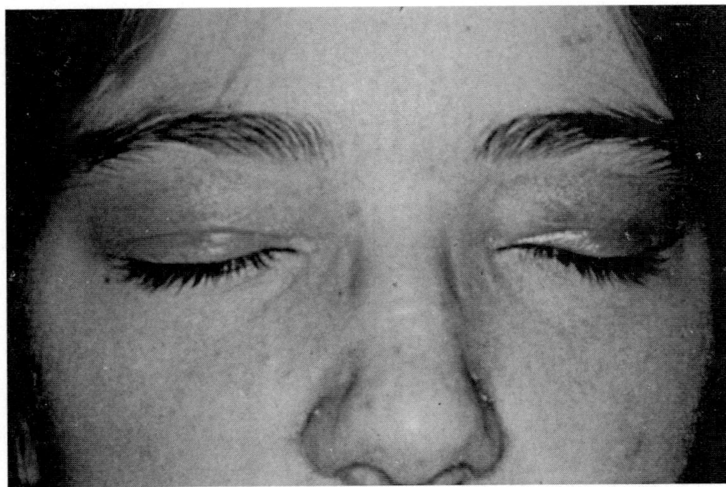

Figure 20–4. Heliotrope discoloration and violaceous suffusion with edema of the upper eyelids in an 11-year-old with acute dermatomyositis.

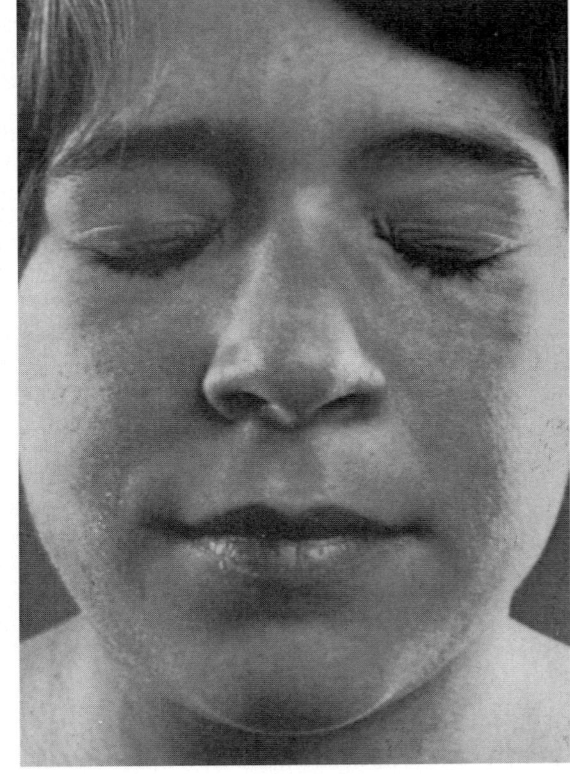

Figure 20–5. Erythematous, scaly rash in a malar distribution with an associated heliotrope discoloration and violaceous suffusion of the upper eyelids. Facial edema is marked.

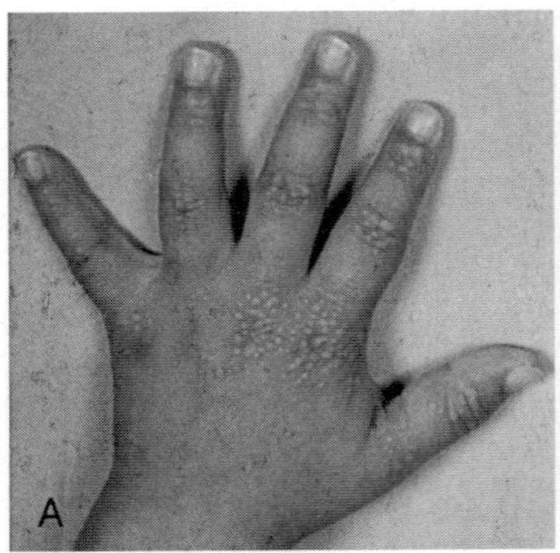

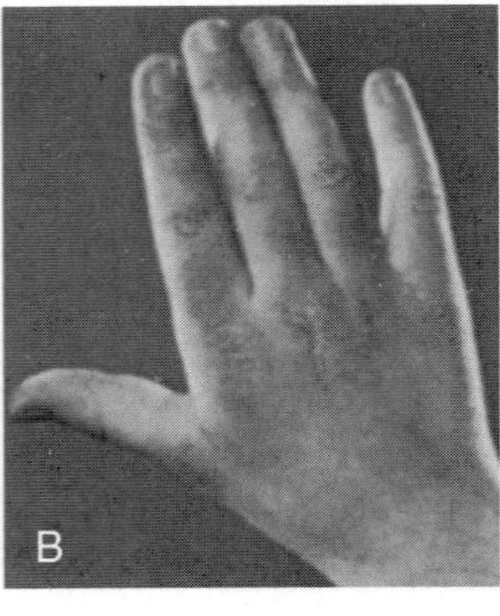

Figure 20–6. *A,* Gottron's papules. *B,* Symmetric, scaly, erythematous papules over the metacarpophalangeal and proximal interphalangeal joints of the hand in an 8-year-old girl with dermatomyositis.

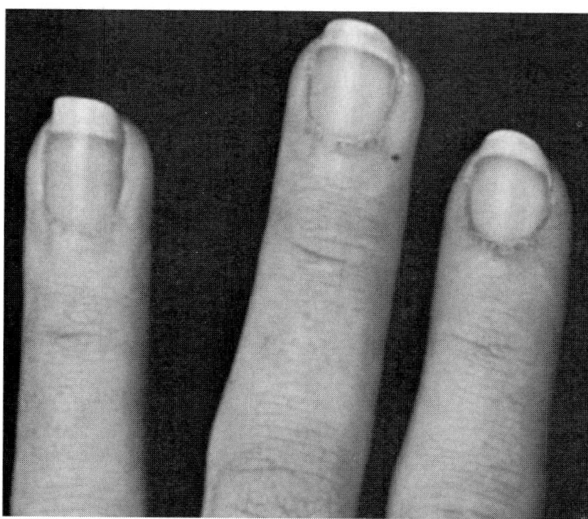

Figure 20–7. Nailfold telangiectases in a girl with acute dermatomyositis.

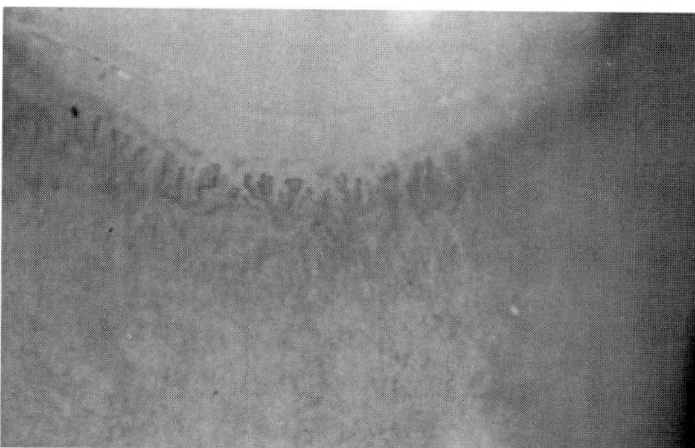

Figure 20–9. Abnormal nailfold capillary pattern with the classic changes of dermatomyositis. The capillaries are thickened and tortuous with the typical peripheral "bushy" pattern. (Courtesy of Dr. Jay Kenik.)

documents the presence of nailfold telangiectases (Fig. 20–7). Dilatation of isolated loops, thrombosis and hemorrhage (often visible), dropout of surrounding vessels,[150a] and arborized clusters of giant capillary loops that are distinctive, if not pathognomonic, of JDM are present (Figs. 20–8 to 20–10). Similar changes occur in other connective tissue diseases, especially systemic scleroderma but are seldom as dramatic as those seen in the child with JDM. These abnormalities, like the noninflammatory vasculopathy, correlate with a more severe chronic disease course, cutaneous ulceration, or the development of calcinosis.[151–154] The acute nailfold abnormalities may abate with resolving illness or remission, in our experience.

Cutaneous involvement in JDM can vary from the slightest erythematous tinge over the knuckles or eyelids to a generalized scaly rash. At onset, edema and induration of skin and subcutaneous tissues, especially in the periorbital areas and face, are common; less frequently, the extremities and trunk are affected.[154a] Extensive rashes often take on an infiltrative character with hyperemic borders in addition to the acute intradermal and subcutaneous edema. Photosensitivity occurs in up to one third of patients.[145, 155] Sun exposure has been associated with onset of the disease and exacerbations. Gingival and buccal ulcerations develop in 10 to 45 percent of children with JDM and are associated with pain on swallowing.[156, 156a] Oral ulcers may precede or accompany the onset of the disease.

Cutaneous ulceration occurred relatively frequently in the series of Crowe and coworkers[24] and was associated with severe and prolonged disease in 11 of 42 patients. Vasculitic ulcers at the corners of the eyes, in the axillae, over the elbows or pressure points, and over stretch marks may become a serious problem (Figs. 20–11*A–D* and 20–12*A–C*). Children who display the generalized rash and cutaneous ulcerations may have the poorest prognosis,[24, 157] but this is not always the case.[158]

Late in the course of JDM, other cutaneous and subcutaneous changes occur. Thinning and atrophy of the skin and supporting structures may supervene, and alterations in pigmentation become more common. Although individual lesions may be hypopigmented, the child may exhibit generalized hyperpigmentation. Hyperkeratosis of the palms and the soles has been described in one 11-year-old girl.[38]

Controversy has continued as to whether dermatomyositis sine myositis exists in children (amyopathic dermatomyositis). If it exists, it is rare,[159–162] although JDM may present with rash alone,[163] or muscle disease may not be initially documented.[163a] It is our opinion that these children eventually develop overt myositis if followed for long enough. There are a few children with JDM who have persistently normal levels of serum muscle enzymes.

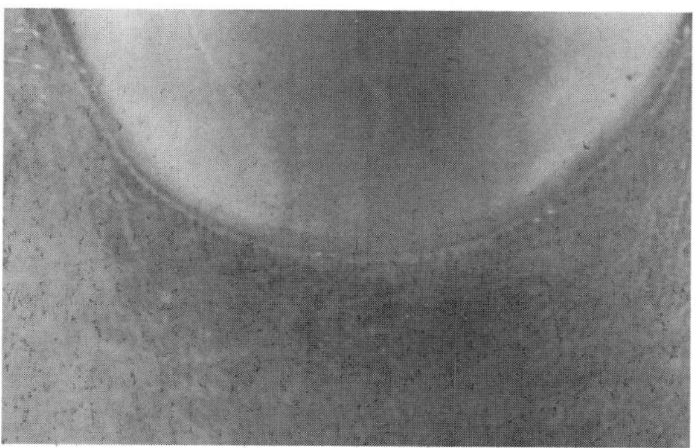

Figure 20–8. Normal nailfold capillary pattern, ×100. (Courtesy of Dr. Jay Kenik.)

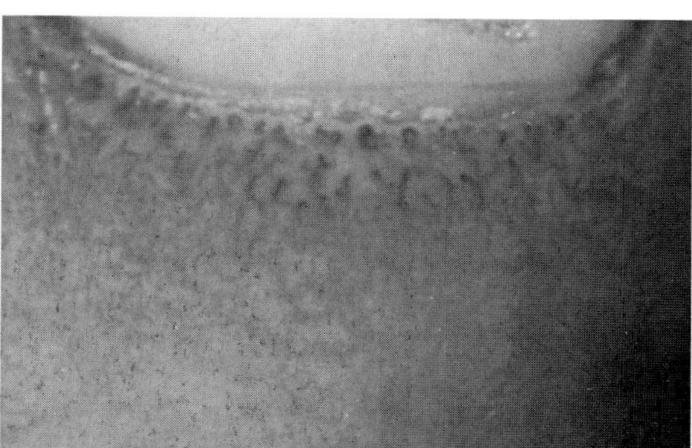

Figure 20–10. Advanced changes of the nailfold capillaries with gross thickening and dropout areas in a child with dermatomyositis. (Courtesy of Dr. Jay Kenik.)

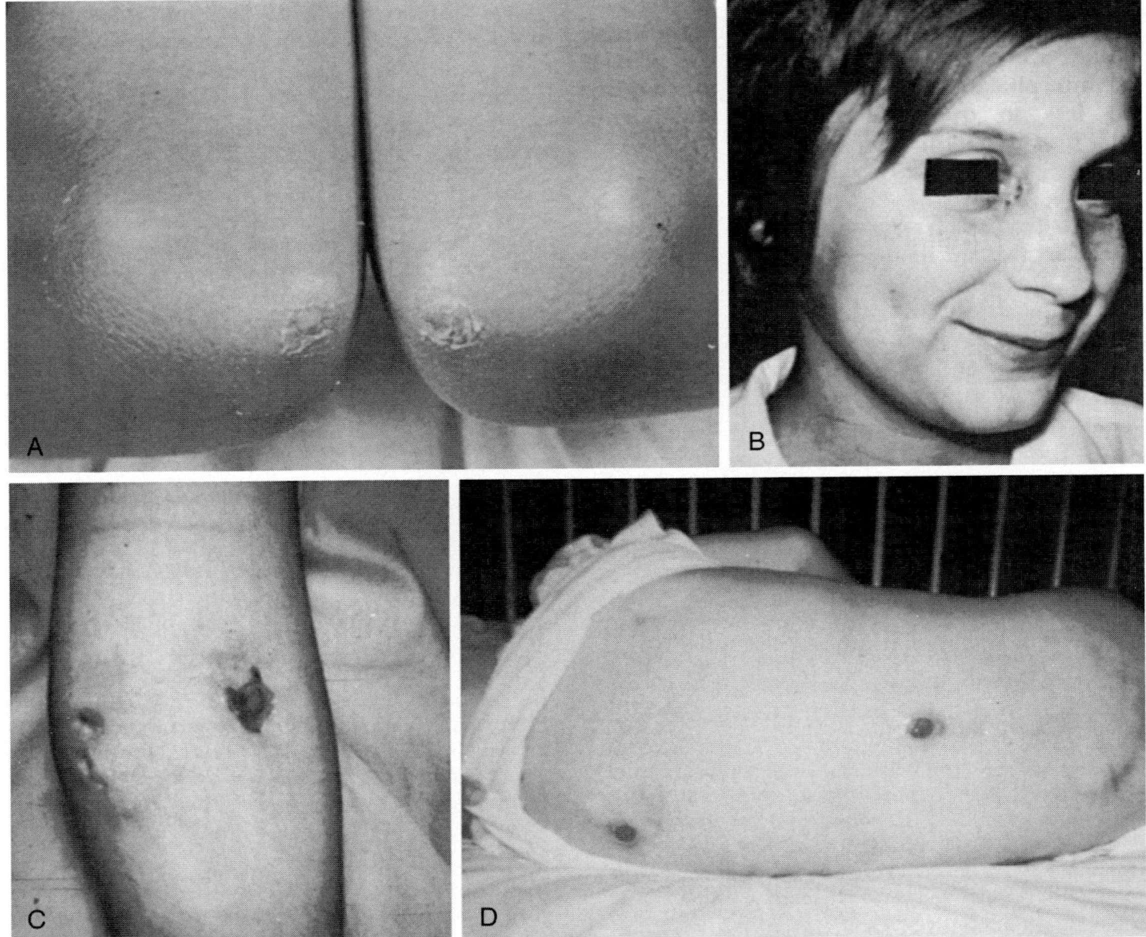

Figure 20–11. Acute dermatomyositis. *A,* Acute ulcerations over the olecranon processes in a child. *B,* Cutaneous ulcerations involving the inner canthal area of the face in a girl. *C,* Vasculitic ulcers over the elbow. *D,* Acute cutaneous ulcerations over pressure points in a 1½-year-old boy.

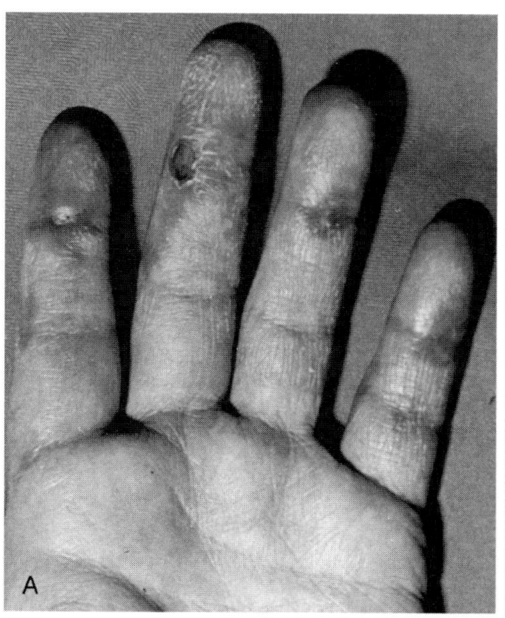

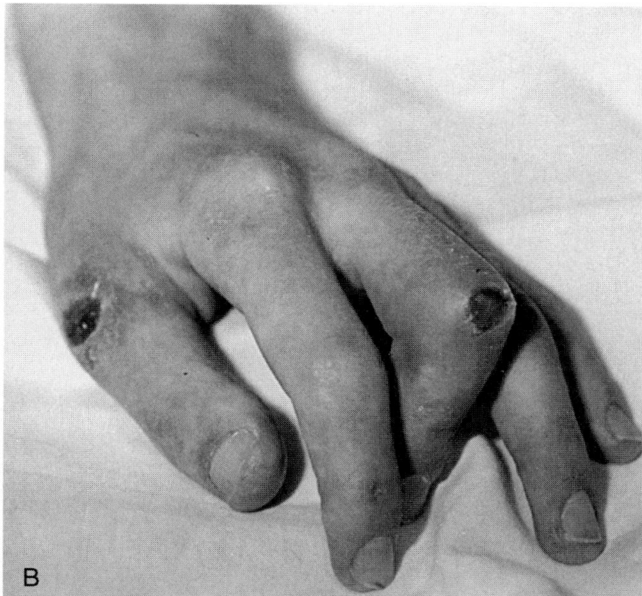

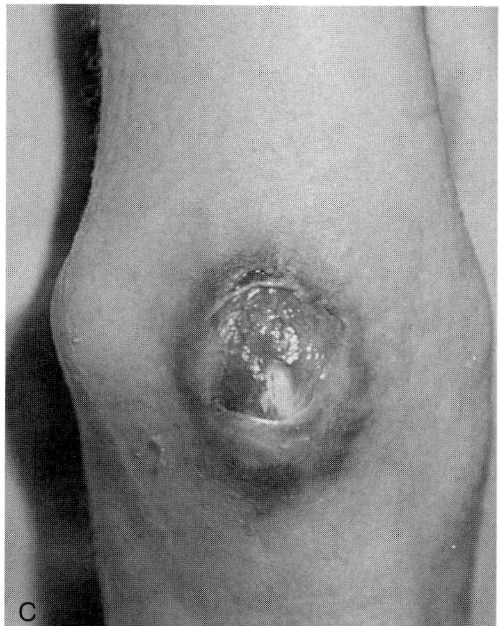

Figure 20–12. *A,* Vasculitic ulcers on fingers of a young boy with severe dermatomyositis. Ulcers on knuckles (*B*) and on elbow (*C*). These open ulcerations led to a *Staphylococcus aureus* bacteremia and endocarditis.

Calcinosis

Dystrophic calcification occurs in approximately 40 percent of children with JDM, often within 6 months of onset.[164] Occasionally, a child will present with calcinosis before it is realized that he has or had JDM.[165] We have seen one such patient. The various types of calcium deposition in children with JDM include subcutaneous plaques or nodules (Fig. 20–13*A* and *B*), large tumorous clumps in muscle groups (Table 20–7; Fig. 20–14*A* and *B*) or bridging joints, calcification within fascial planes, or an extensive subcutaneous exoskeleton (Fig. 20–15*A–C*).[157, 166] Calcinosis affecting the subcutaneous tissues can result in painful superficial ulceration of the overlying skin, with recurrent extrusion of small flecks of calcium salts. Calcinotic deposits may slowly resolve with time (Fig. 20–16*A–C*). If deposition in subcutaneous tissues, along fascial planes, and within muscles is extreme, the child may literally be encased within a shell of calcium salts. This type of calcinosis is unlikely to resolve completely, and results in severe disability.

Vasculitis

Visceral vasculitis occurs in a minority of children, usually soon after disease onset. It signifies a poor prognosis and sometimes rapidly leads to death.[24, 140, 167, 168] This complication is characterized by diffuse abdominal pain, pancreatitis, melena, and hematemesis, representing diffuse vasculitis of the mucosa of the gastrointestinal tract or an acute mesenteric infarction.[169–174] Free intraperitoneal air demonstrated radiographically indicates the presence of a perforation

Table 20–7

Forms of Dystrophic Calcification in Children with Dermatomyositis

FORM	FREQUENCY (%)
Superficial plaques or nodules, usually on the extremities	33
Deep, large, tumorous deposits, generally in the proximal muscles (calcinosis circumscripta)	20
Intermuscular fascial plane deposition (calcinosis universalis)	16
Severe, subcutaneous, reticular exoskeleton-like deposits	10
Mixed forms: superficial plaques or nodules, tumorous deposits, intermuscular fascial plane deposition	22

Modified from Bowyer SL, Blane CE, Sullivan DB, et al: Childhood dermatomyositis: Factors predicting functional outcome and development of dystrophic calcification. J Pediatr 103: 882–888, 1983.

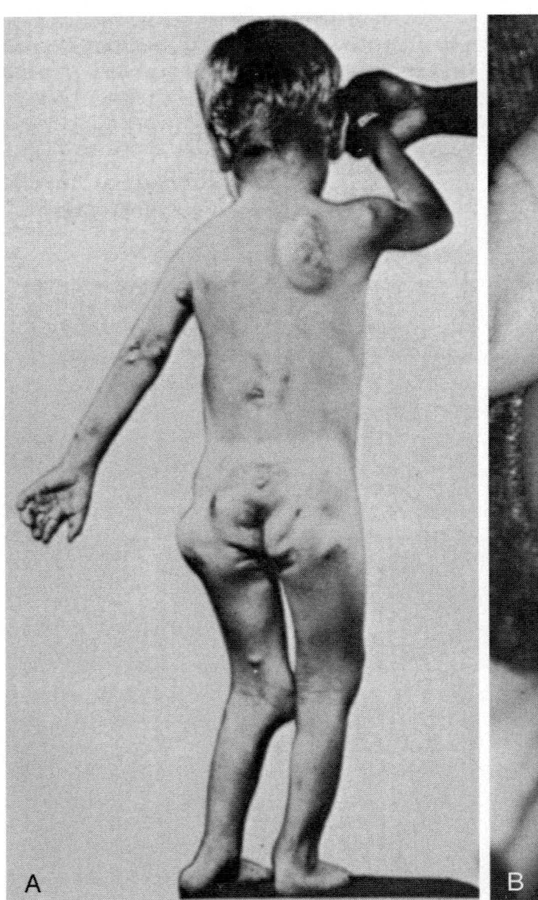

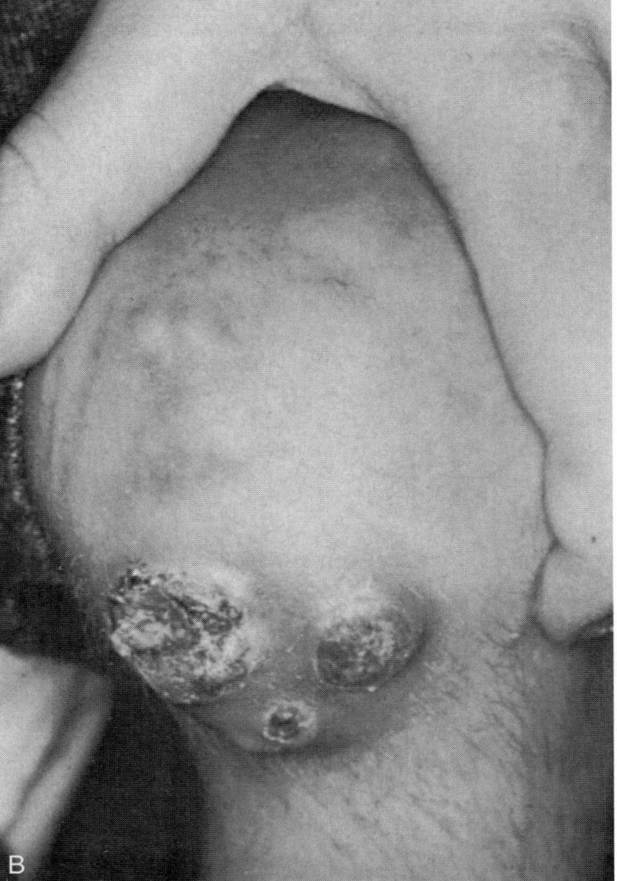

Figure 20–13. *A,* Widespread subcutaneous calcium deposits of varying size in a 6-year-old boy with dermatomyositis for 4 years. This is the same youngster shown in Figure 20–11*D*. *B,* A large area of tumorous calcification over the knee with cutaneous ulceration and drainage in the same boy shown in Figures 20–11*D* and 20–13*A*.

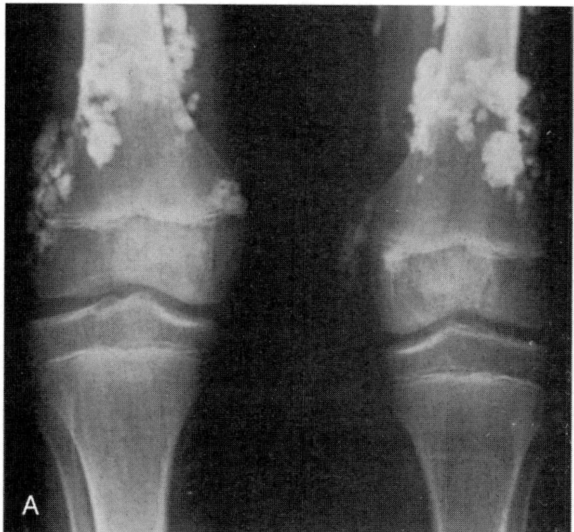

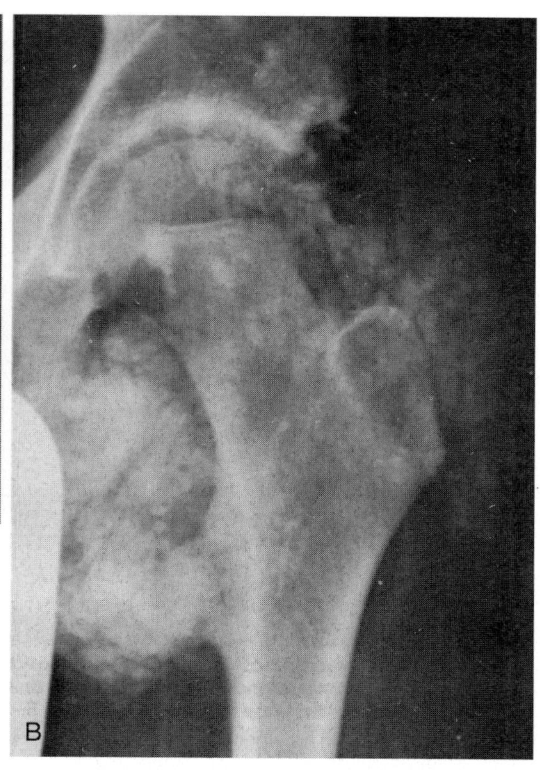

Figure 20–14. *A,* Calcinosis circumscripta in the supracondylar areas of the knees. *B,* Massive tumorous calcium deposits appeared unilaterally around the hip in a 7-year-old boy with onset of dermatomyositis at age 3 years.

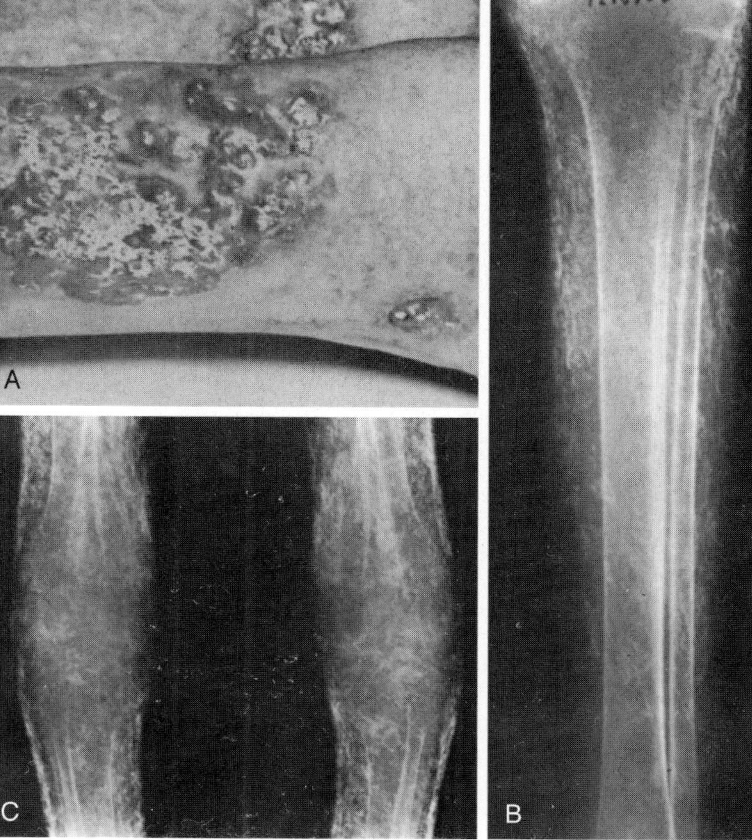

Figure 20–15. *A,* Calcinosis universalis in a 15-year-old girl with diffuse cutaneous ulcerations over the legs. Spicules of calcium salts were constantly extruded from these lesions. *B,* Interfascial deposition of calcium salts during the healing phases in the leg of a child with dermatomyositis. *C,* Radiograph of a 12-year-old girl with onset of acute, unremitting dermatomyositis at age 10. Extensive radiopaque deposits of calcium salts are observed throughout the interfascial planes of the musculature of the entire body.

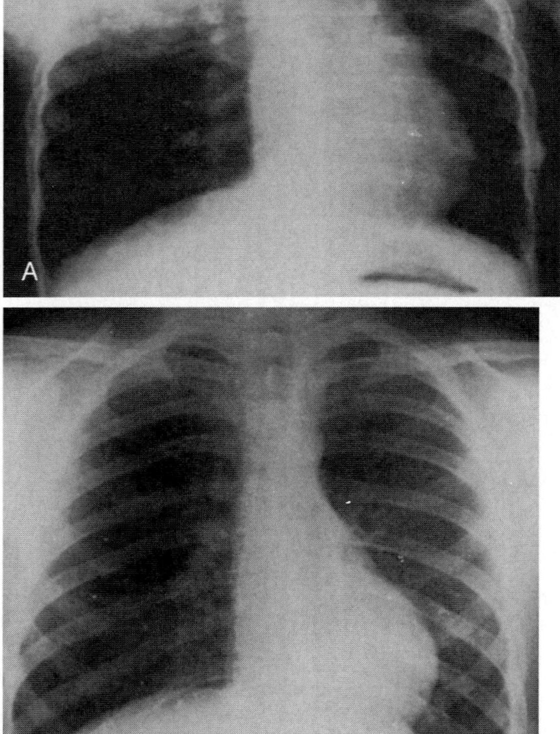

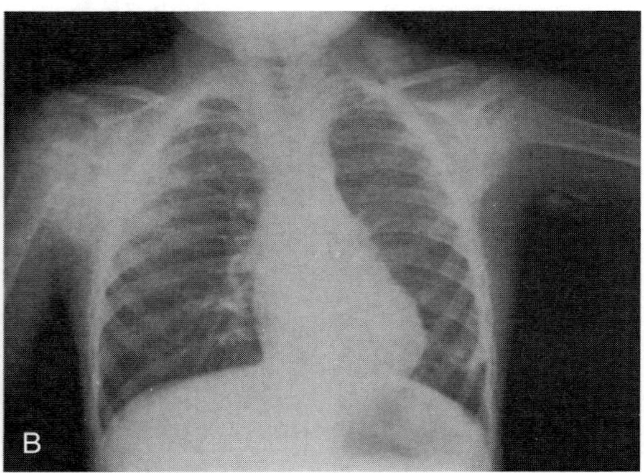

Figure 20–16. Radiographs of the chest of the same child in Figures 20–11*D* and 20–13*A* and *B*. *A,* Massive deposits of calcium salts around the right shoulder and in subcutaneous tissues of the chest. *B,* Partial resolution of the calcium deposits 2 years later. *C,* Almost complete resolution of the calcification about the left shoulder; residual calcium deposits still exist in the subcutaneous areas of the left lateral thorax.

of the gastrointestinal tract. Multiple perforations of the duodenum are particularly difficult to recognize.[170–174] Vasculitis of the gallbladder, urinary bladder, uterus, vagina, and testes can also occur.[24, 175–177] Widespread vascular disease can also involve both the central and the peripheral sensorimotor nervous systems.[24, 175, 176] Other evidence of vasculitis includes retinitis characterized by cotton-wool exudates (cytoid bodies).[178] A number of children have been reported to have repeated episodes of microscopic hematuria at onset that may represent mild glomerulitis.[11] Progression to renal insufficiency has not been described.

Cardiopulmonary Disease

The most frequently detected cardiac abnormalities are nonspecific murmurs and cardiomegaly, with or without electrocardiographic changes.[75, 179] Pericarditis has also been described. Serious cardiac involvement (e.g., acute myocarditis, conduction defects, and first-degree heart block) is rare but has been associated with death and may be delayed in onset until years after the diagnosis of the disease.[24, 75, 179–181] Radioisotopic studies suggest that subclinical involvement of cardiac muscle may be more common than has been appreciated.[182] Hypertension can also be present and may be severe.[10, 18, 24] It occurred in 25 percent of patients in the series reported by Crowe and associates[24] and is sometimes, but not always, associated with or exacerbated by glucocorticoid therapy. Raynaud's phenomenon is unusual in JDM but has been described in 2 to 15 percent of patients.[24, 146] Respiratory muscle weakness leads to restrictive pulmonary disease in a majority of moderately to severely affected children. Interstitial pneumonitis is rare.[183–187]

Lipodystrophy

The association of lipodystrophy and JDM has only recently been fully appreciated, but it may actually be quite common (20 percent of patients).[188, 189] Commens and colleagues[190] reported a 10-year-old boy with JDM who developed multiple areas of lipodystrophy over the buttocks and thighs. We have seen one such patient, a girl with mild JDM who had two areas of localized lipodystrophy. Generalized lipodystrophy has also been described in children with JDM.[191, 192] It is characterized by marked loss of subcutaneous tissue, often most noticeable over the face, hirsutism, acanthosis nigricans, clitoral enlargement, hepatomegaly, insulin resistance,[193] and hypertriglyceridemia (Fig. 20–17*A* and *B*). Tucker and colleagues[191] described the syndrome in three girls with JDM. Huemer and colleagues[194] reported two other patients with the com-

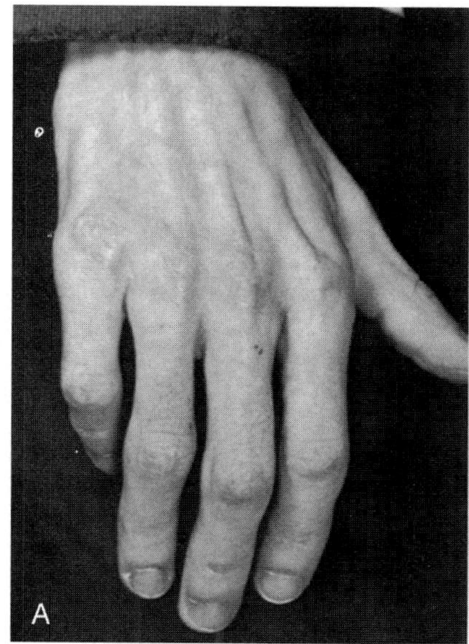

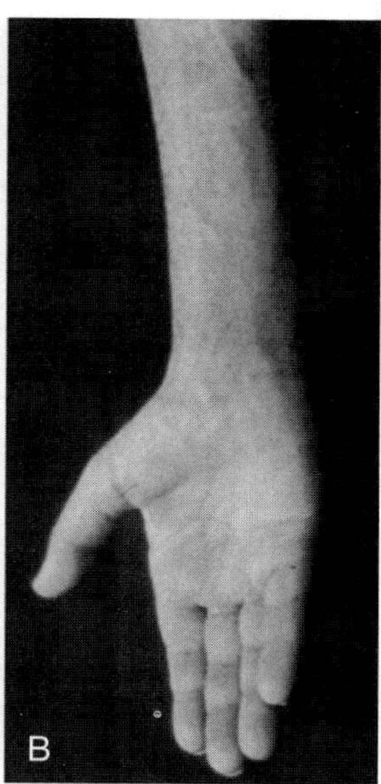

Figure 20–17. Paucity of subcutaneous tissue in two children with partial generalized lipoatrophy associated with dermatomyositis. *A,* Gottron's papules, periungual capillary changes, and interosseous muscle atrophy are evident in the hand. *B,* Loss of subcutaneous fat is indicated by prominence of the veins on the volar surface of the forearm.

plete syndrome and have found insulin resistance in three others. The significance of this complication and its relation to the pathogenesis of JDM are not known.

PATHOLOGY

The distinctive pathologic lesions of JDM involve the striated muscles, skin, and gastrointestinal tract. The severity of clinical disease may or may not be correlated with the intensity of the findings on microscopic examination.[164, 195] The histologic characteristics of JDM are contrasted with those in muscular dystrophy and neurogenic atrophy in Table 20–8.

Skeletal Muscle

Muscle fibers characteristically demonstrate group atrophy or necrosis at the periphery of the fascicle (Fig. 20–18*A* and *B*).[24] This perifascicular myopathy is characteristic of JDM and is often associated with a noninflammatory capillaropathy.[24, 196] Nonspecific changes of myopathy include disruption of the myofibrils and tubular systems, central nuclear migration, prominent nuclei, and basophilia.[95, 164] Concomitant degeneration and regeneration of muscle fibers are seen and result in moderate variation in fiber size. Areas of focal necrosis are replaced during the healing phase by an interstitial proliferation of connective tissue and fat.

The majority of specimens from muscle biopsies contain an inflammatory exudate. The inflammatory cells, which are often sparse and are principally lymphocytes and mononuclear cells, are located predominantly in the perimysium and perivascularly around the septae or in the fascicles (Fig. 20–19*A*–*C*). Macrophages, plasma cells, mast cells, and, rarely, eosinophils or basophils are also present.[59, 197, 198]

Electron microscopy may demonstrate focal degeneration of the myofibrils, cytoplasmic masses, disorganization of sarcomeres, disruption of the Z lines and Z-disc streaming, actin-myosin filament disorganization, thickening of the capillary basement membranes, mitochondrial abnormalities, or an increase in vacuole formation (Fig. 20–20*A* and *B*).[199–201] Lysosomes are more frequent in inflammatory myopathy than in normal

Table 20–8

Comparison of Muscle Histopathology in Juvenile Dermatomyositis, Muscular Dystrophy, and Neurogenic Muscle Atrophy

	DERMATOMYOSITIS	MUSCULAR DYSTROPHY	NEUROGENIC ATROPHY
Focal necrosis and phagocytosis of muscle fibers	++	±	–
Fiber regeneration	++	±	–
Endomysial proliferation	++	++	–
Random fiber atrophy	++	++	–
Inflammatory cell infiltrates	++	±	–
Vasculitis	++	–	–
Central migration of nuclei	+	++	±
Fat cell hyperplasia	+	+	–
Fiber atrophy	±	++	±
Motor unit atrophy	–	–	++

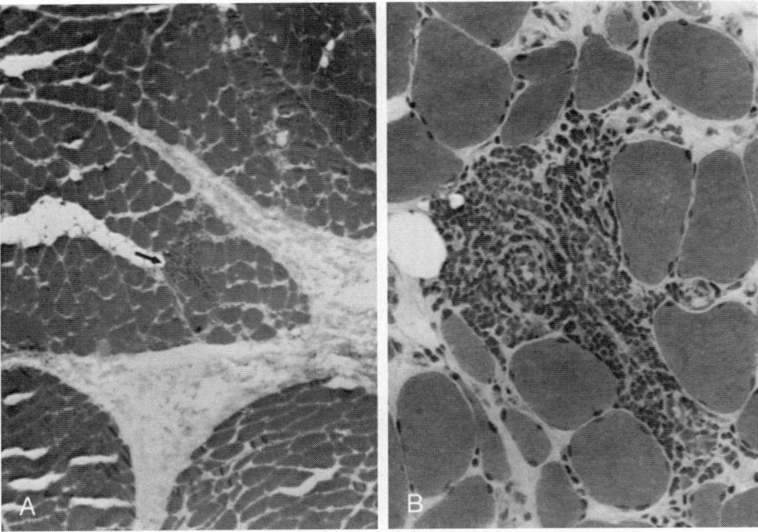

Figure 20–18. *A,* Muscle biopsy (H&E, ×40). Scattered foci (*arrow*) of perivascular inflammation. *B,* Enlargement (H&E, ×250) of central area of *A.* Perivascular mononuclear inflammatory infiltrate, arterial wall thickening, and endothelial prominence.

muscle. The relation between these organelles and muscle necrosis is uncertain.

The regenerative phase is probably dependent on the mononuclear myoblast that is derived from satellite cells.[202] Regenerating fibers contain increased oxidative enzyme and alkaline phosphatase activities.[202–204] Immunoglobulins can often be demonstrated on the sarcolemmal membrane by immunofluorescence microscopy, but this finding is of doubtful pathogenic significance.[70, 205] Damaged muscle fibers have an increase in calcium content,[206, 207] which may explain the uptake of technetium-99m diphosphonate by the muscles in inflammatory myopathy.

Blood Vessels

JDM should be considered primarily as a systemic vasculopathy rather than simply an inflammation of muscle and skin. Vasculitis and noninflammatory vasculopathy are hallmarks of JDM. A necrotizing vasculitis, presumably resulting from immune-complex deposition, affects arterioles, capillaries, and venules of the striated muscles, gastrointestinal tract, skin, and subcutaneous tissues. Especially in the gastrointestinal tract, vasculitis leads to infarction and results in ulceration and diffuse bleeding. The early studies of Banker and Victor[140] identified this type of vasculitis as an important prognostic factor in the survival of children with JDM. Studies by Crowe and associates[24] identified distinctive features associated with persistent morbidity, adding to the understanding of this complication. In their patients, muscle infarction and ulceration of the cutaneous and gastrointestinal tissues were associated with a zonal loss of the capillary bed, areas of focal infarction of muscle, non-necrotizing lymphocytic vasculitis, and noninflammatory endarteropathy (Fig. 20–

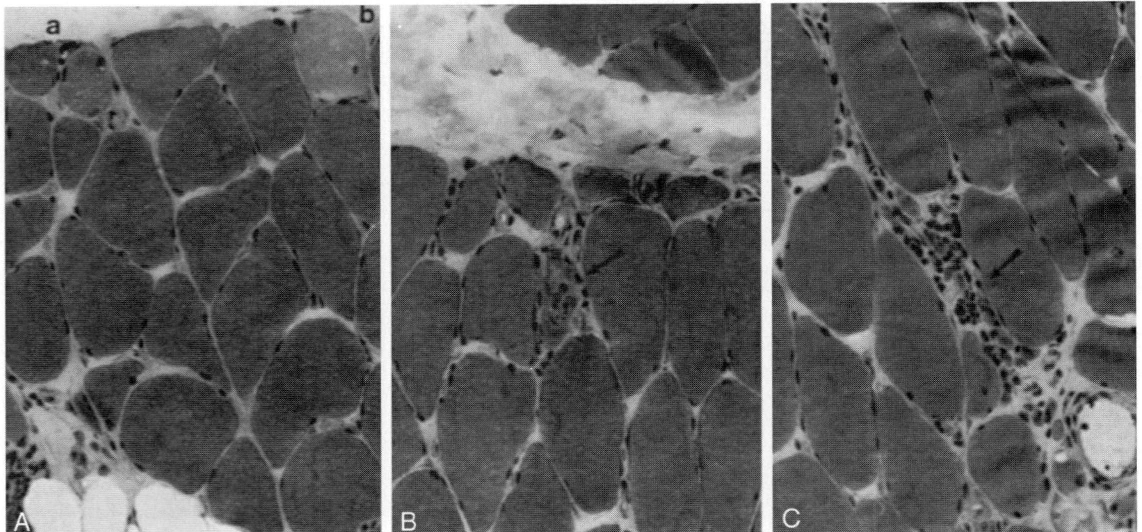

Figure 20–19. *A,* Muscle biopsy (H&E, ×250). Atrophic muscle fibers (a), and pale necrotic fiber (b). *B,* Muscle biopsy (H&E, ×430). Partially necrotic myofiber with phagocytosis. *C,* Muscle biopsy (H&E, ×250). Endomysial mononuclear cell inflammatory infiltrate.

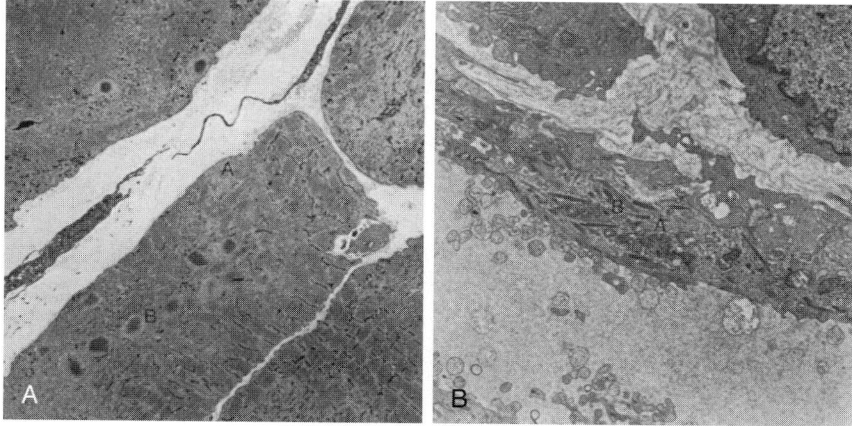

Figure 20–20. *A,* Electron microscopic section of muscle from a 5-year-old girl with acute dermatomyositis shows myofibrillar disarray (A) and filamentous dense bodies (B) (×5525). *B,* Electron microscopic section of muscle from an 8-year-old boy with tubulovesicular inclusions (A) and elongated mitochondria with parallel cristae (B) in endothelial cells of a small blood vessel (×15,000).

21*A–C*). Conversely, severe vasculopathy was absent from the muscle specimens of children with limited disease.[24] This spectrum of capillary endothelial damage had also been suggested in previous studies.[70, 140, 208]

Capillaries

Widespread capillaropathy leads to intravascular coagulation, microvascular occlusion and infarction, and associated perifascicular myopathy.[24, 208] These capillary changes, although characteristic, are not specific for JDM and have been described in other connective tissue diseases, viral and rickettsial infections, malignancy, and normal wound healing.[208, 209]

Changes in the capillaries can be seen in JDM in the nailfold areas (see Figs. 20–7, 20–9, and 20–10) and in tissues by light and electron microscopy.[24, 140] Endothelial swelling and necrosis, capillary thrombosis and obliteration, and endoplasmic tubuloreticular inclusions are present (see Fig. 20–3).[140, 210–212] The latter are sometimes associated with endothelial damage and are

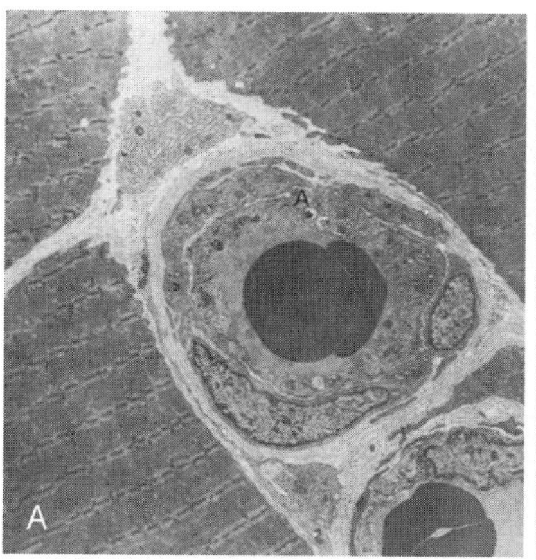

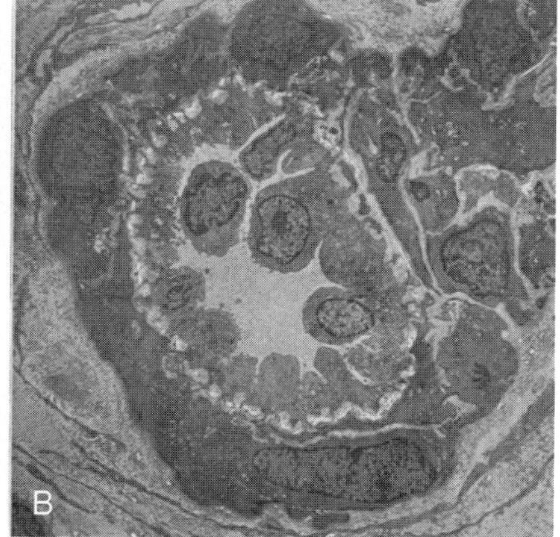

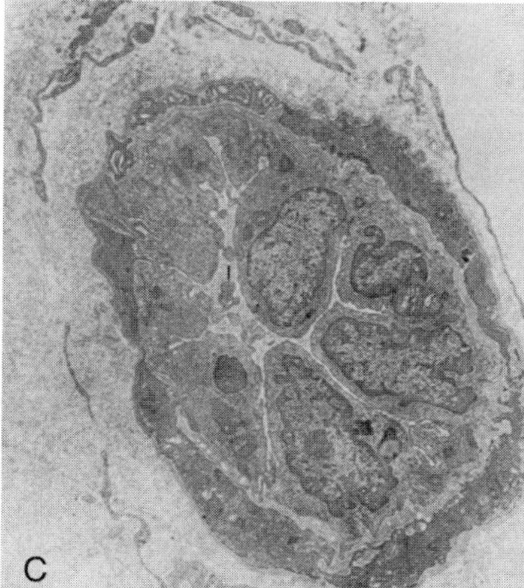

Figure 20–21. Electron microscopic section of muscle from patient in Figure 20–20*B. A,* Slight degree of endothelial cells swelling (A) in an arteriole (×63,337). *B,* More marked endarteropathy (×5200). *C,* Virtual occlusion of the lumen (1) of a small arteriole by extreme swelling of the endothelial cells (×10,968). Thrombosis and inflammation are not present.

most common early in the disease.[24, 208] These undulating tubules may be present in the cytoplasm of 98 percent of the endothelial cells[140] and are regarded by some as abnormally thick myofilaments.[213]

Arteries

Small muscular arteries may be involved by an immune-complex vasculitis that leads to infarction of muscle.[24] Other arterial lesions are unassociated with an actual inflammatory cell infiltrate. These changes do not always correspond to those present in the capillaries, and severe capillaropathy may not be associated with discernible endarteropathy.

IgM, IgG, and C3 were deposited in the perimysial veins in 9 of the 11 cases studied by Whitaker and Engle.[70] Crowe and associates[24] described similar changes but did not find IgG in the lesions. Diffuse linear and occasionally granular vascular wall deposits of IgM, C3d, and fibrin were also observed in the areas of noninflammatory vasculopathy. Electron microscopy has not provided evidence of subendothelial deposition of immunoglobulins within vessel walls, as might have been expected in classic immune-complex disease, although circulating complexes and anticomplementary activity are often present in the blood.[75, 214]

Veins

Intramural and perivascular mononuclear cell inflammatory infiltrates are often identified in the veins and may or may not be associated with immunoglobulin deposition.[24, 70] The endothelial cells may contain inclusions.

Connective Tissues

It is not known whether autoimmunity to connective tissues or collagen is involved in the pathogenesis of JDM. In human muscle, types I and III collagens are found in the endomysium and perimysium, although the endomysium predominantly contains type I collagen.[215, 216] Basement membranes contain type IV collagen. Type V collagen is present in the small blood vessels and endomysium. The synthesis of collagen appears to be excessive in myositis.

Skin

A capillary endothelial change similar to that in muscle is almost always present in involved skin.[24] Histopathologic examination of the skin of patients with dermatomyositis may demonstrate epidermal atrophy, liquefaction degeneration of basal cells, vascular dilatation, and lymphocytic infiltration of the dermis.[217] An increase in acid mucopolysaccharides has been found in both involved and uninvolved skin in approximately one third of patients.[218] In a study of the histopathology of Gottron's papules,[219] basal layer vasculopathy, periodic acid-Schiff–positive basement membrane thickening, upper dermal mucin deposition, and a diffuse upper dermal mononuclear infiltrate were frequently found. Epidermal hyperplasia, consisting of acanthosis or papillomatosis, was often present. Epidermal atrophy was rare.

In the healing phase of the disease, calcium salts, hydroxyapatite or fluorapatite,[220, 221] may be identified in the skin and subcutaneous tissues as well as in the interfascial planes of the muscle. With calcinosis, there may be persistence of fibrosis as well as some degree of round cell and giant cell infiltration. Mechanisms for the excessive accumulation of hydroxyapatite are unknown.[75]

Gastrointestinal Tract

Ulceration or perforation resulting from vasculopathy can occur in any part of the gastrointestinal tract, including the esophagus.[24, 140] Serious disease of this type develops in approximately 10 percent of patients.[75] Pneumatosis intestinalis has been described in JDM.[170, 171] Except for the vascular disease, smooth muscle is not generally a site of involvement. Pancreatitis and hepatitis are extremely rare.[139] Hepatosplenomegaly and lymphadenopathy occur in fewer than 5 percent of children with JDM. Hepatomegaly may be associated with lipoatrophy and insulin resistance.

Heart

Cardiac muscle is seldom clinically affected by the primary pathologic process.[222, 223] A few cases of carditis have been described, with areas of focal myocardial fibrosis and contraction-band necrosis. Interstitial myocarditis and narrowing of the coronary arteries have been reported.[24]

Kidneys

Although renal abnormalities have occasionally been noted in JDM, they appear to be rare.[11, 140] In one report, however, histopathologic findings in five of six renal biopsies were abnormal.[11] The changes that were described included cellular hyperplasia, capillary thickening, capsular adhesions, and hyperplasia involving the small blood vessels. Renal abnormalities have not been common in postmortem reports,[16, 24, 176] and the possibility that overlap syndromes were responsible for some of the renal abnormalities that have been described cannot be excluded.

DIFFERENTIAL DIAGNOSIS

The five criteria outlined in Table 20–9 can be applied to the diagnosis of JDM, although their sensitivity and specificity have not been validated in children with myopathies. In pediatric rheumatology, a diagnosis of

Table 20–9

Criteria Used for Diagnosis of Juvenile Dermatomyositis

1. Symmetric weakness of the proximal musculature
2. Characteristic cutaneous changes consisting of heliotrope discoloration of the eyelids with periorbital edema, and an erythematous, scaly rash over the dorsal aspects of the metacarpophalangeal and proximal interphalangeal joints (Gottron's papules)
3. Elevation of the serum level of one or more of the skeletal muscle enzymes: creatine kinase, aspartate aminotransferase, lactic dehydrogenase, and aldolase
4. Electromyographic demonstration of the characteristics of myopathy and denervation
5. Muscle biopsy documenting histologic evidence of necrosis and inflammation

Data from Bohan A, Peter JB: Polymyositis and dermatomyositis. N Engl J Med 292: 344, 403, 1975.

JDM requires the presence of the pathognomonic rash and two of the other criteria.[167, 168, 224] In general, the first two criteria (proximal muscle weakness and classic rash) are almost always present; criteria number 3 (elevated serum levels of muscle enzymes), number 4 (electromyographic changes), and number 5 (histopathologic changes) provide laboratory support for the diagnosis. A diagnosis of JDM is not necessarily excluded by failure to meet one or more of these criteria, except for that related to the dermatitis.

The differential diagnosis of JDM includes juvenile polymyositis, postinfectious myositis, primary myopathies, and inflammatory myositis accompanying other connective tissue diseases such as scleroderma or mixed connective tissue disease. In the presence of the characteristic rash and weak, painful, or tender proximal muscles, the correct diagnosis is usually straightforward. Early in the disease course, however, especially in the absence of the characteristic rash, the differential diagnosis can be challenging.

Juvenile Polymyositis

Juvenile polymyositis has been very uncommon in our experience.[23, 25, 45] Age at onset and sex ratio are comparable to those for JDM. The same environmental triggers and immunogenetic risk factors have been associated with onset, along with administration of D-penicillamine and growth hormone or following bone marrow transplantation.[2] Weakness of both proximal and distal muscles occurs at presentation. The nailfold capillary pattern is normal. In most patients, the disease has a chronic course, often relatively unresponsive to glucocorticoids. Infantile polymyositis during the first year of life may in some cases be secondary to maternal in utero infection.[225] Severe muscle weakness with hypotonia and dysphagia are present at onset. Muscle biopsy is usually necessary for accurate diagnosis.

Postinfectious Myositis

Acute transient myositis can follow certain viral infections, especially influenza A and B,[82] and coxsackievirus B.[77, 78, 80, 116] Although myalgia is a characteristic complaint of acute influenza, myositis per se is rare (Table 20–10). Coxsackie B virus causes epidemic pleurodynia (*Bornholm disease*) characterized by fever and sharp pain in the muscles of the chest and abdominal wall. This syndrome is sometimes preceded by a moderate to severe headache, nausea, vomiting, and pharyngitis. The illness is most common in children and adolescents and usually lasts for 3 to 5 days. Treatment is supportive.

Other infectious causes of myositis include toxoplasmosis, trichinosis, staphylococcal bacteremia, schistosomiasis, and trypanosomiasis.[226, 227] Toxoplasmosis may be associated with a syndrome that resembles dermatomyositis.[91, 93, 227] Trichinosis, caused by ingestion of the larval cyst of the nematode *Trichinella spiralis,* is characterized initially by fever, diarrhea, and abdominal pain, followed in 1 week by periorbital edema and swelling and tenderness of muscles, especially those of the face, neck, and chest. Peripheral blood eosinophilia is often striking, and biopsy of affected muscles confirms the presence of the larvae and, later, calcified cysts. Treatment includes glucocorticoids to diminish inflammation and agents such as mebendazole and thiabendazole.

Staphylococcal *pyomyositis* is an abscess in skeletal muscle following local muscle injury. It occurs at all ages and is more common in boys than in girls. Lesions may be solitary or multiple and are usually located in the thigh, calf, buttock, arm, scapular areas, or chest wall. The abscess is tender and, if not too deep, warm. Low-grade fever is usually present. Symptoms last for up to a week. Ultrasonography or gallium 67 citrate scanning helps to localize the lesion. Severe pustular acne may occasionally be associated with inflammatory disease of muscle as well as an arthritis.[228] Treatment includes intravenous antistaphylococcal antibiotics. Acute myopathy may also follow the use of isotretinoin for treatment of acne.[229]

In 1957, Lundberg[83] described a contagious illness that occurred most commonly in preadolescent boys and was characterized by fever, headache, rhinitis, cough, nausea, and vomiting that lasted 2 to 3 days. This was followed by severe proximal calf pain and tenderness (*myalgia cruris epidemica*) that was exacerbated by movement. Complete recovery occurred after approximately 3 days. Laboratory studies demonstrated a slightly elevated erythrocyte sedimentation rate, moderate leukopenia with relative lymphocytosis, and a concomitant elevation of the serum levels of creatine kinase (CK) and aspartate aminotransferase (AST). Although no specific infectious agent was identified in this classic study, subse-

Table 20–10

Acute Myositis Associated With Influenza B Infection

Onset during recovery phase of the viral illness
Predominant severe bilateral pain and tenderness of the gastrocnemius and soleus muscles
Elevated serum muscle enzyme concentrations (creatine kinase, aspartate aminotransferase)
Recovery in 3 to 5 days

Table 20–11

Classification of the Major Neuromuscular Disorders of Infancy and Childhood

- I. Primary myopathies
  - A. The muscular dystrophies
    - 1. Sex-linked recessive
      - a. Duchenne's muscular dystrophy
      - b. Becker's muscular dystrophy
    - 2. Autosomal dominant
      - a. Facioscapulohumeral (Déjérine-Landouzy)
      - b. Distal myopathy (Welander's)
      - c. Ocular myopathy
      - d. Oculopharyngeal muscular dystrophy
    - 3. Autosomal recessive
      - a. Limb-girdle (Erb's)
  - B. Congenital myopathies
    - 1. Congenital muscular dystrophy
    - 2. Benign congenital myopathy
    - 3. Central core disease
    - 4. Nemaline myopathy
    - 5. Myotubular myopathy
  - C. Myotonic disorders
    - 1. Myotonia congenita (Thomsen's disease)
    - 2. Dystrophia myotonia (Steinert's disease)
  - D. Metabolic disorders
    - 1. Glycogen storage disease (myophosphorylase deficiency)
    - 2. Familial periodic paralysis
    - 3. Carnitine deficiency
    - 4. Carnitine palmitoyl-transferase deficiency
    - 5. Secondary to endocrinopathies
      - a. Addison's disease
      - b. Cushing's syndrome
      - c. Hypopituitarism
      - d. Hypothyroidism
    - 6. Myoadenylate deaminase deficiency
    - 7. Chronic hemodialysis
  - E. Inflammatory diseases
    - 1. Postinfectious
      - a. Viral syndromes
        - i. Influenza B
        - ii. Coxsackie B virus
        - iii. Echovirus
        - iv. Poliomyelitis
      - b. Toxoplasmosis, sarcosporidiosis
      - c. Trichinosis, cysticercosis
      - d. Septic (staphylococci and other pyogenic organisms)
      - e. Tetanus
      - f. Gas gangrene
    - 2. Connective tissue diseases
  - F. Genetic abnormalities
    - 1. Osteogenesis imperfecta
    - 2. Ehlers-Danlos syndrome
    - 3. Mucopolysaccharidoses
  - G. Trauma
    - 1. Physical (Crush, rhabdomyolysis)
    - 2. Toxic (Snakebite)
    - 3. Drugs
      - a. Glucocorticoids
      - b. Hydroxychloroquine
      - c. Diuretics, licorice
      - d. Amphotericin B
      - e. Alcohol
      - f. Vincristine
      - g. D-Penicillamine
      - h. Cimetidine
- II. Neurogenic atrophies
  - A. Spinal muscular and anterior horn-cell dysfunction
    - 1. Infantile and juvenile muscle atrophy
    - 2. Arthrogryposis multiplex congenita
    - 3. Amyotrophic lateral sclerosis
  - B. Peripheral nerve dysfunction
    - 1. Peroneal muscular atrophy (Charcot-Marie-Tooth disease)
    - 2. Neurofibromatosis
    - 3. Guillain-Barré syndrome
  - C. Disorders of neuromuscular transmission
    - 1. Congenital myasthenia gravis
    - 2. Botulism
    - 3. Tick paralysis
    - 4. Organophosphate poisoning

Adapted from The Research Group on Neuromuscular Diseases: Classification of the neuromuscular disorders. J Neurol Sci 6: 165, 1968.

quent reports have confirmed influenza B as the most common causative agent.[84] Treatment is supportive.

Neuromuscular Diseases and Myopathies

In the absence of characteristic skin changes, the differential diagnosis of JDM includes a wide variety of neuromuscular disorders in children (Tables 20–11 to 20–14).[145] From a practical point of view, the diagnostic possibilities listed in Table 20–11 rarely enter into the differential diagnosis. Early in the disease, or before the development of cutaneous changes, muscular dystrophy, myotonia, myoadenylate deaminase deficiency, or acute rhabdomyolysis may be confused with JDM.

The possibility of *muscular dystrophy* is suggested by a family history of myopathy and an insidious onset of slowly progressive, predominantly proximal muscle weakness. Constitutional signs, muscle tenderness, and cutaneous abnormalities are absent. In Duchenne's muscular dystrophy, there is a characteristic hypertrophy of the calves, a sign that occurs in other myopathies and occasionally in long-standing JDM as well. The hereditary nature of Duchenne's muscular dystrophy is demonstrated by the presence of markedly elevated levels of serum CK in the patient and the patient's mother. Hypotonia in infancy, often associated with projectile vomiting, is a characteristic of the mitochondrial disorders involving the branched chain amino acids. Paroxysmal myoglobinuria may occasionally be encountered. Certain drugs or toxins, including alcohol, clofibrate, D-penicillamine, glucocorticoids, and hydroxychloroquine, can induce a myopathy.[230, 231]

Myoadenylate deaminase deficiency (MDD) (Table 20–15)[232, 233] occurs in an autosomal recessive primary form and as an acquired disorder associated with rheumatic and neuromuscular diseases. Current data suggest that homozygous MDD is relatively common in that 2 percent of muscle biopsies have been found to be deficient in enzyme activity (<2 percent in the primary, <15 percent in the secondary form).

Table 20–12

Classification of Neuromuscular Disorders by Course

Acute
- Muscular dystrophy
- Paroxysmal myoglobinuria

Chronic
- Dermatomyositis
- Muscular dystrophy (Duchenne's, Déjérine-Landouzy)
- Central core disease and nemaline myopathy
- Congenital hypotonia
- Glycogen storage disease
- Myoadenylate deaminase deficiency
- Endocrine myopathy
- Nutritional myopathy
- Amyloidosis

Episodic
- Paramyotonia congenita
- Familial periodic paralysis
- Hypokalemia
- Myasthenia gravis
- Myasthenia of malignancy

Muscle fatigue, stiffness, and cramping after exercise may be noted, beginning in childhood (23 percent) or adolescence (26 percent) in some, but not all, deficient individuals. Patients with MDD may demonstrate a decreased muscle mass, hypotonia, and weakness. With forearm exercise, there is a failure of plasma ammonia to rise along with inosine monophosphate. Electromyographic findings are nonspecific. The muscle biopsy specimen in primary MDD is normal except for the absence of adenosine monophosphate deaminase. Activity of this enzyme is normal in other tissues.

Endocrinopathies, especially hyper- and hypothyroidism, hyper- and hypoparathyroidism, diabetes mellitus, and myopathy associated with idiopathic or iatrogenic Cushing's syndrome, should be considered in the differential diagnosis of JDM without evidence of cutaneous disease.[234] Myasthenia gravis is rare, and the diagnosis is suggested by a decremental response to repetitive nerve stimulation, involvement of ocular and distal muscles, and improvement of the weakness after administration of cholinergic drugs. Primary neurogenic atrophies, including infantile and juvenile spinal muscular atrophy, are associated with proximal muscle weakness and, rarely, may be confused with inflammatory myositis.

Table 20–13

Classification of Neuromuscular Disorders by Predominant Site of Involvement

Proximal
- Dermatomyositis
- Steroid myopathy
- Thyrotoxic myopathy
- Sarcoid myopathy
- Muscular dystrophy
- Proximal familial neuromuscular diseases

Distal
- Myotonic dystrophy
- Distal muscular dystrophy
- Peroneal muscular atrophy
- Motor system diseases

Proximal or distal
- Floppy infant syndrome
- Myotonia congenita
- Dystrophic ophthalmoplegia
- Myasthenia gravis
- Periodic paralysis

Table 20–14

Classification of Neuromuscular Disorders by Age of Onset

Congenital
- Congenital muscular dystrophy
- Central core disease
- Nemaline myopathy
- Congenital hypoplasia
- Benign hypotonia

Childhood
- Muscular dystrophy (Duchenne's)
- Glycogen storage diseases
- Myoadenylate deaminase deficiency

Late childhood and adolescence
- Muscular dystrophy (Déjérine-Landouzy)
- Myotonia congenita
- Periodic paralysis

Any age
- Dermatomyositis
- Steroid and hydroxychloroquine myopathies
- Myasthenia gravis
- Trichinosis

Myositis With Other Connective Tissue Diseases

Children with systemic scleroderma (see Chapter 21), mixed connective tissue disease (see Chapter 23), or, occasionally, SLE (see Chapter 18), may have skin and muscle abnormalities at onset that suggest a diagnosis of JDM.[32] The differentiation of these diseases is usually not difficult, however, because clinical features unique to each are almost always present as well. The laboratory evaluation provides supportive or definitive diagnostic information in most instances.

The child with JDM may have a malar dermatitis that is similar in distribution to the butterfly rash of SLE but often lacks relatively well-defined borders. Furthermore, heliotrope suffusion and periorbital edema are not characteristic of SLE, as they are of

Table 20–15

Myoadenylate Deaminase Deficiency

- Male:female ratio 2:1
- Muscle fatigue, stiffness, or cramping after exercise in some but not all
- Decreased muscle mass, hypotonia, and weakness, often since childhood
- Failure of plasma ammonia to rise with forearm exercise
- Nonspecific electromyographic abnormalities
- Frequently normal muscle biopsy histopathology except absent adenylate deaminase
- Autosomal recessive (?); acquired (associated with rheumatic and neuromuscular disorders)

JDM. Periungual capillary changes are characteristic of various connective tissue diseases, but Gottron's papules are present only in children with JDM. Although early cutaneous abnormalities of scleroderma and JDM are quite different, during the courses of these diseases the skin changes sometimes tend to become similar to each other.

Myositis occurs in systemic scleroderma and mixed connective tissue disease, and, to a limited extent, in SLE and systemic-onset juvenile rheumatoid arthritis (JRA). The myositis of JDM can be differentiated from that of other connective tissue diseases by its severity, by the greater elevation of serum levels of muscle enzymes, and by the results of histologic examination of muscle obtained by biopsy. In uncomplicated JRA, acute rheumatic fever, SLE, or scleroderma, muscle biopsy demonstrates focal accumulations of lymphocytes, patchy fiber atrophy, and increased interstitial connective tissue but no significant vasculopathy.[235–237] Perifascicular atrophy has been described in SLE. In Sjögren's syndrome, muscle fiber degeneration and atrophy, sarcoplasmic degeneration, and microcyst formation have been noted.[238] In polyarteritis, a necrotizing vasculitis with muscle fiber degeneration may be identified, along with areas of neurogenic atrophy. Laboratory evaluation confirms normal or only slightly elevated serum levels of the muscle enzymes in SLE and other connective tissue diseases, compared with marked elevations in JDM. Systemic features of SLE, such as pericarditis and pleural effusions, are rare in JDM. The arthritis of JDM is uncommon and usually mild; that of SLE is much more frequent and, although nonerosive, may be quite florid at onset and extremely painful. Occasionally, an overlap syndrome between JDM and JRA occurs.[33] Although rare, it was present in two children we have seen. One girl appeared to have the simultaneous onset of both diseases accompanied by subcutaneous rheumatoid nodules. A steroid-responsive myositis, differentiated from dermatomyositis by the absence of cutaneous disease and of vasculopathy on muscle biopsy, occurs in infancy.[239]

Miscellaneous Disorders

Rare causes of myositis in children include multicentric reticulohistiocytosis,[240] giant cell myositis,[241] and sarcoidosis.[242] A number of uncommon forms of myositis have been described especially in adults,[242a] including inclusion body myositis,[243–245] eosinophilic myositis,[246] and disease restricted to one muscle group or extremity, such as localized nodular myositis[247, 248] and proliferative myositis.[249] Inclusion body myositis is resistant to all forms of therapy. Rhabdomyolysis may follow an upper respiratory infection, trauma, or extreme muscular exertion.[250] Onset is generally acute and is characterized by profound weakness, myoglobulinuria, very high levels of serum muscle enzymes, and, occasionally, oliguria and renal failure. It may also occur after a snakebite, in heatstroke, and in the familial malignant hyperpyrexia syndrome.

Myositis ossificans progressiva (fibrodysplasia ossificans progressiva) is a rare autosomal dominant inflammatory disorder that results in painful swelling of muscle and fascia, followed by fibrosis and calcification (Fig. 20–22).[251–253] The child may present with a spontaneous joint contracture. The clinical diagnosis is often elusive until calcification and, later, ossification, are evident on the radiograph. Biopsy findings of affected sites at an early stage may be misleading and misinterpreted as a malignant sarcoma. The back of the neck and posterior trunk are often involved initially, followed by the muscles of the limbs. Palmar and plantar fascia may be affected as well. The great toes are often congenitally short, and the thumbs are sometimes involved. The disease early in its course is characterized by exacerbations and remissions and slowly progresses to severe debility. Diphosphonate therapy has been effective in some patients (see Fig. 20–22).

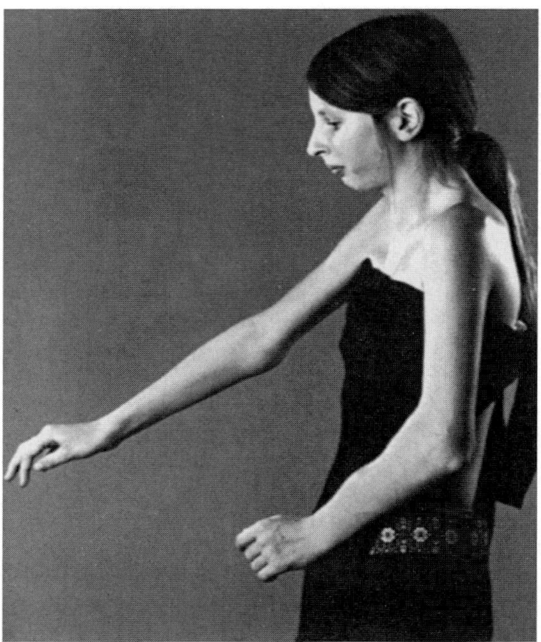

Figure 20–22. Myositis ossificans progressiva. This young girl presented with an extension contracture of the left wrist and later developed the diagnostic features of this disorder. In this photograph, the fixed deformity is visible, along with tumorous ossification of the forearm and a fixed contracture of the elbow. Movement of the left shoulder is greatly restricted, and muscle atrophy around that joint is present. A characteristic receding chin and short thumbs are present.

LABORATORY EXAMINATION

General Findings

Nonspecific indicators of inflammation, such as the erythrocyte sedimentation rate and C-reactive protein level, tend to correlate with the degree of clinical inflammation and are of diagnostic utility in differentiating inflammatory myopathies such as JDM from noninflammatory disorders of muscle such as muscular dystrophy or myotonia.[254, 255] Leukocytosis and anemia are uncommon at onset, except in the child with associated gastrointestinal bleeding. Urinalysis is usually normal, although a few children have microscopic hematuria.[11]

There are few specific abnormalities of immunoglobulin levels.[254, 256] A dermatomyositis-like disease has been observed in children with agammaglobulinemia and common variable immune deficiency (see Chapter 35).[75, 96, 257–259] Elevated IgE levels were found in one study of 22 Japanese children with JDM.[260]

Serum levels of Factor VIII–related antigen (von Willebrand factor) reflect endothelial damage and have been reported to be elevated in children with JDM.[135, 261–264] Although abnormal Factor VIII–related antigen levels are present in most children with active JDM, as is neopterin,[265] they were not found in one study to be of value in predicting a flare of the disease.[262] Neopterin is a derivative of pyrimidine metabolism and its serum concentration has been considered a marker of interferon-activated monocytes and macrophages. Levels are raised in inflammation, infections, and malignant diseases. Determination of its concentration has been proposed as a useful laboratory marker of immune activation and disease activity in JDM.[264, 265] Insulin resistance is characteristic of children who fail to remit or develop calcinosis and also of those with lipodystrophy.[193]

The serum level of myoglobin, a normal constituent of cardiac and skeletal muscle with a molecular weight of approximately 17 kD, is increased in serum in approximately 50 percent of patients with inflammatory myositis.[266, 267] This elevation is not always correlated with an increase in serum CK levels. Antibodies to myoglobin are found in 70 percent of patients and may interfere with its quantitation.[268] Studies by Dickerson and Widdowson[269] and by Hallgren and coworkers[270] estimated that a normal adult with 30 kg of muscle mass releases 0.3 mg of myoglobin per day. Although myoglobin is much more nephrotoxic than hemoglobin, myoglobinuria in JDM seldom reaches levels that are associated with renal damage.

Autoantibodies

The results of tests for rheumatoid factors in children with JDM are almost always negative. Antinuclear antibodies (ANAs) have been reported in a variable frequency of 10 to 85 percent.[13, 15, 48, 271, 272] Specific ANAs have been described, however, in dermatomyositis and polymyositis (Table 20–16). Particularly important are those directed against one of a number of extractable nuclear antigens that are soluble in saline at neutral or acid pH.[273] *Myositis-specific antibodies* (MSAs) such as to the aminoacyl transfer RNA (tRNA) synthetases have been described in only a minority of children.[2, 272, 274] The importance of MSAs has been emphasized by their inclusion in newly proposed criteria for the diagnosis of adult dermatomyositis/polymyositis.[139, 273, 275–280] *Myositis-associated antibodies* occur in variants of JDM, often in association with overlap syndromes. Approximately 80 percent of children are negative for either MSAs and myositis-associated antibodies.[2]

Table 20–16

Autoantibodies in Dermatomyositis/Polymyositis

SEROLOGIC GROUP	SPECIFICITY
Myositis-Specific Antibodies (MSAs)	
Anti-synthetases	
Jo-1	Histidyl-tRNA synthetase
PL-7	Threonyl-tRNA synthetase
PL-12	Alanyl-tRNA synthetase
Anti-Mi-2	206/218 kD nuclear histone deacetylase complex
Anti-SRP	Signal recognition ribonucleopeptide
Myositis-Associated Antibodies (MAAs)	
Anti-PM-Scl	Nucleolar protein complex
Anti-Ku	Acidic nuclear DNA-binding protein dimer
Anti-annexin XI	56 kD nuclear protein
Anti-U (1, 2, 3, 5) RNPs	Small nuclear RNP associated peptides
Anti-SSA/Ro	Nuclear protein complex

Myositis-Specific Antibodies

MSAs are antibodies targeted to RNAs or proteins involved in protein synthesis. They usually occur as a single entity in any one patient. Patients with a specific MSA are relatively homogeneous in clinical manifestations and prognosis.[274] The antisynthetase antibodies are usually present in adults with an acute onset and rapid progression of disease, but they have also been identified in others with very slow progression, and also in asymptomatic adults.[275] The antisynthetases are associated with an increased frequency of HLA-DR3 and DRw52.[139] DQA1*0501 or *0401 may also be present in patients with antibodies to Jo-1, PL-12, and other MSAs.

MSAs have been uncommon in childhood-onset disease and have only been described in approximately 10 percent of patients. Specificities identified in children include antibodies to the Jo-1,[281] Mi-2,[282, 283] and PL-7 antigens. Anti-Jo-1 is the most common antisynthetase antibody. It occurs in approximately 20 percent of adults and has been described in at least 10 children.[281] It is specific for histadyl-transfer RNA synthetase, a cytoplasmic enzyme that catalyzes the esterification of histidine to its cognate tRNA. Patients who are anti-Jo-1 positive demonstrate a subset of multisystemic features that have been termed the *antisynthetase syndrome.* Onset of disease is often acute, with fever and Raynaud's phenomenon, and the myositis can be very severe. Interstitial pulmonary fibrosis often becomes the dominant feature of the course.[275] Although polyarthritis, when it occurs, is generally mild, it can result in erosions and subluxations. A hyperkeratotic nonpruritic fissuring rash of the palms and lateral aspects of the fingers called *mechanic's hands* is another feature of this syndrome, especially in adults.

Anti-Mi-2 has been identified in approximately 22 children with JDM and in adults is strongly associated with a distinct pattern of rash.[2, 282, 283] The area of most intense involvement is often the V of the neck and the anterior chest area, and the shawl area with involvement of the upper back and shoulders. The majority of affected children have not displayed this characteristic area of involvement, although malar erythema and Gottron's papules have been present. The disease has been responsive to glucocorticoid therapy. Mi-2 is a 218 kD nuclear helicase that is involved in transcriptional activation. The HLA associations tend to be with DR7 and DR53.

Another distinct subset of patients with myositis is associated with antibodies to the signal recognition peptide, which has been present in at least four children.[2, 276] Onset of disease is often severe and acute, with polymyositis of both proximal and distal muscles predominating. These patients may have a higher frequency of cardiac disease and respond poorly to glucocorticoid therapy. The signal recognition peptide is a cytoplasmic ribonucleolar protein complex that directs the passage of newly synthesized protein from the ribosome through to the endoplasmic reticulum. ANA immunofluorescent tests may therefore demonstrate anticytoplasmic staining. HLA-DR5 and DRw52 are associated with this syndrome.

Myositis-Associated Antibodies

The myositis-associated antibodies occur in somewhat less than 10 percent of children with idiopathic myositis and involve a number of distinct entities.[2] Anti-PM-Scl is suggested by a nucleolar pattern on ANA testing.[34, 278] It occurs in the overlap syndrome of inflammatory myopathy and systemic scleroderma (scleromyositis) and has been found in at least 39 children. The clinical features include myositis, arthritis, digital sclerosis, and Raynaud's phenomenon. The course of the disease is often benign and prolonged but with a good prognosis. This antibody is associated with HLA-DR3. Antibodies reactive with PM-1 antigens are found in up to 60 percent of adults with polymyositis[284] but in only a minority of affected children.[75] PM-1 antibodies were present in 4 of 18 patients in Pachman's series,[75, 285–287] and in 3 of 21 in the series by Crowe and associates.[24]

Other Antibody Activities

Anti-U1RNP is one of the classic antibodies that is characteristic of the overlap syndrome of mixed connective tissue disease (see Chapter 23). It is suggested by the presence of a high-titered speckled ANA pattern. Anti-SSA/Ro antibody often occurs in association with anti-Jo-1 and other MSAs. The anti-Ku antibody has not often been described in patients from North America[288] but was reported from Japan in approximately 50 percent of patients with an overlap syndrome. It has been found in approximately 10 children with overlap syndromes.[274] The antigen is a protein kinase that is involved in the phosphorylation of a number of transcription factors. Anti-annexin XI has been reported frequently in children with JDM as well as in other connective tissue diseases and is associated with no particular clinical manifestations.[274] Reactivity is against a 56 kD nuclear protein.

Antibodies to endothelial cell antigens have been demonstrated in children with JDM,[289] although such antibodies are present in other vasculopathies.[290] The frequency of antibodies to myosin and muscle is the same for patients with inflammatory myopathy, muscular dystrophy, or denervation atrophy.[291, 292] Therefore, these antibodies may be secondary to muscle damage rather than primary phenomena.

Half of the children with JDM show evidence of circulating immune complexes that may be involved in the pathogenesis of the vascular injury.[64, 75, 293] It is possible that they may also interfere with the accurate serologic detection of other antibodies and potential antigens. Serum complement determinations are normal.[74, 293] Antibodies to cardiolipin, found in a minority of patients with JDM, may also reflect the underlying vasculopathy.[272]

Specific Laboratory Diagnostic Studies

The three investigations that are most useful in making a diagnosis of JDM are measurement of serum levels of the muscle enzymes, electromyography, and histopathologic examination of a muscle specimen obtained by needle or open biopsy (Table 20–17).

Muscle Enzymes

The serum levels of the sarcoplasmic muscle enzymes are important for diagnosis and for monitoring the effectiveness of therapy. Considerable individual variation in the pattern of enzyme elevation is observed; therefore, it is recommended that, at least early in JDM, CK, AST, lactic dehydrogenase (LDH), and aldolase be measured to obtain a reliable baseline evaluation.[12] The degree of elevation in serum concentration ranges from 20 to 40 times normal for CK or AST. The CK level does not always correlate with disease activity.[262] Rarely, some children have normal serum levels of CK during the acute phase of the illness, and others have a persistent elevation late in the course without any other clinical indication of muscle inflammation.[294] In the latter instance, evaluation of serum CK levels in family members may suggest an unrelated, but unsuspected, genetic abnormality. LDH and alanine aminotransferase levels are increased in many children with JDM. Although relatively less specific, these enzymes often best reflect global disease activity. Elevated ala-

Table 20–17

Specific Diagnostic Studies at Onset of Juvenile Dermatomyositis

STUDY	PERCENTAGE
Elevation of serum levels of the muscle enzymes	90–98
Aspartate aminotransferase	87
Creatine kinase	85
Aldolase	65
Lactic dehydrogenase	64
Abnormal electromyography	93–96
Abnormal muscle biopsy (inflammation)	79

nine aminotransferase and LDH activities may also reflect liver disease associated with partial generalized lipodystrophy and insulin resistance.[191] Serum levels of all muscle enzymes usually decrease 3 to 4 weeks before improvement in muscle strength and rise 5 to 6 weeks before clinical relapse. As a general rule, changes in CK levels occur first, often falling to the normal range within several weeks of instituting therapy; aldolase levels are the last to respond. Guzman and colleagues[262] reported that flares of disease are best predicted by a combination of AST and LDH, and that CK functions poorly as a predictor of exacerbation of myositis.

Creatine Kinase. CK catalyzes the transfer of a phosphoryl group from creatine phosphate to adenosine diphosphate to regenerate adenosine triphosphate in the mitochondria of muscle, brain, and heart. The adenosine triphosphate available to muscle is sufficient to sustain contractile activity for only a fraction of a second. In skeletal muscle, CK constitutes up to 20 percent of the soluble sarcoplasmic protein, and total CK activity is 225 to 12,000 units per gram of muscle. CK is a dimeric molecule with two subunits: M (muscle) and B (brain). Both consist of 360 amino acids with a molecular weight of 41 kD. Three isoenzymes exist. MM (CK-3) is found in muscle and myocardium, BB (CK-1) in brain, and MB (CK-2) in myocardium but also in regenerating muscle.[295] Therefore, in muscle inflammation, there may be a persistent elevation of the MB band. The adult pattern of isozymes is achieved by the age of 4 years.

Serum CK concentration is elevated in many cases of muscle injury, motor neuron diseases, vasculitis, metabolic disorders, endocrinopathies, toxic reactions, and infections. Very high levels are most commonly associated with muscular dystrophy and, somewhat less commonly, with JDM. Abnormalities of the junctional sites between the T-tubules and the sarcoplasmic reticulum in muscle cells of children with JDM may be the primary sites of leakage of the enzymes. These abnormal anastomoses are far more extensive in the perifascicular than in the centrofascicular myofibers. Enzyme levels are not increased in diseases in which there is no loss of sarcolemmal integrity (e.g., glucocorticoid myopathy, disuse atrophy).

Transaminases. AST and alanine aminotransferase are cytosolic and mitochondrial enzymes with a wide tissue distribution. AST has two dimeric isoenzymes; one in the cytosol and the other in the mitochondria. The half-life in human plasma is 47 hours for alanine aminotransferase, 6 hours for mitochondrial AST, and 12 to 17 hours for cytosolic AST. Plasma levels decrease to normal adult ranges by 1 year of age.

Aldolase. Aldolase (1,6-diphosphofructoaldolase) is found in myocardium, liver, cerebral cortex, kidneys, and erythrocytes but is present in much higher concentration in skeletal muscle. Aldolase is one of the principal glycolytic enzymes that catalyze the conversion of fructose-1,6-diphosphate to dihydroxyacetone phosphate and D-glyceraldehyde-3-phosphate. There are three cytosolic isoenzymes: aldolase A, which predominates in muscle; aldolase B in liver; and aldolase C in brain. It is aldolase A that is increased in the serum of children with active JDM.

Lactic Dehydrogenase. LDH is abundant in myocardium and skeletal muscle. There are five isoenzymes: I (30 percent), II (40 percent), III (20 percent), IV (6 percent), and V (4 percent). In acute adult polymyositis, there is relatively less isoenzyme I and relatively more isoenzymes II, III, IV, and V. In chronic disease, only isoenzymes I and II are disproportionately elevated. In contrast, patients with active muscular dystrophy exhibit an increase in isoenzymes I and II and a decrease in isoenzymes III, IV, and V, especially in the younger patient.[296]

Creatine/Creatinine Ratio

Creatine is synthesized in the liver from arginine and glycine by an aminotransferase to form ornithine and guanidoacetic acid. The latter is transmethylated by interaction with *S*-adenosylmethionine to form creatine and *S*-adenosylhomocysteine. Creatine circulates in the plasma in relatively low concentrations (less than 0.6 mg/dl in adults). It is stored in muscle as creatine phosphate and serves as the reserve energy pool for muscular activity. In muscle, creatine is converted to the anhydride creatinine at a constant rate of approximately 2 percent per day. Creatinine diffuses passively into the plasma and is excreted by the kidney. If the body pool of creatine decreases, the creatinine excretion per unit of time is also decreased. Therefore, endogenous creatinine excretion is an important index of body creatine stores and total muscle mass. Creatinuria in JDM is not simply a matter of failure of uptake by an inflamed muscle or a decreased muscle mass, but rather an inability to maintain normal membrane permeability.

The age-related urinary creatine/creatinine ratio is increased in children with JDM.[297] In those younger than 12 years of age, however, it is not a reliable guide to the activity of the inflammatory muscle disease. A 24-hour creatinine excretion measurement is an excellent indicator of muscle mass in children between the ages of 3 and 18 years. Boys begin to excrete significantly larger amounts of creatinine than girls at puberty. In males, it increases from approximately 0.36 g/day at 5 years of age to 1.6 g/day at 17 years of age. Creatine excretion, however, is much higher in the younger child. At no age in childhood is there a significant sex difference in the excretion of creatine. A 24-hour urine collection would have to document extremely large or infinitesimally small amounts of creatine before a creatine/creatinine ratio could be judged to be abnormal in children.

Electromyography

Electromyography (EMG) occasionally is useful in confirming the diagnosis of JDM and in selecting the best site for performing a muscle biopsy (along with localization of magnetic resonance imaging [MRI] abnormalities). The electromyogram should be evaluated on one side of the body only, so that the muscle biopsy, if necessary, can be obtained on the opposite extremity without any artifact created by a needle puncture. EMG can be troublesome in the young child, and sedation is often necessary. An EMG is not mandatory and need not be done unless the diagnosis is in doubt.

The characteristic electromyographic changes are those of myopathy and denervation (Table 20–18). These findings are associated with membrane instability (increased insertional activity, fibrillations, positive sharp waves) and random fiber destruction (decreased amplitude and duration of action potentials). The electrical changes in denervation probably result from seg-

Table 20–18

Electromyography in Juvenile Dermatomyositis

Myopathic motor units (decreased amplitude, short duration, polyphasic)
Denervation potentials (positive sharp waves), spontaneous fibrillations, and insertional activity
High-frequency repetitive discharges

mental myonecrosis of the end-plate, although the terminal axons may also be affected.[198] Reinnervation following the acute phase of the disease may occur.[298] Nerve conduction velocities and latencies are normal in JDM, unless severe muscle atrophy is present with a decrease in the number of muscle fibers in a motor unit and with electrical irritability of the sarcolemmal membrane or terminal axonal fibers.

The value of EMG in identifying continuing inflammatory activity of muscle during the course of JDM has not been adequately documented. Quantitative EMG may be more informative in this regard.[295, 299–301] In following the course of the disease, increasing muscle strength correlates with less spontaneous activity and a decreasing proportion of high-frequency components. Early in the initial period of treatment, however, a temporary increase in high-frequency signals is expected.

Muscle Biopsy

A muscle biopsy is indicated in the initial assessment of a child if the diagnosis is in any way uncertain, to evaluate "activity" of the disease, especially late in its course, or if histopathologic support for instituting long-term glucocorticoid therapy or immunosuppressive drugs is deemed necessary.[302] Occasionally, a biopsy is indicated in children who have failed to respond therapeutically to rule out disorders such as inclusion body myositis.[25, 36, 244, 303] A muscle biopsy provides valuable prognostic information, based on the studies of Banker and coworkers[140] and Crowe and coworkers.[24] The muscles to be biopsied, usually the deltoid or quadriceps, should be clinically involved as demonstrated by muscle testing on physical examination, EMG, or MRI, but not atrophied. MRI can be used to select an area of muscle that is likely to be affected by the disease and thereby decrease the possibility of obtaining uninformative tissue. If an electromyogram has been obtained within the previous 6 weeks, the biopsy should be performed on the opposite side of the body. Since muscle involvement in JDM is often spotty, a generous specimen should be obtained for examination. Care should be taken to prepare the tissue in accordance with the instructions of the pathologist.

A generous specimen on open muscle biopsy should be obtained in a muscle clamp (12 mm long, 4 mm wide, 2 mm thick). This is placed in a transport container to be taken immediately to the pathology laboratory. One specimen is frozen in isopentane for immunofluorescent and enzyme studies. Another on a separate pediatric clamp is fixed in glutaraldehyde for electron microscopy. Histopathology is more likely to be negative if the muscle specimen is inadequate in size, obtained from an inappropriate muscle, or taken late in the disease when the pathologic changes may no longer be specific. Occasionally, there is no evidence of inflammatory change even though characteristic abnormalities such as perifascicular atrophy are present.[195] Although an open biopsy is most often performed, needle biopsy is preferred in some centers. Needle biopsy with a spring-activated 14-gauge needle may offer a convenient and cost-effective alternative to a surgical procedure.[304] Three to four cores can be obtained with only surface anesthesia by this procedure. The middle deltoid and vastus lateralis are the safest areas to biopsy by this technique from the standpoint of avoiding vascular or neurologic damage.

RADIOLOGIC EXAMINATION

Radiographs in early JDM demonstrate increased soft tissue density caused by edema of the muscle and subcutaneous tissues and, somewhat later, atrophy of muscle.[305–309] In chronic disease, areas of deposition of calcium in soft tissues can be documented by plain radiographs (see Figs. 20–13 to 20–16). Osteoporosis of long bones and of the vertebral bodies is often marked (Fig. 20–23). Ultrasonographic studies of muscle demonstrate increased echogenicity (Fig. 20–24).[310]

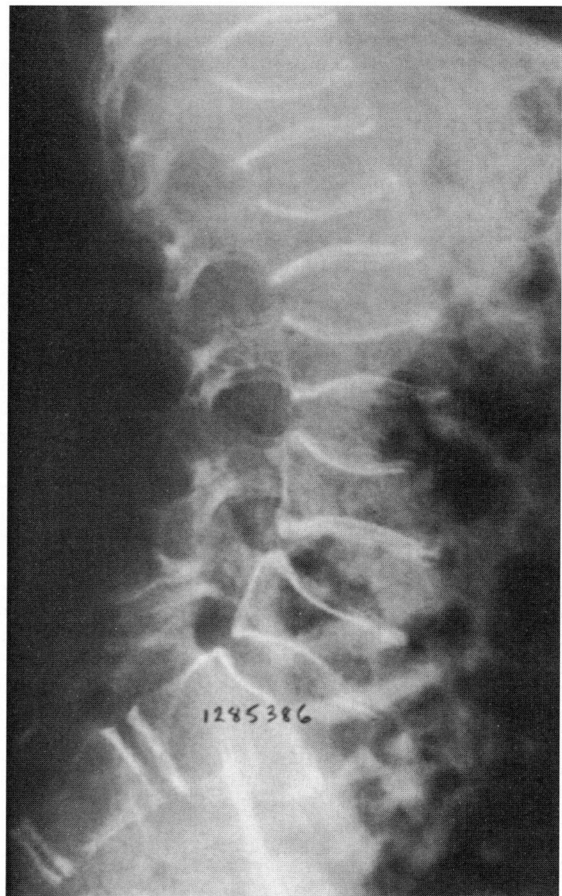

Figure 20–23. Extreme osteopenia of the lumbar spine with multiple vertebral compression fractures in a 15-year-old girl with a long history of chronic polycyclic dermatomyositis and steroid treatment.

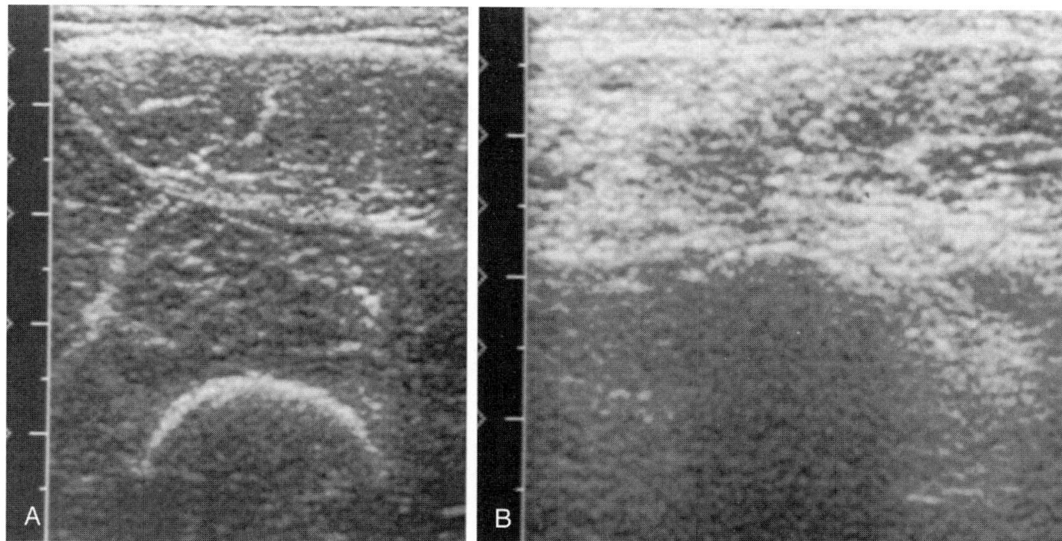

Figure 20–24. *A,* Ultrasound through the mid-thigh of a normal child. The skin surface is at the top; the convex arc is the femoral shaft. Fascial planes are visible in the muscle between the skin and bone. *B,* The same ultrasound view of the mid-thigh of a child with active dermatomyositis. The convex arc of the femoral shaft is difficult to see, and the fascial planes in the muscle are obliterated because of the intense increase in echogenicity in the inflamed muscle. (*A* and *B,* Courtesy of Dr. D. Stringer.)

MRI dramatically documents the extent and focal nature of the muscle abnormalities (Fig. 20–25*A* and *B*).[310–314] The T_1-weighted image demonstrates fibrosis, atrophy, and fatty infiltration. An increased signal is characteristic of fat, blood, edema, or other proteinaceous material. The short tau inversion recovery (STIR) image or T_2-weighted image with fat suppression demonstrates muscle edema and inflammatory changes by a hyperintense signal.[315–317, 317a] Active myositis in general is best documented by the T_2-weighted image even when not reflected in enzyme elevation.

Studies by Hernandez and associates[309, 312, 313] confirmed the value of MRI in the demonstration of myositis in children with JDM. In these studies, abnormalities in the T_2-weighted images correlated with disease activity. Reversal of these changes occurred in response to treatment. The authors suggested that MRI may be useful as a guide to monitor disease course or to delineate an area of affected muscle for surgical biopsy. Radionuclide scanning can detect early abnormal changes in blood flow in diseased muscles.[318–321] This technique has limited clinical application, however, and will likely be superseded by MRI, which has greater capacity for localization of inflamed muscle. One report has suggested that the course of children with JDM can be monitored with P-31 magnetic resonance spectroscopy as an indicator of biochemical defects in energy metabolism and mitochondrial oxidation phosphorylation.[316]

TREATMENT

In the presteroid era, approximately one third of children with JDM died, one third recovered, and one third were disabled to a moderate or severe extent.[11, 13, 22] The introduction of glucocorticoids has revolutionized the treatment and prognosis for children with JDM.[8, 13–15, 40, 142–148, 271, 322–325] In addition, the team approach and general supportive care, including bed rest and positioning early in the disease and individualized physical therapy, are essential. There is general agreement that glucocorticoids are always required, but the specifics of management vary considerably from physician to physician and patient to patient.[147]

The response of the child to the treatment program

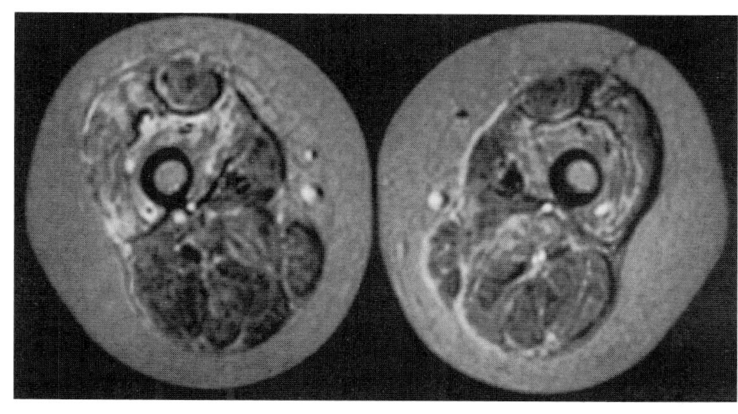

Figure 20–25. Cross-sectional magnetic resonance images of the proximal thigh of a child with chronic severe dermatomyositis. The increase in adipose tissue is evident and the increased signal from the quadriceps muscles is highly suggestive of the diagnosis. (Courtesy of Dr. R. Cairns.)

is judged on the basis of (1) systemic signs and symptoms such as fever, general malaise, muscle tenderness, and pain (if present); (2) repeated muscle examinations by the same observer (see Table 20–6); (3) sequential serum levels of selected muscle enzymes,[326, 327] acute-phase reactants, and other laboratory examinations if indicated (e.g., factor VIII–related antigen),[262, 263] (4) and occasionally other studies, such as MRI of muscle and ultrasonography.[316, 317, 328, 329] Disease activity indices are being validated.[330–332] Assessment of therapy in JDM is difficult, as appropriately controlled clinical studies have not been done. There are only four controlled studies in adults.[333–336]

General Supportive Care

The approach to the management of the child with JDM should be based on the knowledge that in most instances, the disease is a chronic one, but it may remit in 2 to 3 years. There is no evidence that any therapy currently available is curative; rather, treatment is aimed at suppression of the immunoinflammatory response, prevention of loss of muscle function and joint range of motion, and maintenance of general health and normal growth and development.

In acute disease, attention must be directed at the adequacy of ventilatory effort and swallowing. Occasionally, weakness is so profound that respiratory assistance, nasogastric feeding, and frequent oral suctioning are required. Each patient should be monitored carefully for swallowing, adequacy of airway, and depth of breathing. Hypoxia may supervene insidiously. In the older child, vital capacity measurements can be a valuable objective measure of response to therapy. Although respiratory problems occur in approximately one third of severely affected children, ventilatory assistance is seldom required. Profound involvement of the thoracic and respiratory muscles is seen in a few children and leads rapidly to increasing dyspnea at rest, agitation, respiratory insufficiency, aspiration, or death.[183]

Skin care is especially important in children who develop fissures in the axillae and groin or ulcers of the skin over pressure points. Emollients and padding of pressure areas may help prevent breakdown and ulceration (Fig. 20–26). These ulcerations become sites for secondary infections and abscesses, complications that are abetted by the administration of the glucocorticoid drugs. Late in the disease, the dermatitis may become markedly photosensitive, and water-based sun screens with high SPF numbers (30+) are necessary. The rash may or may not respond to the use of low-potency topical glucocorticoid creams. They are generally not recommended because of the secondary atrophic effects that result from long-term application.

Frequent counseling and education of patient and parents are necessary to help allay anxiety and permit understanding of the necessarily slow pace of treatment and recovery. Systemic complications, particularly abdominal pain or gastrointestinal bleeding, require urgent surgical consultation and may be life-threatening, especially early in the disease. Attention to nutritional status and intake of potassium and limitation of total caloric and sodium intake may help minimize the side effects of the glucocorticoid drugs.

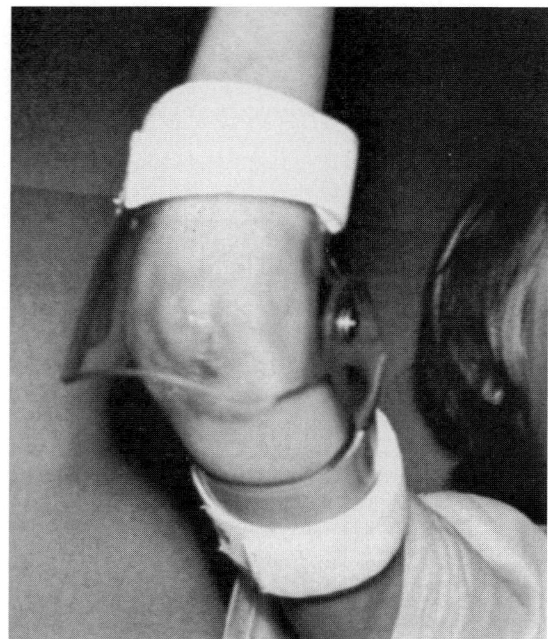

Figure 20–26. Elbow protector.

Glucocorticoid Drugs

Early and adequate treatment of JDM with glucocorticoids is probably the single most important factor in improved prognosis during the last 50 years. Acute disease is treated with suppressive doses of the synthetic glucocorticoids (Table 20–19).[13, 15] Prednisone is preferred to other analogues, such as dexamethasone and triamcinolone, because these steroids may have a more potent myopathic effect (see Chapter 7). Prednisone is given in a dosage of approximately 2 mg/kg/day

Table 20–19

Medical Treatment of Juvenile Dermatomyositis

Glucocorticoids
- *Initial*: oral prednisone 2 mg/kg/d for 1 mo; *or*:
  - IV methylprednisolone 30 mg/kg/d for 1–3 d; *then*: oral prednisone 1 mg/kg/d followed by a gradual taper in dose over approximately 2 yr

Hydroxychloroquine
- 6 mg/kg/d in addition to prednisone for control of skin disease

Immunosuppressives
- Methotrexate: 0.35–0.65 mg/kg/wk
- Cyclosporin: 3–5 mg/kg/d
- Cyclophosphamide: 1 mg/kg/d orally or 500–750 mg/M^2/mo
- Azathioprine: 1–3 mg/kg/d

Intravenous immunoglobulin
- 2 g/kg/mo

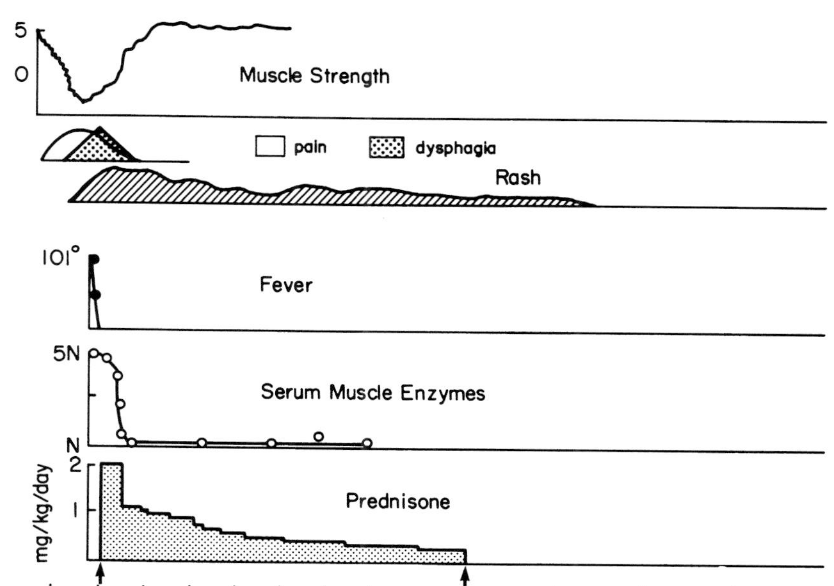

Figure 20–27. Course of a 5-year-old girl with acute onset of dermatomyositis and eventual complete recovery. Dysphagia resolved within the first month, muscle strength returned to normal during the first year, and the rash ultimately subsided by 3 years, as did all other signs of the disease. (Courtesy of Dr. D. B. Sullivan.)

in two to three divided doses for the first month of the disease and then, if indicated by the clinical response and a fall in the serum levels of the muscle enzymes, is reduced toward a dosage of 1 mg/kg/day, also given initially in divided doses. Thereafter, the drug is gradually tapered, as permitted by careful monitoring of improvement in muscle weakness and symptoms and by assay of serum levels of the muscle enzymes. In our experience, alternate-day glucocorticoid therapy is useful only late during the recovery phase of the disease. It is axiomatic that satisfactory clinical control is not attained until the serum enzymes have returned to normal or nearly normal levels and have remained there during continued tapering of the steroids and a gradual increase in the level of physical activity of the child.

The clinical response of the child to glucocorticoid management is not entirely predictable. The fever should abate within a few days, and the serum levels of muscle enzymes should show an appreciable decrease in the first 1 to 2 weeks of therapy (Figs. 20–27 and 20–28). There may be no significant improvement in muscle strength, however, for 1 to 2 months after instituting glucocorticoid drugs. Improvement in the

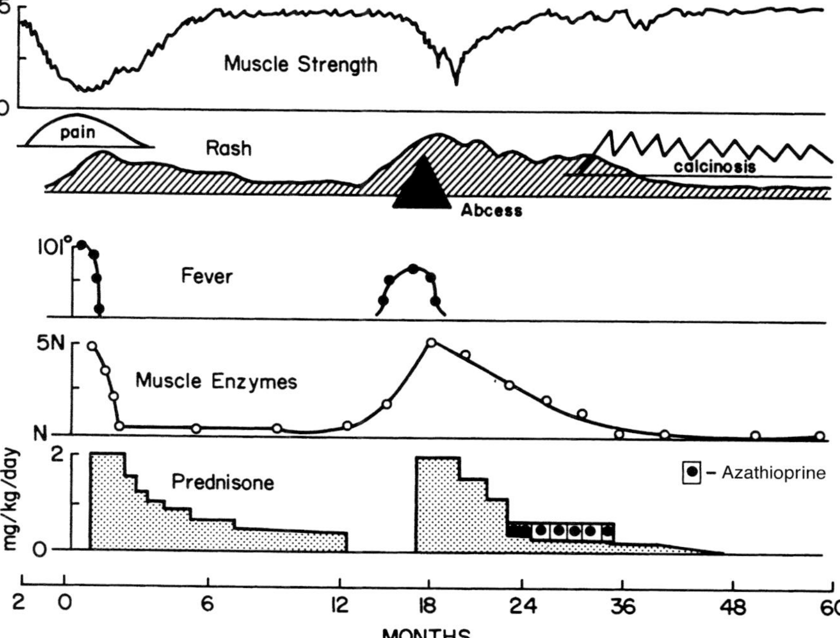

Figure 20–28. Course of an 8-year-old boy who initially responded to steroid treatment that was discontinued after 12 months. At 18 months, a gluteal abscess developed and an acute relapse occurred, which required combined immunosuppressive therapy because of the development of clinically significant steroid toxicity. (Courtesy of Dr. D. B. Sullivan.)

dermatitis is unpredictable. The status of the rash at any point is generally not an indication for a change in steroid therapy, since its course does not parallel that of the inflammatory myopathy. An extensive rash at onset or a generalized progression of the dermatitis is, however, a poor prognostic sign.[15] It is difficult to be certain when glucocorticoids can be totally discontinued without risking an exacerbation of the disease. It is apparently necessary to maintain a few children on very low-dose glucocorticoids even many years after "control" of myositis.

Children who require high-dose steroids for long periods develop severe osteopenia and osteoporosis, sometimes with vertebral compression fractures.[337] It is unsettled whether supplementation with dietary calcium and vitamin D or administration of calcitonin can prevent this complication. The efficacy and long-term safety of alendronate are being evaluated.[337a] Cushing's syndrome and growth retardation result in any child placed on suppressive doses for a period of months. The dosage of the glucocorticoid drug and duration of its use should, therefore, be kept as low as possible, commensurate with the clinical and laboratory responses to therapy.

The pediatric rheumatologist must be wary of the unusual but possible development of *steroid myopathy,* which might be misinterpreted as an exacerbation of the basic disease process (Table 20–20) (see Chapter 7). The manifestations of this syndrome are insidious onset of hip flexor weakness and atrophy, with normal assays of the serum muscle enzymes and minimal myopathic changes on EMG. In our experience, steroid myopathy is rare.

Intravenous pulse glucocorticoid therapy has been used to gain rapid control of muscle inflammation and vasculitis while minimizing the exposure of the child to long-term, high-dose daily steroids.[2, 338–341, 341a, 341b] An initial publication by Laxer and associates[341] indicated a satisfactory response in six children with JDM to steroid-pulse therapy. Subsequently, two additional patients were treated. Both were boys who had fairly mild early disease; a single intravenous pulse of methylprednisolone, 30 mg/kg, led to a fall in the enzyme levels, and improved muscle strength over 2 months.

There may be a subgroup of children with JDM in whom this initial approach to management of the disease will be successful and will abrogate the need for long-term daily glucocorticoid treatment. This approach to therapy in JDM must be evaluated further. In addition, Pachman and colleagues[49] have advanced the concept that early use of intravenous pulse therapy reduces future disability and extent of calcinosis. As with any form of therapy, this approach to glucocorticoid administration is not always effective.[342]

Table 20–20

Characteristics of Steroid-Induced Myopathy

Insidious onset
Hip-flexor weakness and atrophy
Normal serum concentrations of muscle enzymes
Minimal myopathic changes on electromyography
Type II fiber atrophy on muscle biopsy

Hydroxychloroquine

Hydroxychloroquine has been recommended as a steroid-sparing agent and as a drug that is effective in treating the dermatitis of JDM.[343, 344] Olson and Lindsley[344] reported significant improvement of the rash after 3 months and of muscle weakness after 6 months of treatment in a dose of 2 to 5 mg/kg/day in nine children with JDM. Evaluation of additional anecdotal experience suggests that the addition of hydroxychloroquine to a glucocorticoid regimen is warranted but has modest efficacy.

Immunosuppressive Therapy

Primary indications for the use of immunosuppressive drugs include *glucocorticoid resistance or dependence.* In steroid-resistant disease, there is inadequate improvement in muscle strength and a persistence of elevated serum levels of muscle enzymes in response to a closely monitored glucocorticoid program (prednisone 1 to 2 mg/kg/day for at least 3 to 4 months). Steroid dependence occurs later in the course of the disease and is characterized by failure of the manifestations of disease to remain suppressed during a gradual reduction of the glucocorticoid dose to an acceptable level, recurrence of progressive muscle weakness in spite of continuing therapy, or unacceptable steroid toxicity.

At least four immunosuppressive agents have been employed in the treatment of JDM in resistant disease[80–82]: methotrexate,[341b, 345–349] azathioprine,[349, 350] cyclophosphamide,[351] and cyclosporine.[26, 27, 50, 352–355] The efficacy of these drugs is difficult to evaluate because, as with glucocorticoids or hydroxychloroquine, there have been no controlled trials.

Of the immunosuppressive drugs, weekly oral or subcutaneous methotrexate is currently the preferred second-line agent. Benefit is usually evident within 1 to 2 months. No controlled study has been published on the consistency of response to this drug; however, a report of 22 adult patients suggested a favorable improvement in more than 75 percent without major toxicity or hepatic disease.[347] An experimental protocol was evaluated in adults that consisted of intravenous methotrexate, 500 mg/M^2, followed in 24 hours by oral leucovorin, 50 mg/M^2 every 6 hours for four doses. This was repeated every 2 weeks for 6 months. Preliminary data did not suggest that this regimen was superior to oral therapy with methotrexate and azathioprine.[336]

There is little published experience of the use of either azathioprine or cyclophosphamide in JDM. Crowe and colleagues[24] recommended cyclophosphamide in children with a chronic ulcerative course that is unresponsive to glucocorticoids (Table 20–21). Although there are no studies of the management of

Table 20–21

Course of Juvenile Dermatomyositis (Up to 1982)

TYPE OF COURSE	EXTENT OF INVOLVEMENT	STEROID RESPONSE	RESIDUAL DISEASE	NUMBER	(%)	DEATHS (N)
Monocyclic	Limited disease	Responsive	None	9/33	27	0
Chronic ulcerative	Cutaneous and gastrointestinal ulcerations Active disease present for years	Unresponsive	Long-term severe calcinosis and residual disability	11/33	33	3 (1 respiratory failure: 2 gastrointestinal ulcerations)
Chronic nonulcerative	Progressive weakness Limitation of motion	Good initial response Relapses	Permanent disability, calcinosis, severe weakness	13/33	40	1

Modified from Crowe WE, Bove KE, Levinson JE, et al: Clinical and pathogenetic implications of histopathology in childhood polydermatomyositis. Arthritis Rheum 25: 126–139, © 1982 Wiley-Liss, Inc. Reprinted by permission of Wiley-Liss, Inc., a subsidiary of John Wiley & Sons, Inc.

gastrointestinal ulceration in JDM, children with this complication warrant consideration of intravenous cyclophosphamide in addition to high-dose glucocorticoids. Intravenous cyclophosphamide therapy is difficult to use, however, and not always successful.[356] Chlorambucil has been suggested as an alternative by some investigators but has its own toxicities.[357]

There have been several case reports and reviews of successful cyclosporin therapy in JDM.[2, 352–355, 358, 359] Some investigators have suggested that this drug should be considered as first-line therapy in the treatment of inflammatory muscle disease.[360] The efficacy of cyclosporin in the treatment of steroid-resistant or -dependent JDM has been reported by Heckmatt and associates.[352] In this study, 14 children who had failed to respond fully to glucocorticoids and immunosuppressives were given cyclosporin in a dose of 2.5 to 7.5 mg/kg/day (younger children require increased dosage because drug clearance is age dependent). The authors reported considerable benefit, with reduced prednisolone requirements in all, including discontinuation of glucocorticoid in six patients. Two of three nonambulatory patients were able to walk after treatment, and six with limited ambulation subsequently regained good independent ambulation. Muscle strength improved but remained significantly reduced. The only significant side effects were hypertension and reversible decreases in renal function.[361] Our own limited experience is less optimistic. However, except for renal impairment, cyclosporin appears to have less long-term toxicity than the traditional immunosuppressive drugs, and for this reason its use should perhaps be considered earlier, rather than later, in the child who is nonresponsive to steroids or steroid-dependent.

Intravenous Immunoglobulin

A number of studies[362, 362a] and several anecdotal reports describe the efficacy of intravenous immunoglobulin (IVIG) in the management of JDM.[362–366] Clinical experience in children has been summarized in the review by Rider and Miller.[2] Lang and coworkers reported the results of administration of IVIG to five children who were steroid-resistant or -dependent.[362] All patients exhibited improved muscle strength and diminished rash over a 9-month period with infusions every 4 weeks of IVIG 1 g/kg/day on each of 2 consecutive days. Controlled studies in adults have been published, including those by the National Institutes of Health.[367, 368] In these reports, IVIG was of significant benefit, particularly if used early in the disease course, and especially with respect to the skin changes. However, without controlled clinical trials of this therapeutic approach in children, no firm conclusions can be reached regarding efficacy. Toxicity of IVIG is probably more common than was first believed. A syndrome of headache, vomiting, and fever, resembling aseptic meningitis, has been reported in a number of children with connective tissue diseases who have received this form of therapy.[369, 370]

Plasmapheresis

Plasmapheresis has been reported to be of some benefit in a few children with JDM.[195, 371–374] Recent studies in adults with dermatomyositis and polymyositis[334] suggest that the therapeutic effect may be minimal to nonexistent. A report of a single patient with JDM who was treated by extracorporeal photopheresis (ultraviolet activation of methoxypsoralen to covalently cross-link lymphocyte DNA) is an experimental approach of interest.[375]

Physical and Occupational Therapy

Physiotherapy should be initiated at the time of diagnosis. While the skeletal muscles are actively inflamed, the focus of attention should be on preventing loss of range of motion by giving twice- to thrice-daily passive range of motion exercises to all joints, with gentle stretching to regain lost range. Splinting of knees, elbows, or wrists at night or during periods of rest helps to achieve these goals. During the healing phase, the physical therapy program is increased to normalize function as nearly as possible and to minimize development of contractures secondary to muscle weakness or atrophy. Muscle strengthening should be added to the exercise program only after clinical evidence of acute inflammation has subsided.

Management of Calcinosis

None of the many approaches to the treatment of calcinosis has been consistently effective.[220, 221, 376–389] Therapy has included colchicine, aluminum hydroxide, probenecid, diphosphonates, diltiazem, intravenous ethylenediaminetetraacetic acid, and warfarin. Colchicine may suppress local and systemic signs of inflammation associated with calcinosis.[381] Recent experimental data suggest that tumor necrosis factor (TNF) blockade may be beneficial: overexpression of the TNF-α-308A allele is associated with a long duration of active disease and pathologic calcifications.[389a] Surgical excision of calcifications that mechanically interfere with function or have resulted in breakdown of skin may be indicated.[390] Although infections in such sites are a risk,[391] they are rare occurrences in our experience. It should be noted that the natural history of many of these calcific deposits is that they spontaneously begin to disappear after months or years, coincident with inactivity of the muscle disease and increasing mobility of the patient. The one fourth of children who have calcinosis in interfascial planes tend, however, to have persistent lesions.[157] Hypercalcemia and hypercalciuria have been reported during spontaneous resolution of calcinosis in two children with JDM.[376, 392]

COURSE OF THE DISEASE AND PROGNOSIS

The course of JDM in children can be divided into four clinical phases (Table 20–22).[158] The early prodromal phase is supplanted by a period of progressive muscle weakness and rash that then stabilizes for 1 to 2 years before recovery (Table 20–23). In our experience, the majority of children pursue a uniphasic course.[13, 15] The entire disease duration can be as brief as 8 months with complete recovery, or it can last 2 or more years with a continuing requirement for treatment with glucocorticoids. Acute exacerbations and remissions without any stabilization of the initial course of the disease have occurred in our experience in approximately 20 percent of children.

Table 20–22

Clinical Phases of Juvenile Dermatomyositis in Childhood

1. Prodromal period with nonspecific symptoms (weeks to months)
2. Progressive muscle weakness and rash (days to weeks)
3. Persistent weakness, rash, and active myositis (up to 2 years)
4. Recovery with or without residual muscle atrophy, contractures, and calcinosis

Modified from Spencer CH, Hanson V, Singsen BH, et al: Course of treated juvenile dermatomyositis. J Pediatr 105: 399–408, 1984

Table 20–23

Clinical Features of Juvenile Dermatomyositis During the Course of the Disease

- Constitutional signs and symptoms (100%)
- Muscle weakness (90–95%)
  - Proximal pelvic girdle (95%)
  - Proximal shoulder girdle (75%)
  - Neck flexors (60%)
  - Pharyngeal muscles (12–45%)
  - Distal muscles (30%)
  - Facial and extraocular muscles (5%)
- Muscle contractures and atrophy (62–90%)
- Muscle pain and tenderness (30–80%)
- Induration of muscle (50–100%)
- Skin lesions (85–100%)
  - Heliotrope rash of eyelids (10–15%)
  - Erythematous rash of malar area and V of chest (30–60%)
  - Subcutaneous and periorbital edema (60–90%)
  - Periungual and periarticular rash (Gottron's papules) (80–100%)
  - Photosensitive rash (5–40%)
  - Ulcerations (25%)
  - Lipodystrophy (5–15%)
  - Raynaud's phenomenon (2–15%)
  - Acute arthritis and arthralgia (7–38%)
  - Gastrointestinal signs and symptoms (10–60%)
  - Mucosal ulcerations and pharyngitis (10–45%)
  - Calcinosis (20–40%)
- Pulmonary disease (80%)
  - Restrictive defect (80%)
  - Fibrosis (<1%)

Risk factors for a poor prognosis include unremitting severe disease activity, cutaneous ulcerations, extensive calcinosis, distal muscle involvement, dysphagia or dysphonia, advanced nailfold capillary abnormalities, a noninflammatory vasculopathy on muscle biopsy, and the presence of specific MSAs. Delay in treatment and inadequate treatment are also very important.

The studies of Crowe and associates[24] identified a group of children with noninflammatory vasculopathy who had extensive and chronic ulcerative cutaneous disease (see Table 20–21). These children and a similar group reported earlier by Banker and Victor[9] were characterized by significant systemic complications, including fatal gastrointestinal hemorrhage. At a minimum, children with severe generalized erythroderma and cutaneous ulcerations often develop extensive calcinosis and significant overall functional impairment. Approximately 5 percent of children with JDM eventually develop a clinical disease that is more typical of systemic vasculitis.[24, 140] A small number of children late in the course may assume more of the characteristics of scleroderma with sclerodactyly and cutaneous atrophy[15] or develop lipodystrophy with insulin resistance, acanthosis nigricans, or a recurrence of arthritis.[193]

Late progression of JDM has been reported with a recurrence of active disease after a prolonged remission,[393, 394] or smoldering persistent activity many years after onset,[395] with multiple physical or dermatologic sequelae.[396] Of interest in this regard is the risk from pregnancy in women who have had or have JDM.[397–399] Depending on the activity of the disease, residual muscle weakness, calcinosis, and general debility, pregnancy should be considered high-risk for both mother and baby.

Calcinosis

Approximately 20 to 40 percent of children develop calcinosis during the course of the disease (see Tables 20–7 and 20–24).[15, 157, 399a] Children with extensive calcinosis are often those who have suffered from a severe and unremitting course.[157] In those children, and to a lesser extent in others, calcinosis may be responsible for more long-term disability with limitation of movement of involved muscles or contiguous joints than the residual effects of acute myositis. Calcific deposits may appear as early as 6 months or as late as 10 to 20 years after onset. Calcinosis is occasionally present at the time of the first presentation of the child to a physician. In this situation, it is surmised that the child had a prolonged but mild, and therefore undiagnosed, myositis before development of the calcinosis.[165] Rarely, calcinosis is accompanied by hypercalcemia.[376] Trauma has been thought to play a role in the generation of calcific deposits, because they tend to occur in surgical incisions and over pressure points. A study by Moore and coworkers[391] concluded that calcinosis was associated with preceding staphylococcal infection, high levels of IgE and IgE anti-staphylococcal antibodies. Granulocyte chemotaxis to staphylococci was depressed in children with calcinosis, an effect that was mediated by unidentified factors in the patients' sera.

Functional Disability

In children with a typical uniphasic course, functional outcome is usually excellent, although minor flexion contractures and residual skin changes may persist (Table 20–24). In others in whom the disease remains active beyond 3 years, there may be smoldering myositis and dermatitis with deposition of calcium salts and progressive loss of function. Adverse factors that influence the outcome of JDM are shown in Table 20–25. The factor with greatest impact on a favorable outcome is early and adequate steroid treatment.[12, 15] Functional outcome appears best in children who have been seen early and treated vigorously. The majority of survivors are able to function independently as adults, although some have flexion contractures and residual atrophy of skin or muscle.[399b, 399c]

Table 20–24

Prognosis of Juvenile Dermatomyositis

OUTCOME	%
Normal to good functional outcome	64–78
Minimal atrophy or contractures	24
Calcinosis*	20–40
Wheelchair dependence	5
Death	7–10

*Children with calcinosis were also included in the other categories.

Table 20–25

Factors That Adversely Influence Outcome of Juvenile Dermatomyositis

Disease-related
- Rapid onset and extensive weakness
- Extensive cutaneous vasculitis with ulceration
- Gastrointestinal vasculitis
- Severe endarteropathy and infarction in muscle biopsy specimen

Therapy-related
- Delay in diagnosis and institution of therapy
- Inadequate dose or duration of glucocorticoid therapy
- Minimal response to initial glucocorticoid therapy

Psychosocial Outcome

A study by Miller and associates[400] suggested that a number of children with JDM who enter adulthood continue to have psychological problems and learning disabilities based on unrecognized cerebral abnormalities that occurred at onset of disease. Another review of late outcome in JDM indicated that educational achievement and employment status of 18 patients were better than those of the general adult population or a comparable group who had had JRA.[401] Significant disability related to calcinosis or contractures was present in 3 patients, 6 had persistent muscle weakness, and 7 had recurrent rash. Raynaud's phenomenon (33 percent), arthritis (22 percent), and subcutaneous nodules were present in others, and minor increases in the serum concentrations of CK that did not correlate with the presence of muscle weakness or rash were observed in 7.

Death

At present, long-term survival in JDM is somewhat better than 90 percent, but in the presteroid era, this disease was associated with a mortality rate that approached 40 percent.[15, 24, 400, 402, 403] Children who survived often had devastating residual problems of contractures and muscular atrophy.

Fatalities most often occur within 2 years after onset and are often associated with progressive involvement of skin or muscle that is unresponsive to steroids. This observation suggests that the basic nature of the inflammatory disease, its early treatment and response, the presence of widespread vasculitis, and involvement of other organ systems such as the gastrointestinal or pulmonary tracts, are major factors that should be assessed in estimating prognosis. Death most often results from respiratory insufficiency or pneumonitis, or from acute gastrointestinal ulceration and bleeding. Surgical intervention in the group of children with the latter complications has generally not been of benefit.

There were 6 deaths in the Ann Arbor series of 71 children with JDM. One young girl died 5 years after onset as a result of cardiorespiratory collapse. Necropsy examination documented no active myositis. Three patients died at 2 months, 6 months, and 4 years after onset from multiple sites of gastrointestinal hemorrhage. Another girl died from a subdural hematoma caused by a fall from a wheelchair. A boy succumbed shortly after onset of disease from respiratory insufficiency and hypoxia. In the series of Spencer and colleagues,[158] 7 of 66 patients died. Five deaths occurred early during the course of the disease (1 to 11 months from diagnosis) and were related to sepsis (1), gastrointestinal perforation (2), and unresponsive muscle weakness and pneumonitis (2). One patient died 9 years after onset from pulmonary fibrosis with cor pulmonale, and one patient committed suicide 16 years after onset.

In the report of 39 patients with JDM by Miller and associates,[400] there were 10 deaths (26 percent); 8 of these occurred in children seen before 1972. No child who had received intensive glucocorticoid treatment (and, in some cases, azathioprine) died. All deaths were associated with bowel perforation or aspiration pneumonitis and occurred an average of 2½ years after onset. The improved outcome since 1972 (92 percent survival rate) was judged to be related to early and appropriate steroid regimens, better clinical assessment, and follow-up with sequential serum muscle enzyme determinations, and management of complications. Five of the 24 surviving patients were still receiving glucocorticoids at follow-up.

References

1. Pachman LM: Juvenile dermatomyositis. Pathophysiology and disease expression. Pediatr Clin North Am 42: 1071–1098, 1995.
2. Rider LG, Miller FW: Classification and treatment of the juvenile idiopathic inflammatory myopathies. Rheum Dis Clin North Am 23: 619–655, 1997.
3. Hepp P: Uber einen Fall von acuter parenchymatoser myositis, welche Geschwulste bildete und Fluctuation vortauschte. Klin Wochenschr 24: 389, 1887.
4. Jackson H: Myositis universalis acuta infectiosa, with a case. Boston Med Surg J 116: 498, 1887.
5. Wagner E: Ein Fall von acuter Polymyositis. Dtsch Arch Klin Med 40: 241, 1887.
6. Unverricht H: Uber eine eigentumliche Form von acuter Muskelentzundung mit einem der Trichinose ahnelnden Krankheitsbilde. Munch Med Wochschr 34, 1887.
7. Karelitz S, Welt SK: Dermatomyositis. Am J Dis Child 43: 1134, 1932.
8. Wedgwood RJ, Cook C, Cohen J: Dermatomyositis: Report of 26 cases in children with a discussion of endocrine therapy in 13. Pediatrics 12: 447, 1953.
9. Roberts HM, Brunsting LA: Dermatomyositis in childhood. A summary of 40 cases. Postgrad Med 16: 396, 1954.
10. Carlisle JW, Good RA: Dermatomyositis in childhood: report of studies on 7 cases and a review of literature. Lancet 79: 266, 1959.
11. Bitnun S, Daeschner CW Jr, Travis LB, et al: Dermatomyositis. J Pediatr 64: 101, 1964.
12. Hanson V, Kornreich H: Systemic rheumatic disorders ("collagen disease") in childhood: lupus erythematosus, anaphylactoid purpura, dermatomyositis, and scleroderma. I. Bull Rheum Dis 17: 435–440, 1967.
13. Sullivan DB, Cassidy JT, Petty RE, Burt A: Prognosis in childhood dermatomyositis. J Pediatr 80: 555–563, 1972.
14. Rose AL: Childhood polymyositis: A follow-up study with special reference to treatment with corticosteroids. Am J Dis Child 127: 518–522, 1974.
15. Sullivan DB, Cassidy JT, Petty RE: Dermatomyositis in the pediatric patient. Arthritis Rheum 20: 327–331, 1977.
16. Hanson V: Dermatomyositis, scleroderma, and polyarteritis nodosa. Clin Rheum Dis 2: 445, 1976.
17. Scheuermann H: Zur Klinik und Pathogenese der Dermatomyositis (Polymyositis). Arch Dermatol U Syph 178: 414, 1939.
18. Hecht MS: Dermatomyositis in childhood. J Pediatr 17: 791, 1940.
19. Selander P: Dermatomyositis in early childhood. Acta Med Scand 246(Suppl): 187, 1950.
20. Batten FE: Case of dermatomyositis in a child, with pathological report. Br J Child Dis 9: 247, 1912.
21. Pearson CM: Polymyositis. Annu Rev Med 17: 63–82, 1966.
22. Cook WE, Rosen FS, Banker BQ: Dermatomyositis and focal scleroderma. Pediatr Clin North Am 10: 979, 1963.
23. Hanissian AS, Masi AT, Pitner SE, et al: Polymyositis and dermatomyositis in children: an epidemiologic and clinical comparative analysis. J Rheumatol 9: 390–394, 1982.
24. Crowe WE, Bove KE, Levinson JE, Hilton PK: Clinical and pathogenetic implications of histopathology in childhood polydermatomyositis. Arthritis Rheum 25: 126–139, 1982.
25. Serratrice G, Schiano A, Pellissier JF, Desnuelle C: Anatomoclinical expressions of polymyositis in the child. 23 cases. Ann Pediatr (Paris) 36: 237–243, 1989.
26. Sherry DD, Haas JE, Milstein JM: Childhood polymyositis as a paraneoplastic phenomenon. Pediatr Neurol 9: 155–156, 1993.
27. Falcini F, Taccetti G, Trapani S, et al: Acute lymphocytic leukemia with dermatomyositis-like onset in childhood. J Rheumatol 20: 1260–1262, 1993.
28. Page AR, Hansen AE, Good RA: Occurrence of leukemia and lymphoma in patients with agammaglobulinemia. Blood 21: 197, 1963.
29. Solomon SD, Maurer KH: Association of dermatomyositis and dysgerminoma in a 16-year-old patient. Arthritis Rheum 26: 572–573, 1983.
30. Hatada T, Aoki I, Ikeda H, et al: Dermatomyositis and malignancy: case report and review of the Japanese literature. Tumori 82: 273–275, 1996.
31. Bartley GB, Gibson LE: Blepharochalasis associated with dermatomyositis and acute lymphocytic leukemia. Am J Ophthalmol 113: 727–728, 1992.
32. Rider LG, Okada S, Sherry DD: Epidemiologic features and environmental exposures associated with illness onset in juvenile idiopathic inflammatory myopathy. Arthritis Rheum 38(suppl): 362, 1995.
33. Allen RC, St-Cyr C, Maddison PJ, Ansell BM: Overlap connective tissue syndromes. Arch Dis Child 61: 284–288, 1986.
34. Blaszczyk M, Jablonska S, Szymanska-Jagiello W, et al: Childhood scleromyositis: an overlap syndrome associated with PM-Scl antibody. Pediatr Dermatol 8: 1–8, 1991.
35. Lang BA, Laxer RM, Thorner P, et al: Pediatric onset of Behçet's syndrome with myositis: case report and literature review illustrating unusual features. Arthritis Rheum 33: 418–425, 1990.
36. Riggs JE, Schochet SS Jr, Gutmann L, Lerfald SC: Childhood onset inclusion body myositis mimicking limb-girdle muscular dystrophy. J Child Neurol 4: 283–285, 1989.
37. Shapiro MJ, Applebaum H, Besser AS: Cervical focal myositis in a child. J Pediatr Surg 21: 375–376, 1986.
38. Isaacson G, Chan KH, Heffner RR Jr: Focal myositis: a new cause for the pediatric neck mass. Arch Otolaryngol Head Neck Surg 117: 103–105, 1991.
39. Agrawal BL, Giesen PC: Eosinophilic myositis. An unusual cause of pseudotumor and eosinophilia. JAMA 246: 70–71, 1981.
40. Rose AL, Walton JN: Polymyositis: a survey of 89 cases with particular reference to treatment and prognosis. Brain 89: 747–768, 1966.
41. Medsger TA Jr, Dawson WN Jr, Masi AT: The epidemiology of polymyositis. Am J Med 48: 715–723, 1970.
42. Oddis CV, Conte CG, Steen VD, Medsger TA Jr: Incidence of polymyositis-dermatomyositis: A 20-year study of hospital diagnosed cases in Allegheny County, PA 1963–1982. J Rheumatol 17: 1329–1334, 1990.
43. Benbassat J, Geffel D, Zlotnick A: Epidemiology of polymyositis-dermatomyositis in Israel, 1960–76. Isr J Med Sci 16: 197–200, 1980.
44. Barwick DD, Walton JN: Polymyositis. Am J Med 35: 646, 1963.
45. Symmons DP, Sills JA, Davis SM: The incidence of juvenile

dermatomyositis: results from a nation-wide study. Br J Rheumatol 34: 732–736, 1995.
46. Kaipiainen-Seppanen O, Savolainen A: Incidence of chronic juvenile rheumatic diseases in Finland during 1980–1990. Clin Exp Rheumatol 14: 441–444, 1996.
47. Fujikawa S, Okuni M: A nationwide surveillance study of rheumatic diseases among Japanese children. Acta Paediatr Jpn 39: 242–244, 1997.
48. Thompson CE: Polymyositis in children. Clin Pediatr (Phila) 7: 24–28, 1968.
49. Pachman LM: Inflammatory myopathy in children. Rheum Dis Clin North Am 20: 919–942, 1994.
50. Symmons DP, Jones M, Osborne J, et al: Pediatric rheumatology in the United Kingdom: data from the British Pediatric Rheumatology Group National Diagnostic Register. J Rheumatol 23: 1975–1980, 1996.
51. Pachman LM, Hayford JR, Hochberg MC, et al: New-onset juvenile dermatomyositis: comparisons with a healthy cohort and children with juvenile rheumatoid arthritis. Arthritis Rheum 40: 1526–1533, 1997.
52. Shehata R, al-Mayouf S, al-Dalaan A, et al: Juvenile dermatomyositis: clinical profile and disease course in 25 patients. Clin Exp Rheumatol 17: 115–118, 1999.
53. Whitaker JN: Inflammatory myopathy: a review of etiologic and pathogenetic factors. Muscle Nerve 5: 573–592, 1982.
54. Denman AM: Inflammatory disorders of muscle. Aetiology. Clin Rheum Dis 10: 9–33, 1984.
55. Plotz PH, Dalakas M, Leff RL, et al: Current concepts in the idiopathic inflammatory myopathies: polymyositis, dermatomyositis, and related disorders. Ann Intern Med 111: 143–157, 1989.
56. Saunders M, Knowles M, Currie S: Lymphocyte stimulation with muscle homogenate in polymyositis and other muscle-wasting disorders. J Neurol Neurosurg Psychiatry 32: 569–571, 1969.
57. Currie S, Saunders M, Knowles M, Brown AE: Immunological aspects of polymyositis. The in vitro activity of lymphocytes on incubation with muscle antigen and with muscle cultures. Q J Med 40: 63–84, 1971.
58. Esiri MM, MacLennan IC, Hazleman BL: Lymphocyte sensitivity to skeletal muscle in patients with polymyositis and other disorders. Clin Exp Immunol 14: 25–35, 1973.
59. Mastaglia FL, Currie S: Immunological and ultrastructural observations on the role of lymphoid cells in the pathogenesis of polymyositis. Acta Neuropathol (Berl) 18: 1–16, 1971.
60. Lisak RP, Zweiman B: Mitogen and muscle extract induced in vitro proliferative responses in myasthenia gravis, dermatomyositis, and polymyositis. J Neurol Neurosurg Psychiatry 38: 521–524, 1975.
61. Currie S: Destruction of muscle cultures by lymphocytes from cases of polymyositis. Acta Neuropathol (Berl) 15: 11–19, 1970.
62. Dawkins RL, Mastaglia FL: Cell-mediated cytotoxicity to muscle in polymyositis. Effect of immunosuppression. N Engl J Med 288: 434–438, 1973.
63. Johnson RL, Fink CW, Ziff M: Lymphotoxin formation by lymphocytes and muscle in polymyositis. J Clin Invest 51: 2435–2449, 1972.
64. Haas DC, Arnason BG: Cell-mediated immunity in polymyositis. Creatine phosphokinase release from muscle cultures. Arch Neurol 31: 192–196, 1974.
65. Iannaccone ST, Bowen DE, Samaha FJ: Cell-mediated cytotoxicity and childhood dermatomyositis. Arch Neurol 39: 400–402, 1982.
66. Miller ML, Lantner R, Pachman LM: Natural and antibody-dependent cellular cytotoxicity in children with systemic lupus erythematosus and juvenile dermatomyositis. J Rheumatol 10: 640–642, 1983.
67. Haas DC: Absence of cell-mediated cytotoxicity to muscle cultures in polymyositis. J Rheumatol 7: 671–676, 1980.
67a. Abramson LS, Albertini RJ, Pachman LM, Finette BA: Association among somatic HPRT mutant frequency, peripheral blood T-lymphocyte clonality, and serologic parameters of disease activity in children with juvenile onset dermatomyositis. Clin Immunol 91: 61–67, 1999.
68. McDouall RM, Dunn MJ, Dubowitz V: Nature of the mononuclear infiltrate and the mechanism of muscle damage in juvenile dermatomyositis and Duchenne muscular dystrophy. J Neurol Sci 99: 199–217, 1990.
69. Giorno R, Barden MT, Kohler PF, Ringel SP: Immunohistochemical characterization of the mononuclear cells infiltrating muscle of patients with inflammatory and noninflammatory myopathies. Clin Immunol Immunopathol 30: 405–412, 1984.
69a. Falcini F, Calzolari A, Generini S, et al: Bcl-2, p53 and c-myc expression in juvenile dermatomyositis. Clin Exp Rheumatol 18: 643–646, 2000.
70. Whitaker JN, Engel WK: Vascular deposits of immunoglobulin and complement in idiopathic inflammatory myopathy. N Engl J Med 286: 333–338, 1972.
71. Spencer CH, Jordon SC, Hanson V: Circulating immune complexes in juvenile dermatomyositis. Arthritis Rheum 23: 750, 1980.
72. Iannaccone ST, Bowen D, Yarom A, Ciraolo G: In vitro study of cytotoxic factors against endothelium in childhood dermatomyositis. Arch Neurol 41: 862–864, 1984.
73. Kissel JT, Mendell JR, Rammohan KW: Microvascular deposition of complement membrane attack complex in dermatomyositis. N Engl J Med 314: 329–334, 1986.
74. Scott JP, Arroyave C: Activation of complement and coagulation in juvenile dermatomyositis. Arthritis Rheum 30: 572–576, 1987.
75. Pachman LM, Cooke N: Juvenile dermatomyositis: a clinical and immunologic study. J Pediatr 96: 226–234, 1980.
76. Reed AM, Diegelj M, Kredich D, et al: Geographic clustering of juvenile dermatomyositis in subjects. Arthritis Rheum 41(Suppl): S265, 1998.
77. Ruff RL, Secrist D: Viral studies in benign acute childhood myositis. Arch Neurol 39: 261–263, 1982.
78. Bowles NE, Dubowitz V, Sewry CA, Archard LC: Dermatomyositis, polymyositis, and Coxsackie-B-virus infection. Lancet 1: 1004–1007, 1987.
79. Christensen ML, Pachman LM, Maryjowski MC: Antibody to coxsackie B virus: increased incidence in sera from children with recently diagnosed juvenile dermatomyositis. Arthritis Rheum 26: S24, 1983.
80. Christensen ML, Pachman LM, Schneiderman R, et al: Prevalence of Coxsackie B virus antibodies in patients with juvenile dermatomyositis. Arthritis Rheum 29: 1365–1370, 1986.
81. Pachman LM, Nigro R, Rowley A, et al: Polymerase chain reaction does not detect enteroviral or coxsackievirus B mRNA in fresh frozen muscle biopsies from 20 children with juvenile dermatomyositis. Arthritis Rheum 35(Suppl): S65, 1992.
82. Middleton PJ, Alexander RM, Szymanski MT: Severe myositis during recovery from influenza. Lancet 2: 533–535, 1970.
83. Lundberg A: Myalgia crures epedemica. Acta Paediatr 46: 18, 1957.
84. Dietzman DE, Schaller JG, Ray CG, Reed ME: Acute myositis associated with influenza B infection. Pediatrics 57: 255–258, 1976.
84a. Mackay MT, Kornberg AJ, Shield LK, Dennet X: Benign acute childhood myositis: laboratory and clinical features. Neurology 53: 2127–2131, 1999.
85. Landry M, Winkelmann RK: Tubular cytoplasmic inclusion in dermatomyositis. Mayo Clin Proc 47: 479–492, 1972.
86. Cotterill JA, Shapiro H: Dermatomyositis after immunisation. Lancet 2: 1158–1159, 1978.
87. Ehrengut W: Dermatomyositis and vaccination. Lancet 1: 1040–1041, 1978.
88. Hanissian AS, Martinez AJ, Jabbour JT, Duenas DA: Vasculitis and myositis secondary to rubella vaccination. Arch Neurol 28: 202–204, 1973.
89. Kass E, Straume S, Munthe E: Dermatomyositis after B.C.G. vaccination. Lancet 1: 772, 1978.
90. Martini A, Ravelli A, Albani S, et al: Recurrent juvenile dermatomyositis and cutaneous necrotizing arteritis with molecular mimicry between streptococcal type 5 M protein and human skeletal myosin. J Pediatr 121: 739–742, 1992.
90a. Martini A, Revelli A, Albani S, et al: Recurrent juvenile dermatomyositis and cutaneous necrotizing arteritis with molecular mimicry between streptococcal type 5 M protein and human skeletal myosin. J Pediatr 121; 739–742, 1992.
90b. Albani S: Infection and molecular mimicry in autoimmune diseases of childhood. Clin Exp Rheumatol 12(Suppl 10): S35–S41, 1994.

91. Hendrickx GF, Verhage J, Jennekens FG, van Knapen F: Dermatomyositis and toxoplasmosis. Ann Neurol 5: 393–395, 1979.
92. Phillips PE, Kassan SS, Kagen LJ: Increased toxoplasma antibodies in idiopathic inflammatory muscle disease: a case-controlled study. Arthritis Rheum 22: 209–214, 1979.
93. Pollock JL: Toxoplasmosis appearing to be dermatomyositis. Arch Dermatol 115: 736–737, 1979.
94. Kagen LJ, Kimball AC, Christian CL: Serologic evidence of toxoplasmosis among patients with polymyositis. Am J Med 56: 186–191, 1974.
95. Schroter HM, Sarnat HB, Matheson DS, Seland TP: Juvenile dermatomyositis induced by toxoplasmosis. J Child Neurol 2: 101–104, 1987.
96. Webster AD: Inflammatory disorders of muscle. Echovirus disease in hypogammaglobulinaemic patients. Clin Rheum Dis 10: 189–203, 1984.
97. Carroll JE, Silverman A, Isobe Y, et al: Inflammatory myopathy, IgA deficiency, and intestinal malabsorption. J Pediatr 89: 216–219, 1976.
98. Leddy JP, Griggs RC, Klemperer MR, Frank MM: Hereditary complement (C2) deficiency with dermatomyositis. Am J Med 58: 83–91, 1975.
99. Grimley PM, Friedman RM: Arboviral infection of voluntary striated muscles. J Infect Dis 122: 45–52, 1970.
100. Melnick JL, Godman GC: Pathogenesis of coxsackie virus infections: Multiplication of virus and evolution of the muscle lesion in mice. J Exp Med 93: 247, 1951.
101. Ytterberg SR, Mahowald ML, Messner RP: T cells are required for coxsackievirus B1 induced murine polymyositis. J Rheumatol 15: 475–478, 1988.
102. Craighead JE: Pathogenicity of the M and E variants of the encephalomyocarditis (EMC) virus. I. Myocardiotropic and neurotropic properties. Am J Pathol 48: 333–345, 1966.
103. Seay AR, Griffin DE, Johnson RT: Experimental viral polymyositis: age dependency and immune responses to Ross River virus infection in mice. Neurology 31: 656–660, 1981.
104. Chou SM, Miike T: Ultrastructural abnormalities and perifascicular atrophy in childhood dermatomyositis with special reference to transverse tubular system-sarcoplasmic reticulum junctions. Arch Pathol Lab Med 105: 76–85, 1981.
105. Chou SM: Myxovirus-like structures in a case of human chronic polymyositis. Science 158: 1453–1455, 1967.
106. Burch GE, Sohal RS, Colcolough HL, Sun SC: Virus-like particles in skeletal muscle of a heat stroke victim. Arch Environ Health 17: 984–985, 1968.
107. Baringer JR, Swoveland P: Tubular aggregates in endoplasmic reticulum: evidence against their viral nature. J Ultrastruct Res 41: 270–276, 1972.
108. Katsuragi S, Miyayama H, Takeuchi T: Picornavirus-like inclusions in polymyositis—aggregation of glycogen particles of the same size. Neurology 31: 1476–1480, 1981.
109. Fidzianska A, Goebel HH: Tubuloreticular structures (TRS) and cylindric confronting cisternae (CCC) in childhood dermatomyositis. Acta Neuropathol (Berl) 79: 310–316, 1989.
110. Hashimoto K, Robison L, Velayos E, Niizuma K: Dermatomyositis. Electron microscopic, immunologic, and tissue culture studies of paramyxovirus-like inclusions. Arch Dermatol 103: 120–135, 1971.
111. Norton WL: Comparison of the microangiopathy of systemic lupus erythematosus, dermatomyositis, scleroderma, and diabetes mellitus. Lab Invest 22: 301–308, 1970.
112. Ben-Bassat M, Machtey I: Picornavirus-like structures in acute dermatomyositis. Am J Clin Pathol 58: 245–249, 1972.
113. Chou SM, Gutmann L: Picornavirus-like crystals in subacute polymyositis. Neurology 20: 205–213, 1970.
114. Fukuyama Y, Ando T, Yokota J: Acute fulminant myoglobinuric polymyositis with picornavirus-like crystals. J Neurol Neurosurg Psychiatry 40: 775–781, 1977.
115. Mastaglia FL, Walton JN: Coxsackie virus-like particles in skeletal muscle from a case of polymyositis. J Neurol Sci 11: 593–599, 1970.
116. Gyorkey F, Cabral GA, Gyorkey PK, et al: Coxsackievirus aggregates in muscle cells of a polymyositis patient. Intervirology 10: 69–77, 1978.
117. Webb JN: Experimental immune myositis in guinea pigs. J Reticuloendothel Soc 7: 305–316, 1970.
118. Suenaga Y: Experimental pathological studies on homologous immunization with the skeletal muscle tissue of the rabbit. Zasshi Tokyo Ika Daigaku 25: 975–1007, 1967.
119. Morgan G, Peter JB, Newbould BB: Experimental allergic myositis in rats. Arthritis Rheum 14: 599–609, 1971.
120. Smith PD, Butler RC, Partridge TS, et al: Current progress in the study of allergic polymyositis in the guinea pig and man. *In* Rose FC (ed): Clinical Neuroimmunology. Oxford, England, Blackwell Scientific Publications, 1979, p. 146.
121. Kakulas BA: In vitro destruction of skeletal muscle by sensitized cells. Nature 210: 1115–1118, 1966.
122. Currie S: Experimental myositis: the in-vivo and in-vitro activity of lymph-node cells. J Pathol 105: 169–185, 1971.
123. Hathaway PW, Engel WK, Zellweger H: Experimental myopathy after microarterial embolization: comparison with childhood x-linked pseudohypertrophic muscular dystrophy. Arch Neurol 22: 365–378, 1970.
124. Mendell JR, Engel WK, Derrer EC: Duchenne muscular dystrophy: functional ischemia reproduces its characteristic lesions. Science 172: 1143–1145, 1971.
125. Lambie JA, Duff IF: Familial occurrence of dermatomyositis. Ann Intern Med 59: 839, 1963.
126. Lewkonia RM, Buxton PH: Myositis in father and daughter. J Neurol Neurosurg Psychiatry 36: 820–825, 1973.
127. Christianson HB, Brunsting LA, Perry HO: Dermatomyositis: unusual features, complications and treatment. Arch Dermatol 74: 581, 1956.
128. Harati Y, Niakan E, Bergman EW: Childhood dermatomyositis in monozygotic twins. Neurology 36: 721–723, 1986.
129. Rose T, Nothjunge J, Schlote W: Familial occurrence of dermatomyositis and progressive scleroderma after injection of a local anaesthetic for dental treatment. Eur J Pediatr 143: 225–228, 1985.
130. Rider LG, Gurley RC, Pandey JP, et al: Clinical, serologic, and immunogenetic features of familial idiopathic inflammatory myopathy. Arthritis Rheum 41: 710–719, 1998.
131. Andrews A, Hickling P, Hutton C: Familial dermatomyositis. Br J Rheumatol 37: 231–232, 1998.
131a. Plamondon S, Dent PB, Reed AM: Familial dermatomyositis. J Rheumatol 26: 2691–2692, 1999.
132. Friedman JM, Pachman LM, Maryjowski ML, et al: Immunogenetic studies of juvenile dermatomyositis. HLA antigens in patients and their families. Tissue Antigens 21: 45–49, 1983.
133. Friedman JM, Pachman LM, Maryjowski ML, et al: Immunogenetic studies of juvenile dermatomyositis: HLA-DR antigen frequencies. Arthritis Rheum 26: 214–216, 1983.
134. Hirsch TJ, Enlow RW, Bias WB, Arnett FC: HLA-D related (DR) antigens in various kinds of myositis. Hum Immunol 3: 181–186, 1981.
135. Reed AM, Pachman LM, Hayford J, Ober C: Immunogenetic studies in families of children with juvenile dermatomyositis. J Rheumatol 25: 1000–1002, 1998.
136. Reed AM, Pachman L, Ober C: Molecular genetic studies of major histocompatibility complex genes in children with juvenile dermatomyositis: increased risk associated with HLA-DQA1*0501. Hum Immunol 32: 235–240, 1991.
137. Reed AM, Stirling JD: Association of the HLA-DQA1*0501 allele in multiple racial groups with juvenile dermatomyositis. Hum Immunol 44: 131–135, 1995.
137a. West JE, Reed AM: Analysis of HLA-DM polymorphism in juvenile dermatomyositis (JDM) patients. Hum Immunol 60: 255–258, 1999.
138. Vavrincova P, Havelka S, Cerna M, Stastny P: HLA class II alleles in juvenile dermatomyositis. J Rheumatol 20(Suppl 37): 17–18, 1993.
139. Arnett FC, Targoff IN, Mimori T, et al: Interrelationship of major histocompatibility complex class II alleles and autoantibodies in four ethnic groups with various forms of myositis. Arthritis Rheum 39: 1507–1518, 1996.
140. Banker BQ, Victor M: Dermatomyositis (systemic angiopathy) of childhood. Medicine (Baltimore) 45: 261–289, 1966.
141. Hill RH, Wood WS: Juvenile dermatomyositis. Can Med Assoc J 103: 1152–1156, 1970.

142. Schaller JG: Dermatomyositis. J Pediatr 83: 699–702, 1973.
143. Kornreich HK, Hanson V: The rheumatic diseases of childhood. Curr Probl Pediatr 4: 3–40, 1974.
144. Goel KM, Shanks RA: Dermatomyositis in childhood. Review of eight cases. Arch Dis Child 51: 501–506, 1976.
145. Dubowitz V: Muscle disorders in childhood. Major Probl Clin Pediatr 16: iii–282, 1978.
146. Winkelman RK: Dermatomyositis in childhood. J Dermatol 18: 13, 1979.
147. Malleson PN: Controversies in juvenile dermatomyositis. J Rheumatol Suppl 23: 1–2, 1990.
148. Goel KM, King M: Dermatomyositis-polymyositis in children. Scott Med J 31: 15–19, 1986.
149. Resnick JS, Mammel M, Mundale MO, Kottke FJ: Muscular strength as an index of response to therapy in childhood dermatomyositis. Arch Phys Med Rehabil 62: 12–19, 1981.
150. National Foundation: Publication No. 60. National Foundation, 1946.
150a. Scheja A, Elborgh R, Wildt M: Decreased capillary density in juvenile dermatomyositis and in mixed connective tissue disease. J Rheumatol 26: 1377–1381, 1999.
151. Maricq HR, Spencer-Green G, LeRoy EC: Skin capillary abnormalities as indicators of organ involvement in scleroderma (systemic sclerosis), Raynaud's syndrome and dermatomyositis. Am J Med 61: 862–870, 1976.
152. Spencer-Green G, Schlesinger M, Bove KE, et al: Nailfold capillary abnormalities in childhood rheumatic diseases. J Pediatr 102: 341–346, 1983.
153. Nussbaum AI, Silver RM, Maricq HR: Serial changes in nailfold capillary morphology in childhood dermatomyositis. Arthritis Rheum 26: 1169–1172, 1983.
154. Silver RM, Maricq HR: Childhood dermatomyositis: serial microvascular studies. Pediatrics 83: 278–283, 1989.
154a. Ghali FE, Reed AM, Groben PA, McCauliffe DP: Panniculitis in juvenile dermatomyositis. Pediatr Dermatol 16: 270–272, 1999.
155. Woo TR, Rasmussen J, Callen JP: Recurrent photosensitive dermatitis preceding juvenile dermatomyositis. Pediatr Dermatol 2: 207–212, 1985.
156. Hamlin C, Shelton JE: Management of oral findings in a child with an advanced case of dermatomyositis: Clinical report. Pediatr Dent 6: 46–49, 1984.
156a. Ghali FE, Stein LD, Fine JD, et al: Gingival telangiectases: an underappreciated physical sign of juvenile dermatomyositis. Arch Dermatol 135: 1370–1374, 1999.
157. Bowyer SL, Blane CE, Sullivan DB, Cassidy JT: Childhood dermatomyositis: factors predicting functional outcome and development of dystrophic calcification. J Pediatr 103: 882–888, 1983.
158. Spencer CH, Hanson V, Singsen BH, et al: Course of treated juvenile dermatomyositis. J Pediatr 105: 399–408, 1984.
159. Euwer RL, Sontheimer RD: Amyopathic dermatomyositis (dermatomyositis sine myositis). Presentation of six new cases and review of the literature. J Am Acad Dermatol 24: 959–966, 1991.
160. Cosnes A, Amaudric F, Gherardi R, et al: Dermatomyositis without muscle weakness. Long-term follow-up of 12 patients without systemic corticosteroids. Arch Dermatol 131: 1381–1385, 1995.
161. Schmid MH, Trueb RM: Juvenile amyopathic dermatomyositis. Br J Dermatol 136: 431–433, 1997.
162. Eisenstein DM, Paller AS, Pachman LM: Juvenile dermatomyositis presenting with rash alone; late onset of myositis. Arthritis Rheum 39(Suppl): 192, 1996.
163. Eisenstein DM, Paller AS, Pachman LM: Juvenile dermatomyositis presenting with rash alone. Pediatrics 100: 391–392, 1997.
163a. Plamondon S, Dent PB: Juvenile amyopathic dermatomyositis: results of a case finding descriptive survey. J Rheumatol 27: 2031–2034, 2000.
164. Walton J: The inflammatory myopathies. J R Soc Med 76: 998–1010, 1983.
165. Wananukul S, Pongprasit P, Wattanakrai P: Calcinosis cutis presenting years before other clinical manifestations of juvenile dermatomyositis: report of two cases. Australas J Dermatol 38: 202–205, 1997.
166. Blane CE, White SJ, Braunstein EM, et al: Patterns of calcification in childhood dermatomyositis. AJR Am J Roentgenol 142: 397–400, 1984.
167. Bohan A, Peter JB: Polymyositis and dermatomyositis (first of two parts). N Engl J Med 292: 344–347, 1975.
168. Bohan A, Peter JB: Polymyositis and dermatomyositis (second of two parts). N Engl J Med 292: 403–407, 1975.
169. Thompson JW: Spontaneous perforation of the esophagus as a manifestation of dermatomyositis. Ann Otol Rhinol Laryngol 93: 464–467, 1984.
170. Fischer TJ, Cipel L, Stiehm ER: Pneumatosis intestinalis associated with fatal childhood dermatomyositis. Pediatrics 61: 127–130, 1978.
171. Braunstein EM, White SJ: Pneumatosis intestinalis in dermatomyositis. Br J Radiol 53: 1011–1012, 1980.
172. Schullinger JN, Jacobs JC, Berdon WE: Diagnosis and management of gastrointestinal perforations in childhood dermatomyositis with particular reference to perforations of the duodenum. J Pediatr Surg 20: 521–524, 1985.
173. Magill HL, Hixson SD, Whitington G, et al: Duodenal perforation in childhood dermatomyositis. Pediatr Radiol 14: 28–30, 1984.
174. Inamdar S, Slim MS, Bostwick H, Godine L: Treatment of duodenocutaneous fistula with somatostatin analog in a child with dermatomyositis. J Pediatr Gastroenterol Nutr 10: 402–404, 1990.
175. Farber S, Vawter GF: Clinical pathological conference. J Pediatr 57: 784, 1960.
176. Boylan RC, Sokoloff L: Vascular lesions in dermatomyositis. Arthritis Rheum 3: 379, 1960.
177. Jalleh RP, Swift RI, Sundaresan M, et al: Necrotising testicular vasculitis associated with dermatomyositis. Br J Urol 66: 660, 1990.
178. Fruman LS, Ragsdale CG, Sullivan DB, Petty RE: Retinopathy in juvenile dermatomyositis. J Pediatr 88: 267–269, 1976.
179. Schaumburg HH, Nielsen SL, Yurchak PM: Heart block in polymyositis. N Engl J Med 284: 480–481, 1971.
180. Lynch PG: Cardiac involvement in chronic polymyositis. Br Heart J 33: 416–419, 1971.
181. Fernandez-Herlihy L: Heart block in polymyositis. N Engl J Med 284: 1101, 1971.
182. Buchpiguel CA, Roizenblatt S, Lucena-Fernandes MF, et al: Radioisotopic assessment of peripheral and cardiac muscle involvement and dysfunction in polymyositis/dermatomyositis. J Rheumatol 18: 1359–1363, 1991.
183. Dubowitz LM, Dubowitz V: Acute dermatomyositis presenting with pulmonary manifestations. Arch Dis Child 28: 293, 1964.
184. Dickey BF, Myers AR: Pulmonary disease in polymyositis/dermatomyositis. Semin Arthritis Rheum 14: 60–76, 1984.
185. Duncan PE, Griffin JP, Garcia A, Kaplan SB: Fibrosing alveolitis in polymyositis. A review of histologically confirmed cases. Am J Med 57: 621–626, 1974.
186. Singsen BH, Tedford JC, Platzker AC, Hanson V: Spontaneous pneumothorax: a complication of juvenile dermatomyositis. J Pediatr 92: 771–774, 1978.
187. Schwarz MI, Matthay RA, Sahn SA, et al: Interstitial lung disease in polymyositis and dermatomyositis: analysis of six cases and review of the literature. Medicine (Baltimore) 55: 89–104, 1976.
188. Huang JL: Juvenile dermatomyositis associated with partial lipodystrophy. Br J Clin Pract 50: 112–113, 1996.
189. Quecedo E, Febrer I, Serrano G, et al: Partial lipodystrophy associated with juvenile dermatomyositis: report of two cases. Pediatr Dermatol 13: 477–482, 1996.
190. Commens C, O'Neill P, Walker G: Dermatomyositis associated with multifocal lipoatrophy. J Am Acad Dermatol 22: 966–969, 1990.
191. Tucker LB, Sadegi-Neged A, Schaller JG: The association of acquired lipodystropy with juvenile dermatomyositis. Arthritis Rheum 33: S146, 1990.
192. Kavanagh GM, Colaco CB, Kennedy CT: Juvenile dermatomyositis associated with partial lipoatrophy. J Am Acad Dermatol 28: 348–351, 1993.
193. Adams BS, Cemeeroglu AP, Haftel HM, et al: Prevalence of insulin resistance in juvenile dermatomyositis. Arthritis Rheum 39(Suppl): 192, 1985.
194. Huemer C, Kitson H, Malleson PN, et al: Lipodystrophy in juvenile dermatomyositis patients: evaluation of clinical and metabolic abnormalities. Arthritis Rheum 40(Suppl): 140, 1997.

195. Bennington JL, Dau PC: Patients with polymyositis and dermatomyositis who undergo plasmapheresis therapy. Pathologic findings. Arch Neurol 38: 553–560, 1981.
196. Carpenter S, Karpati G, Rothman S, Watters G: The childhood type of dermatomyositis. Neurology 26: 952–962, 1976.
197. Hughes JT, Esiri MM: Ultrastructural studies in human polymyositis. J Neurol Sci 25: 347–360, 1975.
198. Matsubara S, Mair WG: Ultrastructural changes in polymyositis. Brain 102: 701–725, 1979.
199. Rose AL, Walton JN, Pearce GW: Polymyositis: an ultramicroscopic study of muscle biopsy material. J Neurol Sci 5: 457–472, 1967.
200. Shafiq SA, Milhorat AT, Gorycki MA: An electron-microscope study of muscle degeneration and vascular changes in polymyositis. J Pathol Bacteriol 94: 139–147, 1967.
201. Whitaker JN, Bertorini TE, Mendell JR: Immunocytochemical studies of cathepsin D in human skeletal muscle. Trans Am Neurol Assoc 106: 219–221, 1981.
202. Mastaglia FL, Kakulas BA: A histological and histochemical study of skeletal muscle regeneration in polymyositis. J Neurol Sci 10: 471–487, 1970.
203. Cros D, Pearson C, Verity MA: Polymyositis-dermatomyositis: diagnostic and prognostic significance of muscle alkaline phosphatase. Am J Pathol 101: 159–176, 1980.
204. Engel WK, Cunningham GG: Alkaline phosphatase-positive abnormal muscle fibers of humans. J Histochem Cytochem 18: 55–57, 1970.
205. Oxenhandler R, Adelstein EH, Hart MN: Immunopathology of skeletal muscle. The value of direct immunofluorescence in the diagnosis of connective tissue disease. Hum Pathol 8: 321–328, 1977.
206. Bodensteiner JB, Engel AG: Intracellular calcium accumulation in Duchenne dystrophy and other myopathies: a study of 567,000 muscle fibers in 114 biopsies. Neurology 28: 439–446, 1978.
207. Oberc MA, Engel WK: Ultrastructural localization of calcium in normal and abnormal skeletal muscle. Lab Invest 36: 566–577, 1977.
208. Banker BQ: Dermatomyostis of childhood, ultrastructural alterations of muscle and intramuscular blood vessels. J Neuropathol Exp Neurol 34: 46–75, 1975.
209. Eady RA, Odland GF: Intraendothelial tubular aggregates in experimental wounds. Br J Dermatol 93: 165–173, 1975.
210. Oshima Y, Becker LE, Armstrong DL: An electron microscopic study of childhood dermatomyositis. Acta Neuropathol (Berl) 47: 189–196, 1979.
211. Mastaglia FL, Walton JN: An ultrastructural study of skeletal muscle in polymyositis. J Neurol Sci 12: 473–504, 1971.
212. Chou SM, Nonaka I, Voice GF: Anastomoses of transverse tubules with terminal cisternae in polymyositis. Arch Neurol 37: 257–266, 1980.
213. Yunis EJ, Samaha FJ: Inclusion body myositis. Lab Invest 25: 240–248, 1971.
214. Jerusalem F, Rakusa M, Engel AG, MacDonald RD: Morphometric analysis of skeletal muscle capillary ultrastructure in inflammatory myopathies. J Neurol Sci 23: 391–402, 1974.
215. Duance VC, Black CM, Dubowitz V, et al: Polymyositis: an immunofluorescence study on the distribution of collagen types. Muscle Nerve 3: 487–490, 1980.
216. Foidart M, Foidart JM, Engel WK: Collagen localization in normal and fibrotic human skeletal muscle. Arch Neurol 38: 152–157, 1981.
217. Bowyer SL, Clark RA, Ragsdale CG, et al: Juvenile dermatomyositis: histological findings and pathogenetic hypothesis for the associated skin changes. J Rheumatol 13: 753–759, 1986.
218. Janis JF, Winkelmann RK: Histopathology of the skin in dermatomyositis. A histopathologic study of 55 cases. Arch Dermatol 97: 640–650, 1968.
219. Hanno R, Callen JP: Histopathology of Gottron's papules. J Cutan Pathol 12: 389–394, 1985.
220. Loewi G, Dorling J: Calcinosis. Histological and chemical analysis. Ann Rheum Dis 23: 272, 1964.
221. Sewell JR, Liyanage B, Ansell BM: Calcinosis in juvenile dermatomyositis. Skeletal Radiol 3: 137, 1978.
222. Denbow CE, Lie JT, Tancredi RG, Bunch TW: Cardiac involvement in polymyositis: a clinicopathologic study of 20 autopsied patients. Arthritis Rheum 22: 1088–1092, 1979.
223. Haupt HM, Hutchins GM: The heart and cardiac conduction system in polymyositis-dermatomyositis: a clinicopathologic study of 16 autopsied patients. Am J Cardiol 50: 998–1006, 1982.
224. Bohan A, Peter JB, Bowman RL, Pearson CM: Computer-assisted analysis of 153 patients with polymyositis and dermatomyositis. Medicine (Baltimore) 56: 255–286, 1977.
225. Roddy SM, Ashwal S, Peckham N, Mortensen S: Infantile myositis: a case diagnosed in the neonatal period. Pediatr Neurol 2: 241–244, 1986.
226. Levin MJ, Gardner P, Waldvogel FA: An unusual infection due to *Staphylococcus aureus*. N Engl J Med 284: 196–198, 1971.
227. Topi GC, D'Alessandro L, Catricala C, Zardi O: Dermatomyositis-like syndrome due to toxoplasma. Br J Dermatol 101: 589–591, 1979.
228. Noseworthy JH., Heffernan LP, Ross JB, Sangalang VE: Acne fulminans with inflammatory myopathy. Ann Neurol 8: 67–69, 1980.
229. Fiallo P, Tagliapietra AG: Severe acute myopathy induced by isotretinoin. Arch Dermatol 132: 1521–1522, 1996.
230. Schraeder PL, Peters HA, Dahl DS: Polymyositis and penicillamine. Arch Neurol 27: 456–457, 1972.
231. Zucker J: Drug-induced myopathies. Semin Arthritis Rheum 19: 259, 1990.
232. Gross M: Clinical heterogeneity and molecular mechanisms in inborn muscle AMP deaminase deficiency. J Inherit Metab Dis 20: 186–192, 1997.
233. Ashwal S, Peckham N: Myoadenylate deaminase deficiency in children. Pediatr Neurol 1: 185–191, 1985.
234. Newman AJ, Lee C: Hypothyroidism simulating dermatomyositis. J Pediatr 97: 772–774, 1980.
235. Brooke MH, Kaplan H: Muscle pathology in rheumatoid arthritis, polymyalgia rheumatica, and polymyositis: a histochemical study. Arch Pathol 94: 101–118, 1972.
236. Medsger TA Jr, Rodnan GP, Moossy J, Vester JW: Skeletal muscle involvement in progressive systemic sclerosis (scleroderma). Arthritis Rheum 11: 554–568, 1968.
237. Graudal H: Myopathy in rheumatoid arthritis. Rheumatism 17: 81, 1961.
238. Denko CW, Old JW: Myopathy in the sicca syndrome (Sjögren's syndrome). Am J Clin Pathol 51: 631–637, 1969.
239. Thompson CE: Infantile myositis. Dev Med Child Neurol 24: 307–313, 1982.
240. Anderson TE, Carr AJ, Chapman RS, et al: Myositis and myotonia in a case of multicentric reticulohistiocytosis. Br J Dermatol 80: 39–45, 1968.
241. Burke JS, Medline NM, Katz A: Giant cell myocarditis and myositis. Associated with thymoma and myasthenia gravis. Arch Pathol 88: 359–366, 1969.
242. Silverstein A, Siltzbach LE: Muscle involvement in sarcoidosis. Asymptomatic, myositis, and myopathy. Arch Neurol 21: 235–241, 1969.
242a. Wortmann RL (ed): Diseases of Skeletal Muscle. Philadelphia, Lippincott Williams & Wilkins, 2000, pp 45–252.
243. Carpenter S, Karpati G, Heller I, Eisen A: Inclusion body myositis: a distinct variety of idiopathic inflammatory myopathy. Neurology 28: 8–17, 1978.
244. Griggs RC, Askanas V, DiMauro S, et al: Inclusion body myositis and myopathies. Ann Neurol 38: 705–713, 1995.
245. Illa I, Dalakas MC: Dermatomyositis, polymyositis and inclusion body myositis: current concepts. Rev Neurol (Paris) 154: 13–16, 1998.
246. Layzer RB, Shearn MA, Satya-Murti S: Eosinophilic polymyositis. Ann Neurol 1: 65–71, 1977.
247. Cumming WJ, Weiser R, Teoh R, et al: Localised nodular myositis: a clinical and pathological variant of polymyositis. Q J Med 46: 531–546, 1977.
248. Heffner RR Jr, Barron SA: Polymyositis beginning as a focal process. Arch Neurol 38: 439–442, 1981.
249. Enzinger FM, Dulcey F: Proliferative myositis. Report of thirty-three cases. Cancer 20: 2213–2223, 1967.
250. Savage DC, Forbes M, Pearce GW: Idiopathic rhabdomyolysis. Arch Dis Child 46: 594–607, 1971.

251. Smith R, Russell RG, Woods CG: Myositis ossificans progressiva. Clinical features of eight patients and their response to treatment. J Bone Joint Surg Br 58: 48–57, 1976.
252. Hentzer B, Jacobsen HH, Asboe-Hansen G: Fibrodysplasia ossificans progressiva. Scand J Rheumatol 6: 161–171, 1977.
253. Wu T, Chen SS: Differential diagnosis between fibrodysplasia ossificans progressiva and childhood dermatomyositis with calcinosis. J Formos Med Assoc 92: 569–576, 1993.
254. Vignos PJ Jr, Goldwyn J: Evaluation of laboratory tests in diagnosis and management of polymyositis. Am J Med Sci 263: 291–308, 1972.
255. Haas RH, Dyck RF, Dubowitz V, Pepys MB: C-reactive protein in childhood dermatomyositis. Ann Rheum Dis 41: 483–485, 1982.
256. Lisak RP, Zweiman B: Serum immunoglobulin levels in myasthenia gravis, polymyositis, and dermatomyositis. J Neurol Neurosurg Psychiatry 39: 34–37, 1976.
257. Gotoff SP, Smith RD, Sugar O: Dermatomyositis with cerebral vasculitis in a patient with agammaglobulinemia. Am J Dis Child 123: 53–56, 1972.
258. Giuliano VJ: Case report: polymyositis in a patient with acquired hypogammaglobulinemia. Am J Med Sci 268: 53–56, 1974.
259. Bardelas JA, Winkelstein JA, Seto DS, et al: Fatal ECHO 24 infection in a patient with hypogammaglobulinemia: relationship to dermatomyositis-like syndrome. J Pediatr 90: 396–399, 1977.
260. Ishida T, Ohashi M, Matsumoto Y, et al: Connection of atopic disease in Japanese patients with juvenile dermatomyositis based on serum IgE levels. Clin Rheumatol 12: 41–48, 1993.
261. Bowyer SL, Ragsdale CG, Sullivan DB: Factor VIII–related antigen and childhood rheumatic diseases. J Rheumatol 16: 1093–1097, 1989.
262. Guzman J, Petty RE, Malleson PN: Monitoring disease activity in juvenile dermatomyositis: the role of von Willebrand factor and muscle enzymes. J Rheumatol 21: 739–743, 1994.
263. Bloom BJ, Tucker LB, Miller LC, Schaller JG: von Willebrand factor in juvenile dermatomyositis. J Rheumatol 22: 320–325, 1995.
264. Kobayashi S, Higuchi K, Tamaki H, et al: Characteristics of juvenile dermatomyositis in Japan. Acta Paediatr Jpn 39: 257–262, 1997.
265. De Benedetti F, De Amici M, Aramini L, et al: Correlation of serum neopterin concentrations with disease activity in juvenile dermatomyositis. Arch Dis Child 69: 232–235, 1993.
266. Askmark H, Osterman PO, Roxin LE, Venge P: Radioimmunoassay of serum myoglobin in neuromuscular diseases. J Neurol Neurosurg Psychiatry 44: 68–72, 1981.
267. Nishikai M, Reichlin M: Radioimmunoassay of serum myoglobin in polymyositis and other conditions. Arthritis Rheum 20: 1514–1518, 1977.
268. Nishikai M, Homma M: Circulating autoantibody against human myoglobin in polymyositis. JAMA 237: 1842–1844, 1977.
269. Dickerson JW, Widdowson EM: Chemical changes in skeletal muscle during development. Biochem J 74: 247, 1960.
270. Hallgren R, Karlsson FA, Roxin LE, Venge P: Myoglobin turnover: influence of renal and extrarenal factors. J Lab Clin Med 91: 246–254, 1978.
271. Ansell BM, Hamilton E, Bywaters EG: Course and prognosis in juvenile dermatomyositis. *In* Kakulas BA (ed): Second International Congress on Muscle Disease, Part 2. Amsterdam, The Netherlands, Excerpta Medica, 1973.
272. Montecucco C, Ravelli A, Caporali R, et al: Autoantibodies in juvenile dermatomyositis. Clin Exp Rheumatol 8: 193–196, 1990.
273. Feldman BM, Reichlin M, Laxer RM, et al: Clinical significance of specific autoantibodies in juvenile dermatomyositis. J Rheumatol 23: 1794–1797, 1996.
274. Rider LG, Miller FW, Targoff IN, et al: A broadened spectrum of juvenile myositis. Myositis-specific autoantibodies in children. Arthritis Rheum 37: 1534–1538, 1994.
275. Friedman AW, Targoff IN, Arnett FC: Interstitial lung disease with autoantibodies against aminoacyl-tRNA synthetases in the absence of clinically apparent myositis. Semin Arthritis Rheum 26: 459–467, 1996.
276. Targoff IN, Johnson AE, Miller FW: Antibody to signal recognition particle in polymyositis. Arthritis Rheum 33: 1361–1370, 1990.
277. Targoff IN, Miller FW, Medsger TA Jr, Oddis CV: Classification criteria for the idiopathic inflammatory myopathies. Curr Opin Rheumatol 9: 527–535, 1997.
278. Garcia-Patos V, Bartralot R, Fonollosa V, et al: Childhood sclerodermatomyositis: report of a case with the anti-PM/Scl antibody and mechanic's hands. Br J Dermatol 135: 613–616, 1996.
279. Cambridge G, Ovadia E, Isenberg DA, et al: Juvenile dermatomyositis: serial studies of circulating autoantibodies to a 56kD nuclear protein. Clin Exp Rheumatol 12: 451–457, 1994.
280. Tanimoto K, Nakano K, Kano S, et al: Classification criteria for polymyositis and dermatomyositis [published erratum appears in J Rheumatol 22: 1807, 1995]. J Rheumatol 22: 668–674, 1995.
281. Nishikai M, Reichlin M: Heterogeneity of precipitating antibodies in polymyositis and dermatomyositis. Characterization of the Jo-1 antibody system. Arthritis Rheum 23: 881–888, 1980.
282. Nishikai M, Reichlin M: Purification and characterization of a nuclear non-histone basic protein (Mi-1) which reacts with anti-immunoglobulin sera and the sera of patients with dermatomyositis. Mol Immunol 17: 1129–1141, 1980.
283. Reichlin M, Mattioli M: Description of a serological reaction characteristic of polymyositis. Clin Immunol Immunopathol 5: 12–20, 1976.
284. Wolfe JF, Adelstein E, Sharp GC: Antinuclear antibody with distinct specificity for polymyositis. J Clin Invest 59: 176–178, 1977.
285. Pachman LM, Maryjowski MC: Juvenile dermatomyositis and polymyositis. Clin Rheum Dis 10: 95–115, 1984.
286. Pachman LM, Friedman JM, Maryjowski-Sweeney ML, et al: Immunogenetic studies of juvenile dermatomyositis. III. Study of antibody to organ-specific and nuclear antigens. Arthritis Rheum 28: 151–157, 1985.
287. Pachman LM: Juvenile dermatomyositis. Pediatr Clin North Am 33: 1097–1117, 1986.
288. Mimori T, Akizuki M, Yamagata H, et al: Characterization of a high molecular weight acidic nuclear protein recognized by autoantibodies in sera from patients with polymyositis-scleroderma overlap. J Clin Invest 68: 611–620, 1981.
289. Cervera R, Ramirez G, Fernandez-Sola J, et al: Antibodies to endothelial cells in dermatomyositis: association with interstitial lung disease. Br Med J 302: 880–881, 1991.
290. Edelsten C, D'Cruz D, Hughes GR, Graham EM: Anti-endothelial cell antibodies in retinal vasculitis. Curr Eye Res 11(Suppl): 203–208, 1992.
291. Stern GM, Rose AL, Jacobs K: Circulating antibodies in polymyositis. J Neurol Sci 5: 181–183, 1967.
292. Caspary EA, Gubbay SS, Stern GM: Circulating antibodies in polymyositis and other muscle-wasting disorders. Lancet 2: 941, 1964.
293. Behan WM, Behan PO: Complement abnormalities in polymyositis. J Neurol Sci 34: 241–246, 1977.
294. Pachman LM, Hayford JR, Chung A, et al: Juvenile dermatomyositis at diagnosis: clinical characteristics of 79 children. J Rheumatol 25: 1198–1204, 1998.
295. Sandstedt PE, Henriksson KG, Larrsson LE: Quantitative electromyography in polymyositis and dermatomyositis. Acta Neurol Scand 65: 110–121, 1982.
296. Wilkinson JH: The Principles and Practice of Diagnostic Enzymology. Chicago, Year Book Medical, 1976, pp. 303.
297. Clark LC Jr, Thompson HL, Beck EL, et al: Excretion of creatine and creatinine by children. Am J Dis Child 81: 774, 1951.
298. Mechler F: Changing electromyographic findings during the chronic course of polymyositis. J Neurol Sci 23: 237–242, 1974.
299. Haridasan G, Sanghvi SH, Jindal GD, et al: Quantitative electromyography using automatic analysis. A comparative study with a fixed fraction of a subject's maximum effort and two levels of thresholds for analysis. J Neurol Sci 42: 53–64, 1979.
300. Partanen J, Lang H: EMG dynamics in polymyositis. A quantitative single motor unit potential study. J Neurol Sci 57: 221–234, 1982.
301. Smyth DP: Quantitative electromyography in babies and young children with primary muscle disease and neurogenic lesions. J Neurol Sci 56: 199–207, 1982.

302. Calore EE, Cavaliere MJ, Perez NM: Muscle pathology in juvenile dermatomyositis. Rev Paul Med 115: 1555–1559, 1997.
303. Tome FM, Fardeau M, Lebon P, Chevallay M: Inclusion body myositis. Acta Neuropathol Suppl (Berl) 7: 287–291, 1981.
304. Campellone JV, Lacomis D, Giuliani MJ, Oddis CV: Percutaneous needle muscle biopsy in the evaluation of patients with suspected inflammatory myopathy. Arthritis Rheum 40: 1886–1891, 1997.
305. Steiner RM, Glassman L, Schwartz MW, Vanace P: The radiological findings in dermatomyositis of childhood. Radiology 111: 385–393, 1974.
306. Ozonoff MB, Flynn FJ Jr: Roentgenologic features of dermatomyositis of childhood. Am J Roentgenol Radium Ther Nucl Med 118: 206–212, 1973.
307. Fishel B, Diamant S, Papo I, Yaron M: CT assessment of calcinosis in a patient with dermatomyositis. Clin Rheumatol 5: 242–244, 1986.
308. Fleckenstein JL, Reimers CD: Inflammatory myopathies: radiologic evaluation. Radiol Clin North Am 34: 427–39, xii, 1996.
309. Hernandez RJ, Sullivan DB, Chenevert TL, Keim DR: MR imaging in children with dermatomyositis: musculoskeletal findings and correlation with clinical and laboratory findings. Am J Roentgenol 161: 359–366, 1993.
310. Stonecipher MR, Jorizzo JL, Monu J, et al: Dermatomyositis with normal muscle enzyme concentrations. A single-blind study of the diagnostic value of magnetic resonance imaging and ultrasound. Arch Dermatol 130: 1294–1299, 1994.
311. Kaufman LD, Gruber BL, Gerstman DP, Kaell AT: Preliminary observations on the role of magnetic resonance imaging for polymyositis and dermatomyositis. Ann Rheum Dis 46: 569–572, 1987.
312. Hernandez RJ, Keim DR, Sullivan DB, et al: Magnetic resonance imaging appearance of the muscles in childhood dermatomyositis. J Pediatr 117: 546–550, 1990.
313. Keim DR, Hernandez RJ, Sullivan DB: Serial magnetic resonance imaging in juvenile dermatomyositis. Arthritis Rheum 34: 1580–1584, 1991.
314. Hernandez RJ, Keim DR, Chenevert TL, et al: Fat-suppressed MR imaging of myositis. Radiology 182: 217–219, 1992.
315. Park JH, Olsen NJ, King L Jr, et al: Use of magnetic resonance imaging and P-31 magnetic resonance spectroscopy to detect and quantify muscle dysfunction in the amyopathic and myopathic variants of dermatomyositis. Arthritis Rheum 38: 68–77, 1995.
316. Park JH, Niermann KJ, Ryder NM, et al: Muscle abnormalities in juvenile dermatomyositis patients: P-31 magnetic resonance spectroscopy studies. Arthritis Rheum 43: 2359–2367, 2000.
317. Summers RM, Brune AM, Choyke PL, et al: Juvenile idiopathic inflammatory myopathy: exercise-induced changes in muscle at short inversion time inversion-recovery MR imaging. Radiology 209: 191–196, 1998.
317a. Kimball AB, Summers RM, Turner M, et al: Magnetic resonance imaging detection of occult skin and subcutaneous abnormalities in juvenile dermatomyositis. Implications for diagnosis and therapy. Arthritis Rheum 43: 1866–1873, 2000.
318. Guillet GY, Guillet JA, Blanquet P, Maleville J: A new noninvasive evaluation of muscular lesions in dermatomyositis: thallium 201 muscle scans. J Am Acad Dermatol 5: 670–672, 1981.
319. Guillet J, Blanquet P, Guillet G, et al: The use of technetium Tc 99m medronate scintigraphy as a prognostic guide in childhood dermatomyositis. Arch Dermatol 117: 451, 1981.
320. Yonker RA, Webster EM, Edwards NL, et al: Technetium pyrophosphate muscle scans in inflammatory muscle disease. Br J Rheumatol 26: 267–269, 1987.
321. Smith WP, Robinson RG, Gobuty AH: Positive whole-body 67Ga scintigraphy in dermatomyositis. Am J Roentgenol 133: 126–127, 1979.
322. Dubowitz V: Treatment of dermatomyositis in childhood. Arch Dis Child 51: 494–500, 1976.
323. Winkelmann RK: Dermatomyositis in childhood. Clin Rheum Dis 8: 353–368, 1982.
324. Ansell BM: Management of polymyositis and dermatomyositis. Clin Rheum Dis 10: 205–213, 1984.
325. Cassidy JT: Dermatomyositis in children. *In* Hicks RV (ed): Vasculopathies of Childhood. Littleton, MA, PSG Publishing, 1988, p. 205.
326. Van Rossum MA, Hiemstra I, Prieur AM, et al: Juvenile dermato/polymyositis: a retrospective analysis of 33 cases with special focus on initial CPK levels. Clin Exp Rheumatol 12: 339–342, 1994.
327. Rider LG: Assessment of disease activity and its sequelae in children and adults with myositis. Curr Opin Rheumatol 8: 495–506, 1996.
328. Huppertz HI, Kaiser WA: Serial magnetic resonance imaging in juvenile dermatomyositis: delayed normalization. Rheumatol Int 14: 127–129, 1994.
329. Chapman S, Southwood TR, Fowler J, Ryder CA: Rapid changes in magnetic resonance imaging of muscle during the treatment of juvenile dermatomyositis. Br J Rheumatol 33: 184–186, 1994.
330. Rider LG, Feldman BM, Perez MD, et al: Development of validated disease activity and damage indices for the juvenile idiopathic inflammatory myopathies: I. Physician, parent, and patient global assessments. Juvenile Dermatomyositis Disease Activity Collaborative Study Group. Arthritis Rheum 40: 1976–1983, 1997.
331. Feldman BM, Ayling-Campos A, Luy L, et al: Measuring disability in juvenile dermatomyositis: validity of the childhood health assessment questionnaire. J Rheumatol 22: 326–331, 1995.
332. Lovell DJ, Lindsley CB, Rennebohm RM, et al: Development of validated disease activity and damage indices for the juvenile idiopathic inflammatory myopathies. II. The Childhood Myositis Assessment Scale (CMAS): a quantitative tool for the evaluation of muscle function. The Juvenile Dermatomyositis Disease Activity Collaborative Study Group. Arthritis Rheum 42: 2213–2219, 1999.
333. Bunch TW, Worthington JW, Combs JJ, et al: Azathioprine with prednisone for polymyositis. A controlled, clinical trial. Ann Intern Med 92: 365–369, 1980.
334. Miller FW, Leitman SF, Cronin ME, et al: Controlled trial of plasma exchange and leukapheresis in polymyositis and dermatomyositis. N Engl J Med 326: 1380–1384, 1992.
335. Dalakas MC, Illa I, Dambrosia JM, et al: A controlled trial of high-dose intravenous immune globulin infusions as treatment for dermatomyositis. N Engl J Med 329: 1993–2000, 1993.
336. Villalba L, Hicks JE, Adams EM, et al: Treatment of refractory myositis: a randomized crossover study of two new cytotoxic regimens. Arthritis Rheum 41: 392–399, 1998.
337. Perez MD, Abrams SA, Koenning G, et al: Mineral metabolism in children with dermatomyositis. J Rheumatol 21: 2364–2369, 1994.
337a. Bianchi ML, Cimaz R, Bardare M, et al: Efficacy and safety of alendronate for the treatment of osteoporosis in diffuse connective tissue diseases in children: a prospective multicenter study. Arthritis Rheum 43: 1960–1966, 2000.
338. Miller JJ III: Prolonged use of large intravenous steroid pulses in the rheumatic diseases of children. Pediatrics 65: 989–994, 1980.
339. Yanagisawa T, Sueishi M, Nawata Y, et al: Methylprednisolone pulse therapy in dermatomyositis. Dermatologica 167: 47–51, 1983.
340. Wollina U, Schreiber G: Prednisolone pulse therapy for childhood systemic lupus erythematosus with prominent dermatomyositis. A case report. Dermatologica 171: 45–48, 1985.
341. Laxer RM, Stein LD, Petty RE: Intravenous pulse methylprednisolone treatment of juvenile dermatomyositis. Arthritis Rheum 30: 328–334, 1987.
341a. Huang JL: Long-term prognosis of patients with juvenile dermatomyositis initially treated with intravenous methylprednisolone pulse therapy. Clin Exp Rheumatol 17: 621–624, 1999.
341b. Al-Mayouf S, Al-Mazyed A, Bahabri S: Efficacy of early treatment of severe juvenile dermatomyositis with intravenous methylprednisolone and methotrexate. Clin Rheumatol 19: 138–141, 2000.
342. Lang B, Dooley J: Failure of pulse intravenous methylprednisolone treatment in juvenile dermatomyositis. J Pediatr 128: 429–432, 1996.
343. Woo TY, Callen JP, Voorhees JJ, et al: Cutaneous lesions of dermatomyositis are improved by hydroxychloroquine. J Am Acad Dermatol 10: 592–600, 1984.

344. Olson NY, Lindsley CB: Adjunctive use of hydroxychloroquine in childhood dermatomyositis. J Rheumatol 16: 1545–1547, 1989.
345. Malaviya AN, Many A, Schwartz RS: Treatment of dermatomyositis with methotrexate. Lancet 2: 485–488, 1968.
346. Sokoloff MC, Goldberg LS, Pearson CM: Treatment of corticosteroid-resistant polymyositis with methotrexate. Lancet 1: 14–16, 1971.
347. Metzger AL, Bohan A, Goldberg LS, et al: Polymyositis and dermatomyositis: combined methotrexate and corticosteroid therapy. Ann Intern Med 81: 182–189, 1974.
348. Fischer TJ, Rachelefsky GS, Klein RB, et al: Childhood dermatomyositis and polymyositis. Treatment with methotrexate and prednisone. Am J Dis Child 133: 386–389, 1979.
349. Jacobs JC: Methotrexate and azathioprine treatment of childhood dermatomyositis. Pediatrics 59: 212–218, 1977.
350. Benson MD, Aldo MA: Azathioprine therapy in polymyositis. Arch Intern Med 132: 447–451, 1973.
351. Niakan E, Pitner SE, Whitaker JN, Bertorini TE: Immunosuppressive agents in corticosteroid-refractory childhood dermatomyositis. Neurology 30: 286–291, 1980.
352. Heckmatt J, Hasson N, Saunders C, et al: Cyclosporin in juvenile dermatomyositis. Lancet 1: 1063–1066, 1989.
353. Zabel P, Leimenstoll G, Gross WL: Cyclosporin for acute dermatomyositis. Lancet 1: 343, 1984.
354. Girardin E, Dayer JM, Paunier L: Cyclosporine for juvenile dermatomyositis. J Pediatr 112: 165–166, 1988.
355. Dantzig P: Juvenile dermatomyositis treated with cyclosporine. J Am Acad Dermatol 22: 310–311, 1990.
356. Cronin ME, Miller FW, Hicks JE, et al: The failure of intravenous cyclophosphamide therapy in refractory idiopathic inflammatory myopathy. J Rheumatol 16: 1225–1228, 1989.
357. Sinoway PA, Callen JP: Chlorambucil. An effective corticosteroid-sparing agent for patients with recalcitrant dermatomyositis. Arthritis Rheum 36: 319–324, 1993.
358. Zeller V, Cohen P, Prieur AM, Guillevin L: Cyclosporin A therapy in refractory juvenile dermatomyositis. Experience and long-term follow-up of 6 cases. J Rheumatol 23: 1424–1427, 1996.
359. Reiff A, Rawlings DJ, Shaham B, et al: Preliminary evidence for cyclosporin A as an alternative in the treatment of recalcitrant juvenile rheumatoid arthritis and juvenile dermatomyositis. J Rheumatol 24: 2436–2443, 1997.
360. Grau JM, Herrero C, Casademont J, et al: Cyclosporine A as first choice therapy for dermatomyositis. J Rheumatol 21: 381–382, 1994.
361. Peters AM, Heckmatt JZ, Hasson N, et al: Renal haemodynamics of cyclosporin A nephrotoxicity in children with juvenile dermatomyositis. Clin Sci (Colch) 81: 153–159, 1991.
362. Lang BA, Laxer RM, Murphy G, et al: Treatment of dermatomyositis with intravenous gammaglobulin. Am J Med 91: 169–172, 1991.
362a. Al-Mayouf SM, Laxer RM, Schneider R, et al: Intravenous immunoglobulin therapy for juvenile dermatomyositis: efficacy and safety. J Rheumatol 27: 2498–2503, 2000.
363. Roifman CM: Use of intravenous immune globulin in the therapy of children with rheumatological diseases. J Clin Immunol 15: 42S–51S, 1995.
364. Tsai MJ, Lai CC, Lin SC, et al: Intravenous immunoglobulin therapy in juvenile dermatomyositis. Chung Hua Min Kuo Hsiao Erh Ko I Hsueh Hui Tsa Chih 38: 111–115, 1997.
365. Sansome A, Dubowitz V: Intravenous immunoglobulin in juvenile dermatomyositis: four year review of nine cases. Arch Dis Child 72: 25–28, 1995.
366. Collet E, Dalac S, Maerens B, et al: Juvenile dermatomyositis: treatment with intravenous gammaglobulin. Br J Dermatol 130: 231–234, 1994.
367. Cherin P, Herson S, Wechsler B, et al: Efficacy of intravenous gammaglobulin therapy in chronic refractory polymyositis and dermatomyositis: an open study with 20 adult patients. Am J Med 91: 162–168, 1991.
368. Cherin P, Piette JC, Wechsler B, et al: Intravenous gamma globulin as first line therapy in polymyositis and dermatomyositis: an open study in 11 adult patients. J Rheumatol 21: 1092–1097, 1994.
369. Kato E, Shindo S, Eto Y, et al: Administration of immune globulin associated with aseptic meningitis. JAMA 259: 3269–3271, 1988.
370. Goldsmith A, Feldman B, Singh G, et al: Aseptic meningitis following intravenous immune globulin in children. Arthritis Rheum 34: S121, 1991.
371. Brewer EJ Jr, Giannini EH, Rossen RD, et al: Plasma exchange therapy of a childhood onset dermatomyositis patient. Arthritis Rheum 23: 509–513, 1980.
372. Anderson L, Ziter FA: Plasmapheresis via central catheter in dermatomyositis: a new method for selected pediatric patients. J Pediatr 98: 240–241, 1981.
373. Dau PC, Bennington JL: Plasmapheresis in childhood dermatomyositis. J Pediatr 98: 237–240, 1981.
374. Dau PC: Plasmapheresis in idiopathic inflammatory myopathy. Experience with 35 patients. Arch Neurol 38: 544–552, 1981.
375. De Wilde A, DiSpaltro FX, Geller A, et al: Extracorporeal photochemotherapy as adjunctive treatment in juvenile dermatomyositis: a case report. Arch Dermatol 128: 1656–1657, 1992.
376. Wilsher ML, Holdaway IM, North JD: Hypercalcaemia during resolution of calcinosis in juvenile dermatomyositis. Br Med J (Clin Res Ed) 288: 1345, 1984.
377. Lian JB, Pachman LM, Gundberg CM, et al: Gamma-carboxyglutamate excretion and calcinosis in juvenile dermatomyositis. Arthritis Rheum 25: 1094–1100, 1982.
378. Ames EL, Posch JL: Calcinosis of the flexor and extensor tendons in dermatomyositis: case report. J Hand Surg Am 9: 876–879, 1984.
379. Nassim JR, Connolly CK: Treatment of calcinosis universalis with aluminium hydroxide. Arch Dis Child 45: 118–121, 1970.
380. Taborn J, Bole GG, Thompson GR: Colchicine suppression of local and systemic inflammation due to calcinosis universalis in chronic dermatomyositis. Ann Intern Med 89: 648–649, 1978.
381. Fuchs D, Fruchter L, Fishel B, et al: Colchicine suppression of local inflammation due to calcinosis in dermatomyositis and progressive systemic sclerosis. Clin Rheumatol 5: 527–530, 1986.
382. Skuterud E, Sydnes OA, Haavik TK: Calcinosis in dermatomyositis treated with probenecid. Scand J Rheumatol 10: 92–94, 1981.
383. Dent CE, Stamp TC: Treatment of calcinosis circumscripta with probenecid. Br Med J 1: 216–218, 1972.
384. Uttley WS, Belton NR, Syme J, Sheppard H: Calcium balance in children treated with diphosphonates. Arch Dis Child 50: 187–190, 1975.
385. Herd JK, Vaughan JH: Calcinosis universalis complicating dermatomyositis: its treatment with Na2EDTA. Report of two cases in children. Arthritis Rheum 7: 259, 1964.
386. Metzger AL, Singer FR, Bluestone R, Pearson CM: Failure of disodium etidronate in calcinosis due to dermatomyositis and scleroderma. N Engl J Med 291: 1294–1296, 1974.
387. Miller G, Heckmatt JZ, Dubowitz V: Drug treatment of juvenile dermatomyositis. Arch Dis Child 58: 445–450, 1983.
388. Martinez-Cordero E, Lopez-Zepeda J, Choza-Romero F: Calcinosis in childhood dermatomyositis. Clin Exp Rheumatol 8: 198–200, 1990.
389. Nakagawa T, Takaiwa T: Calcinosis cutis in juvenile dermatomyositis responsive to aluminum hydroxide treatment. J Dermatol 20: 558–560, 1993.
389a. Pachman LM, Liotta-Davis MR, Hong DK, et al: TNF-alpha-308A allele in juvenile dermatomyositis: association with increased production of tumor necrosis factor alpha, disease duration, and pathologic calcifications. Arthritis Rheum 43: 2368–2377, 2000.
390. Shearin JC, Pickrell K: Surgical treatment of subcutaneous calcifications of polymyositis or dermatomyositis. Ann Plast Surg 5: 381–385, 1980.
391. Moore EC, Cohen F, Douglas SD, Gutta V: Staphylococcal infections in childhood dermatomyositis: association with the development of calcinosis, raised IgE concentrations and granulocyte chemotactic defect. Ann Rheum Dis 51: 378–383, 1992.
392. Ostrov BE, Goldsmith DP, Eichenfield AH, Athreya BH: Hypercalcemia during the resolution of calcinosis universalis in juvenile dermatomyositis. J Rheumatol 18: 1730–1734, 1991.
393. Miller JJ III: Late progression in dermatomyositis in childhood. J Pediatr 83: 543–548, 1973.
394. Lovell HB, Lindsley CB: Late recurrence of childhood dermatomyositis. J Rheumatol 13: 821–822, 1986.

395. Miller JJ III, Koehler JP: Persistence of activity in dermatomyositis of childhood. Arthritis Rheum 20: 332–337, 1977.
396. Collison CH, Sinal SH, Jorizzo JL, et al: Juvenile dermatomyositis and polymyositis: a follow-up study of long-term sequelae. South Med J 91: 17–22, 1998.
397. Barnes AB, Link DA: Childhood dermatomyositis and pregnancy. Am J Obstet Gynecol 146: 335–336, 1983.
398. Gutierrez G, Dagnino R, Mintz G: Polymyositis/dermatomyositis and pregnancy. Arthritis Rheum 27: 291–294, 1984.
399. Pinheiro GD, Goldenberg J, Atra E, et al: Juvenile dermatomyositis and pregnancy: report and literature review. J Rheumatol 19: 1798–1801, 1992.
399a. Huber AM, Lang B, LeBlanc CM, et al: Medium- and long-term functional outcomes in a multicenter cohort of children with juvenile dermatomyositis. Arthritis Rheum 43: 541–549, 2000.
399b. Collison CH, Sinal SH, Jorizzo JL, et al: Juvenile dermatomyositis and polymyositis: a follow-up study of long-term sequelae. South Med J 91: 17–22, 1998.
399c. Huber AM, Lang B, LeBlanc CM, et al: Medium- and long-term functional outcomes in a multicenter cohort of children with juvenile dermatomyositis. Arthritis Rheum 43: 541–549, 2000.
400. Miller LC, Michael AF, Kim Y: Childhood dermatomyositis. Clinical course and long-term follow-up. Clin Pediatr (Phila) 26: 561–566, 1987.
401. Chalmers A, Sayson R, Walters K: Juvenile dermatomyositis: medical, social and economic status in adulthood. Can Med Assoc J 126: 31–33, 1982.
402. Hochberg MC, Lopez-Acuna D, Gittelsohn AM: Mortality from polymyositis and dermatomyositis in the United States, 1968–1978. Arthritis Rheum 26: 1465–1471, 1983.
403. Taieb A, Guichard C, Salamon R, Maleville J: Prognosis in juvenile dermatopolymyositis: a cooperative retrospective study of 70 cases. Pediatr Dermatol 2: 275–281, 1985.

21

The Systemic Sclerodermas and Related Disorders

James T. Cassidy and Ross E. Petty

DEFINITION AND CLASSIFICATION

The word *scleroderma* means "hard skin." The diseases grouped under this term mean a great deal more, although hardening of the skin is a feature that is common to all types of the disorder and is the most signal characteristic of these entities. A classification of the systemic and localized sclerodermas is given in Table 21–1. Systemic scleroderma is subdivided by the extent of the skin disease into *diffuse cutaneous systemic scleroderma* and *limited cutaneous systemic scleroderma.* The localized forms of the disease, such as morphea or linear scleroderma, often are regarded as more dermatologic than rheumatologic (see Chapter 22).

Table 21–1

Classification of Systemic and Local Sclerodermas and Scleroderma-Like Disorders

- Systemic disease
  - Scleroderma
    - Diffuse
    - Limited
  - Overlap syndromes
    - Sclerodermatomyositis or other connective tissue diseases
    - Mixed connective tissue disease
- Localized disease
  - Morphea
  - Generalized morphea
  - Linear scleroderma
  - Eosinophilic fasciitis
- Graft-versus-host disease
- Chemically induced scleroderma-like disease
  - Polyvinyl chloride
  - Bleomycin
  - Pentazocine
  - Toxic oil syndrome
  - Human adjuvant disease
- Pseudosclerodermas
  - Phenylketonuria
  - Syndromes of premature aging
  - Localized idiopathic fibroses
  - Scleredema
  - Porphyria cutanea tarda
  - Diabetic cheiroarthropathy

Historical Review

The early literature presents a confusing picture of scleroderma in the child because many cases are more compatible with the diagnosis of scleredema. In 1895, Lewin and Heller[1] compiled 505 cases of scleroderma, mainly from the European literature. Goodman[2] noted that 88 occurred in children from birth to 19 years but that the vast majority were examples of circumscribed disease. Only 1 of the 12 cases reported as diffuse scleroderma was compatible with current concepts of this entity, the rest being the "acute form," probably scleredema.[3] A survey concluded that only 12 children with generalized scleroderma had been reported in the world literature through 1960.[4] In 1961, the Mayo Clinic added 63 additional pediatric cases in summarizing their experience with 727 patients.[5] Since then, there have been a number of reports based on relatively small numbers of children, emphasizing the infrequency of this disorder in pediatric rheumatology clinics (Table 21–2). Some reports bracket the linear and generalized disorders: as a rule, the localized disease is limited to the skin and underlying structures, but involvement of other organ systems has been described (see Chapter 22).[6]

Pathologic studies lagged behind the clinical reports, so that there were no comprehensive descriptions until 1924, when Kraus[7] noted both pulmonary and cardiac fibrosis in a patient with scleroderma and Matsui[8] detailed the necropsy findings in five patients with scleroderma and the cutaneous histologic characteristics in another. In 1969, D'Angelo and colleagues[9] compared the postmortem findings of 48 cases of scleroderma with 58 matched control cases, reporting involvement as percentages in excess of control subjects. These percentages were as follows: skin, 98; esophagus, 74; lungs, 59; kidneys, 49; small intestine, 46; pericardium, 41; large intestine, 39; pleura, 29; and myocardium, 26. Other organs with less frequent involvement were adrenal glands, lymph nodes, thyroid, and peripheral arteries.

DIFFUSE CUTANEOUS SYSTEMIC SCLERODERMA

Diffuse cutaneous systemic scleroderma (DCSS), or progressive systemic sclerosis, is a chronic multisystem connective tissue disease characterized by sclerodermatous skin changes and widespread abnormalities of the viscera. Rodnan[10] defined DCSS as a disease in which

Table 21–2

Scleroderma in Childhood

STUDY	PATIENTS (n) Total	Male	Female	AGE AT ONSET (yr)
Jaffe and Winkelmann[3]	5	3	2	3–11
Kass et al.[4]	7	3	4	5–15
Kornreich et al.[22]	13†	4	9	3–12
Cassidy et al.[23]	15	0	15	3–15
Kennedy et al.[24]	1	0	1	6
Mukherjee et al.[25]	1	1	0	6
Velayos and Cohen[26]	1	0	1	4
Szymanska-Jagiello et al.[27]	12	2	10	6–14
Goel and Shanks[28]	4	1	3	2*–10.5
Ansell et al.[29]	1	0	1	13
Gray and Altman[30]	1	1	0	6
Schlesinger and Schaller[31]	11	3	8	N/A
Girouard et al.[32]	3	0	3	6‡–12
Spencer-Green et al.[33]	9	0	9	3–17
Larrègue et al.[34]	3	1	2	8–11
Burge et al.[35]	2	0	2	6–7
Suárez-Almazor et al.[36]	4	1	3	8–10
Lababidi et al.[37]	5	1	4	4–13
Martinez-Cordero et al.[38]	7	1	6	5–16
Vancheeswaran et al.[39]	11	4	7	3–13

*Patient has linear scleroderma with radiologic evidence of esophageal involvement.
†This series presumably includes children in an earlier report from the same institution (Kass et al.[4]).
‡Two of these patients had serum anti-RNP antibodies.

"symmetrical fibrous thickening and hardening (sclerosis) of the skin is combined with fibrous and degenerative changes in synovium, digital arteries, and certain internal organs, most notably the esophagus, intestinal tract, heart, lungs and kidneys." Systemic sclerosis sine scleroderma has been described.[10a]

Epidemiology

DCSS has been described worldwide and in all races.[11–18] It has an estimated annual incidence from 4.5 to 14 per million.[12, 13, 18] The frequency of the disease increases with age and is maximal in the 30- to 50-year-old age group. Childhood onset is very uncommon. It is estimated that approximately 3 percent of all patients with DCSS are children.[23] Children under 10 years account for less than 2 percent of all cases; and patients between 10 and 20 years make up from 1.2 to 9 percent.[14–17, 18a, 18b, 19–22, 22a] DCSS constitutes approximately 1 percent of major connective tissue disorders in pediatric rheumatology clinics (see Table 1–3). There is no racial predilection or peak age of onset.

There are several small series of children with DCSS, and a number of case reports totaling just over 100 patients, although there are undoubtedly many unreported patients. Those children in whom the diagnosis of DCSS is clear, and for whom appropriate data are available in the larger series, are summarized in Table 21–2.[3, 4, 21, 23–39] DCSS occurs with equal frequency in boys and girls younger than 8 years of age, whereas girls outnumber boys 3:1 when disease onset is in patients more than 8 years of age. In adults, the ratio of females:males from the ages of 15 to 44 years is 15:1, whereas after the age of 45 years, it is 1.8:1.[20, 40]

Etiology and Pathogenesis

The cause of DCSS is unknown, and although metabolic, vascular, and immunologic hypotheses all have a degree of scientific support, they should not be considered in isolation from each other. It is probable that there are many relevant interactions among these abnormalities (Fig. 21–1), all of which could have a role in the pathogenesis of this disease.

Abnormalities of Collagen

The excessive accumulation of collagen in affected skin has led to the hypothesis that there may be abnormalities of collagen type or metabolism.[12, 40a] There is an increased number of high collagen-producing fibroblasts in the skin[41]; however, the ratios of various collagen types in skin are normal.[42] Although reduced collagenase activity was found in one study,[43] it was normal in another.[44] Abnormalities of glycosylation[45] and hydroxylation[46] of the collagen molecule may prevent normal feedback mechanisms from being effective in controlling collagen synthesis[47] and thus permit excessive deposition of collagen.

Serum Factors

Serum factors, largely uncharacterized, may contribute to abnormalities in fibroblast function and cytokine

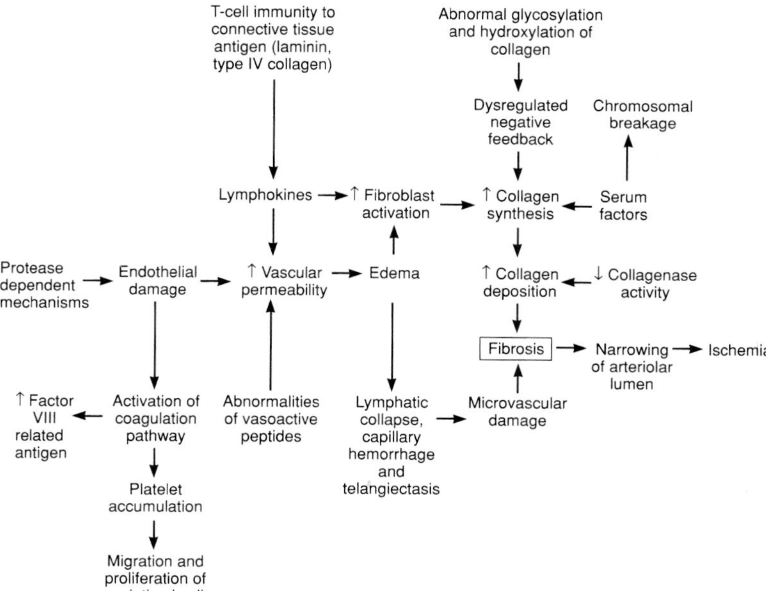

Figure 21–1. Possible pathogenic mechanisms in scleroderma.

regulation by stimulating collagen synthesis or endothelial cell function by initiating endothelial cell damage.[48–50, 50a, 50b] The frequency of occurrence of these serum factors and their specificity are disputed, however, and whether they are responsible for endothelial damage in DCSS is not known. One factor, *endothelin,* an endothelial-dependent vasoconstrictor,[51] is increased in DCSS.[49] *Granzyme 1,* probably a product of activated cytolytic T cells,[52] is a type IV collagenase that may cause endothelial cell damage by destruction of basal lamina. The high frequency of chromosomal breakage in cells of patients with DCSS and their relatives is associated with a serum "breakage" factor that induces chromosome breaks in cultured normal lymphocytes.[53]

Vascular Factors

The vascular hypothesis of pathogenesis is based on the clinical observation of the high frequency of Raynaud's phenomenon in DCSS and the presence of structural histopathologic vascular abnormalities. According to some authorities, endothelial cell injury is the central pathogenic event and predates fibrotic changes. The endothelial cell may be damaged by protease-dependent mechanisms that are independent of complement and immunoglobulin.[54] Abnormalities of cutaneous mast cell number and type, and of mast cell activation as a prefibrotic event, have also been documented.[55] Damage to the endothelial cell results in increased vascular permeability that is responsible for the edematous phase of the illness, which in turn leads to activation of fibroblasts, increased collagen production, and resultant fibrosis. It also initiates activation of the coagulation pathway, contributing to an accumulation of platelets that release factors leading to proliferation and migration of myointimal cells. Clinical evidence of vascular activation in DCSS of childhood onset may be less certain.[56]

Abnormalities of Endothelial Cells

Evidence that the endothelial cell is damaged in DCSS is provided not only by studies of the histology of the lesions in this disease but also by demonstration of elevated levels of factor VIII–related antigen,[57] although this has not been a consistent observation.[58] Endothelial cell apoptosis is accelerated.[59] The initial event in endothelial cell damage may be vasoregulatory failure mediated by abnormalities in the secretion of serotonin and other vasoactive peptides, permitting the transmission of increased arterial pressures to more fragile vessels with resulting exudation of fluid and proteins.[60] As a result of this increased tissue pressure, lymphatics collapse and capillaries hemorrhage and form telangiectases. According to this hypothesis, microvascular injury leads to arteriolar intimal fibrosis and narrowing of the vascular lumen, which results in ischemic damage.[61]

Immunologic Factors

The immunologic hypothesis for the pathogenesis of DCSS suggests that T lymphocyte–mediated autoimmunity to connective tissue or other antigens results in release of cytokines that stimulate fibroblasts to increased collagen production.[61–63, 63a, 63b] Anti–endothelial cell antibodies are also present.[64] Endothelial damage, vascular hyperpermeability, and myointimal cell proliferation result. Cell-mediated immunity to laminin, a constituent of basement membrane, and to a lesser extent, to type IV collagen has been demonstrated in patients with DCSS.[65]

Genetic Background

The rare familial occurrence of DCSS has been noted in a mother and her 6-year-old son,[30] and in a second family with two affected sisters aged 12 and 16 years.[66] These reports and others have been summarized by Gray and Altman.[30] There have been many reports of, but little agreement on, potential associations of histocompatibility antigens with DCSS. Initial studies indicated associations with class I alleles of human leukocyte antigen (HLA)-A9,[67] B8,[68, 69] and Bw35,[70] and class II alleles DR3,[69] DR5,[71] and DRw15.[56] Associations with DR and DQ alleles (DQB3.1, DQB1.1, DQB1.2, DQB1.3) have been reviewed by Whiteside and colleagues[72] and Fox and Kang.[73]

Nelson and coworkers[74] studied 40 mothers and documented high persistent concentrations of male DNA in their circulation years after giving birth to a son. They also found that HLA class II compatibility of the child was more common in DCSS patients than in control subjects. These data support the hypothesis that microchimerism may be involved in the pathogenesis of this disorder. Another investigation by Artlett and colleagues[75] also concluded that fetal antimaternal graft-versus-host reactions may be involved in pathogenesis.

Clinical Manifestations

Early Signs and Symptoms

The presenting signs and symptoms in children are shown in Table 21–3. The onset of the disease is usually insidious and the course prolonged, punctuated by periods of inactivity or episodes of severe systemic complications, occasionally ending in remission or, more often, debility or death.[76] The onset is often characterized by the development of Raynaud's phenomenon; tightening, thinning, and atrophy of the skin of the hands and face; or the appearance of cutaneous telangiectases about the face, upper trunk, and hands. There is often a diagnostic delay of years because of the subtle nature of this presentation. The systemic character of DCSS cannot be too strongly stressed because the ultimate prognosis of the patient depends primarily on the extent and nature of visceral involvement.

Skin Disease

The onset of cutaneous abnormalities may be very insidious. Cutaneous changes characteristically evolve in a sequence beginning with edema, followed by induration and sclerosis resulting in marked tightening and contracture, and finally eventuating in atrophy.

Edema

Tense, nonpitting swelling of the skin and subcutaneous tissues of the digits, hands, face, and arms, or localized areas on the trunk may be the initial manifestations of the disease. Edematous areas of involvement may be warm and tender with an erythematous border, but they are often completely asymptomatic. Swelling may persist for weeks or months before subsiding or being replaced by sclerosis.

Sclerosis

During the sclerotic phase, the skin becomes waxy in texture, tight, hard, and bound to subcutaneous structures. This is particularly noticeable in skin of the dorsal surfaces of the digits, so-called *acrosclerosis* (Fig. 21–2*A* and *B*), and face (Fig. 21–3*A* and *B*), where the characteristic immobile, expressionless, unwrinkled appearance of the skin may be the first clue to the diagnosis to an experienced observer. The absence of forehead wrinkling and the presence of circumoral furrowing or diminished aperture of the mouth are particularly characteristic. Sclerotic changes usually follow

Table 21–3

Presenting Signs and Symptoms in Children With Scleroderma

	STUDY						
SIGN	Goel et al.[28] (n = 4)	Jaffe and Winkelman[3] (n = 5)	Cassidy et al.[23] (n = 15)	Suárez-Almazor et al.[36] (n = 4)	Hanson[21] (n = 13)	Larrègue et al.[34] (n = 3)	Lababidi et al.[37] (n = 5)
Skin tightening	4	4	15	4	13	3	3
Raynaud's phenomenon	2	5	11	4	5	3	3
Soft tissue contracture	1	2	10	4	—	2	3
Arthralgia	3	—	9	1	—	2	5
Muscle weakness and pain	1	—	4	2	—	—	2
Subcutaneous calcification	—	—	3	1	—	—	—
Dysphagia	—	—	3	1	—	—	2
Dyspnea	—	—	3	1	—	—	2

—, Information not provided.

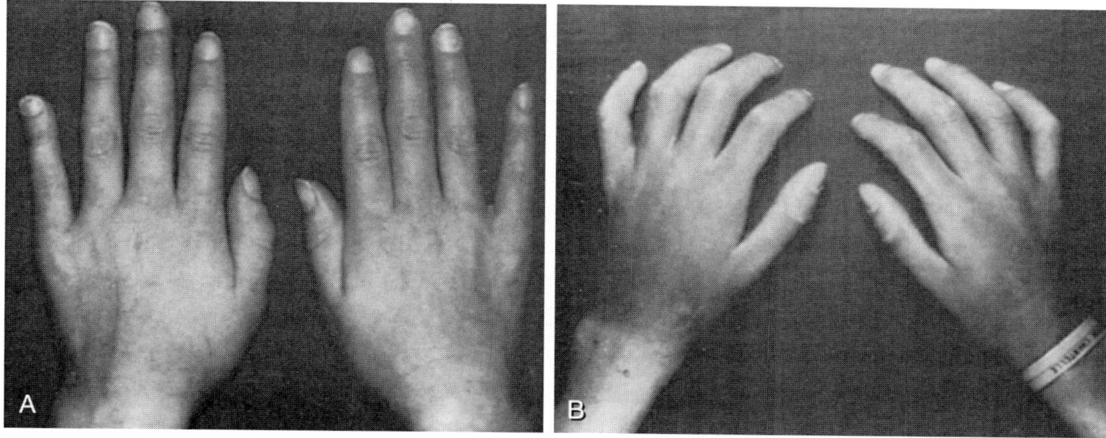

Figure 21–2. *A,* The hands of a 9-year-old girl with systemic scleroderma. The skin over the dorsum of the fingers is taut and shiny. *B,* Five years later, the tightening is more evident and flexion contractures have developed. (*A* and *B,* Courtesy of Dr. K. Oen.)

a temporal sequence of development beginning with bilateral, symmetric acrosclerosis, followed by involvement of the face, and finally by changes in the skin of the trunk and proximal limbs.

Atrophy

The long-term consequence of edema and sclerosis is atrophy of the skin and adnexa. These superficial abnormalities result in a shiny appearance of the skin accompanied by areas of hypopigmentation or hyperpigmentation and, often, by deposition of calcium salts in the subcutaneous tissues. Cutaneous lesions in all stages of evolution may be observed at the same time in the same child.

Telangiectases

Telangiectases are characteristic signs of DCSS (Fig. 21–4). Such lesions are fine macular dilatations of cutaneous or mucous-membrane blood vessels. Unlike "spider" angiomata, which fill rapidly from central arterioles, telangiectatic vessels fill slowly and lack the characteristic central vessel. The periungual nailfold is often the most obvious early location of abnormal vessels (Fig. 21–5) and on examination with the +40 lens of an ophthalmoscope demonstrates capillary dropout, together with tortuous dilated loops and, occasionally, distorted capillary architecture (Table 21–4, Fig. 21–6*A* and *B*).[33, 77] There is often redundant cuticular growth, and dystrophic changes in the nails have also been reported.[78] Digital pitting, sometimes with ulceration, occurs in the pulp of the fingertips as a result of ischemia and is one of the minor criteria for the diagnosis of DCSS (Fig. 21–7*A* and *B*). Digital gangrene may supervene.

Calcinosis

Subcutaneous calcification, especially over the elbows, metacarpophalangeal joints, and knees, may occur,

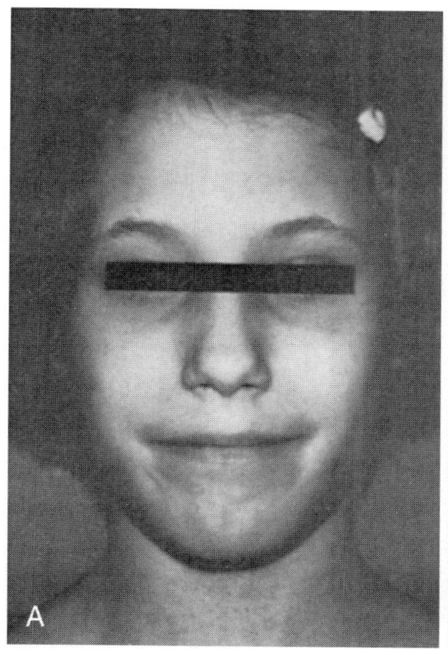

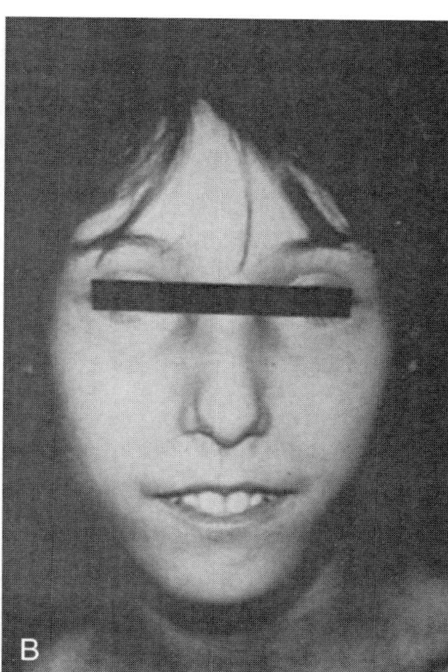

Figure 21–3. *A,* The face of a 9-year-old girl with systemic scleroderma. The face is smooth and unwrinkled but otherwise normal. *B,* Five years later, tightening of the skin is more evident. The patient is no longer able to close her lips. (*A* and *B,* Courtesy of Dr. K. Oen.)

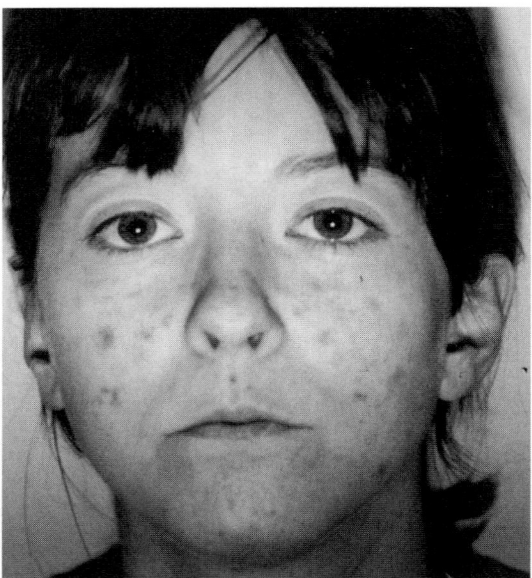

Figure 21–4. Classic round telangiectases on face.

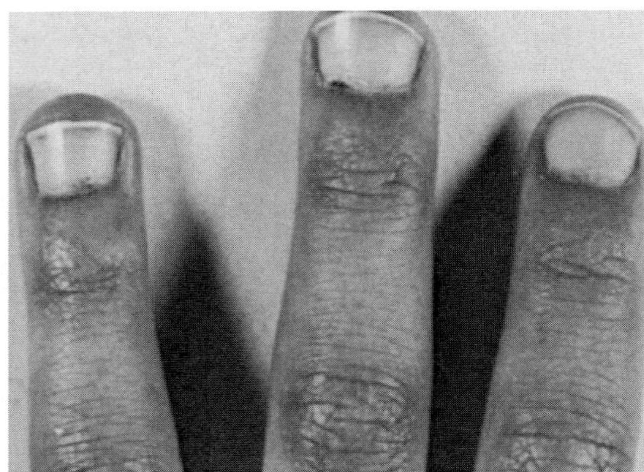

Figure 21–5. Changes in the nailfold vessels with visible tortuosity, thickening, and pigmentary extrusion onto the cuticles.

sometimes with ulceration of surrounding skin. Extensive periarticular calcification (*calcinosis circumscripta*) may be a late complication of scleroderma (Figs. 21–8 and 21–9). These lesions, if extensive, lead to severe reduction in joint mobility. Small, hard, subcutaneous nodules are sometimes present over the extensor surfaces of joints of the fingers. They differ histologically from rheumatoid nodules by the absence of fibrinoid necrosis.[79]

Raynaud's Phenomenon

The triple-phase sequence of blanching, cyanosis, and erythema, occurring spontaneously or in response to cold or physical or emotional stress, was described by Raynaud, a French medical student, in 1862.[80, 81] The term *Raynaud's phenomenon* is used to denote the tricolor change in patients with an underlying disorder such as DCSS. The term *Raynaud's disease* is applied to patients in whom no underlying structural vascular disease can be detected.

Raynaud's phenomenon occurs in 90 percent of children with DCSS and is often the initial symptom of the disease, preceding other manifestations in some instances by years.[82, 83] It is characterized by obstructive digital arterial disease and sympathetic hyperactivity. The blanching phase of the disorder, in particular, is well demarcated and uniformly white, beginning at the distal end of a digit and ending abruptly in the proximal digit or at the metacarpophalangeal joint (Fig. 21–10).[84] Raynaud's phenomenon is much more common in the fingers than elsewhere, but it can be observed in toes and, occasionally, ears, tip of the nose, lips, or tongue. These changes may be restricted to a single digit, may be unilateral or bilateral, and usually spare the thumb. The color changes may be accompanied by paresthesias, numbness, or pain (especially during the erythematous phase). Vascular spasm

Table 21–4

Abnormalities of Nailfold Capillaries in Various Disorders of Children

DISORDER	DECREASED DENSITY	DILATATION & TORTUOSITY	THICKENING	ARBORIZATION	DROPOUT
Systemic scleroderma	+ + +	+ + +	+ + +	+	+ + +
Localized scleroderma	−	−	−	−	−
Eosinophilic fasciitis	−	+	+	−	−
Mixed connective tissue disease*	+ +	+ +	+ +	+	+ +
Raynaud's disease†	−	+	−	−	−
Acrocyanosis	+	+	−	−	−
Juvenile dermatomyositis‡	+	+ + +	+ +	+ + +	+ +
Systemic lupus erythematosus	+	+ +	+	−	−
Juvenile rheumatoid arthritis	−	−	−	−	−

−, Normal; + to + + + = degree of abnormality.
*Markedly abnormal pattern correlates with development of pulmonary hypertension.
†Rare in children; abnormal patterns may predict future development of connective tissue disease.
‡Abnormal patterns correlate with histopathologic lesions of noninflammatory vasculopathy and chronic ulcerative course of the disease.
Data from references 33, 77, 88, 93, 306, 307.

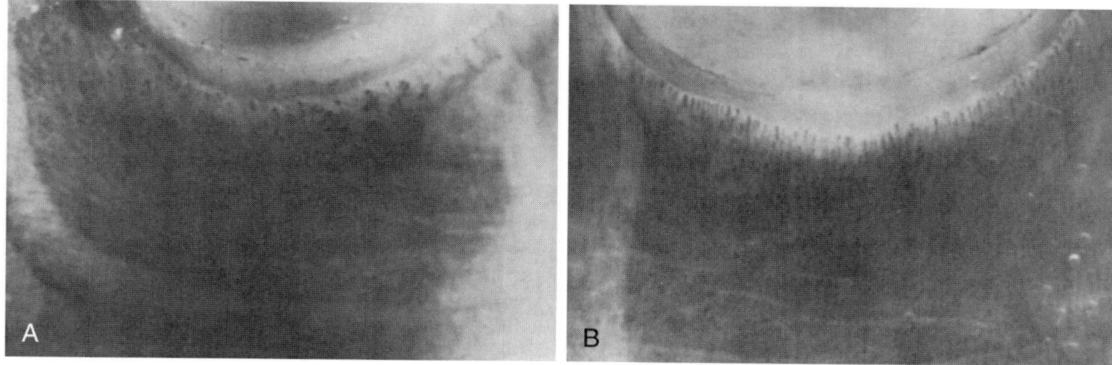

Figure 21–6. *A,* There is a reduction in the number of capillaries and tortuosity of the remaining vessels in the microvasculature viewed with a microscope (×100). *B,* Normal vessels. (*A* and *B,* Courtesy of Dr. J. Kenik.)

within viscera such as the esophagus and heart may accompany the peripheral anoxia.[85]

Idiopathic Raynaud's disease is uncommon in childhood, with the exception of the familial benign variety.[86, 87] Even in those instances in which skin changes of DCSS have not been demonstrated, antinuclear antibodies or abnormalities of esophageal motility have been observed[87] and suggest the possibility of disease progression to systemic scleroderma.[88] Table 21–5 represents the relative proportions of children and adults with Raynaud's phenomenon and Raynaud's disease.

The pathogenesis of Raynaud's phenomenon is not entirely clear. The initial event is arterial vasoconstriction with resultant decrease in cutaneous blood flow leading to pallor of the affected part, often followed by systemic reduction in perfusion of vital organs.[89] Cyanosis results from venous stasis; erythema is the result of reflex vasodilatation caused by mediators released during the ischemic phase. Under experimental conditions, vasoconstriction of the digital arterioles of patients with Raynaud's phenomenon can be induced by immersion of the hand in ice water and relieved by warming. This reversibility is highly characteristic, although the cutaneous circulation may require minutes to hours to return to normal. Factors other than cold may also induce the phenomenon, however, and it may occur spontaneously. The changes in digital arteriolar blood flow can be documented by Doppler-flow studies, plethysmography (Fig. 21–11), or arteriography (the last not usually necessary or indicated in DCSS, and performed with some danger of precipitating catastrophic arteriolar spasm) (Fig. 21–12).

Raynaud suggested in 1862 that the vasospasm resulted from increased sympathetic tone, but surgical sympathectomy results in short-term benefit at best. Furthermore, it has been demonstrated that capillary blood flow in the fingers and the fingerpad temperature of DCSS patients with Raynaud's phenomenon are reduced in both warm and cool environments.[90, 91] The phenomenon is not always reversible, and structural disease may be documented by arteriography,[92] capillary microscopy,[93] or histology.[94] A local vascular abnormality has been postulated, and smooth muscle from arteries of patients with scleroderma is hypersensitive to 5-hydroxytryptamine[95] and demonstrates a temperature-dependent loss of reactivity to catecholamine.[96] Locally repeated episodes of intravascular microcoagulation,[97] with release of prostaglandins such as thromboxane A_2 and prostaglandin E_1, may also contribute to vasospasm.[98]

Raynaud's phenomenon should be distinguished from normal vasomotor instability, especially in young girls. *Acrocyanosis*, first described by Crocq in 1896,[99] is a rare vasospastic disorder in which persistent coldness and bluish discolor-

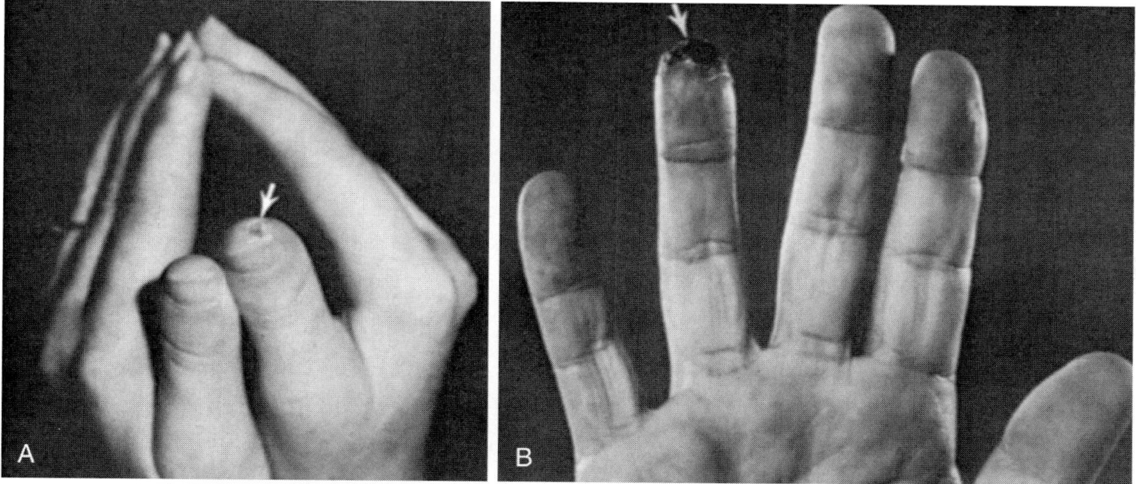

Figure 21–7. *A,* Pitting of the fingertips. Note ulceration of tip of the right thumb (*arrow*) and shiny, tightly stretched skin over the fingertips bilaterally with pronounced flexion contractures at the metacarpophalangeal joints. *B,* Digital gangrene of the fourth right finger (*arrow*).

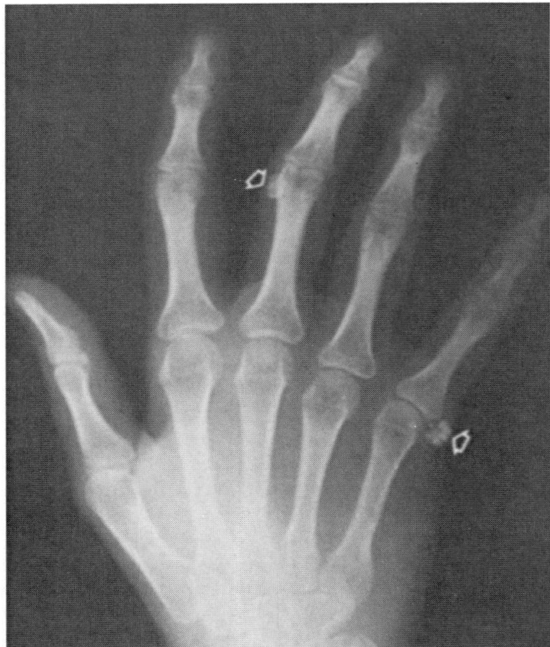

Figure 21–8. Small subcutaneous calcifications near joints (*arrows*) are visible in this radiograph of the hand of a young man with systemic scleroderma.

ation of the hands (and, less commonly, the feet) are present.[100–104] Occasionally, excessive perspiration and edema of the hands and feet may occur. The condition is exacerbated by cold but is essentially benign, unresponsive to treatment. The nailfold capillaries have dilated loops, however, and may be decreased in number.

Musculoskeletal Disease

Musculoskeletal symptoms are common in DCSS and characteristically occur at or near onset of the dis-

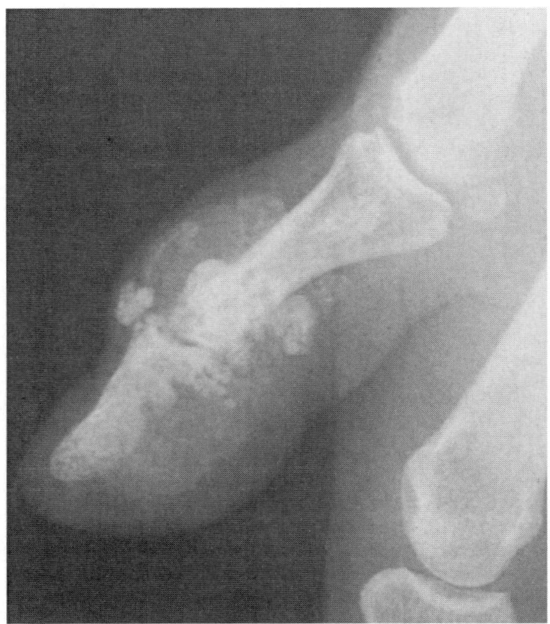

Figure 21–9. Calcinosis circumscripta affecting the thumb.

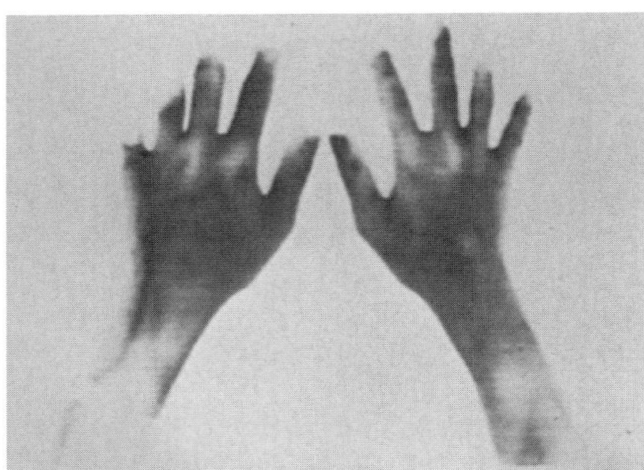

Figure 21–10. Thermographic documentation of Raynaud's phenomenon. The apparent "amputation" of the distal portions of the digits indicates the abrupt transition from normal tissue to cold, blanched skin that is characteristic of this disorder.

ease.[105] Morning stiffness and pain of the small joints of the hands, knees, and ankles may be initial manifestations of the disease. In addition, creaking of a thickened tendon as it moves through its sheath, which is covered with fibrinous deposits, can often be palpated or detected with a stethoscope as an audible, coarse crepitus.[106]

A description of musculoskeletal abnormalities in 12 children with DCSS indicated that all had contractures and limitation of motion.[27] Two thirds had joint pain that was usually mild and transient. Joint contractures of insidious onset were most common at the proximal interphalangeal joints and elbows, but other joints were also affected. Objective evidence of intra-articular inflammation was absent or mild in most instances, although small, bland synovial effusions occurred. Muscle inflammation characterized by pain and tenderness occurs in up to one third of children, and proximal or distal muscle atrophy may be marked. Differentiating affected children from those with early juvenile dermatomyositis or mixed connective tissue disease may be difficult.

Although pertinent studies are lacking in children, Clements and colleagues,[107] in a group of 24 adults with DCSS, described "simple myopathy" in 20 patients and complicated

Table 21–5

Raynaud's Phenomenon and Raynaud's Disease in Children and Adults

CATEGORY	PERCENT	
	Children	Adults
Raynaud's disease	5	70
Raynaud's phenomenon with		
Nonconnective tissue diseases	1	15
Juvenile rheumatoid arthritis	1	7
Systemic lupus erythematosus	60	4
Scleroderma	30	3
Dermatomyositis	3	1
	100	100

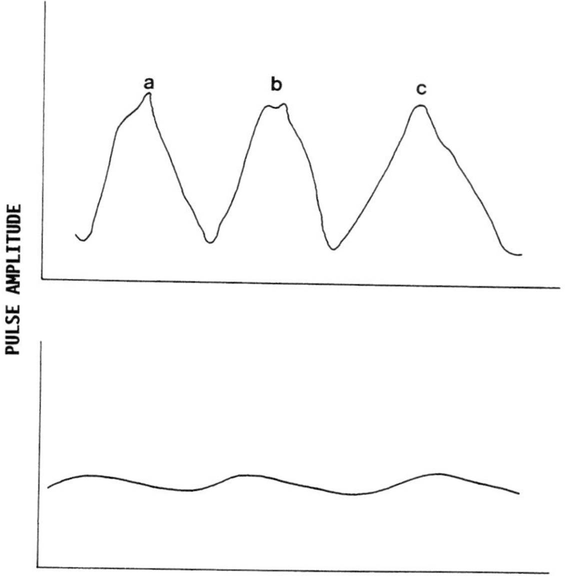

Figure 21–11. Plethysmographic study of the index finger of a child with Raynaud's phenomenon. *Upper tracing* demonstrates pulse amplitude at room temperature. Three abnormal wave forms are shown: (a) anachrotic notching; (b) peak notching; and (c) high dichrotic notching (diminished). *Lower tracing* demonstrates the effect of immersion of the finger in an ice-water bath. The resultant changes persisted for more than 30 minutes.

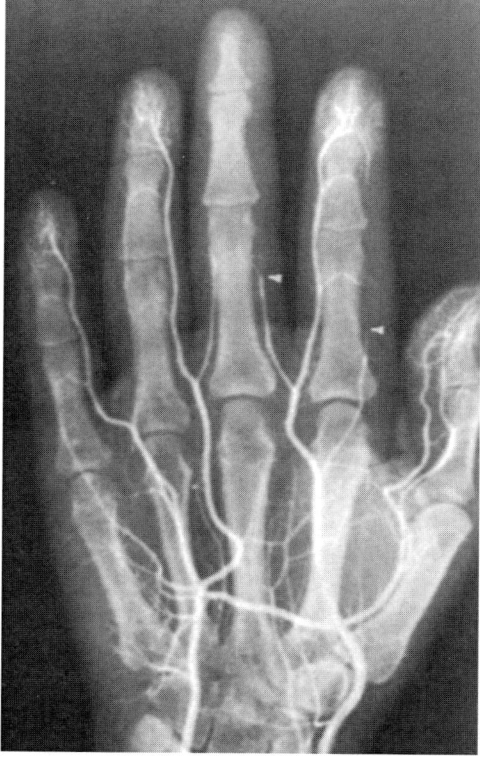

Figure 21–12. Digital arteriography outlines occlusions of proper digital arteries (*arrowheads*).

myopathy (resembling dermatopolymyositis or mixed connective tissue disease) in the remainder. In the simple myopathy group, weakness of the hip and shoulder girdle musculature was demonstrated in 81 percent; serum creatine kinase and aldolase were modestly elevated in fewer than half. In patients with complicated myopathy, enzyme levels were similar to values found in patients with polydermatomyositis. Electromyography documented polyphasic motor unit potentials of normal duration and amplitude in 18 of 19 patients, a decreased number of motor units in 5 of 19, but no insertional irritability, denervation, or diminished size or duration of motor unit potentials. In contrast, patients with dermatopolymyositis exhibited polyphasic motor unit potentials that were short and of low amplitude, and all had insertional irritability or fibrillations and positive sharp waves.

Gastrointestinal Disease

Lesions of the mouth include mucosal telangiectases, reduced interincisor distance secondary to skin thickening and tightness, parotitis as part of the sicca syndrome, and loosening of the teeth secondary to changes in the periodontal membrane. The esophagus is involved in the majority of children,[23] often quite early in the disease. Although many patients are asymptomatic, symptoms in order of decreasing frequency include heartburn with postural aggravation, dysphagia, delayed emptying, regurgitation with reflux into the throat, nocturnal aspiration, and cough with swallowing.[108] Esophagitis, ulceration, and stricture may occur. Progressive weight loss as a consequence of voluntary restriction of food intake may follow. Dilatation of the stomach or duodenum occur uncommonly. Small bowel involvement develops in up to 50 percent of patients,[9] usually in association with esophageal or colonic disease. Abdominal distention and pain with nausea and vomiting result from gut hypotonia that may occasionally be so severe that intestinal pseudo-obstruction occurs.[109] Malabsorptive diarrhea usually reflects long-standing disease. Pneumatosis intestinalis may occur.[110] Large bowel disease, although not uncommon, is usually asymptomatic; however, it may cause severe constipation, bloating, or diarrhea. Primary biliary cirrhosis has not been reported in children.[111, 112]

Cardiac Disease

Cardiopulmonary disease is a primary cause of morbidity among children with DCSS.[36] Pericardial effusions are usually small and asymptomatic, although fever and retrosternal pain may accompany acute disease.[113] Changes in cardiac hemodynamics reflected by the presence of pedal edema, jugular venous distension, hepatomegaly, pulsus paradoxus, and pulsus alternans may be present in patients with chronic effusions. Tamponade and pericardial constriction are rare.

Cardiac anoxia may result from the equivalent of Raynaud's phenomenon of the coronary arteries and is a potential precursor of myocardial fibrosis. Although fixed coronary artery disease is infrequent, electrocardiographic changes and even angina pectoris may occur as a result of disease of the myocardial microvasculature.[114] Systemic and pulmonary hypertension may also contribute to myocardial ischemia.

Pulmonary Disease

Trell and Lindstrom[115] described three types of pulmonary disease in DCSS involving pulmonary vasculature and parenchyma: predominant interstitial fibrosis with gradual obliteration of the vascular bed and slowly progressive cor pulmonale; combined pulmonary parenchymal and vascular lesions; and predominant pulmonary vascular involvement associated with rapidly lethal right ventricular failure. Pulmonary parenchymal disease is almost universal in DCSS, and although frequently asymptomatic, patients often have a dry, hacking cough or dyspnea on exertion.[116] Occasionally, rales or a pleural friction rub are present on auscultation. The risk of alveolar and bronchiolar carcinoma is increased in adults.[117]

It has been postulated that pulmonary fibrosis also results from pulmonary vascular changes similar to Raynaud's phenomenon. Furst and associates[118] demonstrated decreased pulmonary perfusion as measured by krypton 81m scans after cold challenge to the hands. An increased pulmonary uptake of gallium 67 was present in the majority of patients with early disease, a finding that suggested an inflammatory process. Fahey and coworkers[119] noted low diffusing capacity for carbon monoxide (DLCO) in patients with DCSS and Raynaud's phenomenon, but failed to demonstrate a decrease with cold challenge as found in patients with idiopathic Raynaud's disease.

Renal Disease

Renal disease is one of the most ominous features of DCSS. Little information is available from pediatric series, but it is our impression that children may do better than adults in this regard.[4, 23, 36, 40] Medsger and colleagues[120] found that almost 50 percent of adult patients who developed renal disease did so within the first year after onset. As is the case in nephropathy from other causes, symptoms were usually absent initially. Proteinuria, the most common indicator of involvement of the kidneys in DCSS, is often minimal and may be the only evidence of disease in half of the patients.[5, 121, 122] Systemic hypertension occurs in up to half of adult patients and is usually associated with proteinuria.[121, 122] The degree of hypertension ranges from mild or moderate in the majority to "malignant" hypertension in approximately 25 percent. This complication begins most often during the colder months of the year[121] and may be heralded by the development of microangiopathic hemolytic anemia.[123] Onset is followed rapidly in the majority of patients by death within a few weeks in the absence of intensive intervention. Renal or prerenal azotemia occurs in at least 25 percent of patients with DCSS in the presence or absence of hypertension or proteinuria.[122]

Renovascular "Raynaud's phenomenon," demonstrated by decreased cortical blood flow, may be induced by immersion of the hands in cold water.[121] Even in the absence of angiographic evidence of vascular disease, cortical blood flow as measured by xenon 133 may be impaired.[121] These reversible changes are mediated by the renin-angiotensin system, and plasma renin levels have been found to correlate with the presence of malignant hypertension in DCSS.[124]

Central Nervous System Disease

The most frequently described central nervous system abnormality is cranial nerve involvement, especially of the sensory branch of the trigeminal nerve.[125–127] In contrast, peripheral neuropathies are uncommon.[128] A more subtle abnormality, diminished perception of vibration, probably reflects the damping effect of the cutaneous sclerosis on the transmission of the sensation from the vibrations of a tuning fork.[129] Clinical involvement of the central nervous system per se is usually a reflection of renal or pulmonary disease[130]; however, cerebral arteritis has been described.[131]

Sicca Syndrome

The *xerostomia* (dry mouth) and *keratoconjunctivitis sicca* (dry eyes) of Sjögren's syndrome are quite common in DCSS. Histologic evidence of salivary gland involvement was uniformly demonstrable in lip biopsies in a prospective study of Sjögren's syndrome in 17 patients with DCSS and 8 patients with limited DCSS (CREST [*c*alcinosis cutis, *R*aynaud's phenomenon, *e*sophageal dysfunction, *s*clerodactyly, and *t*elangiestasia] syndrome).[132] Xerostomia and salivary gland enlargement were present in 84 percent. Scintigraphy of the salivary glands was abnormal in 88 percent and sialography in 75 percent. Ocular symptoms of dryness, or a foreign body sensation, were present in 76 percent. Schirmer's test was abnormal in 40 percent, and Rose-Bengal staining of the cornea was positive in 55 percent. (See Chapter 23 for a full discussion of other features of this syndrome.)

Pathology

An angiitis is regarded as the basic initial lesion in DCSS. Histologic examination early in disease demonstrates increased hydrophilic glycosaminoglycan in the dermis that may account in part for the accumulation of edema in such sites.[133] There are increased numbers of T lymphocytes, plasma cells, and macrophages in the deep dermis and subcutaneous tissue and around small blood vessels, nerves, the pilosebaceous apparatus and sweat glands.[134, 135] Marked hyalinization of blood vessel walls and proliferation of endothelium occur later. Raynaud's phenomenon, scleroderma renal crisis, and pulmonary hypertension are all associated with this distinctive arteriosclerotic fibrotic lesion (Fig. 21–13*A*). Another characteristic finding is mast cell hyperplasia in both skin and viscera.[136]

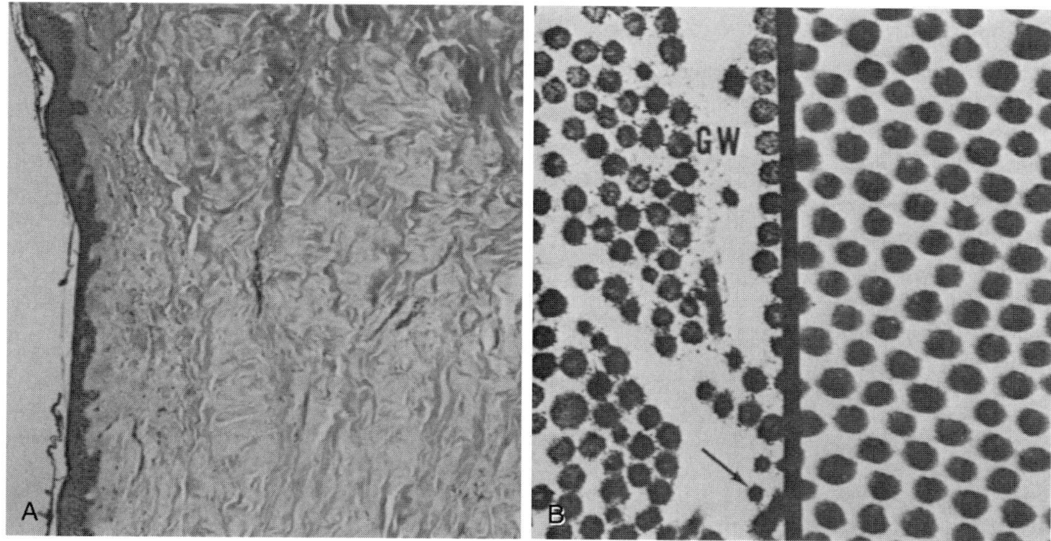

Figure 21–13. *A,* The classic histopathologic features of the cutaneous disease are visible in this full-thickness section of skin from a patient with diffuse cutaneous systemic scleroderma. The epidermis is thin, and there is atrophy of the dermal appendages. The rete pegs are relatively obliterated. H&E, ×480. *B,* Electron microscopic studies in scleroderma show a relative reduction in the fiber size of newly synthesized collagen. Transverse sections of collagen fibers from the skin of a patient with scleroderma are visible on the *left.* A marked variation in fiber size is apparent when compared with healthy skin (*right*). Furthermore, many smaller collagen fibers are observed (*arrow*) (normal diameter, 1200 Å). The fine granular and whiskery material (GW) surrounding the sclerodermal collagen probably represents mucopolysaccharides, their visibility enhanced by staining with ruthenium red. Lead citrate and uranyl acetate, ×38,610. (*A* and *B,* Courtesy of Dr. C. R. Wynne-Roberts.)

Later in the course, biopsies document homogenization of collagen fibers with loss of structural detail and an increased density and thickness of collagen deposition.[65, 137] With electron microscopy, the collagen appears embryonic with narrow fibrils and an immature cross-banding pattern (see Fig. 21–13*B*).[138] The histologic characteristics of the skin in late disease include thinning of the epidermis and loss of the rete pegs, and atrophy of dermal appendages often with a persistent inflammatory infiltrate of T lymphocytes.[139] The synovial membrane histologically resembles that of rheumatoid arthritis except for the abundance of fibrin and dense fibrosis.[68, 140, 141]

Biopsy specimens of muscle are abnormal in approximately half of the patients.[142] The most prominent abnormalities are increased deposition of collagen and fat in interstitial perivascular sites of the perimysium and epimysium and focal, predominantly lymphocytic, perivascular infiltration. There is a relative loss of type II fibers.[143] Blood vessels are thickened and vessel lumens narrowed.[144] Immunofluorescence studies have demonstrated no abnormalities.[143]

Histopathologic changes are similar throughout the gastrointestinal tract but are most prominent in the esophagus, where atrophic muscle is replaced by fibrous tissue.[9, 145, 146] The smooth muscle of the lower two thirds of the esophagus is most commonly affected, but in some patients, striated muscle of the upper third may also be involved. The lamina propria and Auerbach plexus are infiltrated with mononuclear cells.[147] Arterial walls are thickened.

Similar changes of fibrosis are found in the heart. Half of the patients in one necropsy series had evidence of myocardial fibrosis that was unrelated to coronary artery disease (Fig. 21–14).[148] Other findings included contraction band necrosis (myofibrillar degeneration) secondary to transient ischemia in 31 percent (possibly the equivalent of Raynaud's phenomenon of the coronary arteries and a precursor to myocardial fibrosis). Necropsies in adults with DCSS have demonstrated effusions or fibrous, fibrinous, and adhesive pericarditis in approximately 40 percent,[145] a frequency similar to that detected by echocardiography.[149] Convincing

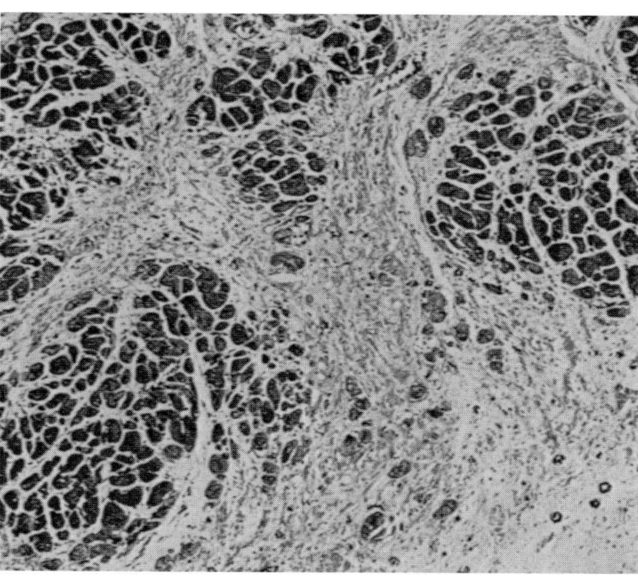

Figure 21–14. Fibrosis of the myocardium. H&E, ×480.

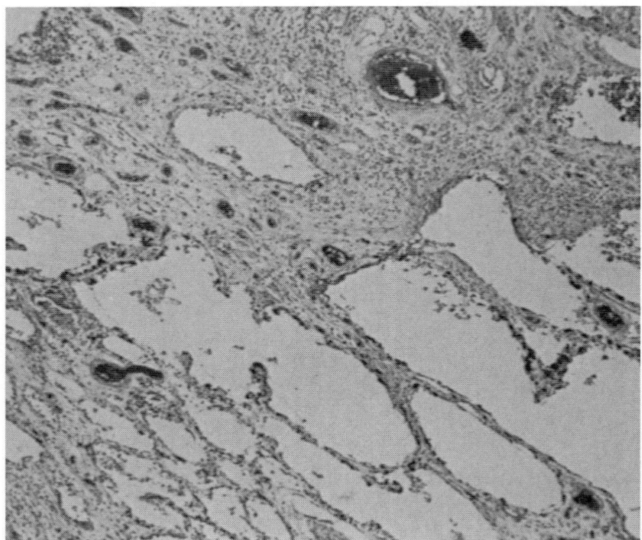

Figure 21–15. Biopsy of lung illustrates striking fibrosis and disruption of alveoli. H&E, ×480.

clinical evidence of pericarditis was less frequent, however, being present in only 3 to 16 percent of patients.[145, 150]

The main histologic abnormality in the lungs is diffuse alveolar, interstitial, and peribronchial fibrosis. The thickened walls may result in reduction of alveolar space (compact sclerosis). Rupture of alveolar septae results in small areas of bullous emphysema (cystic sclerosis) (Fig. 21–15).[151] Extensive bronchiolar hyperplasia, arteriolar endothelial proliferation, fibrous pleuritis, and pleural adhesions are also present. Young and Mark[152] found that 14 of 30 patients had moderate or marked abnormalities in the pulmonary vasculature at necropsy, and postulated that malignant pulmonary hypertension analogous to malignant renal hypertension was the cause of the rapidly progressive pulmonary failure that culminated in death of three patients.

The characteristic histopathologic change in the renal vasculature is concentric intimal proliferation of the interlobar and arcuate arteries, together with cortical infarcts and fibrinoid necrosis of the media.[153, 154] Vasculitis (other than the changes of malignant hypertension) is uncommon. The glomeruli exhibit a wide spectrum of abnormalities (Fig. 21–16*A* and *B*), ranging from acute ischemic necrosis to thickening and sclerosis of the basement membrane. On electron microscopy, intimal thickening of the vessels is associated with the presence of myointimal cells resembling those of smooth muscle but having the capability to produce collagen and elastin.[155] Swelling of the endothelial cells results in vascular narrowing.[156] Deposition of immunoglobulin and complement in the renal vasculature has been reported by some investigators[156–158] but is generally sparse.

Differential Diagnosis

According to criteria of the American College of Rheumatology for the classification of DCSS in adults,[159] definite DCSS requires the presence of the major criterion or two minor criteria (Table 21–6). Proximal scleroderma is the most important characteristic of early disease. Raynaud's phenomenon is almost always present and accompanied by pronounced abnormalities of the nailfold capillaries. Esophageal dysmotility and abnormal pulmonary diffusion and function are often present at onset. The myopathy of early scleroderma

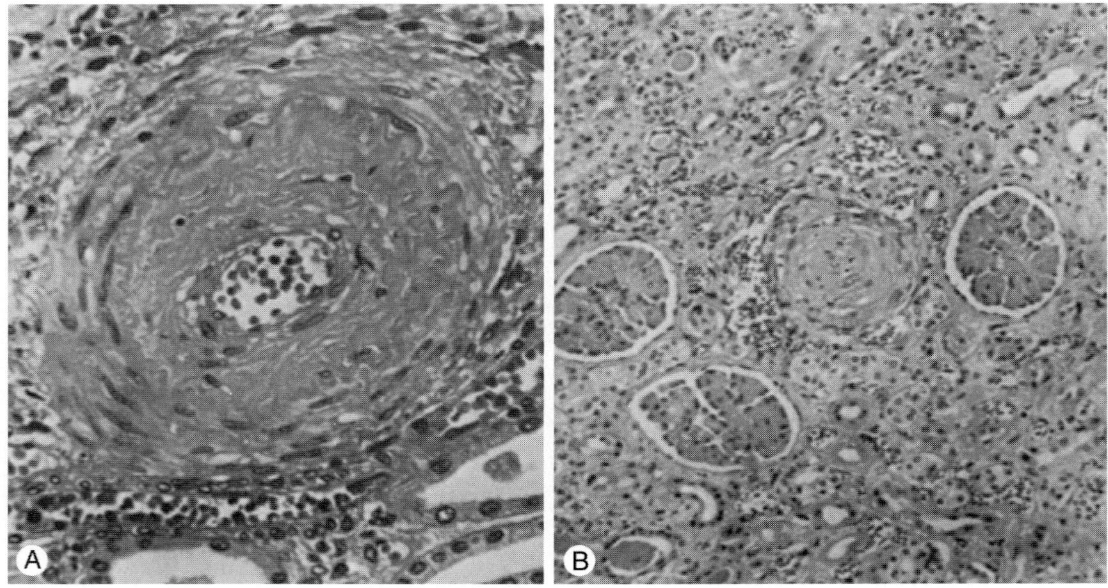

Figure 21–16. Necropsy specimen from a patient with scleroderma of the kidney who died of renal failure and hypertension during the first few months of the disease. *A,* Virtual obliteration of the lumen of an arteriole by subintimal proliferation, thrombus formation, and mucoid hyperplasia of the media. *B,* Glomerulus from the same patient. Fibrinoid necrosis and effacement of capillary loops without significant inflammatory cell infiltration. H&E, ×480.

Table 21–6

Preliminary Criteria for the Classification of Systemic Sclerosis (Scleroderma)

Major Criterion

Proximal scleroderma: typical sclerodermatous skin changes (tightness, thickening, and nonpitting induration, excluding localized forms of scleroderma) involving areas proximal to the metacarpophalangeal or metatarsophalangeal joints

Minor Criteria

Sclerodactyly: sclerodermatous skin changes limited to digits
Digital pitting scars resulting from digital ischemia
Bibasilar pulmonary fibrosis not attributable to primary lung disease

Adapted from Subcommittee for Scleroderma Criteria of the American Rheumatism Association Diagnostic and Therapeutic Criteria Committee: Preliminary criteria for the classification of systemic sclerosis (scleroderma). Arthritis Rheum 23: 581–590, 1980.

must be distinguished from that observed in juvenile dermatomyositis (see Chapter 20). Mixed connective tissue disease and other undifferentiated connective tissue diseases mimic scleroderma both early and late (see Chapter 23).

Chronic Graft-Versus-Host Disease

The similarities of scleroderma to graft-versus-host disease (GVHD) has led to investigation of the hypothesis that prolonged persistence of fetal progenitor cells and microchimerism may be involved in pathogenesis.[45, 74, 75] Chronic GVHD is a complication of allogeneic bone marrow transplantation performed for the treatment of marrow aplasia, leukemia, or malignant diseases.[160, 161] GVHD results from the interaction between immunocompetent T lymphocytes from the donor and host cells bearing histocompatibility antigens that are recognized as foreign. The graft attempts to "reject" the host because, under the circumstances of the transplantation, the recipient is rendered immunologically incompetent by immunosuppression and x-irradiation. The resulting scleroderma-like disease may follow acute GVHD or occur de novo up to 100 days after transplant. It is characterized by immunologically mediated dermatitis, usually beginning with erythema of the face, palms, soles, and other regions, sometimes involving only half of the body, a Harlequin syndrome. This is followed by hyperpigmentation and hypopigmentation. The sclerodermatous changes may be distal in location or generalized. A hidebound skin and extreme tightening of the tendons, subcutaneum, and periarticular structures may severely limit motion. Gastrointestinal disease with severe diarrhea, hepatitis, and other visceral involvement is common.[162] A comparison of the salient features of chronic GVHD and DCSS is shown in Table 21–7. D-Penicillamine has been claimed to be beneficial in these patients, and modifications of the chemotherapeutic preparation of the graft recipient may offer some hope of prevention of this complication.[162]

Chemically Induced Scleroderma-Like Disease

Several chemicals have been implicated in the induction of individual cases of scleroderma.[163] Polyvinyl chloride that was initially used as an anesthetic agent[164, 165] is now known to cause a scleroderma-like disease, primarily among workers in the polyvinyl chloride industries. It is characterized by Raynaud's phenomenon; localized papular skin lesions, especially on fingers and hands, excluding the face and trunk; and osteolysis of the distal phalanges. Bleomycin, an antineoplastic agent, commonly causes skin changes resembling scleroderma[166] and pulmonary fibrosis.[167] This syndrome is not accompanied by Raynaud's phenomenon and may improve on cessation of the drug.[168] Pentazocine, a nonnarcotic analgesic drug, has been reported to cause cutaneous sclerosis with or without ulceration.[169] Predisposing factors may include diabetes mellitus and alcohol abuse.

The *toxic oil syndrome*, caused by ingestion of rapeseed cooking oil that presumably contained unidentified contaminants, occurred in epidemic proportions in Spain in early 1981,[170–173] affecting approximately 20,000 persons and resulting in at least 350 deaths. A report of the disease in 21 children indicated that complications may have been less severe in the younger age group, and that the sex ratio was closer to equal (female:male, 2.5:1) than was the ratio in adults (female:male, 6:1).[174] The onset of the disease was characterized by fever, eosinophilia, dyspnea secondary to pulmonary edema, pruritic rash, and malaise. Sclerodermatous skin lesions, alopecia, conjunctivitis sicca, Raynaud's phenomenon, myositis, neuropathy, joint contractures, dysphagia, and liver disease evolved over a period of months.

Adjuvant disease, a systemic scleroderma-like condition, has been reported to follow cosmetic surgery involving injection of paraffin or silicone.[175, 176] An inflammatory reaction in surrounding tissue occurs when silicone gel leaks from implants used for augmentation mammoplasty. A granulomatous reaction can also be demonstrated in regional lymph nodes. Silicone synovitis is well documented in patients after arthroplasty.[177] A variety of atypical "connective tissue diseases," principally scleroderma-like, with chronic fatigue, myalgia, arthralgia, and arthritis, had been reported in women who have undergone silicone implants.[178, 179] The systemic illnesses described had been based on epidemiologic data and extrapolations,[180] and recent observations[180a, 180b] have not conclusively demonstrated a causal relationship (U.S. Institute of Medicine).

Table 21–7

Comparison of Diffuse Cutaneous Systemic Scleroderma (DCSS) and Chronic Graft-Versus-Host Disease (GVHD)

	PERCENT		
SYSTEM AFFECTED	DCSS (Early) n=13	DCSS (Late) n=36	GVHD n=12
Skin	100	100	100
Raynaud's phenomenon	100	92	42
Lungs	77	96	58
Esophagus	77	86	17
Small bowel	8	92	0
Heart	69	61	42
Kidney	15	75	8
Keratoconjunctivitis sicca	15	69	50

Adapted from Clements PJ, Furst DE, Ho W, et al: Progressive systemic sclerosis-like disease following bone marrow transplantation. *In* Black CM, Myers AR (eds): Systemic Sclerosis (Scleroderma). New York, Gower Medical, 1985, p 376.

Pseudosclerodermas

The term *pseudoscleroderma* is used to describe a diverse group of disorders that are characterized by scleroderma-like fibrotic changes in the skin in association with other nonrheumatic diseases. This brief discussion is restricted to those disorders of significance in the pediatric population.

Phenylketonuria

A small minority of children with phenylketonuria (phenylalanine hydroxylase deficiency) develop sclerodermatous skin lesions.[181–184] These lesions, which usually appear within the first year of life, are symmetric and poorly demarcated and resemble morphea. They occur most frequently on the lower extremities and trunk. It is believed that the lesions regress on introduction of a low-phenylalanine diet.[185, 186] Although no differences with respect to serum phenylalanine or tryptophan levels were found between children with phenylketonuria who did or did not have sclerodermatous changes, urinary excretion of 5-hydroxyindoleacetic acid, indoleacetic acid, and tryptamine was much higher in children with skin changes.[186] The relationship of these biochemical abnormalities to the pathogenesis of the accompanying skin lesions, or to that of the other sclerodermas, is not known. The experimental use of a low-phenylalanine diet in patients with DCSS produced inconclusive results.[186]

Syndromes of Premature Aging

Two rare autosomal recessive disorders accompanied by dwarfing, premature aging, and early death from atherosclerotic heart disease are associated with sclerodermatous skin changes. *Progeria* is characterized by alopecia, nail dystrophy, and thickened, bound-down skin on the abdomen, flanks, proximal thighs, and upper buttocks.[187, 188] The cutaneous changes usually appear before 1 year of age. *Werner's syndrome* most often presents in adolescence with generalized atrophy of muscle and subcutaneous tissue, graying hair, baldness, and scleroderma-like skin changes and ulcers involving the extremities.[188–190] The histologic features of this disorder mimic those of scleroderma. Metastatic calcification may also develop.[191]

Localized Idiopathic Fibroses

A number of relatively rare disorders in children result in fibrosis of specific organs or structures.[192–194] Keloids are an obvious example.[195] Retroperitoneal fibrosis usually occurs in the region of the sacral promontory and affects vital structures in this area, notably the great vessels and ureters.[196] It is more common in males than in females and occurs in children as well as in adults. The syndrome may be idiopathic or associated with administration of the serotonin inhibitor methysergide. Retractile mesenteritis, mediastinal fibrosis, fibrosing pericarditis, fibrosing carditis, and peritoneal fibrosis may represent similar disorders and have been related to administration of certain drugs, notably methysergide and some antihypertensives and anticonvulsants.[197, 198]

There are variants of fibromatosis restricted to childhood that are distinctive pathologically.[193, 199–201] Congenital torticollis or *fibromatosis colli* affects the lower sternomastoid muscle and is present at birth or shortly thereafter. It is associated with other congenital anomalies such as congenital dislocations of the hip. *Fibromatosis hyalinica multiplex* is a morphologically distinctive type of familial multiple fibromatosis affecting children but not present at birth. *Infantile digital fibromatosis* affects the distal fingers or toes but may develop elsewhere. A distinctive microscopic feature is the presence of eosinophilic cytoplasmic inclusions. *Infantile myofibromatosis* presents as solitary or multiple nodules in superficial soft tissues, either limited to those sites or associated with internal organ involvement.[202] This disorder probably represents an inborn error of metabolism and has possible autosomal dominant transmission. It is characterized microscopically by hyalinization of connective tissues of the skin, oral cavity, joint capsules, and bones. Microscopically peripheral areas that resemble smooth muscle alternate with hemangiopericytoma-like foci with a more typical fibroblastic configuration. Central necrosis and intravascular growth may be present. The *stiff skin syndrome* represents congenital scleroderma-like indications of fascia, predominantly of the buttocks and thighs.[202a]

Gardner's syndrome is a form of fibrosis associated with multiple colonic polyps and osteomas.[203] The fibrosis has a tendency to involve intra-abdominal structures, such as the omentum and mesentery, or to occur after an operative procedure. *Dupuytren's contracture* is a nodular thickening of the palmar fascia and flexion contractures of the digits.[204] Idiopathic disease, unassociated with other disorders such as diabetes, is exceedingly rare in children. *Lipogranulomatosis subcutanea of Rothmann-Makai* produces scleroderma-like changes in the skin of the lower extremities with subcutaneous nodules.[205] Morphea or linear scleroderma may be the initial diagnostic consideration. Systemic involvement is absent.

Scleromyxedema is characterized by papular cutaneous lesions with induration of underlying subcutaneous tissues.[206] The lesions occur predominantly on the hands, forearms, trunk, face, and neck. Histologic characteristics include a prominent fibrohistiocytic infiltrate and dense acid mucopolysaccharide deposits in the upper dermis. The disease in adults has been associated with monoclonal gammopathies.

Scleredema

Scleredema, a disorder primarily of historical interest, classically followed β-hemolytic streptococcal infection and was characterized by edematous induration of the face, neck, shoulders, thorax, and proximal extremities, but not of the hands.[207, 208] It was often of insidious onset and had a prolonged course of 6 to 12 months. It characteristically was subtle in presentation and resolved spontaneously. Cardiac abnormalities suggesting the concurrence of acute rheumatic fever have been reported.

The diagnosis of scleredema is based on documentation of nonpitting, indurated edema or stiffness of the skin in the typical locations. Dysphagia may be present, but Raynaud's phenomenon and telangiectases are not. Some children have poorly controlled insulin-dependent diabetes, but this syndrome is presumably distinct from diabetic cheiroarthropathy. Histologically, the dermis is thickened, there are multiple fenestrations between swollen collagen bundles, and a scant perivascular lymphocytic infiltrate. Minimal deposits of acid mucopolysaccharides are present within the fenestrations. Immunofluorescent staining is negative.

Porphyria Cutanea Tarda

The development of scleroderma in adults with porphyria cutanea tarda has been reviewed.[209, 210] The skin changes were described as plaquelike and occurred predominantly on the face, neck, upper chest, and back. Some patients had features of other connective tissue diseases such as discoid lupus. There are no reports of this association in children.

Diabetic Cheiroarthropathy

A syndrome of juvenile-onset diabetes mellitus, short stature, and tightening of the skin and soft tissues leading to contractures of the finger joints has been described by Rosenbloom and associates.[211] In their survey, 29 percent of diabetic children were found to have one or more flexion contractures (see Chapter 36).

Laboratory Examination

Anemia, although not a common feature of DCSS, is present in approximately one quarter of patients[212] and may be characteristic of the anemia of chronic inflammation or, less commonly, reflect vitamin B_{12} or folate deficiency resulting from chronic malabsorption.[213] Anemia resulting from microangiopathic hemolysis[123, 214] or bleeding from mucosal telangiectases also occurs. Autoimmune hemolytic anemia is rare.[215, 216] Leukocytosis is not prominent but correlates in degree with advanced visceral or muscle disease. Eosinophilia ($>300/mm^3$; $>3 \times 10^9/L$) occurs in approximately 15 percent of patients with DCSS.[217] Synovial fluid was reported in one study to contain large amounts of protein and high numbers of polymorphonuclear leukocytes that had inclusions similar to those seen in rheumatoid arthritis.[105] Pericardial fluid in DCSS has the characteristics of an exudate.[218]

High-titered antinuclear antibodies are frequently present in the sera of children with DCSS.[219, 220] The predominant patterns are speckled and nucleolar on HEp-2 cell substrate. A large study of adults with DCSS confirmed that 26 percent had antibody to Scl-70 (DNA-topoisomerase 1) and 22 percent had antibody to centromere (kinetochore).[221] No patient had antibodies to both antigens. Antibody to Scl-70 occurred most frequently in patients with diffuse scleroderma, in whom it was associated with peripheral vascular disease (digital pitting) and pulmonary interstitial fibrosis. The anticentromere antibody occurred almost exclusively in patients with limited cutaneous systemic scleroderma (LCSS), in association with calcinosis and telangiectases. A correlation was also demonstrated between anticentromere antibody and HLA-DR1, and between antibody to Scl-70 and DR5. A second study confirmed similar disease-antibody correlations, although patients with antibodies to both centromere and Scl-70 were occasionally encountered.[222] An association between the presence of antibody to Scl-70 and malignancy was also noted.[222] Antibodies that are specific for a 70 kD mitochondrial antigen have been described in a small proportion of patients with DCSS,[223] and the occurrence of antibodies to the PM-Scl antigen has recently been reviewed.[224]

Cardiac Function

Electrocardiographic abnormalities include first-degree heart block, right and left bundle branch block, premature atrial and ventricular contractions, nonspecific T-wave changes, and evidence of ventricular hypertrophy.[225] Disturbances of rhythm are probably secondary to myocardial fibrosis or to fibrosis of the sinus node and bundle branches.[226] With Holter monitoring, Clements and associates[227] noted paroxysmal supraventricular tachycardia in 13 of 46 patients, although 11 of 13 had no cardiovascular symptoms. Ventricular tachycardia and premature atrial or ventricular contractions were less common. Radionuclide scans with thallium 201 often document abnormalities of myocardial perfusion, ventricular wall motion, chamber size, and left ventricular ejection fraction.[228] Echocardiographic abnormalities in addition to effusions include thickening of the wall of the left ventricle in 57 percent and diminished left ventricular compliance in 42 percent.[229]

Pulmonary Function

Pulmonary diffusion and spirometry are sensitive measures of involvement of the respiratory tract. Characteristic findings include a decrease in the timed vital capacity and forced expiratory flow, an early decrease in diffusion, and an increase in functional residual volume.[230, 231] Steen and colleagues[232] reported that only 38 percent of 77 adults with DCSS and 28 percent of 88 with LCSS had normal studies of pulmonary function. Restrictive lung disease and isolated reduction of DLCO were the most common abnormalities, occurring respectively in 34 (18 percent) of DCSS patients and in 23 (26 percent) of patients with LCSS. The earliest change was a decrease in the forced vital capacity, with an FEV_1/FVC of less than 70 percent. This was present in 8 percent of patients with diffuse disease and 16 percent of those with limited disease. Guttadauria and associates[233] noted, in addition, a high prevalence of small airways disease (42 percent), usually in the absence of symptoms, chest radiographic changes, or other abnormalities of pulmonary function. In one series, 11 of 15 children with DCSS had diminished pulmonary diffusion.[23]

The two-dimensional echocardiogram is important in confirming early pulmonary hypertension by documentation of a dilated right ventricle with thickening of the ventricular wall and straightening of the septum. One-dimensional (M-mode) echocardiography is characterized by changes in the midsystolic movement of the pulmonary valve. Right heart catheterization provides definitive confirmation but is often unnecessary.

Renal Function

Renal plasma flow is decreased in most patients with DCSS, especially in the cortex, although normal glomerular filtration may be preserved by intrarenal shifts in blood flow.[121] Even in patients without clinical evidence of renal disease, plasma renin levels correlate with the degree of histologic abnormality of the renal arteries and arterioles.[234] Renal arteriography may document irregular arterial narrowing, tortuosity of the interlobular and arcuate arterioles, cortical hypoperfusion, and other changes of malignant hypertension. The kidneys are small to normal in size.[235]

Radiologic Examination

The most characteristic radiologic findings in the hands are a marked decrease in soft tissue and resorption of the tufts of the distal phalanges (*acro-osteolysis*), particularly in patients with severe Raynaud's phenomenon (Fig. 21–17*A* and *B*).[236] Resorption of the distal tufts is particularly common in children.[23, 237] Resorption of bone may also occur in ribs, clavicles, distal radius and ulna, and other sites.[238] Periarticular or subcutaneous calcification, especially in the dominant hand, occurs in 15 to 25 percent of patients (see Figs. 21–8 and 21–9).[23, 239] Bony erosions can also develop at the distal interphalangeal and proximal interphalangeal joints, and involvement of the first carpometacarpal joint is said to be particularly characteristic of DCSS.[240] An increase in the thickness of the periodontal membrane results in radiolucent widening between the teeth and the jaw.[241]

Radiologic studies of the gastrointestinal tract may demonstrate characteristic abnormalities even in the absence of symptoms. A ciné-esophagogram may document decreased or absent peristalsis in the lower part of the esophagus with distal dilatation and, frequently, a hiatus hernia with stricture and shortening of the esophagus (Fig. 21–18*A* and *B*). The presence of air in the distal esophagus on the lateral chest radiograph is suggestive of the diagnosis of DCSS.[242] Esophageal motility studies by manometry and pH probe monitoring of the distal esophagus over 12 to 24 hours provide more sensitive indicators of diminished sphincter tone and the presence of reflux. The most frequent radiographic changes in the small bowel are dilatation of the second and third parts of the duodenum and the proximal jejunum (Fig. 21–19). Abnormalities in the colon are characterized by loss of colonic haustrations[243] and the presence of wide-mouthed diverticula or pseudosacculations on the antimesenteric border.[147]

Radiographic changes on chest films correlate poorly with pulmonary function studies. Radiologic bibasilar pulmonary fibrosis is one of the minor criteria for classification of DCSS (Fig. 21–20*A* and *B*). It may be accompanied by rib notching and calcified pulmonary "granulomata" in limited DCSS.[232] High-resolution (thin-slice) computed tomography may confirm pulmonary disease even in the presence of a normal chest radiograph.[244]

Treatment

No uniformly effective therapy is available.[10] Management of patients with DCSS presents one of the most difficult and frustrating challenges in all of rheumatology. Disease severity ranges from mild and stable to rapidly progressive and fatal. Management of the child with DCSS can be divided into three general areas: general supportive measures, therapy directed at controlling the underlying disease process, and management of complications.

General Supportive Measures

Supportive therapy is of utmost importance in the management of any child with a chronic, unpredictable, and potentially debilitating or fatal disease. Education of the patient and parents should be undertaken early in an attempt to prevent unnecessary psychological trauma. In general, "optimistic veracity" regarding complications, outcome, and treatment is appropriate.

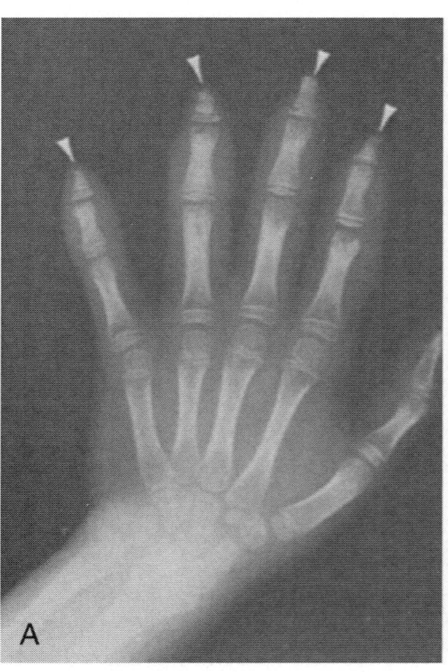

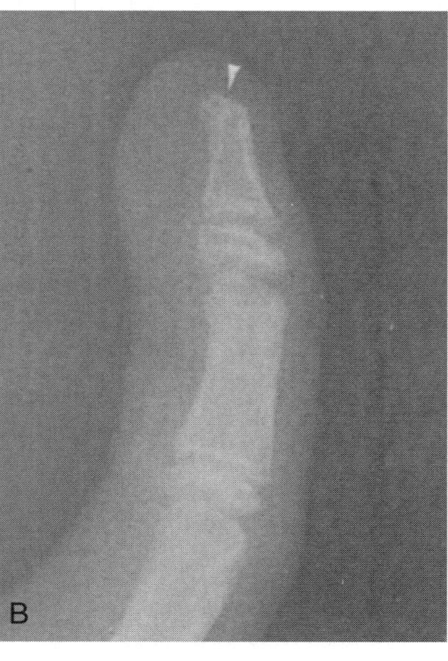

Figure 21–17. *A,* Radiograph of a boy with systemic scleroderma with early resorption of the tufts of the distal phalanges (*arrowheads*). *B,* Magnified view of acro-osteolysis of index finger (*arrowhead*).

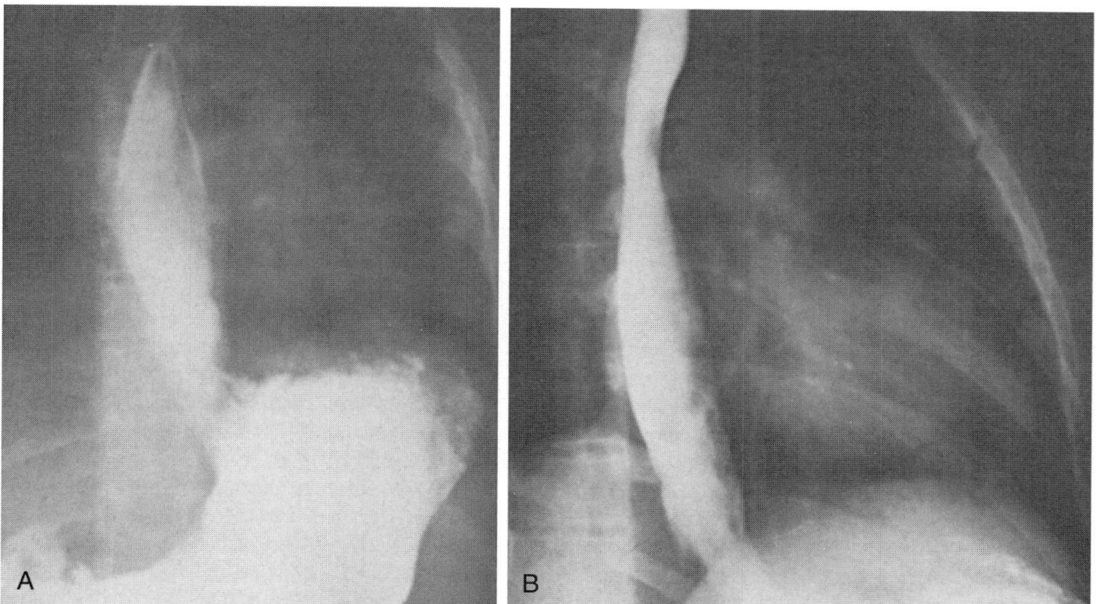

Figure 21–18. Barium-contrast examinations of the esophagus illustrate moderate dilatation and lack of a normal peristaltic pattern. *A,* Supine anteroposterior view. *B,* Lateral view.

Patient support groups may be helpful and important, albeit difficult to assemble for such a rare disease. The therapeutic team, including pediatric rheumatologist, nurse, social worker, physical and occupational therapists, dermatologist, nephrologist, and other healthcare professionals, should be involved in the patient's care where appropriate from the beginning. Patients should be instructed to avoid cold and trauma. Especially in cold climates, the family should be reminded to keep the child warm both by maintaining a satisfactory household temperature and by ensuring use of appropriate clothing, including well-insulated mittens (not gloves), boots, and a hat. On the other hand, the child should avoid excessive sun exposure and heat in the summer because of the susceptibility to hyperpigmentation of the skin and a relative inability to dissipate sufficient heat through sclerotic skin.

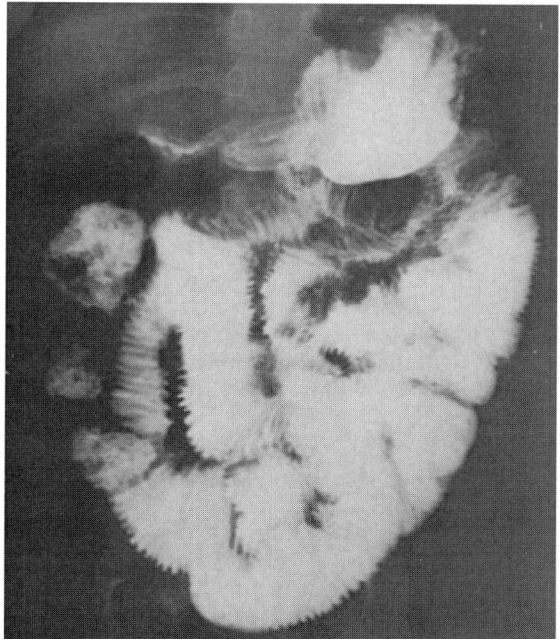

Figure 21–19. Upper gastrointestinal barium series with small bowel follow-through in a 3-year-old girl who had scleroderma with dilatation of the jejunum and closely approximated valvulae conniventes (the "closed accordion" sign) due to thickening of the ileal mucosa.

General skin care should include avoidance of drying or irritating substances and application of lanolin or water-soluble cream as an emollient once or several times daily. The child should be encouraged to be as physically active as possible within the constraints of the disease. Daily active and gentle passive range of motion exercises are essential to preserve maximal function. Dynamic splints may be necessary to treat or prevent contractures. Nonsteroidal anti-inflammatory drugs may relieve some of the musculoskeletal symptoms. Subcutaneous calcifications, if ulcerating, may respond well to incision and drainage.

Therapy of the Disease Process

The large number and variety of pharmacologic agents that have been recommended to treat DCSS are testimony to their relative inefficacy.[245] Drugs that are in current use are directed at breaking down or preventing collagen cross-linkage (D-penicillamine), inhibiting the fibroproliferative process (colchicine), and suppressing the immune response (immunosuppressants).[246]

D-Penicillamine

D-Penicillamine has been the drug most commonly used to treat DCSS, in both children and adults, al-

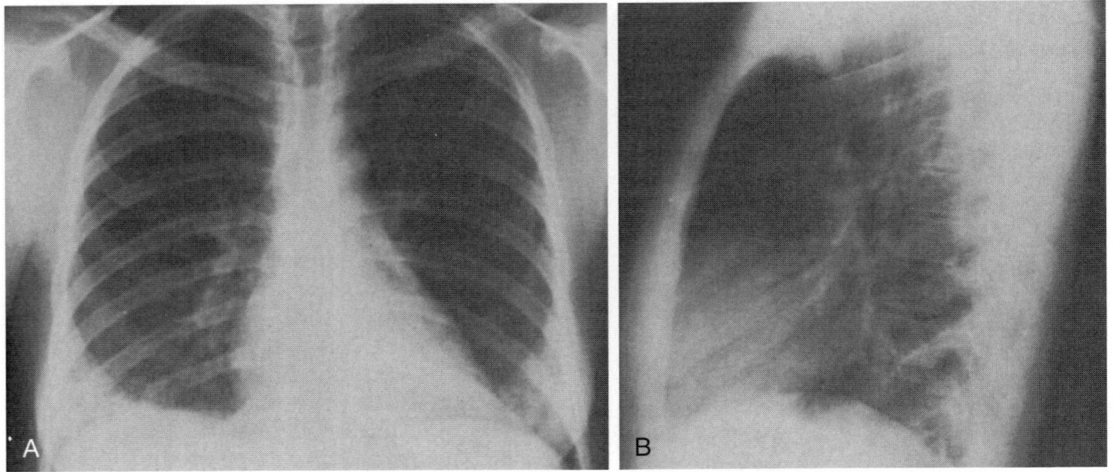

Figure 21–20. *A,* Posteroanterior radiograph of chest illustrates a fine reticular pattern in both lower lobes. *B,* Lateral view of chest.

though published results have been inconsistent.[247–249] There is, however, general agreement that if employed early, D-penicillamine may benefit the skin disease. It may also be of considerable help in preventing or retarding the progress of pulmonary involvement.

One report compared D-penicillamine (n = 17) with low-dose prednisone or no treatment (n = 6) in patients with diffuse DCSS (n = 17), LCSS (n = 2), or mixed connective tissue disease (n = 4). With a mean follow-up of 4.5 years, DLCO/LV and DLCO remained stable in the D-penicillamine–treated group but decreased in patients receiving steroids or no treatment.[250] These results, together with the observation that FVC did not improve, suggested that this chelating agent could reverse vascular endothelial thickening but not interstitial fibrosis.[251] In vitro evidence that synthetic vitamin A analogues (retinoids) suppress synthesis of pro-α_1 (I) and pro-α_1 (III) collagen molecules by fibroblasts obtained from patients with DCSS suggests that these agents may be useful in treatment,[252, 252a] but experience is extremely limited.[253]

Colchicine

There have been several reports that long-term colchicine administration (up to 0.5 mg four times a day in adults) results in softening of the skin in patients with DCSS.[254, 255] Sustained improvement in visceral disease is inconsistent.

Immunosuppressants

There have been no controlled trials of immunosuppressive drugs in the treatment of DCSS in adults or children. In spite of this, belief that immunologic mechanisms are perpetuators, if not initiators, of the disease process has prompted the use of drugs such as azathioprine, chlorambucil, methotrexate, cyclosporin, and cyclosporin with iloprost.[256–260, 260a] Other therapeutic trials predominantly in adults include evaluations of ketotifen,[261] apheresis,[262] extracorporeal photochemotherapy,[263] recombinant human relaxin,[263a] and interferon-α.[263b] Anecdotal reports suggest that such agents have had no demonstrable, or limited, benefit. Autologous stem cell transplantation has led to sustained improvement in at least one child with DCSS.[264, 264a] Glucocorticoids, the mainstay of treatment in many of the connective tissue disorders, are generally ineffective in the management of DCSS, except for the early inflammatory stage of muscle involvement or in the edematous phase of the cutaneous disease.[107] They may be contraindicated in the presence of renovascular hypertension.

Therapy of Specific Complications

Raynaud's Phenomenon

Specific treatment of Raynaud's phenomenon may be necessary, in addition to avoidance of precipitating circumstances such as cold or stress. Useful agents for amelioration of this complication include drugs that inhibit or suppress the sympathetic nervous system, thereby indirectly causing vasodilatation, and those that act directly on the smooth muscle of the vessel wall.[265, 266] Reserpine, methyldopa, captopril, and ketanserin have been used.[267–272] One drug may be effective in one patient, whereas a different agent is effective in another. It is therefore worth trying several, one at a time, until the desired effect is hopefully obtained (Table 21–8). Griseofulvin has been used in a few resistant patients, as have surgical approaches, prostaglandin E_1 infusions, and prostacyclin.[273–277] Oral iloprost (a prostacyclin analogue) has been recommended as beneficial in one study,[277a] but in another was no more effective than placebo.[278]

Nifedipine is probably the current drug of choice in management of Raynaud's phenomenon, although this priority may change as new agents are developed. Nifedipine is a calcium channel blocker and has been

Table 21–8

Pharmacologic Agents Used in Treatment of Raynaud's Phenomenon

DRUG	ACTION	REFERENCES
Drugs Affecting the Sympathetic Nervous System		
Tolazoline	Blocks alpha-adrenergic receptors	266
Phenoxybenzamine	Blocks alpha-adrenergic receptors	283
Prazosin	Blocks alpha-1 receptors	283, 284
Reserpine	Depletes norepinephrine from sympathetic nerves; IV administration results in short-lived vasodilation	266–268
Methyldopa	Central action	269
Guanethidine	Interferes with norepinephrine release at sympathetic neuroeffector junctions	265
Direct-Acting Drugs		
Captopril	Angiotensin converting enzyme inhibitor	270
Nifedipine	Slow calcium channel blocker	279, 280, 281, 282
Prostaglandin E_1	Vasodilator and platelet inhibitor	276
Prostaglandin I_1	Vasodilator	277
Glyceryl trinitrate (topical)	Vasodilator	285
Ketanserin	Antagonizes vasoconstrictor effects of 5-HT	271, 272
Griseofulvin	Vasodilator	273, 274

well tolerated in several controlled trials. It has significantly reduced the frequency and severity of Raynaud's phenomenon in DCSS and promoted healing of cutaneous ischemic ulcers.[279–282] Nifedipine is best started in a low dose at bedtime. Full dosage (approximately 10 mg two to four times a day in a 50-kg patient) is then achieved gradually to avoid precipitating postural hypotension.

Phenoxybenzamine is effective in doses of 10 to 40 mg per day, divided into three or four doses, although depression may be a significant side effect.[23, 76] Treatment should be initiated with a small dose (10 mg) at bedtime and increased gradually. Prazosin[283, 284] and locally applied nitroglycerin paste[285, 286] may also be helpful. Talpos and colleagues[287] and Winkelmann and coworkers[288] have employed serial plasmaphereses with good effect in some patients but with none in others. Biofeedback has also been used as the primary mode of therapy for some patients.[289] Sympathectomy is currently indicated only in the treatment of gangrene or intractable pain in the digits, and then only if temporary stellate ganglion block produces a beneficial result.

Renal Disease

Until recently, prognosis for DCSS patients with renal crisis was uniformly dismal. Immediate and effective lowering of the blood pressure in patients with malignant hypertension is mandatory. LeRoy and Fleischmann[123] cautioned, however, that any sudden change in plasma volume should be avoided because marked reductions in renal blood flow may precipitate full-blown clinical deterioration. The introduction of inhibitors of angiotensin-converting enzyme (e.g., captopril) has brought about remarkable improvement in the outlook for these patients with effective long-term control of blood pressure and stabilization of renal function.[290–292] It has also been observed, anecdotally, that systemic disease and especially cutaneous scleroderma improved concomitantly in some patients. In irreversible renal failure, or uncontrollable hypertension, some success has followed the use of hemodialysis with or without bilateral nephrectomy and transplantation.[293] Dialysis may also lead to improvement in the cutaneous abnormalities.

Pulmonary Disease

Pulmonary complications in DCSS are very serious, and there may be no long-term effective approach to either fibrosing alveolitis or primary pulmonary hypertension. For the former, night-time positive-pressure ventilation has been advocated to improve oxygenation and lower carbon dioxide levels. For the latter, experimental therapy has included intravenous iloprost, angiotension-2 receptor antagonist, ET-1 antagonist, and thromboxane A_2 antagonist administration.

Course of the Disease and Prognosis

The prognosis of DCSS has been poor but may be improving.[293a] Skin tightness and joint contractures inevitably lead to severe disability in some patients (Fig. 21–21). Progressive visceral involvement is typical, although the disease may stabilize in some patients for long periods of time (Table 21–9). It is a curious but oft-repeated observation that the skin may eventually soften years after onset of the disease.

The most common causes of death in children are related to involvement of the cardiac, renal, and pulmonary systems (Table 21–10). Gastrointestinal complications, including severe inanition, may also become important in some patients.[20] Cardiac arrhythmias may develop during the course of the disease secondary to

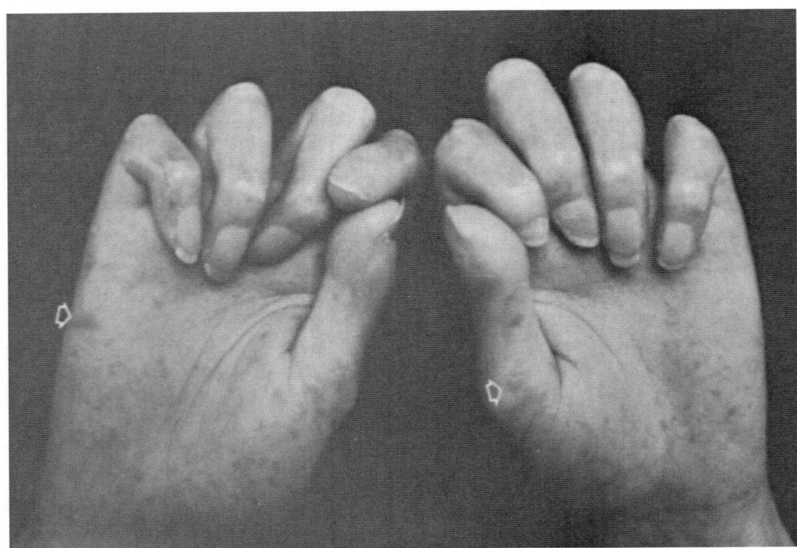

Figure 21–21. Hands of a 27-year-old woman with diffuse cutaneous systemic scleroderma that began in childhood. There was essentially no movement possible in these fingers due to joint contractures. Note also the extensive telangiectases (*arrows*).

myocardial fibrosis. Congestive heart failure is often a terminal event. Pulmonary interstitial disease and vascular lesions are probably universal. Renal failure or acute hypertensive encephalopathy supervenes as a potentially fatal outcome in a few children. At least in adults, this event seems more likely to occur early in the course of the disease.

The frequency of a fatal outcome from DCSS has not been definitively determined in any large series of children because of the rarity of this disease. In a recent multinational survey,[293a] 8 of 135 patients died. However, prognosis is not judged to be any more favorable than in adults, in whom mortality rates are significantly increased (standardized mortality ratio [SMR], 4.5; 95 percent CI, 3.5 to 5.7) or in patients under the age of 35 years (SMR, 13; 95 percent CI, 2.7 to 37).[294] Another recent study cited a survival rate 7 years from diagnosis of 72.5 percent in black women and 77.6 percent in white women.[18] A child may live decades after onset, however; therefore, an optimistic but realistic attitude should be taken in discussions with the parents. The age-specific mortality rate in one epidemiologic study for the age group 0 to 14 years was 0.04 per million person-years.[295] Pulmonary hypertension was associated with death in at least two children.[148, 296] As children with DCSS live into adulthood, complications that might be associated with pregnancy become of concern.[297, 297a]

Table 21–9

Organ System Involvement During the Course of Disease in 15 Children With Scleroderma

ORGAN SYSTEM	NO. WITH INVOLVEMENT/ NO. OBSERVED
Skin	
Subcutaneous calcification	4/15
Ulcerations	9/15
Telangiectases	4/15
Pigmentation	3/15
Digital arteries (Raynaud's phenomenon)	11/15
Musculoskeletal system	
Contractures	11/15
Resorption of digital tufts	9/11
Muscle weakness	6/15
Muscle atrophy	6/15
Gastrointestinal tract	
Abnormal esophageal motility	11/15
Dilatation of duodenum	1/15
Colonic sacculations	3/5
Lungs	
Abnormal diffusion	11/15
Abnormal vital capacity	10/15
Heart	
Cardiomegaly	2/15
Electrocardiographic abnormalities	4/15
Congestive heart failure	2/15

From Cassidy JT, Sullivan DB, Dabich L, et al: Scleroderma in children. Arthritis Rheum 20(Suppl): 351–354, 1977.

Mortality from DCSS seemingly increases throughout life and is higher for males than females, and for nonwhites than whites. Although no specific data on survival rates for children are available, studies of patients of all ages demonstrate mean survival rates of 70 to 94 percent at 1 year, 34 to 73 percent at 5 years, and 35 to 74 percent at 10 years.[120] Cardiac and renal disease were the most common contributors to mortality. Outcome in another study of 48 adults with "early" scleroderma indicated that survivorship at 1 year was 92 percent, at 3 years 75 percent, and at 5 years 68 percent.[298] An overall 10-year survival rate close to 90 percent was reported in a group of 106 patients from Italy who were predominantly female.[16] This improved outcome may reflect the advantage of more current medical therapy. Survival was better in patients with onset before 35 years of age, although this difference could be attributable to other causes. In another study, 20-year mortality in patients with DCSS and renal involvement was 60 percent, compared with 10 percent in those without renal disease.[121] Two additional investigations, one from Spain,[298a] and the other from Denmark,[294] identified the extent of sclerosis of the skin as an important determining factor in prognosis.

Table 21–10

Causes of Death in Children With Scleroderma

STUDY	SEX	AGE AT ONSET (YR)	DISEASE DURATION	CAUSE OF DEATH
Kornreich et al.[22]	M	4	10 yr	Cerebral hemorrhage secondary to thrombocytopenia
	F	6	9 yr	Cardiac failure
	M	7	23 mo	Kidney failure
	F	10	15 mo	Cardiac failure
	F	10	22 mo	Pulmonary emboli
	F	15	5 mo	Cardiac failure
Cassidy et al.[23]	F	12	6 mo	Cardiac failure
	F	11	10 yr	Cardiac failure
	F	8	9 yr	Central nervous system disease, hypertension
Suárez-Almazor et al.[36]	M	10	2 yr	Cardiac failure and pulmonary hypertension
Bulkley[148]	M	13	2 yr	Pulmonary hypertension
	F	16	1 yr	Pulmonary hypertension

LIMITED CUTANEOUS SYSTEMIC SCLERODERMA

Definition

LCSS is the current designation for those patients previously classified as having the *CREST syndrome*. The acronym *CREST* stands for *calcinosis, Raynaud's phenomenon, esophageal dysmotility, sclerodactyly,* and *telangiectases,* a syndrome that was described as acrosclerosis in the older literature. Whether it is a relatively mild form of DCSS or an entirely separate, although related, disorder is uncertain.[10, 299] The combination of scleroderma and calcinosis has also been referred to as the *Thibierge-Weissenbach syndrome.*[300] Winterbauer[301] first described the CREST syndrome as another variant of systemic scleroderma. Very few instances of LCSS in children have been reported (Table 21–11).

Epidemiology

Overall, cases of LCSS account for approximately one third to one half of the adult patients with scleroderma.[302] Limited disease is more frequent among women and tends to occur at an earlier age than DCSS.

Table 21–11

Limited Cutaneous Systemic Scleroderma (CREST Syndrome) and Variants in Children

STUDY	SEX	AGE AT ONSET (YR)	CLINICAL FEATURES
Larrègue et al.[34]	F	6	CRST
Burge et al.[35]	M	6	CREST
Suárez-Almazor et al.[36]	F	10	RST

C, calcinosis; R, Raynaud's phenomenon; E, esophageal dysmotility; S, sclerodactyly; T, telangiectases.

A long interval between the onset of Raynaud's phenomenon and diagnostic skin changes is characteristic.

Clinical Manifestations

Calcinosis is often more severe in patients with LCSS compared with those who have DCSS (Fig. 21–22). Raynaud's phenomenon is more frequently complicated by digital ulceration and gangrene, and telangiectases are more widespread.[301] LCSS is by no means a mild disease, and severe systemic involvement, espe-

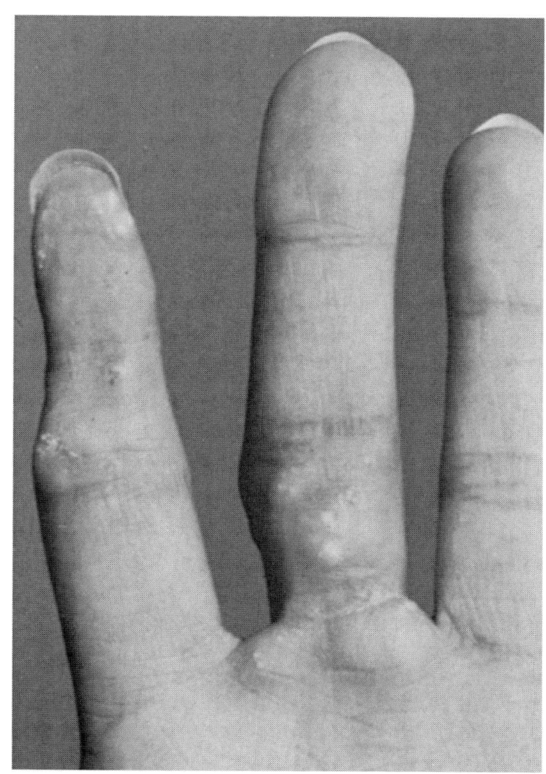

Figure 21–22. Striking subcutaneous calcification with extrusion of calcareous material.

Table 21–12

Comparison of Diffuse Cutaneous Systemic Scleroderma (DCSS), Limited Cutaneous Systemic Scleroderma (LCSS), Eosinophilic Fasciitis (EF), Mixed Connective Tissue Disease (MCTD), Juvenile Dermatomyositis (JDM), and Systemic Lupus Erythematosus (SLE)

CHARACTERISTIC	DCSS	LCSS	EF	MCTD	JDM	SLE
Distal sclerosis	+ + +	+ + + +	+ + +	+ +	−	−
Proximal sclerosis	+ + + +	−	+	+	−	−
Raynaud's phenomenon	+ + + +	+ + + +	−	+ + + +	+	+ +
Telangiectases	+ + +	+ + + +	−	+	−	−
Nailfold capillaropathy	+ + +	+ + +	−	+ +	+ + +	+
Calcinosis	+ +	+ + + +	−	+	+ +	−
Esophageal disease	+ + +	+ + +	−	+ +	−	−
Pulmonary disease	+ + + +	+ + +	−	+ +	+	+
Cardiac disease	+ + + +	−	−	+	±	+ +
Renal disease	+ + +	−	−	+	−	+ + +
Muscle disease	+ +	−	+	+ + +	+ + + +	+
Arthritis	+	+	+	+ + +	+	+ +
Central nervous system disease	+	−	−	+	−	+ + +
Anti-dsDNA antibody	−	−	−	+	−	+ + +
Anti-nucleolar antibody	+ +	−	+	−	−	−
Anticentromere antibody	+	+ + + +	−	−	−	−
Anti-Sm antibody	−	−	−	+	−	+ +
Anti-RNP low titer	−	−	−	+	−	+ +
Anti-RNP high titer	−	−	−	+ + + +	−	−
Thrombocytopenia	−	−	−	+	−	+ +
Peripheral eosinophilia	−	−	+ + + +	−	−	−

−, rare or absent; +, up to 25%; + +, up to 50%; + + +, up to 75%; + + + +, up to 100%.

cially of the parenchyma of the lungs and pulmonary vasculature, occurs, although renal disease is less frequent than in DCSS.

Diagnosis

In LCSS, cutaneous sclerosis is restricted to the distal segments of the digits, and the other elements of the CREST acronym (telangiectases, Raynaud's phenomenon, calcinosis) are more prominent than in diffuse disease (Table 21–12). Isolated proximal scleroderma in a patient would suggest the diagnosis of DCSS rather than limited disease. In other ways, however, these two syndromes closely resemble each other, and *clinical division of the two disorders may be entirely artificial*. Furthermore, incomplete forms (e.g., CRST, CRT) merge with diffuse disease and make differentiation of these two forms of systemic scleroderma difficult, if not impossible, in a number of patients.

Immunologic Characteristics

Antibody to centromere has been described as the serologic hallmark of LCSS, and its discovery historically supported the rationale for clinical differentiation of DCSS from the CREST syndrome.[299, 303] These antibodies are directed at the kinetochore of integral components of the mitotic spindle. It is now understood, however, that anticentromere antibody is associated with diseases other than limited LCSS,[304] notably primary biliary cirrhosis, occasionally DCSS, Sjögren's syndrome, isolated Raynaud's phenomenon, and rarely rheumatoid arthritis, systemic lupus erythematosus, and other connective tissue diseases. Other antinuclear antibodies (anti-ssDNA, anti-RNP) may occasionally occur in patients with LCSS.[305]

Treatment

The management of children with LCSS is not materially different from that for diffuse disease, modified by each patient's specific organ involvement and severity.

Course of the Disease and Prognosis

It was initially believed that patients with this limited variant of scleroderma had a more benign course and a lower mortality rate than patients with diffuse disease, but this distinction has not been entirely substantiated. Mortality in LCSS, although somewhat less than in DCSS, is considerable, with a 10-year survival rate of approximately 75 percent in adults.[302]

References

1. Lewin G, Heller J: Die sclerodermie. Berlin, August Hirschwald, 1895, p 236.
2. Goodman H: A case of scleroderma diffusa in a girl, nine years of age; with a review of the literature. J Cutan Pathol 36: 210, 1918.

3. Jaffe MO, Winkelmann RK: Generalized scleroderma in children. Acrosclerotic type. Arch Dermatol 83: 402, 1961.
4. Kass H, Hanson V, Patrick J: Scleroderma in childhood. J Pediatr 68: 243, 1966.
5. Tuffanelli DL, Winkelmann RK: Systemic scleroderma. A clinical study of 727 cases. Arch Dermatol 84: 359, 1961.
6. Belch JJ: The clinical assessment of the scleroderma spectrum disorders. Br J Rheumatol 32: 353–355, 1993.
7. Kraus EJ: Zur pathogenese der diffusen Sklerodermie. Zugleich ein Beitrag zur Pathologie der Epithelkörperchen. Virchows Archiv Pathol Anat 253: 710, 1924.
8. Matsui S: Anatomie pathologique et pathogénique de la sclérodermie géneralisée. Presse Méd 32: 142, 1924.
9. D'Angelo WA, Fries JF, Masi AT, et al: Pathologic observations in systemic sclerosis (scleroderma). A study of fifty-eight autopsy cases and fifty-eight matched controls. Am J Med 46: 428–440, 1969.
10. Rodnan GP: When is scleroderma not scleroderma? The differential diagnosis of progressive systemic sclerosis. Bull Rheum Dis 31:7–10, 1981.
10a. Poormoghim H, Lucas M, Fertig N, Medsger TA Jr: Systemic sclerosis sine scleroderma: demographic, clinical, and serologic features and survival in forty-eight patients. Arthritis Rheum 43: 444–451, 2000.
11. Caperton EM, Hathaway DE: Scleroderma with eosinophilia and hypergammaglobulinemia: the Shulman syndrome. Arthritis Rheum 18: 391, 1975.
12. Medsger TA Jr, Masi AT: Epidemiology of progressive systemic sclerosis. Clin Rheumat Dis 5: 15, 1979.
13. Kurland LT, Hauser WA, Ferguson RH, et al: Epidemiologic features of diffuse connective tissue disorders in Rochester, Minnesota, 1951 through 1967, with special reference to systemic lupus erythematosus. Mayo Clin Proc 44: 649–663, 1969.
14. Shinkai H: Epidemiology of progressive systemic sclerosis in Japan. *In* Black CM, Myers AR (eds): Systemic Sclerosis (Scleroderma). New York, Gower Medical, 1985, pp 79–81.
15. Asboe-Hansen G: Epidemiology of progressive systemic sclerosis in Denmark. *In* Black CM, Myers AR (eds): Systemic Sclerosis (Scleroderma). New York, Gower Medical, 1985, p 78.
16. Giordano M, Valentini G, Ara M, et al: Epidemiology of progressive systemic sclerosis in Italy. *In* Black CM, Myers AR (eds): Systemic Sclerosis (Scleroderma). New York, Gower Medical, 1985, pp 72–77.
17. Barnett AJ: Epidemiology of systemic sclerosis (scleroderma) in Australia. *In* Black CM, Myers AR (eds): Systemic Sclerosis (Scleroderma). New York, Gower Medical, 1985, pp 82–83.
18. Laing TJ, Gillespie BW, Toth MB, et al: Racial differences in scleroderma among women in Michigan. Arthritis Rheum 40: 734–742, 1997.
18a. Black CM: Scleroderma in children. Adv Exp Med Biol 455: 35–48, 1999.
18b. Medsger TA Jr: Epidemiology of systemic sclerosis. Clin Dermatol 12: 207–216, 1994.
19. Tuffanelli DL, LaPerriere R: Connective tissue diseases. Pediatr Clin North Am 18: 925–951, 1971.
20. Medsger TA Jr, Masi AT: Epidemiology of systemic sclerosis (scleroderma). Ann Intern Med 74: 714–721, 1971.
21. Hanson V: Dermatomyositis, scleroderma, and polyarteritis nodosa. Clin Rheum Dis 2: 445, 1976.
22. Kornreich HK, Koster King K, Bernstein BH: Scleroderma in childhood. Arthritis Rheum 20(Suppl): 343–350, 1977.
22a. Emery H: Pediatric scleroderma. Semin Cutan Med Surg 17: 41–47, 1998.
23. Cassidy JT, Sullivan DB, Dabich L, et al: Scleroderma in children. Arthritis Rheum 20(Suppl): 351–354, 1977.
24. Kennedy WP: Cardiac death from progressive systemic scleroderma in a child. Can Med Assoc J 90: 33–35, 1964.
25. Mukherjee SK, Lahiri K, Sen MK: Scleroderma in a boy of nine. J Indian Med Assoc 47: 132–135, 1966.
26. Velayos EE, Cohen BS: Progressive systemic sclerosis. Diagnosis at the age of 4 years. Am J Dis Child 123: 57–60, 1972.
27. Szymanska-Jagiello W, Rondio H, Jakubowska K: Changes in the locomotor system in progressive systemic sclerosis in children. Mater Med Pol 4: 201–209, 1972.
28. Goel KM, Shanks RA: Scleroderma in childhood. Report of 5 cases. Arch Dis Child 49: 861–866, 1974.
29. Ansell BM, Nasseh GA, Bywaters EG: Scleroderma in childhood. Ann Rheum Dis 35: 189–197, 1976.
30. Gray RG, Altman RD: Progressive systemic sclerosis in a family: case report of a mother and son and review of the literature. Arthritis Rheum 20: 35–41, 1977.
31. Schlesinger M, Schaller JG: Progressive systemic sclerosis of childhood. Arthritis Rheum 24: S104, 1981.
32. Girouard M, Pare C, Camerlain M: La sclerodermie juvenile. Union Med Can 111: 546–551, 1982.
33. Spencer-Green G, Schlesinger M, Bove KE, et al: Nailfold capillary abnormalities in childhood rheumatic diseases. J Pediatr 102: 341–346, 1983.
34. Larrègue M, Canuel C, Bazex J, et al: Sclérodermie systemique de l'enfant. A propos de 5 observations. Révue de la litterature. Ann Dermatol Venereol 110: 317–326, 1983.
35. Burge SM, Ryan TJ, Dawber RP: Juvenile onset systemic sclerosis. J R Soc Med 77: 793–794, 1984.
36. Suárez-Almazor ME, Catoggio LJ, Maldonado-Cocco JA, et al: Juvenile progressive systemic sclerosis: clinical and serologic findings. Arthritis Rheum 28: 699–702, 1985.
37. Lababidi HM, Nasr FW, Khatib Z: Juvenile progressive systemic sclerosis: report of five cases. J Rheumatol 18: 885–888, 1991.
38. Martinez-Cordero E, Fonseca MC, Aguilar Léon DE, et al: Juvenile systemic sclerosis. J Rheumatol 20: 405–407, 1993.
39. Vancheeswaran R, Black CM, David J, et al: Childhood-onset scleroderma: is it different from adult-onset disease. Arthritis Rheum 40: 1041–1049, 1996.
40. Singsen BH: Scleroderma in childhood. Pediatr Clin North Am 33: 1119–1139, 1986.
40a. Kuroda K, Okamoto O, Shinkai H: Dermatopontin expression is decreased in hypertrophic scar and systemic sclerosis skin fibroblasts and is regulated by transforming growth factor-beta1, interleukin-4, and matrix collagen. J Invest Dermatol 112: 706–710, 1999.
41. Jelaska A, Arakawa M, Broketa G, et al: Heterogeneity of collagen synthesis in normal and systemic sclerosis skin fibroblasts. Increased proportion of high collagen-producing cells in systemic sclerosis fibroblasts. Arthritis Rheum 39: 1338–1346, 1996.
42. Lovell CR, Nicholls AC, Duance VC, et al: Characterization of dermal collagen in systemic sclerosis. Br J Dermatol 100: 359–369, 1979.
43. Brady AH: Collagenase in scleroderma. J Clin Invest 56: 1175–1180, 1975.
44. Uitto J, Bauer EA, Eisor AZ: Scleroderma: increased biosynthesis of triple-helical type I and type III procollagens associated with unaltered expression of collagenase by skin fibroblasts in culture. J Clin Invest 64: 921–930, 1979.
45. Peltonen L, Palotie A, Myllyla R, et al: Collagen biosynthesis in systemic scleroderma: regulation of post-translational modifications and synthesis of procollagen in cultured fibroblasts. J Invest Dermatol 84: 14–18, 1985.
46. Blumenkrantz N, Asboe-Hanson G: Subhydroxylated collagen in scleroderma. Acta Derm Venereol (Stockh) 58: 359–361, 1978.
47. Haustein UF, Herrmann K, Bohme HJ: Pathogenesis of progressive systemic sclerosis. Int J Dermatol 25: 286–293, 1986.
48. Cohen S, Johnson AR, Hurd E: Cytotoxicity of sera from patients with scleroderma. Effects on human endothelial cells and fibroblasts in culture. Arthritis Rheum 26: 170–178, 1983.
49. Kahaleh MB: Endothelin, an endothelial-dependent vasoconstrictor in scleroderma. Enhanced production and profibrotic action. Arthritis Rheum 34: 978–983, 1991.
50. Feghali CA, Boulware DW, Levy LS: Mechanisms of pathogenesis in scleroderma. II. Effects of serum and conditioned culture medium on fibroblast function in scleroderma. J Rheumatol 19: 1212–1219, 1992.
50a. Sato S, Nagaoka T, Hasegawa M, et al: Serum levels of connective tissue growth factor are elevated in patients with systemic sclerosis: association with extent of skin sclerosis and severity of pulmonary fibrosis. J Rheumatol 27: 149–154, 2000.
50b. Abraham DJ, Shiwen X, Black CM, et al: Tumor necrosis factor alpha suppresses the induction of connective tissue growth factor by transforming growth factor-beta in normal and scleroderma fibroblasts. J Biol Chem 275: 15220–15225, 2000.
51. Odoux C, Crestani B, Lebrun G, et al: Endothelin-1 secretion by alveolar macrophages in systemic sclerosis. Am J Respir Crit Care Med 156: 1429–1435, 1997.

52. Kaheleh MB, Yin T: The molecular mechanism of endothelial cell injury in scleroderma (SSc): identification of granzyme 1 (a product of cytolytic T cell) in SSc sera. Arthritis Rheum 33(Suppl): S21, 1990.
53. Emerit I, Housset E, Feingold J: Chromosomal breakage and scleroderma: studies in family members. J Lab Clin Med 88: 81–86, 1976.
54. Kahaleh MB, Sherer CK, LeRoy EC: Endothelial injury in scleroderma. J Exp Med 149: 1326–1335, 1979.
55. Irani AM, Gruber BL, Kaufman LD, et al: Mast cell changes in scleroderma. Presence of MCT cells in skin and evidence of mast cell activation. Arthritis Rheum 35: 933–939, 1992.
56. Black CM, Welsh KI, Maddison PJ, et al: HLA antigens in scleroderma. *In* Black CM, Myers AR (eds): Systemic Sclerosis (Scleroderma). New York, Gower Medical, 1985, pp 84–88.
57. Kahaleh MB, Osborn I, LeRoy EC: Increased Factor VIII/von Willebrand factor antigen and von Willebrand factor activity in scleroderma and in Raynaud's phenomenon. Ann Intern Med 94: 482–484, 1981.
58. Woolf AD, Wakerley G, Wallington TB, et al: Factor VIII related antigen in the assessment of vasculitis. Ann Rheum Dis 46: 441–447, 1987.
59. Sgonc R, Gruschwitz MS, Dietrich H, et al: Endothelial cell apoptosis is a primary pathogenetic event underlying skin lesions in avian and human scleroderma. J Clin Invest 98: 785–792, 1996.
60. Fries JF: The microvascular pathogenesis of scleroderma: an hypothesis. Ann Intern Med 91: 788–789, 1979.
61. Sternberg EM: Pathogenesis of scleroderma: the interrelationship of immune and vascular hypotheses. Surv Immunol Res 4: 69–80, 1985.
62. Postethwaite AE, Stuart JM, Kang AH: The cell-mediated immune system in progressive systemic sclerosis: an overview. *In* Black CM, Myers AR (eds): Systemic Sclerosis (Scleroderma). New York, Gower Medical, 1985, pp 319–325.
63. Needleman BW, Wigley FM, Stair RW: Interleukin-1, interleukin-2, interleukin-4, interleukin-6, tumor necrosis factor alpha, and interferon-gamma levels in sera from patients with scleroderma. Arthritis Rheum 35: 67–72, 1992.
63a. Hasegawa M, Sato S, Ihn H, Takehara K: Enhanced production of interleukin-6 (IL-6), oncostatin M and soluble IL-6 receptor by cultured peripheral blood mononuclear cells from patients with systemic sclerosis. Rheumatology (Oxford) 38: 612–617, 1999.
63b. Atamas SP, Yurovsky VV, Wise R, et al: Production of type 2 cytokines by CD8 + lung cells is associated with greater decline in pulmonary function in patients with systemic sclerosis. Arthritis Rheum 42: 1168–1178, 1999.
64. Salojin KV, Le Tonqueze M, Saraux A, et al: Antiendothelial cell antibodies: useful markers of systemic sclerosis. Am J Med 102: 178–185, 1997.
65. Huffstutter JE, DeLustro FA, LeRoy EC: Cellular immunity to collagen and laminin in scleroderma. Arthritis Rheum 28: 775–780, 1985.
66. Burge KM, Perry HO, Stickler GB: "Familial" scleroderma. Arch Dermatol 99: 681–687, 1969.
67. Clements PJ, Opelz G, Terasaki PI, et al: Association of HLA antigen A9 with progressive systemic sclerosis (scleroderma). Tissue Antigens 11: 357–361, 1978.
68. Van der Meulen J, Van der Voort-Beelen JM, D'Amaro J, et al: HLA-B8 in Raynaud's phenomenon. Tissue Antigens 15: 81, 1980.
69. Kallenberg CG, Van der Voort-Beelen JM, D'Amaro J, et al: Increased frequency of B8/DR3 in scleroderma and association of the haplotype with impaired cellular immune response. Clin Exp Immunol 43: 478–485, 1981.
70. Lynch CJ, Singh G, Whiteside TL, et al: Histocompatibility antigens in progressive systemic sclerosis (PSS; scleroderma). J Clin Immunol 2: 314–318, 1982.
71. Gladman DD, Keystone EC, Baron M, et al: Increased frequency of HLA-DR5 in scleroderma. Arthritis Rheum 24: 854–856, 1981.
72. Whiteside TL, Medsger TA Jr, Rodnan G: Studies of HLA antigens in progressive systemic sclerosis. *In* Black CM, Myers AR (eds): Systemic Sclerosis (Scleroderma). New York, Gower Medical, 1985, p 89.
73. Fox RI, Kang HI: Genetic and environmental factors in systemic sclerosis. Curr Opin Rheumatol 4: 857–861, 1992.
74. Nelson JL, Furst DE, Maloney S, et al: Microchimerism and HLA-compatible relationships of pregnancy in scleroderma. Lancet 351: 559–562, 1998.
75. Artlett CM, Smith JB, Jiminez SA: Identification of fetal DNA and cells in skin lesions from women with systemic sclerosis. N Engl J Med 338: 1186–1191, 1998.
76. Dabich L, Sullivan DB, Cassidy JT: Scleroderma in the child. J Pediatr 85: 770–775, 1974.
77. Jacobs MJ, Breslau PJ, Slaaf DW, et al: Nomenclature of Raynaud's phenomenon: a capillary microscopic and hemorrheologic study. Surgery 101: 136–145, 1987.
78. Patterson JW: Pterygium inversum unguis–like changes in scleroderma. Report of four cases. Arch Dermatol 113: 1429–1430, 1977.
79. Moore CP, Willkens RF: The subcutaneous nodule. Its significance in the diagnosis of rheumatic disease. Semin Arthritis Rheum 7: 63–79, 1977.
80. Raynaud M: De l'asphyxie locale et de la gangrene symetrique des extremities. Paris, L Leclerc, Libraire-Editeur, 1862.
81. Raynaud M: On local asphyxia and symmetrical gangrene of the extremities (1862). Arch Gen Med 1:189, 1874.
82. Yarom A, Levinson JE: Vasculopathy in scleroderma. *In* Hicks RV (ed): Vasculopathies in Childhood. Littleton, MA, PSG, 1988, p 243.
83. Duffy CM, Laxer RM, Lee P, et al: Raynaud syndrome in childhood. J Pediatr 114: 73–78, 1989.
84. Allen EV, Brown GE: Raynaud's disease: a critical review of minimal requisites for diagnosis. Am J Med Sci 183: 187, 1932.
85. Follansbee WP, Curtiss EI, Medsger TA Jr, et al: Physiologic abnormalities of cardiac function in progressive systemic sclerosis with diffuse scleroderma. N Engl J Med 310: 142–148, 1984.
86. Gutheroth WG, Morgan BC, Harbinson JA: Raynaud's disease in children. Circulation 36: 724–729, 1967.
87. Jung LK, Dent PB: Prognostic significance of Raynaud's phenomenon in children. Clin Pediatr (Phila) 22: 22–25, 1983.
88. Harper FE, Maricq HR, Turner RE, et al: A prospective study of Raynaud phenomenon and early connective tissue disease. A five-year report. Am J Med 72: 883–888, 1982.
89. Dessein PH, Joffe BI, Metz RM, et al: Autonomic dysfunction in systemic sclerosis: sympathetic overactivity and instability. Am J Med 93: 143–150, 1992.
90. LeRoy EC, Downey JA, Cannon PJ: Skin capillary blood flow in scleroderma. J Clin Invest 50: 930–939, 1971.
91. Fries JF: Physiologic studies in systemic sclerosis (scleroderma). Arch Intern Med 123: 22, 1969.
92. Dabich L, Bookstein JJ, Zweifler A, et al: Digital arteries in patients with scleroderma. Arteriographic and plethysmographic study. Arch Intern Med 130: 708–714, 1972.
93. Maricq HR, Spencer-Green G, LeRoy EC: Skin capillary abnormalities as indicators of organ involvement in scleroderma (systemic sclerosis), Raynaud's syndrome and dermatomyositis. Am J Med 61: 862–870, 1976.
94. Rodnan GP, Myerowitz RL, Justh GO: Morphologic changes in the digital arteries of patients with progressive systemic sclerosis (scleroderma) and Raynaud phenomenon. Medicine (Baltimore) 59: 393–408, 1980.
95. Winkelmann RK, Goldyne ME, Linscheid RL: Influence of cold on catecholamine response of vascular smooth muscle strips from resistance vessels of scleroderma skin. Angiology 28: 330–339, 1977.
96. Winkelmann RK, Goldyne ME, Linscheid RL: Hypersensitivity of scleroderma cutaneous vascular smooth muscle to 5-hydroxytryptamine. Br J Dermatol 95: 51–56, 1976.
97. Kallenberg CG, Vallenga E, Wouda AA, et al: Platelet activation, fibrinolytic activity and circulating immune complexes in Raynaud's phenomenon. J Rheumatol 9: 878–884, 1982.
98. Majerus PW: Arachidonate metabolism in vascular disorders. J Clin Invest 72: 1521–1525, 1983.
99. Crocq C: De L' "acrocyanose." Semaine Méd 16: 208, 1896.
100. Lewis T, Landis EM: Observations upon the vascular mechanism in acrocyanosis. Heart 15: 230, 1930.
101. Stern ES: The aetiology and pathology of acrocyanosis. Br J Derm Syph 49: 100, 1937.

102. Peacock JH: Vasodilatation in the human hand. Observations on primary Raynaud's disease and acrocyanosis of the upper extremities. Clin Sci 17: 575, 1957.
103. Peacock JH: A comparative study of the digital cutaneous temperatures and hand blood flows in the normal hand, primary Raynaud's disease and primary acrocyanosis. Clin Sci 18: 25, 1959.
104. Sivula A: Vascular reactions in acrocyanosis. Angiology 17: 269–274, 1966.
105. Rodnan GP, Medsger TA: The rheumatic manifestations of progressive systemic sclerosis (scleroderma). Clin Orthop 57: 81–93, 1968.
106. Schulman LE, Kurban AK, Harvey AM: Tendon friction rubs in progressive systemic sclerosis (scleroderma). Arthritis Rheum 4: 438, 1961.
107. Clements PJ, Furst DE, Campion DS, et al: Muscle disease in progressive systemic sclerosis. Diagnostic and therapeutic considerations. Arthritis Rheum 21: 62–71, 1978.
108. Orringer MB, Dabich L, Zarafonetis CJ, et al: Gastroesophageal reflux in esophageal scleroderma: diagnosis and implications. Ann Thorac Surg 22: 120–130, 1976.
109. Ortiz-Alvarez O, Cabral D, Prendiville JS, et al: Intestinal pseudo-obstruction as an initial presentation of systemic sclerosis in two children. Br J Rheumatol 36: 280–284, 1997.
110. Meihoff WE, Hirschfield JS, Kern F Jr: Small intestinal scleroderma with malabsorption and pneumatosis cystoides intestinalis. Report of three cases. JAMA 204: 854–858, 1968.
111. Bartholomew LG, Cain JC, Winkelmann RK, et al: Chronic disease of the liver associated with systemic scleroderma. Am J Digest Dis 9: 43, 1964.
112. Reynolds TB, Denison EK, Frankl HD, et al: Primary biliary cirrhosis with scleroderma, Raynaud's phenomenon and telangiectasia. New syndrome. Am J Med 50: 302–312, 1971.
113. Follansbee WP, Zerbe TR, Medsger TA Jr: Cardiac and skeletal muscle diseases in systemic sclerosis (scleroderma): a high risk association. Am Heart J 125: 194–203, 1993.
114. Gupta MP, Zoneraich S, Zeitlin W, et al: Scleroderma heart disease with slow flow velocity in coronary arteries. Chest 67: 116–119, 1975.
115. Trell E, Lindstrom C: Pulmonary hypertension in systemic sclerosis. Ann Rheum Dis 30: 390–400, 1971.
116. Eid NS, Buchino JJ, Schikler KN: Pulmonary manifestations of rheumatic diseases. Pediatr Pulmonol Suppl 18: 91–92, 1999.
117. Zatuchni J, Campbell WN, Zarafonetis CJD: Pulmonary fibrosis and terminal bronchiolar ("alveolar cell") carcinoma in scleroderma. Cancer 6: 1147, 1953.
118. Furst DE, Davis JA, Clements PJ, et al: Abnormalities of pulmonary vascular dynamics and inflammation in early progressive systemic sclerosis. Arthritis Rheum 24: 1403–1408, 1981.
119. Fahey PJ, Utell MJ, Condemi JJ, et al: Raynaud's phenomenon of the lung. Am J Med 76: 263–269, 1984.
120. Medsger TA Jr, Masi AT: Survival with scleroderma. II. A lifetable analysis of clinical and demographic factors in 358 male U.S. veteran patients. J Chronic Dis 26: 647–660, 1973.
121. Cannon PJ, Hassar M, Case DB, et al: The relationship of hypertension and renal failure in scleroderma (progressive systemic sclerosis) to structural and functional abnormalities of the renal cortical circulation. Medicine (Baltimore) 53: 1–46, 1974.
122. Oliver JA, Cannon PJ: The kidney in scleroderma. Nephron 18: 141–150, 1977.
123. LeRoy EC, Fleischmann RM: The management of renal scleroderma: experience with dialysis, nephrectomy and transplantation. Am J Med 64: 974–978, 1978.
124. Whitman HH III, Case DB, Laragh JH, et al: Variable response to oral angiotensin-converting-enzyme blockade in hypertensive scleroderma patients. Arthritis Rheum 25: 241–248, 1982.
125. Teasdall RD, Frayha RA, Shulman LE: Cranial nerve involvement in systemic sclerosis (scleroderma): a report of 10 cases. Medicine (Baltimore) 59: 149–159, 1980.
126. Burke MJ, Carty JE: Trigeminal neuropathy as the presenting symptom of systemic sclerosis. Postgrad Med J 55: 423–425, 1979.
127. Farrell DA, Medsger TA Jr: Trigeminal neuropathy in progressive systemic sclerosis. Am J Med 73: 57–62, 1982.
128. Lee P, Bruni J, Sukenik S: Neurological manifestations in systemic sclerosis (scleroderma). J Rheumatol 11: 480–483, 1984.
129. Dahlgaard T, Nielsen VK, Kristensen JK: Vibratory perception in patients with generalized scleroderma. Acta Derm Venereol 60: 119–122, 1980.
130. Gordon RM, Silverstein A: Neurologic manifestations in progressive systemic sclerosis. Arch Neurol 22: 126–134, 1970.
131. Estey E, Lieberman A, Pinto R, et al: Cerebral arteritis in scleroderma. Stroke 10: 595–597, 1979.
132. Alarcon-Segovia D, Ibanez G, Herandez-Ortiz J, et al: Sjögren's syndrome in progressive systemic sclerosis (scleroderma). Am J Med 57: 78–85, 1974.
133. Braun-Falco O: Über das Verhalten der interfibrillaren Grundsubstanz bei Sklerodermie. Dermatol Wochenschr 136: 1085, 1957. Cited by Rodnan GP: Progressive systemic sclerosis: clinical features and pathogenesis of cutaneous involvement (scleroderma). Clin Rheumat Dis 5: 49, 1979.
134. Fleischmajer R, Perlish JS, West WP: Ultrastructure of cutaneous cellular infiltrates in scleroderma. Arch Dermatol 113: 1661–1666, 1977.
135. Fleischmajer R., Perlish JS, Reeves JR: Cellular infiltrates in scleroderma skin. Arthritis Rheum 20: 975–984, 1977.
136. Claman HN: Mast cells and fibrosis. Rheum Dis Clin North Am 16: 141–151, 1990.
137. Rodnan GP, Lipinski E, Luksick J: Skin thickness and collagen content in progressive systemic sclerosis and localized scleroderma. Arthritis Rheum 22: 130–140, 1979.
138. Hayes RL, Rodnan GP: The ultrastructure of skin in progressive systemic sclerosis (scleroderma). I. Dermal collagen fibers. Am J Pathol 63: 433–442, 1971.
139. Kondo H, Rabin BS, Rodnan GP: Cutaneous antigen-stimulating lymphokine production by lymphocytes of patients with progressive systemic sclerosis (scleroderma). J Clin Invest 58: 1388–1394, 1976.
140. Rodnan GP, Medsger TA Jr: Musculoskeletal involvement in progressive systemic sclerosis (scleroderma). Bull Rheum Dis 17: 419, 1966.
141. Clark JA, Winkelmann RK, Ward LE: Serologic alterations in scleroderma and sclerodermatomyositis. Mayo Clin Proc 46: 104–107, 1971.
142. Medsger TA Jr, Rodnan GP, Moossy J, et al: Skeletal muscle involvement in progressive systemic sclerosis (scleroderma). Arthritis Rheum 11: 554–568, 1968.
143. Lindamood M, Mills D, Steigerwald J: Skeletal muscle abnormalities in progressive systemic sclerosis. Arthritis Rheum 19: 807, 1976.
144. Norton WL, Hurd ER, Lewis DC, et al: Evidence of microvascular injury in scleroderma and systemic lupus erythematosus: quantitative study of the microvascular bed. J Lab Clin Med 71: 919–933, 1968.
145. Russell ML, Friesen D, Henderson RD, et al: Ultrastructure of the esophagus in scleroderma. Arthritis Rheum 25: 1117–1123, 1982.
146. Treacy WL, Baggenstoss AJH, Slocomb CH, et al: Scleroderma of the esophagus. A correlation of histologic and physiologic findings. Ann Intern Med 59: 351, 1963.
147. Meszaroso WT: The colon in systemic sclerosis (scleroderma). Am J Roentgenol 82: 1000, 1959.
148. Bulkley BH: Progressive systemic sclerosis: Cardiac involvement. Clin Rheumat Dis 5: 131, 1979.
149. Smith JW, Clements PJ, Levisman J, et al: Echocardiographic features of progressive systemic sclerosis (PSS). Correlation with hemodynamic and postmortem studies. Am J Med 66: 28–33, 1979.
150. Sackner MA, Heinz ER, Steinberg AJ: The heart in scleroderma. Am J Cardiol 17: 542–559, 1966.
151. Getzowa S: Cystic and compact pulmonary sclerosis in progressive scleroderma. Arch Pathol 40: 99, 1945.
152. Young RH, Mark GJ: Pulmonary vascular changes in scleroderma. Am J Med 64: 998–1004, 1978.
153. Fisher ER, Rodnan GP: Pathologic observations concerning the kidney in progressive systemic sclerosis. Arch Pathol 65: 29, 1958.
154. Sinclair RA, Antonovych TT, Mostofi FK: Renal proliferative arteriopathies and associated glomerular changes: a light and electron microscopic study. Hum Pathol 7: 565–588, 1976.
155. Jarmolych JJ, Daoud AS, Landau J, et al: Aortic media explants. Cell proliferation and production of mucopolysaccharides, collagen and elastic tissue. Exp Mol Pathol 9: 171–188, 1968.

156. Lapenas D, Rodnan GP, Cavallo T: Immunopathology of the renal vascular lesion of progressive systemic sclerosis (scleroderma). Am J Pathol 91:243–258, 1978.
157. Gerber MA: Immunohistochemical findings in the renal vascular lesions of progressive systemic sclerosis. Hum Pathol 6: 343–347, 1975.
158. McGivern AR, DeBoer WG, Barnett AJ: Renal immune deposits in scleroderma. Pathology 3: 145–150, 1971.
159. Subcommittee for Scleroderma Criteria of the American Rheumatism Association Diagnostic and Therapeutic Criteria Committee: Preliminary criteria for the classification of systemic sclerosis (scleroderma). Arthritis Rheum 23: 581–590, 1980.
160. Furst DE, Clements PJ, Graze P, et al: A syndrome resembling progressive systemic sclerosis after bone marrow transplantation. A model for scleroderma? Arthritis Rheum 22: 904–910, 1979.
161. Chosidow O, Bagot M, Vernant JP, et al: Sclerodermatous chronic graft-versus-host disease. Analysis of seven cases. J Am Acad Dermatol 26: 49–55, 1992.
162. Clements PJ, Furst DE, Ho W, et al: Progressive systemic sclerosis-like disease following bone marrow transplantation. *In* Black CM, Myers AR (eds): Systemic Sclerosis (Scleroderma). New York, Gower Medical, 1985, pp 376–381.
163. Owens GR, Medsger TA: Systemic sclerosis secondary to occupational exposure. Am J Med 85: 114–116, 1988.
164. Selikoff IJ, Hammond EC: Toxicity of vinyl chloride polyvinyl chloride. Ann N Y Acad Sci 246: 1, 1975.
165. Lelbach WK, Marsteller HJ: Vinyl chloride associated disease. Ergeb Inn Med Kinderheilkd 47: 1–110, 1981.
166. Cohen IS, Mosher M, O'Keefe EJ, et al: Cutaneous toxicity of bleomycin therapy. Arch Dermatol 107: 553–555, 1973.
167. Luna MA, Bedrossian CW, Lichtiger B, et al: Interstitial pneumonitis associated with bleomycin therapy. Am J Clin Pathol 58: 501–510, 1972.
168. Finch WR, Buckingham RB, Rodnan GP, et al: Scleroderma induced by bleomycin. *In* Black CM, Myers AR (eds): Systemic Sclerosis (Scleroderma). New York, Gower Medical, 1985, pp 114–121.
169. Palestine RF, Millns JL, Sigel GT, et al: Skin manifestations of pentazocine abuse. J Am Acad Dermatol 2: 47–55, 1980.
170. Alonso-Ruiz A, Zea-Mendoza AC, Salazar-Vallinas JM, et al: Toxic oil syndrome: a syndrome with features overlapping those of various forms of scleroderma. Semin Arthritis Rheum 15: 200–212, 1986.
171. Kilbourne EM, Rigau-Perez JG, Heath CW Jr, et al: Clinical epidemiology of toxic-oil syndrome. Manifestations of a new illness. N Engl J Med 309: 1408–1414, 1983.
172. Abaitua Borda I, Philen RM, Posada de la Paz M, et al: Toxic oil syndrome mortality: the first 13 years. Int J Epidemiol 27: 1057–1063, 1998.
173. Diaz-Perez JL, Zubizarreta J, Gardeazabal J, et al: Familial eosinophilic fascitis induced by toxic oil. Med Cut Ibero Lat Am 16: 51–58, 1988.
174. Izquierdo M, Mateo I, Rodrigo M, et al: Chronic juvenile toxic epidemic syndrome. Ann Rheum Dis 44: 98–103, 1985.
175. Miyjoshi K, Shiragami H, Yoshida K: Adjuvant disease of man. Clin Immunol (Tokyo) 5: 785, 1973.
176. Kumagai Y, Shiokawa Y, Medsger TA Jr, et al: Clinical spectrum of connective tissue disease after cosmetic surgery. Observations on eighteen patients and a review of the Japanese literature. Arthritis Rheum 27: 1–12, 1984.
177. Santavirta S, Konttinen YT, Bergroth V, et al: Aggressive granulomatous lesions associated with hip arthroplasty. J Bone Joint Surg Am 72: 252–258, 1990.
178. Bridges AJ, Conley C, Wang G, et al: A clinical and immunologic evaluation of women with silicone breast implants and symptoms of rheumatic disease. Ann Intern Med 118: 929–936, 1993.
179. Germain BF: Silicone breast implants and rheumatic disease. Bull Rheum Dis 41: 1–5, 1991.
180. Bridges AJ, Vasey FB: Silicone breast implants. History, safety, and potential complications. Arch Intern Med 153: 2638–2644, 1993.
180a. Wolfe F: "Silicone related symptoms" are common in patients with fibromyalgia: no evidence for a new disease. J Rheumatol 26: 1172–1175, 1999.
180b. Wolfe F, Anderson J: Silicone filled breast implants and the risk of fibromyalgia and rheumatoid arthritis. J Rheumatol 26: 2025–2028, 1999.
181. Kornreich HK, Shaw KN, Koch R, et al: Phenylketonuria and scleroderma. J Pediatr 73: 571–575, 1968.
182. Lasser AE, Schultz BC, Beaff D, et al: Phenylketonuria and scleroderma. Arch Dermatol 114: 1215–1217, 1978.
183. Coskun T, Ozalp I, Kale G, et al: Scleroderma-like skin lesions in two patients with phenylketonuria. Eur J Pediatr 150: 109–110, 1990.
184. Nova MP, Kaufman M, Halperin A: Scleroderma-like skin lesions in a child with phenylketonuria: a clinicopathologic correlation and review of the literature. J Am Acad Dermatol 26: 329–333, 1992.
185. Drummond KN, Michael AF, Good RA: Tryptophan metabolism in a patient with phenylketonuria and scleroderma: a proposed explanation of the indole defect in phenylketonuria. Can Med Assoc J 94: 834–838, 1966.
186. Nishimura N, Okamtoto M, Yasui M, et al: Intermediary metabolism of phenylalanine and tyrosine in diffuse collagen diseases. II: Influences on the low phenylalanine and tyrosine diet upon patients with collagen diseases. Arch Dermatol 80: 466, 1959.
187. Vilee DB, Nichols G Jr, Talbot NB: Metabolic studies in two boys with classical progeria. Pediatrics 43: 207–216, 1969.
188. Fleischmajer R, Pollock JL: Progressive systemic sclerosis: pseudoscleroderma. Clin Rheumat Dis 5: 243, 1979.
189. Epstein CJ, Martin GM, Schultz AL, et al: Werner's syndrome. A review of its symptomatology, natural history, pathologic features, genetics and relationship to the natural aging process. Medicine (Baltimore) 45: 177–221, 1966.
190. Bauer EA, Uitto J, Tan EM, et al: Werner's syndrome. Evidence for preferential regional expression of a generalized mesenchymal cell defect. Arch Dermatol 124: 90–101, 1988.
191. Rocco VK, Hurd ER: Scleroderma and scleroderma-like disorders. Semin Arthritis Rheum 16: 22–69, 1986.
192. Falanga V: Fibrosing conditions in childhood. Adv Dermatol 6: 145–158, 1991.
193. Rosenberg HS, Stenbeck WA, Spjut HJ: The fibromatoses of infancy and childhood. Perspect Pediatr Pathol 4: 269–348, 1978.
194. Young EM Jr, Barr RJ: Sclerosing dermatoses. J Cutan Pathol 12: 426–441, 1985.
195. Datubo-Brown DD: Keloids: a review of the literature. Br J Plast Surg 43: 70–77, 1990.
196. Higgins PM, Aberm GM: Idiopathic retroperitoneal fibrosis—an update. Dig Dis 8: 206–222, 1990.
197. Ormond JK: Idiopathic retroperitoneal fibrosis: a discussion of the etiology. J Urol 94: 385–390, 1965.
198. Marshall AJ, Baddeley M, Barritt DW, et al: Practolol peritonitis. A study of 16 cases and a survey of small bowel function in patients taking beta-adrenergic blockers. Q J Med 46: 135–149, 1977.
199. Stout AP: The fibromatoses. Clin Orthop 19: 11, 1961.
200. Allen PW: The fibromatoses: A clinicopathologic classification based on 140 cases. Am J Surg Pathol 1: 255–270, 1977.
201. Enzinger FM, Weiss SW: Soft Tissue Tumors. St. Louis, CV Mosby, 1983.
202. Jennings TA, Duray PH, Collins FS, et al: Infantile myofibromatosis. Evidence for an autosomal dominant disorder. Am J Surg Pathol 8: 529–538, 1984.
202a. Jablonska S, Blaszczyk M: Scleroderma-like indurations involving fascias: an abortive form of congenital fascial dystrophy (stiff skin syndrome). Pediatr Dermatol 17: 105–110, 2000.
203. Hajdu SI: Pathology of Soft Tissues Tumors. Philadelphia, Lea & Febiger, 1979.
204. Gelberman RH, Amiel D, Rudolph RM, et al: Dupuytren's contracture. An electron microscopic, biochemical, and clinical correlative study. J Bone Joint Surg Am 62: 425–432, 1980.
205. Layman CW, Peterson WC Jr: Lipogranulomatosis subcutanea (Rothmann-Makai). Arch Dermatol 90: 288, 1964.
206. Helfrich DJ, Walker ER, Martinez AJ, et al: Scleromyxedema myopathy: case report and review of the literature. Arthritis Rheum 31: 1437–1441, 1988.
207. Greenberg LM, Geppert C, Worthen HG, et al: Scleredema "adultorum" in children. Pediatrics 32: 1044, 1963.

208. Vanencie PY, Powell FC, Su WP, et al: Scleroderma: a review of thirty-three cases. J Am Acad Dermatol 11: 128–134, 1984.
209. Doyle JA, Friedman SJ: Porphyria and scleroderma: a clinical and laboratory review of 12 patients. Aust J Dermatol 24: 109–114, 1983.
210. Grossman ME, Bickers DR, Poh-Fitzpatrick MB, et al: Porphyria cutanea tarda. Clinical features and laboratory findings in 40 patients. Am J Med 67: 277–286, 1979.
211. Grgic A, Rosenbloom AL, Weber FT, et al: Joint contracture—common manifestation of childhood diabetes mellitus. J Pediatr 88: 584–588, 1976.
212. Frayha RA, Shulman LE, Stevens MB: Hematological abnormalities in scleroderma. A study of 180 cases. Acta Haematol 64: 25–30, 1980.
213. Doig A, Girdwood RM: The absorption of folic acid and labeled cyanocobalamine in intestinal malabsorption with observations on the fecal excretion of fat nitrogen and the absorption of glucose and xylose. Q J Med 29: 333, 1960.
214. Salyer WR, Salyer DC, Heptinstall RH: Scleroderma and microangiopathic hemolytic anemia. Ann Intern Med 78: 895–897, 1973.
215. Rosenthal DS, Sack B: Autoimmune hemolytic anemia in scleroderma. JAMA 216: 2011–2012, 1971.
216. Doyle JA, Connolly SM, Hoagland HC: Hematologic disease in scleroderma syndromes. Acta Derm Venereol 65: 521–525, 1985.
217. Giordano M, Ara M, Valentini G, et al: Presence of eosinophilia in progressive systemic sclerosis and localized scleroderma. Arch Dermatol Res 271: 411–417, 1981.
218. Gladman DD, Gordon DA, Urowitz MB, et al: Pericardial fluid analysis in scleroderma (systemic sclerosis). Am J Med 60: 1064–1068, 1976.
219. Burgos-Vargas R, Martinez-Cordero E, Reyes PA, et al: Antibody pattern and other criteria for diagnosis and classification in progressive systemic sclerosis. J Rheumatol 15: 153–154, 1988.
220. Bernstein RM, Pereira RS, Holden AJ, et al: Autoantibodies in childhood scleroderma. Ann Rheum Dis 44: 503–506, 1985.
221. Steen VD, Powell DL, Medsger TA Jr: Clinical correlations and prognosis based on serum autoantibodies in patients with systemic sclerosis. Arthritis Rheum 31: 196–203, 1988.
222. Weiner ES, Earnshaw WC, Senécal JL, et al: Clinical associations of anticentromere antibodies and antibodies to topoisomerase. 1. A study of 355 patients. Arthritis Rheum 31: 378–385, 1988.
223. Fregeau DR, Leung PS, Coppel RL, et al: Autoantibodies to mitochondria in systemic sclerosis. Frequency and characterization using recombinant cloned autoantigen. Arthritis Rheum 31: 386–392, 1988.
224. Oddis CV, Okano Y, Rudert WA, et al: Serum autoantibody to the nucleolar antigen PM-Scl. Clinical and immunogenetic associations. Arthritis Rheum 35: 1211–1217, 1992.
225. Armstrong GP, Whalley GA, Doughty RN, et al: Left ventricular function in scleroderma. Br J Rheumatol 35: 983–988, 1996.
226. Ridolfi RL, Bulkley BH, Hutchins GM: The cardiac conduction system in progressive systemic sclerosis. Clinical and pathologic features of 35 patients. Am J Med 61: 361–366, 1976.
227. Clements PJ, Furst DE, Cabeen W, et al: The relationship of arrhythmias and conduction disturbances to other manifestations of cardiopulmonary disease in progressive systemic sclerosis (PSS). Am J Med 71: 38–46, 1981.
228. Alexander EL, Firestein GS, Weiss JL, et al: Reversible cold-induced abnormalities in myocardial perfusion and function in systemic sclerosis. Ann Intern Med 105: 661–668, 1986.
229. Gottdiener JS, Moutsopoulos HM, Decker JC: Echocardiographic identification of cardiac abnormality in scleroderma and related disorders. Am J Med 66: 391–398, 1979.
230. Garty BZ, Athreya BH, Wilmott R, et al: Pulmonary functions in children with progressive systemic sclerosis. Pediatrics 88: 1161–1167, 1991.
231. Falcini F, Pignone A, Matucci-Cerinic M, et al: Clinical utility of noninvasive methods in the evaluation of scleroderma lung in pediatric age. Scand J Rheumatol 21: 82–84, 1992.
232. Steen VD, Owens GR, Fino GJ, et al: Pulmonary involvement in systemic sclerosis (scleroderma). Arthritis Rheum 28: 759–767, 1985.
233. Guttadauria M, Ellman H, Kaplan D: Progressive systemic sclerosis: pulmonary involvement. Clin Rheumat Dis 5: 151, 1979.
234. Kovalchik MT, Guggenheim SJ, Silverman MH, et al: The kidney in progressive systemic sclerosis: a prospective study. Ann Intern Med 89: 881–887, 1978.
235. Lester PD, Koehler PR: The renal angiographic changes in scleroderma. Radiology 99: 517–521, 1971.
236. Scharer L, Smith DW: Resorption of the terminal phalanges in scleroderma. Arthritis Rheum 12: 51–63, 1969.
237. Szymanska-Jagiello W, Rondio H: Clinical picture of articular changes in progressive systemic sclerosis in children in the light of our own observations. Rheumatologia 8: 1–9, 1970.
238. Resnick D, Niwayama G: Scleroderma (progressive systemic sclerosis). *In* Resnick D, Niwayama G (eds): Diagnosis of Bone and Joint Disorders. Philadelphia, WB Saunders, 1988, p 1293.
239. Schlenker JD, Clark DD, Weckesser EC: Calcinosis circumscripta of the hand in scleroderma. J Bone Joint Surg Am 55: 1051–1056, 1973.
240. Resnick D, Greenway G, Vint VC: Selective involvement of the first carpometacarpal joint in scleroderma. Am J Roentgenol 131: 283–286, 1978.
241. Rowell BR, Hopper FE: The periodontal membrane in systemic sclerosis. Br J Dermatol 93(Suppl 2): 23, 1975.
242. Dinsmore RE, Goodman D, Dreyfus JR: The air esophagram: a sign of scleroderma involving the esophagus. Radiology 87: 348–349, 1966.
243. Martel W, Chang SF, Abell MR: Loss of colonic haustration in progressive systemic sclerosis. Am J Roentgenol 126: 704–713, 1976.
244. Seely JM, Jones LT, Wallace C, et al: Systemic sclerosis: using high-resolution CT to detect lung disease in children. Am J Roentgenol 170: 691–697, 1998.
245. Schaller JG: Therapy for childhood rheumatic diseases. Have we been doing enough? Arthritis Rheum 36: 65–70, 1993.
246. Lehman TJ: Aggressive therapy for childhood rheumatic diseases. When are immunosuppressives appropriate? Arthritis Rheum 36: 71–74, 1993.
247. Bluestone R, Grahame R, Holloway V, et al: Treatment of systemic sclerosis with D-penicillamine. A new method of observing the effects of treatment. Ann Rheum Dis 29: 153–158, 1970.
248. Steen VD, Medsger TA Jr, Rodnan GP: D-Penicillamine therapy in progressive sclerosis (scleroderma). A retrospective analysis. Ann Intern Med 97: 652–659, 1982.
249. Jiminez SA, Andrews RP, Myers AR: Treatment of rapidly progressive systemic sclerosis with D-penicillamine: a prospective study. *In* Black CM, Myers AR (eds): Systemic Sclerosis (Scleroderma). New York, Gower Medical, 1985, p 387.
250. DeClerk LS, Dequeker J, Francx L, et al: D-Penicillamine therapy and interstitial lung disease in scleroderma. A long-term followup study. Arthritis Rheum 30: 643–650, 1987.
251. Medsger TA Jr: D-Penicillamine treatment of lung involvement in patients with systemic sclerosis (scleroderma). Arthritis Rheum 30: 832–834, 1987.
252. Ohta A, Uitto J: Procollagen gene expression by scleroderma fibroblasts in culture. Inhibition of collagen production and reduction of pro alpha 1 (I) and pro alpha 1 (III) collagen messenger RNA steady-state levels by retinoids. Arthritis Rheum 30: 404–411, 1987.
252a. Mizutani H, Yoshida T, Nouchi N, et al: Topical tocoretinate improved hypertrophic scar, skin sclerosis in systemic sclerosis and morphea. J Dermatol 26: 11–17, 1999.
253. Uhlmann A, Brauninger W: [Therapeutic results with the aromatic retinoid (Tigason) in Sharp syndrome and progressive scleroderma]. Z Hautkr 60: 774–782, 1985.
254. Steigerwald JC: Colchicine vs. placebo in the treatment of progressive systemic sclerosis. *In* Black CM, Myers AR (eds): Systemic Sclerosis (Scleroderma). New York, Gower Medical, 1985, p 415.
255. Alarcon-Segovia D, Ramos-Niembro F, Ibanez de Kasep G, et al: Long-term evaluation of colchicine in the treatment of scleroderma. J Rheumatol 6: 705–712, 1979.
256. Steigerwald JC: Progressive systemic sclerosis: management. III: Immunosuppressive agents. Clin Rheumat Dis 5: 289, 1979.
257. Steigerwald JC: Chlorambucil in the treatment of progressive systemic sclerosis. *In* Black CM, Myers AR (eds): Systemic Sclerosis (Scleroderma). New York, Gower Medical, 1985, p 423.
258. Furst DE, Clements PJ, Hillis S, et al: Immunosuppression with

chlorambucil, versus placebo, for scleroderma. Results of a three-year, parallel, randomized, double-blind study. Arthritis Rheum 32: 584–593, 1989.

259. Bode BY, Yocum DE, Gall EP, et al: Methotrexate in scleroderma: experience in ten patients. Arthritis Rheum 33: S66, 1990.

260. Clements PJ, Paulus HE, Sterz M, et al: A preliminary report of cyclosporin A in systemic sclerosis. Arthritis Rheum 33: S66, 1990.

260a. Filaci G, Cutolo M, Scudeletti M, et al: Cyclosporin A and iloprost treatment of systemic sclerosis: clinical results and interleukin-6 serum changes after 12 months of therapy. Rheumatology (Oxford) 38: 992–996, 1999.

261. Gruber BL, Kaufman LD: A double-blind randomized controlled trial of ketotifen versus placebo in early diffuse scleroderma. Arthritis Rheum 34: 362–366, 1991.

262. Weiner SR, Kono DH, Osterman HA, et al: Preliminary report on a controlled trial of apheresis in the treatment of scleroderma. Arthritis Rheum 30: S27, 1987.

263. Rook AH, Freundlich B, Jegasothy BV, et al: Treatment of systemic sclerosis with extracorporeal photochemotherapy. Results of a multicenter trial. Arch Dermatol 128: 337–346, 1992.

263a. Seibold JR, Korn JH, Simms R, et al: Recombinant human relaxin in the treatment of scleroderma. A randomized, double-blind, placebo-controlled trial. Ann Intern Med 132: 871–879, 2000.

263b. Black CM, Silman AJ, Herrick AI, et al: Interferon-alpha does not improve outcome at one year in patients with diffuse cutaneous scleroderma: results of a randomized, double-blind, placebo-controlled trial. Arthritis Rheum 42: 299–305, 1999.

264. Martini A, Maccario R, Ravelli A, et al: Marked and sustained improvement two years after autologous stem cell transplantation in a girl with systemic sclerosis. Arthritis Rheum 42: 807–811, 1999.

264a. Locatelli F, Perotti C, Torretta L, et al: Mobilization and selection of peripheral blood hematopoietic progenitors in children with systemic sclerosis. Haematologica 84: 839–843, 1999.

265. Hansteen V, Lorentsen E: Vasodilator drugs in the treatment of peripheral arterial insufficiency. Acta Med Scand 556(Suppl): 3–62, 1974.

266. Coffman JD: Drug therapy: vasodilator drugs in peripheral vascular disease. N Engl J Med 300: 713–717, 1979.

267. McFadyen IJ, Housley E, MacPherson AI: Intraarterial reserpine administration in Raynaud syndrome. Arch Intern Med 132: 526–528, 1973.

268. Kontos HA, Wasserman AJ: Effect of reserpine in Raynaud's phenomenon. Circulation 39: 259–266, 1969.

269. Varadi DP, Lawrence AM: Suppression of Raynaud's phenomenon by methyldopa. Arch Intern Med 124: 13–18, 1969.

270. Miyazaki S, Miura K, Kasai Y, et al: Relief from digital vasospasm by treatment with captopril and its complete inhibition by serine proteinase inhibitor in Raynaud's phenomenon. Br Med J (Clin Res Ed) 284: 310–311, 1982.

271. Seibold JR, Jageneau AH: Treatment of Raynaud's phenomenon with ketanserin, a selective antagonist of the serotonin 2 (5-HT2) receptor. Arthritis Rheum 27: 139–146, 1984.

272. Coffman JD, Clement DL, Creager MA, et al: International study of ketanserin in Raynaud's phenomenon. Am J Med 87: 264–268, 1989.

273. Naidoo P: Griseofulvin in Raynaud's phenomenon. Lancet 2: 1090, 1971.

274. Giordano M, Ara M, Capelli L, et al: Griseofulvin in scleroderma. *In* Black CM, Myers AR (eds): Systemic Sclerosis (Scleroderma). New York, Gower Medical, 1985, pp 446–448.

275. Drake DB, Kesler RW, Morgan RF: Digital sympathectomy for refractory Raynaud's phenomenon in an adolescent. J Rheumatol 19: 1286–1288, 1992.

276. Martin MF, Dowd PM, Ring EF, et al: Prostaglandin E1 infusions for vascular insufficiency in progressive systemic sclerosis. Ann Rheum Dis 40: 350–354, 1981.

277. Belch JJ, McArdle B, McKay A, et al: Epoprostenol (prostacyclin) and severe arterial disease. A double blind trial. Lancet 1: 315–317, 1983.

277a. Vayssairat M: Preventive effect of an oral prostacyclin analog, beraprost sodium, on digital necrosis in systemic sclerosis. French Microcirculation Society Multicenter Group for the Study of Vascular Acrosyndromes. J Rheumatol 26: 2173–2178, 1999.

278. Wigley FM, Korn JH, Csuka ME, et al: Oral iloprost treatment in patients with Raynaud's phenomenon secondary to systemic sclerosis: a multicenter, placebo-controlled, double-blind study. Arthritis Rheum 41: 670–677, 1998.

279. Smith CD, McKendry RJ: Controlled trial of nifedipine in the treatment of Raynaud's phenomenon. Lancet 2: 1299–1301, 1982.

280. Rodeheffer RJ, Rommer JA, Wigley F, et al: Controlled double-blind trial of nifedipine in the treatment of Raynaud's phenomenon. N Engl J Med 308: 880–883, 1983.

281. Sauza J, Kraus A, González-Amaro R, et al: Effect of the calcium channel blocker nifedipine on Raynaud's phenomenon. A controlled double blind trial. J Rheumatol 11: 362–364, 1984.

282. Winston EL, Pariser KM, Miller KB, et al: Nifedipine as a therapeutic modality for Raynaud's phenomenon. Arthritis Rheum 26: 1177–1180, 1983.

283. Gifford RW Jr: The arteriospastic diseases: clinical significance and management. Cardiovasc Clin 3: 127–139, 1971.

284. Russell IJ, Lessard JA: Prazosin treatment of Raynaud's phenomenon: a double blind single crossover study. J Rheumatol 12: 94–98, 1985.

285. Coppock JS, Hardman JM, Bacon PA, et al: Objective relief of vasospasm by glyceryl trinitrate in secondary Raynaud's phenomenon. Postgrad Med J 62: 15–18, 1986.

286. Kleckner MS, Allen EV, Wakim WG: The effect of local application of glyceryl trinitrate (nitroglycerine) on Raynaud's disease and Raynaud's phenomenon. Circulation 3: 684, 1951.

287. Talpos G, Horrocks M, White JM, et al: Plasmapheresis in Raynaud's disease. Lancet 1: 416–417, 1978.

288. Winkelmann RK, McCune MA, Pineda AA, et al: A controlled study of plasma exchange in scleroderma. *In* Black CM, Myers AR (eds): Systemic Sclerosis (Scleroderma). New York, Gower Medical, 1985, pp 449–453.

289. Surwitt RS: Biofeedback: a possible treatment for Raynaud's disease. Semin Psychiatry 5: 483–490, 1973.

290. Beckett VL, Donadio JV Jr, Brennan LA Jr, et al: Use of captopril as early therapy for renal scleroderma: a prospective study. Mayo Clin Proc 60: 763–771, 1985.

291. Whitman HH III, Case DB, LeRoy EC: Management of hypertensive scleroderma patients with converting-enzyme inhibition. *In* Black CM, Myers AR (eds): Systemic Sclerosis (Scleroderma). New York, Gower Medical, 1985, p 428.

292. Steen VD, Costantino JP, Shapiro AP, et al: Outcome of renal crisis in systemic sclerosis: relation to availability of angiotensin converting enzyme (ACE) inhibitors. Ann Intern Med 113: 352–357, 1990.

293. Richardson JA: Hemodialysis and kidney transplantation for renal failure from scleroderma. Arthritis Rheum 16: 265–271, 1973.

293a. Foeldvari I, Zhavania M, Birdi N, et al: Favourable outcome in 135 children with juvenile systemic sclerosis: results of a multi-national survey. Rheumatology (Oxford) 39: 556–559, 2000.

294. Jacobsen S, Halberg P, Ullman S: Mortality and causes of death of 344 Danish patients with systemic sclerosis (scleroderma). Br J Rheumatol 37: 750–755, 1998.

295. Hochberg MC, Lopez-Acuna D, Gittelsohn AM: Mortality from systemic sclerosis (scleroderma) in the United States, 1969–1977. *In* Black CM, Myers AR (eds): Systemic Sclerosis (Scleroderma). New York, Gower Medical, 1985, pp 61–69.

296. Bulkley BH, Ridolfi RL, Salyer WR, et al: Myocardial lesions of progressive systemic sclerosis. A cause of cardiac dysfunction. Circulation 53: 483–490, 1976.

297. Silman AJ: Pregnancy and scleroderma. Am J Reprod Immunol 28: 238–240, 1992.

297a. Buyon JP: The effects of pregnancy on autoimmune diseases. J Leukoc Biol 63: 281–287, 1998.

298. Bulpitt KJ, Clements PJ, Lachenbruch PA, et al: Early undifferentiated connective tissue disease: III. Outcome and prognostic indicators in early scleroderma (systemic sclerosis). Ann Intern Med 118: 602–609, 1993.

298a. Simeon CP, Armadans L, Fonollosa V, et al: Survival prognostic factors and markers of morbidity in Spanish patients with systemic sclerosis. Ann Rheum Dis 56: 723–728, 1997.

299. Fritzler MJ, Kinsella TD: The CREST syndrome: a distinct sero-

logic entity with anticentromere antibodies. Am J Med 69: 520–526, 1980.
300. Thibierge G, Wiessenbach RJ: Concretions calcaires souscutanees et sclerodermie. Ann Dermatol Syph 2: 129, 1911.
301. Winterbauer RH: Multiple telangiectasia, Raynaud's phenomenon, sclerodactyly and subcutaneous calcinosis: a syndrome mimicking hereditary hemorrhagic telangiectasia. Bull Johns Hopkins Hosp 114: 361, 1964.
302. Rodnan GP, Jablonska S: Classification of systemic and localized scleroderma. *In* Black CM, Myers AR (eds): Systemic Sclerosis (Scleroderma). New York, Gower Medical, 1985, pp 3–6.
303. Tan EM, Rodnan GP, Garcia I, et al: Diversity of antinuclear antibodies in progressive systemic sclerosis. Anti-centromere antibody and its relationship to CREST syndrome. Arthritis Rheum 23: 617–625, 1980.
304. Powell FC, Winkelmann RK, Venencie-Lemarchand F, et al: The anticentromere antibody: disease specificity and clinical significance. Mayo Clin Proc 59: 700–706, 1984.
305. Furst DE, Clements PJ, Saab M, et al: Clinical and serological comparison of 17 chronic progressive systemic sclerosis (PSS) and 17 CREST syndrome patients matched for sex, age and disease duration. Ann Rheum Dis 43: 794–801, 1984.

22

Localized Sclerodermas

Audrey M. Nelson

The unifying characteristic of all of the types of scleroderma is an abnormal accumulation of collagen in the tissues.[1, 2] The localized sclerodermas are a group of disorders that are for the most part benign and self-limited, with manifestations confined to the skin and subdermal tissues. They are rare conditions even in childhood, when *linear scleroderma* is more common. The term *morphea* is applied to many of the types of localized scleroderma and, in general, may be preferred because the word scleroderma often leads to consideration of only the ominous consequences of systemic scleroderma.

DEFINITION AND CLASSIFICATION

Localized scleroderma includes a number of conditions that are often grouped together, and therefore the individual syndromes may seem ill defined. Commonly, localized scleroderma has been divided into three groups: (1) morphea, (2) generalized morphea, and (3) linear scleroderma.[3–5] Eosinophilic fasciitis, which was originally considered to be a separate syndrome, may also be classified among the subtypes of localized scleroderma/morphea. Peterson and colleagues[6] have proposed a revised expanded classification that divides localized scleroderma/morphea into five general groups: plaque morphea, generalized morphea, bullous morphea, linear morphea, and deep morphea (Table 22–1).

Table 22–1

Classification of Morphea

Classification
Plaque morphea
Morphea en plaque
Guttate morphea
Atrophoderma of Pasini and Pierini
Keloid morphea (nodular morphea)
[Lichen sclerosus et atrophicus]*
Generalized morphea
Bullous morphea
Linear morphea
Linear morphea (linear scleroderma)
En coup de sabre scleroderma
Progressive hemifacial atrophy
Deep morphea
Subcutaneous morphea
Eosinophilic fasciitis
Morphea profunda
Disabling pansclerotic morphea of childern

*The entry in brackets is not universally accepted.

From Peterson LS, Nelson AM, Su WPD: Classification of morphea (localized scleroderma). Mayo Clin Proc 70: 1068–1076, 1995.

Plaque Morphea

Plaque morphea is the most common and benign form of the morphea syndromes. It is confined to the dermis with only occasional involvement of the superficial panniculus. Subtypes of plaque morphea include morphea en plaque, guttate morphea, atrophoderma of Pasini and Pierini, keloid morphea, and sometimes lichen sclerosus et atrophicus.

Morphea en plaque is the most common subtype and is characterized by the insidious onset of an oval or round circumscribed area of induration with a waxy, ivory color in the center surrounded by a violaceous halo (Fig. 22–1). The plaques are typically several centimeters in diameter and evolve from an erythematous inflammatory stage through a sclerotic indurated phase with surrounding inflammation, and subsequently to softening and dermal atrophy with associated hypopigmentation or hyperpigmentation. These lesions occur most frequently on the trunk and less often on the extremities. The face is usually spared.

Guttate morphea is much less common. These lesions are small, oval areas less than 1 cm in diameter. *Atrophoderma of Pasini and Pierini* is characterized by asymptomatic hyperpigmented atrophic patches with well-demarcated, so-called cliff-drop borders on the trunk. These lesions lack the typical inflammatory changes seen in plaque morphea.

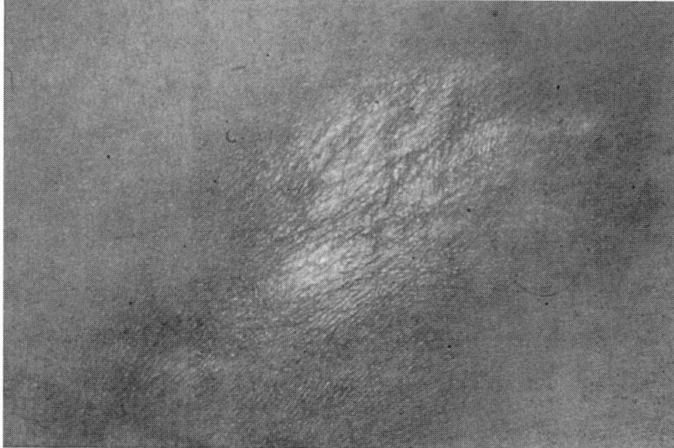

Figure 22–1. Morphea en plaque lesion characterized by a central area of induration with waxy, ivory color surrounded by inflammation and hyperpigmentation.

Generalized Morphea

The term *generalized morphea* is applied when individual plaques of morphea become confluent or multiply and affect more than two anatomic sites.

Bullous Morphea

Bullous morphea can occur with most subtypes, including typical plaque morphea and morphea profunda. The bullous lesions may possibly result from localized trauma or may be related to lymphatic obstruction secondary to the sclerodermatous process.[7, 8]

Linear Scleroderma

Linear scleroderma is the most common subtype of localized scleroderma in children and adolescents[9, 10] and is characterized by one or more linear streaks that typically involve an upper or lower extremity and may be associated with morphea plaques. The streaks become progressively more indurated and can extend through the dermis, subcutaneous tissue, and muscle to the underlying bone (Fig. 22–2*A* and *B*). The lesions frequently follow a dermatomal distribution and are unilateral in 85 to 95 percent of cases.[10, 11]

When a linear lesion involves the face or scalp, it is referred to as *en coup de sabre scleroderma* (Fig. 22–3*A* and *B*). This term was applied historically because the lesion was reminiscent of the depression caused by a dueling stroke from a sword. A number of associated disorders have been reported in such patients, including seizures, uveitis, dental abnormalities, ocular muscle dysfunction, and loss of eyebrows or eyelashes.[12–19] Progressive hemifacial atrophy is frequently a consequence of the linear lesion on the head and scalp. When hemifacial atrophy occurs without a definable lesion of en coup de sabre, the term *Parry-Romberg*

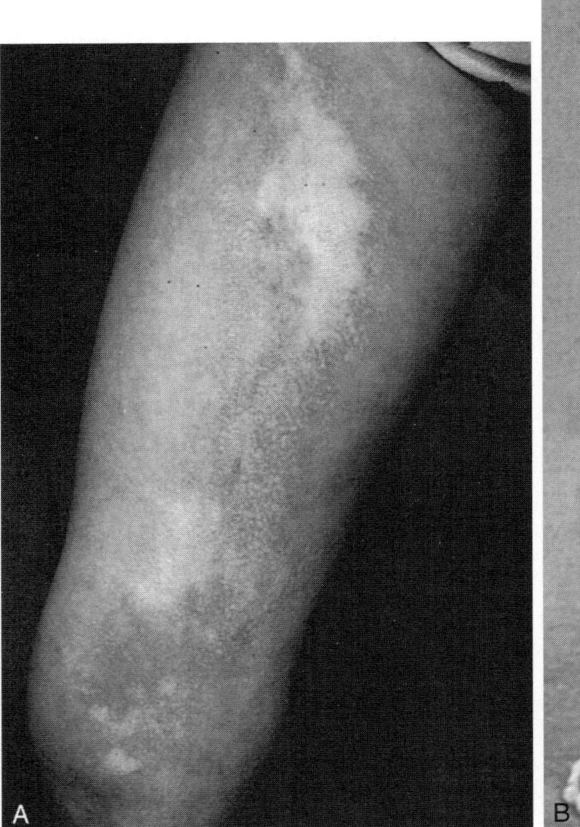

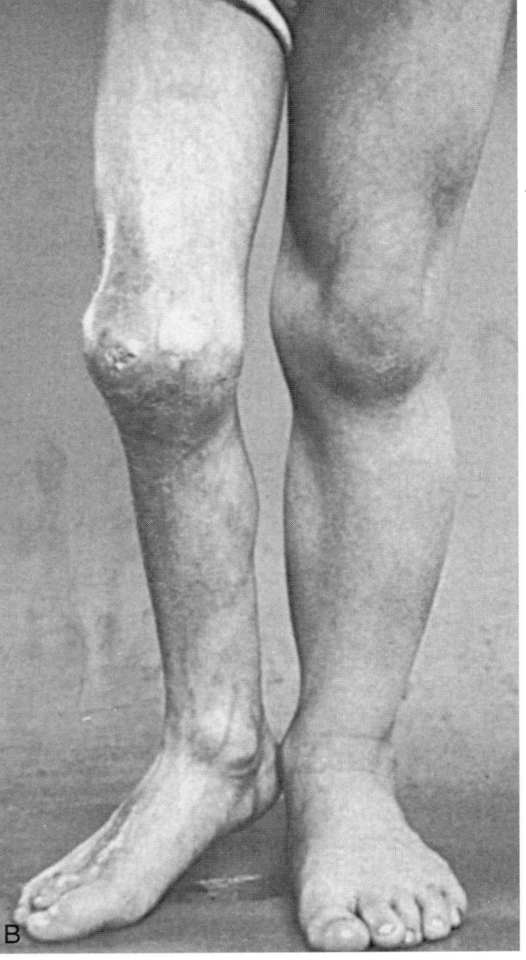

Figure 22–2. *A,* Typical lesion of linear scleroderma involving the lower extremity. The skin changes are characterized by a waxy induration with surrounding inflammation and hyperpigmentation distributed in a linear pattern. *B,* Linear scleroderma resulting in undergrowth of the leg; taut, shiny skin; and shortening of the extensor tendon to the second toe on the right foot.

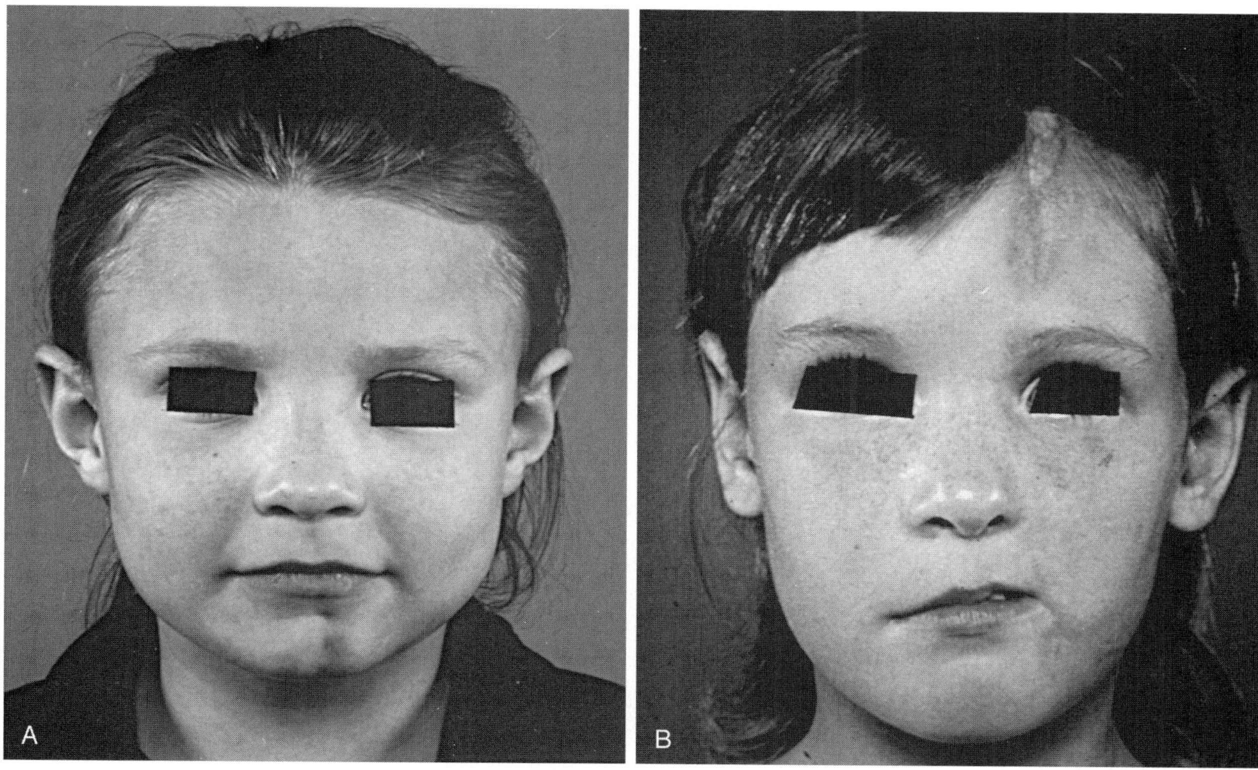

Figure 22–3. *A,* En coup de sabre linear scleroderma of approximately 2 years' duration affecting the chin just to the left of midline, resulting in a depression and mild asymmetry of the jaw. *B,* En coup de sabre linear scleroderma involving the left face with hyperpigmentation, atrophy of subcutaneous tissues, and early hemifacial atrophy.

syndrome is applied.[20] Whether this syndrome exists as a separate entity from localized scleroderma is controversial.

Deep Morphea

The subtypes of deep morphea (Fig. 22–4) are the least common but most disabling variants of the localized sclerodermas and include subcutaneous morphea, eosinophilic fasciitis, morphea profunda, and disabling pansclerotic morphea of children. In *subcutaneous morphea,* the primary site of involvement is in the panniculus or subcutaneous tissue,[21, 22] and the onset of sclerosis is often rapid over a period of several months. The plaques are hyperpigmented, symmetric, and somewhat ill defined, and the degree of inflammation is more pronounced than in the other subtypes of morphea.

In *morphea profunda,* the entire skin feels thickened, taut, and bound down, but it may be more localized to a solitary, indurated plaque that usually involves the upper torso.[23, 24] An extremely rare but severe form of localized scleroderma is *disabling pansclerotic morphea of children,* which was first described in 1980 by Diaz-Perez and colleagues.[25] This disorder typically begins before the age of 14 years and is characterized by generalized full-thickness involvement of the skin of the trunk, extremities, face, and scalp with sparing of the fingertips and toes. The course is relentlessly progressive.

Eosinophilic fasciitis was described in 1974 and 1975 by Shulman[26, 27] and by Rodnan and colleagues,[28] who termed the condition "diffuse fasciitis with eosinophilia" and noted that these patients typically had hypergammaglobulinemia and eosinophilia. The fascia is the predominant site of involvement. These lesions typically involve the extremities but spare the hands and feet and have an appearance that is described as "peau d'orange." Similar histologic changes are found in most of the subtypes of localized scleroderma, however, raising the question as to whether this is indeed a separate subtype of localized scleroderma. Frequently in the pediatric literature, eosinophilic fasciitis is described as involving the hands and feet. Some of these cases may be more consistent with subcutaneous morphea or morphea profunda than eosinophilic fasciitis. Miller[29] has described the combined syndrome of fasciitis and morphea in children and pointed out the linkage of these manifestations.

EPIDEMIOLOGY

Localized scleroderma is a rare condition but is more frequent than systemic scleroderma. Whereas systemic scleroderma is estimated to have an annual incidence between 0.45 and 1.9 per 100,000,[30, 31] the annual inci-

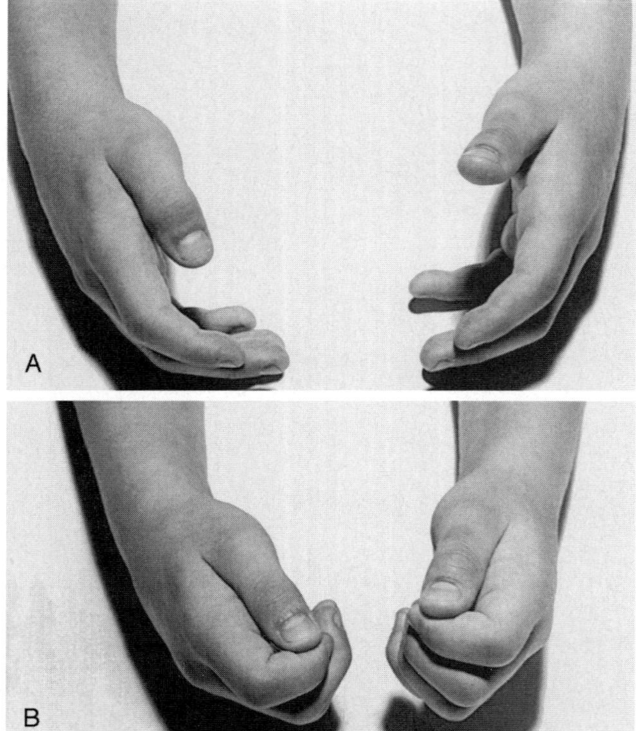

Figure 22–4. Hands of a 7-year-old boy with deep morphea, demonstrating limitation of extension *(A)* and flexion *(B)* of the fingers. (*A* and *B*, From Nelson AM: Localized scleroderma including morphea, linear scleroderma, and eosinophilic fasciitis. Curr Probl Pediatr 26: 318, 1996.)

dence of the localized sclerodermas is 2.7 per 100,000.[10] In a population-based study of localized scleroderma,[10] plaque morphea accounted for 56 percent of the cases, generalized morphea for 13 percent, linear morphea for 20 percent, and deep morphea for 11 percent. Linear and plaque morphea coexisted in 11 percent of the patients. Referral-based studies of localized scleroderma include a higher proportion of linear scleroderma.[4, 9] The female:male ratio of localized scleroderma is 2.5:1, whereas in linear scleroderma the ratio is 1:1.

Linear scleroderma is predominantly a pediatric disease. In a population-based study covering patients of all ages,[10] 67 percent of the individuals with linear scleroderma were diagnosed before the age of 18 years. The prevalence of morphea by 18 years of age was estimated to be 50 per 100,000. The mean age at onset of localized scleroderma in the pediatric population is approximately 7.9 years.[4]

Uziel and colleagues[4] examined 30 patients with localized scleroderma over a 7-year period and noted that this patient group numbered approximately the same as those with a diagnosis of juvenile dermatomyositis, and about half the number of those with systemic lupus erythematosus seen during the same time. In a review of their pediatric rheumatology practice, Levinson and Bove[32] identified 15 children with localized scleroderma, a frequency that was approximately 1 for every 20 diagnoses of juvenile rheumatoid arthritis. A recent study by Woo and colleagues[33] reported that 2 percent of the patients attending their pediatric rheumatology clinic had localized scleroderma.

ETIOLOGY AND PATHOGENESIS

The etiology and pathogenesis of the localized sclerodermas are unknown. The focus of much investigation is on abnormalities of regulation of fibroblasts and production of collagen. In morphea, the collagen fibers become thickened and hyalinized.[34] Multiple studies have demonstrated increased levels of cytokines and other molecules known to influence fibroblasts and collagen synthesis.[35] Autoimmunity, environmental factors, infection, and trauma all have shown some association with localized scleroderma. It seems certain that autoimmunity is important in etiology, given the multiplicity of abnormal antibodies that occurs in patients with localized scleroderma, as well as the association of similar cutaneous abnormalities in patients with chronic graft-versus-host disease.[36, 37]

A number of drugs and environmental toxins have been associated with scleroderma-like reactions, including chemotherapeutic agents such as bleomycin, ergot, bromocriptine, analgesics such as pentazocine, and other drugs such as carbidopa and vitamin K_1.[38] A toxin contained in some lots of L-tryptophan was incriminated in a large epidemic of a syndrome that was similar to eosinophilic fasciitis and morphea, the *eosinophilia-myalgia syndrome*.[39, 40]

Many investigations have examined a putative association of morphea and *Borrelia burgdorferi*, the spirochete that causes Lyme disease. Since this association was reported in 1985,[41] many studies have documented evidence of infection with *B. burgdorferi* in patients with morphea who live in areas endemic for Lyme disease or who have a history of tick bites[42, 43]; however, morphea patients who do not live in endemic areas have no evidence of prior exposure to *B. burgdorferi*.[44, 45] Thus, in the evaluation of patients with morphea, serologic testing for Lyme disease is not likely to be helpful per se, unless the patient has been in an endemic area.

Trauma or physical exertion has been implicated in initiation of lesions and in particular with the onset of eosinophilic fasciitis.[24, 46, 47] A recent review of childhood-onset scleroderma reported a history of trauma at the site of the lesion in 14 of 58 patients[48]; a similar history was not obtained in adult morphea patients. The authors also noted that 3 patients had developed lesions at the site of their measles, mumps, and rubella vaccination.

CLINICAL MANIFESTATIONS

The onset of localized scleroderma is subtle. The first manifestation is usually a localized area of erythema or of waxy induration with a surrounding halo of erythema. A few patients have systemic symptoms such as arthralgias, synovitis, joint contractures, and carpal tunnel syndrome.[10] Plaque morphea mainly appears on the chest, abdomen, and back, whereas generalized morphea involves extremities, chest, and back. Linear morphea affects the lower extremities more commonly than the arms, whereas the deep morphea subtypes affect both upper and lower extremities. The scalp is affected only in the en coup de sabre and Parry-Romberg forms of the disorder and in disabling pansclerotic morphea of childhood.[29]

The majority of patients with generalized or deep morphea have bilateral involvement, whereas unilateral lesions are most frequent in those with plaque and linear disease. Arthralgias and mild synovitis with contractures out of keeping with the degree of synovitis are common presentations in patients with the deep morphea subtypes. Carpal tunnel syndrome has been associated with either linear or deep morphea.[10, 49, 50] Raynaud's phenomenon has also been described, although this is rare, is usually unilateral, and occurs in patients who have extensive sclerosis of the hands and forearms.[4, 9, 21, 46, 51]

The en coup de sabre type presents with a set of unusual manifestations unique to this group, including progressive hemifacial atrophy,[52] ipsilateral uveitis, various dental abnormalities such as separation of the teeth, and involvement of the eyebrows and eyelashes.[53] Central nervous system manifestations including seizures have been reported.[54, 55]

A systematic search for internal organ involvement was conducted by Dehen and colleagues[56] who studied 76 consecutive patients with morphea with or without associated linear scleroderma. They found evidence of visceral involvement in 16 patients. This group included 7 of 41 patients tested who had esophageal abnormalities, and 9 of 53 patients who had pulmonary function abnormalities. Only 2 of the 16 patients with evidence of internal involvement had symptomatic or severe disease and 1 of these patients was determined to have had systemic sclerosis. The esophageal and pulmonary abnormalities were mild and usually asymptomatic and required no interventions. It was concluded that, unless there are symptoms suggesting abnormalities in pulmonary, gastrointestinal, or other systems, there was no need to screen patients for internal organ involvement.[10, 56]

PATHOLOGY

The histologic abnormalities of localized scleroderma and systemic scleroderma are considered by most authors to be indistinguishable. Prior to fibrosis, there may be an intense inflammatory infiltrate with lymphocytes, plasma cells, macrophages, eosinophils, and mast cells. Subsequently, there is an increase in collagen and fibroblasts that leads to increasing sclerosis. In advanced stages, the entire dermis may be replaced by compact collagen fibers.[4]

The depth of involvement is important in differentiating the various morphea subtypes (Fig. 22–5).[6] Plaque morphea is more superficial, with principal involvement in the dermis and occasionally in the panniculus, whereas linear morphea involves the dermis, subcutaneous tissue, muscle, and underlying bone. The deep morphea syndromes tend to spare the superficial dermis and involve the deep dermis, subcutaneous tissue, fascia, or superficial muscle. Eosinophilic fasciitis involves the deep subcutaneous tissues with sclerosis as well as inflammatory infiltrate while sparing the dermis.

In a recent study, Torres and colleagues[57] reviewed a total of 51 skin biopsy samples submitted to their laboratory from 1993 to 1995 with a diagnosis of scleroderma, and classified the cases into systemic scleroderma or localized scleroderma. They concluded that localized and systemic scleroderma could be differentiated by the thickness of the dermis and amount of inflammatory infiltrate, both of which were greater in localized scleroderma.

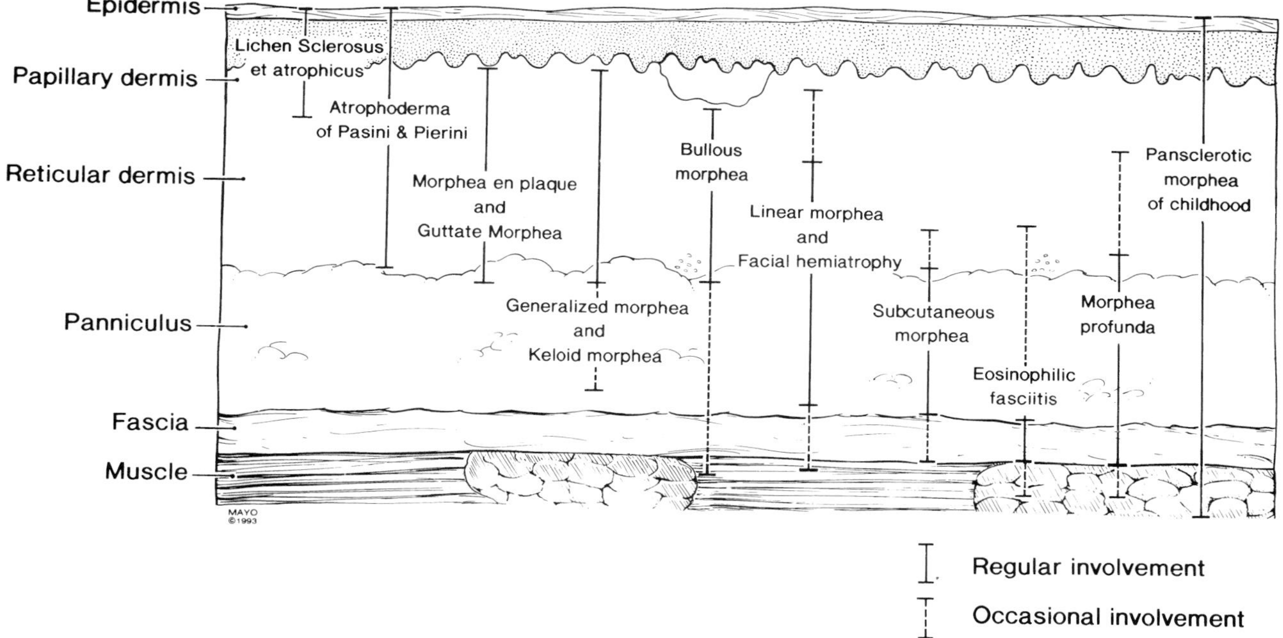

Figure 22–5. Schematic diagram of a full-thickness skin biopsy sample, demonstrating location of tissue involvement by the subtypes of localized scleroderma. (Courtesy of W. P. Daniel Su, M.D.)

DIFFERENTIAL DIAGNOSIS

The most important condition to differentiate from localized scleroderma is systemic scleroderma. The majority of the localized sclerodermas in children are linear scleroderma, in which the lesions are discrete and limited to a single extremity and easily differentiated from systemic scleroderma. The more difficult diagnostic challenge is to differentiate systemic scleroderma from the diffuse deep forms of morphea with distal involvement. These patients, in contrast to those with systemic scleroderma, rarely have Raynaud's phenomenon and do not develop symptomatic evidence of internal organ involvement. Occasionally, the deep forms of morphea may be confused with juvenile rheumatoid arthritis in that they can present with contractures of the hands, arthralgias, and sometimes synovitis and may have a positive rheumatoid factor test. In such cases, however, further testing frequently documents the presence of antinuclear antibodies, antihistone antibodies, hypergammaglobulinemia, and eosinophilia.

A number of other conditions may mimic localized scleroderma (Table 22–2).[6] In addition, morphea has been reported to coexist with systemic scleroderma. Soma and colleagues[58] observed morphea in 9 of 133 patients (6.7 percent) who presented with systemic scleroderma. They considered morphea to be a part of the skin involvement of this disease. Morphea profunda may present as localized areas of induration. In patients in whom little inflammation is apparent, the initial concern may be a localized malignancy.[27, 28] However, histologic examination of biopsy specimens easily differentiates morphea profunda from malignancy.

Table 22–2

Conditions That Mimic Morphea

- Eosinophilia-myalgia syndrome
- Graft-versus-host disease
- Agents that induce scleroderma-like diseases
  - Vinyl chloride
  - Bleomycin
  - Pentazocine
  - L-Tryptophan
- Scleredema adultorum
- Scleromyxedema
- Premature aging (Werner's syndrome)
- Poikiloderma
- Acrodermatitis chronica atrophicans
- Diabetic cheiroarthropathy
- POEMS syndrome (*p*olyneuropathy, *o*rganomegaly, *e*ndocrinopathy, *M* protein, and *s*kin changes)
- Winchester's syndrome
- Pachydermoperiostosis
- Phenylketonuria
- Localized idiopathic fibrosis
- Acromegaly
- Progeria
- Porphyria cutanea tarda
- Amyloidosis
- Carcinoid syndrome
- Connective tissue hamartomas
- Growers' panatrophy
- Connective tissue panniculitis
- Focal lipoatrophy

From Peterson LS, Nelson AM, Su WPD: Classification of morphea (localized scleroderma). Mayo Clin Proc 70: 1068–1076, 1995.

LABORATORY EXAMINATION

The diagnosis of localized scleroderma is established on clinical grounds, usually by the physical appearance of the lesions and sometimes aided by biopsy of the skin or subcutaneous tissues. Results of laboratory studies are frequently abnormal, however, raising the question of an associated systemic rheumatic disease. There is no laboratory study that is diagnostic of localized scleroderma. Results of routine laboratory tests such as a complete blood count, blood chemistries, and urinalysis are normal. The erythrocyte sedimentation rate may be increased in the subtypes of the disease with active inflammation, particularly in eosinophilic fasciitis. Eosinophilia and hypergammaglobulinemia are hallmarks of eosinophilic fasciitis but also occur in linear scleroderma and the other deep subtypes. Eosinophilia and hypergammaglobulinemia tend to be markers of active disease and normalize as the disease becomes less active.[3, 46] The serum level of immunoglobulin G is increased more often in patients with active and extensive disease and in those with joint contractures.[46] Rheumatoid factors are present in 25 to 40 percent of patients.[11, 59] The presence or absence of rheumatoid factors does not correlate significantly with any particular clinical findings, although higher titers are usually associated with more severe cutaneous and articular involvement.[46]

Antinuclear antibodies can be present in any of the morphea subtypes, with a frequency ranging from 23 to 73 percent.[4] Takehara and colleagues[60] noted positive results of antinuclear antibody tests in 50 percent of patients with morphea, 100 percent of those with generalized morphea, and 67 percent of those with linear scleroderma. They did not find antibodies to centromere, Scl-70, nuclear ribonucleoproteins, Sm, or La(SS-B) antigens in any patients with localized scleroderma. Antihistone antibodies were present in patients with more extensive localized disease.[61] Antibodies to denatured DNA were present in 56 percent of children in a study by Rosenberg and colleagues.[62] Deficiency of C2 has been described in patients with en coup de sabre lesions.[63, 64] In their review of 76 patients with morphea, Dehen and colleagues[56] noted that serum complement levels were frequently lower than normal.

Elevations of serum aldolase levels in the presence of normal concentrations of creatine kinase have been observed in patients with eosinophilic fasciitis.[50, 65, 66] These levels of enzyme activity may correlate with activity of the disease.[65] Serum concentrations of soluble interleukin-2 receptor have been noted to be increased in localized scleroderma and may differentiate active from inactive disease.[67, 68]

Magnetic resonance imaging may be helpful in delineating areas of involvement: hyperintensity of signal within the fascia on T_2-weighted images, fascial enhancement on T_1-weighted images, and resolution with clinical improvement in eosinophilic fasciitis.[69–71] Perhaps the most useful application of magnetic resonance imaging is to document evidence of central nervous system or orbital involvement.[72]

TREATMENT

No controlled trials have demonstrated effectiveness of any treatment modalities in patients with localized scleroderma. All therapy to date is based on anecdotal reports and personal experience. Decisions for management must be based on the realization that the condition is benign in the majority of patients and will often spontaneously enter remission after 3 to 5 years.[9, 10, 73, 74]

Morphea en plaque lesions generally are of cosmetic concern only, and therefore treatments with potentially significant toxicity are not justified. In general, these lesions will spontaneously remit with residual pigmentation as the only abnormality. Therefore, treatment should be directed mainly at topical therapies such as moisturizing agents or topical glucocorticoids.

There is, however, significant risk for disability in patients with linear morphea and the deep subtypes; therefore, systemic treatment should be considered.[10] If there is evidence of active disease by laboratory measures such as eosinophilia, hypergammaglobulinemia, or elevated sedimentation rate, and cutaneous evidence of inflammation such as an erythematous halo about the lesions, or rapid progression, treatment with glucocorticoids may be indicated. This is particularly true in children with eosinophilic fasciitis.[26, 74a] There is increasing anecdotal evidence that methotrexate in the range of 0.5 to 1 mg/kg per week is beneficial in morphea.[74a, 75–77] Additional agents to be considered, particularly when the disease is more indolent, include D-penicillamine[78] and hydroxychloroquine or chloroquine.[79, 80]

Therapeutic successes have been reported in the treatment of localized scleroderma with high-dose ultraviolet A_1 radiation therapy,[81] low-dose ultraviolet A_1 phototherapy,[82] and psoralen plus ultraviolet A therapy.[83] Treatment measures such as these, however, must be considered carefully, as the long-term side effects of ultraviolet A_1 and psoralen plus ultraviolet A therapy in children are not known.

Additional agents that have been utilized with anecdotal success include cimetidine,[84] the antiallergenic drug tranilast,[85] and oral calcitriol.[86] A double-blind placebo-controlled study of intralesional interferon gamma has concluded that this agent was ineffective in the treatment of localized scleroderma.[87]

Patients with significant involvement from one of the forms of localized scleroderma should have physical therapy directed at counteracting the tendency for development of flexion contractures. Surgical reconstruction may be considered, usually after the active phase of the disease has abated and the child's growth is complete.[88, 89]

COURSE OF THE DISEASE AND PROGNOSIS

In contradistinction to systemic scleroderma, the prognosis in localized scleroderma is usually benign. The course is that of an early inflammatory phase with progression to multiple or extensive lesions, then stabilization, and finally improvement with softening of the skin and increased pigmentation about the lesions. In most instances, the mean duration of activity of disease is 3 to 5 years.[9, 10, 46]

In a population-based study of localized scleroderma,[10] 50 percent of the patients had documented skin softening of 50 percent or more, or disease resolution by 3.8 years after diagnosis. The 50 percent resolution point occurred at 2.7 years in the plaque group, 5 years in the generalized and linear groups, and 5.5 years in the deep groups. A small number of patients had active disease for more than 20 years. Prolonged disease activity was associated preponderantly with the linear type. During the period of follow-up, 25 percent of the patients with linear scleroderma and 44 percent of those with deep morphea had or developed significant disability. In this series, none of the patients progressed to systemic scleroderma; however, such progression does rarely occur.[9, 47, 59]

Farrington and colleagues[66] reported on the long-term outcome of 21 pediatric patients with biopsy-proven eosinophilic fasciitis. Two-thirds of these patients developed residual cutaneous fibrosis. The authors noted that children under the age of 7 years were at two times greater risk for progression to cutaneous fibrosis than older children. All of the 14 patients who progressed to cutaneous fibrosis had involvement of three to four extremities; 6 had truncal involvement.

Therefore, localized scleroderma should be viewed as a usually benign and self-limited condition with minimal risk of progression to systemic scleroderma. The spectrum of localized scleroderma and systemic scleroderma may be likened to that of discoid lupus erythematosus and systemic lupus erythematosus. It is important to identify the subtypes at risk for disability and to intervene early with appropriate anti-inflammatory medication and physical therapy, in order to minimize the possibility of long-term disability.

References

1. Falanga V: Fibrosing conditions in childhood. Adv Dermatol 6: 145–159, 1991.
2. Doyle JA, Connolly SM, Winkelmann RK: Cutaneous and subcutaneous inflammatory sclerosis syndromes. Arch Dermatol 118: 886–890, 1982.
3. Falanga V: Localized scleroderma. Med Clin North Am 73: 1143–1156, 1989.
4. Uziel Y, Krafchik BR, Silverman ED, et al: Localized scleroderma in childhood: a report of 30 cases. Semin Arthritis Rheum 23: 328–340, 1994.
5. Schachter RK: Localized scleroderma. Curr Opin Rheumatol 1: 505–511, 1989.
6. Peterson LS, Nelson AM, Su WPD: Subspecialty clinics: rheumatology and dermatology. Classification of morphea (localized scleroderma). Mayo Clin Proc 70: 1068–1076, 1995.
7. Daoud MS, Su WP, Leiferman KM, et al: Bullous morphea: clinical, pathologic, and immunopathologic evaluation of thirteen cases. J Am Acad Dermatol 30: 937–943, 1994.
8. Su WP, Greene SL: Bullous morphea profunda. Am J Dermatopathol 8: 144–147, 1986.
9. Christianson HB, Dorsey CS, O'Leary PA, et al: Localized scleroderma: a clinical study of two hundred thirty-five cases. Arch Dermatol 74: 629–639, 1956.
10. Peterson LS, Nelson AM, Su WPD, et al: The epidemiology of morphea (localized scleroderma) in Olmsted County 1960–1993. J Rheumatol 24: 73–80, 1997.
11. Kornreich HK, King KK, Bernstein BH, et al: Scleroderma in childhood. Arthritis Rheum 20(Suppl 2): 343–350, 1977.
12. Chung MH, Sum J, Morrell MJ, et al: Intracerebral involvement

in scleroderma en coup de sabre: report of a case with neuropathologic findings. Ann Neurol 37: 679–681, 1995.
13. Goldenstein-Schainberg C, Pereira RM, Gusukuma MC, et al: Childhood linear scleroderma "en coup de sabre" with uveitis. J Pediatr 117: 581–584, 1990.
14. David J, Wilson J, Woo P: Scleroderma "en coup de sabre." Ann Rheum Dis 50: 260–262, 1991.
15. Seow WK, Young W: Localized scleroderma in childhood: review of the literature and case report. Pediatr Dent 9: 240–244, 1987.
16. Campbell WW, Bajandas FJ: Restrictive ophthalmopathy associated with linear scleroderma. J Neuroophthalmol 15: 95–97, 1995.
17. Tang RA, Mewis-Christmann L, Wolf J, et al: Pseudo-oculomotor palsy as the presenting sign of linear scleroderma. J Pediatr Ophthalmol Strabismus 23: 236–238, 1986.
18. Suttorp-Schulten MS, Koornneef L: Linear scleroderma associated with ptosis and motility disorders. Br J Ophthalmol 74: 694–695, 1990.
19. Serup J, Alsbirk PH: Localized scleroderma "en coup de sabre" and iridopalpebral atrophy at the same line. Acta Derm Venereol 63: 75–77, 1983.
20. Lewkonia RM, Lowry RB: Progressive hemifacial atrophy (Parry-Romberg syndrome): report with review of genetics and nosology. Am J Med Genet 14: 385–390, 1983.
21. Jablonska S: Localized scleroderma. *In* Jablonska S (ed): Scleroderma and Pseudoscleroderma. Warsaw, Polish Medical Publishers, 1975, pp 277–303.
22. Person JR, Su WP: Subcutaneous morphoea: a clinical study of sixteen cases. Br J Dermatol 100: 371–380, 1979.
23. Su WP, Person JR: Morphea profunda: a new concept and a histopathologic study of 23 cases. Am J Dermatopathol 3: 251–260, 1981.
24. Whittaker SJ, Smith NP, Jones RR: Solitary morphoea profunda. Br J Dermatol 120: 431–440, 1989.
25. Diaz-Perez JL, Connolly SM, Winkelmann RK: Disabling pansclerotic morphea in children. Arch Dermatol 116: 169–173, 1980.
26. Shulman LE: Diffuse fasciitis with hypergammaglobulinemia and eosinophilia: a new syndrome? J Rheumatol 1(Suppl 1):46, 1974.
27. Shulman LE: Diffuse fasciitis with eosinophilia: a new syndrome? Trans Assoc Am Physicians 88: 70–86, 1975.
28. Rodnan GP, Di Bartolomeo A, Medsgar TA Jr: Eosinophilic fasciitis. Report of six cases of a newly recognized scleroderma-like syndrome. Arthritis Rheum 18: 525, 1975.
29. Miller JJ III: The fasciitis-morphea complex in children. Am J Dis Child 146: 733–736, 1992.
30. Medsger TA Jr, Masi AT: Epidemiology of systemic sclerosis (scleroderma). Ann Intern Med 74: 714–721, 1971.
31. Mayes MD, Laing TJ, Gillespie BW, et al: Prevalence, incidence and survival rates of systemic sclerosis in the Detroit Metropolitan area. Arthritis Rheum 39: S150, 1996.
32. Levinson JE, Bove KE: Scleroderma. *In* Gershwin ME, Robbins DE (eds): Musculoskeletal Diseases of Children. Orlando, FL, Grune & Stratton, 1983, pp 195–208.
33. Woo P, David J, Vancheeswaran R, et al: Is scleroderma the same disease in childhood? Arthritis Rheum 35: S137, 1992.
34. Kahari VM, Sandberg M, Kalimo H, et al: Identification of fibroblasts responsible for increased collagen production in localized scleroderma by in situ hybridization. J Invest Dermatol 90: 664–670, 1988.
35. Liu B, Connolly MK: The pathogenesis of cutaneous fibrosis. Semin Cutan Med Surg 17: 3–11, 1998.
36. Janin A, Socie G, Devergie A, et al: Fasciitis in chronic graft-versus-host disease: a clinicopathologic study of 14 cases. Ann Intern Med 120: 993–998, 1994.
37. Aractingi S, Socie G, Devergie A: Localized scleroderma-like lesions on the legs in bone marrow transplant recipients: association with polyneuropathy in the same distribution. Br J Dermatol 129: 201–203, 1993.
38. Haustein UF, Haupt B: Drug-induced scleroderma and sclerodermiform conditions. Clin Dermatol 16: 353–366, 1998.
39. Martin RW, Duffy J, Engel AG: The clinical spectrum of the eosinophilia-myalgia syndrome associated with L-tryptophan ingestion. Clinical features in 20 patients and aspects of pathophysiology. Ann Intern Med 113: 124–134, 1990.
40. Mayeno AN, Lin F, Foote CS, et al: Characterization of "peak E," a novel amino acid associated with eosinophilia-myalgia syndrome. Science 250: 1707–1708, 1990.
41. Aberer E, Neumann R, Stanek G: Is localised scleroderma a *Borrelia* infection? Lancet 2: 278, 1985.
42. Aberer E, Stanek G, Ertl M, et al: Evidence for spirochetal origin of circumscribed scleroderma (morphea). Acta Derm Venereol 67: 225–231, 1987.
43. Aberer E, Klade H, Stanek G, et al: *Borrelia burgdorferi* and different types of morphea. Dermatologica 182: 145–154, 1991.
44. Fan W, Leonardi CL, Penneys NS: Absence of *Borrelia burgdorferi* in patients with localized scleroderma (morphea). J Am Acad Dermatol 33: 682–684, 1995.
45. Dillon WI, Saed GM, Fivenson DP: *Borrelia burgdorferi* DNA is undetectable by polymerase chain reaction in skin lesions of morphea, scleroderma, or lichen sclerosus et atrophicus of patients from North America. J Am Acad Dermatol 33: 617–620, 1995.
46. Falanga V, Medsger TA Jr, Reichlin M, et al: Linear scleroderma: clinical spectrum, prognosis, and laboratory abnormalities. Ann Intern Med 104: 849–857, 1986.
47. Curtis AC, Jansen TG: The prognosis of localized scleroderma. Arch Dermatol 78: 749–757, 1958.
48. Vancheeswaran R, Black CM, David J, et al: Childhood-onset scleroderma: is it different from adult-onset disease? Arthritis Rheum 39: 1041–1049, 1996.
49. Michet CJ Jr, Doyle JA, Ginsburg WW: Eosinophilic fasciitis: report of 15 cases. Mayo Clin Proc 56: 27–34, 1981.
50. Winkelmann RK, Connolly SM, Doyle JA: Carpal tunnel syndrome in cutaneous connective tissue disease: generalized morphea, lichen sclerosus, fasciitis, discoid lupus erythematosus, and lupus panniculitis. J Am Acad Dermatol 7: 94–99, 1982.
51. Jarratt M, Bybee JD, Ramsdell W: Eosinophilic fasciitis: an early variant of scleroderma. J Am Acad Dermatol 1: 221–226, 1979.
52. Blaszczyk M, Janniger CK, Jablonska S, et al: Childhood scleroderma and its peculiarities. Cutis 58: 141–144, 148–152, 1996.
53. Barton DH, Henderson HZ: Oral-facial characteristics of circumscribed scleroderma: case report. J Clin Pediatr Dent 17: 239–242, 1993.
54. Littman BH: Linear scleroderma: a response to neurologic injury? Report and literature review. J Rheumatol 16: 1135–1140, 1989.
55. Pupillo G, Andermann F, Dubeau F: Linear scleroderma and intractable epilepsy: neuropathologic evidence for a chronic inflammatory process. Ann Neurol 39: 277–278, 1996.
56. Dehen L, Roujeau J, Cosnes A, et al: Internal involvement in localized scleroderma. Medicine 73: 241–245, 1994.
57. Torres JE, Sanchez JL: Histopathologic differentiation between localized and systemic scleroderma. Am J Dermatopathol 20: 242–245, 1998.
58. Soma Y, Tamaki T, Kikuchi K, et al: Coexistence of morphea and systemic sclerosis. Dermatology 186: 103–105, 1993.
59. Torok E, Ablonczy E: Morphoea in children. Clin Exp Dermatol 11: 607–612, 1986.
60. Takehara K, Moroi Y, Nakabayashi Y, et al: Antinuclear antibodies in localized scleroderma. Arthritis Rheum 26: 612–616, 1983.
61. Sato S, Fujimoto M, Ihn H, et al: Clinical characteristics associated with antihistone antibodies in patients with localized scleroderma. J Am Acad Dermatol 31: 567–571, 1994.
62. Rosenberg AM, Uziel Y, Krafchik BR, et al: Antinuclear antibodies in children with localized scleroderma. J Rheumatol 22: 2337–2343, 1995.
63. Hulsmans RF, Asghar SS, Siddiqui AH, et al: Hereditary deficiency of C2 in association with linear scleroderma "en coup de sabre." Arch Dermatol 122: 76–79, 1986.
64. Venneker GT, van Meegan M, deKok-Nazaruk M, et al: Incomplete functional deficiencies of the fourth (C4) and second (C2) components of complement in a patient with linear frontoparietal scleroderma and his family. Exp Clin Immunogenet 13: 104–111, 1996.
65. Fujimoto M, Sato S, Ihn H, et al: Serum aldolase level is a useful indicator of disease activity in eosinophilic fasciitis. J Rheumatol 22: 563–565, 1995.
66. Farrington ML, Haas JE, Nazar-Stewart V, et al: Eosinophilic fasciitis in children frequently progresses to scleroderma-like cutaneous fibrosis. J Rheumatol 20: 128–132, 1993.
67. Uziel Y, Krafchik BR, Feldman B, et al: Serum levels of soluble

interleukin-2 receptor. A marker of disease activity in localized scleroderma. Arthritis Rheum 37: 898–901, 1994.
68. Ihn H, Sato S, Fujimoto M, et al: Clinical significance of serum levels of soluble interleukin-2 receptor in patients with localized scleroderma. Br J Dermatol 134: 843–847, 1996.
69. Nakajima H, Fujiwara S, Shinoda K, et al: Magnetic resonance imaging and serum aldolase concentration in eosinophilic fasciitis. Intern Med 36: 654–656, 1997.
70. Al-Shaikh A, Freeman C, Avruch L, et al: Use of magnetic resonance imaging in diagnosing eosinophilic fasciitis. Report of two cases. Arthritis Rheum 37: 1602–1608, 1994.
71. Liu P, Uziel Y, Chuang S, et al: Localized scleroderma: imaging features. Pediatr Radiol 24: 207–209, 1994.
72. Ramboer K, Dermaerel P, Baert AL, et al: Linear scleroderma with orbital involvement: follow up and magnetic resonance imaging [letter]. Br J Ophthalmol 81: 90–93, 1997.
73. Chazen EM, Cook CD, Cohen J: Focal scleroderma. J Pediatr 60: 385–393, 1962.
74. Gaffney K, Kearns G, Moraes D, et al: Eosinophilic fasciitis: a good response with conservative treatment. Ir J Med Sci 162: 256–257, 1993.
74a. Uziel Y, Feldman B, Krafchik BR, et al: Methotrexate and corticosteroid therapy for pediatric localized scleroderma. J Pediatr 136: 91–95, 2000.
75. Laxer RM, Feldman BM: General and local scleroderma in children and dermatomyositis and associated syndromes. Curr Opin Rheumatol 9: 458–464, 1997.
76. Janzen L, Jeffery JR, Gough J, et al: Response to methotrexate in a patient with idiopathic eosinophilic fasciitis, morphea, IgM hypergammaglobulinemia, and renal involvement. J Rheumatol 22: 1967–1970, 1995.
77. Seyger MMB, van den Hoogen FHJ, de Boo T, et al: Low-dose methotrexate in the treatment of widespread morphea. J Am Acad Dermatol 39: 220–225, 1998.
78. Krafchik BR: Localized cutaneous scleroderma. Semin Dermatol 11: 65–72, 1992.
79. Lakhanpal S, Ginsburg WW, Michet CJ, et al: Eosinophilic fasciitis: clinical spectrum and therapeutic response in 52 cases. Semin Arthritis Rheum 17: 221–231, 1988.
80. Weiss JS: Antimalarial medications in dermatology: a review. Dermatol Clin 9: 377–385, 1991.
81. Stege H, Berneburg M, Humke S, et al: High-dose UVA_1 radiation therapy for localized scleroderma. J Am Acad Dermatol 36: 938–944, 1997.
82. Kerscher M, Volkenandt M, Gruss C, et al: Low-dose UVA_1 phototherapy for treatment of localized scleroderma. J Am Acad Dermatol 38: 21–26, 1998.
83. Kanekura T, Fukumaru S, Matsushita S: Successful treatment of scleroderma with PUVA therapy. J Dermatol 23: 455–459, 1996.
84. Naschitz JE, Boss JH, Misselevich I, et al: The fasciitis-panniculitis syndromes. Clinical and pathologic features. Medicine 75: 6–16, 1996.
85. Taniguchi S, Yorifuji T, Hamada T: Treatment of linear localized scleroderma with the anti-allergic drug, tranilast. Clin Exp Dermatol 19: 391–393, 1994.
86. Hulshof MM, Pavel S, Breedveld FC, et al: Oral calcitriol as a new therapeutic modality for generalized morphea. Arch Dermatol 130: 1290–1293, 1994.
87. Hunzelmann N, Anders S, Fierlbeck G, et al: Double-blind, placebo-controlled study of intralesional interferon gamma for the treatment of localized scleroderma. J Am Acad Dermatol 36: 433–435, 1997.
88. Sengezer M, Deveci M, Selmanpakoglu N: Repair of "coup de sabre," a linear form of scleroderma. Ann Plast Surg 37: 428–432, 1996.
89. Slavin SA, Gupta S: Reconstruction of scleroderma of the breast. Plast Reconstr Surg 99: 1736–1741, 1997.

23

Overlap Syndromes

James T. Cassidy and Ross E. Petty

A number of relatively rare systemic connective tissue diseases (CTDs) present with signs and symptoms that are characteristic of two or more of the major rheumatic disorders, such as juvenile rheumatoid arthritis (JRA), systemic lupus erythematosus (SLE), juvenile dermatomyositis (JDM), cutaneous systemic scleroderma (CSS), or vasculopathy. Children with these disorders are often difficult to categorize under existing classification criteria and are properly referred to as having "overlap syndromes" or "undifferentiated CTD." Two of the defined disorders in these categories are discussed in this chapter: *mixed connective tissue disease* (MCTD) and *Sjögren's syndrome* (SS). Overlap syndromes specific for the other major CTDs are discussed in their respective chapters: Chapter 12, Juvenile Rheumatoid Arthritis (JRA/SLE overlap); Chapter 18, Systemic Lupus Erythematosus (anti-RNA polymerase syndromes); Chapter 20, Juvenile Dermatomyositis (anti-tRNA synthetase syndromes); and Chapter 22, Localized Scleroderma.

MIXED CONNECTIVE TISSUE DISEASE

Definition and Classification

MCTD was initially reported by Sharp and colleagues in 1972[1] in 25 patients as a disorder of favorable prognosis with an excellent initial response to relatively low-dose glucocorticoid therapy. The syndrome included clinical features of rheumatoid arthritis, scleroderma, lupus, and dermatomyositis occurring in conjunction with a high antibody titer to an extractable nuclear antigen. It was initially believed that these patients had infrequent serious renal disease, that clinical response to glucocorticoids was excellent, and that prognosis was in general favorable. However, a reassessment of the original patients indicated that over time the inflammatory manifestations (arthritis, serositis, fever, myositis) tended to become less evident, while sclerodactyly and esophageal disease, less responsive to treatment with glucocorticoids, persisted and began to dominate the clinical picture.[2] Severe renal disease, however, remained unusual, as only one patient developed membranous glomerulonephritis. Although the concept of MCTD as a clinical entity separate from the other CTDs has remained controversial, classification employing more precise serologic criteria and human leukocyte antigen (HLA) typing have confirmed the uniqueness of this disorder (Table 23–1).[3–6]

Epidemiology

MCTD is one of the least common CTDs in a pediatric rheumatology clinic. It had a frequency of 0.1 percent in a Finnish nationwide prospective study[7] and 0.3 percent in the U.S. Pediatric Rheumatology Data Base.[8] The median age at onset is approximately 11 years (range, 4 to 16 years). MCTD is three times more frequent in girls than in boys. There is one report of the occurrence of this disorder in siblings.[9]

Immunogenetic Background

In white populations, the predominant HLA class II specificities associated with MCTD in children have been DR4 and DR2,[10] as in adults.[6, 11–17] Patients with DR4 or DR2 have a region of homology of seven amino acids (numbers 26, 28, 30, 31, 32, 70, and 73) in the highly polymorphic antigen-binding segment encoded by the DRB1 gene.[16, 18] These HLA specificities are also linked to the anti-U1snRNP antibodies that are characteristic of the disorder. HLA types associated with CSS (DR5) or SLE (DR3) are infrequent.

There are also unique T cell–dependent immune responses in patients with MCTD.[19, 20] T cell clones are directed against the U1 70 kD polypeptide and are

Table 23–1

Clinical Characteristics of Mixed Connective Tissue Disease

Clinical signs of two or more of the following disease
Juvenile rheumatoid arthritis
Systemic lupus erythematosus
Juvenile dermatomyositis
Systemic scleroderma
Serology positive for
High-titer of antibodies to U1snRNP and the 70 kD, A and C polypeptides
Anti-U1RNA antibodies
The presence of HLA-DR4 or -DR2

principally of the CD4-positive, T_H1 type. These data support the role of a specific HLA immunogenetic profile and T cell reactivity in generation of the B cell immune responses.

Clinical Manifestations

MCTD has been recognized with increasing frequency in childhood.[10, 14, 21–30] These children present with features of more than one CTD, a speckled antinuclear antibody (ANA) pattern, and high titers of antibody to ribonucleoprotein (RNP) (see Table 23–1). Clinical characteristics of children from selected studies are summarized in Table 23–2. Polyarthritis (93 percent) and Raynaud's phenomenon (85 percent) are the most common manifestations at onset. The arthritis may be relatively painful. Erosive disease is infrequent, but swan-neck or flexion contraction deformities may develop. The arthritis is often associated with rheumatoid factor (RF) seropositivity. Cutaneous changes include scleroderma-like disease in almost one half, the rash of SLE in one third, and that of JDM in one third. Nailfold capillary abnormalities are similar to those seen in CSS (see Table 21–4).[31–33] Cardiopulmonary disease and esophageal dysmotility are frequent. Although nephritis occurs in about one fourth of the patients, it is less common and usually, but not always, less severe than in patients with SLE.

However, children with MCTD may have more frequent and severe renal disease than adults, more hematologic complications such as thrombocytopenia, and less pulmonary hypertension. In a prospective, longitudinal study, 31 of 34 adults with high titers of RNP antibody had typical MCTD in which pulmonary disease (often initially asymptomatic) was common.[34] Pulmonary hypertension was the most frequent serious complication. A comparison of the clinical and serologic characteristics of diffuse and limited CSS, eosinophilic fasciitis, MCTD, and SLE is given in Table 21–12.

Table 23–2

Disease Characteristics of Children With Mixed Connective Tissue Disease

Characteristic	Reported(n)*	Present(n)†	Percent
Arthritis	72	67	93
Raynaud's phenomenon	72	61	85
Sclerodermatous skin	67	33	49
Rash of systemic lupus erythematosus	67	22	33
Rash of juvenile dermatomyositis	67	22	33
Fever	61	34	56
Abnormal esophageal motility	56	23	41
Cardiac disease	67	20	30
Pericarditis	67	18	27
Muscle disease	72	44	61
Sicca syndrome	66	24	36
Central nervous system disease	61	14	23
Lung			
Abnormal diffusion	56	24	43
Restrictive disease	56	8	14
Hypertension	56	4	7
Effusion	56	13	23
Radiographic changes only	56	1	2
Splenomegaly	63	18	29
Hepatomegaly	68	19	28
Renal disease	72	19	26
Anti-dsDNA positive	64	13	20
Anti-Sm positive	58	6	10
Anti-RNP positive	72	72	100
Rheumatoid factor positive	57	39	68

*The number of children in whom the characteristic was noted.
†The number in whom the abnormality was present.
Data derived from 10 reports with a total of 72 children. Sharp et al,[1] Sanders et al,[21] Singsen et al,[22] Fraga et al,[23] Rosenthal,[24] Peskett et al,[25] Oetgen et al,[28] Eberhardt et al,[29] Cassidy et al,[43] and Savouret et al.[44]

Pathology

Singsen and colleagues[35] described widespread intimal proliferation and medial hypertrophy of vascular walls in four children with MCTD who died. Renal biopsies in eight additional patients confirmed abnormalities of the glomerular basement membranes or vascular sclerosis. These authors commented that although the histopathology of MCTD resembled that of CSS, the extent of fibrosis was less, and intimal vascular abnormalities in larger vessels such as the aorta and the coronary, pulmonary, and renal arteries were more prominent. Another study reported pulmonary hypertension and proliferative vasculopathy in the virtual absence of interstitial fibrosis in patients with MCTD in contrast to CSS.[34]

Differential Diagnosis

As with the disorder in adults, MCTD in children is a syndrome that evolves over time from a more limited presentation of clinical disease to one with overlapping features of JRA, SLE, CSS, or JDM. Initial abnormalities are likely to include polyarthritis and Raynaud's phenomenon. These may be accompanied by fever. Other manifestations develop sequentially but not in any predictable order or over any circumscribed period of time. The rashes of SLE or JDM are common at onset. Moderately symptomatic involvement, such as myositis with minimal weakness, mild atrophy, and minimal to moderate increases in the serum levels of muscle enzymes, is also frequent. Dysphagia and bowel dysmotility may also be present. Manifestations of the sicca syndrome with xerostomia, keratoconjunctivitis sicca, or parotid gland enlargement occur in one third of children.[36] Although children do not usually complain of shortness of breath (depending on cognitive development or unconsciously self-imposed restriction of activity), pulmonary functional impairments are often present. Sclerodermatous skin changes are slow to develop but may become the most prominent feature of the disease late in its course.

Serologic findings may also evolve over time. ANAs

Table 23–3

Diagnostic Criteria for Mixed Connective Tissue Disease

Major Criteria	Minor Criteria	Diagnosis	Exclusion
1. Severe myositis 2. Pulmonary involvement, with one or more of the following: DLco < 70% normal, pulmonary hypertension, or proliferative vascular lesions on lung biopsy 3. Raynaud's phenomenon or esophageal hypomotility 4. Swollen hands or sclerodactyly 5. Highest observed anti-ENA ≥ 1:10,000 and anti-RNP positive	1. Alopecia 2. Leukopenia (<4000 WBC/mm³) 3. Anemia (≤10 g/dl women, ≤12 g/dl men) 4. Pleuritis 5. Pericarditis 6. Arthritis 7. Trigeminal neuropathy 8. Malar rash 9. Thrombocytopenia (<100,000/mm³) 10. Mild myositis 11. History of swollen hands	**Definite** A. 4 major criteria Anti-U1RNP+ with anti-ENA ≥ 1:4000 **Probable** A. 3 major criteria B. 2 major criteria (including 1 or more from #1, #2, #3) and 2 minor criteria Anti-U1RNP+ with anti-ENA ≥ 1:1000 **Possible** A. 3 major criteria B. 2 major criteria plus Anti-U1RNP+ with anti-ENA ≥ 1:100 C. 1 major criteria and 3 minor criteria plus Anti-U1RNP+ with anti-ENA ≥ 1:100	**Definite** anti-Sm+(by immunodiffusion) **Probable** None **Possible** None

ENA, extractable nuclear antigens; RNP, ribonucleoproteins; Sm, Smith antigen.

Modified from Sharp GC: Diagnostic criteria for classification of MCTD. *In* Kasukawa R, Sharp GC: Mixed Connective Tissue Disease and Anti-Nuclear Antibodies. Amsterdam, The Netherlands, Excerpta Medica, 1987, pp 23–32.

may be absent at onset or in very low titer in a speckled pattern. The development of high-titer anti-RNP antibodies that are RNAse sensitive should alert the pediatric rheumatologist to the probable evolution of the child's illness into the pattern of MCTD. RF seropositivity is often present early and occurs in approximately two thirds of the children.

Criteria for MCTD have been evaluated in adults but not in children (Table 23–3).[37] These criteria are summarized in the review by Smolen and colleagues.[17, 37–40] A study by Shen and coworkers[41] in 50 patients from China during a 2- to 8-year period indicated that the criteria of Sharp[37] were the most reliable for a diagnosis of MCTD. Among 23 patients fulfilling these criteria, only 1, or 4.3 percent, developed scleroderma. Among 23 patients satisfying the criteria of Kasukawa and colleagues,[38] 7, or 30.4 percent, developed another CTD. Of the 27 who met the criteria of Alarcon-Segovia and colleagues,[36] 12, or 44 percent, went on to fulfill criteria for another major rheumatic disease. The frequencies of HLA-DR4 and -DR5 were significantly higher in the patients whose disease fulfilled Sharp's criteria.[37] Differing conclusions were reached, however, in a comparative study of four diagnostic criteria from France by Amigues and coworkers.[42] These investigators analyzed the criteria of Sharp,[37] Kasukawa and colleagues,[38] Alarcon-Segovia and coworkers,[39] and Kahn and associates[40] in 45 patients with anti-U1RNP antibodies who were classified as MCTD. They found that the criteria of Alarcon-Segovia and coworkers[39] had the highest sensitivity (62.5 percent) and specificity (86.2 percent), with an overlap of 16 percent with other major CTDs. These results were comparable to those obtained with the criteria of Kahn and associates.[40]

Laboratory Examination

Very high titers of ANAs are usually present initially, often in a speckled pattern on the HEp-2 cell substrate. They react specifically with an RNAse-sensitive component of extractable nuclear antigen (ENA) and RNP: *Anti-RNP antibodies in high titer have been the serologic hallmark of MCTD.* These antibodies may, however, be present in low titer in other diseases such as SLE.[17, 22, 43] Further investigations confirmed that the most characteristic specificities of the anti-RNP antibodies in MCTD were directed against a uridine rich (U1) small nuclear RNP (snRNP) complex of the spliceosome consisting of U1RNA and the associated 70 kD, A and C polypeptides (Fig. 23–1).[44–46] The anti-U1snRNP profile in patients with MCTD is characterized by a high-titer antibody response, predominantly if not solely of immunoglobulin (Ig) G antibodies, and specificity for an epitope different from that of SLE sera.[17] Thus, a false-positive anti-U1snRNP antibody response may be observed in SLE.[47] More recently, it has been reported that antibodies to U1RNA are even more closely associated with disease activity in MCTD than are U1RNP antibodies.[48–50]

Substantial advances have now been made in employing these specific autoantibody activities against the U1snRNP polypeptides for classification of disease.[16, 51] Among adult patients with high titers of autoantibodies against the U1-70 kD antigen, in contradistinction to patients with CTDs who did not demonstrate these antibody activities, there were significant clinical associations with the presence of Raynaud's phenomenon, swollen hands, sclerodactyly, telangiectasia, and abnormal esophageal motility.[15] In the study by DeRooij and colleagues,[14] all five children who had antibodies against the U1-70 kD antigen had clinical disease characterized by arthralgia or arthritis, swollen hands, Raynaud's phenomenon, and abnormalities of pulmonary function.

Children with antibodies against the 70 kD polypeptide uncommonly have diffuse glomerulonephritis, cardiac disease, widespread cutaneous sclerosis, or central nervous sys-

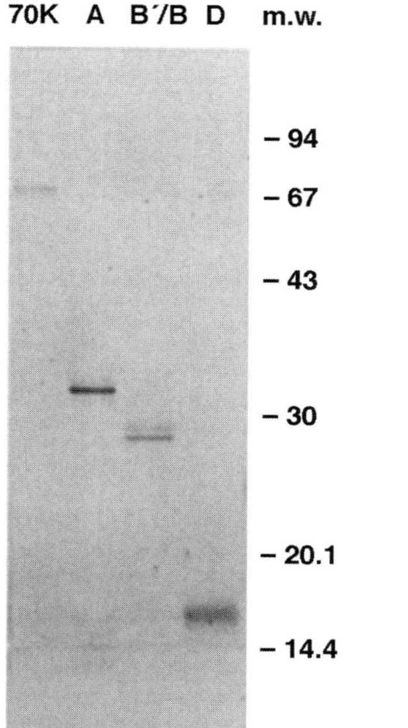

Figure 23–1. Western blot with patient sera delineating reaction with the 70 kD, A, B′/B, and D polypeptides. (Courtesy of Dr. R. Hoffman.)

tem disease. Clinical renal disease occurred, however, in 3 of the 11 patients reported by Hoffman and colleagues[10] and was confined to a subset of children who had IgG autoantibodies against the D polypeptide of the U1snRNP. These children were also HLA-DR2 positive. These were the same patients who progressed clinically to develop an adverse or fatal outcome associated with anti-dsDNA antibodies. Children with anti-Sm antibodies may go on to develop reactivity to the D polypeptide and clinically important renal disease. Their course may be accompanied by hypocomplementemia and other features of nephritis more characteristic of SLE (see Table 23–2). It is noteworthy that such sera may not be positive for anti-Sm antibodies by the relatively insensitive techniques of double immunodiffusion or counterimmunoelectrophoresis.

Some MCTD sera, including those from patients without renal disease, also react with B/B′ polypeptides, but probably to one or more epitopes different from those characteristic of the anti-Sm antibody activity found in patients with SLE.[51, 52] Some patients have marked elevations of serum immunoglobulin levels, especially of IgG,[23, 28] and two children with selective IgA deficiency have been reported.[21, 43]

In a study of adults with MCTD,[53] 48 anti-U1-70 kD antibody-positive patients with MCTD were compared with 59 anti-U1-70 kD antibody-negative patients with classic SLE. Although antiphospholipid antibodies were increased in the patients with MCTD compared with control subjects, these antibodies were even more frequent in the patients with SLE in whom deep vein thrombosis, pulmonary embolism, recurrent fetal loss, chorea, livedo reticularis, severe thrombocytopenia, and avascular necrosis occurred. These clinical manifestations of the antiphospholipid antibody syndrome were absent from the MCTD group of patients.

In a prospective investigation of 11 children with MCTD,[10] antibodies to U1snRNP polypeptides were compared sequentially with the course of the disease. All of the patients had high-titer anti-ENA antibodies by hemagglutination (>1:1,000,000) and positive anti-RNP reactivity by immunodiffusion. Antibody specificity identified by immunoblot analysis and enzyme-linked immunosorbent assay was to the 70 kD polypeptide in 11, A in 10, C in 2, B/B′ in 9, and D in 3. Four children had both IgG and IgM antibodies to the 70 kD protein, 5 to the A peptide, 2 to the B/B′, and only 1 to the D. One patient developed low-titer anti-Sm antibodies and 3 had low-titer, transient anti-dsDNA seropositivity. Three had anti-Ro antibodies. Anti-ENA titers and 70 kD reactivity decreased in patients in prolonged remission; positive reactions remained in those with continuing active disease and in patients receiving only symptomatic treatment. The predominant HLA antigens were DR2 in 6 of 9 and DR4 in 4 of 9; all patients were either DR2 or DR4 positive, similar to findings in adults with MCTD.

Treatment

There is no specific treatment for children with MCTD. The management program should address the predominant problems of the child, be they arthritis, cutaneous disease, or visceral involvement. Many children respond satisfactorily to low-dose glucocorticoids, nonsteroidal anti-inflammatory drugs, or hydroxychloroquine, or a combination of these drugs.[43] Patients with severe myositis or renal or visceral disease require high-dose glucocorticoids and sometimes cytotoxic drugs such as cyclophosphamide, especially for life-threatening complications such as pulmonary hypertension. Low-dose methotrexate has also been advocated.[54]

Course of the Disease and Prognosis

The long-term outcome of MCTD in children is varied and unpredictable.[43, 55–59] Deaths have been reported from disease resembling SLE, accompanied by renal failure. In contrast to SLE, however, morbidity and mortality in MCTD is more often associated with the development of pulmonary hypertension (7 percent),[26, 29, 34, 43, 60] or gradually evolving restrictive disease (15 percent) with minimal fibrosis.[22, 26] Pulmonary dysfunction in children may be underestimated clinically because it tends to develop insidiously.[34] Another ominous development is severe thrombocytopenia (20 percent) that is often resistant to conventional therapy. This complication is more common in children than in adults.[43]

Tiddens and colleagues,[55] in a retrospective review, reported 14 children with MCTD who met the criteria of Kasukawa and coworkers,[38] with a mean follow-up of 9.3 years (range, 3.8 to 14.1 years) and a mean age at onset of 10.6 years (range, 5.2 to 15.6 years). Features of the disease characteristic of SLE and JDM tended to disappear over time, whereas those of CSS, Raynaud's phenomenon, and JRA persisted. At follow-up, thrombocytopenia was still present in 3 children, 4 had extensive limitation of range of joint movement, all had abnormal esophageal function, and none had active renal disease. No pulmonary hypertension was documented, although half had restrictive disease on function studies. Glucocorticoids were judged to be successful in managing MCTD but were associated with osteonecrosis in 3 children and growth retardation in 1 child.

The outcome of children with MCTD was evaluated in a study in three U.S. Midwestern clinics.[43] There were 21 girls and 6 boys, with a mean age at onset of 13 years (range, 5 to 18 years) and a mean duration of disease of 8 years (range, 1 to 18 years). Organ systems predominantly involved at onset and then at follow-up at 8 years or more were joints (24 and 11, respectively), muscles (8 and 9), skin (16 and 8), lungs (10 and 13), heart (7 and 4), gastrointestinal tract (5 and 5), and kidneys (3 and 4). A characteristic onset involved Raynaud's phenomenon, arthritis, swollen hands, myositis, and the cutaneous features of JDM or SLE. Cutaneous disease, esophageal dysfunction, myositis, and arthritis were prominent during the course of the disease. These clinical features were similar to those of adults with MCTD, with less frequent and severe pulmonary disease and only one instance of pulmonary hypertension. Five patients developed severe thrombocytopenia. All patients had positive immunodiffusion for anti-RNP antibodies. Anti-ENA antibodies were found in titers up to 1:16,000,000 by hemagglutination and were often maintained at high levels for many years, but ultimately declined if the course stabilized or the patient entered remission. Transient, low-titer anti-dsDNA antibodies were present in 8 patients. Hypocomplementemia occurred in 8 and high titers of RF in 7 children. Outcome was good or stable in 12 and prolonged remissions occurred in 5 patients. Progressive disease developed in 7 patients; 4 died of renal disease, diffuse intravascular coagulation, or cardiopulmonary failure.

MCTD in the 66 children from Japan studied by Yokota and colleagues[58] also presented a homogeneous course and had both clinical and laboratory characteristics that were different from those of children with SLE or other defined CTDs. These authors confirmed the diagnostic importance of Raynaud's phenomenon and high-titered anti-RNP antibodies. Additional frequent clinical characteristics included swelling of the hands, polyarthralgia, facial erythema, RF seropositivity, hypergammaglobulinemia, and increased serum levels of the muscle enzymes.

Michels[59] reviewed the course of MCTD in 224 children reported up until 1996, including 33 patients from the Rheumatic Children's Hospital in Garmisch-Partenkirchen, Germany. Because this review involved a number of studies over many years, often retrospective and without serologic or genetic characterization by current standards, it predominantly reflects the clinical classifications and historical conclusions of the various authors and centers. Nevertheless, this meta-analysis indicated that most of the children improved over time and remissions occurred in 3 to 27 percent of the subjects in the series. Raynaud's phenomenon and scleroderma-like skin changes were reported in up to 86 percent of the patients. Long-term problems included loss of range of joint motion in 29 percent, renal disease in up to 47 percent, pulmonary restrictive disease in up to 24 percent, and esophageal dysmotility in up to 29 percent. Cardiovascular disease included cardiomyopathy, pericarditis, and pulmonary hypertension. Central nervous system involvement was rare, but when it occurred it could be severe. Seventeen of the 224 patients, or 7.6 percent, died from sepsis ($n = 7$), cerebral disease (3), heart failure (2), pulmonary hypertension (2), renal failure (2), and gastrointestinal bleeding (1). It was concluded that this mortality rate was in the range of that from the other major systemic CTDs and that otherwise the long-term problems seen in patients who survived appeared minor. These conclusions are similar to observations from our clinic in children[10] and in adults.[60]

Kotajima and colleagues[56] compared two groups of Japanese patients with MCTD, one with onset under 16 years of age, and another with onset at 16 years of age or older. These investigators confirmed that signs typical of SLE, such as facial erythema, photosensitivity, the presence of lupus erythematosus cells, lymphadenopathy, and cellular casts, were more frequent in the juvenile onset group. Conversely, scleroderma-like symptoms such as esophageal dysmotility, sclerodactyly, and pulmonary disease were less common in the younger group. The authors also noted that swelling of the hands was less frequent in the juvenile patients. The mortality rate was approximately 2.8 percent in the children. Compared with other CTDs, the authors interpreted these outcomes as relatively favorable.

The long-term outcome of MCTD in adults and children was studied by Burdt and colleagues[60] in 47 patients who met the criteria of Kasukawa and coworkers[38] and were followed at one university center for 3 to 29 years. All patients had antibodies to the 70 kD polypeptide of U1RNP, 81 percent to A, 79 percent to B/B′, 48 percent to C, and 14 percent to D. Anti-U1RNA was positive in 89 percent of the patients, and these antibody levels correlated with the activity of the disease. Initially, epitope spreading was noted as a feature of active MCTD. With time, antibody reactivity was selectively reduced in patients in remission (epitope contraction). HLA-DR4 and -DR2 were present in 23 of 27 patients who were typed (85 percent). Inflammatory features of the disease such as Raynaud's phenomenon and esophageal hypomotility diminished over time, whereas pulmonary hypertension and central nervous system disease persisted in spite of treatment. Sclerodactyly was frequent (49 percent), but diffuse cutaneous sclerosis occurred in only 19 percent of patients. Antibodies to centromere, Scl-70, and PM1/PM-Scl were not detected. Renal disease developed in 5 patients (11 percent: World Health Organization class III in 2, class IV in 2, and classes III and V in 1). Eleven patients died 3 to 25 years after onset of MCTD with pulmonary hypertension the major contributory factor in 9, often associated with the presence of anticardiolipin antibodies. A favorable outcome was documented in 62 percent of the patients, with 17 percent in remission (11 off therapy) and leading normal lives without functional disabilities at the time of the study.

SJÖGREN'S SYNDROME

Definition and Classification

SS is a disorder in which decreased secretion of saliva and tears results in dryness of the mouth (xerostomia) and eyes (xerophthalmia or keratoconjunctivitis sicca).[61] It is characterized serologically by the presence of autoantibodies to the nuclear antigens Ro/SS-A and La/SS-B (Table 23–4). There are no validated classification criteria for SS, although a number have been proposed.[62–66] Recently, criteria have been evaluated for children.[67] If SS occurs as an isolated disorder, it is referred to as *primary SS*, which is very rare in children. A more frequent occurrence in childhood, *secondary SS*, most commonly accompanies SLE, as it does in adults,[41] or less commonly another CTD. Children with primary or secondary SS reported up to 1988 have been reviewed by Deprettere and associates.[68–77] Eleven of 28 children had secondary SS, most commonly associated with SLE or MCTD, and only rarely with JRA or CSS. The remaining 17 children had primary SS.

Table 23–4

Sjögren's Syndrome in Children

Definition	Keratoconjunctivitis sicca (dry eyes secondary to decreased tear production by lacrimal glands) and xerostomia (dry mouth secondary to decreased saliva production by salivary glands)
Primary Sjögren's syndrome	Not associated with any other disease; rare in childhood
Secondary Sjögren's syndrome	Associated with a connective tissue disease, most often systemic lupus erythematosus or mixed connective tissue disease; uncommon in childhood
Autoantibodies	Ro/SS-A (95%) and La/SS-B (85%)

Clinical Manifestations

The initial characteristics of SS are quite variable at onset. SS often presents as recurrent parotid swelling that may be unilateral or bilateral, painful or painless (Fig. 23–2).[78–81] Deficiency of saliva results in difficulty chewing and swallowing, abnormalities of taste, and severe dental caries.[82] Photophobia or irritation of the eyes results from involvement of the lacrimal glands with insufficiency of tears. Dryness of other mucosal surfaces, including nose, pharynx, and vagina, occurs. About 25 percent of adults with primary SS develop other systemic complications, such as interstitial pneumonitis, interstitial nephritis, myositis, achalasia with achlorhydria, isosthenuria or renal tubular acidosis, Hashimoto's thyroiditis,[83] or splenic vasculitis.[84] Severe involvement of the central nervous system has been described in children and adults.[85–87] Optic neuropathy has occurred[88] and in some patients may be associated with antiphospholipid antibodies.[89]

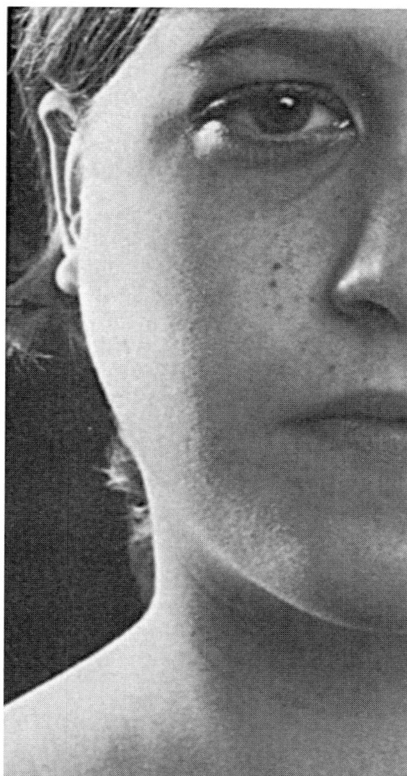

Figure 23–2. Swelling of the parotid gland *(arrow)* is present at onset of Sjögren's syndrome in this young girl. Within 2 years, she developed the clinical features of systemic lupus erythematosus.

Pathology

Histologic changes include widespread infiltration of lymphocytic cells and, to a lesser extent, of plasma cells and reticulum cells in parenchymal organs and the salivary and lacrimal glands. In some cases, germinal follicle formation occurs. There is subsequently secondary atrophy and obliteration of secretory acini. Lymphoma may develop secondary to primary SS.[90] Particularly in the salivary glands, there is a proliferation of ductal lining cells to form epimyoepithelial islands. This latter histologic finding is one of the important diagnostic features of SS (Fig. 23–3). The diagnosis may be confirmed if necessary by biopsy of a minor salivary gland from the lower lip demonstrating periductal lymphocytic infiltrates.[91] The nailfold capillaries are normal unless another CTD is present,[92] but may be abnormal in adults depending on the presence of Raynaud's phenomenon.[93]

Laboratory Examination

The most striking laboratory abnormalities include polyclonal hypergammaglobulinemia, high-titer RFs, and ANAs directed to Ro/SS-A (95 percent) and La/SS-B (85 percent). Anti-Ro antibodies in patients with

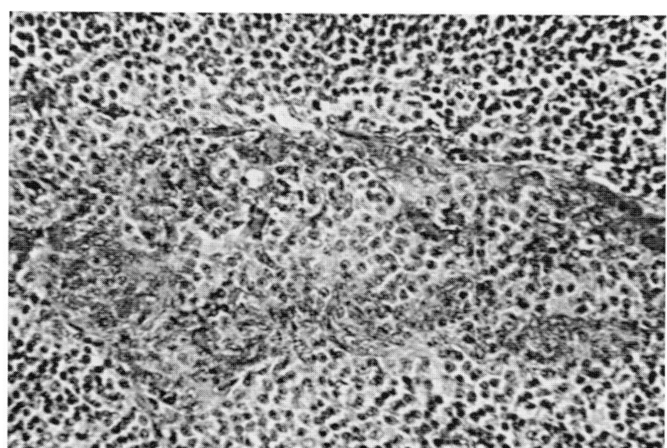

Figure 23–3. Parotid gland (H&E ×40). There is obliteration of the normal acinar architecture by lymphocytes. A regenerative epimyoepithelial island occupies the center of the field.

SS are frequently accompanied by anemia, leukopenia, lymphopenia, cryoglobulinemia, and vasculitis.[94–96] Specific HLA class II alleles are associated with the development of anti-Ro/La antibodies (DR3, DQw1, DQw2).[97–99] Antiphospholipid antibodies have been described in children but are usually of low titer and not associated with thrombotic phenomena.[100]

A positive Schirmer test indicates deficient tear flow (<5 mm wetting of a filter paper strip in 15 minutes), and Rose-Bengal or fluorescein staining of the cornea may demonstrate superficial erosions. A study of Spath and associates[95] documented the usefulness of magnetic resonance imaging of the parotid gland in patients with SS. Demonstration of ectasia of the parotid ducts by sialography[101] or decreased uptake of technetium-99m pertechnetate supports the diagnosis.

Treatment

Treatment is nonspecific and not curative.[102] The systemic manifestations of SS are treated with nonsteroidal anti-inflammatory drugs or glucocorticoids. The sicca component is managed with attention to environmental humidity, artificial tears, nasal saline douches, and sour lemon drops to stimulate production of saliva. Recently, pilocarpine tablets have been recommended for the sicca symptoms in the eyes and mouth.[103, 104] The drug is well tolerated and safe, but with significant parasympathomimetic side effects.

References

1. Sharp GC, Irvin WS, Tan EM, et al: Mixed connective tissue disease: an apparently distinct rheumatic syndrome associated with a specific antibody to an extractable nuclear antigen. Am J Med 52: 148–159, 1972.
2. Nimelstein SH, Brody S, McShane D, et al: Mixed connective tissue disease: a subsequent evaluation of the original 25 patients. Medicine (Baltimore) 59: 239–248, 1980.
3. Mukherjee SK, Lahiri K, Sen MK: Scleroderma in a boy of nine. J Indian Med Assoc 47: 132–135, 1966.
4. Bennett RM, O'Connell DJ: Mixed connective tissue disease: a clinicopathologic study of 20 cases. Semin Arthritis Rheum 10: 25–51, 1980.
5. Lundberg I, Hedfors E: Clinical course of patients with anti-RNP antibodies. A prospective study of 32 patients. J Rheumatol 18: 1511–1519, 1991.
6. Hoffman RW, Sharp GC: Is anti-U1-RNP autoantibody positive connective tissue disease genetically distinct? J Rheumatol 22: 586–589, 1995.
7. Pelkonen PM, Jalanko HJ, Lantto RK, et al: Incidence of systemic connective tissue diseases in children: a nationwide prospective study in Finland. J Rheumatol 21: 2143–2146, 1994.
8. Bowyer S, Roettcher P, and the members of the Pediatric Rheumatology Database Research Group: Pediatric rheumatology clinic populations in the United States: results of a 3 year study. J Rheumatol 23: 1968–1974, 1996.
9. Horn JR, Kapur JJ, Walker SE: Mixed connective tissue disease in siblings. Arthritis Rheum 21: 709–714, 1978.
10. Hoffman RW, Cassidy JT, Takeda Y, et al: U1-70-kd autoantibody-positive mixed connective tissue disease in children: a longitudinal clinical and serologic analysis. Arthritis Rheum 36: 1599–1602, 1993.
11. Genth E, Zarnowski H, Mierau R, et al: HLA-DR4 and Gm(1,3;5,21) are associated with U1-nRNP antibody positive connective tissue disease. Ann Rheum Dis 46: 189–196, 1987.
12. Black CM, Maddison PJ, Welsh KI, et al: HLA and immunoglobulin allotypes in mixed connective tissue disease. Arthritis Rheum 31: 131–134, 1988.
13. Harley JB, Sestak AL, Willis LG, et al: A model for disease heterogeneity in systemic lupus erythematosus. Relationships between histocompatibility antigens, autoantibodies, and lymphopenia or renal disease. Arthritis Rheum 32: 826–836, 1989.
14. DeRooij DJ, Fiselier TH, van de Putte LB, et al: Juvenile-onset mixed connective tissue diseases: clinical, serologic and follow-up data. Scand J Rheumatol 18: 157–160, 1989.
15. Hoffman RW, Rettenmaier LJ, Takeda Y, et al: Human autoantibodies against the 70-kD polypeptide of U1 small RNP are associated with HLA-DR4 among connective tissue disease patients. Arthritis Rheum 33: 666–673, 1990.
16. Kaneoka H, Hsu K, Takeda Y, et al: Molecular genetic analysis of HLA-DR and HLA-DQ genes among anti-U1-70 kD autoantibody-positive connective tissue disease patients. Arthritis Rheum 35: 83–94, 1992.
17. Smolen JS, Steiner G: Mixed connective tissue disease: to be or not to be? Arthritis Rheum 41: 768–777, 1998.
18. Lanchburg JS, Hall MA, Welsh KI, et al: Sequence analysis of HLA-DR4 B1 subtypes: additional first domain variability is detected by oligonucleotide hybridization and nucleotide sequencing. Hum Immunol 27: 136–144, 1990.
19. Hoffman RW, Takeda Y, Sharp GC, et al: Human T cell clones reactive against U-small nuclear ribonucleoprotein autoantigens from connective tissue disease patients and healthy individuals. J Immunol 151: 6460–6469, 1993.
20. Talken BL, Lee DR, Caldwell CW, et al: Analysis of T cell receptors specific for U1-70kD small nuclear ribonucleoprotein autoantigen: the alpha chain complementarity determining region three is highly conserved among connective tissue disease patients. Hum Immunol 60: 200–208, 1999.
21. Sanders DY, Huntley CC, Sharp GC: Mixed connective tissue disease in a child. J Pediatr 83: 642–645, 1973.
22. Singsen BH, Kornreich HK, Koster-King K, et al: Mixed connective tissue disease in children. Arthritis Rheum 20(Suppl): 355–360, 1978.
23. Fraga A, Gudino J, Ramos-Niembro F, et al: Mixed connective tissue disease in childhood. Am J Dis Child 132: 263–265, 1978.
24. Rosenthal M: Sharp-Syndrom (mixed connective tissue disease) bei Kindern. Helv Paediatr Acta 33: 251–258, 1978.
25. Peskett SA, Ansell BM, Fizzman P, et al: Mixed connective tissue disease in children. Rheumatol Rehabil 17: 245–248, 1978.
26. Rosenberg AM, Petty RE, Cumming GR, et al: Pulmonary hypertension in a child with mixed connective tissue disease. J Rheumatol 6: 700–704, 1979.
27. Allen RC, St-Cyr C, Maddison PJ, et al: Overlap connective tissue syndromes. Arch Dis Child 61: 284–288, 1986.
28. Oetgen WJ, Boice JA, Lawless OJ: Mixed connective tissue disease in children and adolescents. Pediatrics 67: 333–337, 1981.
29. Eberhardt K, Svantesson II, Svensson B: Follow-up study of 6 children presenting with a MCTD-like syndrome. Scand J Rheumatol 10: 62–64, 1981.
30. Allen R: Overlap syndrome. *In* Woo P, White PH, Ansell BM (eds): Pediatric Rheumatology Update. Oxford, England, Oxford University Press, 1990, pp 209–216.
31. Maricq HR, LeRoy EC, D'Angelo WA, et al: Diagnostic potential of in vivo capillary microscopy in scleroderma and related disorders. Arthritis Rheum 23: 183–189, 1980.
32. Maricq HR: Widefield capillary microscopy. Technique and rating scale for abnormalities seen in scleroderma and related disorders. Arthritis Rheum 24: 1159–1165, 1981.
33. Gendi NS, Welsh KI, Van Venrooij WJ, et al: HLA type as a predictor of mixed connective tissue disease differentiation. Ten-year clinical and immunogenetic followup of 46 patients. Arthritis Rheum 38: 259–266, 1995.
34. Sullivan WD, Hurst DJ, Harmon CE, et al: A prospective evaluation emphasizing pulmonary involvement in patients with mixed connective tissue disease. Medicine (Baltimore) 63: 92–107, 1984.
35. Singsen BH, Swanson VI, Bernstein BH, et al: A histologic evaluation of mixed connective tissue disease in childhood. Am J Med 68: 710–717, 1980.
36. Alarcon-Segovia D: Symptomatic Sjögren's syndrome in mixed connective tissue disease. J Rheumatol 11: 582–583, 1984.

37. Sharp GC: Diagnostic criteria for classification of MCTD. *In* Kasukawa R, Sharp GC (eds): Mixed Connective Tissue Disease and Anti-Nuclear Antibodies. Amsterdam, The Netherlands, Excerpta Medica, 1987, pp 23–32.
38. Kasukawa R, Tojo T, Miyawaki S, et al: Preliminary diagnostic criteria for classification of mixed connective tissue disease. *In* Kasukawa R, Sharp GC (eds): Mixed Connective Tissue Disease and Anti-Nuclear Antibodies. Amsterdam, The Netherlands, Excerpta Medica, 1987, pp 41–48.
39. Alarcon-Segovia D, Villarreal M: Classification and diagnostic criteria for mixed connective tissue disease. *In* Kasukawa R, Sharp GC (eds): Mixed Connective Tissue Disease and Anti-Nuclear Antibodies. Amsterdam, The Netherlands, Excerpta Medica, 1987, pp 33–40.
40. Kahn MF, Appelboom T: Syndrome de Sharp. *In* Kahn MF, Peltier AP, Meyer O, et al (eds): Les Maladies Systémiques. Paris, Flammarion, 1991, pp 545–556.
41. Shen N, Chen S, Yang H, et al: Mixed connective tissue disease: a disease entity? Chin Med J (Engl) 111: 214–217, 1998.
42. Amigues JM, Cantagrel A, Abbal M, et al: Comparative study of 4 diagnosis criteria sets for mixed connective tissue disease in patients with anti-RNP antibodies. Autoimmunity Group of the Hospitals of Toulouse. J Rheumatol 23: 2055–2062, 1996.
43. Cassidy JT, Hoffman RW, Wortmann DW, et al: Long-term outcome of children with mixed connective tissue disease (MCTD). J Rheumatol 27(Suppl 58): 100, 2000.
44. Savouret J-F, Chudwin DS, Wara DW, et al: Clinical and laboratory findings in childhood mixed connective tissue disease: presence of antibody to ribonucleoprotein containing the small nuclear ribonucleic acid U_1. J Pediatr 102: 841–846, 1983.
45. Pettersson I, Wang G, Smith EI, et al: The use of immunoblotting and immunoprecipitation of (U) small nuclear ribonucleoproteins in the analysis of sera of patients with mixed connective tissue disease and systemic lupus erythematosus. Arthritis Rheum 29: 986–996, 1986.
46. Margaux J, Hayem G, Palazzo E, et al: Clinical usefulness of antibodies to U1snRNP proteins in mixed connective tissue disease and systemic lupus erythematosus. Rev Rhum Engl Ed 65: 378–386, 1998.
47. Habets WJ, Hoet MH, Sillekens PT, et al: Detection of autoantibodies in a quantitative immunoassay using recombinant ribonucleoprotein antigens. Clin Exp Immunol 76: 172–177, 1989.
48. Deutscher SL, Keene JD: A sequence-specific conformational epitope on U1 RNA is recognized by a unique autoantibody. Proc Natl Acad Sci U S A 85: 3299–3303, 1988.
49. Van Venrooij WJ, Hoet R, Castrop J, et al: Anti (U_1) small nuclear RNA antibodies in anti-small nuclear ribonucleoprotein sera from patients with connective tissue diseases. J Clin Invest 86: 2154–2160, 1990.
50. Hoet RM, Koornneef I, de Rooij DJ, et al: Changes in anti-U_1RNA antibody levels correlate with disease activity in patients with systemic lupus erythematosus overlap syndrome. Arthritis Rheum 35: 1202–1210, 1992.
51. Takeda Y, Wang GS, Wang RJ, et al: Enzyme-linked immunosorbent assay using isolated (U) small nuclear ribonucleoprotein polypeptides as antigens to investigate the clinical significance of autoantibodies to these polypeptides. Clin Immunol Immunopathol 50: 213–230, 1989.
52. Takano M, Golden SS, Sharp GC, et al: Molecular relationships between two nuclear antigens, ribonucleoprotein and Sm: purification of active antigens and their biochemical characterization. Biochemistry 20: 5929–5936, 1981.
53. Komatireddy GR, Wang GS, Sharp GC, et al: Antiphospholipid antibodies among anti-U1-70 kDa autoantibody positive patients with mixed connective tissue disease. J Rheumatol 24: 319–322, 1997.
54. Nakata S, Uematsu K, Mori T, et al: Effective treatment with low-dose methotrexate pulses of a child of mixed connective tissue disease with severe myositis refractory to corticosteroid. Nihon Rinsho Meneki Gakkai Kaishi 20: 178–183, 1997.
55. Tiddens HAWM, van der Net JJ, de Graeff-Meeder ER, et al: Juvenile-onset mixed connective tissue disease: longitudinal follow-up. J Pediatr 122: 191–197, 1993.
56. Kotajima L, Aotsuka S, Sumiya M, et al: Clinical features of patients with juvenile onset mixed connective tissue disease: analysis of data collected in a nationwide collaborative study in Japan. J Rheumatol 23: 1088–1094, 1996.
57. Mier R, Ansell B, Hall MA, et al: Long term follow-up of children with mixed connective tissue disease. Lupus 5: 221–226, 1996.
58. Yokota S, Imagawa T, Katakura S, et al: Mixed connective tissue disease in childhood: a nationwide retrospective study in Japan. Acta Paediatr Jpn 39: 273–276, 1997.
59. Michels H: Course of mixed connective tissue disease in children. Ann Med 29: 359–364, 1997.
60. Burdt MA, Hoffman RW, Deutscher SL, et al: Long-term outcome in mixed connective tissue disease: longitudinal clinical and serologic findings. Arthritis Rheum 42: 899–909, 1999.
61. Talal N: Sjögren's syndrome: historical overview and clinical spectrum of disease. Rheum Dis Clin North Am 18: 507–515, 1992.
62. Vitali C, Bombardieri S: Diagnostic criteria for Sjögren's syndrome: the state of the art. Clin Exp Rheumatol 8(Suppl 5): 13–16, 1990.
63. Vitali C, Bombardieri S, Moutsopoulos HM, et al: Preliminary criteria for the classification of Sjögren's syndrome. Results of a prospective concerted action supported by the European Community. Arthritis Rheum 36: 340–347, 1993.
64. Fox RI, Saito I: Criteria for diagnosis of Sjögren's syndrome. Rheum Dis Clin North Am 20: 391–407, 1994.
65. Vitali C, Moutsopoulos HM, Bombardieri S: The European Community Study Group on diagnostic criteria for Sjögren's syndrome. Sensitivity and specificity of tests for ocular and oral involvement in Sjögren's syndrome. Ann Rheum Dis 53: 637–647, 1994.
66. Thomas E, Hay EM, Hajeer A, Silman AJ: Sjögren's syndrome: a community-based study of prevalence and impact. Br J Rheumatol 37: 1069–1076, 1998.
67. Bartunkova J, Sediva A, Vencovsky J, et al: Primary Sjögren's syndrome in children and adolescents: proposal for diagnostic criteria. Clin Exp Rheumatol 17: 381–386, 1999.
68. Deprettere AJ, Van Acker KJ, De Clerck LS, et al: Diagnosis of Sjögren's syndrome in children. Am J Dis Child 142: 1185–1187, 1988.
69. Cosif C: Pathologie salivaire de l'enfant. Rev Stomatol Chir Maxillofac 77: 337–340, 1976.
70. Athreya BH, Norman ME, Myers AR, et al: Sjögren's syndrome in children. Pediatrics 59: 931–938, 1977.
71. Romero RW, Nesbitt LT, Ichinose H: Mikulicz disease and subsequent lupus erythematosus development. JAMA 237: 2507–2510, 1977.
72. Simila S, Kokkonen J, Kaski M, et al: Achalasia sicca: juvenile Sjögren's syndrome with achalasia and gastric hyposecretion. Eur J Pediatr 129: 175–181, 1978.
73. Chudwin DS, Daniels TE, Wara DW, et al: Spectrum of Sjögren syndrome in children. J Pediatr 98: 213–217, 1981.
74. Palcoux JB, Janin-Mercier A, Campagne D, et al: Sjögren's syndrome and lupus erythematosus nephritis. Arch Dis Child 59: 175–177, 1984.
75. Vermylen C, Meurant A, Noel H, et al: Sjögren's syndrome in a child. Eur J Pediatr 144: 266–269, 1985.
76. Siamopoulou-Mavridou A, Drosos AA, Andonopoulos AP: Sjögren syndrome in childhood: report of two cases. Eur J Pediatr 148: 523–524, 1989.
77. Rocha G, Kavalec C: Sjögren's syndrome in a child. Can J Ophthalmol 29: 234–237, 1994.
78. Bernstein BH, Koster-King K, Singsen BH, et al: Sjögren's syndrome in childhood. Arthritis Rheum 20: 361–362, 1977.
79. Krause A, Alarcón-Segovia D: Primary juvenile Sjögren's syndrome. J Rheumatol 15: 803–806, 1988.
80. Hara T, Nagata M, Mizuno Y, et al: Recurrent parotid swelling in children: clinical features useful for differential diagnosis of Sjögren's syndrome. Acta Paediatr 81: 547–549, 1992.
81. Fox RI, Michelson P, Törnwall J: Approaches to the treatment of Sjögren's syndrome. *In* Ruddy S, Harris ED Jr, Sledge CB, et al (eds): Kelley's Textbook of Rheumatology, 6th ed. Philadelphia, WB Saunders, 2000, pp 1027–1037.
82. Nathavitharana KA, Tarlow MJ, Bedi R, et al: Primary Sjögren's syndrome and rampant dental caries in a 5-year-old child. Intern Paediatr Dent 5: 173–176, 1995.

83. Mirante A, Salgado M, Moura L, et al: Hashimoto's thyroiditis and mixed connective tissue disease in an 11 year-old girl. Pediatr Endocrinol Metabol 10: 77–78, 1997.
84. Akin E, Tucker LB, Miller LC, et al: Splenic vasculitis in juvenile onset mixed connective tissue disease. J Rheumatol 25: 1444–1445, 1998.
85. Ohtsuka T, Saito Y, Hasegawa M, et al: Central nervous system disease in a child with primary Sjögren syndrome. J Pediatr 127: 961–963, 1995.
86. Niemela RK, Hakala M: Primary Sjögren's syndrome with severe central nervous system disease. Semin Arthritis Rheum 29: 4–13, 1999.
87. Ioannidis JP, Moutsopoulos HM: Sjögren's syndrome: too many associations, too limited evidence. The enigmatic example of CNS involvement. Semin Arthritis Rheum 29: 1–3, 1999.
88. Rojas-Rodriguez J, Garcia-Carrasco M, Ramirez ES, et al: Optic neuropathy in a child with primary Sjögren's syndrome. Rev Rhum Engl Ed 65: 355–357, 1998.
89. Leo-Kottler B, Klein R, Berg PA, et al: Ocular symptoms in association with antiphospholipid antibodies. Graefes Arch Clin Exp Ophthalmol 236: 658–668, 1998.
90. Tapinos NI, Polihronis M, Moutsopoulos HM: Lymphoma development in Sjögren's syndrome: novel p53 mutations. Arthritis Rheum 42: 1466–1472, 1999.
91. Daniels TE: Labial salivary gland biopsy in Sjögren's syndrome. Arthritis Rheum 27: 147–156, 1984.
92. Terreri MT, Andrade LE, Puccinelli ML, et al: Nail fold capillaroscopy: normal findings in children and adolescents. Semin Arthritis Rheum 29: 36–42, 1999.
93. Tektonidou M, Kaskani E, Skopouli FN, et al: Microvascular abnormalities in Sjögren's syndrome: nailfold capillaroscopy. Rheumatology (Oxford) 38: 826–830, 1999.
94. Tan EM: Antinuclear antibodies: diagnostic markers and clues to the basis of systemic autoimmunity. Pediatr Infect Dis J 7(5 Suppl): S3–S9, 1988.
95. Spath M, Kruger K, Dresel S, et al: Magnetic resonance imaging of the parotid gland in patients with Sjögren's syndrome. J Rheumatol 18: 1372–1378, 1991.
96. Provost TT, Watson R, Simmons-O'Brien E: Anti-Ro (SS-A) antibody positive Sjögren's/lupus erythematosus overlap syndrome. Lupus 6: 105–111, 1997.
97. Harley JB, Reichlin M, Arnett FC, et al: Gene interaction at HLA-DQ enhances autoantibody production in primary Sjögren's syndrome. Science 232: 1145–1147, 1986.
98. Reveille JD, Macleod MJ, Whittington K, et al: Specific amino acid residues in the second hypervariable region of HLA-DQA1 and DQB1 chain genes promote the Ro (SS-A)/La (SS-B) autoantibody responses. J Immunol 146: 3871–3876, 1991.
99. Harley JB, Scofield RH, Reichlen M: Anti-Ro in Sjögren's syndrome and systemic lupus erythematosus. Rheum Dis Clin North Am 18: 337–358, 1992.
100. Gattorno M, Buoncompagni A, Molinari AC, et al: Antiphospholipid antibodies in paediatric systemic lupus erythematosus, juvenile chronic arthritis and overlap syndromes: SLE patients with both lupus anticoagulant and high-titre anticardiolipin antibodies are at risk for clinical manifestations related to the antiphospholipid syndrome. Br J Rheumatol 34: 873–881, 1995.
101. Bloch KJ, Buchanan WW, Wohl MJ, et al: Sjögren's syndrome. A clinical, pathological, and serological study of sixty-two cases. Medicine (Baltimore) 44: 187–231, 1965.
102. Bell M, Askari A, Bookman A, et al: Sjögren's syndrome: a critical review of clinical management. J Rheumatol 26: 2051–2061, 1999.
103. Vivino FB, Al-Hashimi I, Khan Z, et al: Pilocarpine tablets for the treatment of dry mouth and dry eye symptoms in patients with Sjögren syndrome: a randomized, placebo-controlled, fixed-dose, multicenter trial. Arch Intern Med 159: 174–181, 1999.
104. Talal N (ed): Sjögren's syndrome: expanding concept and new treatment. J Rheumatol 27(Suppl 61): 1–21, 2000.

24

Uncommon Chronic Systemic Inflammatory Diseases

Anne-Marie Prieur and Ross E. Petty

This chapter discusses a number of unrelated chronic inflammatory diseases of unknown etiology. Many of them may, at least initially, be confused with systemic-onset juvenile rheumatoid arthritis. They include the chronic infantile neurologic, cutaneous, and articular (CINCA) syndrome, Castleman's disease, familial Mediterranean fever (FMF), the hyper-immunoglobulin D (IgD) syndrome, and the syndrome of periodic fever, aphthous stomatitis, pharyngitis, and adenitis (PFAPA).

CHRONIC INFANTILE NEUROLOGIC CUTANEOUS AND ARTICULAR SYNDROME

CINCA syndrome (also known as *neonatal-onset multisystem inflammatory disease*—NOMID) was probably described for the first time in 1950 as familial toxoplasmosis.[1] The propositus was a 19-year-old man with recurrent headaches, papilledema, deafness, a fixed rash, and polyarthritis. His mother and sister had the same disease. Since then, several publications[2–17] have documented the disorder in more than 30 patients and have permitted a more accurate and complete description of the syndrome.

Etiology, Pathogenesis, and Genetics

The etiology of the CINCA syndrome is obscure. There is evidence of systemic inflammation, but the main target organ, cartilage, does not appear to be inflamed. Instead, there is disordered growth of cartilage indicating that, at least in part, the syndrome has a genetic or metabolic basis. Serum from some patients with the CINCA syndrome has been reported to have a toxic effect on normal cartilage in vitro,[18] but the nature of this abnormality is unknown. The role of genetics is uncertain, although there have been some familial descriptions including the initial cases.[1] Siblings were reported later,[3] and one of us (AMP) is personally following four patients in two families. Consanguinity has not been observed. The disorder occurs with approximately equal frequency in males and females.

Clinical Manifestations

Perinatal Events

The symptoms and signs were usually present at birth. Half of the infants were born prematurely after uneventful pregnancies and had low birth weights. Umbilical cord anomalies were observed in a few children. In one, a histologic study of the placenta showed thickened vessel walls with thrombosis, microcalcifications, and infiltration by neutrophils. No infections were present in these infants.

Clinical Presentation

Patients with the CINCA syndrome have blond hair and a characteristic facial appearance of frontal bossing and a hypoplastic midface. In adults, a saddle nose is common. There is progressive growth retardation, and height often tracks below the 3rd percentile for age. The hands appear short and thick; in older patients, there may be clubbing of fingers and toes and a wrinkled appearance of the palms and soles. The CINCA syndrome is also characterized by the triad of rash, joint abnormalities, and central nervous system (CNS) involvement. These manifestations have been proposed as diagnostic criteria (Table 24–1).

Cutaneous Disease

A rash is present at birth in three quarters of affected infants and develops in others within the first few months of life (Fig. 24–1). It is characteristically nonpruritic and papular and varies in intensity from patient to patient, with time, and with disease activity. Histologically, the epidermis is normal and there is

Table 24–1

Proposed Diagnostic Criteria for CINCA Syndrome

A diagnosis of CINCA syndrome can be made in a patient with a persisting urticarial rash that is migrating, of variable intensity and often present at birth, plus at least one of the following:

- Symmetric arthropathy with epiphyseal and/or metaphyseal changes (early ossification of patella, with irregular ossification pattern and/or growth plate irregularities and/or irregular epiphyseal overgrowth)
- Chronic meningitis with neutrophils in the cerebrospinal fluid

CINCA, chronic infantile neurologic, cutaneous, and articular.

mild dermal inflammation and perivascular neutrophil infiltration.

Musculoskeletal Disease

Bone and joint involvement varies greatly. In approximately half of the patients, joint manifestations are limited to arthralgia and transient swelling without effusion during flare-ups. Such patients have no morning stiffness, no joint deformities, and normal-appearing radiographs on long-term follow-up. In the other half, however, joint abnormalities usually begin in the first year of life. The knees, ankles, wrists, and elbows are most commonly affected in a symmetric pattern, but small joints can also be involved. The metaphyses and epiphyses of long bones are affected, resulting in marked "overgrowth" of the joint, articular and bone pain, and loss of range of motion. Patellar overgrowth can result in a gross deformity of the knee (Fig. 24–2).

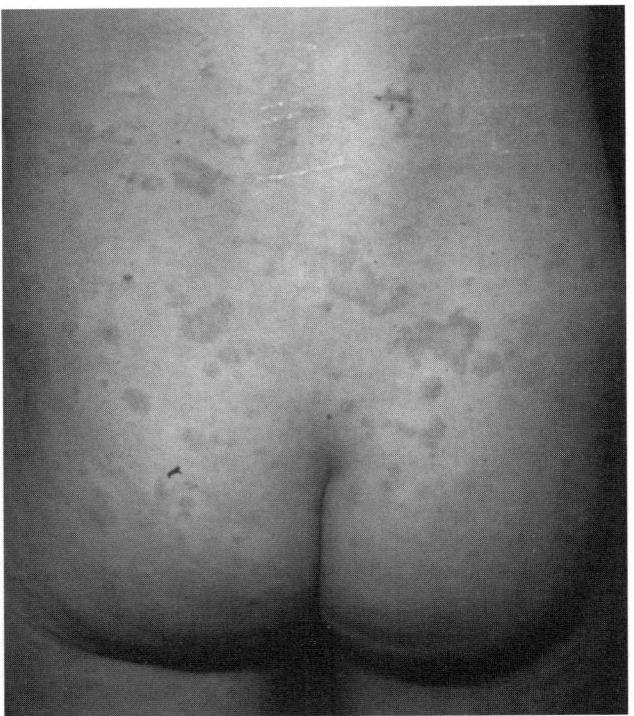

Figure 24–1. The rash of the chronic infantile neurologic, cutaneous, and articular (CINCA) syndrome. The appearance of the rash is variable both in character and in severity. It usually appears within the first few months of life.

Radiologic manifestations, when present, are distinctive.[11] The most characteristic changes occur in the metaphyses and epiphyses (Fig. 24–3). The principal findings are overgrowth of the epiphyses with irregularity of ossification. There may be bowing, shortening, and widening of long bones with a periosteal reaction. There may also be multiple erosions around the phalanges and metacarpals.[14] Disordered cartilage growth can result in an irregular, tumor-like appearance. There is complete disorganization of cartilage histology with disturbance of the normal orderly columns of chondrocytes, and irregular metachromatic coloration of the ground substance, but no inflammatory cells.

Central Nervous System Disease

Abnormalities of the CNS are present in almost all patients.[15] Chronic headaches, sometimes with vomiting and seizures, result from chronic meningeal inflammation. Spastic diplegia may develop. Progressive cognitive impairment occurs in some patients. The skull is slightly increased in size, and there is delayed closure of the anterior fontanelle. Computed tomography or magnetic resonance imaging often demonstrates mild ventricular dilatation and enlarged subdural fluid spaces, suggesting mild cerebral atrophy. Some patients have progressive calcifications of the falx cerebri and dura mater.

Sensory Abnormalities

Abnormalities of the eyes occur in 90 percent of patients.[17] Ocular disease consists of anterior uveitis in half and posterior uveitis in another 20 percent. The most striking abnormalities are papilledema and optic atrophy in more than 80 percent of patients. Ocular manifestations can progress to blindness, and one patient in four has a significant ocular disability. Perceptive deafness (in varying degrees) is present in older patients. Hoarseness of the voice is frequent.

Laboratory Examination

There are nonspecific indications of inflammation, with hypochromic anemia, leukocytosis (with a predominance of neutrophils and eosinophils), thrombocytosis, and an increase in the erythrocyte sedimentation rate (ESR) and acute-phase reactants.[2, 12, 13] A polyclonal increase in immunoglobulin levels is present in all patients. The frequency of antinuclear antibodies is not increased; rheumatoid factor tests are seldom positive.[7] No specific immunodeficiency has been reported. Synovial fluid contains a few neutrophils, but the findings are nonspecific. The cerebrospinal fluid is usually char-

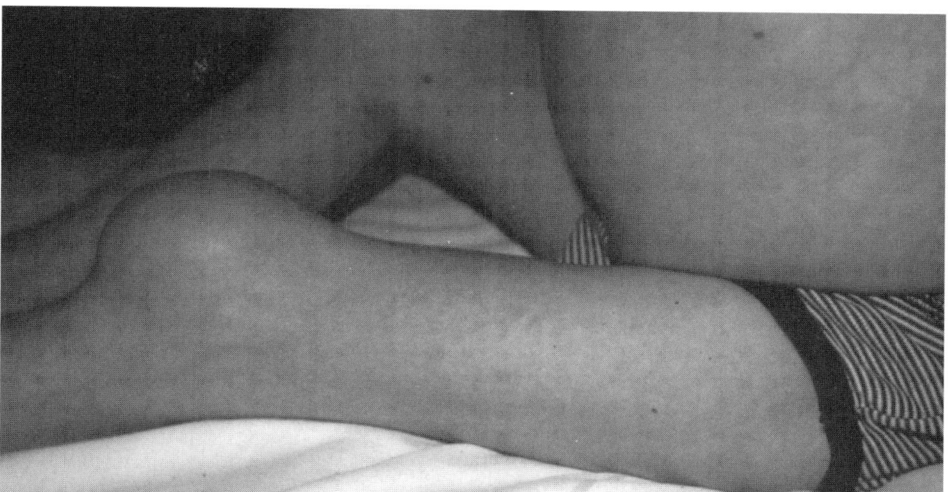

Figure 24–2. The large knee reflects in part the enlarged patella in this child with arthritis associated with CINCA. Note also the flexion contracture, loss of muscle bulk, the distended abdomen, and rash.

acterized by an increased protein level and the presence of neutrophils.

Treatment

No therapeutic approach has been effective in altering the course of disease. Treatment is aimed at minimizing symptoms. Nonsteroidal anti-inflammatory drugs (NSAIDs) provide some pain relief. Glucocorticoids may be partially effective in management of the rash. Immunosuppressive and disease-modifying drugs have been ineffective in the experience of one of us (AMP). Physiotherapy may improve the functional status in patients with chronic arthropathy.

Course of the Disease and Prognosis

The course is one of persisting chronic inflammation with relapsing fever, progressive joint deformity, and CNS deterioration.[12, 15] Some patients reach adulthood, however. Death results from leukemia (possibly related to immunosuppressive therapy),[5] necrotizing leukoencephalopathy,[4] sepsis,[6] or secondary amyloidosis.[12]

FAMILIAL MEDITERRANEAN FEVER

FMF is a periodic disease of unknown etiology. The diagnostic criteria most frequently used are listed in Table 24–2.

Epidemiology

FMF is common in countries surrounding the eastern Mediterranean and is particularly frequent in Sephardic and Iraqi Jews, Armenians, and Levantine Arabs.[19] It is rare in most areas of North American and in northern Europeans. The disease is slightly more com-

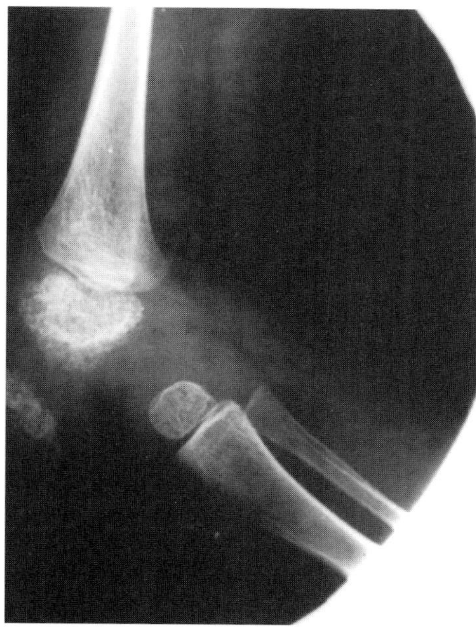

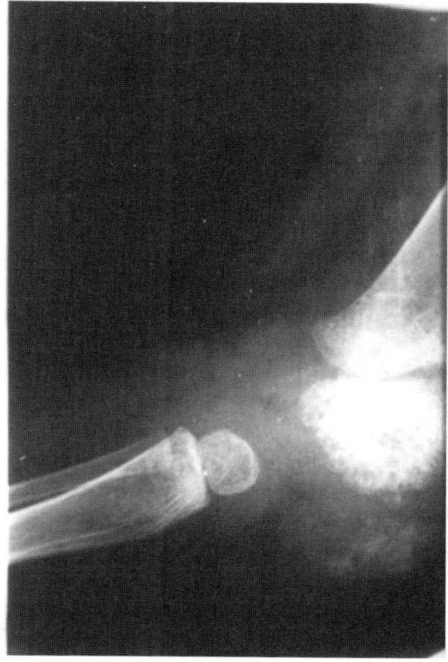

Figure 24–3. Radiographic enlargement and irregularity of calcification of the metaphyses and epiphyses around the knee in a child with CINCA. Histologically, there is disordered cartilage growth in these sites.

Table 24–2

Familial Mediterranean Fever (FMF): Diagnostic Criteria

Major Criteria

1. Recurrent febrile episodes accompanied by peritonitis, synovitis, or pleuritis
2. Amyloidosis of the AA-type without predisposing disease
3. Favorable response to continuous colchicine treatment

Minor Criteria

1. Recurrent febrile episodes
2. Erysipelas-like erythema
3. FMF in a first-degree relative

Definite FMF: 2 major criteria or 1 major and 2 minor criteria
Probable FMF: 1 major and 1 minor criterion

From Pras M, Kastner DL: Familial mediterranean fever. *In* Klippel JH, Dieppe PA (eds): Rheumatology, 2nd ed. St. Louis, Mosby, 1998, pp 5-23-1 to 5-23-4.

mon in boys than in girls.[20] Most patients with FMF experience onset of clinical disease in childhood.

Genetics and Etiology

FMF is strongly familial, and inheritance is autosomal recessive. Estimates of carrier frequency in the Mediterranean population range from 1 in 5 to 1 in 16.[21] The gene responsible for this disease is located on chromosome 16 (16p13.3).[22] Its product (pyrin or marenostrin) is expressed predominantly by polymorphonuclear leukocytes and myeloid bone marrow precursors. At least 28 mutations have been identified.

Clinical Manifestations

Typical episodes of FMF are characterized by fever, abdominal or pleuropericardial pain, arthritis, or cutaneous erythema about the ankles (Table 24–3). An attack begins abruptly and lasts for 12 to 72 hours before slowly subsiding. These episodes occur at intervals of days to months; between attacks, the patients are asymptomatic. Symptoms usually start between 5 and 15 years of age but may start in infancy.

Table 24–3

Familial Mediterranean Fever: Clinical and Other Characteristics

Clinical characteristics	Acute, self-limited episodes of fever, peritonitis, pleuritis, arthritis and dermatitis; onset < 15 years of age in two thirds of patients
Genetics	Autosomal recessive; defective gene at chromosome 16p13.3
Laboratory abnormalities	Abnormal acute-phase reactants; no specific diagnostic test
Complications	Amyloidosis
Treatment	Colchicine

Abdominal Pain

Abdominal pain caused by inflammation of the peritoneum is a manifestation of FMF in almost all patients. It varies in intensity from generalized or localized aching to severe peritonitis with direct and rebound tenderness and paralytic ileus. The abdominal pain usually runs its course in 24 to 72 hours, but may mimic an acute surgical abdomen. Occasionally, inflammation of the tunica vaginalis results in pain and swelling of the scrotum that may be misdiagnosed as testicular torsion.[23]

Pleuropericardial Pain

Pleuritis causes unilateral or bilateral chest pain in 25 to 50 percent of patients. These symptoms last for 24 to 72 hours before abating. A small pleural effusion (usually unilateral) may be present. Clinically evident pericarditis is rare, although when it occurs it may be complicated by tamponade.[24] Echocardiographic evidence of pericarditis has been noted in approximately 25 percent of patients.[25]

Arthritis

Joint symptoms include arthralgias, recurrent oligoarthritis, and (in approximately 5 percent of patients) prolonged chronic arthritis. Swelling and pain are prominent, but erythema and increased heat are absent. Residual joint damage is most serious in the hips, where secondary degenerative arthritis may develop. As a general rule, radiographs show juxta-articular osteoporosis but no evidence of erosive disease. The sacroiliac joints are occasionally involved.[26, 27] Severe prolonged myalgia may occur.[28]

Several patterns of arthritis were observed in a group of 133 children with FMF followed for a mean of 5.5 years.[26] Monarthritis affecting the knee or ankle occurred in 71 percent; arthritis in both knees or both ankles in 18 percent; JRA-like symmetric polyarthritis in 4 percent; and asymmetric oligoarthritis in 4 percent. Between attacks, the joints were normal. The overall outcome was good, except for residual damage in the hip joint of one patient and the shoulder joint in another.

Cutaneous Lesions

A highly characteristic "erysipelas-like" lesion develops in 20 percent of children with FMF.[29] These well-demarcated, tender, swollen, erythematous lesions range from 5 to 15 cm in diameter and occur most frequently around the ankle or on the dorsum of the foot. Purpura and other types of lesions have also been reported.[26, 29] In the series of Saatci and colleagues,[20] Henoch-Schönlein purpura developed in 2 percent; polyarteritis nodosa occurred with a similar frequency.

Differential Diagnosis

Other forms of periodic disease have been described by Reimann.[30] Their relation to FMF is unclear. A syndrome that resembles FMF, except in its mode of inheritance (which is autosomal dominant), has been reported in three members of a family in two successive generations.[31] Although the clinical presentation strongly resembled FMF, the attacks were more persistent, lasting up to 5 weeks and recurring every 6 to 24 months. Miller and Emery described a syndrome of migrating arthritis in unrelated children of nonconsanguinous Assyrian ancestry living in California.[32] These children had protracted courses of arthritis in the ankle or knee, with a proliferative synovium and rapid destruction of bone and cartilage in affected joints. Although this syndrome resembles FMF, the articular outcome is usually severe and other features of FMF are lacking in most patients. With the identification of the genetic mutations responsible for FMF, such patients can now be re-evaluated and the relationship to FMF clarified. The hyper-IgD syndrome should also be considered in the differential diagnosis (see later).

Pathology and Laboratory Examination

The inflammatory cells in the synovial, cutaneous, and visceral lesions are characteristically polymorphonuclear. Similarly, the synovial fluid cell count may range from a few hundred to a million cells per cubic millimeter, depending on the severity of the attack, and consists predominantly of neutrophils. Inflammatory indices are elevated. Autoantibodies are absent.

Treatment

Colchicine, which inhibits leukocyte chemotaxis, is effective in treating or aborting the acute, recurrent exacerbations of the disease and in preventing amyloidosis.[33–36] Colchicine is given throughout life in a dose of 1 to 2 mg/day regardless of weight.[37] Although diarrhea, nausea, bone marrow suppression, and other dose-related short-term complications may occur, significant long-term sequelae to chronic colchicine therapy appear to be rare. Two children with reversible myoneuropathy have been reported, however.[38] NSAIDs may be required for symptomatic management of the musculoskeletal symptoms.

Course of the Disease and Prognosis

The outcome of FMF is determined largely by the occurrence of amyloidosis, which in turn is related in part to ethnic origin (Sephardic Jews are most susceptible) and to inadequate treatment with colchicine. In patients treated with colchicine, however, the incidence of amyloidosis is low (2 to 3 percent). In a Turkish series, amyloidosis occurred in 32 children and was somewhat more common in boys than in girls.[20] Amyloidosis accompanying FMF in children in North America is very rare. Amyloidosis primarily affects the kidney, leading to the nephrotic syndrome and eventually to end-stage renal disease.[39, 40] It uncommonly results in splenomegaly or affects the gastrointestinal tract, heart, or adrenal glands. The diagnosis of amyloidosis is confirmed by demonstration of the AA protein on a rectal biopsy specimen by immunofluorescence microscopy or Congo red stains.

CASTLEMAN'S DISEASE

Castleman's disease, also called *angiofollicular lymph node hyperplasia*, is a histologically well-defined disorder with a widely divergent clinical spectrum.[41] There are two main clinical forms, *localized* and *multicentric*. Localized Castleman's disease is usually observed in young patients; the multicentric form occurs in older persons and is often associated with other systemic disorders (Tables 24–4; and 24–5).

Epidemiology and Genetics

Castleman's disease is rare; 83 cases were identified in the pediatric literature in a 1999 review.[42] The disease was somewhat more common in females and had an onset between 2 months and 17 years of age, with 14 percent of cases occurring before 4 years of age, a further 14 percent with onset between 4 and 10 years of age, and the remaining 72 percent with onset between 10 and 17 years of age. Eighty-seven percent of patients had the localized form. Familial cases were not noted.

Etiology and Pathogenesis

The etiology of Castleman's disease is unknown; although infection with Epstein-Barr virus[43] or herpesvi-

Table 24–4

Comparison of Localized and Multicentric Castleman's Disease

	LOCALIZED	MULTICENTRIC
Mean age (yr)	20	57
Fever	+	+ +
Anemia	+	+ +
Polyclonal hypergammaglobulinemia	+	+ +
Lymph-node location	Internal	Peripheral
Visceral manifestations	Absent	Frequent
Autoimmune manifestations	Absent	Possible
Associated diseases	Absent	Frequent
Treatment	Surgery	Glucocorticoids Cytotoxics

Table 24–5

Diseases Associated With Multicentric Castleman's Disease

Kaposi's sarcoma	Sjögren's syndrome
AIDS	Mixed connective tissue disease
Malignant lymphoma	Neurofibromatosis
Rheumatoid arthritis	Pheochromocytoma

rus type 8[44] has been suspected, confirmation is lacking. The pathogenesis of Castleman's disease, particularly in the localized form, is related to increased levels of circulating interleukin (IL)-6, IL-8, IL-1β, tumor necrosis factor α (TNF-α), IL-1Ra, and TNF-Rp75, which return to normal after surgical removal of the affected tissue.[45] IL-6 gene expression is very high in the interfollicular areas of lymph nodes but is expressed within the follicles only in the localized disease with systemic manifestations.[46]

Clinical Manifestations

Almost one fourth of children with Castleman's disease have no symptoms, and the diagnosis is made fortuitously.[42] Systemic symptoms occur in almost one half and include fever, failure to thrive, weight loss, fatigue, and pain. In one quarter, the presenting complaint is the presence of a slowly growing mass, which occurs in the peripheral lymph nodes in one third, in the abdomen in another third, and in the chest in the remainder. In the series of Parez and colleagues,[42] two patients also had glomerulonephritis. Castleman's disease has been noted in a number of rheumatic diseases, including rheumatoid arthritis,[47] sicca syndrome,[48] and mixed connective tissue disease.[49]

Laboratory Examination

Evidence of inflammation (elevated ESR, elevated immunoglobulins, anemia, hypoalbuminemia) is more common in children with multicentric Castleman's disease. Autoantibodies are not detected.

Diagnosis and Pathology

In the localized forms, the affected lymph node may be in the abdomen (mostly retroperitoneal) or the thoracic or cervical regions. The condition may be difficult to localize and requires careful diagnostic studies with ultrasound imaging, magnetic resonance imaging, and radionuclide scanning.

There are two characteristic histologic patterns, which sometimes overlap. The *hyaline vascular type* has well-preserved lymph-node architecture with germinal centers often traversed by a thick-walled blood vessel surrounded by a cuff of concentrically arranged lymphocytes, giving an "onion ring" appearance. The *plasma-cell type* of morphology is characterized by large follicles with preserved node architecture and dilated sinuses. There is massive plasma-cell infiltration of the interfollicular areas. Both types of histology can be observed in localized and multicentric forms of the diseases.

Management

The key to management is localization of the affected node or nodes and their surgical excision. Rapid resolution of symptoms follows. The efficacy of interferon-α therapy has been suggested in some reports,[50, 51] and the possible association with human herpesvirus 8 raises the prospect of therapy with anti-herpesvirus drugs.[52]

Course of the Disease and Prognosis

The prognosis is generally good with the localized form, in which surgical removal of the mass leads to the disappearance of all symptoms.[45, 53–55] The prognosis in the multicentric forms depends on the underlying associated disease.[47–49, 56] Surgical excision of the lesion may result in resolution of systemic reactive amyloidosis associated with localized Castleman's disease.[57]

HYPER-IgD SYNDROME (RECURRENT FEVER WITH ELEVATED IgD)

The clinical characteristics of this syndrome were described in eight French children in 1983.[58] Although resembling FMF, this disease is distinguishable from FMF, as stressed in a study of six patients of Dutch ancestry and 44 patients reported previously.[59] A comprehensive description of the spectrum of this disorder has therefore emerged.[60, 61] An increased serum level of IgD is by definition necessary to make the diagnosis. However, this increase in IgD is not pathognomic because increases in IgD can occur in other disorders and the significance of such increases is not yet established.

Genetic Background

In some families, several siblings were affected, indicating an autosomal recessive mode of transmission of this disease. Mutations of the gene encoding mevalonate kinase have been identified in this syndrome and differ from the genetic mutations responsible for FMF.[62, 63]

Clinical Manifestations

Most reported patients are of European ancestry. The first symptoms are recognized in childhood before the age of 10 years; in two thirds of the patients, symptoms

Table 24–6

Characteristics of Hyper-IqD Syndrome

General

High IgD (>100 U/ml on two occasions at least 1 month apart)
Elevated IgA (>2.6 g/L)
Recurrent attacks

During Attacks

Elevated erythrocyte sedimentation rate and white blood cell count
Abrupt onset of fever (>38°C)
Cervical lymphadenopathy
Abdominal distress
  Vomiting
  Diarrhea
  Pain
Rash
Arthralgia, arthritis
Splenomegaly

Adapted from Drenth JPH, Haagsma CJ, Vander Meer JW, et al: Hyperimmunoglobulinemia D and periodic fever syndrome. The clinical spectrum in a series of 50 patients. Medicine 73: 133, 1994.

occur during the first year of life. The clinical features described by Drenth and associates[60] are summarized in Table 24–6. Premonitory symptoms of pharyngitis, headache, fatigue, and irritability are frequent. Fever starts abruptly, often accompanied by chills, reaching 40°C within a few hours, and remaining elevated for 3 to 7 days. In half of the cases, a febrile attack is triggered by antigen stimulation such as vaccination, viral infection, or immunoglobulin administration. During the febrile period, arthralgia is common; in two thirds of the patients, transient nondestructive arthritis with objective joint swelling is observed.

Abdominal pain with diarrhea and vomiting is frequent. The severity of the abdominal manifestations, together with the presence of fever, has led to celiotomy in some patients, documenting the presence of lymphadenopathy and adhesions, which may be the result of peritoneal inflammation.[60] Cutaneous manifestations are frequent during attacks.[61] Erythematous macules and papules, urticarial lesions, and nodular lesions may occur. Tender, enlarged lymph nodes, usually cervical in location, occur during attacks.

Laboratory Examination

During an attack, evidence of inflammation is documented by an increased ESR, leucocytosis, thrombocytosis, and increased acute-phase reactants. Between attacks, these abnormalities disappear. There are no known autoantibodies, complement levels are normal, and no immunodeficiency has been identified. By definition, IgD serum levels are increased, but hyper-IgD can also occur in other conditions such as immune deficiencies,[64, 65] during chemotherapy for cancer,[66] in Hodgkin's disease,[67] and in healthy subjects.[64] The level of IgD does not correlate with the intensity of the clinical disease. IgG and IgM levels are usually in the normal range or only slightly increased; however, most patients have increased levels of IgA. Mevalonic acid can be detected in the urine during episodes of disease activity.[63]

Cytokine abnormalities have also been documented. IgD induces in vitro release of IL-1β and IL-1Ra, but not TNF-α, by monocytes.[69] Increased interferon-γ levels were observed during febrile episodes as well as increased urine neopterin excretion, reflecting activation of cellular immunity.[68] During attacks, ex vivo production of TNF-α, IL-1β and IL-1Ra is significantly increased, suggesting that monocytes/macrophages are already primed in vivo to produce increased levels of these cytokines. Circulating IL-6 levels are high during attacks, correlating with the levels of C-reactive protein. The levels of the anti-inflammatory cytokines IL-1Ra, sTNF-Rp55, and sTNF-Rp75 are higher during febrile attacks.[70] These findings indicate an activation of the cytokine network, possibly correlated with the effect of IgD on the monocytes/macrophages.

The subject of hyper-IgD syndrome and *mevalonate kinase deficiency* has been recently reviewed by Frenkel and colleagues.[71] More than 150 patients with hyper-IgD syndrome have been diagnosed, half of whom are Dutch, and one quarter of whom are French. Almost all patients have polyclonal elevation of serum IgD levels at some time during the disease course, although it may be normal for up to 3 years in young children. At least 2 children with this syndrome have had persistently normal IgD levels, however. Mevalonate kinase levels are 1 to 7 percent of normal in fibroblasts and leukocytes of patients with this syndrome. As a result of the enzyme deficiency, mevalonic acid levels increase in the urine, especially with febrile episodes. The mutations responsible for the defective enzyme occur on chromosome 12q24.

Prognosis and Treatment

Attacks generally decrease in intensity with time; however, the interval between attacks varies from patient to patient. Therapeutic attempts are disappointing. In some cases, low-dose glucocorticoids can reduce clinical symptoms, particularly arthritis. Intravenous immunoglobulins have no effect. Secondary amyloidosis has not been observed. The frequency of attacks decreases during pregnancy and the offspring of affected women are normal.[72]

PERIODIC FEVER, APHTHOUS STOMATITIS, PHARYNGITIS, AND ADENITIS (PFAPA SYNDROME)

In 1987, Marshall and coworkers described a group of 12 children with unexplained periodic fever, pharyngitis, and aphthous stomatitis.[73] The fever was preceded by chills and rose to more than 40°C. The main clinical signs were cervical adenopathy, aphthous stomatitis, pharyngitis, headaches, and abdominal pain with vomiting. During the attacks, laboratory studies showed an elevated ESR and leukocytosis. All signs and symp-

Table 24–7

Criteria used for Diagnosis of Periodic Fever, Aphthous Stomatitis, Pharyngitis, and Adenitis

Regularly recurring fevers with onset < 5 yr of age
Constitutional symptoms in the absence of upper respiratory infection with at least one of the following clinical signs:
  Aphthous stomatitis
  Cervical lymphadenitis
  Pharyngitis
Exclusion of cyclic neutropenia
Completely asymptomatic interval between episodes
Normal growth and development

Adapted from Abramson JS, Givner LB, Thompson JN: Possible role of tonsillectomy and adenoidectomy in children with recurrent fever and tonsillopharyntitis. Pediatr Infect Dis J 8: 119, 1989.

toms disappeared between attacks. Although the authors excluded the possibility of hyper-IgD syndrome because the IgD levels were normal, the similarities with that syndrome are striking. This syndrome lasted from 1 to 15 years and may be confused with systemic-onset juvenile rheumatoid arthritis.[74–76]

Subsequently, there have been two large series of patients with this syndrome,[77, 78] and diagnostic criteria have been proposed[78] (Table 24–7). Arthralgia is reported in a minority of patients in some series[77] but has not been noted in others.[78] The etiology is unknown, and the pathogenesis is obscure.[79] The syndrome does not appear to be of infectious origin.

A variety of treatments have been used.[79] NSAIDs are of limited benefit. Acyclovir and colchicine are ineffective. Cimetidine may be useful in up to 50 percent of patients.[80] Most patients respond symptomatically to prednisone. Tonsillectomy and adenoidectomy has also been reported as effective therapy.[81]

RECURRENT INFLAMMATORY SYNDROMES

A familial syndrome of periodic fever associated with a mutation of the TNF receptor 1 (TNFR1) has been described.[82] TNFR1 levels in plasma were approximately half of normal. The mechanism proposed for this febrile syndrome is diminished shedding of the TNFR1 into the soluble phase, thereby allowing TNF to bind to cell-bound receptors. It is inherited as an autosomal dominant disorder.

Familial Hibernian fever, a rare autosomal dominant disorder, has been reported in only a few families of Irish or Scottish origin. Intermittent febrile attacks, abdominal pain, and myalgia are common. Episodes of rash, conjunctivitis, and unilateral periorbital edema also occur.[83] The defect in familial Hibernian fever has been mapped to chromosome 12p13.[84] Reviews of familial periodic fevers have recently been published.[85, 86]

References

1. Campbell AMG, Clifton F: Adult toxoplasmosis in one family. Brain 73: 281, 1950.
2. Lorber J: Syndrome for diagnosis. Proc R Soc Med 66: 1070, 1973.
3. Ansell BM, Bywaters EGL, Elderkin FM: Familial arthropathy with rash, uveitis, and mental retardation. Proc R Soc Med 68: 584, 1975.
4. Lampert F, Belohradsky BH, Forster C, et al: Infantile chronic relapsing inflammation of the brain, skin and joints. Lancet 1:1250, 1975.
5. Prieur AM, Griscelli C: Arthropathy with rash, chronic meningitis, eye lesions and mental retardation. J Pediatr 99: 79, 1981.
6. Farjardo JE, Geller TJ, Koenig HM, et al: Chronic meningitis, polyarthritis, lymphadenitis and pulmonary hemosiderosis. J Pediatr 101: 738, 1982.
7. Hassink SG, Goldsmith DJ: Neonatal onset multisystem inflammatory disease. Arthritis Rheum 26: 668, 1983.
8. Yarom A, Rennebohm RM, Levinson JE: Infantile multisystem inflammatory disease: a specific syndrome? J Pediatr 106: 390, 1985.
9. Lovell DJ, Kaufman R, Brewer EF, et al: Radiographic manifestations of infantile onset multisystem inflammatory disease. Arthritis Rheum 29: 525, 1986.
10. Goldsmith DP, Dent PB, Lishner HW, et al: Neonatal onset multisystemic inflammatory disease (NOMID): long term follow-up. Arthritis Rheum 29: 567, 1986.
11. Kaufman RA, Lovell DJ: Infantile-onset multisystem inflammatory disease: radiologic findings. Radiology 160: 741, 1986.
12. Prieur AM, Griscelli C, Lampert F, et al: A chronic, infantile, neurological cutaneous and articular (CINCA) syndrome. A specific entity analyzed in 30 patients. Scand J Rheumatol 66: 57, 1987.
13. Mallouh A, Abu-Osba YK, Talar Y: Infantile-onset arthritis and multisystem inflammatory disease: a new syndrome. J Pediatr Orthop 7: 227, 1987.
14. Brueton LA, Sanderson IR, Jadresi C, et al: An infant with chronic articular and cutaneous manifestations: a new syndrome? J R Soc Med 82: 223, 1989.
15. Torbiak RP, Dent PB, Cockshott WP: NOMID, a neonatal syndrome of multisystem inflammation. Skeletal Radiol 81: 359, 1989.
16. Huttenlocher A, Frieden IJ, Emery H: Neonatal onset multisystem inflammatory disease. J Rheumatol 22: 1171, 1995.
17. Dollfus H, Häfner R, Hofmann HM, et al: Chronic infantile neurological and articular/neonatal onset multisystem inflammatory disease syndrome: ocular manifestations in a recently recognized chronic inflammatory disease of childhood. Arch Ophthalmol 118:1396, 2000.
18. Prieur AM, Cournot-Witmer G, Plachot JJ, et al: In vitro study of growth cartilage in children with the infantile onset neurologic, cutaneous and articular syndrome. Inhibitory effect of patient's sera on cultured normal chondrocyte metabolism. Arthritis Rheum 31: 578, 1988.
19. Sohar E, Gafni J, Pras M, et al: Familial Mediterranean fever. Am J Med 43: 227, 1967.
20. Saatci U, Ozen S, Ozdemir S, et al: Familial Mediterranean fever in children: report of a large series and discussion of the risk and prognostic factors of amyloidosis. Eur J Pediatr 156: 619, 1997.
21. Daniels M, Shohar T, Brennar-Ullman A, Shohar M: Familial Mediterranean fever: high gene frequency among the non-Ashkenazy and Ashkenazic Jewish populations in Israel. Am J Med Genet 55: 311, 1995.
22. Pras E, Aksentijevich I, Gruberg L, et al: Mapping of a gene causing familial Mediterranean fever to the short arm or chromosome 16. N Engl J Med 326: 1509, 1992.
23. Eshel G, Vinograd I, Barr J, Zemer D: Acute scrotal pain complicating familial Mediterranean fever in children. Br J Surg 81: 894, 1994.
24. Zimand S, Tauber T, Hegesch T, Aladjem M: Familial Mediterranean fever presenting with massive cardiac tamponade. Clin Exp Rheumatol 12: 67, 1994.
25. Dabestani A, Noble LM, Child JS, et al: Pericardial disease in familial Mediterranean fever. An echocardiographic study. Chest 81: 592, 1982.
26. Majeed HA, Rawashdeh M: The clinical patterns of arthritis in children with familial Mediterranean fever. Q J Med 90: 37, 1997.
27. Lehman TJA, Hanson V, Kornreich H, et al: HLA-B27–negative sacroiliitis: a manifestation of familial Mediterranean fever in childhood. Pediatrics 61: 423, 1978.

28. Langevitz P, Zemer D, Livneh A, et al: Protracted febrile myalgia in patients with familial Mediterranean fever. J Rheumatol 21: 1708, 1994.
29. Gedalia A, Adar A, Gorodischer R: Familial Mediterranean fever in children. J Rheumatol 19(Suppl 35): 1, 1992.
30. Reimann HR: Periodic disease: a probable syndrome including periodic fever, benign paroxysmal peritonitis, cyclic neutropenia and intermittent arthralgia. JAMA 136: 239, 1948.
31. Mache CJ, Goriup U, Fischel-Ghodsian N, et al: Autosomal dominant familial Mediterranean fever–like syndrome. Eur J Pediatr 155: 787, 1996.
32. Miller JJ III, Emery HM: Migrating monopredominant arthritis in children of Assyrian ancestry. J Rheumatol 23: 178, 1996.
33. Lerner D, Revach M, Pras M, et al: A controlled trial of colchicine in preventing attacks of familial Mediterranean fever. N Engl J Med 291: 93, 1974.
34. Ben-Chetrit E, Levy M: Colchicine prophylaxis in familial Mediterranean fever: reappraisal after 15 years. Semin Arthritis Rheum 20: 241, 1991.
35. Zemer D, Livneh A, Danon YL, et al: Long-term colchicine treatment in children with familial Mediterranean fever. Arthritis Rheum 34: 973, 1991.
36. Lehman TJA, Peters RS, Hanson V, et al: Long-term colchicine therapy of familial Mediterranean fever. J Pediatr 93: 876, 1978.
37. Arav-Boger R, Spirer Z: Periodic syndromes of childhood. Adv Pediatr 44: 389, 1997.
38. Harel L, Mukamel M, Amir J, et al: Colchicine-induced myoneuropathy in childhood. Eur J Pediatr 157: 853, 1998.
39. Ludominsky A, Passwell J, Boichis H: Amyloidosis in children with familial Mediterranean fever. Arch Dis Child 56: 464, 1981.
40. Bakir F, Murtadha M, Issa N: Amyloidosis and periodic peritonitis (familial Mediterranean fever). West J Med 131: 193, 1979.
41. D'Agay MF, Miclea JM, Clauvel JP, et al: Castleman's disease: a well defined histological pattern for a widely divergent clinical spectrum. Nouv Rev Fr Hematol 31: 145, 1989.
42. Parez N, Bader-Meunier B, Roy CC, Dommergues JP: Paediatric Castleman disease: report of seven cases and review of the literature. Eur J Pediatr 158: 631, 1999.
43. Murray PG, Deacon E, Young LS, et al: Localization of Epstein-Barr virus in Castleman's disease by in situ hybridization and immunocytochemistry. Hematol Pathol 9: 17, 1995.
44. Gaidano G, Castanos-Velez E, Biberfeld P: Lymphoid disorders associated with HHV-8/KSHV infection: facts and contentions. Med Oncol 16: 8, 1999.
45. Herbelin C, Roux-Lombard P, Herbelin A, et al: Inflammation: a new natural experiment on the systemic pathogenicity of cytokines. Eur Cytokine Rev 9: 57, 1998.
46. Leger-Ravet MB, Peuchmaur M, Devergne O, et al: Interleukin-6 gene expression in Castleman's disease. Blood 78: 2923, 1991.
47. Ben-Chetrit E, Flusser D, Okon E, et al: Multicentric Castleman's disease associated with rheumatoid arthritis: a possible role of hepatitis B antigen. Ann Rheum Dis 48: 326, 1989.
48. Kingsmore SF, Silva OE, Hall BD, et al: Presentation of multicentric Castleman's disease with sicca syndrome, cardiomyopathy, palmar and plantar rash. J Rheumatol 20: 1588, 1993.
49. Nanki T, Tomioyama J, Arai S: Mixed connective tissue disease associated with multicentric Castleman's disease. Scand J Rheumatol 23: 215, 1994.
50. Tamayo M, Gonzalez C, Majado MJ, et al: Long-term complete remission after interferon treatment in a case of multicentric Castleman's disease. Am J Hematol 49: 359, 1995.
51. Stoha R, Tschachler E, Breyer S, et al: Reactivation of Behçet's disease in the course of multicentric HHV8-positive Castleman's disease: long-term complete remission by a combined chemoradiation and interferon-alpha therapy regimen. Br J Hematol 104: 788, 1998.
52. Boulanger E: Human herpes virus 8 (HHV8): II. Pathogenic role and sensitivity to antiviral drugs. Ann Biol Clin 57: 19, 1999.
53. el Messaoudi A, el Edghiri H, Lazraka M, et al: La maladie de Castleman. A propos de deux localizations cervicales. Rev Laryngol Oto Rhinol 114: 189, 1993.
54. Gheyssens B, Baste JC, Midy D, et al: Retroperitoneal Castleman disease. A propos of a new case. J Chir 131: 492, 1994.
55. Winter SS, Howard TA, Ritchey AK, et al: Elevated levels of tumor necrosis factor-beta, gamma-interferon, and IL-6 mRNA in Castelman's disease. Med Pediatr Oncol 26: 48: 1996.
56. Brouet JC, Levy Y: IL-6 and lymphoproliferative disorders. Nouv Rev Fr Hematol 33: 433, 1991.
57. Ikeda S, Chisuwa H, Kawasaki S, et al: Systemic reactive amyloidosis associated with Castleman's disease: serial changes of the concentration of acute phase serum amyloid A and interleukin 6 in serum. J Clin Pathol 50: 965, 1997.
58. Prieur AM, Griscelli C: Aspects nosologiques des formes systemiques d'arthrite chronique juvenile à début très précoce. A propos de dix sept observations. Ann Pediatr 30: 565, 1983.
59. Van der Meer JWM, Vossen JM, Radl J, et al: Hyperimmunoglobulinaemia D and periodic fever: a new syndrome. Lancet 1: 1087, 1994.
60. Drenth JPH, Haagsma CJ, van der Meer JW, and the International Hyper IgD Study Group: Hyperimmunoglobulinemia D and periodic fever syndrome. The clinical spectrum in à series of 50 patients. Medicine 73: 133, 1994.
61. Drenth JPH, Boom BW, Toonstra J, van der Meer JW: Cutaneous manifestations and histologic findings in the hyperimmunoglobulinemia D syndrome. Arch Dermatol 130: 59, 1994.
62. Drenth JPH, Mariman ECM, van der Velde-Visser SD, et al: Location of the gene causing hyperimmunoglobulinemia D and periodic fever syndrome differs from that for familial Mediterranean fever. Hum Genet 94: 616, 1994.
63. Houten SM, Kuis W, Duran M, et al: Mutations in the gene encoding mevalonate kinase cause hyperimmunoglobulinemia D and periodic fever syndrome. Nature Genet 22: 175, 1999.
64. Hiemstra I, Vossen JM, van der Meer JW, et al: Clinical and immunological studies in patients with an increased IgD level. J Clin Immunol 9: 393, 1989.
65. Mizuma H, Zolla-Pazner S, Litwin S, et al: Serum IgD elevation is an early marker of B cell activation during infection with the human immunodeficiency viruses. Clin Exp Immunol 68: 5, 1987.
66. Azuma E, Masuda S, Hanada M, et al: Hyperimmunoglobulinemia D following cancer chemotherapy. Oncology 48: 387, 1991.
67. Corte G, Ferraris AM, Rees JK, et al: Correlation of serum IgD level with clinical and histological parameters in Hodgkin disease. Blood 52: 905, 1978.
68. Drenth JPH, Powell RJ, Brown NS, et al: Interferon-gamma and urine neopterin in attacks of the hyperimmunoglobulinaemia D and periodic fever syndrome. Eur J Clin Invest 25: 683, 1995.
69. Drenth JPH, Goertz J, Daha MR, van der Meer JW: Immunoglobulin D enhances the release of tumor necrosis factor gamma and interleukin beta as well as interleukin 1 receptor antagonist from human mononuclear cells. Immunology 88: 355, 1996.
70. Drenth JPH, van Deuren M, van der Ven-Jongekri JG, et al: Cytokine activation during attacks of the hyperimmunoglobulin D and periodic fever syndrome. Blood 85: 3586, 1995.
71. Frenkel J, Houten SM, Waterham HR, et al: Mevalonate kinase deficiency and Dutch type periodic fever. Clin Exp Rheumatol 18: 525, 2000.
72. De Hullu JA, Drenth JPH, Struyk AP, van der Meer JW: Hyper IgD syndrome and pregnancy. Eur J Obstet Gynecol Reprod Biol 88: 355, 1996.
73. Marshall GS, Edwards KM, Butler J, et al: Syndrome of periodic fever, pharyngitis and aphthous stomatitis. J Pediatr 110: 43, 1987.
74. Rubin LG, Kamani N: Syndrome of periodic fever and pharyngitis. J Pediatr 111: 307, 1987.
75. Nelson JD, McCracken GH: The MEBL syndrome. Pediatr Infect Dis J 13: 3, 1987.
76. Feder HM, Bialeck CA: Periodic fever associated with aphthous stomatitis, pharyngitis and cervical adenitis. Pediatr Infect Dis J 8: 186, 1989.
77. Padeh S, Brezniak N, Zemer D, et al: Periodic fever, aphthous stomatitis, pharyngitis, and adenopathy syndrome: clinical characteristics and outcome. J Pediatr 135: 98, 1999.
78. Tyson KT, Feder HM Jr, Lawton AR, Edwards KM: Periodic fever syndrome in children. J Pediatr 135: 15, 1999.
79. Long SS: Syndrome of periodic fever, apthous stomatitis, pharyngitis, and adenitis (PFAPA)—what it isn't. What is it? J Pediatr 135: 1, 1999.
80. Feder HM: Cimetidine treatment for periodic fever associated with aphthous stomatitis, pharyngitis, and cervical adentitis. Pediatr Infect Dis J 11: 348, 1992.
81. Abramson JS, Givner LB, Thompson JN: Possible role of tonsillectomy and adenoidectomy in children with recurrent fever and tonsillopharyngitis. Pediatr Infect Dis J 8: 119, 1989.
82. McDermott MF, Aksentijevich I, Galon J, et al: Germline muta-

tions in the extracellular domains of the 55 kDa TNF receptor, TNFR1, define a family of dominantly inherited autoinflammatory syndromes. Cell 9: 133, 1999.
83. McDermott EM, Smillie DM, Powell RJ: Clinical spectrum of familial Hibernian fever: a 14-year follow-up study of the index case and extended family. Mayo Clin Proc 72: 806, 1997.
84. McDermott MF, Ogunkolade BW, McDermott EM, et al: Linkage of familial Hibernian fever to chromosome 12p13. Am J Hum Genet 62: 1446, 1998.
85. Centola M, Aksentijevich I, Kastner DL: The hereditary periodic fever syndromes: molecular analysis of a new family of inflammatory diseases. Hum Mol Genet 7: 1581, 1998.
86. Grateau G, Drenth JP, Delpech M: Hereditary fevers. Curr Opin Rheumatol 11: 75, 1999.

Systemic Vasculitis

4

25

Vasculitis and Its Classification

Ross E. Petty and James T. Cassidy

DEFINITIONS

The term *vasculitis* indicates the presence of inflammation in a blood-vessel wall. The inflammatory infiltrate may be one that is predominantly neutrophilic, eosinophilic, or mononuclear. *Perivasculitis* describes inflammation around the blood-vessel wall but without involvement of the mural structure itself. *Vasculopathy*, a broader term, indicates an abnormality of blood vessels that may be inflammatory but may also be degenerative or may result from intimal proliferation.

CLASSIFICATION

The vasculitides are the most difficult of all rheumatic diseases to classify. A number of attempts have been made, and none has completely succeeded.[1, 2] In part, this has resulted from inconsistent use of definitions of individual vasculitides, a problem that was addressed by a committee of the American College of Rheumatology (ACR).[3] In this publication and in an accompanying series of papers, individual diseases were defined in some detail. Subsequently, the Chapel Hill Consensus Conference refined and modified the ACR classification (Table 25–1).[4] Neither of these studies specifically addressed vasculitis in childhood; therefore, from a practical point of view, they are of limited usefulness to the pediatrician or pediatric rheumatologist.

In these and other classifications, diseases are grouped by the size of the vessel affected. A more comprehensive list of vasculitides (many of which are very rare in childhood) is given in Table 25–2.[5] In other classifications, the character of the vascular lesion or a combination of vessel size and histologic characteristics is considered. In a classification proposed by Savage and colleagues in 1997,[6] a combination of dominant size of the affected vessel and the presence or absence of granulomata was used to classify vasculitis in childhood (Table 25–3).

The consistency of histopathologic findings within any clinical diagnostic category of vasculitis is often limited. Some disorders, such as Henoch-Schönlein purpura (HSP) and Kawasaki disease, have consistent pathologic pictures; however, in polyarteritis nodosa, microscopic polyarteritis, the granulomatous vasculitides, and giant-cell arteritides, the histologic picture is often mixed, with lesions of differing types occurring in patients with similar clinical syndromes or in individual patients. Indeed, the term *polyangiitis overlap syndrome* has been suggested in recognition of the high frequency (40 percent) of patients who exhibit features of more than one distinct vasculitis syndrome.[7]

Hoffman eloquently points out the many pitfalls in classifications of vasculitis and notes that "there is one certainty about vasculitis classification systems. They will continue to change until these diseases can be categorized by a more complete understanding of their etiology and pathogenesis."[2] Until that time, the choice of a system of classification of vasculitis is somewhat arbitrary and a matter of personal preference. The classification used in the third edition of this book accommodated the most significant histopathologic and clinical findings of the common vasculitides of childhood and, with slight modifications (Table 25–4), will continue to be used in this edition of the textbook.

GENERAL CLINICAL ASPECTS OF VASCULITIS

Childhood vasculitis is a difficult but fascinating area of pediatric rheumatology. It is an area that is often shared with other pediatric subspecialists, such as dermatologists, cardiologists, and nephrologists, a fact that emphasizes the multisystem nature of these diseases. The type of pathologic change, site of involvement, size of vessel, and systemic extent of the vascular injury determine the clinical expression of the disease and its severity. Table 25–5 summarizes features that suggest a vasculitis syndrome. The onset of some vasculitides (Kawasaki disease, HSP) is usually abrupt, and diagnostic characteristics of the disease become apparent in a few days to a week. In many of the other vasculitides, however, the presentation is more indolent, and varying signs and symptoms over weeks to months are more characteristic (see Table 25–5). In this case, diag-

Table 25–1

Chapel Hill Consensus Conference on Nomenclature of Systemic Vasculitis

Large-Vessel Vasculitis	
Giant cell (temporal) arteritis	Granulomatous arteritis of the aorta and its major branches, with a predilection for the extracranial branches of the carotid artery. *It often involves the temporal artery. Usually occurs in patients older than 50 and is often associated with polymyalgia rheumatica.*
Takayasu's arteritis	Granulomatous inflammation of the aorta and its major branches. *Usually occurs in patients younger than 50 yr.*
Medium-Vessel Vasculitis	
Polyarteritis nodosa	Necrotizing inflammation of medium-sized or small arteries without glomerulonephritis or vasculitis in arterioles, capillaries, or venules.
Kawasaki disease	Arteritis involving large, medium-sized, and small arteries and associated with mucocutaneous lymph node syndrome. *Coronary arteries are often involved. Aorta and veins may be involved. Usually occurs in children.*
Small-Vessel Vasculitis	
Wegener's granulomatosis*	Granulomatous inflammation involving the respiratory tract and necrotizing vasculitis affecting small to medium-sized vessels. *Necrotizing glomerulonephritis is common.*
Churg-Strauss syndrome*	Eosinophil-rich and granulomatous inflammation involving the respiratory tract and necrotizing vasculitis affecting small- to medium-sized vessels and associated with asthma and eosinophilia.
Microscopic polyangiitis*	Necrotizing vasculitis with few or no immune deposits, affecting small vessels. *Necrotizing arteritis involving small- and medium-sized arteries may be present. Necrotizing glomerulonephritis is very common. Pulmonary capillaritis often occurs.*
Henoch-Schönlein purpura	Vasculitis, with IgA-dominant immune deposits, affecting small vessels. *Typically involves skin, gut, and glomeruli and is associated with arthralgias or arthritis.*
Essential cryoglobulinemic vasculitis	Vasculitis with cryoglobulin immune deposits, affecting small vessels and associated with cryglobulins in serum. *Skin and glomeruli are often involved.*
Cutaneous leukocytoclastic angiitis	Isolated cutaneous leukocytoclastic angiitis without systemic vasculitis or glomerulonephritis.

Large vessels: aorta and the larger branches directed toward major body regions
Medium vessels: renal, hepatic, coronary, and mesenteric arteries
Small vessels: venules, capillaries, arterioles, and intraparenchymal distal arteries that connect with arterioles
Essential components are shown in normal type; *italicized type* represents usual, but not essential, components.

*Strongly associated with antinuclear cytoplasmic antibodies.

Modified from Jennette JC, Falk RJ, Andrassy K, et al: Nomenclature of systemic vasculitides. Proposal of an international consensus conference. Arthritis Rheum 37: 187, 1994.

Table 25–2

Classification of Vasculitis by Vessel Size

Large-vessel vasculitis
- Giant cell (temporal) arteritis
- Takayasu's arteritis

Medium-sized vessel vasculitis
- Polyarteritis nodosa
- Kawasaki disease
- Primary granulomatous central nervous system vasculitis

Small-vessel vasculitis
- ANCA-associated small-vessel vasculitis
  - Microscopic polyangiitis
  - Wegener's granulomatosis
  - Churg-Strauss syndrome
  - Drug-induced, ANCA-associated vasculitis
- Immune complex small-vessel vasculitis
  - Henoch-Schönlein purpura
  - Essential cryoglobulinemic vasculitis
  - Hypocomplementemic urticarial vasculitis
  - Vasculitis with lupus, rheumatoid arthritis, or Sjögren's syndrome
  - Behçet's syndrome
  - Goodpasture's syndrome
  - Serum sickness
  - Drug-associated, immune complex vasculitis
  - Infection-associated immune complex vasculitis
- Paraneoplastic small-vessel vasculitis
  - Lymphoproliferative neoplasm–induced vasculitis
  - Myeloproliferative neoplasm–induced vasculitis
  - Carcinoma-induced vasculitis
- Inflammatory bowel disease vasculitis

ANCA, antinuclear cytoplasmic antibody.
From Jennette JC, Falk, RJ: Small-vessel vasculitis. N Engl J Med 337: 1512, 1997.

nosis is often difficult and requires both a high index of suspicion and a thorough investigation of symptomatic and asymptomatic (but potentially affected) organs such as the heart, lungs, liver, and kidneys. Frequently, definitive diagnosis requires a biopsy of one or more sites. Table 25–6 summarizes the clinical and pathologic characteristics of the vasculitides in childhood that are discussed in greater detail in subsequent chapters.

Table 25–3

Classification of Primary Systemic Vasculitis by Vessel Size and Presence of Granulomata

VESSEL SIZE	GRANULOMATOUS	NONGRANULOMATOUS
Large	Temporal arteritis Takayasu's arteritis	
Medium		Polyarteritis nodosa Kawasaki disease
Small	Wegener's granulomatosis Churg-Strauss syndrome	Microscopic polyangiitis Henoch-Schönlein purpura Cutaneous leukocytoclastic vasculitis Essential cryoglobulinemic vasculitis

From Savage COS, Harper L, Adu D: Primary systemic vasculitis. Lancet 349: 554, 1997.

Table 25–4

A Classification of Primary Systemic Vasculitis in Children

Polyarteritis
- Polyarteritis nodosa
- Kawasaki disease
- Microscopic polyangiitis
- Cutaneous polyarteritis
- Cogan's syndrome

Leukocytoclastic vasculitis
- Henoch-Schönlein purpura
- Hypersensitivity angiitis
- Hypocomplementemic urticarial vasculitis
- Mixed cryoglobulinemia

Granulomatous vasculitis
- Churg-Strauss syndrome (allergic granulomatosis)
- Wegener's granulomatosis
- Lymphomatoid granulomatosis
- Primary angiitis of the central nervous system

Giant cell arteritis
- Takayasu's arteritis
- Temporal arteritis

Other vasculitides
- Behçet's syndrome
- Mucha-Habermann disease
- Köhlmeier-Degos syndrome

EPIDEMIOLOGY

The precise incidence and prevalence of vasculitis in the population are not known. The relative frequencies of selected vasculitides among a group of 1000 patients (mostly adults) with vasculitis are shown in Table 25–7.[8] The distribution is very different in the pediatric population, as shown in Table 25–8. Without doubt, Kawasaki disease and HSP are the most common childhood vasculitides in North America and Europe. In Asia, however, Takayasu's arteritis is also common. In the British Paediatric Rheumatology Group National

Table 25–5

Features That Suggest a Vasculitis Syndrome

A combination of several clinical and laboratory features:

Clinical

Fever, weight loss, fatigue of unknown origin
Skin lesions (palpable purpura, vasculitic urticaria, livedo reticularis, nodules, ulcers)
Neurologic lesions (headache, mononeuritis multiplex, focal central nervous system lesions)
Arthralgia or arthritis, myalgia or myositis, serositis
Hypertension
Pulmonary infiltrates or hemorrhage

Laboratory

Increased erythrocyte sedimentation rate or C-reactive protein
Leukocytosis, anemia
Eosinophilia
Antineutrophil cytoplasmic antibodies
Elevated factor VIII–related antigen (von Willebrand factor)
Cryoglobulinemia
Circulating immune complexes
Hematuria

Table 25–6

Clinical and Pathologic Characteristics of Some of the Vasculitides in Childhood

SYNDROME	FREQUENCY	VESSELS AFFECTED	CHARACTERISTIC PATHOLOGY
Polyarteritis			
Polyarteritis nodosa	Rare	Medium and small muscular arteries and sometimes arterioles	Focal segmental (often near bifurcations); fibrinoid necrosis; GI, renal, microaneurysms; lesions at various stages of evolution
Kawasaki disease	Common	Coronary and other muscular arteries	Thrombosis, fibrosis, aneurysms, especially coronaries
Leukocytoclastic vasculitis			
Henoch-Schönlein purpura	Common	Arterioles and venules, often small arteries and veins	Leukocytoclasis; mixed cells, eosinophils; IgA deposits in affected vessels (GI tract)
Hypersensitivity angiitis	Rare	Arterioles and venules	Leukocytoclastic or lymphocytic, varying eosinophils, occasionally granulomatous; widespread lesions at same stage of evolution
Granulomatous vasculitis			
Allergic granulomatosis	Very rare	Small arteries and veins, often arterioles and venules	Necrotizing extravascular granulomata; lung involvement; eosinophilia
Wegener's granulomatosis	Rare	Small arteries and veins, occasionally larger vessels	Upper and lower respiratory tract, necrotizing granulomata, glomerulonephritis
Giant cell arteritis			
Takayasu's arteritis	Uncommon	Muscular and elastic arteries	Granulomatous inflammation, giant cells; aortic arch and branches; aneurysms, dissection
Temporal arteritis	Very rare	Medium and large arteries	Granulomatous inflammation, giant cell arteritis; carotid and branches

GI, gastrointestinal.

Diagnostic Register, the various forms of vasculitis accounted for only 1 percent of rheumatic diseases in almost 5000 children.[9] In the Canadian Pediatric Rheumatic Diseases Registry,[10] 225 children with vasculitis accounted for 6.1 percent of all children entered into the registry in a 2-year period. In a similar study of children in the United States, newly diagnosed children with vasculitis accounted for 3.4 percent of those entered into the registry.[11] The proportions of children from the two registries that identified specific vasculitides are shown in Table 25–8.

The wide differences in frequencies noted probably reflect differences in referral patterns rather than any real geographic differences. Large comprehensive studies of the frequencies of vasculitides in Asia are not available, but it would be expected that Kawasaki disease and Takayasu's arteritis would constitute a larger proportion of childhood vasculitis in that area of the world. Polyarteritis nodosa and cutaneous polyarteritis also appear to be more frequent in Japan and Turkey.

Although childhood vasculitis is uncommon, it occupies an important place in the spectrum of childhood

Table 25–7

Categories and Frequencies of Vasculitis in 1000 Patients

TYPE OF VASCULITIS	%
Giant cell (temporal) arteritis	21.4
Vasculitis with a connective tissue disease	14.1
Vasculitis of unknown type	12.9
Polyarteritis nodosa	11.8
Hypersensitivity vasculitis	9.3
Wegener's granulomatosis	8.5
Henoch-Schönlein purpura	8.5
Takayasu's arteritis	6.3
Kawasaki disease	5.2
Churg-Strauss syndrome	2.0

Data from Bloch DA, Michel BA, Hunder GG, et al. The American College of Rheumatology 1990 criteria for the classification of vasculitis. Arthritis Rheum 33: 1068, 1990.

Table 25–8

Relative Frequencies of Vasculitides in Childhood

	CANADIAN REGISTRY*		U.S. REGISTRY†	
TOTAL	225	%	434	%
Kawasaki disease	147	65.3	97	22.4
Henoch-Schönlein purpura	38	16.9	213	49.1
Wegener's granulomatosis	5	2.2	6	1.4
Polyarteritis nodosa	4	1.8	14	3.2
Behçet's disease	2	0.9	—	—
Takayasu's arteritis	2	0.9	8	1.8
Unclassified	27	12.0	96	22.1

*Data from Malleson PN, Fung MY, Rosenberg AM: The incidence of pediatric rheumatic diseases: results from the Canadian Pediatric Rheumatology Association Disease Registry. J Rheumatol 23: 1981–1987, 1996.

†Data from Bowyer S, Roettcher P: Pediatric rheumatology clinic populations in the United States: results of a 3 year survey. J Rheumatol 23: 1968–1974, 1996.

rheumatic diseases and often demands a disproportionately large amount of the clinician's time and expertise. Diagnosis can be difficult, monitoring disease activity is problematic, and the outcome in some of the vasculitides may be serious. In the ensuing chapters, the important vasculitides of childhood and their management are described.

References

1. Lie JT: Nomenclature and classification of vasculitis: plus ca change, plus c'est la meme chose. Arthritis Rheum 37: 181, 1994.
2. Hoffman GS: Classification of the systemic vasculitides: antinuclear cytoplasmic antibodies, consensus and controversy. Clin Exp Rheumatol 16: 111, 1998.
3. Hunder GG, Arend WP, Block DA, et al: The American College of Rheumatology 1990 criteria for the classification of vasculitis. Arthritis Rheum 33: 1065, 1990.
4. Jennette JC, Falk RJ, Andrassy K, et al: Nomenclature of systemic vasculitides. Proposal of an international consensus conference. Arthritis Rheum 37: 187, 1994.
5. Jennette J, Falk RJ: Medical progress: small-vessel vasculitis. N Engl J Med 337: 1512, 1997.
6. Savage COS, Harper L, Adu D: Primary systemic vasculitis. Lancet 349: 554, 1997.
7. Leavitt RY, Fauci AS: Polyangiitis overlap syndrome. Am J Med 81: 79, 1986.
8. Bloch DA, Michel BA, Hunder GG, et al: The American College of Rheumatology 1990 criteria for the classification of vasculitis. Arthritis Rheum 33: 1068–1073, 1990.
9. Symmons DPM, Jones M, Osborne J, et al: Pediatric rheumatology in the United Kingdom: data from the British Pediatric Rheumatology Group National Diagnostic Register. J Rheumatol 23: 1975, 1986.
10. Malleson PN, Fung MY, Rosenberg AM: The incidence of pediatric rheumatic diseases: results from the Canadian Pediatric Rheumatology Association Disease Registry. J Rheumatol 23: 1981–1987, 1996.
11. Bowyer S, Roettcher P, and members of the Pediatric Rheumatology Database Research Group: Pediatric rheumatology clinic populations in the United States: results of a 3 year survey. J Rheumatol 23: 1968–1974, 1996.

26

Leukocytoclastic Vasculitis

Arvind Bagga and Michael J. Dillon

OVERVIEW

Leukocytoclastic vasculitis is characterized by inflammation and necrosis involving small vessels, chiefly the postcapillary venules, capillaries, and arterioles. Neutrophils infiltrate the necrotic vessel wall, and scattered nuclear debris (leukocytoclasia), hemorrhage, and fibrin deposits are found.[1] Immunofluorescence microscopic examination documents deposits of immunoglobulin, complement, and fibrin. Palpable purpura is the most common clinical pattern; edema, urticaria, nodules, and bullae are less common.

The two most important disorders associated with leukocytoclastic vasculitis in children are Henoch-Schönlein purpura (HSP) and hypersensitivity vasculitis (Table 26–1).[2] This type of vasculitis occurs occasionally in some children with connective tissue disorders, Wegener's granulomatosis, and the Churg-Strauss syndrome. Cutaneous polyarteritis is limited to the skin without evidence of systemic vasculitis or glomerulonephritis. Leukocytoclastic vasculitis may also be a manifestation of an ongoing infection or an underlying malignancy. Urticarial and cryoglobulinemic vasculitis are rare in children. Management of leukocytoclastic vasculitis requires as specific a diagnosis as possible, assessment of prognosis, and initiation of therapy.

Table 26–1

Conditions Associated With Leukocytoclastic Vasculitis

Condition
Henoch-Schönlein purpura
Hypersensitivity angiitis
Cutaneous polyarteritis
ANCA-associated vasculitis*
Wegener's granulomatosis
Microscopic polyarteritis
Churg-Strauss syndrome
Connective tissue disorders*
Systemic lupus erythematosus
Dermatomyositis
Juvenile rheumatoid arthritis
Miscellaneous
Urticarial vasculitis
Essential mixed cryoglobulinemia
Malignancy-associated
Erythema elevatum diutinum

ANCA, antinuclear cytoplasmic antibody.

*Leukocytoclastic vasculitis may occur in cutaneous lesions found in some patients with ANCA-associated vasculitis and collagen vascular diseases.

Pathogenesis

Immune complex deposition is central to the pathogenesis of most types of leukocytoclastic vasculitis. The postcapillary venule is an important site of initiation of damage. Immune complexes, formed in a state of antigen excess, circulate in the vascular compartment until some event precipitates their deposition in the walls of blood vessels. The trapping of immune complexes in vessel walls initiates local complement activation and adhesion molecule expression that result in migration and adhesion of neutrophils and macrophages to endothelial cells.[1, 3] The subsequent release of proteolytic enzymes, leukotrienes, nitric oxide, and reactive oxygen molecules damage the vessel walls and surrounding tissues.[4, 5]

The precise role of antineutrophilic cytoplasmic antibodies (ANCAs), antiendothelial cell antibodies (AECAs), and anticardiolipin antibodies in the pathogenesis of vasculitis is not clear. ANCAs can activate neutrophils, promote their adhesion to the endothelium, and induce neutrophil-mediated endothelial injury.[6, 7] AECAs, on the other hand, although reportedly present in a number of vasculitides, are not so clearly identified as major contributors to vascular damage.[7] Adhesion molecules and cytokines released by endothelial cells and activated neutrophils are key factors in the interaction between vascular endothelium and leukocytes.[8]

HENOCH-SCHÖNLEIN PURPURA

HSP is the most common systemic vasculitis in children. It is characterized by nonthrombocytopenic purpura, arthritis and arthralgia, abdominal pain, gastrointestinal (GI) hemorrhage, and glomerulonephritis. Immunoglobulin A (IgA)–dominant immune deposits are found in small vessels, chiefly postcapillary venules. Schönlein[9] and Henoch[10] are credited with describing the condition. However, the earliest report of the syndrome was probably that in 1801 by Heberden, who described a 5-year-old boy with abdominal and joint pains, vomiting, blood-stained stools, petechial hemorrhages on the legs, and hematuria.[11] HSP is often regarded as a special form of allergic vasculitis (anaphylactoid purpura).

Table 26–2

Clinical Features of Henoch-Schönlein Purpura

CLINICAL FEATURE	SAULSBURY, 1984[28] (%) (n = 25)	ROSENBLUM & WINTER, (%) 1987[29] (n = 43)	EMERY ET AL, 1977[30] (%) (n = 43)	BAGGA ET AL, 1991[31] (%) (n = 47)
Purpura	100*	97	100*	96
Arthralgia/arthritis	84	65	79	47
Abdominal pain	76	100*	63	64
Gastrointestinal bleeding	40	26		26
Renal involvement	44		37	51
Subcutaneous edema			63	21
Encephalopathy	8			
Orchitis	4			6

*Criterion used for inclusion in the series.

Epidemiology

HSP is predominantly a disease of childhood, with a reported incidence of 13.5 per 100,000.[12] It occurs most frequently between the ages of 3 and 15 years and is more common in boys than in girls (1.5:1.0).[13] Onset is more common in winter,[14] often following an upper respiratory tract infection.[15] Many reports have proposed infection, particularly β-hemolytic streptococcal disease, as a trigger for HSP.[16] Other associations include those related to varicella,[17] rubella and rubeola,[18] and infection with hepatitis B,[19] parvovirus B19,[20] *Mycoplasma pneumoniae*,[21] *Helicobacter pylori*,[22] *Staphylococcus aureus*,[23] and *Campylobacter jejuni*.[24] HSP may occasionally occur after insect bites,[25] drug use, and intake of specific dietary allergens.[26] Familial clustering of the disease has been reported with siblings affected either simultaneously or sequentially.[14] No definite human leukocyte antigen associations are documented. The condition has been described in patients with complement C2 or C4 deficiency.[27]

Clinical Manifestations

Clinical characteristics of HSP are listed in Table 26–2.[28–31] The onset of HSP is often acute, with the principal features unfolding over a period of days to weeks. Nonspecific manifestations such as low-grade fever and malaise may occur.

Cutaneous Involvement

The appearance of palpable purpuric lesions on dependent or pressure-bearing areas—especially around the malleoli of the ankle, dorsal surface of the legs, and buttocks—is characteristic (Fig. 26–1).[28, 32] Involvement of the face and scalp is extremely uncommon in older children. Skin involvement usually begins with an acute, symmetric, erythematous macular or urticarial rash. After 12 to 24 hours, the lesions coalesce to form palpable purpura or ecchymosis. They tend to occur in crops and change color from red to purple to brown. Ulceration may occasionally develop in large ecchymotic areas. Hemorrhagic bullae have also been described.[33]

In children younger than 3 years, the clinical picture may be dominated by subcutaneous edema of the scalp, periorbital area, dorsa of the hands and feet, and scrotum.[34] The edema correlates with the activity of the vasculitis and not with the degree of proteinuria.

Gastrointestinal Disease

GI symptoms occur in approximately two thirds of children with HSP within 1 to 4 weeks of the onset of the rash.[29, 31, 35] Abdominal pain, thought to be caused by submucosal and subserosal hemorrhage and edema, may occur in more than 50 percent of children. The

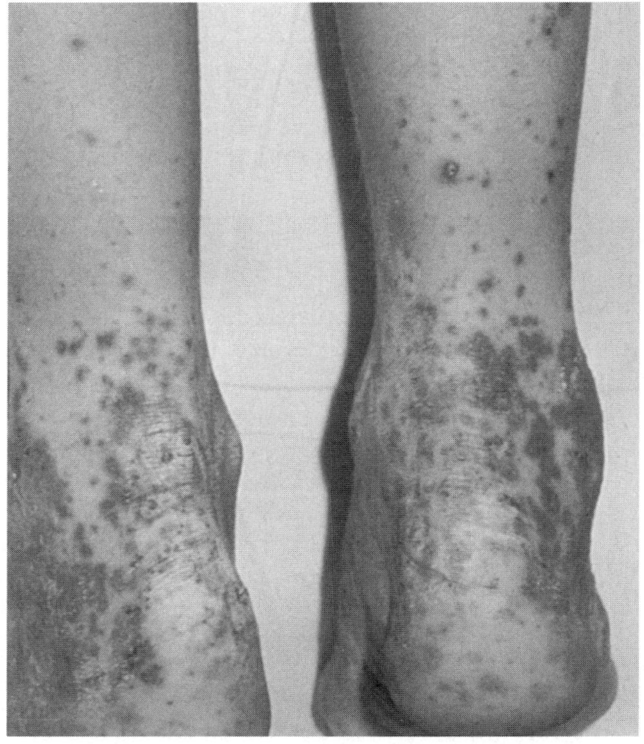

Figure 26–1. Palpable purpuric lesions involving the heels and ankles in Henoch-Schönlein purpura.

pain is usually colicky, periumbilical, and accompanied by mild abdominal distention and vomiting.[29] Occult or symptomatic GI hemorrhage (presenting as hematemesis, melena, or bleeding per rectum) is common but usually self-limiting. Occasionally, massive GI hemorrhage occurs.[35]

Abdominal pain may precede the typical purpuric rash of HSP in 14 to 36 percent of patients; the symptoms may mimic an acute surgical abdomen and result in unnecessary celiotomy. Major complications of GI involvement, of which intussusception is the most common, develop in 4.6 percent (range, 1.3 to 13.6 percent). The intussusceptum is confined to the small bowel in most cases.[35] Bowel ischemia and infarction, intestinal perforation, fistula formation, late ileal stricture, hemorrhagic pancreatitis, hydrops of the gallbladder, and pseudomembranous colitis occur infrequently.[35–37] Early diagnosis and treatment of intra-abdominal complications have significantly improved the outcome of HSP.

Renal Disease

Renal involvement can occur in 20 to 34 percent of children with HSP.[12, 25, 38, 39] The spectrum of renal manifestations ranges from the more usual microscopic hematuria and mild proteinuria to the less common nephrotic syndrome, acute nephritic syndrome, hypertension, and renal failure. Age at onset of more than 7 years, presence of persistent purpuric lesions and severe abdominal symptoms, and low factor XIII activity are associated with an increased risk of renal disease.[40] In most instances, renal disease develops within a month of onset of purpura; the initial 3 months of disease usually determines the eventual extent of the illness. In a few children, however, urinary abnormalities may not be evident until much later, sometimes after a number of recurrences of purpura. Renal disease, like abdominal pain, seldom precedes the purpura.

Extrarenal Genitourinary Complications

Orchitis with associated epididymitis is reported in 2 to 38 percent of patients.[28, 30, 41, 42] Periureteral vasculitis and ureteral ischemia may result in ureteral obstruction that presents as gross hematuria, hydronephrosis, and renal failure.[43]

Joint Involvement

The joints are involved in 50 to 80 percent of patients. The knees and ankles, and less often the wrists, elbows, and small joints of the fingers, are most commonly affected.[28–31] Characteristic findings include periarticular swelling and tenderness, usually without erythema, warmth, or effusions but with considerable pain and limitation of movement. The joint symptoms are transient and resolve within a few days without residual abnormalities. Occasionally, arthritis may precede the appearance of rash by a few days.[30]

Other Features

Central nervous system vasculitis may present with seizures and coma.[44, 45] Magnetic resonance imaging in these patients may delineate bilateral multifocal cerebral lesions that gradually resolve. Rare complications include subarachnoid hemorrhage, Guillain-Barré syndrome,[46] ocular involvement, intramuscular or subconjunctival hemorrhage, recurrent epistaxis, parotitis, and carditis.[25, 47] Pulmonary hemorrhage is rare but often fatal.[48, 49]

Pathology

Skin biopsy documents leukocytoclastic vasculitis with IgA deposits in dermal capillaries and postcapillary venules (Fig. 26–2). In the kidney, a proliferative glomerulonephritis that ranges in severity from focal and segmental mesangial proliferation to severe crescentic disease is characteristic. The most severe lesions consist of diffuse proliferation of endothelial and mesangial cells with infiltration of neutrophils (Fig. 26–3). Proliferation of epithelial cells may develop with crescents. Marked infiltration of the interstitium with mononuclear cells occurs; vasculitis per se is usually not detected. Immunofluorescence microscopy documents the presence of IgA in the mesangium and walls of the peripheral capillaries (Fig. 26–4).[50, 51] The IgA deposited is mainly of the IgA_1 subclass, although the presence of IgA_2 has also been reported.[52] In addition, the deposits frequently contain C3, IgG, properdin, and fibrin.

Laboratory Examination

There are no diagnostic laboratory abnormalities.[28, 30, 32] The platelet count is normal or increased, thus differentiating this form of purpura from that caused by thrombocytopenia. A moderate leukocytosis of up to 20,000 white blood cells (WBC)/mm^3 (20×10^9/L) with a left shift occurs in some children. Normochromic anemia is often related to GI blood loss, confirmed by guaiac-positive stools.

There is a direct correlation between the clinical features of the renal disease and the findings on renal histopathology.[50] Patients with microscopic hematuria or mild proteinuria usually have only mild mesangial proliferation. Those with nephrotic syndrome, hypertension, and a rapid deterioration of renal function frequently demonstrate medium to large circumferential crescents in a majority of the glomeruli. However, renal abnormalities on biopsy occasionally are present without overt urinary findings. A decreased concentrating ability and creatinine clearance occasionally occur. Although serum levels of C1q, C3, and C4 are usually normal,[15, 53] activation of the alternate complement pathway is demonstrated by the presence of acti-

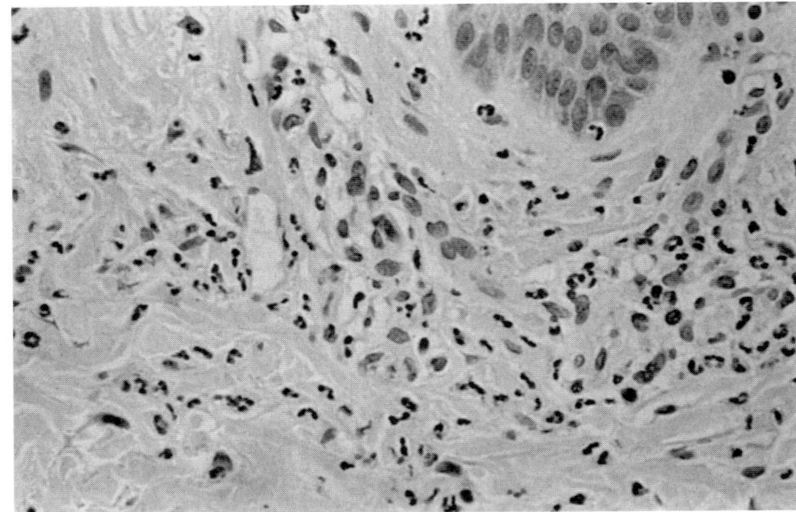

Figure 26–2. Leukocytoclastic vasculitis in the skin of a patient with Henoch-Schönlein purpura.

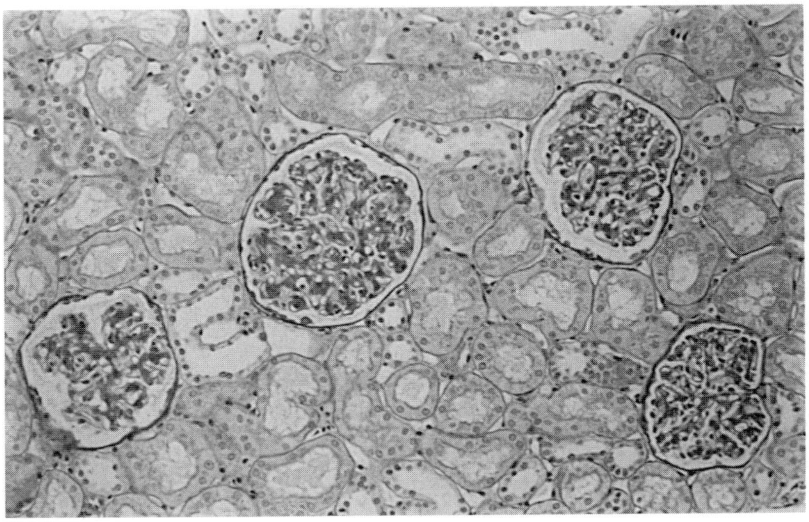

Figure 26–3. Renal biopsy demonstrates the diffuse mesangial proliferative changes in Henoch-Schönlein purpura.

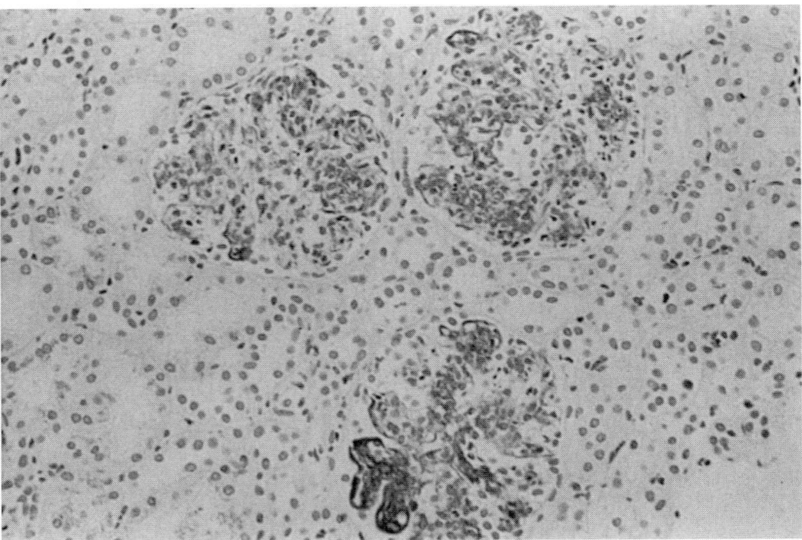

Figure 26–4. Renal biopsy with the mesangial and capillary wall deposition of immunoglobulin A in Henoch-Schönlein purpura. (Lowest glomerulus immunoperoxidase stain.)

vated C3 (C3d), decreased CH50, and low levels of properdin and factor B.[53, 54]

Circulating IgA-containing immune complexes may be present.[55, 56] Serum IgA and IgM concentrations are increased in 50 percent of patients during the acute phase of the disease.[57] One study reported an increased number of circulating IgA-producing B cells.[58] Raised titers of IgA ANCA have been demonstrated in some patients.[59–62] However, the immunofluorescence pattern of ANCAs is atypical, and the target antigen remains undefined. Other workers have not confirmed the presence of ANCAs in patients with HSP.[63] Abnormally large von Willebrand factor multimers may be found in the plasma, and their levels correlate with disease severity.[56, 64]

Radiologic Examination

Ultrasonography is useful in confirming bowel involvement and diagnosing intussusception.[35] It delineates dilated bowel loops and decreased motility and may document abnormally thickened walls of the small intestine. Ultrasonography has a high sensitivity and specificity in the diagnosis of intussusception and for following its clinical course. Plain abdominal films may delineate dilated, thickened bowel loops with or without air-fluid levels; pneumoperitoneum is detected in cases with perforation. Contrast enema studies have been used to confirm and treat intussusception that extends into the large bowel; their role in diagnosing small bowel involvement is limited.[28]

The diagnosis of orchitis may be confirmed on scrotal ultrasonography by the presence of marked cutaneous and subcutaneous edema, an enlarged epididymis, and a hydrocele with intact testicular blood flow. Testicular torsion can thus be excluded, avoiding the need for testicular exploration.

Diagnosis

The American College of Rheumatology (ACR) criteria are given in Table 26–3.[32] Punch biopsy is usually not necessary but, by demonstrating leukocytoclastic vasculitis with deposition of IgA and C3, can assist in the identification of patients with HSP when the clinical manifestations are atypical. HSP must be differentiated from immune thrombocytopenic purpura, acute poststreptococcal glomerulonephritis, systemic lupus erythematosus, septicemia, disseminated intravascular coagulation, the hemolytic uremic syndrome, and other types of vasculitis.

The majority of children do not require renal biopsy.[39, 50] A biopsy is not necessary in patients with microscopic hematuria with low-grade proteinuria (who usually have only mild renal histologic changes). Renal biopsy should usually be performed in children with increasing proteinuria, nephrotic or nephritic syndrome, or renal insufficiency. These patients are likely to show severe histologic alterations and are at risk for poorer long-term outcome.

Table 26–3

Criteria for Classification of Henoch-Schönlein Purpura

CRITERION	DEFINITION
Palpable purpura	Slightly raised "palpable" hemorrhagic skin lesions not related to thrombocytopenia
Age ≤20 yr at onset	Patient ≤20 yr old at onset of first symptoms
Bowel angina	Diffuse abdominal pain, worse after meals, or the diagnosis of bowel ischemia, usually including bloody diarrhea
Wall granulocytes on biopsy	Histologic changes showing granulocytes in the walls of arterioles or venules

For purposes of classification, a patient shall be said to have Henoch-Schönlein purpura if at least two of these criteria are present. The presence of any two or more criteria yields a sensitivity of 87.1% and specificity of 87.7%.

From Mills JA, Michel BA, Bloch DA, et al: The American College of Rheumatology 1990 criteria for the classification of Henoch-Schönlein purpura. Arthritis Rheum 33: 1114–1121, 1990.

Other causes of an acute surgical abdomen in children with abdominal pain and GI tract bleeding must be considered. Palpation of a tender abdominal mass indicative of intussusception or suspicion of pancreatitis associated with a raised serum amylase level may be important. The sudden onset of cough, pallor, dyspnea, and hemoptysis suggests pulmonary hemorrhage. A chest radiograph in such a patient may document bilateral lung opacities or infiltration consistent with intra-alveolar hemorrhage.

Acute Hemorrhagic Edema

Acute hemorrhagic edema, first described by Snow in 1913,[65] is usually considered a variant of HSP that presents in children between the ages of 4 months and 2 years. The clinical features are marked by sudden onset of fever, purpuric skin lesions with a target-like pattern, and peripheral edema affecting the face, ear lobes, and extremities.[34, 66, 67] Involvement of the kidneys or the GI tract is usually mild or absent. The course of the illness is essentially benign, with spontaneous remission in 1 to 3 weeks. Recurrent attacks may occur, however. A leukocytoclastic vasculitis with perivascular IgA deposits in 10 to 35 percent of cases is a characteristic finding on biopsy of the skin.

HSP in Adults

HSP is uncommon in adults, with a reported incidence of 0.12 per 100,000.[68] Males are affected as commonly as females. One study compared the clinical features and outcome in an unselected population of 46 adults and 116 children with HSP.[69] At onset of symptoms, cutaneous lesions were the main manifestation in both groups. However, adults had a lower frequency of abdominal pain and fever and a higher frequency of joint symptoms and severe renal involvement. Adults also required more aggressive therapy, consisting of glucocorticoids, cytotoxic agents, or both. The outcome was relatively good in both groups, with complete recovery in 94 percent of children and 89 percent of adults. Another study found that leukocytosis, thrombocytosis, and elevated levels of serum C-reactive protein were more common in children, whereas elevated serum IgA and cryoglobulin levels were more frequent in adults.[70] HSP in adults may represent a more severe form of the disease with a higher frequency of significant renal involvement.[70] However, the final outcome is usually satisfactory. Berger's nephropathy in adults may represent an identical IgA nephropathy without the other manifestations of HSP.

Treatment

Treatment of HSP is supportive, with attention to maintenance of good hydration, nutrition, and electrolyte balance; control of pain with simple analgesics (such as acetaminophen); and if necessary, control of hypertension. Although glucocorticoids dramatically decrease joint and skin findings, they are not usually required for the management of these manifestations. Systemic steroids, however, are indicated in patients with severe GI disease or hemorrhage.[16, 29] Prednisone may be used in a dose of 1 to 2 mg/kg/day for 7 days followed by a gradual reduction in dosage over 2 to 3 weeks. A short-term course of steroids is also effective in alleviating edema and relieving pain associated with orchitis.[71] Some investigations have examined the role of short-term glucocorticoids in the prevention of nephritis. The results of these studies vary, and precise recommendations are currently lacking.[40, 72, 73]

Children with HSP who have clinical features and histology suggestive of severe renal disease may be treated with glucocorticoids with or without cytotoxic drugs. However, there are currently no prospective controlled studies that clearly define the approach to treatment in these patients. Administration of intravenous "pulse" methylprednisolone may be effective if started early in the course of the disease.[74] Combined therapy with prednisolone, cyclophosphamide, heparin or warfarin, and dipyridamole is also reported to result in clinical and histologic benefit in severe cases.[75] The use of intravenous immunoglobulin and plasma exchange has resulted in encouraging outcomes in individual cases but has not been confirmed in large trials.[76, 77] Patients with persistent proteinuria may be treated with angiotensin-converting enzyme inhibitors.

Course and Prognosis

In two thirds of children, HSP runs its entire course within 4 weeks of onset.[78, 79] Younger children generally experience a shorter course and fewer recurrences than older patients. Approximately 16 to 40 percent have at least one recurrence, which most commonly consists of rash and abdominal pain, each episode usually being similar but briefer and milder than the preceding one. The majority of these exacerbations take place within the initial 6-week period but may occur as late as 2 years after onset. These episodes may be spontaneous or coincide with repeated respiratory tract infections.

The overall prognosis is excellent, and supportive care suffices in most patients. Significant morbidity is associated with disease of the GI tract in the short term and with nephritis in the long term. The reported outcome in children with renal disease varies.[80] The clinical and pathologic features are to some extent predictive of the long-term outcome. In patients who present with a nephritic, nephrotic, or nephritic-nephrotic syndrome, 44 percent have hypertension or impaired renal function on long-term follow-up, whereas 82 percent who present with hematuria (with or without mild proteinuria) are normal. Children with renal manifestations in the acute phase, particularly with extensive crescents on biopsy, require prolonged follow-up with regular monitoring of blood pressure and proteinuria.

Long-term studies confirm that renal failure or hypertension can develop up to 10 years after onset of the disease. Overall, 1 to 5 percent of children with HSP progress to end-stage renal failure. These patients account for approximately 10 percent of children with renal failure.[25, 38] Renal transplantation has been successful. Although histologic features recur in one third to one half of all patients, clinical recurrence and graft loss are uncommon.[81, 82]

HYPERSENSITIVITY VASCULITIS

Historically, serum sickness, one of the best examples of immune complex–mediated disease in humans, was encountered after the administration of heterologous antiserum to treat or prevent specific infections such as diphtheria and tetanus. Although this is rarely encountered today, polyangiitis due to hypersensitivity to drugs and other antigens (including infections) is an important cause of small-vessel vasculitis in children.[83, 84] A report of serum sickness–like arthritis in Finland estimated its frequency at 4.7 per 100,000 children younger than 16 years, making it one of the most common causes of acute arthritis in childhood.[83] Drugs that have been implicated include penicillins, sulfonamides, quinolones, allopurinol, thiazide diuretics, nonsteroidal anti-inflammatory drugs (NSAIDs), and phenytoin.[85] Other foreign proteins, such as antisera, streptokinase, recombinant human growth hormone, cytokines, and monoclonal antibodies, may also cause immune complex formation and vasculitis. Infection with hepatitis B or C, human immunodeficiency virus, and streptococci may result in similar clinical features.

The syndrome of hypersensitivity vasculitis begins 7 to 14 days after primary exposure to the antigen and is characterized by fever, arthralgia, sometimes frank arthritis, myalgia, lymphadenopathy, and a rash. The chief cutaneous manifestations include palpable nodules, urticaria, and purpura. These skin lesions are distributed predominantly over the lower legs, although the trunk and upper limbs may also be affected (Fig. 26–5). The disease runs a variable course, usually lasting a few weeks. Kunnamo and colleagues[83] described the presence of patchy discoloration over the affected joints, with urticaria predominantly on the trunk. In this study, the arthritis was transient and

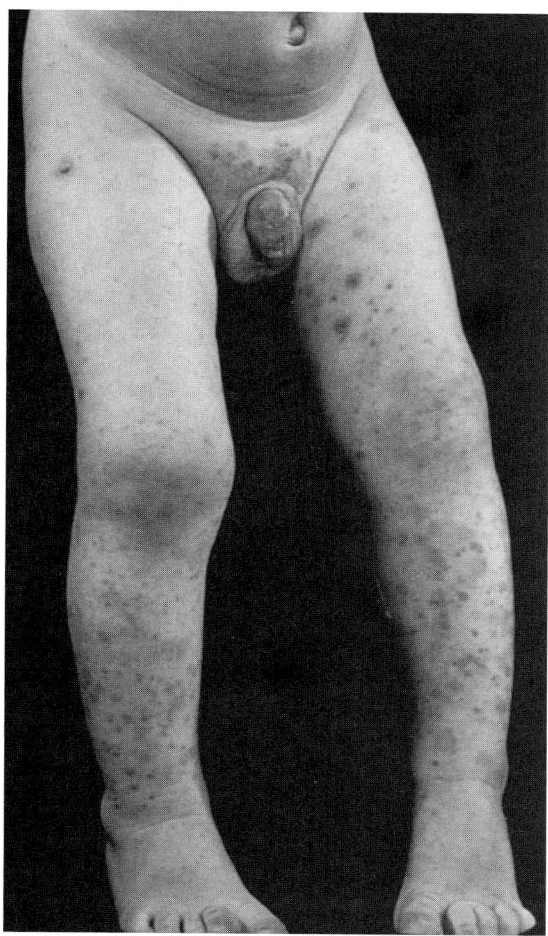

Figure 26–5. Skin lesions in hypersensitivity vasculitis.

most commonly affected the ankles, metacarpophalangeal joints, wrists, and knees. Occasionally, other organs can be affected, and the condition can evolve into systemic necrotizing vasculitis, with involvement of the GI and respiratory tract and kidneys.[86]

Diagnosis

The ACR criteria for the diagnosis of hypersensitivity vasculitis are listed in Table 26–4.[87] These criteria overlap with those of HSP, and distinction between the two conditions is sometimes difficult.[88] Leukocytosis is usually present, sometimes accompanied by eosinophilia and circulating immune complexes.[83] The erythrocyte sedimentation rate (ESR) is usually raised but may be normal, and C3 may be reduced. IgG antibodies to the inciting antigen may be found. Skin biopsy documents a leukocytoclastic vasculitis chiefly involving capillaries and small venules, and the inflammatory lesions are at a similar stage of development in all vessels. The cellular infiltrate contains large numbers of neutrophils and eosinophils. In one report, synovial fluid examination demonstrated the presence of 9000 to 59,000 WBC/mm^3 (9 to 59 $\times$ 10^9/L), of which 38 to 80 percent were polymorphonuclear neutrophils.[83]

The Chapel Hill International Consensus Conference did not use the term *hypersensitivity vasculitis.* They proposed that the categories of microscopic polyarteritis and cutaneous leukocytoclastic vasculitis best equated with the most common usage of hypersensitivity vasculitis.[89]

Treatment

This disorder is often acute and self-limiting but may pursue a relapsing or chronic course. Removal of the precipitating agent, if identified, is the first step in treatment. In the absence of systemic features, management is usually symptomatic. Antihistamines and NSAIDs alleviate cutaneous symptoms and arthralgias, respectively. Glucocorticoid therapy may be indicated in children showing severe cutaneous symptoms or systemic vasculitis.

OTHER LEUKOCYTOCLASTIC VASCULITIDES

In a number of other types of vasculitis, the histopathology of the lesions has a leukocytoclastic element. Some of these types, such as cutaneous polyarteritis, are discussed in detail in Chapters 28 and 29.

Cutaneous Polyarteritis

Cutaneous polyarteritis is limited to the skin and muscle.[90–92] It is relatively rare in childhood. Livedo reticularis—a red-blue mottling of the skin—is reported in some cases. There is often a history of a preceding sore throat or otitis. Raised

Table 26–4

Criteria for Diagnosis of Hypersensitivity Vasculitis

CRITERION	DEFINITION
Age at onset >16 yr	Development of symptoms after age 16 yr
Medication at disease onset	Medication that may have been a precipitating factor was taken at the onset of symptoms
Palpable purpura	Slightly elevated purpuric rash over one or more areas of skin; does not blanch with pressure and is not related to thrombocytopenia
Maculopapular rash	Flat and raised lesions of various sizes over one or more areas of the skin
Biopsy (including arteriole and venule)	Histologic changes showing granulocytes in a perivascular or extravascular location

For purposes of classification, a patient shall be said to have hypersensitivity vasculitis if at least three of these criteria are present. The presence of any three or more criteria yields a sensitivity of 71.0% and specificity of 83.9%. *The age criterion is not applicable for children.*

From Calabrese LH, Michel BA, Bloch DA, et al: The American College of Rheumatology 1990 criteria for the classification of hypersensitivity vasculitis. Arthritis Rheum 33: 1108–1113, 1990.

antistreptolysin and antihyaluronidase titers may be found. Mild fever, malaise, and myalgias are often present. In the report of David and colleagues, all patients had evanescent arthritis affecting the knees and ankles.[92] More than half had brawny edema of muscles and periorbital edema.

Skin biopsy demonstrates necrotizing panarteritis with deposition of fibrinoid material, presence of neutrophils, and leukocytoclasia.[93, 94] The most common noncutaneous finding is a mononeuritis multiplex.[91] Progression to polyarteritis nodosa is rare.[91, 92] The acute symptoms resolve within a few weeks, but relapses, particularly in association with streptococcal infection, can affect 25 percent of patients.[95]

This condition responds to penicillin, NSAIDs, and steroids. Penicillin prophylaxis may be considered in patients with multiple recurrences. (See also Chapter 28.)

ANCA-Associated Small-Vessel Vasculitis

The presence of ANCAs is associated with three major vasculitides, all of which are uncommon in children: *Wegener's granulomatosis, microscopic polyarteritis,* and the *Churg-Strauss syndrome.*[96–98] Wegener's granulomatosis and the Churg-Strauss syndrome are characterized by granulomatous inflammation involving the respiratory tract and necrotizing vasculitis affecting medium- and small-sized vessels (capillaries, venules, arterioles, veins, and arteries).[96, 99]

Cutaneous involvement may occur in 40 to 60 percent of cases and consists of palpable purpura, skin ulcers, papules, and nodules.[89, 100] Skin lesions rarely precede the appearance of other features of these illnesses. The typical findings of leukocytoclastic vasculitis are present on biopsy specimens of cutaneous lesions. Similar cutaneous lesions may occur in cases of microscopic polyarteritis.[101] The management of these disorders is similar and usually employs a combination of glucocorticoids and cytotoxic agents.[89, 100] Antiplatelet drugs such as dipyridamole or aspirin have been used in patients with Wegener's granulomatosis and microscopic polyarteritis. Plasma exchange and high-dose intravenous immunoglobulin may be of benefit in patients in whom standard therapy has been unsuccessful.[102, 103] Rapid diagnosis of ANCA-associated vasculitis is important because appropriate immunosuppressive treatment often limits life-threatening injury to vital organs. For further discussion, see Chapter 29.

Vasculitis Associated With Connective Tissue Disorders

Vasculitis occurs with systemic lupus erythematosus, mixed connective tissue disease, dermatomyositis and scleroderma, and very rarely in juvenile rheumatoid arthritis. Leukocytoclastic vasculitis is particularly well recognized in juvenile dermatomyositis, in which small-vessel vasculitis has been identified in striated muscle, skin, subcutaneous tissue, and the GI tract.[104–106] Muscle infarction and extensive skin ulceration can result because of occlusive endarteropathy.[104] Infarction of the palate, retinal exudates, and GI ulceration with bleeding may occur. Therapy with intravenous methylprednisolone is recommended, especially if there is GI involvement or cutaneous vasculitic ulceration. Persistence of active disease is an indication for treatment with cyclophosphamide. Intravenous immunoglobulin, methotrexate, and plasmapheresis have been used in recalcitrant disease.[107]

Leukocytoclastic vasculitis may also occur in systemic lupus erythematosus, usually presenting as palpable purpuric lesions or urticaria.[108, 109]

Urticarial Vasculitis

Children, usually girls, with the rare syndrome of urticarial vasculitis have recurrent episodes of urticaria that are associated with pruritus and a burning sensation. The urticarial lesions resolve over 2 to 4 days, leaving residual pigmentation. Other skin lesions include purpura, papules, and vesicles. Arthralgias may occur in approximately 60 percent, arthritis (usually of small joints) in 30 percent, abdominal and chest pain in 25 percent, pulmonary disease (cough, dyspnea, and hemoptysis) in 30 percent, and glomerulonephritis in 15 percent of patients. Less commonly, uveitis and episcleritis, fever, angioedema, Raynaud's phenomenon, pseudotumor cerebri, and seizures may be associated manifestations.[110, 111]

Urticarial vasculitis occasionally is the presenting feature of systemic lupus erythematosus.[109, 112] It also has been described in Sjögren's syndrome, hepatitis B and C antigenemia, drug reactions, and exposure to sun.[113, 114] The pathogenesis is related to immune-complex deposition and activation of the classical complement pathway. Levels of C3, C4, and C1q are reduced in 18 to 50 percent. Patients with hypocomplementemia tend to have more severe symptoms; some may later show features of systemic lupus.[112] Skin biopsy documents features of leukocytoclastic vasculitis with abundant neutrophil and occasional eosinophil infiltrates.[112, 114] Immunofluorescence microscopy confirms the deposition of IgM and C3 in the affected vessels.

Management consists of supportive measures and treatment of associated disorders. Antihistamines, dapsone, hydroxychloroquine, colchicine, and indomethacin have been used with variable success. Systemic steroids or other immunosuppressive drugs may be required in severe disease. The course of disease is usually benign but may vary depending on the associated disorders and extent of systemic involvement.

Vasculitis of Mixed Cryoglobulinemia

Cryoglobulinemic vasculitis results in acute vascular inflammation by localization of mixed (types II and III) cryoglobulins in the vessel walls.[115] The prefix "essential" is used if no underlying disorder is found. Infection with hepatitis B or C virus must always be excluded.[116, 117] This condition is extremely rare in children.

The vasculitis presents with purpuric skin lesions that are exacerbated by exposure to cold, polyarthralgia, and weakness. The main cause of long-term morbidity is progressive renal disease that resembles membranoproliferative glomerulonephritis. The presence of high levels of mixed cryoglobulins (IgG and IgM) that reversibly precipitate on cooling is characteristic. Low levels of C4 with normal or slightly low C3 are distinctive. The outcome is related to severity of the systemic disease. Treatment with various combinations of steroids, cyclophosphamide, plasmapheresis, and intravenous immunoglobulin may be of benefit in some patients.[118, 119]

Vasculitis Associated With Malignancy

Lymphoproliferative disease rarely is accompanied by a leukocytoclastic vasculitis limited to the skin. Lymphocytic lymphoma and Waldenström's macroglobulinemia, both very rare in children, can result in a cryoglobulinemic vasculitis.[120] Lymphoma may also be associated with Wegener's granulomatosis and HSP. Occasionally, vasculitis precedes the diagnosis of a lymphoproliferative syndrome.

Miscellaneous Associations

A number of reports describe the occurrence of HSP in patients with familial Mediterranean fever.[121, 122] In some patients, the diagnosis of vasculitis may precede that of Mediterranean fever. Similarly, many patients with Behçet's disease[123, 124] develop papular or pustular lesions that may ulcerate. Skin biopsy documents vasculitis with a predominant lymphocytic infiltrate, but a leukocytoclastic vasculitis may be present. In such circumstances, the vasculitic component may need to be treated in its own right.

Erythema elevatum diutinum is an extremely rare form of localized chronic cutaneous leukocytoclastic vasculitis, characterized by edematous purplish plaques mainly over extensor surfaces. A similar lesion, *granuloma faciale*, is localized to the face. Both conditions entail leukocytoclastic vasculitis with fibrinoid necrosis of the upper and middle dermal vessels. Systemic involvement is extremely unusual. Treatment with dapsone or intralesional steroids may be beneficial.[125, 126]

References

1. Swerlick RA, Lawley TJ: Small vessel vasculitis and cutaneous vasculitis. *In* Churg A, Churg J (eds): Systemic Vasculitides. New York, Igaku-Shoin, 1991, pp 193–201.
2. Blanco R, Martinez-Taboada VM, Rodriguez-Valverde V, Garcia-Fuentes M: Cutaneous vasculitis in children and adults. Associated diseases and etiologic factors in 303 patients. Medicine (Baltimore) 77: 403, 1998.
3. Soter NA, Austen KF: Pathogenic mechanisms in the necrotizing vasculitides. Clin Rheum Dis 6: 233, 1980.
4. Harlan JM: Neutrophil-mediated vascular injury. Acta Med Scand Suppl 71S: 123, 1987.
5. Demircin G, Oner A, Unver Y, et al: Erythrocyte superoxide dismutase activity and plasma malondialdehyde levels in children with Henoch Schönlein purpura. Acta Paediatr 87: 848, 1988.
6. Jennette JC, Falk RJ, Wilkman AS: Anti-neutrophil cytoplasmic autoantibodies—a serologic marker for vasculitides. Ann Acad Med Singapore 24: 248, 1995.
7. Savage CO, Pottinger BE, Gaskin G, et al: Vascular damage in Wegener's granulomatosis and microscopic polyarteritis: presence of anti-endothelial cell antibodies and their relation to anti-neutrophil cytoplasm antibodies. Clin Exp Immunol 85: 14, 1991.
8. Sundy JS, Haynes BF: Pathogenic mechanisms of vessel damage in vasculitis syndromes. Rheum Dis Clin North Am 21: 861, 1995.
9. Schönlein JL: Allegemeine und specielle Pathologie und Therapie, vol 2, 3rd ed. Herisau, Germany, Literatur-Comptoir, 1837, p 48.
10. Henoch EHH: About a peculiar form of purpura. Am J Dis Child 128: 78, 1974 (Translated from Berl Klin Wochenschr 11: 641, 1874.)
11. Heberden W: Commentarii di morboriana-historia et curatione. London, T. Payne, 1801.
12. Stewart M, Savage JM, Bell B, McCord B: Long term renal prognosis of Henoch-Schönlein purpura in an unselected childhood population. Eur J Pediatr 147: 113, 1988.
13. Habib R, Cameron JS: Schönlein-Henoch purpura. *In* Bacon PA, Hadler NM (eds): The Kidney and Rheumatic Diseases. London, Butterworth, 1982, p 178.
14. Farley TA, Gillespie S, Rasoulpour M, et al: Epidemiology of a cluster of Henoch-Schönlein purpura. Am J Dis Child 143: 798, 1989.
15. Atkinson SR, Barker DJ: Seasonal distribution of Henoch-Schönlein purpura. Br J Prev Soc Med 30: 22, 1976.
16. Allen DM, Diamond LK, Howell DA: Anaphylactoid purpura in children: review with a follow-up of the renal complications. Am J Dis Child 99: 833, 1960.
17. Pedersen FK, Petersen EA: Varicella followed by glomerulonephritis. Treatment with corticosteroids and azathioprine resulting in recurrence of varicella. Acta Paediatr Scand 64: 886, 1975.
18. Meadow SR, Glasgow EF, White RH, et al: Schönlein-Henoch nephritis. Q J Med 41: 241, 1972.
19. Maggiore G, Martini A, Grifeo S, et al: Hepatitis B virus infection and Schönlein-Henoch purpura. Am J Dis Child 138: 681, 1984.
20. Minohara Y: Studies on the relationship between anaphylactoid purpura and human parvovirus B19. Kansenshogaku Zasshi 69: 928, 1995.
21. Liew SW, Kessel I: Mycoplasmal pneumonia preceding Henoch-Schönlein purpura. Arch Dis Child 49: 912, 1974.
22. Cecchi R, Torelli E: Schönlein-Henoch purpura in association with duodenal ulcer and gastric *Helicobacter pylori* infection. J Dermatol 25: 482, 1998.
23. Hirayama K, Kobayashi M, Kondoh M, et al: Henoch-Schönlein purpura nephritis associated with methicillin-resistant *Staphylococcus aureus* infection. Nephrol Dial Transplant 13: 2703, 1998.
24. Lind KM, Gaub J, Pedersen RS: Henoch-Schönlein purpura associated with *Campylobacter jejuni* enteritis. Scand J Urol Nephrol 28: 179, 1994.
25. Kobayashi O, Wada H, Okawa K, Takeyama I: Schönlein-Henoch's syndrome in children. Contrib Nephrol 4: 48, 1975.
26. Ackroyd JK: Allergic purpura, including purpura due to foods, drugs and infections. Am J Med 14: 605, 1953.
27. Jin DK, Kohsaka T, Koo JW, et al: Complement 4 locus II gene deletion and DQA1*0301 gene: genetic risk factors for IgA nephropathy and Henoch-Schönlein nephritis. Nephron 73: 390, 1996.
28. Saulsbury FT: Henoch-Schönlein purpura. Pediatr Dermatol 1: 195, 1984.
29. Rosenblum ND, Winter HS: Steroid effects on the course of abdominal pain in children with Henoch-Schönlein purpura. Pediatrics 79: 1018, 1987.
30. Emery H, Larter W, Schaller JG: Henoch-Schönlein vasculitis. Arthritis Rheum 20(Suppl): 385, 1977.
31. Bagga A, Kabra SK, Srivastava RN, Bhuyan UN: Henoch-Schönlein syndrome in northern Indian children. Indian Pediatr 28: 1153, 1991.
32. Mills JA, Michel BA, Bloch DA, et al: The American College of Rheumatology 1990 criteria for the classification of Henoch-Schönlein purpura. Arthritis Rheum 33: 1114, 1990.

33. Saulsbury FT: Hemorrhagic bullous lesions in Henoch-Schönlein purpura. Pediatr Dermatol 15: 357, 1998.
34. Al-Sheyyab M, El-Shanti H, Ajlouni S, et al: The clinical spectrum of Henoch-Schönlein purpura in infants and young children. Eur J Pediatr 154: 969, 1995.
35. Choong CK, Beasley SW: Intra-abdominal manifestations of Henoch-Schönlein purpura. J Paediatr Child Health 34: 405, 1998.
36. Gow KW, Murphy JJ III, Blair GK, et al: Multiple entero-entero fistulae: an unusual complication of Henoch-Schönlein purpura. J Pediatr Surg 31: 809, 1996.
37. Levy-Weil FE, Sigal M, Renard P, et al: Acute pancreatitis in rheumatoid purpura. Apropos of 2 cases. Rev Med Interne 18: 54, 1997.
38. Koskimies O, Mir S, Rapola J, Vilska J: Henoch-Schönlein nephritis: long-term prognosis of unselected patients. Arch Dis Child 56: 482, 1981.
39. Andreoli SP: Chronic glomerulonephritis in childhood. Membranoproliferative glomerulonephritis, Henoch-Schönlein purpura nephritis, and IgA nephropathy. Pediatr Clin North Am 42: 1487, 1995.
40. Kaku Y, Nohara K, Honda S: Renal involvement in Henoch-Schönlein purpura: a multivariate analysis of prognostic factors. Kidney Int 53: 1755, 1998.
41. Clark WR, Kramer SA: Henoch-Schönlein purpura and the acute scrotum. J Pediatr Surg 21: 991, 1986.
42. Mintzer CO, Nussinovitch M, Danziger Y, et al: Scrotal involvement in Henoch-Schönlein purpura in children. Scand J Urol Nephrol 32: 138, 1998.
43. Bruce RG, Bishof NA, Jackson EC, et al: Bilateral ureteral obstruction associated with Henoch-Schönlein purpura. Pediatr Nephrol 11: 347, 1997.
44. Ha TS, Cha SH: Cerebral vasculitis in Henoch-Schönlein purpura: a case report with sequential magnetic resonance imaging. Pediatr Nephrol 10: 634, 1996.
45. Lewis ID, Philpot MG: Neurological complications of the Schönlein-Henoch syndrome. Arch Dis Child 31: 369, 1956.
46. Goraya JS, Jayashree M, Ghosh D, et al: Guillain-Barré syndrome in a child with Henoch-Schönlein purpura. Scand J Rheumatol 27: 310, 1998.
47. Imai T, Matsumoto S: Anaphylactoid purpura with cardiac involvement. Arch Dis Child 45: 727, 1970.
48. Chaussain M, de Boissieu D, Kalifa G, et al: Impairment of lung diffusion capacity in Schönlein-Henoch purpura. J Pediatr 121: 12, 1992.
49. Paller AS, Kelly K, Sethi R: Pulmonary hemorrhage: an often fatal complication of Henoch-Schoenlein purpura. Pediatr Dermatol 14: 299, 1997.
50. White RHR: Henoch-Schönlein purpura. *In* Churg A, Churg J (eds): Systemic Vasculitides. New York, Igaku-Shoin, 1991, pp 203–217.
51. Nakamoto Y, Asamo Y, Dohi K, et al: Primary IgA glomerulonephritis and Schönlein-Henoch purpura nephritis: clinicopathological and immunohistological characteristics. Q J Med 47: 495, 1978.
52. Conley ME, Cooper MD, Michael AF: Selective deposition of immunoglobulin A1 in immunoglobulin A nephropathy, anaphylactoid purpura nephritis, and systemic lupus erythematosus. J Clin Invest 66: 1432, 1980.
53. Garcia-Fuentes M, Martin A, Chantler C, Williams DG: Serum complement components in Henoch-Schönlein purpura. Arch Dis Child 53: 417, 1978.
54. Spitzer RE, Urmson JR, Farnett ML, et al: Alteration of the complement system in children with Henoch Schönlein purpura. Clin Immunol Immunopathol 11: 52, 1978.
55. Kauffmann RH, Herrmann WA, Meyer CJ, et al: Circulating IgA-immune complexes in Henoch-Schönlein purpura. A longitudinal study of their relationship to disease activity and vascular deposition of IgA. Am J Med 69: 859, 1980.
56. De Mattia D, Penza R, Giordano P, et al: von Willebrand factor and factor XIII in children with Henoch-Schönlein purpura. Pediatr Nephrol 9: 603, 1995.
57. Trygstad CW, Stiehm ER: Elevated serum IgA globulin in anaphylactoid purpura. Pediatrics 47: 1023, 1971.
58. Casanueva B, Rodriguez-Valverde V, Luceno A: Circulating IgA producing cells in the differential diagnosis of Henoch-Schönlein purpura. J Rheumatol 15: 1229, 1988.
59. Ronda N, Esnault VL, Layward L, et al: Antineutrophil cytoplasm antibodies (ANCA) of IgA isotype in adult Henoch-Schönlein purpura. Clin Exp Immunol 95: 49, 1994.
60. Fujieda M, Oishi N, Naruse K, et al: Soluble thrombomodulin and antibodies to bovine glomerular endothelial cells in patients with Henoch-Schönlein purpura. Arch Dis Child 78: 240, 1998.
61. Coppo R, Cirina P, Amore A, et al: Properties of circulating IgA molecules in Henoch-Schönlein purpura nephritis with focus on neutrophil cytoplasmic antigen IgA binding (IgA-ANCA): new insight into a debated issue. Nephrol Dial Transplant 12: 2269, 1997.
62. Lin JJ, Stewart CL, Kaskel FJ, Fine RN: IgG and IgA classes of anti-neutrophil cytoplasmic autoantibodies in a 13-year-old girl with recurrent Henoch-Schönlein purpura. Pediatr Nephrol 7: 143, 1993.
63. Robson WL, Leung AK, Woodman RC: The absence of anti-neutrophil cytoplasmic antibodies in patients with Henoch-Schönlein purpura. Pediatr Nephrol 8: 295, 1994.
64. Casonato A, Pontara E, Bertomoro A, et al: Abnormally large von Willebrand factor multimers in Henoch-Schönlein purpura. Am J Hematol 51: 7, 1996.
65. Snow IM: Purpura, urticaria and angioneurotic edema of the hands and feet in a nursing baby. JAMA 61: 18, 1913.
66. Krause I, Lazarov A, Rachmel A, et al: Acute haemorrhagic oedema of infancy, a benign variant of leucocytoclastic vasculitis. Acta Paediatr 85: 114, 1996.
67. Gonggryp LA, Todd G: Acute hemorrhagic edema of childhood. Pediatr Dermatol 15: 91, 1998.
68. Watts RA, Carruthers DM, Scott DG: Epidemiology of systemic vasculitis: changing incidence or definition? Semin Arthritis Rheum 25: 28, 1995.
69. Blanco R, Martinez-Taboada VM, Rodriguez-Valverde V, et al: Henoch-Schönlein purpura in adulthood and childhood: two different expressions of the same syndrome. Arthritis Rheum 40: 859, 1997.
70. Lin SJ, Huang JL: Henoch-Schönlein purpura in Chinese children and adults. Asian Pac J Allergy Immunol 16: 21, 1998.
71. Ben-Chaim J, Korat E, Shenfeld O, et al: Acute scrotum caused by Henoch-Schönlein purpura, with immediate response to short-term steroid therapy. J Pediatr Surg 30: 1509, 1995.
72. Mollica F, Li Volti S, Garozzo R, Russo G: Effectiveness of early prednisone treatment in preventing the development of nephropathy in anaphylactoid purpura. Eur J Pediatr 151: 140, 1992.
73. Saulsbury FT: Corticosteroid therapy does not prevent nephritis in Henoch-Schönlein purpura. Pediatr Nephrol 7: 69, 1993.
74. Niaudet P, Habib R: Methylprednisolone pulse therapy in the treatment of severe forms of Schönlein-Henoch purpura nephritis. Pediatr Nephrol 12: 238, 1998.
75. Iijima K, Ito-Kariya S, Nakamura H, Yoshikawa N: Multiple combined therapy for severe Henoch-Schönlein nephritis in children. Pediatr Nephrol 12: 244, 1998.
76. Rostoker G, Desvaux-Belghiti D, Pilatte Y, et al: High-dose immunoglobulin therapy for severe IgA nephropathy and Henoch-Schönlein purpura. Ann Intern Med 120: 476, 1994.
77. Rostoker G, Desvaux-Belghiti D, Pilatte Y, et al: Immunomodulation with low-dose immunoglobulins for moderate IgA nephropathy and Henoch-Schönlein purpura. Preliminary results of a prospective uncontrolled trial. Nephron 69: 327, 1995.
78. Counahan R, Winterborn MH, White RH, et al: Prognosis of Henoch-Schönlein nephritis in children. Br Med J 2: 11, 1977.
79. Coakley JC, Chambers TL: Should we follow up children with Henoch-Schönlein syndrome? Arch Dis Child 54: 903, 1979.
80. Goldstein AR, White RH, Akuse R, Chantler C: Long-term follow-up of childhood Henoch-Schönlein nephritis. Lancet 339: 280, 1992.
81. Meulders Q, Pirson Y, Cosyns JP, et al: Course of Henoch-Schönlein nephritis after renal transplantation. Report on ten patients and review of the literature. Transplantation 58: 1179, 1994.
82. Cameron JS: Recurrent primary disease and de novo nephritis following renal transplantation. Pediatr Nephrol 5: 412, 1991.
83. Kunnamo I, Kallio P, Pelkonen P, Viander M: Serum-sickness–

like disease is a common cause of acute arthritis in children. Acta Paediatr Scand 75: 964, 1986.
84. Michel BA, Hunder GG, Bloch DA, et al: Hypersensitivity vasculitis and Henoch-Schönlein purpura: a comparison between the 2 disorders. J Rheumatol 19: 721, 1992.
85. Haber MM, Marboe CC, Fenoglio JJ Jr: Vasculitis in drug reactions and serum sickness. *In* Churg A, Churg J (eds): Systemic Vasculitides. New York, Igaku-Shoin, 1991, pp 305–313.
86. Fauci AS, Haynes B, Katz P: The spectrum of vasculitis: clinical, pathologic, immunologic and therapeutic considerations. Ann Intern Med 89: 660, 1978.
87. Calabrese LH, Michel BA, Bloch DA, et al: The American College of Rheumatology 1990 criteria for the classification of hypersensitivity vasculitis. Arthritis Rheum 33: 1108, 1990.
88. Watts RA, Jolliffe VA, Grattan CE, et al: Cutaneous vasculitis in a defined population—clinical and epidemiological associations. J Rheumatol 25: 920, 1998.
89. Jennette JC, Falk RJ, Andrassy K, et al: Nomenclature of systemic vasculitides. Proposal of an international consensus conference. Arthritis Rheum 37: 187, 1994.
90. Mocan H, Mocan MC, Peru H, Ozoran Y: Cutaneous polyarteritis nodosa in a child and a review of the literature. Acta Paediatr 87: 351, 1998.
91. Daoud MS, Hutton KP, Gibson LE: Cutaneous periarteritis nodosa: a clinicopathological study of 79 cases. Br J Dermatol 136: 706, 1997.
92. David J, Ansell BM, Woo P: Polyarteritis nodosa associated with streptococcus. Arch Dis Child 69: 685, 1993.
93. Thomas RH, Black MM: The wide clinical spectrum of polyarteritis nodosa with cutaneous involvement. Clin Exp Dermatol 8: 47, 1983.
94. Ginarte M, Pereiro M, Toribio J: Cutaneous polyarteritis nodosa in a child. Pediatr Dermatol 15: 103, 1998.
95. Albornoz MA, Benedetto AV, Korman M, et al: Relapsing cutaneous polyarteritis nodosa associated with streptococcal infections. Int J Dermatol 37: 664, 1998.
96. Jennette JC, Falk RJ: Small-vessel vasculitis. N Engl J Med 337: 1512, 1997.
97. Wong SN, Shah V, Dillon MJ: Antineutrophil cytoplasmic antibodies in Wegener's granulomatosis. Arch Dis Child 79: 246, 1998.
98. Nash MC, Dillon MJ: Antineutrophil cytoplasm antibodies and vasculitis. Arch Dis Child 77: 261, 1997.
99. Rottem M, Fauci AS, Hallahan CW, et al: Wegener granulomatosis in children and adolescents: clinical presentation and outcome. J Pediatr 122: 26, 1993.
100. Davis MD, Daoud MS, McEvoy MT, Su WP: Cutaneous manifestations of Churg-Strauss syndrome: a clinicopathologic correlation. J Am Acad Dermatol 37: 199, 1997.
101. Savage CO, Winearls CG, Evans DJ, et al: Microscopic polyarteritis: presentation, pathology and prognosis. Q J Med 56: 467, 1985.
102. Gianviti A, Trompeter RS, Barratt TM, et al: Retrospective study of plasma exchange in patients with idiopathic rapidly progressive glomerulonephritis and vasculitis. Arch Dis Child 75: 186, 1996.
103. Jordan SC: Treatment of systemic and renal-limited vasculitic disorders with pooled human intravenous immune globulin. J Clin Immunol 15: 76S, 1995.
104. Banker BQ, Victor M: Dermatomyositis (systemic angiopathy) of childhood. Medicine (Baltimore) 45: 261, 1966.
105. Dillon MJ, Ansell BM: Vasculitis in children and adolescents. Rheum Dis Clin North Am 21: 1115, 1995.
106. Crowe WE, Bove KE, Levinson JE, Hilton PK: Clinical and pathogenetic implications of histopathology in childhood polydermatomyositis. Arthritis Rheum 25: 126, 1982.
107. Miller LC, Sisson BA, Tucker LB, et al: Methotrexate treatment of recalcitrant childhood dermatomyositis. Arthritis Rheum 35: 1143, 1992.
108. Gyselbrecht L, De Keyser F, Ongenae K, et al: Etiological factors and underlying conditions in patients with leucocytoclastic vasculitis. Clin Exp Rheumatol 14: 665, 1996.
109. Provost TT, Zone JJ, Synkowski D, et al: Unusual cutaneous manifestations of systemic lupus erythematosus: I. Urticaria-like lesions. Correlation with clinical and serological abnormalities. J Invest Dermatol 75: 495, 1980.
110. Martini A, Ravelli A, Albani S, et al: Hypocomplementemic urticarial vasculitis syndrome with severe systemic manifestations. J Pediatr 124: 742, 1994.
111. Gibson LE, Su WP: Cutaneous vasculitis. Rheum Dis Clin North Am 21: 1097, 1995.
112. Davis MD, Daoud MS, Kirby B, et al: Clinicopathologic correlation of hypocomplementemic and normocomplementemic urticarial vasculitis. J Am Acad Dermatol 38: 899, 1998.
113. Hamid S, Cruz PD Jr, Lee WM: Urticarial vasculitis caused by hepatitis C virus infection: response to interferon alpha therapy. J Am Acad Dermatol 39: 278, 1998.
114. O'Donnell B, Black AK: Urticarial vasculitis. Int Angiol 14: 166, 1995.
115. Cattaneo R, Fenini MG, Facchetti F: The cryoglobulinemic vasculitis. Ric Clin Lab 16: 327, 1986.
116. Levo Y, Gorevic PD, Kassab HJ, et al: Association between hepatitis B virus and essential mixed cryoglobulinemia. N Engl J Med 296: 1501, 1977.
117. Revenga Arranz F, Diaz R, Iglesias Diez L, et al: Cryoglobulinemic vasculitis associated with hepatitis C virus infection. A report of eight cases. Acta Derm Venereol 75: 234, 1995.
118. Tavoni A, Mosca M, Ferri C, et al: Guidelines for the management of essential mixed cryoglobulinemia. Clin Exp Rheumatol 13(Suppl 13): S191, 1995.
119. Boom BW, Brand A, Bavinck JN, et al: Severe leukocytoclastic vasculitis of the skin in a patient with essential mixed cryoglobulinemia treated with high-dose gamma-globulin intravenously. Arch Dermatol 124: 1550, 1988.
120. Wooten MD, Jasin HE: Vasculitis and lymphoproliferative diseases. Semin Arthritis Rheum 26: 564, 1996.
121. Tinaztepe K, Gucer S, Bakkaloglu A, Tinaztepe B: Familial Mediterranean fever and polyarteritis nodosa: experience of five paediatric cases. A causal relationship or coincidence? Eur J Pediatr 156: 505, 1997.
122. Ozdogan H, Arisoy N, Kasapcapur O, et al: Vasculitis in familial Mediterranean fever. J Rheumatol 24: 323, 1997.
123. Plotkin GR, Patel BR, Shah VN: Behçet's syndrome complicated by cutaneous leukocytoclastic vasculitis. Response to prednisone and chlorambucil. Arch Intern Med 145: 1913, 1985.
124. Chen KR, Kawahara Y, Miyakawa S, Nishikawa T: Cutaneous vasculitis in Behçet's disease: a clinical and histopathologic study of 20 patients. J Am Acad Dermatol 36: 689, 1997.
125. Katz SI, Gallin JI, Hertz KC, et al: Erythema elevatum diutinum: skin and systemic manifestations, immunologic studies, and successful treatment with dapsone. Medicine (Baltimore) 56: 443, 1977.
126. Rodriguez-Serna M, Fortea JM, Perez A, et al: Erythema elevatum diutinum associated with celiac disease: response to a gluten-free diet. Pediatr Dermatol 10: 125, 1993.

27

Kawasaki Disease

Ross E. Petty and James T. Cassidy

INTRODUCTION AND HISTORICAL BACKGROUND

Since its first formal description in 1967 in the Japanese literature,[1] Kawasaki disease (KD), or mucocutaneous lymph node syndrome (as Professor Kawasaki first named it), has become one of the most commonly recognized of the childhood vasculitides. It was not until 1974 that the first description of this disorder was published in the English language literature.[2] Although the frequency of the disease has undoubtedly increased since then, it is also likely that KD existed before that time. In a review of published cases of infantile polyarteritis nodosa (IPN) in 1959, Munro-Faure identified a systemic clinical syndrome that characterized infants who died: fleeting macular skin eruptions, fever, conjunctivitis, pharyngitis, cervical adenitis, and occasionally other signs or symptoms.[3] The striking similarity of these clinical characteristics to those described by Kawasaki, together with the similarity in the pathologic lesions of IPN and KD, has led to the belief that patients with IPN had the most severe sequelae of KD, resulting in death. The history of KD has been recently documented.[4]

DEFINITION AND DIAGNOSTIC CRITERIA

KD is a multisystem inflammatory syndrome of unknown etiology and variable clinical expression, characterized histologically by the presence of vasculitis resulting in stenosis and aneurysms. The proximal coronary arteries are particularly likely to be affected.

The principal clinical presentations of KD are included in the criteria listed in Table 27–1.[5] For a diagnosis of KD to be confirmed, five of the six criteria must be documented or, if only four criteria are present, coronary aneurysms must be demonstrable by echocardiography. These criteria are most applicable to patients in the second week of disease and for therapeutic and other studies; however, from the viewpoint of the clinician attempting to make an early accurate diagnosis of KD (and therefore be in a position to initiate appropriate therapy), these criteria are often difficult to apply.

As clinicians become more aware of the disease and suspect a diagnosis of KD early in the disease course, it has become common to base a presumptive diagnosis of incomplete KD on the highly characteristic clinical and laboratory findings and to initiate therapy before fulfillment of the required five criteria. It is clear that a re-evaluation of the diagnostic criteria and their application is in order.

EPIDEMIOLOGY

KD is probably the most common vasculitis of childhood and may well be the most common vasculitis at any age.[6–9] The frequency of the disease varies from one part of the world to another; the highest frequency is still recorded in Japan, where there is an annual incidence of 90 per 100,000 children under 5 years of

Table 27–1

Kawasaki Disease: Frequency and Characteristics of Diagnostic Criteria

CRITERION	FREQUENCY (%)	CHARACTERISTICS
1. Fever	100	Duration 5 days or more; 39–40°C; unresponsive to antibiotics
2. Conjunctivitis	85	Bilateral, bulbar, nonsuppurative
3. Lymphadenopathy	70	Cervical, tender, often unilateral, acute, nonpurulent, >1.5 cm in diameter
4. Rash	80	Polymorphous, no vesicles or crusts
5. Changes in lips or oral mucosa	90	Dry, swollen, red, vertically cracked lips; "strawberry" tongue Diffusely erythematous oropharynx
6. Changes in extremities	70	*Acute:* erythema of palms or soles; indurative edema of hands or feet *Convalescent:* membranous desquamation from fingertips

Diagnosis requires 5 of 6 criteria, or 4 criteria plus coronary artery aneurysms shown on echocardiography. For criteria 5 and 6, any one of the 3 findings is sufficient to fulfill the criterion

From Centers for Disease Control: Multiple outbreaks of Kawasaki syndrome—United States. MMWR 34: 33, 1985.

age.[10] A minimum annual incidence of 5.95 per 100,000 children younger than 5 years has been estimated for the metropolitan Chicago area in the United States. The highest frequencies were found in children of Asian origin, boys, and younger children.[11]

KD is typically a disease of the young, and in Japan, the disease is more common in boys than in girls (1.36:1) and peaks in frequency between 6 and 11 months of age. In boys the highest incidence is in the 9- to 11-month age group (227.3 per 100,000 children), and in girls the highest incidence is between 3 and 8 months of age (133.9 per 100,000 children).[10] In North America, the peak age distribution is somewhat older than in Japan, and children in the 2- to 3-year age group are most frequently affected. Although the disease typically affects young children, it has been described in older children[12] and occasionally in adults.[13] An even wider and older range of age at onset was reported in a study from Australia.[14] In this nationwide survey, incidences were 3.7 per 100,000 for children under 5 years of age and 0.59 per 100,000 for children over 5 years of age. Only 20 percent of the children were under 1 year of age at the time of diagnosis, and 25 percent were over 5 years of age. The reasons for these geographic differences in age at onset are not clear.

There have been several reports of seasonal peaks of incidence,[15, 16] and in North America most cases occur between February and May.[17] In Hawaii, there has been some clustering in time and geographic area, suggesting an unrecognized vector, although cases among children sharing the same home are uncommon.[18–20] A hospital survey[21] documented the previously reported cyclic occurrence[22] of the disease. Three distinct epidemics of KD were recorded in Japan up to 1987, but none since that time.[15] In North America, it is our current experience that KD occurs year-round, but clusters of the disease occur in the late winter and spring.

ETIOLOGY AND PATHOGENESIS

The etiology of KD is unknown. Many of its clinical manifestations suggest an infectious etiology: the fever, exanthem, lymphadenopathy, conjunctivitis, and lesions of the oral mucosa are all reminiscent of a bacterial or viral illness. A close resemblance to scarlet fever is evident. Clusters of cases grouped in time and geographic location have been reported, but the incidence of familial occurrence in most studies is low, and the inconsistency of clear-cut epidemics of the disease make an infectious etiology uncertain. If an infectious agent causes KD, either it is of very low communicability or almost all cases of infection are subclinical.

An association with mycobacterial antigens has been suggested because of the inflammatory change that occurs at the site of a previous bacillus Calmette-Guérin (BCG) immunization in children with KD[23, 24] and the temporarily positive response to mycobacterial antigens, both in vivo and in vitro in children with acute KD.[25] Whether these responses represent a specific reaction to mycobacterial antigens, or represent a more general response to bacterial or other heat-shock proteins cross-reactive with those in the test antigens, is not clear. The 65-kD heat-shock protein of mycobacteria is recognized by lymphocytes from patients convalescing from KD, and such patients also have antibodies to this antigen.[26] Furthermore, it has been reported that children with KD have increased expression of the 63-kD human heat-shock protein in peripheral blood lymphocytes compared with febrile controls patients or normal controls.[27]

Superantigens, capable of stimulating large numbers of T cells by interaction with the β chain of the T-cell receptor, are produced by several organisms, notably certain strains of *Staphylococcus* and *Streptococcus*. Controversial studies have linked staphylococcal toxins to KD but have not convincingly demonstrated a cause-and-effect relationship. In 1993, toxic shock syndrome toxin type 1 (TSST-1) from *Staphylococcus aureus* was isolated by Leung and associates[28] from patients with KD. Further studies by the same group[29] demonstrated *S. aureus* secreting TSST-1 or exfoliative toxin A in three acutely ill KD patients with coronary artery lesions. These findings have been refuted by others, however.[30] The question of toxin-induced KD is not yet settled.[31] The role of one or more superantigens in the etiology of KD is hotly debated, but the inconsistency of its demonstration, although not excluding an etiologic role, has made it difficult to ascribe most cases of KD to this mechanism.

A study published in 1997 demonstrated the predominance of immunoglobulin A (IgA)–secreting plasma cells in vasculitic tissues taken from children with acute fatal KD.[32] The authors suggested that the presence of IgA in the vessel walls indicated an antigen-driven immune response to an organism that gained entry through the mucosal surfaces. High levels of serum IgE in children with IPN and KD have been construed as evidence of an allergic basis for this disorder.[33]

The viral genome of the Epstein-Barr virus has been isolated from the renal tubule cells of a child with KD[34] and from the cardiac and aortic tissues from patients with a KD-like illness,[35] but convincing evidence of a causal relationship between Epstein-Barr virus and KD is lacking. Associations with rotavirus,[36] other viruses,[37–41] or infectious agents spread by carpet shampooing[42, 43] have been noted inconsistently.

GENETIC BACKGROUND

KD is seldom familial, and the extent of a genetic predisposition to KD is not certain. At a time when the overall incidence of KD in Japan was 0.19 percent, Fujita and associates[19] used a questionnaire to determine that the second-case rate for siblings in a family was 2.1 percent. The authors acknowledged that, because of the study design, this probably represented a maximum frequency. In a later and larger study, the proportion of patients with a family history of a sibling with KD was estimated at approximately 1 percent.[10]

In the study of Fujita and colleagues,[19] three of 30 twin pairs (10 percent) were concordant for KD; in each instance, both twins experienced the disease at the same time. Harada and colleagues[44] have documented concordance for KD in 14.1 percent in monozygotic twins and 13.3 percent in dizygotic twins in Japan. They noted that the disease usually occurred in the second twin within 2 weeks of onset of disease in the first twin. There have been few other reports of KD in twins[45–47] or siblings.[48, 49] Although the incidence of KD is undoubtedly higher in siblings of affected children than in the population at large, the fact that second cases tend to occur at or close to the time of the first suggests that, although there may be a genetic factor, age-dependent and environmental factors probably play a more important role in causation.

Rarely, KD has been reported in two generations of one family. In one report,[50] the 5-year-old son of a mother who had died at his birth and who, at the age of 16 years, had a KD-like illness with resulting coronary artery aneurysms, developed KD with coronary artery involvement. In a second report, a father and child had KD 21 years apart.[51] There has been no convincing association between KD and genes of the human leukocyte antigen (HLA) system.[44, 52–55] HLA-Bw51 was reported to be increased in Israeli patients with KD.[56] DR genomic typing of a group of 62 patients with KD failed to show any significant associations, except for an increase in HLA-DR3*0301 in one group of Caucasian patients (38 percent) compared with controls (11 percent) (relative risk, 5.0). No specific class II allele was associated with coronary artery disease.[55]

Shulman and coworkers[57] noted an increased frequency of the kappa chain allotype Km1 in patients with KD compared with race-matched control children. This light-chain immunoglobulin allotype was present in 25.6 percent of the Caucasian patients with KD but in only 14.4 percent of the control group ($P < .01$). Although there was no difference in distribution of specific Gm gamma-chain markers between patients with KD and controls, the combination of Km1 and heterozygosity for the Gm marker was increased in children with KD (17.9 percent) compared with controls (6.4 percent) ($P < .0001$). These differences were not present in Japanese patients. A study of the frequency of expression of the CDR3 domain in V kappa III–derived immunoglobulin light chains indicated that the 11-amino-acid CDR3 domain may be involved in the pathogenesis of KD.[58] A genetic contribution to the severity of KD is suggested by a study of the angiotensin I converting enzyme genotypes. Genotype II was present in 65 percent of children with coronary artery aneurysms, compared with 12.5 percent of those without aneurysms ($P < .01$; OR, 13.0). Why this genotype should predispose to severe KD is not known.[59]

Overall, the evidence that a specific genetic predisposition plays a major role in the etiology and pathogenesis of KD is supportive but not compelling. The fact remains, however, that this disease is more common in children of Japanese or Korean ancestry, wherever they live, than in other groups. Despite this, twin studies do not convincingly support a genetic basis for the disease, and the studies of known genetic polymorphisms such as in the major histocompatibility complex and immunoglobulin markers have yielded inconsistent results. It must be concluded that the extent and nature of the genetic contribution to KD are unknown and the interaction between genetic predispositions and environmental agents requires closer scrutiny.

CLINICAL MANIFESTATIONS

Disease Course

KD usually begins acutely; its course may be divided into three phases (Fig. 27–1)[8, 22]:

1. Acute febrile period of approximately 10 days
2. Subacute phase of approximately 2 to 4 weeks, ending with a return to normal of the platelet count and erythrocyte sedimentation rate (ESR)
3. Convalescent or recovery period lasting months or perhaps years, during which coronary artery disease may first be noted

There are no precise markers of the progression from one phase to another, but this concept of progression provides a useful framework for considering the course of the untreated disease.

Acute Febrile Phase

KD characteristically begins abruptly, without identifiable preceding events. The child becomes febrile and usually very irritable. Over the next 3 to 4 days (but in no particular order), cervical adenitis, conjunctivitis, changes in the lips and oral mucosa, a pleomorphic skin rash, and erythema and edema in the hands and feet—often with pain—develop. Untreated, these manifestations persist for 7 to 10 days and then subside. If carditis occurs, it often does so early and may be manifested by tachycardia and subtle or occasionally marked signs of congestive heart failure. Abdominal pain and hydrops of the gallbladder may occur at this time.

Subacute Phase

After the acute phase, the child may be entirely asymptomatic if given intravenous immunoglobulin (IVIG). Untreated, the fever gradually resolves by the third or fourth week. Desquamation of the digits or perineum (which may develop earlier) may be the only clinically apparent residual of the illness. Some children experience arthritis of one or several joints during the late acute and subacute phases. Coronary artery aneurysms are most common during the subacute or convalescent phases, occasionally earlier.

Convalescent Phase

Most children with KD are asymptomatic during the convalescent phase. With current therapy, the three-

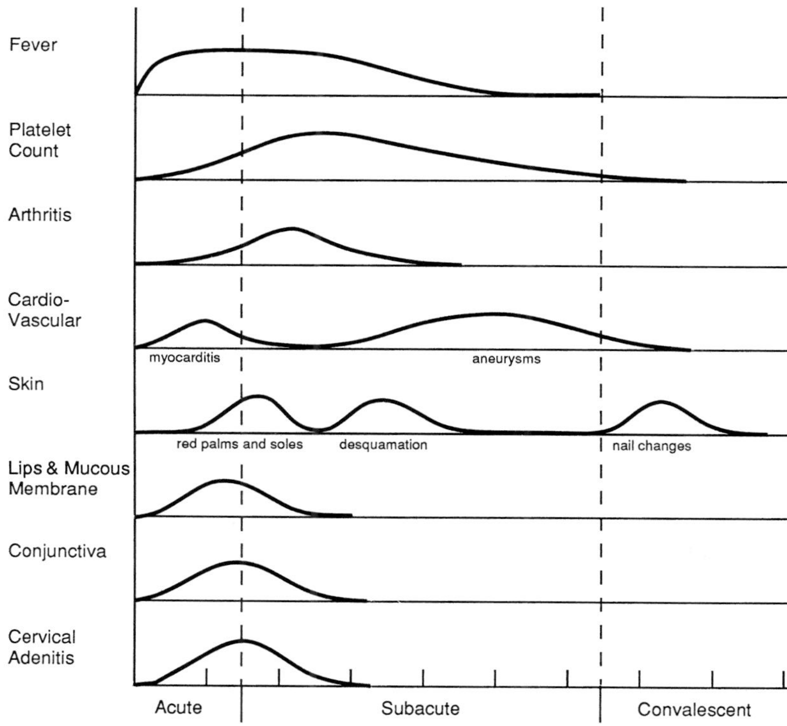

Figure 27–1. Kawasaki disease (KD) can be viewed as an illness with acute, subacute, and recovery phases. The temporal characteristics outlined in this figure are characteristic of the course of the disease.

phase pattern of disease is considerably altered and the first two phases are markedly abbreviated. With treatment, the acute phase usually lasts no more than 1 or 2 days after IVIG, and the subacute phase intervenes for another 3 to 4 weeks. By then, the acute-phase response has returned to normal, unless there are disease complications that indicate a failure of treatment. Beau's lines may appear at that time. Indicators of acute inflammation return to normal.

Classification Criteria

Fever

A remittent fever, often up to 40°C or higher, is characteristic of the acute phase and usually heralds the onset of the illness. This fever is unresponsive to antibiotics but responds partially to antipyretics. In untreated children, the febrile period lasts from 5 to 25 days, with a mean of approximately 10 days.

Conjunctivitis

Conjunctivitis is characteristically bilateral, affects only the bulbar conjunctivae, and is not accompanied by suppuration. The child may be somewhat photophobic, but because of irritability, this is often uncertain. The conjunctivitis may be difficult to differentiate from adenoviral conjunctivitis clinically; when there is doubt, the expertise of an ophthalmologist should be sought. Medium- to large-sized vessels of the conjunctiva are engorged, and the conjunctiva near the limbus may be spared. Subconjunctival hemorrhages occasionally occur. Conjunctivitis usually occurs within the first few days of the illness and may persist for a week or more. Exceptionally, there may be a conjunctival exudate,[60] conjunctival scarring,[61] or changes in the retina and vitreous.[62]

Changes in Lips and Oral Mucosa

The most characteristic changes are the bright red, swollen lips with vertical cracking and bleeding (Fig. 27–2). The mucosa of the oropharynx may be bright red, and the tongue may have a typical "strawberry" appearance. Occasionally, there are petechiae on the palate. The oral lesions persist throughout the febrile period.

Exanthem

The rash of KD begins in the acute febrile phase of the disease and lasts from 1 or 2 days to a week or more (Fig. 27–3). The rash varies over time; it is characteristically located on the trunk and may spread to involve the face, extremities, and perineum. Scarlatiniform, macular, papular, multiforme, and purpuric lesions have all been described. The rash is neither bullous nor vesicular, however, and crusting of the lesions does not occur. The rash is seldom pruritic. It usually fades

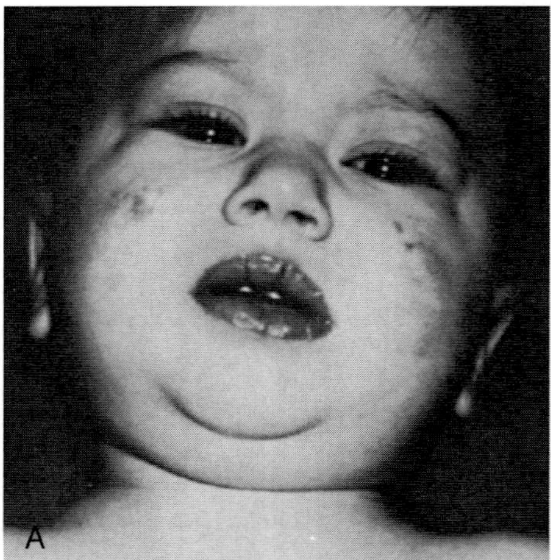

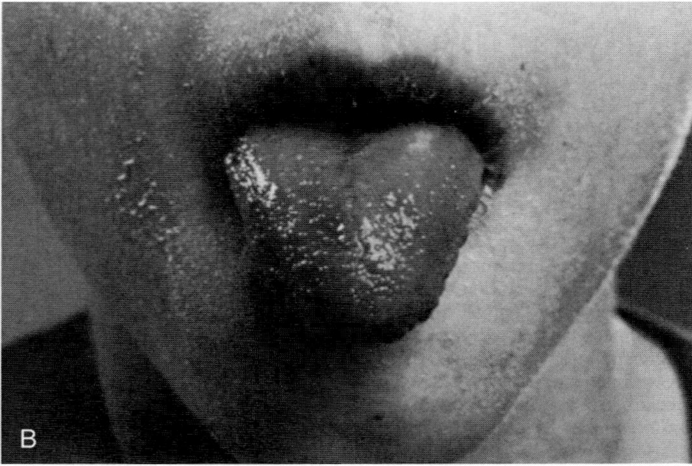

Figure 27–2. *A,* The intense reddening, swelling, and vertical cracking of the lips is characteristic of KD. Bilateral bulbar conjunctivitis and a nonspecific facial rash are also seen in this 2-year-old boy with acute KD. *B,* Strawberry tongue of acute KD with hypertrophied papillae on an erythematous base. Note also peeling of the facial skin.

without residua except for desquamation of the affected areas. Desquamation occurs first in the perineum[63]; flaky desquamation can occur elsewhere as well.

Extremity Changes

Changes in the peripheral extremities include reddish-purple ("magenta") erythema of the palms and soles that is often accompanied by painful, brawny edema of the dorsa of the hands and feet. These changes usually occur early in the course and last for 1 to 3 days. After the acute febrile phase, the fingertips begin to peel. This may involve mild flaking of the tips of the fingers or desquamation of the entire finger, beginning around the fingernail and extending proximally, sometimes to involve the entire palm (Fig. 27–4). Toes are less commonly affected.

Lymphadenopathy

Lymphadenopathy, characteristically of the anterior cervical chain, is usually unilateral and may involve only a single node. Enlargement of lymph nodes, which develops in the initial febrile period of the disease, may be marked, leading to a mistaken decision to incise and drain or excise the node. The duration of enlargement is usually brief (3 to 4 days) and although a *history* of an enlarged node is frequently elicited, it is one of the signs of KD least commonly observed by the physician (which is one of the reasons for abandoning the former designation *mucocutaneous lymph node syndrome*).

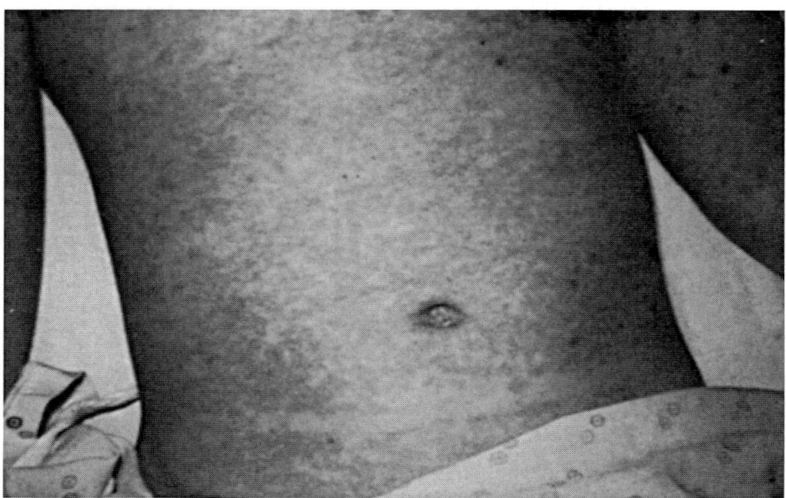

Figure 27–3. The polymorphous exanthem of KD is shown in this photograph taken during the acute phase of the disease. It is not diagnostic in its appearance and may evolve in character as the disease progresses, although it is rarely purpuric and never has vesicles or crusts.

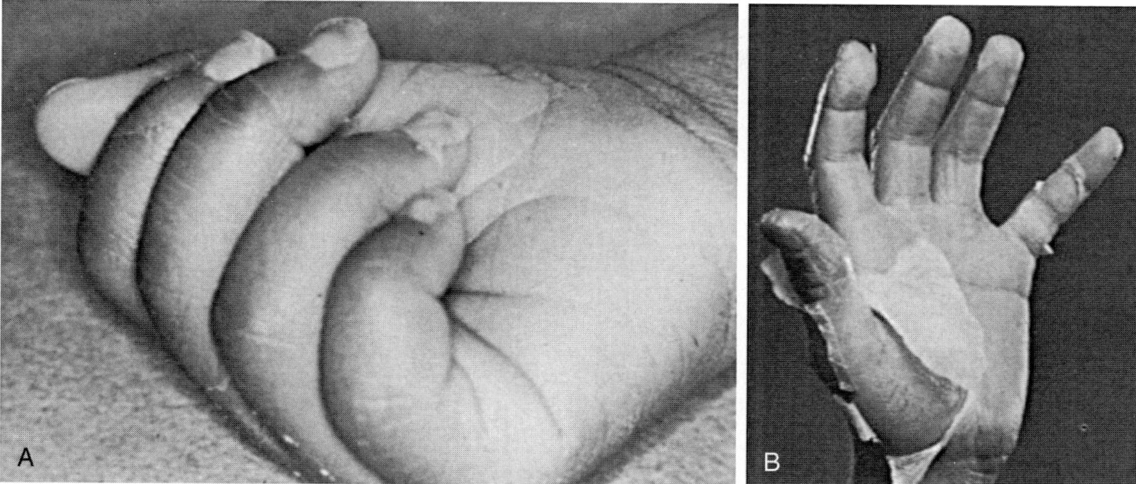

Figure 27–4. *A,* Edema of the hand and early peeling of the skin beginning around the nail margins during the subacute phase of KD. *B,* Desquamation of the skin of the hand later in the subacute and early recovery phase of KD. In many children, the degree of desquamation is much less than is depicted here.

Other Clinical Manifestations of Kawasaki Disease

The clinical features discussed thus far constitute the diagnostic criteria for KD, but the disease frequently has other characteristic manifestations, most importantly those affecting the cardiovascular system.

Cardiac Involvement

Cardiac disease is the most serious manifestation of KD.[64–67] Almost all of the early deaths and most of the long-term disability are related to involvement of the heart. Congestive heart failure may supervene as a result of myocarditis or myocardial infarction. Symptoms or signs of pericarditis (midsternal pain, muffled heart sounds, systolic murmurs or rubs) or arrhythmias may occur. Although detection of coronary artery aneurysms requires two-dimensional echocardiography (Fig. 27–5) or angiography (Fig. 27–6), aneurysms of other vessels such as the brachial and femoral arteries may be either palpable clinically or demonstrable angiographically (Fig. 27–7). Left-ventricular dysfunction should be evaluated by echocardiography along with

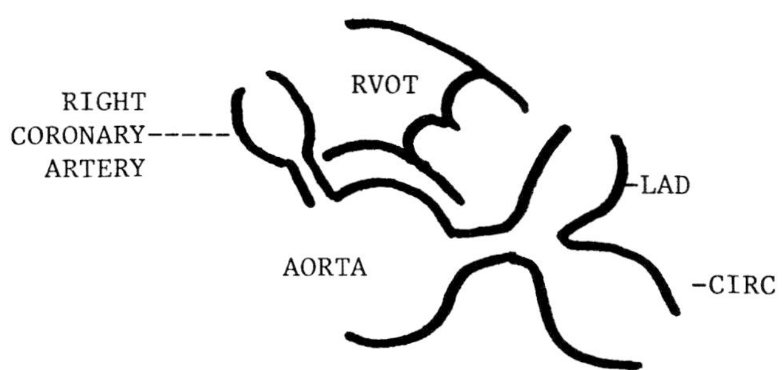

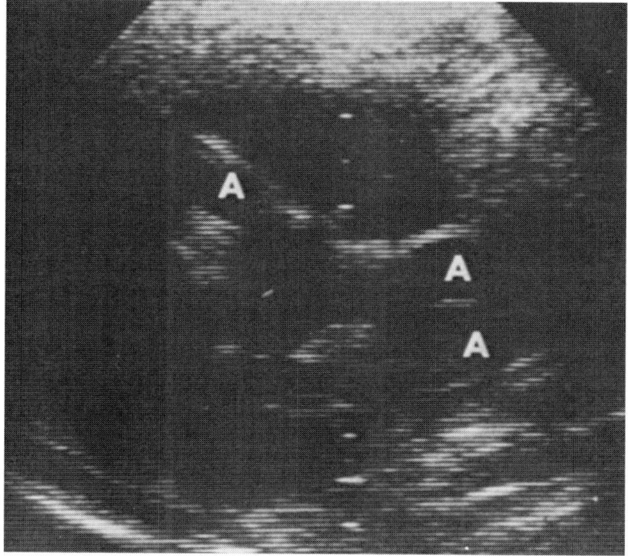

Figure 27–5. Echocardiographic demonstration of aneurysms of three coronary arteries in a child with KD. A, aneurysms; CIRC, circumflex; LAD, left anterior descending coronary artery; RVOT, right ventricular outflow tract. (Courtesy of Dr. Dennis Crowley.)

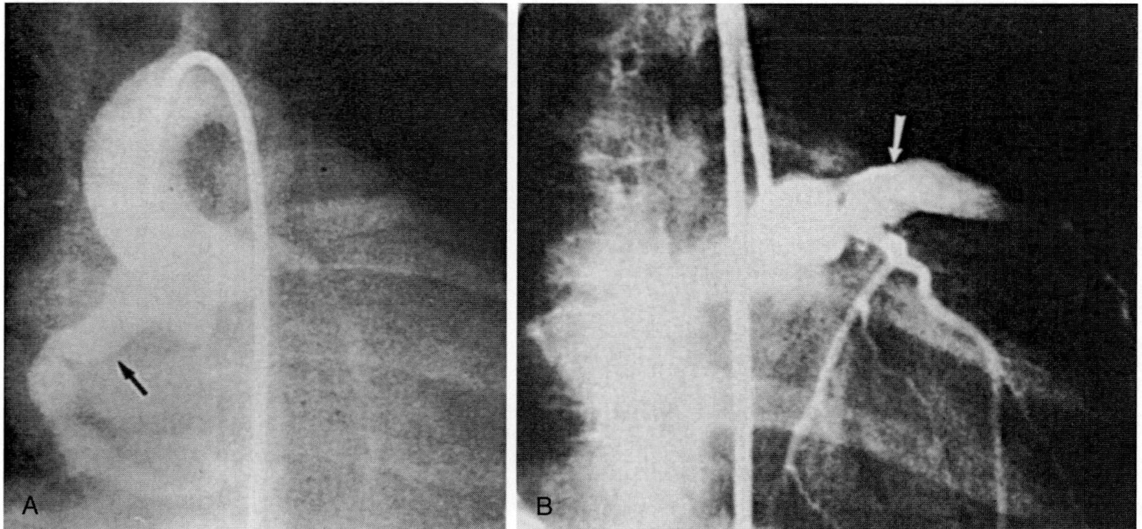

Figure 27–6. *A,* Angiography of coronary vessels in a 7-month-old white boy with KD. Huge aneurysmal dilatation of right coronary artery *(arrow)*. Aneurysms of the left and circumflex arteries were also present. *B,* Aneurysm of left coronary artery in a 3-year-old white girl with KD *(arrow)*. (*A* and *B,* Courtesy of Dr. Zuidi Lababidi.)

abnormalities of echodensity ("coronary artery prominence") that suggest the presence of vasculitis or perivasculitis of the proximal segments of the coronary arteries.

Central Nervous System Abnormalities

One of the most consistent clinical observations of children with KD is their extreme irritability, particularly

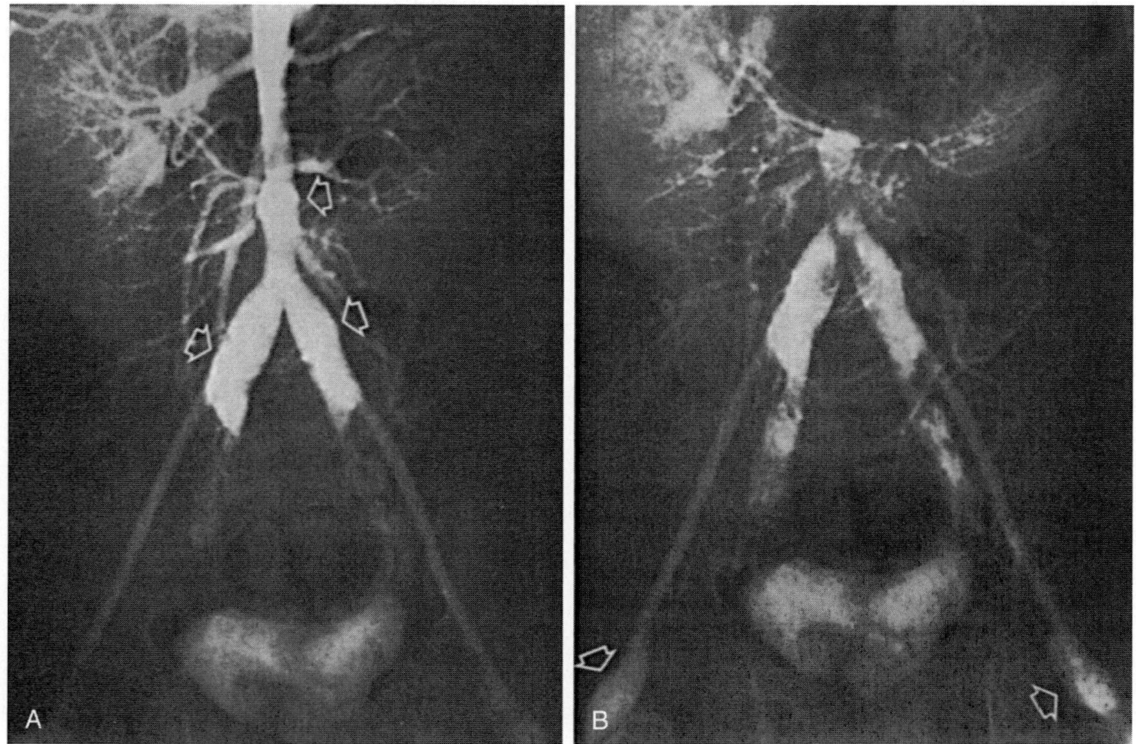

Figure 27–7. Angiographic study of a 2-year-old boy with severe KD resulting in multiple aneurysms of the coronary, axillary, iliac, and femoral arteries. Large aneurysms of the iliac *(A)* and femoral *(B)* arteries are seen *(arrows)*. Aneurysms that were palpable in the axilla and groin in this patient later resolved. (*A* and *B,* Courtesy of Dr. G. Culham.)

in the infant or very young child. This probably represents the effect of aseptic meningitis and associated headache.[68] Cerebrospinal fluid (CSF) is characterized by pleocytosis with a striking mononuclear cell predominance. In a study of 46 children with KD who underwent lumbar puncture, pleocytosis was present in 18 patients (39.1 percent), CSF glucose less than 45 mg/dl in 1 patient, and elevated CSF protein in 8 patients (17.4 percent). Pleocytosis ranged from 7 to 320 cells (median, 22.5 cells), with a median of 6 percent neutrophils and 91.5 percent mononuclear cells.[69] Rarely, central nervous system (CNS) vasculitis results in focal neurologic lesions.[70, 71] Laxer and associates[71] reported two patients with a KD-like illness and acute hemiplegia and reviewed four other reported cases. The authors noted that three of the six patients had received glucocorticoids before the onset of neurologic signs. Inappropriate antidiuretic hormone production with resulting hyponatremia is common in children with KD, probably as a reflection of CNS disease. Seizures, ataxia, and coma are rare manifestations of KD.[69]

Other Ocular Changes

Although conjunctivitis is the most characteristic ocular abnormality in KD and is one of the diagnostic criteria, additional ocular abnormalities are common.[72] Asymptomatic anterior uveitis occurs in approximately three quarters of children with KD. It is more common in those older than 2 years of age, is bilateral, and begins a little later than the conjunctivitis, peaking between days 5 and 8 of the illness.[73] Posterior synechiae are rare.[74] The anterior uveitis and other ocular signs listed in Table 27–2 disappear without visually significant sequelae and require no specific therapy.

Musculoskeletal Disease

Arthralgia and myalgia and, less commonly, arthritis may occur in children with KD. Arthritis usually presents during the recovery period and most commonly affects the large weight-bearing joints, particularly the knee and ankle, but not uncommonly affects the small joints of the hands and may occur in other joints as well. It was described in approximately one quarter of the children from Hawaii as oligoarthritis involving the knees, ankles, or hips.[75] Involvement of the proximal interphalangeal joints may be difficult to differentiate from edema of the digits.

Table 27–2

Frequency of Ocular Signs and Symptoms in Kawasaki Disease

OCULAR SIGN OR SYMPTOM	FREQUENCY (%)
Injection of bulbar conjunctivae	89
Nongranulomatous iridocyclitis	78
Superficial punctate keratitis	22
Vitreous opacities	12
Papilledema	11
Subconjunctival hemorrhage	3

From Kumagai N, Ohno S: Kawasaki disease. *In* Pepose JS, Holland GM, Wilhelmus KR (eds): Ocular Immunity and Infection. St. Louis, Mosby, 1996, pp 391–396.

Respiratory Tract Disease

Cough, coryza, or hoarseness are frequent early in the course of the disease and suggest a viral upper respiratory tract infection. Such symptoms are usually mild and transient and are only occasionally accompanied by pulmonary infiltrates or otitis media.[76, 77] The basis of the persistent sensorineural hearing loss that occurs in some children after KD is unknown.[76]

Gastrointestinal Tract Disease and Other Abnormalities

Abdominal pain is common, and approximately one quarter of children with KD have profuse, watery diarrhea during the acute febrile period. Vomiting is less common. Abdominal distention may occur and may mimic mesenteric vasculitis or intussusception similar to that observed in children with Henoch-Schönlein purpura. The relatively common occurrence of hydrops of the gallbladder demonstrated by ultrasonography[78] sometimes aids diagnosis of incomplete or atypical KD. Occasionally, the gallbladder becomes large enough to be seen as a bulge in the anterior abdominal wall. Hepatosplenomegaly may occur in the absence of heart disease or may reflect cardiac failure. Laboratory evidence of hepatic involvement includes elevation of liver enzymes and occasionally hyperbilirubinemia. Meatitis and dysuria occur frequently, and priapism has been described.[79]

Differential Diagnosis

Early in the illness, KD may be difficult to differentiate from other diseases, particularly when only two or three criteria are present. The differential diagnoses are listed in Table 27–3.

PATHOLOGY

The basic pathologic lesion in KD is necrotizing vasculitis with fibrinoid necrosis of the medium-sized muscular arteries, with coronary arteries the predominant sites of involvement.[80, 81] Histopathologic changes include an acute polymorphonuclear inflammatory infiltrate of all layers of the heart, including the valves.[65] The coronary arteries are characterized by an intense perivascular and intimal inflammation that also involve the vasa vasorum. Plasma cells are present, and the internal elastic lamina is disrupted. Studies have documented the presence of large numbers of IgA-producing plasma cells in the affected arteries.[32]

Evolution of the cardiac lesions is detailed in the

Table 27–3

Kawasaki Disease: Differential Diagnosis

Infectious Agents

Adenovirus
Rubeola
Parvovirus
Epstein-Barr virus
Cytomegalovirus
Rocky mountain spotted fever
Leptospirosis
Streptococcus
Staphylococcus

Toxic Reactions

Antibiotics
Anticonvulsants
Antifungals

Rheumatic Diseases

Systemic-onset juvenile rheumatoid arthritis
Polyarteritis nodosa

study of Fujiwara and Hamashima.[65] In the coronary arteries, vasculitis predominated in children who died early but was absent in those who died after 28 days of illness. Aneurysms, thrombosis, and stenosis did not appear until 12 days of disease or later. Pericarditis, myocarditis, and endocarditis were universal early in disease but diminished as fibrosis of the myocardium became the predominant lesion in children whose death occurred 40 days or more after onset (Table 27–4). The large study of Suzuki and associates[66] documented the location of angiographic findings in 262 children. Aneurysms, dilatations, and local stenoses (those associated with aneurysms) occurred with equal frequency in left and right coronary arteries. The right coronary artery was more frequently the site of segmental stenosis (89 percent) and occlusions (69 percent).

LABORATORY EXAMINATION

Indices of inflammation (ESR, platelet count, white blood cell count) are characteristically elevated early in the course of the disease.[22] Occasionally, significant neutropenia occurs early,[82] possibly signaling the presence of particularly severe disease. Toxic granulation of neutrophils is more frequent in children with KD than in those with other febrile illnesses.[83] Although the platelet count may be abnormally low during the early acute period of the illness, it almost always rises markedly during the subacute phase (>500,000/mm^3) and often exceeds 1,000,000/mm^3 (100×10^9/L). Moderate elevations of serum concentrations of liver enzymes occur, as does mild-to-moderate normocytic, normochromic, or hypochromic anemia, which is often present close to the onset of disease. A sterile pyuria and the presence of occasional erythrocytes may be documented on urinalysis. CSF contains modest increases in numbers of white blood cells, principally lymphocytes, representing aseptic meningitis.[84] The synovial fluid has been described as inflammatory.[80]

Antinuclear antibodies and rheumatoid factor are usually absent, but antibodies to neutrophil cytoplasmic antigens (ANCAs)[85] and to endothelial cells (AECAs)[86] may be present. Although ANCAs have been demonstrated in the sera of some children with KD late in the disease,[87] neither the frequency nor the titer of ANCAs differentiated children with KD from those with nonspecific febrile illnesses within the first 2 weeks of disease.[88] Increased levels of von Willebrand factor (factor VIII–related antigen)[89] indicate the involvement of the endothelium in pathogenesis.[90] Serum levels of C3 and C4 are normal or elevated, but activation products of these complement components have been demonstrated on erythrocytes (C3dg) and in the plasma (C4d),[91, 92] suggesting the participation of the complement pathway in the pathogenesis of the disease. Elevations of levels of tumor necrosis factor α and other cytokines document the systemic inflammatory nature of KD and the role of proinflammatory cytokines in its pathogenesis.[93, 94]

In the third phase of the illness, a number of abnormalities have been observed that may be important with respect to long-term cardiovascular sequelae. Lipid abnormalities occur during the initial phase of the disease and (at least in some studies) may persist for months or years after the inflammatory disease has disappeared. Newburger and colleagues[95] measured the serum levels of total cholesterol, high-density lipoprotein (HDL) cholesterol, and triglycerides in patients with a history of KD at intervals from less than 10 days to more than 3 years after disease onset. The most striking abnormalities were a marked depression of the levels of HDL cholesterol and marked elevation of nonfasting triglyceride levels during the first 10 days of illness. Of interest is the persistence of the low HDL cholesterol levels even at the longest time period studied (3 years or more), a phenomenon that tended to correlate with coronary artery disease. The depressed HDL cholesterol levels during the acute phase of the illness were confirmed in subsequent studies, although prolonged depression was not confirmed.[96, 97] Whether these lipid abnormalities are associated with the development of coronary artery disease or its sequelae is uncertain.

Table 27–4

Kawasaki Disease: Cardiac Pathology

	INTERVAL FROM ONSET TO DEATH (DAYS)			
LESION (%)	0–9	12–25	28–31	40–49
Coronary Artery				
Vasculitis	100	75	0	0
Aneurysms	0	85	100	85
Thrombosis	0	85	100	70
Myocardium				
Pericarditis	100	100	100	70
Myocarditis	100	85	25	0
Endocarditis	100	50	50	15
Myocardial fibrosis	0	0	0	70
Endocardial elastosis	0	0	25	40

Modified from Fujiwara H, Hamashima Y: Pathology of the heart in Kawasaki disease. Pediatrics 61: 100, 1978.

Long-term persistence of abnormalities of vascular reactivity were described in a study of 20 patients who had had KD a mean of 11 years (range, 5 to 17 years) before the investigation.[98] In this study, high-resolution ultrasonography was used to evaluate the response of the brachial artery to reactive hyperemia (endothelium-dependent dilatation) and glyceryl trinitrate (endothelium-independent dilatation). Endothelium-dependent flow-mediated dilatation was markedly reduced in patients with KD compared with control subjects (3.1 percent vs. 9.4 percent, $P < .001$). This study is important from two points of view: none of the patients studied had coronary artery lesions detected, and the fact that abnormalities were seen suggested that even in patients with relatively mild disease, subclinical vascular abnormalities may occur. Furthermore, the long duration of the abnormality suggested a more profound pathology than had heretofore been perceived. This observation calls into question the manner in which patients with KD (even those without coronary artery abnormalities) should be treated and monitored.

CARDIAC INVESTIGATIONS

The electrocardiogram is useful in the initial evaluation to delineate ventricular dysfunction, ischemia, or arrhythmia. Two-dimensional echocardiography is effective in detecting coronary ectasia or aneurysms as small as 0.2 to 0.4 mm in diameter (see Fig. 27–5). Ultrasound studies can also demonstrate aneurysms in the brachial or other peripheral arteries. Arteriography may be necessary to demonstrate peripheral coronary artery narrowing or occlusion or to confirm the presence of aneurysms in other locations if this is clinically indicated (see Fig. 27–7). Magnetic resonance arteriography offers a noninvasive procedure for further documentation of aneurysms.[99]

TREATMENT

General

The child with suspected or definite KD should be admitted to the hospital for observation, monitoring of cardiac status, and management of systemic manifestations (Table 27–5). Unless the diagnosis of KD is in doubt, isolation is not necessary. If the diagnosis is relatively certain (even if diagnostic criteria are not entirely fulfilled), treatment should be initiated with aspirin and IVIG. Although extreme irritability is a common feature of KD, if there is any question of meningitis, CSF should be examined to exclude bacterial infection. Evaluation of the cardiovascular system is essential in order to detect early congestive heart failure and should include an electrocardiogram to identify arrhythmias, signs of ischemia, or myocarditis (which occurs early in the disease course). A baseline echocardiograph is required to detect coronary artery vasculitis, ectasia, or aneurysms.

Table 27–5

Kawasaki Disease: Evaluation and Management

Make Diagnosis

Admit to Hospital

Evaluate	**Treat**
Cardiac status (ECHO, ECG)	Aspirin
CNS status	If platelets <400,000: 80–100 mg/kg/d in 4 doses
Fluid and electrolyte status	If platelets >400,000: 3–5 mg/d
Urinalysis	IVIG 2 g/kg
Ophthalmologic status	Keep in hospital until afebrile for 24 hr or if there are complications. Repeat IVIG once. If no clinical response, consider IV methylprednisolone 30 mg/kg
Monitor cardiac status	Maintain low-dose aspirin until ESR and platelet count are normal if there have been no coronary artery abnormalities; for 2 years, if coronary abnormalities have been but are no longer present; "forever" if coronary artery disease persists
Monitor ESR and platelet count 2-week intervals until stable, then 1-month intervals until normal	
Repeat echocardiograph at 6–8 weeks	

CNS, central nervous system; ECG, electrocardiogram; ECHO, echocardiogram; ESR, erythrocyte sedimentation rate; IVIG, intravenous immunoglobulin.

Aspirin

Aspirin serves two functions in the management of KD. In the early stages when the fever is still present and before the platelet count has risen, aspirin is used at anti-inflammatory doses (80 to 100 mg/kg/day in four divided doses). Several reports have noted difficulty in achieving therapeutic salicylate levels in children with early KD because of impaired absorption.[100–103] Care should be taken not to exceed a dose of 100 mg/kg/day because as the disease comes under control, the salicylate level may suddenly increase to toxic levels. As the fever disappears, and the platelet count rises, the dose is reduced to 3 to 5 mg/kg/day, a dose well below an anti-inflammatory level but one that inhibits platelet adhesion to endothelium by curtailing platelet release of thromboxane A_2 without suppressing prostacyclin production by endothelial cells.[103] Although long-term, low-dose aspirin is recommended for any child in whom cardiac abnormalities have been detected, the efficacy of this approach for the prevention of coronary thrombosis has not been documented in controlled studies.

The role of aspirin in the present-day management of KD is not entirely certain. Whether the aspirin dose should be maintained at the higher level until the platelet count rises or reduced to the low dose when the fever disappears is a matter of opinion. After IVIG, the fever in patients with KD usually subsides rapidly and the requirement for antipyretics is minimal to none. It is our practice to use high-dose aspirin only until the fever disappears. In the event of aspirin sensitivity, another antiplatelet agent such as dipyridamole should be given to inhibit thrombus formation. A meta-analysis of published studies[105] concluded that there was no justification for the use of high-dose rather than low-dose aspirin in conjunction with IVIG with respect to the occurrence of coronary artery disease, although the analysis pointed out that high-dose aspirin could have other benefits. Some clinicians question the necessity of high-dose aspirin at all because the effectiveness of IVIG is so profound and so rapid. Nonetheless, it is important to remember that in the trials that demonstrated the efficacy of IVIG, all patients were receiving aspirin. Other nonsteroidal anti-inflammatory drugs have been little used in treating KD.

Intravenous Immunoglobulin

The administration of IVIG has an established role in the treatment of KD.[106] Several studies have demonstrated its efficacy in suppressing the clinical manifestations of the disease in general and in reducing the severity and frequency of coronary aneurysms.[105, 107–109] A number of regimens have been used: initially, IVIG 400 mg/kg/day was given on 4 consecutive days[110]; in a subsequent study, IVIG was administered once in a dose of 1 g/kg.[111] Currently, it is recommended that IVIG be given at 2 g/kg in a single dose.[108] There is a suggestion that the incidence of coronary artery disease is lowest in those receiving the highest dose of IVIG,[112] and the possibility exists that doses higher than 2 g/kg may be even more effective, although there have been no studies in this regard. The addition of the vasodilating drug pentoxifylline to a regimen of IVIG may have additional benefit but requires more study.[113] Table 27–6 presents a representative protocol for the administration of IVIG.

IVIG is entrenched in the therapeutic armamentarium and generally has few immediate-term or long-term complications. It is a blood product, however, and the risk of transmitting some known or unknown infectious agent should not be ignored. Documentation[114] of the transmission of hepatitis C via IVIG is a reminder to use the product only with appropriate indications. IVIG-related aseptic meningitis is common in children with inflammatory diseases. It is characterized by rapid onset of headache, sometimes with nausea and vomiting, occurring 24 to 36 hours after the initiation of the infusion, and may be difficult to differentiate from a recurrence of the initial illness. It lasts for 12 to 24 hours and disappears without known residua. Hyperviscosity syndrome, a theoretical risk (particularly in those who require retreatment with IVIG), is exceedingly rare. Nakamura and Yanagawa reported that children with KD who were treated with IVIG were 2.66 times as likely to experience recurrence of disease within 12 months as those who did not receive IVIG.[115] This curious phenomenon has not been further studied, and because almost all patients with recognized KD are treated with IVIG, it will be difficult to evaluate.

Table 27–6

Protocol for Administration of Intravenous Immunoglobulin (IVIG)

1. Admit to hospital.
2. Start IV with normal saline.
3. Infuse IVIG (5%) in a dose of 2 g/kg body weight. Give over 8–12 hr, beginning at a rate of 0.1 to 0.2 ml/kg/hr for the first 30 minutes and increasing gradually over the next hour to a rate of not more than 2 ml/kg/hr for the remainder of the infusion.
4. Monitor blood pressure and heart rate:
   Every 15 minutes for first hour,
   Every 30 minutes for second hour,
   Every hour thereafter, if stable.
5. Monitor temperature every hour during infusion, every 4 hours thereafter.
6. If blood pressure or heart rate fluctuate significantly, change infusion to normal saline and reevaluate.
7. Observe for at least 24 hours for evidence of benefit or side effect of IVIG:
   Benefit: fall in temperature, increased well-being, decreased irritability, decreased rash
   Side effect: anaphylaxis, headache, vomiting (aseptic meningitis), signs of hypervolemia or heart failure.

Note: This outline is a guide only.

In controlled studies of the efficacy of IVIG, treatment was initiated within the first 10 to 12 days of illness. For a number of reasons, this is not always possible,[14, 116] and it is not certain if therapy begun after this time is as effective. It is our practice, however, to give IVIG in the usual manner to any patient with KD at any time after disease onset if symptoms or laboratory evaluations (ESR, platelet count, white blood cell count) suggest ongoing inflammation.

Glucocorticoids

The role of glucocorticoids in the treatment of KD remains controversial, although it is standard practice to avoid their use as first-line management. Among the vasculitides, KD stands alone as a disease that is allegedly made worse by the use of glucocorticoids. This conclusion was first reached in a clinical trial by Kato and colleagues,[117] in which the frequency of aneurysms was much higher in those treated with prednisolone (65 percent) than in children treated only with aspirin (11 percent). This study has been criticized because of its design, the small number of patients in the prednisolone-treated group, and the high frequency of aneurysms, but it has profoundly influenced the treatment of this disease. An uncontrolled study published in 1996[118] reported a frequency of aneurysms of 17.8 percent (giant aneurysms in 2.4 percent) in children treated with a combination of glucocorticoid and aspirin. Another small study has reported the efficacy of intravenous pulse methylprednisolone (30 mg/kg) given with heparin for 3 consecutive days in prevention of coronary artery disease.[119]

Thus, reliable data are few and largely uncontrolled, and current evidence is that glucocorticoids do not have a place in the management of KD in most children. In children who are unresponsive to one or at most two full doses of IVIG, however—or in whom severe active myocarditis is present—intravenous methylprednisolone should be considered. Wright and colleagues[120] reported the results of therapy with intravenous methylprednisolone in four patients with KD who experienced no response to two or three doses of IVIG and who had progressing coronary artery dilatation on echocardiography. In all patients, the fever disappeared after glucocorticoid use (although in one patient it recurred and responded to a third course of IVIG). Occasionally, IVIG and intravenous methylprednisolone produce no response in children. Such children should be suspected of having polyarteritis nodosa and treated with oral prednisone in a dose of 2 mg/kg/day initially. A role for cyclophosphamide has been suggested in a recent study of children with persistent KD.[119a]

Monitoring Cardiac Status

There is considerable disagreement as to the timing and frequency of echocardiographic monitoring in patients with KD. Most protocols are somewhat arbitrary but account for the timing of the development of coronary artery aneurysms that occur most frequently between the second and the eighth weeks. However, aneurysms can be present in the first week of the illness, and the recommendations of the Committee on Rheumatic Fever, Endocarditis, and Kawasaki Disease of the American Heart Association[121] are that *the initial echocardiograph should be performed at the time a diagnosis of KD is suspected* and that each child with KD should undergo a second echocardiograph 6 to 8 weeks after disease onset. If both examinations yield normal results, no further echocardiographic studies are routinely necessary. If ectasia is present on the first echocardiograph but has disappeared by the time of the second study, no further studies are needed. However, if a solitary small aneurysm is detected on either study, the patient should undergo echocardiography annually until the age of 10 years and thereafter as indicated by the cardiologist. If multiple small aneurysms, or one or more giant aneurysms, are detected on either the initial or the 6- to 8-week study, echocardiographs should be repeated annually. If coronary artery obstruction is detected on either of the two initial studies, echocardiographs should be repeated at 6-month intervals. Electrocardiographs are recommended annually in the first decade of life, and stress testing should be performed for children in the second decade of life in risk groups III and IV (Table 27–7) and every 6 months in group V. Angiography is indicated if stress testing or echocardiography suggests stenosis in order to delineate the patency and extent of the smaller branches of the coronary system.

Kitamura and coworkers reported a large series of Japanese children requiring coronary artery bypass grafting for coronary artery disease secondary to KD.[122] Half of the patients had had myocardial infarcts. The peak age for performance of the procedure was 5 to 7 years, although infants under 1 year of age have undergone bypass grafts for KD-related coronary artery disease.[123] A number of children with coronary artery disease secondary to KD have required cardiac transplantation.[124] Many of these patients underwent transplantation within a year of KD because of severe left-ventricular dysfunction secondary to infarction, intractable arrhythmias, and extensive distal coronary artery involvement.

COURSE OF THE DISEASE AND PROGNOSIS

Recurrences

In most instances, the course of KD is uniphasic. Occasionally, however, there are recurrences. In the Japanese survey,[115] there were recurrences in 3 percent of patients and the rate of recurrence was highest in children who were older at disease onset, reaching approximately 6 percent in those older than 6 years. Two or more recurrences were noted in only 0.2 percent of these patients. Second episodes were observed within the first 12 months in almost half, but in 7 percent the recurrence did not appear until at least 48 months later.[115] Recurrences among North American patients seem to be less frequent,[125] although children of Japanese extraction living in the United States are reported to be more susceptible to recurrences than Caucasian children.[126]

Late Mortality

There are numerous reports of sudden unexpected death in older children or young adults who have had

Table 27–7

Recommendations for Long-Term Management of Kawasaki Disease Based on Echocardiographic Findings

	RISK LEVEL	DRUGS	PHYSICAL RESTRICTIONS
I	Normal	None after 1st 6–8 wk	None beyond 1st 6–8 wk
II	Transient ectasia	None after 1st 6–8 wk	None beyond 1st 6–8 wk
III	Small-medium solitary aneurysm	Aspirin 3–5 mg/kg/d until abnormalities resolve	None beyond 1st 6–8 wk under 11 yr of age After 11 yr of age activity guided by results of annual stress test; competitive contact sports with endurance training discouraged
IV	Multiple small to medium or one or more giant aneurysms	Aspirin 3–5 mg/kg/d long-term ± warfarin	As for III All strenuous sports strongly discouraged
V	Obstruction	Aspirin 3–5 mg/kg/d long-term ± warfarin ? Calcium channel blockers	As for III and IV; avoid contact sports, isometrics, weight training

Modified from Dajani AS, Taubert KA, Takahashi M, et al: Guidelines for long-term management of patients with Kawasaki disease. Circulation 89: 916, 1994.

KD in infancy.[127–130] The exact risk of this event is not known, however. There are many other reports of persons who died suddenly in the second or third decades of life who had had a history of what was almost certainly KD as infants. It has been estimated that in the United States, acquired coronary artery disease accounts for 12 percent of cardiac causes of sudden death associated with physical exertion or sports in persons between 11 and 35 years of age.[131] It is probable that most if not all of these patients had KD earlier in life.

In a survey of cases published in the Japanese or English language literature, Burns and associates[132] identified 74 patients who presented with cardiac disease at a mean of almost 25 years after KD. Symptoms at presentation included chest pain or myocardial infarction (60.8 percent), arrhythmia (10.8 percent), and sudden death (16.2 percent). Ring calcification of a coronary vessel was documented on chest radiographs in one third of the patients studied. Angiographic studies demonstrated coronary artery occlusion in two thirds. At necropsy, coronary artery aneurysms were present in all patients, and coronary artery occlusion in 72 percent. Supraventricular tachycardia is another late sequela.[133]

In a large Japanese study,[134] 797 of 6585 patients (12.1 percent) examined within the first 15 days of illness had cardiac sequelae after an average of 5.7 years of follow-up. It is not clear how these patients were treated. Mortality was higher for boys than girls. Nineteen patients (0.3 percent) died, 7 of them during the acute phase of cardiac disease[6] or encephalopathic disease[1] or as the result of an accident.[1] Eleven patients died after the acute phase: 2 of coronary artery disease, 2 of congenital cardiac anomalies, 2 of malignant neoplasms, and 5 of other causes. Death from KD was rare after the first 2 months of disease.

PERSPECTIVE

In recent decades, KD has emerged as a major health problem in young children throughout the world, but particularly in Japan, North America, and parts of Europe. Its early diagnosis, so essential to effective management, is often difficult. Treatment with IVIG is effective, but its mode of action is still unclear. The development of biologic agents that bind or block specific inflammatory mediators offers hope for improved therapy for what is usually a unicyclic inflammatory disease of limited duration, but one which has life-threatening long-term complications.

References

1. Kawasaki T: Acute febrile mucocutaneous syndrome with lymphoid involvement with specific desquamation of the fingers and toes in children. Jpn J Allergy 16: 178, 1967.
2. Kawasaki T, Kosaki F, Okawa S, et al: A new infantile acute febrile mucocutaneous lymph node syndrome (MLNS) prevailing in Japan. Pediatrics 54: 271, 1974.
3. Munro-Faure H: Necrotising arteritis of the coronary vessels in infancy. Pediatrics 23: 914, 1959.
4. Burns JC, Kushner HI, Bastian JF, et al: Kawasaki disease. A brief history. Pediatrics 106: E27, 2000 [electronic citation].
5. Dajani AS, Taubert KA, Gerber MA, et al: Diagnosis and therapy of Kawasaki disease in children. Circulation 87: 1776, 1993.
6. Yanagawa H, Kawasaki T, Shigematsu I: Nationwide survey on Kawasaki disease in Japan. Pediatrics 80: 58, 1987.
7. Cook DH, Antia A, Attie F, et al: Results from an international survey of Kawasaki disease in 1979–1982. Can J Cardiol 5: 389, 1989.
8. Schackelford PG, Strauss AW: Kawasaki syndrome. N Engl J Med 324: 1664, 1991.
9. Watanabe N: Kawasaki disease (MCLS). Jpn J Rheumatol 1: 3, 1986.
10. Yanagawa H, Yashiro M, Nakamura Y, et al: Epidemiologic pictures of Kawasaki disease in Japan: From the nationwide incidence survey in 1991 and 1992. Pediatrics 95: 475, 1995.
11. Shulman ST, McAuley JB, Pachman LM, et al: Risk of coronary abnormalities due to Kawasaki disease in urban area with small Asian population. Am J Dis Child 141: 420, 1987.
12. Momenah T, Sanatani S, Potts J, et al: Kawasaki disease in the older child. Pediatrics 102: E7, 1998 (www.pediatrics.org). [electronic citation.]
13. Jackson JL, Kunkel MR, Libow L, Gates RH: Adult Kawasaki disease. Report of two cases treated with intravenous gamma globulin. Arch Intern Med 154: 1398, 1994.
14. Royle JA, Williams K, Elliott E, et al: Kawasaki disease in Australia, 1993–95. Arch Dis Child 78: 33, 1998.
15. Yanagawa H, Nakamura Y, Kawasaki T, et al: Nationwide epidemic of Kawasaki disease in Japan during winter of 1985–86. Lancet 2: 1138, 1986.
16. Salo E, Pelkonen P, Pettay O: Outbreak of Kawasaki syndrome in Finland. Acta Pediatr Scand 75: 75, 1986.
17. Bell DM, Morens DM, Holman RC, et al: Kawasaki syndrome in the United States 1976–1980. Am J Dis Child 137: 211, 1983.
18. Dean AG, Melish ME, Hicks R, et al: An epidemic of Kawasaki disease in Hawaii. J Pediatr 100: 552, 1982.
19. Fujita Y, Nakamura Y, Sakata K, et al: Kawasaki disease in families. Pediatrics 84: 666, 1989.
20. Hewitt M, Smith LJ, Joffe HS, et al: Kawasaki disease in siblings. Arch Dis Child 64: 398, 1989.
21. Taubert KA, Rowley AH, Shulman ST: Nationwide survey of Kawasaki disease and acute rheumatic fever. J Pediatr 119: 279, 1991.
22. Wortmann DW, Nelson AM: Kawasaki syndrome. Rheum Dis Clin North Am 16: 363, 1990.
23. Kuniyuki S, Asada M: An ulcerated lesion at the BCG vaccination site during the course of Kawasaki disease. J Am Acad Dermatol 37: 303, 1997.
24. Hsu Y-H, Wang Y-H, Hsu W-Y, Lee Y-P: Kawasaki disease characterized by erythema and induration of the Bacillus Calmette-Guérin and purified protein derivative inoculation sites. Pediatr Infect Dis J 6: 576, 1987.
25. Bertotto A, Spinozzi F, Radicioni M, Vaccaro R: Mantoux test in Kawasaki disease. Pediatrics 98: 161, 1996.
26. Yokota S, Tsubaki K, Kuriyama T, et al: Presence in Kawasaki disease of antibodies to mycobacterial heat-shock protein HSP 65 and autoantibodies to epitopes of human HSP65 cognate antigen. Clin Immunol Immunopathol 67: 163, 1993.
27. Takeshita S, Kawase H, Yamamoto M, et al: Increased expression of human 63-kD heat shock protein gene in Kawasaki disease determined by quantitative reverse transcription-polymerase chain reaction. Pediatr Res 35: 179, 1994.
28. Leung DYM, Meissner HC, Fulton DR, et al: Toxic shock syndrome toxin-secreting *Staphylococcus aureus* in Kawasaki syndrome. Lancet 342: 1385, 1993.
29. Leung DY, Sullivan KE, Brown-Whitehorn TF, et al: Association of toxic shock syndrome toxin-secreting and exfoliative toxin-secreting *Staphylococcus aureus* with Kawasaki syndrome complicated by coronary artery disease. Pediatr Res 42: 268, 1997.
30. Terai M, Miwa K, Williams T, et al: The absence of evidence of staphylococcal toxin involvement in the pathogenesis of Kawasaki disease. J Infect Dis 172: 558, 1995.
31. Meissner HC, Leung DY: Superantigens, conventional antigens and the etiology of Kawasaki syndrome. Pediatr Infect Dis J 19: 91, 2000.
32. Rowley AH, Eckerley CA, Jack HM, et al: IgA plasma cells in vascular tissue of patients with Kawasaki syndrome. J Immunol 159: 5946, 1997.

33. Kraus HF, Clausen CR, Roy CG: Elevated immunoglobulin E in infantile polyarteritis nodosa. J Pediatr 84: 841, 1974.
34. Muso E, Fujiwara H, Yoshida R, et al: Epstein-Barr virus genome positive tubulointerstitial nephritis associated with Kawasaki disease-like coronary artery aneurysms. Clin Nephrol 40: 7, 1993.
35. Kikuta H, Sakiyaja Y, Matsumoto S, et al: Detection of Epstein-Barr virus DNA in cardiac and aortic tissues from chronic, active Epstein-Barr virus infection associated with Kawasaki disease–like coronary artery aneurysms. J Pediatr 123: 90, 1993.
36. Matsuno S, Utagawa E, Sugiura A: Association of rotavirus infections with Kawasaki syndrome. J Infect Dis 148: 177, 1983.
37. Melish ME, Marchette NJ, Kaplan JC, et al: Absence of significant RNA-dependent DNA polymerase activity in lymphocytes from patients with Kawasaki syndrome. Nature 337: 288, 1989.
38. Kikuta H, Taguchi Y, Tomizawa K, et al: Epstein-Barr virus genome-positive T lymphocytes in a boy with chronic active EBV infection associated with Kawasaki disease. Nature 333: 455, 1988.
39. Okano M, Hase N, Sakiyama Y, et al: Long term observation in patients with Kawasaki syndrome and their relation to Epstein-Barr infection. Pediatr Infect Dis J 9: 139, 1990.
40. Marchette NJ, Melish ME, Hicks R, et al: Epstein-Barr virus and other herpesvirus infections in Kawasaki syndrome. J Infect Dis 161: 680, 1990.
41. Okano M, Thiele GM, Sakiyama Y, et al: Adenovirus infection in patients with Kawasaki disease. J Med Virol 32: 53, 1990.
42. Patriarca PA, Rogers MF, Morens DM, et al: Kawasaki syndrome: association with the application of rug shampoo. Lancet 2: 578. 1982.
43. Daniels SR, Specker B: Association of rug shampooing with Kawasaki disease. J Pediatr 118: 485, 1991.
44. Harada F, Sada M, Kamiya T, et al: Genetic analysis of Kawasaki syndrome. Am J Hum Genet 39: 537, 1986.
45. Kaneko K, Unno A, Takagi M, et al: Kawasaki disease in dizygotic twins. Eur J Pediatr 154: 868, 1995.
46. Fink HW: Kawasaki syndrome in twins. Pediatr Infect Dis 33: 372, 1984.
47. Fink HW: Simultaneous Kawasaki disease in identical twins: case report. Virginia Med 112: 248, 1985.
48. Matsubara T, Furukawa S, Ino T, et al: A sibship with recurrent Kawasaki disease and coronary artery lesion. Acta Paediatrica 83: 1002, 1994.
49. Lyen KR, Brook CG: Mucocutaneous lymph node syndrome in two siblings. Br Med J 1: 1187, 1978.
50. Bruckheimer E, Bulbul Z, McCarthy P, et al: Kawasaki disease: coronary aneurysms in mother and son. Circulation 97: 410, 1998.
51. Iwata F, Hanawa Y, Takashima H, et al: Kawasaki disease in a father and son. Acta Paediatr Jpn 34: 84, 1992.
52. Kato S, Kimura M, Tsuji K, et al: HLA antigens in Kawasaki disease. Pediatrics 61: 252, 1978.
53. Matsuda I, Hayttori S, Nagata JL, et al: HLA antigens in mucocutaneous lymph node syndrome. Am J Dis Child 131: 1417, 1977.
54. Krensky AM, Berenberg W, Shanley K, et al: HLA antigens in mucocutaneous lymph node syndrome in New England. Pediatrics 67: 741, 1981.
55. Barron KS, Silverman ED, Gonzales JC, et al: Major histocompatibility complex class II alleles in Kawasaki syndrome—lack of consistent correlation with disease or cardiac involvement. J Rheumatol 19: 1790, 1992.
56. Keren G, Danon YL, Orgad S, et al: HLA Bw51 is increased in mucocutaneous lymph node syndrome in Israeli patients. Tissue Antigens 20: 144, 1982.
57. Shulman ST, Melish M, Inoue O, et al: Immunoglobulin allotypic markers in Kawasaki disease. J Pediatr 122: 84, 1993.
58. Kim DS, Han BH, Lee SK, et al: Evidence for selection of 11 amino acid CDR3 domains in V kappa III-derived immunoglobulin light chains in Kawasaki disease. Scand J Rheumatol 26: 350, 1997.
59. Takeuchi K, Yamamoto K, Kataoka S, et al: High incidence of angiotensin I converting enzyme genotype II in Kawasaki disease patients with coronary aneurysms. Eur J Pediatr 156: 266, 1997.
60. Ammerman SD, Rao MS, Shope TC, et al: Diagnostic uncertainty in atypical Kawasaki disease and a new finding: exudative conjunctivitis. Pediatr Infect Dis J 4: 210–211, 1985.
61. Ryan EH, Walton DS: Conjunctival scarring in Kawasaki disease: a new finding? J Pediatr Ophthalmol Strabismus 20: 106, 1983.
62. Jacob J, Polomeno R, Chad Z, et al: Ocular manifestations of Kawasaki's disease (mucocutaneous lymph node syndrome). Can J Ophthalmol 17: 199, 1982.
63. Urbach AH, McGregor RS, Malatack JJ, et al: Kawasaki disease and perineal rash. Am J Dis Child 142: 1174, 1988.
64. Fujiwara H, Kawai C, Hamashima Y: Clinicopathologic study of the conduction systems in 10 patients with Kawasaki's disease (mucocutaneous lymph node syndrome). Am Heart J 96: 744, 1978.
65. Fujiwara H, Hamashima Y: Pathology of the heart in Kawasaki disease. Pediatrics 61: 100, 1978.
66. Suzuki A, Kamiya T, Kuwahara N, et al: Coronary artery lesions of Kawasaki disease: cardiac catheterization findings of 1100 cases. Pediatr Cardiol 7: 3, 1986.
67. Honda S, Sunagawa H, Mizogushi Y, et al: Left ventricular performance and compliance following acute febrile mucocutaneous lymph node syndrome. Jpn Circ J 44: 848, 1980.
68. McIlroy MA, Fisher EJ, Saravolatz LD, et al: Aseptic meningitis complicating adult Kawasaki disease. Am J Med 87: 106, 1989.
69. Dengler LD, Capparelli EV, Bastian JF, et al: Cerebrospinal fluid profile in patients with acute Kawasaki disease. Pediatr Infect Dis J 17: 478, 1998.
70. Amano S, Hazama F: Neural involvement in Kawasaki disease. Acta Pathol Jpn 30: 265, 1980.
71. Laxer RM, Dunn HG, Flodmark O: Acute hemiplegia in Kawasaki disease and infantile polyarteritis nodosa. Dev Med Child Neurol 26: 814, 1984.
72. Kumagai N, Ohno S: Kawasaki disease. *In* Pepose JS, Holland GN, Wilhelmus KR (eds): Ocular Immunity and Infection. St. Louis, Mosby, 1996, pp 391–396.
73. Burns JC, Joffe L, Sargent RA, Glode MP: Anterior uveitis associated with Kawasaki syndrome. Pediatr Infect Dis 4: 258, 1985.
74. Blatt AN, Vogler L, Tychsen L: Incomplete presentations in a series of 37 children with Kawasaki disease: the role of the pediatric ophthalmologist. J Pediatr Ophthalmol Strabismus 33: 114, 1996.
75. Melish ME, Hicks RM, Larson EJ: Mucocutaneous lymph node syndrome in the United States. Am J Dis Child 130: 599, 1976.
76. Sundel RP, Newburger JW, McGill T, et al: Sensorineural hearing loss associated with Kawasaki disease. J Pediatr 117: 371, 1990.
77. Suzuki J, Yanagawa T, Kihira S: Two cases of hearing loss associated with Kawasaki disease. Clin Pediatr 41: 167, 1988.
78. Magilavy DB, Speert DP, Silver TM, et al: Mucocutaneous lymph node syndrome: report of two cases complicated by gallbladder hydrops and diagnosed by ultrasound. Pediatrics 61: 699, 1978.
79. Waring NP, Ortemberg J, Galen WK, et al: Priapism in Kawasaki disease. JAMA 261: 1730, 1989.
80. Amano S, Hazama F, Hamashima Y: Pathology of Kawasaki disease I. Pathology and morphogenesis of the vascular changes. Jpn Cir J 43: 633, 1979.
81. Amano S, Hazama F, Hamashima Y: Pathology of Kawasaki disease II. Distribution and incidence of the vascular lesions. Jpn Cir J 43: 741, 1979.
82. Hara T, Mizuno Y, Ueda K, et al: Neutropenia in Kawasaki disease. Eur J Pediatr 148: 580, 1989.
83. Rowe PC, Quinlan A, Luke BKH: Value of degenerative change in neutrophils as a diagnostic test for Kawasaki syndrome. J Pediatr 119: 370, 1991.
84. April MM, Burns JC, Newburger JW, et al: Kawasaki disease and cervical adenopathy. Arch Otolaryngol Head Neck Surg 116: 512, 1989.
85. Soppi E, Salp E, Pelkonnen P: Antibodies against neutrophil cytoplasmic components in Kawasaki disease. Acta Pathol Micro Immunol Scand 100: 269, 1992.
86. Tizard EJ, Baguley E, Hughes GR, et al: Antiendothelial cell antibodies detected by a cellular based ELISA in Kawasaki disease. Arch Dis Child 66: 189, 1991.

87. Savage COS, Tizard J, Jayne D, et al: Antineutrophil cytoplasm antibodies in Kawasaki disease. Arch Dis Child 64: 360, 1989.
88. Guzman J, Fung M, Petty RE: Diagnostic value of serum antineutrophil cytoplasmic and anti-endothelial antibodies in Kawasaki disease. J Pediatr 124: 917, 1994.
89. Irazuzta JE, Elbl F, Rees AR: Factor VIII related antigen (von Willebrand's factor) in Kawasaki disease. Clin Pediatr 29: 347, 1990.
90. Nonoyama S: Immunological abnormalities and endothelial cell injury in Kawasaki disease. Acta Paediatr Jpn 33: 752, 1991.
91. Laxer RM, Schaffer FM, Myones BL, et al: Lymphocyte abnormalities and complement activation in Kawasaki disease. Prog Clin Biol Res 250: 175, 1987.
92. Myones BL, Tomita S, Corydon K, Shulman ST: Intravenous IgG administration is associated with a decrease in classical pathway complement activation products in patients with Kawasaki disease. Arthritis Rheum 34: S44, 1991.
93. Suzuki H, Uemura S, Tone S, et al: Effects of immunoglobulin and gamma interferon on the production of tumor necrosis factor α and interleukin 1 β by peripheral blood mononuclear cells in the acute phase of Kawasaki disease. Eur J Pediatr 155: 291, 1996.
94. Eberhard BA, Andersson U, Laxer RM, et al: Evaluation of the cytokine response in Kawasaki disease. Pediatr Infect Dis J 14: 199, 1995.
95. Newburger JW, Burns JC, Beiser AS, Loscalzo J: Altered lipid profile after Kawasaki syndrome. Circulation 84: 625, 1991.
96. Cabana VG, Gidding SS, Getz GS, et al: Serum amyloid A and high density lipoprotein participate in the acute phase response of Kawasaki disease. Pediatr Res 42: 651, 1997.
97. Chiang AN, Hwang B, Shaw GC, et al: Changes in plasma levels of lipids and lipoprotein composition in patients with Kawasaki disease. Clin Chim Acta 260: 15, 1997.
98. Dhillon R, Clarkson P, Donald AE, et al: Endothelial dysfunction late after Kawasaki Disease. Circulation 94: 2103, 1996.
99. Bisset GS, Strife JL, McCloskey J: MR imaging of coronary artery aneurysms in a child with Kawasaki disease. Am J Radiol 152: 805, 1989.
100. Koren G, MacLeod SM: Difficulty in achieving therapeutic serum concentrations of salicylate in Kawasaki disease. J Pediatr 105: 991, 1984.
101. Koren G, Schaffer F, Silverman E, et al: Determinants of low serum concentrations of salicylates in patients with Kawasaki disease. J Pediatr 112: 663, 1988.
102. Koren G, Silverman E, Sundel R, et al: Decreased protein binding of salicylate in Kawasaki disease. J Pediatr 118: 456, 1991.
103. Akagi T, Kato H, Inoue O, et al: A study of the optimal dose of aspirin therapy in Kawasaki disease: clinical evaluation and arachidonic acid metabolism. Kurume Med J 37: 203, 1990.
104. Pedersen AK, FitzGerald GA: Dose-related kinetics of aspirin. Presystemic acetylation of platelet cyclooxygenase. N Engl J Med 311: 1206, 1984.
105. Durongpisitkul K, Gururaj VJ, Park JM, Martin CF: The prevention of coronary artery aneurysm in Kawasaki disease: a meta-analysis on the efficacy of aspirin and immunoglobulin treatment. Pediatrics 96: 1057, 1995.
106. Shulman ST: Recommendations for intravenous immunoglobulin therapy of Kawasaki disease. Pediatr Infect Dis J 11: 985, 1992.
107. Furusho K, Kamiya T, Nakano H, et al: High-dose intravenous gamma globulin for Kawasaki disease. Lancet 2: 1055, 1984.
108. Newburger JW, Takahashi M, Burns JC, et al: The treatment of Kawasaki syndrome with intravenous gammaglobulin. N Engl J Med 315: 341, 1986.
109. Nagashima M, Matsushima M, Matsuoka H, et al: High-dose gammaglobulin therapy for Kawasaki disease. J Pediatr 110: 710, 1987.
110. Newburger JW, Takahashi M, Burns JC, et al: The treatment of Kawasaki syndrome with intravenous gamma globulin. N Engl J Med 315: 341, 1986.
111. Barron KS, Murphy DJ Jr, Silverman ED: Treatment of Kawasaki syndrome: a comparison of two dosage regimens of intravenously administered immune globulin. J Pediatr 117: 638, 1990.
112. Terai M, Shulman ST: Prevalence of coronary artery abnormalities in Kawasaki disease is highly dependent on gamma globulin dose but independent of salicylate dose. J Pediatr 131: 888, 1997.
113. Furukawa S, Matsubara T, Umezawa Y, et al: Pentoxifylline and intravenous gamma globulin combination therapy for acute Kawasaki disease. Eur J Pediatr 153: 664, 1994.
114. Bjoro K, Froland SS, Yun Z, et al: Hepatitis C infection in patients with primary hypogammaglobulinemia after treatment with contaminated immune globulin. N Engl J Med 331: 1607, 1994.
115. Nakamura Y, Yanagawa H: A case-control study of recurrent Kawasaki disease using the database of the nationwide surveys in Japan. Eur J Pediatr 155: 303, 1996.
116. Dhillon R, Newton L, Rutt PT, et al: Management of Kawasaki disease in the British isles. Arch Dis Child 69: 631, 1993.
117. Kato H, Koike S, Yokoyama T: Kawasaki disease: effect of treatment on coronary artery involvement. Pediatrics 63: 175, 1979.
118. Shinohara M, Sone K, Kobayashi T, et al: Treatment of Kawasaki disease with corticosteroid. J Pediatr 129: 483, 1996.
119. Kijima Y, Kamiya T, Suzuki A, et al: A trial procedure to prevent aneurysm formation of the coronary arteries by steroid pulse therapy in Kawasaki disease. Jpn Circ J 46: 1239, 1982.
119a. Wallace CA, French JW, Kahn SJ, Sherry DD: Initial gamma globulin treatment failure in Kawasaki disease. Pediatrics 105: E78, 2000 [electronic citation].
120. Wright DA, Newburger JW, Baker A, et al: Treatment of immune globulin resistant Kawasaki disease with pulsed doses of corticosteroids. J Pediatr 128: 146, 1996.
121. Dajani AS, Taubert KA, Takahashi M, et al: Guidelines for long-term management of patients with Kawasaki disease. Circulation 89: 916, 1994.
122. Kitamura S, Kamedo Y, Sekit S, et al: Long-term outcome of myocardial revascularization in patients with Kawasaki coronary artery disease. J Thorac Cardiovasc Surg 107: 663, 1994.
123. Dalzell V, Gottheiner NL, Duffy CE, et al: Coronary artery bypass grafting for Kawasaki disease. Pediatr Res 41: 118A, 1997.
124. Checchia PA, Pahl E, Shaddy RE, Shulman ST: Cardiac transplantation for Kawasaki disease. Pediatrics 100: 695, 1997.
125. Davis RL, Waller PL, Mueller BA, et al: Kawasaki syndrome in Washington state. Race-specific incidence rates and residential proximity to water. Arch Pediatr Adolesc Med 149: 66, 1995.
126. Mason WH, Takahashi M, Schneider T: Recurrence of Kawasaki disease in a large urban cohort in the United States. *In* Takahashi M, Taubert K (eds): Proceedings of the Fourth International Symposium on Kawasaki Disease, 1991. Dallas, American Heart Association, 1993, pp 21–26.
127. Kegel SM, Dorsey TJ, Rowen M, Taylor WF: Cardiac death in mucocutaneous lymph node syndrome. Am J Cardiol 40: 282, 1977.
128. Kohr RM, McCowen C, Henderson DC: Sudden death in incomplete Kawasaki's disease. Arch Dis Child 63: 1254, 1988.
129. Runge MS, Stouffer GA, Sheahan RG, et al: Sudden cardiac death in a teenager: A review of Kawasaki disease. Am J Med Sci 315: 273, 1998.
130. McConnell ME, Hannon DW, Steed RD, Gilliland MG: Fatal obliterative coronary vasculitis in Kawasaki disease. J Pediatr 133: 259, 1998.
131. Liberthson RR: Sudden death from cardiac causes in children and young adults. N Engl J Med 334: 1039, 1996.
132. Burns JC, Shike H, Gordon JB, et al: Sequelae of Kawasaki disease in adolescents and young adults. J Am College Cardiol 28: 253, 1996.
133. Seymour JJ, Dickinson ET: Delayed cardiovascular sequelae from Kawasaki syndrome. Am J Emerg Med 16: 579, 1998.
134. Nakamura Y, Yanagawa H, Kato H, Kawasaki T: Mortality rates for patients with a history of Kawasaki disease in Japan. J Pediatr 128: 75, 1996.

28

Polyarteritis Nodosa and Related Vasculitides

Ross E. Petty and James T. Cassidy

Polyarteritis nodosa (PAN) and cutaneous polyarteritis (CPA) are rare vasculitides in childhood. They may represent diverse manifestations of the same disease, although some authorities regard them as separate entities linked by similarities of cutaneous lesions and histopathology. PAN is typically a multisystem disease resulting from vascular inflammation in skin, abdominal viscera, kidneys, central nervous system, muscles, and other locations. CPA is restricted to vessels of the skin, muscle, joints, and peripheral nerves.

POLYARTERITIS NODOSA

Definition

The classic form of PAN, initially described in 1866 by Küssmaul and Maier as periarteritis nodosa,[1] is a chronic, relapsing, febrile disease with protean clinical manifestations resulting from inflammation of small- and medium-sized muscular arteries ("nodose lesions"), often leading to aneurysm formation. Jennette and colleagues[2] defined PAN as necrotizing inflammation of medium- or small-sized arteries without glomerulonephritis or vasculitis in arterioles, capillaries, or venules. The American College of Rheumatology (ACR) criteria for the diagnosis of PAN are given in Table 28–1.[3] Some of the individual criteria are inappropriate for use in children, and the criteria have not been evaluated in children or adolescents. Using the clinical findings in a group of 31 Turkish children aged 1 to 14 years, Ozen and colleagues[4] have proposed age-specific diagnostic criteria for PAN (Table 28–2). These criteria lack specificity, however, and although they describe the disease in a substantial number of patients, no control group was included in their analysis. The criteria require further refinement and validation before they can be used as diagnostic criteria.

Epidemiology

Frequency

PAN is uncommon at any age but occurs most frequently in the fifth and sixth decades of life; it is rare in childhood, particularly in North America. The correct diagnosis in reported cases is often uncertain, and interpretation of published reports is sometimes difficult. Early review of the subject usually included children with infantile PAN, which is now viewed as a severe manifestation of Kawasaki disease rather than PAN. This chapter focuses on more recent studies,[4–11] but the interested reader is referred to the early important reports of Fager and associates[12] and Frohnert

Table 28–1

American College of Rheumatology 1990 Criteria for the Classification of Polyarteritis Nodosa

CRITERION	DEFINITION
1. Weight loss	Loss of 4 kg or more of body weight not caused by dieting or other factors
2. Livedo reticularis	Mottled reticular pattern of the skin of portions of the extremities or torso
3. Testicular pain	Pain or tenderness of testicles not due to other causes
4. Myalgia	Diffuse myalgia excluding shoulder and hip girdle, or muscle weakness, or tenderness of leg muscles
5. Mono- or polyneuropathy	Mononeuropathy, multiple mononeuropathies or polyneuropathy
6. Diastolic BP >90	
7. ↑ Blood urea nitrogen (BUN) or creatinine	BUN >40 mg/dl or creatinine >1.5 mg/dl not due to other causes
8. Hepatitis B virus	Presence of hepatitis B surface antigen or antibody in serum
9. Arteriographic change	Aneurysms or occlusions of visceral arteries not due to other causes
10. Biopsy	Granulocytes and mononuclear leukocytes in wall of small or medium-sized artery

For classification purposes, a patient is said to have polyarteritis nodosa if at least three criteria are met (sensitivity 82.2%; specificity 86.6% in adult population).

From Lightfoot RW Jr, Michel BA, Bloch DA, et al: The American College of Rheumatology 1990 criteria for the classification of polyarteritis nodosa. Arthritis Rheum 33: 1088, 1990.

Table 28–2

Proposed Criteria for a Diagnosis of Polyarteritis Nodosa

Major Criteria

Renal disease
Musculoskeletal findings

Minor Criteria

Cutaneous findings
Gastrointestinal involvement
Peripheral neuropathy
Central nervous system disease
Hypertension
Cardiac disease
Lung disease
Constitutional symptoms
Increased acute-phase reactants
Presence of hepatitis B surface antigen

Diagnosis of PAN requires the presence of five criteria, including at least one major criterion. Antinuclear antibody and anti-dsDNA must be absent.

From Ozen S, Besbas N, Saatci U, et al: Diagnostic criteria for polyarteritis nodosa in childhood. J Pediatr 120: 206, 1992.

and Sheps.[13] Reimold and colleagues[5] estimated that fewer than 150 cases of PAN in infants and children had been reported up to 1976. Since that time, there have been several additional small series.[4, 6–11]

Sex, Age, and Geography

PAN occurs with approximately equal frequency in boys and girls and has a peak age at onset of 9 to 11 years, although it can occur in very young children. It is probably the childhood equivalent of PAN in the adult. It is worldwide in distribution, but the largest and most recent reports come from Turkey[4] and Japan.[11]

Genetic Background

Genetic factors do not appear to constitute an important risk for PAN, and familial occurrence is rare. The disease is so uncommon that studies of human leukocyte antigens and other genetic markers have not been reported.

A possible association between PAN and familial Mediterranean fever (FMF), a disease with a clear genetic basis, has been reported.[14–17] Tinaztepe and colleagues[16] noted 16 cases of FMF and PAN in the literature, and described a further five patients with both disorders. It is interesting that all of the reports of coincidence of FMF and PAN have come from Turkey, where both FMF and PAN appear to be more common than in North America or Northern Europe. It is not clear whether vasculitis is part of FMF (at least in the Middle East) or whether the two disorders have occurred by coincidence in the same individual. The identification of the gene causing FMF should permit screening in patients with PAN to further delineate this association.

Etiology and Pathogenesis

The etiology of PAN is unknown, but infectious processes are sometimes implicated. In adults with PAN, an association with hepatitis B infection has been described in 10 to 54 percent of patients, with the highest frequencies among inner-city populations.[18] In some patients with a clinical picture of classic polyarteritis, a relation between hepatitis B–associated antigen and immune complex formation has been proved.[19] PAN occurring after infection with hepatitis C has also been reported.[20, 21] To the best of our knowledge, these associations have not been recognized in children, although a child with severe PAN-like vasculitis occurring after infection with parvovirus B19 has been described.[22] The relation of PAN to preceding group A streptococcal infection remains a matter of interest.[5, 7, 23] In some series, upper airway infection with group B *Streptococcus* is a frequent event before the onset of PAN[7] or CPA[23]; in other series, such an association is not apparent. PAN as a paraneoplastic event has not been reported in children, although it occasionally occurs in adults.[24] In animals, infectious agents, particularly viruses, have been shown to produce polyarteritis-like lesions (see Chapter 2).[25] This finding supports the view that vasculitis in humans may be related to an initial or a sustained infectious process.

Clinical Manifestations

No single pattern of clinical presentation characterizes this disease, but the insidious onset of unexplained fever, weight loss, skin lesions, abdominal pain, and musculoskeletal pain should suggest the diagnosis of PAN (Table 28–3). The fever is usually remittent and may be low or high grade. Musculoskeletal pain with tenderness of muscle, and in two thirds of patients

Table 28–3

Frequency of Clinical Abnormalities in 81 Children With Polyarteritis Nodosa

CLINICAL FINDING	%
Fever	84
Arthritis/arthralgia	74
Abdominal pain	68
Myalgia	67
Skin abnormalities	
Rash	69
Edema	20
Petechiae	17
Mucous membrane abnormalities	9
Nervous system abnormalities	
Seizures	16
Other (including peripheral neuropathy)	10
Cardiac disease	21
Respiratory disease	7
Cervical lymphadenopathy	<5
Splenomegaly	<5
Renal	25

Compiled from data in references 4, 8–13.

overt arthritis, may be localized or diffuse. Secondary hypertrophic osteoarthropathy is a rare cause of musculoskeletal pain in patients with PAN.[26]

Nonspecific abdominal pain occurs in two thirds of patients, presumably related to ischemia caused by vasculitis of mesenteric and other intra-abdominal arteries. Infarction of the gut, gallbladder, or pancreas has been noted.[27] One young patient with PAN and abdominal pain had an aneurysm of the suprarenal artery.[28] Renal involvement (proteinuria, nephrotic syndrome, nephritis, hypertension) has been described in 26 children with PAN.[29]

Central nervous system involvement ultimately develops in 50 to 70 percent of children. Clinical findings include organic brain syndrome, psychosis, focal neurologic defects, unilateral blindness, seizures, and hemiparesis. Isolated central nervous system vasculitis and that related to Henoch-Schönlein purpura produce similar findings. A 1999 case report documents monocular blindness in a 9-year-old girl. Magnetic resonance imaging demonstrated multiple focal cortical and subcortical ischemic changes. Arteriography showed small aneurysms located at bifurcations of small- and medium-sized arteries.[30] A severe sensorimotor peripheral neuropathy (mononeuritis multiplex) may occur and is characteristic.

Cutaneous involvement includes painful subcutaneous nodules (particularly in the calf and foot), purpura, splinter hemorrhages (Fig. 28–1), livedo reticularis (Fig. 28–2), edema, peripheral gangrene, and ulceration. A multiplicity of other signs—including testicular or epididymal swelling, pain, or tenderness, and serous otitis media—rarely occur.

Cardiovascular abnormalities identified in one study of children with PAN included mild mitral or tricuspid valve regurgitation, diminished left-ventricular systolic function, and (in one patient) pericardial thickening.[31] None of the 15 children in this study had symptoms referable to the cardiovascular system, and electrocardiographs were normal. When the renal vasculature is inflamed, patients with PAN may have signs that suggest primary renal disease or renovascular hypertension.[32]

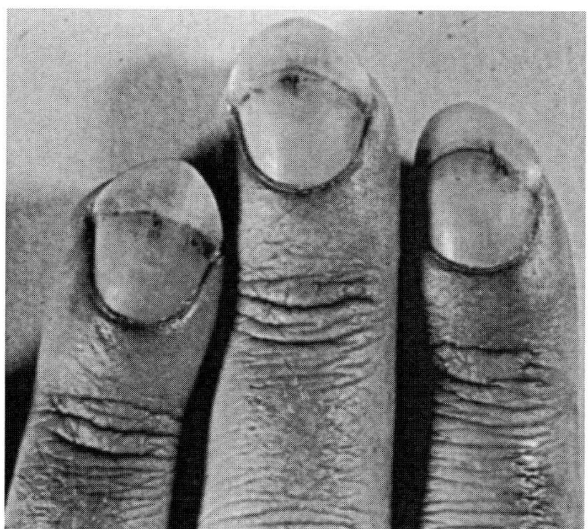

Figure 28–1. Splinter hemorrhages under the nails in a teenage girl with polyarteritis nodosa.

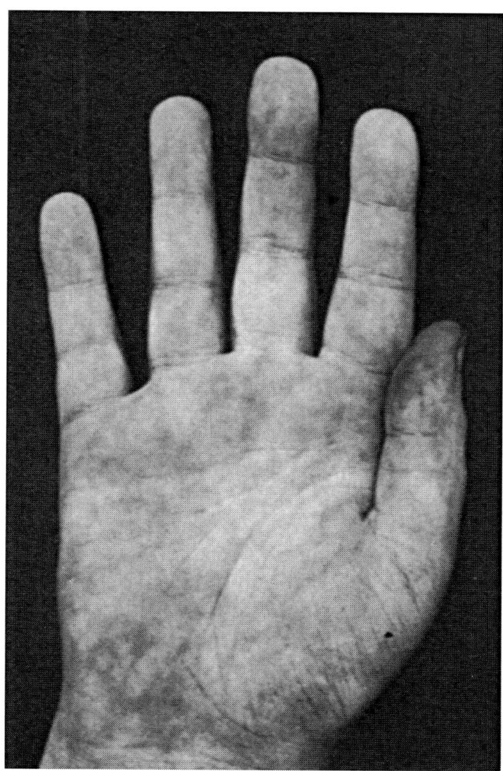

Figure 28–2. Marked digital cyanosis, livedo reticularis, and pain were characteristics of acute polyarteritis nodosa in this 9-year-old boy. Although muscle and kidney involvement were present, he made a complete recovery over a 5-year period of follow-up.

Pathology

As described by Küssmaul and Maier,[1] the characteristic pathologic features included necrotizing arteritis with the formation of nodules along the walls of medium- and small-sized muscular arteries, especially in the mesenteric vasculature. The lesions of necrotizing vasculitis tend to be segmental, with a predilection for bifurcations of vessels. Biopsy specimens show vasculitis in all stages of development, from acute to chronic, interspersed with areas of normal vessel wall. Aneurysm formation is highly characteristic of this type of vasculitis. Histopathologic diagnosis depends on identification of fibrinoid necrosis of the entire thickness of the walls of the medium- and small-sized muscular arteries (Fig. 28–3). Destruction of the internal elastic lamina is common. Immunofluorescence microscopy usually documents little evidence of complement or immunoglobulin deposition. In necrotizing arteritis, destruction of the vascular wall may be the direct consequence of immune complex deposition and complement activation.[33]

Laboratory Examination

Anemia, leukocytosis, thrombocytosis, and marked elevation of the erythrocyte sedimentation rate, C-reactive

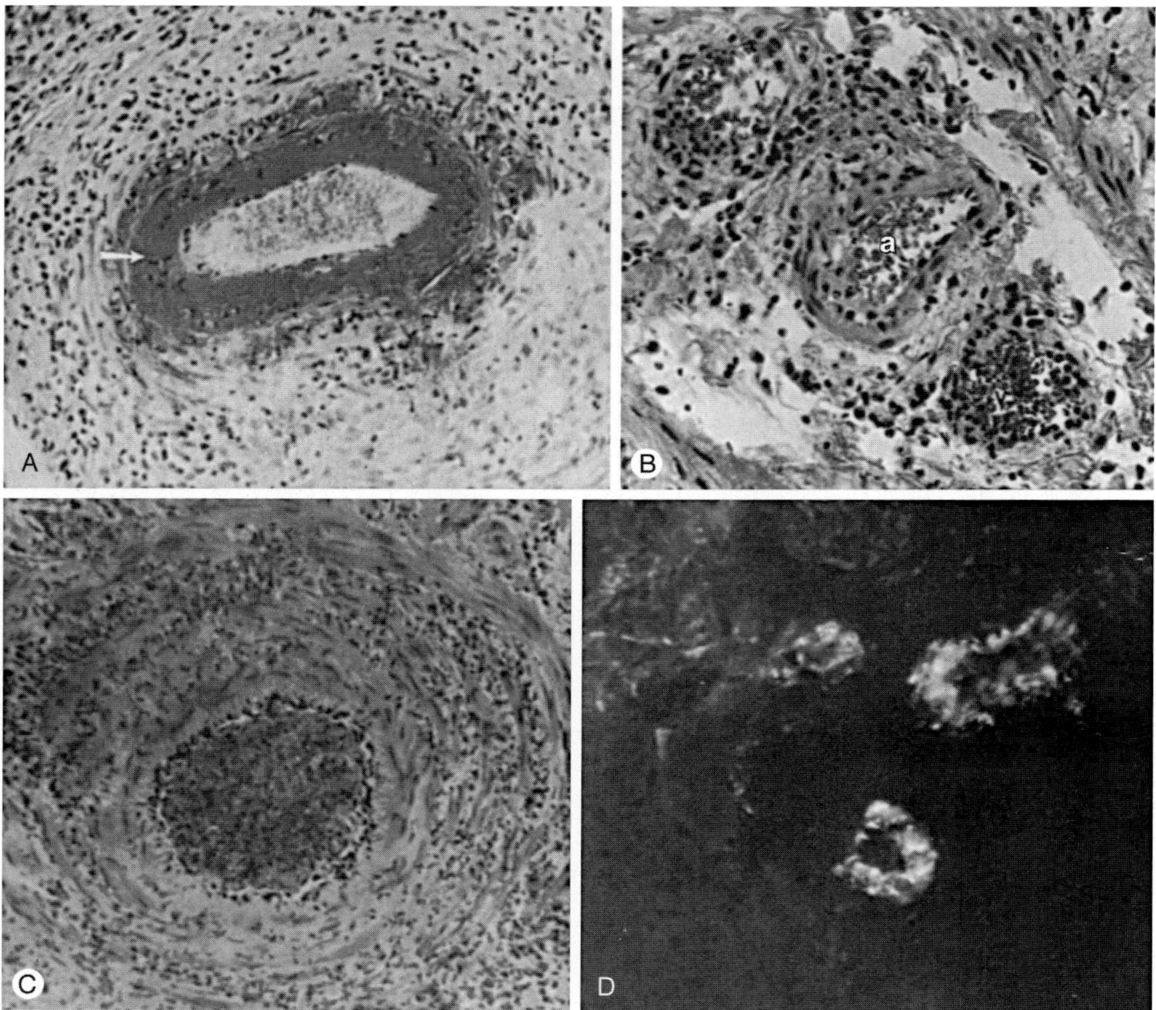

Figure 28–3. *A,* This biopsy shows a medium-sized muscular artery that exhibits marked fibrinoid necrosis of the vessel wall (*arrow*). This lesion is characteristic of polyarteritis nodosa. *B,* Muscle biopsy specimen from a 6-year-old boy with polyarteritis nodosa. Vasculitis with marked mixed cellular infiltration is seen in and around the walls of arteriole (a) and venules (v). Fibrinoid necrosis of the arteriole is visible. *C,* Infiltration of mononuclear cells around the central arteriole, which is surrounded by a dense fibrous scar. The lumen is occluded by a dense thrombus. H&E, ×480. *D,* Polyarteritis nodosa in a 19-year-old male with hematuria that developed 3 years after the onset of disease. Renal biopsy specimen demonstrated deposits of immunoglobulin G (IgG) in the media of the afferent arterioles (glomerulus at the upper left corner) (×480).

protein, and serum immunoglobulins, together with urinary sediment changes, are frequent (Table 28–4). Rheumatoid factor and antinuclear antibody are seldom detected. Immune complexes may be present.[34] Antineutrophil cytoplasmic antibodies may be present, but they are more frequently detected in Wegener's granulomatosis or microscopic polyarteritis (polyangiitis).[35] Levels of factor VIII–related antigen[36] and β-thromboglobulin[37] reflect the activity of the vascular inflammation and may be useful in following the effects of treatment. Dillon noted the presence of a greenish color of the plasma secondary to a ceruloplasmin-like acute-phase protein in patients with PAN.[38] The ischemic effects of coronary arteritis may be evident on electrocardiography.

Radiologic Examination

Demonstration by angiography of small aneurysms involving the renal, celiac, or mesenteric arteries is highly suggestive of PAN (Figs. 28–4 and 28–5).[39, 40] Magnetic resonance angiography may confirm the presence of abnormalities of the vascular system without the need for contrast studies. Unusual but characteristic abnormalities of intravenous excretory urography, including fixed segmental ureteral obstruction, have been reported in at least four children with PAN.[41–43]

Diagnosis

Although PAN can be suspected from a typical clinical presentation, diagnosis can be secured only by patho-

Table 28–4

Laboratory Abnormalities in Polyarteritis Nodosa

LABORATORY FINDING	%
Elevated erythrocyte sedimentation rate	75
Elevated C-reactive protein	90
Leukocytosis	90
Anemia	60
Proteinuria	80
Hematuria	65
↑ Blood urea nitrogen or creatinine	50
Antinuclear antibody present	25
ANCA present	~15
Rheumatoid factor present	0

ANCA, antineutrophil cytoplasmic antibody.
Estimated from published cases and series.

logic demonstration of characteristic lesions or by radiologic documentation of aneurysms.[44, 45] The ACR criteria shown in Table 28–1 clearly describe the character of the disease. The onset is often insidious, and a high index of suspicion is needed to make a timely diagnosis of PAN. The presence of a cutaneous lesion or subcutaneous nodule should prompt careful excisional (not punch) biopsy. These lesions may be transient, and should undergo biopsy early in their course. In the presence of peripheral neuropathy, muscle or nerve biopsy may be useful. Selective angiography of the celiac, mesenteric, or renal vasculature is likely to demonstrate one or many aneurysms, characteristically located at the bifurcations of small- to medium-sized arteries (see Fig. 28–5).

Treatment

Glucocorticoid therapy is indicated in most children with systemic PAN. Prednisone (1 to 2 mg/kg/day) improves life expectancy and decreases the frequency of hypertension and renal involvement.[32, 46] Oral cyclophosphamide (2 mg/kg/day)[47] or azathioprine (2 mg/kg/day) may be useful if glucocorticoids fail. Intravenous cyclophosphamide may be indicated in the more severe forms of the disease with aneurysmal involvement of the celiac and mesenteric vessels.[47] Plasmapheresis has not improved survival.[48]

Conflicting data regarding the effectiveness of glucocorticoid therapy have resulted in part from failure to distinguish among the several forms of polyarteritis in reports of therapeutic responsiveness. There was concern that glucocorticoids could suppress the inflammatory vasculitis without permitting adequate coincident wound healing, with the resultant formation of aneurysms, or that rapid healing of the vascular lesions could lead to occlusion and peripheral anoxia or necrosis of tissue. Direct evidence that these potential actions of glucocorticoids affect outcome in PAN is lacking, although the apparently deleterious effect of glucocorticoids in children with Kawasaki disease suggests continued caution in their use.

Although the evidence is very limited, the efficacy of intravenous immunoglobulin in the management of Kawasaki disease suggests that this treatment might also have a role in the management of children with PAN in whom glucocorticoids fail, before cytotoxic agents are used. A case report supports this possibility: Intravenous immunoglobulin was effective in treatment of a 2-year-old boy with necrotizing vasculitis.[49] Severe vascular insufficiency affecting the extremities and causing gangrene may respond to iloprost.[22] In

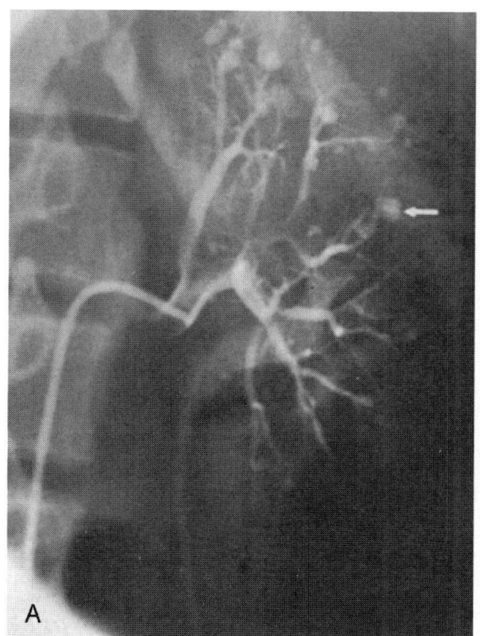

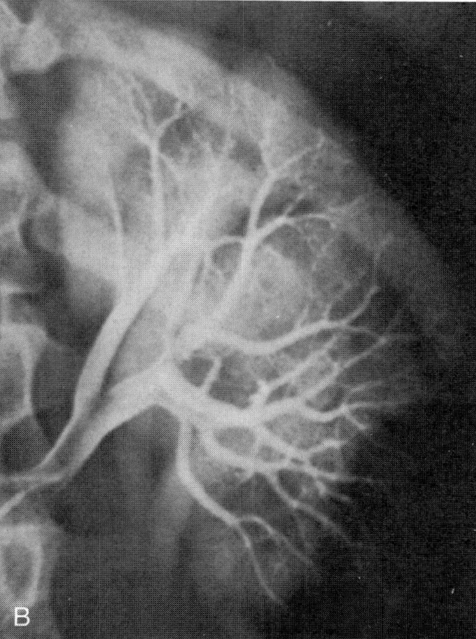

Figure 28–4. *A,* Characteristic renal aneurysms *(arrow)* visualized by angiography in a 15-year-old boy with polyarteritis nodosa who presented with hypertension, myocardial infarction, and hematuria. *B,* These lesions eventually disappeared as shown on this repeat angiogram some years after a course of prednisone therapy.

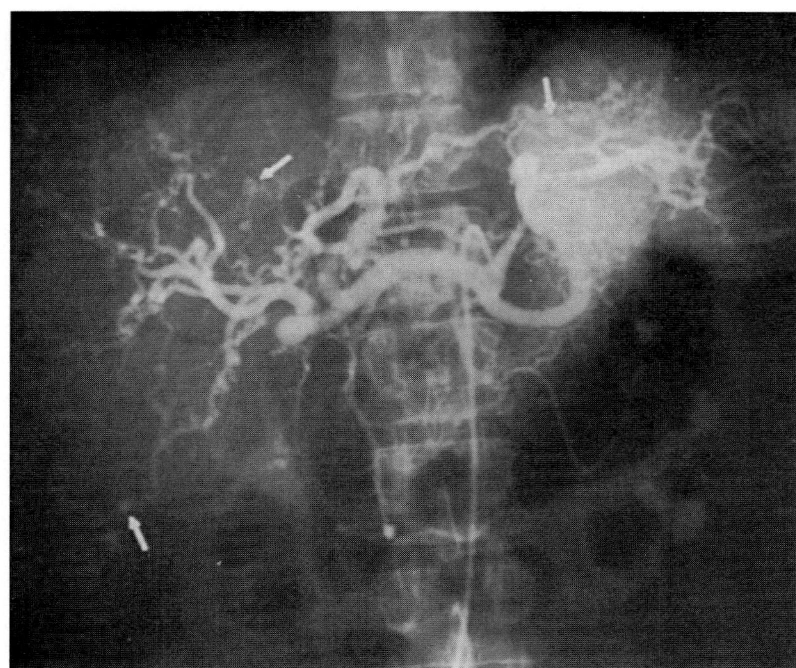

Figure 28–5. Celiac angiography documents aneurysms *(arrow)* in multiple vessels of 18-year-old boy with polyarteritis nodosa.

patients in whom there is an association with streptococcal infection, prophylaxis with penicillin for prevention of recurrences has been advocated.[7]

Course and Prognosis

The reported outcome for children with PAN varies a great deal from study to study. This reflects not only improvement in prognosis with more recent treatment protocols but also, apparently, differences in the severity of the disease recognized in different series. It is difficult to rationalize these differences but important to bear them in mind when considering any individual child.

Even in children with definite systemic involvement[8] characterized by fever, calf pain, subcutaneous nodules, elevated acute-phase reactants, and multisystem vasculitis demonstrated by biopsy or arteriography, the outcome is often satisfactory. In one study of nine children, most of whom had classic PAN, subjects were followed for a mean of 4 years and were treated with high-dose prednisone (approximately 2 mg/kg/day PO). Although serious complications (myocardial infarction, systemic hypertension, impaired renal function) occurred, the course was in general chronic with no mortality. In contrast, the report of Fink[7] described eight children with polyarteritis, seen between 1959 and 1974, who suffered severe hypertension, seizures, renal failure, and (in three) death. All of the 10 patients in the recent series from Japan[11] were alive, although serious sequelae were observed in one third.

CUTANEOUS POLYARTERITIS

There is no strict definition of CPA, and therefore, no accurate estimate of the numbers of reported cases, although it appears to be rare in children. In a 1998 case report and literature review, Ginarte and colleagues[50] noted 45 cases of CPA in childhood. Mocan and colleagues[51] identified only 15 cases that met their definition of CPA: tender subcutaneous nodules with high fever, arthralgias, and myalgias without major organ system involvement. Kumar and coworkers[52] reported 10 children from India with what they called benign cutaneous PAN who ranged in age from 1 to 10 years. The disease was limited to skin and joints.

The most characteristic clinical findings are purpura (Fig. 28–6) and multiple tender subcutaneous nodules, particularly on the lower extremities and sometimes on the soles of the feet. Ulceration may occur and is associated with a more protracted course and periph-

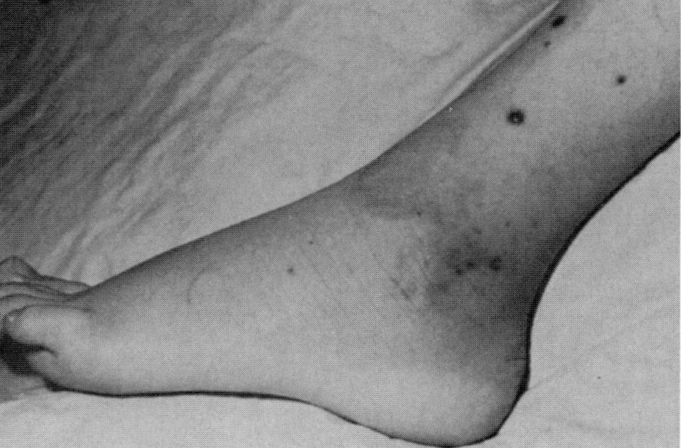

Figure 28–6. Cutaneous polyarteritis. Acute arthritis involving the ankle and tarsometatarsal joints and vascular necrotic purpura in a 5-year-old girl.

eral neuropathy, at least in adults.[53] Livedo reticularis is common. Biopsy of the dermis and subdermal structures demonstrates panarteritis.

There are three reports of neonates with CPA born to mothers with the disease.[54–56] All three had livedo reticularis and cutaneous nodules. Necrosis of fingers and toes occurred in two patients.[55, 56] Treatment with glucocorticoids was advocated, but heparin may be required in the face of acral arterial insufficiency.[56] The transient nature of the infants' lesions suggests an unknown transplacental effect rather than a genetic pathogenic influence.

CPA usually responds to glucocorticoids (prednisone, 0.5 to 1.0 mg/kg/day), although the course may be prolonged and recurrences are frequent, sometimes over a decade or more.[57, 58] When streptococcal infection is implicated as a triggering event,[8, 59–61] prophylaxis with penicillin may be effective.[57] Intravenous immunoglobulin has been used successfully to treat a 9-year-old boy[59] and a 2-year-old boy[49] with poststreptococcal CPA. Children with CPA usually have a very good outlook, although the disease is often characterized by relapses over a period of many years. In the series of children with CPA described by Kumar and colleagues,[52] most of the patients had digital gangrene but otherwise did well.

OTHER RARE VASCULITIDES

Cogan's Syndrome

Cogan's syndrome (nonsyphilitic interstitial keratitis with vestibuloauditory dysfunction)[62] is a rare disease that most frequently affects young adults of either sex. It has been identified in a number of children.[63–71] The cause is unknown, and associations with infection with *Borrelia burgdorferi*,[63] *Chlamydia trachomatis*,[64] or *Chlamydia psittaci*[65] are unconvincing. The ocular and auditory-vestibular abnormalities may be caused by organ-specific autoimmune processes.[72]

The major clinical features are listed in Table 28–5.

Table 28–5

Clinical Manifestations of Cogan's Syndrome

Inflammatory eye disease*
Interstitial keratitis
Other (conjunctivitis, episcleritis/scleritis, vitritis, retinal vasculitis, retinitis/choroiditis)
Vestibuloauditory dysfunction*
Hearing impairment, vertigo, tinnitus, ear pain
Systemic vasculitis
Aortitis
Aortic valve insufficiency
Vasculitis of small- and medium-sized arteries
Constitutional
Fever, weight loss, arthritis, abdominal pain, hepatosplenomegaly, lymphadenopathy

*Both elements are required to make the diagnosis.

Modified from St. Clair EW, McCallum RM: Cogan's syndrome. Curr Opin Rheumatol 11: 47, 1999.

In addition to photophobia, vertigo, and hearing loss, patients with Cogan's syndrome have evidence of widespread vasculitis,[66] including aortitis and aortic valve insufficiency, resembling that occurring in Takayasu's arteritis; both disorders have been reported in the same adult patient.[73] In some patients, involvement of other vessels such as the renal artery may suggest a similarity to PAN.[74]

Early treatment with systemic glucocorticoids is beneficial, although hearing loss may persist. Methotrexate has been advocated as an effective agent in some patients who have experienced an unsatisfactory response to glucocorticoids.[75, 76] The subject is thoroughly reviewed by St. Claire and McCallum.[72]

Soter's Syndrome

Soter and colleagues[77] described two males with cystic fibrosis who experienced palpable purpura on the basis of a cutaneous necrotizing venulitis. A confirmatory report has been published.[78]

REFERENCES

1. Küssmaul A, Maier K: Über eine bisher nicht beschriebene eigenthümliche Arterienerkrankung (Periarteritis nodosa), die mit Mörbus Brightii und rapid fortshreitender allgemeiner Muskellähmung einhergeht. Dsch Arch Klin Med 1: 484, 1866. (Translated into English by Matteson EL: On a previously undescribed peculiar arterial disease (periarteritis nodosa) accompanied by Bright's disease and rapidly progressive muscle weakness. Rochester, MN, Mayo Foundation, 1996.)
2. Jennette JC, Falk RJ, Andrassy K, et al: Nomenclature of systemic vasculitides: proposal of an international consensus conference. Arthritis Rheum 37: 187, 1994.
3. Lightfoot RW Jr, Michel BA, Bloch DA, et al: The American College of Rheumatology 1990 criteria for the classification of polyarteritis nodosa. Arthritis Rheum 33: 1088, 1990.
4. Ozen S, Besbas N, Saatci U, et al: Diagnostic criteria for polyarteritis nodosa in childhood. J Pediatr 120: 206, 1992.
5. Reimold EW, Weinberg AF, Fink CW, et al: Polyarteritis in children. Am J Dis Child 130: 534, 1976.
6. Blau EB, Morris RF, Yunis EJ: Polyarteritis nodosa in older children. Pediatrics 60: 227, 1977.
7. Fink CW: Polyarteritis and other diseases with necrotizing vasculitis in childhood. Arthritis Rheum 20(Suppl): 392, 1977.
8. Petty RE, Magilavy DB, Cassidy JT, et al: Polyarteritis in childhood. A clinical description of eight cases. Arthritis Rheum 20(Suppl): 392, 1977.
9. Magilavy DB, Petty RE, Cassidy JT, et al: A syndrome of childhood polyarteritis. J Pediatr 91: 25, 1977.
10. Ettlinger RE, Nelson AM, Burke EC, et al: Polyarteritis nodosa in childhood. A clinical pathologic study. Arthritis Rheum 22: 820, 1979.
11. Maeda M, Kobayashi M, Okamoto S, et al: Clinical observation of 14 cases of childhood polyarteritis nodosa in Japan. Acta Paediatr Jpn 39: 277, 1997.
12. Fager DB, Bigler JA, Simonds JP: Polyarteritis nodosa in infancy and childhood. J Pediatr 39: 65, 1951.
13. Frohnert PP, Sheps SG: Long-term follow-up study of periarteritis nodosa. Am J Med 43: 8, 1967.
14. Glikson M, Galun R, Schlesinger M, et al: Polyarteritis nodosa and familial Mediterraean fever: report of 2 cases and review of the literature. J Rheumatol 16: 536, 1989.
15. Kocak H, Cakar N, Hekimoglu B, et al: The coexistence of familial Mediterranean fever and polyarteritis nodosa: report of a case. Pediatr Nephrol 10: 631, 1995.

16. Tinaztepe K, Gucer S, Bakkaloglu A, Tinaztepe B: Familial Mediterranean fever and polyarteritis nodosa: experience of five paediatric cases. A causal relationship or coincidence? Eur J Pediatr 156: 505, 1997.
17. Ozdogan H, Arisoy N, Kasapcapur O, et al: Vasculitis in familial Mediterranean fever. J Rheumatol 24: 323, 1997.
18. Guillevin L, Lhote F, Cohen P, et al: Polyarteritis nodosa related to hepatis B virus: a prospective study with long-term observations of 41 patients. Medicine 74: 238, 1995.
19. Gocke DJ, Hsu K, Morgan C, et al: Association of polyarteritis and Australia antigen. Lancet 2: 1149, 1970.
20. Cacoub P, Lunel-Fabiani F, Le thi Huong D: Polyarteritis nodosa and hepatitis C virus infection. Ann Intern Med 116: 605, 1992.
21. Deny P, Bonacorsi S, Guillevin L, Quint L: Association between hepatitis C virus and polyarteritis nodosa. Clin Exp Rheumatol 10: 319, 1992.
22. Zulian F, Costantini C, Montesco MC, et al: Successful treatment of gangrene in systemic necrotizing vasculitis with iloprost. Br J Rheumatol 37: 228, 1998.
23. Sheth AP, Olson JC, Esterly NB: Cutaneous polyarteritis nodosa of childhood. J Am Acad Dermatol 31: 561, 1994.
24. Seelen MAJ, de Meijer PHEM, Arnoldus EPJ, et al: A patient with multiple myeloma presenting with severe polyneuropathy caused by necrotizing vasculitis. Am J Med 102: 485, 1997.
25. Jones TC, Doll ER, Bryans JT: The lesions of equine viral arteritis. Cornell Vet 47: 52, 1957.
26. Woodward AH, Andreini PH: Periosteal new bone formation in polyarteritis nodosa. A syndrome involving the lower extremities. Arthritis Rheum 17: 1017, 1974.
27. Adu D, Bacon PA: Classical polyarteritis nodosa, microscopic polyarteritis, and Churg-Strauss syndrome. *In* Maddison PJ, Isenberg DA, Woo P, Glass DN (eds): Oxford Textbook of Rheumatology, 2nd ed. Oxford, England, Oxford University Press, 1998, p 1351.
28. Ogazkurt L, Cekirge S, Balkanoi F: Inferior suprarenal artery aneurysm in polyarteritis nodosa. Pediatr Radiol 27: 234, 1997.
29. Besbas N, Ozen S, Saatci U, et al: Renal involvement in polyarteritis nodosa: evaluation of 26 Turkish children. Pediatr Nephrol 14: 325, 2000.
30. Bert RJ, Antonacci VP, Berman L, Melhem ER: Polyarteritis nodosa presenting as temporal arteritis in a 9-year-old child. AJNR Am J Neuroradiol 20: 167, 1999.
31. Gunal N, Kara N, Cakar N, et al: Cardiac involvement in childhood polyarteritis nodosa. Int J Cardiol 60: 257, 1997.
32. Furlong TJ, Ibels LS, Eckstein RP: The clinical spectrum of necrotizing glomerulonephritis. Medicine (Baltimore) 66: 192, 1987.
33. McCluskey RT, Fienberg R: Vasculitis in primary vasculitides, granulomatoses and connective tissue diseases. Hum Pathol 14: 305, 1983.
34. Levin M: Platelet immune complex interaction in pathogenesis of Kawasaki disease and childhood polyarteritis. Br Med J 290: 1456, 1985.
35. Nash MC, Dillon MJ: Antineutrophil cytoplasm antibodies and vasculitis. Arch Dis Child 77: 261, 1997.
36. Woolf AD, Wakerley G, Wallington TB, et al: Factor VIII related antigen in the assessment of vasculitis. Ann Rheum Dis 46: 441, 1987.
37. Burns JC, Glode MP, Clarke SH, et al: Coagulopathy and platelet activation in Kawasaki syndrome. Identification of patients at high risk for development of coronary artery aneurysms. J Pediatr 105: 206, 1983.
38. Dillon MJ: Primary vasculitis in children. *In* Maddison PJ, Isenberg DA, Woo P, Glass DN (eds): Oxford Textbook of Rheumatology, 2nd ed. Oxford, England, Oxford University Press, 1998, pp 1402–1413.
39. McLain LG, Bookstein JJ, Kelsch RC: Polyarteritis nodosa diagnosed by renal arteriography. J Pediatr 80: 1032, 1972.
40. Yousefzadeh DK, Chow KC, Benson CA: Polyarteritis nodosa: regression of arterial aneurysms following immunosuppressive and corticosteroid therapy. Pediatr Radiol 10: 139, 1981.
41. Fisher RS, Howard HH: Unusual ureterograms in a case of periarteritis nodosa. J Urol 60: 398, 1948.
42. Glanz I, Grunebaum M: Ureteral changes in polyarteritis nodosa as seen during excretory urography. J Urol 116: 731, 1976.
43. Khanfar NM, Morgenstern BZ: 15-year-old-boy with abdominal pain and hypertension. Mayo Clin Proc 71: 713, 1996.
44. Hunder GG, Arend WP, Block DA, et al: The American College of Rheumatology 1990 criteria for the classification of vasculitis. Arthritis Rheum 33: 1065, 1990.
45. Lie JT: American College of Rheumatology Subcommittee for Classification of Vasculitis: illustrated histopathologic classification criteria for selected vasculitic syndromes. Arthritis Rheum 33: 1074, 1990.
46. Sack M, Cassidy JT, Bole GG: Prognostic factors in polyarteritis. J Rheumatol 2: 411, 1976.
47. Fauci AS, Katz P, Haynes BF, et al: Cyclophosphamide therapy of severe necrotizing vasculitis. N Engl J Med 301: 235, 1979.
48. Guillevin L, Fain O, Lhote F, et al: Lack of superiority of steroids plus plasma exchange to steroids alone in the treatment of polyarteritis nodosa and Churg-Strauss syndrome. A prospective, randomized trial in 78 patients. Arthritis Rheum 35: 208, 1992.
49. Gedalia A, Correa H, Kaiser M, Sorensen R: Case report: steroid-sparing effect of intravenous gamma globulin in a child with necrotizing vasculitis. Am J Med Sci 309: 226, 1995.
50. Ginarte M, Pereiro M, Toribio J: Cutaneous polyarteritis nodosa in a child. Pediatr Dermatol 15: 103, 1998.
51. Mocan H, Mocan MC, Peru H, Ozoran Y: Cutaneous polyarteritis nodosa in a child and a review of the literature. Acta Paediatr 87: 351, 1998.
52. Kumar L, Thapa BR, Sarkar B, Walia BN: Benign cutaneous polyarteritis nodosa in children below 10 years of age—a clinical experience. Ann Rheum Dis 54: 134, 1995.
53. Daoud MS, Hutton KP, Gibson LE: Cutaneous periarteritis nodosa: a clinicopathological study of 79 cases. Br J Dermatol 136: 706, 1997.
54. Boren RJ, Everett MA: Cutaneous vasculitis in mother and infant. Arch Dermatol 92: 568, 1965.
55. Miller JJ, Fries JF: Simultaneous vasculitis in a mother and newborn infant. J Pediatr 87: 443, 1975.
56. Stone MS, Olson RR, Weismann DN, et al: Cutaneous vasculitis in the newborn of a mother with cutaneous polyarteritis nodosa. J Am Acad Dermatol 28: 101, 1993.
57. Till SH, Amos RS: Long-term follow-up of juvenile-onset cutaneous polyarteritis nodosa associated with streptococcal infection. Br J Rheumatol 36: 909, 1997.
58. Albornoz MA, Benedetto AV, Korman M, et al: Relapsing cutaneous polyarteritis nodosa associated with streptococcal infections. Int J Dermatol 37: 664, 1998.
59. Uziel Y, Silverman ED: Intravenous immunoglobulin therapy in a child with cutaneous polyarteritis nodosa. Clin Exp Rheumatol 16: 767, 1998.
60. David J, Ansell BM, Woo P: Polyarteritis nodosa associated with streptococcus. Arch Dis Child 69: 685, 1993.
61. Sibery GK, Cohen BA, Johnson B: Cutaneous polyarteritis nodosa. Report of two cases in children and review of the literature. Arch Dermatol 130: 884, 1994.
62. Cogan DG: Syndrome of nonsyphilitic interstitial keratitis and vestibuloauditory symptoms. Arch Ophthalmol 33: 144, 1945.
63. Schwegmann JP, Enzenauer RJ: Cogan's syndrome mimicking acute Lyme arthritis. Am J Orthop 24: 426, 1995.
64. Haynes BF, Kaiser-Kupfer MI, Mason P, Fauci AS: Cogan syndrome: studies in thirteen patients, long-term follow-up and review of the literature. Medicine (Baltimore) 59: 426, 1980.
65. Darougar S, John AC, Viswalingam N, et al: Isolation of *Chlamydia psittaci* from a patient with interstitial keratitis and uveitis associated with otological and cardiovascular lesions. Br J Ophthalmol 62: 709, 1978.
66. Kundell SP, Ochs HD: Cogan syndrome in childhood. J Pediatr 97: 96, 1980.
67. Cheson BD, Bluming AZ, Alroy J: Cogan's syndrome: a systemic vasculitis. Am J Med 60: 549, 1976.
68. Podder S, Shepherd RC: Cogan's syndrome: a rare systemic vasculitis. Arch Dis Child 71: 163, 1994.
69. Bachynski B, Wise J: Cogan's syndrome: a treatable cause of neurosensory deafness. Can J Ophthalmol 19: 145, 1984.
70. Andler W, Hulse M, Bruch PM, Partsch CJ: Cogan's syndrome in childhood. Monatsschr Kinderheilkd 125: 161, 1977.
71. Podder S, Shepherd RC: Cogan's syndrome: a rare systemic vasculitis. Arch Dis Child 71: 163, 1994.
72. St. Clair EW, McCallum RM: Cogan's syndrome. Curr Opin Rheumatol 11: 47, 1999.

73. Raza K, Karokis D, Kitas GD: Cogan's syndrome with Takayasu's arteritis. Br J Rheumatol 37: 369, 1998.
74. Vella JP, O'Callaghan J, Hickey D, Walshe JJ: Renal artery stenosis complicating Cogan's syndrome. Clin Nephrol 47: 407, 1997.
75. Richardson B: Methotrexate therapy for hearing loss in Cogan's syndrome. Arthritis Rheum 37: 1559, 1994.
76. Riente L, Taglione E, Berrettini S: Efficacy of methotrexate in Cogan's syndrome. J Rheumatol 23: 1830, 1996.
77. Soter NA, Mihm MC, Colten HR: Cutaneous necrotizing venulitis in patients with cystic fibrosis. J Pediatr 95: 197, 1979.
78. Fradin MS, Kalb RE: Recurrent cutaneous vasculitis in cystic fibrosis. Pediatr Dermatol 4: 108, 1987.

29

Granulomatous Vasculitis, Giant Cell Arteritis, and Sarcoidosis

Carol B. Lindsley

GRANULOMATOUS VASCULITIDES

The granulomatous vasculitides include Wegener's granulomatosis (WG), Churg-Strauss syndrome, lymphomatoid granulomatosis, and primary angiitis of the central nervous system (CNS). These diseases are categorized as histiocytic disorders in a pathophysiologic model of macrophage-monocyte proliferation. All are rare in childhood and adolescence, and much of what we know about them comes from studies of adults with the diseases. Of these four, WG is the most common.

Wegener's Granulomatosis

WG was first described in the 1930s.[1, 2] It is a systemic disease characterized by granulomatous vasculitis involving the upper and lower respiratory tracts associated with glomerulonephritis. Although rare and occurring predominantly in middle-aged adults, the disease has been reported in a number of children.[3, 4]

Classification

The 1990 American College of Rheumatology (ACR) criteria for the classification of WG are given in Table 29–1.[5] If lesions are limited to the upper respiratory passages and the manifestations of vasculitis are minimal, the syndrome is called *localized WG* or *midline granuloma*. A limited form of WG does not include glomerulonephritis.[6]

Epidemiology

Very little is known about the incidence, prevalence, or demographic characteristics of WG in children and adolescents. In a large study of patients who were hospitalized for WG between 1986 and 1990,[7] the 5-year incidence was 3.2 per 100,000. Those with onset under 20 years of age accounted for 3.3 percent, an incidence in that age group of approximately 0.1 per 100,000. In the pediatric patient, WG is generally a disease of the second decade of life, with a mean age at onset of 15.4 years in one of the largest studies.[4] There is no clear sex predominance in the pediatric age range,[8] although in adults males outnumber females 1.7:1.[5] In a prospective study of 23 children aged 9 to 19 years at onset, 61 percent had generalized disease and 39 percent had a limited form of the disease.[4]

Etiology and Genetic Factors

The etiology of WG is unknown. Theories of causation have included autoimmune, hypersensitivity, or aller-

Table 29–1

Four Criteria for Classification of Wegener's Granulomatosis

Nasal or oral inflammation	Painful or painless oral ulcers or purulent or bloody nasal discharge
Abnormal-appearing chest radiograph	Nodules, fixed infiltrates or cavities
Abnormal urinary sediment	Microhematuria (>5 RBC/hpf) or RBC casts
Granulomatous inflammation	Granulomatous inflammation within the wall of an artery or in the perivascular or extravascular area of an artery or arteriole

Diagnosis of Wegener's granulomatosis requires the presence of two of the four criteria. The presence of any two or more criteria has a sensitivity of 88.2% and a specificity of 92.0%.

RBC, red blood cell.

Adapted from Leavitt RY, Fauci AS, Bloch DA, et al: The American College of Rheumatology 1990 criteria for the classification of Wegener's granulomatosis. Arthritis Rheum 33: 1101, © 1990. Wiley-Liss, Inc. Reprinted by permission of Wiley-Liss, Inc., a subsidiary of John Wiley & Sons, Inc.

gic reactions to unknown antigens and sensitization of the respiratory tract to bacterial pathogens. Nasal carriage of *Staphylococcus aureus* has been associated in adults with high rates of relapse.[9] Using T-lymphocyte clones derived from two patients with WG, reactivity to *S. aureus* but not to other bacteria was demonstrated, suggesting a role for this organism in the pathogenesis of the disease.[10]

The familial occurrence of WG has only occasionally been reported.[11–13] Associations with antigens of the histocompatibility system (human leukocyte antigen [HLA]) have been inconsistent. A large study from the Netherlands reported a highly significant decrease in the frequency of DR13/DR6.[14] Increased expression of some of the polymorphic forms of the Fc γ receptors have been associated with WG in some studies but not in others: Homozygosity for both the R131 form of Fc γ RIIa and the F158 form of Fc γ RIIIa were associated with an increased risk of relapse in adults with WG.[15] These forms of the Fc γ receptors limit antigen clearance and may therefore predispose to disease associated with chronic infection with organisms such as *S. aureus*.

Clinical Manifestations

The triad of paranasal sinus involvement, pulmonary infiltration, and renal disease is characteristic of WG (Table 29–2).[4, 7, 16–18] At onset, nonspecific complaints—including fever, malaise, and weight loss—are common, and the majority of patients present with upper and lower respiratory disease. Upper respiratory tract signs and symptoms such as rhinorrhea, nasal mucosal ulcerations and epistaxis, persistent cough, hoarseness, and paranasal sinus pain or drainage are frequent. Damage to the nasal cartilage, characteristic of longstanding disease, may result in a "saddle-nose" deformity, suggesting the possible diagnosis of relapsing polychondritis (Fig. 29–1). Overall, nasal, sinus, tracheal, or ear abnormalities were reported in 91 percent of patients with childhood onset of the disease.[4] Lower respiratory tract symptoms include dyspnea and hemoptysis.

Lung disease occurs in 74 percent of children with WG.[4] Nodular pulmonary infiltrates are often visible on radiographs.[19] Blurred vision, conjunctivitis, episcleritis, persistent otitis media, hearing loss, arthralgia, and myalgia are also common.[20] Renal disease occurs in 61 percent of children[4] and often leads to renal failure.[19] Skin lesions may resemble Henoch-Schönlein purpura[17] or may be ulcerative, vesicular, papular, or nodular; these lesions occur in 9 percent of patients at disease onset and in up to one half during the course of the disease.[4] CNS involvement (neuropathy, cranial nerve palsies, seizures) is less frequent than in adult patients.[21] Cardiac disease is infrequent but may include myocardial infarction, arrhythmias, and valvulitis; in one 16-year-old boy a right ventricular granuloma, was reported.[22] Gastrointestinal symptoms include nonspecific pain, nausea, and vomiting.[17] Mild, transient arthralgia occurs in 30 to 78 percent of patients.[4]

Table 29–2

Manifestations of Wegener's Granulomatosis in Childhood

ABNORMALITY	PATIENTS AFFECTED (%) (n = 23) Onset	Total
Ear, nose, throat	*87*	*91*
Sinusitis	61	83
Nasal disease	48	65
Otitis media	39	48
Subglottic stenosis	4	48
Hearing loss	26	39
Ear pain	22	22
Oral lesions	4	9
Arthralgia/arthritis	*30*	*78*
Pulmonary disease	*22*	*74*
Infiltrates	9	61
Nodules	13	43
Hemoptysis	9	26
Pleuritis	9	13
Glomerulonephritis	*9*	*61*
Rash (purpura, vesicles, papules, nodules)	*9*	*52*
Ocular disease	*13*	*48*
Dacrocystitis	4	26
Eye pain	4	17
Proptosis	0	17
Scleritis/episcleritis	4	13
Conjunctivitis	0	9
Visual loss	0	9
Corneal ulcers	0	4
Fever	*22*	*43*
Weight loss	*13*	*26*
CNS disease (cranial nerve palsy, seizure)	*4*	*17*
Peripheral neuropathy	*0*	*9*
Pericarditis	*9*	*9*

CNS, central nervous system.

Data from Rottem M, Fauci AS, et al: Wegener granulomatosis in children and adolescents: clinical presentation and outcome. J Pediatr 122: 26, 1993.

Diagnosis

A definite diagnosis of WG requires demonstration of typical changes on biopsy of lung, skin, or kidney. The differential diagnosis includes other causes of granulomatous vasculitis such as mycobacteria, fungi, or helminths.[19] Other forms of vasculitis such as Goodpasture's syndrome, systemic lupus erythematosus, or polyarteritis nodosa should be considered. In young children, chronic granulomatous disease may also need to be excluded.

Laboratory Examination

White blood cell counts are usually normal or moderately elevated. Anemia, thrombocytosis, and marked elevation of the erythrocyte sedimentation rate (ESR) or C-reactive protein are usually present. Elevation of blood urea nitrogen and serum creatinine indicates the

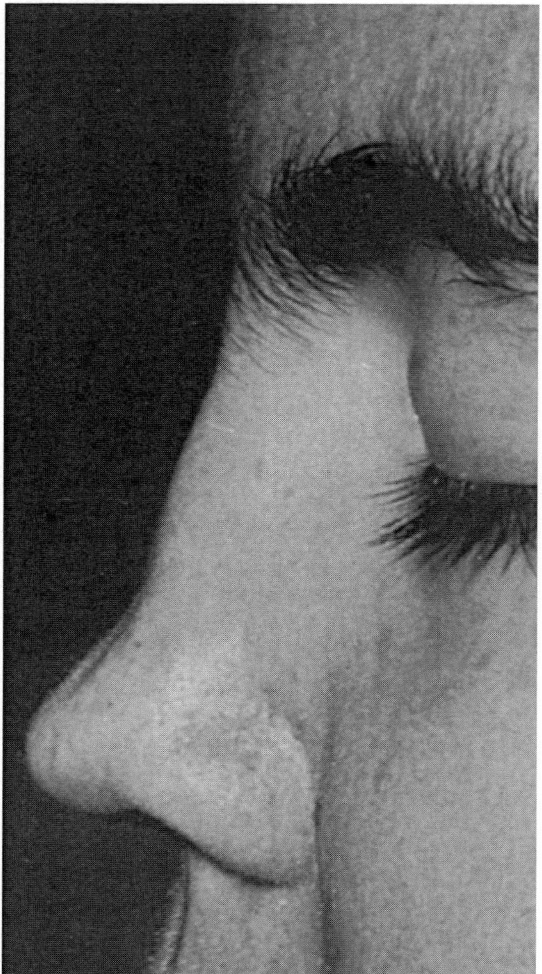

Figure 29–1. "Saddle nose" deformity resulting from granulomatous destruction of the nasal cartilage in this 14-year-old girl with Wegener's granulomatosis. The process was painless and occurred over several months. Later, she experienced pulmonary hemorrhage and radiologic changes that led to the diagnosis.

presence of significant renal disease. Urinalysis characteristically demonstrates proteinuria, microscopic hematuria, and red blood cell casts in up to 50 percent of patients.[5, 19] Gross hematuria is uncommon.[4]

The most important autoantibodies in WG are those directed to neutrophil cytoplasmic antigens (ANCAs). ANCAs may be either cytoplasmic (cANCA) or perinuclear (pANCA) on immunofluorescence microscopy (Fig. 29–2). Each pattern has a different antigenic specificity and correlates somewhat with the type of vascular injury.[26] ANCAs directed to neutrophil cytoplasmic enzyme protein PR3 (cANCA) were present in more than 90 percent of patients.[23–25] Although these antibodies have not been associated with other types of connective tissue disease, they have been demonstrated in inflammatory bowel diseases, infection-associated vasculitis, and paraneoplastic syndromes[25–27] (Table 29–3).

Antinuclear antibodies (ANAs) of unknown specificity are uncommon. Rheumatoid factors (RFs) are present in approximately 50 percent of adult patients.[19] Serum levels of immunoglobulin A (IgA) may be increased.[7]

Pathology

Granulomatous involvement of medium-size arteries and veins is characteristic. Arteritis per se is rare. Granulomata show acute and chronic inflammation with central necrosis and histiocytes, lymphocytes, and giant cells (Fig. 29–3).[19] Renal glomeruli are infiltrated with lymphocytes and histiocytes (Fig. 29–4). The most commonly reported renal lesions are extracapillary proliferation (with or without fibrinoid necrosis) and crescent formation, followed by necrotizing glomerulonephritis.[28, 29] Renal granulomata are rare.[30] Immunofluorescence microscopy is characteristic of a "pauci-immune" pattern with scanty deposition of immunoglobulins and complement.[7, 28] Dense subendothelial deposits are visible on electron microscopy.[20]

Radiologic Examination

Approximately two thirds of children with WG have abnormalities on chest radiographs, including nodules (granulomata), cavitation, and infiltrates[31, 32] (Fig. 29–5). The lesions may be solitary or bilateral. Infiltrates are often fleeting and may be asymptomatic. In one study,[4] one third of all abnormal radiographs were those of patients without pulmonary symptoms. Pleural effusions and pneumothorax may also occur. Sinus radiographs may demonstrate thickening of the sinus lining or opacification of the frontal or maxillary sinuses.

Treatment

Once a firm diagnosis of WG is established, treatment with glucocorticoids in combination with cyclophosphamide is indicated. The disease was fatal in almost all children reported before the use of a combination of glucocorticoid and cytotoxic agents.[16] This protocol has induced remission in over 90 percent of patients.[16, 19, 20, 33] In critically ill patients, intravenous methylprednisolone followed by daily high-dose glucocorticoids and cyclophosphamide should be used initially.[34] Cyclophosphamide (2 mg/kg/day) with prednisone initially at a dose of 1 mg/kg/day for 4 weeks, then tapered to an alternate-day regimen, induced remission in 97 percent of patients in one large series.[4] This regimen was continued for approximately 1 year past remission and then the cyclophosphamide was tapered by 25-mg decrements every 2 months if there was no relapse. The median requirement for cytotoxic therapy was 28 months. Studies of therapy are summarized in Table 29–4.

Therapy with a combination of glucocorticoid and methotrexate resulted in remission in 69 percent of adults with WG that was not immediately life threatening.[23] Methotrexate has also been suggested as an alter-

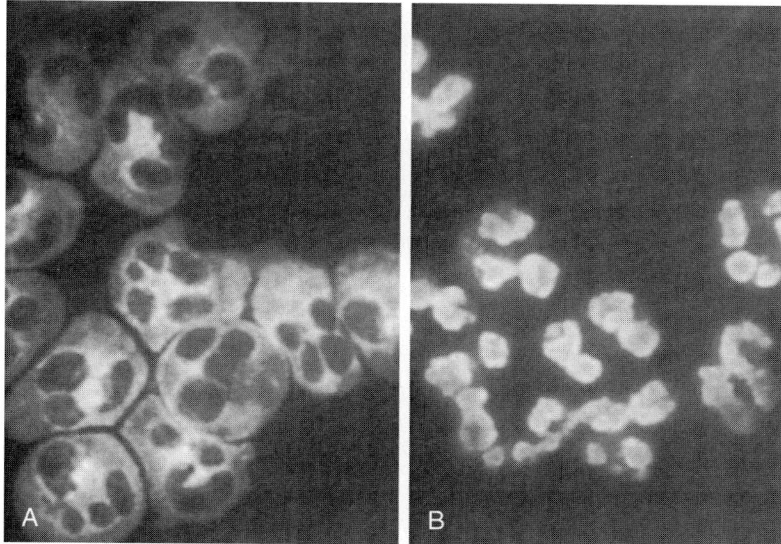

Figure 29–2. Indirect immunofluorescence microscopy staining patterns produced by cANCA (*A*) and pANCA (*B*) on alcohol-fixed neutrophils. (*A* and *B*, From Jennette JC, Falk RJ: Antineutrophil cytoplasmic autoantibodies and associated diseases: A review. Am J Kidney Dis 15: 517, 1990.)

Table 29–3

Common Disease Associations With Neutrophil Cytoplasmic Antigens (ANCAs)

ANTIGEN	ANCA PATTERN	DISEASE ASSOCIATION	FREQUENCY (%)
PR3	cANCA	Wegener's granulomatosis	30–90
		Churg-Strauss syndrome	25–50
MPO	pANCA	Microscopic polyarteritis	25–75
		Churg-Strauss syndrome	50–75
		Ulcerative colitis	40–80
		Sclerosing cholangitis	65–85
		Crohn's disease	10–40
BPI	pANCA	Cystic fibrosis	80–90
Actin	pANCA	Autoimmune hepatitis type I	70–75

The *p* and *c* before "ANCA" stand for *perinuclear* and *cytoplasmic*, respectively.
Data from Hoffman et al[23] and Specks et al.[24]

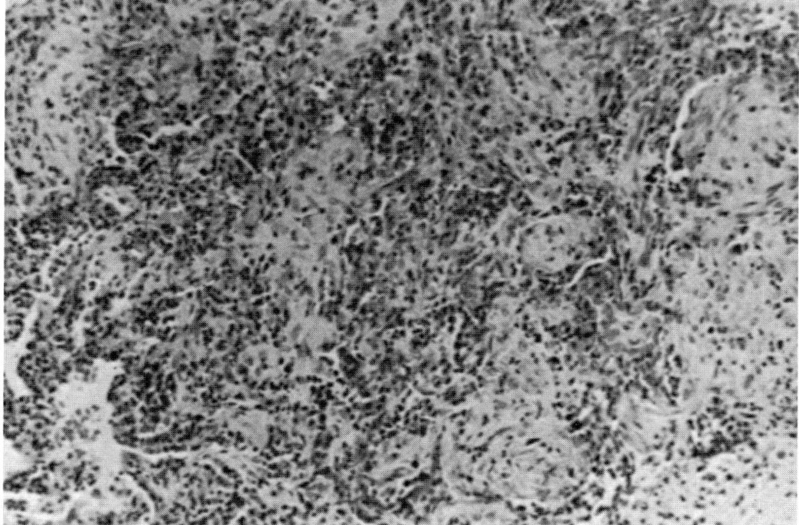

Figure 29–3. Lung biopsy specimen in Wegener's granulomatosis. Necrotizing granulomata and fibrous tissue have obliterated the normal alveolar architecture. H&E, ×480.

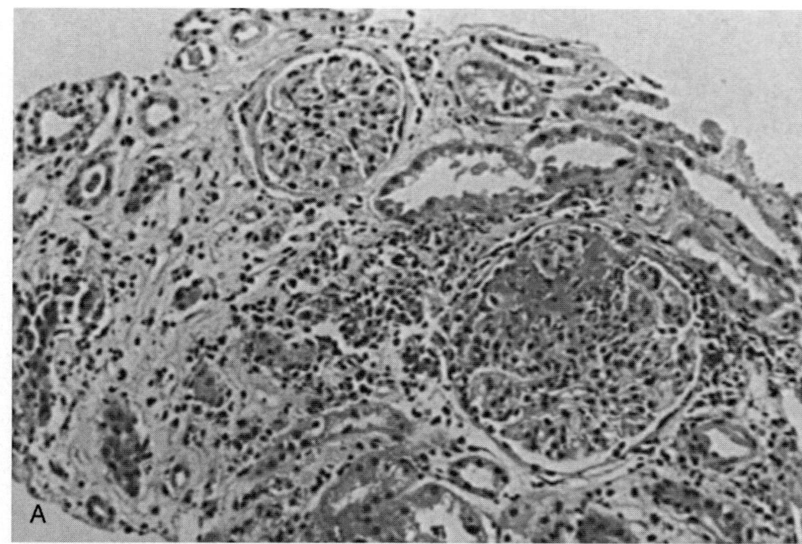

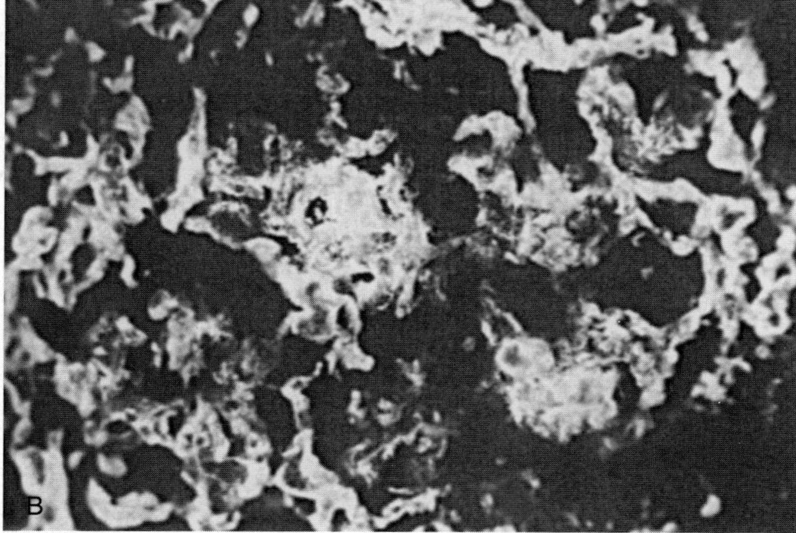

Figure 29–4. *A,* Renal biopsy specimen from a child with Wegener's granulomatosis. The glomerulus on the right shows areas of hypercellularity and fibrinoid necrosis with interstitial inflammation. H&E, ×480. *B,* Positive immunofluorescent stain for fibrin in a renal biopsy specimen from a patient with Wegener's granulomatosis (×480).

native to cyclophosphamide in children with WG.[35] Because of long-term toxicity of cyclophosphamide, the use of methotrexate for maintenance should be considered. Trimethoprim-sulfamethoxazole has been reported to be effective in some patients[36, 37] and should be considered as adjunctive therapy. Current therapeutic recommendations are summarized in Table 29–5.

Course of the Disease and Prognosis

Approximately 25 percent of children with WG have at least one serious infection during the course of the illness.[4] Subglottic stenosis is four times as common, and nasal deformity twice as common, in children as in adults; surgical intervention may be necessary to maintain the airway. In one third of children, irreversible renal insufficiency develops. Treatment-related morbidity includes cystitis and infertility in 22 percent.[4] Malignancies did not occur in any of 23 children followed for a mean of 8.7 years.[4] Relapses of disease requiring retreatment occurred in approximately one half of the patients. Persistent sinus pain and dysfunction, hearing loss, and pulmonary insufficiency may ensue. Twenty-two children under the age of 15 years died of the disease in a 10-year period ending in 1988 in the United States.[7] In the series reported by Rottem and associates,[4] one patient died from severe lung disease and cor pulmonale, and one died from sepsis.

Churg-Strauss Syndrome (Allergic Granulomatosis)

Churg and Strauss originally described this disorder in 1951[42] in a report of 13 patients with severe asthma associated with fever, eosinophilia, and vasculitis affecting various organ systems. They later broadened the initial description to include eosinophilic pneumonitis, angiitis, allergic granulomata, and necrotizing angiitis. Granulomatous extravascular and vascular changes are characteristic.

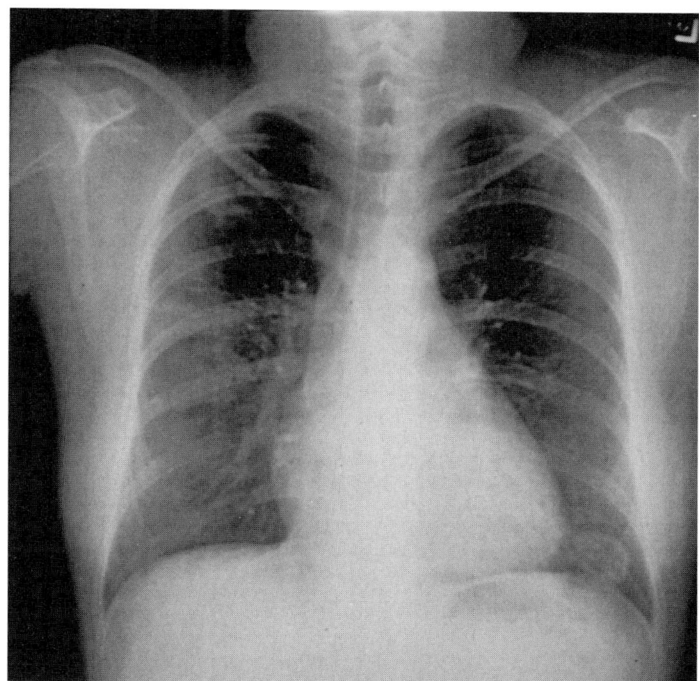

Figure 29–5. Patchy lower lobe infiltrates and several well-defined granulomata (left lower lobe, right upper and middle lobes) are evident in the lungs of this adolescent with Wegener's granulomatosis.

Table 29–4

Studies of the Treatment of Wegener's Granulomatosis

STUDY	REGIMEN	RESULT
Fauci et al, 1983[19]	CTX 2 mg/kg/d PO Prednisone 1 mg/kg/d PO	Remission in 93%
Hoffman et al, 1990[35]	CTX every month IV	Response followed by relapse in 72%
Hoffman et al, 1992[36]	TMP-SMX	Improvement in 1 of 9
de Groot et al, 1996[37]	*Induction*: CTX 2 mg/kg/d PO or IV Prednisone 1 mg/kg/d PO *Maintenance*:	
	MTX 0.3 mg/kg/wk SC	86% responded
	or TMP-SMX 960 mg BID PO	58% responded
	or MTX + prednisone	91% responded
	or TMP-SMX + prednisone	0% responded
Guillevin et al, 1997[38]	*Induction*: CTX 0.7 g/M[2] Methylprednisolone IV × 3 d followed by oral prednisone 1 mg/kg/d *Maintenance*:	
	CTX IV + prednisone	59% relapsed
	CTX PO + prednisone	13% relapsed
Langford et al, 1999[38a]	*Induction*: CTX 2 mg/kg/d PO Prednisone 1 mg/kg/d PO *Maintenance*: MTX 0.3 mg/kg/wk PO increasing to maximum of 20–25 mg/wk Prednisone tapered to alternate-day dose	100% responded

CTX, cyclophosphamide; MTX, methotrexate; TMP-SMX, trimethoprim-sulfamethoxazole.

Table 29–5

Current Therapy of Wegener's Granulomatosis

PHASE	DRUG	REGIMEN
Induction	Prednisone	1 mg/kg/d PO (exceptionally ill patients receive methylprednisolone 30 mg/kg/d for 1–3 d IV)
		plus
	Cyclophosphamide	2 mg/kg/d PO (exceptionally ill patients may receive 3–5 mg/kg/d PO for 3 d, followed by 2 mg/kg/d)
Maintenance	Prednisone	After 4 wk, prednisone is tapered to an every-other-day schedule over 3–4 mo
		plus either
	Cyclophosphamide	2 mg/kg/d PO (taper after 1 yr of disease control or remission)
		or
	Methotrexate	0.3–0.6 mg/kg SC once a week

Table 29–6

American College of Rheumatology Criteria for Classification of the Churg-Strauss Syndrome

CRITERION	DESCRIPTION
Asthma	History of wheezing or diffuse high-pitched rales on expiration
Eosinophilia	Eosinophils >10% of white blood cell differential count
History of allergy	History of seasonal allergy (e.g., allergic rhinitis) or other documented allergies, including food, contactants, and others (except for drug allergies)
Mononeuropathy or polyneuropathy	Mononeuropathy, multiple mononeuropathies or polyneuropathy (i.e., glove/stocking distribution) attributable to a systemic vasculitis
Pulmonary infiltrates	Migratory or transitory pulmonary infiltrates on radiographs attributable to a systemic vasculitis
Paranasal sinus abnormality	History of acute or chronic paranasal sinus pain or tenderness or radiographic opacification of the paranasal sinuses
Extravascular eosinophils	Biopsy including artery, arteriole, or venule, showing accumulation of eosinophils in extravascular areas

For classification purposes, a patient shall be said to have Churg-Strauss syndrome if at least four of these criteria are present. The presence of any four or more criteria has a sensitivity of 85% and a specificity of 99.7%.

From Masi AT, Hunder GG, Lie JT, et al: The American College of Rheumatology 1990 criteria for the classification of Churg-Strauss syndrome (allergic granulomatosis and angiitis). Arthritis Rheum 33: 1094, © 1990. Wiley-Liss, Inc. Reprinted by permission of Wiley-Liss, Inc., a subsidiary of John Wiley & Sons, Inc.

Definition and Diagnostic Criteria

Criteria for the classification of Churg-Strauss syndrome were developed by the ACR in a study of 20 patients with the disease and 787 controls (Table 29–6).[43] The disease characteristically affects middle-aged males[44] and is rare in children. To date, 10 patients age 16 years and younger have been reported[42, 45–52] (Table 29–7). The etiology is unknown.

Clinical Manifestations

Churg-Strauss syndrome usually occurs in conjunction with a long history of asthma. Other allergic manifestations such as chronic allergic rhinitis may be present, particularly in the prodromal or early phase, that may last several years.[2] Eosinophilia, pulmonary infiltrates, and finally, vasculitis follow with varying speed. Not all components may be present at one time; the disease may first occur as a localized disorder early on. In the ACR classification study[43] (see Table 29–6), all patients had pulmonary infiltrates and neuropathy (especially mononeuritis multiplex) and 83 percent had paranasal sinus infection. The vasculitis may be clinically indistinguishable from polyarteritis nodosa or hypersensitivity angiitis.[53] In one pediatric patient, microaneu-

Table 29–7

Reported Cases of Churg-Strauss Syndrome in Childhood

REFERENCE	SEX	AGE (yr)	CLINICAL MANIFESTATIONS
Churg & Strauss[42]	F	7	Asthma, eosinophilia, pneumonitis, hypertension, skin nodules and purpura, cardiac failure, nephritis, death
	M	9	Asthma, eosinophilia, pneumonitis, hypertension, skin nodules and purpura, cardiac failure, nephritis, peripheral neuropathy
Farooki et al[45]	M	12	Pericarditis, myocarditis, eosinophilia, history of wheezing, death
Petty et al[46]	M	16	Fever, asthma, painful calf nodules, peripheral neuropathy, hypertension, eosinophilia
Frayha[47]	F	13	Fever, asthma, peripheral neuropathy, celiac aneurysms, paresthesias, eosinophilia, death
Treitman et al[48]	M	14	Asthma, sinusitis, pulmonary basilar infiltrates, cardiomegaly, eosinophilia, death
Heine et al[49]	F	4	Fever, pneumonia, pseudotumor, eosinophilia
Jessuran et al[50]	M	14	Cough, weight loss, skin lesions, eosinophilia, mediastinal granulomata with central necrosis, eosinophils; arteries infiltrated with histiocytes, eosinophils, and giant cells
Rabusin et al[51]	M	2	Asthma, eosinophilia, food allergies, eosinophilic myocarditis, eosinophilic infiltrates in skin, lung; death
Mpofu et al[52]	M	7	Fever, asthma, eosinophilia, skin lesions, proteinuria, pulmonary infiltrates

rysms typical of those occurring in polyarteritis nodosa were present in the hepatic artery and celiac axis.[47] Overlap features have been described in other pediatric patients, including the presence of pANCA in a patient with ocular pseudotumor.[49]

Additional skin manifestations include purpura (representing leukocytoclastic vasculitis), maculopapular rash, and cutaneous nodules (extravascular granulomata),[45] livedo reticularis, ulcers, and bullae.[54] Cardiac involvement was prominent in the patients described by Churg and Strauss and included granulomatous pericardial disease[55] and eosinophilic myocarditis. Renal disease is usually mild and rarely progresses.[44, 56] Myalgia, arthralgia, and arthritis can occur. Hypertension and ocular involvement in addition to pseudotumor cerebri occur in some patients.[57] Gastrointestinal ulceration and granulomata of the omentum have been reported.[47]

Pathology

Histopathologic studies confirm vasculitis of small arteries and veins associated with necrotizing extravascular granulomata and eosinophilic infiltrates. These eosinophilic exudates with necrosis, fibrinoid changes, and granulomatous proliferation of epithelioid and giant cells are characteristic[55] (Fig. 29–6).

Differential Diagnosis

The differential diagnosis includes other forms of vasculitis such as WG, polyarteritis nodosa, and Henoch-Schönlein purpura. The diagnosis is based on the presence of two or more of the clinical criteria described in Table 29–3 and confirmed by biopsy of renal, skin, or lung tissue. (Transbronchial biopsy is less invasive than transthoracic biopsy for obtaining lung tissue.[48]) The diagnosis should be considered in an asthmatic patient with fever, deteriorating clinical course, and eosinophilia.

A syndrome similar to the Churg-Strauss syndrome has been reported following the use of the leukotriene antagonist zafirlukast in adult patients with asthma.[58] This disorder was characterized by pulmonary infiltrates, eosinophilia, neuropathy, sinusitis, rash, fever, and muscle pain. Acute dilated cardiomyopathy was also characteristic of the zafirlukast-associated syndrome but is not a typical feature of the Churg-Strauss syndrome.

Laboratory Examination

Elevation of acute-phase reactants accompanies active disease. There is almost always a peripheral blood eosinophilia (with eosinophils accounting for 10 percent or greater of the leukocytes) and elevation of serum levels of IgE. Chest radiographs may reveal diffuse pulmonary infiltrates (Fig. 29–7), and pulmonary function tests demonstrate poor lung diffusing capacity and low P_{O_2}. ANCA and other autoantibodies are usually not present.

Treatment

There is at least an initial response to high-dose glucocorticoids, but often immunosuppressive agents such

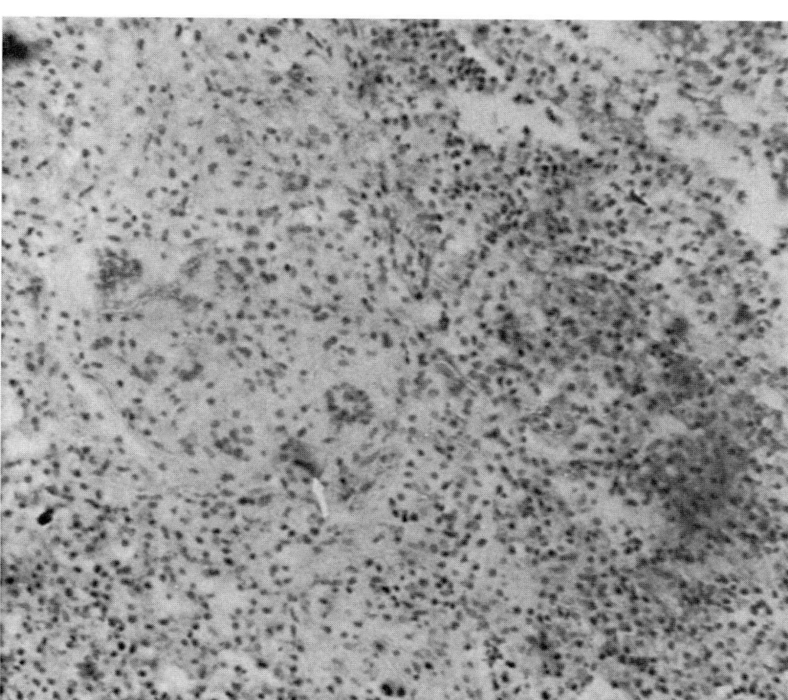

Figure 29–6. Lung biopsy specimen from a young girl with allergic granulomatosis. No definite vasculitis is present, but there are necrotizing granulomata with giant cells (*arrow*). H&E, ×480.

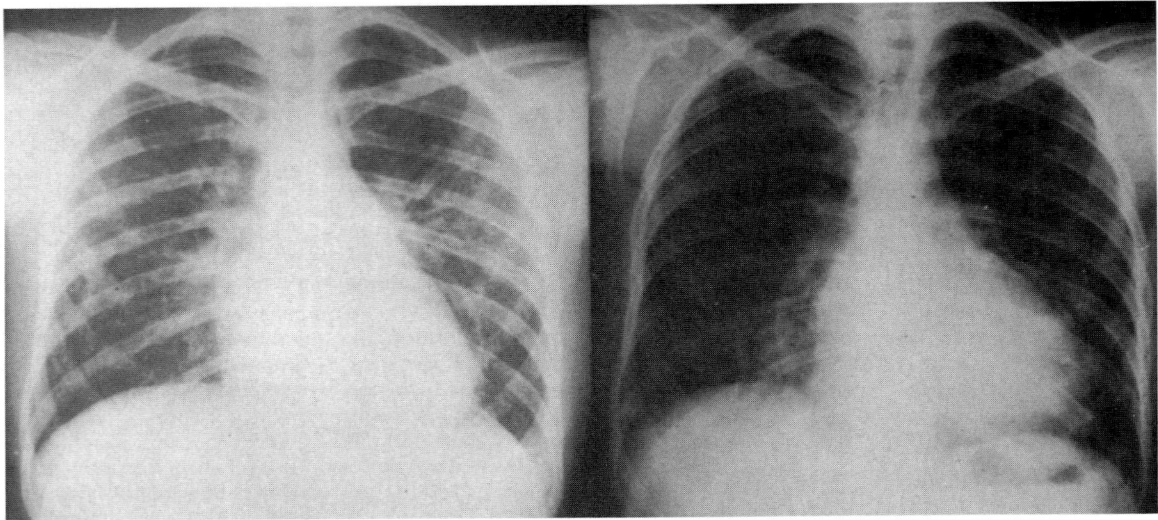

Figure 29–7. Chest roentgenograms in a young man with allergic granulomatosis. The initial film on the left demonstrates an enlarged cardiac silhouette and relatively normal pulmonary fields. The film on the right was taken during an acute episode of left- and right-sided heart failure. Note further cardiac enlargement and disappearance of the normal pulmonary vascular markings, indicating acute pulmonary hypertension and cor pulmonale, in this case on the basis of vasculitis.

as cyclophosphamide or methotrexate are required.[53] The use of interferon-α was reported to be beneficial in four patients with Churg-Strauss syndrome that was resistant to a combination of glucocorticoids and cyclophosphamide or methotrexate.[59] Plasmapheresis may also have a role in the management of the Churg-Strauss syndrome.[60]

Course of the Disease and Prognosis

The long-term follow-up of 96 patients with the Churg-Strauss syndrome reported by Guillevin and colleagues[60] noted a 24 percent mortality. In this study, development of severe myocardial or gastrointestinal disease was associated with a poor outcome. The disease course is often very prolonged, however, and therapy with glucocorticoids with or without other drugs is usually required for years.

Lymphomatoid Granulomatosis

Lymphomatoid granulomatosus, first described in 1972 by Liebow and coworkers,[61] is a rare necrotizing pulmonary vasculitis that is often fatal. It may initially resemble WG but then progress to lymphoma.[61–64] It is sometimes associated with immunodeficiencies (Wiskott-Aldrich syndrome, X-linked lymphoproliferative syndrome), HIV infection, and malignancy.[65–69] The disease has been reported in several adult patients who had undergone renal transplantation.[70–72] Descriptions of this disease in children have been extremely rare and include an infant,[65] a 16-year-old boy,[62] a child with leukemia in remission,[69] and a child with the Wiskott-Aldrich syndrome.[67]

The primary clinical manifestations include fever, pneumonia, lymphadenopathy, and (particularly in children) failure to thrive and recurrent infections, including otitis media and sinusitis. Other organs and systems involved include kidneys, liver, skin, and the CNS. Midline sinus or upper respiratory disease is rare. The characteristic lesions are angiocentric necrotizing granulomata with cellular infiltrates consisting of immunoblasts, lymphocytes, histiocytes, plasma cells, and eosinophils.[44] There is thrombosis and necrosis of the adjacent parenchyma (necrotic nodules involving vascular infiltration surrounded by areas of parenchymal necrosis).

Primary Angiitis of the Central Nervous System

Primary angiitis of the central nervous system (PACNS), first called *granulomatous angiitis*,[73] is now recognized as a distinct form of vasculitis.[74] It occurs predominantly in Caucasians of either sex between 35 and 50 years of age. There are fewer than 50 reports of children with this disorder. The marked variation observed in disease course led Calabrese and associates[75] to subdivide the disease into PACNS and benign angiitis of the central nervous system (BACNS). The benign form is a mild monophasic illness that usually responds well to glucocorticoids and resolves with minimal residua over a period of several weeks. BACNS is extremely rare in children.

Clinical Manifestations

The clinical signs and symptoms are variable. Headache occurs in up to 75 percent of patients at onset.[76] Other common neurologic manifestations include transient ischemic attacks, paresis, seizures, visual loss, neurocognitive impairment, and progressive encephalopathy. Systemic signs and symptoms are absent. The majority of patients have an abrupt onset of symptoms several weeks before diagnosis.[76] The study of Calabrese and Mallek[77] included a 10-year-old girl and a 10-year-old boy, both with hemiparesis. Intracranial hemorrhage may be the initial presentation.[78, 79] There appears to be an increased risk in the postpartum period.[76, 80]

Laboratory Examination

Leukocytosis is common, occasionally associated with thrombocytosis and the presence of antinuclear antibodies. Antiphospholipid antibodies do not occur. Complement activation has been reported.[81] Cerebrospinal fluid analysis is usually characterized by an increased protein level and mild pleocytosis.[76] Disease is restricted to small- and medium-sized arteries and venules of the brain and spinal cord.[82] Infiltration of mononuclear cells and granuloma formation have been found.

Radiologic Examination

The diagnosis is usually made by angiography, which demonstrates beading or alternating ectasia and stenosis of intracranial arteries (Fig. 29–8).[83] Abu-Shakra[76] found abnormalities in 73 percent of patients by computed tomography, in 77 percent by magnetic resonance imaging (MRI), and in three of four patients studied by single photon emission computed tomography and pertechnetate isotope brain scans. Other studies have shown a higher frequency of MRI abnormalities.[84]

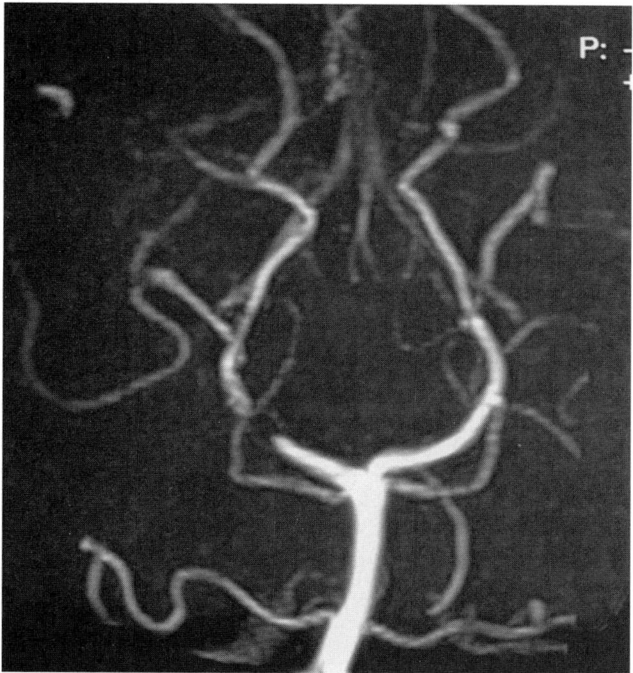

Figure 29–8. Magnetic resonance angiogram of a 12-year-old girl who presented with mild right-sided hemiparesis and headache. Antinuclear antibody was strongly positive, anti-dsDNA antibody was negative, and antibody to myeloperoxidase (pANCA) was positive. An obstruction to flow was demonstrated in the right posterior cerebral artery. The patient had no evidence of extracerebral vasculitis. She was treated with intravenous methylprednisolone and cyclophosphamide and has remained asymptomatic without progression of the vascular lesion.

Treatment and Outcome

PACNS was initially thought to be uniformly fatal, but with the availability of improved imaging techniques allowing earlier diagnosis, an improved outcome has been reported.[85, 86] Nonetheless, morbidity is significant and recurrences are frequent. When patients were treated with glucocorticoids and cyclophosphamide, Woolfenden and colleagues[84] reported that although patients developed no new lesions, old lesions did not resolve. In another study, glucocorticoids alone or in combination with cyclophosphamide were used if visual loss, stroke, or severe neurocognitive disease developed.[76] Eighty percent of this group stabilized, but 12 percent experienced relapse after a median of 2 months. Two recent studies[76, 84] showed significant permanent neurologic deficits including paresis, visual loss, and seizures in patients treated with glucocorticoids or glucocorticoids and cyclophosphamide.

Moyamoya Disease

First described in 1969, moyamoya[87] ("puff of smoke" in Japanese) is a term applied to the appearance of the cerebral angiograms in patients with hemiplegia associated with supraclinoid carotid stenosis and multiple cerebral telangiectasia. Approximately 25 percent of patients are under 10 years of age.[88] Ninety percent present with hemiplegia.[88, 89] Other manifestations include alteration of consciousness, speech or visual disturbances, and seizures.[90] Characteristic vessel abnormalities apparent on angiography include multiple collateral vessels and anastomoses of meningeal vessels with internal carotid vessels (rete mirabile) (Fig. 29–9). Diffusion-weighted MRI offers a noninvasive means of early detection of ischemic lesions and monitoring of the clinical course.[91] Surgical extracranial-intracranial bypass procedures have been reported to be useful.[92] Calcium channel blockers may be helpful in some patients.[93] The prognosis may be worse in patients under 16 years of age, and recovery or stabilization was observed in only 40 percent of that age group.[88]

Both congenital arterial dysplasia and changes secondary to nonspecific vascular injury have been hypothesized as causes.[94–96] A number of clinical associations have been described, including Down syndrome,[88, 97] occlusive peripheral vascular disease,[96] primary pulmonary hypertension,[98] and other cerebrovascular malformations.[99] The familial occurrence of moyamoya disease has been described.[100] In adults, further associations include myopathy, renal artery stenosis, Fanconi's anemia, hemoglobinopathies, meningitis, and arteritis.[88]

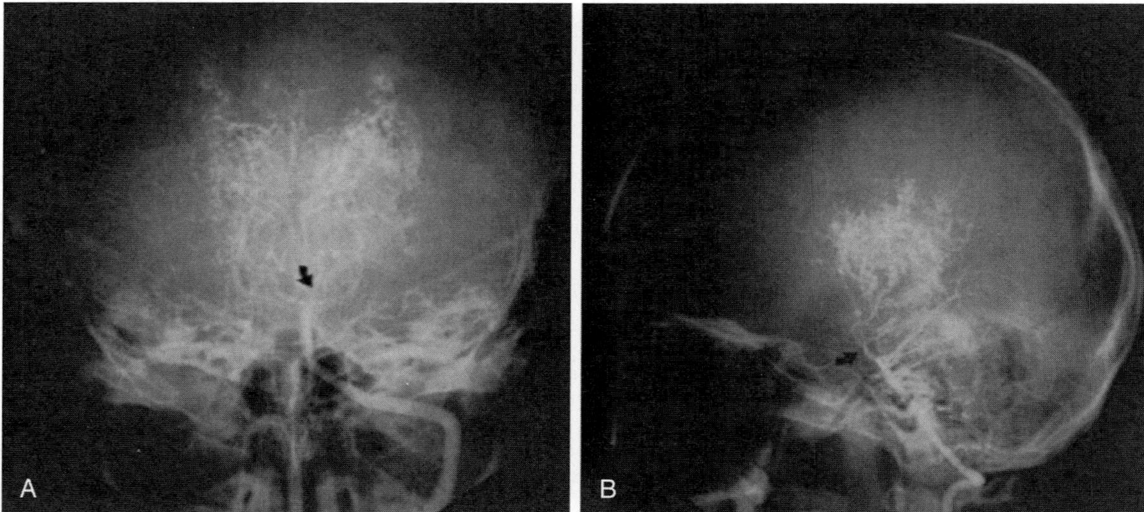

Figure 29–9. Arteriography of left vertebral artery shows stenosis of the basilar artery (*arrow*) just above the tentorium. The extensive collaterals are the characteristic "puff of smoke"—moyamoya. *A,* Anteroposterior view. *B,* Lateral view. (*A* and *B,* Courtesy of Dr. O. Flodmark.)

GIANT CELL ARTERITIS

A number of clinically different diseases are characterized by identical histologic abnormalities of a giant cell arteritis. The two major vasculitides of this type that occur in childhood and adolescence are Takayasu's arteritis (TA) and temporal arteritis.

Takayasu's Arteritis

TA, a chronic inflammatory vasculitis affecting the aorta and its major branches, is most common in young women, particularly of Japanese origin. It was first described as *pulseless disease*.[101, 102] Takayasu, a Japanese ophthalmologist, first described the characteristic arteriovenous abnormalities of the retina in 1908.[103]

Definition and Classification

The ACR classification criteria are shown in Table 29–8.[104] The presence of all six criteria has a sensitivity of 90.5 percent and a specificity of 97.8 percent for TA. In the patient population analyzed for validation of these criteria, 18 of 63 patients (29 percent) were younger than 20 years at diagnosis. TA is categorized according to the distribution of affected vessels (Table 29–9).[105, 106] Type I affects the aortic arch; type II the thoracic and abdominal aorta; type III the aorta both above and below the diaphragm; and type IV the aorta and the pulmonary artery.

Epidemiology

Although rare before the age of 16 years, TA is the most common giant cell arteritis of childhood; worldwide, it follows Kawasaki disease and Henoch-Schönlein purpura as the most frequent of the vasculitides of childhood. In Japan, 20 percent of patients with TA are younger than 19 years, and 2 percent are younger than 10 years of age. Reports from South Africa,[110] Canada,[111] and Mexico[112] document its occurrence in children around the world. Blacks, Asians, Hispanic Americans,

Table 29–8

Classification Criteria for Takayasu's Arteritis

Subclavian or aortic bruit
Age <40 yr at onset
Decreased brachial artery pulse
Blood pressure difference of >10 mm between arms
Claudication of extremities
Arteriographic evidence of narrowing or occlusion of aorta, its primary branches or large arteries in the proximal, upper, or lower extremities

From Arend WP, Michel BA, Bloch DA, et al: The American College of Rheumatology 1990 criteria for the classification of Takayasu arteritis. Arthritis Rheum 33: 1129, 1990.

Table 29–9

Takayasu's Arteritis in Childhood—Patterns of Involvement

TYPE	AFFECTED VESSELS	PERCENTAGE
I	Aortic arch only	5
	Aortic arch and decending thoracic aorta	19
	Aortic arch, thoracic and abdominal aorta	16
	Aortic arch and abdominal aorta	19
II	Descending thoracic aorta only	7
	Descending thoracic and abdominal aorta	19
III	Diffuse aortic involvement	0
IV	Diffuse aortic and pulmonary artery involvement	2

Data derived from published reports of TA in children.

and Sephardic Jews are most at risk. The female:male ratio is about 8:1 in adults but closer to 2:1 in children.[109, 113]

There are, however, unexplained geographic variations in the presentation of TA. Obstructive lesions are the most common in the United States, Europe, and Japan, whereas aneurysms appear to be more common in India, Thailand, and Africa. Involvement of the brachiocephalic arteries occurs in patients in most geographic areas; the abdominal aorta is most often involved in reports from Thailand[114] and the descending aorta in those from India.[115, 116] The significance of these differences, if real, is unknown.

Genetic Background

TA has been reported in families and in monozygotic twin sisters.[117] Associations with specific HLA antigens in different racial groups have been reported. In Japanese patients, the haplotype A11 B40,[118] the complotype Aw24-DW52-C4A2-C4BQ0-Dw12,[118] and B5201 and B3902[119] have been noted, whereas in patients from northern India, there is a marked increase in the frequency of B5 compared with an ethnically matched control population (relative risk, 4.3). B51 and B52 were equally represented in this population.[120] A weaker association with DR8 was found in the same group. Possible associations with DR6 (DRB1*1301) were observed in a Mexican population.[121]

Etiology and Pathogenesis

The etiology of TA is not known. An association with tuberculosis in some areas of the world has been suggested but not proved.[122–124] In India, patients with TA have an increased humoral immune response to the 65 kD heat shock protein from *Mycobacterium tuberculosis*.[125] Whether this indicates a role for tuberculosis in the etiopathogenesis of TA or is an indication that there is cross-reactivity with other heat shock proteins or cross-reacting self-antigens is not clear.

Laboratory Examination

Laboratory findings are nonspecific and include elevation of the ESR, moderate anemia, mild leukocytosis, and hypergammaglobulinemia. ANAs are rare, and RFs are only occasionally present. ANCAs are seldom found,[126, 127] but antibodies to endothelial cells are frequently present.[126] Electrocardiographs may confirm left ventricular hypertrophy, which is strongly associated with the presence of hypertension.[128]

Radiologic Examination

Chest radiographs may demonstrate cardiomegaly or an irregular contour of the aortic arch and descending aorta. There may be areas of calcification or widening related to prestenotic dilatation (Figs. 29–10 and 29–11). Arteriography of the aorta and its major branches may demonstrate multiple sites of segmental involvement.[129] Transfemoral digital subtraction angiography avoids the risk of catheter manipulation in the presence of severe aortic disease.[130] The usefulness of such studies may be limited by cardiac failure and motion artifacts. Sonography and Doppler echocardiography may be useful in demonstrating flow turbulence.[131, 132] Echocardiography may be needed to assess the aortic root in coronary artery disease. In one study, duplex color-flow Doppler demonstrated decreased pulses and vascular bruits and was superior to MRI in defining mural thickening in involved vessels.[133]

Treatment

Treatment requires high-dose glucocorticoids (1 to 2 mg/kg/d) for an initial period of 4 to 8 weeks followed by a judicious reduction of the dose. The response to glucocorticoids depends on the activity of the disease; not all patients respond.[134] Cytotoxic drug therapy has been used, but its efficacy has not been established.[135] Low-dose oral methotrexate may be an effective steroid-sparing agent.[135a] Aggressive treatment of hypertension is critical. Use of angiotensin-converting enzyme (ACE) inhibitors should be withheld unless other antihypertensive therapy has failed, because these drugs may diminish renal function. Antiplatelet agents (low-dose aspirin or dipyridamole) may be helpful in preventing thrombosis in abnormal vessels.

Surgical interventions for severe renal hypertension, cerebral hypoperfusion, claudication, or aneurysm formation have led to varying success. Percutaneous transluminal renal angioplasty was successful in 80 percent of Indian children subjected to the procedure.[136] Percutaneous expandable renal and aortic stents have been placed with success.[134, 137, 138, 138a] When feasible, renal autotransplantation may be the definitive procedure for some patients if other measures fail to control renovascular hypertension.[124, 134]

Course of the Disease and Prognosis

The course is prolonged and variable, and relapses occur in spite of therapy. A prospective study in adults demonstrated an 83 percent 5-year survival rate and a 58 percent 10-year survival rate.[106] In a study of 11 patients who met ACR criteria for the diagnosis of TA, 1 patient died and 5 patients required renal artery transplantation, resulting in preserved renal function in 4.[135] The length of time between disease onset and institution of therapy is critical to the outcome because glucocorticoid therapy is unlikely to alter vascular lesions in which fibrosis with narrowing has already taken place.

Temporal (Cranial) Arteritis

Classic giant cell arteritis affecting the temporal artery is a common form of vasculitis in elderly patients but

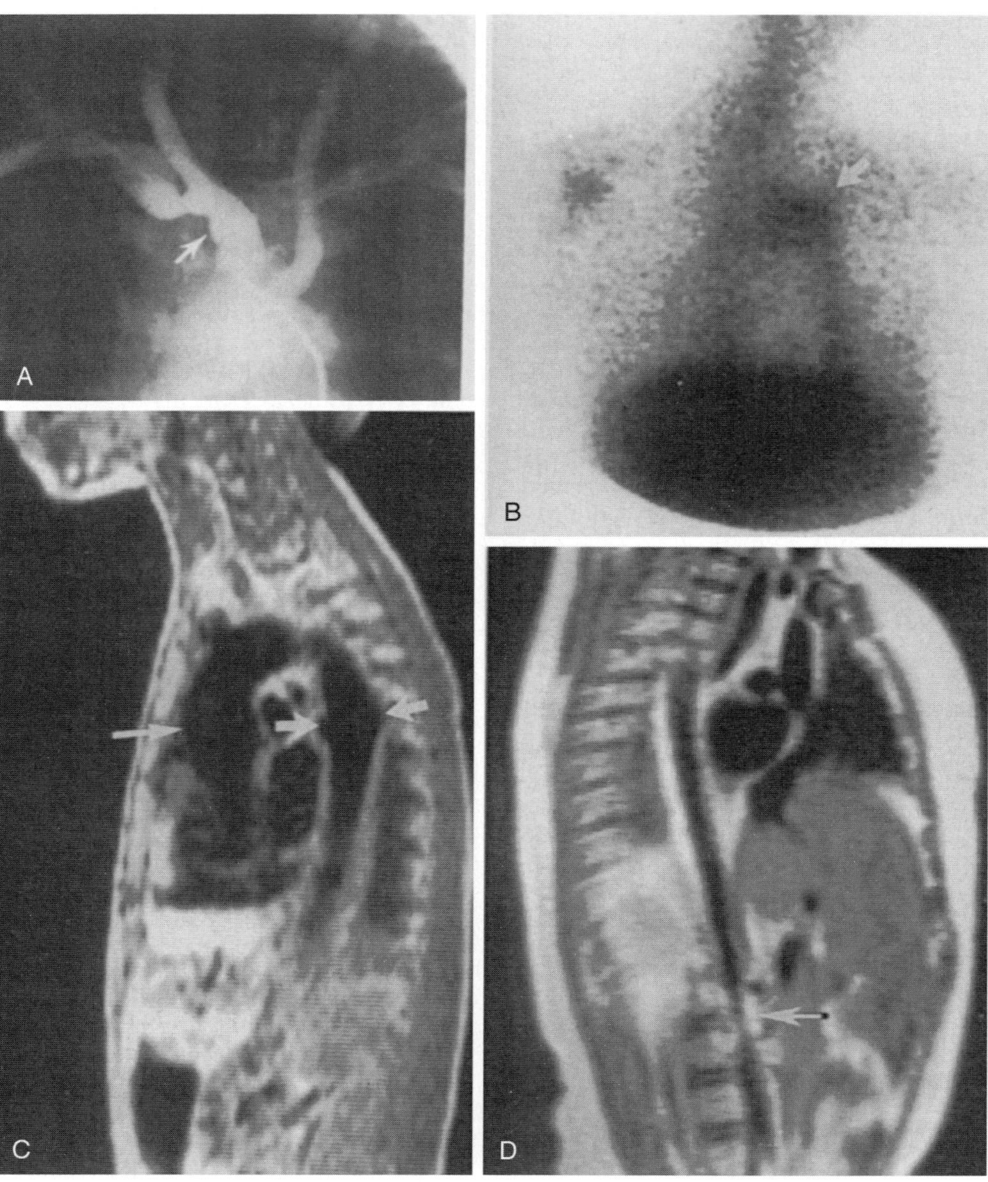

Figure 29–10. Four different studies document the lesions of Takayasu's arteritis. *A,* There is dilatation, irregularity, and stenosis of the right innominate artery and its branches on angiography (*arrow*). The left subclavian artery is not visualized owing to occlusion. *B,* This gallium scan shows increased uptake of the isotope in the region of the aortic arch (*arrow*), supporting the diagnosis of inflammation of this structure. *C,* Magnetic resonance image shows the dilated aortic arch and localized aneurysms of the thoracic portion of the descending aorta (*arrow*). *D,* Stenotic region of the abdominal aorta (*arrow*). (*B,* Courtesy of Dr. H. Nadel. *D,* Courtesy of Dr. G. Culham.)

is rare in childhood and adolescence. Inflammation involves primarily the carotid artery and its branches. Headache, localized pain and tenderness over the temporal arteries, and occasionally, jaw or face claudication are present. Disease of the ophthalmic and central retinal vessels may cause blindness. Studies suggest that the arterial damage is secondary to an antigen-driven immune response.[139] Temporal arteritis is often associated with polymyalgia rheumatica in the adult population but not in children.

Juvenile temporal arteritis is a non–giant cell, nonnecrotizing vasculitis of the temporal arteries of unknown cause, initially described by Lie and associates in 1975.[140] It is a specific form of temporal arteritis that differs from the classic disease. It has been reported in seven children[140, 141] and occasionally in adults.[142] There are no systemic symptoms. The lesions are noted accidentally as pea-sized nodules in the temporal area. The condition is usually bilateral. Patients with juvenile temporal arteritis have a benign course that does not require glucocorticoid therapy. This disease has been cured by excisional biopsy with no evidence of recurrence. Similar involvement of the occipital artery has also been described.[143]

SARCOIDOSIS

Sarcoidosis is an uncommon multisystem disease of unknown etiology. Two patterns of clinical manifestations are reported in children. Early descriptions of the disorder were primarily of older children or adolescents who had lung disease, lymphadenopathy, weight loss, fever, and hypercalcemia but little no joint disease.[144–150] In 1966, Harris and colleagues[151] described patients with onset under 4 years of age characterized

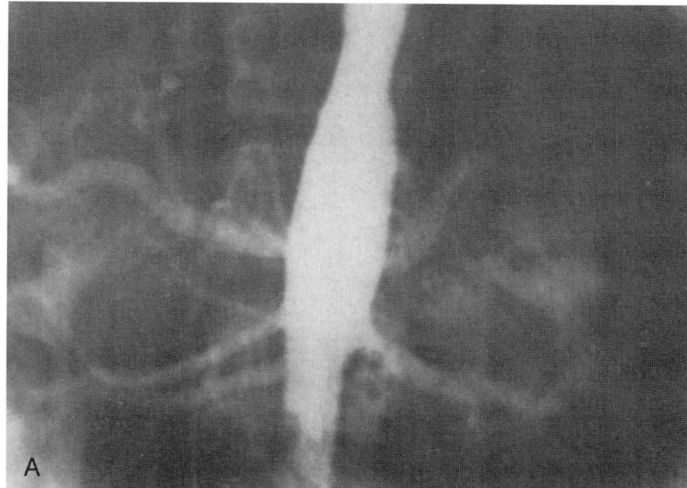

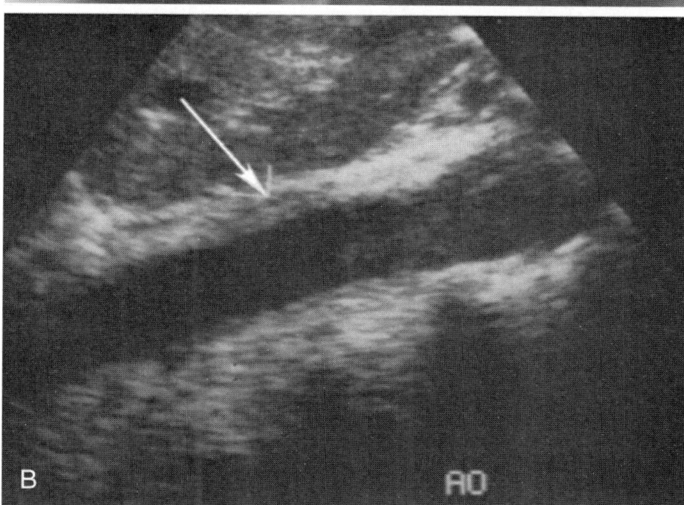

Figure 29–11. *A,* Dilatation of the abdominal aorta. *B,* Ultrasound study (sagittal section) shows thickening of the aortic wall *(arrow)* in a child with active Takayasu's aortitis. (*A,* Courtesy of Dr. G. Culham. *B,* Courtesy of Dr. A. R. Buckley.)

by the clinical triad of skin, joint, and eye disease. Subsequent series have to a large extent confirmed these two distinct patterns of disease,[152–155] although many exceptions have been noted.[156, 157]

Epidemiology

Sarcoidosis is primarily a disease of adults in the 20- to 40-year age range and is almost twice as common in women as in men.[158, 159] Approximately 3 percent of cases in a 1953 study were in patients under 15 years of age.[144] In a study from eastern Hungary, however, 15 percent of patients were children between 8 and 14 years of age.[150] In 1983, there were 325 pediatric cases in the English language literature, 15 of which (5 percent) included arthritis.[160] In an international registry study of children with sarcoidosis associated with joint disease, the mean age at onset was 10.6 years (range, 0.1 to 16 years). Thirty-eight of 53 patients (72 percent) had onset before 5 years of age.[161]

The prevalence of sarcoidosis is high in Japanese children,[158, 162] and the disease is more common in black children than in white children, although the racial distribution varies with geographic location.[144, 146, 149, 155, 163–167] Within the United States, approximately 80 percent of reported patients live in the southeastern part of the country, particularly in rural areas.[146, 148, 155] An increased incidence of the onset of sarcoidosis between December and May has been noted.[155]

Genetic Background

There have been numerous reports of a familial occurrence of sarcoidosis in parent-offspring or sibling pairs.[168–174] In an international registry, a familial pattern was noted in 11 of 53 children with sarcoid arthritis.[161] Patterns of inheritance in a study from the United Kingdom of 80 black patients from 11 families supported multigenic inheritance.[175] The incidence of familial disease was three times greater in Los Angeles than in London, and a pattern consistent with autosomal recessive inheritance was evident.[176] Studies of HLA antigens suggest associations of sarcoidosis with DQB1*0603, DQB1*0604, and DPB1*0201 (Glu positive).[177]

Clinical Manifestations

Sarcoidosis may be asymptomatic, and diagnosis may therefore be delayed. Only 11 of 18 children in one study were symptomatic: Hilar adenopathy seen on routine chest radiographs was the first indication of the disease.[146] Symptomatic children were younger, had more extensive disease, and experienced a more complicated course. Duration of symptoms before diagnosis in one study was 7.6 months.[155] In this group, 75 percent had more than one area of involvement. Six of the seven asymptomatic children were well at follow-up.

Lymphadenopathy and Hepatosplenomegaly

Lymphadenopathy is the most common initial manifestation. The lymph nodes are usually firm, mobile, and nontender.[146, 155] Retroperitoneal adenopathy is common.[178] In a study of children with sarcoid arthritis, 9 of 12 children had hepatosplenomegaly.[156]

Skin Disease

Skin disease occurs in approximately 30 percent of children with sarcoidosis.[148, 179] The lesions may be maculopapular, vesicular, papular, or nodular (including erythema nodosum). An association between ichthyosiform cutaneous lesions and severe joint disease has been made.[180] Nodular subcutaneous sarcoid lesions also occur.[181] Sarcoidosis should always be included in the differential diagnosis of unusual skin lesions (Fig. 29–12).

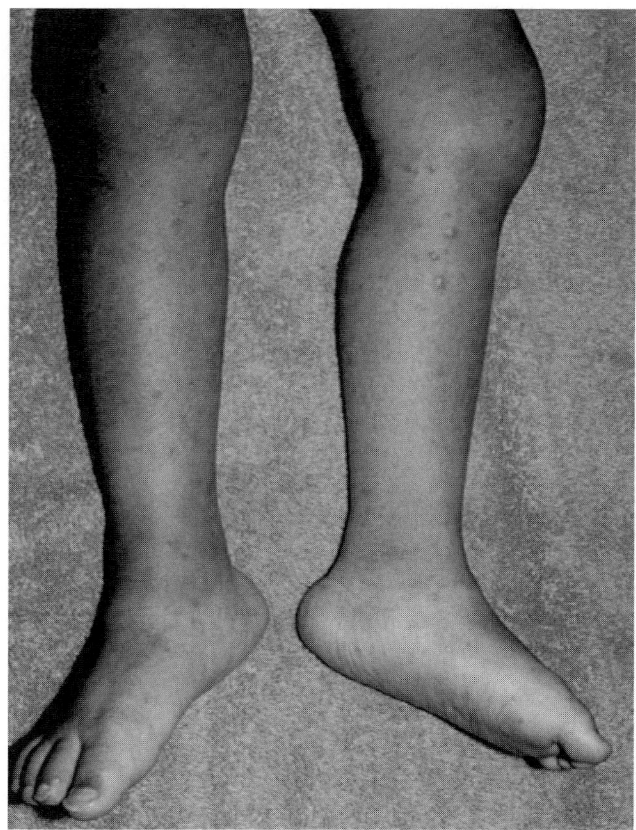

Figure 29–12. Many of the lesions visible on the legs of this child with sarcoidosis are nodular. The child also has sarcoid arthritis in the knees and ankles.

Eye Disease

Ocular abnormalities are common causes of morbidity in sarcoidosis and may be the presenting manifestations.[182] In a study of uveitis associated with systemic diseases, 3 of 340 children were found to have sarcoidosis.[183] However, in a population of children with sarcoidosis and joint disease, the incidence of eye involvement is higher. All of the 12 patients reported by Hafner and associates[156] had iridocyclitis; 8 had residual eye damage. Uveitis may be more common in early-onset disease than in later-onset disease. In children between 8 and 15 years of age, 32 percent had eye involvement.[145, 146, 148] In another study,[184] 77 percent of children with sarcoidosis under 5 years of age had eye disease. Posterior uveitis also occurs. In the sarcoid registry, 44 of 53 children had uveitis, which was bilateral in 43. The anterior uveal tract,[42] posterior uveal tract,[23] or both[21] were involved.[161] Posterior or panuveitis may be associated with CNS involvement.[185]

Other manifestations are diverse and include lacrimal gland swelling, orbital granulomata, conjunctival granulomata (Fig. 29–13), vitritis, chorioretinitis, optic nerve involvement, and proptosis.[184, 186–188] Interstitial keratitis is uncommon. Eye involvement may precede joint or pulmonary manifestations.[189] It should be emphasized that young children may be asymptomatic, even though blind at the time of diagnosis![145, 146, 190] The pattern of eye involvement differs from that of juvenile rheumatoid arthritis (JRA). The tightly packed corneal accumulations of lymphocytes (keratic precipitates) are often larger and in the peripheral cornea may be confluent ("snowbank").[191] Similar accumulations may be present at the iris-pupil margin (Koeppe's nodules).[191]

Pulmonary Disease

Chronic cough is the second most common presenting symptom of sarcoidosis.[155] Of 53 children in the international registry, 5 (9 percent) had lung disease.[161] Although bronchopulmonary disease is less common in children under 4 years of age, 22 percent had lung disease in one study.[154] In children with sarcoid arthritis, pulmonary disease occurred in almost one half, and in about 15 percent it was severe.[156] Hilar and paratracheal adenopathy, together with parenchymal involvement, is common.[163] Parenchymal disease, characterized by small irregular interstitial infiltrates, pleural effusions, and atelectasis,[192] is less common in chil-

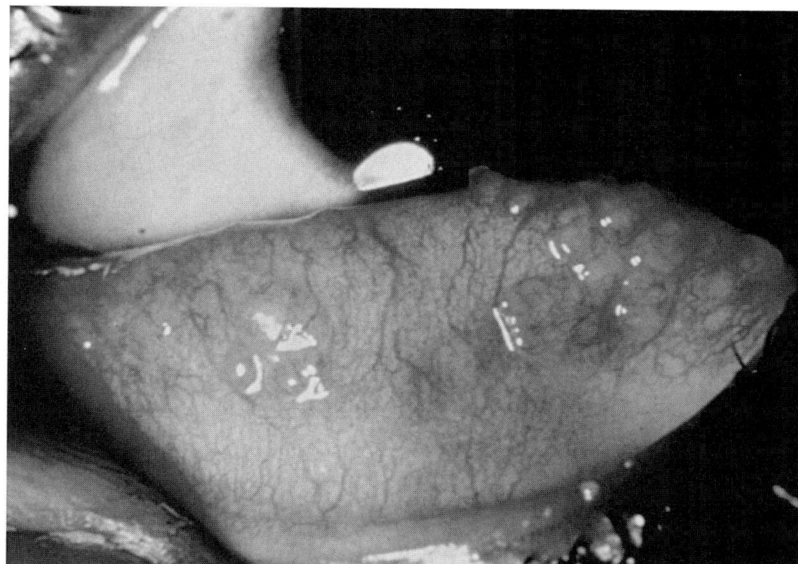

Figure 29–13. Conjunctival nodules are evident in this everted lower eyelid of a child with sarcoidosis.

dren than in adults, in whom it occurs in one quarter of patients.[163] Restrictive disease is most characteristic.[155]

Neurologic Abnormalities

There is a plethora of neurologic manifestations of sarcoidosis.[193] In one study of children with sarcoid arthritis, 30 percent had CNS abnormalities, including encephalopathy and seizures.[156] In adults, CNS involvement is reported in 5 to 10 percent,[194–196] most commonly affecting the brain and peripheral nerves.[197–199] Of the cranial nerves, the seventh is most frequently affected, but involvement of the optic, acoustic, vagus, and glossopharyngeal nerves has been described.[200, 201] Mass lesions are much more common in the cerebrum than in the posterior fossa.[193, 201] Obstructive hydrocephalus, aseptic meningitis, myelopathy, general and focal seizures, pituitary-hypothalamic lesions, and spinal cord involvement also occur.[201–203] Three cases of intraspinal sarcoid without systemic manifestations have been described.[194]

Musculoskeletal Disease

Musculoskeletal involvement varies from less than 5 percent to 50 percent in reported series of children with sarcoidosis.[155] Fewer than a dozen cases of sarcoid arthritis were described in children before 1970.[204] Musculoskeletal manifestations of sarcoidosis include arthralgia, arthritis, bone abnormalities, and muscle involvement. The arthritis is characterized by a boggy synovial thickening with large effusions of joints and tendon sheaths. There is often minimal pain, stiffness, or limitation of motion.[204] Prolonged synovitis may not be associated with radiographic evidence of erosion or osteoporosis. Although initial joint involvement may be transient and affect only a few joints, a polyarticular pattern generally evolves over a period of several years.[180, 204] As the duration of disease increases, the arthritis more closely resembles that of JRA with increasing limitation of motion, stiffness, fusiform swelling of the fingers, and a high frequency of cervical spine involvement. This type of deforming polyarthritis has been described with increasing frequency.[191, 205] Eight of 12 patients in one study had progressive articular disease.[156] Transient polyarthritis occurs in 6 to 25 percent of adults but later may become chronic and destructive (Fig. 29–14).[206]

Osseous sarcoid is uncommon in children, although small bones of the hands and feet may be involved. Vertebral sarcoid can occur and may present as back pain.[207] Up to 50 percent of adults have muscle disease,[208, 209] although it may be symptomatic in less than 5 percent.[210] Muscle involvement in children is rare but was described as a cause of myalgia with associated electromyographic abnormalities in a 9-year-old boy with symptoms for 5 years.[211] The spectrum of muscle involvement includes nodular lesions and inflammatory myositis.[159, 212, 213]

Other Manifestations

Gastrointestinal tract involvement is uncommon, but when it occurs, the stomach is most frequently affected.[214] Intestinal obstruction with gastric and small bowel involvement[215] and rectal prolapse[192] have been reported. Bilateral parotid swelling is described,[216] and in one study,[156] one third of patients had a sicca syndrome including lacrimal and submandibular involvement. Sarcoidosis can present as a testicular mass.[217]

In one study,[156] 8 of 12 children had pericardial effusions and chronic pericarditis. Involvement of the myocardium can also occur.[132, 218, 219] Renal involvement is rare in both adults and children.[146, 152–154, 157, 220–228] It may be asymptomatic or present as polyuria or even eneuresis.[224, 225] These signs have been associated with

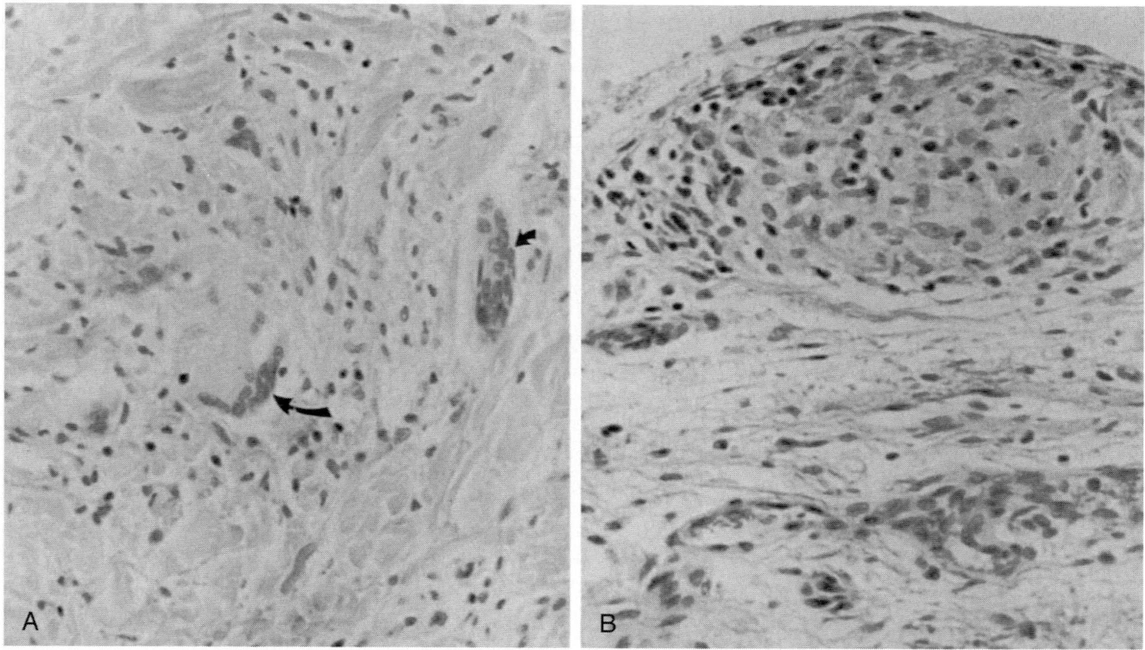

Figure 29–14. Synovial biopsy from a child with sarcoid arthritis. H&E, ×480. *A*, Giant cells (*arrows*). *B*, Noncaseating granuloma.

bilateral enlargement of the kidneys.[226] Nephrocalcinosis may be precipitated by hypercalciuria.[155, 228]

Differential Diagnosis

Sarcoidosis should be suspected in any child with unexplained lymphadenopathy, hepatomegaly, uveitis, enlargement of the salivary or lacrimal glands, cystic bone lesions of the hand and feet, or cutaneous infiltrates or papules, especially if the patient has an associated arthritis.

Several rare autosomal dominant familial syndromes should be considered in the differential diagnosis.[229, 230] Blau[231] described 11 family members with a multisystem granulomatous disease characterized by uveitis, joint and skin disease, and camptodactyly associated with elevation of serum levels of ACE. They had negative Kveim-Siltzbach skin tests and no lung disease. Later studies disclosed "comma" and "wormlike" bodies on electron microscopy of the granulomas.[232] Additional similar families have been reported.[230, 233–236] Linkage analysis studies have demonstrated a susceptibility locus for Blau's disease on the pericentromere region of chromosome 16 (16p12-16q21).[237, 238] Jabs[239] described familial granulomatous synovitis associated with uveitis and cranial neuropathies, but without skin disease, in four members of one family. The relationship of this syndrome to that described by Blau, and of both syndromes to sarcoidosis, is not certain. They may be variants of the same disorder.

A wide spectrum of vasculitides including small, medium, and large vessel disease, granulomatous vasculitis, and leukocytoclastic vasculitis has been associated with sarcoidosis.[239–241] Aortic arch disease identical to that of TA,[239] carotid and subclavian arteritis,[242] and abdominal aortic aneurysms have been reported in patients with sarcoidosis.[243]

Laboratory Examination

No laboratory test is diagnostic of sarcoidosis. Leukopenia, eosinophilia, increased levels of immunoglobulins and elevated acute-phase reactants are common. Hypercalciuria occurs in the majority of patients, with or without nephrocalcinosis.[155] Serum calcium may be normal even in multisystem disease, however.[156] Hoffman[244] described a 15-year-old who presented with hypercalcemic crisis, and hypercalcemia has also been reported in an infant with sarcoidosis.[245] Hypercalciuria can occur with normal serum levels of calcium.[246] Hypercalcemia appears to result from abnormal pulmonary alveolar macrophages: Both the cells and homogenates of lymph nodes are capable of synthesizing 1,25-dihydroxyvitamin D from 25-hydroxyvitamin D, and these cells appear to be insensitive to regulatory feedback by hypercalcemia.[247, 248]

Serum levels of ACE produced by epithelial cells in granulomata[249] are elevated in up to 80 percent of children with sarcoidosis,[250] a frequency similar to that seen in adults.[251–254] ACE is less frequently elevated in very young children with sarcoidosis. Serum levels appear to correlate with disease activity and may be helpful in adjusting therapy.[250, 255] Levels of ACE in normal children are higher than in adults, and pediatric standards are important in assessing results.[256] The Kveim-Siltzbach skin test (sarcoid granulomata resulting from intradermal injection of extract of spleen from a patient with sarcoidosis) is antiquated, and the standard test reagent is no longer available.[257, 258] Cutaneous delayed-type hypersensitivity to previously administered antigens is not present in approximately one half of patients. Such anergy is characteristic but not diagnostic of sarcoidosis. Anergy to purified protein derivatives of *M. tuberulosis* is often present.

Investigation of Pulmonary Disease

Measurement of pulmonary function indicates that up to 50 percent of patients with sarcoidosis have restrictive lung disease, even if asymptomatic.[155] Bronchial alveolar lavage (BAL) yields a three-fold to five-fold increase in the number of lymphocytes and macrophages in children with sarcoidosis.[155, 259] There is an elevated CD4-positive:CD8-positive ratio. Macrophages demonstrate an increased release of hydrogen peroxide. With glucocorticoid therapy, the mononuclear cell abnormalities slowly normalize.[260, 261] Tessier and colleagues[262] reported 11 children with pulmonary sarcoidosis who underwent BAL. Elevated levels of interleukin (IL)-1β, IL-6, tumor necrosis factor α, and tumor growth factor β mRNA corresponded with disease activity and severity.

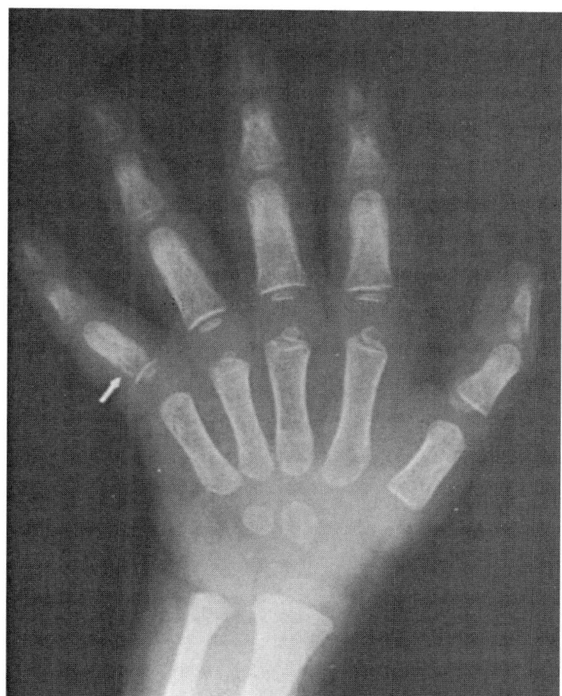

Figure 29–15. Sarcoid arthritis involving the wrists and proximal interphalangeal joints in a 2-year-old black boy. There is a destructive lacelike permeative lesion in the proximal end of the left fifth proximal phalanx consistent with the osseous changes of sarcoidosis (*arrow*).

Radiologic Examination

Chest radiography is the standard screening procedure for sarcoidosis of the lungs, although computed tomography may better define details of specific lesions.[263, 264] Plain radiographs identify characteristic lytic bone lesions, which have been reported in up to 19 percent of patients[146, 149, 166, 167] and are most common in the metacarpal bones or vertebrae (Figs. 29–15 and 29–16). Computed tomography and ultrasonography are helpful in defining the nature and extent of orbital lesions.[187, 265] Demineralization of the orbital wall with bony destruction indicates sinus extension. MRI is particularly useful for the detection of basilar and meningeal abnormalities and also nodular lesions in the bone marrow.[266, 267] A common pattern of involvement includes both orbits, parotids, and submandibular glands ("panda pattern").[268] A combination of gallium and thallium-201 myocardial scintigraphy is best for defining cardiac disease.[269]

Treatment

Glucocorticoids have been the standard treatment for patients who are symptomatic and have significant organ involvement.[145] In one study of sarcoid arthritis,[156] glucocorticoids were effective in 11 of 12 patients, but most required 0.2 to 0.3 mg/kg of prednisolone per day as a maintenance dose, and all required either azathioprine or methotrexate in addition. Low-dose methotrexate was reported to be effective, safe, and glucocorticoid-sparing in a study of seven children.[205] No adverse effects were noted in this study. Other immunomodulating drugs, including cyclosporin, cyclophosphamide, and chloroquine, have demonstrated some benefit in adults.[219, 270–272] Ocular involvement with sarcoidosis usually responds well to glucocorticoids administered topically, locally, or systemically.

Course of the Disease and Prognosis

Mortality from sarcoidosis varies with the geographic region, sex of the patient, and race. Mortality in most studies was higher in females than in males,[265] and in African Americans than in Caucasians.[219, 273, 274] Japanese children with bilateral hilar adenopathy had complete clearing of these abnormalities over a 2-year period.[162] At follow-up, children with sarcoidosis often had significant residual disease. In Kendig's series[275] of 28 children, 5 had severe sequelae: restrictive lung disease occurred in 3 (1 died) and blindness in 2. Of 60 children and youths with sarcoidosis reported by Patishall and colleagues,[155] 47 percent had persistent abnormalities on chest radiograph at 5-year follow-up. A further 35 percent had physical abnormalities, and 40 percent were normal. Abnormal lung function was demonstrated in 68 percent of 19 patients with childhood-onset sarcoidosis followed for a mean of 21 years; 5 patients were blind, had Bell's palsy, vertebral lesions causing back pain, or cor pulmonale.[276]

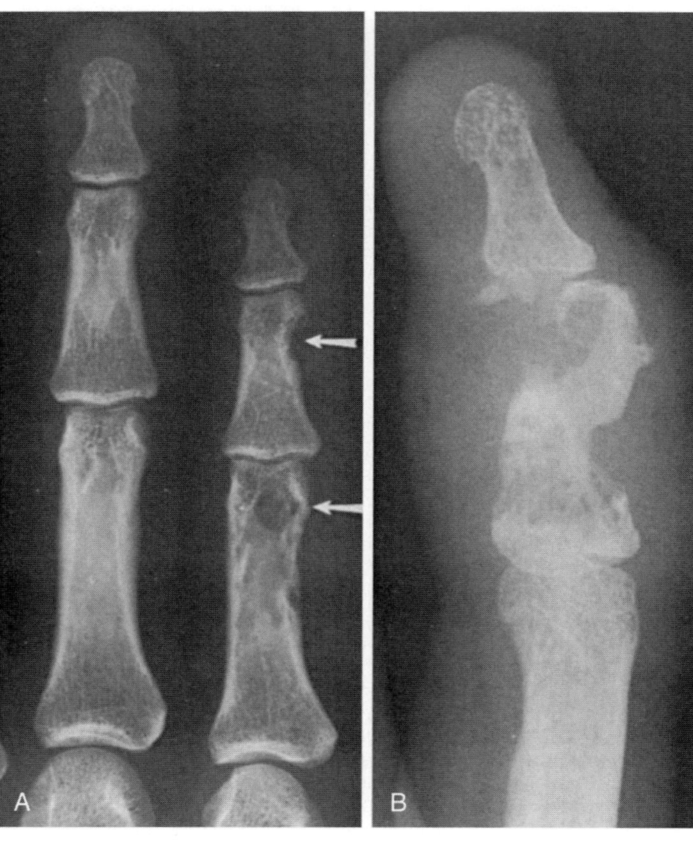

Figure 29–16. Sarcoid arthritis. *A,* Fenestrated lesions of bone and scalloping of osseous defects (*arrow*). *B,* Profound granulomatous destruction of phalanx resembling changes seen in tuberculosis.

A number of studies have noted severe growth delay in children with both early- and late-onset joint disease.[157, 277] Sarcoid arthritis may result in minimal morbidity and residual disease[204] or may cause destructive polyarthritis.[156] The latter group of patients also had a high fequency of cardiac, lung, and CNS involvement at 8 to 19 years of follow-up.[156] Ocular sequelae are often very significant, and synechiae and band keratopathy may be present early.

References

1. Wegener F: Uber generalisierte septische Gefasserkrankungn. Verh Dtsch Ges Pathol 29: 202, 1936.
2. Klinger H: Grenzformen der Periarteritis nodosa. Z Pathol 42: 455, 1931.
3. Fahey J, Leonard E, Churg J, et al: Wegener's granulomatosis. Am J Med 17: 168, 1954.
4. Rottem M, Fauci AS, Hallahan CW, et al: Wegener's granulomatosis in children and adolescents: clinical presentation and outcome. J Pediatr 122: 26, 1993.
5. Leavitt RY, Fauci AS, Bloch DA, et al: The American College of Rheumatology 1990 criteria for the classification of Wegener's granulomatosis. Arthritis Rheum 33: 1101, 1990.
6. Carrington CB, Liebow AA: Limited forms of angiitis and granulomatosis of Wegener's type. Am J Med 41: 497, 1968.
7. Cotch MF, Hoffman GS, Yerg DE, et al: The epidemiology of Wegener's granulomatosis. Estimates of the five-year period prevalence, annual mortality, and geographic disease distribution from population-based data sources. Arthritis Rheum 39: 87, 1996.
8. Orlowski JP, Clough JD, Dyment PG: Wegener's granulomatosis in the pediatric age group. Pediatrics 61: 83, 1978.
9. Stegeman CA, Travaert JW, Sluiter WJ, et al: Association of chronic nasal carriage of *Staphylococcus aureus* and higher relapse rates in Wegener's granulomatosis. Ann Intern Med 120: 12, 1994.
10. Mayet WJ, Marker-Hermann E, Schlaak J, et al: Irregular cytokine pattern of CD4+ T lymphocytes in response to staphylococcus aureus in patients with Wegener's granulomatosis. Scand J Immunol 49: 585, 1999.
11. Stoney PJ, Davies W, Ho SF, et al: Wegener's granulomatosis in two siblings: a family study. J Laryngol Otol 105: 123, 1991.
12. Hay EM, Beaman M, Ralston AJ, et al: Wegener's granulomatosis occurring in siblings. Br J Rheumatol 30: 144, 1991.
13. Nowack R, Lehmann H, Flores-Suarez LF, et al: Familial occurrence of systemic vasculitis and rapidly progressive glomerulonephritis. Am J Kidney Dis 34: 364, 1999.
14. Hagen EC, Stegeman CA, D'Amaro J, et al: Decreased frequency of HLA-DR13DR6 in Wegener's granulomatosis. Kidney Int 48: 801, 1995.
15. Dijstelbloem HM, Scheepers RH, Oost WW, et al: Fc gamma receptor polymorphisms in Wegener's granulomatosis: risk factors for disease relapse. Arthritis Rheum 42: 1823, 1999.
16. Moorthy AV, Cheswney RW, Segar WE, et al: Wegener's granulomatosis in childhood: prolonged survival following cytotoxic therapy. J Pediatr 91: 616, 1977.
17. Hall SL, Miller LC, Duggan E, et al: Wegener's granulomatosis in pediatric patients. 106: 739, 1985.
18. Isaeva LA, Fedorova AN, Lysenka GA: Wegener's granulomatosis in children. Pediatriia 51: 67, 1972.
19. Fauci AS, Haynes BF, Katz P, et al: Wegener's granulomatosis: prospective clinical and therapeutic experience with 85 patients for 21 years. Ann Intern Med 98: 76, 1983.
20. Wolff SM, Fauci AS, Horn HG, et al: Wegener's granulomatosis. Ann Intern Med 81: 513, 1974.
21. Drachman DA: Neurological complications of Wegener's granulomatosis. Arch Neurol 8: 145, 1963.
22. Kosovsky PA, Ehlers KH, Rafal RB, et al: Case report: MR imaging of cardiac mass in Wegener's granulomatosis. J Comput Assist Tomogr 15: 1028, 1991.

23. Hoffman GS, Leavitt RY, Kerr GS, et al: Treatment of Wegener's granulomatosis with glucocorticoids and methotrexate. Arthritis Rheum 35: 1322, 1992.
24. Specks U, Wheatley CL, McDonald TJ, et al: Anticytoplasmic autoantibodies in the diagnosis and follow-up of Wegener's granulomatosis. Mayo Clin Proc 64: 28, 1989.
25. Nolle B, Specks U, Ludermann J, et al: Anticytoplasmic autoantibodies: their immunodiagnostic value in Wegener's granulomatosis. Ann Intern Med 111: 28, 1989.
26. Jennette JC, Falk RJ: Diagnostic classification of anti-neutrophil cytoplasmic autoantibody–associated vasculitides. Am J Kidney Dis 18: 184, 1991.
27. Third International Workshop on ANCA. Am J Kidney Dis 18: 148, 1991.
28. Roback SA, Herdman RC, Hoyer J, et al: Wegener's granulomatosis in a child. Am J Dis Child 118: 608, 1969.
29. Rubin DF, Peterson P, Meltzer JI: Renal lesions in Wegener's granulomatosis. Ann Intern Med 82: 849, 1975.
30. Bajema IM, Hagen EC, van der Woude FJ, Bruijn JA: Wegener's granulomatosis: a meta-analysis of 349 literary case reports. J Lab Clin Med 129: 17, 1997.
31. Felson B: Less familiar roentgen patterns of pulmonary granulomas. Am J Roentgenol Radium Ther Nucl Med 81: 211, 1959.
32. McGregor MBB, Sandler G: Wegener's granulomatosis: a clinical and radiological survey. Br J Radiol 37: 430, 1964.
33. Baliga R, Chang CH, Bidani AK: A case of generalized Wegener's granulomatosis in childhood: successful therapy with cyclophosphamide. Pediatrics 61: 286, 1978.
34. Harrison HL, Linshaw MA, Lindsley CB, et al: Bolus corticosteroids and cyclophosphamide for initial treatment of Wegener's granulomatosis. JAMA 244: 1599, 1980.
35. Hoffman GS, Leavitt RY, Fleisher TA, et al: Treatment of Wegener's granulomatosis with intermittent high dose intravenous cyclophosphamide. Am J Med 89: 403, 1990
36. Hoffman GS, Kerr GS, Leavitt RY, et al: Wegener's granulomatosis: an analysis of 158 patients. Ann Intern Med 116: 488, 1992.
37. de Groot K, Reinhold-Keller E, Tatsis E, et al: Therapy for the maintenance of remission in sixty-five patients with generalized Wegener's granulomatosis. Arthritis Rheum 39: 2052, 1996.
38. Guillevin L, Cordier JF, Lhote F, et al: A prospective randomized trial comparing steroids with pulse cyclophosphamide versus steroids and oral cyclophosphamide in the treatment of generalized Wegener's granulomatosis. Arthritis Rheum 40: 2187, 1997.
38a. Langford CA, Taler-Williams C, Barron KS, Sneller MC: A staged approach to the treatment of Wegener's granulomatosis: induction of remission with glucocorticoids and daily cyclophosphamide switching to methotrexate for remission maintenance. Arthritis Rheum 42: 2666, 1999.
39. Gottlieb BS, Miller LC, Ilowite NT: Methotrexate treatment of Wegener's granulomatosis in children. J Pediatr 129: 604, 1996.
40. DeRemee RA: The treatment of Wegener's granulomatosis with trimethoprim/sulfamethoxazole: illusion or vision? Arthritis Rheum 31: 1068, 1988.
41. Leavitt RY, Hoffman GS, Fauci AS: Response: the role of trimethoprim/sulfamethoxazole in the treatment of Wegener's granulomatosis. Arthritis Rheum 31: 1073, 1988.
42. Churg J, Strauss L: Allergic granulomatosis, allergic angiitis, and periarteritis nodosa. Am J Pathol 27: 277, 19.
43. Masi AT, Hunder GG, Lie JT, et al: The American College of Rheumatology 1990 criteria for the classification of Churg-Strauss syndrome (allergic granulomatosis and angiitis). Arthritis Rheum 33: 1094, 1990.
44. Lanhan JG, Elkon KB, Pusey CD, Hughes GR: Systemic vasculitis with asthma and eosinophilia: a clinical approach to the Churg-Strauss syndrome. Medicine (Baltimore) 62: 142, 1983.
45. Farooki ZQ, Brough AJ, Green EW: Necrotizing arteritis. Am J Dis Child 128: 837, 1974.
46. Petty RE, Magilavy DB, Cassidy JT, et al: Polyarteritis in childhood. A clinical description of eight cases. Arthritis Rheum 20(Suppl): 392, 1977.
47. Frayha RA: Churg-Strauss syndrome in a child. J Rheumatol 9: 807, 1982.
48. Treitman P, Herskowitz JL, Bass HN: Churg-Strauss syndrome in a 14-year-old boy diagnosed by transbronchial lung biopsy. Clin Pediatr 30: 502, 1991.
49. Heine A, Beck R, Stropahl G, et al: Inflammatory pseudotumor of the anterior orbit. A symptom of allergic granuloma. Ophthalmologe 92: 870, 1995.
50. Jessurun J, Azevedo M, Saldan M: Allergic angiitis and granulomatosis (Churg-Strauss syndrome): report of a case with massive thymic involvement in a nonasthmatic patient. Hum Pathol 17: 637, 1986.
51. Rabusin M, Lepore L, Constantinides F, Bussani R: A child with severe asthma. Lancet 351: 32, 1998.
52. Mpofu C, Bakalinova D, Kazi MA, Dawson KP: Churg-Strauss syndrome in childhood. Ann Trop Paediatr 15: 341, 1995.
53. Lie JP: The classification of vasculitis and a reappraisal of allergic granulomatosis and angiitis (Churg-Strauss syndrome). Mt Sinai J Med N Y 53: 429, 1986.
54. Davis MD, Daoud MS, McEvoy MT, Su WP: Cutaneous manifestations of Churg-Strauss syndrome: a clinicopathologic correlation. J Am Acad Dermatol 37: 199, 1997.
55. Churg J, Strauss L: Case 46-1980: interstitial eosinophilic pneumonitis, pleuritis and angiitis. N Engl J Med 304: 611, 1981.
56. Chumbley LC, Harrison EG Jr, DeRemee RA: Allergic granulomatosis and angiitis (Churg-Strauss syndrome): report and analysis of 30 cases. Mayo Clin Proc 52: 477, 1977.
57. Cury D, Braekley AS, Payne BF: Allergic granulomatous angiitis associated with posterior uveitis and papilloedema. Arch Ophthalmol 55: 261, 1956.
58. Wechsler ME, Garpestad E, Flier SR, et al: Pulmonary infiltrates, eosinophilia and cardiomyopathy following corticosteroid withdrawal in patients with asthma receiving zafirlukast. JAMA 279: 455, 1998.
59. Tatsis E, Schnabel A, Gross WL: Interferon-alpha treatment of four patients with the Churg-Strauss syndrome. Ann Intern Med 129: 370, 1998.
60. Guillevin L, Cohen P, Gayraud M, et al: Churg-Strauss syndrome. Clinical study and long-term follow-up of 96 patients. Medicine (Baltimore) 78: 26, 1999.
61. Liebow AA, Carrington CRB, Friedman PJH: Lymphomatoid granulomatosis. Hum Pathol 3: 457, 1972.
62. Fauci AS, Haynes BF, Costa J, et al: Lymphomatoid granulomatosis: prospective clinical and therapeutic experience over 10 years. N Engl J Med 306: 68, 1987.
63. Koss MN Liselotte H, Langloss JM, et al: Lymphomatoid granulomatosis: a clinicopathologic study of 42 patients. Pathology 18: 283, 1986.
64. Katzenstein AA, Carrington CB, Liebow AA: Lymphomatoid granulomatosis. A clinicopathologic study of 152 cases. Cancer 43: 360, 1979.
65. Lehman TJ, Church JA, Isaacs H: Lymphomatoid granulomatosis in a 13-month-old infant. J Rheumatol 16: 235, 1989.
66. Grierson H, Purtilo DT: Epstein-Barr virus infections in males with the X-linked immunoproliferative syndrome. Ann Intern Med 106: 538, 1987.
67. Ilowite NT, Fligner CL, Ochs HD, et al: Pulmonary angiitis with atypical lymphoreticular infiltrates in Wiskott-Aldrich syndrome: possible relationship of lymphomatoid granulomatosis and EBV infection. Clin Immunol Immunopathol 41: 479, 1986.
68. Anders KH, Guerra WF, Tomiyasu U, et al: The neuropathology of AIDS. ULCA experience and review. Am J Pathol 124: 537, 1986.
69. Shen SC, Heuser ET, Landing NH, et al: Lymphomatoid granulomatosis–like lesions in a child with leukemia in remission. Hum Pathol 12: 276, 1981.
70. Gardiner GW: Lymphomatoid granulomatosis of the larynx in a renal transplant recipient. J Otolaryngol 8: 549, 1979.
71. Waltern M, Thomson NM, Dowling J, et al: Lymphomatoid granulomatosis in a renal transplant recipient. Aust N Z J Med 9: 434, 1979.
72. Hammer S, Mennemeyer R: Lymphomatoid granulomatosis in a renal transplant recipient. Hum Pathol 7: 111, 1976.
73. Newman W, Wolf A: Non-infectious granulomatous angiitis involving the central nervous system. Trans Am Neurol Assoc 77: 114, 1952.
74. Cravioto H, Feigin I: Noninfectious granulomatous angiitis with a predilection for the nervous system. Neurology 9: 599, 1959.
75. Calabrese LH, Furlan AJ, Gragg LA, Popos TJ: Primary angiitis of the central nervous system: diagnostic criteria and clinical approach. Cleveland Clin J Med 59: 293, 1992.

76. Abu-Shakra M, Khraishi M, Grosman H, et al: Primary angiitis of the CNS diagnosed by angiography. Q J Med 87: 351, 1994.
77. Calabrese LH, Mallek JA: Primary angiitis of the central nervous system: report of 8 new cases, review of the literature and proposal for diagnostic criteria. Medicine (Baltimore) 67: 20, 1988.
78. Biller J, Loftus CM, Moore SA, et al: Isolated central nervous system angiitis first presenting as spontaneous intracranial hemorrhage. Neurosurgery 20: 310, 1987.
79. Forman HP, Levin S, Stewart B, et al: Cerebral vasculitis and hemorrhage in an adolescent taking diet pills containing phenylpropanolamine: case report and review of literature. Pediatrics 83: 737, 1989.
80. Farine D, Andreyko J, Lysikiewicz A, et al: Isolated angiitis of brain in pregnancy and puerperium. Obstet Gynecol 63: 586, 1984.
81. Langlois PF, Sharon GE, Gawryl MS: Plasma concentrations of complement-activation complexes correlate with disease activity in patients diagnosed with isolated central nervous system vasculitis. J Allergy Clin Immunol 83: 11, 1989.
82. Hellman DB, Roubenoff R, Healy RA, et al: Central nervous system angiography: safety and predictors of a positive result in 125 consecutive patients evaluated for possible vasculitis. J Rheumatol 19: 568, 1992.
83. Moore PM: Diagnosis and management of isolated angiitis of the central nervous system. Neurology 39: 167, 1989.
84. Woolfenden AR, Tong DC, Marks MP, et al: Angiographically defined primary angiitis of the CNS. Is it really benign? Neurology 51: 183, 1998.
85. Cupps TR, Moore PM, Fauci AS: Isolated angiitis of the CNS: prospective diagnostic and therapeutic experience. Am J Med 74: 97, 1983.
86. Sigal LH: Therapy of isolated angiitis of the central nervous system. Neurology 39: 164, 1989.
87. Suzuki J, Takaku A: Cerebrovascular "moyamoya" disease: disease showing abnormal net-like vessels in base of brain. Arch Neurol 20: 288, 1962.
88. Van Erven PM, Gabreels FJ, Thijssen HO, Renier WO: The Moya-Moya syndrome: a report of two children. Clin Neurol Neurosurg 84: 179, 1982.
89. Carlson CB, Harvey FH, Loop J: Progressive alternating hemiplegia in early childhood and basal arterial stenosis and telangiectasia (moyamoya syndrome). Neurology 23: 734, 1973.
90. Magee R, Marshall M, Schaub M, Terrio L: Speech-language patterns in a child with moya moya disease. Percept Mot Skills 79: 1183, 1994.
91. Chabbert V, Ranjeva JP, Sevely A, et al: Diffusion and magnetisation transfer weighted MRA in childhood moya-moya. Neuroradiology 40: 267, 1998.
92. Suzuki Y, Negoro M, Shibuya M, et al: Surgical treatment for pediatric moyamoya disease: use of the superficial artery for both areas supplied by the anterior and middle cerebral arteries. Neurosurgery 40: 324, 1997.
93. McLean MJ, Gebarski SS, van der Spek AFL, Goldstein GW: response of moyamoya disease to verapamil. Lancet 1: 163, 1985.
94. Harvey FH, Alvord EC Jr: Juvenile arteriosclerosis and other cerebral arteriopathies of childhood. Acta Neurol Scand 48: 479, 1972.
95. Galligioni F, Andrioli GC, Marin G, et al: Hypoplasia of the internal carotid artery associated with cerebral pseudoangiomatosis: report of four cases. Am J Roentgenol Radium Ther Nucl Med 112: 251, 1971.
96. Goldberg HJ: Moyamoya associated with peripheral vascular occlusive disease. Arch Dis Child 49: 964, 1974.
97. Schrager GO, Cohen SJ, Vigman MP: Acute hemiplegia and cortical blindness due to moya moya disease: report of a case in a child with Down's syndrome. Pediatrics 60: 33, 1977.
98. Kapusta L, Daniels O, Renier WO: Moya-Moya syndrome and primary pulmonary hypertension in childhood. Neuropediatrics 21: 162, 1990.
99. Kowada M, Momma F, Kikuchi K: Intracranial aneurysm associated with cerebrovascular moyamoya disease. Report of a case and review of 13 cases. Br J Radiol 52: 236, 1979.
100. Kitahara T, Ariga N, Yamaura A, et al: Familial occurrence of moya-moya disease: report of three Japanese families. J Neurol Neurosurg Psychiatry 42: 208, 1979.
101. Shimizu K, Sano K: Pulseless disease [in Japanese]. Clin Surg (Tokyo) 3: 377, 1948.
102. Shimizu K, Sano K: Pulseless disease. J Neuropathol Clin Neurol 1: 37, 1951.
103. Takayasu M: Case with unusual changes of the central vessels in the retina. Acta Soc Ophthalmol Jpn 12: 554, 1908
104. Arend WP, Michel BA, Bloch DA, et al: The American College of Rheumatology 1990 criteria for the classification of Takayasu arteritis. Arthritis Rheum 33: 1129, 1990.
105. Lupi-Herrera E, Sanches-Torres G, Marushamer J, et al: Takayasu's arteritis. Clinical study of 107 cases. Am Heart J 93: 94, 1977.
106. Ishikawa K: Survival and morbidity after diagnosis of occlusive thromboaortopathy (Takayasu's disease). Am J Cardiol 48: 1026, 1981.
107. Wagenvoort CA, Harris LE, Brown AL, et al: Giant cell arteritis with aneurysm formation in children. Pediatrics 32: 861, 1963.
108. Warshaw JB, Spach MS: Takayasu's disease (primary aortitis) in childhood: case report with a review of the literature. Pediatrics 35: 620, 1965.
109. Hong CY, Yun YS, Choi JY, et al: Takayasu arteritis in Korean children: clinical report of seventy cases. Heart Vessels 71(Suppl): 91, 1992.
110. Hahn D, Thomson PD, Kala U, et al: A review of Takayasu's arteritis in children in Gauteng, South Africa. Pediatr Nephrol 12: 668, 1998.
111. D'Souza SJ, Tsai WS, Silver MM, et al: Diagnosis and management of stenotic aorto-arteriopathy in childhood. J Pediatr 132: 1016, 1998.
112. Dabague J, Reyes PA: Takayasu arteritis in Mexico: a 38-year clinical perspective through literature review. Int J Cardiol 54(Suppl): S103, 1996.
113. Hall S, Barr W, Lie JT, et al: Takayasu arteritis: a study of 32 North American patients. Medicine (Baltimore) 64: 89, 1985.
114. Vinijchaikul AJ: Primary arteritis of the aorta and its main branches (Takayasu's arteriopathy). Medicine (Baltimore) 43: 15, 1967.
115. Gupta S: Surgical and haemodynamic considerations in middle aortic syndrome. Thorax 34: 470, 1979.
116. Gupta S, Goswami B, Ghosh DC, et al: Middle aortic syndrome as a cause of heart failure in children and its management. Thorax 36: 63, 1981.
117. Numano R, Isohisa I, Kishi U, et al: Takayasu's disease in twin sisters. Possible genetic factors. Circulation 58: 173, 1978.
118. Numano F: Hereditary factors of Takayasu arteritis. Heart Vessels Suppl 7: 68, 1992.
119. Kimura A, Kitamura H, Date Y, Numano F: Comprehensive analysis of HLA genes in Takayasu arteritis in Japan. Int J Cardiol 54(Suppl): S61, 1996.
120. Mehra NK, Rajalingam R, Sagar S, et al: Direct role of HLA-B5 in influencing susceptibility to Takayasu aortoarteritis. Int J Cardiol 54(Suppl): S71, 1996.
121. Girona E, Yamamoto-Furusho JK, Cutino T, et al: HLA-DR6 (possibly DRB1*1301) is associated with susceptibility to Takayasu arteritis in Mexicans. Heart Vessels 11: 277, 1996.
122. Pantell RH, Goodman BW Jr: Takayasu's arteritis: the relationship with tuberculosis. Pediatrics 67: 84, 1981.
123. Morales E, Pineda C, Martinez-Lavin M: Takayasu's arteritis in children. J Rheumatol 18: 1081, 1991.
124. Milner LS, Jacobs DW, Thomson PD, et al: Management of severe hypertension in childhood Takayasu's arteritis. Pediatr Nephrol 5: 38, 1991.
125. Aggarwal A, Chag M, Sinha N, Naik SP: Takayasu's arteritis: role of *Mycobacterium tuberculosis* and its heat shock protein. Int J Cardiol 55: 49, 1996.
126. Eichorn J, Sima D, Thiele B, et al: Anti-endothelial cell antibodies in Takayasu arteritis. Circulation 94: 2396, 1996.
127. Garcia-Torres R, Noel LH, Reyes PA, et al: Absence of ANCA in Mexican patients with Takayasu's arteritis. Scand J Rheumatol 26: 55, 1997.
128. Wiggelinkhuizen J, Cremin BJ: Takayasu arteritis and renovascular hypertension in childhood. Pediatrics 62: 209, 1978.
129. Hall S, Nelson AM: Takayasu's arteritis and juvenile rheumatoid arthritis. J Rheumatol 13: 431, 1986.

130. Yamato M, Kecky JW, Hiramatsu K, et al: Takayasu arteritis: radiographic and angiographic findings in 59 patients. Radiology 161: 329, 1986.
131. Fournier AM, Dickinson ZC, Kelly R: Doppler ultrasonography as a guide to management of Takayasu's arteritis. J Rheumatol 15: 527, 1988.
132. Hunder GG, Weyland CM: Sonography in giant-cell arteritis. N Engl J Med 337: 1385, 1997.
133. Buckley A, Southwood T, Culham G, et al: The role of ultrasound in evaluation of Takayasu's arteritis. J Rheumatol 18: 1073, 1991.
134. D'Souza SJA, Tsai WS, Silver MM, et al: Diagnosis and management of stenotic aorto-arteriopathy in childhood. J Pediatr 132: 1016, 1998.
135. Shelhamer JH, Volkman DJ, Parillo JE, et al: Takayasu's arteritis and its therapy. Ann Intern Med 103: 121, 1985.
135a. Shetty AK, Stopa AR, Gedalia A: Low-dose methotrexate as a steroid-sparing agent in a child with Takayasu's arteritis. Clin Exp Rheumatol 16: 335, 1998.
136. Sharma S, Rajani M, Shrivastava S, et al: Non-specific aorto-arteritis (Takayasu's disease) in children. Br J Radiol 64: 690, 1991.
137. Becker GJ: Intravascular stents. General principles and status of lower-extremity arterial applications. Circulation 83: 1, 1991.
138. Palmaz JC: Intravascular stents: tissue-stent interactions and design considerations. Am J Roentgenol 160: 613, 1993.
138a. Tyagi S, Sharma VP, Arora R: Stenting of the aorta for recurrent, long stenosis due to Takayasu's arteritis in a child. Pediatr Cardiol 20: 215, 1999.
139. Weyand CM, Wagner AD, Bjornson J, et al: Correlation of the topographical arrangement and the functional pattern of tissue-infiltrating macrophages in giant cell arteritis. J Clin Invest 98: 1642, 1996.
140. Lie JT: Bilateral juvenile temporal arteritis. J Rheumatol 22: 774, 1995.
141. Lie JT, Gordon LP, Titus JL: Juvenile temporal arteritis: biopsy study of four cases. JAMA 234: 496, 1975.
142. Fujimoto M, Sato S, Hayashi N, et al: Juvenile temporal arteritis with eosinophilia: a distinct clinicopathological entity. Dermatology 192: 32, 1996.
143. Bollinger A, Leu H-J, Brunner U: Juvenile arteritis of extracranial arteries with hypereosinophilia. Klin Wochenschr 64: 526, 1986.
144. McGovern JP, Merritt DH: Sarcoidosis in childhood. Adv Pediatr 8: 97, 1956.
145. Jasper PL, Denny FW: Sarcoidosis in children with special emphasis on the natural history and treatment. J Pediatr 73: 499, 1968.
146. Siltzbach LE, Greenberg GM: Childhood sarcoidosis—a study of 18 patients. N Engl J Med 279: 1239, 1968.
147. Kendig EL: Sarcoidosis among children: a review. J Pediatr 61: 269, 1962.
148. Kendig EL: The clinical picture of sarcoidosis in children. Pediatrics 54: 289, 1974.
149. Beier FR, Lahey ME: Sarcoidosis among children in Utah and Idaho. J Pediatr 65: 350, 1964.
150. Mandi L: Thoracic sarcoidosis in childhood. Acta Tuberc Scand 45: 256, 1964.
151. Harris C, Gibson WM, Schuchter SL, et al: Rare diagnosis: sarcoid arthritis in four children. JAMA 197: 31, 1966.
152. Sahn EE, Hampton MT, Garen PD, et al: Preschool sarcoidosis masquerading as juvenile rheumatoid arthritis: two case reports and a review of the literature. Pediatr Dermatol 7: 208, 1990.
153. Gluck J, Miller JJ III, Summerlin WT: Sarcoidosis in a young child. J Pediatr 81: 354, 1972.
154. Hetherington S: Sarcoidosis in young children. Am J Dis Child 136: 13, 1982.
155. Pattishall EN, Strope GL, Spinola SM, et al: Childhood sarcoidosis. J Pediatr 109: 169, 1986.
156. Hafner R, Vogel P: Sarcoidosis of early onset. A challenge for the pediatric rheumatologist. Clin Exp Rheumatol 11: 685, 1993.
157. Cron RQ, Wallace CA, Sherry DD: Childhood sarcoidosis—does age of onset predict clinical manifestations? J Rheumatol 24: 1654, 1997.
158. Bresnitz EA, Strom BL: Epidemiology of sarcoidosis. Epidemiol Rev 5: 124, 1956.
159. Fanburg BL, Pitt EA: Sarcoidosis. *In* Murray JF, Nadel JA (eds): Textbook of Respiratory Medicine. Philadelphia, WB Saunders, 1988, p 1495.
160. Rosenberg AM, Yee EH, MacKenzie JW: Arthritis in childhood sarcoidosis. J Rheumatol 19: 987, 1983.
161. Lindsley CB, Petty RE: Childhood sarcoid arthritis registry. Arthritis Rheum 36: S123, 1993.
162. Niitu Y, Horikawa M, Suetake T, et al: Pulmonary sarcoidosis among children. Sai Shin Med 27: 1347, 1972.
163. Merten DF, Kirks DR, Grossman HP: Pulmonary sarcoidosis in children. Am J Roentgenol 135: 673, 1980.
164. Kendig EL Jr: Sarcoidosis in children: personal observations on age distribution. Pediatr Pulmonol 6: 69, 1989.
165. Schabel SI, Stanley HJ, Shelley BE Jr: Pediatric sarcoidosis. J South Carolina Med Assoc 76: 419, 1980.
166. Reed WB: Sarcoidosis: a review and report of eight cases in children. J Tenn Med Assoc 62: 27, 1969.
167. Schmitt ES, Appelman H, Threatt BL: Sarcoidosis in children. Radiology 106: 621, 1973.
168. Beskow R, Wiman LG: Familial occurrence of sarcoidosis. *In* Levinsky L, MacHolda F (eds): Proceedings of the Fifth International Conference on Sarcoidosis, Universita Karlova, Prague, Czechoslovakia, 1971, p 280.
169. James DG, Piyasena HG, Neville E, et al: Possible genetic influences in familial sarcoidosis. Postgrad Med J 50: 664, 1974.
170. Jorgensen G: Untersuchungen zur Genetik der Sarkoidose. Göttingen, Germany, Habil Schrift, 1965.
171. Buck AA, McKusick VA: Epidemiologic investigations of sarcoidosis. Am J Hygiene 74: 174, 1961.
172. Keating JP, Weissbluth M, Ratzan SK, et al: Familial sarcoidosis. Am J Dis Child 126: 644, 1973.
173. Schweizer AT, Kanaar P: Sarcoidosis with polyarthritis in a child. Arch Dis Child 42: 671, 1967.
174. Prieur AM, Henkes CJ, Bessis JL, et al: Sarcoidose articulaire familiale. Arch Fr Pediatr 39: 311, 1982.
175. Headings VE, Weston D, Young RC Jr, et al: Familial sarcoidosis with multiple occurrences in eleven families: a possible mechanism of inheritance. Ann N Y Acad Sci 278: 377, 1976.
176. Sharma OP, Neville E, Walker AN, et al: Familial sarcoidosis: a possible genetic influence. Ann N Y Acad Sci 278: 386, 1976.
177. Schurmann M, Bein G, Kirsten D, et al: HLA-DQB1 and HLA-DPB1 genotypes in familial sarcoidosis. Respir Med 92: 649, 1998.
178. Zsolway K, Sinai LN, Magnusson M, Tunnessen WW Jr: Two unusual pediatric presentations of sarcoidosis. Arch Pediatr Adolesc Med 152: 410, 1998.
179. Clark SK: Sarcoidosis in children. Pediatr Dermatol 4: 291, 1987.
180. Mallory SB, Paller AS, Ginsburg BC, et al: Sarcoidosis in children: differentiation from juvenile arthritis. Pediatr Dermatol 4: 313, 1987.
181. Kuramoto Y, Shindo Y, Tagami H: Subcutaneous sarcoidosis with extensive caseation necrosis. J Cutan Pathol 15: 188, 1988.
182. Obenauf CD, Shaw HE, Sydnor CR, Klintworth GK: Sarcoidosis and its ophthalmic manifestations. Am J Ophthalmol 86: 648, 1978.
183. Kansi JJ, Shun-Shin GA: Systemic uveitis syndromes in childhood: an analysis of 340 cases. Ophthalmology 91: 1247, 1984.
184. Khan JA, Hoover DL, Giangiacomo J, et al: Orbital and childhood sarcoidosis. J Pediatr Ophthalmol Strabismus 23: 190, 1986.
185. Brinkman CJJ, Pogany KP: Neurosarcoidosis and uveitis. *In* Dernouchamps JP, Veroughstraete L, Caspers-Velu L, Tassignon MJ (eds): Recent Advances in Uveitis. Proceedings of the Third International Symposium on Uveitis, Brussels, Belgium, 1992, p 375.
186. Hoover DL, Khan J, Giangiacomo J: Pediatric ocular sarcoidosis. Surv Ophthalmol 30: 215, 1986.
187. Bronson LJ, Fisher YL: Sarcoidosis of the paranasal sinuses with orbital extension. Arch Ophthalmol 95: 243, 1976.
188. Srinivasan E: A case of Boeck's sarcoidosis involving the orbit. Arch Ophthalmol 25: 493, 1941.
189. Lennarson P, Barney NP: Interstitial keratitis as presenting ophthalmic sign of sarcoidosis in a child. J Pediatr Ophthalmol Strabismus 32: 194, 1995.
190. Leigh MW: Sarcoidosis. *In* Behrman RE (eds): Nelson's Textbook of Pediatrics, 16th ed. Philadelphia, WB Saunders, 2000, p 2143.

191. Lindsley CB, Godfrey WA: Childhood sarcoidosis manifesting as juvenile rheumatoid arthritis. Pediatrics 76: 765, 1985.
192. Harris RO III, Spock A: Childhood sarcoidosis: pulmonary infiltrates as an early sign in a very young child. Clin Pediatr 17: 119, 1978.
193. Aszkanazy CL: Sarcoidosis of the central nervous system. J Neuropathol Exp Neurol 11: 392, 1952.
194. Jallo GI, Zagzag D, Lee M, et al: Intraspinal sarcoidosis: diagnosis and management. Surg Neurol 48: 514, 1997.
195. Bernstein J, Rival J: Sarcoidosis of the spinal cord as the presenting manifestation of the disease. South Med J 71: 1571, 1978.
196. Campbell JN, Black P, Ostrow PT: Sarcoid of the cauda equina: case report. J Neurosurg 47: 109, 1977.
197. Stern BJ, Krumholz A, Johns C, et al: Sarcoidosis and its neurological manifestations. Arch Neurol Psychiatry 42: 909, 1985.
198. Wood EH, Bream CA: Spinal sarcoidosis. Radiology 73: 226, 1959.
199. Rubinstein I, Hiss J, Baum GL: Intramedullary spinal cord sarcoidosis. Surg Neurol 21: 272, 1984.
200. Leiba H, Siatkowski RM, Culbertson WW, Glaser JS: Neurosarcoidosis presenting as an intracranial mass in childhood. J Neuro-Ophthalmol 16: 268, 1996.
201. Weinberg S, Bennett H, Weinstock I: Central nervous system manifestations of sarcoidosis in children: case report and review. Clin Pediatr 22: 477, 1983.
202. Day AL, Sypert GW: Spinal cord sarcoidosis. Ann Neurol 1: 79, 1977.
203. Caroscio J, Yahr MD: Progressive myelopathy due to sarcoid. Clin Neurol Neurosurg 84: 217, 1980.
204. North FA, Fink CW, Gibson WM, et al: Sarcoid arthritis in children. Am J Med 48: 449, 1970.
205. Gedalia A, Molina JF, Ellis GS, et al: Low-dose methotrexate therapy for childhood sarcoidosis. J Pediatr 130: 25, 1997.
206. Gumpel JM, Johns CJ, Shulman LE: The joint disease of sarcoidosis. Ann Rheum Dis 26: 194, 1967.
207. Stump K, Spock A, Grossman H: Vertebral sarcoidosis in adolescents. Pediatr Radiol 121: 153, 1976.
208. Silverstein A, Siltzbach LE: Muscle involvement in sarcoidosis. Arch Neurol 21: 235, 1969.
209. Stjernberg N, Cajander S, Truedsson H, et al: Muscle involvement in sarcoidosis. Acta Med Scand 209: 213, 1981.
210. Mayock RL, Bertrand P, Morrison DE, Scott JH: Manifestations of sarcoidosis: analysis of 145 patients with a review of nine series selected from the literature. Am J Med 35: 67, 1963.
211. Celle ME, Veneselli E, Rossi GA, et al: Childhood sarcoidosis presenting with prevalent muscular symptoms: report of a case. Eur J Pediatr 156: 340, 1997.
212. Banker BQ: Other inflammatory myopathies. *In* Engel AG, Banker BQ (eds): Myology. New York, McGraw-Hill, 1986, p 1507.
213. Dubowitz V: Inflammatory myopathies. *In* Dubowitz V (ed): Muscle Biopsy: A Practical Approach. London, Bailliere Tindall, 1985, p 605.
214. Levine MS, Ekberg O, Rubesin SE, et al: Gastrointestinal sarcoidosis: radiographic findings. Am J Roentgenol 153: 293, 1989.
215. Noel JM, Katona IM, Pineiro-Carrero VM: Case report: sarcoidosis resulting in duodenal obstruction in an adolescent. J Pediatr Gastroenterol Nutr 24: 594, 1997.
216. Cohen DL: Sicca syndrome: an unusual manifestation of sarcoidosis in childhood. Am J Dis Child 137: 289, 1983.
217. Evans SS, Fisher RG, Scott MA, et al: Sarcoidosis presenting as bilateral testicular masses. Pediatrics 100: 392, 1978.
218. Mastui Y, Iwai K, Tachibana T, et al: Clinicopathological study of fatal myocardial sarcoidosis. Ann N Y Acad Sci 80: 1179, 1988.
219. Demeter SL: Myocardial sarcoidosis unresponsive to steroids. Treatment with cyclophosphamide. Chest 94: 202, 1988
220. Muther RS, McCarron DA, Bennett WM: Renal manifestations of sarcoidosis. Arch Intern Med 141: 643, 1981.
221. Morris KP, Coulthard MG, Smith PJ, et al: Renovascular and growth effects of childhood sarcoid. Arch Dis Child 75: 74, 1996.
222. McDonald CH: Renal sarcoidosis. J Clin Pathol 9: 136, 1956.
223. Keech MR: Generalized sarcoidosis with renal involvement. Proc R Soc Med 44: 728, 1951.
224. Berger KW, Arnold SR: Renal impairment due to sarcoid infiltration of the kidney: report of a case proved by renal biopsies before and after treatment with cortisone. N Engl J Med 252: 44, 1955.
225. Longcope TW, Freeman CD: A study of sarcoidosis. Medicine 31: 132, 1952.
226. Bautista A: Childhood sarcoidosis involving joints and kidneys. Am J Dis Child 119: 259, 1970.
227. Correa P: Sarcoidosis: association with glomerulonephritis. Arch Pathol 57: 523, 1954.
228. Nocton JJ, Stork JE, Jacobs G, Newman AJ: Sarcoidosis associated with nephrocalcinosis in young children. J Pediatr 121: 937, 1992.
229. James DG: A comparison of Blau's syndrome and sarcoidosis. Sarcoidosis 11: 100, 1994.
230. Manouvrier-Hanu S, Puech B, Piette F, et al: Blau syndrome of granulomatous arthritis, iritis, and skin rash: a new family and review of the literature. Am J Med Genet 76: 217, 1998.
231. Blau EB: Familial granulomatous arthritis, iritis and rash. J Pediatr 107: 689, 1985.
232. De Chadaverian JP, Raphael SA, Murphy GF: Histologic, ultrastructural, and immunocytochemical features of the granulomas seen in a child with the syndrome of familial granulomatous synovitis, uveitis and rash. Arch Pathol Lab Med 117: 1050, 1993.
233. Raphael SA, Blau EN, Zhang WH, et al: Analysis of a large kindred with Blau syndrome for HLA, autoimmunity and sarcoidosis. Am J Dis Child 147: 842, 1993.
234. Moraillon J, Hayem F, Bourrillon A, et al: Syndrome de Blau ou forme infantile de sarcoidose a debut infantile. Ann Dermatol Venereol 123: 29, 1996.
235. Pastores GM, Michels VV, Stickler GB, et al: Autosomal dominant granulomatous arthritis, uveitis, skin rash, and synovial cysts. J Pediatr 117: 403, 1990.
236. Mau U, Baykal HE, Erb C, et al: Blau syndrome (familial non HLA-B27–associated acute anterior uveitis with arthritis and skin manifestations): a rare syndrome in a family with 10 members over 4 generations. Med Genet 7: 180, 1995.
237. Tgromp G, Kuivaniemi H, Raphael S, et al: Molecular characterization of Blau syndrome: genetic linkage to chromosome 16. Am J Hum Genet Suppl 55: 205, 1994.
238. Tromp Kuivaniemi H, Raphael S, et al: Genetic linkage of familial granulomatous inflammatory arthritis, skin rash and uveitis to chromosome 16. Am J Hum Genet 59: 1097, 1996.
239. Bottcher E: Disseminated sarcoidosis with a marked granulomatous arteritis. Arch Pathol 68: 419, 1959.
240. Churg A, Carrington CB, Gupta R: Necrotizing sarcoid granulomatosis. Chest 76: 406, 1979.
241. Gross KR, Malleson PN, Culham G, et al: Vasculopathy with renal artery stenosis in a child with sarcoidosis. J Pediatr 108: 724, 1986.
242. Rose CD, Eichenfield AH, Goldsmith DP, et al: Early onset sarcoidosis with aortitis—"juvenile systemic granulomatosis"? J Rheumatol 17: 102, 1990.
243. Gedalia A, Shetty AK, Ward K, et al: Abdominal aortic aneurysm associated with childhood sarcoidosis. J Rheumatol 23: 757, 1996.
244. Hoffmann AL, Milman N, Nielson HE, et al: Childhood sarcoidosis presenting with hypercalcaemic crisis. Sarcoidosis 11: 141, 1994.
245. Stanworth SJ, Kennedy CTC, Chetcuti PAJ, et al: Hypercalcaemia and sarcoidosis in infancy. J R Soc Med 85: 177, 1992.
246. James DG, Kendig EL Jr: Childhood sarcoidosis. Sarcoidosis 5: 57, 1988.
247. Mason RS, Frankel T, Chan Y-L, et al: Vitamin D conversion by sarcoid lymph node homogenate. Ann Intern Med 100: 59, 1984.
248. Reichel H, Koeffler HP, Barbers R: Regulation of 1,25-dihydroxyvitamin D3 production by cultured alveolar macrophages from normal human donors and from patients with pulmonary sarcoidosis. J Clin Endocrinol Metab 65: 1201, 1987.
249. Bresnihan B: Sarcoidosis. *In* Maddison PJ, Isenberg DA, Woo P, Glass DN (eds): Oxford Textbook of Rheumatology. New York, Oxford University Press, 1993, p 928.
250. Rodriguez DE, Shin BC, Abernathy RS, Kendig EL: Serum angiotensin-converting enzyme activity in normal children and in those with sarcoidosis. J Pediatr 99: 68, 1981.
251. Studdy P, Bird R, James DG, et al: Serum angiotensin converting

enzyme (SACE) in sarcoidosis and other granulomatous disorders. Lancet 2: 1332, 1978.

252. Silverstein E, Friedland J, Lyons HA, et al: Elevation of angiotensin converting enzyme in granulomatous lymph nodes and serum in sarcoidosis: clinical and possible pathogenic significance. Ann N Y Acad Sci 278: 498, 1976.
253. DeRemee RA, Rohrbach MS: Serum angiotensin-converting enzyme activity in evaluating the clinical course of sarcoidosis. Ann Intern Med 92: 361, 1980.
254. Lieberman J: Elevation of serum angiotensin-converting enzyme (ACE) level in sarcoidosis. Am J Med 59: 365, 1976.
255. Katz P, Fauci AS, Yeager H, et al: Serum angiotensin-converting enzyme in granulomatous diseases of unknown cause. Ann Intern Med 94: 359, 1981.
256. Beneteau-Burnate B, Baudin B, Morgant G, et al: Serum angiotensin-converting enzyme in healthy and sarcoidotic children: comparison with the reference interval for adults. Clin Chem 36: 344, 1990.
257. Mitchell DN, Cannon P, Dyer NH, et al: Further observations on Kveim test in Crohn's disease. Lancet 2: 496, 1970.
258. Siltzbach LE: An international Kveim test study. Acta Med Scand 176(Suppl 425): 178, 1964.
259. Hunninghak GW, Kawanami O, Ferrans VJ, et al: Characterization of the inflammatory and immune effector cells in the lung parenchyma of patients with interstitial lung disease. Am Rev Respir Dis 123: 407, 1981.
260. Baughman RP, Lower EE: The effects of corticosteroid or methotrexate therapy on lung lymphocytes and macrophages in sarcoidosis. Am Rev Respir Dis 142: 1268, 1990.
261. Chadelat K, Baculard A, Grimfeld A, et al: Pulmonary sarcoidosis in children: serial evaluation of bronchoalveolar lavage cells during corticosteroid treatment. Pediatr Pulmonol 16: 41, 1993.
262. Tessier V, Chadelat K, Baculard A, et al: BAL in children: a controlled study of differential cytology and cytokine expression profiles by alveolar cells in pediatric sarcoidosis. Chest 109: 1430, 1996.
263. Brauner MW, Crenler P, Mompoint D, et al: Pulmonary sarcoidosis: evaluation with high-resolution CT. Radiology 172: 467, 1989.
264. Keesling CA, Frush DP, O'Hara SM, Fordham LA: Clinical and imaging manifestations of pediatric sarcoidosis. Acad Radiol 5: 122, 1998.
265. Nichols CW, Mishkin M, Yanoff M: Presumed orbital sarcoidosis: report of a case followed by computerized axial tomography and conjunctival biopsy. Trans Am Ophthalmol Soc 66: 67, 1978.
266. Gedalia A, Shetty AK, Ward KJ, et al: Role of MRI in diagnosis of childhood sarcoidosis with fever of unknown origin. J Pediatr Orthop 17: 460, 1997.
267. Haynes W, Sherman J, Stern B, et al: MR and CT evaluation of intracranial sarcoidosis. Am J Neuroradiol 8: 841, 1987.
268. Sakuari Y, Nakajima M, Kamisue S, et al: Preschool sarcoidosis mimicking juvenile rheumatoid arthritis. The significance of gallium scintigraphy and skin biopsy in the differential diagnosis. Acta Paediatr Jpn 39: 74, 1997.
269. Hirase Y, Ishida Y, Hayashida K, et al: Myocardial involvement in patients with sarcoidosis: an analysis of 75 patients. Clin Nucl Med 19: 522, 1994.
270. Martinet Y, Pinkston P, Saltini C, et al: Evaluation of the *in vitro* and *in vivo* effects of cyclosporine on the lung T-lymphocyte alveolitis of active pulmonary sarcoidosis. Am J Respir Crit Care Med 138: 1242, 1988.
271. The Research Committee of the British Tuberculosis Association. Chloroquine in the treatment of sarcoidosis. Tubercle 48: 257, 1967.
272. Mathur AM, Kremer JM: Immunopathology, rheumatic features and therapy of sarcoidosis. Curr Opin Rheumatol 4: 76, 1992.
273. Young RC Jr, Hackney RL, Harden KA: Epidemiology of sarcoidosis: ethnic and geographic considerations. J Natl Med Assoc 66: 386, 1974.
274. Gillum RF: Sarcoidosis in the United States—1968–1984. Hospitalization and death. J Natl Med Assoc 80: 1179, 1988.
275. Kendig EL Jr, Brummer DL: The prognosis of sarcoidosis in children. Chest 70: 351, 1976.
276. Marcille R, McCarthy M, Barton JW, et al: Long-term outcome of pediatric sarcoidosis with emphasis on pulmonary status. Chest 102: 1444, 1992.
277. Fink CW, Cimaz R: Early onset sarcoidosis: not a benign disease. J Rheumatol 24: 174, 1997.

30

Behçet's Disease and Other Vasculitides

Ross E. Petty and James T. Cassidy

BEHÇET'S DISEASE

In 1937, the Turkish dermatologist Hulusi Behçet[1] described the syndrome that bears his name: the clinical triad of *aphthous stomatitis, genital ulceration,* and *uveitis.* Occurrences of Behçet's disease (BD) retrace the historical route of the ancient Silk Road from Japan to the eastern edge of the Mediterranean Sea.[2] The history of this disorder was reviewed in 1998 by Kaklamani and colleagues.[3]

Definition and Classification

There is still no unanimous agreement about the definition of this syndrome,[4, 5] and complete and incomplete forms have been described. Several sets of diagnostic criteria have been proposed for BD. Those of the International Study[6] are most widely used and are listed in Table 30–1. Criteria proposed by Mason and Barnes[7] are also frequently cited and are listed in Table 30–2. Like those of Mason and Barnes, the criteria proposed by O'Duffy and Goldstein[8] emphasize the broader spectrum of disease and require, in addition to the presence of aphthous stomatitis, the presence of two of the following criteria:

- Aphthous genital ulcers
- Uveitis
- Cutaneous pustular vasculitis
- Synovitis
- Meningoencephalitis

In addition to the clinical triad that was originally described, the presentation and course of this syndrome often include other signs; therefore, the criteria proposed by Mason and Barnes may more accurately reflect the entire spectrum of the disease. The International Study Group criteria have a specificity of 96 percent and sensitivity of 91 percent; the Mason and Barnes criteria[9] have a specificity of 84 percent and sensitivity of 86 percent. All have been applied to the diagnosis of BD in children.

Epidemiology

BD is most common in Japan and countries of the eastern Mediterranean Sea; it is rare in children in North America[10] and Northern Europe.[11] A frequency of 1 in 600,000 French children under 15 years of age was estimated by Koné-Paut and Bernard.[12] There have been several reviews of childhood BD. In 1990, Lang and colleagues[13] reviewed 37 cases of BD beginning before 17 years of age published in the English language literature. Thirty-five of the patients met criteria for complete BD by the criteria of Mason and Barnes. An international study of the clinical features of BD in 65 children from France, Turkey, Iran, and Saudi Arabia used the International Study Group criteria.[14] Eighteen

Table 30–1

Criteria of the International Study Group for the Diagnosis of Behçet's Disease

CRITERION	DESCRIPTION
Recurrent oral ulceration	Minor aphthous, major aphthous, or herpetiform ulceration recurring at least three times in one 12-mo period, observed by physician or patient
Plus two of:	
Recurrent genital ulcers	Aphthous ulceration or scarring observed by physician or patient
Eye lesions	Anterior uveitis, posterior uveitis, or cells in vitreous on slit-lamp examination, or retinal vasculitis observed by an ophthalmologist
Skin lesions	Erythema nodosum observed by physician or patient; pseudofolliculitis or papulopustular lesions; or acneiform nodules observed by physician in postadolescent patient not on corticosteroid treatment
Pathergy	Skin reaction to a needle prick observed by physician at 24–48 hr

From Criteria for the diagnosis of Behçet's disease. International Study Group for Behçet's Disease, vol 335, issue no 8697, pp 1078–1080, © by The Lancet Ltd, 1990.

Table 30–2

Mason and Barnes Criteria for a Diagnosis of Behçet's Disease

MAJOR CRITERIA	MINOR CRITERIA
Buccal ulceration	Gastrointestinal lesions
Genital ulceration	Thrombophlebitis
Eye lesions	Cardiovascular lesions
Skin lesions	Arthritis
	Central nervous system lesions
	Family history of Behçet's disease

Diagnosis requires the presence of at least three major criteria, or two major and two minor criteria.

From Mason RM, Barnes CG: Behçet's syndrome with arthritis. Ann Rheum Dis 28: 95, 1969.

Greek children who met the International Study Group criteria for BD were described by Vaiolopolos and colleagues in 1999.[15] There have also been a number of series reported from Saudi Arabia,[16] Turkey,[17] Korea,[18] Italy,[19] Japan,[20] and Israel.[21] In most series, boys and girls are affected with equal frequency in contrast to BD in adults, in which males are affected almost twice as frequently as females. Of all reported cases of BD, childhood onset ranges from 4 to 8 percent[19, 22] to 26 percent.[15] The age at onset of disease ranges widely (Table 30–3). BD has been reported in neonates born to mothers with BD.[23–25]

Genetic Background

The higher frequency of BD in Japan and the countries of the Middle East suggest that there may be a genetic or environmental component to the disease. Large population surveys in the United Kingdom[26] and Japan[27] have shown that familial BD is rare. However, in a recent international study of BD in children, 15 percent had parents or siblings with the disease.[14] It has been reported in a mother and her two adolescent daughters,[28] and in three siblings with disease onset at 2 months to 2 years of age.[29] Human leukocyte antigen (HLA)-B5 has been associated with the syndrome in adults in the Turkish,[30] Japanese,[31] Italian,[32] and Mexican Mestizo populations[33] but not in Caucasian North American[4] or English patients.[34] B5 was increased in children from Israel.[21] B51 (a split of B5) has been reported to be increased in patients from Turkey,[35] Ireland,[36] and Spain.[37] It is likely that B51 confers significant risk of BD (relative risk, 6.3 to 6.44), particularly in patients with a family history of the disease.[38] A study of microsatellite markers in Japanese and European adults with BD suggested that the pathogenic gene is HLA-B51 and not other genes located in its vicinity.[38a] No associations with DR or RD + DQ antigens were demonstrable in a North American study[39] or in studies from Europe.[35, 36]

Etiology and Pathogenesis

The cause of BD disease is unknown. Despite several studies suggesting a role for herpes simplex virus-1, parvovirus B19, and streptococci, no microbial etiology has been established. An antibody-mediated process may be responsible, as suggested by the observation of transient neonatal BD in offspring of mothers with the disorder.[23–25] Lehner[40] has suggested that immunity to microbial heat-shock proteins that share homology with human 65 kD mitochondrial heat-shock protein may be important in pathogenesis. Gamma-delta T cells from patients with BD are highly responsive to four peptides from human 60-kD heat-shock protein compared with healthy controls, patients with systemic illnesses, or patients with recurrent oral ulcers but no other manifestations of the disease.[41]

Clinical Manifestations

The clinical manifestations of BD are varied and often emerge over a period of several years. In a study of 40 Korean children, the mean interval between the first and the second major manifestations was 7 years.[18] The

Table 30–3

Behçet's Disease in Childhood

REFERENCE	n	M:F	ONSET (yr)	CRITERIA (%)				
				OU	GU	Skin	Uveitis	Pathergy
Lang et al[13]	37	19:18	8.7	100	75	84*	30	?
Bahabri et al[16]	12	7:5	11.5	100	65	83	92	57
Koné-Paut et al[14]	65	33:32	8.4	100	96	92	45	80
Eldem et al[17]	20	15:5	15.1	100	65	35	80	?
Kim et al[18]	40	16:24	10.6	100	82	72	27	?
Pivetti-Pezzi et al[19]	16	9:7						
Fujikawa & Suemitsu[20]	31	14:17						
Uziel et al[21]	15	7:8	6.6	100	33	100	53	40
Total	*199*	*101:98*						

GU, genital ulceration; OU, oral ulceration.

*Includes pathergy.

frequency of the major and minor manifestations are given in Table 30–3.[7, 10, 13, 32, 42]

Mucocutaneous Disease

Oral ulceration is almost always present, usually occurs at disease onset, and may be persistent for much of the course of the disease.[42] Crops of extremely painful ulcers appear on lips, tongue, palate, and elsewhere in the gastrointestinal tract (Fig. 30–1). They last for 3 to 10 days, sometimes longer, and usually heal without scarring. The exception to this is neonatal disease, in which extensive scarring may result.[24]

Recurrent painful ulcerations of the glans penis, prepuce, scrotum, and perianal area in the male, and of the vulva and vagina in the female, are characteristic. These ulcers usually occur after oral ulcers and, unlike them, may scar with healing.

Other skin lesions include ulceration, erythema nodosum, erythema multiforme, and other rashes including psoriasis.[7] Pathergy, an unusual cutaneous pustular reaction occurring 24 to 48 hours after a needle puncture, is highly characteristic but not pathognomonic of the syndrome.[30] Pathergy test positivity varies considerably from one series to another and occurs most commonly (50 to 70 percent) in patients from the Middle East.[3]

Ocular Disease

The classic ocular lesion of BD is acute uveitis, which is almost always bilateral and involves both the anterior and the posterior uveal tracts.[43] Hypopyon may occur, and severe uveitis may lead to blindness. In older studies,[44] blindness in untreated patients exceeded 90 percent. Complications of uveitis (glaucoma, cataract) may occur. Corneal ulceration, cystoid macular degeneration, retinal vasculitis, and retinal detachment are rare events. Retrobulbar neuritis has been

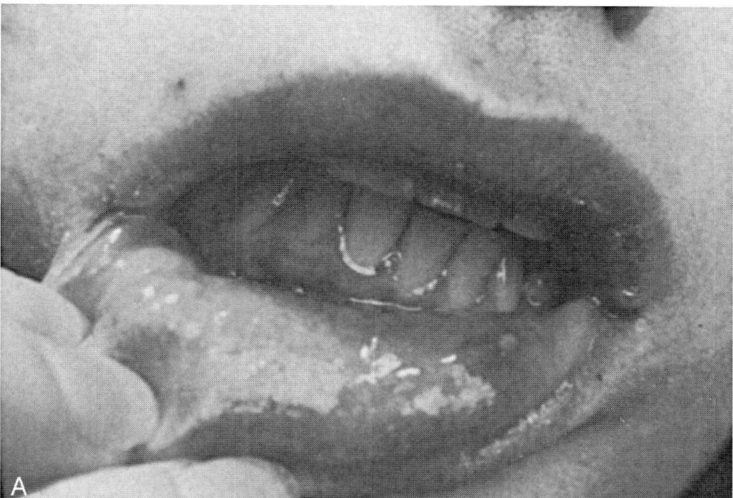

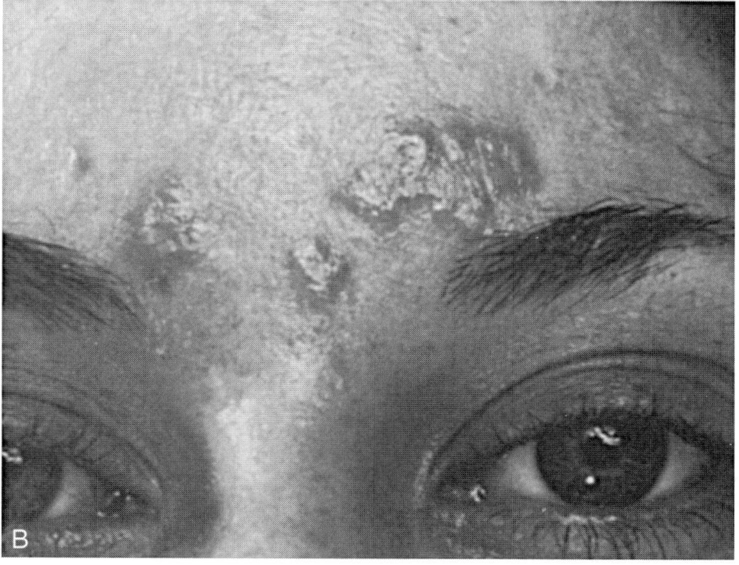

Figure 30–1. *A,* Mucous membrane ulceration in a young girl with Behçet's disease. *B,* Vesicular rash over the forehead of the same girl.

reported.[7] Ocular disease was much more common in boys than girls in one large study.[14]

Central Nervous System Disease

Four neurologic syndromes are recognized in patients with BD[45]:

- Encephalomyelitis (pyramidal, extrapyramidal, cerebellar, spinal cord abnormalities, seizures)
- Aseptic meningitis (headaches, meningitis)
- Benign intracranial hypertension (pseudotumor cerebri, papilledema)
- Organic psychiatric disturbances (psychoses, depression, dementia)

Several of these manifestations may occur simultaneously. The most common central nervous system (CNS) disorder at presentation is meningoencephalitis with headache, stiff neck, focal neurologic abnormalities, and pleocytosis of the cerebrospinal fluid.[8] Neuro-BD develops in 5 to 15 percent of children with BD.[14]

Musculoskeletal Disease

Polyarthritis or oligoarthritis occurs in 50 percent[14] to 75 percent[21] of children with BD. It most commonly affects the knees, ankles, wrists, and elbows but may occur in other joints as well.[7, 14, 21] The disease is usually oligoarticular, but polyarthritis is observed in at least one third of patients.[14] The disease does not usually result in erosions or joint destruction. There is probably no association of BD with sacroiliac arthritis, at least in childhood.[14, 46]

Acute, localized myositis is very uncommon, is rarely multifocal,[47] and has been reported in only a few children.[13, 21] It may be confused with vasculitis or venous thrombosis, especially when it affects the gastrocnemius muscle.[13]

Vascular Disease

Superficial or deep venous thromboses are common in adults[7] but occur only in 5 to 15 percent of children.[14] Most thromboses develop in veins, especially those of the lower extremities, but involvement of the pulmonary artery and central retinal artery has been reported.[14] Arteritis and arterial aneurysms may occur.[48–50] Dilatation and dropout of periungual capillaries was reported in the majority of adults in one study.[51]

Other Uncommon Manifestations

A number of cardiac complications (endocarditis, myocarditis, pericarditis, arrhythmias) have been reported in adults[3] but are rare in children. Recurrent dyspnea, cough, chest pain, and hemoptysis suggest pulmonary hemorrhage.[52] Diarrhea, abdominal pain, and ulceration of the colon appear to be more common in Japanese patients.[5] Gastrointestinal tract lesions indistinguishable from those of Crohn's disease[53, 54] or ulcerative colitis[7] may develop in patients with BD. Renal disease (including glomerulonephritis) has been rarely reported,[55] but a 1998 review[56] suggests that it may be under-recognized.

Pathology

The underlying pathologic lesion is an occlusive vasculitis in arterioles and veins. In the skin, the lesions may be necrotizing but do not exhibit fibrinoid degeneration.[6, 48] Synovial histology is characterized by only nonspecific inflammation, often predominantly with neutrophils. Muscle biopsies have demonstrated a wide range of abnormalities, from perivascular infiltrates and fibrosis[13] to muscle necrosis.[47]

Laboratory Examination

No laboratory findings are diagnostic of BD. There is a generalized increase in acute phase reactants. Levels of immunoglobulins and circulating immune complexes are increased.[57] Autoantibodies such as antinuclear antibody and rheumatoid factor are absent, but antibodies to ocular and oral mucosal antigens have been observed.[58] Anticardiolipin antibodies are rare, although their presence may correlate with the presence of retinal vascular disease.[59] Markers of vasculitis, such as elevated von Willebrand factor[60] and antibodies to neutrophil cytoplasmic antigen,[61] are uncommon and, when present, are associated with vasculitis.

Abnormalities of T cells and cytokines have also been noted. Increased serum levels of tumor necrosis factor (TNF)-α[62] and soluble TNF-α receptor[63] may serve as markers of active disease. The pathogenic significance of elevated sIL-2R,[62] interleukin (IL)-10,[63] IL-12,[63] and IL-8[64] requires further evaluation.

Neutrophils are prominent infiltrating cells in the skin and eye lesions of BD and inconsistent abnormalities of their function have been reported. Carletto and colleagues[65] studied neutrophil function in 15 adults and found that although superoxide production and adhesion were normal, migration was significantly increased in patients with active disease compared with those with inactive disease or controls. The enhanced migration into inflammatory sites would facilitate their participation in the leukocytoclastic vasculitis or neutrophilic vasculitis that may occur in BD and may be at least partly responsible for pathergy. It should be noted that in other studies,[66] levels of reactive oxygen species were increased. The role of neutrophil abnormalities in the pathogenesis of BD is not clear and requires further study. Synovial fluid analysis is characterized by a predominance of neutrophils in relatively low numbers ($<15,000/mm^3$ [$<15 \times 10^9/L$]) and low glucose levels, but no other distinguishing features.[67]

Diagnosis

In general, aphthous stomatitis is the presenting sign; other components of the syndrome may not appear for decades. The diagnosis is principally clinical, with the laboratory supplying only supporting evidence. The differential diagnosis includes inflammatory bowel disease; aphthous stomatitis, erythema nodosum, arthritis, and uveitis occur in both diseases. In BD, the likelihood of occurrence of posterior uveitis is greater than in inflammatory bowel disease.

Treatment

BD is difficult to treat, and treatment depends largely on the site and severity of involvement. Yazici and colleagues[68] suggest that young males have the worst prognosis and should be treated most aggressively. Whether this applies to the pediatric age range is not certain. Some patients are glucocorticoid-responsive,[21] and prednisone is usually chosen as the initial therapy, although some studies have reported disappointing results, especially for CNS and ocular disease.[8] The addition of cyclosporin to glucocorticoids has been recommended for the treatment of sight-threatening uveitis in adults.[69] The results of cyclosporin alone (5 mg/kg/d for 2 years) in 16 patients was generally favorable, and complete clinical remission was attained in 14 patients within 6 months.[70]

Colchicine has also been used with success.[21, 71, 72] Low-dose methotrexate may prevent progression of CNS manifestations.[73] Chlorambucil (0.1 mg/kg/d for 1 to 4 years) has been successful in suppressing CNS disease.[74, 75] Short-term high-dose therapy with this drug may be useful in treatment of intractable ocular disease.[76] Thalidomide was given to patients with mucocutaneous BD who did not have major organ involvement in doses of 100 mg/d with significant improvement in oral and genital ulceration within 4 to 8 weeks.[77] Peripheral neuropathy may be a limiting side effect of this drug; of course, thalidomide is a potent teratogen and must not be used in females of child-bearing age without contraception. New approaches to therapy of BD have been recently reviewed.[77a]

Course of the Disease and Prognosis

This disease tends to run a very long, relapsing course.[54, 78] The ocular and CNS manifestations, in particular, can be extremely incapacitating.[11, 21, 43, 55, 78] The young child who presents with only recurrent oral mucocutaneous lesions may develop genital ulcerations and gastrointestinal tract disease during adolescence.[42] Potentially fatal lesions include occlusion or aneurysms of arteries supplying the CNS or heart, pulmonary hemorrhage, and bowel perforation.[10, 54] In a series of 65 patients, the mortality rate was 3 percent.[14]

OTHER VASCULITIDES

Mucha-Habermann Disease

Mucha-Habermann disease, or *pityriasis lichenoides et varioliformis acuta* (PLEVA), is a form of cutaneous vasculitis of unknown etiology. At presentation, the dermatitis has the appearance of chronic or recurrent chickenpox-like lesions that become atrophic and scarred. The rash is accompanied by fever and joint pain and swelling (Fig. 30–2). Histologically, the lesions

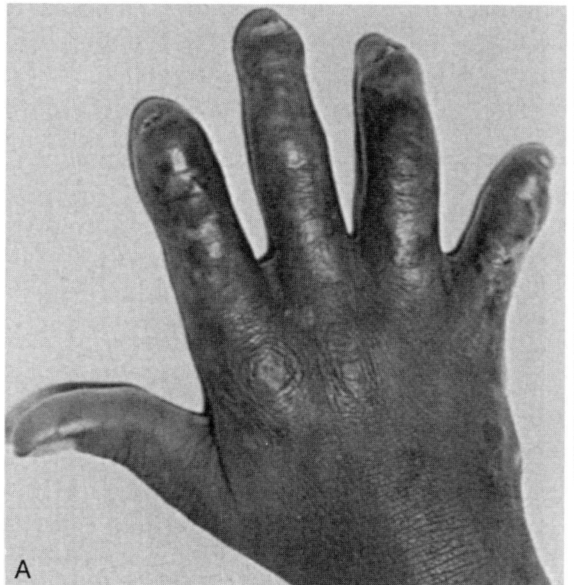

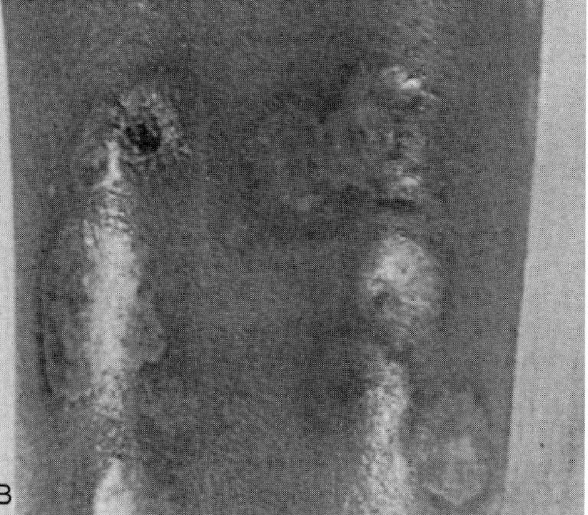

Figure 30–2. An 11-year-old black girl with destructive acrosclerosis and Mucha-Habermann disease. *A*, Hand. *B*, Forearm. Characteristic cutaneous lesions of the latter disorder are visible, along with advanced ischemic digital changes.

are characterized by a lymphocytic inflammation of capillaries and venules of the upper dermis. PLEVA has been observed in two children in association with chronic arthritis resembling juvenile rheumatoid arthritis and with severe acrosclerosis and scleroderma.[79] A third patient with similar cutaneous findings was reported by Lister and Hollingworth,[80] and we have observed two sisters with PLEVA, one of whom also had bland but recurrent arthritis.

Kohlmeir-Degos Syndrome

The Kohlmeir-Degos syndrome has a number of other names, including papulosis atrophicans maligna[81] and progressive arterial occlusive disease.[82] It is a very rare, often fatal vasculitis of cutaneous and gastrointestinal small- and medium-sized arteries that results in progressive occlusion by fibrosis, leading to infarction. It occurs almost exclusively in young to middle-aged men and has been reported in three teenaged boys.[82] Its presentation and course has been reviewed by Snow and Muller.[83]

Cronkhite-Canada syndrome

Juvenile gastrointestinal polyposis is rarely associated with a widespread vasculitis of small and medium-sized arteries, the Cronkhite-Canada syndrome.[84, 85] Cutaneous anergy is present. The disease has a poor prognosis, and few affected children live more than 2 years.[86] Infantile necrotizing enterocolitis may also be associated with vasculitis.[87]

SYNDROMES THAT RESEMBLE VASCULITIS

A number of unrelated disorders have clinical presentations that may suggest the presence of vasculitis. They include infectious vasculitis, vasculitis associated with malignancy, retroperitoneal fibrosis, and embolism.

Relapsing Polychondritis

Relapsing polychondritis is a rare, widespread inflammation of cartilage that is associated with uveitis, deafness, vestibular involvement, and aortic valve insufficiency. It has seldom been described in children.[88–92] Inflammation affects the cartilage of the ear or hyaline cartilage of the joints and then spreads to involve cartilage of the upper respiratory tract, including the nose, trachea, and bronchi (Fig. 30–3). Episodic oligoarthritis occurs in approximately 80 percent of affected persons. Synovial fluid samples are noninflammatory, and the synovial membrane shows minimal inflammation.[92] Uveitis may occur.[92] Relapsing polychondritis has occurred in a patient with Henoch-Schönlein purpura.[93] The course is initially episodic but becomes progressive in the majority of patients. The cause is unknown. Intrauterine transmission has been suggested in one patient,[94] but this association appears to be exceptional.[95] Glucocorticoids suppress the disease. Death is often the result of respiratory obstruction.[96]

Sweet's Syndrome

Acute febrile neutrophilic dermatosis (Sweet's syndrome) is a rare syndrome in children[97–102] that consists of a perivasculitis characterized clinically by spiking fever and tender, raised pseudovesicular, erythematous plaques or nodules on the face and extremities and sometimes on the trunk. Arthritis occurs in one third of adult patients[103] and has been reported in an 8-month-old boy.[102] Musculoskeletal pain, including multifocal osteomyelitis, has also been reported in children.[104, 105]

Weber-Christian Disease

This rare relapsing panniculitis is characterized by fever, constitutional signs, and subcutaneous ulcerating nodules.[106, 107] Severe disease may involve parenchymal organs (lungs, heart, gastrointestinal tract and omentum, kidneys, spleen, and adrenal glands).

Stevens-Johnson Syndrome

The Stevens-Johnson syndrome is a severe systemic form of mucocutaneous erythema multiforme. Numerous erosive, vesiculobullous, hemorrhagic and papular lesions develop acutely on the mucosa and skin of the face, hands, trunk, and feet (Fig. 30–4). Anal, genital, and ocular orifices are often affected, and scarring may result. Onset is usually abrupt and is associated with fever, profound constitutional symptoms, and the appearance of periarticular swelling and pain or frank arthritis. The respiratory and gastrointestinal tracts can be involved in severe disease.[108]

Histopathologic studies demonstrate perivasculitis within lesions that results in stomatitis, conjunctivitis, or corneal ulcerations with no evidence of actual necrotizing vasculitis. The etiology of the syndrome is unknown, but a preceding infectious illness, particularly with *Mycoplasma pneumoniae*, is frequently documented.[109, 110] Antibiotics, especially trimethoprim-sulfamethoxazole[111] and cefaclor,[112] have also been implicated in the syndrome's cause. Lamotrigine, an anticonvulsant medication, has been associated with Stevens-Johnson syndrome.[113]

Expert supportive care is usually the only treatment needed for this self-limited disease, although in severe cases glucocorticoids are considered necessary.[114] Extensive mucosal and cutaneous disease is best treated in a burn unit.

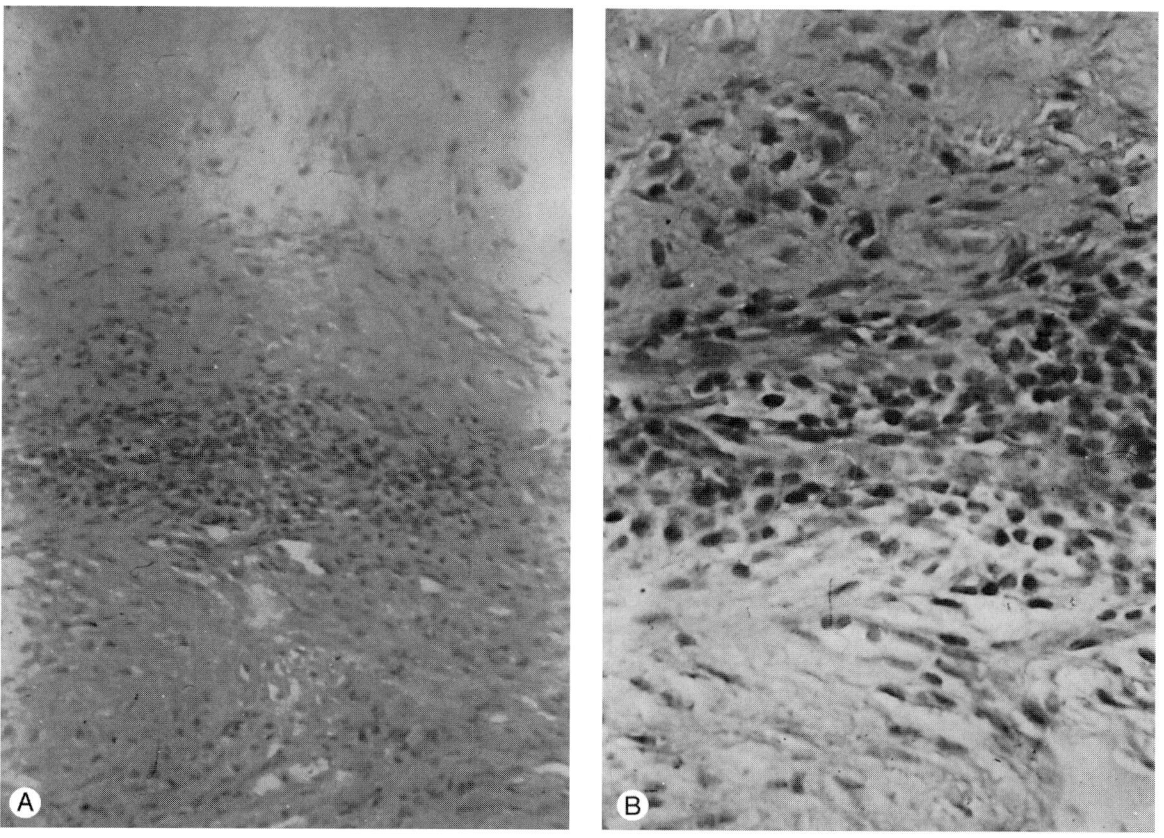

Figure 30–3. Histopathology of relapsing polychondritis. *A,* Biopsy specimen of ear cartilage, ×250. *B,* Close-up view. H&E, ×600. Acute inflammation and perichondritis are present with numerous lymphocytes and plasma cells and smaller numbers of polymorphs. The edge of the aural elastic cartilage is being destroyed by the cellular exudate.

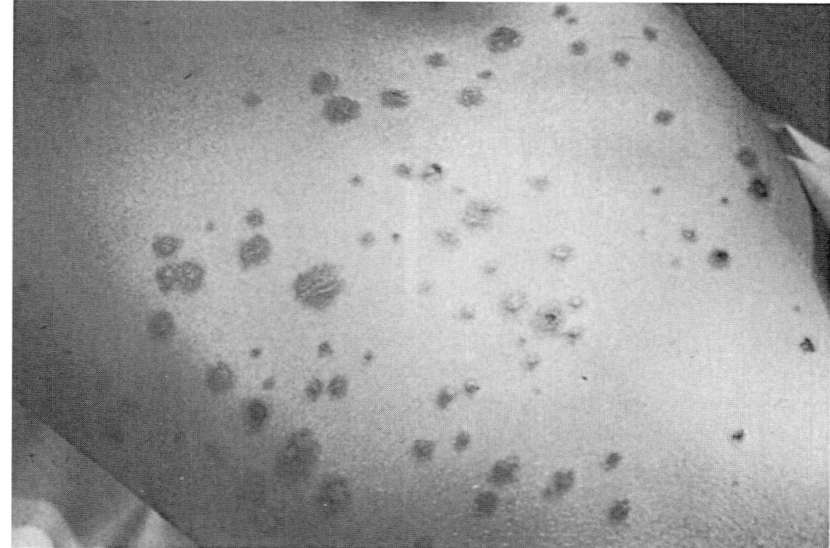

Figure 30–4. Vesicular erythematous lesions of erythema multiforme in a young boy with Stevens-Johnson syndrome. There were also the characteristic bullous lesions around body orifices.

Cardiac Myxoma

An atrial myxoma may simulate vasculitis by embolization[115–117] and should be considered in the diagnosis of an obscure vasculitis-like syndrome. The phenomenon has only rarely been reported in children or adolescents.[118–120] Echocardiography demonstrates the lesion,[120] and surgical removal is curative.

Goodpasture's Syndrome

In 1919, Goodpasture[121] described a patient who experienced pulmonary hemorrhage and severe proliferative glomerulonephritis with crescent formation, leading to death. Constitutional symptoms (e.g., fever, chills, increased sweating) occur in one fourth of patients with this syndrome, and pulmonary complaints (e.g., dyspnea, weakness, chest pain, wheezing) are common.[122] Pulmonary hemorrhage is often the initial manifestation and may precede renal abnormalities by weeks to years. Clinical progression may be rapid. The presence of serum antibodies to the NC1 domain of type IV collagen in alveolar and glomerular basement membranes is diagnostic.[123, 124] These antibodies are present in the serum or can be demonstrated as linear staining of the basement membrane in the lung and glomeruli by immunofluorescence microscopy.

This disease predominantly affects young men, with a male:female ratio of 9:1. Goodpasture's syndrome has only occasionally been reported in children or adolescents.[125–131] In children, idiopathic pulmonary hemosiderosis, Wegener's granulomatosis, hemolytic uremic syndrome, and systemic lupus erythematosus are all considerations in the differential diagnosis. Goodpasture's syndrome has occurred after therapy with D-penicillamine, in heavy metal poisoning, and in patients with a variety of rheumatic diseases.

Treatment includes the prompt use of glucocorticoids, plasmapheresis, and immunosuppressive agents with varying results.[126, 127] The rationale for this combined approach is that circulating anti–basement membrane antibodies are removed from the vascular compartment by plasmapheresis, and their synthesis is limited by immunosuppressive agents. Nonetheless, the survival rate of patients with Goodpasture's syndrome is low.[130] Death is caused by asphyxia, pulmonary hemorrhages, or uremia.

References

1. Behçet H: Über rezidivierende Aphthose, durch ein Virus verursachte Geschwure am Mund, am Auge und an den Genitalien. Dermatol Wochenschr 105: 1151, 1937.
2. Dilsen N: History and development of Behçet's disease. Rev Rhum Engl Ed 63: 512, 1996.
3. Kaklamani VG, Vaiopoulos G, Kaklamanis PG: Behçet's disease. Semin Arthritis Rheum 27: 197, 1998.
4. O'Duffy JD: Summary of international symposium on Behçet's disease. J Rheumatol 5: 229, 1978.
5. Shimizu T, Erhlich GE, Inaba G: Behçet's disease (Behçet's syndrome). Semin Arthritis Rheum 8: 223, 1979.
6. International Study Group for Behçet's Disease: Criteria for the diagnosis of Behçet's disease. Lancet 335: 1070, 1990.
7. Mason RM, Barnes CGL: Behçet's syndrome with arthritis. Ann Rheum Dis 28: 95, 1969.
8. O'Duffy JD, Goldstein NP: Neurologic involvement in seven patients with Behçet's disease. Am J Med 61: 170, 1976.
9. Rigby AS, Chamberlain MA, Bhakta B: Classification and assessment of rheumatic diseases. Part I: Behçet's disease. Baillieres Clin Rheumatol 9: 375, 1995.
10. Ammann AJ, Johnson A, Fyfe G, et al: Behçet syndrome. J Pediatr 107: 41, 1985.
11. Chamberlain MA: Behçet's syndrome in 32 patients in Yorkshire. Ann Rheum Dis 36: 491, 1977.
12. Koné-Paut I, Bernard JL: La maladie de Behçet chez l'enfant en France. Arch Fr Pediatr 50: 561, 1993.
13. Lang BA, Laxer RM, Thorner P, et al: Pediatric onset of Behçet's syndrome with myositis: case report and literature review illustrating unusual features. Arthritis Rheum 33: 418, 1990.
14. Koné-Paut I, Yurdakul S, Bahabri SA, et al: Clinical features of Behçet's disease in children: an international collaborative study of 86 cases. J Pediatr 132: 721, 1998.
15. Vaiolpoulos G, Kaklamani VG, Markomichelakis N: Clinical features of juvenile Adamantiades-Behçet's disease in Greece. Clin Exp Rheumatol 17: 256, 1999.
16. Bahabri SA, Al-Mazyed A, Al-Balaa S, et al: Juvenile Behçet's disease in Arab children. Clin Exp Rheumatol 14: 331, 1996.
17. Eldem B, Onur C, Ozen S: Clinical features of pediatric Behçet's disease. J Pediatr Ophthalmol Strabismus 35: 159, 1998.
18. Kim DK, Chang SN, Bang D, et al: Clinical analysis of 40 cases of childhood-onset Behçet's disease. Pediatr Dermatol 11: 95, 1994.
19. Pivetti-Pezzi P, Accorinti M, Abdulaziz MA, et al: Behçet's disease in children. Jpn J Ophthalmol 39: 309, 1995.
20. Fujikawa S, Suemitsu T: Behçet disease in children: a nationwide retrospective survey in Japan. Acta Paediatr Jpn 39: 285, 1997.
21. Uziel Y, Brik R, Padeh S, et al: Juvenile Behçet's disease in Israel. Clin Exp Rheumatol 16: 502, 1998.
22. Mangelsdorf HC, White WL, Jorizzo JL: Behçet's disease. Report of twenty-five patients from the United States with prominent mucocutaneous involvement. J Am Acad Dermatol 34: 745, 1996.
23. Stark AC, Bhakta B, Chamberlain MA, et al: Life-threatening transient neonatal Behçet's disease. Br J Rheumatol 36: 700, 1997.
24. Fam AG, Siminovitch KA, Carette S, et al: Neonatal Behçet's syndrome in an infant of a mother with the disease. Ann Rheum Dis 25: 1343, 1982.
25. Lewis MA, Priestly BL: Transient neonatal Behçet's disease. Arch Dis Child 61: 805, 1986.
26. Chamberlain MA: A family study of Behçet's syndrome. Ann Rheum Dis 37: 459, 1978.
27. Nishiura K, Kotake S, Ichiishi A, Matsuda H: Familial occurrence of Behçet's disease. Jpn J Ophthalmol 40: 255, 1996.
28. Pitkeathly DA: Discussion on Behçet's syndrome with arthritis. Ann Rheum Dis 28: 102, 1969.
29. Koné I, Palix C, Berbis P, Bernard JL: Familial Behçet's disease in children. A report of 3 cases. Clin Exp Rheumatol 10: 627, 1992.
30. Yazici H, Tuzun Y, Pazarli H, et al: The combined used of HLA-B5 and the pathergy test as diagnostic markers of Behçet's disease in Turkey. J Rheumatol 7: 206, 1980.
31. Ohno S, Narayama E, Sigiura S, et al: Specific histocompatibility antigens associated with Behçet's disease. Am J Ophthalmol 80: 636, 1975.
32. Adorno D, Pezzi PP, Bonini S, et al: HLA-B5 and Behçet's disease. Tissue Antigens 14: 444, 1979.
33. Lavalle C, Alarcon-Segovia D, Del Giudice-Knipping JA, et al: Association of Behçet's syndrome with HLA-B5 in the Mexican Meztiso population. J Rheumatol 8: 325, 1981.
34. Lehner T, Batchelor JR, Challacombe SJ, et al: An immunogenetic basis for the tissue involvement in Behçet's syndrome. Immunology 37: 895, 1979.
35. Alpsy E, Yilmaz E, Coskun M, et al: HLA antigens and linkage disequilibrium patterns in Turkish Behçet's patients. J Dermatol 25: 158, 1998.
36. Kilmartin DJ, Finch A, Acheson RW: Primary association of

HLA-B51 with Behçet's disease in Ireland. Br J Ophthalmol 81: 649, 1997.
37. Gonzalez-Escribano MF, Rodriquez MR, Walter K, et al: Association of HLA-B51 subtypes and Behçet's disease in Spain. Tissue Antigens 52: 78, 1998.
38. Chajek-Shaul T, Pisanty S, Knobler H, et al: HLA-B51 may serve as an immunogenetic marker for a subgroup of patients with Behçet's syndrome. Am J Med 83: 666, 1987.
38a. Mizuki N, Ota M, Yabuki K, et al: Localization of the pathogenic gene of Behçet's disease by microsatellite analysis of three different populations. Invest Ophthalmol Vis Sci 41: 3702, 2000.
39. Moore SB, O'Duffy JF: Lack of association between Behçet's disease and major histocompatibility complex class II antigens in an ethnically diverse North American Caucasoid patient group. J Rheumatol 13: 771, 1986.
40. Lehner T: The role of heat shock protein, microbial and autoimmune agents in the aetiology of Behçet's disease. Int Rev Immunol 14: 21, 1997.
41. Hasan A, Fortune F, Wilson A, et al: Role of gamma delta T cells in pathogenesis and diagnosis of Behçet's disease. Lancet 347: 789, 1996.
42. Mundy TM, Miller JJ III: Behçet's disease presenting as chronic aphthous stomatitis in a child. Pediatrics 62: 205, 1978.
43. Colvard DM, Robertson DM, O'Duffy J: Ocular manifestations of Behçet's disease. Arch Ophthalmol 95: 1813, 1977.
44. Mamo JG: the rate of visual loss in Behçet's disease. Arch Ophthalmol 84: 451, 1970.
45. Koné-Paut I, Chabrol B, Riss J-M, et al: Neurologic onset of Behçet's disease: a diagnostic enigma in childhood. J Child Neurol 12: 237, 1997.
46. Chamberlain MA, Robertson RJ: A controlled study of sacroiliitis in Behçet's disease. Br J Rheumatol 32: 693, 1993.
47. Arkin CD, Rothchild BM, Florendo NT, Popoff N: Behçet syndrome with myositis: a case report with pathologic findings. Arthritis Rheum 23: 600, 1980.
48. Enoch BA, Castillo-Olivares JL, Khoo TCL, et al: Major vascular complications in Behçet's syndrome. Postgrad Med J 44: 453, 1968.
49. Davies JD: Behçet's syndrome with haemoptysis and pulmonary lesions. J Pathol 109: 351, 1973.
50. Grenier P, Bletry O, Cornud F, et al: Pulmonary involvement in Behçet's disease. Am J Roentgenol 137: 565, 1981.
51. Vaiopoulos G, Pangratis N, Samarkos M, et al: Nailfold capillary abnormalities in Behçet's disease. J Rheumatol 22: 1108, 1995.
52. Raz I, Okon E, Chajek-Shaul T: Pulmonary manifestations in Behçet's syndrome. Chest 12: 575, 1989.
53. Lorenzetti ME, Forbes IJ, Roberts-Thomson IC: Oesophageal and ileal ulceration in Behçet's disease. J Gastroenterol Hepatol 5: 714, 1990.
54. O'Duffy JD: Prognosis in Behçet's syndrome. Bull Rheum Dis 29: 972, 1978.
55. Akutsu Y, Itami N, Tanaka M, et al: IgA nephritis in Behçet's disease: case report and review of the literature. Clin Nephrol 34: 52, 1990.
56. Benekli M, Haznedaroglu C, Erdem Y: Glomerular involvement in Behçet's disease. Nephrol Dial Transplant 13: 1351, 1998.
57. Scully C, Boyle P, Yap PL: Immunoglobulins G, M, A, D and E in Behçet's syndrome. Clin Chim Acta 120: 237, 1982.
58. Klok AM, de Vries J, Rothova A, et al: Antibodies against ocular and oral antigens in Behçet's disease associated with uveitis. Curr Eye Res 8: 957, 1989.
59. Hall RG, Harris EN, Gharavi AE, et al: Anticardiolipin antibodies: occurrence in Behçet's syndrome. Ann Rheum Dis 43: 746, 1984.
60. Yazici H, Hekim N, Ozbakir F, et al: Von Willebrand factor in Behçet syndrome. J Rheumatol 14: 305, 1987.
61. Vaiopoulos G, Hatzinicolaou P, Tsiroyanni A, et al: Antineutrophil cytoplasmic antibodies in Adamantiades-Behçet's disease. Br J Rheumatol 33: 406, 1994.
62. Sayinalp N, Ozcebe OI, Tozdemir O, et al: Cytokines in Behçet's disease. J Rheumatol 23: 321, 1996.
63. Turan B, Gallati H, Erdi H, et al: Systemic levels of the T cell regulatory cytokines IL-10 and IL-12 in Behçet's disease; soluble TNFR-75 as a biological marker of disease activity. J Rheumatol 24: 128, 1997.
64. Al-Dalaan A, Al-Sedairy S, Al-Balaa S, et al: Enhanced interleukin 8 secretion in circulation of patients with Behçet's disease. J Rheumatol 22: 904, 1995.
65. Carletto A, Pacor ML, Biasi D, et al: Changes of neutrophil migration without modification of in vitro metabolism and adhesion in Behçet's disease. J Rheumatol 24: 1332, 1997.
66. Takeno M, Kariyone A, Yamashita N, et al: Excessive function of peripheral blood neutrophils from patients with Behçet's disease and from HLA-B51 transgenic mice. Arthritis Rheum 38: 426, 1995.
67. Yurdakul S, Yazici H, Tuzun Y, et al: The arthritis of Behçet's disease: a prospective study. Ann Rheum Dis 42: 505 1983.
68. Yazici H, Yurdakul S, Hamurydan V: Behçet's syndrome. Curr Opin Rheumatol 11: 53, 1999.
69. Whitcup SM, Salvo EC Jr, Nussenblatt RB: Combined cyclosporine and corticosteroid therapy for sight-threatening uveitis in Behçet's disease. Am J Ophthalmol 118: 39, 1994.
70. Pacor ML, Biasi D, Lunardi C, et al: Cyclosporin in Behçet's disease: results in 16 patients after 24 months of therapy. Clin Rheumatol 13: 224, 1994.
71. Mizushima Y, Matsumura N, Mori M: Chemotaxis of leukocytes and colchicine treatment in Behçet's disease. J Rheumatol 6: 108, 1979.
72. Masuda K, Makajima A, Usayama A, et al: Double-masked trial of cyclosporin versus colchicine and long-term open study of cyclosporin in Behçet's disease. Lancet 1: 1093, 1989.
73. Hirohata S, Suda H, Hashimoto T: Low-dose weekly methotrexate for progressive neuropsychiatric manifestations in Behçet's disease. J Neurol Sci 159: 181, 1998.
74. Rakover Y, Adar H, Tal I, et al: Behçet disease: long-term follow-up of three children and review of the literature. Pediatrics 83: 986, 1989.
75. Matteson EL, O'Duffy JD: Treatment of Behçet's disease with chlorambucil. *In* O'Duffy JD, Kokmen E (eds): Behçet's Disease: Basic and Clinical Aspects. Proceedings of the Fifth International Conference on Behçet's Disease. New York, Marcel Dekker, 1992, p 575.
76. Tessler HH, Jennings T: High-dose short-term chlorambucil for intractable sympathetic ophthalmia and Behçet's disease. Br J Ophthalmol 74: 353, 1990.
77. Hamuryudan V, Mat C, Saip S, et al: Thalidomide in the treatment of the mucocutaneous lesions of the Behçet syndrome. A randomized, double-blind, placebo-controlled trial. Ann Intern Med 128: 443, 1998.
77a. Sakane T, Takeno M: Novel approaches to Behçet's disease. Expert Opin Investig Drugs 9: 1993, 2000.
78. Oshima Y, Shimizu T, Hokohari R, et al: Clinical studies on Behçet's syndrome. Ann Rheum Dis 28: 102, 1969.
79. Ellsworth JE, Cassidy JT, Ragsdale CG, et al: Mucha-Habermann disease in children—the association with rheumatic diseases. J Rheumatol 9: 319, 1982.
80. Lister PD, Hollingworth P: Arthritis associated with leukocytoclastic angiitis. Ann Rheum Dis 39: 526, 1980.
81. Degos R, Delort J, Tricot R: Papulose atrophiante maligne (syndrome cutaneo-intestinal mortel). Bull Soc Med Hôp Paris 64: 803, 1948.
82. Strole WE Jr, Clark WH Jr, Isselbacher KJ: Progressive arterial occlusive disease (Kohlmeier-Degos). A frequently fatal cutaneosystemic disorder. N Engl J Med 276: 195, 1967.
83. Snow JL, Muller SA: Degos syndrome: malignant atrophic papulosis. Semin Dermatol 14: 99, 1995.
84. Cronkhite LW Jr, Canada WJ: Generalized gastrointestinal polyposis. An unusual syndrome of polyposis, pigmentation, alopecia and onychatrophia. N Engl J Med 252: 1011, 1955.
85. Parsa C: Cronkhite-Canada syndrome associated with systemic vasculitis—an autopsy study. Hum Pathol 13: 758, 1982.
86. Kuchukaydin M, Patiroglu TE, Okur H, et al: Infantile Cronkhite-Canada syndrome? Case report. Eur J Pediatr Surg 2: 295, 1992.
87. Gray ES, Lloyd DJ, Miller SS, et al: Evidence for an immune complex vasculitis in neonatal necrotizing enterocolitis. J Clin Pathol 34: 759, 1981.
88. McAdam LP, O'Hanlan MA, Bluestone R, et al: Relapsing polychondritis: prospective study of 23 patients and a review of the literature. Medicine (Baltimore) 55: 193, 1976.

89. Blau ED: Relapsing polychondritis and retroperitoneal fibrosis in an 8-year-old boy. Am J Dis Child 130: 1149, 1976.
90. Sacco O, Fregonese B, Oddone M, et al: Severe endobronchial obstruction in a girl with relapsing polychondritis: treatment with Nd YAG laser and endobronchial silicon stent. Eur Respir J 10: 494, 1997.
91. Masaoka A, Yamakawa Y, Niwa H, et al: Pediatric and adult tracheobronchomalacia. Eur J Cardiothorac Surg 10: 87, 1996.
92. Balsa A, Espinosa A, Cuesta M, et al: Joint symptoms in relapsing polychondritis. Clin Exp Rheumatol 13: 425, 1995.
93. Varonos S, Kostaki M, Tsapra H, et al: Polychondritis associated with Schönlein-Henoch purpura: report of a case. Clin Exp Rheumatol 12: 443, 1994.
94. Arundell FW, Haserick JR: Familial chronic atrophic polychondritis. Arch Dermatol 82: 439, 1960.
95. Papo T, Wechsler B, Bletry O, et al: Pregnancy in relapsing polychondritis. Arthritis Rheum 40: 1245, 1997.
96. Michet JM Jr, McKenna CH, Luthra HS, et al: Relapsing polychondritis. Survival and predictive role of early disease manifestations. Ann Intern Med 104: 74, 1986.
97. van-den Driesch P: Sweet's syndrome (acute febrile neutrophilic dermatosis). J Am Acad Dermatol 31: 535, 1994.
98. Bajwa RPS, Marwaka RK, Garewal G, Rajagopalan M: Acute febrile neutrophilic dermatosis (Sweet's syndrome) in myelodysplastic syndrome. J Pediatr Hematol Oncol 10: 343, 1993.
99. Garty BZ, Levy I, Nitzan M, Barak Y: Sweet's syndrome associated with G-CSF treatment in a child with glycogen storage disease type Ib. Pediatrics 97: 401, 1996.
100. Shimizu T, Yoshidea I, Eguchi H, et al: Sweet's syndrome in a child with aplastic anemia receiving recombinant granulocyte colony-stimulating factor. J Pediatr Hematol Oncol 18: 282, 1996.
101. Eghari-Sabet JS, Hartley AH: Sweet's syndrome: an immunologically mediated skin disease? Ann Allergy 72: 125, 1994.
102. Tuerlinckx D, Bodart E, Despontin K, et al: Sweet's syndrome with arthritis in an 8-month-old boy. J Rheumatol 26: 440, 1999.
103. Moreland LW, Brick JE, Kovack RE, et al: Acute febrile dermatosis (Sweet's syndrome): a review of the literature with emphasis on musculoskeletal manifestations. Semin Arthritis Rheum 17: 145, 1988.
104. Nurre LD, Rabalais GP, Callen JP: Neutrophilic dermatosis–associated sterile chronic multifocal osteomyelitis in pediatric patients: case report and review. Pediatr Dermatol 16: 214, 1999.
105. Boatman BW, Taylor RC, Klein LE, Cohen BA: Sweet's syndrome in children. South Med J 87: 193, 1994.
106. Weber EP: A case of relapsing non-suppurative nodular panniculitis showing phagocytosis of subcutaneous fat-cells by macrophages. Br J Dermatol Syph 37: 301, 1925.
107. Christian HA: Relapsing febrile nodular nonsuppurative panniculitis. Arch Intern Med 42: 3338, 1928.
108. Edell DS, Davidson JJ, Muelenaer AA, et al: Unusual manifestation of Stevens-Johnson syndrome involving the respiratory and gastrointestinal tract. Pediatrics 89: 429, 1992.
109. Levy M, Shear NH: Mycoplasma pneumoniae infections and Stevens-Johnson syndrome. Clin Pediatrics 30: 42, 1991.
110. Tay YK, Huff JC, Weston WL: Mycoplasma pneumoniae infection is associated with Stevens-Johnson syndrome, not erythema multiforme (von Hebra). J Am Acad Dermatol 35: 757, 1996.
111. Myers MW, Jick H: Hospitalization for serious blood and skin disorders following use of co-trimoxazole. Br J Clin Pharmacol 43: 446, 1997.
112. Murray DL, Singer DA, Singer AB, et al: Cefaclor—a cluster of adverse reactions. N Engl J Med 303: 1003, 1980.
113. Messenheimer JA: Rash in adult and pediatric patients treated with lamotrigine. Can J Neurol Sci 25: S14, 1998.
114. Prendiville JS, Herbert AA, Greewald MJ, et al: Management of Stevens-Johnson syndrome and toxic epidermal necrolysis in children. J Pediatr 115: 881,1989.
115. Weerasena NA, Groome D, Pollock JG, et al: Atrial myxoma as a cause of acute lower limb ischaemia in a teenager. Scott Med J 34: 440, 1989.
116. Tonz M, Laske A, Carrel T, et al: Convulsions, hemiparesis and central retinal artery occlusion due to left atrial myxoma in child. Eur J Pediatr 151: 652, 1992.
117. Hung PC, Wang HS, Chou ML, et al: Multiple cerebral aneurysms in a child with cardiac myxoma. J Formos Med Assoc 91: 818, 1992.
118. Park JM, Garcia RR, Patrick JK, et al: Right atrial myxoma with a nonembolic intestinal manifestation. Pediatr Cardiol 11: 164, 1990.
119. Couglin WF, Knott PE: Right atrial myxoma. A cause of septic pulmonary emboli in an adolescent female. J Adolesc Health Care 11: 351, 1990.
120. Pasaoglu I, Demircin M, Ozkutlu S, et al: Right atrial myxoma in an infant. Jpn Heart J 32: 263, 1991.
121. Goodpasture EW: The significance of certain pulmonary lesions in relation to the etiology of influenza. Am J Med Sci 158: 863, 1919.
122. Harrity P, Gilbert-Barness E, Cabalka A, et al: Isolated pulmonary Goodpasture syndrome. Pediatr Pathol 11: 635, 1991.
123. Thorner PS, Baumal R, Eddy A, Marrano P: Characterization of the NC1 domain of collagen type IV in glomerular basement membranes (GBM) and of antibodies to GBM in a patient with anti-GBM nephritis. Clin Nephrol 31: 160, 1989.
124. Kalluri R, Melendez E, Rumpf KW, et al: Specificity of circulating and tissue-bound autoantibodies in Goodpasture syndrome. Proc Assoc Am Phys 108: 134, 1996.
125. Levin M, Tigden SPA, Pincott JR, et al: Goodpasture's syndrome: treatment with plasmapheresis, immunosuppression, and anticoagulation. Arch Dis Child 58: 697, 1983.
126. Anand SK, Landing BH, Heuser ET, et al: Changes in glomerular basement membrane antigen(s) with age. J Pediatr 92: 952, 1978.
127. Siegler RL, Bond DP, Morris AH: Treatment of Goodpasture's syndrome with plasma exchange and immunosuppression. Clin Pediatr 19: 488, 1980.
128. Rydel JJ, Rodby RA: An 18-year-old man with Goodpasture's syndrome and ANCA-negative central nervous system vasculitis. Am J Kidney Dis 31: 345, 1998.
129. McCarthy LJ, Cotton J, Danielson C, et al: Goodpasture's syndrome in childhood: treatment with plasmapheresis and immunosuppression. J Clin Apheresis 9: 116, 1994.
130. Gilvarry J, Doyle GF, Gill DG: Good outcome in anti-glomerular basement membrane nephritis. Pediatr Nephrol 6: 244, 1992.
131. Harrity P, Gilbert-Barness E, Cabalka A, et al: Isolated pulmonary Goodpasture syndrome. Pediatr Pathol 11: 635, 1991.

Arthritis Related to Infection

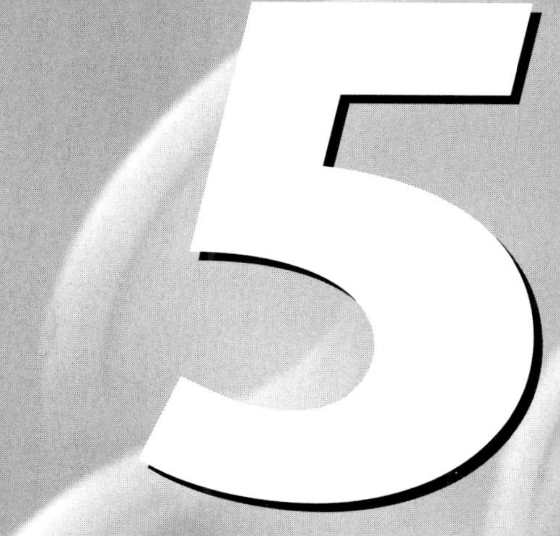

31

Infectious Arthritis and Osteomyelitis

James T. Cassidy and Ross E. Petty

The relation of infectious agents to arthritis is an area of great interest to the rheumatologist.[1] Important discoveries have led to an understanding of the origin, pathogenesis, treatment, and cure of at least one infection-related arthritis—Lyme disease—and have given impetus to investigations of other possible arthritogenic infectious agents. Recovery of viruses such as rubella and parvovirus from synovial fluid of patients with chronic arthritis has strengthened the argument that such agents may have an etiologic role in diseases such as juvenile rheumatoid arthritis (JRA) or rheumatoid arthritis (RA) in adults.

Arthritis related to infection can be regarded as either septic, reactive, or postinfectious.[2] *Septic arthritis* occurs when a viable infectious agent is present or has been present in the synovial space. Although direct bacterial infection of the joint constitutes the most widely recognized form of septic arthritis, direct infection with viruses, spirochetes, or fungi also occurs. *Reactive arthritis* is a response to an infectious agent that is or has been present in some other part of the body, usually the upper airway, the gastrointestinal tract, or the genitourinary tract. By definition, infectious agents are not recoverable from the synovial space in patients with reactive arthritis, which may be regarded as an autoimmune disorder resulting from immunologic cross-reactivity between articular structures and infectious antigens. The reactive arthritis group merges pathogenically with diseases such as the seronegative spondyloarthropathies (Reiter's syndrome and possibly juvenile ankylosing spondylitis). *Postinfectious arthritis* may be considered to be a special type of reactive arthritis in which immune complexes containing nonviable components of an initiating infectious agent may be present in the inflamed joint.

The precise relation of infection to arthritis is complex and by no means completely understood.[3] As techniques for the demonstration of infectious organisms improve, the frequency with which they are detected in synovial fluid or membrane is increasing, thus lending authority to the suspicion that some if not many of the arthritides of children are related to infectious diseases. For the same reasons, it is often difficult to categorize a disease as being postinfectious as opposed to reactive. Perhaps many of the so-called reactive arthritides will be found to represent diseases in which pathogens are actually present in the joint and therefore are, by definition, septic. In some of the viral arthritides that fit the concept of "reactive" arthritis—in that joint disease follows the onset of the acute illness by days or weeks—viral antigen or living virus can actually be isolated from synovial fluid lymphocytes or membrane when appropriate techniques are used. The same has been true for Lyme disease, in which early attempts to demonstrate *Borrelia* were unsuccessful, although the organisms have now been demonstrated by silver stain in several different laboratories. The lesson implicit in all of these observations is that in chronic arthritides that we currently consider aseptic, concerted investigations for infectious agents, using the most powerful techniques of molecular biology, may yet demonstrate the causative agent in the joint space. Although study of infectious agents such as viruses as possible initiators of some forms of arthritis in children has attracted much attention, it is important to remember that bacterial infections, both intra-articular and systemic, remain the most important curable causes of arthritis in childhood.

SEPTIC ARTHRITIS

Epidemiology

Septic arthritis of bacterial origin accounts for approximately 6.5 percent of all childhood arthritis.[4] Septic arthritis is more common in children, and it has been suggested that its frequency may actually be increasing.[5, 5a] However, the retrospective review by Fink and Nelson[6] of 591 cases of septic arthritis in children in Dallas from 1955 to 1984 does not document an increase in incidence. In one 1997 report, 12.7 percent of 1158 patients with septic arthritis were children under the age of 10 years.[7]

Sex Ratio and Age at Onset

Septic arthritis is slightly less common in girls than in boys, who account for 55 to 62 percent of patients in reported series.[8–10] Septic arthritis is found most often in the very young[11] and the very old: septic arthritis may occur in the neonate, is most common in children

Table 31–1

Age of Occurrence of Bacterial Septic Arthritis

	AGE			
	<2 yr	2–5 yr	6–10 yr	11–15 yr
Number	341	167	109	60
Percent of total	50	25	16	9

Data from Fink CW, Nelson JD: Septic arthritis and osteomyelitis in children. Clin Rheum Dis 12: 423, 1986; and Speiser JC, Moore TL, Osborn TG, et al: Changing trends in pediatric septic arthritis. Semin Arthritis Rheum 15: 132, 1985.

younger than 2 years, and diminishes in frequency throughout childhood until adolescence (Table 31–1).[6, 12]

Familial and Geographic Clustering

There does not appear to be a genetic predisposition to septic arthritis. Typical cases of presumed septic arthritis in which no pathogen is identified tend to occur in the summer and fall,[5] but geographic clustering has not been reported. In spirochetal arthritis, such as Lyme disease, there are marked geographic and seasonal outbreaks.

Etiology and Pathogenesis

The organisms that have been most commonly isolated from children with septic arthritis are *Staphylococcus aureus* and *Haemophilus influenzae* (Table 31–2).[5, 6, 9, 10, 13, 14] There are, however, considerable interinstitutional variations in the relative frequencies with which certain pathogens are identified and, more importantly, a strong relation to the age of the patient.[2, 6] *H. influenzae* type B had been the most common infection identified in children younger than 2 years. Routine vaccination of infants for *H. influenzae* has now decreased the frequency of infection with this organism.[14–16, 16a] After the age of 10 years, it is rarely a cause of septic arthritis. *Streptococcus pneumoniae* is a frequent cause of infection in children younger than 2 years and is not uncommon in the older child.[17, 17a] After 2 years of age, *S. aureus* is the most frequently occurring organism.[14] Group A streptococci and enterococci account for a small proportion of all cases of septic arthritis in childhood and are most prevalent in the 6- to 10-year-old age group. *Salmonella* arthritis constitutes approximately 1 percent of all cases of septic arthritis, and it is particularly common in association with sickle cell disease.[18] Infection with *Mycobacterium tuberculosis* is an unusual cause of septic monarthritis in childhood. Other unusual causes of infectious arthritis in children include *Streptobacillus moniliformis* (rat-bite fever), *Pseudomonas aeruginosa*, *Bacteroides* species, *Campylobacter fetus*, *Serratia* species, *Corynebacterium pyogenes*, *Pasteurella multocida*, and *Propionibacterium acnes*.

The neonate presents a somewhat different bacteriologic picture, with the majority of infants younger than 1 month having *S. aureus* (40 to 50 percent) or group B *Streptococcus* (20 to 25 percent) as the causative organisms.[6, 10, 19] Enterobacteriaceae, the gonococcus, and *Candida* species are also significant pathogens in the neonate.

Septic arthritis usually arises by hematogenous spread from a focus of infection elsewhere in the body.[20] Direct extension of an infection from overlying soft tissues (cellulitis, abscess) or bone (osteomyelitis)[21] or traumatic invasion of the joint accounts for only 15 to 20 percent of cases. Proliferation of bacteria in the synovial membrane results in accumulation of polymorphonuclear (PMN) leukocytes with the inflammatory effects outlined in Chapter 4. The ensuing damage to cartilaginous surfaces of the bone and the supporting structures of the joint may be severe and permanent if treatment is not urgently initiated.

Although trauma or extra-articular infection preceding onset of septic arthritis is common in case histories, knowledge of the etiologic significance of these factors is incomplete.[22] In one series, upper respiratory tract infections preceded septic arthritis in approximately 50 percent of patients, and approximately one third had received antibiotics within 1 week of onset.[5] A history of a mild, nonpenetrating injury to the affected extremity was elicited in approximately one third of patients. Intravenous drug users are at particular risk for septic arthritis of the sacroiliac (SI) and sternoclavicular joints, usually caused by gram-negative organisms.[23] Chronic inflammatory arthritis such as JRA may predispose to joint infection.[24]

Clinical Manifestations

Septic arthritis is usually accompanied by systemic signs of illness (e.g., fever, vomiting, headache) and

Table 31–2

Bacterial Species in Septic Arthritis in Children*

	FINK AND NELSON[6] n = 591 (%)	WELKON ET AL[5] n = 95 (%)	SPEISER ET AL[10] n = 86 (%)	WILSON AND DI PAOLA[9] n = 61 (%)
Hemophilus influenzae	25	29	17	16
Staphylococcus aureus	17	13	37	44
Other identified species	25	22	29	32

*Includes only cases in which organism was identified.

Table 31–3

Extra-Articular Sites of Infection in Children with Septic Arthritis

	NELSON AND KOONTZ[8] n = 117 (%)	WELKON ET AL[5] n = 95 (%)	SPEISER ET AL[10] n = 86 (%)
Osteomyelitis	12	12	26
Meningitis	4	4	11
Cellulitis, abscess	—	—	9
Respiratory tract	19	—	9
Middle ear	—	20	3
Urine	—	—	1
Genital tract	4	—	1
Pericardium	—	—	1
Pleura	—	—	1

may be a component of a more generalized infection that may include meningitis, cellulitis, osteomyelitis, or pharyngitis.[25] Joint pain is usually severe, and the infected joint and periarticular tissues are swollen, hot, and sometimes erythematous. Passive and active motion of the joint is severely, often completely, restricted (pseudoparalysis). Osteomyelitis frequently accompanies bacterial arthritis, and the presence of bone pain (as opposed to joint pain) should alert the examiner to this possibility. Other sites of hematogenous spread, although less frequent, are nonetheless important (Table 31–3).[5, 8, 10]

Affected Joints

The joints of the lower extremity are most commonly the sites of infection. Knees, hips, ankles, and elbows account for 90 percent of infected joints in children. Septic arthritis affecting the small joints of the hands or feet is rare (Table 31–4).[5, 6, 9, 10] Pyogenic SI joint disease can occur.[26]

Multiple Infected Joints

Although septic arthritis is most often a monarthritis, two or more joints are infected simultaneously or during the course of the same illness in a few children. In the large clinical experience reported by Fink and Nelson,[6] septic arthritis was monarticular in 93.4 percent but affected two joints in 4.4 percent, three in 1.7 percent, and four in 0.5 percent. Certain immune deficiencies, such as chronic granulomatous disease or AIDS, may predispose to septic arthritis in multiple joints.

Diagnosis

It is essential that every child with acute unexplained monarthritis undergo aspiration of the affected joint immediately because septic arthritis continues to be associated with considerable morbidity and mortality.[13, 27, 28] Synovial fluid should have the following procedures done immediately:

- Aspiration under sterile conditions
- Examination by Gram's stain
- White blood cell (WBC) and differential counts
- Glucose, lactate, and protein determinations
- Culturing on sheep's blood chocolate agar (for *H. influenzae* and *Neisseria gonorrhoeae*) and on MacConkey's agar (for gram-negative organisms)

If an anaerobic organism or mycobacterium is suspected, enriched medium and special anaerobic condi-

Table 31–4

Frequency of Infected Joints in Septic Arthritis

	FINK AND NELSON[6] n = 591 (%)	WELKON ET AL[5] n = 95 (%)	SPEISER ET AL[10] n = 86 (%)	WILSON AND DI PAOLA[9] n = 61 (%)	OVERALL n = 833 (%)
Knee	40	46	30	29	39
Hip	23	25	29	40	25
Ankle	13	15	17	21	14
Elbow	14	5	11	3	12
Shoulder	4	4	2	3	4
Wrist	4	—	1	1	3
PIP, MCP, MTP*	1	—	10	—	2
Other	1	5	—	1	1

*PIP, proximal interphalangeal; MCP, metacarpophalangeal; MTP, metatarsophalangeal.

Table 31–5

Laboratory Confirmation of Septic Arthritis in Children

	FINK AND NELSON[6] n = 591 (%)	WELKON ET AL[5] n = 95 (%)	SPEISER ET AL[10] n = 86 (%)	WILSON AND DI PAOLA[9] n = 61 (%)
Confirmed diagnosis (culture positive)	66	64	84	92
Positive synovial fluid Gram's stain	33	—	19–54*	—
Positive synovial fluid culture	79	84	36–70*	71–80†
Positive blood culture	33	46	46	41

*Dependent on prior administration of antibiotics.
†Dependent on procedure (aspiration = 80; arthrotomy = 71).

tions are necessary. Children in whom septic arthritis is considered should also have cultures of blood and of any potential source of infection (e.g., cellulitis, abscess, cerebrospinal fluid) performed. Rapid antigen latex agglutination tests for *H. influenzae*, group B and C streptococci, *Neisseria meningitidis*, and *S. pneumoniae* are available in most clinics. The polymerase chain reaction (PCR) more recently has proven useful in detecting evidence of infectious agents in synovial fluid.[29–32]

In a group of children with septic arthritis in whom the bacterial agent was identified, Fink and Nelson[6] reported that synovial fluid was culture-positive in 307 of 389 patients (79 percent) (Table 31–5).[5, 9, 10] The remaining 21 percent had positive cultures from sites other than the joint: blood (10 percent), cerebrospinal fluid (3.8 percent), blood and cerebrospinal fluid (2.3 percent), vagina (1.3 percent). Thus, 1 in 5 children with culture-positive septic arthritis had a negative synovial fluid culture but a positive culture from elsewhere, most often the blood. Although an organism can be identified in one third to two thirds or more of patients by culturing of all appropriate sites, no causative organisms are ever identified in approximately one third of children with pyogenic arthritis.[32a] In these patients, the diagnosis of septic arthritis is based on a typical history and the demonstration of frank pus by arthrocentesis.

Synovial Fluid Analysis

The characteristics of the synovial fluid depend somewhat on the duration and severity of the disease and previous administration of antibiotics. Synovial fluid may appear normal, turbid, or grayish green with bloody streaks (see Appendix). The synovial fluid WBC count is often markedly elevated with 90 percent PMNs. Speiser and colleagues[10] reported that synovial WBC counts in septic arthritis were less than 50,000/mm^3 (50 × 10^9/L) in 15 percent of children, 50,000 to 100,000/mm^3 in 34 percent, and more than 100,000/mm^3 in 51 percent. Fink and Nelson[6] noted a relatively low WBC count (<25,000/mm^3) in one third of their patients.

The protein content is high (>2.5 g/dl; >25 g/L) and the glucose concentration compared with plasma glucose is usually low in septic arthritis, although it may be normal. A Gram stain identifies the organism in half of untreated patients but in only one fifth of those who have received antibiotics. The advantage of performing a Gram stain is that it provides rapid confirmation of bacterial infection and tentative identification of the organism (if the findings are positive), thus permitting rational antibiotic therapy. Special procedures such as counterimmunoelectrophoresis, latex agglutination, or evaluation by PCR may sometimes identify bacterial antigens in a culture-negative fluid (blood, urine, or cerebrospinal fluid). These techniques have the advantage of providing antigenic identification much more rapidly than cultures, but they do not provide antibiotic sensitivities.

Blood Studies

At least two blood cultures should always be performed in a child suspected of having septic arthritis. An elevated WBC count with a predominance of PMNs and bands, and a markedly elevated erythrocyte sedimentation rate (ESR) or C-reactive protein—although of limited help in specific diagnosis—provide a baseline whereby the efficacy of subsequent treatment can be judged. Other acute-phase reactants are usually increased as well but provide no additional useful information.

Radiologic Examination

A number of imaging techniques are of value in evaluating a child with septic arthritis (Fig. 31–1).[33, 34] Radiographs of the affected area early in the course may demonstrate only increased soft tissue and capsular swelling but are occasionally useful in excluding the presence of a radiopaque foreign body or unsuspected trauma. Juxta-articular osteoporosis reflects inflammatory hyperemia and is evident within several days after onset of infection. Cartilage loss and narrowing of the joint space develop as the disease progresses. These changes are followed by marginal erosions and eventually by ankylosis (Fig. 31–2*A* and *B*).[33] Computed tomography (CT) and, especially, magnetic resonance imaging (MRI) are additional confirmatory techniques.

In the hip, accumulation of fluid within the joint

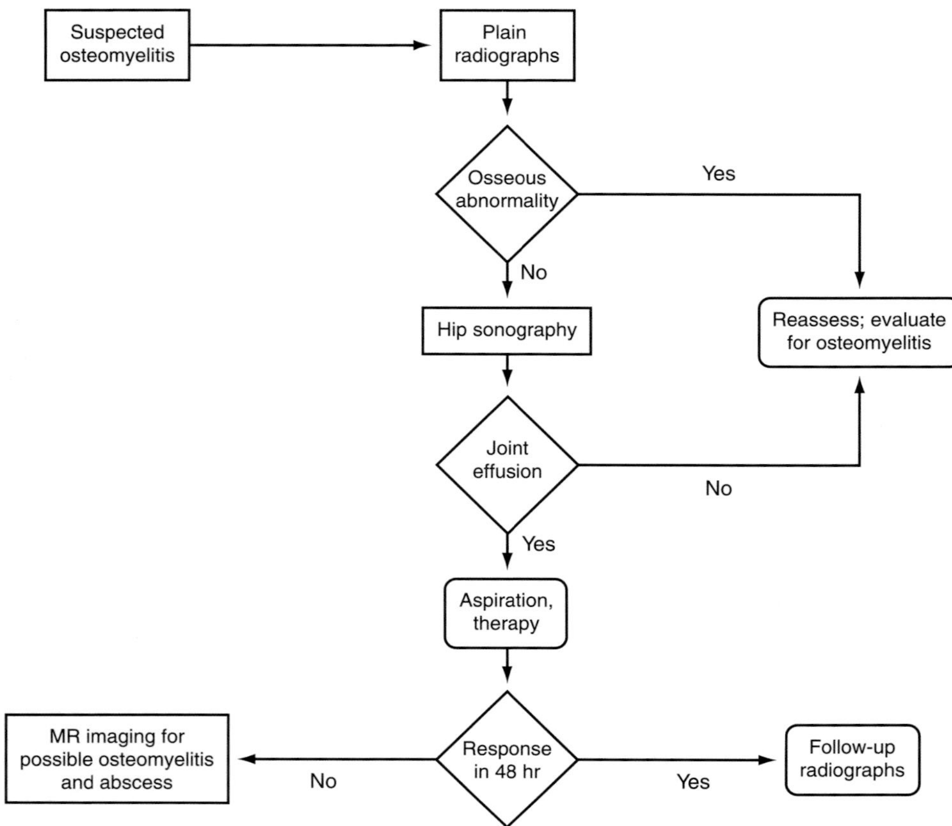

Figure 31–1. Flowchart of recommendations for evaluating septic arthritis in children. (Adapted from Jaramillo D, Treves ST, Kasser JR, et al: Osteomyelitis and septic arthritis in children: appropriate use of imaging to guide treatment. Am J Roentgenol 165:399–403, 1995.)

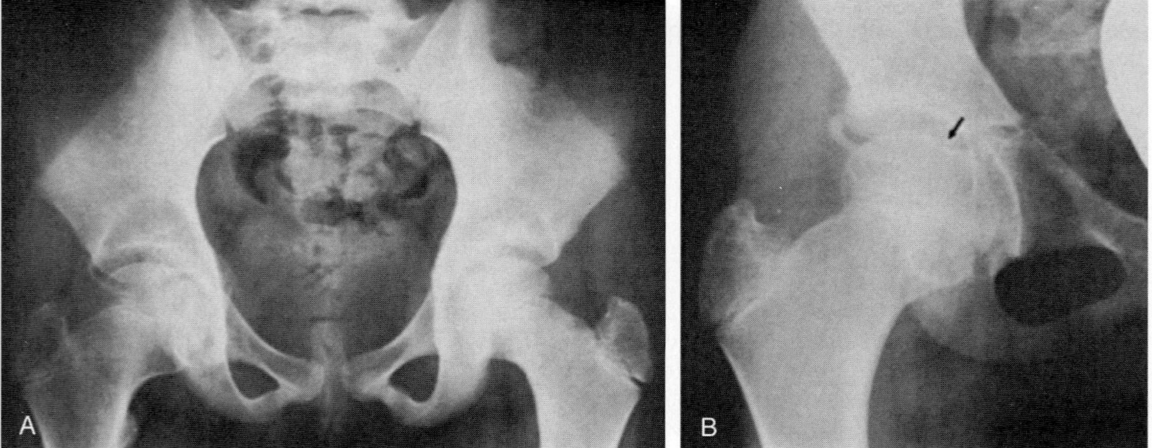

Figure 31–2. *A,* Questionable joint-space widening of the right hip of a 10-year-old girl with fever and an irritable hip. *B,* Repeat film taken 20 days later demonstrated epiphyseal demineralization and erosion (*arrow*).

displaces the gluteal fat lines laterally, or the obturator sign (displacement of the margins of this muscle medially) may be present. Traction applied to the leg during the radiographic procedure normally induces a radiolucent outline of the femoral head, the "vacuum" phenomenon. This lucency does not occur in the presence of increased intra-articular fluid.[33]

Ultrasonography

The ultrasonic detection of an effusion in the hip of a child being treated for osteomyelitis of the femur indicates the presence of septic arthritis of that joint.[33] Although the antibiotics administered for osteomyelitis and septic arthritis are similar, an effusion in the hip joint is sufficiently hazardous to the blood supply of the femoral head that open drainage is indicated.

Radionuclide Scans

During the first few days of disease, when plain radiographs show only soft tissue changes, technetium-99m scans reflect hyperemia of the infected area on blood-flow studies and increased uptake of the isotope on both sides of the joint.[35] This technique is useful in the early detection of joint or bone inflammation or infection,[26] but it does not differentiate the two with certainty. Radionuclide scans with gallium-67 or the patient's indium-111–labeled granulocytes can be used to identify accumulations of PMNs in infected sites, including joints with septic arthritis.

Magnetic Resonance Imaging

Delineation of soft tissue structures by MRI is superior to that provided by CT.[33, 36] Signal-intensity alterations in the bone marrow are characteristic but not diagnostic of septic arthritis (low intensity on fat-suppressed, gadolinium-enhanced, T1-weighted spin-echo images and high signal intensity on fat-suppressed, T2-weighted, fast spin-echo images).[37] Articular cartilage and growth cartilage in children are depicted along with other fibrous structures, muscle, blood vessels, and synovial fluid. An abnormal collection of fluid or debris, often displacing the joint capsule, eroding into other tissues, or in children, leading to subluxation, supports the possibility of septic arthritis.

Treatment

Antibiotics

In a child with septic arthritis, intravenous (IV) antibiotics should be administered as promptly as possible. The choice of antibiotic depends on the presence of predisposing factors, the age of the child, and the organisms that are suspected on the basis of the Gram stain or rapid antigen detection tests (although it is hazardous to narrow initial treatment based solely on these results because either can be wrong). Effective vaccination against *H. influenzae* type B has effectively eliminated approximately one third of the cases of childhood septic arthritis and has permitted initial therapy to be directed principally at Gram-positive cocci.[16] If the Gram stain and results of rapid antigen detection are negative or not available, an approach based on age (outlined in Table 31–6) is suggested.[38] The demonstration of an organism or antigen may support or contradict the generalizations outlined in this table and should influence the physician in selection of the initial antibiotic treatment.[27, 39]

It is prudent to monitor IV antibiotic efficacy with serum bactericidal titer determinations at frequent intervals initially and in follow-up for compliance, especially if home therapy is instituted. Once satisfactory control of the infectious process with IV antibiotic administration is achieved, treatment by the oral route, either in hospital or on an outpatient basis, may be appropriate.[40, 41, 41a] Such a program should be undertaken only after careful consideration and consultation with an expert in pediatric infectious disease.

If the culture is negative, IV antibiotics should be continued for a minimum of 21 days.[2] If the child's clinical state is improving (temperature returning to normal, pain diminishing, range of motion improving) and the WBC count and ESR are falling, the initial antibiotics should be maintained. If the patient does not appear to be responding, however, additional IV antibiotic coverage should be instituted.

Because of varying patterns of antibiotic susceptibility and resistance, guidelines regarding antibiotic choice and duration of treatment are constantly changing, and the physician is urged to review the most current recommendations.[38]

Aspiration and Drainage

The usefulness of repeated aspiration and drainage of an infected joint has been hotly debated. There is no

Table 31–6

Presumed Organisms in Septic Arthritis Based on the Age of the Child

INFANT	2–10 yr	>10 yr
Staphylococcus aureus	*(Hemophilus influenzae)*	*Staphylococcus aureus*
Group B streptococcus	*Staphylococcus aureus*	*Neisseria gonorrhoeae*
	Group A streptococcus	Group A streptococcus
Enterobacteriaceae	Enterobacteriaceae	Enterobacteriaceae

dispute that an initial diagnostic arthrocentesis must be performed. Indeed, any joint that appears to be under pressure from an effusion would probably benefit from aspiration, even if only for pain relief. Studies of the importance of repeated aspirations under other circumstances, however, have failed to show a consistent benefit. Similarly, open drainage is not better than closed needle aspiration (except for specific joints such as the hip) and is attended by significantly increased morbidity. Irrigation of the joint at the time of aspiration has no demonstrated additional benefit. Occasionally, arthroscopic examination is indicated.[42] Intra-articular administration of antibiotic is unnecessary because (1) therapeutic synovial fluid antibiotic levels are readily achieved,[43] and (2) it may actually induce chemical synovitis in the infected joint.

Course of the Disease and Prognosis

The outcome in septic arthritis is somewhat guarded because, even with early and appropriate antibiotic treatment, permanent damage is common. The child almost always recovers from the acute illness, but with the passage of time, reduction in range of motion, pain, and eventually degeneration of the surfaces of the affected joint may require surgical intervention.

Special Cases

Neonatal Septic Arthritis

Group B *Streptococcus* can be the offending organism in the neonate.[44] Septic arthritis in the neonate previously accounted for 16 per 1000 admissions,[45] but this condition may be undetected at onset because of its subtle presentation. The majority of affected newborns show no fever, toxemia, or leukocytosis. Any baby who has swelling in the region of the thigh or holds the leg flexed, abducted, or externally rotated must be investigated promptly. Problems in early recognition of disease undoubtedly contribute to the often disastrous outcome of this involvement.[46, 47]

Hip

Septic arthritis of the hip is such an important problem that it merits special attention.[48, 49] The femoral head is intracapsular, and the arterial supply passes via the ligamentum teres through the intracapsular space. Increased intracapsular pressure can therefore interrupt the blood supply to the femoral head, with disastrous consequences to its viability and the subsequent development of avascular necrosis.[50] Metaphyseal osteomyelitis readily leads to septic arthritis of the hip joint in the infant because nutrient blood vessels pass from the metaphysis through the epiphyseal growth plate and terminate in the distal ossification center.

Septic arthritis of the hip joint is most common in infants and very young children, 70 percent of patients being 4 years of age or younger.[51] The typical clinical picture is that of an infant or young child who has an unexplained fever, is irritable and inconsolable, and refuses to move an extremity, bear weight, or walk (pseudoparalysis). Any movement of the hip is extremely painful, and the affected leg is held in a position of partial flexion, abduction, and external rotation at the hip. Occasionally, the child has lower abdominal pain or tenderness, sometimes with paralytic ileus.

Predisposing factors are common with a septic hip, particularly in very young or premature infants.[52] In a study of septic arthritis of the hip of 16 infants younger than 4 weeks, 11 were premature, 7 had an umbilical catheter, and 12 had septicemia. In contrast, of 13 children aged 1 month to 3 years, none was premature or had an umbilical catheter, and only 5 were septicemic. A high frequency of preceding or accompanying osteomyelitis of the femur or pelvis has also been observed. The association of septic arthritis of the hip and femoral venipuncture has been recorded[53] and may account in part for the high frequency of arthritis of this site in the premature neonate.

Management of septic arthritis of the hip requires open drainage to minimize intra-articular pressure.[54, 54a] Traction and immobilization for the first 2 to 3 days of treatment provides pain relief but should be followed by passive and then active physiotherapy to prevent loss of range of motion. Prognosis is guarded even with the best treatment, especially in the neonate. The anatomy of the shoulder joint is not unlike that of the hip with respect to vascular supply. Septic arthritis of this joint, although rare, should be treated similarly.[55]

Gonococcal Arthritis

Arthritis caused by *N. gonorrhoeae* is most common in the adolescent, although it occasionally occurs in the neonate in association with disseminated infection.[12] It is more common in girls than in boys and is particularly likely just after menstruation or with pregnancy.[56] Gonococcal arthritis usually develops in patients with primary asymptomatic genitourinary gonorrhea or with a gonococcal infection of the throat or rectum. The patient presents with a systemic illness characterized by fever and chills.[57] A vesiculopustular rash, sparsely distributed on the extremities, commonly yields organisms on culture or Gram stain of the smear. Gonococcal arthritis may have an initial migratory phase and may be accompanied by tenosynovitis. In contrast with most patients with septic arthritis, those with gonococcal arthritis may present with a purulent arthritis of several joints. In a patient with suspected gonococcal arthritis, it is important to culture the genital tract, throat, rectum, and any vesicles as well as the affected joint. The possibility of sexual abuse should be considered and appropriately investigated.

Tuberculous Arthritis

Tuberculous arthritis is seldom encountered in North America or Europe, although its frequency may be

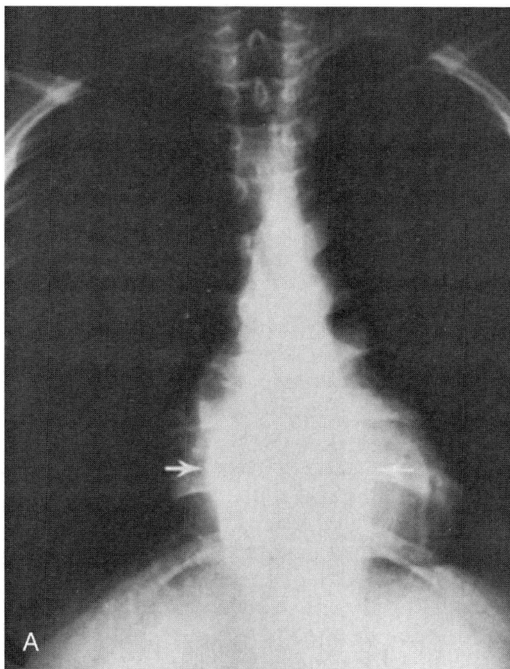

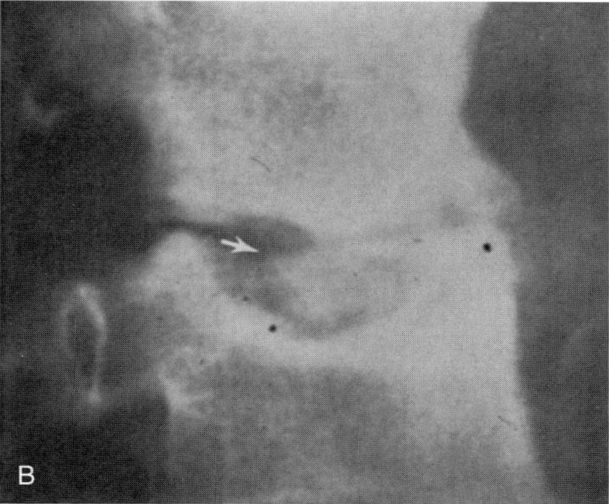

Figure 31–3. *A,* Pott's disease of the vertebral column in an adolescent boy with pulmonary tuberculosis. Extravertebral inflammatory mass (*arrows*). *B,* Destruction of disk space and vertebral end plate erosion (*arrow*).

increasing because of immunosuppressive therapy, drug-resistant strains of tuberculosis, and the HIV epidemic.[58–60] Tuberculous arthritis is by no means rare in other parts of the world. Typically, arthritis arises on a background of pulmonary tuberculosis as indolent, chronic monarthritis, often of the knee or wrist, that eventually results in extreme destruction of the joint and surrounding bones. Rarely, it presents as acute arthritis.[61] Joint infection occurs by hematogenous dissemination of the organism from adjoining osteomyelitis. Pott's disease is a consequence of vertebral osteomyelitis (Fig. 31–3*A* and *B*). Tuberculous dactylitis with cystic expansion and destruction of bone (spina ventosa) may occur (Fig. 31–4*A* and *B*).[62] A family or environmental history of pulmonary tuberculosis, together with a positive purified protein derivative (Mantoux) skin test,[61] should suggest the possibility of tuberculous arthritis. Although synovial fluid cultures are positive in approximately three quarters of patients, synovial membrane biopsy and culture are preferred and confirm the diagnosis in almost all patients (Fig. 31–5). The synovial WBC count is classically less than 50,000/mm^3 (50 $\times$ 10^9/L), with a high proportion of mononuclear cells. Genus-specific PCR is invaluable in

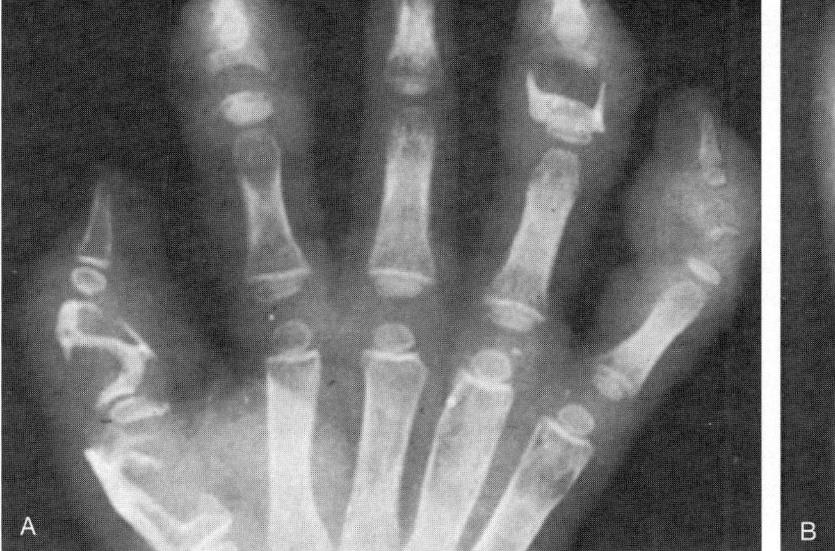

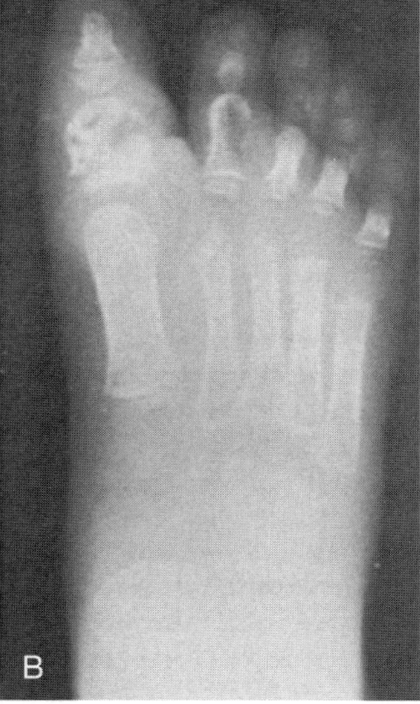

Figure 31–4. *A,* Advanced osseous destruction in the hand of a child with tuberculous dactylitis (spina ventosa). *B,* Similar changes in the foot.

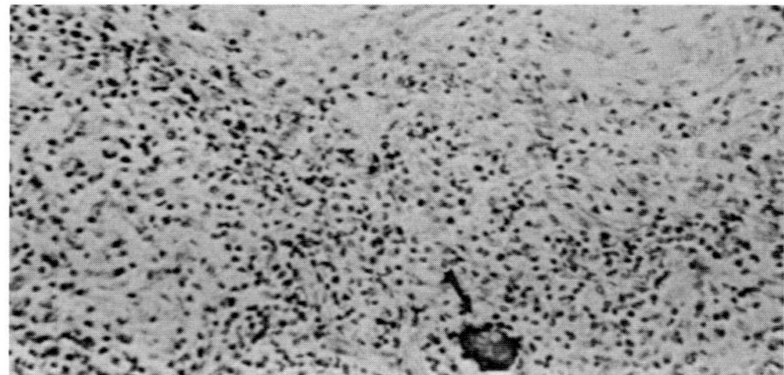

Figure 31–5. Synovial biopsy specimen of chronic inflammation in tuberculous joint disease. A giant cell (*arrow*) is indicated.

diagnosis.[32] Rarely, a polyarthritis accompanies tuberculosis (Poncet's disease); it probably represents a reactive arthritis because culture of the inflamed joints fails to demonstrate tubercle bacilli.[63, 63a]

Leprosy can result in both articular changes and inflammatory disease, including polyarthritis and subcutaneous nodules.[64] Clinical differentiation from JRA may be difficult, especially if the possibility of leprosy is not considered in a nonendemic area.[65] *Mycobacterium leprae* is not always easily identified in synovial biopsies.[66, 67]

Arthritis Associated With Brucellosis

Human *Brucella* infections are uncommon in North America, but there are European[68] and South American[69, 70] reports of substantial numbers of patients with this infection complicated by arthritis. The species most frequently implicated are *B. melitensis*[68–70] and, less commonly, *B. canis*.[71] Unpasteurized milk was a former source of infection.

The systemic illness is often mild in children but is usually characterized by undulant fever, gastrointestinal complaints, lymphadenopathy, and sometimes dermatitis. In 88 children from Israel,[72] clinical presentation of the acute disease varied, but the classic triad of fever (91 percent), arthralgia or arthritis (83 percent), and hepatosplenomegaly (63 percent) was characteristic of most patients. In a large series of cases from Peru,[69] almost one third were children and one third had arthritis. In the birth to 15-year age group, peripheral arthritis of a hip or knee was most common. Spondylitis and SI arthritis became predominant after 15 years of age. Synovial fluid WBC counts were only modestly elevated, with a slight predominance of mononuclear cells. Joint fluid culture was positive for the organism in some patients. Gomez-Reino and colleagues[68] noted that periarthritis without effusion was most common and that small joints and the spine were not affected. Whether this reflects differences in the infecting organism or in ascertainment is not known. Tetracyclines, aminoglycosides, rifampin, and trimethoprim-sulfamethoxazole provide effective treatment of the acute infection, although permanent sequelae may result.[68, 70] These drugs are often used in combination[72]; specific therapy should be addressed for each child.

Mycoplasma and Arthritis

Myalgia and arthralgia are common during pulmonary infection with *M. pneumoniae*. Objective oligoarticular, polyarticular, or migratory arthritis has also been described.[73] Two children have been reported who developed arthritis after an upper respiratory infection.[74] The association with mycoplasmal infection was confirmed in both by enzyme-linked immunosorbent assay (ELISA) and Western blot analysis.

Arthritis in Immunocompromised Patients

Chronic inflammatory arthritis in patients with a primary immunodeficiency is discussed in Chapter 35. Typical septic arthritis has been reported infrequently in immunodeficient children.[75] *Mycoplasma* is the most common cause of severe chronic erosive arthritis in patients with congenital immunodeficiency syndromes[76, 77] and has been recovered from joints of patients with AIDS.[78] *Ureaplasma ureolyticum* has been identified in patients with agammaglobulinemia.[79] *Candida albicans* is occasionally responsible for arthritis in immunosuppressed patients.[80] Patients with systemic lupus erythematosus are susceptible to septic arthritis; whether the arthritis occurs secondary to their disease, to asplenism, or to immunosuppressive treatment is not clear.

OSTEOMYELITIS

Although osteomyelitis is most often encountered and treated by specialists in orthopedics and infectious diseases, its frequent occurrence in association with septic arthritis and the diagnostic problems that it presents require that it be included in this discussion.[5a, 40, 81–84, 84a]

Definition and Classification

Osteomyelitis may be defined as intraosseous infection with bacteria or, rarely, fungi. It is classified as acute, subacute, or chronic. *Acute osteomyelitis* is of recent onset and short duration. It is most often hematogenous in origin but may result from trauma such as a compound fracture or puncture wound. It can be metaphyseal, epiphyseal, or diaphyseal in location. *Subacute osteomyelitis* is of longer duration and is usually caused by less virulent organisms. *Chronic osteomyelitis* results from ineffective treatment of acute osteomyelitis and is characterized by necrosis and sequestration of bone.

Epidemiology

Acute osteomyelitis is somewhat less common than acute septic arthritis. An incidence of 16.7 per 100,000 per year was reported from an institution at which acute septic arthritis occurred at a rate of 28.4 per 100,000 per year.[6] Osteomyelitis is more common than septic arthritis in developing countries of the world.[85] It occurs twice as often in boys as in girls[6, 86] and is more common in younger children. It can occur in the neonate.[44]

S. aureus (50 to 80 percent) and the group A streptococci (5 to 10 percent) are the predominant organisms at all ages.[6, 87] Even before specific immunization, *H. influenzae* seldom caused osteomyelitis (2 to 10 percent) and should now be even less common.[16a, 88] In certain circumstances, specific or unusual organisms (15 percent) are found. For example, infection of the calcaneus or other bone in the foot associated with a puncture wound through athletic footwear is likely to be due to *P. aeruginosa*.[20, 22, 88a, 89] Osteomyelitis caused by *S. pneumoniae*[17, 90] usually occurs in children with associated diseases such as sickle cell anemia,[91, 92, 92a] asplenia,[93] or hypogammaglobulinemia,[94] although it has been observed in young infants without underlying disease.[95] *Salmonella* osteomyelitis is a complication of sickle cell anemia but also occurs in normal children.[96] In the neonate, group B streptococci,[97, 98] gram-negative organisms,[99–101] and *Candida* in addition to *S. aureus* are all potential causes of osteomyelitis. *B. melitensis* uncommonly results in osteomyelitis, but when it does, it has a predilection for the vertebral bodies.[71] Tuberculous osteomyelitis may mimic chronic pyogenic disease, Brodie's abscess, tumor, or other types of granuloma.[102–104] *Bartonella henselae* (the organism of cat-scratch disease) has been identified as the causative agent in a few patients with osteomyelitis.[105–107]

Clinical Manifestations

Fever, severe bone pain, and tenderness with or without local swelling should suggest the possibility of acute osteomyelitis. Although a history of prior trauma is elicited in approximately one third of young patients, its significance is uncertain. In the infant, fever may be minimal and localization of the pain may be difficult on physical examination.[108] Pseudoparalysis of a limb is often evident. Clinical evidence of a preceding systemic infection may be present. The site of infection is usually metaphyseal, and bony tenderness is elicited by pressure near or over the infected area. There may also be an area of overlying cellulitis, especially in the infant, in whom the thin cortex allows pus to erode into the periosteal structures. The presence of a joint effusion adjacent to the site of bone infection may reflect septic arthritis or a sterile noninflammatory "sympathetic" effusion.[108a]

Osteomyelitis in children has a predilection for the metaphysis of rapidly growing bone. Many explanations have been suggested for this tendency. The anatomic differences in vasculature in this area in children and its easily compromised blood supply may in part explain the clinical observation (see Chapter 2). In one anatomic model, bacteremia and, in some cases, preceding microtrauma were sufficient to initiate disease.[109] The bones of the lower extremity are affected in two thirds of patients; those of the upper extremity account for approximately 25 percent; but those of the skull, face, spine, and pelvis are the site of infection in fewer than 10 percent (Table 31–7).[6, 86, 110–113] A small proportion (<10 percent) of children have two or more simultaneously infected bones; in some cases, five or more bones are involved as part of a severe septicemic illness, usually caused by staphylococci. This type of involvement must be distinguished from chronic recurrent multifocal osteomyelitis (discussed later).

Brodie's Abscess

Subacute osteomyelitis, usually of staphylococcal origin, may develop after a penetrating injury or by hematogenous spread of an infection to the metaphysis. It is characterized clinically by localized soft tissue swelling

Table 31–7

Comparison of Affected Sites in Septic Osteomyelitis and Chronic Recurrent Multifocal Osteomyelitis (CRMO)

BONE	OSTEOMYELITIS* (%)	CRMO† (%)
Tibia	25	28
Clavicle	<1	13
Fibula	6	10
Spine	1	10
Femur	27	9
Metatarsus, metacarpus, phalanx	4	9
Radius	4	6
Pelvis	6	4
Humerus	11	3
Ulna	2	3
Sternum	<1	3
Mandible	<1	1
Scapula	<1	1
Rib	<1	1
Talus	1	1
Calcaneus	6	0

*Data from Fink CW, Nelson JD: Septic arthritis and osteomyelitis in children. Clin Rheum Dis 12: 423, 1986, and Cole WG, Dalziel RE, Leitl S: Treatment of acute osteomyelitis in childhood. J Bone Joint Surg 64B: 218, 1982.

†Data from Sonozaki H, Mitsui H, Miyanaga Y, et al: Clinical features of 53 cases with pustulotic arthro-osteitis. Ann Rheum Dis 40: 547, 1981.

Table 31–8
Brodie's Abscess

Symptoms: Pain may be severe; child awakens at night
Signs: Evidence of a penetrating injury of hematogenous spread; first week, soft tissue swelling; second week, metaphyseal osteolytic lesion with surrounding sclerosis
Investigations: Sterile joint effusion; curettage/cultures may be negative
Treatment: Immobilization; NSAIDs; antibiotics

NSAIDs, nonsteroidal anti-inflammatory drugs.

and tenderness with marked pain that may awaken the child at night (Table 31–8). Radiographs demonstrate only soft tissue swelling in the first week, but metaphyseal osteolytic lesions are evident by the second week of the illness. They are most common in the proximal or distal ends of the tibia (Fig. 31–6*A–C*).[114, 115] Culture of the abscess may be negative. Treatment includes IV antibiotics, a nonsteroidal anti-inflammatory drug (NSAID), and immobilization.

Chronic Recurrent Multifocal Osteomyelitis

The syndrome known as *chronic recurrent multifocal osteomyelitis* (CRMO), first described by Giedion in 1972,[114] clinically mimics septic osteomyelitis. The cause is unknown; cultures for bacteria are almost always negative, although it has been speculated that a viral, chlamydial, mycoplasmal, or fastidious slow-growing organism could be responsible for this syndrome.[116–121, 121a]

Clinically, patients with CRMO experience an acute or insidious onset of multifocal bone pain, accompanied by fever (Table 31–9). The course of the disease is characterized by periodic painful relapses and remissions. In a review of the anatomic distribution of 181 lesions in 35 patients, Gamble and Rinsky[118] found that long bones such as the tibia were most often affected. The ribs, clavicles, and vertebral bodies may also be involved.[122] Radiographic changes are similar to those of septic osteomyelitis, with osteolytic lesions identified early in the illness that gradually become surrounded by sclerosis and enlargement of the affected bones (Fig. 31–7). Unusual presentations may lead to diagnostic delay.[77, 122, 122a] Bone scans demonstrate the presence of multiple areas of involvement and occasional involvement of the epiphysis.[123, 124] Biopsy does not confirm an infectious organism but is often necessary to eliminate other diagnostic possibilities. Histologic examination shows necrosis and new bone formation together with acute and chronic inflammatory cells with fibrosis.[117] The lesions of CRMO heal without specific treatment but may recur months or years later. Antibiotics are unnecessary and ineffective. NSAIDs and, occasionally, glucocorticoids bring symptomatic relief. Interferon-γ has been used to treat one child with chronic recurrent multifocal osteomyelitis.[125] Prognosis is uncertain, however, and the course of this painful disorder may be prolonged.

Table 31–9
Multifocal Osteomyelitis

Fever is usually present but may be absent
ESR is usually elevated
Pustular dermatitis is occasionally an antecedent event
Bone scan confirms metaphyseal lesions

ESR, erythrocyte sedimentation rate.

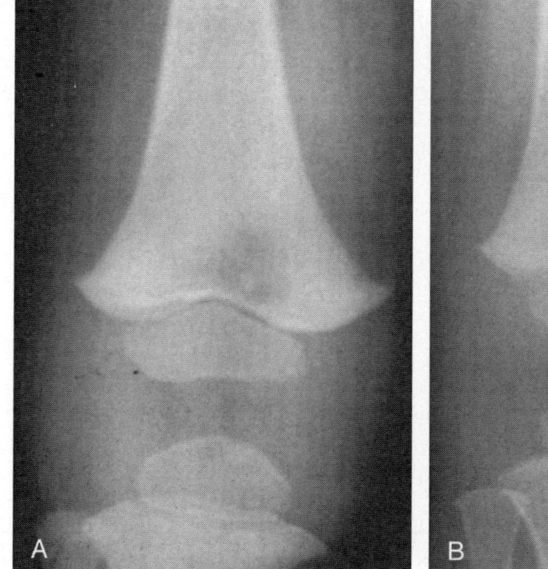

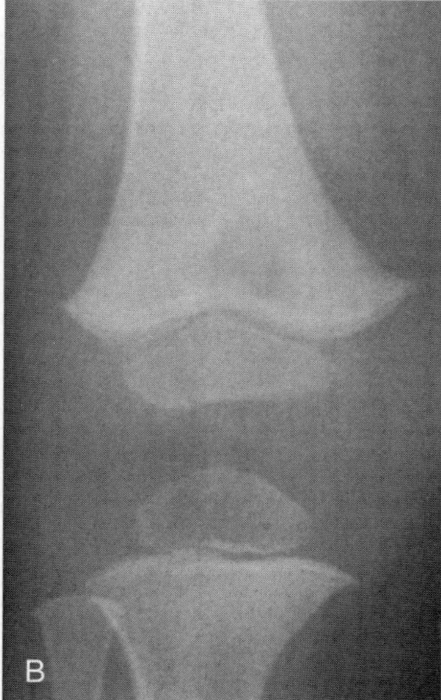

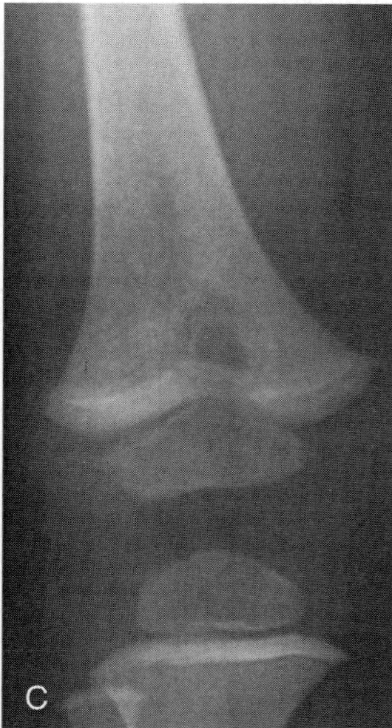

Figure 31–6. Brodie's abscess. Radiographs of knee of 16-month-old boy with inadequately treated acute hematogenous osteomyelitis 1 month previously. *A,* Central sequestration with surrounding ill-defined lytic margin. Patient was appropriately treated with antibiotics at this stage. *B,* One month later, sequestrum has been removed by osteoclasts. *C,* One month later, radiograph shows well-defined lesion with sclerotic borders. (*A–C,* Courtesy of Dr. B. Wood.)

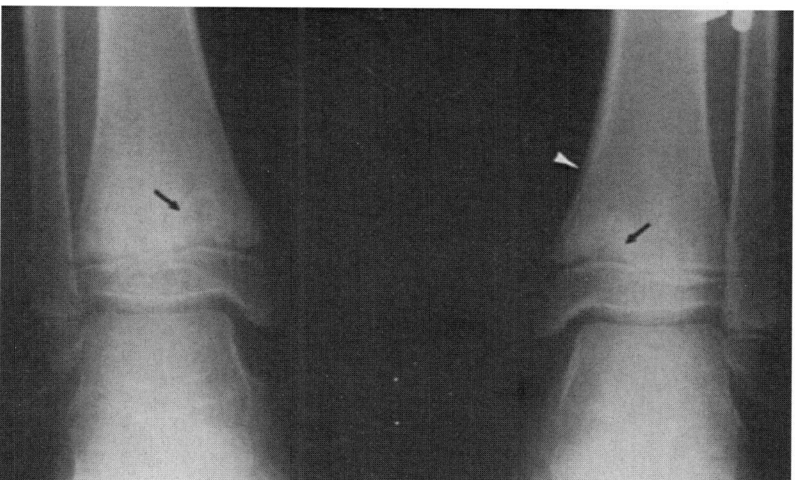

Figure 31–7. Radiographs of a patient with chronic recurrent multifocal osteomyelitis affecting both distal tibiae. There are lytic lesions of both distal tibiae (*arrows*) and periosteal new bone apposition (*arrowhead*).

In a large series from Japan, Sonozaki and coworkers[110] noted inflammatory oligoarthritis in one quarter of patients and SI joint disease resembling ankylosing spondylitis in a small proportion. In contrast with the satisfactory outcome of most patients, two recent reports have documented a less favorable end-result of CRMO, with leg-length discrepancy and valgus deformity.[110, 123, 126] Bjorksten and associates[127] described a cutaneous complication, *palmoplantar pustulosis,* in six of nine patients, and two of the seven patients reported by Laxer and colleagues[117] had palmoplantar pustulosis and psoriasis. The relation of these skin changes to the bony lesions of this syndrome is not known.[128] Pyoderma gangrenosum has been described as a complication of CRMO.[129]

Caffey's disease (infantile cortical hyperostosis), a rare disorder of infancy, may be confused with osteomyelitis. It is characterized by fever, irritability, and swelling associated with hyperostosis of the mandible, clavicles, and long bones (see Chapter 36).[130] The SAPHO (synovitis, acne, pustulosis, hyperostosis, osteomyelitis) syndrome may be another variant.[130a]

Diagnosis

As in septic arthritis, it is essential that every reasonable attempt be made to identify the organism and determine its antibiotic susceptibility.[81] Aspiration of subperiosteal pus is the diagnostic procedure of choice and, together with cultures of the blood, synovial fluid, or infected wound, should yield an organism in approximately 70 to 80 percent of cases.[16] A bone biopsy may be desirable or necessary if other sites of culture prove negative. The WBC and differential counts and the ESR provide little help with diagnosis; they are useful in assessing effectiveness of therapy.

Radiographic evaluation may delineate soft tissue swelling very early, but osteoporosis is not evident until days 10 to 14, and diagnostic findings may not be present until days 10 to 21 (Fig. 31–8*A–D*; Fig. 31–9).[34] Radionuclide scanning (technetium-99m polyphosphonate or diphosphonate) provides a sensitive, if nonspecific, method for the early detection of increased blood flow and uptake in the infected bone (see Fig. 31–8*C*).[20, 35, 130b] A bone scan is particularly helpful in localizing osteomyelitis in the neonate or infection of the axial skeleton.[26, 96] It is also of use in searching for subclinical areas of infection in multifocal osteomyelitis. A positive result is not necessarily diagnostic of osteomyelitis, but a negative scan is unlikely in a child with bacterial osteomyelitis, except in the very early stages of the illness.

MRI is often superior to other modalities in identifying osteomyelitis in the marrow cavity in children (see Fig. 31–8*D*).[26, 131, 132, 132a] T1- or T2-weighted images, fat suppression, and gadolinium enhancement can confirm a focal area of increased inflammatory exudate (protons/water). A major advantage of MRI in early disease—over plain radiographs, ultrasonography,[133, 133a, 133b] or CT—is the delineation of soft tissue or subperiosteal pus.[134, 135]

Treatment

In the absence of specific indications to the contrary,[41] the initial antibiotic choices in the treatment of acute osteomyelitis should be effective against methicillin-resistant *S. aureus* (see Table 31–6). IV antibiotics for 4 to 6 weeks have been traditionally recommended, with subsequent oral coverage if appropriate. Recent recommendations have included a shortened course of IV treatment.[16, 136, 137] Surgical treatment, which should be kept to a minimum,[16, 138] includes drainage of subperiosteal and soft tissue abscesses and débridement of associated lesions. Immobilization of the extremity for relief of pain is often necessary; otherwise, weight bearing may be permitted as tolerated by the patient.

Course of the Disease and Prognosis

The most dreaded complications of acute osteomyelitis are chronic osteomyelitis and impaired bone growth.[139] Chronic osteomyelitis should be suspected in a child whose systemic symptoms have responded slowly or incompletely to antibiotics or in whom there is a late

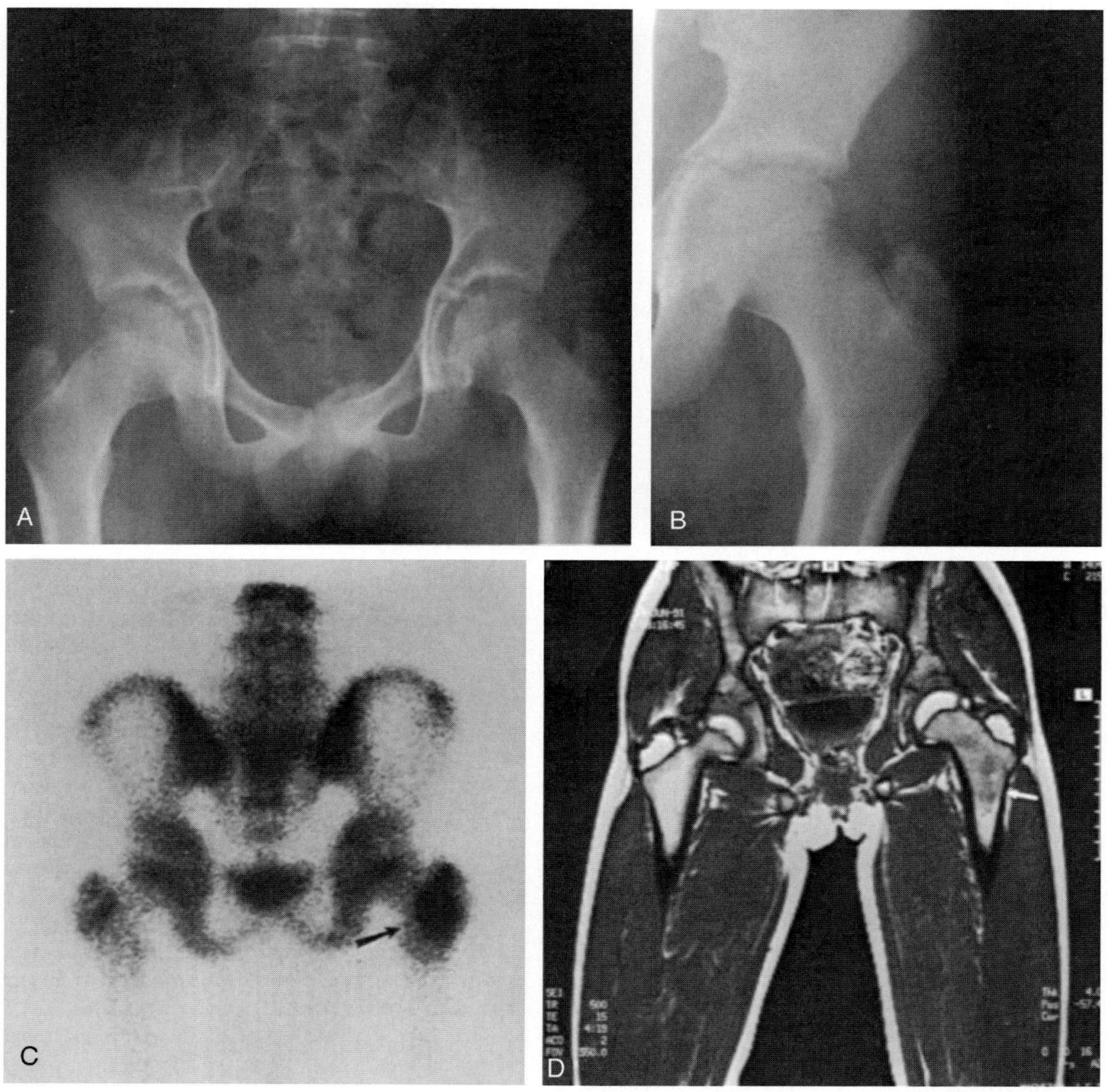

Figure 31–8. *A,* Anteroposterior radiograph of pelvis in a 14-year-old boy with fever and an irritable left hip. This film and close-up of left hip *(B)* are normal. *C,* Bone scan documents increased uptake of technetium-99m in area of left proximal femur (*arrow*). *D,* MRI demonstrates an increased marrow signal in same area of left hip *(arrow)* indicative of acute osteomyelitis.

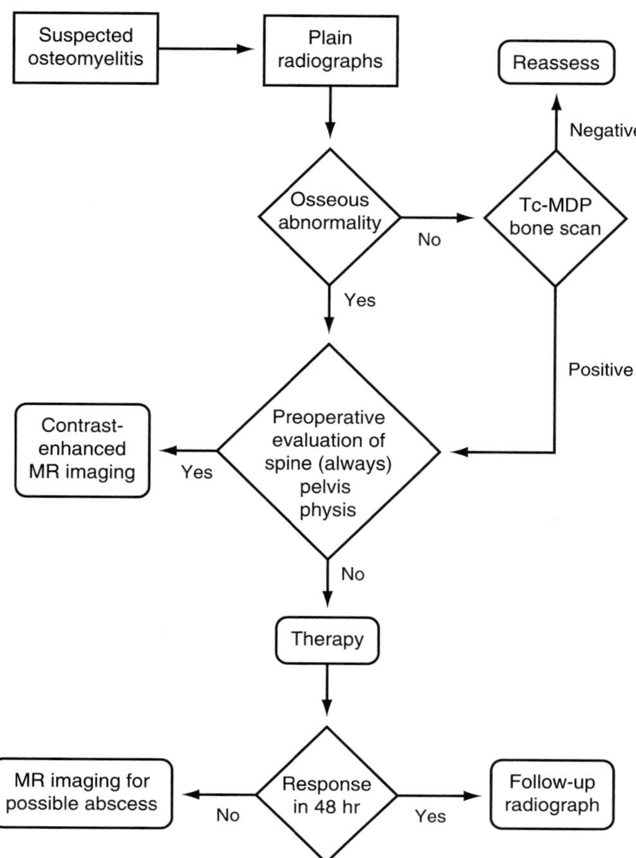

Figure 31–9. Flowchart of recommendations for evaluating acute hematogenous osteomyelitis in children. (Adapted from Jaramillo D, Treves ST, Kasser JR, et al: Osteomyelitis and septic arthritis in children: appropriate use of imaging to guide treatment. Am J Roentgenol 165:399–403, 1995.)

recurrence of pain at the affected site. Radiographic studies at that time show a radiolucent involucrum (granulation tissue) surrounding dead (sclerotic) sequestered bone.

Related Disorders

Diskitis

There is considerable dispute as to whether diskitis is basically an infectious process. Infection of an intervertebral disk space secondary to osteomyelitis of an adjoining vertebral body is rare.[140] However, acute diskitis, unassociated with vertebral osteomyelitis, is a self-limited inflammation of an intervertebral disk that may be caused by pathogens of low virulence, although bacteria or viruses are seldom recovered by aspiration. *S. aureus* and Enterobacteriaceae or *Moraxella* are responsible in some patients. Diskitis occurs throughout childhood, but half of the cases present before 4 years of age (peak age, 1 to 3 years).[141, 142] The sex ratio is approximately equal, although one review noted that diskitis was more frequent in girls.[143]

Clinical signs may be subtle. Diskitis is characterized by vague back pain and stiffness, often resulting in a characteristic tripod position during sitting or other unusual posturing.[144, 145] The child, who almost always has a low-grade fever, usually refuses to walk, stand, or bend over and may complain of abdominal pain. Palpation of the spine produces well-localized tenderness, almost always in the lower lumbar region. The ESR is usually moderately elevated.

Plain radiographs of the affected area often appear normal until late in the disease (Fig. 31–10*A* and *B*). A technetium-99m bone scan is valuable diagnostically (Fig. 31–11). The L4-L5 interspace is most often affected (44 percent), followed by L3-L4 (37 percent), L2-L3 (7 percent), and L5-S1 (6 percent).[141, 142, 146, 147] The cervical spine may also be involved. In one study, disk space narrowing was present in 82 percent of children and a bone scan was positive in 72 percent.[144] MRI may be valuable in differentiating infection from other conditions, including idiopathic disk calcification.[148, 149, 149a] Aspiration of the disk space or disk biopsy should not be routinely necessary. Treatment is supportive with immobilization. If bacterial infection is suspected, IV antibiotics should be instituted until results of blood cultures are available; otherwise, the course of the disease may be prolonged.

Arthritis Associated With Acne

The association between arthritis and acne has been reviewed by Davis and associates.[150] Most patients are male and experience onset of musculoskeletal complications during adolescence. The syndrome includes severe truncal acne followed in several months by fever and arthralgia or arthritis, most often involving hips, knees, and shoulders. Myopathy may also accompany this disorder (see Chapter 20).[151] We have observed one such boy with pain and swelling in the sternoclavicular, knee, and ankle joints and SI tenderness. Synovial histology was characterized by nonspecific proliferative synovitis. SI joint radiographs confirmed early bilateral inflammatory changes. The patient was positive for HLA-B27. It is possible that this syndrome is another example of reactive arthritis. Although arthritis lasts for only a few months in some patients, recurrences over many years have been documented.[150, 152] Treatment with NSAIDs, and antibiotics for control of the acne, is indicated. It should be noted that isotretinoin can cause an acute arthritis.[153–156]

Whipple's Disease

Whipple's disease, first described in 1907,[157] is extremely rare in childhood (approximately five children <15 years of age).[158] It is characterized by abdominal pain, weight loss, diarrhea, and in 65 to 90 percent of patients, arthralgias or arthritis.[159–161] Whipple's disease occurs 10 times more frequently in males than in females and is most common in middle age, although it has been identified in a 3-month-old boy[162] and a 7-year-old boy[163]; there is also one report of central nervous system disease in a young boy.[158] Migratory, peripheral joint pain and inflammation, lasting hours to months, occur over a period of many years, often in association with fatigue, weight loss, and anemia. Joint swelling with increased synovial fluid and restriction of range of motion may occur,[164] although residual deformity does not.[159]

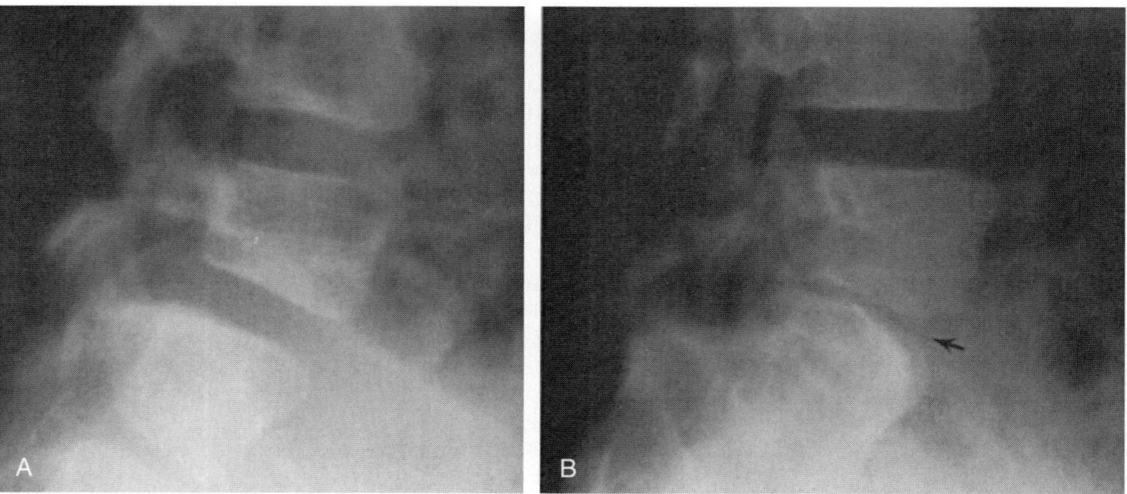

Figure 31–10. *A,* Normal disk space on lateral view of lumbar spine. *B,* Collapse of space from diskitis (*arrow*).

The joints most frequently affected are ankles, knees, shoulders, and wrists,[164] and spondylitis has been reported in 20 percent (see Chapter 13).[165] Periodic acid–Schiff–positive material and bacteria are detectable in macrophages infiltrating the upper small intestine and abdominal lymph nodes. Although the role of the bacterium (*Tropheryma whippelii*), if any, is unknown, antimicrobial therapy (e.g., tetracycline, penicillin, streptomycin) has greatly improved the outcome in this disease.

ARTHRITIS CAUSED BY VIRUSES

A classification of viruses known to be associated with arthritis in humans is shown in Table 31–10.[166] The togaviruses account for most of the viral arthritides. In general, viral arthritides occur much more often in adults than in children.[167] Arthralgia is more common than objective arthritis, and both are usually migratory and of short duration (1 to 2 weeks), disappearing without residual joint disease. Small joints are most often affected by rubella, hepatitis B, and members of the alphavirus group (e.g., Ross River, chikungunya), whereas one or two large joints (usually the knees) are most often affected by mumps, varicella, and other viruses. In some viral arthritides, virus can be isolated from the joint space (rubella, varicella, herpes simplex, cytomegalovirus); in others, only virus-containing immune complexes are found (hepatitis B, adenovirus 7); and in still others, neither virus nor viral antigen can be recovered from the joint.[168] Whether this represents limitations of recovery and culture techniques or the fact that culture-negative viral arthritis is "reactive" rather than "septic" is not known.

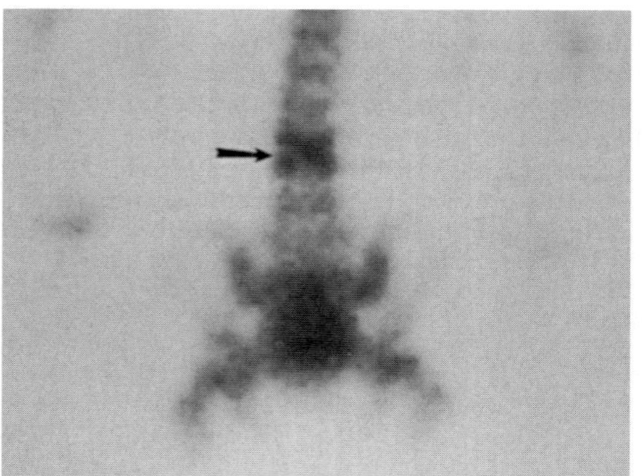

Figure 31–11. Diskitis. Technetium-99m bone scan of 2½-year-old girl with back pain demonstrates increased uptake of isotope in inferior end plate of L2 and superior end plate of L3 (*arrow*) characteristic of diskitis. (Courtesy of Dr. H. Nadel.)

Rubella Virus

Rubella-associated arthropathy was recognized by Osler[169] and was one of the most commonly identified virus-associated arthritides in North America. Musculoskeletal symptoms after natural rubella infection are relatively common in young women. These symptoms are unusual in preadolescent children and in males, however, and are much less frequent after rubella immunization than after natural infection. Not only is arthritis more common after natural infection, it is also more severe and lasts longer (see Chapter 12).[170]

Arthralgia usually begins within 7 days of the appearance of the rash, or 10 to 28 days after immunization. The joints of the fingers, and later the knees, are most frequently affected. Joint pain may be accompanied by warmth, erythema, and effusion, and tenosynovitis is common. Carpal tunnel syndrome has also been reported. These findings usually disappear within 3 to 4 weeks but occasionally persist for months or even years.

In a study of natural rubella infection in 37 teenage students, 52 percent of girls and 8 percent of boys developed objective arthritis,[170] and an additional 13 percent and 48 percent, respectively, experienced arthralgia. In a group of young women who received RA 27/3 rubella vaccine, 14 percent developed an acute polyarthritis.[170] Arthralgia and

Table 31–10

Viruses That Cause Arthritis in Humans

VIRUS	COMMENT
Togaviruses	
Rubivirus	
Rubella	Global; most reports from North America and Europe
Alphaviruses	
Ross River	Australasia
Chikungunya	Africa, Asia
O'nyong-nyong	Africa
Mayaro	South America
Sindbis	Africa, Asia, Australia
Ockelbo	Sweden
Pogosta	Finland
Parvoviruses	B19 associated with fifth disease
Hepadnaviruses	
Hepatitis B	Global
Adenoviruses	
Adenovirus 7	Rare
Herpesviruses	
Epstein-Barr	Rare; suggested role in RA
Cytomegalovirus	Rare
Varicella-zoster	Rare
Herpes simplex	Rare
Paramyxoviruses	
Mumps	Rare
Enteroviruses	
Echovirus	Rare
Coxsackievirus B	Rare
Orthopoxvirus	
Variola virus (Smallpox)	Nonexistent today
Vaccinia virus	Rare

Modified from Petty RE, Tingle AJ: Arthritis and viral infection. J Pediatr 113: 948, 1988.

arthritis are most common in adults, although approximately 25 percent of prepubertal females develop arthralgia and 10 percent an arthritis.[171, 172] Chronic arthritis in adult women has been reported after vaccination in 5 to 11 percent.[173, 174] It has been suggested that reinfection contributes to arthritis in susceptible hosts.[175] Pre-immunization IgG and IgA antirubella antibodies were present in six of six patients who developed vaccine-associated arthropathy.[176] Rubella virus can be recovered from the synovial fluid of patients with rubella arthritis in many[177, 178] but not all instances.[167, 179] In one study of JRA, virus was isolated from synovial or peripheral blood mononuclear cells in 7 of 19 children but from no control subjects.[180] Other investigations have failed to confirm that rubella virus was associated with chronic arthritis.[181]

Parvovirus

Parvoviruses are the latest candidates in the list of viruses putatively involved in the etiology of RA in adults.[182, 183] Parvovirus RA-1 has been isolated from the synovial membrane of one patient with classic RA.[184, 185] A second parvovirus, B19, is now known to be the agent responsible for erythema infectiosum (*fifth disease* or *slapped cheek syndrome*).[186] This illness is sometimes accompanied by an arthritis not unlike that of rubella infection.[36, 167, 185, 187–189]

Arthralgia, symmetric joint swelling, and morning stiffness have been described in adults, especially women, after parvovirus B19 infection.[189] Carpal tunnel syndrome, hepatitis, and angioedema have been noted. This syndrome may be more widespread than previously thought and considerably underdiagnosed. In some patients, symptoms have persisted for years. An early study of erythema infectiosum in 364 patients indicated that joint pain, most often affecting knees and wrists, was present during the first week in 77 percent of adults and 8 percent of patients younger than 20 years.[190] Subsequently, it was determined that arthritis was most common in patients who were HLA-DR4 positive.[191] Whether a chronic arthritis results from parvovirus B19 infection is still controversial.[168, 192]

Parvovirus is an autonomously replicating species first identified in 1975.[193] Infection is common and widespread. Parvovirus B19 genome consists of a linear, 5.6 kD, single-stranded DNA. There is only one serotype of parvovirus B19. Human parvovirus B19 has been implicated as the causative agent in erythema infectiosum, aplastic crises, some cases of hemophagocytic syndrome, and hydrops fetalis.[194] Erythema infectiosum, or fifth disease, is a common exanthem of older children that lasts for a few days to a week and presents with a low-grade fever, an erythematous facial rash ("slapped cheeks"), and a lacy, reticular rash on the extremities. These manifestations often recur with malaise, irritability, and arthralgia.

Only a few cases of children with documented B19-associated arthritis have been reported.[36, 187, 195, 196] Joint symptoms tend to be mild and transient. In the children reported by Reid and coworkers,[187] there was symmetric involvement of the small joints of the hands and feet. In one child, the arthritis preceded development of the rash. In another, the arthritis persisted for 3 months. Antinuclear antibodies (ANAs) and rheumatoid factors (RFs) were absent in all of the patients in this series. Rivier and colleagues[36] described a 5-year-old boy with arthritis of one knee that lasted for 6 weeks after typical erythema infectiosum. In the report by Nocton and associates,[196] 20 of 22 children with parvovirus B19 infection developed acute arthritis, but 2 had only arthralgias. The arthritis was associated with constitutional symptoms in half of the children and was of brief duration (<4 months) in 14. Six children had persistent arthritis lasting up to 13 months: criteria for a diagnosis of JRA would have been met in this group. Laboratory results were generally normal, however, except for serologic evidence of the B19 infection.

The precise relation of the viral infection to arthritis has not been clarified. The virus has not been grown from synovial fluid or blood in patients with joint symptoms, although B19-specific DNA has been identified by hybridization in the synovial fluid of adults[197] and by PCR amplification in synovial tissue.[198] However, Soderlund and colleagues[199] demonstrated genomic B19 DNA in the synovium of joints that had suffered trauma even more frequently than in those of children with chronic arthritis. Inflammatory synovitis may not be identifiable by arthroscopy. Although infection gives rise first to IgM antibodies[200] and then to IgG antibodies, there is no evidence that the arthropathy represents an immune complex disease. Demonstration of IgM antibodies, however, is essential to diagnosis. The prevalence of IgG antibodies in the general population is too high to be diagnostically helpful, unless a fourfold increase concurrent with the clinical symptoms is demonstrated.[201–203]

Hepatitis B Arthritis-Dermatitis Syndrome

In adults, up to 20 percent of infections with hepatitis B virus are characterized by a period of rash and arthritis that resembles serum sickness.[204] In a review of reported cases of arthritis associated with hepatitis B infection,[205] the age of the patients ranged from 14 to 56 years and the sex ratio was 1.5 males:1 female. The dermatitis is characterized by a maculopapular rash, sometimes with petechiae, or urticaria, and is most prominent on the lower extremities. The arthritis usually begins abruptly and symmetrically and affects the interphalangeal joints in 82 percent, knees in 30 percent, and ankles in 24 percent of patients. Although erythema and warmth are present, synovial effusions are uncommon. Joint symptoms last for 4 weeks on average, respond well to NSAIDs, and disappear without sequelae. The ESR is usually normal, although serum and synovial fluid complement levels are low in the early stages of the illness.[206] Synovial fluid has been reported to show a mononuclear cell predominance.[207] Electron microscopic evidence of hepatitis antigen in the synovial membrane has been reported.[208] Hepatitis C virus is lymphotrophic and is associated with rheumatic symptoms secondary to mixed cryoglobulinemia.[167]

Alphaviruses

Epidemic polyarthritis caused by infection with one of the alphaviruses is the most common viral-associated arthritis in Australia, the islands of the South Pacific, Africa, and Asia.[209] These viruses are transmitted by arthropods, usually the mosquito, and incite an illness characterized by arthritis and a rash that may be macular, papular, vesicular, or purpuric. Although there are some virus-specific differences in these illnesses, in general they are mild in children and occur with equal frequency in males and in females.

In Ross River virus disease, the wrist is most commonly affected, often accompanied by tenosynovitis and enthesitis at the insertion of the plantar fascia into the calcaneus.[209, 210] The synovial fluid is said to be highly characteristic, with a predominance of vacuolated macrophages and very few PMNs. In chikungunya, the knee is the most commonly involved joint and back pain and myalgia are prominent. The arthritis lasts 1 to 2 weeks and is followed by complete recovery. Diagnosis rests on the clinical presentation and an elevated level of antibodies to the specific virus. Viral antigen has not been recovered from synovial fluid.

Herpesviruses

Four of the herpesviruses have been associated with arthritis. Herpes simplex virus type 1 has been isolated from the synovial fluid of one patient with arthritis and disseminated herpes simplex infection.[211] Epstein-Barr virus has long been thought by some investigators to have a primary role in the etiology or pathogenesis of RA, although direct evidence is lacking.[212–214] Arthritis is a rare complication of infectious mononucleosis.[215, 216, 216a] Cytomegalovirus is occasionally associated with arthritis and has been isolated from synovial fluid in one instance.[211]

Varicella-zoster infection is uncommonly complicated by arthritis.[217–223, 223a] However, there have been instances of bacterial septic arthritis complicating chickenpox.[222, 224, 225] In one instance, varicella-zoster virus was grown from synovial fluid of an 8-year-old girl with acute, painless monarthritis occurring 3 days after the onset of chickenpox.[219] The synovial fluid cells were predominantly lymphocytes.[217, 219, 226] Occasionally, chickenpox is associated with the emergence of psoriatic arthritis.[227] Acute monarthritis has been reported in association with herpes zoster in two adults.[228, 229]

Mumps Virus

The paramyxovirus (mumps) rarely causes arthritis: In a 1984 review,[230] only 32 cases were well documented. Since then, two additional patients have been briefly reported.[231, 232] The sex ratio is 3.6 males:1 female, and the peak age of occurrence is 21 to 30 years. Four patients younger than 11 years and 7 between the ages of 11 and 20 years have been noted. Arthritis occasionally preceded, but in general followed, parotitis by 1 to 3 weeks. In children, the arthritis was mild, affected few joints, and lasted 1 to 2 weeks. In postadolescent males, arthritis was often accompanied by orchitis and pancreatitis.[230] It is reported that the arthritis responds to ibuprofen or prednisone but not to aspirin.[230] The pathogenesis is unknown, and no attempts at recovery of mumps virus from synovium or synovial fluid have been reported. Arthritis is not known to have occurred after mumps immunization.

Human Immunodeficiency Virus

AIDS secondary to infection with human immunodeficiency virus (HIV) may be complicated by septic arthritis, usually of fungal origin.[233, 234] Although the precise nature of rheumatic syndromes associated with HIV infection remains controversial, a number of stereotypic presentations have been documented in adults.[235] These include the possibility of Reiter's syndrome, reactive arthritis, psoriasiform arthritis, and an undifferentiated spondyloarthropathy,[236–240] often more severe than in patients without HIV infection. Arthralgias occur initially with viremia; lower-extremity oligoarthritis, or persistent polyarthritis, can supervene later.[7] A study of 270 patients concluded that the most frequent pattern of joint involvement was one of an acute onset, short duration, few if any recurrences, and no erosive sequelae.[241] We have observed chronic oligoarthritis in two young children with HIV infection (one transplacental and one related to blood products).

Other Viruses

There are reports of arthritis associated with adenovirus type 7 infections, although virus was not isolated from the synovial fluid and diagnosis was confirmed only on clinical and serologic grounds.[242–244] Echoviruses[245–247] and coxsackie B viruses[243, 248] have been rarely implicated as the cause of arthritis. Smallpox (variola virus infection), now eradicated from the world, was often accompanied by arthritis, especially in children younger than 10 years. Arthritis also followed cowpox vaccination.[249] Human T-cell leukemia virus type I has been associated with a number of rheumatic disorders in adults, including arthritis and Sjögren's syndrome.[250] A 1998 report[251] outlined an outbreak of Sindbis virus–induced Pogosta disease (fever, rash, joint symptoms) in Finland.

Syndromes Presumably Related to Viral Infection

Transient or toxic synovitis of the hip is an idiopathic disorder often preceded by a nonspecific upper respiratory tract infection. It occurs most commonly in boys (70 percent) in the 3- to 10-year-old age group (Table 31–11).[252] Pain in the hip, thigh, or knee may be of sudden or gradual onset and lasts for an average of 6 days. Bilateral involvement occurs in approximately 4 percent of cases. There is loss of internal rotation of the hip, and it may be held in the flexed, abducted position. The ESR and WBC count are usually normal.[252, 253] Radiographs often appear normal or may document widening of the joint space with lateral displacement of the femoral head because of effusion. These findings can be confirmed by CT or ultrasound studies.[252] Radionuclide scanning may demonstrate a transient decrease in uptake of technetium-99m phosphate. Signal intensity is normal with MRI and differentiates toxic synovitis of the hip from a septic process,[37] which is often the principal differential diagnosis.[253a]

After a diagnostic ultrasound scan to confirm the presence of fluid, the hip joint should be aspirated to rule out bacterial sepsis.[254] The synovial fluid has a normal or minimally increased cell count but may be under high pressure.[252] After aspiration, the pain and range of motion are dramatically improved, at least temporarily. Treatment includes the use of analgesics or NSAIDs, bed rest, and skin traction with the hip in 45 degrees of flexion to minimize intracapsular pressure.[252] Long-term sequelae include Legg-Calvé-Perthes disease in about 1.5 percent of cases,[255, 256] coxa magna, and osteoarthritis. Recurrences, often accompanied by low-grade fever, occur.

Table 31–11

Transient Synovitis of the Hip

Age at onset: 3–10 yr
Sex ratio: Boys > girls
Symptoms: Antecedent respiratory infection; limp, knee pain
Signs: Decreased range of motion of hip; low-grade fever
Investigations: ESR slightly elevated to normal; occasional widening of joint space, capsular distention
Treatment: Self-limited course of 1–2 wk; relief with joint aspiration (coxa plana develops in 5%)

ESR, erythrocyte sedimentation rate.

FUNGAL ARTHRITIS

Arthritis caused by fungal infection is rare[257] and is almost unknown in children beyond the neonatal period. Fungi that have been reported as causing arthritis or osteomyelitis are *C. albicans*,[258] *Sporothrix schenkii*,[259, 260] *Actinomyces israelii*,[261] *Aspergillus fumigatus*,[262] *Histoplasma capsulatum*,[263] *Cryptococcus neoformans*,[263] *Blastomyces dermatididis*,[264] *Coccidioides immitis*,[265] *Paracoccidioides brasiliensis*,[266] *Nocardia asteroides*,[267] and *Pseudallescheria boydii*.[268] Candidal arthritis,[258] often with accompanying osteomyelitis, is a recognized entity in the newborn[269, 270] and occurs occasionally in immunocompromised patients[233, 234] and in patients with prosthetic joints.[271]

Sporotrichosis

Infection with *Sporothrix schenckii* is a rare but significant occupational hazard of gardeners, night-crawler farmers, and field workers.[259, 260] Monarthritis or, less commonly, polyarthritis resembling RA has been reported (Fig. 31–12). Synovial biopsy is often necessary in order to make the diagnosis (Fig. 31–13). Other fungal infections are even less common causes of bone

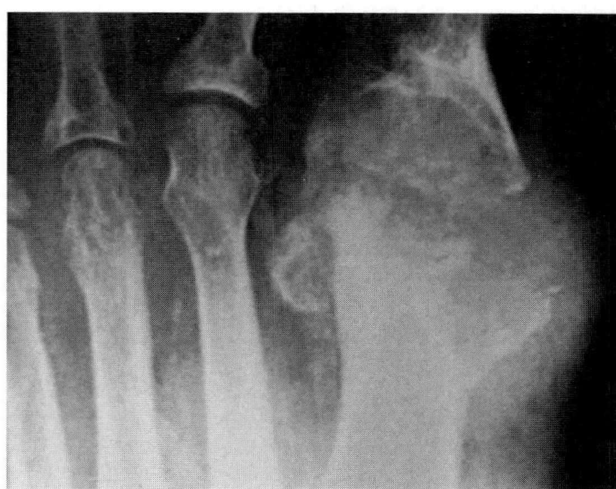

Figure 31–12. Destruction of first metatarsophalangeal joint secondary to sporotrichosis.

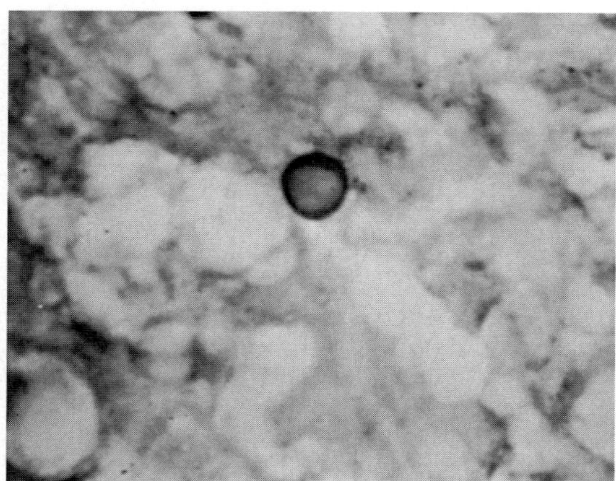

Figure 31–13. *Sporothrix schenckii* in Gram stain preparation of synovial fluid aspirate.

or joint infection in children. The interested reader is referred to the review by Goldenberg and Cohen[260] and to other selected references.[262–268, 270, 271]

Plant Thorn Synovitis

Synovitis caused by the penetration of a plant thorn into the joint space or surrounding structures is probably a reaction to the foreign material rather than an outright infection, although the circumstances of the injury may suggest the latter (Table 31–12). The synovial effusion is inflammatory, and culture occasionally yields a relatively nonvirulent organism. In the case of rose thorn penetration, *S. schenckii* is the probable cause. More commonly, the thorn of the palm tree or blackthorn is implicated.[272] There are local signs of inflammation, and radiographs demonstrate periosteal new bone formation, a radiolucent defect in bone, or the presence of radiopaque foreign material. CT is indicated if plain radiographic results are negative. Because this disorder may develop months after the initial injury, foreign-body synovitis may be ignored as a diagnostic possibility. Treatment should be directed at appropriate surgical exploration and removal of the foreign material.[272]

ARTHRITIS CAUSED BY SPIROCHETES

Lyme Disease

The geographic and temporal clustering of cases of what was thought to be "JRA" in Old Lyme, Connecticut, led Steere, Malawista, and their colleagues in 1977[273–278] to the discovery and description of the etiology, pathogenesis, and cure of what is now known as Lyme disease. This epidemiologic work is one of the most important developments of the last quarter century in rheumatology and provides a model for approaching the question of the infectious etiology of other chronic arthritides of childhood. It has led directly to a vaccine for prevention of the illness. Chapter 32 provides a complete discussion of classic Lyme disease.

Table 31–12

Plant Thorn Synovitis

Onset: Days to months after periarticular injury by penetrating foreign body (palm or blackthorn)
Signs: Local inflammation; joint effusion
Investigations: Lytic lesion on radiographs, periosteal new bone apposition (may need CT scan); synovial fluid culture occasionally positive
Treatment: Surgical removal of foreign material

Variants of Lyme disease are currently being described. An illness nearly indistinguishable from early Lyme disease has been investigated in the United States in Texas, Missouri, North Carolina, Virginia, and Georgia by the Centers for Disease Control and Prevention.[279, 280] Evidence indicates that it is transmitted by the Lone Star tick (*Amblyomma americanum*). *B. burgdorferi* has not been isolated from the tick, patient sera, or lesions. Erythema migrans is the initial presentation of the illness along with mild fever and malaise. There are no long-term sequelae.

Other Spirochetes and Arthritis

Arthritis rarely complicates leptospirosis (*Leptospira icterohemorrhagica*)[281] and syphilis (*Treponema pallidum*).[282, 283] Congenital syphilis causes juxtaepiphyseal osteochondritis and periarthritis in infancy and syphilitic dactylitis in early childhood (Fig. 31–14*A* and *B*). Clutton's joints—relatively painless, recurrent, nonprogressive, symmetric synovitis of the knees—develop later.[284]

POSTINFECTIOUS ARTHRITIS

Arthritis-Dermatitis Syndrome Associated With Small-Bowel Bypass

A syndrome characterized by recurrent episodes of polyarthritis, often with an associated pustular vasculitis, occurred in 5 to 10 percent of adults who had undergone surgical bypass of the distal jejunum and proximal ileum for treatment of morbid obesity.[285] This syndrome included arthritis or arthralgia in all patients, cutaneous lesions in 75 percent, paresthesia in 35 percent, Raynaud's phenomenon in 29 percent, fever in 14 percent, and pericarditis in 3 percent.[286] Morning stiffness occurred, and severe periarthritis with warmth and swelling most commonly affected knees, ankles, fingers, wrists, shoulders, and elbows. The ESR was usually elevated, and cryoglobulins were present in one third of patients. RFs and ANAs were seldom detected, and complement levels were usually normal.[286] The pathogenesis of this syndrome is not certain, although circulating immune complexes have been implicated and sometimes shown to contain antibodies to *Escherichia coli* and *Bacillus fragilis*.[287, 288] Effective treatment included phenylbutazone, prednisone, and (if a blind-loop syndrome was suspected) tetracycline. To our knowledge, this syndrome has not been reported in children.

Musculoskeletal Manifestations of Systemic Bacterial Infections

Bacterial infection of ventricular shunts for the management of hydrocephalus may result in arthritis and nephritis.[289] RFs

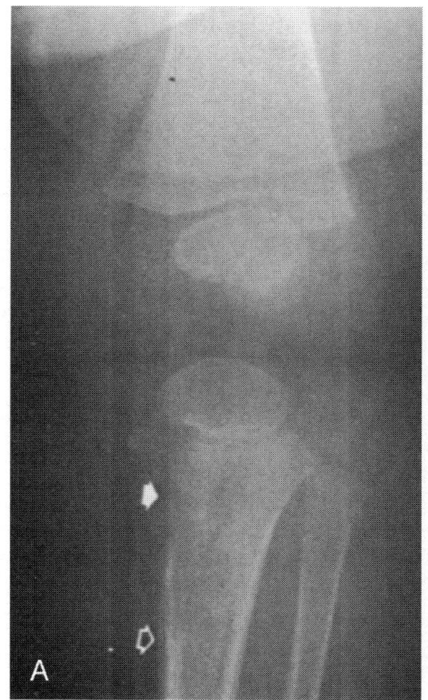

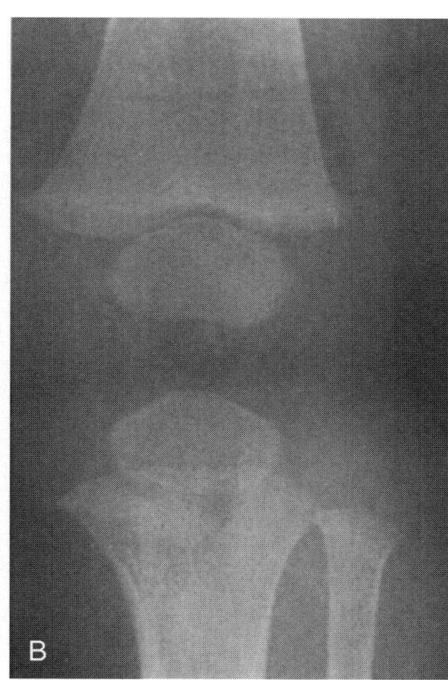

Figure 31–14. Lesions of congenital syphilis in a 6-month-old girl brought to the child abuse clinic because of multiple fractures that occurred during the previous 10 days. Her RPR was 1:256. *A,* There were bilateral symmetric destructive lesions of metaphysitis of the proximal ends of the tibiae (*solid arrow,* Wimberger's sign). Periosteal new bone apposition was also present (*open arrow*). *B,* These lesions have almost healed 2 months later with penicillin therapy.

may be demonstrable in the sera of such patients. Meningococcemia is complicated by arthritis in up to 10 percent of cases.[290] It is usually oligoarticular and occurs most often during the recovery phase, when immune complexes can be demonstrated in the synovium.[291] It can also be complicated by acute septic arthritis in the early stage of the disease. *H. influenzae* type B meningitis may lead to a sterile arthritis.[292]

Infective endocarditis frequently causes arthralgia or arthritis[293, 294] and signs suggesting vasculitis (e.g., Osler nodes, Janeway lesions, Roth spots). The musculoskeletal signs and symptoms (e.g., arthralgia, arthritis, myalgia, low back pain) may precede other manifestations of infective endocarditis by weeks.[294] The arthritis is characteristically polyarticular and symmetric, affecting both large and small joints. An immune complex–mediated pathogenesis is thought to be responsible, and the presence of hypocomplementemia,[295] circulating immune complexes,[296] and sometimes RFs[295] supports this theory. Specificity of the RFs is directed to the patient's IgG in combination with the infecting organism.

REACTIVE ARTHRITIS

By definition, infectious agents are not recoverable in reactive arthritis, which is a response to infection, usually in the sinopulmonary, gastrointestinal, or genitourinary tracts.

Acute Rheumatic Fever

The first complete description of the illness we now identify as acute rheumatic fever is ascribed to Thomas Sydenham in 1848.[297] In recent decades, physicians in the United States, Canada, and Europe had come to believe that acute rheumatic fever was a disease of the past, although it remained a significant health problem elsewhere in the world, where cardiac sequelae from this illness are the most important cause of heart disease.[298, 299] Since 1985, the disease has once again occurred in small epidemics in North America.[300–303] Chapter 34 provides a complete description of acute rheumatic fever.

Arthritis Following Infection With Enteric Bacteria

The reactive arthritides, other than Reiter's syndrome and acute rheumatic fever, are poorly documented in children. Enteric pathogens, such as *Shigella flexneri, Salmonella* species, *Yersinia enterocolitica, Campylobacter jejuni,* and *Clostridium difficile,* give rise to infections that in some children are followed by sterile arthritis. (Chapter 33 provides a discussion of reactive arthritis.)

Parasites and Arthritis

There have been case reports of arthritis accompanying a wide range of parasitic infestations,[304] including *Giardia intestinalis (lamblia),*[305] *Endolimax nana,*[306] *Toxocara canis,*[307] schistosomiasis,[308] and others.[309] In general, the joint disease presumably is reactive or postinfectious rather than septic and pursues a benign course with a good prognosis. The possibility of parasitic disease contributing to the chronic uveitis of JRA has also been raised.[310]

References

1. Rose CD, Eppes SC: Infection-related arthritis. Rheum Dis Clin North Am 23: 677–695, 1997.
2. Krogstad P, Smith AL: Osteomyelitis and septic arthritis. *In* Feigin RD, Cherry JD (eds): Textbook of Pediatric Infectious Diseases, 4th ed. Philadelphia, WB Saunders, 1998, pp 683–704.

3. Koopman WJ: Host factors in the pathogenesis of arthritis triggered by infectious organisms. Overview. Rheum Dis Clin North Am 19: 279–292, 1993.
4. Kunnamo I, Kallio P, Pelkonen P, et al: Clinical signs and laboratory tests in the differential diagnosis of arthritis in children. Am J Dis Child 141: 34–40, 1987.
5. Welkon CJ, Long SS, Fisher MC, et al: Pyogenic arthritis in infants and children: a review of 95 cases. Pediatr Infect Dis 5: 669–676, 1986.
5a. Christiansen P, Frederiksen B, Glazowski J, et al: Epidemiologic, bacteriologic, and long-term follow-up data of children with acute hematogenous osteomyelitis and septic arthritis: a ten-year review. J Pediatr Orthop B 8: 302–305, 1999.
6. Fink CW, Nelson JD: Septic arthritis and osteomyelitis in children. Clin Rheum Dis 12: 423–435, 1986.
7. Ryan MJ, Kavanagh R, Wall PG, et al: Bacterial joint infections in England and Wales: analysis of bacterial isolates over a four year period. Br J Rheumatol 36: 370–373, 1997.
8. Nelson JD, Koontz WC: Septic arthritis in infants and children: a review of 117 cases. Pediatrics 38: 966–971, 1966.
9. Wilson NI, Di Paola M: Acute septic arthritis in infancy and childhood. 10 years' experience. J Bone Joint Surg Br 68: 584–587, 1986.
10. Speiser JC, Moore TL, Osborn TG, et al: Changing trends in pediatric septic arthritis. Semin Arthritis Rheum 15: 132–138, 1985.
11. Wang CH, Huang FY: Septic arthritis in early infancy. Chung Hua Min Kuo Hsiao Erh Ko I Hsueh Hui Tsa Chih 31: 69–75, 1990.
12. Scopelitis E, Martinez-Osuna P: Gonococcal arthritis. Rheum Dis Clin North Am 19: 363–377, 1993.
13. Shetty AK, Gedalia A: Septic arthritis in children. Rheum Dis Clin North Am 24: 287–304, 1998.
14. Luhmann JD, Luhmann SJ: Etiology of septic arthritis in children: an update for the 1990s. Pediatr Emerg Care 15: 40–42, 1999.
15. Bowerman SG, Green NE, Mencio GA: Decline of bone and joint infections attributable to *Haemophilus influenzae* type b. Clin Orthop 341: 128–133, 1997.
16. Peltola H, Kallio MJ, Unkila-Kallio L: Reduced incidence of septic arthritis in children by *Haemophilus influenzae* type-b vaccination. Implications for treatment. J Bone Joint Surg Br 80: 471–473, 1998.
16a. Howard AW, Viskontas D, Sabbagh C: Reduction in osteomyelitis and septic arthritis related to *Haemophilus influenzae* type B vaccination. J Pediatr Orthop 19: 705–709, 1999.
17. Bradley JS, Kaplan SL, Tan TQ, et al: Pediatric pneumococcal bone and joint infections. The Pediatric Multicenter Pneumococcal Surveillance Study Group (PMPSSG). Pediatrics 102: 1376–1382, 1998.
17a. Ispahani P, Weston VC, Turner DP, et al: Septic arthritis due to *Streptococcus pneumoniae* in Nottingham, United Kingdom, 1985–1998. Clin Infect Dis 29: 1450–1454, 1999.
18. Wright J, Thomas P, Serjeant GR: Septicemia caused by *Salmonella* infection: an overlooked complication of sickle cell disease. J Pediatr 130: 394–399, 1997.
19. Dan M: Septic arthritis in young infants: clinical and microbiologic correlations and therapeutic implications. Rev Infect Dis 6: 147–155, 1984.
20. Ezra E, Wientroub S: Primary subacute haematogenous osteomyelitis of the tarsal bones in children. J Bone Joint Surg Br 79: 983–986, 1997.
21. Jackson MA, Burry VF, Olson LC: Pyogenic arthritis associated with adjacent osteomyelitis: identification of the sequela-prone child. Pediatr Infect Dis J 11: 9–13, 1992.
22. Laughlin TJ, Armstrong DG, Caporusso J, et al: Soft tissue and bone infections from puncture wounds in children. West J Med 166: 126–128, 1997.
23. Roca RP, Yoshikawa TT: Primary skeletal infections in heroin users: a clinical characterization, diagnosis and therapy. Clin Orthop 238–248, 1979.
24. Morrey BF, Bianco AJ Jr, Rhodes KH: Septic arthritis in children. Orthop Clin North Am 6: 923–934, 1975.
25. Pioro MH, Mandell BF: Septic arthritis. Rheum Dis Clin North Am 23: 239–258, 1997.
26. Tokuda K, Yoshinaga M, Nishi J, et al: Three cases of pyogenic sacro-iliitis, and factors in the relapse of the disease. Acta Paediatr Jpn 39: 385–389, 1997.
27. Mader JT, Mohan D, Calhoun J: A practical guide to the diagnosis and management of bone and joint infections. Drugs 54: 253–264, 1997.
28. Weston VC, Jones AC, Bradbury N, et al: Clinical features and outcome of septic arthritis in a single UK Health District 1982–1991. Ann Rheum Dis 58: 214–219, 1999.
29. Li F, Bulbul R, Schumacher HR Jr, et al: Molecular detection of bacterial DNA in venereal-associated arthritis. Arthritis Rheum 39: 950–958, 1996.
30. Louie JS, Liebling MR: The polymerase chain reaction in infectious and post-infectious arthritis. A review. Rheum Dis Clin North Am 24: 227–236, 1998.
31. Wilbrink B, van der Heijden I, Schouls LM, et al: Detection of bacterial DNA in joint samples from patients with undifferentiated arthritis and reactive arthritis, using polymerase chain reaction with universal 16S ribosomal RNA primers. Arthritis Rheum 41: 535–543, 1998.
32. van der Heijden I, Wilbrink B, Schouls LM, et al: Detection of mycobacteria in joint samples from patients with arthritis using a genus-specific polymerase chain reaction and sequence analysis. Rheumatology (Oxford) 38: 547–553, 1999.
32a. Lyon RM, Evanich JD: Culture-negative septic arthritis in children. J Pediatr Orthop 19: 655–659, 1999.
33. Poznanski AK, Conway JJ, Shkolnik A, et al: Radiological approaches in the evaluation of joint disease in children. Rheum Dis Clin North Am 13: 57–73, 1987.
34. Jaramillo D, Treves ST, Kasser JR, et al: Osteomyelitis and septic arthritis in children: appropriate use of imaging to guide treatment. Am J Roentgenol 165: 399–403, 1995.
35. Sundberg SB, Savage JP, Foster BK: Technetium phosphate bone scan in the diagnosis of septic arthritis in childhood. J Pediatr Orthop 9: 579–585, 1989.
36. Rivier G, Gerster JC, Terrier P, et al: Parvovirus B19 associated monoarthritis in a 5-year-old boy. J Rheumatol 22: 766–767, 1995.
37. Lee SK, Suh KJ, Kim YW, et al: Septic arthritis versus transient synovitis at MR imaging: preliminary assessment with signal intensity alterations in bone marrow. Radiology 211: 459–465, 1999.
38. American Academy of Pediatrics: Pickering LK, Peter G, Baker CJ, et al: Red Book: report of the Committee on Infectious Diseases, 25th ed. Elk Grove Village, IL, American Academy of Pediatrics, 2000.
39. Cimmino MA: Recognition and management of bacterial arthritis. Drugs 54: 50–60, 1997.
40. Sonnen GM, Henry NK: Pediatric bone and joint infections. Diagnosis and antimicrobial management. Pediatr Clin North Am 43: 933–947, 1996.
41. Wall EJ: Childhood osteomyelitis and septic arthritis. Curr Opin Pediatr 10: 73–76, 1998.
41a. Newton PO, Ballock RT, Bradley JS: Oral antibiotic therapy of bacterial arthritis. Pediatr Infect Dis J 18: 1102–1103, 1999.
42. Stanitski CL, Harvell JC, Fu FH: Arthroscopy in acute septic knees. Management in pediatric patients. Clin Orthop 241: 209–212, 1989.
43. Nelson JD: Antibiotic concentrations in septic joint effusions. N Engl J Med 284: 349–353, 1971.
44. Frederiksen B, Christiansen P, Knudsen FU: Acute osteomyelitis and septic arthritis in the neonate, risk factors and outcome. Eur J Pediatr 152: 577–580, 1993.
45. Morrissy RT: Bone and joint infection in the neonate. Pediatr Ann 18: 33–8, 40, 1989.
46. Ish-Horowicz MR, McIntyre P, Nade S: Bone and joint infections caused by multiply resistant *Staphylococcus aureus* in a neonatal intensive care unit. Pediatr Infect Dis J 11: 82–87, 1992.
47. Betz RR, Cooperman DR, Wopperer JM, et al: Late sequelae of septic arthritis of the hip in infancy and childhood. J Pediatr Orthop 10: 365–372, 1990.
48. Bennett OM, Namnyak SS: Acute septic arthritis of the hip joint in infancy and childhood. Clin Orthop 123–132, 1992.
49. Klein DM, Barbera C, Gray ST, et al: Sensitivity of objective parameters in the diagnosis of pediatric septic hips. Clin Orthop 338: 153–159, 1997.

50. Vidigal EC Jr, Vidigal EC, Fernandes JL: Avascular necrosis as a complication of septic arthritis of the hip in children. Int Orthop 21: 389–392, 1997.
51. Griffin PP, Green WT Sr: Hip joint infections in infants and children. Orthop Clin North Am 9: 123–134, 1978.
52. Fabry G, Meire E: Septic arthritis of the hip in children: poor results after late and inadequate treatment. J Pediatr Orthop 3: 461–466, 1983.
53. Chacha PB: Suppurative arthritis of the hip joint in infancy. A persistent diagnostic problem and possible complication of femoral venipuncture. J Bone Joint Surg Am 53: 538–544, 1971.
54. Campagnaro JG, Donzelli O, Urso R, et al: Treatment of the sequelae of septic osteoarthritis of the hip during pediatric age. Chir Organi Mov 77: 233–245, 1992.

54a. Kim HK, Alman B, Cole WG: A shortened course of parenteral antibiotic therapy in the management of acute septic arthritis of the hip. J Pediatr Orthop 20: 44–47, 2000.

55. Bos CF, Mol LJ, Obermann WR, et al: Late sequelae of neonatal septic arthritis of the shoulder. J Bone Joint Surg Br 80: 645–650, 1998.
56. Brogadir SP, Schimmer BM, Myers AR: Spectrum of the gonococcal arthritis-dermatitis syndrome. Semin Arthritis Rheum 8: 177–183, 1979.
57. Cohen M: Gonococcal arthritis. Bull Rheum Dis 47: 4–6, 1998.
58. Rook G, Lydyard P, Stanford J: Mycobacteria and rheumatoid arthritis. Arthritis Rheum 33: 431–435, 1990.
59. Ruggieri M, Pavone V, Polizzi A, et al: Tuberculosis of the ankle in childhood: clinical, roentgenographic and computed tomography findings. Clin Pediatr (Phila) 36: 529–534, 1997.
60. Shih HN, Hsu RW, Lin TY: Tuberculosis of the long bone in children. Clin Orthop 335: 246–252, 1997.
61. Zahraa J, Johnson D, Lim-Dunham JE, et al: Unusual features of osteoarticular tuberculosis in children. J Pediatr 129: 597–602, 1996.
62. Wessels G, Hesseling PB, Beyers N: Skeletal tuberculosis: dactylitis and involvement of the skull. Pediatr Radiol 28: 234–236, 1998.
63. Southwood TR, Hancock EJ, Petty RE, et al: Tuberculous rheumatism (Poncet's disease) in a child. Arthritis Rheum 31: 1311–1313, 1988.

63a. Sood R, Wali JP, Handa R: Poncet's disease in a north Indian hospital. Trop Doct 29: 33–36, 1999.

64. Pernambuco JC, Cossermelli-Messina W: Rheumatic manifestations of leprosy: clinical aspects. J Rheumatol 20: 897–899, 1993.
65. Markusse HM, Smelt AH, Teepe RG: Unusual arthritis: be on the alert for leprosy. Clin Rheumatol 8: 266–268, 1989.
66. Atkin SL, el-Ghobarey A, Kamel M, et al: Clinical and laboratory studies of arthritis in leprosy. Br Med J 298: 1423–1425, 1989.
67. Louie JS, Kornasky JR, Cohen AH: Lepra cells in synovial fluid of a patient with erythema nodosum leprosum. N Engl J Med 289: 1410–1411, 1973.
68. Gomez-Reino FJ, Mateo I, Fuertes A, et al: Brucellar arthritis in children and its successful treatment with trimethoprim-sulphamethoxazole (co-trimoxazole). Ann Rheum Dis 45: 256–258, 1986.
69. Gotuzzo E, Alarcon GS, Bocanegra TS, et al: Articular involvement in human brucellosis: a retrospective analysis of 304 cases. Semin Arthritis Rheum 12: 245–255, 1982.
70. Thapar MK, Young EJ: Urban outbreak of goat cheese brucellosis. Pediatr Infect Dis 5: 640–643, 1986.
71. Young EJ: Human brucellosis. Rev Infect Dis 5: 821–842, 1983.
72. Gottesman G, Vanunu D, Maayan MC, et al: Childhood brucellosis in Israel. Pediatr Infect Dis J 15: 610–615, 1996.
73. Broughton RA: Infections due to *Mycoplasma pneumoniae* in childhood. Pediatr Infect Dis 5: 71–85, 1986.
74. Cimolai N, Malleson P, Thomas E, et al: *Mycoplasma pneumoniae* associated arthropathy: confirmation of the association by determination of the antipolypeptide IgM response. J Rheumatol 16: 1150–1152, 1989.
75. Arlievsky N, Li KI, Munoz JL: Septic arthritis with osteomyelitis due to *Streptococcus pneumoniae* in human immunodeficiency virus–infected children. Clin Infect Dis 27: 898–899, 1998.
76. Franz A, Webster AD, Furr PM, et al: Mycoplasmal arthritis in patients with primary immunoglobulin deficiency: clinical features and outcome in 18 patients. Br J Rheumatol 36: 661–668, 1997.
77. Quelquejay C, Job-Deslandre C, Hamidou A, et al: [Chronic recurrent multifocal osteomyelitis in children]. J Radiol 78: 115–121, 1997.
78. Gilbert MS, Aledort LM, Seremetis S, et al: Long term evaluation of septic arthritis in hemophilic patients. Clin Orthop 328: 54–59, 1996.
79. Asmar BI, Andresen J, Brown WJ: Ureaplasma urealyticum arthritis and bacteremia in agammaglobulinemia. Pediatr Infect Dis J 17: 73–76, 1998.
80. Swanson H, Hughes PA, Messer SA, et al: *Candida albicans* arthritis one year after successful treatment of fungemia in a healthy infant. J Pediatr 129: 688–694, 1996.
81. Morrissy RT, Shore SL: Bone and joint sepsis. Pediatr Clin North Am 33: 1551–1564, 1986.
82. Scott RJ, Christofersen MR, Robertson WW Jr, et al: Acute osteomyelitis in children: a review of 116 cases. J Pediatr Orthop 10: 649–652, 1990.
83. Hoffman EB, de Beer JD, Keys G, et al: Diaphyseal primary subacute osteomyelitis in children. J Pediatr Orthop 10: 250–254, 1990.
84. Faden H, Grossi M: Acute osteomyelitis in children. Reassessment of etiologic agents and their clinical characteristics. Am J Dis Child 145: 65–69, 1991.

84a. Trobs R, Moritz R, Buhligen U, et al: Changing pattern of osteomyelitis in infants and children. Pediatr Surg Int 15: 363–372, 1999.

85. Nade S: Acute haematogenous osteomyelitis in infancy and childhood. J Bone Joint Surg Br 65: 109–119, 1983.
86. Cole WG, Dalziel RE, Leitl S: Treatment of acute osteomyelitis in childhood. J Bone Joint Surg Br 64: 218–223, 1982.
87. Dahl LB, Hoyland AL, Dramsdahl H, et al: Acute osteomyelitis in children: a population-based retrospective study 1965 to 1994. Scand J Infect Dis 30: 573–577, 1998.
88. Stricker T, Frohlich S, Nadal D: Osteomyelitis and septic arthritis due to *Citrobacter freundii* and *Haemophilus influenzae* type b. J Paediatr Child Health 34: 90–91, 1998.

88a. Jaakkola J, Kehl D: Hematogenous calcaneal osteomyelitis in children. J Pediatr Orthop 19: 699–704, 1999.

89. Elliott SJ, Aronoff SC: Clinical presentation and management of *Pseudomonas* osteomyelitis. Clin Pediatr (Phila) 24: 566–570, 1985.
90. Jacobs NM: Pneumococcal osteomyelitis and arthritis in children. A hospital series and literature review. Am J Dis Child 145: 70–74, 1991.
91. Seeler RA, Metzger W, Mufson MA: *Diplococcus pneumoniae* infections in children with sickle cell anemia. Am J Dis Child 123: 8–10, 1972.
92. Sadat-Ali M: The status of acute osteomyelitis in sickle cell disease. A 15-year review. Int Surg 83: 84–87, 1998.

92a. Narchi H: Osteomyelitis in sickle cell haemoglobinopathy with elevated fetal haemoglobin. Ann Trop Paediatr 20: 70–75, 2000.

93. Mallouh A, Talab Y: Bone and joint infection in patients with sickle cell disease. J Pediatr Orthop 5: 158–162, 1985.
94. Kauffman CA, Watanakunakorn C, Phair JP: Pneumococcal arthritis. J Rheumatol 3: 409–419, 1976.
95. Hadari I, Dagan R, Gedalia A, et al: Pneumococcal osteomyelitis. An unusual cluster of cases. Clin Pediatr (Phila) 24: 143–145, 1985.
96. Sucato DJ, Gillespie R: *Salmonella* pelvic osteomyelitis in normal children: report of two cases and a review of the literature. J Pediatr Orthop 17: 463–466, 1997.
97. Perkins MD, Edwards KM, Heller RM, et al: Neonatal group B streptococcal osteomyelitis and suppurative arthritis. Outpatient therapy. Clin Pediatr (Phila) 28: 229–230, 1989.
98. Barton LL, Villar RG, Rice SA: Neonatal group B streptococcal vertebral osteomyelitis. Pediatrics 98: 459–461, 1996.
99. Knudsen CJ, Hoffman EB: Neonatal osteomyelitis. J Bone Joint Surg Br 72: 846–851, 1990.
100. Gutman LT: Acute, subacute, and chronic osteomyelitis and pyogenic arthritis in children. Curr Probl Pediatr 15: 1–72, 1985.
101. Deshpande PG, Wagle SU, Mehta SD, et al: Neonatal osteomyelitis and septic arthritis. Indian Pediatr 27: 453–457, 1990.
102. Vohra R, Kang HS, Dogra S, et al: Tuberculous osteomyelitis. J Bone Joint Surg Br 79: 562–566, 1997.

103. Chen SC, Huang SC, Wu CT: Nonspinal tuberculous osteomyelitis in children. J Formos Med Assoc 97: 26–31, 1998.
104. Wang MN, Chen WM, Lee KS, et al: Tuberculous osteomyelitis in young children. J Pediatr Orthop 19: 151–155, 1999.
105. Keret D, Giladi M, Kletter Y, et al: Cat-scratch disease osteomyelitis from a dog scratch. J Bone Joint Surg Br 80: 766–767, 1998.
106. Ratner LM, Kesack A, McCauley TR, et al: Disseminated *Bartonella henselae* (cat-scratch disease): appearance of multifocal osteomyelitis with MR imaging. Am J Roentgenol 171: 1164–1165, 1998.
107. Robson JM, Harte GJ, Osborne DR, et al: Cat-scratch disease with paravertebral mass and osteomyelitis. Clin Infect Dis 28: 274–278, 1999.
108. Willis RB, Rozencwaig R: Pediatric osteomyelitis masquerading as skeletal neoplasia. Orthop Clin North Am 27: 625–634, 1996.
108a. Perlman MH, Patzakis MJ, Kumar PJ, et al: The incidence of joint involvement with adjacent osteomyelitis in pediatric patients. J Pediatr Orthop 20: 40–43, 2000.
109. Morrissy RT, Haynes DW: Acute hematogenous osteomyelitis: a model with trauma as an etiology. J Pediatr Orthop 9: 447–456, 1989.
110. Sonozaki H, Mitsui H, Miyanaga Y, et al: Clinical features of 53 cases with pustulotic arthro-osteitis. Ann Rheum Dis 40: 547–553, 1981.
111. Tyrrell PN, Cassar-Pullicino VN, Eisenstein SM, et al: Back pain in childhood. Ann Rheum Dis 55: 789–793, 1996.
112. Chelsom J, Solberg CO: Vertebral osteomyelitis at a Norwegian university hospital 1987–97: clinical features, laboratory findings and outcome. Scand J Infect Dis 30: 147–151, 1998.
113. Krogsgaard MR, Wagn P, Bengtsson J: Epidemiology of acute vertebral osteomyelitis in Denmark: 137 cases in Denmark 1978–1982, compared to cases reported to the National Patient Register 1991–1993. Acta Orthop Scand 69: 513–517, 1998.
114. Giedion A, Holthusen W, Masel LF, et al: [Subacute and chronic "symmetrical" osteomyelitis]. Ann Radiol (Paris) 15: 329–342, 1972.
115. Green NE, Beauchamp RD, Griffin PP: Primary subacute epiphyseal osteomyelitis. J Bone Joint Surg Am 63: 107–114, 1981.
116. Speer DP: Chronic multifocal symmetrical osteomyelitis. Am J Dis Child 138: 340, 1984.
117. Laxer RM, Shore AD, Manson D, et al: Chronic recurrent multifocal osteomyelitis and psoriasis—a report of a new association and review of related disorders. Semin Arthritis Rheum 17: 260–270, 1988.
118. Gamble JG, Rinsky LA: Chronic recurrent multifocal osteomyelitis: a distinct clinical entity. J Pediatr Orthop 6: 579–584, 1986.
119. Van Howe RS, Starshak RJ, Chusid MJ: Chronic, recurrent multifocal osteomyelitis. Case report and review of the literature. Clin Pediatr (Phila) 28: 54–59, 1989.
120. Kourtis AP, Ibegbu CC, Snitzer JA, et al: Recurrent multifocal osteomyelitis due to *Mycobacterium avium* complex. Clin Infect Dis 23: 1194–1195, 1996.
121. Handrick W, Hormann D, Voppmann A, et al: Chronic recurrent multifocal osteomyelitis—report of eight patients. Pediatr Surg Int 14: 195–198, 1998.
121a. Girschick HJ, Huppertz HI, Harmsen D, et al: Chronic recurrent multifocal osteomyelitis in children: diagnostic value of histopathy and microbial testing. Hum Pathol 30: 59–65, 1999.
122. Martin JC, Desoysa R, O'Sullivan MM, et al: Chronic recurrent multifocal osteomyelitis: spinal involvement and radiological appearances. Br J Rheumatol 35: 1019–1021, 1996.
122a. Bousvaros A, Marcon M, Treem W, et al: Chronic recurrent multifocal osteomyelitis associated with chronic inflammatory bowel disease in children. Dig Dis Sci 44: 2500–2507, 1999.
123. Manson D, Wilmot DM, King S, et al: Physeal involvement in chronic recurrent multifocal osteomyelitis. Pediatr Radiol 20: 76–79, 1989.
124. Mandell GA, Contreras SJ, Conard K, et al: Bone scintigraphy in the detection of chronic recurrent multifocal osteomyelitis. J Nucl Med 39: 1778–1783, 1998.
125. Gallagher KT, Roberts RL, MacFarlane JA, et al: Treatment of chronic recurrent multifocal osteomyelitis with interferon gamma. J Pediatr 131: 470–472, 1997.
126. Peters W, Irving J, Letts M: Long-term effects of neonatal bone and joint infection on adjacent growth plates. J Pediatr Orthop 12: 806–810, 1992.
127. Bjorksten B, Gustavson KH, Eriksson B, et al: Chronic recurrent multifocal osteomyelitis and pustulosis palmoplantaris. J Pediatr 93: 227–231, 1978.
128. Ravelli A, Marseglia GL, Viola S, et al: Chronic recurrent multifocal osteomyelitis with unusual features. Acta Paediatr 84: 222–225, 1995.
129. Schaen L, Sheth AP: Skin ulcers associated with a tender and swollen arm. Pyoderma gangrenosum (PG) in association with chronic recurrent multifocal osteomyelitis (CRMO). Arch Dermatol 134: 1146–1150, 1998.
130. Marshall GS, Edwards KM, Wadlington WB: Sporadic congenital Caffey's disease. Clin Pediatr (Phila) 26: 177–180, 1987.
130a. Eyrich GK, Harder C, Sailer HF, et al: Primary chronic osteomyelitis associated with synovitis, acne, pustulosis, hyperostosis and osteitis (SAPHO syndrome). J Oral Pathol Med 28: 456–464, 1999.
130b. Pennington WT, Mott MP, Thometz JG, et al: Photopenic bone scan osteomyelitis: a clinical perspective. J Pediatr Orthop 19: 695–698, 1999.
131. Cohen MD, Cory DA, Kleiman M, et al: Magnetic resonance differentiation of acute and chronic osteomyelitis in children. Clin Radiol 41: 53–56, 1990.
132. Mandell GA: Imaging in the diagnosis of musculoskeletal infections in children. Curr Probl Pediatr 26: 218–237, 1996.
132a. Umans H, Haramati N, Flusser G: The diagnostic role of gadolinium enhanced MRI in distinguishing between acute medullary bone infarct and osteomyelitis. Magn Reson Imaging 18: 255–262, 2000.
133. Howard CB, Einhorn M, Dagan R, et al: Ultrasound in diagnosis and management of acute haematogenous osteomyelitis in children. J Bone Joint Surg Br 75: 79–82, 1993.
133a. Chao HC, Lin SJ, Huang YC, et al: Color Doppler ultrasonographic evaluation of osteomyelitis in children. J Ultrasound Med 18: 729–734, 1999.
133b. William RR, Hussein SS, Jeans WD, et al: A prospective study of soft-tissue ultrasonography in sickle cell disease patients with suspected osteomyelitis. Clin Radiol 55: 307–310, 2000.
134. Azouz EM, Greenspan A, Marton D: CT evaluation of primary epiphyseal bone abscesses. Skeletal Radiol 22: 17–23, 1993.
135. Jurik AG, Egund N: MRI in chronic recurrent multifocal osteomyelitis. Skeletal Radiol 26: 230–238, 1997.
136. Nelson JD: Toward simple but safe management of osteomyelitis. Pediatrics 99: 883–884, 1997.
137. Karwowska A, Davies HD, Jadavji T: Epidemiology and outcome of osteomyelitis in the era of sequential intravenous-oral therapy. Pediatr Infect Dis J 17: 1021–1026, 1998.
138. Hamdy RC, Lawton L, Carey T, et al: Subacute hematogenous osteomyelitis: are biopsy and surgery always indicated? J Pediatr Orthop 16: 220–223, 1996.
139. Gledhill RB: Subacute osteomyelitis in children. Clin Orthop 96: 57–69, 1973.
140. Sapico FL, Montgomerie JZ: Pyogenic vertebral osteomyelitis: report of nine cases and review of the literature. Rev Infect Dis 1: 754–776, 1979.
141. Fischer GW, Popich GA, Sullivan DE, et al: Diskitis: a prospective diagnostic analysis. Pediatrics 62: 543–548, 1978.
142. Hensey OJ, Coad N, Carty HM, et al: Juvenile discitis. Arch Dis Child 58: 983–987, 1983.
143. Alexander CJ: The aetiology of juvenile spondylarthritis (discitis). Clin Radiol 21: 178–187, 1970.
144. Wenger DR, Bobechko WP, Gilday DL: The spectrum of intervertebral disc-space infection in children. J Bone Joint Surg Am 60: 100–108, 1978.
145. Crawford AH, Kucharzyk DW, Ruda R, et al: Diskitis in children. Clin Orthop 266: 70–79, 1991.
146. Spiegel PG, Kengla KW, Isaacson AS, et al: Intervertebral disc-space inflammation in children. J Bone Joint Surg Am 54: 284–296, 1972.
147. Rocco HD, Eyring EJ: Intervertebral disk infections in children. Am J Dis Child 123: 448–451, 1972.
148. Heinrich SD, Zembo MM, King AG, et al: Calcific cervical intervertebral disc herniation in children. Spine 16: 228–231, 1991.
149. Song KS, Ogden JA, Ganey T, et al: Contiguous discitis and osteomyelitis in children. J Pediatr Orthop 17: 470–477, 1997.

149a. Fernandez M, Carrol CL, Baker CJ: Discitis and vertebral osteomyelitis in children: an 18-year review. Pediatrics 105: 1299–1304, 2000.
150. Davis DE, Viozzi FJ, Miller OF, et al: The musculoskeletal manifestations of acne fulminans. J Rheumatol 8: 317–320, 1981.
151. Noseworthy JH, Heffernan LP, Ross JB, et al: Acne fulminans with inflammatory myopathy. Ann Neurol 8: 67–69, 1980.
152. Cros D, Gamby T, Serratrice G: Acne rheumatism. Report of a case. J Rheumatol 8: 336–339, 1981.
153. Hughes RA: Arthritis precipitated by isotretinoin treatment for acne vulgaris. J Rheumatol 20: 1241–1242, 1993.
154. Dubourg G, Koeger AC, Huchet B, et al: Acute monoarthritis in a patient under isotretinoin. Rev Rhum Engl Ed 63: 228–229, 1996.
155. Erhardt E, Harangi F: Two cases of musculoskeletal syndrome associated with acne. Pediatr Dermatol 14: 456–459, 1997.
156. De FV, Stinco G, Campanella M: Acute arthritis during isotretinoin treatment for acne conglobata. Dermatology 194: 195, 1997.
157. Whipple GH: A hitherto undescribed disease characterized anatomically by deposits of fat and fatty acids in the intestinal and mesenteric lymphatic tissues (intestinal lipodystrophy). Bull Johns Hopkins Hosp 18: 382, 1907.
158. Tan TQ, Vogel H, Tharp BR, et al: Presumed central nervous system Whipple's disease in a child: case report. Clin Infect Dis 20: 883–889, 1995.
159. Maizel H, Ruffin JM, Dobbins WO III: Whipple's disease: a review of 19 patients from one hospital and a review of the literature since 1950. Medicine (Baltimore) 49: 175–205, 1970.
160. LeVine ME, Dobbins WO III: Joint changes in Whipple's disease. Semin Arthritis Rheum 3: 79–93, 1973.
161. Misbah SA, Ozols B, Franks A, et al: Whipple's disease without malabsorption: new atypical features. Q J Med 90: 765–772, 1997.
162. Aust CH, Smith EB: Whipple's disease in a three-month-old infant. Am J Clin Pathol 37: 66, 1962.
163. Barakat AY, Bitar J, Nassar VH: Whipple's disease in a seven-year-old child. Report of a case. Am J Proctol 24: 312–315, 1973.
164. Caughey OE, Bywaters EGL: The arthritis of Whipple's syndrome. Ann Rheum Dis 22: 327, 1963.
165. Kelly JJ, Weisiger BB: The arthritis of Whipple's disease. Arthritis Rheum 6: 615, 1963.
166. Petty RE, Tingle AJ: Arthritis and viral infection. J Pediatr 113: 948–949, 1988.
167. Phillips PE: Viral arthritis. Curr Opin Rheumatol 9: 337–344, 1997.
168. Ytterberg SR: Viral arthritis. Curr Opin Rheumatol 11: 275–280, 1999.
169. Osler W: The Principles and Practice of Medicine, 8th ed. New York, Appleton, 1918, p 348.
170. Tingle AJ, Allen M, Petty RE, et al: Rubella-associated arthritis. I. Comparative study of joint manifestations associated with natural rubella infection and RA 27/3 rubella immunisation. Ann Rheum Dis 45: 110–114, 1986.
171. Best JM, Banatvala JE, Bowen JM: New Japanese rubella vaccine. Comparative trials. Br Med J 3: 221–224, 1974.
172. Polk BF, Modlin JF, White JA, et al: A controlled comparison of joint reactions among women receiving one of two rubella vaccines. Am J Epidemiol 115: 19–25, 1982.
173. Tingle AJ, Chantler JK, Pot KH, et al: Postpartum rubella immunization: association with development of prolonged arthritis, neurological sequelae, and chronic rubella viremia. J Infect Dis 152: 606–612, 1985.
174. Grillner L, Hedstrom CE, Bergstrom H, et al: Vaccination against rubella of newly delivered women. Scand J Infect Dis 5: 237–241, 1973.
175. Tingle AJ, Yang T, Allen M, et al: Prospective immunological assessment of arthritis induced by rubella vaccine. Infect Immun 40: 22–28, 1983.
176. Tingle AJ, Pot KH, Yong FP, et al: Kinetics of isotype-specific humoral immunity in rubella vaccine-associated arthropathy. Clin Immunol Immunopathol 53: S99–S106, 1989.
177. Ogra PL, Herd JK: Arthritis associated with induced rubella infection. J Immunol 107: 810–813, 1971.
178. Chantler JK, Ford DK, Tingle AJ: Persistent rubella infection and rubella-associated arthritis. Lancet 1: 1323–1325, 1982.
179. Spruance SL, Metcalf R, Smith CB, et al: Chronic arthropathy associated with rubella vaccination. Arthritis Rheum 20: 741–747, 1977.
180. Chantler JK, Tingle AJ, Petty RE: Persistent rubella virus infection associated with chronic arthritis in children. N Engl J Med 313: 1117–1123, 1985.
181. Bosma TJ, Etherington J, O'Shea S, et al: Rubella virus and chronic joint disease: is there an association? J Clin Microbiol 36: 3524–3526, 1998.
182. Naides SJ: Parvovirus B19 infection. Rheum Dis Clin North Am 19: 457–475, 1993.
183. Ware R: Human parvovirus infection. J Pediatr 114: 343–348, 1989.
184. Simpson RW, McGinty L, Simon L, et al: Association of parvoviruses with rheumatoid arthritis of humans. Science 223: 1425–1428, 1984.
185. White DG, Woolf AD, Mortimer PP, et al: Human parvovirus arthropathy. Lancet 1: 419–421, 1985.
186. Anderson MJ, Jones SE, Fisher-Hoch SP, et al: Human parvovirus, the cause of erythema infectiosum (fifth disease)? Lancet 1: 1378, 1983.
187. Reid DM, Reid TM, Brown T, et al: Human parvovirus-associated arthritis: a clinical and laboratory description. Lancet 1: 422–425, 1985.
188. Semble EL, Agudelo CA, Pegram PS: Human parvovirus B19 arthropathy in two adults after contact with childhood erythema infectiosum. Am J Med 83: 560–562, 1987.
189. Smith CA, Woolf AD, Lenci M: Parvoviruses: infections and arthropathies. Rheum Dis Clin North Am 13: 249–263, 1987.
190. Ager EA, Chin TD, Poland JD: Epidemic erythema infectiosum. N Engl J Med 275: 1326–1331, 1966.
191. Klouda PT, Corbin SA, Bradley BA, et al: HLA and acute arthritis following human parvovirus infection. Tissue Antigens 28: 318–319, 1986.
192. Speyer I, Breedveld FC, Dijkmans BA: Human parvovirus B19 infection is not followed by inflammatory joint disease during long term follow-up. A retrospective study of 54 patients. Clin Exp Rheumatol 16: 576–578, 1998.
193. Cossart YE, Field AM, Cant B, et al: Parvovirus-like particles in human sera. Lancet 1: 72–73, 1975.
194. Anderson LJ: Role of parvovirus B19 in human disease. Pediatr Infect Dis J 6: 711–718, 1987.
195. Schwarz TF, Roggendorf M, Suschke H, et al: Human parvovirus B19 infection and juvenile chronic polyarthritis. Infection 15: 264–265, 1987.
196. Nocton JJ, Miller LC, Tucker LB, et al: Human parvovirus B19–associated arthritis in children. J Pediatr 122: 186–190, 1993.
197. Dijkmans BA, Elsacker-Niele AM, Salimans MM, et al: Human parvovirus B19 DNA in synovial fluid. Arthritis Rheum 31: 279–281, 1988.
198. Foto F, Marsh JL, Scharosch LL: Synovial tissue analysis in patients with chronic parvovirus B19 arthropathy. Arthritis Rheum Suppl 34: S50, 1991.
199. Soderlund M, von Essen R, Haapasaari J, et al: Persistence of parvovirus B19 DNA in synovial membranes of young patients with and without chronic arthropathy. Lancet 349: 1063–1065, 1997.
200. Naides SJ, Scharosch LL, Foto F, et al: Rheumatologic manifestations of human parvovirus B19 infection in adults. Initial two-year clinical experience. Arthritis Rheum 33: 1297–1309, 1990.
201. Erdman DD, Usher MJ, Tsou C, et al: Human parvovirus B19 specific IgG, IgA, and IgM antibodies and DNA in serum specimens from persons with erythema infectiosum. J Med Virol 35: 110–115, 1991.
202. Schwarz TF, Hottentrager B, Roggendorf M: Prevalence of antibodies to parvovirus B19 in selected groups of patients and healthy individuals. Zentralbl Bakteriol 276: 437–442, 1992.
203. Yamashita K, Matsunaga Y, Taylor-Wiedeman J, et al: A significant age shift of the human parvovirus B19 antibody prevalence among young adults in Japan observed in a decade. Jpn J Med Sci Biol 45: 49–58, 1992.
204. Alarcon GS, Townes AS: Arthritis in viral hepatitis. Report of two cases and review of the literature. Johns Hopkins Med J 132: 1–15, 1973.
205. Inman RD: Rheumatic manifestations of hepatitis B virus infection. Semin Arthritis Rheum 11: 406–420, 1982.

206. Alpert E, Isselbacher KJ, Schur PH: The pathogenesis of arthritis associated with viral hepatitis. Complement-component studies. N Engl J Med 285: 185–189, 1971.
207. Duffy J, Lidsky MD, Sharp JT, et al: Polyarthritis, polyarteritis and hepatitis B. Medicine (Baltimore) 55: 19–37, 1976.
208. Schumacher HR, Gall EP: Arthritis in acute hepatitis and chronic active hepatitis. Pathology of the synovial membrane with evidence for the presence of Australia antigen in synovial membranes. Am J Med 57: 655–664, 1974.
209. Fraser JR: Epidemic polyarthritis and Ross River virus disease. Clin Rheum Dis 12: 369–388, 1986.
210. Aaskov JG, Chen JY, Hanh NT, et al: Surveillance for Ross River virus infection using blood donors. Am J Trop Med Hyg 58: 726–730, 1998.
211. Friedman HM, Pincus T, Gibilisco P, et al: Acute monoarticular arthritis caused by herpes simplex virus and cytomegalovirus. Am J Med 69: 241–247, 1980.
212. Bluestein HG, Hasler F: Epstein-Barr virus and rheumatoid arthritis. Surv Immunol Res 3: 70–77, 1984.
213. Lotz M, Roudier J: Epstein-Barr virus and rheumatoid arthritis: cellular and molecular aspects. Rheumatol Int 9: 147–152, 1989.
214. Baboonian C, Halliday D, Venables PJ, et al: Antibodies in rheumatoid arthritis react specifically with the glycine alanine repeat sequence of Epstein-Barr nuclear antigen-1. Rheumatol Int 9: 161–166, 1989.
215. Adebonojo FO: Monarticular arthritis: an unusual manifestation of infectious mononucleosis. Clin Pediatr (Phila) 11: 549–550, 1972.
216. Pollack S, Enat R, Barzilai D: Monoarthritis with heterophil-negative infectious mononucleosis. Case of an older patient. Arch Intern Med 140: 1109–1111, 1980.
216a. Berger RG, Raab-Traub N: Acute monoarthritis from infectious mononucleosis. Am J Med 107:177–178, 1999.
217. Ward JR, Bishop B: Varicella arthritis. JAMA 212: 1954–1956, 1970.
218. Friedman A, Naveh Y: Polyarthritis associated with chickenpox. Am J Dis Child 122: 179–180, 1971.
219. Mulhern LM, Friday GA, Perri JA: Arthritis complicating varicella infection. Pediatrics 48: 827–829, 1971.
220. Brook I: Varicella arthritis in childhood. Reports of 2 cases and 4 others found in the literature. Clin Pediatr (Phila) 16: 1156–1157, 1977.
221. Fierman AH: Varicella-associated arthritis occurring before the exanthem. Case report and literature review. Clin Pediatr (Phila) 29: 188–190, 1990.
222. Schreck P, Bradley J, Chambers H: Musculoskeletal complications of varicella. J Bone Joint Surg Am 78: 1713–1719, 1996.
223. Stebbings S, Highton J, Croxson MC, et al: Chickenpox monoarthritis: demonstration of varicella-zoster virus in joint fluid by polymerase chain reaction. Br J Rheumatol 37: 311–313, 1998.
223a. Chen MK, Wang CC, Lu JJ, et al: Varicella arthritis diagnosed by polymerase chain reaction. J Formos Med Assoc 98: 519–521, 1999.
224. Buck RE: Pyarthrosis of the hip complicating chickenpox. JAMA 206: 135–136, 1968.
225. Sethi AS, Schloff I: Purulent arthritis complicating chickenpox. Clin Pediatr (Phila) 13: 280, 1974.
226. Priest JR, Urick JJ, Groth KE, et al: Varicella arthritis documented by isolation of virus from joint fluid. J Pediatr 93: 990–992, 1978.
227. Shore A, Ansell BM: Juvenile psoriatic arthritis—an analysis of 60 cases. J Pediatr 100: 529–535, 1982.
228. Cunningham AL, Fraser JR, Clarris BJ, et al: A study of synovial fluid and cytology in arthritis associated with herpes zoster. Aust N Z J Med 9: 440–443, 1979.
229. Devereaux MD, Hazelton RA: Acute monarticular arthritis in association with herpes zoster. Arthritis Rheum 26: 236–237, 1983.
230. Gordon SC, Lauter CB: Mumps arthritis: a review of the literature. Rev Infect Dis 6: 338–344, 1984.
231. Fontebasso M: Mumps polyarthritis. J R Coll Gen Pract 35: 152, 1985.
232. Moffatt CD: Mumps arthropathy. J R Coll Gen Pract 36: 230, 1986.
233. Lipstein-Kresch E, Isenberg HD, Singer C, et al: Disseminated *Sporothrix schenckii* infection with arthritis in a patient with acquired immunodeficiency syndrome. J Rheumatol 12: 805–808, 1985.
234. Ricciardi DD, Sepkowitz DV, Berkowitz LB, et al: Cryptococcal arthritis in a patient with acquired immune deficiency syndrome. Case report and review of the literature. J Rheumatol 13: 455–458, 1986.
235. Calabrese LH: Human immunodeficiency virus (HIV) infection and arthritis. Rheum Dis Clin North Am 19: 477–488, 1993.
236. Raphael SA, Wolfson BJ, Parker P, et al: Pyomyositis in a child with acquired immunodeficiency syndrome. Patient report and brief review. Am J Dis Child 143: 779–781, 1989.
237. Labrune P, Blanche S, Catherine N, et al: Human immunodeficiency virus–associated thrombocytopenia in infants. Acta Paediatr Scand 78: 811–814, 1989.
238. Calabrese LH, Estes M, Yen-Lieberman B, et al: Systemic vasculitis in association with human immunodeficiency virus infection. Arthritis Rheum 32: 569–576, 1989.
239. Espinoza LR, Aguilar JL, Berman A, et al: Rheumatic manifestations associated with human immunodeficiency virus infection. Arthritis Rheum 32: 1615–1622, 1989.
240. Steinbach LS, Tehranzadeh J, Fleckenstein JL, et al: Human immunodeficiency virus infection: musculoskeletal manifestations. Radiology 186: 833–838, 1993.
241. Berman A, Cahn P, Perez H, et al: Human immunodeficiency virus infection associated arthritis: clinical characteristics. J Rheumatol 26: 1158–1162, 1999.
242. Panush RS: Adenovirus arthritis. Arthritis Rheum 17: 534–536, 1974.
243. Rahal JJ, Millian SJ, Noriega ER: Coxsackievirus and adenovirus infection. Association with acute febrile and juvenile rheumatoid arthritis. JAMA 235: 2496–2501, 1976.
244. Luder AS, Naphtali V, Ben Porat E, et al: Still's disease associated with adenovirus infection and defect in adenovirus directed natural killing. Ann Rheum Dis 48: 781–786, 1989.
245. Blotzer JW, Myers AR: Echovirus-associated polyarthritis. Report of a case with synovial fluid and synovial histologic characterization. Arthritis Rheum 21: 978–981, 1978.
246. Kujala G, Newman JH: Isolation of echovirus type 11 from synovial fluid in acute monocytic arthritis. Arthritis Rheum 28: 98–99, 1985.
247. Ackerson BK, Raghunathan R, Keller MA, et al: Echovirus 11 arthritis in a patient with X-linked agammaglobulinemia. Pediatr Infect Dis J 6: 485–488, 1987.
248. Roberts-Thomson PJ, Southwood TR, Moore BW, et al: Adult onset Still's disease or coxsackie polyarthritis? Aust N Z J Med 16: 509–511, 1986.
249. Holtzman CM: Postvaccination arthritis. N Engl J Med 280: 111–112, 1969.
250. Nishioka K, Nakajima T, Hasunuma T, et al: Rheumatic manifestation of human leukemia virus infection. Rheum Dis Clin North Am 19: 489–503, 1993.
251. Turunen M, Kuusisto P, Uggeldahl PE, et al: Pogosta disease: clinical observations during an outbreak in the province of North Karelia, Finland. Br J Rheumatol 37: 1177–1180, 1998.
252. Wingstrand H: Transient synovitis of the hip in the child. Acta Orthop Scand Suppl 219: 1–61, 1986.
253. Hardinge K: The etiology of transient synovitis of the hip in childhood. J Bone Joint Surg Br 52: 100–107, 1970.
253a. Kocher MS, Zurakowski D, Kasser JR: Differentiating between septic arthritis and transient synovitis of the hip in children: an evidence-based clinical prediction algorithm. J Bone Joint Surg Am 81: 1662–1670, 1999.
254. Del Beccaro MA, Champoux AN, Bockers T, et al: Septic arthritis versus transient synovitis of the hip: the value of screening laboratory tests. Ann Emerg Med 21: 1418–1422, 1992.
255. Spock A: Transient synovitis of the hip joint in children. Pediatrics 24: 1042, 1959.
256. Wynne-Davies R, Gormley J: The aetiology of Perthes' disease. Genetic, epidemiological and growth factors in 310 Edinburgh and Glasgow patients. J Bone Joint Surg Br 60: 6–14, 1978.
257. Cuellar ML, Silveira LH, Citera G, et al: Other fungal arthritides. Rheum Dis Clin North Am 19: 439–455, 1993.
258. Silveira LH, Cuellar ML, Citera G, et al: Candida arthritis. Rheum Dis Clin North Am 19: 427–437, 1993.

259. Crout JE, Brewer NS, Tompkins RB: Sporotrichosis arthritis: clinical features in seven patients. Ann Intern Med 86: 294–297, 1977.
260. Goldenberg DL, Cohen AS: Arthritis due to tuberculous and fungal microorganisms. Clin Rheum Dis 4: 211, 1978.
261. Hart PD, Russell EJ, Remington JS: The compromised host and infection. II. Deep fungal infection. J Infect Dis 120: 169–191, 1969.
262. Tack KJ, Rhame FS, Brown B, et al: Aspergillus osteomyelitis. Report of four cases and review of the literature. Am J Med 73: 295–300, 1982.
263. Bayer AS, Choi C, Tillman DB, et al: Fungal arthritis. V. Cryptococcal and histoplasmal arthritis. Semin Arthritis Rheum 9: 218–227, 1980.
264. Sanders LL: Blastomycosis arthritis. Arthritis Rheum 10: 91–98, 1967.
265. Bayer AS, Yoshikawa TT, Galpin JE, et al: Unusual syndromes of coccidioidomycosis: diagnostic and therapeutic considerations; a report of 10 cases and review of the English literature. Medicine (Baltimore) 55: 131–152, 1976.
266. Castaneda OJ, Alarcon GS, Garcia MT, et al: *Paracoccidioides brasiliensis* arthritis. Report of a case and review of the literature. J Rheumatol 12: 356–358, 1985.
267. Dinulos JG, Darmstadt GL, Wilson CB, et al: *Nocardia asteroides* septic arthritis in a healthy child. Pediatr Infect Dis J 18: 308–310, 1999.
268. Ansari RA, Hindson DA, Stevens DL, et al: *Pseudallescheria boydii* arthritis and osteomyelitis in a patient with Cushing's disease. South Med J 80: 90–92, 1987.
269. Klein JD, Yamauchi T, Horlick SP: Neonatal candidiasis, meningitis, and arthritis: observations and a review of the literature. J Pediatr 81: 31–34, 1972.
270. Poplack DG, Jacobs SA: Candida arthritis treated with amphotericin B. J Pediatr 87: 989–990, 1975.
271. MacGregor RR, Schimmer BM, Steinberg ME: Results of combined amphotericin B-5-fluorcytosine therapy for prosthetic knee joint infected with *Candida parapsilosis*. J Rheumatol 6: 451–455, 1979.
272. Sugarman M, Stobie DG, Quismorio FP, et al: Plant thorn synovitis. Arthritis Rheum 20: 1125–1128, 1977.
273. Steere AC, Malawista SE, Snydman DR, et al: Lyme arthritis: an epidemic of oligoarticular arthritis in children and adults in three Connecticut communities. Arthritis Rheum 20: 7–17, 1977.
274. Steere AC, Bartenhagen NH, Craft JE, et al: The early clinical manifestations of Lyme disease. Ann Intern Med 99: 76–82, 1983.
275. Eichenfield AH, Goldsmith DP, Benach JL, et al: Childhood Lyme arthritis: experience in an endemic area. J Pediatr 109: 753–758, 1986.
276. Culp RW, Eichenfield AH, Davidson RS, et al: Lyme arthritis in children. An orthopaedic perspective. J Bone Joint Surg Am 69: 96–99, 1987.
277. Williams CL, Strobino B, Lee A, et al: Lyme disease in childhood: clinical and epidemiologic features of ninety cases. Pediatr Infect Dis J 9: 10–14, 1990.
278. Zemel LS: Lyme disease—a pediatric perspective. J Rheumatol Suppl 34: 1–13, 1992.
279. Masters E, Granter S, Duray P, et al: Physician-diagnosed erythema migrans and erythema migrans–like rashes following Lone Star tick bites. Arch Dermatol 134: 955–960, 1998.
280. Swinfard RW, Anderson PC: Erythema chronica migrans (ECM). Ticks and Lyme disease in Missouri. Mo Med 96: 159–161, 1999.
281. Sutliff WD, Shepard R, Dunham WB: Acute *Leptospira pomona* arthritis and myocarditis. Ann Intern Med 39: 134, 1953.
282. Reginato AJ, Schumacher HR, Jimenez S, et al: Synovitis in secondary syphilis. Clinical, light, and electron microscopic studies. Arthritis Rheum 22: 170–176, 1979.
283. Reginato AJ: Syphilitic arthritis and osteitis. Rheum Dis Clin North Am 19: 379–398, 1993.
284. Argen RJ, Dixon AS: Clutton's joints with keratitis and periostitis. A case report with histology of synovium. Arthritis Rheum 6: 341, 1963.
285. Shagrin JW, Frame B, Duncan H: Polyarthritis in obese patients with intestinal bypass. Ann Intern Med 75: 377–380, 1971.
286. Stein HB, Schlappner OL, Boyko W, et al: The intestinal bypass: arthritis-dermatitis syndrome. Arthritis Rheum 24: 684–690, 1981.
287. Wands JR, LaMont JT, Mann E, et al: Arthritis associated with intestinal-bypass procedure for morbid obesity. Complement activation and characterization of circulating cryoproteins. N Engl J Med 294: 121–124, 1976.
288. Ginsberg J, Quismorio FP Jr, DeWind LT, et al: Musculoskeletal symptoms after jejunoileal shunt surgery for intractable obesity. Clinical and immunologic studies. Am J Med 67: 443–448, 1979.
289. Pinals RS, Tinnessen WW Jr: Shunt arthritis. J Pediatr 91: 681, 1977.
290. Schaad UB: Arthritis in disease due to *Neisseria meningitidis*. Rev Infect Dis 2: 880–888, 1980.
291. Greenwood BM, Whittle HC, Bryceson AD: Allergic complications of meningococcal disease. II. Immunological investigations. Br Med J 2: 737–740, 1973.
292. Rush PJ, Shore A, Inman R, et al: Arthritis associated with *Haemophilus influenzae* meningitis: septic or reactive? J Pediatr 109: 412–415, 1986.
293. Churchill MA Jr, Geraci JE, Hunder GG: Musculoskeletal manifestations of bacterial endocarditis. Ann Intern Med 87: 754–759, 1977.
294. Levo Y, Nashif M: Musculoskeletal manifestations of bacterial endocarditis. Clin Exp Rheumatol 1: 49–52, 1983.
295. Williams RC Jr, Kunkel HG: Rheumatoid factor, complement and conglutinin aberrations in patients with subacute bacterial endocarditis. J Clin Invest 41: 666, 1962.
296. Bayer AS, Theofilopoulos AN, Eisenberg R, et al: Circulating immune complexes in infective endocarditis. N Engl J Med 295: 1500–1505, 1976.
297. Sydenham T: The Works of Thomas Sydenham. London Sydenham Soc 1: 254, 1848.
298. El Kholy A, Rotta J, Wannamaker LW: Recent advances in rheumatic fever control and future prospect: a WHO memorandum. Bull WHO 56: 887–912, 1978.
299. World Health Organization: WHO programme for the prevention of rheumatic fever/rheumatic heart disease in 16 developing countries: report from Phase I (1986–90). WHO Cardiovascular Diseases Unit and principal investigators. Bull WHO 70: 213–218, 1992.
300. Denny FW: The streptococcus saga continues. N Engl J Med 325: 127–128, 1991.
301. Bisno AL: Group A streptococcal infections and acute rheumatic fever. N Engl J Med 325: 783–793, 1991.
302. Homer C, Shulman ST: Clinical aspects of acute rheumatic fever. J Rheumatol Suppl 29: 2–13, 1991.
303. Wong D, Bortolussi R, Lang B: An outbreak of acute rheumatic fever in Nova Scotia. Can Commun Dis Rep 24: 45–47, 1998.
304. Bocanegra TS, Vasey FB: Musculoskeletal syndromes in parasitic diseases. Rheum Dis Clin North Am 19: 505–513, 1993.
305. Woo P, Panayi GS: Reactive arthritis due to infestation with *Giardia lamblia*. J Rheumatol 11: 719, 1984.
306. Burnstein SL, Liakos S: Parasitic rheumatism presenting as rheumatoid arthritis. J Rheumatol 10: 514–515, 1983.
307. Williams D, Roy S: Arthritis and arthralgia associated with toxocaral infestation. Br Med J (Clin Res Ed) 283: 192, 1981.
308. Atkin SL, Kamel M, el-Hady AM, et al: Schistosomiasis and inflammatory polyarthritis: a clinical, radiological and laboratory study of 96 patients infected by *S. mansoni* with particular reference to the diarthrodial joint. Q J Med 59: 479–487, 1986.
309. Corman LC: Acute arthritis occurring in association with subcutaneous *Dirofilaria tenuis* infection. Arthritis Rheum 30: 1431–1434, 1987.
310. Wirostko E, Johnson L, Wirostko W: Juvenile rheumatoid arthritis inflammatory eye disease. Parasitization of ocular leukocytes by mollicute-like organisms. J Rheumatol 16: 1446–1453, 1989.

32

Lyme Disease

Hans-Iko Huppertz and Frank Dressler

Lyme arthritis was first described by Steere and colleagues in 1977[1] in a cluster of children thought to have juvenile rheumatoid arthritis (JRA) in and around Old Lyme, Connecticut. Subsequent studies documented that this arthritis was caused by the spirochete *Borrelia burgdorferi*[2, 3] and that arthritis was only one of many possible manifestations of this infection now known as *Lyme borreliosis* or *Lyme disease*.[4–8]

Clinical case descriptions of various manifestations of this disease date back more than a century. Acrodermatitis chronica atrophicans was described in Germany in 1883.[9] Erythema migrans, the early skin manifestation of Lyme borreliosis, was noted in Sweden in 1909.[10] The first case of neuroborreliosis and its association with a tick bite was reported in France in 1922.[11] Among the cases of lymphocytic meningitis and inflammatory polyneuritis studied by Bannwarth in Germany in 1941,[12] several patients were described with "rheumatism," probably the first report of what is now called Lyme arthritis. Successful treatment with penicillin was described in 1946.[13] Erythema migrans was transferred by skin biopsy to healthy human volunteers in 1955.[14] These observations suggested an infectious etiology.

DEFINITION AND CLASSIFICATION

Lyme disease is a complex disease with cutaneous, articular, neurologic, and other systemic manifestations that results from infection with the spirochete *B. burgdorferi* transmitted by the bite of a tick of the genus *Ixodes*. Various components of the disease (e.g., erythema migrans, arthritis, and neuroborreliosis) may occur in isolation. The term *Lyme borreliosis* is often used in Europe; *Lyme disease* is the most frequent term in North America. Clinical and serologic criteria for diagnosis are described later.

EPIDEMIOLOGY

Geographic Distribution

Lyme disease has been documented only in the temperate zones of the Northern Hemisphere.[4, 15] In North America, the disease is recognized most commonly in the northeastern United States, less commonly in the Midwest, South, and West Coast, and in Ontario, Canada.[16, 17] Lyme borreliosis is rare or absent in the other parts of the United States and Canada. In Europe, the disease is most common in central Europe but occurs endemically from southern Sweden to the northern Mediterranean and from Portugal to Russia. Although sporadic cases of Lyme disease have been noted in eastern Russia, China, Korea, and Japan, it appears to be much less common in Asia than in the endemic areas of North America or Europe.

Incidence and Prevalence

The Centers for Disease Control and Prevention has reported a rapid increase in the frequency of Lyme disease in the United States since 1982. Up to 1996, 16,455 cases were reported.[17] In 1997 and 1998, case numbers were 12,801 and 15,934, respectively (D. T. Dennis, personal communication, 1999). The highest incidence (95 per 100,000) was in Connecticut; the highest local incidence (1200 per 100,000) was on the island of Nantucket, Massachusetts.[16, 17] Data from the Slovenian National Registry document annual incidences of Lyme disease of 114 to 155 per 100,000 between 1993 and 1998 (see ref. 18; F. Strle also supplied data via personal communication, 1999). A study in southern Sweden reported an incidence of 69 per 100,000; Lyme arthritis was present in 7 percent of all cases.[19] In a population-based study in Würzburg, Germany, the incidence was 111 per 100,000, with higher rates in children younger than 16 years.[20]

In a community-based Connecticut cohort study of 201 consecutive cases in children in whom Lyme disease had been newly diagnosed, 13 (6 percent) had arthritis and 5 percent had facial palsy.[21] In Europe, Lyme arthritis has been reported slightly less commonly than early neuroborreliosis, although in the Würzburg study, arthritis was more common.[20] Compared with adults, children more frequently had manifestations other than isolated erythema migrans.[20] Early onset of cutaneous disease and neural involvement are closely related to tick activity in the spring to autumn months; there is no seasonal pattern to late manifestations such as Lyme arthritis.[4, 5, 20, 22]

Sex Ratio and Age at Onset

Both sexes are affected equally. Cases have been reported in all ages, with peaks in school-age children and between 40 and 74 years of age.[19–20]

GENETIC BACKGROUND

Although Lyme disease may affect several members of the same family, genetic factors appear to have a limited influence on its development. Nonetheless, host factors influence the course of the disease. In American patients, the development of chronic Lyme arthritis and antibiotic unresponsiveness has been associated with the presence of human leukocyte antigen (HLA)-DR4. DR2 is an additional risk factor, especially in patients who are DR4 negative.[23] These results have not been confirmed in European patients.

ETIOLOGY AND PATHOGENESIS

Etiology

Lyme disease is the most common vector-borne infection in North America and Europe and is transmitted by hard-bodied ticks of the genus *Ixodes*[4, 24] (Fig. 32–1). Transmission by other ticks or flying hematophagous insects has been suggested but not proven. Ticks of the genus *Ixodes* include *I. ricinus* in central Europe, *I. persulcatus* in eastern Europe and Asia, *I. scapularis* in the northeastern and north-central United States and Ontario, and *I. pacificus* in the western United States.[4] Infection is acquired in tick habitats, including forests, gardens, lawns, and inner-city parks. After gaining access to unprotected skin, ticks crawl to the preferred feeding locations on the thigh, groin, breast, axilla, neck, or head. *Ixodes* ticks feed only once during each of the three stages of their life cycle. Most human infections occur after the painless bite of nymphs (Fig. 32–2). *Ixodes* ticks also transmit tickborne encephalitis virus and *Ehrlichia* and *Babesia* organisms. Coinfection of these organisms with *B. burgdorferi* has been reported.[25–27]

Microbiology

Lyme disease is caused by infection with one of several species of *B. burgdorferi sensu lato*. These spirochetes have a protoplasmic cylinder surrounded by a cell membrane, a periplasmic flagellum, and an outer membrane.[28] They are microaerophilic and grow best at 33°C in a special liquid medium. They grow slowly, with doubling times between 12 and 24 hours. *B. burgdorferi sensu lato* has been subdivided into several species, of which only *B. burgdorferi sensu stricto* has been found to cause human disease in North America; in addition, *Borrelia garinii* and *Borrelia afzelii* have been identified regularly in patients in Europe.[4, 5, 29] In general, diversity in *B. burgdorferi* organisms has been greater in Europe and Asia than in North America. Concurrent infection with more than one species of *B. burgdorferi* was described in a patient with acrodermatitis and erythema migrans,[30] as was culture-confirmed reinfection in patients with several episodes of erythema migrans.[31]

B. burgdorferi species differ genomically. Even within a species, different strains express proteins of different molecular weights as identified on gel electrophoresis. The major proteins identified in sonicates of *B. burgdorferi* are the 41 kD flagellar antigen; the 60 kD GroEL heat-shock protein; the three major outer surface proteins (Osp) OspA (30 to 32 kD), OspB (34 to 36 kD), and OspC (21 to 25 kD); the 39 kD BmpA protein; and the 83 to 100 kD antigen. Other proteins remain unidentified. The linear chromosome and 11 plasmids of *B. burgdorferi sensu stricto* strain B31 have been sequenced.[32]

The natural reservoirs of *B. burgdorferi* are mice and voles, although other animals (i.e., hedgehogs, songbirds) may also subserve this function. The life cycle of *Ixodes* ticks lasts 2 years (see Fig. 32–2).[33] The eggs hatch and larvae develop in the spring of the first year. The larvae feed once that summer on their preferred host (i.e., the white-footed mouse) and so become infected with *B. burgdorferi*. The next spring, the larvae molt into nymphs, which feed once again on the preferred host before becoming mature ticks, at which time larger animals (such as deer) act as a host. Mating occurs

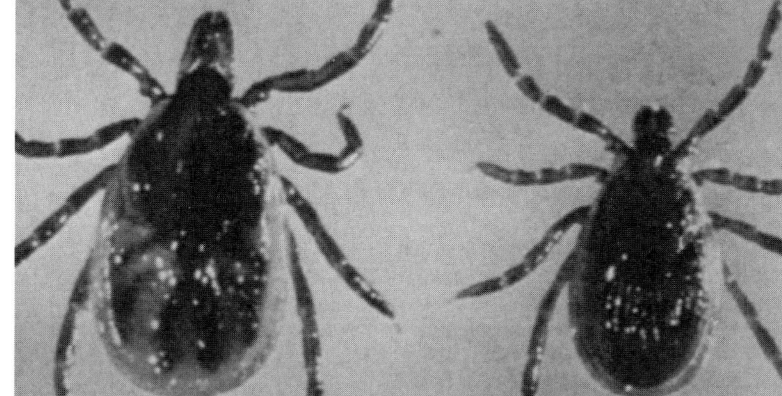

Figure 32–1. *Ixodes scapularis*, a member of the *Ixodes ricinus* complex. *A*, Adult. *B*, Nymph. (From Pfizer Central Research.)

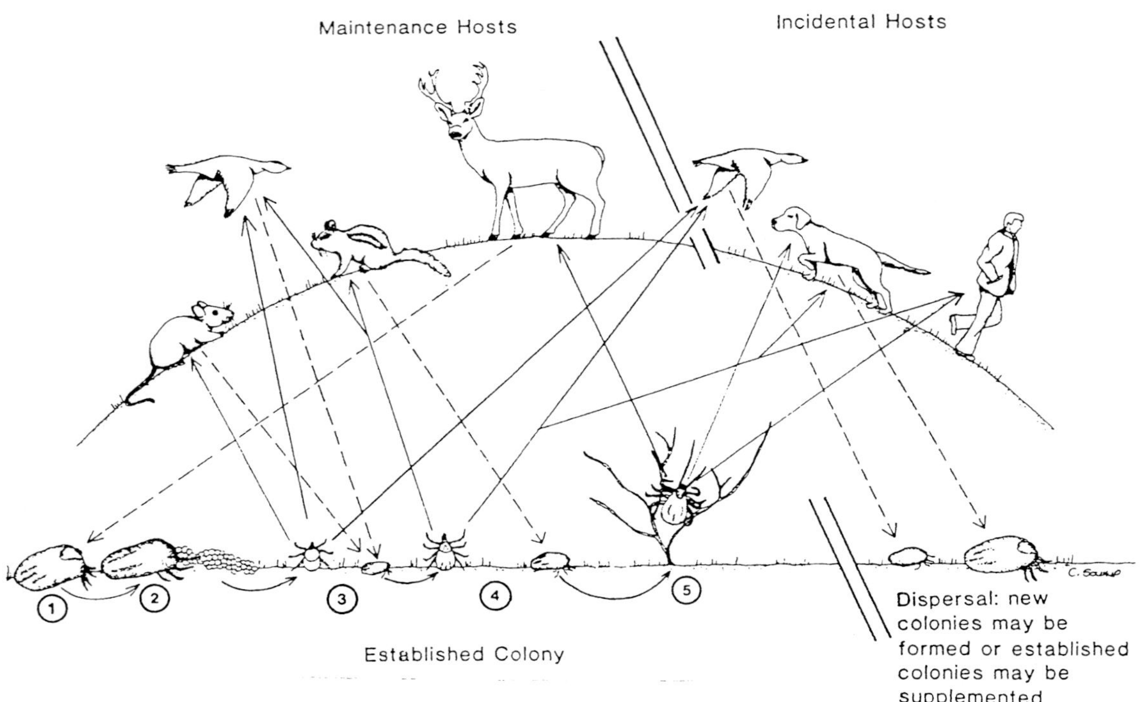

Figure 32–2. Life cycle of *Ixodes scapularis.* 1, Engorged female; 2, adult female laying eggs; 3, questing and engorged larva; 4, questing and engorged nymph; 5, questing adult; *solid arrows,* questing tick successfully finds host; *dashed arrows,* tick engorges and drops from host; *curved arrows,* tick develops to next stage. (From Anderson JF, Magnarelli LA: Avian and mammalian hosts for spirochete-infected ticks and insects in a Lyme disease focus in Connecticut. *In* Steere AC, Malawista AC, Craft JE, et al [eds]: First International Symposium on Lyme Disease, New Haven, CT. Yale J Biol Med 57: 638, 1984.)

while the female tick feeds. The female then detaches and lays her eggs on the ground.

Pathogenesis

Lyme arthritis provides a fascinating model for other arthritides because the causative organism and the clinical picture are well known. However, knowledge of the pathogenesis of this disease remains fragmented. *B. burgdorferi* excreted through tick salivary glands spread locally in the skin and can frequently be found at the advancing edge of erythema migrans. They attach to human cells by binding to various integrins, such as the fibronectin and vitronectin receptors.[34] Binding of the organism to platelets may play a role in its hematogenous spread.[35] *B. burgdorferi* organisms are presumed to reach the synovium through the bloodstream. It is probable that their presence in synovium is required at the onset of arthritis and for the ongoing inflammatory process.

Survival of *B. burgdorferi* for decades in the lesions of acrodermatitis chronica atrophicans indicates that the spirochetes are able to evade the host immune response. There is also evidence that *B. burgdorferi* may survive intracellularly in endothelial cells, fibroblasts, and synovial cells.[36–38] *B. burgdorferi* has stimulatory effects on B cells,[39] and a dominant Th1-cell response has been found in synovial fluid of patients with Lyme arthritis.[40, 41] In addition to these CD4+ T cells, a *B. burgdorferi*–specific CD8+ cytotoxic T-cell response has been confirmed in patients with Lyme arthritis.[42] Interestingly, these cells were found only after the disappearance of arthritis.[42] A number of cytokines are induced, including the interleukins-1 and -6,[43, 44] tumor necrosis factor,[45] and interferon-γ and interleukin-10.[46]

Molecular mimicry might also play a role in the pathogenesis of some of the manifestations of Lyme disease. Sequence homologies have been identified between *B. burgdorferi* flagellin and human myelin basic protein as well as cross-reactivity between flagellin and a human axonal protein.[47, 48] In American patients, antibody reactivity to OspA and OspB occurred late in the course of infection in patients with chronic Lyme arthritis.[49] T-helper cells from patients with treatment-resistant Lyme arthritis demonstrated dominant recognition of an OspA peptide of *B. burgdorferi*.[50] A study published in 1998 implicates the human leukocyte function–associated antigen-1 (LFA-1) as a candidate autoantigen in treatment-resistant Lyme arthritis.[51]

CLINICAL MANIFESTATIONS

Many persons infected with *B. burgdorferi* are asymptomatic. Very often, a tick bite is not recalled. In symptomatic patients, the cutaneous, nervous, and musculoskeletal systems are most commonly involved.[4–7] Symptoms of Lyme disease can be divided into early and late manifestations (Table 32–1). Early signs of

Table 32–1

Major Clinical Manifestations of Lyme Disease in Children and Adolescents

ORGAN SYSTEM	EARLY LYME DISEASE	LATE LYME DISEASE
Skin	Erythema migrans Borrelial lymphocytoma*	Acrodermatits chronica atrophicans*
Nervous system	Cranial nerve palsy Lymphocytic meningitis	Chronic encephalomyelitis*
Musculoskeletal system	Arthralgia	Arthritis Myositis*
Other	Carditis*	

*Rare in childhood.

infection become evident within weeks or a few months of the tick bite, whereas late organ involvement begins several months or even years later. Early symptoms are usually self-limiting, whereas late manifestations may become chronic and occasionally lead to irreversible damage of involved organs. It is important to note that most patients present with disease that affects only one organ system.

Cutaneous Disease

The earliest and most common skin manifestation, *erythema migrans,* typically occurs days to months after infection as an enlarging, warm, but usually painless erythematous rash at the site of the bite that lasts for days or weeks (Fig. 32–3).[4–7, 52] In its classic form, this lesion begins as a red macule or papule and expands peripherally with partial central clearing. In children, the neck and head are the most frequently affected sites. It is also common in the groin, axilla, or thigh and may be quite large (up to 30 cm). Secondary lesions can occur at sites distant from the tick bite. Erythema migrans may be accompanied by flu-like symptoms of fever, chills, arthralgia, musculoskeletal pain, headaches, malaise, and fatigue. Lyme disease may also begin as a flu-like illness in the absence of erythema migrans.[53]

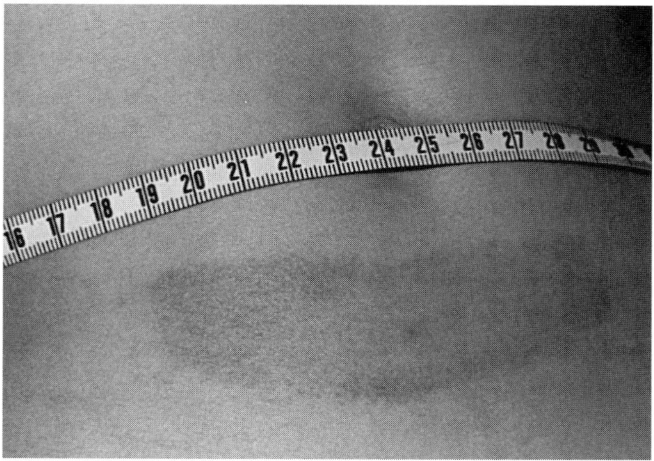

Figure 32–3. Erythema migrans. The site of the tick bite is visible near the center of the lesion.

Weeks to months after infection, borrelial lymphocytoma, also known as *lymphadenosis cutis benigna* (a purple swelling most commonly at an earlobe, the scrotum, or a nipple) is occasionally reported in European patients.[54] *Acrodermatitis chronica atrophicans,* a late skin manifestation, rarely affects European children and then only years after infection.[52, 55] In the early phase of acrodermatitis, the affected limb develops inflammatory changes with a red or bluish discoloration. Later, cutaneous atrophy becomes apparent. A peripheral neuropathy can accompany the skin lesion. Both lymphocytoma and acrodermatitis are extremely uncommon in North America.

Nervous System Disease (Neuroborreliosis)

Early neuroborreliosis most frequently presents as lymphocytic meningitis or a cranial nerve palsy weeks to months after infection.[56–58] It may be accompanied by fever, headache, nausea, vomiting, radicular paresthesias, or pain. Unilateral or bilateral facial nerve palsy is the most common focal neurologic manifestation, but cranial nerves III, IV, VI, or VIII may also be affected. Signs of meningitis may be mild or absent in spite of increased protein and lymphocytes in the cerebrospinal fluid. A painful meningoradiculoneuritis is the most common neurologic manifestation in European adults but is relatively rare in children. Months to years after infection, a relatively few patients will develop progressive encephalomyelitis or an encephalopathy.[57–59] Other rare neurologic manifestations include the Guillain-Barré syndrome,[60, 61] pseudotumor cerebri,[62] optic neuritis,[63] or cerebral vasculitis.[64, 65]

Musculoskeletal Disease

After erythema migrans, arthritis is the most common manifestation of Lyme borreliosis in some series of pediatric patients and is perhaps slightly more common in North America than in Europe.[4–8, 22, 66–69] There is little evidence that the musculoskeletal symptoms of Lyme borreliosis otherwise differ between Europe and North America. Myalgia and myositis occur less often, and enthesitis is not a common feature, although *B. burgdorferi* have been cultured from a few patients with enthesitis.[70] Arthralgia and myalgia develop as early as days to weeks after infection, sometimes concurrent with erythema migrans or flu-like symptoms. However, arthritis appears typically months to years after infection.[71]

The two largest series of pediatric patients with Lyme arthritis include 90 children from Connecticut[68] and 109 from Germany,[71] 62 of whom have been described in detail.[22] Monarthritis of a knee occurred in approximately two thirds of all children.[22, 68] Both knees or other large joints may also be affected.[22, 68, 71] Polyarticular involvement of small joints was rare. At onset, the arthritis was usually episodic with relatively painless swelling lasting only a few days and disappearing without therapy. Recurrent episodes of arthritis may become prolonged, and chronic arthritis (duration >3 months) has been reported in up to 18 percent of patients.[22] Among 109 German children with Lyme arthritis, 70 had monarthritis, 32 oligoarthritis, and 7 polyarthritis.[71] The pattern of oligoarticular involvement differed from that found in patients with early-onset oligoarticular JRA or juvenile spondyloarthropathy. Ocular involvement with keratitis and anterior and intermediate uveitis may occur in children with Lyme arthritis.[71a]

Myositis has only rarely been described in adult patients,[69] and only myalgia has been reported in children.[72] A dermatomyositis-like picture has also occurred in an adult patient.[73] *B. burgdorferi* was isolated from a child with subacute multifocal osteomyelitis.[74] Fibromyalgia may follow Lyme borreliosis and does not respond to antibiotic therapy.[75]

Other Manifestations

Involvement of other organ systems is much more rare. Carditis is very rare in children and most commonly presents as a reversible atrioventricular block.[76] Ocular involvement including conjunctivitis, keratitis, iridocyclitis, intermediate uveitis, choroiditis, or optic neuritis has been described in children with Lyme arthritis.[71a, 77, 78] Even more rarely, patients may develop hepatitis[79] or neurogenic bladder.[80] There have been anecdotal reports of transplacental transmission of *B. burgdorferi*,[81] but this has not been confirmed in controlled studies.[82] The offspring of 5 of 19 pregnant women who had Lyme disease during pregnancy had one or more of the following abnormal outcomes: prematurity, syndactyly, rash, cortical blindness, developmental delay, or intrauterine fetal death.[83, 84] Whether any of these complications is attributable to infection with *B. burgdorferi* or with other spirochetes is not certain. At present, there is no evidence that maternal infection presents a significant risk to the fetus.

PATHOLOGY

The synovitis of Lyme arthritis resembles that of JRA, with villous hypertrophy, synovial cell hyperplasia, and infiltration of lymphocytes and plasma cells.[85] Lymphoid follicles may also be present. Endarteritis is also a characteristic finding in Lyme synovitis. In one study, spirochetes were detected in 2 of 17 synovia, mainly in a perivascular distribution.[85] Other studies using special silver stains have also identified *B. burgdorferi* in synovium or synovial fluid.[86, 87] The organism has also been recovered from the margins of the erythema migrans lesion and cardiac tissue.[88, 89, 90] Although cardiomyopathy may result from the initial myocarditis, valvular endocarditis does not develop. Myositis may in part account for the myalgia and fatigue that occur in this disease, and DNA from *B. burgdorferi* has been identified in the muscle of such patients.[91]

LABORATORY EXAMINATION

Nonspecific Abnormalities

The erythrocyte sedimentation rate is elevated in one half of the patients, especially during the early phase of Lyme arthritis. Meningoencephalitis results in a mild cerebrospinal fluid lymphocytic pleocytosis.[92] The mean synovial fluid white blood cell count ranges from less than 1000 to greater than 50,000/mm^3, with a predominance of neutrophils in samples with high cell counts.[22]

Confirmation of Infection With *B. burgdorferi*

Laboratory methods to document infection with *B. burgdorferi* include direct tests, such as culture or the polymerase chain reaction (PCR) to detect borrelial sequences, and indirect tests such as serology (Table 32–2).[93] The latter tests are most frequently used and universally available. Although attempts have been made to standardize the laboratory evaluation of North American patients with Lyme disease, the approach suggested by the American College of Physicians[94, 95] has not been widely adopted for European patients. Some of the common problems with standardization of test procedures for the diagnosis of Lyme disease have been reviewed.[96]

Direct Methods to Detect Infection

Culture of *B. burgdorferi* usually takes from 2 weeks to a few months, requires immediate suspension of the test material in special medium, and has relatively high

Table 32–2

Laboratory Diagnosis of Lyme Arthritis

METHOD	ASSESSMENT
Culture of *B. burgdorferi*	Requires weeks; rarely successful
Histochemistry using silver stain or monoclonal antibodies	Rarely successful in synovial tissue
Polymerase chain reaction for borrelial DNA	Efficiency varies widely: Urine 5–85% Synovium (6–90%) (Higher in membrane than in fluid)
Enzyme immunoassay or immunofluorescence assay	High sensitivity, low specificity
Immunoblot	Confirmatory test with high specificity
Lymphocyte-proliferation assay with borrelial antigens	Sensitivity and specificity <80% Limited availability

All diagnostic tests bear the risk of false-negative or false-positive results. No test is of value in a patient with low pre-test probability of having Lyme arthritis.

Adapted from Huppertz HI: Lyme arthritis. *In* Wahn U, Seger R, Wahn V (eds): Paediatrische Allergologie and Immunologie. Munich, Urban & Fischer, 1999, pp 598–602.

rates of recovery only in skin biopsies of patients with dermatologic manifestations of the disease.[88] Culture of the organism from blood and synovial fluid has been relatively unsuccessful. The possibility of obtaining positive cultures is somewhat better from the cerebrospinal fluid of patients with early neuroborreliosis.[97] Methods such as silver staining of spirochetes in tissue specimens or staining with monoclonal antibodies are not routinely performed and are relatively prone to artifacts.

The PCR can demonstrate DNA of *B. burgdorferi* in tissues or body fluids including synovial fluid.[98–103] In a large North American study of synovial fluid from patients with Lyme arthritis,[98] PCR was positive in 96 percent of patients not previously treated with antibiotics and in 37 percent of those who had been treated. In a later study from the same group, borrelial sequences were undetectable in synovial specimens from patients with chronic Lyme arthritis following long-term antibiotic therapy.[98a]

The precise role of PCR in routine diagnosis is unclear. False-positive or false-negative results may occur. Optimization of PCR includes using more than one primer pair, targeting genes situated on both the bacterial chromosome and the plasmids, performing nested PCR, and analyzing both synovial fluid and urine.[99] There is evidence that PCR on synovial tissue may have a higher positivity rate than with synovial fluid[102] and may remain positive in patients with ongoing arthritis whose synovial fluid is negative by PCR after antibiotic treatment.[103] PCR in urine may be positive in healthy humans whose sera contain *B. burgdorferi*–specific antibodies.[104]

Indirect Methods to Detect Infection

Specific antibodies can be demonstrated after *B. burgdorferi* infection by a variety of tests including enzyme-immunoassay (EIA), immunofluorescence, hemagglutination, and Western blotting[104a] (Fig. 32–4). It is recommended that a sensitive EIA be used as a screening test and that all results in the indeterminate or low positive ranges be confirmed by Western blotting.[105] Immunoglobulin (Ig) M Western blots are considered positive if at least two of the following three bands are present:

- 21 kD OspC
- 39 kD BmpA
- 41 kD flagellin

IgG blots are considered positive if at least 5 of the following 10 bands are present[105–107]:

- 18 kD
- 21 kD OspC
- 28 kD
- 30 kD
- 39 kD BmpA
- 41 kD flagellin
- 45 kD
- 58 kD
- 66 kD
- 93 kD

Typical IgM and IgG responses of patients with Lyme arthritis are shown in Figure 32–4. It must be noted that antigens from different strains of *B. burgdorf-*

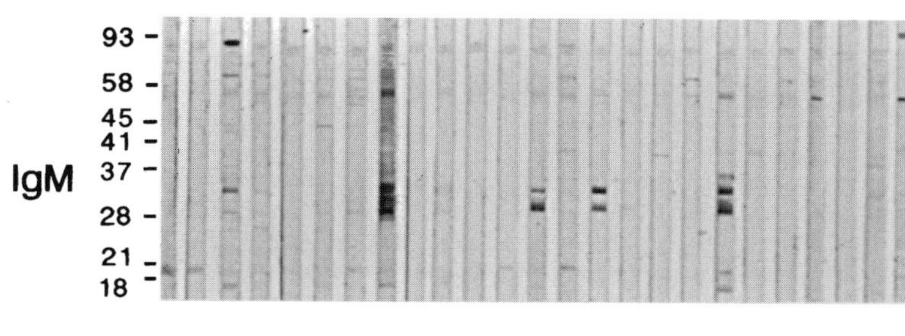

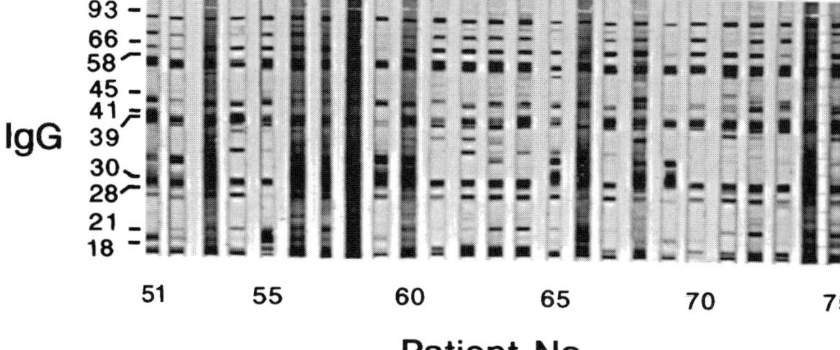

Figure 32–4. Western blots of immunoglobulin M (IgM) and IgG antibody responses of 25 patients with Lyme arthritis to a sonicated whole-cell lysate of *Borrelia burgdorferi sensu stricto* strain G39/40. Molecular weight (in kilodaltons) is indicated on the left side. Characteristic of Lyme arthritis, strong IgG responses against many antigens are demonstrated. In North America, criteria for a positive IgG blot are the detection of least five of the following 10 bands: 18 kD, 21 kD OspC, 28 kD, 30 kD, 39 kD BmpA, 41 kD flagellin, 45 kD, 58 kD, 66 kD, and 93 kD. All patients met these criteria. A minority of patients also have IgM responses to a smaller number of antigens. Molecular weights may vary depending on the strain used for testing. (Adapted from Dressler F, Whalen JA, Reinhardt BN, et al: Western blotting in the serodiagnosis of Lyme disease. J Infect Dis 167: 392, 1993. By permission of the publisher, the University of Chicago.)

eri have different molecular weights. For this reason, North American criteria cannot easily be applied in Europe or Asia, where there is greater strain diversity. Even so, a two-test approach is the best currently available method for diagnosis of Lyme disease in European children.[22] In a German pediatric Lyme arthritis study,[22] at least six specific bands were required for a positive IgG Western blot, similar to the American criteria. Commonly, patients with Lyme disease have 10 or more IgG bands, including the ones mentioned earlier. Specific blot-positivity criteria have been established for each of the three pathogenic species in Europe, with different positivity criteria for each strain.[108, 108a]

Within the first weeks after infection, all serologic results may be negative because specific IgM antibodies usually do not appear until 3 to 4 weeks after infection and IgG antibodies cannot be detected until 4 to 8 weeks after infection. Not infrequently, EIA may give false-positive results related to cross-reactive antibodies such as RFs or after infection with Epstein-Barr virus[109] or other spirochetes, including *Treponema pallidum*, *Treponema denticola*, *Borrelia hermsii*, and leptospirosis.[110] Antibodies to *B. burgdorferi* occasionally are found in children with JRA,[111, 112] systemic lupus erythematosus,[113] and other illness (bacterial endocarditis, mumps, Rocky Mountain spotted fever, other rickettsial diseases).

Serologic tests cannot distinguish patients with active infection from those with a previous infection that has responded to therapy. In particular, about 10 percent of patients with late manifestations of Lyme disease continue to demonstrate both an IgM and an IgG response. Because IgG titers tend to remain elevated for years, serology also cannot be used to monitor treatment success or failure. In an endemic area, serologic tests should be performed only in patients with clinical signs suggestive of the disease because a positive result in a patient with a low pre-test probability of Lyme disease is much more likely to represent a false-positive rather than a true-positive result.[96, 114] Given these restrictions, serology is useful diagnostically in patients with Lyme arthritis because almost all patients are clearly IgG seropositive.[22, 68] Table 32–3 provides a simplified overview of the laboratory evaluation.

"Seronegative" Lyme arthritis has been described[115–117] but must be considered to be so rare that vigorous attempts must be undertaken by centers with special experience with this disease to rule out another diagnosis. In these cases, the cellular immune response induced by *B. burgdorferi* can be evaluated,[36, 115–118] and this is the route that is recommended when clinical symptoms and serologic results are discordant.[117] However, lymphoproliferative assays are not well standardized and have high rates of false positivity and false negativity.[115–117]

Table 32–3

Laboratory Evaluation of Patients With Suspected Lyme Arthritis

- Patient living in or having visited an endemic area
- Presence of arthritis documented
- No other obvious cause of arthritis

Serology positive (enzyme immunoassay [EIA] and Western blot):
No further laboratory test needed
Start therapy

Serology negative (EIA and Western blot):
Rule out other diagnosis
Refer for specialized evaluation

DIAGNOSIS

Clinical characteristics of patients with arthritis that suggest a diagnosis of Lyme arthritis include residence in or travel to an endemic area, a preceding tick bite, the presence of episodic oligoarthritis involving the knee joint, the absence of arthralgias preceding the onset of arthritis, and an adolescent age at onset. Specific criteria have been combined to form a clinical diagnostic score that would confirm or exclude Lyme arthritis in two thirds of children with arthritis[119] (Table 32–4). For a diagnosis of Lyme arthritis, arthritis (swelling and effusion or painful limitation of motion in the absence of trauma) must be observed by a physician. Arthralgias alone or reports by the patient or the parents that the joint was swollen are not "objective" signs of arthritis in this context.

Not infrequently, however, the clinical presentation of Lyme arthritis may be indistinguishable from that of other rheumatic diseases of childhood with arthritis as a principal manifestation, making laboratory tests mandatory in all patients with arthritis living in or having traveled to an endemic area.[96]

The Centers for Disease Control and Prevention has established criteria for the diagnosis of Lyme disease[120]:

- Presence of erythema migrans >5 cm in diameter *or* at least one clinical sign (arthritis, meningitis, radiculoneuritis, mononeuritis, or carditis)
- Presence of specific antibodies to *B. burgdorferi*

However, these criteria were developed for epidemiologic research and may not always be applicable in the clinical setting. For example, borrelial lymphocytoma may initially occur in the absence of specific antibodies. Moreover, the mere combination of an objective sign with specific antibodies may include chance associations between two not-infrequent events: arthritis of some kind may affect 1 in 1000 children, and in endemic areas, up to 3 percent of healthy blood donors may be positive for specific antibodies to *B. burgdorferi*.[121] Serology can provide evidence of present or prior infection but cannot absolutely confirm a pathogenic link between the infection and the clinical manifestation. The child may have been infected with *B. burgdorferi* as documented by serology; however, arthritis may be due not to this infection but to other known or unknown causes.

Synovial fluid analysis is of little help in establishing a diagnosis of Lyme arthritis because the white blood cell count (approximately 30,000/mm^3) and type of cells vary greatly.[101, 122] However, synovial fluid analysis can exclude septic arthritis and other infection-associated arthritides, yields material for testing by PCR, and confirms the presence of inflammation. Although a positive PCR result from an experienced laboratory indicates a persistent infection, a negative result does not exclude the diagnosis. Synovial tissue may be more

Table 32–4

Diagnosis of Lyme Arthritis Using a Clinical Score

CRITERION	SCORE
Episodic arthritis	+4
Arthralgia before onset of arthritis	−3
Age at onset of arthritis	+0.3 × age in yr
Initial arthritis in knee joint	+2
History of tick bite	+2
Number of joints involved	−0.4 × number of large joints affected

If a criterion is found in the patient, its indicated value is added to (or subtracted from) the total score. If it is not found, the item is scored "0." Values of 6 or greater indicate the presence of Lyme arthritis. Values of 2.5 or below exclude the diagnosis.

Example: A 10-year-old developed arthritis in a knee. There was no prior arthralgia and no history of a tick bite. After 10 days, the arthritis resolved, but it recurred after an interval of 3 mo.

Scoring:		
	Episodic arthritis present	+4
	No initial arthralgias	0
	Age at onset × 0.3	+3
	Initial arthritis in knee	+2
	No history of tick bite	0
	1 large joint affected	−0.4
	Total	8.6

This patient's serum contained IgG antibodies to *B. burgdorferi* by enyme immunoassay and immunblot. He was treated with ceftriaxone for 2 wk. Arthritis disappeared during therapy and has not recurred in the subsequent 2 yr.

Adapted from Huppertz HI, Bentas W, Haubitz I, et al: Diagnosis of pediatric Lyme arthritis using a clinical score. Eur J Pediatr 157: 304, Table 3, 1998 Copyright Springer-Verlag.

suitable than synovial fluid for PCR testing, especially after antibiotic treatment has failed to produce a remission of symptoms.[102, 103]

A lumbar puncture should be performed in patients with suspected neuroborreliosis. Characteristically, lymphocytic pleocytosis and elevated cerebrospinal fluid protein are present.[57, 58] The reliable standard in diagnosing neuroborreliosis in European patients remains detection of intrathecal antibody production.[57, 58, 123] However, specific antibody production frequently occurs only after several weeks to months of infection and has been less commonly demonstrable in American patients.

TREATMENT

Antibiotic Regimens

Recommendations for the treatment of Lyme disease (Table 32–5) vary according to disease manifestations. In the treatment of patients with erythema migrans or neuroborreliosis, amoxicillin plus probenecid is as effective as doxycycline.[124] Cephalosporins were only marginally better than penicillin G.[125–130] Whereas doxycycline and ceftriaxone have been equally effective,[131] macrolide antibiotics are inferior to other antibiotics.[132–135] It is not known whether these results are applicable to patients with Lyme arthritis, in whom a variety of antibiotics have been recommended, including parenteral penicillin G, oral penicillins, amoxicillin with or without probenecid, ceftriaxone, cefotaxime, cefuroxime, erythromycin, roxithromycin (plus cotrimoxazole), azithromycin, tetracycline, doxycycline, and others.[22, 136] When initial treatment with ceftriaxone fails, 4 weeks of therapy with amoxicillin, or roxithromycin plus cotrimoxazole in young children, or doxycycline in adolescents, is recommended. Before one assumes failure of antibiotic therapy, at least two courses of sufficient duration and well-documented compliance are required. When confronted with failure of a treatment program with appropriate antibiotics, the correctness of a diagnosis of Lyme arthritis should be questioned and reconfirmed.

Duration of therapy is a matter of debate. Because *B. burgdorferi* is a slow-growing organism, treatment should be continued for at least 10 days. However, there is no proof that treatment extending beyond 1 month is of any additional benefit. The success of antibiotic treatment must be determined clinically because serologic results remain positive for a long time after resolution of all manifestations.[137]

An approach to treatment is shown in Figure 32–5. In young children, erythema migrans is treated with amoxicillin (50 mg/kg/day) in three doses for 10 days to 3 weeks. In children 10 years or older, doxycycline 200 mg/day is given once daily for 10 days to 3 weeks. In all other forms of the disease, including Lyme arthritis, ceftriaxone 50 mg/kg/day is administered intravenously for 14 days. Because only one 20-minute infusion is required per day, treatment can be continued in the outpatient clinic with an indwelling venous access line. Patients with Lyme arthritis have also been treated successfully with oral antibiotics, including amoxicillin or doxycycline, for 4 weeks. This approach to treatment is more convenient for the patient and more cost-effective than intravenous regimens, but it should not be used in patients with a Baker cyst, neuroborreliosis, or carditis.[138] In case of allergy to penicillin, amoxicillin, or cephalosporins, macrolide antibiotics are recom-

Table 32–5

Current Recommendations for Treatment of Lyme Disease in Children and Adolescents

MANIFESTATION	DRUGS*	DOSE*	DURATION
Erythema migrans	Amoxicillin	50 mg/kg/d in 3–4 doses	10–30 d‡
	Doxycycline†	200 mg/d in 1–2 doses	10–30 d‡
Early disseminated and late disease	Ceftriaxone	50–100 mg/kg/d in 1 dose	2–4 wk
	Cefotaxime	50–150 mg/kg/d in 3 doses	2–4 wk
	Amoxicillin	50 mg/kg/d in 3–4 doses	4 wk
	Doxycycline†	100–200 mg/d in 1–2 doses	4 wk
	Roxithromycine	5 mg/kg/d plus cotrimoxazole 6 mg/kg/d in 2 doses	4 wk

*Ceftriaxone and cefotaxime IV; amoxicillin and doxycycline orally. Maximum daily dose of amoxicillin = 2 g; doxycycline = 200 mg; ceftriaxone = 2 g; cefotaxime = 6 g.

†Doxycycline should not be administered to patients <10 yr of age.

‡Continue treatment for another 10 days if erythema migrans is still present at the end of 10 days.

mended in children under 10 years of age, although these drugs are less effective than the β-lactam antibiotics.[132, 135] This disadvantage may be overcome by a combination of roxithromycin and cotrimoxazol.[139] Infection during pregnancy should be treated with antibiotics not posing a risk to the fetus (i.e., amoxicillin or intravenous penicillin G).

During antibiotic treatment, up to 10 percent of patients with arthritis develop a Jarisch-Herxheimer reaction, with fever, a nonpruritic, nonpalpable rash, and severe pain. This complication usually develops after the first few doses of antibiotics but may occur up to 10 days after beginning treatment. It must be distinguished from allergic reactions to the administered drug.[22] In our experience, most reactions thought to be allergic are Jarisch-Herxheimer reactions. Whereas an allergic response to the antibiotic requires immediate interruption of administration of the drug, a Jarisch-Herxheimer reaction is a favorable self-limited sign, and treatment can be continued.

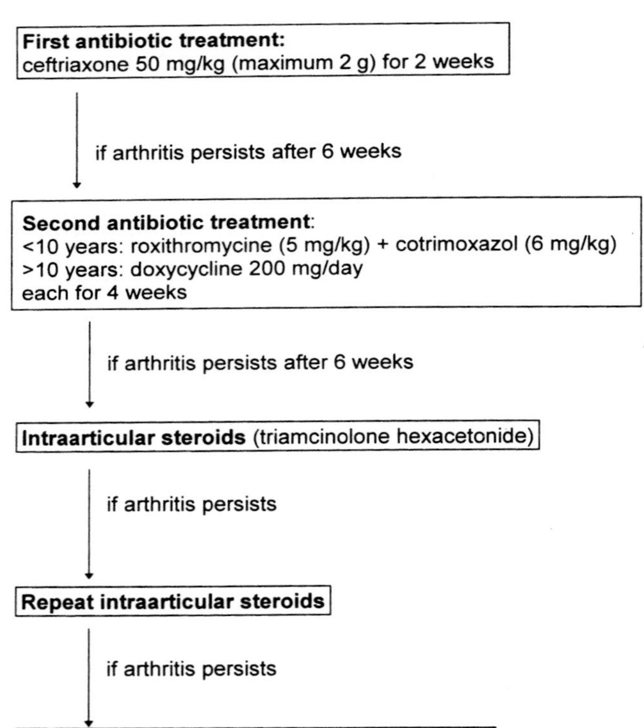

Figure 32–5. Sequential treatment of Lyme arthritis. (Adapted from Huppertz HI: Lyme arthritis. *In* Wahn U, Seger R, Wahn V [eds]: Paediatrische Allergologie und Immunologie. Munich, Urban & Fischer, 1999, pp 598–602.)

Although nonsteroidal anti-inflammatory agents are frequently given to patients with Lyme arthritis, often before the correct diagnosis is made, their efficacy has not been established; however, nonsteroidal anti-inflammatory agents can be used as analgesics or after antibiotics have failed. Treatment failures in patients with Lyme arthritis or late neuroborreliosis are often associated with prior administration of glucocorticoids.[125] In such instances, repetition of antibiotic treatment with the same or another antibiotic is recommended. Intra-articular steroids, sulfasalazine, methotrexate, or arthroscopic synovectomy[140] with a further course of antibiotics—in that order—are treatment options.

Prevention

Recommendations for the prevention of Lyme disease have been published by the American Academy of Pediatrics.[140a]

Avoidance

Avoiding tick bites in endemic areas is difficult. Appropriate clothing with light-colored long trousers tucked into socks makes it more difficult for ticks to attach to a human host. Tick repellents containing N,N-diethylmeta-toluamide (DEET) or permethrin applied to clothing will reduce tick attachment for several hours.[24] DEET may also be applied directly to skin, but the use of repellents on skin should be limited because toxic side effects can occur. Ticks should be removed promptly if present because *B. burgdorferi* resides in the midgut and proliferation starts only after the host's blood has entered the tick's gut. Thereafter, *B. burgdorferi* organisms spread via the acarial hemolymph to the tick's salivary glands. Because this takes 24 to 36 hours, a daily search for and removal of ticks is helpful in endemic areas.[24]

Ticks should be grasped with tweezers as close to their point of attachment as possible and pulled steadily away from the skin to allow the tick to detach its mouth parts.[24] Mouth parts that remain in the skin do not pose a risk for further transmission of *B. burgdorferi* but may lead to a superficial bacterial infection. Therefore, the site of the tick bite should be disinfected after the tick is removed. Prophylactic antibiotics should not be used in the absence of any symptoms because the frequency of their side effects may exceed the estimate of preventable disease manifestations.[141] However, prompt antibiotic treatment of the early manifestations of Lyme disease almost always prevents late manifestations such as arthritis.

Immunization

Two human vaccines have been developed with a recombinant fragment of OspA of *B. burgdorferi sensu stricto*. These vaccines were first evaluated in North American adults and found to be safe. After three injections, vaccine efficacy in adults was 76 to 92 percent.[142, 143] First results of studies of the safety and efficacy of these vaccines in North American children have been reported.[143a] Recommendations for the use of the vaccine have been published.[144, 145] The degree of protection that will be afforded by these vaccines in Europe or Asia, where strain diversity is greater, is unclear.

COURSE OF THE DISEASE AND PROGNOSIS

The prognosis in children with erythema migrans or early neuroborreliosis is excellent when the disease has been promptly treated with appropriate antibiotics.[145, 145a] Even in children with Lyme arthritis who have not been treated, manifestations usually diminish and eventually disappear over time.[78] Among 90 children with Lyme arthritis treated with appropriate antibiotics, 4 had ongoing musculoskeletal complaints 7 years later.[69] Of 51 German children with Lyme arthritis examined 1 year after initiation of antibiotic treatment, 8 patients had chronic arthritis and 4 had persistent arthralgias in joints previously affected by arthritis.[145b] In rare cases, flares of arthritis in a previously affected joint have been observed several years after antibiotic treatment and the initial disappearance of arthritis.

Erosion of cartilage is very rare in children. Arthralgia in joints previously affected by arthritis may persist for several months but, in contrast with similarly affected adults, children generally do not fulfill diagnostic criteria for fibromyalgia, and arthralgias usually do not restrict the physical or educational performance of adolescents. Late neurologic complications have been described in untreated children with Lyme arthritis[78] but have not been observed after appropriate treatment.[146] However, transient neurocognitive abnormalities may occur.[59] Late development of keratitis has occurred in both treated and untreated children.[78] Lyme disease is not fatal and rarely results in significant persistent organ damage, but coinfection with tick-borne encephalitis virus, *Ehrlichia* or *Babesia* organisms may lead to a more severe disease course.[25–27]

A follow-up study in American adult patients found more musculoskeletal disease and verbal memory impairment in patients than in controls.[148] Poor prognosis of Lyme arthritis in American adults has been associated with the presence of antibodies to OspA, HLA-DR2 or DR4, the DRB1*0401 allele, and autoreactivity to LFA-1.[51] The risk of treatment failure seems to increase with increasing age and when intra-articular steroids were given before antibiotics.[125, 145a]

Szer and colleagues[78] studied 46 American children (25 boys) with chronic Lyme arthritis with onset of disease between 1976 and 1979. None had been treated with antibiotics for the first 4 years of disease. Almost all (98 percent) had arthralgias during the early phase, with a median time from onset to development of arthritis of 3 months (range, 2 to 24 months). The number of children with recurrent episodes declined each year. Older children tended to have arthritis of longer duration. At the end of the study, 12 children (31 percent) still had occasional brief episodes of joint pain. One child had marked fatigue, and 2 developed keratitis. All 46 children had persistently positive IgG antibody responses. IgM responses were more frequent and IgG titers higher in children with recurrent symptoms than in those who became asymptomatic.

References

1. Steere AC, Malawista SE, Snydman DR, et al: Lyme arthritis. An epidemic of oligoarticular arthritis in children and adults in three Connecticut communities. Arthritis Rheum 20: 7, 1977.
2. Burgdorfer W, Barbour AG, Hayes SF, et al: Lyme disease—a tick-borne spirochetosis? Science 216: 1317, 1982.
3. Steere AC, Grodzicki RL, Kornblatt AN, et al: The spirochetal etiology of Lyme disease. N Engl J Med 308: 733, 1983.
4. Nadelman RB, Wormser GP: Lyme borreliosis. Lancet 352: 557, 1998.
5. Steere AC: Lyme disease. N Engl J Med 321: 586, 1989.
6. Huppertz HI: Childhood Lyme borreliosis in Europe. Eur J Pediatr 149: 814, 1990.
7. Dressler F: Lyme borreliosis in European children and adolescents. Clin Exp Rheumatol 12(Suppl 10): S49, 1994.
8. Sigal LH: Musculoskeletal manifestations of Lyme arthritis. Rheum Dis Clin North Am 24: 323, 1998.
9. Buchwald A: Ein Fall von diffuser idiopathischer Hautatrophie. Arch Dermatol Syph 10: 553, 1883.
10. Afzelius A: Verhandlungen der dermatologischen Gesellschaft zu Stockholm. Arch Dermatol Syph 101: 404, 1910.
11. Garin C, Bujadoux A: Paralysie par les tiques. J Méd Lyon 71: 765, 1922.
12. Bannwarth A: Chronische lymphocytäre Meningitis, entzündliche Polyneuritis und "Rheumatismus." Arch Psychiatr Nervenkr 113: 284, 1941.
13. Svartz N: Penicillinbehandling vid dermatitis atrophicans Herxheimer. Nord Med 32: 2783, 1946.
14. Binder E, Doepfmer R, Hornstein O: Übertragung des Erythema chronicum migrans von Mensch zu Mensch in zwei Passagen. Klin Wochenschr 33: 727, 1955.
15. Steere AC: Lyme disease: a growing threat to urban populations. Proc Natl Acad Sci U S A 91: 2378, 1994.
16. Lyme disease—United States, 1994. MMWR 44: 459, 1995.
17. Lyme disease—United States, 1996. MMWR 46: 531, 1997.
18. Strle F, Stantic-Pavlinic M: Lyme disease in Europe. N Engl J Med 334: 803, 1996.

19. Berglund J, Eitrem R, Ornstein K, et al: An epidemiologic study of Lyme disease in Southern Sweden. N Engl J Med 333: 1319, 1995.
20. Huppertz HI, Böhme M, Standaert SM, et al: Incidence of Lyme borreliosis in the Würzburg region of Germany. Eur J Clin Microbiol Infect Dis 18: 697–703, 1999.
21. Gerber MA, Shapiro ED, Burke GS, et al: Lyme disease in children in southeastern Connecticut. N Engl J Med 335: 1270, 1996.
22. Huppertz HI, Karch H, Suschke HJ, et al: Lyme arthritis in European children and adolescents. Arthritis Rheum 38: 361, 1995.
23. Steere AC, Dwyer E, Winchester R: Association of chronic Lyme arthritis with HLA-DR4 and HLA-DR2 alleles. N Engl J Med 323: 219, 1990.
24. Fish D: Environmental risk and prevention of Lyme disease. Am J Med 98(Suppl 4A): 2S, 1995.
25. Cimperman J, Maraspin V, Lotric-Furlan S, et al: Concomitant infection with tick-borne encephalitis virus and *Borrelia burgdorferi sensu lato* in patients with acute meningitis or meningoencephalitis. Infection 26: 160, 1998.
26. Krause PJ, Telford SR, Spielman A, et al: Concurrent Lyme disease and babesiosis: evidence for increased severity and duration of disease. JAMA 275: 1657, 1996.
27. Nadelman RB, Horowitz HW, Hsieh T, et al: Simultaneous human granulocytic ehrlichiosis and Lyme borreliosis. N Engl J Med 337: 27, 1997.
28. Barbour AG, Hayes SF: Biology of *Borrelia* species. Microbiol Rev 50: 381, 1986.
29. Huppertz HI, Horneff G, Neudorf U, et al: Acute childhood neuroborreliosis with a selective immune response to a low molecular weight protein expressed by *Borrelia garinii*. Eur J Pediatr 153: 898, 1994.
30. Wienecke R, Neubert U, Volkenandt M: Cross immunity among types of *Borrelia burgdorferi*. Lancet 342: 435, 1993.
31. Nowakowski J, Schwartz I, Nadelman R, et al: Culture-confirmed infection and reinfection with *Borrelia burgdorferi*. Ann Intern Med 127: 130, 1997.
32. Fraser CM, Casjens S, Huang WM, et al: Genomic sequence of a Lyme disease spirochaete, *Borrelia burgdorferi*. Nature 390: 580, 1997.
33. Anderson JF, Magnarelli LA: Avian and mammalian hosts for spirochete-infected ticks and insects in a Lyme disease focus in Connecticut. *In* Steere AC, Malawista AC, Craft JE, et al (eds): First International Symposium on Lyme Disease, New Haven. Yale J Biol Med 57: 638, 1984.
34. Coburn J, Magoun L, Bodary SC, et al: Integrins alpha(v)-beta3 and alpha5beta1 mediate attachment of Lyme disease spirochetes to human cells. Infect Immun 66: 1946, 1998.
35. Coburn JC, Leong JM, Erban JK: Integrin alpha IIb-beta III mediates binding of the Lyme disease agent *Borrelia burgdorferi* to human platelets. Proc Natl Acad Sci U S A 90: 7059, 1993.
36. Ma Y, Sturrock A, Weis JJ: Intracellular localization of *Borrelia burgdorferi* within human endothelial cells. Infect Immun 59: 671, 1991.
37. Klempner M, Noring R, Rogers RA: Invasion of human skin fibroblasts by the Lyme disease spirochete, *Borrelia burgdorferi*. J Infect Dis 167: 1074, 1993.
38. Girschick HJ, Huppertz HI, Rüssmann H, et al: Intracellular persistence of *Borrelia burgdorferi* in human synovial cells. Rheumatol Int 16: 125, 1996.
39. Yang L, Ma Y, Schoenfeld R, et al: Evidence of B-lymphocyte mitogen activity in *Borrelia burgdorferi*–infected mice. Infect Immun 60: 3033, 1992.
40. Yin Z, Braun J, Neure L, et al: T cell cytokine pattern in the joints of patients with Lyme arthritis and its regulation by cytokines and anticytokines. Arthritis Rheum 40: 69, 1997.
41. Gross DM, Steere AC, Huber BT: T helper 1 response is dominant and localized to the synovial fluid in patients with Lyme arthritis. J Immunol 160: 1022, 1998.
42. Busch DH, Jassoy C, Brinckmann U, et al: Detection of *Borrelia burgdorferi*–specific CD8+ cytotoxic T-cells in patients with Lyme arthritis. J Immunol 157: 3534, 1996.
43. Miller LC, Isa S, Vannier E, et al: Live *Borrelia burgdorferi* preferentially activate interleukin-1beta gene expression and protein synthesis over the interleukin-1 receptor antagonist. J Clin Invest 90: 906, 1992.
44. Habicht GS, Katona LI, Benach JL: Cytokines and the pathogenesis of neuroborreliosis: *Borrelia burgdorferi* induces glioma cells to secrete interleukin-6. J Infect Dis 164: 568, 1991.
45. Defosse DL, Johnson RC: In vitro and in vivo induction of tumor necrosis factor alpha by *Borrelia burgdorferi*. Infect Immun 60: 1109, 1992.
46. Pohl-Koppe A, Balashov KE, Steere AC, et al: Identification of a T cell subset capable of both IFN-gamma and IL-10 secretion in patients with chronic *Borrelia burgdorferi* infection. J Immunol 160: 1804, 1998.
47. Weigelt W, Schneider T, Lange R: Sequence homology between spirochaete flagellin and human myelin basic protein. Immunol Today 13: 279, 1992.
48. Sigal LH: Cross-reactivity between *Borrelia burgdorferi* flagellin and a human axonal 64000 molecular weight protein. J Infect Dis 167: 1372, 1993.
49. Kalish R, Leong JM, Steere AC: Association of treatment-resistant chronic Lyme arthritis with HLA-DR4 and antibody reactivity to OspA and OspB of *Borrelia burgdorferi*. Infect Immun 61: 2774, 1993.
50. Kamradt T, Lengl-Janssen B, Strauss AF, et al: Dominant recognition of a *Borrelia burgdorferi* outer surface protein A peptide by T helper cells in patients with treatment-resistant Lyme arthritis. Infect Immun 64: 1284, 1996.
51. Gross DM, Forsthuber T, Tary-Lehmann M, et al: Identification of LFA-1 as a candidate autoantigen in treatment-resistant Lyme arthritis. Science 281: 703, 1998.
52. Malane MS, Grant-Kels JM, Feder HM, et al: Diagnosis of Lyme disease based on dermatologic manifestations. Ann Intern Med 114: 490, 1991.
53. Feder HM, Gerber MA, Krause PJ, et al: Early Lyme disease: a flu-like illness without erythema migrans. Pediatrics 91: 456, 1993.
54. Pohl-Koppe A, Wilske B, Weiss M, et al: *Borrelia* lymphocytoma in childhood. Pediatr Infect Dis J 17: 423, 1998.
55. Nadal D, Gundelfinger R, Flüeler U, et al: Acrodermatitis chronica atrophicans. Arch Dis Child 63: 72, 1988.
56. Huppertz HI, Sticht-Groh V, Schwan T: Borderline antibody response in initial stages of lymphocytic meningitis does not rule out borreliosis. Lancet 2: 1468, 1986.
57. Christen HJ, Hanefeld F, Eiffert H, et al: Epidemiology and clinical manifestations of Lyme borreliosis in childhood. A prospective multicentre study with special regard to neuroborreliosis. Acta Paediatr 82(Suppl 386): 1, 1993.
58. Hansen K, Lebech AM: The clinical and epidemiologic profile of Lyme neuroborreliosis in Denmark 1985–1990. Brain 115: 399, 1992.
59. Bloom BJ, Wyckoff PM, Meissner HC, et al: Neurocognitive abnormalities in children after classic manifestations of Lyme disease. Pediatr Infect Dis J 17: 189, 1998.
60. Shapiro EE: Guillain-Barré syndrome in a child with serologic evidence of *Borrelia burgdorferi* infection. Pediatr Inf Dis J 17: 264, 1998.
61. Horneff G, Huppertz H-I, Muller K et al: Demonstration of *Borrelia burgdorferi* infection in a child with Guillain Barré syndrome. Eur J Pediatr 152: 810, 1993.
62. Kam L, Sood SK, Maytal J: Pseudotumor cerebri in Lyme disease: a case report and review of the literature. Pediatr Neurol 18: 439, 1998.
63. Scott IU, Silva-Lepe A, Siatkowski RM: Chiasmal optic neuritis in Lyme disease. Am J Ophthalmol 123: 136, 1997.
64. Lock G, Berger G, Grobe H: Neuroborreliosis: progressive encephalomyelitis with cerebral vasculitis. Monatsschr Kinderheilkd 137: 101, 1989.
65. Oksi J, Kalimo H, Manttila RJ, et al: Inflammatory brain changes in Lyme borreliosis. A report on three patients and review of literature. Brain 119: 2143, 1996.
66. Huppertz HI, Karch H: Die Lyme-Arthritis im Kindesalter: Monarthritis des Kniegelenks, klinisch nicht unterscheidbar von Monarthritiden unbekannter Ursache. Monatsschr Kinderheilkd 139: 759, 1991.
67. Hammers-Berggren S, Andersson U, Stiernstedt G: *Borrelia* arthritis in Swedish children: clinical manifestations in 10 children. Acta Paediatr 81: 921, 1992.

68. Gerber MA, Zemel LS, Shapiro ED: Lyme arthritis in children: clinical epidemiology and long-term outcomes. Pediatrics 102: 905, 1998.
69. Reimers CD, de Koning J, Neubert U, et al: *Borrelia burgdorferi* myositis: report of eight patients. J Neurol 240: 278, 1993.
70. Häupl T, Hahn G, Rittig M, et al: Persistence of *Borrelia burgdorferi* in ligamentous tissue from a patient with chronic Lyme borreliosis. Arthritis Rheum 36: 1621, 1993.
71. Huppertz HI, Michels H: Pattern of joint involvement in children with Lyme arthritis. Br J Rheumatol 35: 1016, 1996.
71a. Huppertz HI, Münchmeier D, Lieb W: Ocular manifestations in children and adolescents with Lyme arthritis. Br J Ophthalmol 83: 1149–1152, 1999.
72. Christoforo RL, Appel MH, Gelb RF, Williams CL: Musculoskeletal manifestations of Lyme disease in children. J Pediatr Orthop 7: 527, 1987.
73. Hoffmann JC, Stichtenoth DO, Zeidler H, et al: Lyme disease in a 74-year-old forest owner with symptoms of dermatomyositis. Arthritis Rheum 38: 1157, 1995.
74. Oksi J, Mertsola J, Reunanen M, et al: Subacute multiple-site osteomyelitis caused by *Borrelia burgdorferi*. Clin Infect Dis 19: 891, 1994.
75. Sigal LH, Patella SJ: Lyme arthritis as the incorrect diagnosis in pediatric and adolescent fibromyalgia. Pediatrics 90: 523, 1992.
76. Cox J, Krajden M: Cardiovascular manifestations of Lyme disease. Am Heart J 122: 1449, 1991.
77. Aaberg TM: The expanding ophthalmologic spectrum of Lyme disease. Am J Ophthalmol 107: 77, 1989.
78. Szer IS, Taylor E, Steere AC: The long-term course of Lyme arthritis in children. N Engl J Med 325: 159–163, 1991.
79. Edwards KS, Kanengiser S, Li KI, et al: Lyme disease presenting as hepatitis and jaundice in a child. Pediatr Infect Dis J 9: 592, 1990.
80. Chancellor MB, McGinnis DE, Shenot PJ, et al: Urinary dysfunction in Lyme disease. J Urol 149: 26, 1993.
81. Weber K, Bratzke HJ, Neubert U, et al: *Borrelia burgdorferi* in a newborn despite oral penicilline for Lyme borreliosis during pregnancy. Pediatr Infect Dis J 7: 286, 1988.
82. Silver HM: Lyme disease during pregnancy. Infect Dis Clin North Am 11: 93, 1997.
83. Markowitz LE, Steere AC, Benach JL, et al: Lyme disease during pregnancy. JAMA 255: 3394, 1986.
84. Nadal D, Hunziker UA, Bucher HU, et al: Infants born to mothers with antibodies against *Borrelia burgdorferi* at delivery. Eur J Pediatr 148: 426, 1989.
85. Johnson YE, Duray PH, Steere AC, et al: Spirochetes found in synovial microangiopathic lesions. Am J Pathol 118: 26, 1985.
86. Snydman DR, Schenkein DP, Berardi VP, et al: *Borrelia burgdorferi* in joint fluid in chronic Lyme arthritis. Ann Intern Med 104: 798, 1986.
87. De Koning J, Bosma RB, Hoogkamp-Korstanje JAA: Demonstration of spirochaetes in patients with Lyme disease with a modified silver stain. J Med Microbiol 23: 261, 1987.
88. Berger BW, Johnson RC, Kodner C, et al: Cultivation of *Borrelia burgdorferi* from erythema migrans lesions and perilesional skin. J Clin Microbiol 30: 359, 1992.
89. Stanek G, Klein J, Bittner R, et al: Isolation of *Borrelia burgdorferi* from the myocardium of a patient with longstanding cardiomyopathy. N Engl J Med 322: 249, 1990.
90. Lardieri G, Salvi A, Camerini F: Isolation of *Borrelia burgdorferi* from myocardium. Lancet 342: 490, 1993.
91. Frey M, Jaulhac B, Piemont Y, et al: Detection of *Borrelia burgdorferi* DNA in muscle of patients with chronic myalgia related to Lyme disease. Am J Med 104: 591, 1998.
92. Eppes SC, Nelson DK, Lewis LL, Klein JD: Characterization of Lyme meningitis and comparison with viral meningitis in children. Pediatrics 103: 1957, 1999.
93. Golightly M: Laboratory considerations in the diagnosis and management of Lyme borreliosis. Am J Clin Pathol 99: 168, 1993.
94. American College of Physicians: Guidelines for laboratory evaluation in the diagnosis of Lyme disease. Clinical guideline, part 1. Ann Intern Med 127: 1106, 1997.
95. Tugwell P, Dennis DT, Weinstein A, et al: Laboratory evaluation in the diagnosis of Lyme disease. Clinical guideline, part 2. Ann Intern Med 127: 1109, 1997.
96. Sigal LH: Pitfalls in the diagnosis and management of Lyme disease. Arthritis Rheum 41: 195, 1998.
97. Karlsson M, Hovind-Hougen K, Svenungsson B, et al: Cultivation and characterization of spirochetes from cerebrospinal fluid of patients with Lyme borreliosis. J Clin Microbiol 28: 473, 1990.
98. Nocton JJ, Dressler F, Rutledge BJ, et al: Detection of *Borrelia burgdorferi* DNA by polymerase chain reaction in synovial fluid from patients with Lyme arthritis. N Engl J Med 330: 229, 1994.
98a. Carlson D, Hernandez J, Bloom BJ, et al: Lack of *Borrelia burgdorferi* DNA in synovial fluid samples from patients with antibiotic treatment–resistant Lyme arthritis. Arthritis Rheum 42: 2705–2709, 1999.
99. Priem S, Rittig MG, Kamradt T, et al: An optimized PCR leads to rapid and highly sensitive detection of *Borrelia burgdorferi* in patients with Lyme borreliosis. J Clin Microbiol 35: 685, 1997.
100. Huppertz HI, Schmidt H, Karch H: Detection of *Borrelia burgdorferi* by nested polymerase chain reaction in cerebrospinal fluid and urine of children with neuroborreliosis. Eur J Pediatr 152: 414, 1993.
101. Karch H, Huppertz HI: Repeated detection of *Borrelia burgdorferi* DNA in synovial fluid of a child with Lyme arthritis. Rheumatol Int 12: 227, 1993.
102. Jaulhac B, Chary-Valckenaere I, Sibila J, et al: Detection of *Borrelia burgdorferi* by DNA amplification in synovial tissue samples from patients with Lyme arthritis. Arthritis Rheum 39: 736, 1996.
103. Priem S, Burmester GR, Kamradt T, et al: Detection of *Borrelia burgdorferi* by polymerase chain reaction in synovial membrane, but not in synovial fluid from patients with persisting Lyme arthritis after antibiotic therapy. Ann Rheum Dis 57: 118, 1998.
104. Karch H, Huppertz HI, Böhme M, et al: Demonstration of *Borrelia burgdorferi* DNA in urine samples from healthy humans whose sera contain *B. burgdorferi*–specific antibodies. J Clin Microbiol 32: 2312, 1994.
104a. Brown SL, Hansen SL, Langore JJ: Role of serology in the diagnosis of Lyme disease. JAMA 282: 62–66, 1999.
105. Recommendations for test performance and interpretation from the second national conference on serologic diagnosis of Lyme disease. MMWR 44: 590, 1995.
106. Dressler F, Whalen JA, Reinhardt BN, et al: Western blotting in the serodiagnosis of Lyme disease. J Infect Dis 167: 392, 1993.
107. Engstrom SM, Shoop E, Johnson RC: Immunoblot interpretation criteria for serodiagnosis of early Lyme disease. J Clin Microbiol 33: 419, 1995.
108. Hauser U, Lehnert G, Lobentanzer R, et al: Interpretation criteria for standardized Western blots for three European species of *Borrelia burgdorferi sensu lato*. J Clin Microbiol 35: 1433, 1997.
108a. Hauser U, Lehnert G, Wilkske B: Validity of interpretation criteria for standardized Western blots (immunoblots) for serodiagnosis of Lyme borreliosis based on sera collected throughout Europe. J Clin Microbiol 37: 2241–2247, 1999.
109. Levine D, Tilton RC, Parry MF et al: False positive EBNA IgM and IgG antibody tests for infectious mononucleosis in children. Pediatrics 94: 892, 1994.
110. Berardi VP, Weeks KE, Steere AC: Serodiagnosis of early Lyme disease: analysis of IgM and IgG antibody responses by using an antibody-capture enzyme immunoassay. J Infect Dis 158: 754, 1988.
111. Sood SK, Rubin LG, Blader ME, Ilowite NT: Positive serology for Lyme borreliosis in patients with juvenile rheumatoid arthritis in a Lyme borreliosis endemic area: analysis by immunblot. J Rheumatol 20: 739, 1993.
112. Saulsbury FT, Katzmann JA: Prevalence of antibody to *Borrelia burgdorferi* in children with juvenile rheumatoid arthritis. J Rheumatol 17: 1193, 1990.
113. Weiss NL, Sadock VA, Sigel LH, et al: False positive seroreactivity to *Borrelia burgdorferi* in systemic lupus erythematosus: value of immunoblot analysis. Lupus 4: 131, 1995.
114. Nichol G, Dennis DT, Steere AC, et al: Test-treatment strategies for patients suspected of having Lyme disease: a cost-effectiveness analysis. Ann Intern Med 128: 37, 1998.
115. Dressler F, Yoshinari NH, Steere AC: The T-cell proliferative assay in the diagnosis of Lyme disease. Ann Intern Med 15: 533, 1991.
116. Zoschke DC, Skemp AA, Defosse DL: Lymphoproliferative re-

sponses to *B. burgdorferi* in Lyme disease. Ann Intern Med 114: 285, 1991.
117. Huppertz HI, Mösbauer S, Busch DH, et al: Lymphoproliferative responses to *Borrelia burgdorferi* in the diagnosis of Lyme arthritis in children and adolescents. Eur J Pediatr 155: 297, 1996.
118. Rutkowski S, Busch DH, Huppertz HI: Lymphocyte proliferation assay in response to *Borrelia burgdorferi* in patients with Lyme arthritis: analysis of lymphocyte subsets. Rheumatol Int 17: 151, 1997.
119. Huppertz HI, Bentas W, Haubitz I, et al: Diagnosis of pediatric Lyme arthritis using a clinical score. Eur J Pediatr 157: 304, 1998.
120. Case definitions for public health surveillance. MMWR 39: 19–21, 1990.
121. Böhme M, Schweneke S, Fuchs E, et al: Screening of blood donors and recipients for *Borrelia burgdorferi* antibodies: no evidence of *B. burgdorferi* infection transmitted by transfusion. Infusionstherapie 19: 204, 1992.
122. Huppertz HI, Karch H, Heesemann J: Diagnostic value of synovial fluid analysis in children with reactive arthritis. Rheumatol Int 15: 167, 1995.
123. Kaiser R, Rauer S: Analysis of the intrathecal immune response in neuroborreliosis to a sonicate antigen and three recombinant antigens of *Borrelia burgdorferi senso stricto*. Eur J Clin Microbiol Infect Dis 17: 159, 1998.
124. Dattwyler RJ, Volkman DJ, Conaty SM, et al: Amoxicillin plus probenecid versus doxycycline for treatment of erythema migrans borreliosis. Lancet 336: 1404, 1990.
125. Dattwyler RJ, Halperin JJ, Volkman DJ, et al: Treatment of late Lyme borreliosis—randomised comparison of ceftriaxone and penicillin. Lancet 1: 1191, 1988.
126. Weber K, Preac-Mursic V, Wilske B, et al: A randomized trial of ceftriaxone versus oral penicillin for the treatment of early European Lyme borreliosis. Infection 18: 91, 1990.
127. Pfister HW, Preac-Mursic V, Wilske B, et al: Cefotaxime versus penicillin G for acute neurologic manifestations in Lyme borreliosis. A prospective randomized study. Arch Neurol 46: 1190, 1989.
128. Müllegger RR, Millner MM, Stanek G, et al: Penicillin G sodium and ceftriaxone in the treatment of neuroborreliosis in children—a prospective study. Infection 19: 279, 1991.
129. Massarotti EM, Luger SW, Rahn DW, et al: Treatment of early Lyme disease. Am J Med 92: 396, 1992.
130. Nadelman RB, Luger SW, Frank E, et al: Comparison of cefuroxime and doxycycline in the treatment of early Lyme disease. Ann Intern Med 117: 273, 1992.
131. Dattwyler RJ, Luft BJ, Kunkel MJ, et al: Ceftriaxone compared with doxycycline for the treatment of acute disseminated Lyme disease. N Engl J Med 337: 289, 1997.
132. Hansen K, Hovmark A, Lebeque AM, et al: Roxithromycine in Lyme borreliosis: discrepant results of an in vitro and in vivo animal susceptibility study and a clinical trial in patients with erythema migrans. Acta Derm Venerol (Stockh) 72: 297, 1992.
133. Weber K, Wilske B, Preac-Mursic V, et al: Azithromycin versus penicillin V for the treatment of early Lyme borreliosis. Infection 21: 367, 1993.
134. Strle F, Preac-Mursic V, Cimperman J, et al: Azithromycin versus doxycycline for treatment of erythema migrans: clinical and microbiologic findings. Infection 21: 83, 1993.
135. Luft BJ, Dattwyler RJ, Johnson RC, et al: Azithromycin compared with amoxicillin in the treatment of erythema migrans. A double-blind, randomized, controlled trial. Ann Intern Med 124: 785, 1996.
136. Steere AC, Levin RE, Molloy PJ, et al: Treatment of Lyme arthritis. Arthritis Rheum 37: 878, 1994.
137. Rose CD, Fawcett PT, Gibney KM, et al: Residual serologic reactivity in children with resolved Lyme arthritis. J Rheumatol 23: 367, 1996.
138. Eckman MH, Steere AC, Kalish RA, et al: Cost effectiveness of oral as compared with intravenous antibiotic therapy for patients with early Lyme disease or Lyme arthritis. N Engl J Med 337: 357, 1997.
139. Gasser R, Wendelin I, Reisinger E, et al: Roxithromycin in the treatment of Lyme disease—update and perspectives. Infection 23(Suppl): S39, 1995.
140. Schoen RT, Aversa JM, Rahn DW, et al: Treatment of refractory chronic Lyme arthritis with arthroscopic synovectomy. Arthritis Rheum 34: 1056, 1991.
140a. American Academy of Pediatrics, Committee on Infectious Diseases: Prevention of Lyme disease. Pediatrics 105: 142–147, 2000.
141. Warshafsky S, Nowakowski J, Nadelman RB, et al: Efficacy of antibiotic prophylaxis for prevention of Lyme disease. J Gen Intern Med 11: 329, 1996.
142. Steere AC, Sikand VK, Meurice F, et al: Vaccination against Lyme disease with recombinant *Borrelia burgdorferi* outer-surface lipoprotein A with adjuvant. N Engl J Med 339: 209, 1998.
143. Sigal LH, Zahradnik JM, Lavin P, et al: A vaccine consisting of recombinant *Borrelia burgdorferi* outer-surface protein A to prevent Lyme disease. N Engl J Med 339: 216, 1998.
143a. Feder HM, Beran J, van Hoecke C, et al: Immunogenicity of a recombinant *Borrelia burgdorferi* outer surface protein A vaccine against Lyme disease in children. J Pediatr 135: 575–579, 1999.
144. Recommendations for the use of Lyme disease vaccine. Recommendations of the Advisory Committee on Immunization Practices (ACIP). MMWR 48: 1, 1999.
145. Availability of Lyme disease vaccine. MMWR 48: 35, 1999.
145a. Adams WV, Rose CD, Eppes SC, et al: Cognitive effects of Lyme disease in children: a 4 year followup study. J Rheumatol 26: 1190–1094, 1999.
145b. Bentas W, Karch H, Huppertz HI: Lyme arthritis in children and adolescents: outcome 12 months after initiation of antibiotic therapy. J Rheumatol 27: 2025–2030, 2000.
146. Salazar JC, Gerber MA, Goff CW: Long-term outcome of Lyme disease in children given early treatment. J Pediatr 122: 591, 1993.
147. Adams WV, Rose CD, Eppes SC, Klein JD: Cognitive effects of Lyme disease in children. Pediatrics 94: 185, 1994.
148. Shadick NA, Phillips CB, Logigian EL, et al: The long-term clinical outcomes of Lyme disease. A population-based retrospective cohort study. Ann Intern Med 121: 560, 1994.

33

Reactive Arthritis

Rubén Burgos-Vargas and Janitzia Vázquez-Mellado

The reactive arthritides constitute a diverse group of inflammatory arthritides including acute rheumatic fever and arthritis following genitourinary tract or gastrointestinal tract infections with specific organisms. They are probably among the most common of the childhood rheumatic diseases worldwide. Viral and postinfectious arthritides are discussed in Chapter 31. Acute rheumatic fever and poststreptococcal arthritis are considered in Chapter 34. This chapter reviews disorders related to enteric or genitourinary bacterial infections.

DEFINITION AND CLASSIFICATION

In this chapter, use of the term *reactive arthritis* (ReA) is restricted to the human leukocyte antigen (HLA)-B27–associated arthritides, a group of conditions traditionally classified with the spondyloarthropathy (SpA) group and triggered by enteric and genital bacterial infections. ReA is a form of nonseptic arthritis developing after an extra-articular infection with one of the so-called arthritogenic bacteria, particularly *Chlamydia, Yersinia, Salmonella, Shigella,* or *Campylobacter.*[1–3]

Reiter's syndrome is a presentation of ReA defined by the triad of arthritis, conjunctivitis, and urethritis (or cervicitis).[3–5] It was first noted in English medical literature in 1818 by Sir Benjamin Brodie.[6] Almost 100 years later, Hans Reiter, whose name is now associated with this syndrome, published a case report of a 16-year-old boy who developed arthritis, urethritis, and conjunctivitis after dysentery.[7] Later, cutaneous changes were added to form a diagnostic tetrad.

Classification and Diagnostic Criteria

The diagnosis of ReA is a clinical challenge. The criteria used in the literature and in clinical practice to arrive at a diagnosis of ReA have ranged from a brief episode of undifferentiated arthritis to criteria such as those of the 1995 Berlin Third International Workshop on ReA[8] (Table 33–1), which require the presence of typical peripheral arthritis (a predominantly lower limb, asymmetric oligoarthritis) in addition to evidence of a preceding infection (either a history of diarrhea or urethritis within the preceding 4 weeks or laboratory confirmation of infection with an arthritogenic organism in the absence of clinical symptoms) (Table 33–2). The value of these criteria is yet to be determined, particularly with regard to the retrospective diagnosis

Table 33–1

The Berlin Diagnostic Criteria for Reactive Arthritis

Typical Peripheral Arthritis

Predominantly lower limb, asymmetric oligoarthritis

plus

Evidence of Preceding Infection

If there is a clear history of diarrhea or urethritis within the preceding 4 weeks, laboratory confirmation is desirable but not essential

Where no clear clinical infection is identified, laboratory confirmation of infection is essential

Exclusion Criteria

Patients with other known causes of monarthritis or oligoarthritis (such as other defined spondyloarthropathies, septic arthritis, crystal arthritis, Lyme disease, and streptococcal ReA) should be excluded

From Kingsley G, Sieper J: Third International Workshop on Reactive Arthritis: an overview. Ann Rheum Dis 55:564–570, 1996, with permission from the BMJ Publishing Group.

Table 33–2

Laboratory Tests for Documenting Preceding Infection in Reactive Arthritis

Stool culture
Urethral culture
Serology: antibodies against specific arthritogenic bacteria
Urethral swab for detection of bacterial DNA by polymerase chain reaction (PCR)*
Synovial fluid or synovial membrane for detection of bacterial DNA by PCR*
Immunofluorescence microscopy for detection of bacteria in synovium†
Stimulation of synovial fluid lymphocytes with antigens from arthritogenic bacteria†

*A potential diagnostic test.
†Research tools, not suitable for routine diagnostic use.
From Kingsley G, Sieper J: Third International Workshop on Reactive Arthritis: an overview. Ann Rheum Dis 55:564–570, 1996, with permission from the BMJ Publishing Group.

of infection. The problem of definition and classification of ReA has been reviewed by Pacheco-Tena and colleagues.[9]

EPIDEMIOLOGY

The frequency of occurrence of ReA reflects the prevalence of HLA-B27 and the rate of infections by arthritogenic bacteria in the general population. Reports of postinfectious Reiter's syndrome and *Yersinia*-triggered ReA in children have usually come from countries in which *Yersinia* and other infections prevail.

In epidemiologic studies summarized by Keat,[3] ReA was estimated to occur in 1 percent of patients with sexually acquired infections, 2.4 percent of those with either *Shigella* or *Campylobacter* infections, 3.2 percent with *Salmonella* infections, and up to 33 percent of patients with yersiniosis. ReA develops in 5 to 10 percent of children with yersiniosis.[10, 11]

The relative frequency of ReA (including Reiter's syndrome) among patients in four registries of pediatric rheumatology clinics in the United States,[12, 13] United Kingdom,[14] and Canada[15] ranged between 8.6 and 41.1 percent. This wide variation is consistent with differences in the stringency of diagnostic and classification criteria used in each study. The American and Canadian data[12, 13, 15] included four different but related categories: Reiter's syndrome, probable Reiter's syndrome, ReA, and probable ReA. In contrast, the British study[14] included only the Reiter syndrome category. Further reports from other sources suggest that clinical recognition of ReA may be increasing.[16–21]

Most cases of ReA occur in boys between the ages of 8 and 12 years, but sex and age distribution vary according to the causative organism. In an Italian study of children with *Yersinia*-triggered ReA, most cases occurred between 3 and 7 years of age and there was a slight predominance of females.[21] Enteric infections are responsible for ReA at all ages, but ReA following genital infections with *Chlamydia* occurs more frequently during adolescence.

GENETIC BACKGROUND

Although the susceptibility to infection is not related to any genetic marker, ReA frequently occurs in HLA-B27 individuals. This association provides the strongest link between ReA and juvenile ankylosing spondylitis. The frequency of B27 is somewhat lower in patients with ReA (65 to 85 percent) compared with those with ankylosing spondylitis or juvenile ankylosing spondylitis (90 percent).[22] In some children, particularly those with mild forms of *Yersinia-*, *Campylobacter-*, and *Chlamydia*-related ReA, or those with nasopharyngeal infection, an increased frequency of B27 is not found.[10, 11, 23, 24] An association with the tumor necrosis factor c1 allele that is independent of B27 was reported in a predominantly adult Finnish population with ReA.[25] In a similar population, TAP2J, a polymorphism of transporters associated with antigen processing (TAP2), was more frequent in B27 patients with ReA.[26] No other genetic associations have been noted.

ETIOLOGY AND PATHOGENESIS

Arthritogenic Bacteria

Several bacteria are involved in the etiology of ReA, including Reiter's syndrome in children. In preadolescent patients, ReA following *Salmonella*, *Shigella*, *Yersinia*, and *Campylobacter* enteric infections is much more frequent than that following genital infections by *Chlamydia*. A significant proportion of children with ReA may have no recognized prior infection. In children, gastroenteritis precedes the onset of arthritis in 80 percent of instances. *Shigella flexneri*,[27–30] *Yersinia enterocolitica*,[31] *Salmonella enteritidis*,[32] *Salmonella oranienburg*,[30] and *Salmonella typhimurium*[33] have all been isolated from children with postdysenteric Reiter's syndrome. In at least two youths and three children, *Chlamydia trachomatis*[34] has been identified in synovial fluid. Respiratory tract infection with *Mycoplasma pneumoniae*[35] or *Chlamydia pneumoniae*[36] has preceded the development of ReA in a few children, and the latter agent was responsible for approximately 10 percent of cases of ReA in a Finnish study.[36] Enteritis caused by *Clostridium difficile*,[37, 38] the protozoan *Giardia lamblia*,[39] and *Cryptosporidium*[40] has occasionally been associated with ReA, although the extent of these associations and their relationship to HLA-B27 are not known.

Role of HLA-B27

The role of HLA-B27 in the pathogenesis of ReA is still unknown.[41–44] The *arthritogenic peptide theory* postulates a CD8-positive cross-reactive T-cell response to endogenous or exogenous peptides presented by B27-positive antigen-presenting cells.[43, 45–47] These peptides induce a CD8-positive T-cell response that cross-reacts with bacterial epitopes.[48, 49] The role of T cells in the inflammatory process that characterizes ReA is paramount.[48, 50, 51]

The *promiscuous peptide theory* suggests that class II molecules present B27–derived peptides to CD4-positive cells.[42, 46, 52] In this case, these peptides would induce a CD4-positive response, which then cross-reacts with B27 peptides. Although the serum antibody response against arthritogenic bacteria in patients with ReA lasts longer than that in patients with the same infection who do not develop arthritis, the role of antibodies in the pathogenesis of ReA is probably minimal. Other hypotheses include defective oxidation of cysteine at the B27 B pocket and the existence of B27-linked genes.[42, 43, 53] Additional findings suggest a role for heat-shock proteins and bacterial peptidoglycan in the pathogenesis or ReA.[54, 55]

Arthritogenic bacteria invade the mucosa and replicate within polymorphonuclear cells and macrophages.[56–58] The transport of bacteria and their products from the mucosa to the joint is complex and involves adhesion molecules on phagocytic cells. Studies in murine fibroblasts transfected with B27 indicated that the expression of this antigen inhibited invasion by arthritogenic bacteria.[59, 60] This phenomenon could not be replicated in human cells, however,[61–63] although persistence of the organism within the cell was prolonged in cells expressing B27.[64] It has been possible to identify various bacterial components (including lipopolysaccharide, DNA, and RNA) in both synovial fluid cells and synovial membranes of patients with ReA.[65–71]

CLINICAL MANIFESTATIONS

The course and severity of ReA vary considerably. Several stages of ReA may be recognized. A clinical infection precedes the appearance of arthritis, enthesitis, or extra-articular disease (either singly or in combination) by 1 to 4 weeks. After an active period of weeks to months, the arthritis subsides and the patient may then enter a sustained remission or follow a pattern characterized by recurrent episodes of disease activity lasting a number of years.

Characteristics of the Primary Infection

An appreciation of the characteristics of the preceding infectious illness will help to identify patients with ReA. In retrospect, diarrhea had preceded the onset of disease in 69 percent of children with Reiter's syndrome.[63]

Shigella Enteritis

A period of high fever, with or without watery diarrhea and cramping abdominal pain lasting 48 to 72 hours, may be followed in 7 to 21 days by the sudden onset of oligoarthritis, most commonly affecting the knees and ankles. The arthritis is nonmigratory and lasts several weeks to 3 or 4 months. Diagnosis requires a careful history, demonstration of a sterile synovial fluid culture, the presence of agglutinins to *Shigella flexneri* serotype 2 or 2a,[29, 30] and an attempt to isolate the organism from the stool. Because of the long interval between the diarrhea and the joint complaints, blood cultures are positive in fewer than 4 percent of patients.

Salmonella Infection

The acute onset of oligoarthritis, most often affecting the knees and ankles, may follow an enteric infection with *Salmonella typhimurium* or *Salmonella enteritidis* by 1 to 3 weeks.[72, 73] The enteric infection may be mild, but the onset of arthritis is usually accompanied by low-grade fever. Because *Salmonella* infection can result in osteomyelitis and septic arthritis as well as ReA, it is important to make certain that the synovial fluid is sterile. The erythrocyte sedimentation rate (ESR) is usually elevated, and the leukopenia that may accompany the acute infection is generally followed by leukocytosis. Stool cultures are usually positive, even late in the disease course, but seroconversion to *Salmonella* H and O antigens occurs in only 50 percent of patients.

Yersinia Infection

An ReA of peripheral joints or the spine follows infection with *Yersinia* in susceptible children (Table 33–3). The interval between infection and onset of arthritis in 18 children with *Yersinia*-triggered ReA reported by Tacceti and colleagues[21] was 7 to 30 days. Although rarely reported from North America, the disease has been extensively studied in the Scandinavian countries, where serologic surveys indicate a prevalence of *Yersinia* infection of 3 percent in the population.[74] The diarrhea preceding ReA was notably very mild, much more so than in the usual *Yersinia* enterocolitis. Contact with the organism is through infected drinking water or milk. *Yersinia enterocolitica* causes gastroenteritis in young children and a syndrome of abdominal pain similar to that of appendicitis in older children and adolescents. In a study of children who were hospitalized because of *Yersinia* infection, 35 percent had arthritis lasting 3 to 22 months (average, 6.5 months).[10] Of those with arthritis, 85 percent had HLA-B27. *Yersinia* can occasionally cause septic arthritis.

Campylobacter Infection

In an epidemic of *Campylobacter jejuni* enteritis in Finland, 2.3 percent of patients—all adults—developed oligoarthritis or polyarthritis 4 days to 4 weeks after infection. Synovial fluid cultures were negative, and 70 percent of the patients with arthritis were positive for HLA-B27.[75]

Table 33–3

Post-*Yersinia* Arthritis

Organisms	*Yersinia enterocolitica* (Enterobacteriaceae, gram-negative coccobacilli)
Source	Contaminated food, streams, animals
Identification	Stool cultures, *Yersinia* agglutinins
Clinical manifestations	Fever Abdominal pain and diarrhea (may be extremely mild) Mesenteric adenitis and ileitis Erythema nodosum Arthritis and tenosynovitis Myalgia Uveitis, episcleritis, conjunctivitis Electrocardiographic abnormalities
Duration	2 wk–8 mo
Genetic factors	HLA-B27 positivity
Treatment	Aminoglycosides, cefotaxime, tetracycline, trimethoprim-sulfamethoxazole
Differential diagnosis	Acute appendicitis, shigellosis or salmonellosis, acute rheumatic fever, Reiter's syndrome, juvenile rheumatoid arthritis

Chlamydia Infection

Genitourinary tract infection with *Chlamydia trachomatis* is often asymptomatic but may cause dysuria, frequency, and a urethral or vaginal discharge. ReA may also be related to upper respiratory tract infections with *Chlamydia pneumoniae*.[36] Artamonov and colleagues[24] found evidence of nasopharyngeal infection in 45 of 52 children with ReA. Although the prevalence of HLA-B27 was higher than that in the control population (relative risk, 2.5), it was certainly lower than that in those who developed Reiter's syndrome after intestinal infection.

Musculoskeletal Disease

Acute arthritis is characteristic of ReA, but some children present with only slight to moderate joint pain and swelling over several weeks.[10, 21, 34, 72–80] Enthesitis may occur alone or with arthritis, tenosynovitis, or bursitis (Figs. 33–1 and 33–2). In other children, arthralgias antedate the onset of arthritis for a variable period of time. The initial episode of arthritis usually affects the knees or ankles. The pattern of arthritis in the metatarsophalangeal (MTP) joints and the proximal and distal interphalangeal (IP) joints of the feet may be that of a dactylitis and involve two or three joints in one or more digits in combination with tenosynovitis and bursitis. Arthritis of the small joints of the hands has also been described in ReA caused by *Yersinia* and *Salmonella*.[10, 21, 34, 73–77]

The synovial fluid effusion is usually marked, but proliferative synovitis is uncommon. In addition to involvement of peripheral joints and entheses, there may be inflammation of joints of the axial skeleton resulting in spinal and sacroiliac pain, stiffness, and reduced mobility of the lumbar and cervical spine.

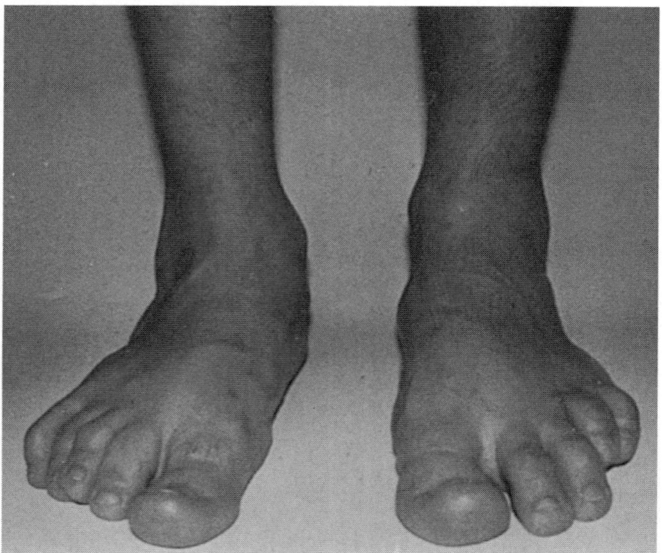

Figure 33–1. There is slight swelling of the midfoot and dactylitis involving the right 2nd toe and the 4th and 5th left toes in an adolescent with *Salmonella*-triggered reactive arthritis of 6 months' duration.

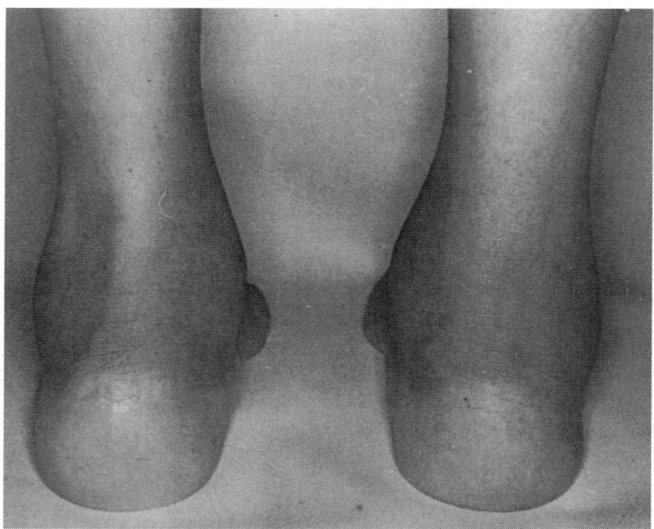

Figure 33–2. Achilles tendinitis and swelling of the retrocalcaneal bursa of the right foot of the patient in Figure 33–1.

In a study of 11 children with ReA followed for 0.9 to 6.7 years, Hussein[72] observed recurrent episodes of arthritis in most patients: 4 children had severe arthritis and 5 had sacroiliitis but none had significant disability. Cuttica and colleagues[78] found that, at a mean follow-up of 28.6 months, 18 of 26 children with Reiter's syndrome developed oligoarthritis, 7 polyarthritis, and 1 monarthritis, with axial symptoms in 6. Five patients followed for a mean of 83.5 months developed radiographic sacroiliitis. Symptoms remitted in most patients, but some had either a sustained or a fluctuating course. In a group of 9 Greek children with *Salmonella*-triggered ReA, disease was active at 4 to 13 months and there were one to four recurrences in 4 patients during 48 to 78 months but no axial symptoms.[78]

Constitutional Signs and Symptoms

Apart from residual disease resulting from the infection itself, children with ReA may continue to have fever, weight loss, fatigue, and muscle weakness during active periods of disease. Polyarthralgia, muscle pain, and joint stiffness affecting peripheral joints and the axial skeleton sometimes accompany these symptoms. Myocarditis and pericarditis have been described during the active phase of the disease in children with *Salmonella enteritidis*–triggered ReA.[81]

Mucocutaneous and Ocular Disease

Painless, shallow ulcers of the oral mucosa and palate are common and often ignored because they are asymptomatic. Aphthous stomatitis occurs in some patients. Urethritis and cervicitis are rare manifestations, occurring more frequently in adolescents with sexually acquired ReA caused by *Chlamydia* but also developing in ReA of other causes.[34] These conditions are often mild and in girls tend to have no symptoms; they are detected only because of the presence of sterile pyuria. Diarrhea occurs in association with bacterial infection but may also be part of a generalized episode of mucositis.

Skin lesions in ReA include erythema nodosum in some children with *Yersinia*-triggered ReA as well as circinate balanitis (Fig. 33–3) and keratoderma blennorrhagicum (Fig. 33–4), with or without other stigmata of Reiter's disease.[11, 34, 73, 82] The latter may be clinically and histologically indistinguishable from psoriasis (Fig. 33–5). Several other nonspecific skin lesions have been described in patients with ReA and Reiter's syndrome. Mucocutaneous involvement in ReA tends to parallel disease activity in the peripheral joints.

Conjunctivitis, one of the components of Reiter's syndrome, occurs in about two thirds of children at onset. In *Yersinia*-triggered ReA, conjunctivitis may be purulent and severe.[83] Acute iridocyclitis in these cases is characterized by aqueous flare and cells, small keratic precipitates, cells in the vitreous, and occasionally fibrinous exudates, posterior synechiae, and macular edema in a unilateral or bilateral pattern. Acute anterior uveitis has also been described in ReA triggered by *Salmonella typhimurium*.[84] Although there are few studies of the visual prognosis in children with ReA, the percentage of patients with permanent ocular sequelae appears to be low.

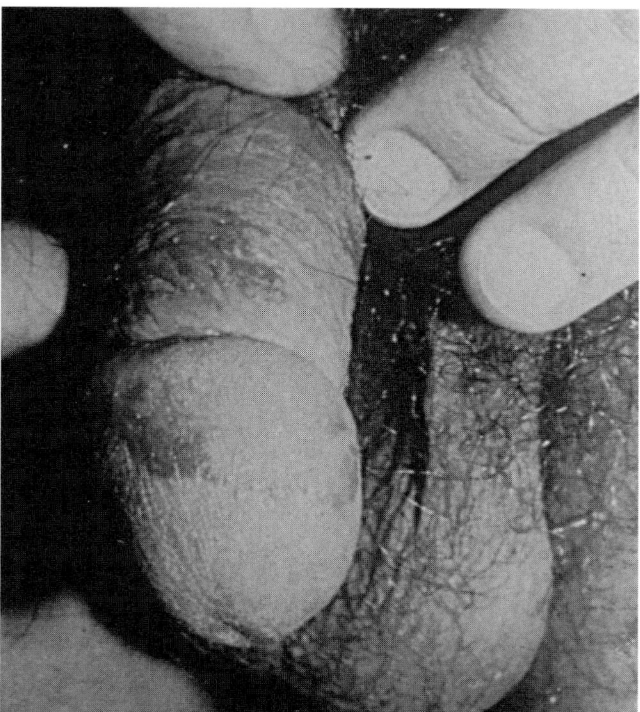

Figure 33–3. Circinate balanitis in an adolescent with *Chlamydia*-triggered reactive arthritis. The shallow ulcers on the glans penis are usually painless.

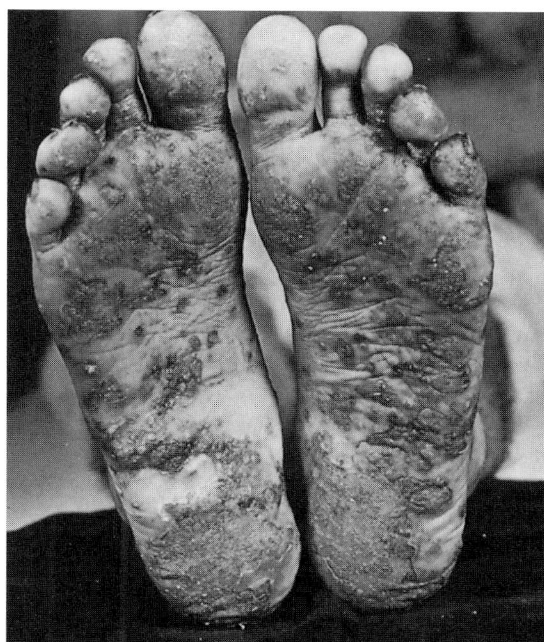

Figure 33–4. Keratoderma blennorrhagicum. This scaly eruption on the soles of the feet of an 18-year-old youth with Reiter's syndrome is difficult to distinguish from psoriasis.

LABORATORY EXAMINATION

In the early inflammatory phase, there may be a slight decrease of hemoglobin and hematocrit as well as mild leukocytosis and neutrophilia. The platelet count and serum levels of immunoglobulins (Ig) M, G, and occa-

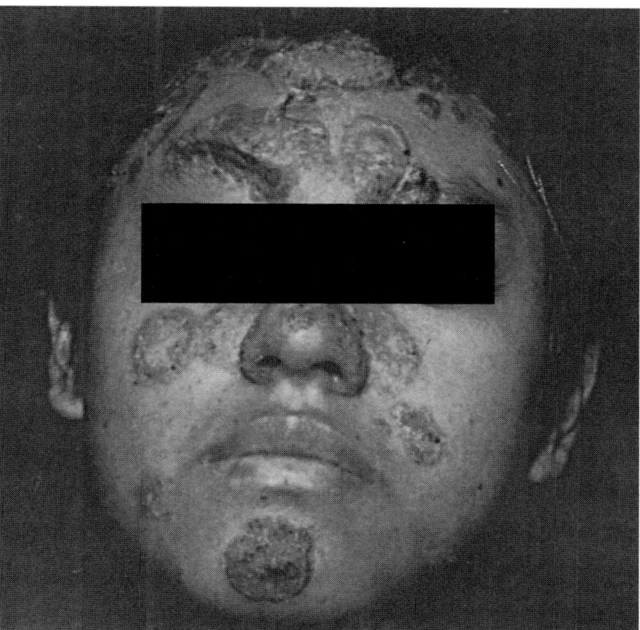

Figure 33–5. Keratoderma blennorrhagicum resembling psoriasis on the face of a 9-year-old girl with *Chlamydia*-induced reactive arthritis.. She had become infected with *Chlamydia* after being sexually abused. (Courtesy of Dr. Mario Magaña-Garcia.)

sionally A may be elevated. The ESR and C-reactive protein correlate with disease activity. In patients with severe disease—particularly in those with polyarthritis and polyenthesitis, fever, weight loss, fatigue, mucositis, or dermatitis—each of the aforementioned laboratory abnormalities may be extreme. In particular, the hemoglobin concentration may fall to 8 to 10 g/dl and the platelet count rise well above 400,000 mm^3. The ESR and C-reactive protein values may remain elevated for a protracted period. Autoantibodies (e.g., rheumatoid factor, antinuclear antibodies) are usually absent. Synovial fluid analysis helps to distinguish between ReA and septic arthritis.[85]

With the exception of epidemics and some isolated reports, the clinical and laboratory confirmations of infection as a trigger in children with ReA are seldom made. When available, cultures obtained at the time of the infection may be helpful: *Salmonella, Yersinia, Shigella,* and *Campylobacter* may be isolated from the gut during an episode of diarrhea or *Chlamydia* may be cultured from the urethra, but negative results do not exclude the diagnosis of infection-related arthritis. Because *Salmonella* and *Chlamydia* may also be present in asymptomatic carriers, these organisms can occasionally be cultured from patients who have arthritis that is not directly related to these organisms.

More frequently, ReA is diagnosed in the appropriate clinical setting because of the presence of high titers of serum antibodies against arthritogenic bacterial antigens.[8, 9] Hemagglutination tests are useful in documenting recent infections with *Salmonella* or *Yersinia*.[10, 21, 34, 73–76] Both the sensitivity and the specificity of circulating IgA and IgM antibodies to *Salmonella, Yersinia,* and *Campylobacter* detected by enzyme-linked immunoassay are acceptable but results must be compared with those in the control population. IgG antibodies are useful if levels change significantly; a rising titer of IgA antibodies may be noted.

Lymphoproliferation assays performed on cells from peripheral blood or synovial fluids also have some utility as diagnostic tools.[8, 9] Unfortunately, these tests are not easy to perform and often demonstrate nonspecific responses to several antigens.

Yersinia or *Chlamydia* antigens may be detected in intestinal or genital smears or biopsies. The ability to identify bacterial structures and antigens in synovial fluid cells or the synovial membrane by electron and immunofluorescence microscopy, immunohistochemistry, and the demonstration of bacterial DNA or RNA by the polymerase chain reaction has been an important advance in the study of ReA. Through these and other techniques, it has been possible to identify intra-articular chlamydial elemental bodies,[34, 65] *Yersinia* 60 kD heat-shock protein and the urease β subunit,[66, 67] and *Salmonella* lipopolysaccharide.[68]

RADIOLOGIC EXAMINATION

Radiographic abnormalities early in the disease consist only of nonspecific soft tissue swelling, juxta-articular osteopenia, and (less frequently) slight periosteal irregularities at tendon attachments.[86] The occurrence of subchondral cysts, erosions, and sometimes extensive destruction of joints such as the hips, proximal and distal IPs of the hands and feet, and less commonly, joints of the wrist indicate the severity of the synovitis that can be present in ReA. Ultrasonographic studies may delineate synovial sheath and tendon thickening and the accumulation of synovial fluid within the tendon sheath and bursae. Magnetic resonance imaging is also an excellent method for studying peripheral and axial joints and entheses.[79]

In certain areas, particularly the foot, osteopenia may be extensive and affect entire bones. Various entheses, especially those at the attachment of the plantar fascia to the calcaneus, develop erosions and marked bony proliferation and spur formation (Fig. 33–6). These abnormalities may also be apparent in the navicular bone, greater trochanter, and ischium. Subchondral cysts and bony erosions of the hip, metacarpophalangeal, MTP, and proximal IP joints of the hands and feet in a unilateral or asymmetric distribution characterize more extensive and unremitting disease. An association between joint erosions and occult inflammation of the gut has been described in patients with ReA.[87]

Sacroiliac and spinal involvement in children with ReA is rare (Fig. 33–7). However, in an extensive study of the utility of magnetic resonance imaging of the sacroiliac joints in children with ReA, but no sacroiliac joint symptoms,[88] approximately one half had acute or chronic sacroiliitis.

DIFFERENTIAL DIAGNOSIS

Differentiation of ReA from other types of arthritis is often difficult. Table 33–4 lists the most common

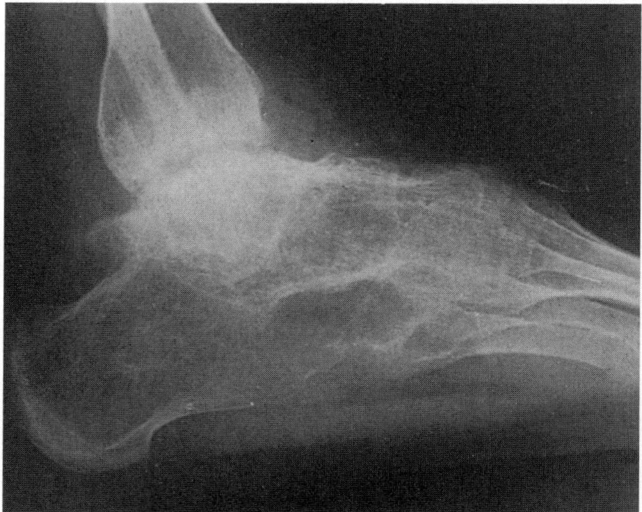

Figure 33–6. Lateral radiograph of a foot of a 16-year-old boy whose first symptom started after a 1-week episode of diarrhea at the age of 8 years. The radiograph demonstrates marked osteopenia and probable ankylosis of the intertarsal joints. During the course of his disease, he experienced recurrent episodes of arthritis and enthesitis, sometimes associated with diarrhea. *Salmonella* organisms were isolated from his stools on two occasions, and bacterial DNA was identified from the knee that was consistent with the stool cultures.

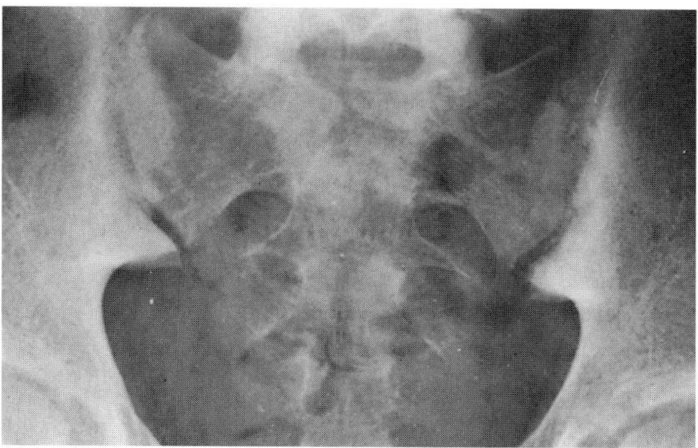

Figure 33–7. Sacroiliac joints of a 16-year-old youth with Reiter's syndrome. On the left, there are erosions and marked reactive sclerosis most prominent on the iliac side of the joints. Changes on the right are minimal.

conditions that need to be excluded. Reactive and infectious arthritides not associated with HLA-B27 share similar symptoms of arthritis after infection, although the primary site of infection is usually the upper airway rather than the gastrointestinal or genitourinary tracts. The second group of diseases possibly related to infection includes those in which mucocutaneous symptoms and arthritis predominate.[89] The third group includes certain orthopedic conditions and pain syndromes that might mimic arthralgias, enthesopathy, and even foot swelling and tenderness. Other forms of childhood arthritis must also be differentiated from ReA. Dactylitis and skin manifestations such as keratoderma blennorrhagicum and nail changes may make it difficult to separate children with ReA from those who have developed psoriatic arthritis.

Table 33–4

Differential Diagnosis of Reactive Arthritis

Infectious Arthritides

Viral arthritis
Poststreptococcal arthritis, rheumatic fever
Lyme disease
Septic arthritis, tuberculosis, gonococcal arthropathy

Disease Possibly Related to Infection

Irritable hip or toxic synovitis of the hip
SAPHO syndrome (synovitis, acne, pustulosis, hyperostosis, and osteomyelitis)
Behçet's disease
Kawasaki disease

Orthopedic and Amplification Pain Syndromes

Legg-Calvé-Perthes, Osgood-Schlatter disease
"Growing pains"
Idiopathic pain syndromes (fibromyalgia, reflex sympathetic dystrophy)

Other Forms of Juvenile Idiopathic Arthritis

Juvenile rheumatoid arthritis
Psoriatic arthritis
Spondyloarthropathies
Crohn's disease and ulcerative colitis

TREATMENT

Disease activity, functional status, and quality of life should be evaluated in children with ReA. Although no specific instruments have been developed for this disease, the use of validated measures of health status designed for other chronic arthritides of childhood should be helpful (see Chapter 9).[90, 91]

In addition to the arthritis, a number of other issues are relevant to quality of life. In developing countries, where ReA is most common, resources for treating ReA are limited. In fact, socioeconomic and educational factors determine the prognosis of many chronic diseases. An understanding of these attributes of each culture will lead to a better understanding of the effects of the disease on the child, family, and society.

There are no special nutritional recommendations for children with ReA. Any measure taken to avoid bacterial contamination of food, from slaughtering of the animals to refrigeration, cooking, and serving, is essential to avoid enteric infections. ReA not only is an epidemic disease but also is endemic to some areas of the world. Programs that improve the sanitary conditions of the community to prevent the spread of infectious diseases are required. Counseling of the family about the risk of recurrences in case of enteric infections is advisable. This applies to adolescents with regard to sexual activities and the risk of sexually transmitted diseases.

Pharmacologic Therapy

The inflammatory manifestations of ReA require the administration of nonsteroidal anti-inflammatory drugs (NSAIDs) in nearly all patients and glucocorticoids in some. The requirement for anti-inflammatory drug treatment of ReA tends to be intermittent rather than constant. However, in patients in whom ReA becomes chronic, medications should be maintained for long periods. Likewise, treatment of ReA often requires the use of sulfasalazine and in some patients, antibiotics. Except for the use of antibiotics in selected cases, there is no clear evidence that any drug alters the course of the disease.

Recommended doses and therapeutic regimens of NSAIDs in children with ReA are similar to those used in other forms of childhood arthritis. Because episodes of ReA tend to be self-limiting, lasting from 3 to 6 months, NSAIDs may be discontinued in many children with onset of a remission. Glucocorticoids may be required for children with severe and disabling polyarthritis and polyenthesitis. Oral or intravenous glucocorticoids generally control arthritis. In contrast, enthesitis responds poorly, may require higher doses of drug than usual, and may demand a longer period of treatment. Fever, fatigue, and anemia tend to disappear, and C-reactive protein levels and ESR tend to improve after several weeks of treatment. In spite of this and perhaps as a consequence of the episodic nature of the disease, glucocorticoid dose reduction and withdrawal in children with ReA are usually easily achieved.

Doses of prednisone or prednisolone may vary between 10 and 20 mg/day and doses of deflazacort between 12 and 24 mg/day. To minimize the risk of adverse events, it is advisable to administer the drug as a single dose in the morning and to start reducing the dose after 2 to 3 weeks. As an alternative to oral therapy, intravenous methylprednisolone offers several advantages. One recommended approach is a step-down regimen of 3 consecutive days of 15 to 30 mg/kg, with a maximum of 1 g to be administered during the first day. Doses on days 2 and 3 are reduced to approximately 75 percent and 50 percent, respectively. Depending on clinical response, this schedule may be repeated at 4-week intervals. The need for this approach to suppression of the disease rarely extends beyond the first 3 months of illness.

Both intra-articular and intralesional administration of glucocorticoids are recommended in special situations. In patients with slight or mild synovitis, the intra-articular administration of triamcinolone hexacetonide or analogues of methylprednisolone or hydrocortisone, produces rapid and sustained relief. It is not unusual, however, for synovial fluid to reaccumulate in less than a week. There is no reported experience regarding the injection of synovial sheaths, bursae, or entheses in children with ReA. Injection of entheses may result in postinjection pain and local soft tissue calcification or atrophy.

Because of the possible presence of occult inflammation of the gut in patients with SpAs, including ReA,[92, 93] and the responsiveness of SpAs in general to sulfasalazine,[94–97] this drug is often recommended in the management of resistant arthritis and enthesitis. The administration of sulfasalazine at doses ranging from 30 to 50 mg/kg/day (maximum 1.5 to 2.0 g/day in adolescents) reduces the number of painful and swollen joints, pain intensity, and ESR.[94–97] The response to sulfasalazine is usually good, and most patients enter remission after 3 to 6 months of therapy. This period of time corresponds, however, to the natural history of the disease, and in many trials, the 6-month placebo response equals that of sulfasalazine. It is advisable to sustain the same dose of the drug (or in some cases a lower dose) through an additional period of 3 to 6 months after remission has been achieved in order to avoid a flare. The frequency of adverse events with sulfasalazine ranges from 10 to 20 percent. These mainly consist of dyspepsia or slight and transitory increases of aspartate transaminase and alanine aminotransferase levels. Very rarely, toxicity necessitates sulfasalazine withdrawal. Some beneficial effect of the drug has also been observed in patients with iritis and skin manifestations such as keratoderma blennorrhagicum.

There is a limited experience with the use of methotrexate in any of the SpAs[98] and only anecdotal reports of good responses to methotrexate at weekly doses ranging from 7.5 to 15 mg in patients with ReA. Our experience with this drug in ReA has not been as favorable. It is possible that the dose of methotrexate needed to reduce disease activity in children with ReA is greater than that used for juvenile rheumatoid arthritis. In contrast, its effects on iritis and keratoderma blennorrhagicum in children have been satisfactory. Iritis usually responds to topical or systemic glucocorticoids, but severe, resistant ocular inflammation occasionally requires other immunosuppressive drugs.

The practice of using antibiotics in ReA is justified (1) by the fact that bacteria may trigger the onset and perhaps relapses of the disease, and (2) because there is evidence of an extended period of persistence of bacteria in these syndromes. No antibiotic regimen has been clearly demonstrated to be efficacious, however. Data from double-blind and open comparative trials of various tetracycline derivatives (except for one using lymecycline) or ciprofloxacin have noted no significant differences when compared with placebo. A double-blind trial comparing lymecycline and placebo[99] demonstrated a significant difference between groups with regard to the time needed to recover from arthritis in patients with *Chlamydia* but not enteritis-related ReA.

Physical Therapy and Rehabilitation

In the acute inflammatory phase, treatment of ReA is similar to that for other forms of chronic arthritis. Rest, ice, or hot packs, as well as aids for walking, may be useful. In children with plantar fasciitis, custom-made insoles relieve pain caused by enthesitis at the heel and metatarsal heads and help preserve the longitudinal arch of the foot. The use of night resting splints helps avoid joint contractures associated with tendonitis or tenosynovitis. Both active and passive stretching of joints as well as muscle strengthening should be prescribed when inflammation is being controlled and pain permits. Children with chronic and recurrent ReA tend to develop fibrous ankylosis first, followed by bone ankylosis of the midtarsal joints and subluxation of the MTP joints, and therefore require special attention to insoles and shoes. Knee, hip, and axial disease benefits from activities such as biking and swimming.

Orthopedic Surgery

Arthroscopic synovectomy is potentially beneficial for children with recurrent synovitis of the knee or small joints of the hands and feet. Early soft tissue release of contractures at the hip, knee, MTP, and IP joints increases functional capacity and may reduce the risk of severe impairment thereafter. Adolescents with severe hip or knee disease may require arthroplasties and joint replacements in the long term.

COURSE OF THE DISEASE AND PROGNOSIS

The course of arthritis in children with ReA varies. Most children have only a single episode of monarthritis or oligoarthritis. Such may typify the case in ReA triggered by *Yersinia*[10, 21, 31, 80] or *Campylobacter*.[23] Others have recurrent episodes of oligoarthritis or an extended form of disease affecting multiple joints and entheses that may account for most of those attending specialized clinics. Although remission may still occur in some patients, many others evolve into an identifiable SpA with sacroiliac arthritis.

Very few data indicate which factors are likely to influence the outcome of ReA or undifferentiated SpA in children. It is a clinical impression that most children with ReA recover in a matter of several months; however, a few go on to develop chronic SpA. There are unfortunately no reports of long-term outcome of ReA in children. Children with ReA (including *Yersinia*- and *Salmonella*-triggered ReA) who carry HLA-B27 have more severe involvement.[21, 24, 34, 77] Extra-articular disease, including iridocyclitis and Reiter's syndrome, also occurs more frequently among children with ReA who are B27 positive. Surprisingly, three of five children who were B27 positive with *Salmonella*-triggered ReA developed psoriasis.[77] The number of joints involved at onset and systemic features such as fever or anemia, the number of episodes of disease activity in a given period of time, and their duration could also influence the outcome of ReA.

The specific infectious agent responsible for the infection may also play a role in determining ultimate outcome. For example, the clinical prognosis of *Chlamydia*- or *Yersinia*-triggered ReA is less severe than that described after *Shigella* or *Salmonella* infection. Whether this is a direct influence of the infectious agent or represents different frequencies of association with HLA-B27 is uncertain.

References

1. Aho K, Leirisalo-Repo M, Repo H: Reactive arthritis. Clin Rheum Dis 11: 25, 1985.
2. Toivanen A: Reactive arthritis. *In* Klippel JH, Dieppe P (eds): Rheumatology. London, Mosby, 1994, pp 4.9.1–4.9.8.
3. Keat A: Reiter's syndrome and reactive arthritis in perspective. N Engl J Med 309: 1606, 1983.
4. Bauer W, Engelman EP: Syndrome of unknown aetiology characterised by urethritis, conjunctivitis and arthritis (so-called Reiter's disease). Trans Assoc Am Phys 57: 304, 1942.
5. Fan PT, Yu DTY: Reiter's syndrome and undifferentiated spondyloarthropathy. *In* Ruddy S, Harris ED Jr, Sledge CB (eds): Kelley's Textbook of Rheumatology, 6th ed. Philadelphia, WB Saunders, 2000, p 1055.
6. Brodie BC: Pathological and Surgical Observations on Diseases of the Joints. London, Longman Hurst Rees, Orme and Brown, 1818.
7. Reiter H: Uber eine bisher unerkannte spirochaeteninfektion (Spirochaetosis arthritica). Dtsch Med Wochenschr 42: 1535, 1916.
8. Kingsley G, Sieper J: Third international workshop on reactive arthritis. An overview. Ann Rheum Dis 55: 564, 1996.
9. Pacheco-Tena C, Burgos-Vargas R, Vázquez-Mellado J, et al: A proposal for the classification of patients for clinical and experimental studies on reactive arthritis. J Rheumatol 26: 1338, 1999.
10. Leino R, Mäkelä AL, Tiilikainen A, et al: *Yersinia* arthritis in children. Scand J Rheumatol 9: 245, 1980.
11. Hoogkamp-Korstanje JA, Stolk-Engelaar VM: *Yersinia enterocolitica* infection in children. Pediatr Infect Dis J 14: 771, 1995.
12. Denardo BA, Tucker LB, Miller LC, et al: Demography of a regional pediatric rheumatology patient population. J Rheumatol 21: 1553, 1994.
13. Bowyer S, Roettcher P, and the members of the Pediatric Rheumatology Database Research Group: Pediatric Rheumatology Clinic populations in the United States: results of a 3 year survey. J Rheumatol 23: 1968, 1996.
14. Symmons DPM, Jones M, Osborne J, et al: Pediatric rheumatology in the United Kingdom: data from the British Pediatric Rheumatology Group National Diagnostic Register. J Rheumatol 23: 1975, 1996.
15. Malleson PN, Fung MY, Rosenberg AM, for the Canadian Pediatric Rheumatology Association: The incidence of pediatric rheumatic diseases: results from the Canadian Pediatric Rheumatology Association Disease Registry. J Rheumatol 23: 1981, 1996.
16. Rosenberg AM: Analysis of a pediatric rheumatology clinic population. J Rheumatol 17: 827, 1990.
17. Gäre BA, Fasth A: The natural history of juvenile chronic arthritis: a population based cohort study: I. Onset and disease process. J Rheumatol 22: 295, 1995.
18. Oen KG, Cheang M: Epidemiology of chronic arthritis in childhood. Semin Arthritis Rheum 26: 575, 1996.
19. Kiessling U, Döring E, Listing J, et al: Incidence and prevalence of juvenile chronic arthritis in East Berlin 1980–88. J Rheumatol 25: 1837, 1998.
20. Ozen S, Karaaslan Y, Ozdemir O, et al: Prevalence of juvenile chronic arthritis and familial Mediterranean fever in Turkey: a field study. J Rheumatol 25: 2445, 1998.
21. Tacceti G, Trapani S, Ermini M, et al: Reactive arthritis triggered by *Yersinia enterocolitica*: a review of 18 pediatric cases. Clin Exp Rheumatol 12: 681, 1994.
22. Vander LS, Vander HDN: Clinical and epidemiologic aspects of ankylosing spondylitis and spondyloarthropathies. Curr Opin Rheumatol 8: 269, 1996.
23. Johnsen K, Ostensen M, Melbye AC, et al: HLA-B27–negative arthritis related to *Campylobacter jejuni* enteritis in three children and two adults. Acta Med Scand 214: 165, 1983.
24. Artamonov VA, Akhmadi S, Polianskaia IS: The clinical and immunogenetic characteristics of reactive arthritis in children. Ter Arkh 63: 22, 1991.
25. Tuokko J, Koskinen S, Westman P, et al: Tumour necrosis factor microsatellites in reactive arthritis. Br J Rheumatol 37: 1203, 1998.
26. Tuokko J, Pushnova E, Yli-Kerttula U, et al: TAP2 alleles in inflammatory arthritis. Scand J Rheumatol 27: 225, 1998.
27. Czonka GW: The course of Reiter's syndrome. Br Med J 1: 1088, 1958.
28. Florman AL, Goldstein HM: Arthritis, conjunctivitis and urethritis (so-called Reiter's syndrome) in a 4-year-old boy. J Pediatr 33: 172, 1948.
29. Davies NE, Haverty JR, Boatwright M: Reiter's disease associated with shigellosis. South Med J 62: 1011, 1969.
30. Singsen BH, Bernstein BH, Koster-King KG, et al: Reiter's syndrome in childhood. Arthritis Rheum 20(Suppl): 402, 1977.
31. Russell AS: Reiter's syndrome in children following infection with *Yersinia enterocolitica* and shigella. Arthritis Rheum 20(Suppl): 471, 1977.
32. Iveson JMI, Nanda BS, Hancock JAH, et al: Reiter's disease in three boys. Ann Rheum Dis 34: 364, 1975.
33. Jacobs AG: A case of Reiter's syndrome in childhood. Br Med J 2: 155, 1961.
34. Rosenberg AM, Petty RE: Reiter's disease in children. Am J Dis Child 133: 394, 1979.
35. Cimolai N, Malleson P, Thomas E, Middleton PJ: *Mycoplasma pneumoniae* associated arthropathy: confirmation of the association by determination of the antipolypeptide IgM response. J Rheumatol 16: 1150, 1989.
36. Hannu T, Puolakkainen M, Leirisalo-Repo M: *Chlamydia pneumoniae* as a triggering infection in reactive arthritis. Rheumatology (Oxford) 38: 411, 1999.
37. Cron RQ, Gordon PV: Reactive arthritis to *Clostridium difficile* in a child. West J Med 166: 419, 1997.
38. Kocar IH, Caliskaner Z, Pay S, Turan M: *Clostridium difficile* infection in patients with reactive arthritis of undetermined etiology. Scand J Rheumatol 27: 357, 1998.
39. Letts M, Davidson D, Lalonde F: Synovitis secondary to giardiasis in children. Am J Orthop 27: 451, 1998.
40. Cron RQ, Sherry DD: Reiter's syndrome associated with cryptosporidial gastroenteritis. J Rheumatol 22: 1962, 1995.

41. Ikeda M, Yu DT: The pathogenesis of HLA-B27 arthritis: role of HLA-B27 in bacterial defense. Am J Med Sci 316: 257, 1998.
42. Wordsworth P, Brown M: HLA-B27, ankylosing spondylitis and the spondyloarthropathies. *In* Calin A, Taurog JD (eds): The Spondyloarthritides. Oxford, England, Oxford University Press, 1998, p 179.
43. Taurog JD: HLA-B27 subtypes, disease susceptibility, and peptide binding. *In* Calin A, Taurog JD (eds): The Spondyloarthritides. Oxford, England, Oxford University Press, 1998, p 267.
44. Wordsworth P: Genes in the spondyloarthropathies. Rheum Dis Clin North Am 24: 845, 1998.
45. Benjamin R, Parham P: Guilt by association: HLA-B27 and ankylosing spondylitis. Immunol Today 11: 137, 1990.
46. Sieper J, Braun J: Pathogenesis of spondyloarthropathies. Persistent bacterial antigen, autoimmunity, or both? Arthritis Rheum 38: 1547, 1995.
47. Sieper J, Braun J: Triggering mechanisms and T-cell responses in the spondyloarthropathies. *In* Calin A, Taurog JD (eds): The Spondyloarthritides. Oxford, England, Oxford University Press, 1998, p 195.
48. Herman E, Yu DTY, Meyer zum Büschenfelde K-H, et al: HLA-B27 restricted CD8 T cells derived from synovial fluids of patients with reactive arthritis and ankylosing spondylitis. Lancet 342: 646, 1993.
49. Sieper J, Kingsley G, Märker-Hermann E: Aetiological agents and immune mechanisms in enterogenic reactive arthritis. Bailliere's Clin Rheumatol 10: 105, 1996.
50. Kingsley G, Panayi GS: Antigenic responses in reactive arthritis. Rheum Dis Clin North Am 18: 49, 1992.
51. Märker-Hermann E, Höhler T: Pathogenesis of human leukocyte antigen B27-positive arthritis: information from clinical materials. Rheum Dis Clin North Am 24: 865, 1998.
52. Davenport MP: The promiscuous B27 hypothesis. Lancet 346: 500, 1995.
53. Scofield RH, Warren WL, Koelsch G, Harley JB: A hypothesis for the HLA-B27 immune dysregulation in spondyloarthropathy: contributions from enteric organism, B27 structure peptides bound by B27, and convergent evolution. Proc Natl Acad Sci U S A 90: 9330, 1993.
54. Burgos-Vargas R, Howard A, Ansell BM: Antibodies to peptidoglycan in juvenile onset ankylosing spondylitis and pauciarticular onset juvenile arthritis associated with chronic iridocyclitis. J Rheumatol 13: 760, 1986.
55. Life P, Hassell A, Williams K, et al: Responses to gram negative enteric bacterial antigens by synovial T cells from patients with juvenile chronic arthritis: recognition of heat shock protein HSP60. J Rheumatol 20: 1388, 1993.
56. Granfors K: Do bacterial antigens cause reactive arthritis? Rheum Dis Clin North Am 18: 37, 1992.
57. Wuorela M, Granfors K: Infectious agents as triggers of reactive arthritis. Am J Med Sci 316: 264, 1998.
58. Uksila J, Toivanen P, Granfors K: Enteric infection and arthritis: Bacteriological aspects. *In* Calin A, Taurog JD (eds): The Spondyloarthritides. Oxford, England, Oxford University Press, 1998, p 167.
59. Kapasi K, Inman RD: HLA B27 expression modulates gram-negative bacterial invasion into transfected L cells. J Immunol 148: 3554, 1992.
60. Kapasi K, Inman RD: ME1 epitope of HLA B27 confers class I–mediated modulation of gram-negative bacterial invasion. J Immunol 153: 833, 1994.
61. Ortiz-Alvarez O, Yu DT, Petty RE, Finlay BB: HLA-B27 does not affect invasion of arthritogenic bacteria into human cells. J Rheumatol 25: 1765, 1998.
62. Huppertz H-I, Heesemann J: The influence of HLA B27 and interferon-γ on the invasion and persistence of yersinia in primary human fibroblasts. Med Microbiol Immunol 185: 163, 1996.
63. Laitio P, Virtala M, Salmi M, et al: HLA-B27 modules intracellular survival of *Salmonella enteritidis* in human monocytic cells. Eur J Immunol 27: 1331, 1997.
64. Granfors K: Host-microbe interaction in reactive arthritis: does HLA-B27 have a direct effect? J Rheumatol 25: 1659, 1998.
65. Schumacher HR, Magge S, Cherian PV, et al: Light and electron microscopic studies on synovial membrane in Reiter's syndrome: immunocytochemical identification of chlamydial antigens in patients with early disease. Arthritis Rheum 31: 937, 1988.
66. Granfors K, Jalkanen S, von Essen R, et al: *Yersinia* antigens in synovial fluid cells from patients with reactive arthritis. N Engl J Med 320: 216, 1989.
67. Hammer M, Zeidler H, Klimsa S, et al: *Yersinia enterocolitica* in the synovial membrane of patients with yersinia induced arthritis. Arthritis Rheum 33: 1795, 1990.
68. Granfors K, Jalkanen S, Lindberg AA, et al: *Salmonella* lipopolysaccharide in the synovial cells from patients with reactive arthritis. Lancet 335: 685, 1990.
69. Taylor-Robinson D, Gilroy CB, Thomas BJ, et al: Detection of *Chlamydia trachomatis* DNA in joints of reactive arthritis patients by polymerase chain reaction. Lancet 340: 81, 1992.
70. García CO, Paira S, Burgos-Vargas R, et al: Detection of *Salmonella* DNA in synovial membrane and synovial fluid from Latin American patients with reactive arthritis using the polymerase chain reaction. Arthritis Rheum 39(Suppl): S185, 1996.
71. Braun J, Tuszewski M, Eggens U, et al: Nested polymerase chain reaction strategy simultaneously targeting DNA sequences of multiple bacterial species in inflammatory joint diseases: I. Screening of synovial fluid samples of patients with spondyloarthropathies and other arthritides. J Rheumatol 24: 1092, 1997.
72. Hussein A: Spectrum of post-enteric reactive arthritis in childhood. Monatsschr Kinderheilkd 135: 93, 1987.
73. Iakovleva AA, Mitchenko AF, Iushchenko GV, et al: *Yersinia* arthritis in children. Vestn Akad Med Nauk S S S R 6: 71, 1989.
74. Jezequel C, Prigent JY, Loiseau-Corvez MN, et al: Reactive arthritis caused by *Yersinia* in children. Report of 4 cases. Ann Pediatr (Paris) 38: 318, 1991.
75. Russell AS: Reiter's syndrome in children following infection with *Yersinia enterocolitica* and *Shigella*. Arthritis Rheum 20(Suppl): 471, 1977.
76. Carroll WL, Balistreri WF, Brilli R, et al: Spectrum of *Salmonella*-associated arthritis. Pediatrics 68: 717, 1981.
77. Kanakoudi-Tsakalidou F, Pardalos G, Prastidou-Gertsi P, et al: Persistent or severe course of reactive arthritis following *Salmonella enteritidis* infection. Scand J Rheumatol 27: 431, 1998.
78. Cuttica RJ, Scheines EJ, Garay SM, et al: Juvenile onset Reiter's syndrome—a retrospective study of 26 patients. Clin Exp Rheumatol 10: 285, 1992.
79. Lockie GN, Hunder GG: Reiter's syndrome in children: a case report and review. Arthritis Rheum 14: 767, 1971.
80. Fris J: Reiter's disease with childhood onset having special reference to HLA B27. Scand J Rheumatol 9: 250, 1980.
81. Huppertz HI, Sandhage K: Reactive arthritis due to *Salmonella enteritidis* complicated by carditis. Acta Paediatr 83: 1230, 1994.
82. Zivony D, Nocton J, Wortmann D, et al: Juvenile Reiter's syndrome: a report of four cases. J Am Acad Dermatol 38: 32, 1998.
83. Saari KM, Mäki M, Päivönsalo T, et al: Acute anterior uveitis and conjunctivitis following *Yersinia* infection in children. Int Ophthalmol 9: 237, 1986.
84. Fischel JD, Lipton J: Acute anterior uveitis in juvenile Reiter's syndrome. Clin Rheumatol 15: 83, 1996.
85. Huppertz HI, Karch H, Heesemann J: Diagnostic value of synovial fluid analysis in children with reactive arthritis. Rheumatol Int 15: 167, 1995.
86. Azouz EM, Duffy CM: Juvenile spondyloarthropathies: clinical manifestations and medical imaging. Skel Radiol 24: 399, 1995.
87. De Keyser F, Elewaut D, De Vos M, et al: Bowel inflammation and the spondyloarthropathies. Rheum Dis Clin North Am 24: 785, 1998.
88. Bollow M, Biedermann T, Kannenberg J, et al: Use of dynamic magnetic resonance imaging to detect sacroiliitis in HLA-B27-positive and negative children with juvenile arthritides. J Rheumatol 25: 556, 1998.
89. Bauman C, Cron RQ, Sherry DD, et al: Reiter syndrome initially misdiagnosed as Kawasaki disease. J Pediatr 128: 366, 1996.
90. Duffy CM, Arsenault L, Duffy KN, et al: The Juvenile Arthritis Quality of Life Questionnaire: development of a new responsive index for juvenile rheumatoid arthritis and juvenile spondyloarthropathies. J Rheumatol 24: 738, 1997.
91. Tucker LB, De Nardo BA, Abetz LN, et al: The childhood arthritis health profile (CAHP): validity and reliability of the condition specific scales. Arthritis Rheum 38: S183, 1995.
92. Mielants H, Veys EM, Joos R, et al: Late onset pauciarticular

juvenile chronic arthritis. Relation to gut inflammation. J Rheumatol 14: 459, 1987.

93. Mielants H, Veys EM, Cuvelier C, et al: Gut inflammation in children with late onset pauciarticular juvenile chronic arthritis and evolution to adult spondyloarthropathy—a prospective study. J Rheumatol 20: 1567, 1993.
94. Joss R, Veys EM, Myelants H, et al: Sulfasalazine treatment in juvenile chronic arthritis: an open study. J Rheumatol 18: 880, 1991.
95. Suschke HJ: Treatment of juvenile spondyloarthritis and reactive arthritis with sulfasalazine. Monatsschr Kinderheilkd 140: 658, 1992.
96. Job-Deslandre C, Menkès CJ: Sulfasalazine treatment for juvenile spondyloarthropathy. Rev Rhum Ed Fr 60: 403, 1993.
97. Leirisalo-Repo M: Prognosis, course of disease, and treatment of the spondyloarthropathies. Rheum Dis Clin North Am 24: 737, 1998.
98. Creemers MC, Franssen MHJ, van de Putte LB, et al: Methotrexate in severe ankylosing spondylitis: an open study. J Rheumatol 22: 1104, 1995.
99. Lauhio A, Leirisalo-Repo M, Landevirta J, et al: Double-blind, placebo-controlled study of three-month treatment with lymecycline in reactive arthritis, with special reference to *Chlamydia* arthritis. Arthritis Rheum 34: 6, 1991.

34

Acute Rheumatic Fever and Poststreptococcal Reactive Arthritis

Elia M. Ayoub

ACUTE RHEUMATIC FEVER

Acute rheumatic fever (ARF) is a connective tissue disease characterized by an inflammatory process that affects several organs of the body. It is one of the few rheumatic diseases in which the cause has been identified. It is well established that tonsillopharyngitis due to the group A β-hemolytic *Streptococcus pyogenes* is the precipitating cause of ARF. The streptococcal infection and the onset of the clinical manifestations of ARF are separated by a period of latency of 2 to 3 weeks. During this time, the patient is asymptomatic. The clinical presentations include arthritis, carditis, inflammation of the basal ganglia of the brain, a characteristic rash, and subcutaneous nodules. Arthritis is the most common but the least specific of these manifestations, whereas carditis is the most specific and serious. The pathologic process underlying the inflammatory reaction in the various organs is a diffuse vasculitis mediated by an immune reaction to the streptococcal infection. This nonpurulent complication of group A streptococcal disease can be prevented by appropriate treatment of the streptococcal pharyngitis.

Epidemiology

ARF was equally prevalent worldwide until the middle part of this century. The advent of industrialization and improved public hygiene in Western Europe and North America was associated with a sharp decline in the incidence of this disease. During the early part of the 20th century, incidence rates of 100 to 200 per 100,000 population were documented in the United States.[1] Although this rate still prevails in developing countries, current estimates of the incidence of ARF in children in the United States provide a markedly lower incidence rate of 0.5 to 3 per 100,000 population.[2] Between 1985 and 1990, a marked resurgence of the disease occurred in several areas in the United States.[3–12] This dramatic reappearance of what had been an increasingly rare disease was followed by a persistently higher rate in the incidence of ARF in these geographic areas.[13–15] The focal nature of these episodes has not significantly affected the overall prevalence of the disease in the United States, however.

The age-related incidence of ARF follows that of group A streptococcal pharyngitis and peaks between the ages of 6 and 15 years. ARF is rarely encountered in the United States in children younger than 5 years.[16–18] Among adults at high risk for streptococcal pharyngitis, such as military recruits and persons working in crowded settings, the incidence of the disease is higher. There is no difference in the incidence of ARF between males and females.

ARF used to be considered a disease of temperate climates but is now more common in tropical climes, particularly in developing countries. In the United States, the highest seasonal incidence is in the spring, following the peak season of streptococcal pharyngitis in the winter. In other countries, a season of peak frequency is less well defined.

Despite the decline of ARF in industrialized countries, its prevalence in developing areas of the world remains very high. About 6 million children suffer from rheumatic heart disease in India and in Sri Lanka, where the annual incidence of the disease is estimated at 100 to 150 cases per 100,000 population.[2, 18] Factors that have been invoked in explaining the decreased incidence of the disease in the United States include less crowding in homes and schools and the increased availability of health care to children.[19, 20] Observations made during the recent resurgence of ARF suggest that these factors may not be of major importance because this disease was now occurring primarily in children from high- to middle-income families with ready access to medical care.[3]

Differences in the incidence of ARF among racial and ethnic groups have been described. In New Zealand, the disease is more common among the Maori population compared with local non-Maoris of similar socioeconomic status.[21] ARF in the United States is more prevalent in African-Americans and Hispanic-Americans than white Americans.[2] Although genetic factors could account for these racial and ethnic differences in incidence, environmental factors may also be instrumental in explaining these differences.

Etiology and Pathogenesis

ARF is a complication of a group A streptococcal infection in a predisposed human host. Other species are not susceptible to this complication, hence the absence of an experimental model for this disease. Specific factors that influence the evolution of this disorder include the characteristics of the etiologic organism, the site of the streptococcal infection, and a genetic predisposition of the host (Fig. 34–1). Group A streptococcal tonsillopharyngitis is the primary inciting infection that precipitates an attack of ARF. Streptococcal pyoderma does not lead to this nonpurulent complication.[22] Fewer than 2 to 3 percent of previously healthy persons who acquire streptococcal pharyngitis develop ARF. This complication can be prevented by treatment of the streptococcal infection.

Etiologic Agent

β-Hemolytic streptococci have been divided into 20 serogroups by Lancefield[23] (A to H and K to V), based on immunochemical differences in their cell-wall polysaccharide. The group A streptococcus is the most common bacterial pathogen that is associated with tonsillopharyngitis and is the only member of these groups of streptococci that can initiate an attack of ARF. Several cellular components and extracellular products produced by the group A streptococcus in vivo and in vitro have been identified (Fig. 34–2).

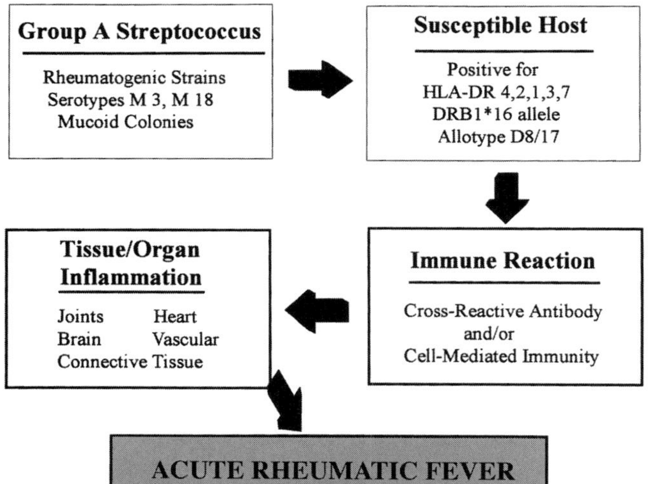

Figure 34–1. Steps in the interactions between the group A *Streptococcus* and the human host leading to acute rheumatic fever. HLA, human leukocyte antigen. (Adapted from Ayoub EM: Acute rheumatic fever. *In* Emmanouilides GC, Riemenschneider TA, Allen HD, et al [eds]: Moss and Adams' Heart Disease in Infants, Children, and Adolescents, Including the Fetus and Young Adult, vol II, 5th ed. Baltimore, Williams & Wilkins, 1995, p 1400.)

The streptococcal bacterium consists of a cytoplasm enclosed in a membrane composed predominantly of lipoproteins. This structure is surrounded by a rigid cell wall made up of three components. The primary component is a peptidoglycan that imparts rigidity to the cell wall. A complex of this component and the cell-wall polysaccharide elicits arthritis and a recurrent nodular reaction when injected into the skin of experimental animals.[24–26] Integrated into the peptidoglycan is the cell-wall polysaccharide or group-specific carbohydrate whose immunochemical structure determines the serogroup specificity. This polysaccharide has been reported to share antigenic determinants with a glycopeptide present in mitral valve tissue.[27] Traversing through and extending outside the cell wall as hairlike fimbriae is the M protein, part of a mosaic that also includes the R and T proteins. The M protein is a coiled protein with an α-helical structure consisting of a free, distal, hypervariable amino terminus and a proximal carboxy terminus anchored to the cell wall.[28] This protein is the type-specific antigen of the group A streptococcus.

About 100 M proteins have been identified by differences in immunochemical composition of the variable amino terminus. This has allowed separation of group A streptococci into about 100 M serotypes. A major biologic property of the M protein resides in its capacity to inhibit phagocytosis of the streptococcus, a property that is neutralized by the antibody to the amino terminal region. Immunity to group A streptococcal infections is type specific and is predicated on formation of antibodies to the various M proteins. Additional attributes that make this molecule a major virulence factor include the association of certain serotypes with potential pathogenicity. Data procured during the recent resurgence of ARF confirmed that serotypes 3 and 18, particularly strains that produced mucoid colonies when cultured on blood agar, were associated with the disease.[29] These two serotypes and the M1 serotype were also associated with severe, invasive group A streptococcal disease, including the streptococcal toxic shock syndrome.[30] Studies have indicated that bacterial strains that have conserved parts of the carboxy terminal portion of the M-protein molecule exposed on their cell surface (class I strains) were associated with ARF, whereas strains that did not have this characteristic (class II) had no such association.[31]

The pathogenetic importance of the M proteins is supported by data indicating that several epitopes of the M-protein molecule cross-react antigenically with human myocardium, myosin, and brain tissue, ostensibly leading to tissue inflammation.[17, 32] M protein also acts as a "superantigen."[33] These findings indicate that this streptococcal molecule can induce an inflammatory response in certain tissues by eliciting "autoimmune" antibodies and can also induce tissue inflammation by nonspecific stimulation of cell-mediated immunity as a superantigen.

The cellular component of the group A streptococcus that has been implicated in the pathogenesis of arthritis is the hyaluronate capsule. Like the M protein, this moiety appears to carry epitopes that elicit antibodies that cross-react with human cartilage and synovial fluid.[34]

In addition to the cellular components, extracellular products of the group A streptococcus have important biologic activities and are of practical value to the diagnosis of group

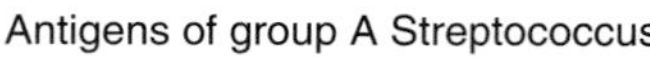

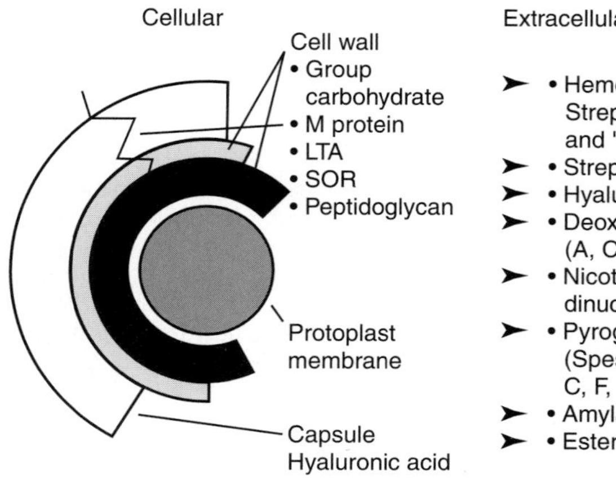

Figure 34–2. Cellular components and extracellular products of the group A *Streptococcus.* LTA, lipoteichoic acid; SOR, serum opacity factor (α-lipoproteinase); Spe, streptococcal pyrogenic exotoxin. (From Ayoub EM: Rheumatic fever. *In* Rich RR, Fleisher TA, Schwartz BD, et al [eds]: Clinical Immunology: Principles and Practice. St. Louis, Mosby–Year Book, 1996, p 1134.)

A streptococcal infections and their nonpurulent complications. Most of these products are proteins with enzymatic properties and as such possess specific biologic and antigenic activity. The streptococcal pyrogenic exotoxins (SPEs) A, B, C, and F (the mitogenic factor MF) and the superantigen SSA are of particular interest because they act as superantigens that induce proliferation of T lymphocytes in vitro and the synthesis and release of several lymphokines in vivo.[35–40] This biologic activity is due to the ability of SPEs to bind simultaneously to the class II major histocompatibility antigens of antigen-presenting cells and to the Vβ region of T cell receptor. The production of these exotoxins is associated in vivo with a febrile response, alteration of membrane permeability, and enhancement of susceptibility to endotoxin-induced lethal shock.[38] Selective activation of lymphocytes has been ascribed to different SPEs. SPE A activates T cells bearing T cell receptor β-chain segments Vβ8, Vβ12, and Vβ14, whereas SPE B activates T cells bearing segments Vβ2 and Vβ8.[41] SPE B has been identified as a cysteine protease that inhibits phagocytosis and enhances dissemination of the organism in vivo. It also induces apoptosis of phagocytic cells.[42]

The frequencies of the *spe* genes and their expression vary among group A streptococci; *speA* is found in 45 percent of strains, *speB* in almost all strains, and *speC* in 30 percent of strains. SPE A is expressed by 43 percent and SPE B by 76 percent of strains.[30, 43, 44] The frequencies of the *speA* genes and their products are similar among M1 and M3 serotypes.[43] The association of certain serotypes with various clinical manifestations of streptococcal infections, such as toxic shock syndrome, has been ascribed to the capacity of the infecting strain to produce one of the SPEs.[30, 41, 43] However, the ubiquity of the production of these toxins makes confirmation of the specificity of these associations questionable.[44]

Streptococcal Antibody Tests

The specific antigenicity of most of the streptococcal extracellular products led to the establishment of antibody tests to these products. These tests are used to provide evidence of group A streptococcal infection, primarily in patients with ARF and glomerulonephritis. The first and still the most universally used of these tests is antistreptolysin O (ASO), which was designed by Todd[44a] to measure neutralizing antibodies to purified streptolysin O in patients with scarlet fever and ARF. This test proved helpful in providing evidence for antecedent group A streptococcal infection, particularly when throat cultures were negative. Subsequently, tests were developed to assay for antibodies to other streptococcal antigens (Table 34–1). Of these tests, anti-DNase B, which assays for antibodies to the most ubiquitous of four deoxyribonuclease isozymes produced by the group A streptococcus (A, B, C, D), proved to be as reliable and reproducible as ASO. The other tests have suffered from the lack of specificity and reproducibility and are not readily available. The streptozyme test, which was widely used at one time, lacked standardization and reproducibility and should not be relied on for evidence of antecedent group A streptococcal infection.[45]

The pattern of the antibody response to the streptococcal antigens is illustrated in Figure 34–3. Antibodies peak approximately 3 weeks after the acute infection. Because of the period of latency between the infection and the onset of the clinical manifestations of ARF, serum obtained at the time of clinical presentation should provide the necessary evidence for antecedent group A streptococcal infection. However, as outlined

Table 34–1

Group A Streptococcal Antigens and Corresponding Antibody Tests

STREPTOCOCCAL ANTIGEN	ANTIBODY TEST
Extracellular Product	
Streptolysin O	Antistreptolysin O (ASO)
Streptokinase	Antistreptokinase
Hyaluronidase	Antihyaluronidase
Deoxyribonuclease B	Anti-DNase B
Nicotinamide adenine dinucleotidase	Anti-NADase
Multiple antigens	Streptozyme
Cellular Component	
M protein	Type-specific antibody
Group-specific polysaccharide	Anti–A-carbohydrate

Adapted from Ayoub EM: Streptococcal antibody tests in rheumatic fever. Clin Immunol Newsl, vol 3, pp 107–111, Copyright 1982, with permission from Elsevier Science.

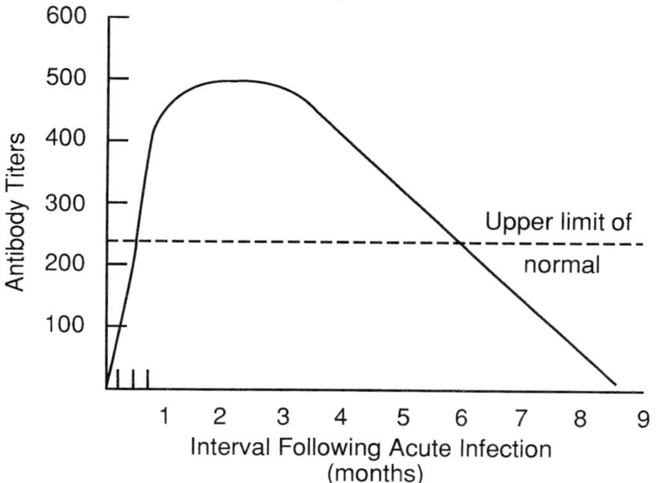

Figure 34–3. Pattern of antibody response to the extracellular antigens of the group A *Streptococcus* after tonsillopharyngeal infection in humans. (Reprinted from Ayoub EM: Streptococcal antibody tests in rheumatic fever. Clin Immunol Newsl, vol 3, pp 107–111, Copyright 1982, with permission from Elsevier Science.)

in Table 34–2, only about 85 percent of patients with ARF mount an ASO response. Another streptococcal antibody test, such as anti-DNase B, can provide such evidence for an antecedent streptococcal infection in patients in whom an ASO response has not been diagnostic.

Tests for antibodies to the cell-wall components of group A streptococcus are available but not widely used. Determination of the antibody to the different M proteins (type-specific antibody) is used in epidemiologic studies to determine previous exposure or immunity to specific M serotypes. Testing for the antibody to the group-specific carbohydrate is available in some laboratories. Because this antibody tends to persist for prolonged periods in patients with rheumatic valvular disease, it may help to confirm the rheumatic etiology of mitral valve disease in a patient without a history of ARF.[46–49]

Table 34–2

Frequency of Patients With Acute Rheumatic Fever With an Elevated ASO and/or Anti-DNase B Titer

	ASO	ANTI-DNASE B	ASO AND ANTI-DNASE B
Normal controls	19	19	30
Acute rheumatic fever	83	82	92
Sydenham's chorea (isolated)	67	40	80

Adapted from Ayoub EM, Wannamaker LW: Evaluation of the streptococcal deoxyribonuclease B and diphosphopyridine nucleotidase antibody tests in acute rheumatic fever and acute glomerulonephritis. Reproduced by permission of Pediatrics, vol 29, pp 527–538, Copyright 1962; Ayoub EM, Wannamaker LW: Streptococcal antibody titers in Sydenham's chorea. Reproduced by permission of Pediatrics, vol 38, pp 946–956, Copyright 1966.

Host Factors

Early postulates regarding the epidemiology of rheumatic fever suggested that persons who acquired this disease had a peculiar susceptibility to it. This suggestion was based on the observation that 30 to 80 percent of patients who had an attack of ARF had a recurrence of the disease after group A streptococcal pharyngitis, whereas only about 2 percent of normal persons would develop ARF after such an infection.[50] In addition, studies by several investigators documented the familial occurrence of the disease.[51–53] Citing their studies, these investigators concluded that susceptibility to ARF is inherited as a single recessive gene.

More substantial evidence for a genetic association was provided by Khanna and associates,[54] who reported that a B-cell alloantigen, designated D8/17, was present in 99 percent of patients with ARF but in only 14 percent of normal controls. Further support for the role of genetic factors in susceptibility was provided by studies on the association of this disease with inheritance of the major histocompatibility antigens (HLAs).[55–64] The results of these investigations, summarized in Table 34–3, document a significant association of susceptibility to ARF with class II HLAs or their alleles.

Early investigators proposed that susceptibility to ARF was related to a state of hyper-reactivity to streptococcal antigens. Studies of hyper-responsiveness to a number of streptococcal and nonstreptococcal antigens suggested a hyperimmune response to streptococcal extracellular products, particularly streptolysin O, although subsequent reports did not confirm these findings.[65, 66] More recent studies on the immune response to the group A streptococcal group-specific carbohydrate documented a peculiar hyperimmune response to this antigen in patients with rheumatic valvular disease.[46–49, 67] This response was associated with inheritance of HLA-DR2 and DR4 antigens.[55] This finding is of particular relevance in view of data that indicate that the immune response to streptococcal cell-wall antigen is under genetic control in experimental animals and humans.[68–70]

Mechanism of Tissue Injury

Initial suggestions that tissue injury in ARF was due to direct invasion by the streptococcus, or the effect of its extracellular toxins, were subsequently replaced by the theory that an immune mechanism was responsible for the inflammatory process in the affected organs. The potential role of an immunologic process as the cause of tissue injury was predicated on the observation that the clinical manifestations of ARF occurred after a period of latency of about 3 weeks from the inciting group A streptococcal infection. Evidence for involvement of an immune mechanism in pathogenesis was first provided by Kaplan and coworkers.[71, 72] These investigators and others described the presence of common antigenic determinants between the cellular components of the group A streptococcus and myocardial tissue. Structures that share cross-reactive antigenic determinants included components of the M protein and

Table 34–3

Reported Associations of HLA-DR Antigens and Alleles With Rheumatic Fever

	LOCATION	NUMBER OF PATIENTS	ETHNICITY	HLA-DR ANTIGEN/ALLELE	PERCENT POSITIVE Controls	PERCENT POSITIVE Patients
Ayoub et al[55]	Florida	24	Caucasian	DRB4*16	32	63
	USA	48	Black	DR2	23	54
Anastasiou-Nana et al[56]	Utah USA	33	Caucasian	DR4	32	52
Jhinghan et al[57]	New Delhi India	134	Indian	DR3	26	50
Rajapakse et al[58]	Riyadh Saudi Arabia	40	Arab	DR4	12	65
Maharaj et al[59]	Durban South Africa	120	Black	DR1	3	13
Taneja et al[60]	New Delhi India	54	Indian	DQw2	32	63
Guilherme et al[61]	São Paulo	40	Brazilian	DR7	26	58
	Brazil		(Mulato)	DRw53	39	73
Ozkan et al[62]	Istanbul	107	Turkish	DR3	23	49
	Turkey			DR7	33	57
Weidebach et al[63]	São Paulo	24	Brazilian	DR16	34	83
	Brazil		(Mulato)	DRw53		
Ahmed et al[64]	Florida USA	18	Caucasian	DRB1*16	4	15

Adapted from Ayoub EM: Rheumatic fever. *In* Rich RR, Fleisher TA, Schwartz BD, et al (eds): Clinical Immunology: Principles and Practice. St. Louis, Mosby–Year Book, 1996, p 1134.

myocardial sarcolemma,[71–76] cell-wall carbohydrate and valvular glycoprotein,[27] streptococcal protoplast membrane and neuronal tissue of the subthalamic and caudate nuclei,[77] and the hyaluronate capsule and articular cartilage.[34] Based on these studies, it was concluded that antibodies formed against these streptococcal antigens cross-reacted with the corresponding tissues and, ostensibly, led to the inflammatory process in the heart, joints, and brain (Fig. 34–4).[17, 32]

As attractive as the process of "antigenic mimicry" is in explaining the inflammatory reaction in ARF, there are several flaws in this hypothesis. The most compelling of these arguments is the presence of high levels of cross-reactive antibodies in the sera of patients who do not have any manifestations of acute carditis or arthritis. An alternative explanation was provided by subsequent studies that documented a potential role for cell-mediated immunity in inducing tissue damage. These studies confirmed that peripheral blood lymphocytes from patients with acute rheumatic carditis were cytotoxic to human myocardial cells grown in tissue culture.[78] Addition of plasma from the same patients abrogated this cytotoxic effect. The latter observation suggested that the cross-reactive antibodies elicited by the group A streptococcus had a protective rather than a detrimental effect on the host. Based on these arguments, the prevalent hypothesis for explaining tissue injury in this disease is that an immunologic mechanism involving either the humoral or the cellular immune system may be responsible for tissue inflammation in ARF.

Pathology

The inflammation that occurs in ARF is the result of a diffuse vasculitis. The organs most commonly affected are the joints, heart, brain, and peripheral vascular system. The vasculitis, which affects the smaller vessels, is characterized by proliferation of endothelial cells. This vasculitic process is reflected in the rash of ARF; inflammation of collagen occurs primarily as an arthritis, valvulitis, and pericarditis. The synovitis of ARF is typified by a mononuclear cell infiltrate with

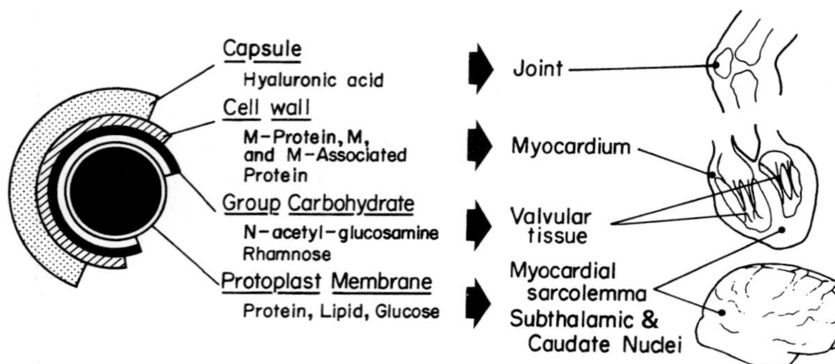

Figure 34–4. Group A streptococcal components and corresponding human tissues that have been reported to exhibit immunologic cross-reactivity. (From Ayoub EM, Schiebler GL: Acute rheumatic fever. *In* Kelley VC [ed]: Practice of Pediatrics, vol 8. New York, Harper & Row, 1987, p 7.)

fibrinoid degeneration. The cartilage is usually not involved.[18, 79]

Inflammation of the heart, the most serious complication of the disease, usually involves the myocardium and endocardium. Unlike other rheumatic diseases, such as systemic lupus erythematosus (SLE) or juvenile rheumatoid arthritis (JRA), sole involvement of the pericardium is uncommon in ARF. Its presence signals the occurrence of a pancarditis with involvement of all cardiac structures by the inflammatory process and is the most life-threatening event in ARF. Valvular endocarditis is the more common and characteristic inflammatory process in the heart and the principal cause of chronic cardiac disease. Acute inflammation leads to valvular insufficiency, and persistence of the inflammation results in scarring and stenosis. The mitral valve is the most commonly involved, and mitral insufficiency is the hallmark of rheumatic carditis. The aortic and tricuspid valves are involved less frequently. A review of the cardiac pathology of ARF by Roberts[80] indicated that isolated mitral valve disease was of rheumatic etiology in 76 percent of cases, whereas aortic valve disease was ascribable to ARF in only 13 percent of cases. The simultaneous presence of mitral and aortic disease was related to a rheumatic etiology in 97 percent of cases.

The histologic changes in acute rheumatic carditis are not particularly specific, and the degree of abnormality does not necessarily correlate with the severity of carditis.[18, 79] In the early stage, when dilatation of the myocardium is present, histologic changes can be minimal. Despite this, cardiac function may be severely impaired and may be associated with a high rate of mortality. Progression of the inflammation leads to an exudative and proliferative reaction in the myocardium characterized by edematous changes followed by a cellular infiltrate of lymphocytes and plasma cells with few granulocytes. CD4-positive cells predominate in the lymphocytic infiltrate.[81] Degenerating collagen fibers are visible throughout the tissue as eosinophilic, granular deposits consisting of a mixture of fibrin, globulin, and other substances. This stage is followed by the formation of the *Aschoff body*.[82, 83] This lesion consists of a perivascular infiltrate of large cells with polymorphous nuclei and basophilic cytoplasm arranged in a rosette around an avascular center of fibrinoid. The Aschoff body is pathognomonic of rheumatic carditis and is most common in patients with subacute or chronic carditis. It may develop in any area of the myocardium but not in other tissues.

Tissue edema and cellular infiltrates characterize inflammation of valvular tissue. This inflammatory process also involves the chordae tendineae. Verrucae may form at the edge of the leaflets, preventing the valves from complete closure. Persistent inflammation for several years leads to fibrosis and calcification of the valve, resulting in stenosis.

Clinical Manifestations

Arthritis, carditis, Sydenham's chorea, erythema marginatum, and subcutaneous nodules constitute the *major* clinical manifestations of ARF based on their specific association with the disease (Fig. 34–5). A patient may present with only one or with two or more of these manifestations, as well as with varying degrees of severity of each. Although the severity and frequency of these manifestations vary considerably from patient to patient, their overall frequency in various populations is similar (Table 34–4). *Minor* or less specific manifestations of ARF include fever, arthralgia, abnormal acute-phase reactants, and a prolonged P-R interval.

Arthritis

Arthritis occurs in about 70 percent of patients with ARF. Although it is the most common of the major manifestations, it is relatively less specific than the others because it is encountered in such a large number of other rheumatic diseases. As such, it is the most common cause of a misdiagnosis of ARF. Despite its

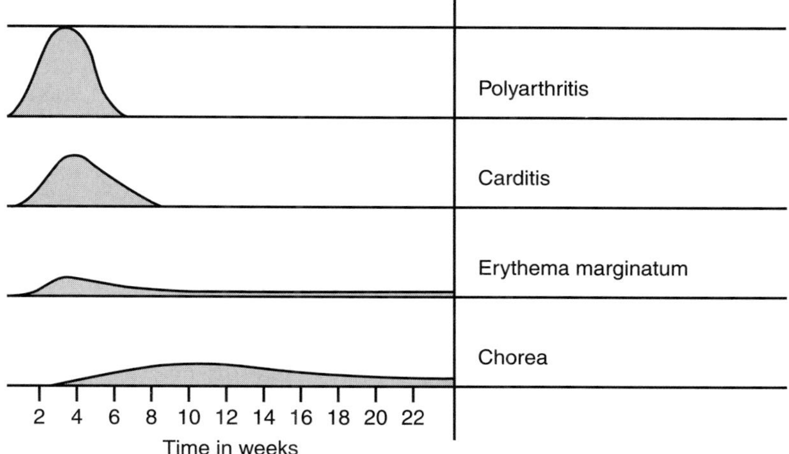

Figure 34–5. The major manifestations of acute rheumatic fever. This diagram illustrates the expected occurrence of each of the major manifestations of acute rheumatic fever. The relative duration in weeks is indicated on the abscissa. In addition, the maximum clinical activity of each finding is represented by the *peak of the shaded area.* The expected frequency of each clinical manifestation is represented by the *relative heights of each of the shaded areas.* Arthritis and carditis in general are manifestations of acute disease. Chorea, although it may be an early manifestation, usually occurs later (3 months) after the inciting episode of pharyngitis. It may be unaccompanied by other manifestations of the disease. Erythema marginatum is present for a longer period during and after the initial acute attack. In addition, this manifestation, although it is often associated with severe disease, is relatively infrequent in children.

Table 34–4

Frequency of Major Manifestations of Acute Rheumatic Fever in Patients in the United States and Patients Outside the United States

	PATIENTS WITH MANIFESTATION (%)			
	US Patients			Non-US Patients
MANIFESTATION	1958–1962	1962–1980	1985–1989	1960–1980
Arthritis	75	53	65	30–79
Carditis	48	78	59	41–93
Sydenham's chorea	16	5	20	1–12
Erythema marginatum	6	2	6	0–16
Subcutaneous nodules	7	5	5	1–9

Adapted from Ayoub EM: Resurgence of rheumatic fever in the United States. The changing pictures of a preventable disease. Postgrad Med 92: 133–142, 1992.

lower specificity, the arthritis of ARF has characteristics that can help in its differentiation from that due to other causes. The arthritis in ARF affects primarily large joints, particularly the knees, ankles, wrists, and elbows. Small peripheral joints are only occasionally involved, and axial disease occurs rarely, if ever. The arthritis of ARF is characteristically migratory and additive. Symptoms in an affected joint may resolve spontaneously within hours of onset, only to reappear in a different joint. The affected joint manifests the cardinal signs of inflammation with swelling, erythema, warmth, and pain. The latter symptom is the most prominent. It occurs at rest and is accentuated by passive or active movement of the joint. The severity of pain induces guarding of the joints, which may lead to a pseudoparalysis.

Carditis

Cardiac inflammation develops in about 50 percent of patients with ARF. The high frequency of this manifestation reported from developing countries probably reflects a bias toward hospitalization of patients with ARF and severe heart disease. Carditis is the most common cause of morbidity and mortality in ARF. As with other manifestations, the severity of the carditis is highly variable. In some patients, such as those with Sydenham's chorea, the signs of carditis may be subtle and cardiac involvement may be missed unless its diagnosis is pursued with echocardiographic examination. Other patients may present with acute pancarditis and severe, life-threatening congestive heart failure. Carditis usually occurs in tandem with other major manifestations, such as arthritis. If it is not present initially, carditis may follow arthritis within 1 week; the onset of carditis beyond this interval is rare.

Inflammation of the heart in ARF usually involves the myocardium and endocardium. Pericarditis is a sign of pancarditis: involvement of all cardiac layers in the inflammatory process. It is an ominous development associated with a high mortality. Unlike its occurrence in other rheumatic diseases, isolated pericarditis is rare in patients with ARF.

Myocarditis occurs during the initial stage of cardiac involvement; it is recognized clinically by the presence of tachycardia at rest in an afebrile patient. Myocarditis may be associated with heart block, cardiac arrhythmias, and a prolonged P-R interval on electrocardiography.

Endocarditis affects principally valvular tissue and leads to the hallmark lesion of rheumatic carditis, valvular insufficiency. The mitral valve is affected either alone or in conjunction with other valves in 94 percent of patients. Isolated mitral valve disease occurs in 65 percent of patients, isolated aortic disease is encountered in 6 percent, and simultaneous involvement of both valves occurs in 29 percent of patients. The pulmonic and tricuspid valves are only occasionally affected.

Mitral insufficiency or regurgitation is identified clinically by the presence on auscultation of a high-frequency, smooth, holosystolic apical murmur. This murmur radiates to the left axilla and is best heard with the patient in a left lateral decubitus position. A mid- to late-diastolic flow murmur of relative mitral stenosis *(Carey-Coombs murmur)* may be present in patients with severe mitral insufficiency.

The murmur of aortic insufficiency is a high-frequency, diastolic murmur that starts with the aortic component of the second heart sound. It is best heard with the diaphragm of the stethoscope over the third left intercostal space with the patient in the upright position and leaning forward. The murmur of mild aortic insufficiency is faint and often difficult to hear. Murmurs of severe insufficiency are loud and accompanied by a diastolic thrill. In these patients, an increased pulse pressure due to aortic runoff is associated with bounding peripheral pulses *(Corrigan pulse)*. Mitral and aortic valve stenoses result from valvular scarring and develop during the chronic stages of the disease.

Acute heart failure due to severe myocarditis or valvular insufficiency occurs in about 5 percent of children with ARF. The clinical manifestations vary greatly and include cough, chest pain, dyspnea, orthopnea, and anorexia. Tachycardia, cardiomegaly, and hepatomegaly with tenderness of the liver are present on physical examination.

Sydenham's Chorea

Also known as *St. Vitus' dance,* this manifestation of inflammatory involvement of the basal ganglia and caudate nucleus of the central nervous system occurs in about 15 percent of patients. A higher frequency was documented by several centers during the recent resurgence of ARF in the United States.[84] The latency period between the inciting streptococcal pharyngitis and the onset of clinical signs of chorea is longer than that of the other major manifestations of the disease, averaging 2 to 4 months and sometimes extending to 12 months.

The patient with Sydenham's chorea presents with persistent involuntary and purposeless movements of the extremities, muscular incoordination, and emotional lability. The symptoms disappear during sleep. On examination, the patient grimaces and fidgets constantly. The protruded tongue darts in and out and resembles a bag of worms (*wormian tongue*). Speech is halting and explosive, and a steady tone cannot be maintained for even a short time. Extension of the arms above the head leads to pronation of the hands (*pronator sign*); extension of the arms anteriorly results in hyperextension of the fingers (*spoon* or *dishing sign*). When the patient is asked to squeeze the examiner's fingers, the examiner feels irregular contractions of the hand muscles (*milkmaid's grip* or *milking sign*). Handwriting, particularly drawing vertical straight lines, is clumsy and irregular because of the loss of fine-muscle coordination. The patient has difficulty putting on clothes or buttoning a shirt. Such attempts lead to easy frustration and emotional upsets. Parents and teachers often complain about the child's clumsiness or inability to concentrate on tasks. Some patients are misdiagnosed as having a behavior problem, an attention-deficit disorder, or a "tic." These symptoms usually resolve spontaneously in 2 to 3 weeks but may persist for several months and sometimes years in severe cases.

Erythema Marginatum

Erythema marginatum is characteristic of rheumatic fever and occurs in about 5 percent of patients. The rash is nonpruritic and macular with a serpiginous erythematous border (Fig. 34–6). The individual lesions are about 1 inch in diameter and usually located on the trunk and proximal inner aspects of the limbs, particularly where they are in juxtaposition to the trunk. The rash is rare on the face or other exposed areas. It is accentuated by warmth, such as the application of warm towels or a bath. Erythema marginatum is difficult to detect in patients with dark skin.

Subcutaneous Nodules

The subcutaneous nodules of ARF that were most common in patients with chronic rheumatic heart disease are now rare. They are usually located on the extensor surfaces of the joints, particularly the elbows, knees, ankles, and knuckles, and occasionally on the occiput and spine. The overlying skin is not discolored. Their size varies from 0.5 to 2 cm, and they are freely movable. In many respects, they resemble benign rheumatoid nodules.

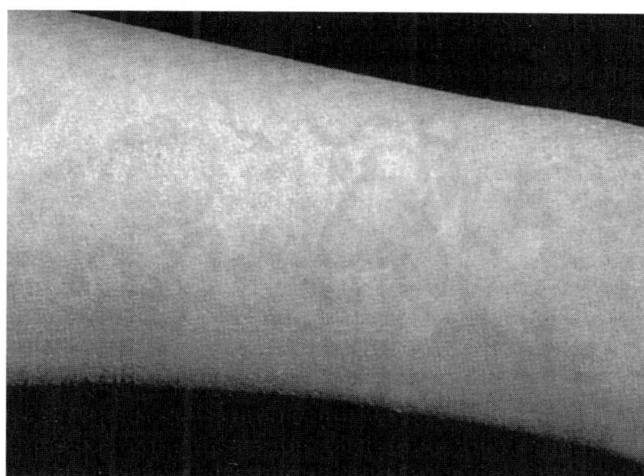

Figure 34–6. Rash of erythema marginatum on the forearm of a patient with acute rheumatic fever with the characteristic serpiginous (erythematous) margins surrounding normal skin areas.

Minor Manifestations of the Disease

The nonspecific minor manifestations of fever, arthralgia, and elevated acute-phase reactants are also encountered in a variety of other rheumatic diseases. Fever is variable in severity and duration; a temperature of 38.5° to 40°C may be present during the acute phase of the disease. Arthralgia—pain without objective changes in the joint—should be differentiated from arthritis. Abnormally elevated acute-phase reactants are indicators of tissue inflammation and are present during the acute stage of the disease. A prolonged P-R interval on electrocardiography occurs in patients with acute rheumatic carditis.

Diagnosis

No specific test is available for the definitive diagnosis of ARF: the diagnosis continues to be based on guidelines using clinical and laboratory criteria that were initially promulgated by T. Duckett Jones and subsequently revised by several committees of the American Heart Association. The latest modification of the Jones criteria[85] is outlined in Table 34–5. The purpose of these guidelines is to assist in the diagnosis of an initial attack of rheumatic fever and to minimize overdiagnosis of this disease. As stated under these guidelines, the presence of two major manifestations or one major plus two minor manifestations provides the basis for the diagnosis of ARF—if supported by evidence of antecedent group A streptococcal infection. The latter is a sine qua non for establishing the diagnosis.

Table 34–5

Guidelines for the Diagnosis of an Initial Attack of Rheumatic Fever (Modified Jones Criteria, 1992)

MAJOR MANIFESTATIONS	MINOR MANIFESTATIONS
Carditis	*Clinical*
Polyarthritis	Fever
Sydenham's chorea	Arthralgia
Erythema marginatum	*Laboratory*
Subcutaneous nodules	Elevated acute phase reactants:
	Erythrocyte sedimentation rate
	C-reactive protein
	Prolonged P-R interval

Supporting Evidence of Antecedent Group A Streptococcal Infection

Elevated or rising streptococcal antibody titer(s)
Positive throat culture or rapid streptococcal antigen test

The presence of two major manifestations or of one major and two minor manifestations indicates a high probability of acute rheumatic fever, if supported by evidence of preceding group A streptococcal infection.

Adapted from Dajani AS, Ayoub EM, Bierman FZ, et al: Guidelines for the diagnosis of rheumatic fever: Jones Criteria, updated 1992. JAMA 87: 302–307, 1992.

A positive throat culture or rapid antigen test can confirm an antecedent group A streptococcal pharyngitis. However, the period of latency between the inciting pharyngitis and the onset of ARF reduces the frequency of positive cultures to less than one third of patients.[86]

More reliable evidence can be obtained by the use of the streptococcal antibody tests listed in Table 34–1. Because of the latency period, a serum obtained at the time of the initial evaluation of the patient will coincide with the peak of the antibody response (see Fig. 34–2). An elevated ASO or anti-DNase B level is expected in about 85 percent of patients (see Table 34–2). When both tests are performed (considered by many to be a reasonable approach to diagnostic specificity), more than 90 percent of patients show an elevated titer for one of these tests. If the ASO is negative, a DNase B test should be performed. Furthermore, a fourfold (two-tube) increase or decrease in titers should be demonstrated over time. It should be noted that these antibody tests may be normal in the majority of patients with chronic rheumatic heart disease and that a high proportion of patients with Sydenham's chorea may have normal ASO or anti-DNase B titers (see Table 34–2).

Thus, neither the ASO nor the other streptococcal antibody tests are diagnostic of ARF per se; they are used to provide supportive evidence for antecedent streptococcal infection. Therefore, one should seriously question the diagnosis of ARF if these antibody tests yield normal values.

The three acute-phase reactant tests most commonly used in the diagnosis of ARF are the peripheral blood leukocyte count, the erythrocyte sedimentation rate (ESR), and the C-reactive protein (CRP). The leukocyte count is the most variable and least dependable of these tests. It is normal in about half of the patients with ARF. The ESR is markedly elevated in patients with acute disease but may be normal in patients with severe congestive failure.[87] The CRP is also elevated in patients with acute disease, and unlike the ESR, it is not affected by congestive heart failure. These tests are most useful in following the course of the disease and its response to treatment.

Other studies that are useful in the diagnosis of ARF include chest radiography, electrocardiography, and echocardiography. A chest radiograph can detect cardiac enlargement or pericardial fluid. These findings are best confirmed by echocardiographic studies, which can also define the presence of myocarditis by assessing myocardial contractility and the nature and extent of valvular lesions. Electrocardiography is most useful in confirming abnormalities in conduction and rhythm during acute myocardial inflammation.

Differential Diagnosis

Other rheumatic diseases account for most of the conditions that are misdiagnosed as ARF. JRA is not uncommonly confused with ARF without carditis. Characteristics that would indicate a diagnosis of JRA rather than ARF include an onset of oligoarticular arthritis in a child before the age of 5 years; absence of erythema of the joint; a protracted, recurrent course with a poor response to nonsteroidal anti-inflammatory drug (NSAID) therapy; and particularly the absence of evidence for antecedent group A streptococcal infection.

Poststreptococcal reactive arthritis poses some difficulty in differentiation from ARF. Clinical findings that should assist in the differentiation of these entities are discussed later. Other conditions in which joint involvement is common and should be differentiated from ARF include SLE, mixed connective tissue disease, other reactive arthritides, and serum sickness. Infectious arthritis, particularly gonococcal arthritis, may cause a problem in differential diagnosis. Leukemia and cases of hemoglobinopathy with bone infarcts can be mistaken for ARF. Appropriate evaluations and laboratory studies should assist proper diagnosis.

Patients with carditis and pericarditis may develop infections by a variety of bacterial, viral, rickettsial, or mycoplasmal agents. Endocardial disease occurs in patients with bacterial endocarditis and older patients with SLE and Libman-Sacks endocarditis. A murmur and systolic clicks are present in patients with mitral valve prolapse. Patients with hyperthyroidism often present diagnostic dilemmas. Some children with Kawasaki disease develop clinically obvious myocarditis and valvular disease during the early stages of illness. In these patients, the lack of evidence for antecedent group A streptococcal infection allows an initial differentiation from ARF.

The differentiation of Sydenham's chorea from other neurologic disorders requires careful evaluation. Imaging studies of the central nervous system are usually normal in patients with Sydenham's chorea. Other neurologic conditions that appear to be related to Sydenham's chorea include congenital or acquired "habitual" tic disorders, attention-deficit disorders, and obsessive-compulsive behavior conditions.[88] ASO and anti-DNase B tests should provide evidence for antecedent streptococcal infection in more than 80 percent of children with Sydenham's chorea and assist in its differentiation from other neurologic disorders.

Treatment

The initial treatment of ARF should address the eradication of streptococci that initiated this complication as well as the inflammatory process that has affected the various organs. Patients with ARF should be hospitalized and evaluated for cardiac involvement. Subsequent management includes prophylaxis to prevent recurrence of streptococcal infections and the treatment of residual cardiac disease when present.

Eradication of Streptococci

Patients should receive a streptococcal eradicating regimen of antimicrobials even though their throat culture or rapid antigen test is negative. Various regimens that can be used to eradicate streptococci from host tissue are listed in Table 34–6. Penicillin is the primary agent of choice and can be administered intramuscularly as a single dose or orally for 10 days. The former dosing is preferable in patients with cardiac involvement because of its greater dependability and efficacy. Patients allergic to penicillin should receive erythromycin orally for 10 days.

Treatment of Clinical Manifestations

Carditis

Treatment of acute carditis, if present, requires immediate attention. For mild to moderate carditis, anti-inflammatory agents are administered in the form of aspirin at a dose of 80 to 100 mg/kg/day in four divided doses. This dose is maintained for 4 to 8 weeks depending on clinical response and then reduced gradually and discontinued over the following 4 weeks. Glucocorticoid therapy is reserved for patients with severe carditis and congestive heart failure— particularly those with pancarditis, in whom it may be life saving. The use of glucocorticoids rather than aspirin in patients with heart failure is also justified to avoid solute overload from aspirin. It should be emphasized that neither form of therapy has been shown to influence the subsequent evolution of valvular disease.[89–91]

Prednisone is given orally in a dose of 2 mg/kg once daily. Duration of steroid therapy should rarely exceed 2 weeks. It should be tapered and withdrawn over the following 2 to 3 weeks. One week before termination of steroid therapy, aspirin should be instituted (following the regimen described earlier) in order to avoid the rebound of symptoms and acute-phase reactants that occurs when steroid therapy is abruptly terminated. As stated earlier, the ESR and CRP are of value in monitoring the response to anti-inflammatory therapy. In patients with heart failure and falsely low ESR, a rise in this reactant may occur with recovery; the CRP is more useful in monitoring response in these patients. Ancillary therapy for cardiac failure includes the judicious use of cardiotonics such as digitalis; inotropic agents such as dobutamine, dopamine, or amrinone; vasodilators (captopril or enalapril); and diuretics.

General aspects of the acute management include bed rest for patients with acute carditis. This recommendation was overly emphasized in the past and led to prolonged confinement in bed and cardiac neurosis. Gradual resumption of normal activity should be allowed after the acute carditis subsides. Prolonged confinement in bed should be discouraged.

Arthritis

The course of the arthritis in ARF is self-limiting, rarely lasting more than 1 week in any one joint. A hallmark

Table 34–6

Antibiotic Regimens for Primary Prevention (Streptococcal Eradication) and Secondary Prevention of Rheumatic Fever

ANTIBIOTIC	DOSE	ROUTE	DURATION
Primary Prevention			
Benzathine penicillin G	600,000–1,200,000 U*	Intramuscular	Single dose
Penicillin V	250 mg TID	Oral	10 days
Erythromycin (estolate or ethylsuccinate)	20–40 mg/kg/d (maximum, 1.0 g/d) in 2–4 divided doses	Oral	10 days
Secondary Prevention			
Benzathine penicillin G	600,000–1,200,000 U every 4 wk†	Intramuscular	
Penicillin V	250 mg BID	Oral	
Sulfadiazine	1.0 g once daily	Oral	
Erythromycin ethyl succinate	250 mg BID	Oral	

*See text for details.

†May be given every 3 weeks in high-risk situations.

Adapted from Dajani A, Taubert K, Ferrieri P, et al: Treatment of acute streptococcal pharyngitis and prevention of rheumatic fever: a statement for health professionals. Reproduced by permission of Pediatrics, vol 96, pp 758–764, Copyright 1995.

characteristic of the arthritis in this disease is its exquisite sensitivity to salicylates. A dose of aspirin of 50 to 75 mg/kg/day given in three to four daily doses is usually effective. This therapy is continued for no more than 2 weeks and is gradually withdrawn thereafter. A rapid resolution of the fever and a decline in the ESR usually parallel the resolution of the arthritis. A lack of resolution of the arthritis within about 5 days of salicylate therapy should prompt one to reconsider the correctness of a diagnosis of ARF. No data are available regarding the efficacy of other NSAIDs in the treatment of ARF. Steroids should not be used in patients with isolated arthritis.

Chorea

Mild manifestations of Sydenham's chorea require only bed rest and avoidance of physical and emotional stress. Although anticonvulsant drugs may help control severe symptoms, the response to these agents is unpredictable. Phenobarbital, haloperidol, and valproate have been used with varying success. Anti-inflammatory agents are not needed for the treatment of Sydenham's chorea.

Prophylaxis of Rheumatic Heart Disease

Medical management after the acute stage of the disease centers on prevention of recurrences of rheumatic fever and continued treatment of residual heart disease, including prevention of bacterial endocarditis in such patients. Antimicrobial prophylaxis against streptococcal pharyngitis has proven highly effective in reducing recurrences of rheumatic fever and preventing cumulative heart damage.

Regimens for streptococcal prophylaxis, recommended by the American Heart Association, are outlined in Table 34–6. Because recurrences of rheumatic fever are most common during the 5 years after the initial attack,[16–18] intramuscular benzathine penicillin prophylaxis is preferable and should be given once monthly in areas of low incidence of rheumatic fever and every 3 weeks in areas endemic to this disease.

Oral prophylaxis is acceptable for patients without cardiac involvement. Although sulfonamides are ineffective in eradicating streptococcal infections, these agents are as effective, if not more effective, than oral penicillin for prophylaxis against recurrent streptococcal infections. Compliance with prophylaxis should be encouraged through education of the patient and parents.

The American Heart Association has revised recommendations on the duration of prophylaxis. Current protocols are based on the risk of reinfection and the development of streptococcal pharyngitis.[92] This risk is highest in school-aged children and in persons working in crowded conditions, particularly those in close contact with children, such as parents, teachers, health providers, and military recruits. Thus, patients with carditis should receive prophylaxis well into adulthood, preferably for life. Prophylaxis should not be discontinued after surgical valve repair. Patients who had a transient carditis should receive prophylaxis until the age of 40 years, whereas it may be discontinued at the age of 21 years in patients with no cardiac involvement (although all such patients should receive prophylaxis for a minimum of 5 years, regardless of age).[92]

Endocarditis Prophylaxis

For surgical or dental procedures in children with known rheumatic heart disease, supplemental doses of antibiotic should be prescribed. Recommendations vary, depending on the procedure and age of the patient.[92a]

Course of the Disease and Prognosis

Major morbidity in rheumatic fever is associated exclusively with the degree of cardiac damage. Severe carditis, which leads to chronic residual valvular disease (Fig. 34–7), primarily occurs in children in developing countries. The availability of cardiac surgery has alleviated to a considerable extent the crippling effect of this disease. Mortality is rare nowadays and occurs predominantly in patients with pancarditis. Our understanding of the relationship of streptococcal infection to the occurrence of initial attacks and recurrences of rheumatic fever has allowed the institution of prophylactic regimens that have prevented recurrences of the

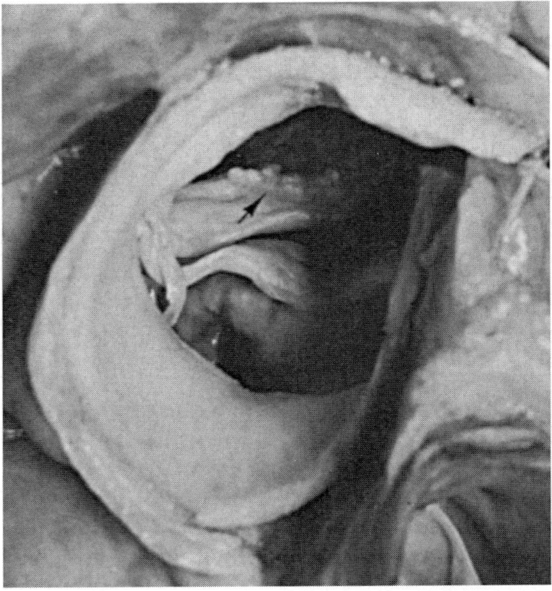

Figure 34–7. Chronic rheumatic valvular heart disease. Verrucal endocardial thickening was present along the line of closure of the valve leaflets (*arrow*).

disease and reduced the cumulative heart damage produced by these recurrences. The study by Tompkins and colleagues[93] emphasizes the singular value of prophylaxis by confirming that signs of rheumatic valvular disease resolve in about 80 percent of patients who receive continuous, long-term prophylaxis. This information is of particular importance in encouraging patients with rheumatic heart disease to adhere to prophylaxis.

Rheumatic arthritis is self-limited. A rare form of nonerosive but deforming arthropathy ascribed to rheumatic fever (*Jaccoud's arthritis*) has been reported in adults but does not occur in children.[94] It is now more commonly associated with SLE. Sydenham's chorea and erythema marginatum are also self-limited, with no permanent residua. Thus, patients who escape severe heart disease can be assured of a benign course and a good prognosis.

POSTSTREPTOCOCCAL REACTIVE ARTHRITIS

The occurrence of arthritis after group A streptococcal infection in children who did not fulfill the criteria for the diagnosis of ARF was described first by Crea and Mortimer in 1959.[95] Subsequently, a number of other studies reported the occurrence of this entity, which was designated *poststreptococcal reactive arthritis*.[64, 96–102] In contrast to the arthritis of ARF, the arthritis observed in these patients was nonmigratory and protracted in course and responded poorly to aspirin and other NSAIDs. Despite these differences, several investigators have claimed that poststreptococcal reactive arthritis is an extension of the spectrum of ARF.[97, 103] Recent studies, however, provide evidence to the contrary and suggest that poststreptococcal reactive arthritis differs significantly in pathogenesis and clinical characteristics from the arthritis of rheumatic fever.

Epidemiology

To date, 86 patients with poststreptococcal reactive arthritis have been described. Although it is difficult to assess accurately, the incidence of poststreptococcal reactive arthritis in north-central Florida is estimated to be 1 to 2 per 100,000 children at risk per year. In our clinic, 17 of 455 patients with rheumatic diseases seen over a period of 2 years had poststreptococcal reactive arthritis.[64] This incidence was twice that encountered for ARF during the same time. The age of the patients varied from 5 to 16 years, with a mean of 9.7 years. A slightly but not significantly higher incidence of the disease occurred in males (56 percent vs. 44 percent). There was no ethnic preponderance of the disease.

Etiology and Pathogenesis

Based on its designation, group A streptococcal infection is the inciting cause for this form of arthritis. Evidence for such an infection should be documented in all patients. In contrast to ARF, in which throat cultures or rapid antigen tests are positive in only one third of patients, results are positive in about 75 percent of patients with poststreptococcal reactive arthritis. This difference can be ascribed to the shorter latency (<10 days) for this disease.[98, 99, 102] Streptococcal pharyngitis is associated with an ASO and an anti-DNase B response in the majority of patients.[104] Skin infection does not elicit an ASO response. The high frequency of elevated ASO titers in patients with poststreptococcal reactive arthritis suggests, therefore, that streptococcal pharyngitis is the primary inciting cause of this disease.

Genetic Background

Studies of the relationship of poststreptococcal reactive arthritis with HLA-B27 failed to document a significant association[64]: only 3 of 18 white American patients (16.7 percent) were positive. This frequency contrasts with Reiter's disease in children, in which 93 percent of patients are B27 positive.[105] Further studies, however, documented a significant association of poststreptococcal reactive arthritis with HLA class II alleles.[64] Compared with normal controls and patients with ARF, these patients had a significant increase in frequency of DRB1*01.[64] This result differs from patients with ARF, who have an increased frequency of the DRB1*16 allele. This association with DRB1 alleles, albeit with different alleles in each disease, suggests a common pathogenetic mechanism for poststreptococcal reactive arthritis and ARF. The lack of an association between poststreptococcal reactive arthritis and B27 indicates that its pathogenetic mechanism differs from that of the reactive arthritides that follow infection by enteric bacteria or chlamydia.

Clinical Manifestations

In addition to a pharyngitis that is present in 66 percent of patients,[64, 106] about 30 percent report the occurrence of a low-grade febrile episode, and a similar number describe a nonscarlatinal rash that precedes onset of the arthritis. About half of the patients complain of morning stiffness of varying duration.

The majority of the patients present with arthritis involving one or more joints. About 10 percent complain of arthralgia only. The frequency of joint involvement is illustrated in Figure 34–8. In 70 to 80 percent, the arthritis is asymmetric and nonmigratory, and in almost all patients, the arthritis involves the joints of the lower extremities. Half of patients also have arthritis involving the upper extremities.[64] Axial disease is present in 25 percent; in our experience, these patients account for any possible association with HLA-B27.

Cardiac disease was present in 5.8 percent of the 86 patients described in the literature.[64] In almost all cases, valvular disease was only detected several months after the onset of arthritis. Most of these patients had not been placed on penicillin prophylaxis. The delay in

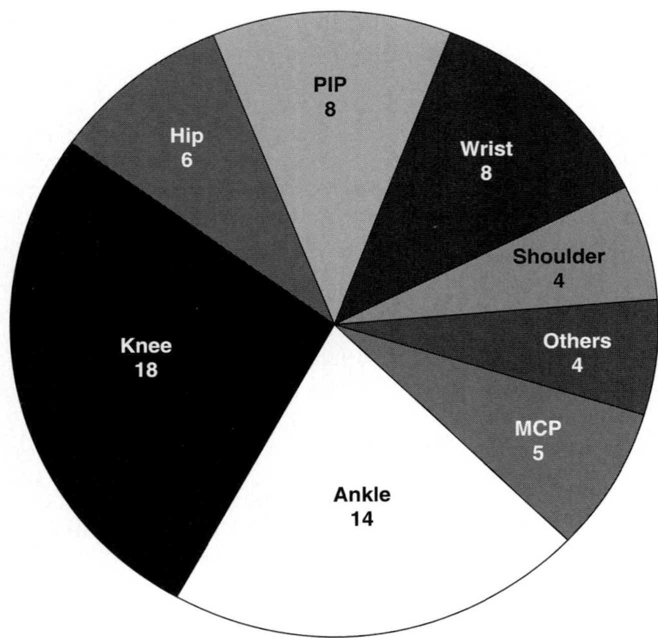

Figure 34–8. Frequency of joint involvement in patients with poststreptococcal reactive arthritis. Values represent the number of patients with involvement of that joint. MCP, metacarpopharyngeal; PIP, proximal interpharyngeal. (From Ahmed S, Ayoub EM, Scornik JC, et al: Poststreptococcal reactive arthritis: clinical characteristics and association with HLA-DR alleles. Arthritis Rheum 41[6]: 1096–1102, 1998.)

onset of cardiac abnormalities should be contrasted with the carditis associated with ARF, wherein cardiac involvement usually occurs during the acute stage of the disease and in tandem with the arthritis. Some authors have described patients who presented with "silent carditis," indicating that this complication was not clinically detectable and required echocardiographic studies for confirmation.[99] This suggests that the incidence of carditis in this disease may be higher than that reported to date.

Diagnosis and Differential Diagnosis

Criteria for the diagnosis of poststreptococcal reactive arthritis are shown in Table 34–7. The differential diagnosis includes most of the same arthritides outlined for ARF. The similarity in etiology and some of the features of both diseases pose unresolved difficulty in differentiating the two entities. However, as outlined in Table 34–8, clinical and laboratory differences should permit the separation of this entity from ARF and other reactive arthritides in the majority of children.

Laboratory Examination

The leukocyte count in poststreptococcal reactive arthritis is normal in the majority of patients. However, the ESR is elevated in 75 percent. As in ARF, this test is helpful in assessing the course of arthritis.

As stated previously, streptococcal antibody tests are more dependable than those in ARF for procuring evidence for an antecedent group A streptococcal infection. The ASO is elevated in 88 percent and the anti-DNase B in 80 percent of patients. At least one of these antibodies should be elevated in almost all patients, either at the time of presentation or shortly thereafter.[64] Because of the shorter period of latency between the streptococcal infection and the onset of arthritis, these patients show a higher frequency of positive throat cultures or reactive rapid antigen tests for group A streptococci than patients with ARF. Tests for antinuclear antibodies and rheumatoid factor are negative in the majority of patients.

Table 34–7

Proposed Criteria for the Diagnosis of Poststreptococcal Reactive Arthritis

A. Characteristics of arthritis:
   1. Acute-onset arthritis, symmetric or asymmetric, usually nonmigratory, can affect any joint
   2. Persistent or recurrent
   3. Poorly responsive to salicylates or nonsteroidal anti-inflammatory drugs
B. Evidence of antecedent group A streptococcal infection
C. Does not fulfill the modified Jones criteria for the diagnosis of acute rheumatic fever

Adapted from Ayoub EM, Ahmed S: Update on complications of group A streptococcal infections. Curr Probl Pediatr 27: 90–101, 1997.

Treatment

The NSAIDs are the principal drugs used in the treatment of poststreptococcal reactive arthritis (naproxen, ibuprofen, tolmetin). Aspirin offers no particular advantage. The value of disease-modifying drugs, such as methotrexate, has not been assessed. Physical therapy

Table 34–8

Clinical and Laboratory Characteristics of Poststreptococcal Reactive Arthritis (PSRA)

	PSRA	RHEUMATIC FEVER
Antecedent group A streptococcal infection	Yes	Yes
Onset of arthritis after infection	<2 wk	2–3 wk
Migratory arthritis	No	Yes
Axial arthritis	Yes	No
Heart involvement	6%	50%
Response to ASA	Not dramatic	Dramatic
Association with HLA-B27	No	No
Association with HLA-DRβ alleles	DRβ1*01	DRβ1*16

Adapted from Ahmed S, Ayoub EM, Scornick JC, et al: Poststreptococcal reactive arthritis: clinical characteristics and association with HLA-DR alleles. Arthritis Rheum 41(6): 1096–1102, 1998.

should be recommended for relief of joint pain and stiffness.

As recommended for patients with group A streptococcal pharyngitis and its complications, antimicrobial therapy should be prescribed at the time of initial diagnosis to eradicate streptococci from the tonsillopharyngeal tissue (see Table 34–6). Antimicrobial prophylaxis to prevent recurrences and possibly subsequent cardiac disease has been recommended by some investigators, but this issue is controversial. Because carditis can occur in this disease, albeit at a lower rate than that in patients with rheumatic fever, the American Heart Association has suggested prophylaxis for 1 year.[92] If carditis is not detected by then, prophylaxis is discontinued. If carditis occurs during this interval, the patient is considered to have had ARF and should continue to receive prophylaxis in accordance with previously stated recommendations. However, discontinuing prophylaxis after only 1 year potentially leaves the patient at risk for development of carditis. Our preference is to institute a prophylactic regimen similar to that proposed by the American Heart Association for patients with ARF who have arthritis but no carditis—that is, to continue prophylaxis until the patient reaches the age of 21 years but for a minimum of 5 years.[92] All patients should be evaluated for the appearance of carditis for a period extending over 5 years.

Course of the Disease and Prognosis

Unlike the arthritis of ARF, the course of poststreptococcal reactive arthritis is protracted, lasting from 5 days to 8 months, with a mean duration of 66 days from onset to resolution of symptoms.[64] In addition, some patients continue to have arthralgia for several months after remission of the arthritis. This prolonged course is not altered significantly by the administration of NSAIDs or antimicrobials.

References

1. Stollerman GH: Rheumatogenic group A streptococci and the return of rheumatic fever. Adv Intern Med 35: 1–26, 1990.
2. Markowitz M: The decline of rheumatic fever: role of medical intervention. The Lewis W. Wannamaker Memorial Lecture. J Pediatr 106: 545–550, 1985.
3. Veasy LG, Wiedmeier SE, Orsmond GS, et al: Resurgence of acute rheumatic fever in the intermountain area of the United States. N Engl J Med 316: 421–427, 1987.
4. Wald ER, Dashefsky B, Feidt C, et al: Acute rheumatic fever in western Pennsylvania and the tristate area. Pediatrics 80: 371–374, 1987.
5. Congeni B, Rizzo C, Congeni J: Outbreak of acute rheumatic fever in northeast Ohio. J Pediatr 111: 176–179, 1987.
6. Hosier DM, Craenen JM, Teske DW: Resurgence of rheumatic fever. Am J Dis Child 141: 730–733, 1987.
7. Griffiths SP, Gersony WM: Acute rheumatic fever in New York City (1969 to 1988): a comparative study of two decades. J Pediatr 116: 882–887, 1990.
8. Westlake RM, Graham TP, Edwards KM: An outbreak of acute rheumatic fever in Tennessee. Pediatr Infect Dis J 9: 97–100, 1990.
9. Eckerd JM, McJunkin JE: Recent increase in incidence of acute rheumatic fever in southern West Virginia. W V Med J 85: 323–325, 1989.
10. Mason T, Fisher M, Kujala G: Acute rheumatic fever in West Virginia. Arch Intern Med 151: 133–136, 1991.
11. Papadinos T, Escanmilla J, Garst P, et al: Acute rheumatic fever at a Navy training center San Diego, California. MMWR 37: 101–104, 1988.
12. Sampson GL, Williams RG, House MD, et al: Acute rheumatic fever among Army trainees—Fort Leonard Wood, Missouri, 1987–1988. MMWR 37: 519–522, 1988.
13. Zangwill KM, Wald ER, Londino AV Jr: Acute rheumatic fever in western Pennsylvania: a persistent problem into the 1990s. J Pediatr 118: 561–563, 1991.
14. Loeffler AM, Neches WH, Ortenzo M, et al: Identification of cases of acute rheumatic fever managed on an outpatient basis. Pediatr Infect Dis J 14: 975–978, 1995.
15. Veasy LG, Tani LY, Hill HR: Persistence of acute rheumatic fever in the intermountain area of the United States. J Pediatr 124: 9–16, 1994.
16. Bland EF, Jones KF: Rheumatic fever and rheumatic heart disease: a twenty-year report on 1000 patients followed since childhood. Circulation 4: 836–843, 1951.
17. Ayoub EM: Cross-reacting antibodies in the pathogenesis of rheumatic myocardial and valvular disease. *In* Wannamaker LW, Matsen JM (eds): Streptococci and Streptococcal Diseases. Recognition, Understanding and Management, 1st ed. New York, Academic Press, 1972, pp 451–464.
18. Taranta A: Rheumatic fever. *In* McCarty DJ (ed): Arthritis and Allied Conditions: A Textbook of Rheumatology. Philadelphia, Lea & Febiger, 1979, pp 825–870.
19. Gordis L: Changing risk of rheumatic fever. *In* Shulman S (ed): Management of Pharyngitis in an Era of Declining Rheumatic Fever. 86th Conference on Pediatric Research. Columbus, OH, Ross Laboratories, 1983, pp 7–13.
20. Gordis L: The virtual disappearance of rheumatic fever in the United States: lessons in the rise and fall of disease. Circulation 72: 1155–1162, 1985.
21. Caughey DE, Douglas R, Wilson W, Hassall IB: HLA antigens in Europeans and Maoris with rheumatic fever and rheumatic heart disease. J Rheumatol 2: 319–322, 1975.
22. Wannamaker LW: Differences between streptococcal infections of the throat and of the skin. N Engl J Med 282: 78–85, 1970.
23. Lancefield RC: A serological differentiation of human and other groups of hemolytic streptococci. J Exp Med 57: 571–595, 1933.
24. Schwab JH, Cromartie WJ: Immunological studies on a C polysaccharide complex of group A streptococci having a direct toxic effect on connective tissue. J Exp Med 111: 295–307, 1960.
25. Cromartie WJ, Craddock JG, Schwab JH, et al: Arthritis in rats after systemic injection of streptococcal cells or cell walls. J Exp Med 146: 1585–1602, 1977.
26. Esser RE, Stimpson SA, Cromartie WJ, Schwab JH: Reactivation of streptococcal cell wall-induced arthritis by homologous and heterologous cell wall polymers. Arthritis Rheum 28: 1402, 1985.
27. Goldstein I, Halpern B, Robert L: Immunologic relation between streptococcus A polysaccharide and the structural glycoproteins of heart valve. Nature 213: 44–47, 1967.
28. Fischetti VA: Streptococcal M protein. Sci Am 264: 58–65, 1991.
29. Johnson DR, Stevens DL, Kaplan EL: Epidemiologic analysis of group A streptococcal serotypes associated with severe systemic infections, rheumatic fever or uncomplicated pharyngitis. J Infect Dis 166: 374–382, 1992.
30. Talkington DF, Schwartz B, Black CM, et al: Association of phenotypic and genotypic characteristics of invasive *Streptococcus pyogenes* isolates with clinical components of streptococcal toxic shock syndrome. Infect Immun 61: 3369–3374, 1993.
31. Bessen D, Jones KF, Fischett VA: Evidence for two distinct classes of streptococcal M protein and their relationship to rheumatic fever. J Exp Med 169: 269–283, 1989.
32. Ayoub EM, Kaplan EL: Host-parasite interaction in the pathogenesis of rheumatic fever. J Rheumatol 18(Suppl 30): 6–13, 1991.
33. Tomai M, Kotb M, Majundar G, Beachey EH: Superantigenicity of streptococcal M protein. J Exp Med 172: 359–362, 1990.

34. Sandson J, Hamerman D, Janis R, et al: Immunologic and chemical similarities between the streptococcus and human connective tissue. Trans Assoc Am Physicians 81: 249–257, 1968.
35. Hauser AR, Stevens DL, Kaplan EL, Schlievert PM: Molecular analysis of pyrogenic exotoxins from *Streptococcus pyogenes* isolates associated with toxic shock syndrome. J Clin Microbiol 29: 1562–1567, 1991.
36. Norrby-Teglund A, Newton D, Kotb M, et al: Superantigenic properties of the group A streptococcal exotoxin SpeF (MF). Infect Immun 62: 5227–5233, 1994.
37. Mollick JA, Miller GG, Musser JM, et al: A novel superantigen isolated from pathogenic strains of *Streptococcus pyogenes* with aminoterminal homology to staphylococcal enterotoxins B and C. J Clin Invest 92: 710–719, 1993.
38. Stevens DL: Streptococcal toxic-shock syndrome: spectrum of disease, pathogenesis, and new concepts in treatment. Emerg Infect 1: 69–78, 1995.
39. Fast DJ, Schlievert PM, Nelson RD: Toxic shock syndrome–associated staphylococcal and streptococcal pyrogenic toxins are potent inducers of tumor necrosis factor production. Infect Immun 57: 291–294, 1989.
40. Hackett SP, Schlievert PM, Stevens DL: Cytokine production by human mononuclear cells in response to streptococcal exotoxins. Clin Res 39: 189A, 1991.
41. Murray DL, Ohlendorf DH, Schlievert PM: Staphylococcal and streptococcal superantigens: their role in human diseases. ASM News 61: 229–235, 1995.
42. Kuo CF, Wu JJ, Tsai PJ, et al: Streptococcal pyrogenic exotoxin B induces apoptosis and reduces phagocytic activity in U937 cells. Infect Immun 67: 126–130, 1999.
43. Yu CE, Ferretti JJ: Molecular epidemiologic analysis of the type A streptococcal exotoxin (erythrogenic toxin) gene (*speA*) in clinical *Streptococcus pyogenes* strains. Infect Immun 57: 3715–3719, 1989.
44. Chaussee MS, Liu J, Stevens DL, Ferretti JJ: Genetic and phenotypic diversity among isolates of *Streptococcus pyogenes* from invasive infections. J Infect Dis 173: 901–908, 1996.
44a. Todd EW: Antihaemolysin titers in haemolytic streptococcal infections and their significance in rheumatic fever. Br J Exp Pathol 13: 248–259, 1932.
45. Gerber MA, Wright LL, Randolph MF: Streptozyme test for antibodies to Group A streptococcal antigens. Pediatr Infect Dis J 6: 36–40, 1987.
46. Dudding BA, Ayoub EM: Persistence of streptococcal group A antibody in patients with rheumatic valvular disease. J Exp Med 128: 1081–1098, 1968.
47. Ayoub EM, Shulman ST: Pattern of antibody response to the streptococcal group A carbohydrate in rheumatic patients with or without carditis. *In* Read SE, Zabriskie JB (eds): Streptococcal Disease and the Immune Response. New York, Academic Press, 1980, pp 649–659.
48. Appleton RS, Victorica BE, Ayoub EM: Specificity of persistence of antibody to the streptococcal group A carbohydrate in rheumatic valvular heart disease. J Lab Clin Med 105: 114–119, 1985.
49. Ayoub EM: Immune response to group A streptococcal infections. Pediatr Infect Dis J 10(Suppl): S15–S19, 1991.
50. Rammelkamp CHJ: Epidemiology of streptococcal infections. Harvey Lecture Series 51: 113–142, 1956.
51. Read SE, Reid H, Poon-King T: HLAs and predisposition to the non-suppurative sequelae of group A streptococcal infections. Transplant Proc 9: 543–546, 1977.
52. Wilson MG, Schweitzer MD, Lubschez R: The familial epidemiology of rheumatic fever: genetic and epidemiologic studies. J Pediatr 22: 468–492, 1943.
53. Wilson MG, Schweitzer M: Pattern of hereditary susceptibility in rheumatic fever. Circulation 10: 699–704, 1954.
54. Khanna AK, Buskirk DR, Williams RC, et al: Presence of a non-HLA B cell antigen in rheumatic fever patients and their families as defined by a monoclonal antibody. J Clin Invest 83: 1710–1716, 1989.
55. Ayoub EM, Barrett DJ, Maclaren NK, Krischer JP: Association of class II human histocompatibility leukocyte antigens with rheumatic fever. J Clin Invest 77: 2019–2025, 1986.
56. Anastasiou-Nana MI, Anderson JL, Carlquist JF, Nanas JN: HLA-DR typing and lymphocyte subset evaluation in rheumatic heart disease: a search for immune response factors. Am Heart J 112: 992–997, 1986.
57. Jhinghan B, Mehra NK, Reddy KS, et al: HLA, blood groups and secretor status in patients with established rheumatic fever and rheumatic heart disease. Tissue Antigens 27: 172–178, 1986.
58. Rajapakse CNA, Halim K, Al-Orainey I, et al: A genetic marker for rheumatic heart disease. Br Heart J 58: 659–662, 1987.
59. Maharaj B, Hammond MG, Appadoo B, et al: HLA-A, B, DR, and DQ antigens in black patients with severe chronic rheumatic heart disease. Circulation 76: 259–261, 1987.
60. Taneja V, Mehra NK, Reddy KS, et al: HLA-DR/DQ and reactivity to B cell alloantigen D8/17 in Indian patients with rheumatic heart disease. Circulation 80: 335–340, 1989.
61. Guilherme L, Weidebach W, Kiss MH, et al: Association of human leukocyte class II antigens with rheumatic fever or rheumatic heart disease in a Brazilian population. Circulation 83: 1995–1998, 1991.
62. Ozkan M, Carin M, Sonmez G, et al: HLA antigens in Turkish race with rheumatic heart disease. Circulation 87: 1974–1978, 1993.
63. Weidebach W, Goldberg AC, Chiarella JM, et al: HLA class II antigens in rheumatic fever: analysis of the DR locus by restriction fragment polymorphism and oligotyping. Hum Immunol 40: 253–258, 1994.
64. Ahmed S, Ayoub EM, Scornick JC, et al: Poststreptococcal reactive arthritis: clinical characteristics and association with HLA-DR alleles. Arthritis Rheum 41: 1096–1102, 1998.
65. Stetson CA: The relation of antibody response to rheumatic fever. *In* McCarty M (ed): Streptococcal Infections. New York, Columbia University Press, 1954.
66. Ayoub EM, Wannamaker LW: Evaluation of the streptococcal deoxyribonuclease B and diphosphopyridine nucleotidase antibody tests in acute rheumatic fever and acute glomerulonephritis. Pediatrics 29: 527–538, 1962.
67. Shulman ST, Ayoub EM, Victorica BE: Differences in antibody response to streptococcal antigens in children with rheumatic and non-rheumatic mitral valve disease. Circulation 50: 1244–1251, 1974.
68. Braun DG, Eichmann K, Krause RM: Rabbit antibodies to streptococcal carbohydrates: influence of primary and secondary immunization and of possible genetic factors on the antibody response. J Exp Med 129: 809–830, 1969.
69. Klapper DG, Kindt TJ: Idiotypic cross-reactions among anti-streptococcal antibodies in an inbred rabbit population. Scand J Immunol 3: 483–490, 1974.
70. Saszuki T, Kaneoka H, Nishimura Y, et al: An HLA-linked immune suppression gene in man. J Exp Med 152: 297S–313S, 1980.
71. Kaplan MH, Meyeserian M: An immunological cross reaction between group A streptococcal cells and human heart tissue. Lancet 1: 706–710, 1962.
72. Kaplan MH, Svec KH: Immunological relation of streptococcal and tissue antigens. J Exp Med 119: 651–666, 1964.
73. Widdowson JP, Maxted WR, Pinney AM: An M-associated protein antigen (MAP) of group A streptococci. J Hyg (Lond) 69: 553–564, 1971.
74. Zabriskie JB, Freimer EH: An immunological relationship between group A streptococci and mammalian muscle. J Exp Med 124: 661–668, 1966.
75. Van de Rijn I, Zabriskie JB, McCarty M: Group A streptococcal antigens cross reactive with myocardium. Purification of heart reactive antibody and isolation and characterization of the streptococcal antigen. J Exp Med 146: 579–599, 1977.
76. Dale JB, Beachey EH: Multiple heart-cross-reactive epitopes of streptococcal M proteins. J Exp Med 161: 113–122, 1985.
77. Husby G, Van de Rijn I, Zabriskie JB, et al: Antibodies reacting with cytoplasm of the subthalamic and caudate nuclei neurons in chorea and acute rheumatic fever. J Exp Med 144: 1094–1110, 1976.
78. Hutto J, Ayoub EM: Cytotoxicity of lymphocytes from patients with rheumatic carditis to cardiac cells in vitro. *In* Read SE, Zabriskie JB (eds): Streptococcal Disease and Immune Response. New York, Academic Press, 1980, pp 733–738.
79. Markovitz M, Gordis IJ: Rheumatic Fever. Philadelphia, WB Saunders, 1972.

80. Roberts WC: Anatomically isolated aortic valvular disease: the case against it being of rheumatic etiology. Am J Med 49: 151–159, 1970.
81. Raizada V, Williams RC, Chopra P, et al: Tissue distribution of lymphocytes in rheumatic heart valves as defined by monoclonal anti-T cell antibodies. Am J Med 74: 90–96, 1983.
82. Aschoff L: Zur myocarditisfrage. Dtsch Ges 8: 46–53, 1904.
83. Murphy GE: Nature of rheumatic heart disease. With special reference to myocardial disease and heart failure. Medicine 39: 289–340, 1960.
84. Ayoub EM: Resurgence of rheumatic fever in the United States. The changing picture of a preventable disease. Postgrad Med J 92: 133–142, 1992.
85. Dajani AS, Ayoub EM, Bierman FZ, et al: Guidelines for the diagnosis of rheumatic fever: Jones Criteria, updated 1992. JAMA 87: 302–307, 1992.
86. Ayoub EM: Streptococcal antibody tests in rheumatic fever. Clin Immunol Newsl 3: 107–111, 1982.
87. Haber HL, Leavy JA, Kessler PD, et al: Erythrocyte sedimentation rate in congestive heart failure. N Engl J Med 324: 353–358, 1991.
88. Swedo SE, Rappoport JL, Cheslow DL, et al: High prevalence of obsessive-compulsive symptoms in patients with Sydenham's chorea. Am J Psychiatry 145: 246, 1989.
89. United Kingdom and United States Joint Report: The treatment of acute rheumatic fever in children: a cooperative clinical trial of ACTH, cortisone and aspirin. Circulation 11: 343–371, 1955.
90. United Kingdom and United States Joint Report: The natural history of rheumatic fever and rheumatic heart disease: ten year report of a cooperative clinical trial of ACTH, cortisone, and aspirin. Circulation 32: 457–476, 1965.
91. United Kingdom and United States Joint Report: The evolution of rheumatic heart disease in children: five year report of a cooperative clinical trial of ACTH, cortisone and aspirin. Circulation 22: 503–515, 1960.
92. Dajani A, Taubert K, Ferrieri P, et al: Treatment of acute streptococcal pharyngitis and prevention of rheumatic fever: a statement for health professionals. Pediatrics 96: 758–764, 1995.
92a. American Academy of Pediatrics: Red Book 2000, 25th ed. Elk Grove Village, IL, AAP, 2000, pp 735–740.
93. Tompkins DG, Boxerbaum B, Liebman J: Long-term prognosis of rheumatic fever patients receiving regular intramuscular benzathine penicillin. Circulation 45: 543–551, 1972.
94. Zvaifler NJ: Chronic postrheumatic-fever (Jaccoud's) arthritis. N Engl J Med 267: 10–14, 1962.
95. Crea MA, Mortimer EA Jr: The nature of scarlatinal arthritis. Pediatrics 23: 879–884, 1959.
96. Goldsmith DP, Long SS: Streptococcal disease of childhood—a changing syndrome. Arthritis Rheum 25(Suppl): S18, 1982.
97. De Cunto CL, Giannini EH, Fink CW, et al: Prognosis of children with poststreptococcal reactive arthritis. Pediatr Infect Dis J 7: 683–686, 1988.
98. Gibbas DL, Broussard DA: Post streptococcal reactive polyarthritis (PSRA)—rheumatic fever or not? Arthritis Rheum 29(Suppl): S92, 1986.
99. Schaffer FM, Agarwal R, Helm J, et al: Poststreptococcal reactive arthritis and silent carditis: a case report and review of the literature. Pediatrics 93: 837–839, 1994.
100. Fink CW: The role of the streptococcus in poststreptococcal reactive arthritis and childhood polyarteritis nodosa. J Rheumatol 18: 14–20, 1991.
101. Hubbard WN, Hughes GR: Streptococci and reactive arthritis. Ann Rheum Dis 41: 435, 1982.
102. Birdi N, Allen U, D'Astous J: Poststreptococcal reactive arthritis mimicking acute septic arthritis: a hospital-based study. J Pediatr Orthop 15: 661–665, 1995.
103. Denny FW: The mystery of acute rheumatic fever and poststreptococcal glomerulonephritis. J Lab Clin Med 108: 523–524, 1986.
104. Kaplan EL, Anthony BF, Chapman SS, et al: The influence of the site of infection on the immune response to group A streptococci. J Clin Invest 49: 1405–1414, 1970.
105. McDermott M, McDevitt H: The immunogenetics of rheumatic diseases. Bull Rheum Dis 38: 1–10, 1988.
106. Ayoub EM, Ahmed S: Update on complications of group A streptococcal infections. Curr Probl Pediatr 27: 90–101, 1997.

35

Immunodeficiencies and the Rheumatic Diseases

Nico M. Wulffraat, Lieke A. M. Sanders, and Wietse Kuis

Genetic disorders of the immune system enable us to study the relation between the clinical expression of immunodeficiencies and the underlying immune defect. Although infections are the most common and early clinical expressions of primary immunodeficiencies, autoimmune diseases (as well as malignancies) often occur in immunodeficient patients. In recent years, knowledge of the genetic basis of immunodeficiencies has increased and the molecular abnormalities of these diseases have started to be unraveled. An increasing number of associated genetic defects have been identified by a variety of techniques such as positional cloning and complementation.

Through better understanding of the molecular basis of immunodeficiencies and the consequences for the immune system, we can better understand why autoimmune diseases develop under these circumstances. This knowledge permits the linking of observations in immunodeficient patients with autoimmune diseases and a known gene defect to patients with comparable autoimmune diseases in whom there is no clear understanding of pathogenesis. In this paradigm, autoimmune diseases are regarded as subtle immunodeficiencies. The expectation is that this approach will help clarify the pathogenesis of many autoimmune diseases. This chapter focuses on genetically determined primary immunodeficiencies in which autoimmune disorders may occur.

DISORDERS OF INNATE IMMUNITY ASSOCIATED WITH RHEUMATIC DISEASES

Defective Control of Lymphocyte Survival

Apoptosis (or *programmed cell death*) is one of most essential physiologic mechanisms to regulate embryonic development, cell differentiation, and tissue turnover. Of the several mechanisms leading to apoptosis, that best studied is the death pathway initiated by the interaction of CD95 (Fas/APO-1) and its ligand.[1–4] MRL-lpr/lpr mice have mutations in the Fas-encoding gene leading to faulty Fas (CD95) expression on T cells.[5] This mutation results in a syndrome characterized by lymphoproliferation of $CD4^-CD8^-$ T cells, associated with autoimmune manifestations (Table 35–1). The severity of the disease depends not only on mutations on the Fas-encoding gene but also on the genetic background of the mice. Mutations of the Fas-ligand gene (gld mutation) also result in lymphoproliferation.[5]

The *Canale-Smith syndrome,* the human counterpart of this murine abnormality, is a recently described lymphoproliferative disorder with accumulation of $CD4^-CD8^-$ T cells and B cells, as well as variable autoimmunity.[6, 7] In this homozygous Fas deficiency, lymphoproliferation is already present at birth. Stimulated lymphocytes do not express Fas and are insensitive to treatment by an agonist anti-Fas antibody.[6, 7] Interestingly, apoptotic lymphocytes can be detected in the peripheral blood as well as in the spleen, indicating that other death pathways are operating. The therapy of choice is allogeneic bone marrow transplantation.[7, 7a]

Heterozygous Fas gene mutations are more common.[8, 9] These patients are characterized by lymphadenopathy at an early age, autoimmune hemolytic anemia, and thrombocytopenia. Less frequently, glomerulonephritis, the Guillain-Barré syndrome, and urticaria are also described in this group of patients. Variable heterozygous Fas mutations are present, leading to defective Fas-mediated apoptosis. Parents of affected children have Fas mutations without clinical

Table 35–1

Classification of Immunodeficiency Disorders

Disorders of Innate Immunity

Abnormalities of Fas-mediated apoptosis
Phagocytic abnormalities
Complement abnormalities

Disorders of Adaptive Immunity

Abnormalities of both T and B lymphocytes
Abnormalities of T lymphocytes
Abnormalities of B lymphocytes

symptoms of lymphoproliferation or autoimmunity. This important observation indicates that for the disease to be expressed, the single-allele Fas mutation must be combined with another gene defect (digenic disease).[7] Candidate genes include those encoding proteins downstream of Fas (Mort 1/FADD, RIP, MACH/FLICE, or ICE).

Mutations in the Fas-ligand gene can also result in lymphoproliferative diseases associated with autoimmunity. Mutations have been detected in a patient with systemic lupus erythematosus (SLE).[10] Molecular cloning and sequencing indicated that the genomic DNA of this patient contained an 84-bp deletion within exon 4 of the Fas-ligand gene, resulting in a predicted 28-amino acid in-frame deletion. To complicate the picture further, patients are described with lymphoproliferation and autoimmunity with normal Fas expression and Fas-induced apoptosis of lymphocytes,[11] indicating the presence of defects in other death pathways.

In conclusion, knowledge of the basic mechanisms controlling cell survival or death and the identification of genetic defects in death pathways have led to new concepts of the pathogenesis of autoimmune disease. In addition to Fas-induced apoptosis, a rapidly increasing number of other death pathways are being discovered. It will be a challenge for future research to evaluate the role of these pathways in preventing autoimmune disease and to recognize defects leading to disease.

Rheumatic Diseases Associated With Disorders of Phagocytes

There is an increasing awareness of the association of rheumatic diseases with abnormalities of phagocytic cell function and the complement pathways (Table 35–2).

Chronic Granulomatous Disease

Chronic granulomatous disease (CGD) is a rare (1 in 250,000), inherited primary immunodeficiency of phagocytic leukocytes characterized by recurrent, life-threatening bacterial, fungal, and yeast infections of the subcutaneous tissues, airways, lymph nodes, liver, and bones.[12] The disorder results from absence or malfunction of the reduced form of the nicotinamide-adenine dinucleotide phosphate (NADPH) oxidase enzyme system that produces superoxide in the professional phagocytic cells (neutrophils, monocytes, macrophages, and eosinophils). Deficiency of this oxidase (which is required for the production of microbicidal oxygen metabolites) renders the phagocytes unable to kill ingested microorganisms. NADPH oxidase consists of several subunits, each encoded by a separate gene.[12]

The majority of patients (70 percent) suffer from the X-linked form of the disease, caused by mutations in *CYBB*, the gene that encodes the beta-subunit of cytochrome b558, also called gp91phox. Mutations in three other subunits cause autosomally inherited forms of CGD. This concerns the alpha-subunit of cytochrome b558 (p22phox), needed for stabilization of the cytochrome in the plasma membrane of phagocytes, and the cytoplasmic proteins p47phox and p67phox that translocate to the cytochrome during cell activation, a process needed for induction of the bactericidal enzymatic activity after phagocytosis of microorganisms.[13] The molecular basis of CGD has been extensively reviewed.[14] Clinical variability in CGD is considerable and mainly associated with the degree of residual respiratory burst activity.

A mucocutaneous syndrome characterized by discoid lupus erythematosus (DLE), photosensitive dermatitis, and recurrent aphthous stomatitis occurs in up to one third of carriers of the CGD gene.[15–21] Occasionally, other rheumatic complaints are noted, and some mothers of patients with CGD have autoantibodies to nuclear antigens. One report describes a child with CGD who developed convincing clinical, serologic, and pathologic evidence of SLE[18]; other children have features of discoid lupus and photosensitivity.[17, 19] However, the frequency of defects in neutrophil function among patients with DLE who lack a family history of CGD appears to be very low.[19] The pathogenesis of these cutaneous lesions of lupus in patients with CGD or carriers is unknown. It has been proposed that a partial defect in bactericidal ability leads to chronic antigen persistence and immune activation, possibly provoking autoantibody formation. Ultraviolet irradiation seems to be an environmental trigger.

A girl of Chinese ancestry with autosomal recessive CGD (p47phox) was described as having polyarthritis since the age of 4 years, involving the large joints (wrists, ankles, knees, hip) as well as the small joints (metacarpophalangeal and metatarsophalangeal joints).[22] There was early-morning stiffness and joint swelling with synovial thickening, stiffness, and tenderness. Infections were excluded. Serologic markers included several autoantibodies, such as rheumatoid factor (RF), antinuclear antibodies (ANAs), and anti-dsDNA antibodies. Serum complement factors were not depressed. The patient did not develop SLE-like symptoms in the 22-month period of follow-up,[22] although such symptoms occurred later (R. E. Petty, personal communication, 1998). Bland peripheral arthritis and bursitis in two boys with CGD and erosive polyarthritis in a young girl with the disease have been reported.[23] However, apart from susceptibility to septic arthritis and osteomyelitis, children with CGD have only rarely had a rheumatic disease.

Suppurative and granulomatous infections in CGD patients are established soon after birth, first at body surfaces normally in contact with bacteria and fungi (e.g., the skin, the airways, and the gut).[12] From these areas, infectious organisms may be carried to lymph nodes and internal organs such as the liver. Failure to contain the infection may result in bacteremia that enables further infectious foci to develop. The major clinical manifestations of CGD are thus pyoderma, pneumonia, gastrointestinal involvement, lymphadenitis, liver abscesses, and osteomyelitis.[12, 24] In contrast with normal children, in whom osteomyelitis usually involves the metaphyseal areas of long bones, patients with CGD more often develop infections of the small

Table 35–2

Classification of Deficiencies of Innate Immunity Associated With Rheumatic Disease

DISORDERS OF INNATE IMMUNITY	RHEUMATIC DISEASE ASSOCIATION
Phagocytic Defects	
Chronic granulomatous disease	DLE, SLE
Familial lipochrome histiocytosis	Arthritis
Chédiak-Higashi disease	SLE-like disease in animals
Streaking leukocyte syndrome	Polyarthritis
Complement Deficiencies	
Deficiency of C1q	SLE-like GTN, RTS
Deficiency of C1r	SLE, DLE, GTN
Deficiency of Cls	SLE, DLE
Deficiency of C1 INH	SLE, DLE
Deficiency of C4	SLE, Sjögren's syndrome
Deficiency of C2	SLE, DLE, PM, HSP, vasculitis, GTN, Hodgkin's disease, JRA, RA
Deficiency of C3	SLE, vasculitis, GTN, arthralgias, SLE
Deficiency of C5	SLE
Deficiency of C6	SLE, DLE
Deficiency of C7	SLE, sclerodactyly, RA, vasculitis
Deficiency of C8	SLE, JRA

DLE, discoid lupus erythematosus; SLE, systemic lupus erythematosus; GTN, glomerulotubulonephritis; HSP, Henoch-Schönlein purpura; JRA, juvenile rheumatoid arthritis; RA, rheumatoid arthritis; RTS, Rothmund-Thomson syndrome (congenital poikiloderma); PM, polymyositis.

Adapted in part from Ruddy S: Complement deficiencies and rheumatic diseases. *In* Kelley WN, Harris ED Jr, Ruddy S, Sledge CB (eds): Textbook of Rheumatology, 4th ed. Philadelphia, WB Saunders, 1993, p 1283.

bones of the hands and feet.[12, 24, 25] Multiple sites are often infected. Aspiration of pus is mandatory for identification of the pathogenic microorganism.

A variety of bacterial pathogens have been isolated from the lesions of CGD.[12] *Staphylococcus aureus, Staphylococcus epidermidis,* and enterobacteria predominate. Common gram-negative organisms include *Escherichia coli, Salmonella, Pseudomonas aeruginosa* and *cepacia, Klebsiella-Aerobacter, Proteus, Serratia marcescens, Arizona,* and *Legionella.* Infections with *Nocardia* species and *Mycobacteria* (BCG strain) are of special importance. Fungal pathogens isolated most commonly in CGD are *Aspergillus* species and, to a lesser extent, *Candida albicans.* The response to viral pathogens is normal, and parasitic infections, except for *Pneumocystis carinii,* are rare.

Patients with CGD may be considerably shorter than expected based on parental height.[12, 26] This phenomenon is not fully explained. Infections often suppress growth temporarily, but catch-up growth is normal. Protein-calorie malnutrition does not seem to explain the shorter stature. Patients have a normal pubertal growth spurt.

Familial Lipochrome Histiocytosis

A syndrome of familial lipochrome histiocytosis has been described in three female siblings: one developed migratory polyarthritis, RF seropositivity, and rheumatoid nodules at the age of 15 years; a second had recurrent episodes of monarthritis of brief duration; two had a photosensitive rash.[27, 28] All had increased susceptibility to bacterial infection, hypergammaglobulinemia, and lipochrome pigment in histiocytes of lymph nodes and liver. Subsequent studies revealed defects in polymorphonuclear neutrophil function that were identical to those of patients with CGD.[29] Unlike children with typical CGD, however, these girls did not develop granulomata, and in this way they resembled girls with *Job's syndrome.*[30] The two most severely affected girls died of pulmonary infection at 19 and 34 years of age. The exact relation of this disorder to CGD remains to be determined.

Chédiak-Higashi syndrome

The rare Chédiak-Higashi syndrome is characterized by susceptibility to bacterial infection beginning in early childhood and associated with the presence of large cytoplasmic granules in neutrophils.[31] Although there have been no reports of rheumatic disease in patients with this disorder or their relatives, it is intriguing that the same leukocyte anomaly occurs in Aleutian mink that develop a spontaneous lupus-like disease.[32]

Arthritis, Pyoderma Gangrenosum, and Streaking Leukocyte Factor

A 2-year-old boy developed massive monarticular joint effusions and later severe pyoderma gangrenosum after minor trauma.[33] The sterile pyoarthritic episodes, leading to the repetitive erroneous diagnosis of septic arthritis, were ultimately self-limited or could be controlled by prednisone. The pyoderma responded to FK 506.[34] A second case has been reported by Jacobs.[34] The mechanisms of this disorder remain unknown, although a serum factor that enhanced random migration of leukocytes with a secondary increase in chemotaxis was described.

Rheumatic Diseases Associated With Complement Deficiencies

Primary genetic deficiencies of complement are inherited as autosomal recessive traits with the exception of

C1 inhibitor deficiency (causing hereditary angioneurotic edema [HANE], an autosomal dominant disease, and properdin deficiency, an X-linked disorder). The heterozygous state can usually be detected by measuring the complement protein in serum.

The clinical manifestations of complement deficiencies vary.[35–42] Some patients are asymptomatic, but most suffer from rheumatic diseases, particularly a syndrome resembling SLE. The clinical findings include early onset of skin lesions resembling discoid lupus, alopecia, photosensitivity, and mild renal and pleuropericardial involvement. The two other main clinical presentations are increased susceptibility to infection (repeated bacterial infections with pathogens such as *Streptococcus pneumoniae* and *Neisseria meningitidis* and viral infections),[43] and angioedema in the case of HANE.[44] Frequent infections are the predominant manifestation of deficiencies of C3 and factors I and H, the absence of which leads to consumption of C3. Primary or secondary C3 deficiency leads to infections with encapsulated bacteria such as *S. pneumoniae*, underlining the importance of C3 as a mediator of opsonization. Deficiencies of components of the membrane attack complex C5-C8 particularly predispose to recurrent infections with *Neisseria* species.[37, 42, 45, 46]

SLE-like rheumatic disorders are the major clinical manifestations of classical pathway complement deficiencies.[35–42] The frequency and severity of disease vary with each deficiency. SLE was observed in 28 of 30 C1q-deficient persons, 12 of 16 with C4 deficiency, approximately one third with C2 deficiency, but in only 4 of 24 patients with C3 deficiency. These observations imply a physiologic protective activity of the early activation of the classical complement pathway against the development of the immune complex–mediated syndrome SLE.

Binding of C1 to immune complexes activates the classical complement pathway, resulting in the cleavage of C4 and C3 to C4b and C3b, which bind covalently to immune complexes, thus leading to two important effects.[37, 42, 47] First, binding of C3b (and, to a lesser extent, of C4b) promotes the solubility of immune complexes. Second, immune complexes are bound via C3b and C4b to CR1 receptors on peripheral blood cells, mainly erythrocytes, and transported to the liver and spleen; there immune complexes are transferred to fixed macrophages, after which the erythrocytes return to the circulation.[47, 48] The observation that erythrocytes transport immune complexes in lupus is demonstrated by the depression of CR1 numbers in active disease. This defect is also found in other diseases that are accompanied by complement fixation on red blood cells, whether by immune complexes or directly by red blood cell antibodies.[47, 48]

It has been proposed that failure of the mononuclear phagocytic system to effectively remove immune complexes from the circulation and tissues allows a cycle to develop in which immune complexes deposit in tissue, causing inflammation and release of autoantigens, which in turn stimulate the production of autoantibodies and the production of more immune complexes. Thus autoantibody synthesis in lupus may be primarily antigen-driven rather than due to polyclonal activation of B cells. The specific autoantibodies are formed against defined antigens such as DNA, histones, and nonhistone proteins in the DNA nucleoprotein particle.[35, 37] There is a less frequent disease association with C2 deficiency than with deficiencies of C1 and C4; this is because in C2-deficient subjects, complement fixation proceeds as far as C4, which (albeit to a lesser degree) subserves functions otherwise carried out by fixed C3.

Lesser degrees of defective complement function, either genetic or acquired, may also predispose to lupus.[49–52] In the case of the relatively common heterozygous C4 deficiency, the increase in SLE is associated with deficiency of C4A (C4AQ0 allele) (relative risk, 2 to 5) but not the C4B allele. C4A is the isotype of C4 that is more effective in inhibiting immunoprecipitation and, compared with C4B, binds much more effectively to CR1.[47]

The hypothesis that the complement component deficiency per se is not responsible for the increased incidence of SLE, but that it is merely a marker for a true susceptibility gene, seems unlikely because C1q encoded on chromosome 1, C1r and C1s on chromosome 12, and C4 and C2 in the major histocompatibility complex (MHC) on chromosome 6 are all associated with the same disease. Even for the MHC-linked complement loci, the marker gene role seems to be excluded because Caucasian C2 deficiency is nearly always found as part of one particular haplotype (A10, B18, C4A2B4, DR2), whereas the complete C4 deficiency haplotypes are variable and quite different. Finally, C1 inhibitor deficiency, which results in a secondary subtotal deficiency of C2 and C4, is also associated with an increased incidence of autoimmune immune-complex disease.[42, 44]

The frequency of complement deficiencies in the general population is probably very low. C2 deficiency is still the most frequently recognized component deficiency.[53] Heterozygous deficiency for C2 is estimated to be 1 percent. In patients with SLE, homozygous complement component deficiency is also low (estimated to be about 1 in 2000 for women in the United Kingdom).[53] Nevertheless, particularly in children with early-onset (preschool age) SLE-like disease and in instances of familial SLE, hereditary primary deficiencies of complement should be considered.

C1 Deficiency

The absence of C1q is the most common abnormality of the first component of complement.[48] About 30 patients with homozygous C1q deficiency have been reported in the literature.[54] Of these, 28 subjects suffered from SLE, 1 had discoid lupus alone, and a 38-year-old male was healthy. A number of characteristic clinical features of SLE are associated with C1q deficiency.[48, 54] Disease onset tends to be early, with a median age at onset of 7 years (range, 6 months to 42 years). Skin rash was present in 25 cases. The SLE may be severe; 6 patients had central nervous system disease (5 of 6 with grand mal seizures) and 11 had glomerulonephritis. Seventeen of 23 patients had ANA, and autoantibodies to extractable nuclear antigens were reported in 10 patients (anti-RNP in 6; anti-Sm in 6; anti-Ro in 4). Anti-dsDNA antibodies are unusual in the context of C1q deficiency. Therapy with hydroxychloroquine and oral steroids may relieve some symptoms. Thalidomide may benefit the skin lesions.[55]

Case Report

We have treated a C1q-deficient girl with homozygous nonfunctional C1q with weekly infusions of fresh-frozen plasma for 7 years. She was born of healthy nonconsanguinous Caucasian parents. She began having recurrent otitis and tonsillitis, recurrent fever, and arthralgia at the age of 3 years. At 5 years of age, she had aseptic meningitis and a few months later developed nephrotic syndrome. A kidney biopsy revealed mesangioproliferative glomerulonephritis with granular deposits of immunoglobulin (Ig) M, IgG, C3, and C5—but not C1q—along the basement membrane. Apart from a malar rash after sun exposure, the patient had no other lupus-like symptoms. The nephrotic syndrome responded rapidly to prednisone.

However, in the following years, despite therapy with prednisone and hydroxychloroquine, she developed a severe malar rash even after the mildest sun exposure; alopecia; oral ulcerations; Raynaud's phenomenon; livedo reticularis; and severe vasculitis of the palms and fingers, soles, and toes, making it impossible to write, walk, or wear shoes. Recurrent respiratory tract infections provoked exacerbations of vasculitis, arthralgia, headaches, and depression. Intravenous immunoglobulin (IVIG) every 3 weeks prevented recurrent infections and SLE exacerbations but failed to achieve clinical remission. The girl developed anemia, leukopenia with lymphopenia, and thrombocytopenia. She had ANAs, and tests for anti-dsDNA, anti-Sm, and anti-RNP were positive. RFs were present, and slightly raised levels of anticardiolipin antibodies were detected. Hemolysis of sensitized sheep erythrocytes was defective (CH50 <5 percent), but the functional activity of the alternative complement pathway was intact. Levels of complement factors C3 and C4 were increased even during active disease; C2 was normal. Family investigation confirmed the patient to be homozygous for a gene that resulted in the production of low-molecular-weight C1q that was unable to activate the classical complement pathway.[56] Both parents were heterozygous for the abnormality and asymptomatic.

Fresh-frozen plasma infusions (initially, 2 L every 3 weeks; later, 800 ml once a week) started in 1991 resulted in clinical remission and normalization of hemoglobin, white blood cell count, and platelet count until the onset of menarche, when severe headaches, vasculitis of hands and feet, malar rash, alopecia, and arthralgias required reinstitution of prednisone and treatment with thalidomide, 100 mg/day. In 1999, the patient was well on this regimen. During the entire illness, results of tests for ANA and other autoantibodies have remained positive, despite clinical remission. Antibodies to C1q have not been observed.

Inherited deficiency of C1r, often with a concomitant deficiency of C1s, has been reported in eight children, five of whom had SLE and many of whom also had multiple episodes of upper respiratory tract infections, skin infections, meningitis, unexplained fevers, and glomerulonephritis.[39, 40, 48]

HANE, caused by a deficiency in Cl esterase inhibitor, has no known HLA association but is associated with a lupus-like disease in some families.[38–40, 44]

C2 Deficiency

Lack of the second component of complement is the most common genetic deficiency of complement.[53, 57, 58] Heterozygous C2 deficiency may occur in approximately 1 percent of the normal population, 1.4 percent of adults with rheumatoid arthritis, 3.7 percent of children with juvenile rheumatoid arthritis (JRA), and 6 percent of patients with SLE.[58] About 60 percent of homozygous and 13 percent of heterozygous C2-deficient persons have been found to have associated autoimmune disease, most commonly SLE. These patients usually exhibit a restricted set of clinical manifestations, including sun-sensitive skin lesions, alopecia, febrile episodes, arthritis, and renal disease. The lupus-like disease, particularly in association with heterozygous C2 deficiency, tends to be somewhat milder than one would otherwise expect, with less clinically significant nephritis but more florid cutaneous lesions.[43, 57] Steinsson and colleagues[53] successfully treated a 43-year-old woman with homozygous C2 deficiency and SLE with infusions of fresh-frozen plasma and were able to discontinue previously required medications (prednisone and azathioprine).

C3 Deficiency

Almost all reported patients with homozygous C3 deficiency have been infants or young children with severe bacterial infections (meningitis, pneumonitis, peritonitis, osteomyelitis).[57, 59–61] Other associations described in children have included SLE, vasculitis, arthralgia, and glomerulonephritis. Successful renal transplantation in a C3-deficient patient with glomerulonephritis has been reported.[62]

C4 Deficiency

At least seven homozygous C4-deficient children have been recorded.[37, 41, 42, 57] Five had SLE, one had glomerulonephritis, and three had serious infections. SLE is associated with an extended human leukocyte antigen (HLA) haplotype that includes the C4A null allele.[49–52]

Deficiency of Late Complement Components

Deficiency of C5, although unusual, is more common in adults and older children.[63] Both of the reported C5-deficient adolescents had *Neisseria meningitidis* meningitis, but neither had rheumatic complaints. Absence of C6 has been reported in six children younger than 18 years, most of whom had *N. meningitidis* meningitis.[64] Although no child with C6, C7, or C8 deficiency and a rheumatic disease has been reported, adults with these deficiencies have developed discoid lupus erythematosus, Sjögren's syndrome, or SLE.[64–67] We reported a 13-year-old boy who presented with a 6-month history of recurrent fever; an exanthem involving the trunk and extremities; and arthritis of the wrists, knees, and the metacarpophalangeal and proximal interphalangeal joint of both hands.[68] The patient was found to have deficiency of the β-subunit of C8. Infection, particularly meningococcal infection, was excluded. Deficiencies of C9 and of components of the alternate complement pathway are very rare.[40, 45, 57, 58]

Table 35–3
Disorders of Adaptive Immunity Associated With Rheumatic Disease

DISORDERS OF ADAPTIVE IMMUNITY	RHEUMATIC DISEASE ASSOCIATIONS
Combined Immunodeficiencies	
Wiskott-Aldrich syndrome	Chronic arthritis, vasculitis
Immunodeficiency with thymoma (Good's syndrome)	Chronic arthritis
Nezelof's syndrome	Chronic arthritis, SLE
Humoral Immunodeficiencies	
Selective IgA deficiency	JRA, SLE, RA, others
Hypogammaglobulinemia	Chronic arthritis, SLE
IgG subclass deficiencies	JRA, SLE

JRA, juvenile rheumatoid arthritis; RA, rheumatoid arthritis; SLE, systemic lupus erythematosus.

DISORDERS OF ADAPTIVE IMMUNITY ASSOCIATED WITH RHEUMATIC DISEASES

Adaptive immunity is mediated by lymphocytes and their products. Deficiencies are classified according to abnormalities of T and/or B lymphocytes. Acquired abnormalities of adaptive immunity are common in children with rheumatic diseases. It is thought that these laboratory abnormalities (e.g., hypergammaglobulinemia, altered lymphocyte numbers) reflect a response to the disease rather than a primary abnormality, although the validity of this conclusion is by no means certain. Rare but instructive examples of the association of primary immunodeficiencies and rheumatic diseases are discussed in these paragraphs (Table 35–3). The association of immunodeficiency and rheumatic disease has been reviewed by several authors.[69–72]

Primary Abnormalities of T and B Lymphocytes

This part of the chapter discusses diseases characterized clinically and immunologically by defects in both T and B lymphocytes (Tables 35–4 and 35–5).[73–77] Research has led to gene identification in a substantial number of these disorders.

Severe Combined Immunodeficiency

Severe combined immunodeficiency (SCID) is a rare disorder characterized by severe congenital defects in cellular and humoral immunity.[75–77] The incidence is approximately 1 in 75,000 births. Because of absent T cell–mediated immunity, affected children develop severe lung infections with *Pneumocystis carinii*, chronic candidiasis, persistent diarrhea, and failure to thrive, usually within the first year of life. There is lymphoid aplasia, and the thymus usually cannot be detected radiographically. Laboratory tests confirm the presence of agammaglobulinemia (although some maternal IgG can be detected in the first months of life) and T cell lymphopenia with absent in vitro responses to mitogens.

In the X-linked form of SCID, which accounts for 50 to 60 percent of cases, B lymphocytes are present but natural killer (NK) cells are absent. In these patients (T^-B^+ SCID), the agammaglobulinemia is a direct consequence of deficient T cell help. The X-linked form

Table 35–4
Primary Immunodeficiencies of T and B Lymphocytes

DISEASE	INHERITANCE	GENE
SCID	XL	γ Chain
SCID	AR	JAK-3, RAG-1–2, DNA-PK
Adenosine deaminase deficiency	AR	Adenosine deaminase
Purine nucleoside phosphorylase deficiency	AR	Purine nucleoside phosphorylase
MHC class II deficiency	AR	C II TA, RFX 5
Wiskott-Aldrich syndrome	XL	WASP
Reticular dysgenesis	AR	?
Ataxia telangiectasia	AR	ATM
Omenn's syndrome	AR	RAG-1–2
CD3γ and CD3ε deficiency	AR	?
CD8 deficiency	AR	ZAP-70 kinase
DiGeorge syndrome	AR	Candidate gene exists
Cartilage-hair hypoplasia	AR	Candidate gene exists

MHC, major histocompatibility complex; SCID, severe combined immune deficiency; XL, X-linked; AR, autosomal recessive.

Table 35–5

Evaluation of Potential Immunodeficiency in a Patient With a Rheumatic Disease

Complete blood count: hemoglobin, red blood cell morphology and indices, white blood cell count, differential count, lymphocyte count, platelet count
Quantitative serum immunoglobulins—IgG, IgA, IgM, IgE, IgD
Salivary IgA
Specific serum antibody titer—to diphtheria, tetanus, pneumococcus, *Haemophilus influenzae* (if titers abnormal, repeat after immunization), isohemagglutinins, autoantibodies, anti–streptolysin O
Complement components (CH50 and specific essays)
Delayed hypersensitivity skin tests—*Candida, Trichophyton,* mumps
Quantitation of B- and T-cell subsets (CD assignment)
Chest radiograph for thymic shadow, lateral pharyngeal film
Histologic examination of lymph node, rectal biopsy
Specific studies of phagocytosis (nitroblue tetrazolium test, chemotaxis)

results from a gene defect located at Xq12–13.1.[78, 79] This gene encodes for the common γ chain, present in the interleukin receptors IL-2R, IL-4R, IL-7R, IL-9R, and IL-15R. In the autosomal recessive form of SCID, B cells are lacking and NK cells may be present (T^-B^- SCID). In *adenosine deaminase (ADA) deficiency,* a variety of ADA gene mutations have been described. A lack of ADA in precursor lymphocytes results in a maturation arrest by accumulation of deoxy ATP, which inhibits cell division.[75, 80, 81] The clinical course is fatal within the first 2 years of life. Another form of autosomal recessive SCID is caused by a mutation in the JAK-3 kinase gene.[75] This enzyme mediates post-IL-2R signaling.

The only curative treatment for SCID is allogeneic hemopoietic stem cell transplantation. As in patients with ADA deficiency, patients with the X-linked IL-2R deficiency may potentially benefit from gene therapy; this modality has been successful in mice.[81a]

There are no reports of rheumatic diseases in children with SCID. This may be due to the fact that they usually die before the age of 2 years unless they undergo transplantation, but it may also illustrate the essential role of T cells in the initiation of an autoimmune disorder. After stem cell transplantation, autoimmune hematologic phenomena have been described in patients with graft-versus-host disease (GVHD), a positive Coombs' test result, and autoimmune hemolytic anemia. Chronic GVHD of the skin leads to skin changes that resemble those that occur in systemic scleroderma.

Combined Immunodeficiency

The term *combined immunodeficiency* is applied to a group of disorders of variable clinical severity associated with defects in both cellular and humoral immunity.[72, 82] The *Wiskott-Aldrich syndrome* (WAS) is characterized by a progressive abnormality in both T- and B-lymphocyte function.[83] It is thought to be caused by defects in immunoregulatory peptides involved in cell–cell interactions. There is a low expression of sialophorin (CD43). The syndrome is associated with mutations of the gene located at Xp11.23.[84] The precise function of the protein (the WAS protein) that this gene encodes is uncertain. Interestingly, a female WAS patient has been described in whom the gene mutation was discovered to be present on one of the X chromosomes. The fact that she was nevertheless affected was explained by a nonrandom inactivation of the X chromosomes. Discovery of the gene mutation has also led to the identification of related male adults with only thrombocytopenia.

Children with the Wiskott-Aldrich syndrome have persistent eczema, thrombocytopenia with a low platelet volume, and recurrent ear, nose, and throat infections. They often have chronic cytomegalovirus infection. Laboratory abnormalities vary widely. The characteristic immunoglobulin pattern includes normal IgG and elevated IgA and IgE levels, with absence of antibodies to polysaccharide antigens (such as pneumococcal capsular antigen) and absent blood group isohemagglutinins. There is a high incidence of Coombs'-positive hemolytic anemia, vasculitis, and (mostly transient) arthritis.[85–87] The syndrome is a premalignant condition with a high frequency of thymomas and sarcomas later in life, although the precise incidence of these malignancies is unknown, because persons with the WAS gene mutation may be asymptomatic.

T Cell Immunodeficiencies

In the T cell immunodeficiencies, T lymphocytes are, in contrast with SCID, present in the peripheral blood, although in reduced numbers. This is a heterogeneous and often poorly defined group of disorders. Various functional and genetic defects have been described (see Table 35–4). Clinically, these diseases do not have life-threatening infections in the first months of life but show a more gradually developing immunodeficiency. An imbalance between T and B lymphocytes may explain the high incidence of autoimmune disorders, as well as infections, allergies, and malignancies. Severe and chronic autoimmune manifestations, mostly involving blood cells, develop between 1 and 12 years of age.[82] In addition, vasculitis, autoimmune hepatitis, and thyroiditis have been described. In younger patients, without severe ongoing infections, bone marrow transplantation may be performed.[82]

Cartilage-hair hypoplasia consists of bony dysplasia, short-limbed dwarfism, fine hair, short fingernails, and neutropenia.[88, 89] Affected infants have generalized hypermobility. However, inflammatory rheumatic diseases have not been reported.

Primary Humoral Immunodeficiencies

These antibody deficiency syndromes result from either impaired intrinsic B cell development or ineffective B

Table 35–6

Primary Humoral Immunodeficiencies

X-linked agammaglobulinemia (Bruton's)
X-linked hypogammaglobulinemia with growth hormone deficiency
X-linked hyper IgM
Autosomal recessive hyper IgM
IgG subclass deficiencies
Selective IgA deficiency
Kappa light chain deficiency
Antibody deficiency with normal immunoglobulins (Nezelof's)
Common variable immunodeficiency
Hyper IgD syndrome
Hyper IgE syndrome

cell responses to T cell–derived signals (Table 35–6). The association of primary humoral immunodeficiencies and rheumatic disease is a well-known phenomenon.

Selective IgA Deficiency

Selective IgA deficiency (sIgA-D) is the most common primary immunodeficiency. In Western countries, the prevalence ranges between 1 in 330 and 1 in 2200 persons.[90–92] It is characterized by serum IgA levels of less than 0.01 to 0.05 g/L.[92] IgA is also absent in secretions, although the secretory component of IgA is normally present in saliva. Patients with sIgA-D identified by routine immunodiffusion assays[93] have trace amounts of circulating IgA detectable by the more sensitive radioimmunoassay. Although the term *sIgA-D* denotes an isolated deficiency of IgA, this immunoglobulin is also deficient in 20 percent of patients with IgG subclass deficiency and in 40 percent with a defective antipolysaccharide antibody response. Antibodies of the IgM or the IgG class directed against IgA are commonly found in sera from patients with sIgA-D.[94, 95]

The etiology of sIgA-D is largely unknown. Anti-IgA autoantibodies may play a role in the induction of IgA deficiency (Table 35–7). This is supported by the observation that IgA deficiency is more common in children of affected mothers than in children of affected fathers.[90, 98] Transplacental passage of maternal anti-IgA antibodies might interfere with the developing IgA system. The fact that plasma cells producing anti-IgA could not be detected locally along the mucosal linings has led to the hypothesis that sIgA-D results from systemic exposure to endogenous IgA. sIgA-D with anti-IgA antibodies could thus be regarded as an autoimmune disorder.[96] Moreover, such antibodies are more common in IgA-deficient patients with autoimmune and rheumatic diseases than in asymptomatic IgA-deficient patients.[97] In the majority of patients, B cells expressing IgA on their surface and in the cytoplasm are still present in the blood, albeit in low numbers.[99] Exposure to an oral vaccine induces a normal mucosal immune response by B cells that secrete antigen-specific IgG or IgM.[100] Nevertheless, a B cell maturation defect may be present because, in contrast with B cells of normal persons, B cells from IgA-deficient persons also express surface IgM and IgD.

Comparable to common variable immunodeficiency (CVID), T cellular proliferative responses to mitogens are depressed in a proportion of patients with IgA deficiency.[99] Both defective T-helper cell function and suppressor T cells inhibiting IgA production have been described. sIgA-D can be familial, and in some families an autosomal dominant inheritance pattern is found. The mother and three siblings of an IgA-deficient girl with JRA lacked serum IgA.[23] The mother had very high levels of anti-IgA antibodies detected by a hemagglutination assay. The incidence of sIgA-D is increased in families of persons with CVID or hypogammaglobulinemia. sIgA-D may also precede CVID. As in CVID, the putative gene defect resides on chromosome 6 between the HLA-B and the HLA-DQ regions (see later).[101–103]

sIgA-D is usually congenital and permanent, although transient cases have been described.[99] In some patients with JRA and sIgA-D, the IgA deficiency developed before antirheumatic drugs were prescribed.[98, 104] Drug-induced IgA deficiency is well known, however. In particular, nonsteroidal anti-inflammatory drugs such as diclofenac and sulfasalazine, parenteral gold, and D-penicillamine are associated with IgA deficiency that is sometimes reversible on discontinuation of the drug.[105–110, 110a]

Table 35–7

Frequency of Anti-IgA Antibodies in Selective IgA Deficiency

DIAGNOSIS	NUMBER	ANTI-IgA ANTIBODIES Number	Percent
Asymptomatic blood donors	27	5	19
Miscellaneous diseases	8	2	25
Recurrent infections	10	3	30
RA-like arthritis	4	2	50
JRA-like arthritis	13	10	77
SLE-like disease	10	10	100

JRA, juvenile rheumatoid arthritis; RA, rheumatoid arthritis; SLE, systemic lupus erythematosus.
Modified from Petty RE, Palmer NR, Cassidy JT, et al: The association of autoimmune diseases and anti-IgA antibodies in patients with selective IgA deficiency. Clin Exp Immunol 37: 83, 1979.

Table 35–8

Selective IgA Deficiency: Disease Associations

Recurrent bacterial sinopulmonary, gastrointestinal, or urogenital infections
Rheumatic diseases
  Chronic arthritis (JRA-like), systemic lupus erythematosus, dermatomyositis, scleroderma, ankylosing spondylitis, mixed connective tissue disease, chronic active hepatitis, pernicious anemia, autoimmune hemolytic anemia, and thrombocytopenia
Autoimmune disorders
  Thyroiditis, pulmonary hemosiderosis, sarcoidosis
Gastrointestinal diseases
  Nodular lymphoid hyperplasia, celiac disease, inflammatory bowel disease
Central nervous system disease
  Ataxia-telangiectasia
Drug-induced IgA deficiency
  Dilantin, hydroxychloroquine, gold compounds, D-penicillamine, sulfasalazine, nonsteroidal anti-inflammatory drugs
Malignancy
Chromosome 18 deletions
Other immunodeficiencies
  Chronic mucocutaneous candidiasis, chronic granulomatous disease, neutropenia

Data from Amman AJ, Hong R: Selective IgA deficiency: presentation of 30 cases and a review of the literature. Medicine (Baltimore) 50: 223, 1971; Plebani A, Monafo V, Ugazio AG, et al: Clinical heterogeneity and reversibility of selective immunoglobulin A deficiency in 80 children. Lancet 1: 829, 1986; and Cassidy JT: Selective IgA deficiency anti chronic arthritis in children. *In* Moore TD (ed): Arthritis in Childhood. Report of the Eightieth Ross Conference in Pediatric Research. Columbus, Ross Laboratories, 1981, p 82.

Disease Associations

The clinical spectrum varies from asymptomatic healthy persons to those with recurrent respiratory and gastrointestinal infections. The heterogeneity of this disorder is further illustrated by a variety of associated diseases (Table 35–8). Organ-specific autoimmune diseases are more frequent in patients with sIgA-D, with the exception of those rheumatic diseases listed in the table. The frequency of autoimmune disease as reported in large studies of IgA-deficient individuals ranges between 7 and 36 percent. It has been established that among the rheumatic diseases JRA, SLE, and rheumatoid arthritis are most frequent (Table 35–9). Associations of sIgA-D with other rheumatic diseases such as sarcoidosis, scleroderma, dermatomyositis, and Kawasaki disease are more sporadic and may reflect an ascertainment bias. In general, the rheumatic disease in these patients responds to the conventional antirheumatic therapy.

Chronic Arthritis. The prevalence of sIgA-D in JRA varies from 2 to 4 percent.[87, 93, 98, 101–104] In general, the clinical picture, sex ratio, and age at onset of arthritis do not differ from those in children with JRA and normal or elevated levels of IgA (Table 35–10). The distribution of onset types is also similar: oligoarticular onset in 64 percent, polyarticular onset in 32 percent, and systemic onset in 4 percent[111, 115, 116] (Figs. 35–1 to 35–3). In the majority of patients, the course of the disease is mild and remains oligoarticular with little or no functional limitations. Erosive arthritis, however, has been described in up to 28 percent.[112, 117] In one study, the arthritis appeared more severe in patients with transient IgA deficiency or in patients with borderline IgA values.[99] Patients with sIgA-D associated with oligoarticular JRA may be more prone to chronic uveitis and they have ANAs more frequently,[116, 117] although this could not be confirmed in a study by Pelkonen and colleagues.[115]

Systemic Lupus Erythematosus. The prevalence of sIgA-D in patients with SLE is 1 to 4 percent, which is 20 to 30 times higher than that in the normal population.[92, 118] In general, the clinical manifestations of SLE

Table 35–9

Selective IgA Deficiency and Rheumatic Diseases

AUTHOR	RHEUMATIC DISEASE ASSOCIATIONS	NO./TOTAL*
Cassidy et al, 1977,[111] 1979[93]	Chronic arthritis (JRA-like)	18/477
Huntley et al, 1967[114]	Chronic arthritis (JRA-like)	2/23
Panush et al, 1972[113]	Chronic arthritis (JRA-like)	3/176
Pelkonen et al, 1975[115]	Chronic arthritis (JRA-like)	11/300
Barkley et al, 1979[104]	Chronic arthritis (JRA-like)	2/582
Salmi et al, 1973[104a]	Chronic arthritis (JRA like)	5/115
Cassidy et al, 1969[116]	SLE	10/50
Cleland and Bell, 1978[118]	SLE	2
Cassidy et al, 1969[116]	Dermatomyositis	3
Cassidy, 1981[120a]	Scleroderma (systemic)	1/15
Jay et al, 1981[121]	Scleroderma (systemic)	1
Spirer et al, 1979[122]	Scleroderma (local)	1
Cassidy, 1981[123]	Ankylosing spondylitis	2
Good et al, 1977[123]	Ankylosing spondylitis	1
Barkley et al, 1979[104]	Juvenile ankylosing spondylitis	1
Cassidy et al, 1969[116]	Mixed connective tissue disease	1/14

JRA, juvenile rheumatoid arthritis; SLE, systemic lupus erythematosus.
*No./Total = number of IgA-deficient patients over number of patients with specific rheumatic disease.

Table 35–10

Clinical Manifestations of 18 Children With Chronic Arthritis and Selective IgA Deficiency*

CHARACTERISTIC	PERCENT
Sex	
Female	78
Male	22
Age at onset of arthritis	
≤4 yr	50
5–9 yr	45
10–12 yr	5
Characteristics of arthritis	
Oligoarticular	61
Polyarticular	39
Systemic	0
Erosions	28
Extra-articular manifestations	
Rheumatoid nodules	11
Chronic uveitis	22
Functional capacity at follow-up	
Class I	28
Class II	50
Class III	22
Class IV	0
Laboratory abnormalities	
Antinuclear antibodies present	72
Rheumatoid factors present	6
Anti-IgA antibodies present	79

*Eighteen of 477 children with JRA seen at the University of Michigan, 1961–1979.

From Cassidy JT, Petty RE: Textbook of Pediatric Rheumatology, 3rd ed. Philadelphia, WB Saunders, 1995.

and the response to therapy do not differ in patients with or without sIgA-D, although in a series of 10 children with sIgA-D and SLE, there was more neuropsychiatric disease but nephritis was absent.[94] Interestingly, resolution of the sIgA-D has been described under intensive immunosuppressive therapy, similar to a girl with sIgA-D–associated JRA who was treated with plasma infusions.[119]

Other Rheumatic Diseases. sIgA-D has been described sporadically in other systemic rheumatic diseases such as dermatomyositis,[111] sarcoidosis,[120] scleroderma,[121, 122] and ankylosing spondylitis.[123] However, these associations may merely reflect an ascertainment bias.

Hypogammaglobulinemia

The term *hypogammaglobulinemia* is applied to a number of disorders characterized by decreased levels of serum IgG and the inability to produce specific antibodies when exposed to an antigen. Unlike SCID and combined immunodeficiency, there are generally no specific T cell abnormalities. Among the primary hypogammaglobulinemias are X-linked agammaglobulinemia (Bruton's agammaglobulinemia), CVID (also called *late-onset hypogammaglobulinemia*), autosomal early-onset agammaglobulinemia, and the hyper-IgM syndrome (Table 35–11; see also Table 35–6). Drug-induced hypogammaglobulinemia has been reported in patients exposed to various anticonvulsants and antirheumatic drugs.

X-Linked Agammaglobulinemia

X-linked agammaglobulinemia is characterized by recurrent severe bacterial infections from the age of 6 to 12 months onward.[124] Only males are affected with recurrent otitis media, pneumonia, meningitis, and septic arthritis from extracellular encapsulated organisms such as *Streptococcus pneumoniae* and *Haemophilus influenzae*. The defective gene resides at Xq21.3–22[125] and causes a block in differentiation at the pre–B-cell stage. B cells are therefore absent. Serum IgG is usually less than 2 g/L; IgM, IgA, and IgE are absent. Patients should be treated vigorously with antibiotics and with life-long IVIG.

Common Variable Immunodeficiency

CVID is a heterogeneous primary immunodeficiency characterized by hypogammaglobulinemia and recurrent infections, predominantly by bacterial agents. Recurrent sinopulmonary infections often cause bronchiectasis. There is a high frequency of gastrointestinal disease, such as giardiasis, and autoimmune diseases. Patients with CVID have an increased risk (up to 10 percent) of malignancies of the lymphoid system or the gastrointestinal tract.[126, 127] The incidence of CVID is about 5 per million. The age at onset varies from 1 to 71 years,[126–128] the majority of patients being between 30 and 45 years of age at the onset of their disease. About 25 percent have onset before the age of 15 years.[126, 128]

The number of B lymphocytes in the peripheral blood of

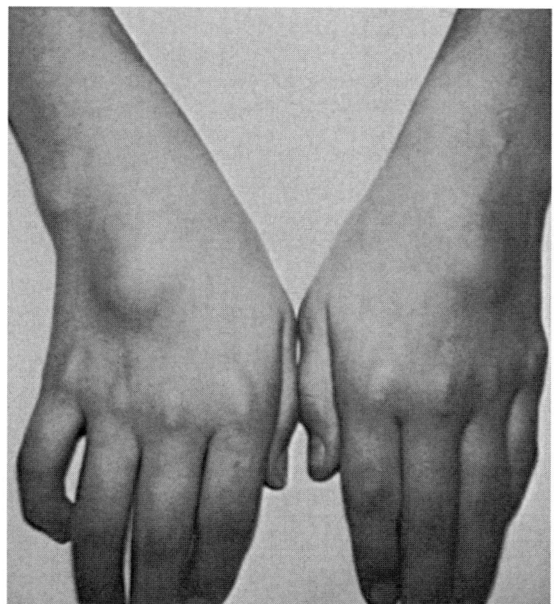

Figure 35–1. Hands of an 11-year-old girl with chronic arthritis, tenosynovitis, and selective immunoglobulin A deficiency (sIgA-D). Hand and wrist involvement gradually returned to normal, but a minimally symptomatic effusion of her right knee persisted.

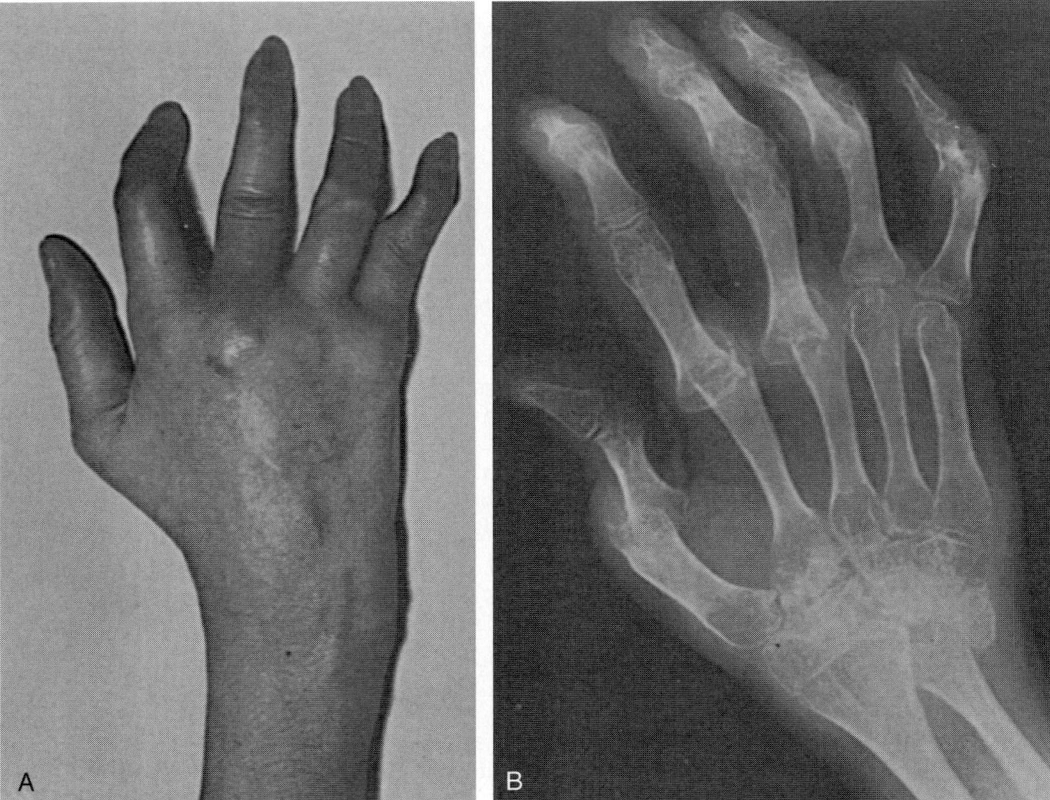

Figure 35–2. *A*, Hand of T. P. at 27 years of age. A chronic, deforming, erosive arthritis of the wrists and small joints of the hands was slowly progressive from onset. These deformities and subluxation of metacarpophalangeal (MCP) joints are evident. The second proximal interphalangeal (PIP) joint had been surgically fused in a functional position. *B*, Hand of an 18-year-old girl with sIgAD and systemic lupus erythematosus (SLE), with onset of arthritis at the age of 7 years. Destruction of joints is already far advanced, with subluxations of ulnar side of wrist, MCP joints 1 to 3, and PIP joints 4 and 5. Erosions, destruction of articulating surfaces, microfractures and bony collapse, and extreme juxta-articular osteoporosis are present.

patients with CVID may be normal or decreased. When purified B cells from patients with CVID were cultured in the presence of normal allogeneic T cells, the defect in immunoglobulin production could not be corrected.[126, 129] When T cells from patients with CVID were co-cultured with normal B cells, normal immunoglobulin secretion was generally not depressed. Studies using B cell mitogens or soluble T cell factors confirmed that most B cells from patients with CVID can synthesize at least some immunoglobulin in the presence of an appropriate in vitro stimulus. Although this disease is regarded as an intrinsic B cell defect, in vitro T lymphocyte proliferative responses to mitogens are decreased or absent in about half of patients.[126, 129, 130]

The precise B cell defect is still unknown, and the hypogammaglobulinemia may also result from a lack of appropriate T cell–derived stimulation necessary for normal B cell maturation. Such a T cell abnormality may account for the observed predisposition of patients with CVID to malignancies and autoimmune disorders. Specifically, patients' $CD4^+$ cells produce less IL-2, possibly because of a selective defect in the ability to activate the IL-2 gene normally.[129, 130] In addition, some patients with CVID have expanded activated (i.e., $CD57^+$ and DR^+) $CD8^+$ populations, a pattern comparable to that in patients infected with cytomegalovirus, Epstein-Barr virus, or human immunodeficiency virus. It was thus speculated that a chronic viral infection in a genetically predisposed person could induce CVID (see later). A similar pathogenesis is thought to apply to the X-linked lymphoproliferative syndrome.[131]

Genetic studies of patients with CVID and sIgA-D and their relatives point to susceptibility to CVID and sIgA-D determined by a gene located at 6p21.3. This region of chromosome 6 contains the 21-hydroxylase A and tumor necrosis factor genes and lies between the HLA-B and HLA-DQ domains.

Autoimmune Disease

Autoimmune disease occurs in 20 to 30 percent of patients with CVID,[126, 127] whereas there are only a few reports of autoimmune disease in X-linked agammaglobulinemia.[121–123] Thrombocytopenia and hemolytic anemia are most common. The association of antibody-mediated autoimmunity and hypogammaglobulinemic states might seem contradictory but could be explained by defects in the anti-idiotypic network, which normally regulates expression of naturally occurring autoantibodies.[135] The prevalence of arthritis in hypogammaglobulinemia ranges from 10 to 30 percent. It is divided into septic and aseptic forms.

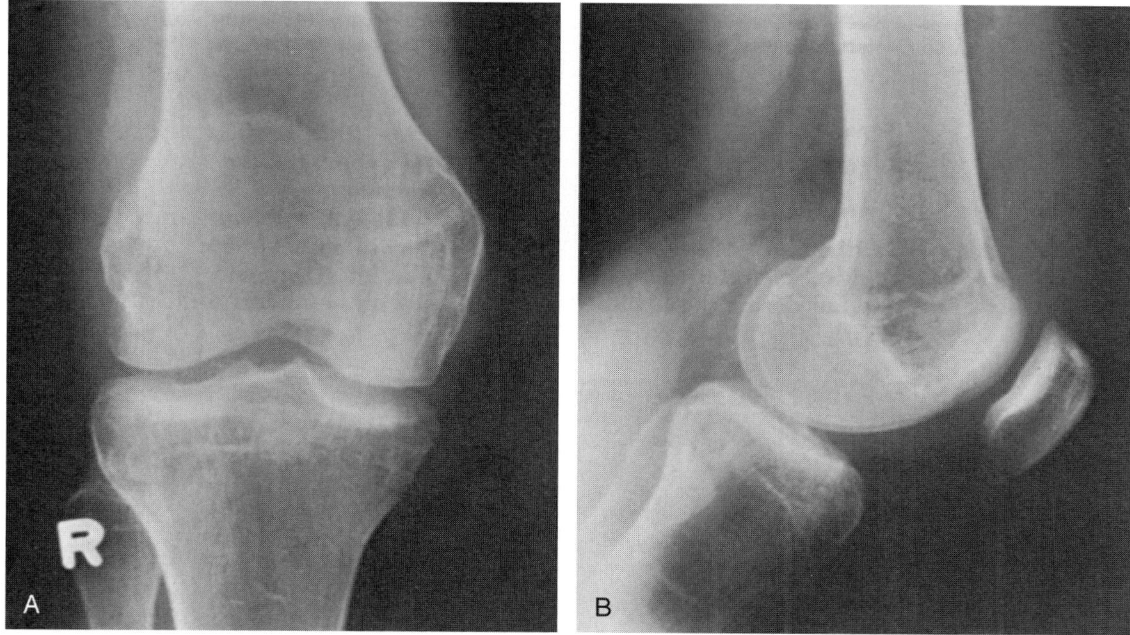

Figure 35–3. Knee films of a patient with sIgA-D at 25 years of age. *A*, Anteroposterior view. *B*, Lateral view. Coarsening of the trabecular architecture and slight osteoporosis are evident, along with a moderate decrease in the cartilaginous space. There is sharpening of the tibial tubercles and the posterior aspect of the lateral femoral condyle. Erosions are not present in spite of 16 years of continuous joint effusion.

Septic Arthritis. Septic arthritis, both with common and with rare microorganisms, occurs relatively frequently in patients with hypogammaglobulinemia.[105] Causative microorganisms are *Staphylococcus aureus*, *Streptococcus pneumoniae*, *Haemophilus influenzae*, *Mycobacteria* species, and *Mycoplasma* species (including *Ureaplasma*). *Mycoplasma* species are difficult to culture. Improved detection techniques (such as specific culture fluids, electron microscopy, polymerase chain reactions) may identify the presence of these microorganisms in a substantial number of cases that have heretofore been regarded as aseptic.[105, 127]

Aseptic Arthritis. The association of rheumatic diseases and CVID or X-linked agammaglobulinemia is firmly established, with reported frequencies varying

Table 35–11

Characteristics of Hypogammaglobulinemia

CHARACTERISTIC	X-LINKED	COMMON VARIABLE
Sex	Males	Equal sex distribution
Genetics	X-linked recessive (Xq21.3-22)	Variable (? 6p21.3)
Age at onset of symptoms	6 mo to 2 yr	2 yr to adulthood
B lymphocytes	(pre-B cell)	B cell
Peripheral lymphoid tissue	Hypoplastic	Normal to enlarged
Plasma cells in nodes	Very rare	Decreased or none
Surface immunoglobulins	Absent	Present
Serum IgG	<1 g/L	<5 g/L
Serum IgA, IgM	Very low	Variable
Natural antibodies	Very low	Variable
Specific antibodies	Absent	Variable (autoantibodies)
T lymphocytes	Numbers increased, subsets normal	Variable number and function
Clinical characteristics		
Severe bacterial infections	Yes	Sometimes; less severe
Viral infections	Yes	Yes
Malabsorption	Sometimes	Frequent
Autoimmune diseases	No	Frequent
JRA-like arthritis	30%	Infrequent; frequency unknown
Control with Ig replacement	Partial	Partial

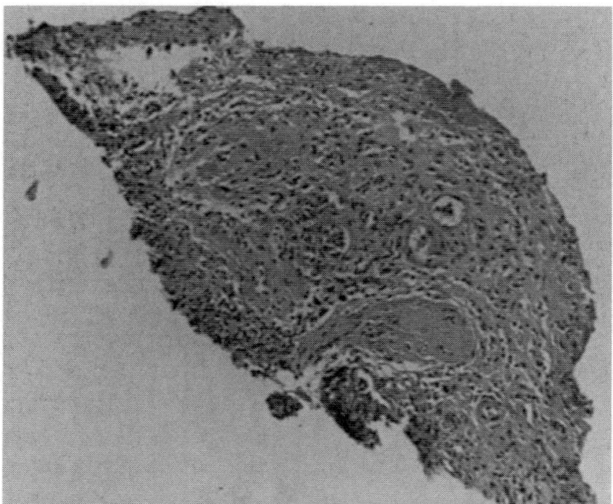

Figure 35–4. Needle biopsy of synovium of R. B., who developed chronic synovitis of the left knee and was found to have common variable immunodeficiency. There is marked hypertrophy of the subsynovial layers with hyperplasia of vascular endothelium and compaction of collagen. A nonspecific infiltrate of mononuclear cells is visible, but there are no aggregations of round cells. Plasma cells are absent. Fibrin is present on the synovial surface. (From Petty RE, Cassidy JT, Tubergen DG: Association of arthritis with hypogammaglobulinemia. Arthritis Rheum 20[Suppl]: 441, 1977.)

between 7 and 42 percent (Table 35–12). In a large series of 103 patients with CVID, 3 were reported as having chronic arthritis similar to JRA, affecting one to four large peripheral joints.[126] Onset of arthritis is between 3 and 15 years of age, is often subtle, and is characterized by small to moderate effusions, soft tissue thickening, and limitation of motion[136] (Figs. 35–4 and 35–5). In about 50 percent of patients, arthritis is the presenting symptom.[134] In the remainder, arthritis is preceded by several years of infectious complications. Uluhan and associates[137] described a patient with a systemic-onset JRA and CVID. This patient later developed neutropenia (found in up to 10 percent of patients with CVID and X-linked agammaglobulinemia), autoimmune hemolytic anemia, and a cellular immune deficiency. Despite immunoglobulin infusions, the patient died at the age of 22 years from infection.

Table 35–12

Hypogammaglobulinemia and Arthritis: A Case History

History

6 mo	Recurrent skin infections, otitis media, poor wound healing
5 yr	Tonsillectomy
6 yr	Painful, stiff shoulders
7 yr	Chronic swelling of the left knee, rhinorrhea, wheezing, pneumonitis
14 yr	Left mastoidectomy; frequent, bulky stools

Received all routine immunizations, including live virus vaccines

Physical Examination at 15 yr of Age

Draining left otitis media, axillary lymphadenopathy, moderate effusion, and warmth of the knee

Investigations at 15 yr of Age

Radiographs
- Sinus wall thickening and clouding
- Abnormal left mastoid
- Left knee: epiphyseal overgrowth and joint effusion, abnormal thermography

Laboratory studies
- IgG 1.4 g/L; IgA 0, IgM 0.6 g/L, IgE 0
- No isohemagglutinins, absent serum antibodies to polio viruses, diphtheria, tetanus; Schick skin test positive
- Negative delayed skin tests to PPD, mumps, *Candida,* SK/SD
- Impaired in vitro lymphocyte response to phytohemagglutinin
- Circulating lymphocytes: T cells 52%, B cells 40%
- Hemolytic complement: normal

Other Rheumatic Diseases. Whereas the prevalence of sIgA-D in patients with SLE is 20 to 30 times higher than that in the normal population, there is no marked association of hypogammaglobulinemia and SLE. To date, only nine cases of SLE with CVID have been described.[138, 139] This low number suggests that the association of SLE and CVID is purely coincidental. It is also difficult to understand an association of an autoimmune disease such as SLE, where B cell activation, elevated serum IgG, and circulating immune complexes are prominent, with another disorder characterized by deficient antibody production.

Dermatomyositis-Like Syndrome. There is considerable doubt that the dermatomyositis-like syndrome

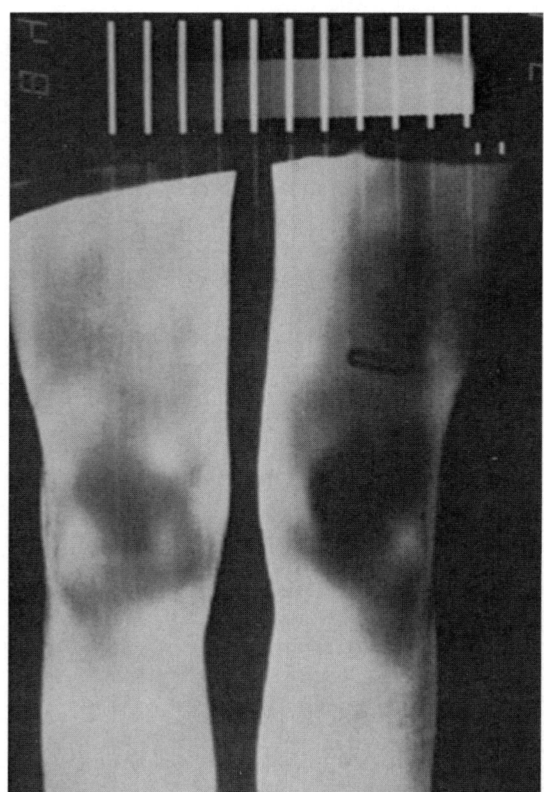

Figure 35–5. Thermograph of the knees of R. B. at 20 years of age show increased heat production on the left knee, the site of the inflammatory arthritis. (The paper clip on the left leg is for standardization in thermography.)

Table 35–13

Dermatomyositis-Like Disease and Hypogammaglobulinemia

REFERENCE	SEX	AGE	CLINICAL DESCRIPTION
139a	M	2 yr	Brawny edema of distal extremities; leg stiffness, contractures; gastrocnemius biopsy specimen consistent with dermatomyositis
139b	?	?	Patient with classic dermatomyositis and hypogammaglobulinemia
139c	?	?	Dermatomyositis, lymphoma
139d	?	?	Adenovirus 12 isolated
139d	?	?	Echovirus 9 isolated
140	M	2 yr	Intermittent arthritis (knees) since 2 yr; at 17 yr, heliotrope rash on eyelids, MCP and PIP rash, muscle weakness, contractures, elevated LDH. *Biopsy:* perivascular, endomysial, perimysial lymphocytic infiltrate; negative immunofluorescence; cerebral vasculitis. Death.
141	M	5 yr	Brawny edema of extremities; violaceous, telangiectatic rash over extensor aspects of legs; muscle wasting, contractures of elbows, wrists, knees. Elevated ALT and AST. CK normal. *Muscle biopsy:* perivascular lymphocytic infiltration. Death.
143	M	24 yr	Muscle weakness, edema, rash on extensor surface of joints; contractures of elbows, knees. *CSF:* echovirus 9. *Muscle biopsy:* perivascular round cell infiltration. Death.
143	M	12 yr	Joint stiffness, contractures; weakness and atrophy of muscles; deafness. *Muscle biopsy:* perivascular lymphocytic infiltration.
143	M	3 yr	Arthritis in knees and ankles, myalgia; ↑ AST, elevated aldolase. *EMG:* myopathy. *ECG:* right bundle branch block. *CSF:* echovirus 33.
144	M	11 yr	Polyarthritis, edema, encephalitis. *Muscle biopsy:* mononuclear infiltration. Leukocyte migration inhibited by echovirus-11 vaccine.
144a	F	3 mo	Fever, muscle weakness, cellulitis, violaceous edematous eyelids, musosal ulceration; elevated CK. *Skin biopsy:* leukocytoclastic vasculitis.
146	M	29 yr	Chronic arthritis at 19 mo; in adulthood myalgia, proximal muscle weakness, elevated CK. *Gastrocnemius biopsy:* active inflammatory myopathy. Echovirus 11 from blood, urine, CSF, muscle.

ALT, alanine transaminase; AST, aspartate transaminase; CK, creatine kinase; CSF, cerebrospinal fluid; ECG, electrocardiogram; EMG, electromyogram; LDH, lactate dehydrogenase; MCP, metacarpophalangeal; PIP, proximal interphalangeal.

that sometimes complicates hypogammaglobulinemia has the same pathogenesis as idiopathic dermatomyositis of childhood. Clinical characteristics of the reported cases of this syndrome are summarized in Table 35–13. It is characterized by subcutaneous edema, myalgia, muscle wasting, and sometimes polyarthritis followed by contractures of large joints. It is not clear whether the myopathy is proximal, distal, or diffuse in most instances. Cutaneous manifestations include heliotrope discoloration of the eyelids in one child, rash on the extensor surfaces of the metacarpophalangeal and proximal interphalangeal joints in two patients, and nonspecific rashes in two other patients.[140, 141] Electromyographic evidence of a myopathy was documented in one patient, and abnormalities on muscle biopsy consistent with a diagnosis of dermatomyositis were present in seven. Focal calcification was present in one. Central nervous system disease and deafness frequently accompanied the myositis, and a fatal outcome was common. Other associations have also been described, including leukemia and lymphoma.[142] Viral isolations (e.g., echovirus, adenovirus) from the cerebrospinal fluid and sometimes from muscle and other sites raise the question of a viral etiology of this syndrome and support a role for persistent latent viral infection in its pathogenesis.[143–146] A direct relation to idiopathic dermatomyositis remains unproven, however, in spite of speculations on its viral cause. One patient was successfully treated with IVIG.

IgG Subclass Deficiencies and Rheumatic Diseases

The availability of specific antisera for the IgG subclasses has enabled the detection of subclass deficiencies in a wide variety of normal and abnormal conditions.[147, 148] A 10-year-old boy with JRA and Hodgkin's disease had low concentrations of IgA (0.19 g/L) and IgG2 (0.02 g/L). Another 10-year-old boy had SLE, undetectable IgA, and an IgG2 concentration of 0.02 g/L.[149] Oxelius also reported IgG2 subclass deficiency in SLE.[150] Heiner and colleagues[151] found low IgG4 levels (<30 mg/L) in 12 of 112 patients with "disseminated collagen vascular disease" but provided no further details. Aucouturier and associates[152] reported 450 patients with subclass deficiencies. IgG2 deficiency was associated most frequently with vasculitis and cytopenias. Another study found an increased frequency of Henoch-Schönlein purpura and glomerulonephritis.[153]

References

1. Dhein J, Walczak H, Baümler C, et al: Autocrine T-cell suicide mediated by APO-1/Fas (D95). Nature 373: 438, 1995.
2. Chinnaiyan AM, O'Rourke K, Tewari M, et al: FADD, a novel death domain-containing protein, interacts with the death domain of Fas and initiates apoptosis. Cell 81: 505, 1995.
3. Stanger BZ, Leder P, Lee T-H, et al: RIP: a novel protein con-

taining a death domain that interacts with Fas/APO-1 (CD95) in yeast and causes cell death. Cell 81: 513, 1995.
4. Hsu H, Xiong J, Goeddel DV: The TNF receptor 1–associated protein TRADD signals cell death and NF-kB activation. Cell 81: 495, 1995.
5. Merino R, Fossati L, Izui S: The lupus-prone BXSB strain: the Yaa gene model of systemic lupus erythematosus. Springer Semin Immunopathol 14: 141, 1992.
6. Rieux-Laucat F, Le Deist F, Hivroz C, et al: Mutations in Fas associated with human lymphoproliferative syndrome and autoimmunity. Science 268: 1347, 1995.
7. Fischer A, Cavazzana-Calvo M, De Saint Basile G, et al: Naturally occurring primary deficiencies of the immune system. Annu Rev Immunol 15: 93, 1997.
7a. Sleight BJ, Prasad VS, de Latt C, et al: Correction of autoimmune lymphoproliferative syndrome by bone marrow transplantation. Bone Marrow Transplant 22: 375, 1998.
8. Sneller MC, Wang J, Dale JK, et al: Clinical, immunologic, and genetic features of an autoimmune lymphoproliferative syndrome associated with abnormal lymphocyte apoptosis. Blood 89: 1341, 1997.
9. Drappa J, Vaishnaw AK, Sullivan KE, et al: Fas gene mutations in the Canale-Smith syndrome, an inherited lymphoproliferative disorder associated with autoimmunity. N Engl J Med 335: 1643, 1996.
10. Dianzani U, Bragardo M, DiFranco D, et al: Deficiency of the Fas apoptosis pathway without Fas gene mutations in pediatric patients with autoimmunity/lymphoproliferation. Blood 89: 2871, 1997.
11. Wu J, Wilson J, He J, et al: Fas ligand mutation in a patient with systemic lupus erythematosus and lymphoproliferative disease. J Clin Invest 98: 1107, 1996.
12. Seger RA, Ezekowitz RAB: Treatment of chronic granulomatous disease. Immunodeficiency 5: 113, 1994.
13. Roos D: X-CGD: a database of X-CGD-causing mutations. Immunol Today 17: 517, 1996.
14. Meisch C, Roos D: The molecular basis of chronic granulomatous disease. Springer Semin Immunopathol 19: 417, 1998.
15. Schaller J: Illness resembling lupus erythematosus in mothers of boys with chronic granulomatous disease. Ann Intern Med 76: 747, 1972.
16. Finlay AY, Johnson CR: Chronic granulomatous disease carrier genodermatosis. Clin Genet 23: 276, 1983.
17. Barton LL, Johnson CR: Discoid lupus erythematosus and X-linked chronic granulomatous disease. Pediatr Dermatol 3: 376, 1986.
18. Manzi S, Urbach AH, McCine AB, et al: Systemic lupus erythematosus in a boy with chronic granulomatous disease: case report and review of the literature. Arthritis Rheum 134: 101, 1991.
19. Humbert JR, Fishman CB, Weston WL, et al: Frequency of the carrier state for X-linked chronic granulomatous disease among females with lupus erythematosus. Clin Genet 10: 16, 1976.
20. Brandrup F, Koch C, Petri M, et al: Discoid lupus erythematosus lesions and stomatitis in female carriers of X-linked chronic granulomatous disease. Br J Dermatol 104: 495, 1981.
21. Stalder JF, Dreno B, Bureau B, Hakim J: Discoid lupus erythematosus like lesions in a patient with autosomal recessive chronic granulomatous disease. Br J Dermatol 114: 251, 1986.
22. Lee BW, Yap HK: polyarthritis resembling juvenile rheumatoid arthritis in a girl with chronic granulomatous disease. Arthritis Rheum 37: 773, 1994.
23. Cassidy JT, Petty RE: Immunodeficiencies and the rheumatic diseases. *In* Textbook of Pediatric Rheumatology, 3rd ed. Philadelphia, WB Saunders, 1995, p 467.
24. Sponseller PD, Malech HL, McCarthy EF, et al: Skeletal involvement in children who have chronic granulomatous disease. J Bone Joint Surg Am 74: 37, 1991.
25. Wolfson JJ, Kane WJ, Laxdal SD, et al: Bone findings in chronic granulomatous disease of childhood. A genetic abnormality of leukocyte function. J Bone Joint Surg Am 51:1573, 1969.
26. Payne NR, Hays NT, Regelmann WE, et al: Growth in patients with chronic granulomatous disease. J Pediatr 102: 397, 1983.
27. Landing BH, Shirkey HS: A syndrome of recurrent infection and infiltration of the viscera by pigmented lipid histiocytes. Pediatrics 20: 431, 1957.
28. Ford DK, Price GE, Culling CFA, et al: Familial lipochrome pigmentation of histiocytes, with hyperglobulinemia, pulmonary infiltration, splenomegaly, arthritis and susceptibility to infection. Am J Med 33: 478, 1962.
29. Rodey GE, Park BH, Ford DK, et al: Defective bactericidal activity of peripheral blood leukocytes in lipochrome histiocytosis. Am J Med 49: 322, 1970.
30. Davis SD, Schaller JG, Wedgwood RJ: Job's syndrome. Recurrent "cold" staphylococcal abscesses. Lancet 1: 1013, 1966.
31. Barak Y, Nir E: Chédiak-Higashi syndrome. Am J Pediatr Hematol Oncol 9: 42, 1987.
32. Windhorst DB, White JG, Dent PB, et al: The Chédiak-Higashi anomaly and the Aleutian trait in mink. Ann N Y Acad Sci 155: 818, 1968.
33. Jacobs JC, Goetzl EJ: "Streaking Leucocyte factor," arthritis and pyoderma gangrenosum. Pediatrics 56: 570, 1975.
34. Jacobs JC: The differential diagnosis of arthritis in childhood. *In* Pediatric Rheumatology for the Practitioner, 2nd ed. New York, Springer-Verlag, 1993, p 153.
35. Ratnoff DR: Inherited deficiencies of complement in rheumatic diseases. Rheum Dis Clin North Am 22: 75, 1998.
36. Fries LF, O'Shea JJ, Frank MM: Inherited deficiencies of complement and complement-related problems. Clin Immunol Immunopathol 40: 37, 1986.
37. Walport MJ, Davies KA, Botto M: C1q and systemic lupus erythematosus. Immunobiology 199: 265, 1998.
38. Atkinson JP: Complement deficiency: predisposing factor to auto-immune syndromes. Clin Exp Rheumatol 53(Suppl 7): 95, 1989.
39. Agnello V: Complement deficiency states. Medicine (Baltimore) 57: 1, 1987.
40. Agnello V: Lupus diseases associated with hereditary and acquired deficiencies of complement. Springer Semin Immunopathol 9: 161, 1986.
41. Ruddy S: Complement deficiencies and rheumatic diseases. *In* Keely WN, Harris ED Jr, Ruddy S, et al (eds): Textbook of Rheumatology, 4th ed. Philadelphia, WB Saunders, 1993, p 1283.
42. Lachman PJ: Complement deficiency and the pathogenesis of autoimmune immune complex disease. *In* Walksman BH (ed): 1939–1989: Fifty Years Progress in Allergy. Chem Immunol 49: 245, 1990.
43. Ross SC, Densen P: Complement deficiency states and infection. Epidemiology, pathogenesis and consequences of neisserial and other infections in an immune deficiency. Medicine (Baltimore) 63: 243, 1984.
44. Rosenfeld GB, Partridge REH, Barholomew W, et al: Hereditary angioneurotic edema (HANE) and systemic lupus erythematosus (SLE) in one of identical twin girls. J Allergy Clin Immunol 53: 68, 1974.
45. Nagata M, Hara T, Aoki T, et al: Inherited deficiency of the ninth component of complement: an increased risk of meningococcal meningitis. J Pediatr 114: 260, 1989.
46. Leggiadro RJ, Winkelstein JA: Prevalence of complement deficiencies in children with systemic meningococcal infections. Pediatr Infect Dis 6: 75, 1987.
47. Gatenby PA, Barbosa JE, Lachmann PJ: Differences between C4A and C4B in the handling of immune complexes: the enhancement of CR1 binding is more important than the inhibition of immunoprecipitation. Clin Exp Immunol 79: 158, 1990.
48. Reid KBM: Deficiency of the first component of human complement. Immunodef Rev 1: 247, 1989.
49. Reveille JD, Arnett FC, Wison RW, et al: Null alleles of the fourth component of complement and HLA-haplotypes in familial systemic lupus erythematosus. Immunogenetics 21: 299, 1985.
50. Fielder AH, Walport MJ, Batchelor JR, et al: Family study of the major histocompatibility complex in patients with systemic lupus erythematosus: importance of null alleles of C4A and C4B in determining disease susceptibility. Br Med J 286: 425, 1983.
51. Goldstein R, Arnett FC, McClean RH, et al: Molecular heterogeneity of complement component C4-null and 21-hydroxylase genes in systemic lupus erythematosus. Arthritis Rheum 31: 736, 1988.
52. Kumar A, Kumar P, Schur PH: DR3 and nonDR3 associated complement component C4A deficiency in systemic lupus erythematosus. Clin Immunol Immunopathol 60: 55, 1991.

53. Steinsson K, Erlendsson K, Valdimarsson H: Successful plasma infusion treatment of a patient with C2 deficiency and systemic lupus erythematosus: clinical experience over forty-five months. Arthritis Rheum 32: 906, 1989.
54. Bowness P, Davies KA, Norsworthy PJ, et al: Hereditary C1q deficiency and systemic lupus erythematosus. Q J Med 87: 455, 1994.
55. Sato EI, Assis LS, Laurenzi VP, et al: Long-term thalidomide in refractory cutaneous lesions of systemic lupus erythematosus. Rev Assoc Med Bras 44: 298, 1998.
56. Hoekzema R, Brouwer MC, de Graeff-Meeder ER, et al: Biosynthesis of normal and low-molecular-mass complement component C1q by cultured human monocytes and macrophages. Biochem J 257: 477, 1989.
57. Agnello V, deBracco MME, Kunkel HG: Hereditary C2 deficiency with some manifestations of systemic lupus erythematosus. J Immunol 108: 837, 1972.
58. Glass D, Raum D, Gibson D, et al: Inherited deficiency of the second component of complement. Rheumatic disease associations. J Clin Invest 58: 853, 1976.
59. Osofsky SG, Thompson BH, Lint TF, et al: Hereditary deficiency of the third component of complement in a child with fever, skin rash and arthralgias, and response to whole blood transfusion. J Pediatr 90: 180, 1977.
60. Roord JJ, Daha M, Kuis W, et al: Hereditary deficiency of the third component of complement in two sisters with systemic lupus erythematosus-like symptoms. Arthritis Rheum 24: 1255, 1981.
61. Mclean RH, Weinstein A, Chapitis J, et al: Familial partial deficiency of the third component of complement and the hypocomplementemic cutaneous vasculitis syndrome. Am J Med 68: 549, 1980.
62. Winkelstein JA, Fivush B, Amerantunga R, et al: Successful renal transplantation in C3 deficiency. Mol Immunol 35: 760, 1998.
63. Rosenfeld SI, Kelly ME, Leddy JP: Hereditary deficiency of the fifth component of complement in man: I. Clinical, immunochemical, and family studies. J Clin Invest 57: 1626, 1976.
64. Leddy JP, Frank MM, Gaither TA, et al: Hereditary deficiency of the sixth component of complement in man: I. Clinical, immunochemical, and family studies. J Clin Invest 53: 44, 1974.
65. Boyer JT, Gall EP, Norman ME, et al: Hereditary deficiency of the seventh component of complement. J Clin Invest 56: 905, 1975.
66. Zeitz HJ, Miller GW, Lint TF, et al: Deficiency of C7 with systemic lupus erythematosus: solubilization of immune complexes in complement deficiency sera. Arthritis Rheum 24: 87, 1981.
67. Jasin HE: Absence of the eighth component of complement in association with systemic lupus erythematosus-like disease. J Clin Invest 60: 709, 1977.
68. Wulffraat NM, Sanders EAM, Fijen CAP, et al: Deficiency of the β subunit of the eighth component of complement presenting as arthritis and exanthem. Arthritis Rheum 37: 1704, 1994.
69. Espinoza LR, Gutierrez S, Berman A: Immunodeficiency states and associated rheumatic manifestations. Curr Opin Rheumatol 7: 65, 1995.
70. Sleasman JW: The association between immunodeficiency and the development of autoimmune disease. Adv Dent Res 10: 57, 1996.
71. Stein CM: Immunodeficient states and associated rheumatic manifestations. Curr Opin Rheumatol 8: 52, 1996.
72. Tucker LB, Miller LC, Schaller JG: Rheumatic disorders. *In* Stiehm R (ed): Immunologic Disorders in Infants and Children, 4th ed. Philadelphia, WB Saunders, 1996, p 742.
73. WHO Scientific Group: Primary immunodeficiency diseases. Clin Exp Immunol 109(Suppl 1): 1, 1997.
74. Rosen FS, Cooper MD, Wedgwood RJP: The primary immunodeficiencies. N Engl J Med 333: 431, 1995.
75. Fischer A, Cavazzana-Calvo M, De Saint Basile G, et al: Naturally occurring primary deficiencies of the immune system. Annu Rev Immunol 15: 93, 1997.
76. Buckley RH, Schiff E, Schiff SE, et al: Human severe combined immunodeficiency: genetic, phenotypic, and functional diversity in one hundred eight infants. J Pediatr 130: 378, 1997.
77. Stephan JL, Vlekova V, Le Deist F, et al: A severe combined immunodeficiency: a retrospective single-center study of the clinical presentation and outcome in 117 cases. J Pediatr 123: 564, 1993.
78. De Saint Basile G, Arveiler R, Oberlé I, et al: Close linkage of the locus for X chromosome linked severe combined immunodeficiency to polymorphic DNA markers in Xq11-13. Proc Natl Acad Sci U S A 84: 7576, 1987.
79. Noguchi M, Yi H, Rosenblatt HM, et al: Interleukin-2 receptor γchain mutation results in X-linked severe combined immunodeficiency in humans. Cell 3: 147, 1993.
80. Markert ML: Molecular basis of adenosine deaminase deficiency. Immunodeficiency 5: 141, 1993.
81. Hirschhorn R: Adenosine deaminase deficiency. Immunodef Rev 2: 175, 1990.
81a. Cavazzana-Calvo M, Hacein-Bey S, de Sainte Basile G, et al: Gene therapy of severe combined immunodeficiency (SCID)-XL disease. Science 288: 669, 2000.
82. Berthet F, Le Deist F, Duliege AM, et al: Clinical consequences and treatment of primary immunodeficiency syndromes characterized by functional T and B lymphocyte anomalies (combined immune deficiency). Pediatrics 93: 265, 1994.
83. Cooper M D, Chase HP, Lowman JT, et al: Wiskott-Aldrich syndrome: an immunologic deficiency disease involving the afferent limb of immunity. Am J Med 44: 499, 1968.
84. Kwan S, Hageman TL, Radtke BE, et al: Identification of mutations in the Wiskott-Aldrich syndrome gene and characterization of a polymorphic dinucleotide repeat at DXS6940, adjacent to the disease gene. Proc Natl Acad Sci U S A 92: 4706, 1995.
85. Perry GS, Spector BD, Schuman LM, et al: The Wiskott-Aldrich syndrome in the United States and Canada (1892–1979). J Pediatr 7: 72, 1980.
86. Schaller JG: Immunodeficiency and autoimmunity. *In* Bergsma D (ed): Immunodeficiency in Man and Animals. Birth Defects 11: 173, 1975.
87. Lau YL, Wong SN, Lawton WM: Takayasu's arteritis associated with Wiskott-Aldrich syndrome. J Paediatr Child Health 28: 407, 1992.
88. Gatti RA, Platt N, Pomerance HH, et al: Hereditary, lymphopenic agammaglobulinemia associated with a distinctive form of short-limbed dwarfism and ectodermal dysplasia. J Pediatr 75: 675, 1969.
89. Polmar SH, Pierce GF: Cartilage hair hypoplasia: immunological aspects and their clinical implications. Clin Immunol Immunopathol 40: 87, 1986.
90. Oen F, Petty RE, Schroeder ML: Immunoglobulin A deficiency: genetic studies. Tissue Antigens 19: 174, 1982.
91. Cassidy JT, Nordby GL: Human serum immunoglobulin concentrations: prevalence of immunoglobulin deficiencies. J Allerg Clin Immunol 55: 35, 1975.
92. Liblau RS, Bach JF: Selective IgA deficiency and autoimmunity. Int Arch Allergy Immunol 99: 16, 1992.
93. Cassidy JT, Oldham G, Platts-Mills TAE: Functional assessment of a B-cell defect in patients with selective IgA deficiency. Clin Exp Immunol 35: 296, 1979.
94. Petty RE, Palmer NR, Cassidy JT, et al: The association of autoimmune diseases and anti-IgA antibodies in patients with selective IgA deficiency. Clin Exp Immunol 37: 83, 1979.
95. Warrington RJ, Rutherford M, Sauder PJ, et al: Homologous antibody to human immunoglobulin IgA suppresses in vitro mitogen-induced IgA synthesis. Clin Immunol Immunopathol 23: 698, 1982.
96. Mochizuki S, Smith CIE, Hallgren R, Hammarstrom L: Systemic immunization against IgA immunoglobulin deficiency. Clin Exp Immunol 94: 334, 1993.
97. Gershwin ME, Blaese RM, Steinberg AD, et al: Antibodies to nucleic acids in congenital immune deficiency states. J Pediatr 89: 377, 1976.
98. Petty RE, Sherry, DD, Johannson J: Anti-IgA antibodies in pregancy. N Engl J Med 313: 1620, 1985.
99. Pelkonen P, Savilahti E, Mäkelä AL: Persistent and transient IgA deficiency in juvenile rheumatoid arthritis. Scand J Rheumatol 12: 273, 1983.
100. Friman V, Quiding M, Czerkinsky C, et al: Intestinal and circulating antibody-forming cells in IgA deficient individuals after oral cholera vaccination. Clin Exp Immunol 95: 222, 1994.

101. Cobain TJ, Stuckey MC, McCluskey J, et al: The coexistence of IgA deficiency and 21-hydroxylase deficiency marked by specific MHC supratypes. Ann N Y Acad Sci 458: 76, 1985.
102. French MA, Dawkins RL: Central MHC genes, IgA deficiency and autoimmune diseases. Immunol Today 11: 271, 1990.
103. Howe HS, So AKL, Farrant J, et al: Common variable immunodeficiency is associated with polymorphic markers in the human major histocompatibility complex. Clin Exp Immunol 84: 387, 1991.
104. Barkley DO, Hohermuth HJ, Howard A, et al: IgA deficiency in juvenile chronic arthritis. J Rheumatol 6: 219, 1979.
104a. Salmi TT, Schmidt E, Laaksonen AL, et al: Levels of immunoglobulins in juvenile rheumatoid arthritis. Ann Clin Res 5: 395, 1973.
105. Itescu S: Adult immunodeficiency and rheumatic disease. Rheum Dis Clin North Am 22: 53, 1996.
106. Stanworth DR, Johns P, Williamson N, et al: Drug-induced IgA deficiency in rheumatoid arthritis. Lancet 1: 1001, 1977.
107. van Riel PLCM, van de Putte LBA, Gribnau AJ, et al: IgA deficiency during aurothioglucose treatment. Scand J Rheumatol 13: 334, 1984.
108. Delamere JP, Farr M, Grindulis KA: Sulphasalazine induced selective IgA deficiency in rheumatoid arthritis. Br Med J 286: 1547, 1983.
109. Savilahti E: Sulphasalazine induced immunodeficiency. Br Med J 287: 759, 1983.
110. Leickly FE, Buckley RH: Development of IgA and IgG2 subclass deficiency after sulfasalazine therapy. J Pediatr 108: 481, 1986.
110a. van Rossum MAJ, Fiselier TJW, Franssen MJAM, et al: Effects of sulfasalazine treatment on serum immunoglobulin levels in children with juvenile chronic arthritis. Scand J Rheumatol (in press).
111. Cassidy JT, Petty RE, Sullivan DB: Occurrence of selective IgA deficiency in children with juvenile rheumatoid arthritis. Arthritis Rheum 20(Suppl): 181, 1977.
112. Cassidy, JT, Petty RE, Sullivan DB: Abnormalities in the distribution of serum immunoglobulin concentrations in juvenile rheumatoid arthritis. J Clin Invest 52: 1931, 1973.
113. Panush RS, Bianco NE, Schur PH, et al: Juvenile rheumatoid arthritis. Cellular hypersensitivity and selective IgA deficiency. Clin Exp Immunol 10: 103, 1972.
114. Huntley CC, Thorpe DP, Lyerly AD, et al: Rheumatoid arthritis with IgA deficiency. Am J Dis Child 113: 411, 1967.
115. Pelkonen P, Salilahti E, Westeren L, et al: IgA deficiency in juvenile rheumatoid arthritis. Scand J Rheumatol 8(Suppl): 4, 1975.
116. Cassidy JT, Burt A, Petty RE, et al: Prevalence of selective IgA deficiency in patients with connective tissue disease. N Engl J Med 280: 275, 1969.
117. Goshen E, Livne A, Krupp M, et al: Antinuclear and related autoantibodies in sera of healthy subjects with IgA deficiency. J Autoimmun 2: 51, 1989.
118. Cleland LG, Bell DA: The occurrence of systemic lupus erythematosus in two kindreds in association with selective IgA deficiency. J Rheumatol 5: 3, 1978.
119. Petty RE, Cassidy JT, Sullivan DB: Reversal of selective IgA deficiency in a child with juvenile rheumatoid arthritis after plasma transfusions. Pediatrics 51: 44, 1973.
120. Thomas LLM, Alberts C, Pegels JG, et al: Sarcoidosis associated with autoimmune thrombocytopenia and selective IgA deficiency. Scand J Haematol 28: 357, 1982.
120a. Cassidy JT: Selective IgA deficiency and chronic arthritis in children. *In* Moore TD (ed): Arthritis in Childhood. Report of the Eightieth Ross Conference on Pediatric Research. Columbus, OH, Ross Laboratories, 1981, p 82.
121. Jay S, Helm S, Wray BB: Progressive systemic scleroderma with IgA deficiency in a child. Am J Dis Child 135: 965, 1981.
122. Spirer Z, Ilie I, Pick A, et al: Localized scleroderma following varicella in a 3-year-old girl with IgA deficiency. Acta Paediatr Scand 68: 783, 1979.
123. Good AE, Cassidy JT, Mutchnick MG, et al: Ankylosing spondylitis with selective IgA deficiency and a circulating anticoagulant. J Rheumatol 4: 297, 1977.
124. Bruton OC: Agammaglobulinemia. Pediatrics 9: 722, 1952.
125. Kwan SP, Kunkel L, Bruns G: Mapping of the X-linked agammaglobulinemia locus by use of restriction fragment-length polymorphism. J Clin Invest 77: 649, 1986.
126. Cunningham-Rundles C: Clinical and immunological analyses of 103 patients with common variable immunodeficiency. J Clin Immunol 9: 22, 1989.
127. Lee AH, Levinson AI, Schumacher HR: Hypogammaglobulinemia and rheumatic disease. Semin Arthritis Rheum 22: 252, 1993.
128. Conley ME, Park L, Douglas SD: Childhood common variable immunodeficiency with autoimmune disease. J Pediatr 108: 915, 1986.
129. Sneller MC, Strober W, Eisenstein E, et al: New insights into common variable immunodeficiency. Ann Intern Med 118: 720, 1993.
130. Kruger G, Welte K, Ciobanu N, et al: Interleukin-2 correction of defective in vitro T cell mitogenesis in patients with common variable immunodeficiency. J Clin Immunol 4: 295, 1984.
131. Grierson H, Purtillo DT: Epstein-Barr virus infections in males with the X-linked lymphoproliferative syndrome. Ann Intern Med 106: 538, 1987.
132. McLaughlin JF, Schaller JG, Wedgwood RJ: Arthritis and immunodeficiency. J Pediatr 81: 801, 1972.
133. Schaller JG: Arthritis and immunodeficiency. Arthritis Rheum 20: 443, 1977.
134. Lederman HM, Winkelstein J: X-linked agammaglobulinemia: an analysis of 96 patients. Medicine (Baltimore) 64: 145, 1985.
135. Jerne NK: Towards a network theory of the immune system. Ann Immunol (Paris) 125c: 373, 1974.
136. Petty RE, Cassidy JT, Tubergen DG: Association of arthritis with hypogammaglobulinemia. Arthritis Rheum 20: 441, 1977.
137. Uluhan A, Sager D, Jasin HE: Juvenile rheumatoid arthritis and common variable hypogammaglobulinemia. J Rheumatol 25:1205, 1998.
138. Swaak AJG, van der Brink HG: Common variable immunodeficiency in a patient with systemic lupus erythematosus. Lupus 5: 242, 1996.
139. Düzgün N, Duman M, Sonel B, et al: Lupus vulgaris in a patient with systemic lupus erythematosus and persistent IgG deficiency. Rheumatol Int 16: 213, 1997.
139a. Janeway CA, Gitlin D, Craig JM, et al: "Collagen disease" associated with congenital agammaglobulinemia. Trans Assoc Am Physicians 69: 93, 1956.
139b. Good RA, Rotstein J, Mazzitello WF: The simultaneous occurrence of rheumatoid arthritis and agammaglobulinemia. J Lab Clin Med 49: 343, 1957.
139c. Page AR, Hansen AE, Good RA: Occurrence of leukemia and lymphoma in patients with agammaglobulinemia. Blood 21: 197, 1963.
139d. Janeway CA, Rosen FS, Merler E, et al: The antibody deficiency syndromes. *In* Janeway CA, Rosen FS, Merler E (eds): The Gamma Globulins. Boston, Little, Brown, 1967, p 75.
140. Gotoff SP, Smith RD, Sugar O: Dermatomyositis with cerebral vasculitis in a patient with agammaglobulinemia. Am J Dis Child 123: 53, 1972.
141. Bardelas JA, Winkelstein JA, Seto DS, et al: Fatal ECHO 24 infection in a patient with hypogammaglobulinemia. Relationship to dermatomyositis-like syndrome. J Pediatr 90: 396, 1977.
142. Page AR, Hansen AE, Good RA: Occurrence of leukemia and lymphoma in patients with agammaglobulinemia. Blood 21: 197, 1963.
143. Wilfert CM, Buckley RH, Mahanakumar T, et al: Persistent and fatal central-nervous-system echovirus infections in patients with agammaglobulinemia. N Engl J Med 296: 1485, 1977.
144. Webster AD, Tripp JH, Hayward AR, et al: Echovirus encephalitis and myositis in primary immunoglobulin deficiency. Arch Dis Child 53: 33, 1978.
144a. Maguire JR, Perez-Atayde AR, Geha RS: Vasculitis presenting in an infant with agammaglobulinemia. Ann Allergy 57: 14, 1986.
145. Mease PJ, Ochs HD, Wedgwood RJ: Successful treatment of echovirus meningoencephalitis and myositisfasciitis with intravenous immune globulin therapy in a patient with X-linked agammaglobulinemia. N Engl J Med 304: 1278, 1984.
146. Crennan JM, Van Scoy RE, McKenna CH, et al: Echovirus poly-

myositis in patients with hypogammaglobulinemia. Am J Med 81: 35, 1986.
147. Plebani A, Ugazio AG, Avanzini MA, et al: Serum IgG subclass concentrations in healthy subjects at different age: age normal percentile chart. Eur J Pediatr 149: 164, 1989.
148. Shackelford PG, Granoff DM, Polmar SH, et al: Subnormal serum concentrations of IgG2 in children with frequent infections associated with varied patterns of immunologic dysfunction. J Pediatr 116: 529, 1990.
149. Cunningham-Rundles C: Antibodies to phosphorylcholine in sera of patients with humoral immunodeficiency disease. Monogr Allergy 20: 42, 1985.
150. Oxelius VA: IgG subclasses and human disease. Am J Med 76: 7, 1985.
151. Heiner DC, Lee SI, Short JA: IgG4 subclass deficiency syndromes. Monogr Allergy 20: 149, 1986.
152. Aucouturier P, Lacombe C, Bremard C, et al: Serum IgG subclass levels in patients with primary immunodeficiency syndromes or abnormal susceptibility to infections. Clin Immunol Immunopathol 51: 22, 1989.
153. Rostoker G, Peck MA, Del Prato S, et al: Serum IgG subclasses and IgM imbalances in adult IgA mesangial glomerulonephritis and idiopathic Henoch-Schönlein purpura. Clin Exp Immunol 75: 30, 1989.

Primary and Acquired Disorders of Bone and Connective Tissue

6

36

Musculoskeletal Manifestations of Systemic Disease

James T. Cassidy and Ross E. Petty

A great many systemic disorders cause musculoskeletal signs or symptoms. Sometimes these are trivial; occasionally, they are the predominant presentations of the underlying disease. This chapter outlines the most significant systemic disorders that may present in the guise of an inflammatory rheumatic disease. It is not our intent to describe comprehensively the clinical and laboratory manifestations or management of such disorders; for this, the reader is referred to standard textbooks dealing with the specific diseases.

NUTRITIONAL ABNORMALITIES

The category of nutritional musculoskeletal disease encompasses a variety of disorders in which there is a defined or suspected nutritional deficiency or excess that results in signs or symptoms suggesting a rheumatic disease.

Rickets

Rickets is an ancient term introduced into the English literature around 1650 that includes several diseases associated with defective ossification of bone matrix (Table 36–1).[1] Rickets can result from deficiency of the active form of vitamin D (1,25-dihydroxyvitamin D_3), from a deficiency of phosphate, or (very rarely) from a deficiency of calcium. Some types (hypophosphatemic rickets and rickets associated with hypophosphatasia) are classified as osteochondrodysplasias associated with defective mineralization and are discussed in Chapter 37.

The affected child presents with pain in the joints and tenderness over the bones. Bowing of the long bones and splaying of the rib cage are characteristic features. Proximal muscle weakness, particularly of the lower extremities, occasionally is dramatic. Defective bone growth results from suppression of calcification and maturation of epiphyseal cartilage. The result is a wide, frayed, irregular zone of uncalcified osteoid at the epiphyseal line—the rachitic metaphysis (Fig. 36–1).

Vitamin D–deficiency rickets has been recognized since ancient times. In humans, the normal source of vitamin D_3 is the skin, where the ultraviolet rays of sunlight convert 7-dehydrocholesterol into the prohormone. This is subsequently transformed to the 25-hydroxy form in the liver and to the active 1,25-dihydroxyvitamin in the kidney (Fig. 36–2). A deficiency of 1,25-dihydroxyvitamin D_3 may result from a nutritional deficiency, from failure of the liver to convert vitamin D to 25-hydroxyvitamin D, or from failure of the kidney to convert 25-hydroxyvitamin D to 1,25-dihydroxyvitamin D_3.

Worldwide, most cases of rickets result from exclu-

Table 36–1

Causes of Rickets

TYPE	CAUSE OR BIOCHEMICAL ABNORMALITY
Vitamin D deficiency	Exclusion from light or insufficient dietary vitamin D
Calcium deficiency	Impaired calcium absorption in celiac disease, inflammatory bowel disease, scleroderma, or liver disease
Vitamin D resistance	Impaired parathormone-dependent proximal renal tubular reabsorption of phosphate
Vitamin D dependence	
Type 1	Defect in renal 1-α-hydroxylase
Type 2	End-organ unresponsiveness to 1,25-dihydroxyvitamin D_3
Hypophosphatasia	Decreased serum alkaline phosphatase

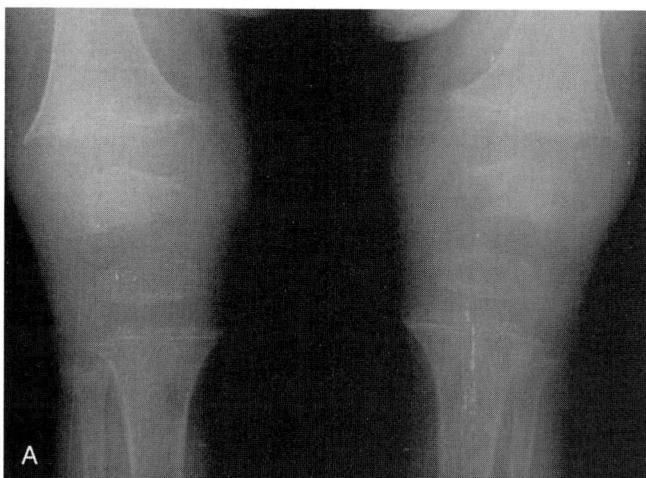

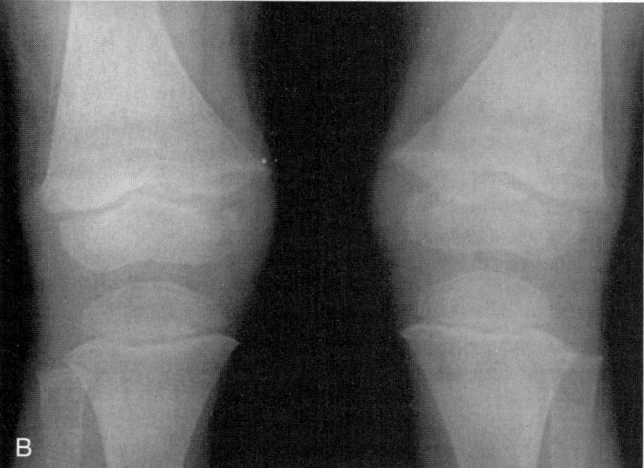

Figure 36–1. Vitamin D–deficient rickets in a toddler. *A*, Radiographs of knees demonstrate rachitic metaphyseal changes, indistinct cortices, and poorly defined trabeculation. The zone of provisional calcification is almost completely absent, the axial height of the epiphyseal plate is markedly increased, and cupping is evident. *B*, Films taken 6 months later demonstrate progressive healing with replacement of vitamin D.

sion from the sun for social or cultural reasons or from insufficient dietary intake of vitamin D. Vitamin D–deficiency rickets is seldom encountered in developed countries but may occur in infantile and adolescent forms in the rest of the world.[2] In the presence of sufficient dietary vitamin D, impaired absorption secondary to celiac disease, inflammatory bowel disease, scleroderma, or liver disease may lead to vitamin D–deficiency rickets. Renal disease or the administration of anticonvulsant medications in children deprived of sunlight may also cause rickets. Glucocorticoids are antagonistic to vitamin D for calcium transport.

Hypophosphatemic vitamin D–resistant rickets, when expressed in infancy, leads to short stature and bowing of the legs.[1, 3] Ectopic calcification may occur. A low serum phosphate concentration with a normal calcium level is characteristic. This disorder is inherited as an X-linked recessive or autosomal dominant trait, although sporadic cases occur. The basic defect is impaired parathormone-dependent proximal renal tubular reabsorption of phosphate.

Type I vitamin D–dependent rickets is an autosomal recessive defect in renal 1-alpha hydroxylase that results in failure of hydroxylation of 25-hydroxyvitamin D to 1,25-dihydroxyvitamin D_3. The onset of typical features of rickets occurs before the age of 2 years. *Type II vitamin D–dependent rickets* is very rare and is characterized by defective intracellular interaction between 1,25-dihydroxyvitamin D_3 and its receptor. Symptoms of rickets begin in early infancy before 1 year of age. Alopecia and absence of eyelashes occur frequently in this disorder.

Hypophosphatasia, a rare autosomal recessive disorder, presents as severe rickets and fractures.[1, 4] Band keratopathy, proptosis, and papilledema develop. There may be early loss of teeth. Marked depression in the concentration of alkaline phosphatase occurs. Chondrocalcinosis and pseudogout may be associated features. No treatment is effective.

Disorders that result in *renal tubular acidosis* may

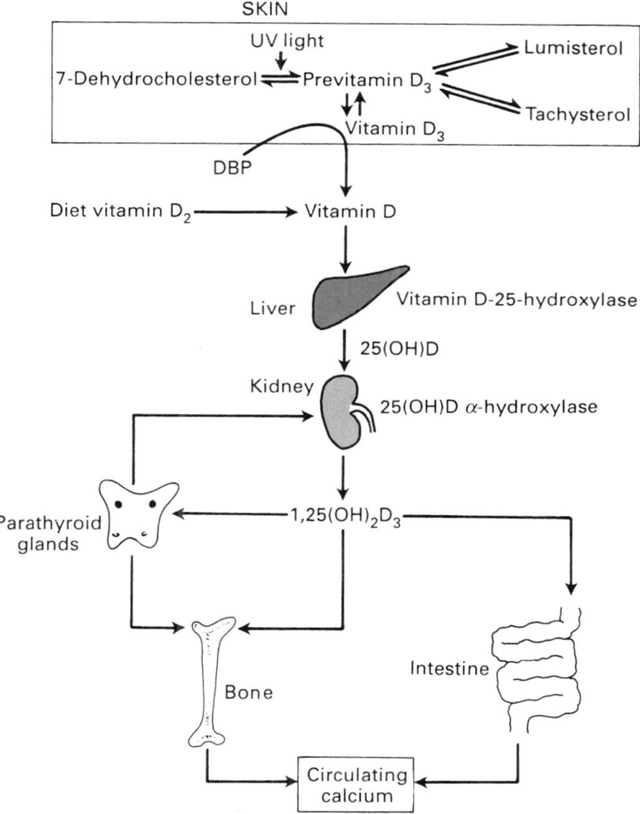

Figure 36–2. Metabolism of vitamin D. Previtamin D_3 is formed in the skin and isomerizes to vitamin D_3 or other biologically inert isomers. Vitamin D binding protein (DBP) has an affinity only for vitamin D_3, which is translocated to the circulation. Vitamin D is then hydroxylated in the liver and kidney to the active metabolite $1,25(OH)_2D_3$. (From Bhalla AK: Osteoporosis and osteomalacia. *In* Maddison PJ, Isenberg DA, Woo P, Glass DN [eds]: Oxford Textbook of Rheumatology. Oxford, England, Oxford University Press, 1993, p 1005.)

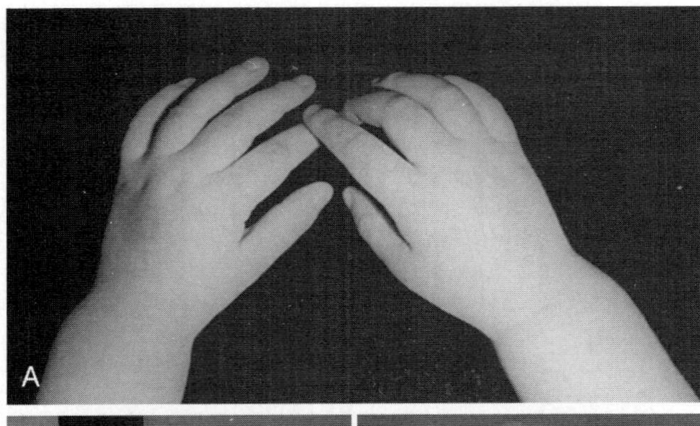

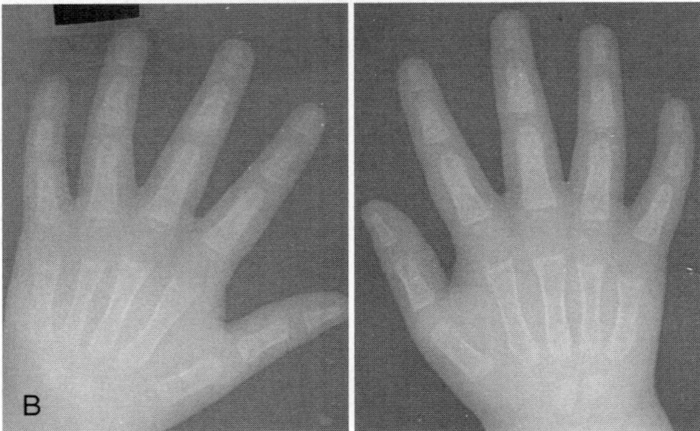

Figure 36–3. Cystinosis. An 18-month-old girl presented with joint pain primarily involving the large joints and profound muscle weakness due to cystinosis. *A*, Hands with swelling predominantly in the metaphyseal area of the radius and ulna—not the wrist joint proper. *B*, Radiographs demonstrate metaphyseal resorption typical of rickets.

present as rickets with pain in the joints and metaphyseal enlargement. We have encountered three children with *cystinosis* with this problem (Fig. 36–3).

Scurvy

Ascorbic acid (vitamin C) is required for the formation of normal collagen and chondroitin sulfate.[5] In scurvy, poor collagen synthesis leads to a tendency to intradermal and subperiosteal hemorrhage. Subperiosteal hemorrhage causes bone pain; the child, usually an infant, assumes the flexed posture of "pseudoparalysis" and is irritable when picked up. Hemarthroses may also occur. In severe cases, "scorbutic beads," resulting from subluxation of the sternum at the costochondral junctions, may be visible. Radiographs demonstrate subperiosteal new bone apposition.

Hypervitaminosis A

Excess intake of vitamin A causes pain in the extremities, irritability, apathy, alopecia, and delayed growth.[6,7] Cortical hyperostosis, particularly of the metatarsal bones and ulnas, is a typical radiographic finding. Abnormal epiphyseal growth and periosteal new bone apposition occur occasionally.

Endemic Osteoarthritis

Kashin-Beck disease and *Mseleni joint disease* are two examples of an early-onset polyarticular arthritis that are little known in the Western world. These disorders may represent the result of a geographically restricted nutritional deficiency or toxin, or they may be related to a heritable epiphyseal dysplasia in a genetically isolated population.

Kashin-Beck (Urov) Disease

Reports from northeastern Russia, Siberia, northern China, and North Korea have described an endemic arthritis in children, unassociated with systemic or visceral manifestations, that presumably develops as a result of eating bread baked from fungus-infected grain or from an epiphyseal dysplasia associated with selenium deficiency.[8–13] If the former is the case, unidentified mycotoxins produce a zonal necrosis of chondrocytes of the epiphyses and metaphyses of the bones. This disorder continues to increase in severity as long as the child lives in the endemic area and eats foods made with the infected grain. Excessive amounts of iron in the water and diet may contribute further to the polyarthritis. Experimental animals fed grain infected with *Fusarium* species have a similar form of epiphyseal dysplasia.[9]

Kashin-Beck disease causes symmetric polyarthritis and progressive enlargement and limitation of motion involving multiple joints (interphalangeal, wrist, knee, and ankle joints).[14] In the school-age child, aching and muscle weakness are the initial symptoms. Joint effusions and laboratory indices of inflammation are absent early in the disease. The eventual dwarfing, bone dysplasia with epiphyseal deformity, and short digits resemble those encountered in the lysosomal storage diseases.

Mseleni Joint Disease

A chronic polyarthritis affects a large proportion of the Tsonga population of the Mseleni area of northern Zululand on the eastern seaboard of South Africa.[15–17] The diagnosis is usually obvious in the geographic and racial context, but the differential diagnosis includes cretinism, brucellosis, hemochromatosis, alkaptonuria, and Legg-Calvé-Perthes disease. Hips, knees, and ankles are the predominant sites of involvement in 66 percent of the women, 25 percent of the men, 7 percent of the girls, and 4 percent of the boys. Hands, wrists, shoulders, and elbows are less commonly affected. The onset of joint pain in childhood or adolescence is the first symptom of disease. Restriction of movement and limitation of mobility develop at a variable rate. Mild stunting of growth is common, and a few patients develop severe dwarfing (Table 36–2). The life span is not shortened. Characteristic radiographic abnormalities include irregularity of the surface, density, and shape of the epiphyses progressing to a secondary

Table 36–2

Mseleni Joint Disease and Kashin-Beck Disease

	MSELENI JOINT DISEASE	KASHIN-BECK DISEASE
First noted	6 yr—adult	6–10 yr
Inherited	Probably not	Probably not
Sex ratio	More females	More males
Stunting of growth	Slight to severe	Moderate
Posture	Lumbar lordosis, genu valgum	Lumbar lordosis, neck extended, knees flexed
Precocious osteoarthritis	Yes	Yes
Radiology	Fragmented epiphyses, flared metaphyses, brachymetacarpia, protrusio acetabuli, platyspondyly	Dysplastic interphalangeal, wrist, knee, ankle joints; intra-articular loose bodies

osteoarthritis in both sexes; in the hips, which bear the brunt of the disease, protrusio acetabuli occurs in females (Fig. 36–4).[18] Short metacarpals, ulna, and radius and deformity of the distal end of the ulna are also present.

Fluorosis

Fluorosis is endemic in certain areas of the world and can cause chronic rheumatic symptoms in children.[19] High levels of fluoride may be found naturally in the water supply or may result from industrial pollution. Knee pain is often an early symptom, followed by limb, hand, or spinal abnormalities that suggest chronic inflammatory arthropathy. Radiographs demonstrate increased bone density, and later there is calcification of the spinal ligaments, intervertebral disks, and entheses.[20] Cord compression can result from narrowing of the spinal canal.

METABOLIC DISEASES

Abnormalities of Uric Acid Metabolism

Gout

The term *gout* refers to a group of disorders characterized by hyperuricemia and deposition of monosodium urate monohydrate crystals in tissues.[21–23] Its major clinical manifestations include acute monarthritis, most commonly in the first metatarsophalangeal (MTP) joint; chronic erosive arthritis associated with subcutaneous periarticular deposits of urate (tophi); and nephrolithiasis, often with chronic renal failure. Normal serum urate levels increase at puberty, particularly in males, from approximately 3.5 mg/dl (0.21 mmol/L) in childhood to an upper normal limit of 7 mg/dl (0.42 mmol/L) in adult males and 6 mg/dl (0.36 mmol/L) in adult

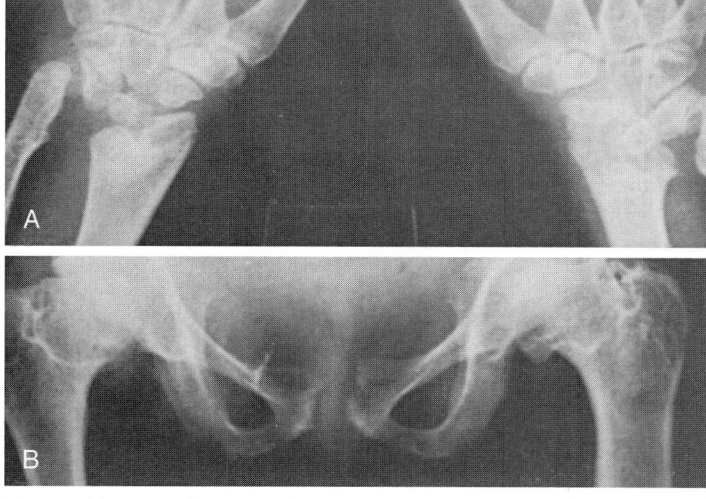

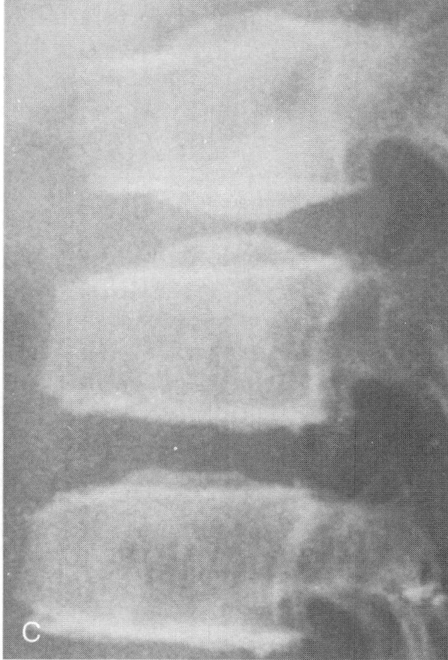

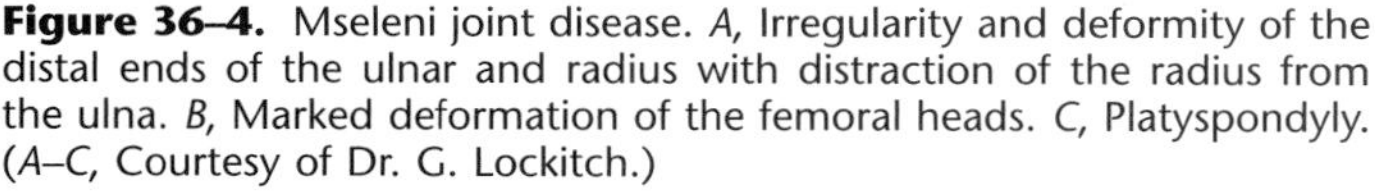

Figure 36–4. Mseleni joint disease. *A*, Irregularity and deformity of the distal ends of the ulnar and radius with distraction of the radius from the ulna. *B*, Marked deformation of the femoral heads. *C*, Platyspondyly. (*A–C*, Courtesy of Dr. G. Lockitch.)

Table 36–3

Causes of Hyperuricemia and Gout

Increased Uric Acid Production

Primary
- Lesch-Nyhan syndrome
- Becker's syndrome (phosphoribosyl pyrophosphate synthetase superactivity)

Secondary
- Glycogenosis type I (G6PD deficiency)
- Myeloproliferative disorders
- Lymphoproliferative disorders
- Severe psoriasis
- Gaucher's disease
- Cytotoxic drugs
- Hypoxia
- Chronic hemolysis
- Secondary polycythemia

Decreased Uric Acid Excretion

Reduced glomerular filtration rate

Reduced fractional urate excretion
- Down syndrome
- Lead nephropathy
- Analgesic nephropathy
- Amyloidosis
- Sickle cell anemia
- Sarcoidosis
- Hypothyroidism
- Hyperparathyroidism

Increased levels of organic acids
- Type I glycogen storage disease
- Maple syrup urine disease

Drugs
- Diuretics
- Salicylates (low-dose)
- Levodopa

females. Above these concentrations, the serum is saturated with urate. Gout may result from either increased production or decreased excretion of uric acid (Table 36–3).

Gouty arthropathy is very rare in children. In a comprehensive review of alleged cases of juvenile gout, Treadwell[24] found 66 patients younger than 20 years who were reported between 1769 and 1960, and added two additional cases. In many early publications, the exact diagnosis is in doubt. The onset of gouty arthritis in a 14-year-old boy as a result of chronic compensated hemolysis of unknown cause has been described.[25] Yarom and colleagues[26] reported two children with marked hyperuricemia, mild renal failure, and acute, episodic, painful swelling of one joint, often the first MTP joint, knee, ankle, elbow, or a proximal interphalangeal (PIP) joint of the hand. Gout has also been reported in children with glycogen storage disease,[27] malignancy,[28] and renal failure.[29–31] The diagnosis of gout is confirmed by the demonstration of negatively birefringent, needle-shaped monosodium urate crystals in synovial fluid via compensated polarized light microscopy. Treatment of the acute attack with nonsteroidal anti-inflammatory drugs (NSAIDs) such as indomethacin or with colchicine is usually effective. After the acute attack has subsided, allopurinol is the drug of choice for prevention of recurrences.[32, 33]

Lesch-Nyhan Syndrome

The *Lesch-Nyhan syndrome* was described in 1967 as an X-linked recessive disorder of uric acid metabolism and central nervous system dysfunction. It results from a deficiency of the enzyme hypoxanthine-guanine phosphoribosyltransferase (HPRT) (Table 36–4).[34–36] It is characterized by the childhood onset of choreoathetosis, spasticity, mental retardation, severe growth retardation, self-mutilation, hyperuricemia with increased uric acid synthesis, and uric acid crystalluria. Severity of the disorder is determined by the degree of HPRT deficiency based on unique mutations in each family.[37] Affected boys, however, do not develop acute gouty arthritis, at least not until the adolescent or adult years. Treatment with allopurinol effectively prevents the rheumatic complaints but does not alter the central nervous system disease, for which there is currently no effective therapy. An incomplete hereditary deficiency of the enzyme (the *Kelley-Seegmiller syndrome*) may occur in adolescent or adult males as severe gouty arthritis with renal calculi, but it lacks the dramatic neurologic and mutilating characteristics of the complete enzyme deficiency.

Phosphoribosyl Pyrophosphate Synthetase (PPRPS) Superactivity

An X-linked mutation resulting in excessive activity of PPRPS, the enzyme that converts ribose-5-phosphate to PP-ribose-phosphate, results in increased purine production and gout, sometimes with neurologic deficits and sensorineural deafness, in children and young adults.[38, 39] Allopurinol effectively controls this disorder.

Glucose-6-Phosphatase Deficiency

Glycogen storage disease type I *(von Gierke's disease)* may be associated with the onset of gouty arthritis in childhood.[40] Children with this disorder are stunted and have marked hepatosplenomegaly, progressive mental retardation, abnormalities of platelet function, and hypoglycemia. Hyperuricemia results from both increased catabolism of adenosine triphosphate and decreased urate excretion.

Table 36–4

Lesch-Nyhan Syndrome

Clinical characteristics	Progressive development of choreoathetosis, spasticity, and mental retardation with self-mutilation
Genetics	X-linked recessive
Biochemical defect	Deficiency of hypoxanthine-guanine phosphoribosyltransferase
Laboratory findings	Hyperuricemia and uric acid crystalluria

Calcium Pyrophosphate Deposition Disease (Pseudogout)

Crystals of calcium pyrophosphate dihydrate (CPPD) in synovial fluid and joint structures are associated with chronic inflammatory and degenerative joint disease.[22, 41] The wrists, knees, shoulders, and ankles are most commonly affected. *Chondrocalcinosis,* the deposition of CPPD crystals in hyaline cartilage and fibrocartilage, is a disease of the mature adult. In familial chondrocalcinosis, however, there have been rare reports of affected adolescents[42] in whom the disease presented as an acute, self-limited polyarthritis, often precipitated by exercise or trauma. The clinical disease has varied, however, depending on the kindred, age of onset, severity, and presence of an associated osteoarthritis or chondrodysplasia. Synovial fluid CPPD crystals are positively birefringent when viewed through a compensated polarized light microscope, and are much shorter than urate crystals. Radiographs delineate linear calcifications in the menisci of the knee and in other cartilagenous structures such as the triangular cartilage of the wrist.[43, 44]

Ochronosis

Ochronosis *(alkaptonuria)* is inherited as an autosomal recessive disorder.[45] A defect in homogentisic acid oxidase in phenylalanine and tyrosine metabolism leads to the accumulation of homogentisic acid in tissues and pigmentation of cartilage (ears, sclerae, heart valves), calcification and ossification of the intervertebral discs, accelerated osteoporosis and osteoarthritis, and vascular disease.[46] A secondary defect, inhibition of lysyl hydroxylation, leads to impairment of collagen cross-linking. Arthritis becomes symptomatic only in mid-adult life and has not been reported in children. Black urine or staining of the diapers is often the sign that prompts referral of the child with this metabolic defect.

Hyperlipoproteinemia

Defects in lipoprotein metabolism lead to a high premature risk of atherosclerosis and coronary artery disease and secondarily to musculoskeletal abnormalities.[47] Articular and tendinous swelling accompany essential familial hypercholesterolemia and hypertriglyceridemia. Both of these conditions are inherited as autosomal dominant traits.[47–49] Homozygotes are most severely involved. In type II hyperlipoproteinemia *(familial hypercholesterolemia),* the Achilles and patellar tendons and the extensor tendons of the hands are the principal locations of the xanthomata.[50] These lesions are associated with recurrent episodes of an acute migratory polyarthritis. In type IV hyperlipoproteinemia *(hypertriglyceridemia),* the hands, knees, and ankles are primarily affected by mild chronic or migratory oligoarthritis.[51] The onset is often acute, and fever and an elevated white blood cell count may occur. The arthritis is self-limited but may be misdiagnosed as acute rheumatic fever, especially if the tendon xanthomata are mistaken for nodules. Both large and small joints may also be involved by symmetric oligoarthritis. Disability from the joint disease is minimal.

Xanthomata of the tendons also occur in *sitosterolemia,* a syndrome resulting from accumulation of sterols derived from vegetable sources. The xanthomata initially appear in childhood and usually involve the extensor tendons of the hands and, later, the patellar, Achilles, and plantar tendons. Plasma sterol levels are elevated, and cholesterol levels may also be increased.[52, 53]

MUSCULOSKELETAL MANIFESTATIONS OF HEMATOLOGIC DISORDERS

Hemoglobinopathies

Homozygous sickle cell disease[54] and β-thalassemia[55, 56] can result in severe rheumatic disease. Musculoskeletal symptoms are caused by secondary skeletal changes that accompany hematopoietic expansion of the bone marrow and repeated episodes of avascular necrosis. *Sickle cell anemia* is inherited as an autosomal dominant trait and occurs almost exclusively in black children.[57] Acute arthritis and long bone pain may be severe and incapacitating during sickle cell crises. In the infant, dactylitis and periostitis of the small bones of the hands may cause painful swollen extremities and the hand-foot syndrome.[54] Each acute episode lasts 1 to 3 weeks and is characterized by diffuse, symmetric, painful swelling of the hands or feet. In a 1997 review, dactylitis occurred before 1 year of age in 41 of 392 children (10 percent) and was a predictor of severe disease in later life.[58] Osteonecrosis may occur in any bone and leads to marked abnormalities of growth and deformity. The hip is particularly vulnerable. It is also the usual site of the septic arthritis caused by *Salmonella* or other species to which these children are unduly susceptible. Differentiation of sickle cell bone infarction from osteomyelitis is sometimes difficult and is aided by scintigraphy and ultrasonography.[59] *Thalassemia minor* is characterized by anemia, hepatosplenomegaly, and recurrent brief episodes of joint pain, swelling, and effusion, especially in the ankles.[55, 56, 60]

Hemophilia

Recurrent intra-articular hemorrhage is a hallmark of classic hemophilia A (Factor VIII deficiency) and is one of the most important causes of morbidity in this X-linked recessive coagulopathy. The frequency of episodes of hemarthrosis is related to the concentration of Factor VIII in the vascular compartment. Levels higher than 5 percent of normal are associated with hemarthrosis in approximately half of the cases, whereas in children with lower levels of Factor VIII, hemarthroses almost invariably occur.[61] A similar association is found in *von Willebrand's disease*.[62]

Hemarthrosis can occur even before the child starts walking, and the frequency of episodes increases during the early childhood years. The most frequently affected joints are the knees, elbows, and ankles.[63] Bleeding into the small joints of the hands, feet, or spine is unusual. Hemorrhage into soft tissues, especially muscle, may be severe and can mimic hemarthrosis. Acute hemarthrosis is signaled by the onset over a few minutes to an hour of increasing pain, a feeling of fullness in the joints, and loss of range of motion. The joint is warm and distended. Resorption of the hemarthrosis takes place over several days with effective Factor VIII replacement. Intra-articular bleeds, however, tend to be recurrent and to lead to secondary proliferation of synovium with hemosiderosis that produces a diffuse increase in the density of the soft tissues on radiographs that is highly suggestive of the diagnosis. These debilitating changes may develop in as little time as 1 to 2 years.

Radiographic findings range from changes in the density of soft tissues to epiphyseal overgrowth, osteoporosis, subchondral cyst formation and bony sclerosis, squaring of the patella, narrowing of the joint space, and, eventually, osteoarthritis (Fig. 36–5).[64] Widening of the femoral intercondylar notch is characteristic.

Intensive physical therapy with strengthening of the muscles around affected joints helps to prevent hemarthroses.[58, 65] Management of the acute bleed consists of Factor VIII replacement,[63] application of ice to the affected joint, splinting, and rest. Agents that affect coagulation (such as NSAIDs) should be avoided. Joint aspiration has only a limited therapeutic role and must be preceded by Factor VIII administration.[64] Arthrocentesis accompanied by intra-articular glucocorticoid is sometimes dramatically effective in reducing the severity and frequency of hemarthroses,[66] as is prophylactic administration of Factor VIII. Surgical or radiation synovectomy may have a place in treating the older child with early destructive changes.

MUSCULOSKELETAL MANIFESTATIONS OF DISORDERS OF ENDOCRINE AND EXOCRINE GLANDS

Diabetes Mellitus

With the exception of diabetes mellitus, musculoskeletal disease is rarely associated with endocrinopathies in childhood. Rosenbloom and coworkers[67–70] drew attention to a syndrome of juvenile-onset insulin-dependent diabetes mellitus, short stature, and contractures of the finger joints (*diabetic cheiroarthropathy* or *stiff-hand syndrome*) (Fig. 36–6 and Table 36–5). In a survey of 229 diabetics aged 7 to 18 years, 29 percent were found to have flexion contractures of one or more joints of the fingers, most often the PIP joints of the fifth or fourth fingers.[68] In a few children, flexion contractures occurred in other joints as well (e.g., wrists, elbows, ankles, toes, knees) and spinal motion was decreased. In most instances, the child was unaware of any joint limitations and pain was absent. Functional disability was uncommon. The prevalence of joint contractures increased from less than 10 percent in those with diabe-

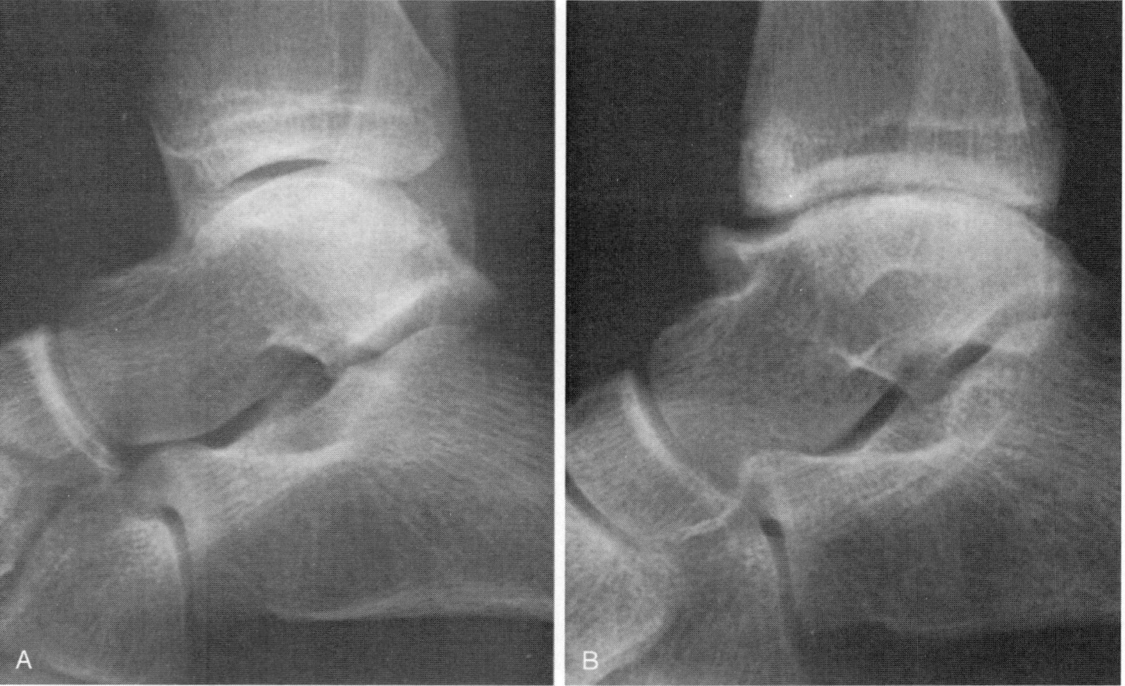

Figure 36–5. Hemophilic arthropathy. *A*, Normal ankle. *B*, Recurrent hemarthroses have resulted in arthritis characterized by a loss of joint space and development of a talar osteophyte. (*A* and *B*, Courtesy of Dr. R. Cairns.)

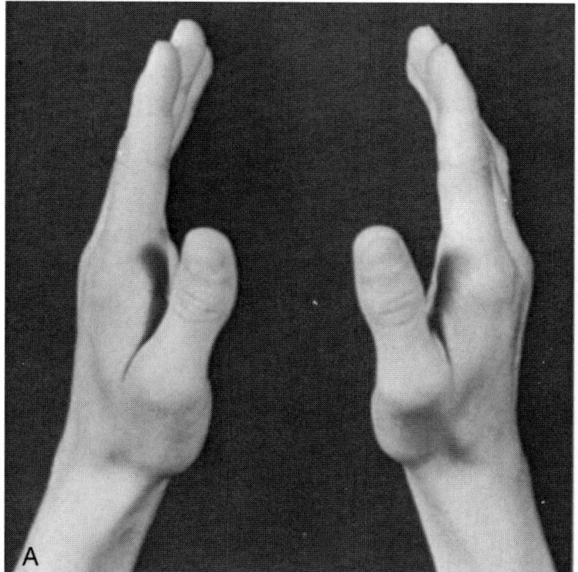

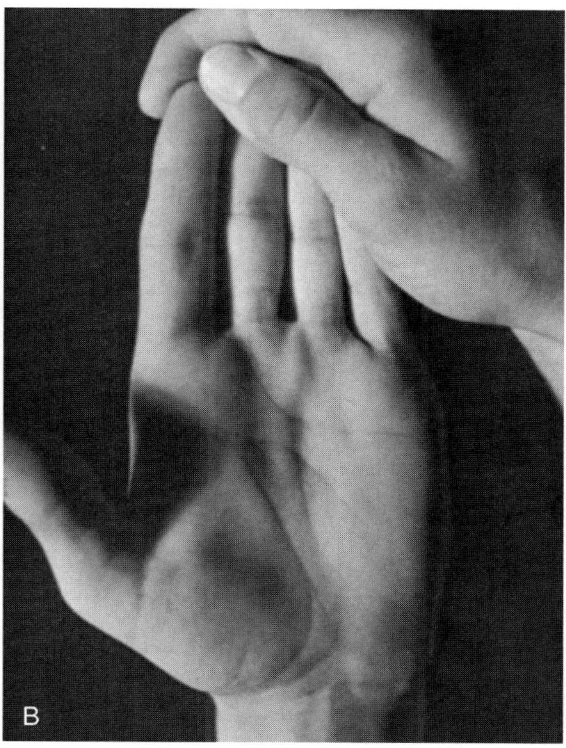

Figure 36–6. Diabetic cheiroarthropathy demonstrates soft tissue contractures that limit extension of the metacarpophalangeal and interphalangeal joints of the hands *(A)* and *(B)* flexor tendon contractures in the palm *(B)*. This was a 16-year-old boy in whom multiple flexion contractures without evidence of intra-articular or muscle inflammation had failed to respond to intense physical therapy over a 2-year period. Routine urinalysis demonstrated glucosuria, and further investigation led to a diagnosis of insulin-dependent diabetes mellitus. Two months after institution of insulin therapy, flexion contractures were considerably improved.

tes for less than 1 year to close to 50 percent in children with disease for longer than 9 years.[68] However, there did not appear to be a correlation with the severity of the diabetes or adequacy of its control. Tightening of the skin over the distal phalanges mimicked the acrosclerosis of scleroderma.

The frequency of juvenile rheumatoid arthritis (JRA) may be increased in children with diabetes mellitus (see Chapter 12).[71] Although Rosenbloom and his colleagues[67] noted that their patients did not have thickening of the palmar fascia, the incidence of *Dupuytren's contractures* is increased in adults with diabetes mellitus.[72] The precise relation of diabetes mellitus to contractures is unknown. Studies have demonstrated increased glucosylation of collagen in this syndrome.[73] Perhaps increased cross-linking of collagen leads to the contractures. NSAIDs have no beneficial effect on this particular disorder.

Occasionally, *hemochromatosis* occurs with diabetes mellitus and leads to an arthropathy that results in a characteristic firm bony enlargement of the second and third metacarpophalangeal (MCP) joints; other joints are affected less commonly.[74] This disorder has not been documented in childhood. *Diabetic osteopathy* is characterized by pain and osteoporosis of the distal metatarsal heads that may progress to erosion or even complete resorption of the ends of the bones.[75] This phenomenon is of unknown cause and has also not been recorded in childhood.

Table 36–5

Musculoskeletal Complications of Diabetes Mellitus

Rosenbloom's syndrome	Short stature, tight skin over distal digits, diabetic cheiroarthropathy
Dupuytren's contracture	Rare in childhood
Hemochromatosis	Rare in childhood
Diabetic osteolysis	Not recorded in childhood

Other Disorders of Endocrine Glands

Hyperparathyroidism is extremely rare in children; in adults, it may be characterized by fever, abdominal pain, musculoskeletal pain, osteoporosis,[76] mental disturbances, and headaches. Elevation of serum parathormone levels confirms the diagnosis.[77] *Pseudohypoparathyroidism* and *pseudopseudohypoparathyroidism* are classified as forms of acromelic dysplasia (see Chapter 37).

Both hyperthyroidism and hypothyroidism can be

associated with diffuse musculoskeletal pain and muscle weakness, although these disorders and their complications appear to be very rare in childhood. *Hashimoto's thyroiditis* can complicate systemic lupus erythematosus.[78] *Thyroid acropachy* is a rare form of hyperostosis of the phalanges, metacarpals, and metatarsals that is associated with hyperthyroidism, pretibial myxedema, exophthalmos, and clubbing.[79]

MUSCULOSKELETAL MANIFESTATIONS OF CYSTIC FIBROSIS

Musculoskeletal disease develops in a small proportion of children with cystic fibrosis (Table 36–6). Some children develop hypertrophic osteoarthropathy, others episodic arthritis, and less commonly, erosive arthritis. Approximately 5 percent of children with cystic fibrosis develop secondary hypertrophic osteoarthropathy.[80, 81] The occurrence of JRA, including rheumatoid factor–positive disease, has been reported in children with cystic fibrosis.[82] Episodic arthritis appears to be the most common musculoskeletal complication of cystic fibrosis.[83–86] In one study,[83] three boys and two girls, aged 2 to 20 years, had episodes of arthritis lasting from 1 to 10 days that occurred at intervals of weeks to months. One or more joints were affected during each episode. A pruritic nodular rash occurred in all five children. Results of serologic studies for rheumatoid factor and antinuclear antibody were negative, and radiographs demonstrated no abnormalities. The etiology and pathogenesis of this self-limited arthropathy are unknown, but it may be a reaction to chronic bacterial infection in the lung. There is no current evidence that fluoroquinolones used in the management of cystic fibrosis lead to arthropathy.[87] A child with cystic fibrosis complicated by sarcoidosis affecting the knee joints has been reported.[88]

PANCREATITIS WITH ARTHRITIS

Acute or chronic pancreatitis or pseudocyst formation from trauma to the pancreas may be accompanied by disseminated fat necrosis, leading to the development of subcutaneous nodules and osteolytic lesions resembling multicentric osteomyelitis or arthritis.[89–92] The nodules are tender, erythematous, and widely disseminated and are similar to those of erythema nodosum. They are often accompanied by systemic illness and fever. Joint pains and effusions may develop 2 to 3 weeks after the initial insult. The arthropathy is self-limited in most cases and remits spontaneously. Soft tissue swelling is evident on radiographs, with multiple sites of periosteal new bone apposition and diaphyseal lytic lesions. Because the bony lesions are delayed in appearance by a few months, the initiating abdominal trauma may have been forgotten. Diagnosis is confirmed during the acute illness by elevation of the serum lipase and amylase concentrations. A bone scan may demonstrate increased uptake of isotope in the metaphyses or diaphyses because of the infarctions that have resulted from the disseminated intravascular fat.

Table 36–6

Musculoskeletal Disorders Reported in Cystic Fibrosis

- Hypertrophic osteoarthropathy
- Episodic arthritis with rash
- Juvenile rheumatoid arthritis
- Sarcoidosis

Table 36–7

Causes of Secondary Hypertrophic Osteoarthropathy

- Malignant metastases to chest (lungs, pleura, mediastinum)
  - Osteosarcoma
  - Neuroblastoma
  - Lymphoma
- Chronic suppurative pulmonary disease
  - Cystic fibrosis
- Cyanotic congenital heart disease
- Gastrointestinal disease
  - Inflammatory bowel disease
  - Biliary cirrhosis/ductal atresia
- Thyroid acropachy

HYPEROSTOSIS

Hyperostosis, the abnormal subperiosteal or endochondral deposition of bone, is characteristic of a number of unrelated disorders (Table 36–7). *Hypertrophic osteoarthropathy* is a type of hyperostosis in which there is clubbing of the fingers and toes, painful subperiosteal apposition of new bone along the shafts of the long bones, and occasionally, arthritis. In children, it may be a primary sporadic or hereditary disease or it may develop secondary to suppurative lung disease, inflammatory bowel disease, malignancy, or tumor metastatic to lung, pleura, or mediastinum (see Chapter 38). Radiographs show distinctive periosteal new bone apposition, soft tissue swelling, and joint effusions. Bone scintigraphy demonstrates increased isotope uptake in the areas of new bone formation. Asymptomatic isolated clubbing can occur in children with cyanotic congenital heart disease. Familial clubbing can develop without associated systemic disease and is usually asymptomatic.

The *Goldbloom syndrome* is a form of idiopathic periosteal new bone formation associated with fever, constitutional symptoms, severe pain in the extremities, and elevated serum immunoglobulin levels and erythrocyte sedimentation rate.[93, 94] Radiographs demonstrate typical periosteal new bone apposition along the long bones. The child may develop limited motion in contiguous joints and refuse to walk if the lower extremities are involved. The disorder runs a chronic course over several months, with a spontaneous recovery. NSAIDs are sometimes useful for control of symptoms. There is no known cause, but the disorder may follow an infectious disease or viral syndrome.

Several of the *osteochondrodysplasias* characterized by increased bone density should be considered in the differential diagnosis of hyperostosis. These include *diaphyseal dysplasia (Camurati-Engelmann disease), craniodiaphyseal dysplasia (leontiasis ossea), cherubism, familial infantile cortical hyperostosis (Caffey's disease),* and *melorheostosis* (see Chapter 37). Children may also develop localized areas of periostitis secondary to repeated episodes of musculoskeletal trauma.[95, 96] *Pachydermoperiostosis* is a rare familial disorder characterized by digital clubbing, enlargement of the extremities, painful and swollen joints, hypertrophic skin changes (cutis verticis gyrata), and hypertrophic osteoarthropathy.[97, 98] It has been suggested that it represents generalized enthesopathy.

SPHINGOLIPIDOSES

In the sphingolipidoses, lipid accumulates in cells as a result of specific enzyme deficiencies.[99] Of the many different sphingolipidoses, three have musculoskeletal signs and symptoms (Table 36–8). *Farber's lipogranulomatosis* is an autosomal recessive sphingolipidosis marked in the neonatal period by a hoarse cry and irritability.[100, 101] Painful red masses develop along tendon sheaths and over pressure points as well as around the joints, especially the wrists, small joints of the hands and feet, elbows, knees, and ankles. Nodules have also been described in conjunctivae, ears, and nares. Epiglottal and laryngeal swelling results in repeated pulmonary infections, leading to death by about 2 years of age. Delayed motor development and mental retardation are prominent. The basic process underlying this disease is the cytoplasmic accumulation of a glycolipid ceramide in fibroblasts, histiocytes, macrophages, and neurons, an accumulation attributable to a deficiency of lysosomal acid ceramidase. The central nervous system, retina, respiratory tract, heart, liver, spleen, lymph nodes, synovium, and bone are all affected to varying degrees. Radiographic changes in the skeleton consist of osteoporosis, juxta-articular erosions, and disruption of the normal trabecular pattern.

In *Gaucher's disease*, glucocerebroside accumulates in the reticuloendothelial cells of the bone marrow, spleen, liver, lymph nodes, and viscera as a result of the autosomal recessive inheritance of a deficiency of glucocerebrosidase. Hepatosplenomegaly and pathologic fractures of the femur or vertebrae suggest the diagnosis. Premature osteoarthritis of weight-bearing joints is an important feature of the juvenile form of this disease. One of the diagnostic features of Gaucher's disease is widening of the distal femur. Characteristic areas of rarefaction and osteoporosis are visible in the other bones of the peripheral and axial skeleton, including the skull.

Fabry's disease is inherited as an X-linked recessive disorder.[1] It is characterized by the progressive accumulation of birefringent deposits of triglycosylceramide in the endothelial, perithelial, and smooth muscle cells of blood vessels and in ganglion and perineural cells of the autonomic nervous system. The disease results from deficiency of ceramide trihexoside α-galactosidase. Affected boys have recurrent attacks of fever and severe arthritis and a characteristic burning, tingling pain in the extremities that is aggravated by hot weather or exercise. The fingers, elbows, and knees may become swollen, and a characteristic deformity limiting extension of the fingers develops. Other bones may also be involved, and secondary effects of osteonecrosis may become increasingly important, especially in weight-bearing joints such as the hips. A typical rash consisting of purple papules, *angiokeratoma corporis diffusum universale,* accompanies the other features of Fabry's disease. Female heterozygotes may develop milder forms of this disorder. Renal, cardiac, or cerebral disease leads to death in the midadult years in untreated patients. Enzyme replacement therapy and renal allograft transplantation are experimental attempts to correct the metabolic defect.[102]

A number of other rare disorders present in a man-

Table 36–8
Sphingolipidoses

DISORDER	GENETICS	MUSCULOSKELETAL ABNORMALITIES
Farber's disease	AR	Painful red masses along tendons at wrists, elbows, knees, and ankles
Gaucher's disease	AR	Osteoporosis with pathologic fractures of femur and vertebrae
Fabry's disease	XR	Recurrent fever and severe distal arthritis with burning pain; rash

AR, autosomal recessive; XR, X-linked recessive.

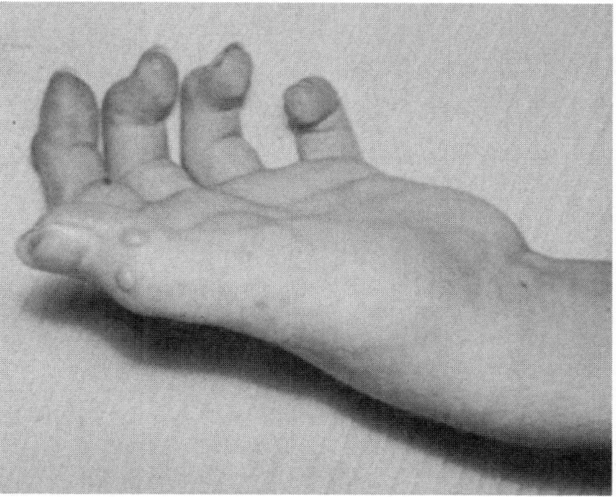

Figure 36–7. Multicentric reticulohistiocytosis. There is marked swelling and subluxation of the wrist, and swelling of the distal interphalangeal joints of the fingers and the interphalangeal joint of the thumb of this 14-year-old boy. Cutaneous nodules are visible over the thumb.

ner similar to that of the diseases discussed earlier but have not been clearly identified as involving an abnormality of a lysosomal degradative enzyme. One such disorder, *multicentric reticulohistiocytosis*, or *lipoid dermatoarthritis*, is a very rare, mutilating, symmetric polyarthritis that mimics JRA when it occurs in a child.[103, 104] An important diagnostic clue is the presence of clear histiocytic cutaneous nodules (Fig. 36–7). Stiffness and contractures appear early, and the joints (with a predilection for the interphalangeal and metacarpophalangeal joints) are swollen and tender. Biopsy of the lesions of the skin, mucous membranes, or synovium reveals lipid-laden histiocytes and foamy multinucleated giant cells. Most described cases have been in adults and are not familial.

References

1. Scriver CR, Beaudet AL, Sly WS, et al (eds): The Metabolic and Molecular Basis of Inherited Disease, 7th ed. New York, McGraw-Hill, 1995.
2. Mishra S, Yadav TP, Nangia S, et al: Vitamin-D dependent rickets type II. Ind Pediatr 33: 334–336, 1996.
3. Ono T, Seino Y: Medical management and complications of X-linked hypophosphatemic vitamin D resistant rickets. Acta Paediatr Jpn 39: 503–507, 1997.
4. Sato S, Matsuo N: Genetic analysis of hypophosphatasia. Acta Paediatr Jpn 39: 528–532, 1997.
5. Jacob RA: Three eras of vitamin C discovery. Subcell Biochem 25: 1–16, 1996.
6. Pease CN: Focal retardation and arrestment of growth of bones due to vitamin A intoxication. JAMA 182: 980, 1962.
7. Christensen WR, Liebman C, Sosman MC: Skeletal and periarticular manifestations of hypervitaminosis. Am J Roentgenol 65: 27, 1951.
8. Sokoloff L: Endemic forms of osteoarthritis. Clin Rheum Dis 11: 187–202, 1985.
9. Lee YW, Mirocha CJ, Shroeder DJ, et al: TDP-1, a toxic component causing tibial dyschondroplasia in broiler chickens, and trichothecenes from *Fusarium roseum* "Graminearum." Appl Environ Microbiol 50: 102–107, 1985.
10. Nesterov AI: The clinical course of Kashin-Beck disease. Arthritis Rheum 7: 29, 1964.
11. Takamori T: Kashin-Beck's Disease. University School of Medicine, Japan, The Professor Tokio Takamori Foundation, 1968.
12. Sokoloff L: Kashin-Beck disease. Rheum Dis Clin North Am 13: 101–104, 1987.
13. Tomlinson R: Beijing conference reviews Kashin-Beck disease [news]. Br Med J 318: 485, 1999.
14. Mathieu F, Begaux F, Lan ZY, et al: Clinical manifestations of Kashin-Beck disease in Nyemo Valley, Tibet. Int Orthop 21: 151–156, 1997.
15. Lockitch G, Fellingham SA, Wittman W, et al: Mseleni joint disease: the pilot clinical survey. S Afr Med J 47: 2283–2293, 1973.
16. Lockitch G, Fellingham SA, Elphinstone CD: Mseleni joint disease: a radiological study of two affected families. S Afr Med J 47: 2366–2376, 1973.
17. Rodriguez-Merchan EC: Effects of hemophilia on articulations of children and adults. Clin Orthop 7–13, 1996.
18. Miller ST, Sleeper LA, Pegelow CH, et al: Prediction of adverse outcomes in children with sickle cell disease. N Engl J Med 342: 83–89, 2000.
19. Barot VV: Occurrence of endemic fluorosis in human population of North Gujarat, India: human health risk. Bull Environ Contam Toxicol 61: 303–310, 1998.
20. Fisher RL, Medcalf TW, Henderson MC: Endemic fluorosis with spinal cord compression. A case report and review. Arch Intern Med 149: 697–700, 1989.
21. Becker MA: Clinical aspects of monosodium urate monohydrate crystal deposition disease (gout). Rheum Dis Clin North Am 14: 377–394, 1988.
22. Agudelo CA, Wise CM: Crystal-associated arthritis. Clin Geriatr Med 14: 495–513, 1998.
23. Simkin PA: Gout and hyperuricemia. Curr Opin Rheumatol 9: 268–273, 1997.
24. Treadwell BL: Juvenile gout. Ann Rheum Dis 30: 279–284, 1971.
25. Liberman UA, Samuel R, Halabe A, et al: Juvenile metabolic gout caused by chronic compensated hemolytic syndrome. Arthritis Rheum 25: 1264–1266, 1982.
26. Yarom A, Rennebohm RM, Strife F, et al: Juvenile gouty arthritis. Two cases associated with mild renal insufficiency. Am J Dis Child 138: 955–957, 1984.
27. Hoyningen-Huene CB: Gout and glycogen storage disease in preadolescent brothers. Arch Intern Med 118: 471–477, 1966.
28. Morley CJ, Houston IB, Morris-Jones P: Acute renal failure and gout as presenting features of acute lymphoblastic leukaemia. Arch Dis Child 51: 723–725, 1976.
29. Warren DJ, Simmonds HA, Gibson T, et al: Familial gout and renal failure. Arch Dis Child 56: 699–704, 1981.
30. Calabrese G, Simmonds HA, Cameron JS, et al: Precocious familial gout with reduced fractional urate clearance and normal purine enzymes. Q J Med 75: 441–450, 1990.
31. Foreman JW, Yudkoff M: Familial hyperuricemia and renal insufficiency. Child Nephrol Urol 10: 115–118, 1990.
32. Wortmann RL: Effective management of gout: an analogy. Am J Med 105: 513–514, 1998.
33. Emmerson BT: The management of gout. N Engl J Med 334: 445–451, 1996.
34. Lesch M, Nyhan WL: A familial disorder of uric acid metabolism and central nervous system function. Am J Med 26: 561, 1964.
35. Seegmiller JE, Rosenbloom FM, Kelley WN: Enzyme defect associated with a sex-linked human neurological disorder and excessive purine synthesis. Science 155: 1682–1684, 1967.
36. Kelley WN, Greene ML, Rosenbloom FM, et al: Hypoxanthine-guanine phosphoribosyltransferase deficiency in gout. Ann Intern Med 70: 155–206, 1969.
37. Nyhan WL: The recognition of Lesch-Nyhan syndrome as an inborn error of purine metabolism. J Inherit Metab Dis 20: 171–178, 1997.
38. Becker MA, Puig JG, Mateos FA, et al: Inherited superactivity of phosphoribosylpyrophosphate synthetase: association of uric acid overproduction and sensorineural deafness. Am J Med 85: 383–390, 1988.
39. Ahmed M, Taylor W, Smith PR, et al: Accelerated transcription of PRPS1 in X-linked overactivity of normal human phosphoribosylpyrophosphate synthetase. J Biol Chem 274: 7482–7488, 1999.
40. Alepa FP, Howell RR, Klinenberg JR, et al: Relationships between glycogen storage disease and tophaceous gout. Am J Med 42: 58–66, 1967.
41. Rosenthal AK: Calcium crystal-associated arthritides. Curr Opin Rheumatol 10: 273–277, 1998.
42. Richardson BC, Chafetz NI, Ferrell LD, et al: Hereditary chondrocalcinosis in a Mexican-American family. Arthritis Rheum 26: 1387–1396, 1983.
43. Reginato AJ, Reginato AM: Diseases associated with deposition of calcium pyrophosphate or hydroxyapatite. *In* Ruddy S, Harris ED Jr, Sledge CB (eds): Kelley's Textbook of Rheumatology, 6th ed. Philadelphia, WB Saunders, 2000, pp 1377–1390.
44. Steinbach LS, Resnick D: Calcium pyrophosphate dihydrate crystal deposition disease revisited. Radiology 200: 1–9, 1996.
45. O'Brien WM, LaDu BN, Bunim JJ: Biochemical, pathologic and clinical aspects of alcaptonuria, ochronosis and ochronotic arthropathy. Review of the world literature (1584–1962). Am J Med 34: 813, 1963.
46. Dom K, Pittevils T: Ochronotic arthropathy: the black hip. Case report and review of the literature. Acta Orthop Belg 63: 122–125, 1997.
47. Davignon J, Genest J Jr: Genetics of lipoprotein disorders. Endocrinol Metab Clin North Am 27: 521–550, 1998.
48. Franklin FA Jr, Dashti N, Franklin CC: Evaluation and management of dyslipoproteinemia in children. Endocrinol Metab Clin North Am 27: 641–654, 1998.

49. Cleeman JI: Detection and evaluation of dyslipoproteinemia. Endocrinol Metab Clin North Am 27: 597–611, 1998.
50. Shapiro JR, Fallat RW, Tsang RC, et al: Achilles tendinitis and tenosynovitis. A diagnostic manifestation of familial type II hyperlipoproteinemia in children. Am J Dis Child 128: 486–490, 1974.
51. Buckingham RB, Bole GG, Bassett DR: Polyarthritis associated with type IV hyperlipoproteinemia. Arch Intern Med 135: 286–290, 1975.
52. Björkem I, Boberg KM: Inborn errors in bile acid biosynthesis and storage of sterols other than cholesterol. *In* Scriver CS, Beaudet AL, Sly WS, et al (eds): The Metabolic and Molecular Basis of Inherited Disease, 7th ed. New York, McGraw-Hill, 1995, pp 2073–2102.
53. Belamarich PF, Deckelbaum RJ, Starc TJ, et al: Response to diet and cholestyramine in a patient with sitosterolemia. Pediatrics 86: 977–981, 1990.
54. Weinberg AG, Currarino G: Sickle cell dactylitis: histopathologic observations. Am J Clin Pathol 58: 518–523, 1972.
55. Gerster JC, Dardel R, Guggi S: Recurrent episodes of arthritis in thalassemia minor. J Rheumatol 11: 352–354, 1984.
56. Arman MI, Butun B, Doseyen A, et al: Frequency and features of rheumatic findings in thalassaemia minor: a blind controlled study. Br J Rheumatol 31: 197–199, 1992.
57. Lane PA: Sickle cell disease. Pediatr Clin North Am 43: 639–664, 1996.
58. Gilbert MS, Radomisli TE: Therapeutic options in the management of hemophilic synovitis. Clin Orthop 343: 88–92, 1997.
59. Rifai A, Nyman R: Scintigraphy and ultrasonography in differentiating osteomyelitis from bone infarction in sickle cell disease. Acta Radiol 38: 139–143, 1997.
60. Vichinsky EP: The morbidity of bone disease in thalassemia. Ann N Y Acad Sci 850: 344–348, 1998.
61. Arnold WD, Hilgartner MW: Hemophilic arthropathy. Current concepts of pathogenesis and management. J Bone Joint Surg Am 59: 287–305, 1977.
62. Ahlberg A, Silwer J: Arthropathy in von Willebrand's disease. Acta Orthop Scand 41: 539–544, 1970.
63. Ljung RC: Can haemophilic arthropathy be prevented? Br J Haematol 101: 215–219, 1998.
64. Handelsman JE: The knee joint in hemophilia. Orthop Clin North Am 10: 139–173, 1979.
65. Buzzard BM: Physiotherapy for the prevention of articular contraction in haemophilia. Haemophilia 5(Suppl)1: 10–15, 1999.
66. Kisker CT, Burke C: Double-blind studies on the use of steroids in the treatment of acute hemarthrosis in patients with hemophilia. N Engl J Med 282: 639–642, 1970.
67. Rosenbloom AL, Silverstein JH, Lezotte DC, et al: Limited joint mobility in childhood diabetes mellitus indicates increased risk for microvascular disease. N Engl J Med 305: 191–194, 1981.
68. Grgic A, Rosenbloom AL, Weber FT, et al: Joint contracture—common manifestation of childhood diabetes mellitus. J Pediatr 88: 584–588, 1976.
69. Sherry DD, Rothstein RR, Petty RE: Joint contractures preceding insulin-dependent diabetes mellitus. Arthritis Rheum 25: 1362–1364, 1982.
70. Verrotti A, Chiarelli F, Morgese G: Limited joint mobility in children with type 1 diabetes mellitus. A critical review. J Pediatr Endocrinol Metab 9: 3–8, 1996.
71. Rudolf MC, Genel M, Tamborlane WV Jr, et al: Juvenile rheumatoid arthritis in children with diabetes mellitus. J Pediatr 99: 519–524, 1981.
72. Vijanto JA: Dupuytren's contracture: a review. Semin Arthritis Rheum 3: 155–176, 1973.
73. Buckingham BA, Uitto J, Sandborg C, et al: Scleroderma-like syndrome and the non-enzymatic glucosylation of collagen in children with poorly controlled insulin dependent diabetes. Pediatr Res 15: 626, 1981.
74. De Seze S, Solnica J, Mitrovic D, et al: Joint and bone disorders and hypoparathyroidism in hemochromatosis. Semin Arthritis Rheum 2: 71–94, 1972.
75. Clouse ME, Gramm HF, Legg M, et al: Diabetic osteoarthropathy. Clinical and roentgenographic observations in 90 cases. Am J Roentgenol Radium Ther Nucl Med 121: 22–34, 1974.
76. Mazzuoli GF, D'Erasmo E, Pisani D: Primary hyperparathyroidism and osteoporosis. Aging (Milano) 10: 225–231, 1998.
77. Bhalla AK: Musculoskeletal manifestations of primary hyperparathyroidism. Clin Rheum Dis 12: 691–705, 1986.
78. Eberhard BA, Laxer RM, Eddy AA, et al: Presence of thyroid abnormalities in children with systemic lupus erythematosus. J Pediatr 119: 277–279, 1991.
79. Kinsella RA Jr, Back DK: Thyroid acropachy. Med Clin North Am 52: 393–398, 1968.
80. Athreya BH, Borns P, Rosenlund ML: Cystic fibrosis and hypertrophic osteoarthropathy in children. Report of three cases. Am J Dis Child 129: 634–637, 1975.
81. Nathanson I, Riddlesberger MM Jr: Pulmonary hypertrophic osteoarthropathy in cystic fibrosis. Radiology 135: 649–651, 1980.
82. Sagransky DM, Greenwald RA, Gorvoy JD: Seropositive rheumatoid arthritis in a patient with cystic fibrosis. Am J Dis Child 134: 319–320, 1980.
83. Newman AJ, Ansell BM: Episodic arthritis in children with cystic fibrosis. J Pediatr 94: 594–596, 1979.
84. Schidlow DV, Goldsmith DP, Palmer J, et al: Arthritis in cystic fibrosis. Arch Dis Child 59: 377–379, 1984.
85. Dixey J, Redington AN, Butler RC, et al: The arthropathy of cystic fibrosis. Ann Rheum Dis 47: 218–223, 1988.
86. Pertuiset E, Menkes CJ, Lenoir G, et al: Cystic fibrosis arthritis. A report of five cases. Br J Rheumatol 31: 535–538, 1992.
87. Warren RW: Rheumatologic aspects of pediatric cystic fibrosis patients treated with fluoroquinolones. Pediatr Infect Dis J 16: 118–122, 1997.
88. Soden M, Tempany E, Bresnihan B: Sarcoid arthropathy in cystic fibrosis. Br J Rheumatol 28: 341–343, 1989.
89. Shackelford PG: Osseous lesions and pancreatitis. Am J Dis Child 131: 731–732, 1977.
90. Goluboff N, Cram R, Ramgotra B, et al: Polyarthritis and bone lesions complicating traumatic pancreatitis in two children. Can Med Assoc J 118: 924–928, 1978.
91. Buntain WL, Wood JB, Woolley MM: Pancreatitis in childhood. J Pediatr Surg 13: 143–149, 1978.
92. Lopez A, Garcia-Estan J, Marras C, et al: Pancreatitis associated with pleural-mediastinal pseudocyst, panniculitis and polyarthritis. Clin Rheumatol 17: 335–339, 1998.
93. Goldbloom RB, Stein PB, Eisen A, et al: Idiopathic periosteal hyperostosis with dysproteinemia. A new clinical entity. N Engl J Med 28: 873, 1966.
94. Kuwashima S, Nishimura G, Harigaya A, et al: A young infant with Goldbloom syndrome. Pediatr Int 41: 110–112, 1999.
95. Grossfeld SL, Van Heest A, Arendt E, et al: Pitcher's periostitis. A case report. Am J Sports Med 26: 303–307, 1998.
96. Craver RD, Correa-Gracian H, Heinrich S: Florid reactive periostitis. Hum Pathol 28: 745–747, 1997.
97. Sinha GP, Curtis P, Haigh D, et al: Pachydermoperiostosis in childhood. Br J Rheumatol 36: 1224–1227, 1997.
98. Loredo R, Pathria MN, Salonen D, et al: Magnetic resonance imaging in pachydermoperiostosis. Clin Imaging 20: 212–218, 1996.
99. Kolter T, Sandhoff K: Recent advances in the biochemistry of sphingolipidoses. Brain Pathol 8: 79–100, 1998.
100. Farber S, Cohen J, Uzman JL: Lipogranulomatosis. A new lipoglycoprotein "storage" disease. J Mt Sinai Hosp 24: 816, 1957.
101. Toppet M, Vamos-Hurwitz E, Jonniaux G, et al: Farber's disease as a ceramidosis: clinical, radiological and biochemical aspects. Acta Paediatr Scand 67: 113–119, 1978.
102. Brady RO: Therapy for the sphingolipidoses. Arch Neurol 55: 1055–1056, 1998.
103. Zayid I, Farraj S: Familial histiocytic dermatoarthritis. A new syndrome. Am J Med 54: 793–800, 1973.
104. Uhl M, Gutfleisch J, Rother E, et al: Multicentric reticulohistiocytosis. A report of 3 cases and review of literature. Bildgebung 63: 126–129, 1996.

37

Primary Disorders of Bone and Connective Tissues

Judith G. Hall

A variety of relatively rare primary disorders of bone or connective tissue may present in childhood with symptoms that suggest a diagnosis of one of the inflammatory arthritides, although they do not have a primary inflammatory etiology. They are genetically determined disorders with swelling and prominence of joints, hypermobility, or joint contractures, and they are often associated with disproportionately short or tall stature. This chapter is not intended to be comprehensive but provides an approach to the identification and differential diagnosis of those conditions most likely to present in childhood with musculoskeletal pain or degenerative joint disease. Many excellent reference books include differential diagnoses.[1–4] In addition, an international working group frequently updates a classification of osteochondrodysplasias.[5] These disorders are identified numerically (McKusick numbers). The latest primary references are also listed in Online Mendelian Inheritance in Man (OMIM), to which there is access through the Internet.[6]

ESTABLISHING A DIAGNOSIS

In an excellent review, Chalom and associates[7] suggested that the clinical characteristics in Table 37–1 should alert the physician to the possible diagnosis of a congenital or familial arthropathy, rather than inflammatory arthritis. Useful parameters that help to differentiate among the primary disorders of bone and connective tissues include age at onset, natural history, distribution of affected bones and joints, radiographic abnormalities, presence of other organ involvement, hereditary pattern, and pathologic changes on examination of tissues. Because specific genes for some of these diseases have been identified, mutational analysis may also contribute to diagnosis.

Table 37–1

Characteristics That Suggest the Presence of Congenital or Familial Arthropathy

Presence of alleged juvenile rheumatoid arthritis in more than one family member
Presence of two or more dysmorphic features
Absence of rheumatoid factor and antinuclear antibody
Absence of evidence of systemic or synovial inflammation (normal erythrocyte sedimentation rate, normal synovial fluid cell count)

From Chalom EC, Ross J, Athreya BH: Syndromes and arthritis. Rheum Dis Clin North Am 23: 709, 1997.

Age at Onset

Those disorders already present at birth, such as spondyloepiphyseal dysplasia congenita and diastrophic dysplasia, can be distinguished from those with onset later in childhood, such as Stickler's syndrome or progressive pseudorheumatoid arthropathy of childhood. The age at which abnormalities first become evident is characteristic of each disorder (e.g., Hurler's syndrome in the first year, pseudoachondroplasia in the second year). Not only is the age at which abnormalities first appear characteristic, but the order in which various body parts become involved is also characteristic of individual syndromes.

Distribution of Involvement

The distribution of affected bones, joints, or other connective tissues can usually be determined by physical examination. The presence of abnormalities of joint range of motion, disproportion between the trunk and the limb, and disproportion within segments of the limb should be noted. Relative shortness of the most proximal segment of the limb is called *rhizomelic shortening;* when the middle segment is involved, it is called *mesomelic shortening;* when the most distal segment is affected, *acromelic shortening* is present.

Radiographic Abnormalities

A radiographic approach to the differential diagnosis is to determine what part of the bone (epiphysis, metaphysis, diaphysis) is involved and whether the spine is affected. Very frequently, the radiographic changes are not present at birth. They may become much more prominent with age or, as in pseudoachondroplasia, may disappear with time. Many of the bony dysplasias are named according to the area of bone affected (e.g., multiple epiphyseal dysplasias or spondyloepiphyseal dysplasias).

Involvement of Other Organs

Some of the primary disorders of bones and connective tissues have specific associated congenital anomalies, such as structural heart abnormalities in Ellis–van Creveld syndrome or cleft palate in spondyloepiphyseal dysplasia congenita and diastrophic dysplasia. Others develop complications such as retinal detachment, deafness, or storage disorders with time.

MOLECULAR MECHANISMS OF DISEASE

Pathologic Changes and Pathogenic Mechanisms

The pathologic changes in tissues have helped to define the metabolic pathways involved in many of these disorders. In general, they have been separated into

- Abnormalities of connective tissues (fibers or matrix changes)
- Abnormalities in growth factors and their receptors
- Abnormalities of transmembrane regulation
- Abnormalities of transcription factors

Frequently, the disease in question may be known to have a genetic basis, but there may be no family history of the disorder. Thus, in reviewing the family history, careful questioning about consanguinity (suggesting an autosomal recessive disorder) and about advanced paternal age (suggesting a new dominant mutation) should be undertaken.

Mutations

Most types of bone and connective tissue disorders have a genetic basis and represent somatic mutations, new dominant mutations, dominantly inherited conditions, autosomal recessively inherited disorders, or X-linked disorders (both recessive and dominant). Different disorders can arise from different mutations in a single gene. In osteogenesis imperfecta, almost every new mutation has its own particular site along the type I collagen gene. However, in some genes there are "hot spots" where more than one new mutation occurs. For instance, in achondroplasia, more than 95 percent of all new mutations occur at exactly the same nucleotide within the transmembrane part of the fibroblast growth factor 3 receptor gene. In addition, the rate of mutation at this site is almost 1000 times that at other sites.

Mosaicism

With new molecular techniques, it is possible to distinguish whether a mutation is present in all cells within an individual or in only a proportion of cells (mosaicism). Thus, a person may have patchy involvement and be relatively mildly affected, whereas the offspring can have every cell in the body involved and be much more severely affected. This phenomenon has occurred in mutations of type II collagen in which the parent is described clinically as having Stickler's syndrome and the child as having Kniest's syndrome. It is therefore important to examine both parents to identify minor changes suggestive of mosaicism.[8]

Parent of Origin

Parent-of-origin effects (genomic imprinting) may occur in bony disorders in which a child is more severely affected when the disease-associated gene is inherited from the mother or from the father. For instance, in Albright's hereditary osteodystrophy, children are more severely affected when they inherit the condition from their mother.[9]

COMMON CLINICAL CONCERNS

Arthritis

Children with a wide range of primary disorders of connective tissue may present with arthritis or what appears to be arthritis (Table 37–2).[10–15] Others develop arthritis as a result of degenerative changes in the joints. The development of "wear and tear" degenerative joint disease is related to abnormal alignment, irregular joint surfaces, ligamentous laxity, and abnormal cartilage. In conditions such as achondroplasia, asymmetric growth (i.e., overgrowth of the fibula) leads to bowing of the fibula, as a result of which weight (if unevenly distributed across the knee joint) leads to wear and tear on the cartilaginous surface of the tibia. Furthermore, when there are biochemical abnormalities of the connective tissues themselves, cartilage or supporting structures may be unable to withstand even normal weight-bearing and movement. If the bones of the skull or face are affected, malalignment of teeth may result and there may be abnormal stresses on the temporomandibular joints. Some patients with disproportionately short stature tend to be obese, which further contributes to the risk of degenerative joint disease (especially in achondroplasia). Joint contractures may resemble arthritis but there is generally no enlargement of the joints. They are characteris-

Table 37–2

Primary Disorders of Connective Tissues That May Present as Arthritis

DISORDER	JOINT ABNORMALITIES	OTHER FEATURES
CACP syndrome[9]	Polyarthritis with contractures, camptodactyly at birth	Pericarditis
		Coxa vara
Arthritis with scoliosis[10]	Polyarthritis; finger flexion contractures	Thoracic scoliosis
Hereditary osteolysis[11]	"Arthritis" in wrists, ankles, elbows, metacarpophalangeal, interphalangeal joints; limitation of elbow range, ulnar deviation of wrist; painless deformity of wrists and feet	Marfan-like syndrome
Nail-patella syndrome[12]	Polyarthritis; restricted elbow range	Hypoplastic patellae and thumbnails, radial head dislocations, iliac horns, clubfeet
Stickler's syndrome[13]	Symmetric polyarthritis	Flat facies, long philtrum, epicanthal folds, myopia, hypermobility, kyphosis, cleft palate
Trichorhinophalangeal dysplasia[14]	Enlarged proximal interphalangeal joints, short fourth and fifth metacarpals, progressive hip arthritis	Bulbous nose, thin hair, large ears, micrognathia

CACP, camptodactyly, arthropathy, coxa vara, pericarditis.

tic of a number of primary disorders of connective tissues (Table 37–3).[16–54] For a more detailed account of these disorders, the reader is referred to the review by Chalom and colleagues.[7]

Effects of Ligamentous Laxity

Many children with ligamentous laxity have hypermobility of joints of the extremities and complain of musculoskeletal pain. Recurrent subluxations of joints may occur. Children with many types of spondyloepiphyseal dysplasias have poor odontoid development and, because of loose ligaments, may have subluxation of C1 on C2 with spinal cord compression. Congenital and familial disorders characterized by joint hypermobility are shown in Table 37–4.[16, 55–69]

Surgical and Anesthetic Concerns

Because many persons with osteochondrodystrophy require surgery, particular attention must be paid to anesthetic risks. As is the case in children with juvenile rheumatoid arthritis (JRA), preanesthetic radiographic evaluation of the cervical spine and protection of the neck during surgery avoid neurologic damage resulting from cervical instability. Similarly, intubation may be difficult because of micrognathia or restriction of spinal movement; in conditions such as diastrophic dysplasia, pressure on the tracheal cartilages can cause swelling and obstruction of the airway. Spinal anesthesia may be difficult in children with spondyloepiphyseal dysplasias, and great care should be taken when using spinal anesthesia in any patient with disproportionately short stature. Intravenous access may be difficult in children with incomplete extension of the elbows.

OSTEOCHONDRODYSPLASIAS

Definition and Classification

The osteochondrodysplasias are developmental disorders of chondral and osseous tissue that are often accompanied by short stature.[70] They include defects of tubular and flat bones or of the axial skeleton, disorganized development of cartilaginous and fibrous components of the skeleton, and idiopathic osteolyses. As genetic abnormalities responsible for these disorders are identified, the traditional classification shown in Table 37–5 will be modified.

Mechanisms of Disease

A number of osteochondrodysplasias have autosomal dominant inheritance, but most occur as the result of new mutations. For example, 85 to 90 percent of cases of achondroplasia and pseudoachondroplasia result from new mutations. Some disorders in this group have a nongenetic basis. Warfarin-induced embryopathy, maternal lupus embryopathy, and congenital rubella syndrome are associated with abnormal bone growth and chondrodysplasia punctata.

Achondroplasia Family

Members of the achondroplasia family have mutations of the fibroblast growth factor receptor 3 gene (FGFR3) on chromosome 4p16.3. Achondroplasia and hypochondroplasia can present as possible inflammatory arthritis because of degenerative joint changes in weight-bearing joints and limitation of range of motion, but their disproportionately short stature is strik-

Table 37–3

Congenital and Familial Disorders With Contractures or Stiff Joints

SYNDROME	CHARACTERISTIC JOINT ABNORMALITIES
Aarskog's syndrome[16]	Hyperextensible proximal interphalangeal (PIP) joints with distal joint restriction; short fifth finger with clinodactyly
Achondroplasia[17]	Incomplete extension of the elbow
Antley-Bixler syndrome[18]	Congenital contractures wrist, finger, hip, knee, ankle
Apert's syndrome[19]	Ankylosis of elbow, shoulder, hip
Arthrogryposis[20, 21]	Stiffness, multiple contractures of large and small joints
Beals' syndrome[22]	Contractures knee, elbow, hand; arachnodactyly
Gangliosidosis I[23]	Contractures elbow, knee, claw hands
Chromosome 2p deletion[24]	Contractures of hip, knee, ankle
Cockayne's syndrome[25]	Mild contractures knee, elbow, ankle
Conradi-Hunermann[26]	Variable contractures; punctate bone mineralization
Farber's disease[27, 28]	Symmetric polyarthritis
Multicentric osteolysis[12]	"Arthritis" of wrist, ankles, elbows, metacarpophalangeal and interphalangeal joints; limited elbow motion, ulnar deviation of involved hand; painless deformity of wrist and feet
Cornelia de Lange syndrome[29]	Flexion contractures of elbows
Diastrophic dwarfism[30]	Limited flexion of PIP joints and elbow; clubfoot
Ectrodactyly-ectodermal dysplasia syndrome[31]	Limited extension of elbows; abnormal third digit
Fabry's disease[32]	(Angiokeratoma corporis diffusum) Bony swelling, distal interphalangeal joints, flexion deformity
Pena-Shokier syndrome[33]	Multiple joint contractures, camptodactyly
GEMSS syndrome[34]	(Glaucoma, lens ectopia, microspherophakia, short stature) Reduced mobility of large joints
Homocystinuria[35]	Enlarged joints with reduced mobility
Hypochondroplasia[36]	Mild reduction of elbow mobility
Jansen's dysostosis[37]	(Jansen's metaphyseal chondrodysplasia) Contractures of hips and knees
Leri pleonosteosis[38]	Limited mobility; flexion contractures of digits, broad thumb
Leri-Weill dyschondrosteosis[39]	Limitation of mobility at wrist and elbow
Marden-Walker syndrome[40]	Multiple congenital contractures, micrognathia
Metatrophic dwarfism[41]	Limited movement at knee, hip; hypermobile fingers
Mucolipidoses (MLSs)[42]	
I-cell disease	(MLS II) Limited hip flexion; hips dislocated
Pseudo-Hurler's syndrome	(MLS III) Limited motion of hands, elbows, knees, shoulders, claw hand
Mucopolysaccharidoses (MPSs)[43]	
Hunter's syndrome	(MPS II) Joint contractures, claw hand
Hurler's syndrome	(MPS I-H) Limitation of extension, claw hand
Maroteau-Lamy syndrome	(MPS VI) Limited motion of knee, hip, elbow
San Filippo syndrome	(MPS III) Mild joint stiffness
Scheie's syndrome	(MPS I-S) Limitation of motion in hands and feet; claw hand
Riley-Day syndrome[44]	(Familial dysautonomia) Neuropathic joint (knee)
Schmid's syndrome[45]	(Metaphyseal chondrodysplasia syndrome) Mild decrease in finger, wrist, and elbow extension; genu varum
Schwartz-Jampel syndrome[46]	Limited motion at hip, wrist, fingers, toes, spine
Seckel's syndrome[47]	Limited motion at elbows; dislocated hips
Spondyloepiphyseal dysplasia[48]	Contractures at elbows, knees, hips; pain, soft tissue swelling PIP joints, hips and elbows
Spondylometaphyseal dysplasia[49]	(Kozlowski's syndrome) Limited mobility of hips, elbows
Trisomy 5q[50]	Contractures at hips, elbows
Trisomy 8[51]	Limited elbow supination
Weaver syndrome[52]	Limited extension of elbow and knee; camptodactyly
Weill-Marchesani syndrome[53]	Progressive joint stiffness
Winchester's syndrome[54]	Symmetric flexion contractures with pain at fingers, elbows, hips, knees, ankles
Zellweger's syndrome[55]	Variable contractures especially of knees, fingers; ulnar deviation of hand

Modified from Chalom EC, Ross J, Athreya BH: Syndromes and arthritis. Rheum Dis Clin North Am 23: 709, 1997.

ing and the diagnosis is unlikely to be missed after the newborn period.

Classic Achondroplasia

The classic disorder of achondroplasia (McKusick 100800) is the most common form of viable disproportionate short stature. It occurs with a frequency of 1 in 20,000 births. The distinguishing features are present at birth, although the diagnosis is not always made at that time. The head is large with frontal bossing, midface hypoplasia, and prognathism. There is rhizomelic shortening of arms and legs, increased lumbar lordosis, bowing of the legs, overgrowth of the fibula, and a trident-shaped hand with short broad phalanges. Kyphosis at L1 occurs because of hypotonia of the trunk in the first few years of life.

Radiographs show a very small sacrosciatic notch of the pelvis, chevron changes of the epiphyses of the distal femur, and constriction at the base of the skull. The pedicles of the vertebrae are short, leading to symptomatic spinal stenosis in many affected persons.

Prenatal diagnosis is possible, both through DNA

Table 37–4

Congenital and Familial Syndromes Associated With Hypermobility

Aarskog's syndrome[16]
Coffin-Lowry syndrome[56]
Coffin-Siris syndrome[57]
Cohen's syndrome[58]
Costello's syndrome[59]
Cutis laxa–growth deficiency syndrome[60]
Dubowitz's syndrome[61]
Ehler-Danlos syndrome type II[62]
Hajdu-Cheney syndrome (acro-osteolysis, arthrodentodysplasia)[63]
Kabuki makeup syndrome[64]
Larsen's syndrome[65]
Marfan syndrome[66]
Cartilage-hair hypoplasia[67]
Morquio's syndrome (MPS IV)[68]
Velofacioskeletal syndrome[69]

From Chalom EC, Ross J, Athreya BH: Syndromes and arthritis. Rheum Dis Clin North Am 23: 709, 1997.

testing and through sequential ultrasound measurement of the growth of the long bones. The natural history and optimal medical supervision of patients with achondroplasia have been well defined by the American Academy of Pediatrics.[71] Adult life is shortened when spinal stenosis causes spinal cord compression, but otherwise most of those persons live a healthy, productive, and independent life.

Table 37–5

International Classification of Osteochondrodysplasias

Defects of Tubular and Flat Bones and/or Axial Skeleton

Achondroplasia group
Achondrogenesis
Spondylodysplastic group
Metatropic dysplasia group
Short-rib dysplasia group
Atelosteogenesis/diastrophic dysplasia group
Kniest-Stickler dysplasia group
Spondyloepiphyseal dysplasia congenita group
Other spondyloepiphyseal and metaphyseal dysplasias
Dysostosis multiplex group
Spondylometaphyseal dysplasias
Epiphyseal dysplasias
Chondrodysplasia punctata group
Metaphyseal dysplasias
Brachyrachia
Mesomelic dysplasias
Acro/acromesomelic dysplasias
Dysplasias with significant membranous bone involvement
Bent-bone dysplasia group
Multiple dislocations with dysplasias
Osteodysplastic primordial dwarfism group
Dysplasias with decreased bone density
Dysplasias with defective mineralization
Dysplasias with increased bone density

Disorganized Development of Cartilaginous and Fibrous Components of the Skeleton

Idiopathic Osteolysis

Predominantly phalangeal
Predominantly carpal/tarsal
Multicentric
Other

From Spranger EJP for the International Working Group on Constitutional Disease of Bone: International classification of osteochondrodysplasias. Eur J Pediatr 151: 407, 1992 Copyright Springer-Verlag.

Hypochondroplasia

Hypochondroplasia (McKusick 146000) is a milder form of disproportionate short stature involving several different mutations of the FGFR3 gene. Affected persons are often slightly taller and have less enlargement of the head than those with achondroplasia.[36]

Collagen Disorders

The number of primary disorders of bones and connective tissues that are associated with identified defects in collagen synthesis is steadily increasing. They include most of the Ehlers-Danlos syndromes (EDSs) and a number of others (Table 37–6). At least five different types of collagen are found in articular cartilage (types II, IV, IX, X, and XI), and genetically determined defects in these molecules might be expected to be associated with joint disease.[72]

Ehlers-Danlos Syndromes

EDSs are disorders of connective tissue characterized by hypermobility, easy bruising, hyperextensibility of the skin, and sometimes atrophic scars, molluscoid pseudotumors, and epicanthal folds (Table 37–7; see also Fig. 37–5) (McKusick 120215, 120160, 120180, 225410, 225320, 130000-90).[62, 72, 73] The nine types of EDS have traditionally been considered as a group, but as their genetic and biochemical abnormalities are eluci-

Table 37–6

Classification of Genetic Disorders of Collagen

COLLAGEN TYPE	DISORDER
I	Osteogenesis imperfecta
	Idiopathic juvenile osteoporosis
	Ehlers-Danlos type VII
II	Stickler's syndrome
	Kniest's syndrome
	Spondyloepiphyseal dysplasia congenita
	Spondyloepiphyseal dysplasia tarda
III	Ehlers-Danlos type III
	Ehlers-Danlos type IV
	Ehlers-Danlos type VIII
IV	Ehlers-Danlos type VI
V	Ehlers-Danlos type I
	Ehlers-Danlos type II
VI	Cutis laxa
IX	Fairbank's multiple epiphyseal dysplasia
X	Schmid's type metaphyseal dysplasia
XI	Stickler's syndrome type II
	Otospondylomegaepiphyseal dysplasias

Table 37–7
The Ehlers-Danlos Syndromes

TYPE	GENETICS	BIOCHEMICAL DEFECT	CLINICAL CHARACTERISTICS: Hyperextensibility — Skin	Joints	Other Features
I (gravis)	AD	Type V collagen	+ + +	+ + +	Severe disease, fragile vasculature, molluscoid pseudotumors
II (mitis)	AD	Type V collagen	+ +	+ +	Mild disease
III (benign)	AD	Type III collagen	±	+ + +	Benign hypermobility
IV (arterial)	AD, AR, sporadic	Type III collagen	+	+	Ecchymoses, rupture of vessels, GI tract, "china doll" appearance
V	XR	Lysyl oxidase deficiency	+ +	+	Ecchymoses, atrophic scars
VI (ocular)	AR	Type IV collagen	+ + +	+ + +	Retinal detachment joint dislocations, scoliosis, hypotonia
VII	AD, AR	Defective conversion of type I procollagen to collagen	+ +	+ + +	Congenital hip dislocations, short stature
VIII	AD	Type III collagen	+ +	+ +	Periodontitis
X	AR	Fibronectin functional deficiency	+	+ + +	Ecchymoses, scarring mitral valve prolapse

AD, autosomal dominant; AR, autosomal recessive; GI, gastrointestinal.

dated, it is more appropriate to consider them in terms of the specific biochemical abnormalities of collagen that they represent. Two others are no longer included in this disease category: that previously designated as type IX (occipital horn syndrome) (McKusick 304150) is now grouped with disorders of copper metabolism (Menkes' syndrome); the former type XI has been grouped with the benign hypermobility syndromes (McKusick 130020). A classification of disorders of collagen based on their known biochemical abnormalities in shown in Table 37–6.

Disorders of Type I Collagen

Mutations of the type I collagen genes (McKusick 120150 and 120160) cause a spectrum of abnormalities from familial osteoarthritis and osteoporosis to severe osteogenesis imperfecta. Each family appears to have its own mutation. Severely affected persons have short stature, blue sclerae, dentinogenesis imperfecta, and osteoporosis with breakable bones. In these patients, joint laxity, cardiac valve regurgitation, myopia, and degenerative joint changes may occur with age. Type I collagen mutations should be considered when any of these features are present.

Osteogenesis Imperfecta

Osteogenesis imperfecta, one of the most common heritable disorders of connective tissue (1:20,000 births), is inherited in either an autosomal recessive or an autosomal dominant manner, depending on the disease subtype (Table 37–8).[74] The various subtypes of osteogenesis imperfecta are related to the site of the

Table 37–8
Classification of Osteogenesis Imperfecta

TYPE	INHERITANCE	SCLERA	DEAFNESS	SKELETAL ABNORMALITIES
I	AD	Blue	50%	Normal stature, little or no deformity
II	AD	Blue	No	Congenital fractures, marked long bone abnormalities, platyspondyly, beaded ribs; lethal in perinatal period
III	AD	Variable	Common	Progressive deformity of bones, usually with moderate deformity at birth; very short stature; dentinogenesis imperfecta
IV	AD	Normal	Uncommon	Variable short stature, mild to moderate bone deformity; dentinogenesis imperfecta

AD, autosomal dominant; AR, autosomal recessive.
Modified from Sillence DO, Senn A, Banks DM: Genetic heterogeneity in osteogenesis imperfecta. J Med Genet 16: 101, 1979.

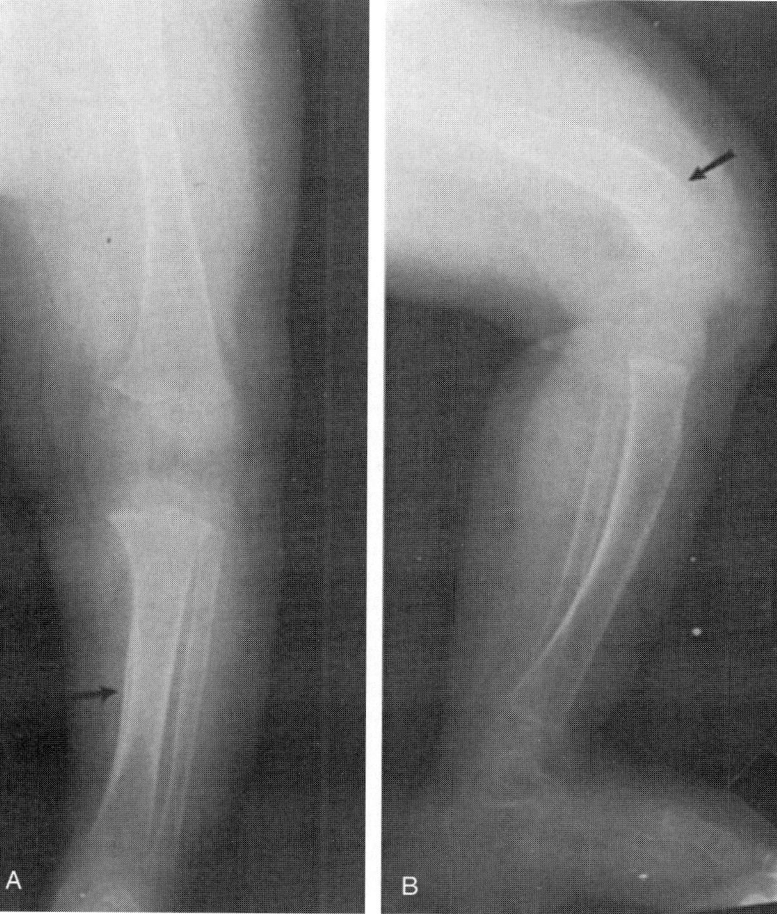

Figure 37–1. Radiographs of the legs of an 8-month-old boy with osteogenesis imperfecta who has experienced many fractures. *A, Arrow* indicates area of periosteal new bone along the tibia. *B, Arrow* indicates the location of a supracondylar fracture.

mutation that affects the chains of the collagen triple helix.[74] The severity of the disease ranges from slight increase in susceptibility to fractures of bones with improvement in adolescence (type I) to forms that are lethal in utero or in the neonatal period (type II). In type III, fractures occur throughout life (Fig. 37–1). In some children, blue sclerae, otosclerosis, and dentinogenesis imperfecta occur. The skin is excessively thin, with abnormal scar formation. The joints are often hyperextensible. In addition to multiple fractures and progressive osteoporosis, radiographs reveal a large skull with wormian bones in the suture lines.

Increased bone turnover and resorption are characteristic; plasma osteocalcin levels are elevated, although serum calcium, phosphorus, and alkaline phosphatase concentrations are normal.[75] Treatment with calcitonin[76, 77] or biphosphonates[78] has been suggested. Long-term management requires expert physical therapy and orthopedic surgery.[79, 80]

Idiopathic Juvenile Osteoporosis

Many forms of osteoporosis (McKusick 114130, 166710, 120160, 259750) are associated with type I collagen mutations. Idiopathic juvenile osteoporosis presents late in childhood or at puberty with pain in the joints, usually the ankles or knees, and is characterized by the development of metaphyseal fractures resulting from osteopenia.[81] Back pain may result from vertebral fractures. Severely affected children develop protrusio acetabuli. All biochemical investigations are normal except for the presence of hypercalciuria. The metabolic abnormalities disappear after completion of growth.[82] Minor fractures around joints may simulate arthritis.

Ehlers-Danlos Syndrome Type VII

EDS type VII (*arthrochalasis multiplex congenita*) is characterized by extreme laxity of the joints that results in early dislocations of the hips, short stature, and mandibular hypoplasia, together with the characteristics of EDS type I. It results from a splicing defect that causes a deletion of a peptidase cleavage site on either the α_1(I) or the α_2(I) genes of type I collagen, thus preventing the normal processing of type I procollagen (McKusick 130060, 225410).[83, 84]

Disorders of Type II Collagen

Type II collagen is found primarily in hyaline cartilage, the nucleus pulposus, and the vitreous of the eye. Mutations of the type II collagen gene lead to osteoarthritis and abnormal growth and often affect the eye and the spine. Diversity within the spectrum seems to be related to mutations in different domains of the gene (i.e., particular domains relate to degrees of severity). Because of hyperextensibility and abnormal cartilage, degenerative changes in the joints often occur at an early age. Occasionally, a parent is affected in a mosaic form with much milder involvement. The child in whom all tissues are involved is likely to be more severely affected.

Stickler's Syndrome

Stickler's syndrome (McKusick 184840) is a heterogeneous group of disorders with an autosomal dominant pattern of inheritance. Children with this syndrome may have a marfanoid body habitus, with hyperextensibility of the joints.[85] Enlargement of the knees, ankles, and wrists—often congenital—can be misdiagnosed as JRA or the chronic infantile neurocutaneous and articular syndrome (CINCA). Associated but variable features include deafness, myopia, cataracts, and retinal degeneration and detachment. Midfacial hypoplasia, a cleft palate, and micrognathia are common. Intelligence is normal. Radiographs in the newborn show characteristic "dumbbell-shaped" long bones with enlarged epiphyses and metaphyses. With increasing age, the epiphyses become fragmented and degenerative arthritis develops (Fig. 37–2). There may be mild platyspondyly and steeply sloping ribs. In Stickler's syndrome type I, the defects in the COL2A1 gene for type II collagen have been localized to the long arm of chromosome 12 (12q13.1–13.3).[86]

Kniest Syndrome

The Kniest, or *Swiss-cheese cartilage,* syndrome (McKusick 156550), inherited as an autosomal dominant disorder of type II collagen, is characterized by congenitally short limbs and trunk as well as macrocephaly with a round face and a depressed nasal bridge.[87] Progressive stiffness of the fingers, dislocation of the hips, and kyphoscoliosis develop. A cleft palate, hypertelorism, myopia, retinal detachment, deafness, and hernias are characteristic. Later, enlargement of the joints and severe contractures interfere significantly with mobility and are associated with pain. Radiographs reveal platyspondyly, flared metaphyses, and epiphyseal deformity in the tubular bones (Fig. 37–3). The cartilaginous growth plate is abnormal, with poorly calcified matrix (Swiss-cheese cartilage). The differences between the Stickler and the Kniest syndromes represent effects of mosaicism.

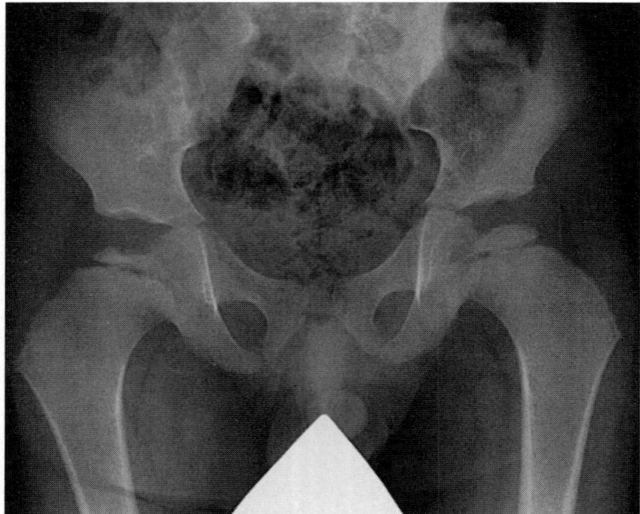

Figure 37–2. Fragmentation of the femoral epiphysis in a child with Stickler's syndrome.

Spondyloepiphyseal Dysplasias

The spondyloepiphyseal dysplasias (SEDs) constitute a group of closely related disorders characterized by short stature and a disproportionately short trunk (Table 37–9). Infants with the most severe forms of SEDs within the type II collagen spectrum are obviously dwarfed at birth. Many other, less severely affected patients may not present until later in life, and their symptoms can easily be confused with those of osteoarthritis. They present with short stature and symmetric joint pain secondary to epiphyseal changes. The possibility of an inborn error of connective tissue metabolism should be considered whenever there is symmetric involvement or epiphyseal fragmentation or both associated with arthritis.

In *SED congenita* (McKusick 183900), the limbs are short and equinovarus deformities of the feet are common. Radiographs show dysplastic and late-developing femoral heads, marked platyspondyly, and characteristic abnormalities of the pelvis and vertebral bodies, especially in the cervical and lumbosacral regions.[48, 88] This autosomal dominant condition reflects mutations in the COL2A1 gene located on the long arm of chromosome 12 (12q13.1–13.3). An associated immunodeficiency has been reported in some patients.

In the X-linked recessive form of *SED tarda* (McKusick 313400), there is moderate shortness of stature, principally secondary to platyspondyly, with onset of hip or back pain and stiffness by 5 to 10 years of age.[89, 90] Radiographic changes include a characteristic posterior hump on the vertebral bodies, which eventually become fused to each other, and mild fragmentation of the epiphyses of the hips and shoulders (Fig. 37–4).

The milder SEDs with coxa vara are often characterized by an autosomal dominant inheritance. A progressive "pseudorheumatoid" arthritis has been described in some children with SED tarda,[91, 92] and pseudogout has also been observed.[93] Hypoplasia of the odontoid, when present, predisposes the child to cervical cord injury from mild trauma.

Disorders of Type III Collagen

Ehlers-Danlos Syndrome Type III

EDS type III (McKusick 225350) is inherited as an autosomal dominant trait or results from a new mutation.

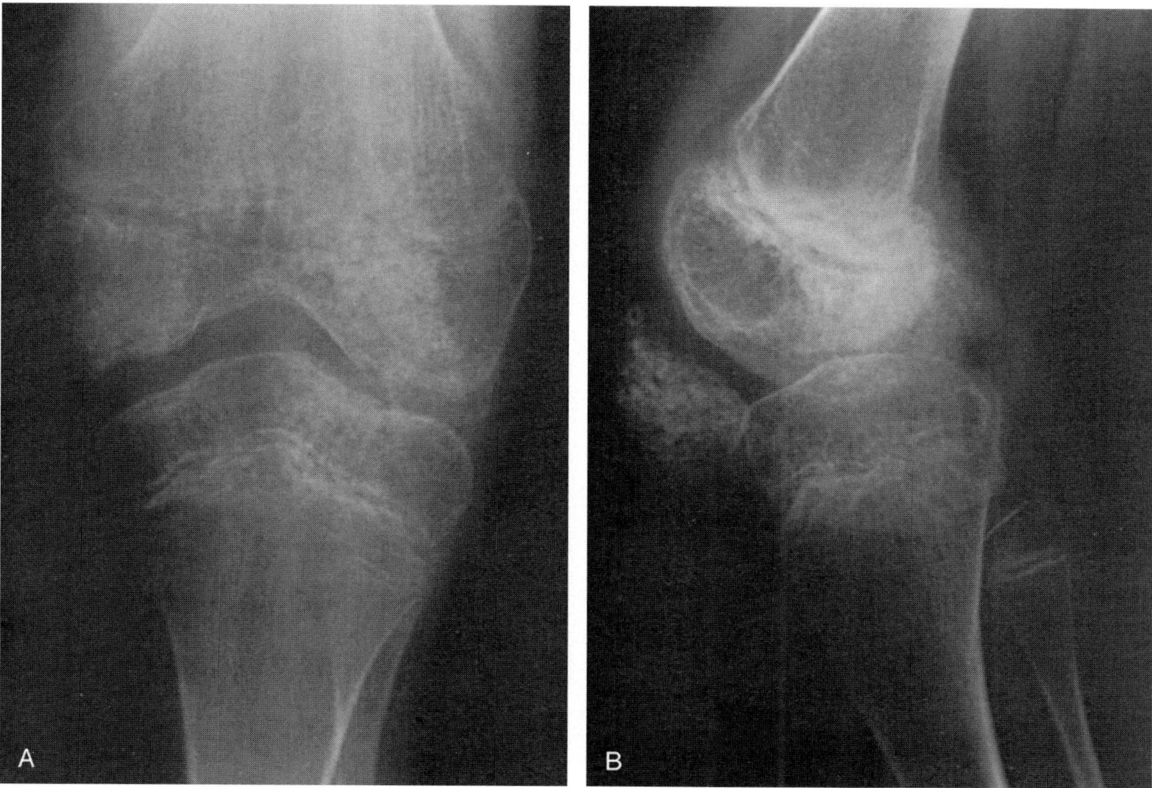

Figure 37–3. *A* and *B*, Radiographs of a knee of a 9-year-old boy with Kniest syndrome show irregular calcification of cartilage, giving a "Swiss-cheese" appearance. The metaphyses are flared, and the epiphyses are deformed. (*A* and *B*, Courtesy of Dr. R. Cairns.)

The distinguishing features are minimal and the child often has only hypermobility, although some patients have hyperelasticity of the skin and cutaneous striae over the lower back. A mutation in COL3A1 has been demonstrated in a patient with EDS type III.[94]

Ehlers-Danlos Syndrome Type IV

The distinguishing features of EDS type IV (McKusick 130050, 225350), of which there are at least four subtypes, are the marked vascular fragility and aneurysms that mainly affect the aorta, medium-sized muscular arteries, and cerebral arteries. Other characteristics include prematurely aged and thin skin over the dorsa of the hands (acrogeria) (types IVA and IVB), sparse scalp hair, large eyes (china doll appearance), and lobeless ears. Ruptures of pleura, peritoneum, or intestinal diverticulae may occur. Musculoskeletal abnormalities include acro-osteolysis of the fingertips, bilateral club feet, and dislocated hips. A variety of mutations of the COL3A1 gene on the long arm of chromosome 2 cause abnormalities of type III collagen in patients with EDS type IV.[95] Histologic examination of the skin shows characteristic collagen depletion and elastin proliferation.

Ehlers-Danlos Syndrome Type VIII

The outstanding characteristics of EDS type VIII (McKusick 130080) include periodontal disease, with

Table 37–9

Spondyloepiphyseal Dysplasias

TYPE	ONSET	INHERITANCE	ASSOCIATED FEATURES
Congenita	Birth	AD	Short limbs, equinovarus feet, myopia, retinal detachment
Tarda	Late childhood	XLR	Moderate short stature, platyspondyly, onset of pain in hips and back at around 10 yr of age; progressive deformity

AD, autosomal dominant; XLR, X-linked recessive.

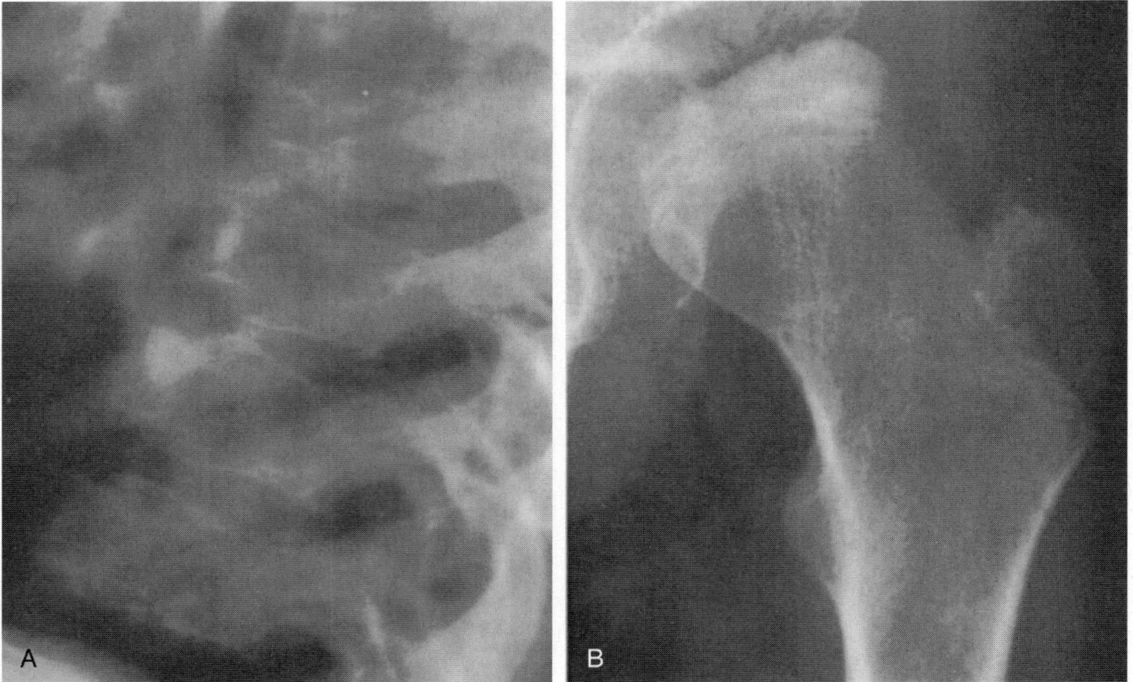

Figure 37–4. Spondyloepiphyseal dysplasia. *A,* Radiograph of the spine demonstrates the characteristic "humps" on the vertebral bodies. *B,* Flattening and sclerosis of the femoral capital epiphysis. (*A* and *B,* Courtesy of Dr. R. Cairns.)

alveolar bone resorption and early loss of teeth, and thickened scars in the pretibial areas. It is an autosomal dominant defect possibly involving the synthesis of type III collagen.[96]

Disorders of Type IV Collagen

An autosomal recessive disorder,[97] EDS type VI (McKusick 130050, 225350) is characterized by neonatal hypotonia and, later, by retinal detachment, thin sclerae, scleral herniation, ligamentous laxity, tendency to late aortic rupture, short stature, kyphoscoliosis, and features of EDS type I. It is associated with abnormalities of lysyl hydroxylase that result in a deficiency of hydroxylysine in type IV collagen.[98]

Disorders of Type V Collagen

EDS types I and II (McKusick 305200), the most common of the EDS variants, closely resemble each other but vary in severity. These disorders are inherited as autosomal dominant traits or occur as new mutations. A defect in type V collagen, a mutation in the COL5AI gene encoding the pro-α_1(V) fibrillar collagen chain, has been identified in type I and type II EDS.[99] In EDS type I, the hyperextensible skin tends to split over bony prominences, with tissue paper scars occurring over the shins (Fig. 37–5). The hands, face, and feet are usually broad. Pectus excavatum is not present, and the palate is normal. Shoulder dislocations can occur. Mitral valve prolapse and, rarely, aortic rupture occur.[62, 100] Fibrous nodules (molluscoid tumors) occur over the elbows, knees, and heels. EDS type II has all of the manifestations of type I but to a much milder degree.

Disorders of Type VI Collagen

Cutis laxa (McKusick 123700) is characterized by hyperextensibility of the skin. Excessive production of type VI collagen and increased expression of mRNA for type VI collagen has been demonstrated in fibroblasts from patients with this rare disorder.[101]

Disorders of Type IX Collagen

Persons with *Fairbank's multiple epiphyseal dysplasia* (McKusick 120260) often appear normal until they experience joint pain and symmetric epiphyseal changes are detected radiographically. These persons may be of normal height and have progressive degenerative joint changes that may require joint replacement.

Disorders of Type X Collagen

In the *Schmid type of metaphyseal dysplasia* (McKusick 120110), an autosomal dominant disorder in which children appear normal at birth, there is progressive enlargement of joints with a waddling gait and limitation of joint movement. The limbs are relatively shortened. Osteoarthritis is progressive.

Disorders of Type XI Collagen

Mutations in three genes coding for type XI collagen result in syndromes that resemble Stickler's syndrome type I.[102]

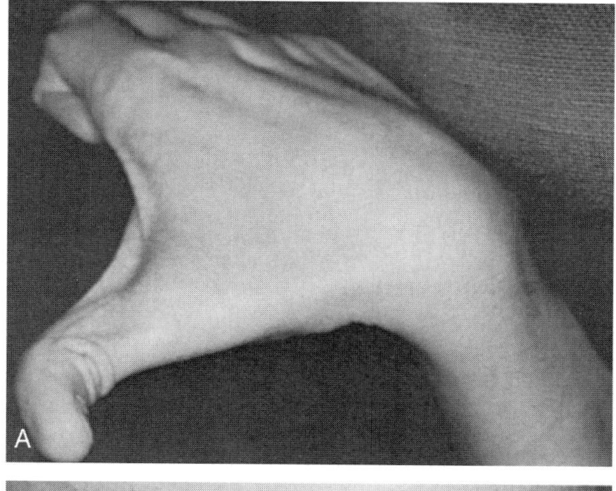

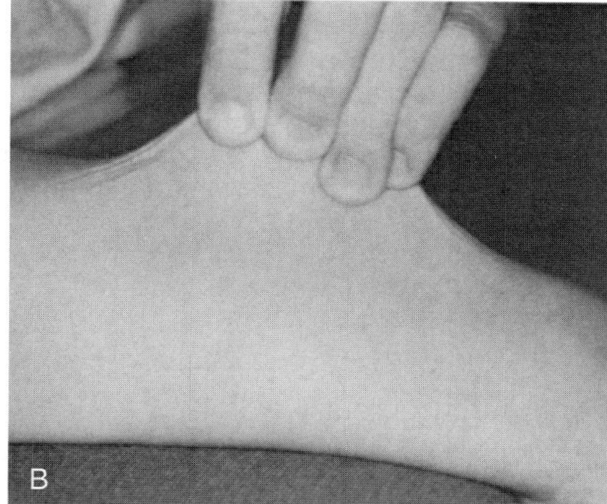

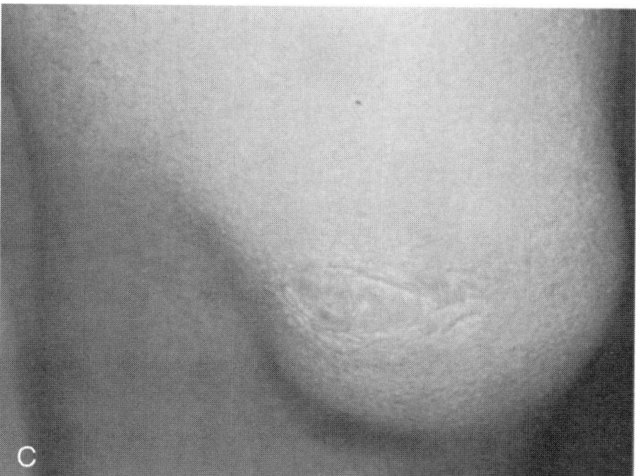

Figure 37–5. A child with Ehlers-Danlos type I shows hypermobility of the thumb (*A*), hyperextensibility of the skin of the forearm (*B*), and a "fish-mouthed" scar over the knee (*C*). (*A–C*, Courtesy of Dr. J. Prendiville.)

Ehlers-Danlos Syndromes Types V and X

EDS type V (McKusick 153455) resembles EDS types II and III and has been associated with deficiency of lysyl oxidase, although the relation of this biochemical defect is not certain.[103]

In addition to joint hypermobility and hyperextensibility of skin, as occurs in patients with EDS type II, patients with the extremely rare EDS type X have abnormal platelet aggregation associated with a fibronectin abnormality.[104] In addition, a variety of other abnormalities of hemostasis have been reported in patients with several types of EDS.[105]

Disorders Characterized by Stiff Joints

Diastrophic Dysplasias

Diastrophic dysplasia (McKusick 222600, 600972) and its variants are characterized by enlarged joints (particularly the knees), clubbing of the feet, and limitation of finger movement. There are often progressive changes in the cartilage with fragmentation, calcification, swelling, and eventually fusion of the joints, particularly the small joints of the phalanges. Pressure on the cartilage leads to cell death with calcification of the cartilage. This occurs in many parts of the body, including the ears, trachea, and costochondral junctions. Diastrophic dysplasia is an autosomal recessive disorder and has been found to be a mutation in the sulfate transporter gene.[106]

Dyggve-Melchior-Clausen Dysplasia

Dyggve-Melchior-Clausen dysplasia (McKusick 223800) is an autosomal recessive disorder. The gene has not yet been found. Affected newborns always present with some limitation of movement. Patients are often short, have an exaggerated lumbar lordosis and sternal protrusion, and have progressive mental retardation. They experience claw-hand deformities. Radiographs show platyspondyly and small sacrosciatic notches. Biopsy shows degenerative chondrocytes without storage.[107]

Progressive Pseudorheumatoid Arthropathy

Infants and young children with this autosomal recessive disorder (McKusick 208230) are often thought to be completely normal, but with time they develop swollen joints with progressive stiffness and kyphoscoliosis.[108] Radiographs show platyspondyly (narrowing of joint spaces) and widening of the metaphyses (Fig. 37–6). This disorder mimics JRA but shows none of the laboratory abnormalities of that disease. The specific gene has not been found, although a locus on chromosome 6q22 has been suggested.[109] At least six genes involved in collagen synthesis are also located in this region.

Wolcott-Rallison Dysplasia

In Wolcott-Rallison dysplasia, an autosomal recessive disorder (McKusick 226980), there is stiffness and pain in the joints, leading to difficulty walking. The spine may also be affected. Infancy-onset diabetes mellitus is usually present; with time, affected persons experience renal insufficiency and hepatomegaly.[110] Collagen fibrils in cartilage are abnormal in appearance.

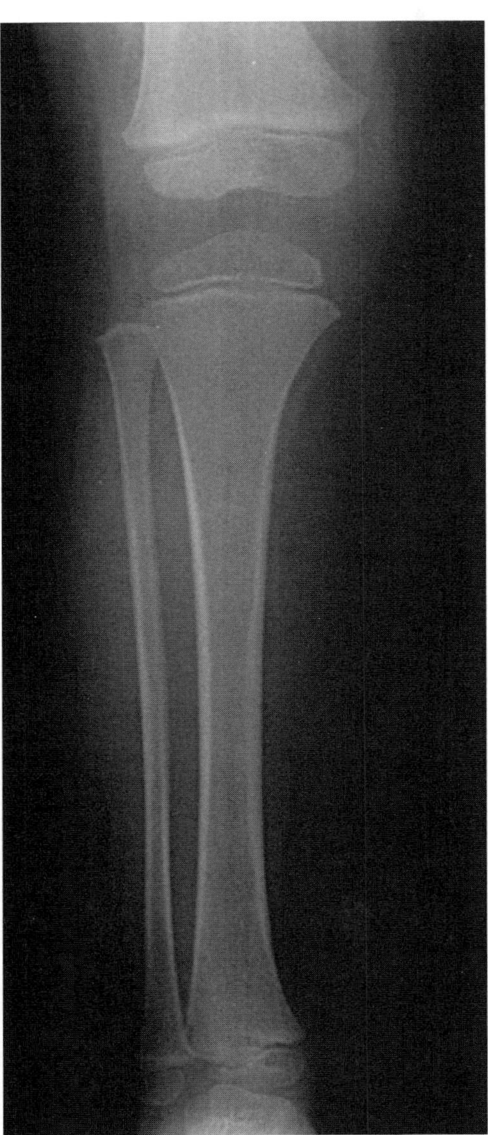

Figure 37–6. Widening of the metaphyses in a child with platyspondyly and progressive pseudorheumatoid arthropathy.

Short Trunk

A short trunk can be a part of any condition with platyspondyly and is often accompanied by back pain. Brachyolmias of the Hobaek type (McKusick 271530) and Maroteaux type (McKusick 217530) are characterized by severe shortening of the trunk caused by platyspondyly that becomes evident during childhood. These autosomal recessive disorders present with back pain, sometimes with scoliosis or spinal stenosis. Radiographs reveal characteristic lateral extension of the vertebral bodies.[111]

Mesomelic Dysplasias

Mesomelic dysplasias are characterized by shortening of the middle segments of the limbs. The most common one is *Leri-Weill dysostosis* (McKusick 127300) (Fig. 37–7). It is present at birth and, particularly in girls, is characterized by a Madelung deformity (hypoplasia and dorsal subluxation of the distal ulna with shortening and bowing of the radius, which can be quite painful). It was thought to be an autosomal dominant disorder, but the gene has recently been found to be X-linked, and specific mutations in the short stature homeobox (SHOX)–containing gene have been described.[112] A patient with both Leri-Will dysostosis and systemic lupus erythematosus has been reported.[113]

Acromelic Dysplasias

A number of acromelic and acro/mesomelic dysplasias, including various types of brachydactyly, are associated with short stature. All patients have disproportionate shortening of the hands and feet. Many have enlargement of the joints associated with limitation of movement and sometimes pain.

Trichorhinophalangeal Dysplasia

Trichorhinophalangeal dysplasia, an autosomal dominant disorder (McKusick 190350), is characterized by a bulbous nose and hypoplastic nares, short stature, sparse hair, and enlarged interphalangeal joints with broad fingers (Fig. 37–8). Cone-shaped epiphyses, short metacarpals and metatarsals, and small, flat, fragmented capital femoral epiphyses suggestive of Legg-Calvé-Perthes disease are characteristic radiologic findings.[15, 114] There are several forms of this disorder, one of which, the *Langer-Gideon syndrome* (McKusick 150230), is also associated with mental retardation and multiple exostoses. The exostoses may cause pain when they occur around joints and are often associated

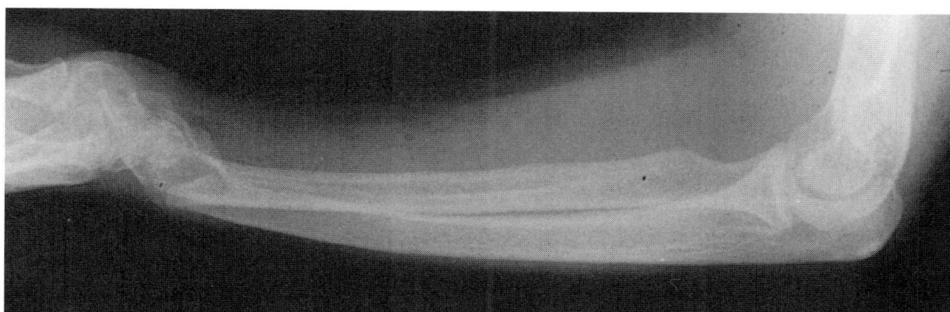

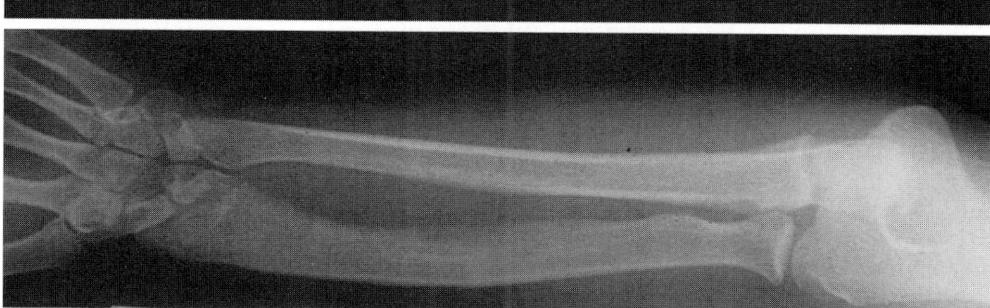

Figure 37–7. Radiographs of the forearm of a young boy with Leri-Weill dyschondrosteosis show the typical Madelung deformity.

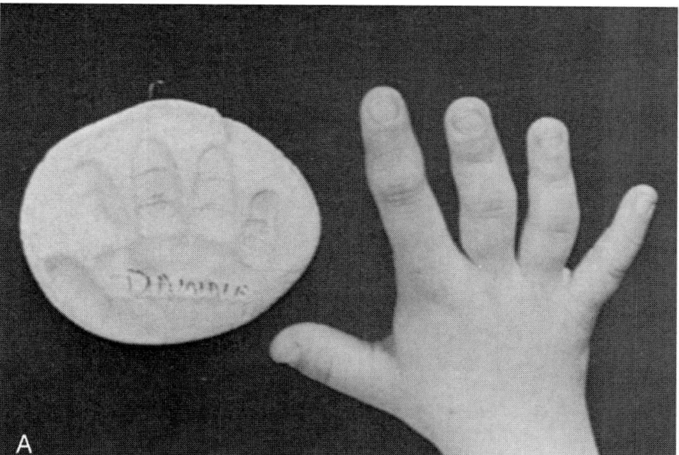

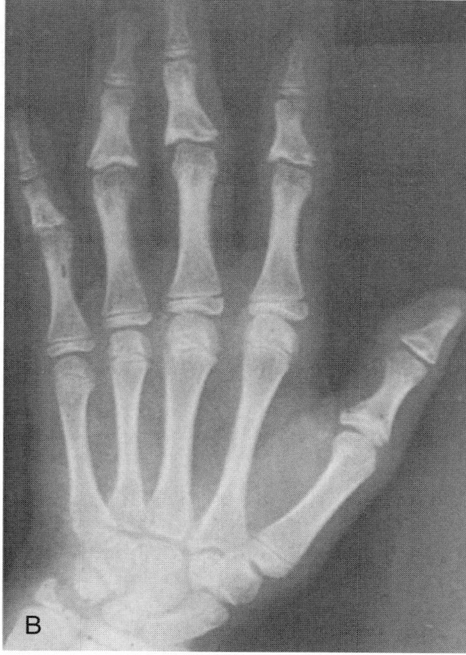

Figure 37–8. Trichorhinophalangeal dysplasia. *A,* The right hand of a 12-year-old girl with trichorhinophalangeal dysplasia, shown beside a plaster imprint made of her hand when she was in kindergarten, illustrates the progressive nature of this deformity. *B,* Radiograph of the hand of a 10-year-old girl with trichorhinophalangeal dysplasia who complained of pain in her finger joints without morning stiffness. Epiphyseal abnormalities are visible at all proximal interphalangeal joints.

with prominence of the joint. The condition involves a deletion of multiple genes at 8q24.11–13.

Metaphyseal Dysplasias

The metaphyseal dysplasias include those associated with *adenosine deaminase deficiency*[115, 116] and the *Schwachman-Diamond syndrome* (pancreatic insufficiency and neutropenia).[117] They are characterized by generalized changes (flaring, irregular ossification) in the metaphyses of tubular bone. Children with adenosine deaminase deficiency have deficient B- and T-lymphocyte function and low levels of immunoglobulins. Metaphyseal dysplasia primarily affects the ribs and long bones. Both the bony and the immunologic abnormalities have been reversed by bone marrow transplantation or enzyme replacement.[118] Children with Schwachman-Diamond syndrome are of low birth weight, have malabsorption because of deficiency of enzymes produced by the exocrine pancreas, and have frequent bacterial infections as a result of neutropenia and defects in neutrophil chemotaxis. There are irregularities in ossification, most commonly noted in the ribs, femurs, and tibias.

Epiphyseal Dysplasias

The epiphyseal dysplasias have in common the progressive emergence of abnormalities of the epiphyses of the axial or peripheral skeleton, resulting in joint pain, stiffness, and usually marked degenerative joint disease. Most cases are not evident at birth but become clinically apparent in infancy and childhood. They are classified according to the pattern of epiphyseal involvement.

Multiple epiphyseal dysplasia is one of the most common skeletal dysplasias and is inherited as an autosomal dominant trait. It is characterized by short stature and short limbs; it presents in childhood with pain and stiffness in affected joints, leading to joint contractures and occasionally scoliosis.[119, 120] There are progressive irregularities of the end-plates of the midthoracic vertebral bodies on radiographs; short metacarpals and terminal phalanges; and flattening, sclerosis, and fragmentation of the epiphyses of the hips, knees, and other joints.

MARFAN SYNDROME

In the Marfan syndrome[66, 121] (McKusick 154700), clinical abnormalities are most prominent in the skeletal, ocular, cardiovascular, and cutaneous systems. In the presence of congenital contractures of digits and elbows, the diagnosis may be made in infancy[122]; in fact, the syndrome was first described by Marfan in a 5-year-old girl. Joint hypermobility, pain and effusion, and arachnodactyly become increasingly obvious by the second decade of life,[66] although many patients are only mildly affected and the diagnosis can be difficult.

Children with the Marfan syndrome are tall, their arm span exceeds their height, and the pubis-to-heel measurement is greater than the crown-to-pubis distance. The palate is high and arched, and there may be other skeletal abnormalities such as moderate-to-severe kyphoscoliosis, pectus carinatum, slipped capital femoral epiphysis, and talipes equinovarus. Muscular hypotonia is common. Skin lesions include striae distensae and elastosis perforans serpiginosa. Ectopia lentis, with upward dislocation of the lens and iridodonesis, and cardiovascular abnormalities occur in about one third of patients. Cardiovascular involvement includes aortic root dilation and aneurysm formation, mitral valve prolapse, and conduction defects.

Affected patients often die unexpectedly from cardiac complications, and the value of pharmacologic approaches to the prevention of such developments is uncertain.[123] Criteria for the diagnosis of Marfan syndrome have been proposed.[124] A definite diagnosis requires the presence of an abnormality in at least three of the categories listed in Table 37–10. Collagen turnover is increased, and a crosslinking defect has been proposed. The defective type 1 fibrillin gene has been localized to chromosome 15, and the disease is inherited in an autosomal dominant manner. A number of variants of the Marfan syndrome have been associated with different mutations in the fibrillin gene

Table 37–10

Diagnosis of Marfan Syndrome

Abnormalities of Skeletal and Connective Tissue
Tall stature
Long limbs (dolichostenomelia)
Long fingers (arachnodactyly)
High arched palate
Joint laxity
Congenital contractures (digits and elbows)
Pectus deformity (carinatum or excavatum)
Scoliosis
Pes planus
Ocular Abnormalities
Myopia
Upward subluxation of the lens
Flat cornea
Retinal detachment
Cardiovascular Abnormalities
Aortic root dilatation
Mitral valve prolapse
Mitral valve regurgitation
Aortic valve regurgitation
Aortic dissection
Abnormalities of Skin and Integument
Striae distensae
Inguinal hernia
Pneumothorax
Central Nervous System Abnormalities
Dural ectasia
Sacral meningocele
Dilated cisterna magna
Family History
Marfan syndrome in a first-degree relative

Data from Pyeritz RE, McKusick VA: The Marfan syndrome: diagnosis and management. N Engl J Med 300: 772, 1979.

FBN1.[125] An excellent overview of the Marfan syndrome is provided by Pyeritz.[126]

Objective measurements that are of some use in the diagnosis of the Marfan syndrome include the ratio of the upper segment (vertex to pubis, or *US*) to the lower segment (top of the pubis to floor, or *LS*) and the metacarpal index. The US:LS ratio is usually increased to greater than 0.85 in children with the Marfan syndrome, but normal age-related changes and complications such as kyphoscoliosis make it difficult to apply and the overall excessive height is a more important indicator.[127] The metacarpal index, a radiographic measurement of arachnodactyly, is the ratio of the length to the width of the midshaft of metacarpals (2–5). The normal value ranges from 5.4 to 7.9. In children with the Marfan syndrome, the ratio ranges from 8.4 to 10.4.[128]

Congenital Contractural Arachnodactyly

Congenital contractural arachnodactyly (McKusick 121020) may be confused with the Marfan syndrome.[129] There are congenital contractures of the knees, elbows, and proximal interphalangeal joints, but the hands and the feet are long as in the Marfan syndrome and the head is elongated. Linear growth is accelerated. Early and progressive kyphoscoliosis may develop. The helix of the ear is abnormal. The defect is associated with a defect in the type 2 fibrillin gene (FBN2) localized to 5q23–q31, and the disorder in inherited as an autosomal dominant.[130] The contractures tend to improve as the child grows older.

Homocystinuria

Patients with type I homocystinuria resemble those with the Marfan syndrome: they are tall, have long limbs, and may have a high arched palate, arachnodactyly, myopia, peripheral retinal degeneration, and inferior (rather than superior) displacement of the lens.[35] Affected children are light skinned and fair haired. Cutaneous ulcerations and livedo reticularis are common. Hypotonia is present, but the joints are usually stiff rather than hyperextensible. Progressive severe osteoporosis and mental retardation are characteristic. The basic biochemical defect is a deficiency of cystathionine synthetase that is inherited as an autosomal recessive trait. There is an accumulation in tissues of the sulfur-containing amino acids homocystine, homocysteine, serine, and methionine. There may also be a defect in collagen crosslinking. Demonstration of homocystine in the urine clearly differentiates children with homocystinuria from those with the Marfan syndrome. Treatment includes methionine restriction and pyridoxine supplementation.[131] Without therapy, arterial or venous thromboses lead to premature death.

Types II and III homocystinuria differ from type I homocystinuria in the nature of the biochemical defect and in the absence of skeletal abnormalities and occlusive arterial disease.[132]

DYSOSTOSIS MULTIPLEX

This group of disorders includes the mucopolysaccharidoses (MPSs), the mucolipidoses (MLs), mannosidosis, fucosidosis, gangliosidosis, sialidosis, sialic storage disease, galactosialidosis, and mucosulfatidosis. Deficiency of a lysosomal degradative enzyme leads to an accumulation of its substrate within the lysosomes of the cell.[43] The phenotype of the specific disease depends on the tissue distribution of the enzyme deficiency. The resulting multisystem degenerative disorders are progressive and unremitting. Skeletal changes include dwarfism, joint contractures, and dysostosis multiplex. Although these disorders are classified as osteochondrodysplasias, they differ from all other members of that group in that they are storage disorders.

Mucopolysaccharidoses

The MPSs are genetically determined deficiencies of enzymes involved in the metabolism of glycosaminoglycans (Table 37–11).[43] Progressive skeletal dysplasia particularly affects the vertebrae, hips, and hands.[43, 133] In the more severe types, such as *Hurler's syndrome* (MPS type I H), dwarfism and marked coarsening of the facial features are present. In addition, deposition of mucopolysaccharide leads to mental retardation and corneal clouding. A claw-hand deformity is often the first clue to the diagnosis.

Two of these storage diseases particularly mimic inflammatory arthritis. The comparatively mild dysostosis but severe dwarfing of *Morquio's syndrome* (MPS type IV) (McKusick 253000, 252300, 230500) may suggest JRA. Children with this syndrome, who have normal intelligence, may present with an effusion of a large joint (particularly the knee) or with progressive musculoskeletal stiffness, usually by 3 or 4 years of age. The small joints of the hands become enlarged and stiff, a valgus deformity of the knees develops, and the gait becomes stiff and waddling. The joints are not always stiff, however, and some joints (such as the wrists), although enlarged, may be hypermobile. A pectus deformity and barrel chest are usual. Characteristic radiographic findings include platyspondyly and odontoid hypoplasia and should help differentiate this disorder from the various forms of spondyloepiphyseal dysplasia.[164] Urinary excretion of keratan sulfate is increased.

In *Scheie's syndrome* (MPS type I S) (McKusick 252800), intelligence is normal and stature is preserved. However, there is progressive stiffening of the joints of the hands, elbows, and knees without swelling or pain. Corneal clouding occurs. All acute-phase reactants are normal, but urinary excretion of dermatan sulfate is increased.

Mucolipidoses

The term *mucolipidosis* is applied to a group of four disorders that are characterized by the intracellular

Table 37–11

Mucopolysaccharidoses

TYPE	NAME	INHERITANCE	MPS	ENZYME DEFECT	CLINICAL FEATURES
IH	Hurler	AR	DS, HS	α-L-Iduronidase	Corneal clouding, dysostosis multiplex, heart disease, severe mental retardation, death in childhood
IS	Scheie*	AR	DS, HS	α-L-Iduronidase	Milder skeletal disease, normal intelligence, normal life span (?)
II	Hunter	XR	DS, HS	Iduronate sulfatase	Milder than type I; no corneal clouding
IIIA	Sanfilippo	AR	HS	Heparan-*N*-sulfatase	Mild skeletal, severe CNS abnormalities
IIIB				*N*-Acetyl-α-D-glucosaminidase	
IIIC				Acetyl-CoA-glucosaminidase acetyltransferase	
IIID				*N*-Acetyl-glucosamine 6-sulfatase	
IVA	Morquio	AR	KS	*N*-AG-6-Sulfatase	Severe skeletal changes; corneal clouding; normal intelligence
IVB				β-Galactosidase	
VI	Maroteaux-Lamy	AR	DS	*N*-AG-4-Sulfatase	Severe skeletal changes, corneal clouding, heart disease, normal intelligence
VII	Sly	AR	DS, HS	β-Glucuronidase	Dysostosis multiplex, variable intelligence, hepatosplenomegaly, white blood cell inclusions

*Formerly classified as type V.
MPS, mucopolysaccharide found in urine; DS, dermatan sulfate; GS, heparan sulfate; KS, keratan sulfate.
Modified from Beighton P: McKusick's Heritable Disorders of Connective Tissue, 5th ed. St. Louis, Mosby-Year Book, 1993.

accumulation of both glycosaminoglycans and sphingolipids but without excess urinary glycosaminoglycan excretion. Progressive neurologic and ocular abnormalities occur in all of these autosomal recessive disorders (Table 37–12).[42]

ML type I, isolated neuraminidase (sialidase) deficiency, causes a Hurler-like syndrome with joint contractures, short trunk and stature, and dysostosis multiplex (vertebral anomalies, hypoplastic odontoid and ilia, coxa valga, and deformed capital femoral epiphyses). Urinary excretion of sialated urinary oligosaccharides (bound sialic acid) is markedly elevated (McKusick 256550).

I-cell disease (ML type II) also causes a Hurler-like syndrome with progressive limitation of joint range of motion; the name is derived from the presence of prominent intracytoplasmic (I) inclusions in cultured fibroblasts. The biochemical defect is not clearly understood but appears to involve an abnormality in the cellular localization of acid hydrolases.

Pseudo–Hurler's polydystrophy is a term applied to ML type III (McKusick 252500). Restriction of joint mobility becomes apparent by 2 years of age, but there is no inflammatory arthritis. Radiologic findings are those of dysostosis multiplex. By 6 years of age, features of Hurler's syndrome dominate the clinical picture. Prognosis for life is good. Inclusions are also found in cultured fibroblasts from some patients with this disease; they probably represent a milder form of ML type II. In ML type IV, there are no characteristic skeletal abnormalities (McKusick 252600).

OTHER DISORDERS

A great many disorders of cartilage and bone defy classification. Some appear to have a genetic basis; others have an inflammatory component as well. Those likely to be of interest to the pediatric rheumatologist are briefly summarized in this section.

Table 37–12

Mucolipidoses

TYPE	NAME	DEFECT	MUSCULOSKELETAL FEATURES
I	Sialidase deficiency	Sialidase deficiency	Contractures, short stature, dysostosis multiplex
II	I-cell disease	Phosphotransferase deficiency	Progressive limitation of range of motion
III	Pseudo-Hurler's polydystrophy	Phosphotransferase deficiency	Progressive limitation of range of motion; dysostosis multiplex
IV	Sialolipidosis	Uncertain	No characteristic skeletal changes

Pseudopseudohypoparathyroidism

Pseudopseudohypoparathyroidism, also known as *Albright's hereditary osteodysplasia,* is characterized by short fourth metacarpals, short stature, and sometimes mental retardation, round face, and subcutaneous calcifications. Hypocalcemia and hyperphosphatemia may occur. The condition results from defects in the alpha-subunit of the G protein.[135] There is an unusual pattern of inheritance in that children who inherited the gene from the mother are more severely affected than those who inherited the gene from the father (genomic imprinting).[136]

Pseudoachondroplasia

Pseudoachondroplasia, a relatively common form of disproportionate short stature (McKusick 177170), is not present at birth but becomes obvious between the ages of 1 and 2 years. There is mild shortening of the trunk, shortening of limbs with hyperextensible joints, but normal face and skull. The spectrum of short stature is very broad, and it has been suggested that mosaicism plays a role in determining severity.[137] Radiographs show platyspondyly and delay in maturation of epiphyses. Because of ligamentous laxity, degenerative arthritis develops and joint replacement may become necessary. Pseudoachondroplasia is due to mutations in the cartilage oligomeric matrix protein.[138]

Chondrodysplasia Punctata

The term *chondrodysplasia punctata* describes a radiologic appearance rather than a specific disease and occurs in a number of conditions. In the autosomal recessive rhizomelic type of chondrodysplasia punctata, there are joint contractures, large head, cataracts, and ichthyosis-like skin changes (McKusick 215100). Most infants with this syndrome die within the first year of life.[139] Chondrodysplasia punctata is a peroxisomal disorder. A milder form (McKusick 302960) is associated with deletion of the distal short arm of the X chromosome and presents as an X-linked recessive disorder. In the X-linked dominant *Conradi-Hünermann* disease (McKusick 302960), the limbs are characteristically affected asymmetrically, and contractures or deformities of the feet may be present. Radiologic abnormalities include stippling of the vertebrae and epiphyses representing disturbed epiphyseal maturation that leads to asymmetric growth. The skin often has patches of ichthyotic change. Only females are affected; it appears to be lethal in males. Genetically determined abnormalities in sterol metabolism may be pathogenically related.[140]

Chondrodysplasia punctata has been observed in one infant with neonatal lupus.[141, 142] It is also associated with the maternal use of warfarin[143] and maternal vitamin K deficiency.[144]

Osteopetrosis

Osteopetrosis (McKusick 166600, 259700) is a rare disorder that may present at birth with frontal bossing, hypertelorism, exophthalmos, nasal obstruction, and cranial nerve palsies. It progresses in severity during infancy and early childhood with repeated fractures, abnormal bleeding, seizures, and early death. The density of all bones is increased, and the metaphyses are flared. Bone marrow transplantation offers hope of effective treatment.[145] *Albers-Schönberg disease* is a form of osteopetrosis with late onset that is milder in degree than the early-onset form. It is inherited as an autosomal dominant trait.[146]

Melorheostosis

Patchy disorders such as melorheostosis (McKusick 155950) and *McCune-Albright syndrome* (McKusick 174800) appear to result from somatic mutations. Melorheostosis develops after the neonatal period and commonly affects only one limb. Clinically, there may be intermittent swelling and pain around joints, with loss of range of motion and development of contractures at the wrists, elbows, hips, and knees.[147] Skin changes may precede contractures and include tense, red, shiny skin with edema of the subcutaneous tissues. Melorheostosis may occur together with other radiographic abnormalities such as *osteopoikilosis* (Fig. 37–9).[148, 149] Melorheostosis of the iliac bone has been described in a boy with linear scleroderma.[150] Radiographs show cortical hyperostosis in a "dripping candle wax" pattern, sometimes with endosteal hyperostosis and prominent soft tissue calcification.

Engelmann's Syndrome

Engelmann's syndrome, or *progressive diaphyseal dysplasia* (McKusick 131300), presents early in childhood with leg pain, abnormalities of gait, muscle weakness, and pain. Radiographs reveal thickening and sclerosis of the cortex of long bones (Fig. 37–10). It is an autosomal dominant disorder, although the gene is not known. Glucocorticoid therapy was reported to be successful in one patient.[151] The abnormalities may resolve spontaneously in adolescence.[152]

Osteolyses

There are several disorders in which bone dissolves or disappears (McKusick 166300, 259600). The idiopathic osteolyses are grouped according to the area predominantly affected: phalangeal, carpal/tarsal, or multicentric. *Familial acro-osteolysis* is inherited as an autosomal dominant trait and becomes apparent at about 3 years of age (Fig. 37–11).[153, 154] The carpus or tarsus alone may be affected, or the bones of the hands, feet, elbows,

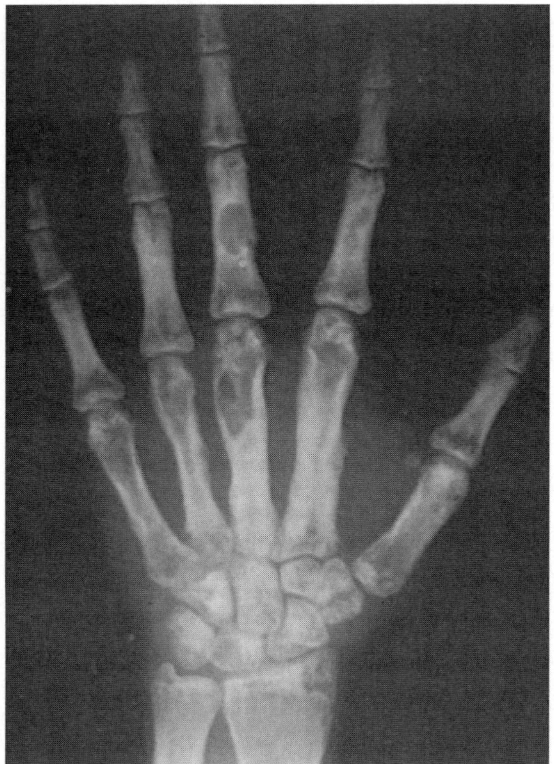

Figure 37–9. Radiograph of the hand of a 15-year-old girl with a history of fractures in her toes and diffuse musculoskeletal pain. All bones except the skull were affected by osteopoikilosis, melorheostosis, and fibrous dysplasia. These abnormalities may occur in isolation, with café-au-lait spots and sexual precocity (fibrous dysplasia in McCune-Albright syndrome), or—as in this patient—as multiple sclerosing bone dysplasia. (Courtesy of Dr. R. Cairns.)

and knees may be involved. The onset can mimic JRA in that affected areas are swollen and warm. Eventually, radiographs show progressive bone lysis and destruction of the involved joints. Spontaneous remissions during the young adult years are characteristic.[155, 156] The osteolysis is often associated with pain or neuropathic changes and may lead to skin ulcerations that overlie the bony abnormalities. *Hereditary distal osteolysis*, inherited as an autosomal dominant trait, involves the phalanges and metacarpal or metatarsal bones, and it produces recurrent ulcerations at the affected sites. It presents generally during late childhood. Spontaneous remission is usual, but unfortunately not before there is loss of digits.[157]

Disorders such as *Winchester's syndrome* (McKusick 277950), a form of multicentric osteolysis, begin at about 6 weeks of age with restricted joint mobility, swelling, and pain of the proximal interphalangeal joints and enlargement of the wrists.[54, 158, 159] Later, corneal clouding, coarsening of the face, and joint contractures occur. Osteoporosis, bone erosion, and atlantoaxial subluxation are characteristic radiographic findings.

Phantom bone disease (Gorham's disease) occurs between the ages of 5 and 10 years and is not hereditary.[160] A carpal/tarsal osteolysis is usual. Carpal/tarsal osteolysis associated with nephropathy has also been described.[155, 156]

Arthrogryposis

Arthrogryposis is the term used to refer to a number of disorders characterized by the presence of multiple congenital contractures. They all appear to result from decreased movement in utero and often produce apparent enlargement of joints, which is actually secondary to loss of connective tissue and muscle.[20, 21] These disorders tend to be nonprogressive and are not usually associated with pain.

Larsen's Syndrome

Larsen's syndrome (McKusick 150250, 145600) is characterized by multiple dislocations of large joints, dysplasias of the spine, and midface hypoplasia. Dislocations cause pain and, if recurrent, may lead to degenerative joint disease. It is inherited as an autosomal dominant condition.[65] Analysis of one family suggests that the responsible gene is located on 3p21.1-14.1—close to, but distinct from, the collagen type VII α_1 chain gene.[161]

Menkes' Syndrome

The skeletal abnormalities of Menkes' syndrome include osteoporosis, repeated fractures, metaphyseal spurring, and wormian bones in the sutures of the

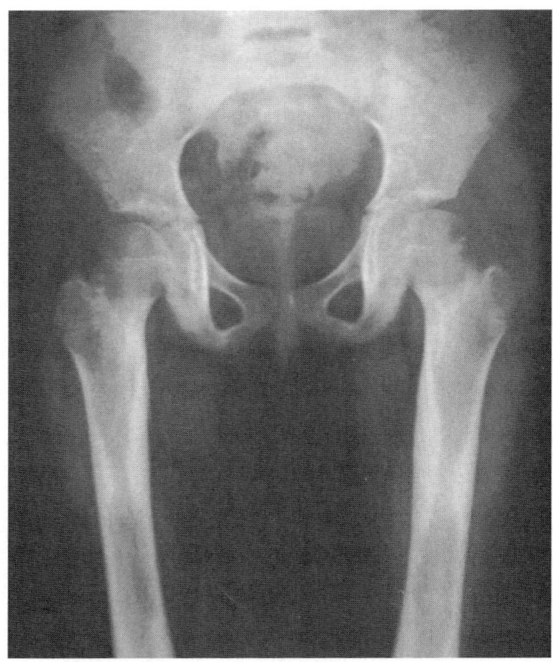

Figure 37–10. Radiograph illustrates the thickening and sclerosis of the diaphyseal cortex of the femurs of a child with diaphyseal dysplasia (Camurati-Engelmann syndrome). (Courtesy of Dr. R. Cairns.)

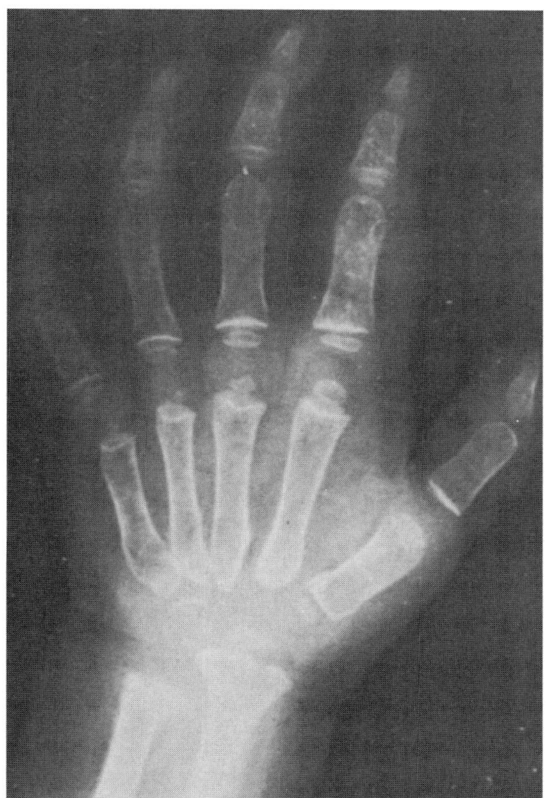

Figure 37–11. Radiograph of the hand of a 3-year-old with familial acro-osteolysis. There is swelling of the wrist and dissolution of the carpal ossification centers. Generalized osteoporosis of the hand is present. The radius has overgrown the ulna. This child died later, probably from associated nephropathy.

skull. These features reflect an abnormality of copper metabolism, with low serum ceruloplasmin and copper but high tissue levels of copper.[162] The *occipital horn syndrome,* formerly classified as EDS type IX, is also thought to be an abnormality of copper metabolism.[163] It is characterized by bony occipital horns, cutaneous hyperextensibility, joint hypermobility, and (in many patients) chronic diarrhea.

Camptodactyly

The term *camptodactyly* refers to the presence of congenital or acquired flexion contractures of the proximal interphalangeal joints, resulting from soft tissue tightening without limitation of flexion.[164] It is most common in the fifth finger but can occur in all digits of the hand except the thumb. The cause is not certain but appears to be related to fibrotic changes in the subcutaneous tissue of the palmar aspect of the joint. Radiographs reveal neither bony nor articular abnormalities per se. Camptodactyly may occur with diseases such as the Marfan syndrome and has been reported in association with familial arthritis by Malleson and associates.[165] Three children in one family had iridocyclitis, and one boy died suddenly at the age of 4 years. Postmortem examination revealed chronic synovitis and granulomatous arteritis affecting the aorta, coronary arteries, myocardium, and pericardium. There have been other reports of familial camptodactyly, and a syndrome of camptodactyly, arthritis, coxa vara, and pericarditis has been described.

The *camptodactyly, arthritis, coxa vara, and pericarditis syndrome* is inherited as an autosomal recessive disorder caused by a defective gene on chromosome 1q25-31.[10] It is characterized by congenital camptodactyly and childhood onset of noninflammatory synovial hyperplasia. Some patients have pericarditis; others have coxa vara.

Cortical Hyperostosis

Pachydermoperiostosis

Pachydermoperiostosis is a rare autosomal dominant disorder characterized by onset (usually in adolescent boys) of "spadelike" enlargement of the hands and feet, sometimes accompanied by pain along the distal long bones.[166–168] In addition to the cylindrical enlargement of the digits, forearms, and lower legs, there may be minimal joint effusions, coarsening of the facial features, excessive oiliness of the skin, and occasionally gynecomastia, female hair distribution, striae, and acne.

Familial Infantile Cortical Hyperostosis (Caffey's Disease)

Caffey's disease is a rare disorder that presents before 4 months of age with fever, irritability, abnormal acute-phase indices, and swelling, tenderness, erythema, or altered contour of the mandible, shoulder girdles, and long bones (Fig. 37–12).[169–171] Bony involvement tends to be asymmetric. The calvarium is never affected. The ribs and clavicles are often involved by marked cortical thickening with altered bone shape. The cause is unknown, although it appears to be inflammatory and may be triggered by an infection. It usually has a self-limited course of weeks to months, after which it subsides without sequelae. Short-term treatment with glucocorticoids may be considered in the infant with severe disease and marked systemic symptoms. There appears to be a familial but nongenetic basis for this disorder (see also Chapter 38).

Disordered Development of Cartilage

Trevor's Disease

In Trevor's disease, there is overgrowth of one of the tarsal or carpal bones or of an epiphysis, often at the knee or ankle. The abnormality is more common in boys than in girls and is self-limited.[172]

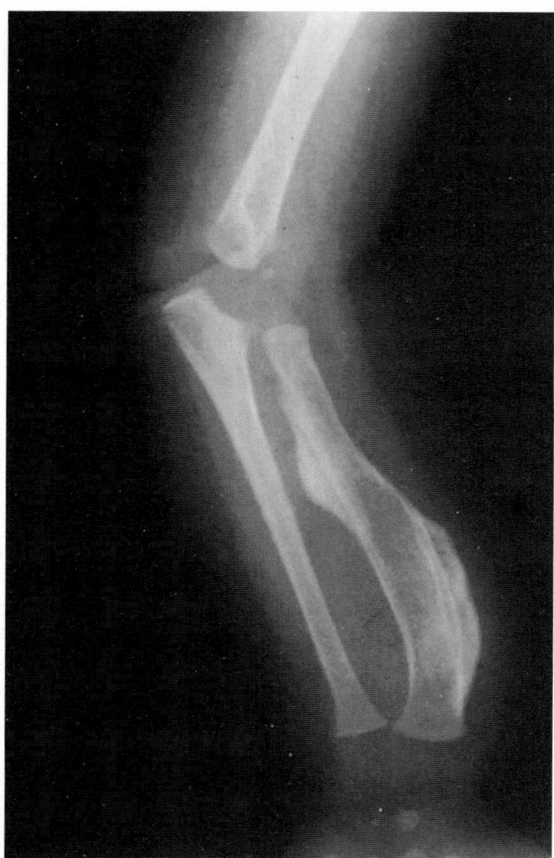

Figure 37–12. Marked hyperostosis of the radius in a 5-month-old boy with Caffey's disease.

Diaphyseal Aclasis

Diaphyseal aclasis is characterized by cartilaginous and bony outgrowths from the metaphyses of long bones, ribs, pelvis, and scapulae. These may interfere with joint function. The gene causing this autosomal dominant condition has been localized to the long arm of chromosome 8 (8q23–a24.1).[5]

Ollier's Disease

Multiple enchondromatosis, or Ollier's disease, becomes evident during childhood, with multiple juxta-articular outgrowths or fractures. Radiographs demonstrate the radiolucent cartilaginous areas in the metaphyseal regions of the tubular and flat bones. Multiple enchondromatosis with hemangiomas is called *Maffucci's syndrome* (see also Chapter 36).

Fetal Alcohol Syndrome

Children with fetal alcohol syndrome have a characteristic facial appearance (flattening of the midface, short palpebral fissures, and smooth, elongated upper lip) but may also have flexion contractures of the elbows, restricted motion of the metacarpophalangeal joints, camptodactyly, and clinodactyly. Developmental delay, impaired linear growth, and cardiac septal defects are associated problems.[173]

References

1. Rimoin DL, Connor JM, Pyeritz RE: Emery and Rimoin's Principles and Practice of Medical Genetics. New York, Churchill Livingstone, 1997.
2. Kozlowski K, Beighton P: Gamut Index of Skeletal Dysplasias. An Aid to Radiodiagnosis. London, Springer-Verlag, 1995.
3. Taybi H, Lachman RS: Radiology of Syndromes, Metabolic Disorders and Skeletal Dysplasia. St. Louis, Mosby–Year Book, 1996.
4. Gorlin RJ, Cohen MM, Levin LS: Syndromes of the Head and Neck. New York, Oxford University Press, 1990.
5. Spranger EJP (for the International Working Group on Constitutional Diseases of Bone): International nomenclature and classification of the osteochondrodysplasias (1997). Am J Med Genet 79: 376, 1998.
6. McKusick V (ed): Online Mendelian Inheritance in Man (*www.nlm.nih.gov/omim*): Mendelian inheritance in man: a catalog of human genes and genetic disorders. Baltimore, Johns Hopkins University Press, 1998.
7. Chalom EC, Ross J, Athreya BH: Syndromes and arthritis. Rheum Dis Clin North Am 23: 709, 1997.
8. Hall JG, Lopez-Rangel E: Bone dysplasias, nontraditional mechanisms of inheritance and monozygotic twins. Pediatr Radiol 27: 422, 1997.
9. Hall JG: Genomic imprinting: nature and clinical relevance. Annu Rev Med 48: 35, 1997.
10. Bahabri SA, Suwairi WM, Laxer RM, et al: The camptodactyly-arthropathy-coxa vara-pericarditis syndrome. Clinical features and genetic mapping to human chromosome I. Arthritis Rheum 41: 730, 1998.
11. Rogers JG, McKusick VA: Dominant familial arthritis with scoliosis. *In* Bergsma D (ed): Disorders of Connective Tissue. New York, Stratton Intercontinental Medical, 1975, pp 75–80.
12. Pai GS, Macpherson RI: Idiopathic multicentric osteolysis: report of two new cases and a review of the literature. Am J Med Genet 29: 929, 1988.
13. Guidera KG, Satterwhite Y, Ogden JA, et al: Nail patella syndrome: a review of 44 orthopaedic patients. J Pediatr Orthop 11: 737, 1991.
14. Stickler GB, Belau PG, Farrell FJ, et al: Hereditary progressive arthro-ophthalmopathy. Mayo Clin Proc 40: 433, 1965.
15. Cope R, Beals RK, Bennett RM: The trichorhinophalangeal syndrome: report of eight kindreds, with emphasis on hip complications, late presentations and premature osteoarthritis. J Pediatr Orthop 6: 133, 1986.
16. Teebi AS, Rucquoi JK, Meyn MS: Aarskog syndrome. A report of a family with review and discussion of nosology. Am J Med Genet 46: 501, 1993.
17. Hecht JT, Butler IJ: Neurologic morbidity associated with achondroplasia. J Child Neurol 5: 84, 1990.
18. Rumball KM, Pang E, Letts RM: Musculoskeletal manifestations of the Antley-Bixler syndrome. J Pediatr Orthop B 8: 139, 1999.
19. Cohen MM Jr, Kreiborg S: Skeletal abnormalities in the Apert syndrome. Am J Med Genet 47: 624, 1993.
20. Gordon N: Arthrogryposis multiplex congenita. Brain Dev 20: 507, 1998.
21. Hall JG: Arthrogryposis multiplex congenita: etiology, genetics, classification, diagnostic approach and general aspects. J Pediatr Orthop B 6: 153, 1997.
22. Viljoen D: Congenital contractural arachnodactyly (Beals syndrome). J Med Genet 31: 640, 1994.
23. O'Brien J: Generalized gangliosidosis. J Pediatr 75: 167, 1969.
24. Neidich J, Zackai E, Aronson M, et al: Deletion of 2p: a cytogenetic and clinical update. Am J Med Genet 27: 707, 1987.
25. Nance MA, Berry SA: Cockayne syndrome: Review of 140 cases. Am J Med Genet 42: 68, 1992.
26. Happle R: X-linked dominant chondrodysplasia punctata: re-

view of the literature and report of a case. Hum Genet 53: 65, 1979.
27. Jameson RA, Holt PJ, Keen JH: Farber's disease. Ann Rheum Dis 46: 559, 1987.
28. Fujiwaki T, Hamanaka S, Koga M, et al: A case of Farber's disease. Acta Paediatr Jpn 34: 72, 1992.
29. Kouseff BG, Newkirk P, Root AW: Brachmann-de Lange syndrome. 1994 update. Arch Pediatr Adolesc Med 148: 749, 1994.
30. Ryoppy S, Poussa M, Merikanto J, et al: Foot deformities in diastrophic dysplasia. An analysis of 102 patients. J Bone Joint Surg Br 74: 441, 1992.
31. Akita S, Kuratomi H, Abe K, et al: EC syndrome in a girl with paracentric inversion (7)(q22.1;q36.3). Clin Dysmorphol 2: 62, 1993.
32. Wallace HJ: Anderson-Fabry disease. Br J Dermatol 88: 1, 1973.
33. Perlman JM, Burns DK, Twickler DM, Weinberg AG: Fetal dyskinesia syndrome in the monochorionic pair of a triplet pregnancy secondary to severe disruptive cerebral injury. Pediatrics 96: 521, 1995.
34. Verloes A, Hermia JP, Galand A, et al: Glaucoma-lens-ectopia-microspherophakia-stiffness-shortness syndrome: a dominant disease with manifestations of Weill-Marchesani syndromes. Am J Med Genet 44: 48, 1992.
35. Mudd SH, Skovby F, Levy HL, et al: The natural history of homocystinuria due to cystathionine beta synthetase deficiency. Am J Hum Genet 37: 1, 1985.
36. Lemyre E, Azouz EM, Teebi AS, et al: Bone dysplasia series. Achondroplasia, hypochondroplasia and thanatophoric dysplasia: review and update. Can Assoc Radiol J 50: 185, 1999.
37. Gordon SL, Varano LA, Alandete A, Maisels MJ: Jansen's metaphyseal dysostosis. Pediatrics 58: 556, 1976.
38. Hilton RC, Wentzel J: Leri pleonosteosis. Q J Med 49: 419, 1980.
39. Felman AH, Kirkpatrick JA: Dyschondrosteoses: mesomelic dwarfism of Leri and Weill. Am J Dis Child 120: 329, 1970.
40. Williams MS, Josephson KD, Wargowski DS: Marden-Walker syndrome: a case report and a critical review of the literature. Clin Dysmorphol 2: 211, 1993.
41. Beck M, Roubicek M, Rogers JG, et al: Heterogeneity of metatropic dysplasia. Eur J Pediatr 140: 231, 1983.
42. Gilbert-Barness EF, Barness LA: The mucolipidoses. Perspect Pediatr Pathol 17: 148, 1993.
43. Wraith JE: The mucopolysaccharidoses: a clinical review and guide to management. Arch Dis Child 72: 263, 1995.
44. Brunt PW, McKusick VA: Familial dysautonomia: a report of genetic and clinical studies with a review of the literature. Medicine 49: 343, 1970.
45. Patel AC, McAlister WH, Whyte MP: Spondyloepimetaphyseal dysplasia: clinical and radiologic investigation of a large kindred manifesting autosomal dominant inheritance, and a review of the literature. Medicine 72: 326, 1993.
46. Pascuzzi RM: Schwartz-Jampel syndrome. Semin Neurol 11: 267, 1991.
47. Harper RG, Orti E, Baker RK: Bird-headed dwarfs (Seckel's syndrome): a familial pattern of developmental, dental, skeletal, genital and central nervous system anomalies. J Pediatr 70: 799, 1967.
48. Wynne-Davis R, Hall C: The clinical variants of spondyloepiphyseal dysplasia. J Bone Joint Surg Br 64: 435, 1982.
49. Nores JM, Dizien O, Remy JM, Maroteaux P: Two cases of spondylometaphyseal dysplasia. Literature review and discussion of the genetic inheritance of the disease. J Rheumatol 20: 170, 1993.
50. Elias-Jones AC, Habibi P, Larcher VF, et al: The trisomy (5)(q31qter) syndrome. Study of a family with a f(5: 14) translocation. Arch Dis Child 63: 427, 1988.
51. Caspersson T, Lindsten J, Zech L, et al: Four patients with trisomy 8 identified by the fluorescence and Giemsa-banding techniques. J Med Genet 9: 1, 1972.
52. Weaver DD, Graham CB, Thomas IT, et al: A new overgrowth syndrome with accelerated skeletal maturation, unusual facies, and camptodactyly. J Pediatr 84: 547, 1974.
53. Haik GM, Terrell WL III, Haik GM Jr: The Weill-Marchesani syndrome: report of two cases and a review. J La State Med Soc 142: 25, 30,1990.
54. Hollister DW, Rimoin DL, Lachman RS, et al: The Winchester syndrome: a nonlysosomal connective tissue disease. J Pediatr 84: 701, 1974.
55. Zellweger H, Maertens P, Superneau D, et al: History of the cerebrohepatorenal syndrome of Zellweger and other peroxisomal disorders. South Med J 81: 357, 1988.
56. Procopis PG, Turner B: Mental retardation, abnormal fingers and skeletal anomalies. Coffin's syndrome. Am J Dis Child 124: 258, 1972.
57. Levy P, Baraitser M: Coffin-Siris syndrome. J Med Genet 28: 338, 1991.
58. Cohen MM Jr, Hall BD, Smith DW, et al: A new syndrome with hypotonia, obesity, mental deficiency and facial, oral, ocular, and limb anomalies. J Pediatr 83: 280, 1973.
59. Teebi AS, Shaabani IS: Further delineation of Costello syndrome. Am J Med Genet 47: 166, 1993.
60. Reisner SH, Seelenfreund M, Ben-Bassat M: Cutis laxa associated with severe intrauterine growth retardation and congenital dislocation of the hip. Acta Pediatr Scand 60: 357, 1971.
61. Hansen KE, Kirkpatrick SJ, Laxova R: Dubowitz syndrome: long-term follow-up of an original patient. Am J Med Genet 55: 161, 1995.
62. Pope EM: Ehlers-Danlos syndrome. Baillieres Clin Rheumatol 5: 321, 1991.
63. Crifasi PA, Patterson MC, Bonde D, Michels VV: Severe Hajdu-Cheney syndrome with upper airway obstruction. Am J Med Genet 70: 261, 1997.
64. Ikegawa S, Sakaguchi R, Kimizuka M, et al: Recurrent dislocation of the patella in Kabuki make-up syndrome. J Pediatr Orthoped 13: 265, 1993.
65. Larsen LJ, Schottstaedt ER, Bost FC: Multiple congenital dislocations associated with characteristic facial abnormalities. J Pediatr 37: 574, 1950.
66. Gray JR, Davies SJ: Marfan syndrome. J Med Genet 33: 403, 1996.
67. Makitie O, Kaitila I: Cartilage-hair hypoplasia—clinical manifestations in 108 Finnish patients. Eur J Pediatr 152: 211, 1993.
68. Mikles M, Stanton RP: A review of Morquio syndrome. Am J Orthop 26: 533, 1997.
69. Teebi AAS, Qumsiyeh MB, Meyers-Seifer CH, et al: Velo-facio-skeletal syndrome in a mother and daughter. Am J Med Genet 58: 8, 1995.
70. Bassett GS, Scott CI Jr: The osteochondrodysplasias. *In* Morrisey RT (ed): Pediatric Orthopaedics, 3rd ed. Philadelphia, JB Lippincott, 1990, p 91.
71. American Academy of Pediatrics Committee on Genetics: Health supervision for children with achondroplasia. Pediatrics 95: 443, 1995.
72. Eyre DR: The collagens of articular cartilage. Semin Arthritis Rheum 21: 2, 1991.
73. Beighton P: The Ehlers-Danlos Syndromes. London, William Heinemann Medical, 1970.
74. Sillence DO, Senn A, Banks DM: Genetic heterogeneity in osteogenesis imperfecta. J Med Genet 16: 101, 1979.
75. Castells S, Yasumura S, Fusi MA, et al: Plasma osteocalcin levels in patients with osteogenesis imperfecta. J Pediatr 109: 88, 1986.
76. Castells S, Colbert C, Chakrabarti C, et al: Therapy of osteogenesis imperfecta with synthetic salmon calcitonin. J Pediatr 95: 807, 1979.
77. Nishi Y, Hamamoto K, Kajiyama M, et al: Effect of long-term calcitonin therapy by injection and nasal spray on the incidence of fractures in osteogenesis imperfecta. J Pediatr 1121: 477, 1992.
78. Glorieux FH, Bishop NJ, Plotkin H, et al: Cyclic administration of pamidronate in children with severe osteogenesis imperfecta. N Engl J Med 339: 947, 1998.
79. Engelbert RH, Pruijs HE, Beemer FA, Helders PJ: Osteogenesis imperfecta in childhood: treatment strategies. Arch Phys Med Rehabil 79: 1590, 1998.
80. Kocher MS, Shapiro F: Osteogenesis imperfecta. J Am Acad Orthop Surg 6: 225, 1998.
81. Brenton DP, Dent CF: Idiopathic juvenile osteoporosis. *In* Bickel H, Stern J (eds): Inborn Errors of Calcium and Bone Metabolism. Baltimore, University Press, 1976, p 222.
82. Dent CE, Friedman M: Idiopathic juvenile osteoporosis. Q J Med 34: 177, 1965.
83. Halila R, Steinmann B, Peltonen L: Processing types I and III

procollagen in Ehlers-Danlos syndrome type VII. Am J Hum Genet 39: 222, 1986.
84. Fujimoto A, Wilcox WR, Cohn DH: Clinical, morphological, and biochemical phenotype of a new case of Ehlers-Danlos syndrome type VIIC. Am J Med Genet 68: 25, 1997.
85. Lewkonia RM: The arthropathy of hereditary arthroophthalmopathy (Stickler syndrome). J Rheumatol 19: 1271, 1992.
86. Ahmad NN, Ala-Kokko L, Knowlton RG, et al: A stop codon in the procollagen II gene (COL2A1) in a family with the Stickler syndrome (arthro-ophthalmopathy). Proc Natl Acad Sci U S A 88: 6624, 1991.
87. Sconyers SM, Rimoin DL, Lachman RS, et al: A distinct chondrodysplasia resembling Kniest dysplasia: clinical, roentgenographic, histologic and ultrastructural findings. J Pediatr 12: 898, 1985.
88. Spranger JW, Langer LO: Spondyloepiphyseal dysplasia congenita. Radiology 94: 3113, 1979.
89. Iceton JA, Horne G: Spondyloepiphyseal dysplasia tarda. The X-linked variety in three brothers. J Bone Joint Surg Br 68: 616, 1986.
90. Whyte MP, Gottesman GS, Eddy MC, McAlister WH: X-linked recessive spondyloepiphyseal dysplasia tarda. Clinical and radiographic evolution in a 6-generation kindred and review of the literature. Medicine (Baltimore) 78: 9, 1999.
91. Kozlowski K, Lewis IC, Kennedy J, et al: Progressive pseudorheumatoid arthritis. Paediatr Indones 25: 237, 1985.
92. Wynne-Davis R, Hau C, Ansell BM: Spondylo-epiphyseal dysplasia tarda with progressive arthropathy. J Bone Joint Surg Br 64: 442, 1982.
93. Bradley JD: Pseudoseptic pseudogout in progressive pseudorheumatoid arthritis of childhood. Ann Rheum Dis 46: 709, 1987.
94. Narcisi P, Richards AJ, Ferguson SD, Pope FM: A family with Ehlers-Danlos syndrome type III/articular hypermobility syndrome has a glycine 637 to serine substitution in type III collagen. Hum Mol Genet 3: 1617, 1994.
95. Pyeritz RE, Stolle A, Parfrey NA, Myers JC: Ehlers-Danlos syndrome is due to a novel defect in type III procollagen. Am J Med Genet 19: 607, 1984.
96. Hartsfield JK, Kousseff BG: Phenotypic overlap of Ehlers-Danlos types IV and VIII. Am J Med Genet 37: 465, 1990.
97. Pinnell SR, Krane SM, Kenzora JLE, Glimcher MJ: A heritable disorder of connective tissue—hydroxylysine deficient collagen. N Engl J Med 286: 1013, 1972.
98. Wenstrup J, Murad S, Pinnell SR: Ehlers-Danlos syndrome type VI: clinical manifestations of collagen type IV hydroxylase deficiency. J Pediatr 115: 405, 1989.
99. DePaepe A, Nuytinck L, Hausser I, et al: Mutations in the COL5A1 gene are causal in the Ehlers-Danlos syndromes I and II. Am J Hum Genet 60: 547, 1997.
100. Beighton P, Price A, Lord J, Diskson E: Variants of the Ehlers-Danlos syndrome—clinical, biochemical, haematological features of 100 patients. Ann Rheum Dis 28: 228, 1969.
101. Hatamochi A, Arakawa M, Mori K, et al: Increased expression of type VI collagen genes in cutis laxa fibroblasts. J Dermatol Sci 11: 97, 1996.
102. Spranger J: The type XI collagenopathies. Pediatr Radiol 28: 745, 1998.
103. Siegel RC, Black CM, Bailey AJ: Cross-linking of collagen in the X-linked Ehlers-Danlos type V syndrome. Biochem Biophys Res Commun 88: 281, 1979.
104. Arneson MA, Hammerschmidt DE, Furcht T, King RA: A new form of Ehlers-Danlos syndrome. JAMA 244: 144, 1980.
105. Anstey A, Mayne K, Winter M, et al: Platelet and coagulation studies in Ehlers-Danlos syndrome. Br J Dermatol 125: 155, 1991.
106. Hastbacka J, de la Chapell A, Mahtani MM, et al: The diastrophic gene encodes a novel sulfate transporter. Cell 78: 1078, 1994.
107. Beighton P: Dyggve-Melchior-Clausen syndrome. J Med Genet 27: 512, 1990.
108. el Shanti HE, Omari HZ, Qubain HI: Progressive pseudorheumatoid dysplasia: report of a family and review. J Med Genet 34: 559, 1997.
109. Fischer J, Urtizberea JA, Pavek S, et al: Genetic linkage of progressive pseudorheumatoid dysplasia to a 3-cM interval of chromosome 6q22. Hum Genet 103: 60, 1998.
110. Stoss H, Pesch HJ, Pontz B, et al: Wolcott-Rallison syndrome: diabetes mellitus and spondyloepiphyseal dysplasia. Eur J Pediatr 138: 120, 1982.
111. Horton WA, Langer LO, Collins DL, Dwyer C: Brachyolmia, recessive type (Hobaek): a clinical, radiographic, and histochemical study. Am J Med Genet 16: 201, 1983.
112. Belin V, Cusin V, Viot G, et al: SHOX mutations in dyschondrosteosis (Leri-Weill syndrome). Nat Genet 19: 67, 1998.
113. Laborde H, Rodrigue S, Catoggio PM: Mycobacterium fortuitum in systemic lupus erythematosus. Clin Exp Rheumatol 7: 291, 1989.
114. Carrington PR, Chen H, Altick JA: Trichorhinophalangeal syndrome, type I. J Am Acad Dermatol 31: 331, 1994.
115. Cederbaum SC, Kaitila I, Rimoin DL, Stiehm ER: The chondro-osseous dysplasia of adenosine deaminase deficiency with severe combined immunodeficiency. J Pediatr 89: 737, 1976.
116. MacDermot KD, Winter RM, Wigglesworth JS, Strobel S: Short stature/short limb skeletal dysplasia with severe combined immunodeficiency and bowing of the femora: report of two patients and review. J Med Genet 28: 10, 1991.
117. McLennan TW, Steinbach HL: Schwachman's syndrome: the broad spectrum of bony abnormalities. Radiology 112: 167, 1974.
118. Yulish BS, Stern RC, Polmar SH: Partial resolution of bone lesions. A child with severe combined immunodeficiency disease and adenosine deaminase deficiency after enzyme-replacement therapy. Am J Dis Child 134: 61, 1980.
119. Patrone NA, Kredich DW: Arthritis in children with multiple epiphyseal dysplasia. J Rheumatol 12: 145, 1985.
120. Shapiro F: Epiphyseal disorders. N Engl J Med 317: 1702, 1987.
121. Marfan AB: Un cas de déformation congénitale des quatre membres, plus prononcee aux extrémités charaterisée par l'allongement des os, avec un certain degre d'amancissement. Bull Mém Soc Méd Hôp (Paris) 13: 220, 1896.
122. Morse RPP, Rockenmacher S, Pyeritz RE, et al: Diagnosis and management of infantile Marfan syndrome. Pediatrics 86: 888, 1990.
123. Reed CM, Fox ME, Alpert BS: Aortic biomechanical properties in pediatric patients with Marfan syndrome, and the effects of atenolol. Am J Cardiol 71: 606, 1993.
124. Pyeritz RE, McKusick VA: The Marfan syndrome: diagnosis and management. N Engl J Med 300: 772, 1979.
125. Montgomery RA, Geraghty MT, Bull E, et al: Multiple molecular mechanisms underlying subdiagnostic variants of Marfan syndrome. Am J Hum Genet 63: 1703, 1998.
126. Pyeritz RE: The Marfan syndrome. Am Fam Physician 34: 83, 1986.
127. Pyeritz RE, Murphy EA, Lin SJ, Rosell EM: Growth and anthropometrics in the Marfan syndrome. Prog Clin Biol Res 200: 355, 1985.
128. Sinclair RTG, Kitchin AH, Turner RWD: The Marfan syndrome. Q J Med 53: 19, 1960.
129. Mirise RT, Shear S: Congenital contractural arachnodactyly: description of a new kindred. Arthritis Rheum 22: 542, 1979.
130. Park ES, Putnam EA, Chitayat D, et al: Clustering of FBN2 mutations in patients with congenital contractural arachnodactyly indicates an important role of the domains encoded by exons 24 through 34 during human development. Am J Med Genet 78: 350, 1998.
131. Boers GHJ, Smals AGH, Trijbels FJM, et al: Heterogeneity for homocystinuria in premature peripheral and cerebral occlusive arterial disease. N Engl J Med 313: 709, 1985.
132. Mudd SH, Skovby F, Levy HL, et al: The natural history of homocystinuria due to cystathionine beta synthase deficiency. Am J Hum Genet 37: 1, 1985.
133. Fisher RC, Horner RI, Wood VE: The hand in mucopolysaccharide disorders. Clin Orthoped 104: 191, 1974.
134. Mikles M, Stanton RP: A review of Morquio syndrome. Am J Orthop 26: 533, 1997.
135. Ringel MD, Schwindinger WF, Levine MA: Clinical implications of genetic defects in G proteins. The molecular basis of McCune-Albright syndrome and Albright hereditary osteodystrophy. Medicine (Baltimore) 75: 171, 1996.
136. Davies SJ, Hughes HE: Imprinting in Albright's hereditary osteodystrophy. J Med Genet 30: 101, 1993.
137. Ferguson HL, Deere M, Evans R, et al: Mosaicism in pseudoachondroplasia. Am J Med Gent 70: 287, 1997.

138. Deere M, Sanford T, Ferguson HL: Identification of twelve mutations in cartilage oligomeric matrix protein (COMP) in patients with pseudoachondroplasia. Am J Med Genet 28: 80, 1998.
139. Spranger J, Opitz JM, Bidder U: Heterogeneity of chondrodysplasia punctata. Humangenetik 11: 190, 1971.
140. Kelley RI, Wilcox WG, Smith M, et al: Abnormal sterol metabolism in patients with Conradi-Hunermann-Happle syndrome and sporadic lethal chondrodysplasia punctata. Am J Med Genet 83: 213, 1999.
141. Kelly TE, et al: Chondrodysplasia punctata stemming from maternal lupus erythematosus. Am J Med Genet 83: 397, 1999.
142. Austin-Ward E, Castillo S, Cuchacovich M, et al: Neonatal lupus syndrome: a case with chondrodysplasia punctata and other unusual manifestations. J Med Genet 35: 695, 1998.
143. Savarirayan R: Common phenotype and etiology in warfarin embryopathy and X-linked chondrodysplasia punctata. Pediatr Radiol 29: 322, 1999.
144. Menger H, Lin AE, Toriello HV, et al: Vitamin K deficiency embryopathy: a phenocopy of the warfarin embryopathy due to a disorder of embryonic vitamin K metabolism. Am J Med Genet 72: 129, 1997.
145. Eapen M, Davies SM, Ramsay NK, Orchard PJ: Hematopoietic stem cell transplantation for infantile osteopetrosis. Bone Marrow Transplant 22: 941, 1998.
146. Johnston CC, Lavy N, Lord T, et al: Osteopetrosis: a clinical, genetic, metabolic, and morphologic study of the dominantly inherited benign form. Medicine (Baltimore) 47: 149, 1968.
147. Beauvais P, Faure C, Montagne JP, et al: Leri's melorheostosis: three pediatric cases and a review of the literature. Pediatr Radiol 6: 153, 1977.
148. Nevin NC, Thomas PS, Davis RI, Cowie GH: Melorheostosis in a family with autosomal dominant osteopoikilosis. Am J Med Genet 82: 409, 1999.
149. Foeldvari I, Cairns RA, Petty RE, Cabral DA: An unusual case of mixed sclerosing bone dystrophy presenting with morning stiffness and joint swelling in childhood: a case report. Clin Exp Rheumatol 13: 525, 1995.
150. Moreno Alvarez MJ, Lazaro MA, Espada G, et al: Linear scleroderma and melorheostosis: case presentation and literature review. Clin Rheumatol 15: 389, 1996.
151. Bourantas K, Tsiara S, Drosos AA: Successful treatment with corticosteroid in a patient with progressive diaphyseal dysplasia. Clin Exp Rheumatol 14: 485, 1995.
152. Fallon MD, Whyte NP, Murphy WA: Progressive diaphyseal dysplasia (Engelmann's disease). J Bone Joint Surg Am 62: 465, 1980.
153. Gluck J, Miller JJ III: Familial osteolysis of the carpal and tarsal bones. J Pediatr 81: 506, 1972.
154. Erickson CM Hirschberger M, Stickler GB: Carpal-tarsal osteolysis. J Pediatr 93: 779, 1978.
155. Brown DN, Bradford DS, Gorlin RJ, et al: The acroosteolysis syndrome: morphologic and biochemical studies. J Pediatr 88: 573, 1976.
156. Beals RK, Bird CB: Carpal and tarsal osteolysis: a case report and review of the literature. J Bone Joint Surg Am 57: 681, 1975.
157. Elias AN, Pinals RS, Anderson HC, et al: Hereditary osteodysplasia with acro-osteolysis (the Hajdu-Cheney syndrome). Am J Med 65: 627, 1978.
158. Winchester PH, Grossman H, Wan NL, et al: A new acid mucopolysaccharidosis with skeletal deformities simulating rheumatoid arthritis. Am J Roentgenol 106: 121, 1969.
159. Costa MM, Santos H, Santos MJ, et al: Idiopathic multicentric osteolysis: a rare disease mimicking juvenile chronic arthritis [letter]. Clin Rheumatol 15: 97, 1996.
160. Gorham LW, Stout AP: Massive osteolysis (acute spontaneous absorption of bone, phantom bone, disappearing bone): its relationship to hemangiomatosis. J Bone Joint Surg Am 37: 985, 1955.
161. Vujic M, Hallstensson K, Wahlstrom J, et al: Localization of a gene for autosomal dominant Larsen syndrome to chromosome region 3p21.1-14.1 in the vicinity of, but distinct from, the COL7A1 locus. Am J Hum Genet 57: 1104, 1995.
162. Scriver CR, Beaudet AL, Sly WS, Valle D (eds): The Metabolic Basis of Inherited Disease, 6th ed. New York, McGraw-Hill, 1989.
163. Kuivaniemi H, Peltonen I, Kivirikko KI: Type IX Ehlers-Danlos syndrome and Menkes syndrome: the decrease in lysyl oxidase activity is associated with a corresponding deficiency in the enzyme protein. Am J Hum Genet 37: 798, 1985.
164. Welch JP, Temtamy SA: Hereditary contractures of the fingers (camptodactyly). J Med Genet 3: 103, 1966.
165. Malleson P, Schaller JG, Dega F, et al: Familial arthritis and camptodactyly. Arthritis Rheum 24: 1199, 1981.
166. Vogl A, Goldfisher S: Pachydermoperiostosis. Primary or idiopathic hypertrophic osteoarthropathy. Am J Med 33: 166, 1962.
167. Rimoin DL: Pachydermoperiostosis (idiopathic clubbing and periostosis). Genetics and physiologic considerations. N Engl J Med 272: 923, 1965.
168. Calabro JE, Marchesano JM, Abruzzo JL: Idiopathic hypertrophic osteoarthropathy (pachydermoperiostosis): onset before puberty. Arthritis Rheum 9: 496, 1966.
169. Caffey J, Silverman WA: Infantile cortical hyperostosis: preliminary report of a new syndrome. Am J Roentgenol 54: 1, 1945.
170. Caffey J: Infantile cortical hyperostosis. J Pediatr 29: 541, 1946.
171. Wilson AK: Infantile cortical hyperostosis. Review of the literature and report of a case without mandibular involvement. Clin Orthop 62: 209, 1969.
172. Azouz EM, Slomic AM, Marton D, et al: The variable manifestations of epiphysealis hemimelica. Pediatr Radiol 15: 44, 1985.
173. Smith DF, Sandor GG, MacLeod PM, et al: Intrinsic defects in the fetal alcohol syndrome: studies on 76 cases from British Columbia and Yukon Territory. Neurobehav Toxicol Teratol 3: 145, 1981.

38

Skeletal Malignancies and Related Disorders

James T. Cassidy and Ross E. Petty

Occasionally, a child in whom arthritis has been erroneously diagnosed is found to have a bone tumor. Although this unfortunate occurrence is rare, one must bear it in mind when examining any child with musculoskeletal pain. Musculoskeletal manifestations of malignancy in childhood may take one of four forms:

- Primary benign or malignant tumors of bone, cartilage, fibrous or soft tissue, or of miscellaneous origin
- Metastatic bone tumors
- Malignant infiltration of bone marrow: leukemia
- Secondary effects of malignancy

Table 38–1 provides a classification of common bone tumors of childhood. This list is not comprehensive, and the interested reader is referred to textbooks on the subject.[1–3] Overall, approximately half of the bone tumors in each of the first two decades of life are malignant.[4] This proportion contrasts sharply with the ratio in adulthood, when malignant tumors are much more common. Except for parosteogenic sarcoma, which is more common in girls, malignant bone tumors are more frequent in boys than in girls, with a ratio of approximately 1.5:1. The ratio is approximately 3:1 in osteoid osteomas and osteoblastomas.[1, 2, 5]

Bone tumors may be completely asymptomatic until a mass is detected by the patient or noticed by a parent. However, they usually present with the insidious onset of tenderness, swelling, and localized pain that is accentuated at night or by weight bearing (Table 38–2). Local tenderness or bony swelling in the absence of trauma strongly suggests this diagnosis. Systemic symptoms such as fever and weight loss are nonspecific and support a diagnosis of a malignant rather than a benign tumor.

A plain radiograph of the affected area is the best initial diagnostic evaluation.[6, 7] It is important to note whether the lesion is osteolytic or osteogenic and whether there is a soft tissue reaction. Each tumor occurs in characteristic bones and locations (Tables 38–3 and 38–4). Most tumors of a long bone, benign or malignant, arise in the metaphysis. Malignant tumors of the epiphysis are rare, and Ewing's sarcoma is the only malignant tumor commonly arising in the diaphysis.

The extent of the lesion can be estimated by computed tomography (CT). Magnetic resonance imaging (MRI) delineates the soft tissue extent of early lesions, including bone marrow involvement.[8] Ultrasonography is also valuable in assessing the extraosseous extension of a tumor.[9] Radionuclide scanning is useful in localizing a tumor or tumors, rather than in assisting with specific diagnosis. Definitive diagnosis of a bone

Table 38–1

Classification of Common Bone Tumors of Childhood

HISTOLOGIC TYPE	BENIGN	MALIGNANT
Osteogenic	Osteoid osteoma	Osteosarcoma
	Osteoblastoma	Parosteal osteosarcoma
Chondrogenic	Osteochondroma	Chondrosarcoma
	Chondroma	—
	Chondroblastoma	—
	Chondromyxoid fibroma	—
Fibrogenic	Fibrous defect	Fibrosarcoma
Uncertain	Giant cell tumor	Ewing's sarcoma
Hematopoietic	—	Reticulum cell sarcoma

Table 38–2

General Clinical Characteristics of Bone Tumors

Pain	May be absent Usually steady, "boring" ache Often worse at night
Tenderness	Overlying soft tissues and affected bone are tender
Swelling	May be localized, palpable, or visible swelling in large tumors
Systemic symptoms	Absent in benign tumors If fever, weight loss, pallor, suspect malignant tumor Hypertrophic osteoarthropathy suggests pleuropulmonary metastases
Laboratory studies	All normal in benign tumors ↑ ESR, abnormal CBC in malignant tumors
Radiographs	Often diagnostic at initial presentation

CBC, complete blood count; ESR, erythrocyte sedimentation rate.

Table 38–3

Most Common Types of Tumors in Specific Bones*

BONE	BENIGN	MALIGNANT
Femur	Osteochondroma	Osteosarcoma
Tibia	Osteoid osteoma	Osteosarcoma
	Osteochondroma	—
	Giant cell tumor	—
Innominate	Osteochondroma	Osteosarcoma
Humerus	Osteochondroma	Osteosarcoma
Vertebra	Osteoid osteoma	Reticulum cell sarcoma
Rib	Osteochondroma	Chondrosarcoma
Hand	Chondroma	Chondrosarcoma
Radius	Giant cell tumor	Osteosarcoma

*Listed in order of decreasing frequency.

Data from Dahlin DC, Unni KK: Bone Tumors: General Aspects and Data on 8,542 Cases, 4th ed. Springfield, IL, Charles C Thomas, 1986. (By permission of the Mayo Foundation.)

tumor rests on the histologic evaluation of a bone biopsy. The laboratory otherwise provides little assistance because anemia, leukocytosis, elevation of the erythrocyte sedimentation rate (ESR), and other indicators of inflammation are all nonspecific and may be absent even in the presence of osseous malignancy. Serum alkaline phosphatase levels may be elevated beyond those normally associated with growth.

PRIMARY TUMORS OF BONE, CARTILAGE, FIBROUS OR SOFT TISSUE, OR OF MISCELLANEOUS ORIGIN

Benign Tumors

Benign Tumors of Bone

Of the benign tumors, osteoid osteomas, osteochondromas, and chondromas are most common in the first two decades of life.[10] Approximately half of all of these lesions occur before the age of 20 years (Table 38–5).

Table 38–4

Typical Anatomic Sites of Tumors in Long Bones

LOCATION	BENIGN	MALIGNANT
Epiphysis	Chondroblastoma	—
	Giant cell tumor	—
Metaphysis	Fibrous defect	Osteosarcoma
	Osteochondroma	Parosteal osteosarcoma
	Chondromyxoid fibroma	Chondrosarcoma
	Chondroma	—
Diaphysis	Osteoid osteoma	Ewing's sarcoma
	Osteoblastoma	—

Osteoid Osteoma

Osteoid osteomas are benign tumors that are most common between the ages of 10 and 20 years, although they are not infrequent in children younger than 10 years (Table 38–6).[11, 12] The most common sites are the proximal femur, often in the neck and greater trochanter; the pedicles, facets, and spinous processes of the vertebrae; and the proximal tibia.

Pain is the typical symptom of osteoid osteoma. It is described as a deep and penetrating ache that is usually worse at night and may be dramatically responsive to low-dose aspirin or other nonsteroidal anti-inflammatory drugs (NSAIDs). The site of the lesion is tender, and there may be marked muscle atrophy, weakness of that limb, or a limp. Lesions in the vertebrae may be associated with scoliosis, with the concavity to the tumor site.[13] Occasionally, a synovial effusion is present if the tumor is adjacent to the hip or knee joint within the confines of the capsule. Signs of systemic illness are absent.

There are no abnormalities on laboratory evaluation; the diagnosis is based principally on radiologic findings. On a plain radiograph, the typical lesion is a nidus of increased density within a ring of decreased density, which is in turn surrounded by bone of increased density (Fig. 38–1). Histologically, the nidus is a mixture of osteoid, bone, and blood vessels surrounded by a fibrovascular layer that separates it from the surrounding sclerotic bone. This lesion is often

Table 38–5

Age Distribution of Benign Bone Tumors of Childhood

TUMOR	PERCENTAGE OF TUMORS ACCOUNTED FOR BY THIS TYPE IN: 1st Decade	2nd Decade	PERCENTAGE OF TUMORS OF THIS TYPE OCCURRING IN: 1st Decade	2nd Decade
Osteoid osteoma	18	17	12	54
Osteoblastoma	3	4	8	44
Giant cell tumor	2	8	1	15
Osteochondroma	44	46	10	49
Chondroma	15	8	10	26
Chondroblastoma	1	6	2	55
Chondromyxoid fibroma	3	13	13	25
Fibrous defect	11	8	19	67

Table 38–6
Osteoid Osteoma

Age at onset	Childhood to young adulthood
Sex ratio	Boys > girls
Symptoms	Localized aching or boring pain, mild at first, increasing in severity
	Worse at night, with rest or elevation
	Limp, stiffness, or weakness
	Long history
Signs	Joint effusion occasionally
	Localized swelling or tenderness
Investigations	Solitary, lucent nucleus surrounded by sclerosis on radiographs
	Positive bone scan
Treatment	Pain is dramatically relieved by aspirin or nonsteroidal anti-inflammatory drug
	Excision

difficult to identify by standard radiographic examination, especially in nondiaphyseal sites; other imaging techniques may be required for identification.[12] If an osteoid osteoma is suspected, even if it is not demonstrable on plain radiographs, technetium-99m bone scintigraphy is the procedure of choice (Fig. 38–2). CT documents the precise extent of the lesion and its characteristic structure and is invaluable in planning a surgical approach. MRI may identify the nature of a soft tissue mass that is associated with an early lesion.[14, 15]

The untreated course of osteoid osteoma varies. This tumor is not malignant, does not metastasize or cause death, and may spontaneously heal radiographically without surgical or other treatment.[11, 16, 17] However, the debility induced by the associated pain usually requires that the lesion be removed. Excision is curative and the recurrence rate is low. Aspirin or another NSAID can provide symptomatic relief and is occasionally justified on a long-term basis if the lesion is surgically inaccessible.

Osteoblastoma

The osteoblastoma is usually regarded as an osteoid osteoma larger than 1 to 2 cm in diameter.[17] It occurs much more often in boys and is more frequent in adolescence than childhood. Pain is the presenting symptom. This tumor is most common in a vertebral arch and has an aggressive radiographic appearance with circumscribed erosion of the cortex. Surgical resection may be difficult because of the site or size of the lesion. Malignant transformation of osteoblastomas has been reported.[18]

Benign Tumors of Cartilaginous Origin

Osteochondroma

Osteochondroma is the most common benign bone tumor between the ages of 5 and 15 years.[1, 2] It occurs with equal frequency in boys and girls. This tumor is often asymptomatic and presents as a painless exostotic

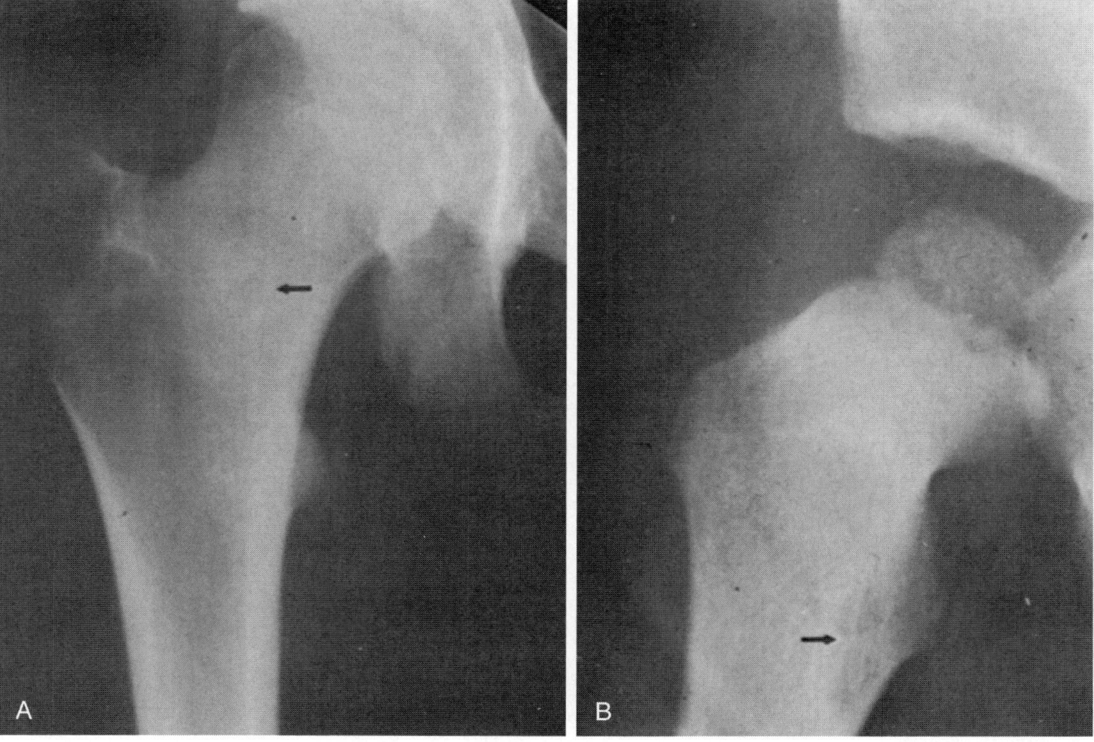

Figure 38–1. *A,* Osteoid osteoma at a radiolucent area in the femoral neck (*arrow*). *B,* Radiographically more apparent osteoid osteoma (*arrow*) in a typical location in femoral neck.

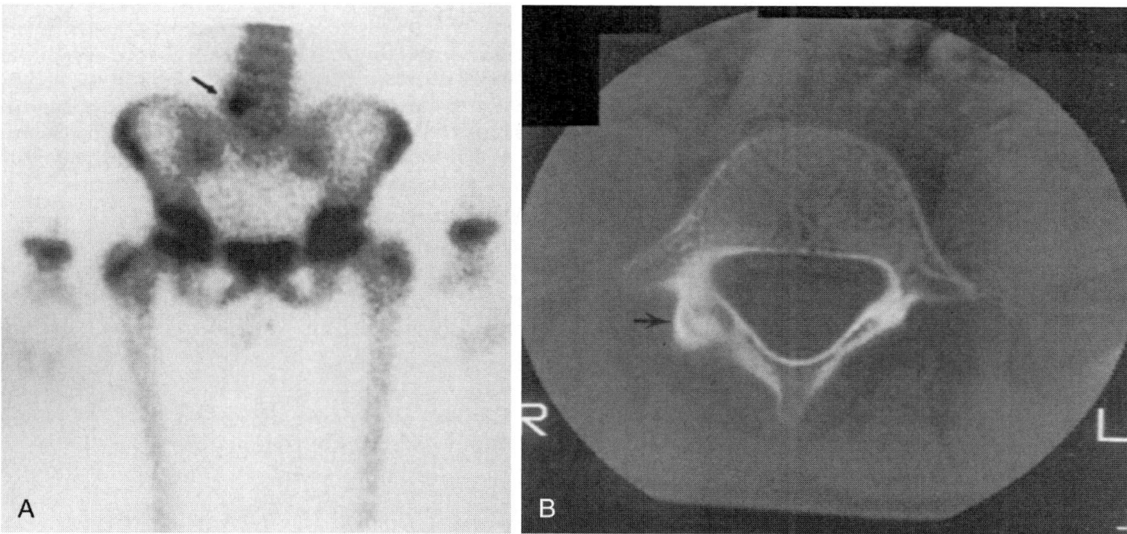

Figure 38–2. *A,* Technetium-99m bone scan demonstrates increased uptake in the region of an osteoid osteoma of the spine (*arrow*). *B,* Computed tomography (CT) scan of the fourth lumbar vertebra delineates the characteristics of the osteoid osteoma of the vertebral arch. Note the sclerotic central nidus, surrounded by radiolucent granulation tissue (*arrow*), which, in turn, is surrounded by sclerotic reactive bone.

mass that, by virtue of location and size, may induce local functional changes or result in pain because of pressure on neurovascular structures. An osteochondroma generally affects the metaphysis of a long bone and often arises at the site of a tendon insertion (most commonly around the knee in the distal femur or proximal tibia) or in the distal humerus. The osteochondroma extends away from the epiphysis as a bony outgrowth capped with cartilage up to 1 cm thick (Fig. 38–3). Some children with multiple lesions exhibit an autosomal dominant pattern of inheritance *(multiple hereditary exostoses)* (Fig. 38–4).[18a] Treatment consists of surgical excision. Malignant change may occur in either solitary or multiple osteochondromas.

Chondroma

Chondromas (enchondromas) make up about 10 percent of benign bone tumors. They occur with equal frequency in boys and girls and may affect young children as well as those in the second decade of life.[1, 2] This cartilaginous tumor, which may represent overgrowth of normal epiphyseal hyaline cartilage, occurs most commonly in the small tubular bones of the hand and foot, although other sites may be involved (Fig. 38–5). It is usually a single, asymptomatic mass.

The radiographic appearance of a chondroma is that of a well-demarcated metaphyseal lesion of central destruction that may protrude from the surface of the bone or be confined within the medullary canal *(enchondroma),* usually with linear or speckled calcification. It often presents as a solitary lesion with a pathologic fracture or as an incidental radiologic finding. Prophylactic resection after biopsy confirmation is not usually considered appropriate. Careful follow-up is warranted, however, because there is a very low rate of malignant transformation (chondrosarcoma).

Multiple enchondromatosis, or *Ollier's disease* commonly affects the hands and feet (see Chapter 37). Joint range of motion may be impaired, and the clinical presentation can be mistaken for arthritis. Growth deformities are common and require surgical management. Endochondromatosis in the presence of multiple cavernous hemangiomas is called *Maffucci's syndrome*

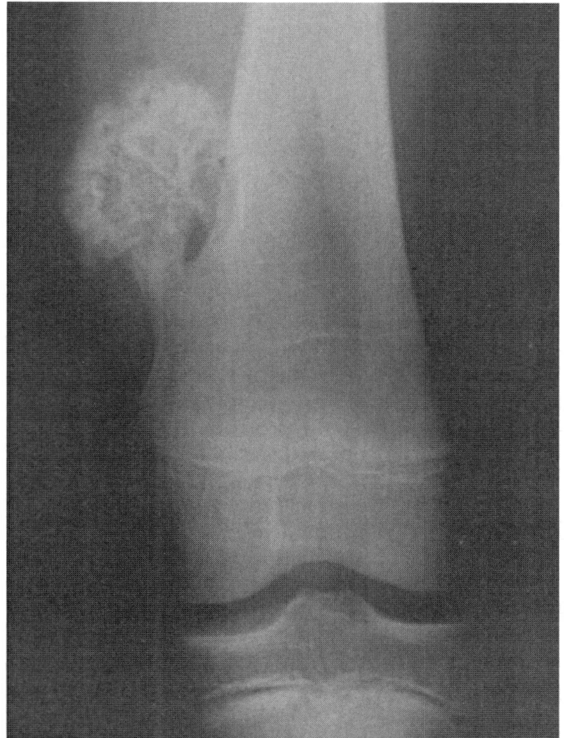

Figure 38–3. Osteochondroma of the distal femoral metaphysis. The tumor is directed away from the joint.

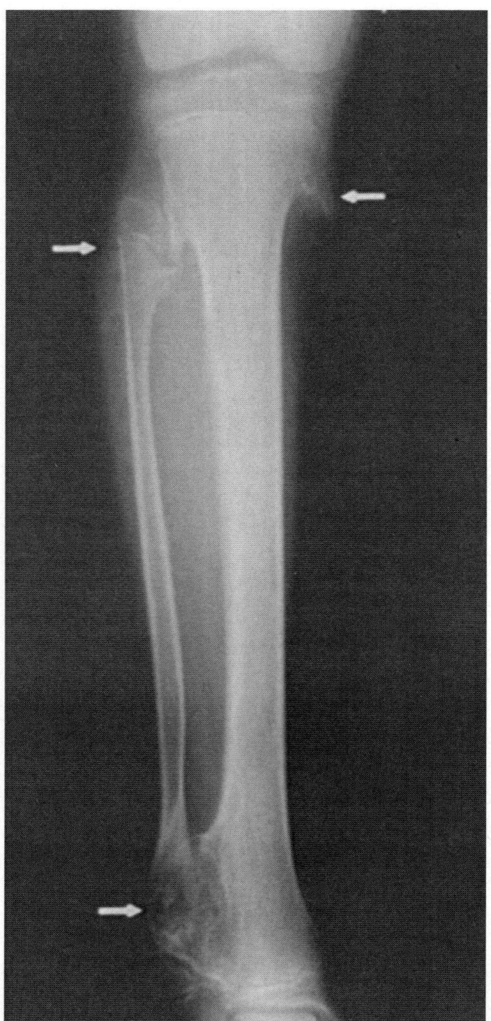

Figure 38–4. Radiograph of the tibia and fibula with multiple osteochondromas (*arrows*).

(Fig. 38–6).[19] The frequency of malignant sarcomatous change is quite high (50 percent) in patients with either Ollier's or Maffucci's syndrome.[2]

Periosteal Chondroma

Periosteal chondroma arises from the cortical surface and is most common in the proximal humerus and other long bones. Although the lesion is nontender, pain is often the presenting symptom. Wide excision is the treatment of choice.

Chondroblastoma

Chondroblastoma is a relatively rare epiphyseal cartilaginous tumor of children (hip, shoulder, knee) that is most common in the second and third decades of life (Fig. 38–7).[19a] The histopathology consists of polyhedral and giant cells with areas of fine calcifications. Foci of osteoid and bone may resemble a chondromyxoid fibroma. Most lesions are cured by excision and bone graft, but recurrences are a major concern. Growth disturbances and loss of function occur but are not common.

Chondromyxoid Fibroma

A chondromyxoid fibroma arises usually in the metaphyseal area with pain and tenderness as the most common presenting symptoms. It is an uncommon lesion and begins to occur in children at about 10 years of age.[19b] The radiographic appearance is one of an eccentric, sharply circumscribed zone of rarefaction, often with expansion of surrounding bone.

Benign Tumors of Fibrous Tissue

Fibrous Cortical Defect (Nonossifying Fibroma)

Fibromas are common between the ages of 10 and 15 years, are more frequent in males, and may affect up to 40 percent of children. They are significant in that they may be mistaken for more serious disease. There

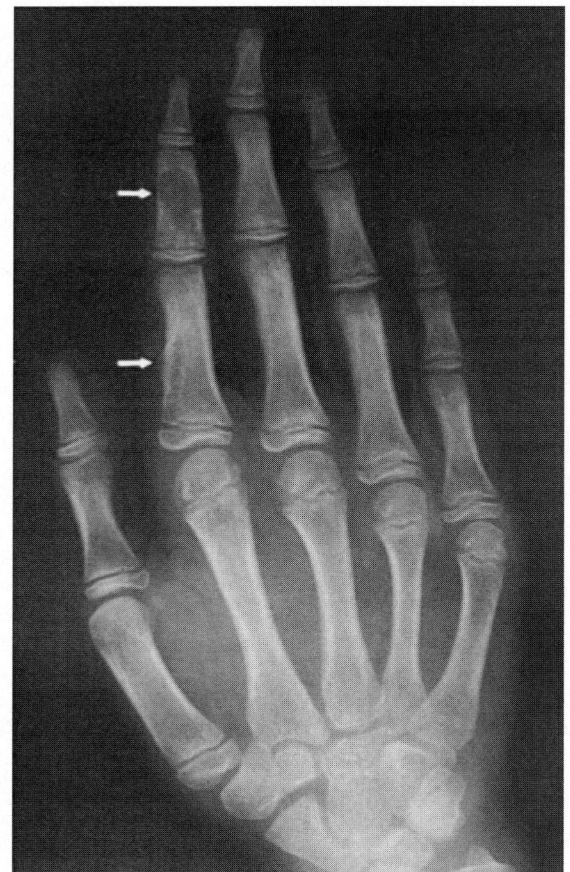

Figure 38–5. Radiograph of the hand of a child with enchondromas of the middle and proximal phalanges of the second finger (*arrows*).

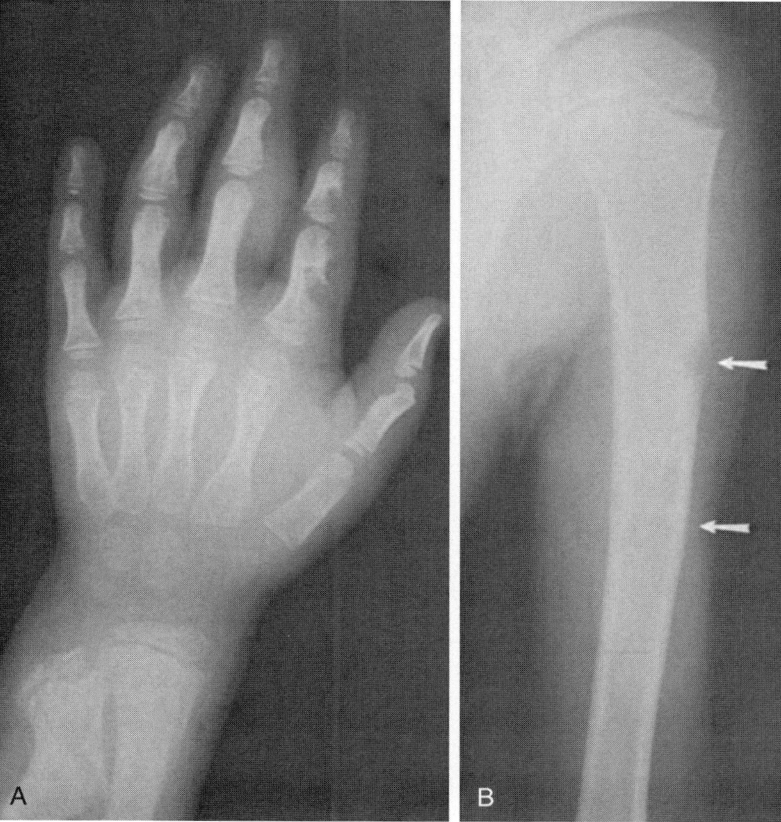

Figure 38–6. *A,* Characteristic changes of Maffucci's syndrome. Note the enchondromas of the proximal and middle phalanges of the second finger in particular. In addition, the fusiform swelling of the third finger represents the soft tissue swelling of the hemangioma. *B,* Radiograph of the humerus with the multiple enchondromas (*arrows*) of Maffucci's syndrome.

may be two or more fibromas, and they are usually found on radiographic evaluation (most often in the distal femur and proximal tibia) as an incidental finding.[6, 7] The radiologic appearance is virtually diagnostic, with a sharply marginated eccentric lucency in the metaphyseal cortex (Fig. 38–8). These tumors rarely cause symptoms, and treatment is conservative; occasionally, pathologic fractures occur. These lesions disappear with increasing age, leaving no significant residual defect.

Juvenile Fibromatosis

The disorders known as the *juvenile fibromatoses* are very rare and include *juvenile aponeurotic fibroma,*[20] ex-

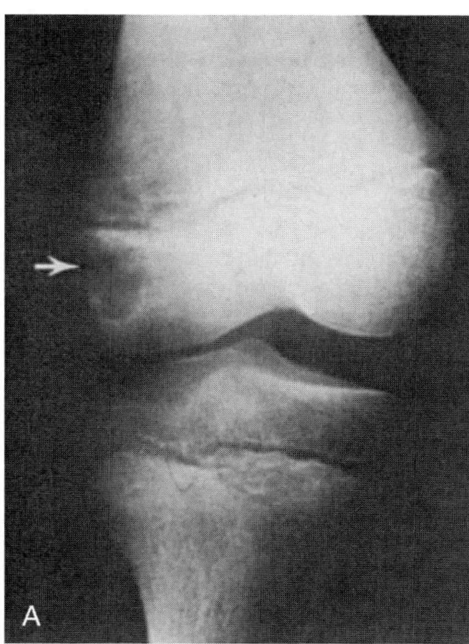

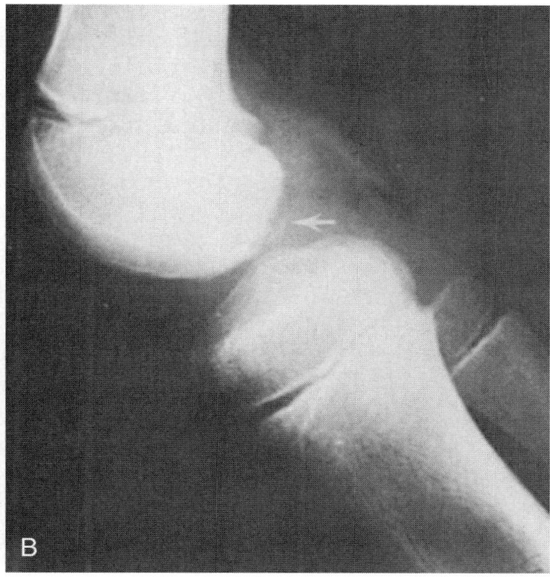

Figure 38–7. Chondroblastoma presenting as pain and effusion of the right knee of a 9-year-old boy. *A,* Anteroposterior view of a well-defined, oval lytic lesion (*arrow*). *B,* Lateral radiograph indicates that the lesion has eroded through the epiphysis (*arrow*) with small foci of calcification.

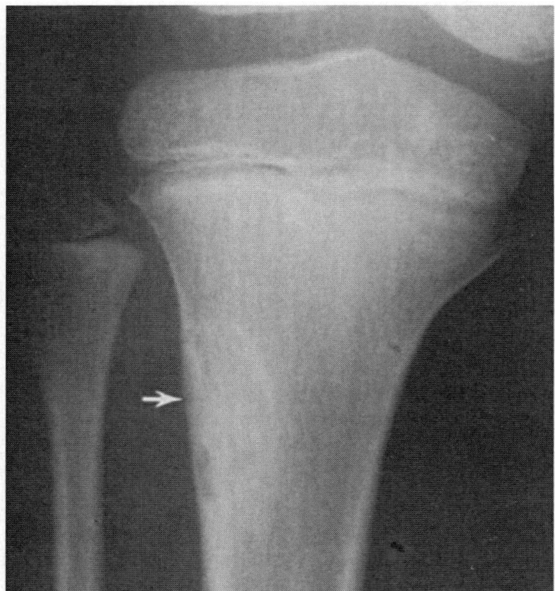

Figure 38–8. Benign fibrous cortical defect of the metaphysis of the tibia (*arrow*). This lesion was detected as an incidental finding in a radiograph taken for evaluation of trauma.

tra-abdominal desmoid tumor,[21] and *diffuse infantile fibromatosis.* Lipomas and neurofibromas are occasionally associated with musculoskeletal symptoms, often related to scoliosis. A variety of other forms of fibromatous soft tissue lesions have been described in children. A further discussion of this topic is presented in Chapter 21.

Fibrous Dysplasia

Fibrous dysplasia is difficult to classify and probably represents a developmental abnormality or a benign neoplastic fibrous tissue lesion.[21a] It is a relatively common disorder with a variable presentation mimicking that of almost any bone lesion. Monostotic disease occurs in approximately 85 percent of patients, most commonly in a rib. Polyostotic fibrous dysplasia may be limited to two or three sites or result in extensive skeletal abnormalities: It is also part of *Albright's syndrome* in association with multiple endocrine abnormalities.

The classic radiologic appearance of fibrous dysplasia is an intramedullary diaphyseal lesion with a thinned, sometimes bulging cortex. An angular deformity of the bone is often present at the site of the lesion and may require surgical intervention, depending on severity and potential for pathologic fracture. Resection is not indicated because most monostotic lesions present no problem to the child. The recurrence rate is high, even with curettage.

Ossifying Fibroma

Ossifying fibroma, or *osteofibrous dysplasia,* is almost always found in the mandible or tibia.[21b] Although benign, it may be locally aggressive. Symptoms are often absent, and bony deformity leads to the consultation. Curettage is often unsuccessful, and observation alone is usually recommended.

Benign Tumors of Soft Tissue

Pigmented Villonodular Synovitis

Pigmented villonodular synovitis (PVS) may represent a benign neoplasia of uncertain etiology, be caused by an infectious process, or be associated with repeated episodes of intra-articular hemorrhage. This condition is rare in childhood (it is most common between 20 and 40 years of age) but may present as a recurrent swelling in the knee, the ankle, or a tendon sheath. PVS affects both sexes equally. The disorder may be nodular or diffuse.[22, 22a, 22b] Nodular disease affects joints, bursae, or tendon sheaths; in diffuse PVS, a monarthritis of the knee, ankle, or (less frequently) the hip is most common. Only rarely is the upper extremity affected.

The disorder is characterized by recurrent painless effusions and a slowly progressive destruction of cartilage and erosion of bone. A boggy fullness about the joint is present on clinical examination. The most striking feature is the presence of blood-stained dark-brown synovial fluid on joint aspiration. The synovium is dark and is characterized by nodular areas of hypertrophy and hemosiderin-laden macrophages. In addition, there are proliferating synovial cells and fibroblasts, stromal cell masses with frequent mitoses, and multinucleated giant cells.[23] A characteristic finding on MRI is a very low signal density on both T_1- and T_2-weighted studies.

Treatment of this lesion often requires surgical excision; this is difficult with the nodular variety because of the extension of the lesion into tendon sheaths. NSAIDs are useful in suppressing the inflammatory disease, and intra-articular glucocorticoids may have a role in the management of this disorder. Malignant PVS is rare, and its precise classification is controversial.[24]

Synovial Hemangioma

The synovial hemangioma is most common in the knee but is an uncommon lesion. It may present as intermittent hemarthrosis simulating monarticular juvenile rheumatoid arthritis (JRA). Synovial hemangioma may be associated with contiguous cutaneous hemangiomas, varicose veins, and bone and soft tissue hypertrophy (*Klippel-Trenaunay-Weber syndrome*)[25] or with capillary hemangiomas, thrombocytopenia, and depressed coagulation pathway components (*Kasabach-Merritt syndrome*).[26] Bleeding from the hemangioma results in the sudden onset of painful joint swelling with effusion, often after minor local trauma. Recurrences are common and may result in chronic inflammatory synovitis and joint damage. Aspiration of synovial fluid at the onset of an effusion produces frank blood; later, the fluid may be xanthochromic and have a high bilirubin content. Radiographs demonstrate soft tissue swelling or a mass and, occasionally, phleboliths. The extent of the lesion is more accurately judged by MRI (Fig. 38–9).

Synovial Chondromatosis

In this unusual condition, synovial cartilaginous and osteocartilaginous bodies develop in the synovium and then are released free into the synovial fluid. Synovial chondromatosis is more common in boys and usually affects the knee. Presenting symptoms are usually those of a loose body with intermittent pain, swelling, locking, and giving way. In early disease, radiographic studies are normal, but as the lesions calcify they may be identified as discrete areas of stippled calcification. Treatment requires surgical excision. Malignant transformation is rare.[26a, 26b]

Benign Tumors of Miscellaneous Origin

Unicameral (Solitary) Bone Cyst

The unicameral bone cyst is rare before 3 years of age, occurs most commonly between the ages of 6 and 10 years, and is more frequent in boys.[27] It usually arises in the metaphysis of a long bone and often is asymptomatic or causes only localized pain.[28] Because of its size, it may result in localized swelling, a pathologic fracture, or growth disturbance.[29] Radiography demonstrates a lucent lesion that adjoins but does not cross the physis, or a fusiform widening of the bone (Fig. 38–10). These cysts almost always require curettage and insertion of bone chips, although injection of the lesion with glucocorticoid is reported to be equally effective.[27, 30]

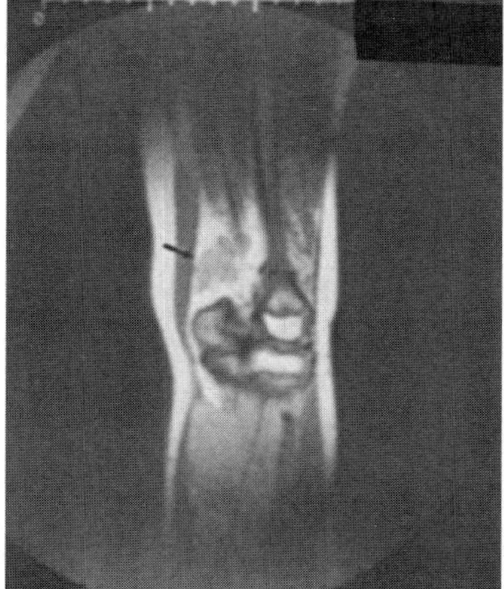

Figure 38–9. Magnetic resonance imaging (MRI) study of the left knee of a 7-year-old boy with recurrent effusion and widespread cutaneous hemangiomata. The study confirms the presence of a vascular mass just proximal to the knee joint (*arrow*).

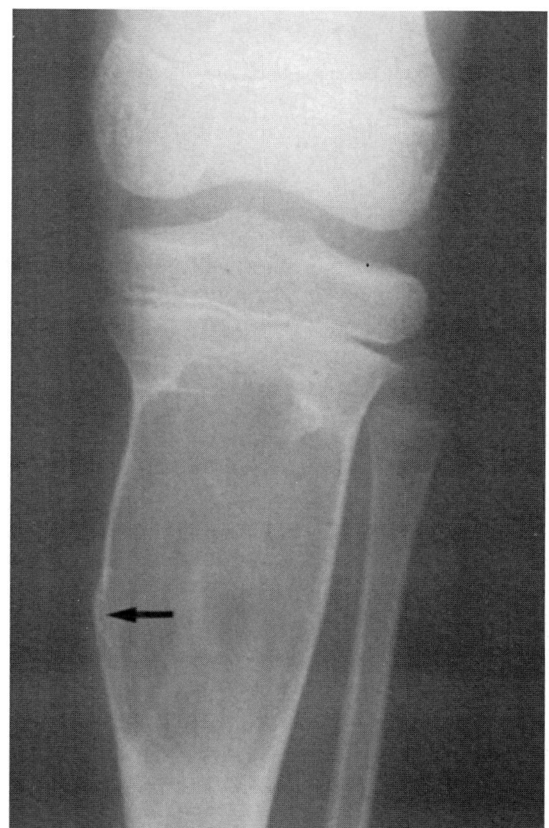

Figure 38–10. Radiograph of a pathologic fracture (*arrow*) through the wall of a unicameral cyst of the tibia.

Aneurysmal Bone Cyst

Aneurysmal bone cyst is far less common than the unicameral cyst, occurs more frequently in girls, and has its peak incidence in adolescence and early adulthood.[30a] It presents most often as a reactive lesion with pain and swelling, commonly in the metaphysis of a long bone or in a posterior element of the spine.[30b] Onset may be insidious and prolonged over weeks to a few years. Radiographically, the lesion appears as a "bubble," with a zone of rarefaction and surrounding destruction of the metaphyseal bone that is usually circumscribed (Fig. 38–11). Differentiation from a unicameral cyst may be aided by MRI.[30c] Treatment requires surgical curettage, sometimes with resection or local irradiation.[27, 30d]

Giant Cell Tumor

Pain is usually the presenting symptom of a giant cell tumor, which most often occurs in the epiphysis of a long bone. This tumor is most common in the second decade of life and is more frequent in girls. On radiographs, an expanding zone of eccentric radiolucency in the end of a long bone is characteristic.[1, 2]

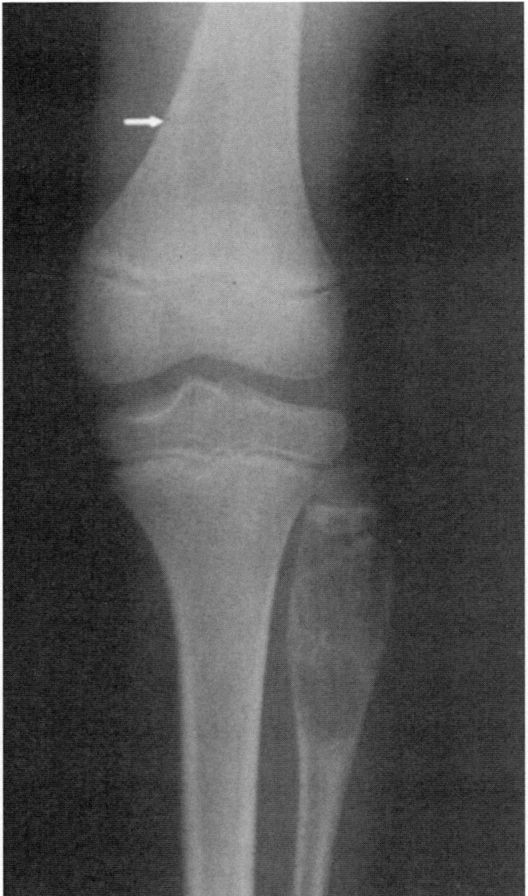

Figure 38–11. Radiograph of an aneurysmal bone cyst of the proximal fibula. Note also the benign cortical defect in the distal femur (*arrow*). The two abnormalities are unrelated.

Eosinophilic Granuloma

Eosinophilic granuloma, a lesion that is classified as a form of localized Langerhans' cell histiocytosis (previously designated histiocytosis X), occurs predominantly in young children between the ages of 5 and 10 years, with a male preponderance. Patients usually present with localized pain and swelling over a solitary mass.[31, 32] The bones of the skull, spine, and pelvis and the diaphysis of the femur are most commonly affected. The radiograph demonstrates a discrete lytic lesion with cortical erosion and periosteal reaction (Fig. 38–12). Percutaneous needle biopsy is useful in establishing the diagnosis.[33] Treatment requires surgical curettage, sometimes with low-dose irradiation. It has been suggested that intralesional glucocorticoid may be a useful adjunct to therapy.[34] Other types of histiocytosis include *Hand-Schüller-Christian disease* and *Letterer-Siwe disease*.

Malignant Tumors

Malignant Tumors of Bone

Malignant musculoskeletal tumors of childhood account for 5 to 10 percent of malignant neoplasms; the most common of these lesions are osteogenic sarcoma, Ewing's sarcoma, and rhabdomyosarcoma.[5] Osteogenic sarcoma is rare in the first decade of life but is the most common malignant bone tumor in the second decade. The mean age of children with Ewing's sarcoma is younger than that for any other primary tumor of bone (Table 38–7). Survival rates have continued to improve modestly for these tumors (60 to 70 percent).[35–37] There has also been progress in understanding their biology and genetic predisposition, especially in Ewing's sarcoma and rhabdomyosarcoma.

Osteosarcoma

Osteosarcoma (osteogenic sarcoma) accounts for 60 percent of all bone tumors in children.[38–41, 41a] It is most common at the time of maximal growth velocity in the second decade of life (75 percent of cases between the ages of 8 and 25 years), especially in taller children.[42] The annual incidence of osteosarcoma is approximately 0.6 to 0.7 per 100,000.[43, 44] It occasionally occurs in siblings.[45] Approximately 3 percent of these tumors develop in a field that has received previous irradiation. Osteosarcomas are also associated with certain acquired or genetic conditions such as retinoblastoma, enchondromatosis, hereditary multiple exostoses, and fibrous dysplasia. An increased risk of osteosarcoma is associated with the *Rothmund-Thomson syndrome*, a rare

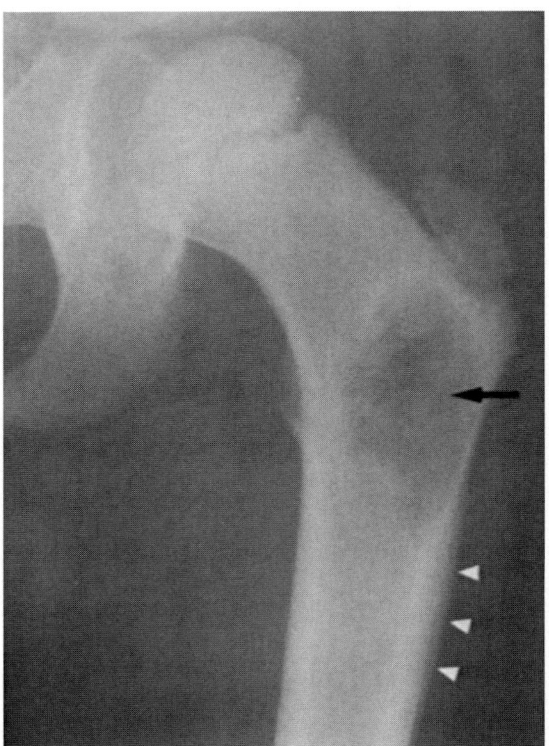

Figure 38–12. Radiograph of the femur with changes (*arrow*) of Langerhans' cell histiocytosis (eosinophilic granuloma). In addition to the lytic lesion, there is marked periosteal new bone apposition (*arrowheads*).

Table 38–7

Age Distribution of Malignant Bone Tumors of Childhood

TUMOR	PERCENTAGE OF TUMORS ACCOUNTED FOR BY THIS TYPE IN:		PERCENTAGE OF TUMORS OF THIS TYPE OCCURRING IN:	
	1st Decade	2nd Decade	1st Decade	2nd Decade
Osteosarcoma	38	60	5	52
Parosteal osteosarcoma	0	1	0	20
Ewing's sarcoma	45	23	18	57
Chondrosarcoma	2	4	1	5
Fibrosarcoma	2	3	2	14
Reticulum cell sarcoma	8	5	3	11

disorder characterized by short stature, telangiectases, small hands and feet, and hypoplastic thumbs.[46, 47]

This tumor usually arises in the medullary canal of the bone and is metaphyseal in location, occurring most often (60 percent) around the knee (e.g., distal femur, proximal tibia) and in the proximal humerus. Osteogenic sarcomas are highly malignant and metastasize early by hematogenous spread to many organs, especially the lungs, where they are a significant cause of secondary hypertrophic osteoarthropathy.[48]

Pain is the most common presenting symptom.[48a] Swelling over the involved bone occurs a few weeks to months later. Secondary signs of local inflammation, involvement of regional lymph nodes, and loss of function of the limb may be present. The presence of systemic signs such as weight loss, fever, or secondary hypertrophic osteoarthropathy suggests that skeletal and pulmonary metastases have already occurred.

Radiologic investigations provide the most meaningful diagnostic information.[49] On plain radiographs, the lesion has a moth-eaten appearance with cortical destruction, periosteal elevation (Codman's triangle), and a soft tissue mass (Fig. 38–13). The differential diagnosis may include osteomyelitis. Occasionally, two or more tumor sites are present, representing either multifocal origin or metastases to bone. Bone scintigraphy, CT, or MRI may be indicated to delineate the extent of the lesion. The diagnosis of osteogenic sarcoma is confirmed by the histologic appearance on biopsy of marked cellular pleomorphism with spindle-shaped cells, chondrocytes, and osteoid. It is commonly divided into four types:

- Osteoblastic
- Chondroblastic
- Fibroblastic
- Telangiectatic

A small-cell type has features overlapping those of Ewing's sarcoma.

The treatment of this tumor has, until recently, included amputation of the limb, with a 5-year survival rate of only 21 percent.[35] Modification of the surgical approach, including segmental resection of the primary tumor[49a] and the addition of adjuvant chemotherapy (including doxorubicin, cisplatinum, and high-dose methotrexate with leucovorin rescue), has led to a disease-free survival of more than 50 percent at 5 years.[42–44] Prognostic features of significance include the histologic grade of the tumor, size of the initial lesion, and its response to preoperative treatment.[50] Metastases at diagnosis are associated with a very poor outcome (<20 percent survival). A rare form of multifocal sclerosing osteosarcoma has a poor prognosis.

Surface osteosarcomas do not involve the medullary cavity and often encircle the entire shaft of the bone.[51] They have been divided into two types: *parosteal* (or *juxtacortical*) and *periosteal*. These tumors behave differently from osteogenic sarcoma. The parosteal variety is more common in girls and occurs most often on the posterior surface of the distal femur. Malignant potential is often low, it tends to metastasize late, and it has a much better prognosis.[52] The periosteal type occurs more commonly in the tibia and contains an abundant proliferation of cartilage.

Malignant Tumors of Cartilage: Chondrosarcoma

Chondrosarcoma is a rare tumor (<5 percent) that develops in children from malignant transformation of a preexisting enchondroma or, later in life, in a patient with multiple heritable exostoses.[52a] The initial symptoms of a chondrosarcoma are localized swelling or pain.[53] Radiographs are usually diagnostic, with destruction of bone combined with mottled densities of calcification and ossification (the "popcorn" appearance). Treatment consists of wide resection, adjuvant chemotherapy, and irradiation.[53a]

Malignant Tumors of Fibrous Tissue: Fibrosarcoma

Fibrosarcoma is an uncommon tumor that occurs most often on a distal part of an extremity as a soft, infiltrative mass with areas of hemorrhage or necrosis.[54] Histopathology confirms fibroblastic or myofibroblastic differentiation of all degrees. There are two major patterns of presentation of this tumor: congenital fibrosarcoma is most frequent in boys younger than 2 years; postpubertal fibrosarcoma is more aggressive.[54, 54a] Onset is characterized in most instances by painful swelling.

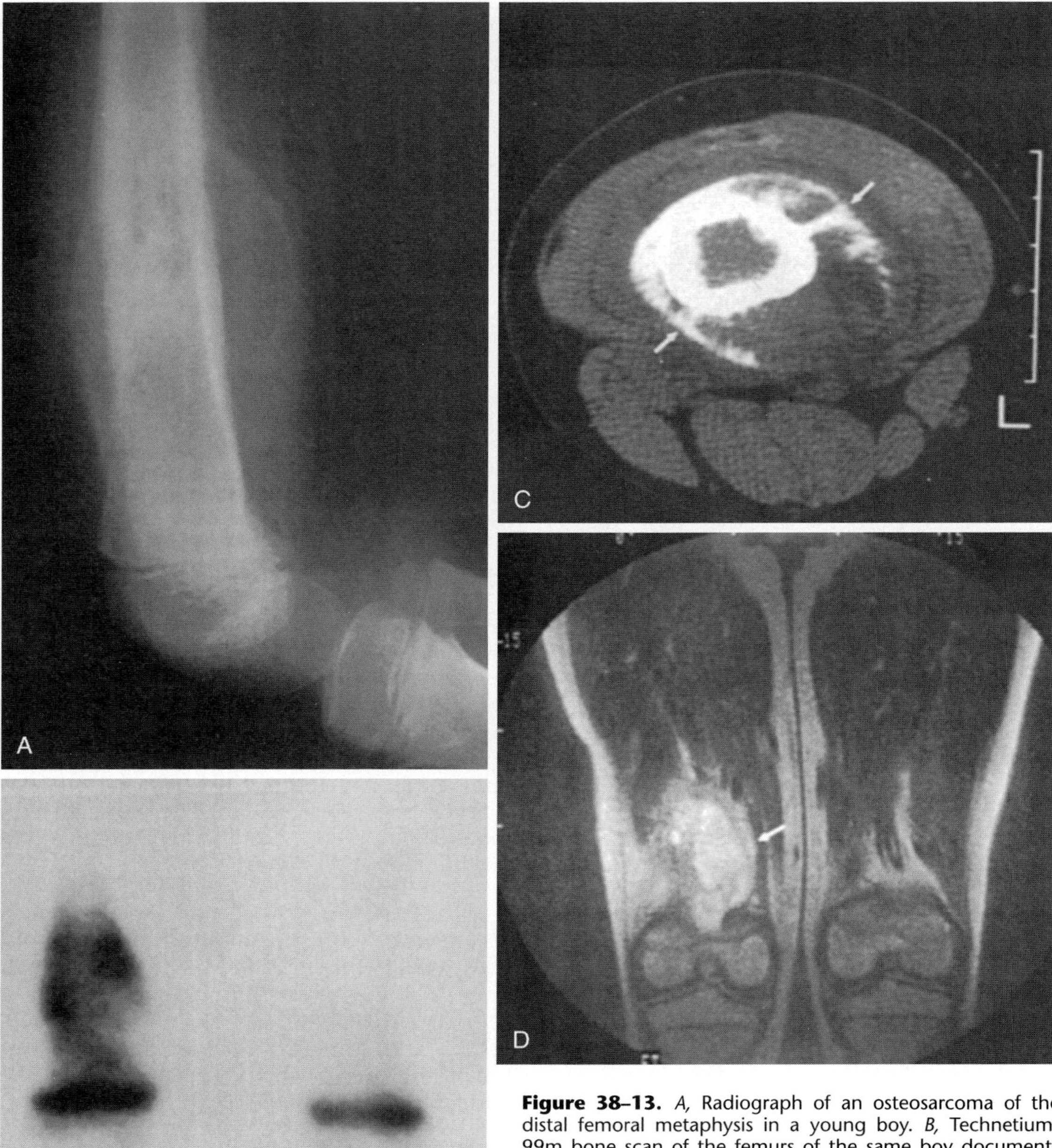

Figure 38–13. *A,* Radiograph of an osteosarcoma of the distal femoral metaphysis in a young boy. *B,* Technetium-99m bone scan of the femurs of the same boy documents increased uptake of isotope by the osteosarcoma. *C,* CT section through the thigh shows the extracortical bony densities (*arrows*) characteristic of osteosarcoma. *D,* MRI study demonstrates the tumor in the right thigh (*arrow*).

There are no diagnostic radiographic features that distinguish this tumor from osteosarcoma. In children younger than 2 to 5 years, congenital fibrosarcomas display rapid growth and extensive local invasion despite a relative lack of distant metastasis (7 percent). In children older than 10 years, the metastatic rate approaches 50 percent. Treatment of the former involves surgical resection; treatment of the latter combines radical excision, postoperative irradiation, and adjuvant chemotherapy. The survival rate in the congenital type is 90 percent and in the postpubertal form 60 percent. The overall survival rate is approximately 40 percent at 5 years and 30 percent at 10 years. Prognosis is obviously best for the more superficial and differentiated tumors.

Malignant Tumors of Soft Tissue

Rhabdomyosarcoma

Rhabdomyosarcomas are the most common soft tissue sarcomas in children and account for half of all soft tissue neoplasms in patients younger than 15 years.[53, 54b–d] They occur most often in children between the ages of 2 and 6 years or during adolescence, with an annual incidence of 0.4 to 0.9 per 100,000,[44] and are rare in older age groups. They present as a localized, painless, soft tissue mass. These tumors are most common in the head and neck region but can arise in any striated muscle. Approximately 20 percent occur in the extremities, especially during adolescence. Rhabdomyosarcoma metastasizes early to lung, bone, and bone marrow and may erode into adjacent bone and produce a radiographic appearance of a soft tissue mass with an underlying periosteal reaction. Treatment includes surgical excision, irradiation, and chemotherapy.[54e, 54f] The 5-year survival is approximately 70 percent.[44]

Synovial Cell Sarcoma

Although rare in childhood, synovial cell sarcoma is the most common soft tissue sarcoma (6 to 10 percent) after the rhabdomyosarcomas.[55, 55a, 55b] This tumor rarely occurs within a joint; it usually develops in the periarticular soft tissue. Lower-extremity involvement is most common, especially around the knee, or in the foot or hand, and the tumor may be associated with calcifications that suggest the diagnosis on radiographs. Tendon sheaths may also be involved.[56] Surgical excision, irradiation, and chemotherapy result in a 7-year survival rate of 60 to 70 percent. Prognosis is related to tumor size and ease of resection.[56a–e] Most synovial sarcomas express a specific chromosomal abnormality: t (x; 18) (p 11.2; q 11.2).[57]

Malignant Tumors of Miscellaneous Origin: Ewing's Sarcoma

The Ewing sarcoma family of tumors probably arises from a primitive multipotential mesenchymal or neural crest cell in the medulla of bone or occasionally in soft tissue.[41, 58, 59] It is the most malignant of bone tumors and the second most common cancer of bone in children.[60] It accounts for 7 to 15 percent of all malignant bone tumors with an annual incidence 0.2 to 0.3 per 100,000.[44, 61] This lesion is most common in white boys in the second decade of life (sex ratio, 1.5:1), although the mean age is somewhat younger than that for osteogenic sarcoma. It is extremely uncommon in children of Asian or African descent. Ewing's sarcoma often occurs in the diaphysis of the long bones (femur, humerus, tibia) or in the innominate but can occur in any bone, including those of the axial skeleton or as an extraskeletal lesion.[61a] Pain and local swelling are present, and systemic signs including fever are common, often with abnormalities of laboratory indices of inflammation.[48a]

The radiographic appearance is characteristically that of an aggressive, elongated, lytic lesion filling the medullary cavity, disrupting the cortex, and causing a roughening of the periosteum described as "onion-skin" or "sunburst" in appearance (Fig. 38–14). This reaction may be easily confused with osteomyelitis. Ewing's sarcoma eventually involves the entire shaft of the long bone and metastasizes to other bones and lungs. The histologic appearance is that of sheets of small round cells that are positive on staining with periodic acid–Schiff reagent, sometimes with a perivas-

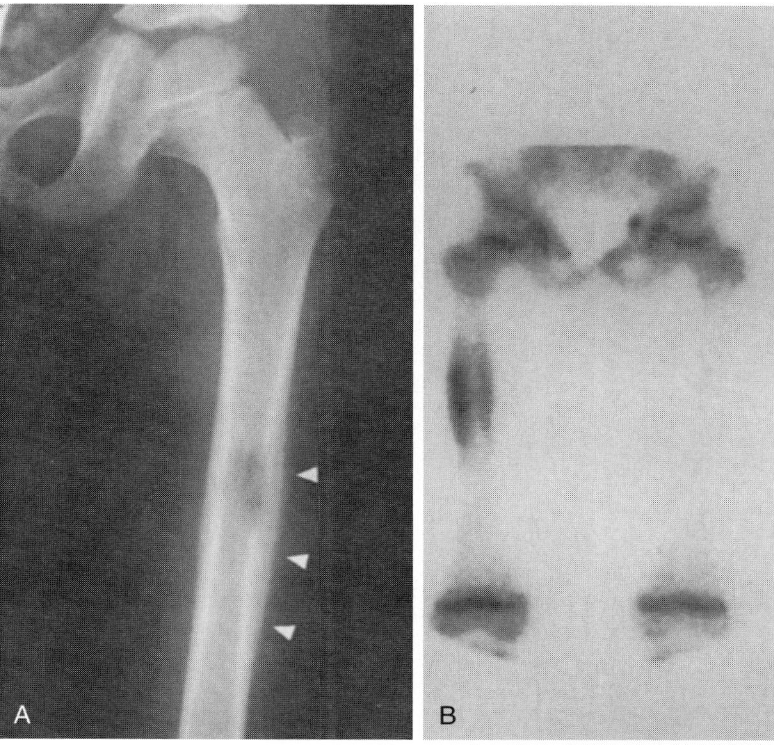

Figure 38–14. *A,* Radiograph of Ewing's sarcoma in the diaphysis of the femur. The central lytic lesion is accompanied by periosteal reaction (*arrowheads*). *B,* Technetium-99m bone scan of the femurs of the same child with localized increased uptake of the isotope in the tumor.

cular "pseudorosette" appearance. Neural markers, chimeric fusion products or a specific chromosomal translocation (t [11;22][q24; q12]) can often be identified to differentiate this tumor from lymphoma, rhabdomyosarcoma, or neuroblastoma. Treatment combines surgical resection with irradiation and adjuvant chemotherapy.[61b] The 5-year survival rate varies from 50 to 80 percent, depending on the site of the primary tumor.[61c, 61d] The presence of metastases to lung or skeleton reduces the survival rate to 20 to 30 percent.[62, 62a]

METASTATIC BONE TUMORS

In childhood, metastatic bone tumors are uncommon except for neuroblastoma. In a retrospective review of metastatic skeletal disease in childhood over a 38-year period, Leeson and coworkers[63] described 39 patients ranging in age from 18 months to 20 years. Tumors most commonly producing skeletal metastases were neuroblastoma (41 percent), rhabdomyosarcoma (18 percent), teratoma-carcinoma (10 percent), Wilms' tumor (8 percent), and retinoblastoma (5 percent).

Neuroblastoma, a tumor of the sympathetic nervous system, has an incidence of 1.6 per 100,000, primarily in young children.[44] Bone metastases usually occur early and may be accompanied by fever but little else in the way of localizing abnormalities. The development of bone pain related to bony metastases or bone marrow infiltration soon follows. Neuroblastoma most commonly metastasizes to the spine (81 percent), skull (69 percent), femur (50 percent), ribs (44 percent), and pelvis (31 percent). Multiple bony metastases are the rule.

The radiographic appearance is that of a lytic lesion arising from the marrow cavity (Fig. 38–15). Bone scintigraphy is the most sensitive technique for determining the site and number of metastases and may document abnormal findings before radiographic changes on plain film are evident. Treatment includes surgical removal of the tumor together with irradiation and chemotherapy.[64] The survival rate at 5 years is approximately 55 percent.[44]

Wilms' tumor is the most common retroperitoneal malignant tumor of childhood (incidence, 2 per 100,000).[44] It occurs most commonly in infants and young children (<4 years old), in whom it usually presents as an abdominal mass. Tumors with a sarcomatous histology are particularly likely to metastasize to bone and may be associated with bone pain. A number of congenital anomalies are frequently associated with Wilms' tumor, including sporadic aniridia, hemihypertrophy, genitourinary anomalies, and a deletion in chromosome 11.[65] Bony changes are detected by radiography and scintigraphy.[66] Treatment includes

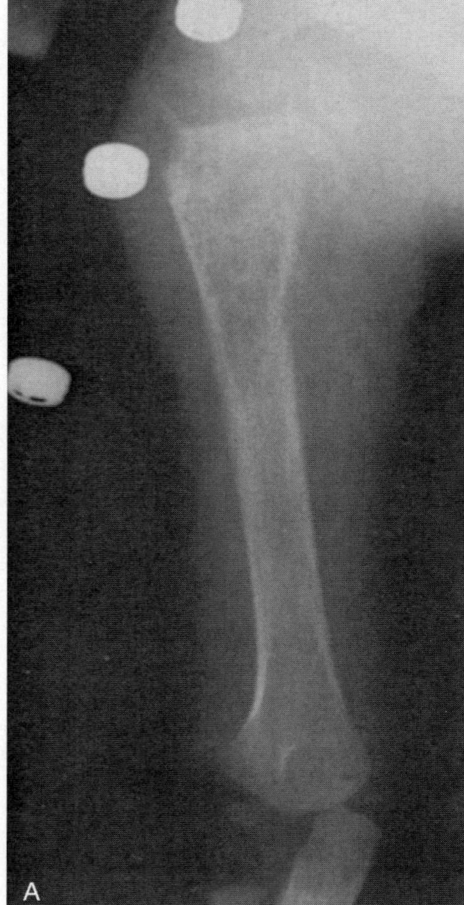

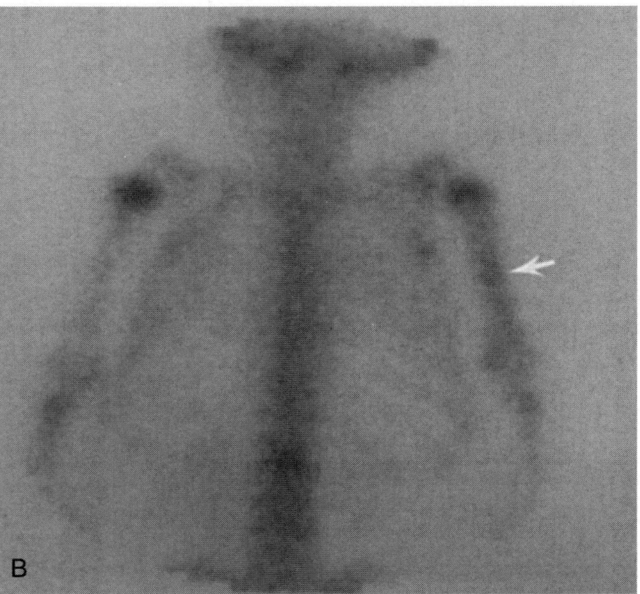

Figure 38–15. *A,* Radiograph of the humerus illustrates the "moth-eaten" appearance of extensive metastatic disease from neuroblastoma in the proximal humerus. *B,* Technetium-99m bone scan of increased uptake in the right humerus of the same child (*arrow*).

Table 38–8

Acute Leukemia in a Child—Clinical Characteristics

Presentation	Low-grade fever, fatigue, pallor, weight loss
Pain	Often disproportionate to objective findings Diffuse musculoskeletal aching or pain and tenderness of metaphyses of long bones May be migratory joint pain or periarticular swelling or joint effusion
Hematologic parameters	May be normal or with ↑ or ↓ WBC count or platelet count, sometimes with blast cells in peripheral smear; ↑ ESR and lactic dehydrogenase
Radiographs	Metaphyseal rarefaction, periosteal new bone apposition

ESR, erythrocyte sedimentation rate; WBC, white blood cell.

nephrectomy, irradiation, and chemotherapy. The 5-year survival rate is approximately 80 percent.[44]

MALIGNANT INFILTRATION OF BONE MARROW: LEUKEMIA

Leukemia is the most common childhood malignancy that results in musculoskeletal pain and arthritis.[67–70] In most instances, the pain is diffusely localized to an area of the body, particularly over the metaphyses of the long bones (Table 38–8). Sometimes a joint effusion occurs. Large joints, especially the knee, are most commonly affected, although small joints of the hands may be involved. The number of affected joints is usually relatively few. Associated periarticular disease is common.

The frequency of musculoskeletal signs or symptoms in childhood leukemia was evaluated in a 2-year prospective study of 28 children.[69] Objective joint findings, often mild, were present in 50 percent of the children, most often at or near onset of the disease. In half of the children, a single joint was involved, most often the knee; in the remainder, two or three joints, rarely more, were affected. Retrospective studies have usually indicated a much lower prevalence of joint disease of 11 to 12 percent.[68, 70]

A high index of suspicion is needed in order to confirm the diagnosis of leukemia in a child presenting with musculoskeletal pain.[71] The most distinctive diagnostic features of leukemia are the degree and location of the pain. In leukemia, pain is much more severe than in JRA and is characteristically metaphyseal in location rather than directly over a joint. Abnormalities in acute-phase indices such as the ESR are out of proportion to the small number of affected joints. In oligoarticular JRA, for example, the ESR is usually only moderately elevated or may be normal. In leukemic joint disease, the ESR is often very high.[67, 70] Dissociation of the inflammatory indices (e.g., an elevated ESR with a normal or low platelet count), a low white blood cell count, or a striking increase in the serum level of lactic dehydrogenase or urate should also alert the physician to the possibility of leukemia. The hematologic findings (complete blood count, white blood cell differential count, and platelet count) may be entirely normal for weeks or months after onset of symptoms, and repeated evaluations are essential. Blast cells in the peripheral blood, virtually pathognomonic for leukemia, may not be present at onset of the musculoskeletal symptoms, in which case diagnostic bone marrow aspiration and biopsy are indicated. Antinuclear antibodies are occasionally detected in children with leukemia, and their presence should not be interpreted as an indication of inflammatory arthritis.[70]

Radiographic changes may be of assistance in diagnosis. In addition to localized metaphyseal rarefaction (Fig. 38–16), there may be subperiosteal elevation or an elongated osteolytic reaction. Such changes, however, may be absent even in the presence of severe symptoms. Bone scintigraphy with technetium-99m documents an increased uptake in bone marrow, metaphyseal, and periosteal areas. Differentiation from osteomyelitis or neoplasm (Ewing's sarcoma) is paramount.

SECONDARY EFFECTS OF MALIGNANCY

Secondary Hypertrophic Osteoarthropathy

The syndrome of secondary hypertrophic osteoarthropathy (SHO) consists of terminal clubbing, painful

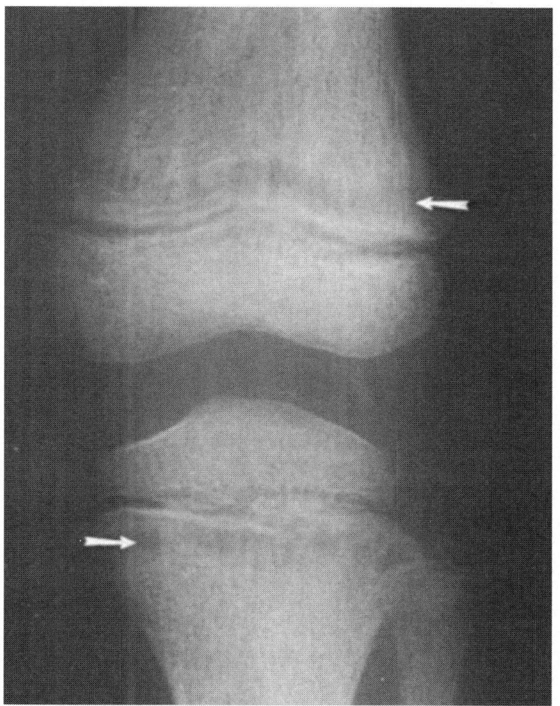

Figure 38–16. Radiograph of metaphyseal rarefaction in a patient with acute lymphoblastic leukemia (*arrows*).

swelling of distal joints and soft tissues, profuse sweating, and radiographic evidence of periosteal new bone formation affecting the bones of the hands, feet, and distal limbs (see Table 38–7). Although periosteal new bone apposition can also be a radiologic characteristic of JRA or juvenile psoriatic arthritis, it is not associated in these children with the severe pain and tenderness of SHO.

Most cases of SHO in childhood are related to chronic pulmonary disease[64] or congenital heart disease, occasionally with the antiphospholipid antibody syndrome,[72, 73] although associations with biliary atresia and regional enteritis have been noted. The pathogenesis of SHO is unknown, although hypoxic, endocrine, and neurogenic mechanisms have been suggested.[72–74] SHO also occurs in the *POEMS syndrome* (polyneuropathy, organomegaly, endocrinopathy, M protein, skin changes).[73] An important cause of SHO in childhood is pulmonary malignancy, most often metastases from osteogenic sarcomas.[48, 75] The typical clubbing and diffuse swelling of the joints and soft tissues of the hands, together with marked periosteal new bone apposition along the proximal phalanges, metacarpals, and distal radius and ulna, are shown in Figure 38–17. Bone scintigraphy with technetium-99m documents increased uptake in areas of periosteal new bone apposition (see Fig. 15–3).

Children with symptomatic SHO are usually profoundly ill. The pain is severe and is usually predominantly distal in location and symmetric in distribution. It is present during the daytime and may waken the child at night. Treatment is usually unsatisfactory, although NSAIDs are sometimes temporarily effective. Resection of the pulmonary or pleural tumor may result in dramatic resolution of all signs and symptoms.

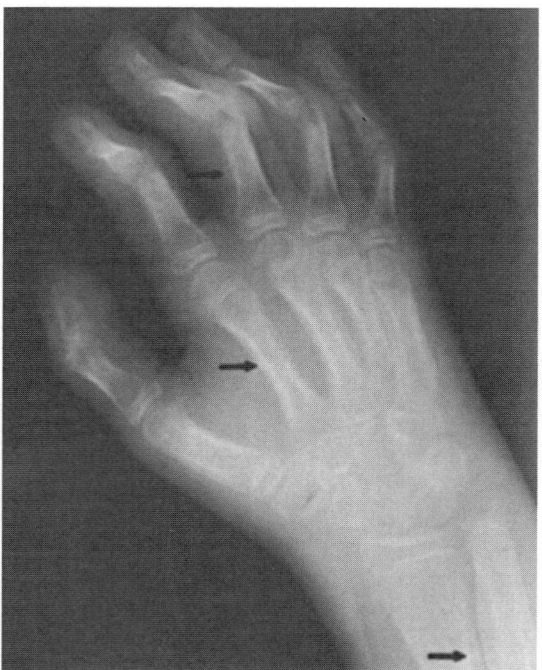

Figure 38–17. Secondary hypertrophic osteoarthropathy in a child with pulmonary metastases from osteosarcoma. Note the marked periosteal new bone apposition along the phalanges, metacarpals, and distal radius and ulna (*arrows*).

Acanthosis Nigricans

Acanthosis nigricans is a rare disorder associated with internal malignancy, diabetes, obesity, various genetic syndromes, connective tissue diseases such as systemic lupus erythematosus, and glucocorticoid administration.[76, 77] It may also occur in children with lipodystrophy or be familial.[78] We have seen several children in our clinics with this disorder and juvenile dermatomyositis, with premature thelarche, lipodystrophy, or insulin resistance.

Acknowledgment

We are grateful for the expert assistance of Dr. Betty Wood, Department of Radiology, British Columbia's Children's Hospital, Vancouver, for selected radiographs.

References

1. Mirra JM, Picci P, Gold RH (eds): Bone Tumors: Clinical, Radiologic, and Pathologic Correlations. Philadelphia, Lea & Febiger, 1989.
2. Dahlin DC, Unni KK: Dahlin's Bone Tumors: General Aspects and Data on 11,087 Cases, 5th ed. Philadelphia, Lippincott-Raven, 1996.
3. Springfield DS, Gebhardt MC: Bone and soft tissue tumors. *In* Morrissy RT, Weinstein SL (eds): Lovell and Winter's Pediatric Orthopaedics, 6th ed. Philadelphia, Lippincott Williams & Wilkins, 2001, pp 507–562.
4. Arndt CA, Crist WM: Common musculoskeletal tumors of childhood and adolescence. N Engl J Med 341: 342–352, 1999.
5. Parkin DM, Stiller CA, Nectoux J: International variations in the incidence of childhood bone tumours. Int J Cancer 53: 371–376, 1993.
6. Silverman FN, Kuhn JP (eds): Essentials of Caffey's Pediatric X-Ray Diagnosis. Chicago, Year Book Medical, 1990, pp 957–980.
7. Resnick D (ed): Diagnosis of Bone and Joint Disorders, 3rd ed. Philadelphia, WB Saunders, 1995, pp 3611–4064.
8. Moore SG, Bisset GS, Siegel MJ, et al: Pediatric musculoskeletal MR imaging. Radiology 179: 345–360, 1991.
9. Saifuddin A, Burnett SJ, Mitchell R: Pictorial review: ultrasonography of primary bone tumours. Clin Radiol 53: 239–246, 1998.
10. Copley L, Dormans JP: Benign pediatric bone tumors. Evaluation and treatment. Pediatr Clin North Am 43: 949–966, 1996.
11. Cohen MD, Harrington TM, Ginsburg WW: Osteoid osteoma: 95 cases and a review of the literature. Semin Arthritis Rheum 12: 265–281, 1983.
12. Davidson RS, Mahboubi S, Heyman S, et al: Nondiaphyseal osteoid osteomas in the pediatric patient. Clin Orthop 243: 230–234, 1989.
13. Keim HA, Reina EG: Osteoid-osteoma as a cause of scoliosis. J Bone Joint Surg Am 57: 159–163, 1975.
14. Woods ER, Martel W, Mandell SH, et al: Reactive soft-tissue mass associated with osteoid osteoma: correlation of MR imaging features with pathologic findings. Radiology 186: 221–225, 1993.
15. Biebuyck JC, Katz LD, McCauley T: Soft tissue edema in osteoid osteoma. Skeletal Radiol 22: 37–41, 1993.
16. Vickers CW, Pugh DC, Ivans JC: Osteoid osteoma: a 15-year follow-up of an untreated patient. J Bone Joint Surg Am 41: 357, 1959.
17. Frassica FJ, Waltrip RL, Sponseller PD, et al: Clinicopathologic

features and treatment of osteoid osteoma and osteoblastoma in children and adolescents. Orthop Clin North Am 27: 559–574, 1996.

18. Seki T, Fukuda H, Ishii Y, et al: Malignant transformation of benign osteoblastoma. A case report. J Bone Joint Surg Am 57: 424–426, 1975.

18a. Porter DE, Emerton ME, Villanueva-Lopez, et al: Clinical and radiographic analysis of osteochondromas and growth disturbance in hereditary multiple exostoses. J Pediatr Orthop 20: 246–250, 2000.

19. Johnson JL, Webster JR, Sippy HY: Maffucci's syndrome (dyschondroplasia with hemangiomas). Am J Med 28: 864, 1960.

19a. Schuppers HA, Van Der Eijken JW: Chondroblastoma during the growing age. J Pediatr Orthop B 7: 293–297, 1998.

19b. Durr HR, Lienemann A, Nerlich A, et al: Chondromyxoid fibroma of bone. Arch Orthop Trauma Surg 120: 42–47, 2000.

20. Keller RB, Baez-Giangreco A: Juvenile aponeurotic fibroma. Report of three cases and a review of the literature. Clin Orthop 106: 198–205, 1975.

21. McDougall A, McGarrity G: Extra-abdominal desmoid tumours. J Bone Joint Surg Br 61: 373–377, 1979.

21a. Stanton RP, Hobson GM, Montgomery BE, et al: Glucocorticoids decrease interleukin-6 levels and induce mineralization of cultured osteogenic cells from children with fibrous dysplasia. J Bone Miner Res 14: 1104–1114, 1999.

21b. Williams HK, Mangham C, Speight PM: Juvenile ossifying fibroma. An analysis of eight cases and a comparison with other fibro-osseous lesions. J Oral Pathol Med 29: 13–18, 2000.

22. Bravo SM, Winalski CS, Weissman BN: Pigmented villonodular synovitis. Radiol Clin North Am 34: 311–326, 1996.

22a. De Visser E, Veth RP, Pruszczynski M, et al: Diffuse and localized pigmented villonodular synovitis: evaluation of treatment of 38 patients. Arch Orthop Trauma Surg 119: 401–404, 1999.

22b. Somerhausen NS, Fletcher CD: Diffuse-type giant cell tumor: Clinicopathologic and immunohistochemical analysis of 50 cases with extraarticular disease. Am J Surg Pathol 24: 479–492, 2000.

23. Schumacher HR, Lotke P, Athreya B, et al: Pigmented villonodular synovitis: light and electron microscopic studies. Semin Arthritis Rheum 12: 32–43, 1982.

24. Bertoni F, Unni KK, Beabout JW, et al: Malignant giant cell tumor of the tendon sheaths and joints (malignant pigmented villonodular synovitis). Am J Surg Pathol 21: 153–163, 1997.

25. Jones KL: Klippel-Trenaunay-Weber syndrome. *In* Jones KL (ed): Smith's Recognizable Patterns of Human Malformation, 5th ed. Philadelphia, WB Saunders, 1997, pp 512–513.

26. Resnick D, Oliphant M: Hemophilia-like arthropathy of the knee associated with cutaneous and synovial hemangiomas. Report of 3 cases and review of the literature. Radiology 114: 323–326, 1975.

26a. Wuisman PI, Noorda RJ, Jutte PC: Chondrosarcoma secondary to synovial chondromatosis. Report of two cases and a review of the literature. Arch Orthop Trauma Surg 166: 307–311, 1997.

26b. Sciot R, Dal Cin P, Bellemans J et al: Synovial chondromatosis: clonal chromosome changes provide further evidence for a neoplastic disorder. Virchows Arch 433: 189–191, 1998.

27. Campanacci M, Capanna R, Picci P: Unicameral and aneurysmal bone cysts. Clin Orthop 204: 25–36, 1986.

28. Lokiec F, Wientroub S: Simple bone cyst: etiology, classification, pathology, and treatment modalities. J Pediatr Orthop B 7: 262–273, 1998.

29. Clayer M, Boatright C, Conrad E: Growth disturbances associated with untreated benign bone cysts. Aust N Z J Surg 67: 872–873, 1997.

30. Gartland JJ, Cole FL: Modern concepts in the treatment of unicameral bone cysts of the proximal humerus. Orthop Clin North Am 6: 487–498, 1975.

30a. Leithner A, Windhager R, Lang S, et al: Aneurysmal bone cyst. A population based epidemiologic study and literature review. Clin Orthop 363: 176–179, 1999.

30b. Rizzo M, Dellaero DT, Harrelson JM, et al: Juxtaphyseal aneurysmal bone cysts. Clin Orthop 364: 205–212, 1999.

30c. Sullivan RJ, Meyer JS, Dormans JP, et al: Diagnosing aneurysmal and unicameral bone cysts with magnetic resonance imaging. Clin Orthop 366: 186–190, 1999.

30d. Ozaki T, Halm H, Hillmann A, et al: Aneurysmal bone cysts of the spine. Arch Orthop Trauma Surg 119: 159–162, 1999.

31. Fowles JV, Bobechko WP: Solitary eosinophilic granuloma in bone. J Bone Joint Surg Br 52: 238–243, 1970.

32. Burgdorf WH, Zelger B: The non-Langerhans' cell histiocytoses in childhood. Cutis 58: 201–207, 1996.

33. Yasko AW, Fanning CV, Ayala AG, et al: Percutaneous techniques for the diagnosis and treatment of localized Langerhans-cell histiocytosis (eosinophilic granuloma of bone). J Bone Joint Surg Am 80: 219–228, 1998.

34. Cohen M, Zornoza J, Cangir A, et al: Direct injection of methylprednisolone sodium succinate in the treatment of solitary eosinophilic granuloma of bone: a report of 9 cases. Radiology 136: 289–293, 1980.

35. Mercuri M, Capanna R, Manfrini M, et al: The management of malignant bone tumors in children and adolescents. Clin Orthop 264: 156–168, 1991.

36. Jaffe N: Advances in the management of malignant bone tumors in children and adolescents. Pediatr Clin North Am 32: 801–810, 1985.

37. Himelstein BP, Dormans JP: Malignant bone tumors of childhood. Pediatr Clin North Am 43: 967–984, 1996.

38. Jaffe N: Osteosarcoma. Pediatr Rev 12: 333–343, 1991.

39. Link MP, Eilber F: Osteosarcoma. *In* Pizzo P, Poplack D (eds): Principles and Practice of Pediatric Oncology, 3rd ed. Philadelphia, JB Lippincott, 1997, pp 889–920.

40. Whelan JS: Osteosarcoma. Eur J Cancer 33: 1611–1618, 1997.

41. Yaw KM: Pediatric bone tumors. Semin Surg Oncol 16: 173–183, 1999.

41a. Rytting M, Pearson P, Raymond AK, et al: Osteosarcoma in preadolescent patients. Clin Orthop 373: 39–50, 2000.

42. Lane JM, Hurson B, Boland PJ, et al: Osteogenic sarcoma. Clin Orthop 204: 93–110, 1986.

43. Goorin AM, Abelson HT, Frei E: Osteosarcoma: fifteen years later. N Engl J Med 313: 1637–1643, 1985.

44. Crist WM, Kun LE: Common solid tumors of childhood. N Engl J Med 324: 461–471, 1991.

45. Colyer RA: Osteogenic sarcoma in siblings. Johns Hopkins Med J 145: 131–135, 1979.

46. Leonard A, Craft AW, Moss C, et al: Osteogenic sarcoma in the Rothmund-Thomson syndrome. Med Pediatr Oncol 26: 249–253, 1996.

47. El-Khoury JM, Haddad SN, Atallah NG: Osteosarcomatosis with Rothmund-Thomson syndrome. Br J Radiol 70: 215–218, 1997.

48. Petty RE, Cassidy JT, Heyn R, et al: Secondary hypertrophic osteoarthropathy. An unusual cause of arthritis in childhood. Arthritis Rheum 19: 902–906, 1976.

48a. Widhe B, Widhe T: Initial symptoms and clinical features in osteosarcoma and Ewing sarcoma. J Bone Joint Surg Am 82: 667–674, 2000.

49. Fletcher BD: Imaging pediatric bone sarcomas. Diagnosis and treatment-related issues. Radiol Clin North Am 35: 1477–1494, 1997.

49a. San Julian M, Aquerreta JD, Benito A, et al: Indications for epiphyseal preservation in metaphyseal malignant bone tumors of children: relationship between image methods and histological findings. J Pediatr Orthop 19: 543–548, 1999.

50. Marcove RC, Mike V, Hajek JV, et al: Osteogenic sarcoma under the age of twenty-one. A review of one hundred and forty-five operative cases. J Bone Joint Surg Am 52: 411–423, 1970.

51. Vander GR: Osteosarcoma and its variants. Orthop Clin North Am 27: 575–581, 1996.

52. Ahuja SC, Villacin AB, Smith J, et al: Juxtacortical (parosteal) osteogenic sarcoma: histological grading and prognosis. J Bone Joint Surg Am 59: 632–647, 1977.

52a. Kivioja A, Ervasti H, Kinnunen J, et al: Chondrosarcoma in a family with multiple hereditary exostoses. J Bone Joint Surg Br 82: 261–266, 2000.

53. Carli M, Gluglielmi M, Sotti G, et al: Soft tissue sarcomas. *In* Plowman PW, Pinkerton CR (eds): Paediatric Oncology: Clinical Practice and Controversies. London, Chapman & Hall, 1992, pp 291–324.

53a. Lee FY, Mankin HJ, Fondren G, et al: Chondrosarcoma of bone: an assessment of outcome. J Bone Joint Surg Am 81: 326–338, 1999.

54. Soule EH, Pritchard DJ: Fibrosarcoma in infants and children: a review of 110 cases. Cancer 40: 1711–1721, 1977.

54a. Trobs R, Meier T, Bennek J, et al: Fibrosarcoma in infants and children: a retrospective analysis–overdiagnosis in earlier years. Pediatr Surg Int 15: 123–128, 1999.
54b. Ruymann FB, Grovas AC: Progress in the diagnosis and treatment of rhabdomyosarcoma and related soft tissue sarcomas. Cancer Invest 18: 223–241, 2000.
54c. Merlino G, Helman LJ: Rhabdomyosarcoma—working out the pathways. Oncogene 18: 5340–5348, 1999.
54d. Dagher R, Helman L: Rhabdomyosarcoma: an overview. Oncologist 4: 34–44, 1999.
54e. Pappo AS, Shapiro DN, Crist WM: Rhabdomyosarcoma. Biology and treatment. Pediatr Clin North Am 44: 953–972, 1997.
54f. Andrassy RJ: Rhabdomyosarcoma. Semin Pediatr Surg 6: 17–23, 1997.
55. Schmidt D, Thum P, Harms D, et al: Synovial sarcoma in children and adolescents. A report from the Kiel Pediatric Tumor Registry. Cancer 67: 1667–1672, 1991.
55a. Ferrari A, Casanova M, Massimino M, et al: Synovial sarcoma: report of a series of 25 consecutive children from a single institution. Med Pediatr Oncol 31: 32–37, 1999.
55b. Skytting B: Synovial sarcoma. A Scandinavian Sarcoma Group project. Acta Orthop Scand 291(Suppl): 1–28, 2000.
56. Hajdu SI, Shiu MH, Fortner JG: Tendosynovial sarcoma: a clinicopathological study of 136 cases. Cancer 39: 1201–1217, 1977.
56a. Bergh P, Meis-Kindblom JM, Gherlinzoni F, et al: Synovial sarcoma: identification of low and high risk groups. Cancer 85: 2596–2607, 1999.
56b. Skytting BT, Bauer HC, Perfekt R, et al: Clinical course in synovial sarcoma: a Scandinavian sarcoma group study of 104 patients. Acta Orthop Scand 70: 536–542, 1999.
56c. Skytting B, Meis-Kindblom JM, Larsson O, et al: Synovial sarcoma—identification of favorable and unfavorable histologic types: a Scandinavian Sarcoma Group study of 104 cases. Acta Orthop Scand 70: 543–554, 1999.
56d. Thompson RC, Jr, Garg A, Goswitz J, et al: Synovial sarcoma. Large size predicts poor outcome. Clin Orthop 373: 18–24, 2000.
56e. Lewis JJ, Antonescu CR, Leung DH, et al: Synovial sarcoma: a multivariate analysis of prognostic factors in 112 patients with primary localized tumors of the extremity. J Clin Oncol 18: 2087–2094, 2000.
57. Fisher C: Synovial sarcoma. Ann Diagn Pathol 2: 401–421, 1998.
58. Dickman PS, Liotta LA, Triche TJ: Ewing's sarcoma. Characterization in established cultures and evidence of its histogenesis. Lab Invest 47: 375–382, 1982.
59. Horowitz ME, Malewer MM, Woo SY, et al: Ewing's sarcoma family of tumors: Ewing's sarcoma of bone and soft tissue and the peripheral primitive neuroectodermal tumors. *In* Pizzo P, Poplack D (eds): Principles and Practice of Pediatric Oncology, 3rd ed. Philadelphia, JB Lippincott, 1997, pp 831–864.
60. Vlasak R, Sim FH: Ewing's sarcoma. Orthop Clin North Am 27: 591–603, 1996.
61. Miser J, Triche T, Kinsella TJ: Other soft tissue sarcomas of childhood. *In* Pizzo P, Poplack D (eds): Principles and Practice of Pediatric Oncology, 3rd ed. Philadelphia, JB Lippincott, 1997, pp 865–888.
61a. Ahmad R, Mayol BR, Davis M, et al: Extraskeletal Ewing's sarcoma. Cancer 85: 725–731, 1999.
61b. Shankar AG, Pinkerton CR, Atra A, et al: Local therapy and other factors influencing site of relapse in patients with localised Ewing's sarcoma. United Kingdom Children's Cancer Study Group (UKCCSG). Eur J Cancer 35: 1698–1704, 1999.
61c. Rosito P, Mancini AF, Rondelli R, et al: Italian Cooperative Study for the treatment of children and young adults with localized Ewing sarcoma of bone: a preliminary report of 6 years of experience. Cancer 86: 421–428, 1999.
61d. McLean TW, Hertel C, Young ML, et al: Late events in pediatric patients with Ewing sarcoma/primitive neuroectodermal tumor of bone: the Dana-Farber Cancer Institute/Children's Hospital experience. J Pediatr Hematol Oncol 21: 486–493, 1999.
62. Mameghan H, Fisher RJ, O'Gorman-Hughes D, et al: Ewing's sarcoma: long-term follow-up in 49 patients treated from 1967 to 1989. Int J Radiat Oncol Biol Phys 25: 431–438, 1993.
62a. Cardenas-Cardos R, Rivera-Luna, Lopez-Facundo NA, et al: Ewing's sarcoma: prognosis and survival in Mexican children from a single institution. Pediatr Hematol Oncol 16: 519–523, 1999.
63. Leeson MC, Makley JT, Carter JR: Metastatic skeletal disease in the pediatric population. J Pediatr Orthop 5: 261–267, 1985.
64. Losty P, Quinn F, Breatnach F, et al: Neuroblastoma—a surgical perspective. Eur J Surg Oncol 19: 33–36, 1993.
65. Breslow NE, Beckwith JB: Epidemiological features of Wilms' tumor: results of the National Wilms' Tumor Study. J Natl Cancer Inst 68: 429–436, 1982.
66. Appell RG, Brandeis WE, Georgi P, et al: Radiographic and scintigraphic appearance of bone metastasizing Wilms' tumour: problems in confirming diagnosis. Ann Radiol (Paris) 25: 14–18, 1982.
67. Schaller J: Arthritis as a presenting manifestation of malignancy in children. J Pediatr 81: 793–797, 1972.
68. Fink CW, Windmiller J, Sartain P: Arthritis as the presenting feature of childhood leukemia. Arthritis Rheum 15: 347–349, 1972.
69. Costello PB, Brecher ML, Starr JI, et al: A prospective analysis of the frequency, course, and possible prognostic significance of the joint manifestations of childhood leukemia. J Rheumatol 10: 753–757, 1983.
70. Saulsbury FT, Sabio H: Acute leukemia presenting as arthritis in children. Clin Pediatr 24: 625–628, 1985.
71. Gallagher DJ, Phillips DJ, Heinrich SD: Orthopedic manifestations of acute pediatric leukemia. Orthop Clin North Am 27: 635–644, 1996.
72. Martinez-Lavin M, Bobadilla M, Casanova J, et al: Hypertrophic osteoarthropathy in cyanotic congenital heart disease: its prevalence and relationship to bypass of the lung. Arthritis Rheum 25: 1186–1193, 1982.
73. Martinez-Lavin M: Hypertrophic osteoarthropathy. Curr Opin Rheumatol 9: 83–86, 1997.
74. Ginsberg J, Brown JB: Increased oestrogen excretion in hypertrophic pulmonary osteoarthropathy. Lancet 2: 1274, 1961.
75. Roebuck DJ: Skeletal complications in pediatric oncology patients. Radiographics 19: 873–885, 1999.
76. Stuart CA, Driscoll MS, Lundquist KF, et al: Acanthosis nigricans. J Basic Clin Physiol Pharmacol 9: 407–418, 1998.
77. Baird JS, Johnson JL, Elliott-Mills D, et al: Systemic lupus erythematosus with acanthosis nigricans, hyperpigmentation, and insulin receptor antibody. Lupus 6: 275–278, 1997.
78. Dhar S, Dawn G, Kanwar AJ, et al: Familial acanthosis nigricans. Int J Dermatol 35: 126–127, 1996.

Appendix

Table A–1

Clinical Manifestations of the Connective Tissue Diseases*

	JUVENILE RHEUMATOID ARTHRITIS	SYSTEMIC LUPUS ERYTHEMATOSUS	POLYARTERITIS	DERMATOMYOSITIS	SCLERODERMA	RHEUMATIC FEVER
Female:male ratio	2:1	5:1	1:3	2:1	2:1	1:1
Constitutional symptoms	+ + +	+ + +	+ + +	+ + +	+	+ + +
Arthritis	+ + +	+ +	+	+	+	+ + +
Skin						
Rash	+	+ + +	+	+ + +	−	+
Photosensitivity	−	+ +	−	+	−	−
Purpura	−	+ + +	+ +	−	−	−
Telangiectases	−	−	−	−	+ + +	−
Pigmentation	−	+	−	+ +	+ +	−
Calcinosis	−	−	−	+ +	+ +	−
Subcutaneous nodules	+	+	+	−	+	+
Alopecia	−	+ +	−	+	+	−
Mucous membranes	−	+ +	−	+	−	−
Raynaud's phenomenon	−	+ +	+	+	+ + +	−
Vasculitis	+	+ + +	+ + +	+ +	+	+
Myositis	+	+	+	+ + +	+ +	−
Serositis	+ +	+ + +	+	+	−	+ +
Cardiac						
Pericardial	+ +	+ + +	+	−	−	+
Myocardial	+	+	+ +	+	+ + +	+
Endocardial	−	+ +	−	−	−	+ + +
Pulmonary disease	+	+ +	+ +	+	+ + +	+
Gastrointestinal						
Dysphagia	−	−	−	+ +	+ + +	−
Abdominal pain	+	+ +	+ + +	+ +	+	+ +
Malabsorption	−	−	−	−	+ + +	−
Hepatomegaly	+	+	−	−	−	+
Splenomegaly	+	+ +	−	−	−	−
Lymphadenopathy	+	+ +	+	+	−	−
Nephritis	+	+ + +	+ + +	+	+ + +	−
Hypertension	−	+ +	+ + +	−	+ +	−
Ocular disease	+ +	+ +	+ +	+	+	−
Nervous system						
Peripheral	−	+	+ + +	−	−	−
Central	−	+ + +	+	−	+	−
Chorea	−	+	−	−	−	+ +

*−, absent; +, minimal; + +, moderate; + + +, severe.

Table A–2

Laboratory Abnormalities in the Rheumatic Diseases of Childhood*

	JUVENILE RHEUMATOID ARTHRITIS							
ABNORMALITY	Polyarthritis	Oligoarthritis	Systemic Onset	SYSTEMIC LUPUS ERYTHEMATOSUS	DERMATOMYOSITIS	SCLERODERMA	VASCULITIS	RHEUMATIC FEVER
Anemia	+	−	+ +	+ + +	+	+	+ +	+
Leukopenia	−	−	−	+ + +	−	−	−	−
Thrombocytopenia	−	−	−	+ +	−	−	−	−
Leukocytosis	+	−	+ + +	−	+	−	+ + +	+
Thrombocytosis	+	−	+ +	−	+	−	+	+
Antinuclear antibodies	+	+ +	−	+ + +	+	+ +	−	−
Anti-dsDNA antibodies	−	−	−	+ + +	−	−	−	−
Rheumatoid factors	+	−	−	+ +	−	+	+	−
Antistreptococcal antibodies	+	−	−	−	−	−	−	+ + +
Hypocomplementemia	−	−	−	+ + +	−	−	+ +	−
Elevated hepatic enzyme levels	+	−	+ +	+	+	+	+	−
Elevated muscle enzyme levels	−	−	−	+	+ + +	+ +	+	−
Abnormal urinalysis	+	−	+	+ + +	+	+	+ +	−

*−, absent; +, minimal; + +, moderate; + + +, severe.

Table A–3

Clinical Manifestations of the Common Forms of Spondyloarthropathy Compared With Juvenile Rheumatoid Arthritis*

	JUVENILE ANKYLOSING SPONDYLITIS	PSORIATIC ARTHROPATHY	REITER'S SYNDROME	JUVENILE RHEUMATOID ARTHRITIS
Clinical course of disease				
Arthritis				
Peripheral	+ +	+ + +	+ + +	+ + +
Axial				
Sacroiliac	+ + +	+ +	+ +	±
Lumbar	+ +	+	+	–
Thoracic	+ +	–	–	+
Cervical	+	+	–	+ + +
Skin and mucous membranes	–	+ + +	+	+
Genital tract	–	+	+ +	–
Ocular disease	+	+	+	+ +
Heart	+	–	+	+
Vasculitis	–	–	–	+
Pulmonary disease	+	–	–	+
Rheumatoid nodules	–	–	–	+
Pathologic findings				
Acute synovitis	+	+	+ + +	+ +
Mononuclear cell infiltrate	+ +	+	+	+ +
Pannus	+	+	+	+ +
Bursitis and tendinitis	+ +	–	+ +	+ +
Ankylosis	+ +	–	+	+ +
Laboratory abnormalities				
Acute phase response	+	+ +	+ +	+ + +
Anemia	+	+	+	+ +
Leukocytosis	–	+	+ +	+ +
Rheumatoid factors	–	–	–	+
Antinuclear antibodies	–	+ +	–	+ +

*–, absent; ± = variable, rare; +, minimal; + +, moderate; + + +, severe.

Table A–4

Characteristics of Synovial Fluid in the Rheumatic Diseases*

GROUP	CONDITION	SYNOVIAL COMPLEMENT	COLOR/ CLARITY	VISCOSITY	MUCIN CLOT	WBC COUNT	PMN (%)	MISCELLANEOUS FINDINGS
Noninflammatory	Normal	N	Yellow Clear	VH	G	<200	<25	
	Traumatic arthritis	N	Xanthochromic Turbid	H	F–G	<2000	<25	Debris
	Osteoarthritis	N	Yellow Clear	H	F–G	1000	<25	
Inflammatory	Systemic lupus erythematosus	↓	Yellow Clear	N	N	5000	10	Lupus erythematosus cells
	Rheumatic fever	N–↑	Yellow Cloudy	↓	F	5000	10–50	
	Juvenile rheumatoid arthritis	N–↓	Yellow Cloudy	↓	Poor	15,000–20,000	75	
	Reiter's syndrome	↑	Yellow Opaque	↓	Poor	20,000	80	Reiter's cells
Pyogenic	Tuberculous arthritis	N–↑	Yellow-white Cloudy	↓	Poor	25,000	50–60	Acid-fast bacteria
	Septic arthritis	↑	Serosanguineous Turbid	↓	Poor	50,000–300,000	>75	Low glucose, bacteria

*WBC, white blood cell; PMN, polymorphonuclear leukocyte; N, normal; VH, very high; H, high; G, good; F, fair; ↓, decreased; ↑, increased.

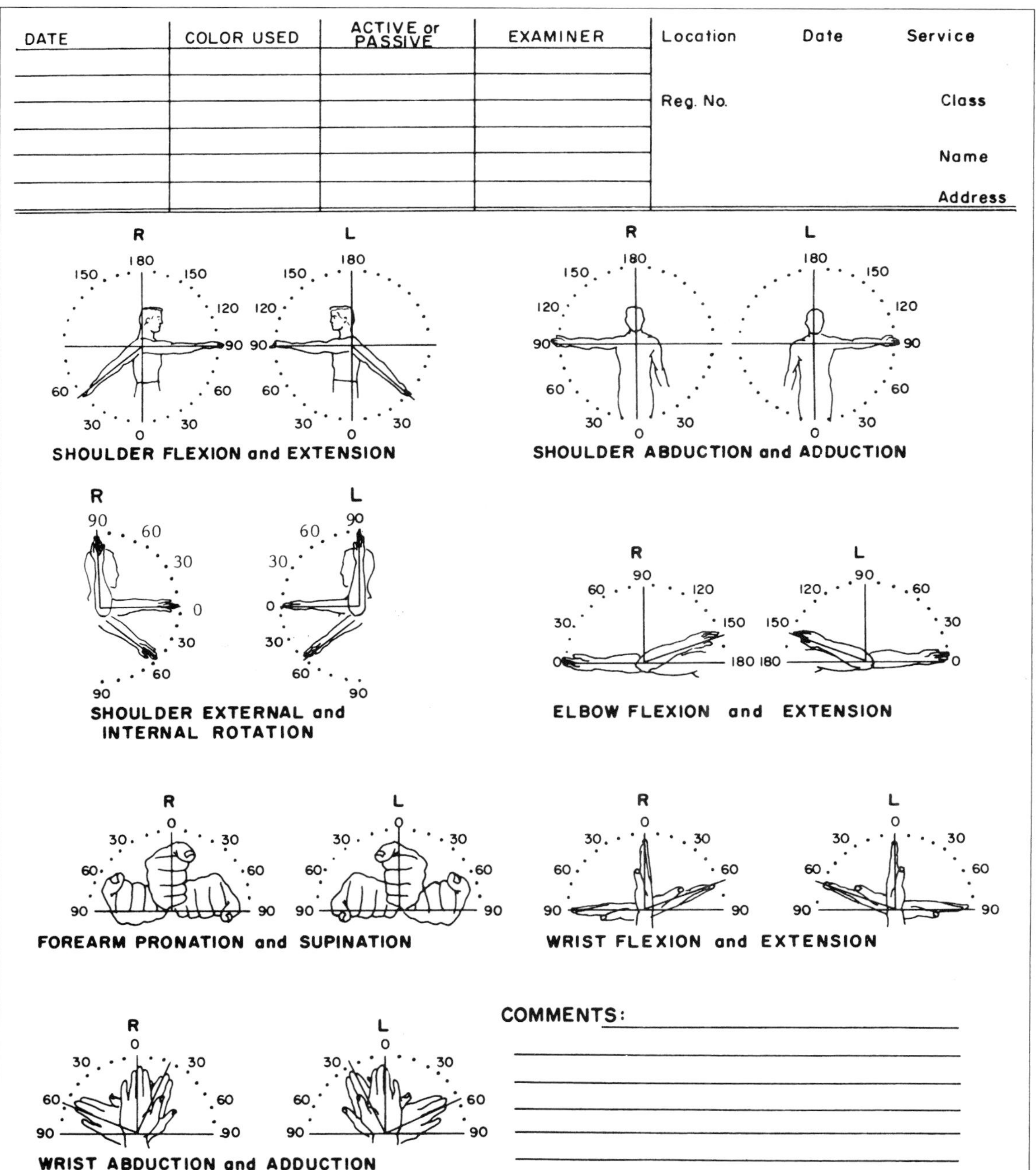

Figure A–1. Range of motion chart.

Illustration continued on following page

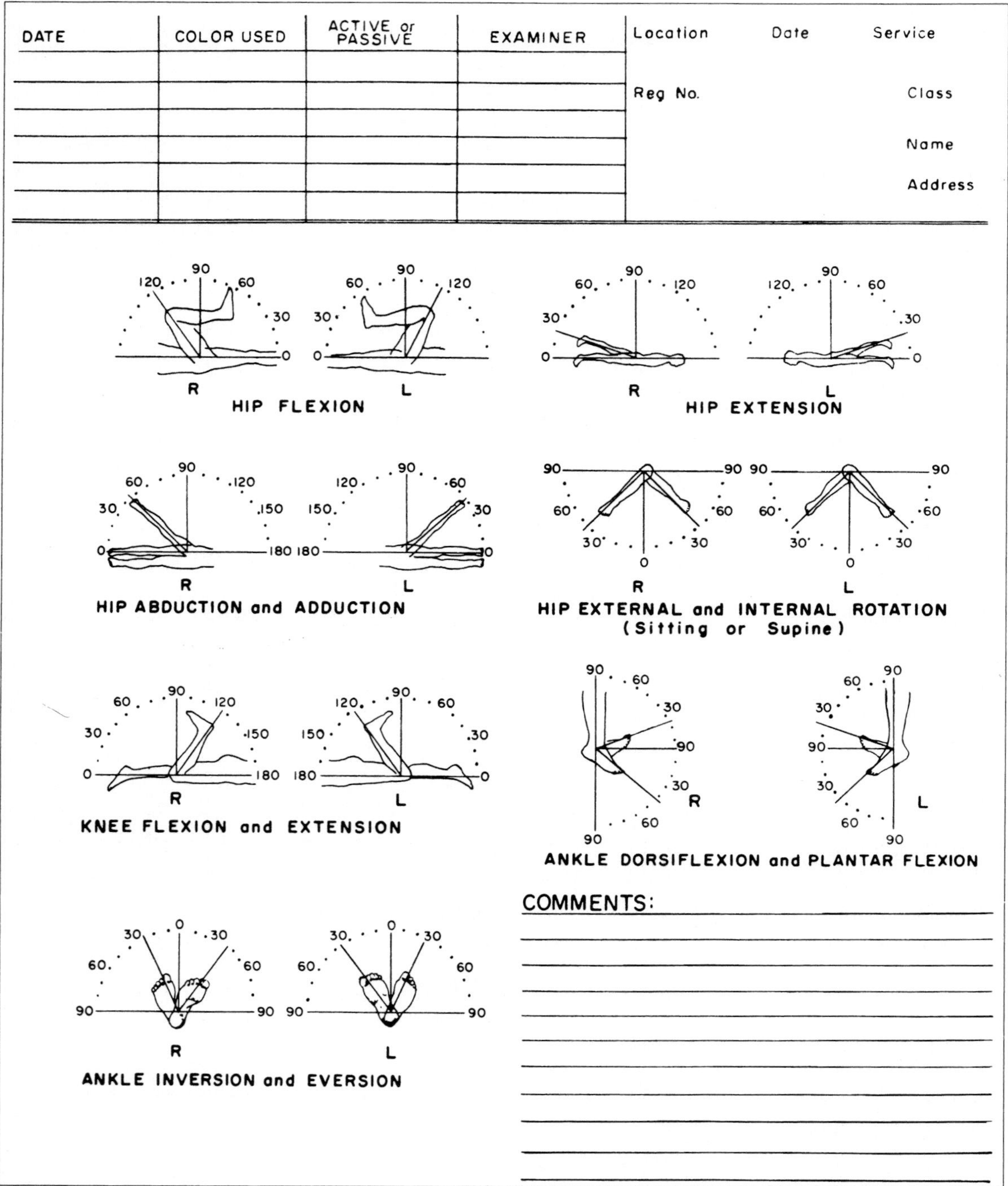

DATE	COLOR USED	ACTIVE or PASSIVE	EXAMINER

Location Date Service

Reg No. Class

Name

Address

COMMENTS:

Figure A–1 *Continued*

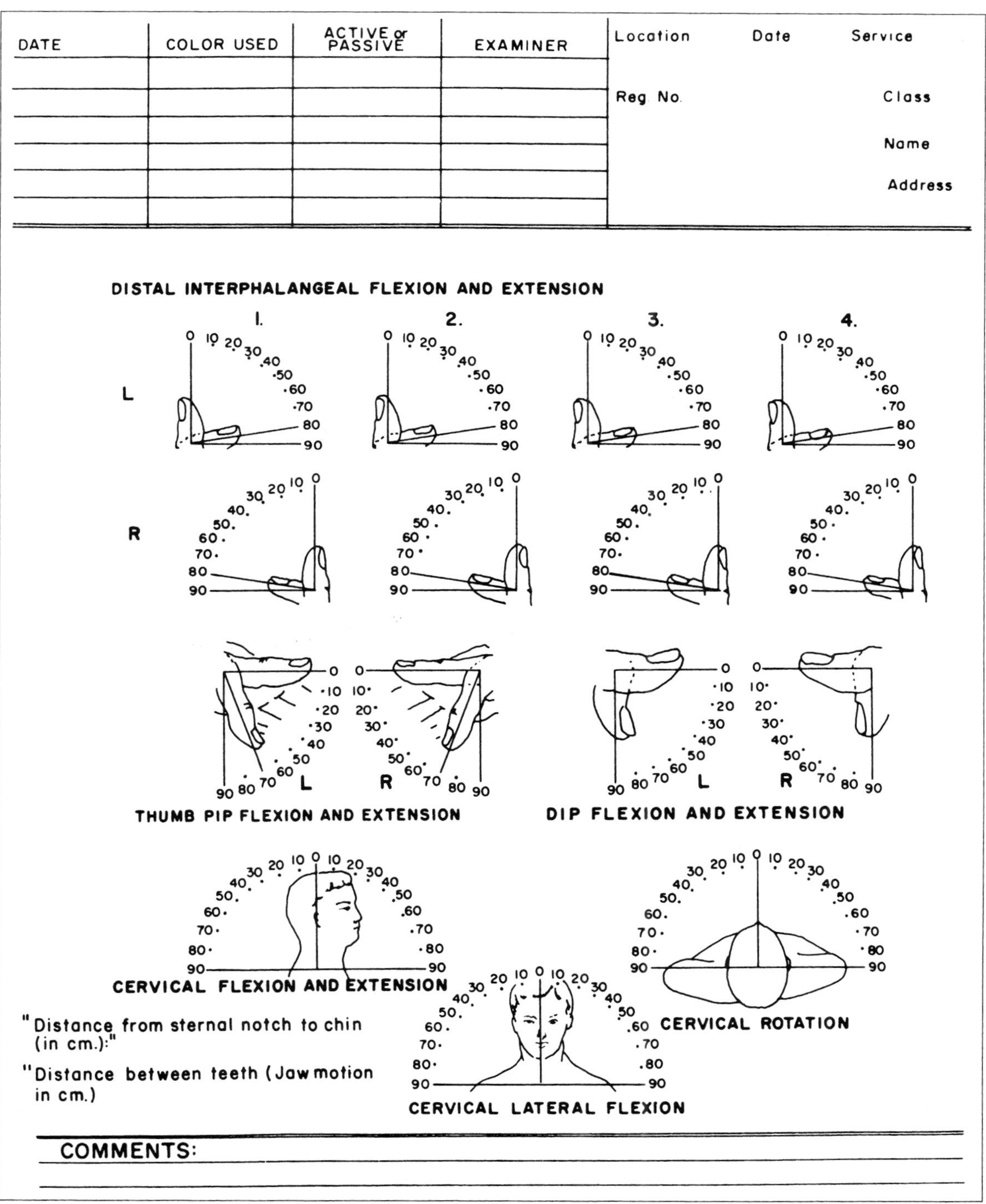

Figure A–1 *Continued*

Illustration continued on following page

DATE	COLOR USED	ACTIVE or PASSIVE	EXAMINER

Location Date Service

Reg. No. Class

Name

Address

METACARPOPHALANGEAL FLEXION AND EXTENSION

1. (Index) 2. 3. 4.

L

R

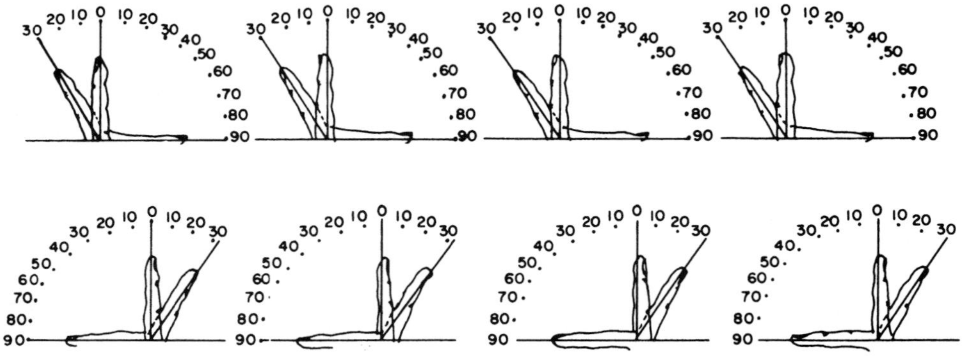

PROXIMAL INTERPHALANGEAL FLEXION AND EXTENSION

L

R

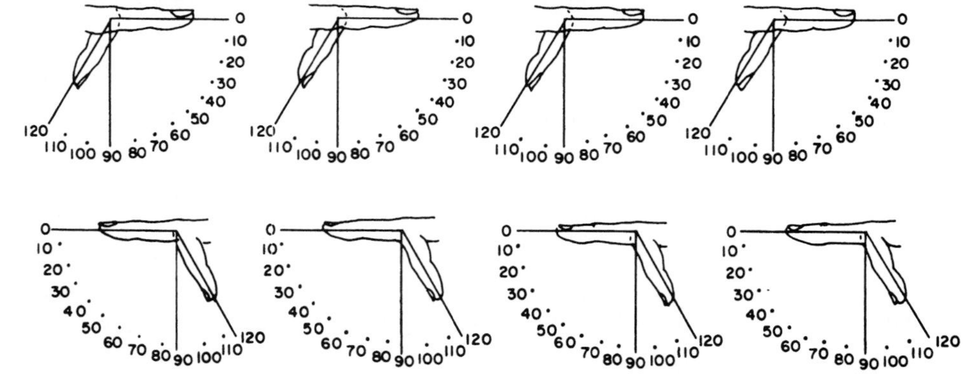

COMMENTS:

Figure A–1 *Continued*

Table A–5

Congenital and Familial Disorders With Arthritis

DISORDER	JOINT FINDINGS	CLINICAL FEATURES
Agammaglobulinemia	Asymmetric arthritis, primarily large joints	Absent tonsils, severe infections
Blau's syndrome	Moderately painful polyarticular arthritis, often leading to camptodactyly	Granulomatous anterior and posteror uveitis, granulomatous intermittent generalized rash, increased serum angiotensin-converting enzyme level, lung involvement
Camptodactyly-arthropathy-pericarditis syndrome	Polyarticular arthritis with contractures, camptodactyly at birth (flexion contractures of PIP joints)	Pericarditis
Cystic fibrosis	Episodic polyarthritis, often associated with erythema nodosum, HPO	Chronic pulmonary disease, failure to thrive, malabsorption
DiGeorge's anomalad (velocardiofacial syndrome, chromosome 22q11.2 deletion syndrome)	Polyarticular arthritis of large and small joints	Immunodeficiency, hypocalcemia, facial and cardiac anomalies
Dominant familial arthritis with scoliosis	Joints: IP and MCP, wrists, elbows; flexion contractures of fingers	Thoracic scoliosis
Familial arthropathy in children ("E" family disease)	Symmetric arthritis of large joints; flexion deformity of PIP joints at birth	Absence of inflammation
Familial histiocytic dermatoarthritis (multicentric reticulohistocytosis)	Symmetric polyarthritis of hands, wrists, elbows, feet	Multiple skin nodules over face, ears, hands, legs, and forearms; subcutaneous plaques over arms and legs; eye anomalies: glaucoma, uveitis, cataract
Familial hypertriglyceridemia	Oligoarticular arthritis or migratory arthralgias and polyarthritis of knees, ankles, hips, elbows, wrists; limitation of movement	Hypercholesterolemia, fever, xanthomata (nodules) in skin and tendons
Familial Mediterranean fever	Episodic arthritis of knees, ankles, hips shoulders, elbows	Periodic fevers, abdominal pain, chest pain, serositis
Farber's disease (disseminated lipogranulomatosis)	Symmetric polyarthritis	Pigmented nodular periarticular swelling, mental retardation, hoarse cry, painful red nodules in tendon sheaths and around joints
Hereditary osteolysis (multicentric idiopathic osteolysis)	"Arthritis" of wrists, ankles, elbows, MCP and IP joints; limitation of elbow extension, supination, and pronation; ulnar deviation of involved hand; painless deformities of wrists and feet	Marfanoid habitus, micrognathia, generalized erythematous rash, nodules over IP joints, generalized wasting of involved limb, bone destruction begins with carpal and tarsal bones and spreads to involve the adjacent long bones, renal failure
Hyperimmunoglobulinemia D	Recurrent arthritis or arthralgias, most commonly knee and ankle, often symmetric	Recurrent fevers, abdominal pain, lymphadenopathy, elevated serum IgD
KID (keratitis, ichthyosis, deafness) syndrome	Jaccoud's arthropathy	Ichthyosis with hyperkeratosis of the palms and soles, keratitis of the cornea causing photophobia, neurosensory deafness
Lesch-Nyhan syndrome	Monarticular arthritis of knees, ankles, toes, or fingers	Self-mutilating behavior, growth and mental retardation; fever, dry skin, tophi of ear; choreoathetosis, spastic cerebral palsy, hyperuricemia
Lowe's syndrome (oculo-cerebro-renal syndrome)	Swelling and contractures of large and small joints, hypermobile joints	Mental retardation, renal tubular dysfunction, hypotonia, cataract
Muckle-Wells syndrome (other mycoidoses)	Periodic arthritis and arthralgias, mainly of knees and ankles	Chronic urticaria, deafness, amyloid nephropathy
Nail-patella syndrome	Polyarticular arthritis Restricted range of movement of elbows	Hypoplastic thumbnails, hypoplastic patellae, radial head dislocations, iliac horns, often clubfoot
Neonatal onset multisystem inflammatory disease (NOMID), (CINCA syndrome, Lorber's syndrome)	Polyarticular arthritis, large patella	Neonatal onset maculopapular rash, hepatosplenomegaly, CNS involvement, severe wasting leading to death
Philadelphia chromosome	Ankylosing spondylitis, rheumatoid arthritis	Myeloproliferative disease
Stickler's syndrome (hereditary arthro-ophthalmopathy)	Symmetric arthritis of large and small joints, hyperextensible joints, spine involvement	Flat facies, epicanthal folds, long philtrum, myopia, cataract, kyphosis
Tricho-rhino-phalangeal syndrome	Enlargement of middle phalangeal joints in fingers and toes, ulnar deviation of fingers, short fourth and fifth metacarpals and metatarsals, progressive arthritis of hips	Pear-shaped nose, thin sparse hair, thin nails, large prominent ears, micrognathia

Table continued on following page

Table A–5

Congenital and Familial Disorders With Arthritis *Continued*

DISORDER	JOINT FINDINGS	CLINICAL FEATURES
Trisomy 21 (Down syndrome)	Polyarticular or oligoarticular arthritis of large and small joints, joint hypermobility, hypoplasia of midphalanx of fifth finger with clinodactyly, hypoplasia of pelvis	Mental retardation, hypotonia, upslanting palpebral fissures, inner epicanthal folds, small ears, flat facies, short stature, brachydactyly, psoriasis
Turner's syndrome	Polyarticular or oligoarticular arthritis	Short stature, broad chest, lymphedema, webbed neck, low hairline, cubitus valgus
18p-syndrome	Arthritis and flexion contractures of knee, ankle, or wrist	Variable mental retardation, growth retardation, ptosis or epicanthal folds, prominent auricles, IgA deficiency
18q-syndrome	Oligoarticular inflammatory arthritis	Mental retardation, short stature, often IgA deficiency

CINCA, chronic infantile neurologic cutaneous and auricular; CNS, central nervous system; HPO, hypertrophic pulmonary osteoarthropathy; Ig, immunoglobulin; IP, interphalangeal; MCP, metacarpophalangeal; PIP, proximal interphalangeal.

From Chalom EC, Ross J, Athreya BH: Syndromes and arthritis. Rheum Dis Clin North Am 23:709–727, 1997.

Table A–6

Congenital and Familial Disorders With Contractures or Stiff Joints

DISORDER	JOINT FINDINGS	CLINICAL FEATURES
Aarskog's syndrome	PIP joint hyperextensibility with distal joint restriction, short fifth finger with clinodactyly	Round face, hypertelorism, short, broad nose, anteverted nostrils, long philtrum, short statue, shawl scrotum, mild interdigital webbings, broad hands
Achondroplasia syndrome	Incomplete extenson of elbow	Short stature, macrocephaly, low nasal bridge, prominent forehead, short limbs
Antley-Bixler syndrome	Joint contractures, present at birth: wrists, fingers, hips, knees, or ankles	Brachycephaly, midface hypoplasia, dysplastic ears, radiohumeral synostosis
Apert's syndrome (acrocephalosyndactyly)	Ankyloses of elbow, shoulder, hip	Craniosynostosis with flat occiput, brachycephaly, midfacial hypoplasia, syndactyly
Arthrogryposis multiplex congenita	Stiffness, multiple contractures of large and small joints, painless deformities	Muscle wasting
Beal's syndrome (contractural arachnodactyly syndrome)	Joint contractures of knees, elbows, hands	Arachnodactyly, crumpled ear
Caffey's pseudo-Hurler syndrome (generalized gangliosidosis syndrome type I, familial neurovisceral lipidosis)	Contractures of elbows and knees, claw hand	Coarse facies, kyphosis
Chromosome 2p terminal deletion	Polyarticular contractures, especially of hips, knees, and ankles	Severe developmental delay, seizures, lack of finger flexion creases
Cockayne's syndrome	Mild to moderate limitation of knees, elbows, ankles	Microcephaly, large ears, loss of facial subcutaneous fat beginning in infancy, growth retardation, impaired hearing, retinal degeneration
Conradi-Hünermann syndrome (X-linked dominant chondrodysplasia punctata)	Variable joint contractures	Asymmetric limb shortness, large skin pores, early punctate mineralization
Cornelia de Lange syndrome	Flexion contracture of elbow	Synophrys (eyebrows run together), thin, down-turning upper lip, micromelia, generalized hirsutism, weak growling cry in infancy, developmental delay
Diastrophic dwarfism syndrome	Limitation of flexion of PIP joints and of extension at elbow; clubfoot	Short tubular bones (especially first metacarpal), hypertrophied auricular cartilage
Ectrodactyly-ectodermal dysplasia-clefting (EEC) syndrome	Limited extension of elbow joints	Abnormality of third digit, cleft lip/palate; ectodermal dysplasia
Fabry's disease (angiokeratoma corporis diffusum)	Bony swelling, all joints may be affected, usually symmetric DIP joints, flexion deformity	Fever, burning pain in fingers or toes, exacerbated by heat or exertion, dark nodular angiectases
Familial blepharophimosis syndrome (Pena-Shokier)	Multiple joint contractures (elbow, wrist, hip, knee, ankle), camptodactyly	Microcephaly, microcornea, cataract, blepharophimosis, micrognathia
Familial (congenital) cold urticaria	Throbbing pain, swelling, stiffness, periarticular erythema	Fever, chills, headache, cold urticaria—pruritic and burning sensation, acrocyanosis
GEMSS syndrome	Progressive joint stiffness	Glaucoma, lens ectopia, microspherophakia, short stature (GEMSS)

Table A–6

Congenital and Familial Disorders With Contractures or Stiff Joints *Continued*

DISORDER	JOINT FINDINGS	CLINICAL FEATURES
Homocystinuria	Reduced joint mobility, enlarged joints	Marfanoid appearance, subluxation of lens, malar flush, osteoporosis, vascular thromboses and embolism, blond hair
Hunter's syndrome (mucopolysaccharidosis II, MPS II)	Reduced joint mobility, joint contractures, claw hand	Coarse facies, deafness, growth deficiency, no corneal clouding
Hurler's syndrome (MPS I-H)	Reduced joint mobility, claw hand, limitation of extension more than flexion	Coarse facies, macrocephaly, mental retardation, cloudy cornea, cardiac involvement
Hypochondroplasia syndrome	Mild limitation of elbow mobility	Short limbs, caudal narrowing of spinal canal, near-normal facies
Jansen's metaphyseal chondrodysplasia syndrome (metaphyseal dysostosis Jansen type)	Flexion deformity of joints, especially of the knees and hips, resulting in a squatting stance	Small thorax (wide, irregular metaphysis)
Kozlowski's syndrome (spondylometaphyseal dysplasia)	Limited mobility in hips and elbows	Short stature, pectus carinatum, mild bowleg deformity
Léri's pleonosteosis syndrome	Limitation of mobility, flexion contractures of the digits	Broad thumb, upward slant of palpebral fissures, short stature
Léri-Weill dyschondrosteosis syndrome	Limitation of mobility at wrist or elbow	Short forearms with Madelung's deformity, with or without short leg
Leroy I cell syndrome (I-cell disease, mucolipidosis II)	Moderate limitation of flexion, especially hips, may have congenital dislocation of the hips	Developmental delay, short stature, early alveolar ridge hypertrophy, thick tight skin in early infancy
Marden-Walker syndrome	Congenital joint contractures	Mental retardation, blepharophimosis, micrognathia, growth delay, decreased muscular mass, immobile facies
Maroteaux-Lamy syndrome (MPS VI)	Limitation of movement of knee, hip, elbow	Coarse facies, short stature, cloudy cornea without mental deterioration, valvular heart disease
Metatrophic dwarfism syndrome	Limitation of movement at knee and hip, hypermobility of fingers	Small thorax, thoracic kyphoscoliosis, metaphyseal flaring
Pseudo-Hurler polydystrophy syndrome (mucolipidosis III)	Limitation of movement of hands, elbows, knees, shoulders, claw hand	Coarse facies, no mucopolysacchariduria, aortic valve involvement
Rhizomelic chondrodysplasia punctata syndrome	Multiple joint contractures	Short humeri and femurs, coronal cleft in vertebrae, saddle nose deformity, punctate epiphyseal mineralization, hypertelorism
Riley-Day syndrome (familial dysautonomia)	Neuropathic joints, commonly the knees	Insensitivity to pain, dysautonomia, lack of tearing, poor coordination
Sanfilippo's syndrome (MP III)	Mildly stiff joints	Mildly coarse faces, mental retardation, hyperactivity, hepatosplenomegaly
Schieie's syndrome (MPS ISS)	Limitation of movement of hands and feet, leading to claw hand	Mildly coarse facies, early corneal opacity, aortic valve disease, normal intelligence
Schmid's metaphyseal chondrodysplasia syndrome (spondyloepimetaphyseal dysplasia)	Mild decrease in extension of fingers and upper limbs, genu varum	Short stature as children (often normal as adults), tibial bowing at the ankle, waddling gait
Schwartz's syndrome (Schwartz-Jampel syndrome)	Limitation of movement at hips, wrists, fingers, toes, spine	Muscle hypertrophy, myotonia, blepharophemosis, short stature
Seckel's syndrome	Limitation of motion of elbows, dislocated hips	Severely short stature, microcephaly, prominent nose, malformed ears
Spondyloepiphyseal dysplasia congenita/ tarda	Limitation of motion at elbows, knees, hips; pain, soft tissue swelling, and contractures of PIP joints, hips, and elbows	Short trunk, myopia, lag in epiphyseal mineralization, immune deficiency
Trisomy 5q	Limitation of movement in hips, elbows, flexion contractures	Mental retardation, short stature, microcephaly, dysmorphic facies, hypertonia, digital anomalies
Trisomy 8	Limited elbow supination	Thick lips, deep-set eyes, prominent ears, camptodactyly
Weaver's syndrome	Limited extension of elbows and knees	Large at birth, camptodactyly, unusual facies (accelerated skeletal maturation)
Weill-Marchesani syndrome	Progressive joint stiffness	Short stature, brachydactyly, ectopia lentis, spherophakia
Winchester's syndrome	Symmetric flexion contractures with pain of fingers, elbows, hips, knees, ankles	Short stature, coarse facies, thickened leathery skin, general osteoporosis with dissolution of carpal and tarsal bones
Zellweger's syndrome (cerebro-hepato-renal syndrome)	Variable contractures, especially of knees and fingers, limited extension of knees, ulnar deviation of hands	High forehead with flat facies, hypotonia, hepatomegaly, micrognathia, abnormal external ears

DIP, distal interphalangeal; PIP, proximal interphalangeal.
From Chalom EC, Ross J, Athreya BH: Syndromes and arthritis. Rheum Dis Clin North Am 23:709–727, 1997.

Table A–7

Congenital and Familial Disorders With Hypermobile Joints

DISORDER	JOINT FINDINGS	CLINICAL FEATURES
Aarskog's syndrome	PIP joint hyperextensibility with distal joint restriction, short fifth finger with clinodactyly	Round face, hypertelorism, short, broad nose, anteverted nostrils, long philtrum, short stature, shawl scrotum, mild interdigital webbing, and broad hands
Coffin-Lowry syndrome	Hypermobile joints	Antimongoloid slanting palpebral fissures, bulbous nose, tapering fingers
Coffin-Siris syndrome	Hypermobile joints with radial dislocation at elbow	Hypoplastic or absent fifth finger and toe nails, coarse facies, sparse scalp hair, developmental delay
Cohen's syndrome	Hypermobile joints	Obesity, hypotonia, retinal degeneration, mental retardation, prominent incisors
Costello's syndrome	Hypermobile joints	Poor growth, "coarse" facies, curly hair, developmental delay, loose skin on hands, feet
Cutis-laxa-growth deficiency syndrome	Hypermobile joints, congenital dislocation of hips	Cutis laxa, growth deficiency
Dubowitz's syndrome	Hypermobile joints	Growth retardation, mild mental retardation, eczema, "characteristic face"
Ehlers-Danlos syndrome II	Hypermobile joints	Hyperextensibility of the skin, poor wound healing, cardiac valvular abnormalities
Hajdu-Cheney syndrome (acro-osteolysis syndrome, arthrodentodysplasia)	Hypermobile joints	Early loss of teeth, acro-osteolysis, generalized skeletal dysplasia
Kabuki make-up syndrome	Generalized ligamentous laxity	Craniofacial abnormalities, including cleft lip and palate, mild to moderate mental retardation, growth deficiency, congenital heart defects
Larsen's syndrome	Hypermobile joints, multiple joint dislocations	Flat facies, broad nasal bridge, cleft palate, hypertelorism, prominent forehead, congenital heart, broad thumbs, cylindrical long fingers, and short stature
Marfan syndrome	Hyperextensible joints	Excessive height, arachnodactyly, lens subluxation, myopia, aortic dilatation
Metaphyseal dysplasia (McKusick-type) (cartilage-hair hypoplasia)	Hypermobile joints, limp hands and feet	Mild bowing of legs, fine sparse hair, wide irregular metaphysis
Morquio's syndrome (MPS IV)	Hypermobile joints	Short stature, spondyloepiphyseal dysplasia, flaring of ribs, pectus carinatum, genu valgum, corneal clouding
Velofacioskeletal syndrome	Hypermobile hand joints	Hypertelorism, broad and high nasal bridge, epicanthal folds, mild mesomelic brachymelia, short hands, small feet

PIP, proximal interphalangeal.
From Chalom EC, Ross J, Athreya BH: Syndromes and arthritis. Rheum Dis Clin North Am 23:709–727, 1997.

DEFINITIONS AND CODES*

A. Chronic Arthritis in Children

Peripheral Arthritis

714.3 *Juvenile rheumatoid arthritis* (JRA)
- (a) Age at onset < 16 years
- (b) Arthritis defined as articular swelling/effusion or the presence of two or more of the following signs:
  - (i) Limitation of range of movement
  - (ii) Joint tenderness or palpation
  - (iii) Pain on joint movement
  - (iv) Increased heat over joint
- (c) Duration of arthritis > 6 weeks
- (d) Exclusion of other causes of arthritis

Onset Pattern During the 6 Months Following Onset of Arthritis

714.30 *Polyarticular:* Five or more joints involved during the first 6 months of the disease.

714.31 *Systemic:* Arthritis (any number of joints involved), with the characteristic rash and at least 2 weeks of high spiking fever. If only one of these two systemic features is present, at least hepatosplenomegaly or pericarditis should be present to make the diagnosis.

714.32 *Oligoarticular:* Four or fewer joints involved during the first 6 months of the disease.

714.33 *Monarticular arthritis*

Other Forms of Chronic Arthritis

713.3 *Juvenile psoriatic arthritis with psoriasis:* Arthritis with typical psoriatic rash.

(713.32) *Juvenile psoriatic arthritis without definite psoriasis:* Arthritis with at least three of the following:
- (1) Dactylitis
- (2) Nail pitting
- (3) Psoriasis-like rash
- (4) Positive family history of psoriasis in a first- or second-degree relative.

(713.33) *Probable juvenile psoriatic arthritis:* Arthritis with at least two of the following:
- (1) Dactylitis
- (2) Nail pitting
- (3) Psoriasis-like rash

720.0 *Juvenile ankylosing spondylitis* (JAS)
- (a) Age of onset before 17 years
- (b) Signs fulfilling New York criteria for ankylosing spondylitis (AS)

Clinical Criteria

- (i) Limitation of motion of lumbar spine in all three planes: anterior flexion, extension, and lateral flexion
- (ii) History of, or the presence of, pain at the dorsolumbar junction or in the lumbar spine
- (iii) Limitation of chest expansion to 1 inch (2.5 cm) or less measured at the level of the 4th intercostal space.

Definite JAS

(a) Grade 3–4 bilateral sacroiliac arthritis with at least one clinical criterion.

(b) Grade 3–4 unilateral or grade 2 bilateral with clinical criterion (i) or clinical criteria (ii) and (iii)

(720.02) *Probable JAS*
- (a) Age of onset before 17 years
- (b) Arthritis affecting one or more joints of lower limb + two or more of the following:
  - (i) Enthesitis
  - (ii) Flattening of normal lumbar curvature on forward flexion
  - (iii) Pain on stressing sacroiliac joints
  - (iv) History of lumbar pain lasting longer than 1 month
  - (v) Radiologic changes of sacroiliac joints (unilateral or bilateral) grade 2 or greater. (Grade 2 = minimal abnormality—small localized areas with erosion or sclerosis without alteration in the joint width.)

(720.03) *Seronegative enthesopathy arthropathy syndrome (SEA)*
- (a) Onset of symptoms before 17 years
- (b) Absence of rheumatoid factors
- (c) Presence of enthesopathic signs
- (d) Presence of arthritis or arthralgia at site separate from site of enthesitis.

711.3 *Reactive arthritis:* Arthritis associated with a proven gastrointestinal or genitourinary infection occurring within the previous 4 weeks.

(711.32) *Probable reactive arthritis:* Arthritis associated with a diarrheal illness or genitourinary discharge probably caused by an infectious agent but in which the infection is unproved.

711.1 *Reiter's syndrome:* Arthritis associated with both urethritis and conjunctivitis.

(711.11) *Probable Reiter's syndrome:* Arthritis associated with either urethritis or conjunctivitis.

713.1 *Arthritis of inflammatory bowel disease:* Arthritis associated with proven inflammatory bowel disease.

Eye Disease

364.0 *Acute anterior uveitis:* Inflammation of the anterior chamber of the eye associated with con-

---

**Note:* Many of these definitions have yet to be validated.

Modified in part from Peter Malleson, MB, Canadian Paediatric Rheumatology Association, 1991; International Classification of Diseases, 9th Revision, Clinical Modification (ICD–9–CM 2001). Numbers in parentheses are not officially sanctioned.

junctival inflammation or pain, which resolves in less than 1 month.

364.10 *Chronic anterior uveitis:* Chronic inflammation of the anterior chamber of the eye (usually asymptomatic), with slit-lamp biomicroscopy findings of an increased number of cells and proteinaceous flare in the anterior chamber or, later, findings of a punctate keratitic precipitate on the posterior surface of the cornea, posterior synechiae, or band keratopathy.

363.1 *Posterior uveitis:* Inflammation involving the posterior uveal tract (chorioretinitis).

B. Connective Tissue Diseases

710.0 *Systemic lupus erythematosus (SLE):* Four of the 11 following criteria present at any time serially or simultaneously during an interval of observation:
- (1) Malar (butterfly) rash
- (2) Discoid-lupus rash
- (3) Photosensitivity
- (4) Oral or nasal mucocutaneous ulcerations
- (5) Nonerosive arthritis
- (6) Nephritis
  - Proteinuria > 0.5 g/d *or*
  - Cellular casts
- (7) Encephalopathy
  - Seizures *or*
  - Psychosis
- (8) Pleuritis or pericarditis
- (9) Cytopenia (anemia, leukopenia [$<4000/mm^3$], lymphopenia [$<1500/mm^3$], *or* thrombocytopenia [$<150{,}000/mm^3$])
- (10) Positive immunoserology
  - Antibodies to dsDNA *or*
  - Antibodies to Sm nuclear antigen *or*
  - Antiphospholipid antibodies based on:
    - a. IgG or IgM anticardiolipin antibodies, *or*
    - b. Lupus anticoagulant, *or*
    - c. False-positive serologic test for syphilis for at least 6 months, confirmed by *Treponema pallidum* immobilization or fluorescent treponemal antibody absorption test
- (11) Positive antinuclear antibody test

(710.01) *Probable SLE:* Any three of the aforementioned 11 criteria present at any time serially or simultaneously during any interval of observation.

(710.02) *Neonatal lupus syndrome:* The occurrence of any of the following in the neonate of a mother with clinical or serological evidence of SLE, RA, MCTD or Sjögren's syndrome:
- (a) Congenital complete heart block
- (b) Thrombocytopenia
- (c) Erythema annulare
- (d) Hepatitis.

710.3 *Dermatomyositis:* Symmetric proximal muscle weakness and a characteristic dermatomyositis rash. If either of these criteria is absent, then at least two of the following must be present:
- (1) Two or more elevated serum muscle enzymes (CK, AST, ALT, LDH, aldolase)
- (2) Characteristic EMG findings
- (3) Characteristic muscle biopsy.

710.1 *Systemic scleroderma:* Generalized diffuse skin thickening or loss of skin elasticity. If there is no scleroderma proximal to the MCP or MTP joints, then at least two of the following must be present:
- (1) Sclerodactyly
- (2) Fingertip scarring or tapering
- (3) Fibrosing alveolitis or pulmonary fibrosis.

(710.8) *CREST syndrome:* Calcinosis, Raynaud's phenomenon, Esophageal dysmotility, Sclerodactyly, and Telangiectasia

701.0 *Morphea:* At least one plaque of inelastic or thickened skin, excluding post-traumatic skin scarring.

(701.01) *Linear scleroderma:* At least one band-like sclerotic lesion involving skin and subcutaneous tissues, excluding post-traumatic skin scarring.

728.89 *Eosinophilic fasciitis:* The combination of (1) skin induration, (2) peripheral and cutaneous eosinophilia, and (3) absence of visceral involvement.

250.9 *Diabetic cheirarthropathy:* Insulin-dependent diabetes mellitus and finger contractures due to tightening of the skin and soft tissues.

710.9 *MCTD:* Arthritis with features of scleroderma, dermatomyositis, and SLE at some time during the illness, in the presence of anti-RNP antibodies without high-titer dsDNA or anti-Sm antibodies.

(710.91) *Other overlap syndromes:* Any overlap among chronic arthritis, scleroderma, dermatomyositis, SLE, and Sjögren's syndrome.

443.0 *Raynaud's phenomenon:* Sudden, reversible "dead-white" uniform pallor of the digits precipitated by cold exposure.

710.2 *Primary Sjögren's syndrome:* Dry eyes (<5 mm wetting of filter paper in conjunctival sac for 5 minutes), dry mouth, and bilateral parotid enlargement in the absence of another defined connective tissue disease, or any one of the these findings with a positive labial biopsy.

729.30 *Panniculitis:* Generalized painful subcutaneous nodules with biopsy evidence of an inflammatory exudate in the subcutaneous tissues.

695.2 *Erythema nodosum:* Painful, erythematous nodules over the anterior surfaces of the lower legs and occasionally the arms.

C. Vasculitis

446.1 *Kawasaki disease:* At least five of the following:
- (1) Fever (>5 days)
- (2) Bilateral conjunctivitis

(3) Changes in the oropharynx (mucosal erythema, dry fissured lips, "strawberry" tongue)
(4) Changes of the extremities (erythema of palms and soles, indurative edema, periungual desquamation)
(5) Polymorphous exanthema of trunk without vesicles or crusts
(6) Acute nonpurulent cervical lymphadenopathy of at least 1.5 cm in diameter.

446.0 *Polyarteritis nodosa:* Either (a) biopsy evidence of necrotizing vasculitis of small and medium sized arteries or (b) arteriography confirming segmental narrowing or aneurysms of small and medium sized arteries in a child who is either systemically unwell (fever, weight loss) or has involvement of at least one organ system other than the skin.

(446.1) *Cutaneous polyarteritis:* Skin biopsy evidence of necrotizing vasculitis of small and medium sized arteries in a child who is otherwise systemically well and who has no organ system involved other than the skin

287.0 *Henoch-Schönlein purpura:* The presence of the classic palpable purpuric rash, with any of the following: arthritis, abdominal pain, or glomerulonephritis.

136.1 *Behçet's syndrome—complete:* The combination of the following (not necessarily coincident):
(1) Recurrent oral aphthous ulcerations
(2) Skin lesions (E. nodosum, phlebitis, folliculitis, or hypersensitivity)
(3) Eye lesions (iridocyclitis, chorioretinitis, or keratoconjunctivitis)
(4) Genital ulceration.

(136.11) *Behçet's syndrome—incomplete:* Either any three of the aforementioned four criteria *or* any two of the aforementioned four plus at least two of
(1) Arthritis—711.2
(2) Gastrointestinal lesions
(3) CNS lesions
(4) Vascular or pulmonary lesions
(5) Epididymitis
(6) Glomerulonephritis

446.7 *Takayasu's arteritis:* Characteristic angiographic findings in a child who either has symptoms or signs of large vessel disease or a systemic illness.

446.4 *Wegener's granulomatosis:* The combination of sinus, lung, and kidney disease with biopsy evidence of a necrotizing arteritis or granuloma.

D. Mechanical/Orthopedic Disorders

727.0 *Toxic synovitis of the hip:* Transient arthritis of the hip (lasting for a maximum of 2 weeks), excluding other diseases associated with hip pain.

732.1 *Legg-Calvé-Perthes disease:* Avascular necrosis of the femoral head of unknown cause.

733.4 *Avascular necrosis:* Avascular necrosis of femoral head or other epiphyses with probable risk factors.

732.2 *Slipped capital femoral epiphysis:* Radiographic evidence of subluxation of the femoral head on the neck of the femur.

717.8 *Anterior patella syndrome:* Anterior knee pain, not associated with persistent synovitis, that can be reproduced by compression and movement of the patella against the femur.

717.7 *Chondromalacia patellae:* arthroscopic evidence of degenerative change of the posterior surface of the patella.

727.83 *Plica syndrome* (see text)

732.9 *Osteochondritis:* Localized pain and tenderness associated with radiologic evidence of separation of a fragment of bone from the joint or bone surface.

732.4 *Osgood-Schlatter disease:* Localized tenderness with or without swelling at one or both tibial tubercles with no evidence of enthesitis at other sites.

728.5 *Generalized joint hypermobility:* A score of at least 4 points:
(1) Passive hyperextension of the 5th MCP joint beyond 90 degrees (1 point for each hand)
(2) Passive apposition of the thumb to the flexor aspect of the forearm (1 point for each thumb)
(3) Hyperextension of the elbow beyond 10 degrees (1 point for each elbow)
(4) Hyperextension of the knee beyond 10 degrees (1 point for each knee)
(5) Placing palms of hands flat on the floor by forward flexion of the trunk while maintaining knee extension (1 point).

728.4 *Localized joint hypermobility:* Increased joint range of movement at least 5 degrees beyond the expected normal range at one or more joints but not fulfilling criteria for generalized joint hypermobility.

724.9 *Back pain not yet specifically diagnosed.*

732.0 *Scheuermann's disease:* Radiographic evidence of anterior wedging of at least one vertebra with associated endplate irregularity or Schmorl's nodes. Exclusion of other causes.

756.11/756.12 *Spondylolysis/spondylolisthesis:* Radiographic evidence of an incompletely ossified, absent, or fractured pars intra-articularis without displacement (with displacement = spondylolisthesis).

723.9 *Neck pain not yet specifically diagnosed.*

959.8 *Trauma:* Including stress fracture or overuse syndromes.

E. Infection

711.0 *Acute septic arthritis:* Specify organism.

730.2 *Recurrent multifocal osteomyelitis:* Multiple recurrent bone lesions resembling osteomyelitis but in the absence of a defined infectious agent.

730.0 *Acute osteomyelitis:* Specify organism.
730.8 *Tuberculosis of bone of joint*
711.5 *Viral arthritis:* Acute arthritis associated with other viral symptoms and laboratory evidence of a specific virus. Specify virus.
(711.51) *Probable viral arthritis:* Arthritis, usually transient, associated with viral symptoms without proven evidence of a viral infection.
088.41 *Lyme arthritis:* Arthritis associated with laboratory evidence of *Borrelia burgdorferi* infection and a specific immune response to *B. burgdorferi.*
390.0 *Rheumatic fever:* Evidence of a preceding streptococcal infection (positive throat culture or raised ASO titer), and at least two of the following:
(1) Carditis—391
(2) Polyarthritis
(3) Chorea without carditis—392.9
(4) Erythema marginatum
(5) Subcutaneous nodules.
Or one of the aforementioned criteria, and at least two of the following:
(1) Fever
(2) Arthralgia
(3) Previous rheumatic fever
(4) Elevated ESR or CRP
(5) Prolonged PR interval on ECG.
(390.01) *Poststreptococcal arthritis:* Arthritis associated with evidence of a preceding streptococcal infection not satisfying criteria for rheumatic fever.

F. Hematologic/Neoplastic Disorders

287.9 *Bleeding disorder:* Specify.
282 *Hereditary hemolytic anemias:* Specify
204 *Leukemia:* Specify.
170.9 *Malignancy—primary bone:* Specify
199 *Malignancy—other.*
213—M9191/0 *Osteoid osteoma:* (a) Compatible radiographic findings in a child with night pain relieved by NSAIDs or (b) proven biopsy.

G. Musculoskeletal Abnormalities

758.0 *Down syndrome:* Trisomy 21.
759.82 *Marfan syndrome:* Autosomal dominant inherited condition of increased height, an arm span that is greater than the height, and an elongation of the distal extremities.
756.83 *Ehlers-Danlos syndrome:* Hypermobility in association with abnormal skin fragility.
756.9 *Bone dysplasias/dysostoses:* Includes primary abnormalities of bone and cartilage growth: Specify.
755.8 *Syndromes with joint contractures:* Includes conditions that are associated with joint contractures not covered elsewhere: Specify.

H. Miscellaneous Disorders

135–713.7 *Sarcoidosis:* Arthritis with
(a) Biopsy evidence of noncaseating epithelioid cell granulomata or
(b) Posterior uveitis or
(c) At least two of the following:
(i) Anterior uveitis
(ii) Bilateral hilar lymphadenopathy
(iii) Erythema nodosum
(iv) Generalized skin rash compatible with sarcoidosis.
277.3 *Amyloidosis:* Primary or secondary amyloidosis, biopsy proven: Specify.
(277.31) *Familial Mediterranean fever:* Recurrent episodes of arthritis, serositis, or fever in a child of Mediterranean extraction for which no other cause can be found.
279 *Immunodeficiency:* Specify.
726.9 *Enthesitis:* Isolated tenderness at any site of insertion of tendon, ligament, or joint capsule into bone.
(714.34) *Benign rheumatoid nodules:* Subcutaneous nodules with characteristic histology in the absence of other rheumatic disease.
277.9 *Metabolic disorder:* Specify.
781.99 *Growing pains:* Recurrent night pain in the lower limbs without daytime pain; pain relieved by simple analgesia or local massage. Exclusion of other causes of limb pain.
729.5 *Limb pains*—not yet diagnosed.
307.80 *Psychogenic pain, site unspecified.*
729.0 *Primary fibromyalgia (fibrositis):* The combination of all of the following:
(1) Widespread musculoskeletal pains for at least 3 months
(2) At least ten specific tender points (base of cervical spine, mid-trapezius ridges, lateral epicondylar regions, costochondral junctions, inner scapular margins, low lumbar spine, upper outer buttocks, inner fat pads of knees)
(3) Normal laboratory and radiologic investigations
(4) Exclusion of systemic and mechanical disorders.
(729.01) *Idiopathic pain syndrome:* Localized or diffuse pain not fulfilling criteria for reflex neurovascular dystrophy or fibromyalgia for which no organic cause can be found after appropriate investigations.
733.7 *Reflex neurovascular dystrophy* (reflex sympathetic dystrophy, algodystrophy): Localized pain lasting > 1 week in the absence of (a) trauma that could reasonably explain the symptoms and (b) other etiologic factors such as local infection, and the presence of at least two of the following:
(1) Soft tissue swelling
(2) Change in skin color or temperature.
(3) Soft tissue tenderness

Index

Note: Page numbers followed by f refer to figures; page numbers followed by t refer to tables.

B

C

D

E

H

I

Q

R

S

X

Y

Z

ISBN 0-7216-8171-9